Clinical Hematology and Oncology

Presentation, Diagnosis, and Treatment

Bruce Furie, MD

Professor of Medicine
Harvard Medical School

Chief, Division of Hemostasis and Thrombosis
Department of Medicine
Beth Israel Deaconess Medical Center
Boston, Massachusetts

Peter A. Cassileth, MD

Professor of Medicine
Division of Hematology and Oncology
Department of Medicine
University of Miami School of Medicine
Miami, Florida

Michael B. Atkins, MD

Professor of Medicine
Harvard Medical School

Deputy Director, Division of Hematology/Oncology
Department of Medicine
Beth Israel Deaconess Medical Center
Boston, Massachusetts

Robert J. Mayer, MD

Professor of Medicine
Harvard Medical School

Vice Chair for Academic Affairs
Department of Medical Oncology
Dana-Farber Cancer Institute
Boston, Massachusetts

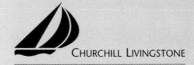

CHURCHILL LIVINGSTONE

An Imprint of Elsevier

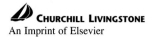

CHURCHILL LIVINGSTONE
An Imprint of Elsevier

The Curtis Center
Independence Square West
Philadelphia, Pennsylvania 19106

CLINICAL HEMATOLOGY AND ONCOLOGY   ISBN 0-443-06556-X

Distributed in the United Kingdom by Churchill Livingstone, Robert Stevenson House, 1–3 Baxter's Place, Leith Walk, Edinburgh EH1 3AF, Scotland, and by associated companies, branches, and representatives throughout the world.

NOTICE

Medicine is an ever-changing field. Standard safety precautions must be followed, but as new research and clinical experience broaden our knowledge, changes in treatment and drug therapy may become necessary or appropriate. Readers are advised to check the most current product information provided by the manufacturer of each drug to be administered to verify the recommended dose, the method and duration of administration, and contraindications. It is the responsibility of the licensed prescriber, relying on experience and knowledge of the patient, to determine dosages and the best treatment for each individual patient. Neither the publisher nor the editors assume any liability for any injury and/or damage to persons or property arising from this publication.

Library of Congress Cataloging-in-Publication Data

Clinical hematology and oncology: presentation, diagnosis, and treatment /
   Bruce Furie . . . [et al.].—1st ed.
      p. ; cm.
   Includes bibliographical references
   ISBN 0-443-06556-X
    1. Cancer—Handbooks, manuals, etc.   2. Blood—Diseases—Handbooks, manuals, etc.
I. Furie, Bruce.
    [DNLM: 1. Hematologic Diseases—diagnosis.   2. Hematologic Diseases—therapy.
3. Hematology—methods.   4. Medical Oncology—methods.   5. Neoplasms—diagnosis.
6. Neoplasms—therapy. WH 120 C6416 2003]
RC262.5.C557 2003
616.99'4—dc21
                             2003043470

International Standard Book Number 0-443-06556-X

Senior Acquisitions Editor: Dolores Meloni
Senior Developmental Editor: Joanne Husovski

Printed in Hong Kong

Last digit is the print number: 9   8   7   6   5   4   3   2   1

To my wife, Barbara C. Furie, my collaborator in everything; and to my sons, Eric and Gregg, who have matured into my collaborators in science and medicine and life.

Bruce Furie

To my wife, Judith, for the love and support that makes work and life so enjoyable, and to our children Jodi, Stuart, Wendy, Peter, Greg, and Jacob.

Peter A. Cassileth

To my wife, Susan, and my children Ben, Melea and Jonathan, for their unfailing love and support.

Michael B. Atkins

To my wife, Jane, and daughters, Erica and Rachel.

Robert J. Mayer

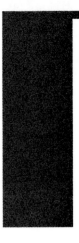

Contributors

James Abbruzzese, MD
Professor of Medicine
Chairman, Department of Gastrointestinal Medical
    Oncology
M. D. Anderson Cancer Center
University of Texas
Houston, Texas

Janet L. Abrahm
Associate Professor of Medicine and Anesthesia
Harvard Medical School
Director, Pain and Palliative Care Program
Dana-Farber Cancer Institute and Brigham and
    Women's Hospital
Boston, Massachusetts

William C. Aird, MD
Associate Professor of Medicine
Harvard Medical School
Attending Physician, Hematology-Oncology Division
Beth Israel Deaconess Medical Center
Boston, Massachusetts

Joseph Aisner, MD
Professor of Medicine
Professor of Environmental and Community
    Medicine
Robert Wood Johnson Medical School
University of Medicine and Dentistry of New Jersey
Associate Director for Clinical Sciences
Cancer Institute of New Jersey
New Brunswick, New Jersey

Corina Akerele, MD
Hematology/Oncology Associates of New Jersey
Paramus, New Jersey

Jeanne E. Anderson, MD
Katmai Oncology Group
Anchorage, Alaska

Nancy C. Andrews, MD, PhD
Professor of Pediatrics
Children's Hospital/Harvard Medical School

Associate Investigator
Howard Hughes Medical Institute
Boston, Massachusetts

Stephen M. Ansell, MD, PhD
Assistant Professor
Division of Hematology
Mayo Clinic
Rochester, Minnesota

Lindsey R. Baden, MD
Instructor of Medicine
Harvard Medical School
Associate Physician
Brigham and Women's Hospital
Dana-Farber Cancer Institute
Boston, Massachusetts

Hasan F. Batirel, MD
Postdoctoral Fellow
Department of Thoracic Surgery
Brigham and Women's Hospital
Boston, Massachusetts

Brent Bauer, MD
Chair, Complementary and Integrative Medicine
    Program
Department of Medicine
Mayo Clinic
Rochester, Minnesota

Pasquale Benedetto, MD
Professor of Medicine
Division of Hematology/Oncology
University of Miami Sylvester Comprehensive
    Cancer Center
Miami, Florida

Robert S. Benjamin, MD
Professor of Medicine
Medical Director
Multidisciplinary Sarcoma Center

Chairman
Department of Sarcoma Medical Oncology
M. D. Anderson Cancer Center
University of Texas
Houston, Texas

Ross S. Berkowitz, MD
William H. Baker Professor of Gynecology
Harvard Medical School
Director of Gynecologic Oncology
Brigham and Women's Hospital
Co-Director
New England Trophoblastic Cancer Center
Boston, Massachusetts

Monica M. Bertagnolli, MD
Associate Professor of Surgery
Harvard Medical School
Brigham and Women's Hospital
Boston, Massachusetts

R. Gregory Bociek, MD
Assistant Professor
Section of Hematology/Oncology
Department of Medicine
University of Nebraska Medical Center
Omaha, Nebraska

Phillip M. Boiselle, MD
Assistant Professor of Radiology
Harvard Medical School
Section Chief, Thoracic Imaging
Co-Director, Resident Training Program
Director, Residency Career Development
Beth Israel Deaconess Medical Center
Boston, Massachusetts

Virginia Borges, MD
Assistant Professor
University of Colorado Health Science Center
Aurora, Colorado

Laurence Alan Boxer, MD
Professor and Director
Pediatric Hematology/Oncology
University of Michigan
Ann Arbor, Michigan

Glenn Bubley, MD
Associate Professor of Medicine
Harvard Medical School
Beth Israel Deaconess Medical Center
Boston, Massachusetts

Craig A. Bunnell, MD, MPH
Assistant Professor of Medicine
Harvard Medical School

Associate Physician
Dana-Farber Cancer Institute
Associate Physician
Brigham and Women's Hospital
Boston, Massachusetts

Harold J. Burstein, MD, PhD
Assistant Professor of Medicine
Harvard Medical School
Department of Medical Oncology
Dana-Farber Cancer Institute
Boston, Massachusetts

Gerald E. Byrne Jr., MD
Professor of Pathology
Director of Hematopathology
University of Miami
Miami, Florida

Beria Cabello Inchausti, MD
Hematopathologist
Department of Pathology and Laboratory Medicine
Mount Sinai Medical Center
Miami, Florida

Stephen A. Cannistra, MD
Associate Professor of Medicine
Harvard Medical School
Director, Program in Gynecologic Medical Oncology
Beth Israel Deaconess Medical Center
Boston, Massachusetts

David S. Caradonna, MD, DMD
Instructor
Department of Otology and Laryngology
Harvard Medical School
Director, Head and Neck Oncology
Beth Israel Deaconess Medical Center
Boston, Massachusetts

Christopher L. Carpenter, MD, PhD
Assistant Professor of Medicine
Harvard Medical School
Clinic Associate in Medicine
Beth Israel Deaconess Medical Center
Boston, Massachusetts

Peter A. Cassileth, MD
Professor of Medicine
Division of Hematology and Oncology
Department of Medicine
University of Miami School of Medicine
Miami, Florida

Bruce D. Cheson, MD
Professor of Medicine
Georgetown University School of Medicine;

Head, Hematology
Georgetown University Hospital
Washington, D.C.

Jeffrey W. Clark, MD
Assistant Professor of Medicine
Harvard Medical School
Massachusetts General Hospital
Boston, Massachusetts

Joseph P. Colgan, MD
Assistant Professor of Medicine
Department of Hematology
Mayo Clinic
Rochester, Minnesota

Steven E. Come, MD
Associate Professor of Medicine
Harvard Medical School
Director, Hematology-Oncology Units
Beth Israel Deaconess Medical Center
Boston, Massachusetts

Larry D. Cripe, MD
Associate Professor of Medicine
Indiana University School of Medicine
Director, Clinical Research Office
Indiana University Cancer Center
Indianapolis, Indiana

Peter T. Curtin, MD
Associate Professor
Department of Medicine
Oregon Health & Science University
Portland, Oregon

Daniel J. DeAngelo, MD, PhD
Instructor in Medicine
Harvard Medical School
Attending Physician
Dana-Farber Cancer Institute
Associate Physician
Brigham and Women's Hospital
Boston, Massachusetts

Reed E. Drews, MD
Assistant Professor of Medicine
Harvard Medical School
Assistant Chief of Medicine for Medical Student
    Education
Beth Israel Deaconess Medical Center
Boston, Massachusetts

John K. Erban, MD
Associate Professor of Medicine
Tufts University School of Medicine

Chief, Division of Hematology/Oncology
Tufts–New England Medical Center
Boston, Massachusetts

Armin Ernst, MD
Director, Interventional Pulmonology
Co-Director, Medical Critical Care
Division of Pulmonary and Critical Care Medicine
Beth Israel Deaconess Medical Center
Boston, Massachusetts

Tracey Evans, MD
Assistant Professor of Medicine
University of Pennsylvania School of Medicine
Philadelphia, Pennsylvania

Robert C. Eyre, MD
Associate Professor of Surgery
Harvard Medical School
Beth Israel Deaconess Medical Center
Boston, Massachusetts

Donald Feinstein, MD
Professor of Medicine
Division of Hematology
University of Southern California Keck School of
    Medicine
Los Angeles, California

Robert W. Finberg, MD
Professor of Medicine
University of Massachusetts Medical School
Chair, Department of Medicine
UMass Memorial Health Care
Worcester, Massachusetts

Lawrence E. Flaherty, MD
Professor of Medicine and Oncology
Karmanos Cancer Institute
Wayne State University
Detroit, Michigan

Stephen J. Forman, MD
Director
Division of Hematology and Bone Marrow
    Transplantation
City of Hope Comprehensive Cancer Center
Duarte, California

Kevin R. Fox, MD
Associate Professor of Medicine
Rowan Breast Center
University of Pennsylvania Cancer Center
University of Pennsylvania School of Medicine
Philadelphia, Pennsylvania

Jonathan W. Freidberg, MD
Assistant Professor of Medicine
Associate Director, Lymphoma Clinical Research
James P. Wilmot Cancer Center
Rochester, New York

Douglas K. Frank, MD
Assistant Professor
Department of Otolaryngology / Head and Neck
   Surgery
Albert Einstein Medical Center
Bronx, New York
Research Scientist
Strang Cancer Prevention Center
New York, New York
Attending Physician
Beth Israel Medical Center
New York, New York

Charles S. Fuchs, MD, MPH
Associate Professor of Medicine
Harvard Medical School
Dana-Farber Cancer Institute
Boston, Massachusetts

Bruce Furie, MD
Professor of Medicine
Harvard Medical School
Chief, Division of Hemostasis and Thrombosis
Department of Medicine
Beth Israel Deaconess Medical Center
Boston, Massachusetts

Judy E. Garber, MD, MPH
Associate Professor of Medicine
Harvard Medical School
Director, Cancer Risk and Prevention
Department of Adult Oncology
Dana-Farber Cancer Institute
Boston, Massachusetts

Kris Ghosh, MD
Assistant Professor of Obstetrics, Gynecology and
   Reproductive Biology
Beth Israel Deaconess Medical Center
Boston, Massachusetts

Ann M. Gillenwater, MD, FACS
Associate Professor
Department of Head and Neck Surgery
M. D. Anderson Cancer Center
University of Texas
Houston, Texas

Donald P. Goldstein, MD
Clinical Professor of Obstetrics, Gynecology, and
   Reproductive Medicine
Harvard Medical School
Brigham and Women's Hospital;
Co-Director
New England Trophoblastic Cancer Center
Boston, Massachusetts

Jared A. Gollob, MD
Associate Professor of Medicine
Duke University
Director, Biologic Therapy Program
Duke University Medical Center
Durham, North Carolina

Susan Goodin, PharmD
Associate Professor of Medicine
Division of Medical Oncology
Robert Wood Johnson Medical School
University of Medicine and Dentistry of New Jersey
Director
Division of Pharmaceutical Science
The Cancer Institute of New Jersey
New Brunswick, New Jersey

AnneKathryn Goodman, MD
Associate Professor
Harvard Medical School
Associate Obstetrician/Gynecologist
Department of Obstetrics and Gynecology
Massachusetts General Hospital
Boston, Massachusetts

Leo I. Gordon, MD
Abby and John Friend Professor of Cancer
   Research
Professor of Medicine and Chief, Division of
   Hematology/Oncology
Northwestern University Feinberg School of
   Medicine
Associate Director for Clinical Research
Robert H. Lurie Comprehensive Cancer Center of
   Northwestern University
Chief, Division of Hematology/Oncology
Northwestern Memorial Hospital
Chicago, Illinois

Philip R. Greipp, MD
Professor of Medicine
Professor of Laboratory Medicine and Pathology
Mayo Medical School
Rochester, Minnesota

Michael L. Grossbard, MD
Associate Professor of Clinical Medicine
Columbia University College of Physicians and
    Surgeons;
Chief, Hematology-Oncology
St. Luke's-Roosevelt Hospital
Beth Israel Medical Center
New York, New York

Stuart A. Grossman, MD
Professor of Oncology, Medicine, and Neurosurgery
The Johns Hopkins University School of Medicine
Attending Physician
Sidney Kimmel Comprehensive Cancer Center
The Johns Hopkins Hospital
Baltimore, Maryland

Thomas M. Habermann, MD
Professor of Medicine
Mayo Clinic
Rochester, Minnesota

William N. Hait, MD, PhD
Robert Wood Johnson Medical School
University of Medicine and Dentistry of New Jersey
The Cancer Institute of New Jersey
New Brunswick, New Jersey

Subramanian Hariharan, MD
Associate Professor
New Jersey Neuroscience Institute
Seton Hall University
Director, Neuro-Oncology
JFK Hospital
Edison, New Jersey

Mohamed Anwar Hau, MD
Orthopaedic Oncology
Department of Pathology
Massachusetts General Hospital
Boston, Massachusetts

George T. Henning, MD
University of Pittsburgh Cancer Center
University of Pittsburgh Medical Center
Pittsburgh, Pennsylvania

Fred H. Hochberg, MD
Associate Professor of Neurology
Harvard Medical School
Attending Physician
Department of Neurology
Massachusetts General Hospital
Boston, Massachusetts

Mohamad A. Hussein, MD
Director, Myeloma Research Program
Cleveland Clinic Taussig Cancer Center
Cleveland, Ohio

David Ilson, MD, PhD
Assistant Professor, Department of Medicine
Cornell University Medical College
Associate Attending Physician, Department of Medicine
Memorial Sloan-Kettering Cancer Center
New York, New York

Barton A. Kamen, MD, PhD
Professor of Pediatrics and Pharmacology
Robert Wood Johnson Medical School
University of Medicine and Dentistry of New Jersey
Division Chief, Pediatric Hematology/Oncology
Cancer Institute of New Jersey
New Brunswick, New Jersey

Daniel Karp, MD
Professor and Deputy Head of Cancer Medicine
M. D. Anderson Cancer Center
University of Texas
Houston, Texas

Joel T. Katz, MD
Assistant Professor of Medicine
Harvard Medical School
Infectious Disease Staff
Brigham and Women's Hospital
Dana-Farber Cancer Institute
Boston, Massachusetts

Lara Kelley, MD
Instructor in Medicine
Harvard Medical School
Director, Dermatologic Surgery
Department of Dermatology
Beth Israel Deaconess Medical Center
Boston, Massachusetts

Craig M. Kessler, MD
Professor of Medicine and Pathology
Chief, Division of Hematology-Oncology
Director, Division of Coagulation
Georgetown University Medical Center
Washington, D.C.

Fadlo R. Khuri, MD
Professor of Medicine, Hematology and Oncology,
    Otolaryngology and Pharmacology
Emory University
Associate Director, Clinical and Translational Research
Winship Cancer Institute
Atlanta, Georgia

Edward S. Kim, MD
Assistant Professor of Medicine
Department of Thoracic / Head and Neck Medical
    Oncology
M. D. Anderson Cancer Center
University of Texas
Houston, Texas

Yoo-Joung Ko, MD
Instructor in Medicine
Harvard Medical School
Beth Israel Deaconess Medical Center
Boston, Massachusetts

Peter Kozuch, MD
Assistant Professor of Clinical Medicine
Columbia University College of Physicians and
    Surgeons
Attending Physician
St. Luke's-Roosevelt Hospital Center
New York, New York

Matthew H. Kulke, MD
Assistant Professor of Medicine
Division of Medical Oncology
Dana-Farber Cancer Institute
Boston, Massachusetts

David J. Kuter, MD, PhD
Associate Professor of Medicine
Harvard Medical School
Chief, Hematology
Massachusetts General Hospital
Boston, Massachusetts

Richard A. Larson, MD
Professor of Medicine
University of Chicago
Chicago, Illinois

Arthur M. Lauretano, MD
Clinical Instructor in Otology and Laryngology
Department of Surgery, Division of Otolaryngology
Beth Israel Deaconess Medical Center
Boston, Massachusetts

Theodore S. Lawrence, MD, PhD
Isadore Lampe Professor and Chair
Department of Radiation Oncology
University of Michigan
Ann Arbor, Michigan

James D. Levine, MD, MS
Assistant Professor of Medicine
Harvard Medical School

Beth Israel Deaconess Medical Center
Boston, Massachusetts

Nancy Lewis, MD
Attending Physician
Department of Medical Oncology
Fox Chase Cancer Center
Philadelphia, Pennsylvania

Howard Liebman, MD
Associate Professor of Medicine and Pathology
University of Southern California
Los Angeles, California

Joseph LoCicero III
Professor and Chair
Department of Surgery
University of South Alabama
Director, Center of Clinical Oncology
University of South Alabama Cancer Research
    Institute
Mobile, Alabama

Patrick J. Loehrer Sr., MD
Professor of Medicine
Chairman, Division of Hematology/Oncology
Indiana University Medical Center
Indianapolis, Indiana

Charles L. Loprinzi, MD
Professor and Chair
Medical Oncology
Mayo Clinic
Rochester, Minnesota

Thomas J. Lynch Jr., MD
Associate Professor of Medicine
Harvard Medical School
Massachusetts General Hospital
Boston, Massachusetts

Jaroslaw Maciejewski, MD
National Heart, Lung, and Blood Institute—
    Hematology Branch
Cleveland Clinics Foundation
Cleveland, Ohio

Henry J. Mankin, MD
Edith M. Ashley Professor of Orthopedic Surgery
    (Emeritus)
Harvard Medical School
Massachusetts General Hospital
Boston, Massachusetts

Peter W. Marks, MD, PhD
Instructor in Medicine
Harvard Medical School
Clinical Director, Hematology

Department of Medicine
Brigham and Women's Hospital
Boston, Massachusetts

Robert J. Mayer, MD
Professor of Medicine
Harvard Medical School
Vice Chair for Academic Affairs
Department of Medical Oncology
Dana-Farber Cancer Institute
Boston, Massachusetts

Minesh P. Mehta, MD
Professor and Chairman
Department of Human Oncology
University of Wisconsin
Madison, Wisconsin

Ann Mellott, MD
Instructor of Medicine
Division of Hematology/Oncology
Northwestern University Feinberg School of
    Medicine
Chicago, Illinois

Joseph J. Merchant, MD
Hematology/Oncology Department
McFarland Clinic
Ames, Iowa

Jeffrey A. Meyerhardt, MD
Instructor in Medicine
Harvard Medical School
Attending Physician
Dana-Farber Cancer Institute
Boston, Massachusetts

Anne Moore, MD
Attending Physician
New York Presbyterian Hospital (Cornell)
Division of Hematology-Oncology
New York, New York

Abraham Morgentaler, MD
Associate Clinical Professor of Surgery (Oncology)
Harvard Medical School
Director
Men's Health Boston
Boston, Massachusetts

Gaston Morillo, MD
Professor of Radiology
University of Miami School of Medicine
Medical Director
Department of Radiology/Imaging Services

University of Miami Hospital and Clinics
Sylvester Comprehensive Cancer Center
Miami, Florida

Martina Morrin, FFRRCSI, FRCR
Assistant Professor of Radiology
Harvard Medical School
Staff Radiologist
Beth Israel Deaconess Medical Center
Boston, Massachusetts

Robert J. Motzer, MD
Attending Physician
Genitourinary Oncology Section
Department of Medicine
Memorial Sloan-Kettering Cancer Center
New York, New York

Hyman B. Muss, MD
Professor of Medicine
University of Vermont
Director, Hematology/Oncology
Fletcher Allen Health Care
Associate Director, Clinical Research
Vermont Cancer Center
Burlington, Vermont

Michael G. Muto, MD
Associate Professor
Obstetrics, Gynecology, and Reproductive Biology
Harvard Medical School
Brigham and Women's Hospital
Boston, Massachusetts

Jonathan M. Niloff, MD
Associate Professor, Obstetrics, Gynecology, and
    Reproductive Biology
Harvard Medical School
Director, Division of Gynecologic Oncology
Beth Israel Deaconess Medical Center
Boston, Massachusetts

Margaret R. O'Donnell, MD
Associate Clinical Director
Division of Hematology and Bone Marrow
    Transplantation
City of Hope National Medical Center
Duarte, California

Michael A. O'Donnell, MD
Associate Professor of Urology
Director of Urologic Oncology
University of Iowa Hospital and Clinics
Iowa City, Iowa

William K. Oh, MD
Assistant Professor of Medicine
Harvard Medical School
The Lank Center for Genitourinary Oncology
Dana-Farber Cancer Insitute
Boston, Massachusetts

Martin M. Oken, MD
Clinical Professor of Medicine
University of Minnesota
Medical Director of Research
Hubert Humphrey Cancer Center
North Memorial Hospital
Robbinsdale, Minnesota

Julie J. Olin, MD
Assistant Professor of Medicine
University of Vermont
Fletcher Allen Health Care
Burlington, Vermont

Aria F. Olumi, MD
Assistant Professor of Surgery/Urology
Harvard Medical School
Attending Urologist
Beth Israel Deaconess Medical Center
Boston, Massachusetts

Shreyaskumar R. Patel, MD
Deputy Chairman
Department of Sarcoma Medical Oncology
M. D. Anderson Cancer Center
University of Texas
Houston, Texas

R. Judith Ratzan, MD
Co-Chief, Division of Hematology/Oncology
Mount Sinai Medical Center
Miami Beach, Florida

Elie E. Rebeiz, MD
Professor of Otolaryngology
Tufts University School of Medicine
Chairman, Department of Otolaryngology / Head
    and Neck Surgery
New England Medical Center
Boston, Massachusetts

Stephen Richman, MD
Professor of Medicine
Division of Hematology/Oncology
University of Miami School of Medicine
Miami, Florida

Bruce J. Roth, MD
The Paul V. Hamilton and Virginia E. Howd
    Professor of Urologic Oncology

Professor of Medicine and Urologic Surgery
Section Chief, Solid Tumor Oncology
Vanderbilt-Ingram Cancer Center
Nashville, Tennessee

Jacob M. Rowe, MD
Professor and Chief
Department of Hematology and Bone Marrow
    Transplantation
Rambam Medical Center and Technion
Haifa, Israel

Eric H. Rubin, MD
Professor
Department of Medicine and Pharmacology
Cancer Institute of New Jersey
Robert Wood Johnson Medical School
University of Medicine and Dentistry of New
    Jersey
Attending Physician
Robert Wood Johnson University Hospital
New Brunswick, New Jersey

David P. Ryan, MD
Assistant Professor of Medicine
Harvard Medical School
Assistant in Medicine
Massachusetts General Hospital
Boston, Massachusetts

Carlos J. Sandoval, MD
Assistant Professor of Clinical Psychiatry and
    Behavioral Sciences
University of Miami School of Medicine
Director
Psychosocial Oncology
Courtelis Center
Miami, Florida

David T. Scadden, MD
Associate Professor
Harvard Medical School
Director, Experimental Hematology
AIDS Research Center
Division of Hematology/Oncology
Massachusetts General Hospital
Boston, Massachusetts

Steven C. Schachter, MD
Professor of Neurology
Harvard Medical School
Beth Israel Deaconess Medical Center
Boston, Massachusetts

Geraldine P. Schechter, MD
Professor of Medicine
George Washington University

Chief, Hematology Section
Veterans Affairs Medical Center
Washington, D.C.

Joan H. Schiller, MD
Professor
University of Wisconsin
Madison, Wisconsin

David P. Schenkein, MD
Associate Professor of Medicine
Tufts University School of Medicine
New England Medical Center
Vice President, Oncology Clinical Development
Millenium Pharmaceuticals
Boston, Massachusetts

Michael V. Seiden, MD, PhD
Associate Physician
Division of Hematology/Oncology
Massachusetts General Hospital
Boston, Massachusetts

Roy B. Sessions, MD
Professor of Otolaryngology-Head and Neck Surgery
Albert Einstein College of Medicine
Bronx, New York
Chairman
Max L. Xom Department of Otolaryngology / Head
    and Neck Surgery
Beth Israel Medical Center
New York, New York

Charles L. Shapiro, MD
Associate Professor of Internal Medicine
Director of Breast Medical Oncology
Arthur G. James Cancer Hospital
Richard J. Solove Research Institute
Columbus, Ohio

Stanley Shapshay, MD
Professor of Otolaryngology
Boston University School of Medicine
Boston, Massachusetts

Leslie E. Silberstein, MD
Professor of Pathology
Harvard Medical School
Director of the Joint Program in Transfusion Medicine
Children's Hospital, Dana-Farber Cancer Institute,
    and Brigham and Women's Hospital
Boston, Massachusetts

Richard T. Silver, MD
Professor of Medicine
Weill Medical College of Cornell University

Director, Leukemia and Myeloproliferative Center
New York Presbyterian-Weill Cornell Medical Center
Attending Physician
New York Presbyterian Hospital
New York, New York

Dinesh Singh, MD
Harvard Medical School
Chief Resident in Urology
Brigham and Women's Hospital
Boston, Massachusetts

Steven R. Sloan, MD, PhD
Assistant Professor of Pathology
Harvard Medical School
Medical Director
Transfusion Medicine
Children's Hospital
Boston, Massachusetts

Elaine Sloand, MD
Assistant to Director
National Heart, Lung, and Blood Institute
National Institutes of Health
Bethesda, Maryland

Barbara L. Smith, MD
Assistant Professor of Surgery
Harvard Medical School
Massachusetts General Hospital
Boston, Massachusetts

Arthur J. Sober, MD
Professor of Dermatology
Harvard Medical School
Associate Chief of Dermatology
Massachusetts General Hospital
Boston, Massachusetts

Joseph A. Sparano, MD
Professor of Medicine
Albert Einstein College of Medicine
Director, Breast Medical Oncology
Montefiore Medical Center
Bronx, New York

Stuart J. Spechler, MD
Professor of Medicine
UT Southwestern Medical Center at Dallas
Chief, Division of Gastroenterology
Dallas VA Medical Center
Dallas, Texas

Jerry L. Spivak, MD
Professor of Medicine and Oncology
Johns Hopkins University School of Medicine

Active Staff
Johns Hopkins Hospital
Baltimore, Maryland

Richard M. Stone, MD
Associate Professor of Medicine
Harvard Medical School
Dana-Farber Cancer Institute
Boston, Massachusetts

Keith E. Stuart, MD
Assistant Professor of Medicine
Division of Hematology/Oncology
Harvard Medical School
Director, Gastrointestinal and Hepatobiliary
    Oncology
Beth Israel Deaconess Medical Center
Boston, Massachusetts

Scott Swanson, MD
Eugene W. Friedman Professor of Surgical Oncology
Mt. Sinai School of Medicine
Chief of Thoracic Surgery
Mt. Sinai Medical Center
New York, New York

Martin S. Tallman, MD
Professor of Medicine
Northwestern University Feinberg School of Medicine
Director, Hematologic Malignancy Program
Robert H. Lurie Comprehensive Cancer Center of
    Northwestern University
Chicago, Illinois

Arafat Tfayli, MD
Assistant Professor of Medicine
Division of Hematology-Oncology
University of Oklahoma Health Sciences Center
Oklahoma City, Oklahoma

Elizabeth M. Thomas, PsyD, PhD
Research Assistant Professor
Psychiatry and Behavioral Sciences
University of Miami
Miami, Florida

Melanie B. Thomas, MD
Assistant Professor
M. D. Anderson Cancer Center
University of Texas
Houston, Texas

Robert L. Thurer, MD
Associate Professor of Surgery
Harvard Medical School

Division of Cardiothoracic Surgery
Department of Surgery
Beth Israel Deaconess Medical Center
Boston, Massachusetts

Ivo Tremont-Lukats, MD
Department of Neurology
M. D. Anderson Cancer Center
University of Texas
Houston, Texas

Robert D. Utiger, MD
Clinical Professor of Medicine
Harvard Medical School
Brigham and Women's Hospital
Boston, Massachusetts

Alan P. Venook, MD
Professor of Clinical Medicine
University of California–San Francisco
San Francisco, California

Jacqueline Vuky, MD
Clinical Instructor
Department of Medicine
University of Washington
Attending Physician
Virginia Mason Medical Center
Section of Hematology/Oncology
Seattle, Washington

Louis M. Weiner, MD
Vice President, Translational Research
Chairman, Department of Medical Oncology
Fox Chase Cancer Center
Philadelphia, Pennsylvania

Sharlene M. Weiss, PhD
Research Associate Professor
Sylvester Comprehensive Cancer Center
University of Miami School of Medicine
Miami, Florida

Jeffrey Weitz, MD
Professor of Medicine
McMaster University
Hamilton, Ontario, Canada

Jeffrey N. Weitzel, MD
Clinical Associate Professor of Preventive Medicine
Keck School of Medicine
University of Southern California
Director, Clinical Cancer Genetics
City of Hope Cancer Center
Duarte, California

Patrick Y. Wen
Associate Professor of Neurology
Harvard Medical School
Medical Director
Center for Neuro-Oncology
Dana-Farber Cancer Institute
Boston, Massachusetts

Clarence C. Whitcomb, MD
Associate Professor of Clinical Pathology
Associate Director of Hematopathology
University of Miami
Miami, Florida

Eric P. Winer, MD
Associate Professor of Medicine
Harvard Medical School
Director, Oncology Center
Dana-Farber Cancer Institute
Boston, Massachusetts

Eric Wong, MD
Assistant Professor of Neurology
Harvard Medical School
Beth Israel Deaconess Medical Center
Boston, Massachusetts

COLOR PLATES

PLATE 1

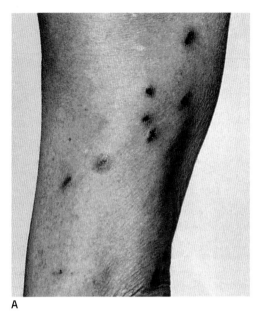 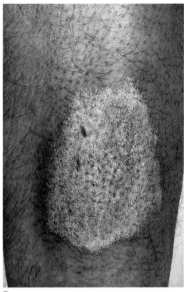

A   B

Figure 3-1 ■ Changes in the skin due to scratching from intense pruritus in a patient with biliary tract obstruction and jaundice. *A,* Excoriations from excavations of the skin by the patient's nails. *B,* Lichenification is thickening of the skin with exaggeration of the skin creases from rubbing the skin in the same site repetitively. (From du Vivier A: Atlas of Clinical Dermatology, 3rd ed. London, Churchill Livingstone, 2002.)

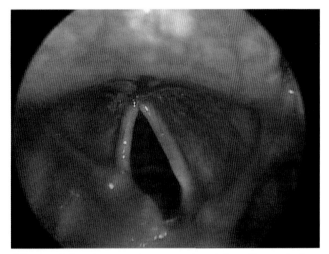 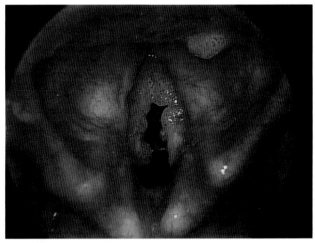

Figure 9-1 ■ Laryngeal cancer involving the anterior commissure and both vocal folds.

Figure 9-2 ■ Vocal fold paralysis. The folds do not meet properly during phonation.

PLATE 2

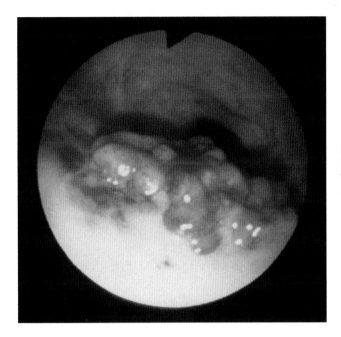

Figure 23-2 ■ Endoscopic photograph showing a nodular carcinoma of the esophagus. (Reprinted, with permission, from the Clinical Teaching Project of the American Gastroenterological Association.)

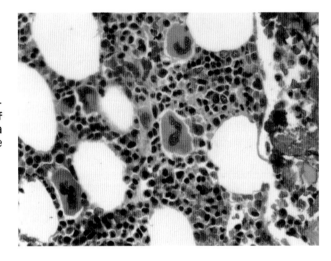

Figure 36-1 ■ Bone marrow megakaryocytes in immune thrombocytopenic purpura. Bone marrow biopsy of patient with chronic immune thrombocytopenic purpura showing a four-fold to five-fold increase in megakaryocyte number.

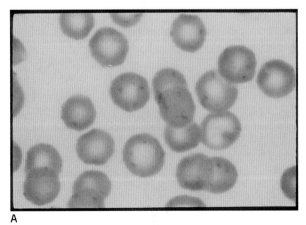

A

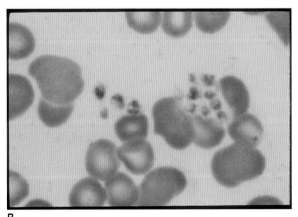

B

Figure 36-2 ■ Platelet clumping. Peripheral blood smear of patient showing no platelets in one field (A) but large platelet clumps in another field (B).

PLATE 3

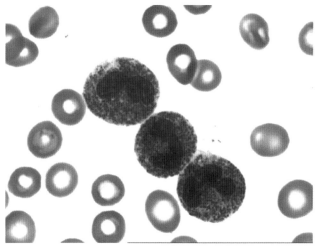

Figure 38-1 ■ Toxic granulation in a patient with neutrophilic leukocytosis.

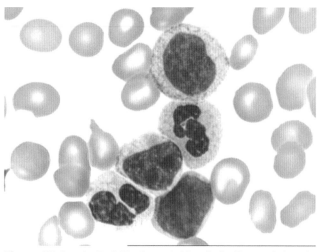

Figure 38-4 ■ Left-shifted myeloid cells in the peripheral blood in a patient with chronic myeloid leukemia.

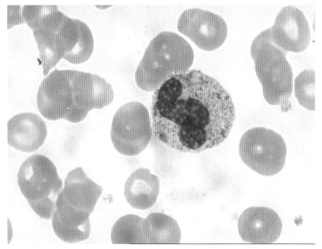

Figure 38-2 ■ Döhle bodies in stress leukocytosis.

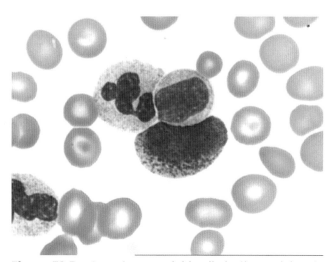

Figure 38-5 ■ Immature myeloid cells in the peripheral blood, including a promyelocyte.

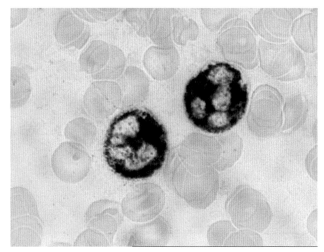

Figure 38-3 ■ Increased leukocyte alkaline phosphatase in a patient with reactive leukocytosis.

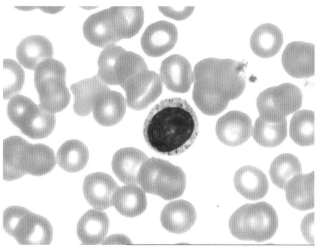

Figure 38-6 ■ Large granular lymphocyte.

PLATE 4

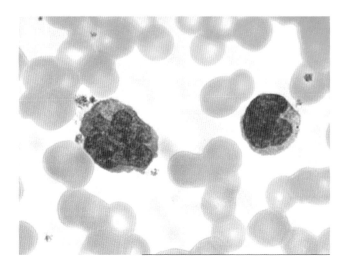

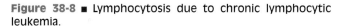

Figure 38-7 ■ Atypical lymphocytes in a patient with infectious mononucleosis.

Figure 38-8 ■ Lymphocytosis due to chronic lymphocytic leukemia.

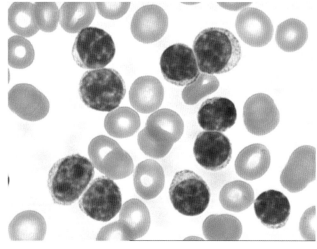

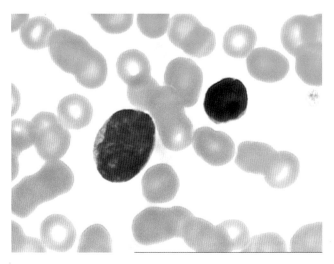

Figure 38-9 ■ Circulating lymphoma cells from a patient with follicular lymphoma.

Figure 38-10 ■ Circulating hairy cells from a patient with hairy cell leukemia.

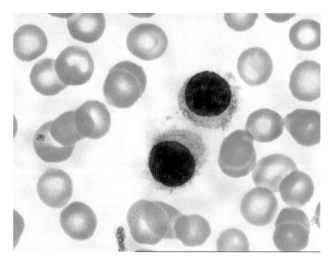

PLATE 5

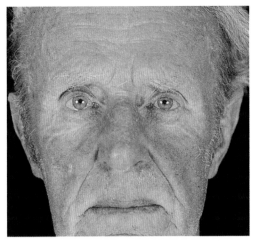

Figure 40-1 ■ Facial plethora in a man with polycythemia vera. (From Hoffbrand AV, Pettit JE: Color Atlas of Clinical Hematology, 3rd ed. St. Louis: Mosby, 2000, p 247.)

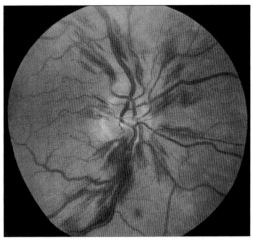

Figure 40-2 ■ Retinal changes in a patient with polycythemia vera. Note distension of retinal vessels and hemorrhage and mild swelling of the optic disc in a patient with a hemoglobin level of 23.5 g/dL, blurred vision, headache, and confusion. (From Hoffbrand AV, Pettit JE: Color Atlas of Clinical Hematology, 3rd ed. St. Louis: Mosby, 2000, p 248.)

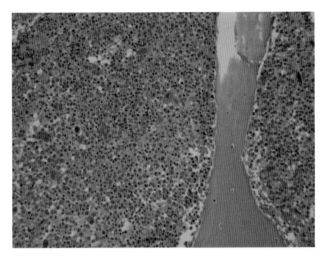

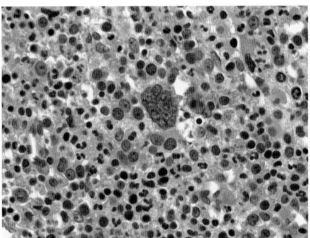

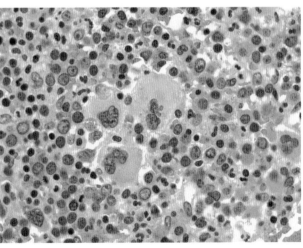

Figure 40-7 ■ Typical bone marrow findings in polycythemia vera include hypercellularity with trilineage hyperplasia (*A*), clustering of megakaryocytes (*B*), and hyperlobated megakaryocytes (*C*).

PLATE 6

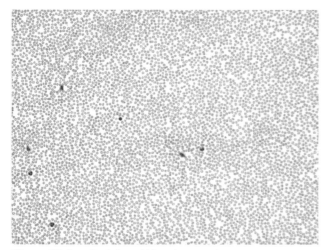

Figure 42-1 ■ Peripheral blood smear. Low-power appearance. Well spread smear with even distribution of cells.

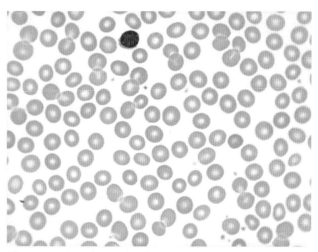

Figure 42-4 ■ The red cells are separated without overlapping. Normal red blood cells with little variation in size and small area of central pallor.

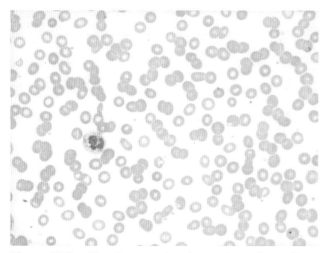

Figure 42-2 ■ Blood smear showing rouleaux formation.

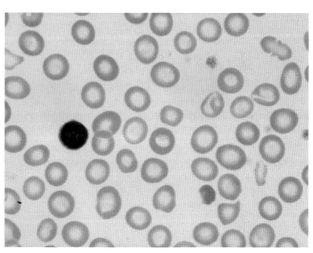

Figure 42-5 ■ Hypochromic red blood cells. Many are also microcytic.

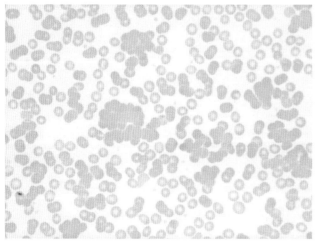

Figure 42-3 ■ Blood smear. Agglutination of red cells in a patient with cold agglutinins.

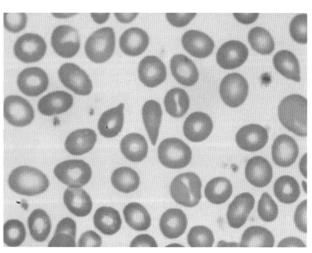

Figure 42-6 ■ Abnormally shaped cell in the form of a teardrop.

PLATE 7

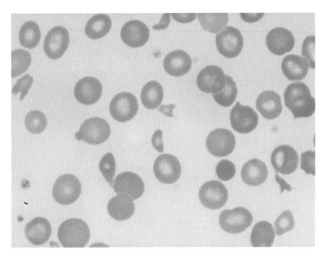

Figure 42-7 ■ Fragmented red cells in a patient with microangiopathic hemolytic anemia.

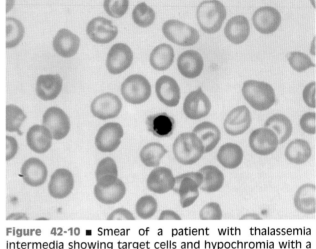

Figure 42-10 ■ Smear of a patient with thalassemia intermedia showing target cells and hypochromia with a nucleated red blood cell.

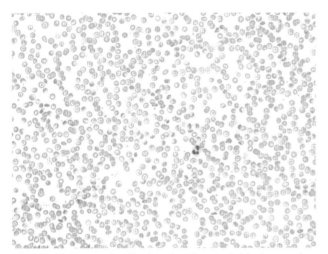

Figure 42-8 ■ Red cells showing hemoglobin in greater concentration at the rim of the cell and at the center producing a "target" appearance.

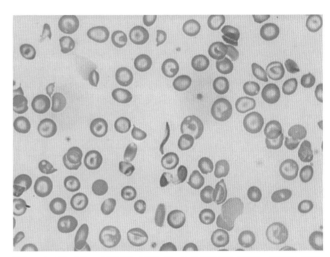

Figure 42-11 ■ Sickle cell in a patient with sickle-cell disease. Target cells and two red cells showing condensation of hemoglobin toward one side of the cell.

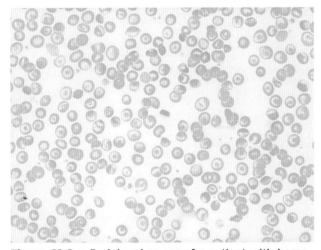

Figure 42-9 ■ Peripheral smear of a patient with hemoglobin C disease. Note elongated structure of hemoglobin crystals within a hypochromic red blood cell and many target cells.

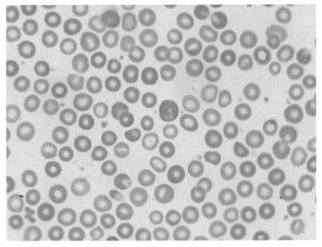

Figure 42-12 ■ Peripheral blood smear showing a polychromatophilic cell in the center of the field. These cells are large and usually lack central pallor.

PLATE 8

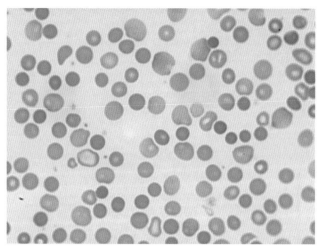

Figure 42-13 ■ Blood smear from a patient with autoimmune hemolytic anemia showing spherocytes, dense staining cells that tend to be microcytic.

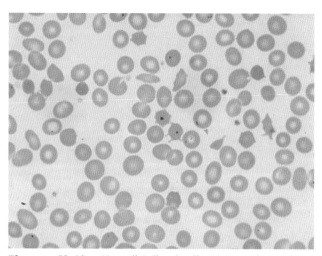

Figure 42-16 ■ Howell-Jolly bodies. Round nuclear remnants in the red cells. There are also acanthocytes (spur cells).

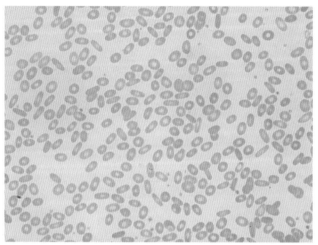

Figure 42-14 ■ Elliptocytes. The red blood cells are pencil or cigar shaped in a typical case of congenital elliptocytosis.

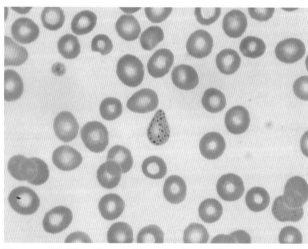

Figure 42-17 ■ Basophilic stippling. Punctate, bluish inclusions throughout the red cell.

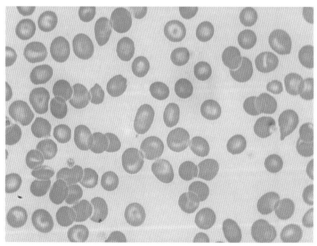

Figure 42-15 ■ Peripheral blood smear showing macroovalocytes (egg-shaped cells). These cells are different from elliptocytes.

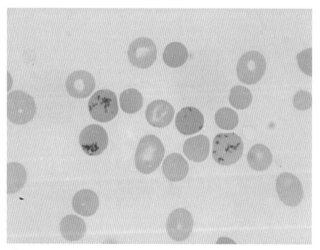

Figure 42-18 ■ Reticulocytes. The structures inside red cells represent precipitated ribonucleoprotein by new methylene blue. On air-dried smears stained with Wright stain, they are polychromatophilic cells.

PLATE 9

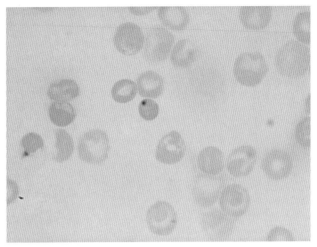

Figure 42-19 ■ Heinz body. Crystal violet stain.

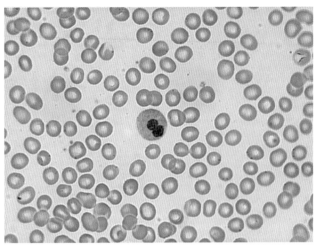

Figure 42-22 ■ Bilobed Pelger-Huet cell.

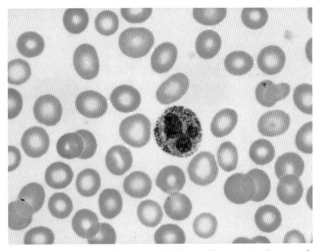

Figure 42-20 ■ Toxic granulation. The cytoplasm of this band neutrophil shows granules diffusely scattered throughout the cytoplasm.

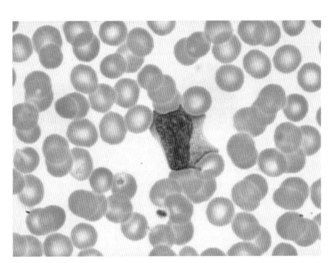

Figure 42-23 ■ Atypical lymphocyte. The morphology of atypical lymphocytes is variable. This one is large with abundant cytoplasm. Young man with infectious mononucleosis.

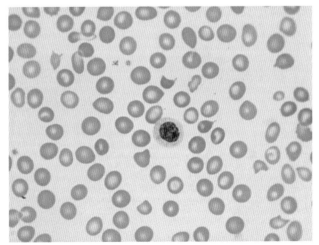

Figure 42-21 ■ Monolobed Pelger-Huet cell. Neutrophil with mature (clumped) chromatin. The nucleus failed to develop lobes.

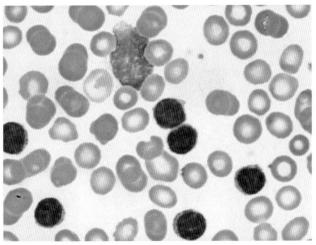

Figure 42-24 ■ Chronic lymphocytic leukemia. Small lymphocytes with dense nuclear chromatin and a very thin rim of cytoplasm. Note smudge cells at top of figure.

PLATE 10

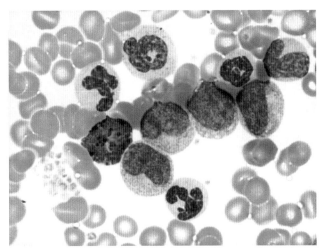

Figure 42-25 ■ Peripheral blood smear. Chronic myeloid leukemia. Spectrum of granulocytic precursors with a basophil (cell with prominent, dark-stained granules).

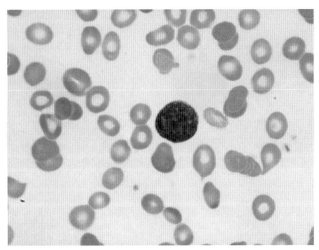

Figure 42-28 ■ Acute lymphocytic leukemia, L1 morphology.

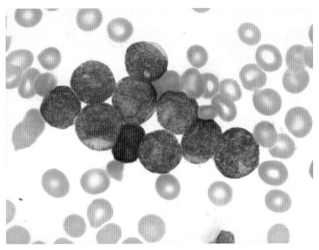

Figure 42-26 ■ Acute myeloid leukemia. These blasts have fine chromatin, prominent nucleolus, and very little cytoplasm.

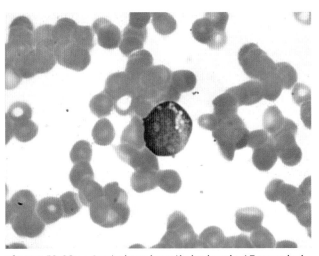

Figure 42-29 ■ Acute lymphocytic leukemia, L3 morphology. This lymphoblast shows a prominent nucleolus and fairly abundant cytoplasm with vacuoles.

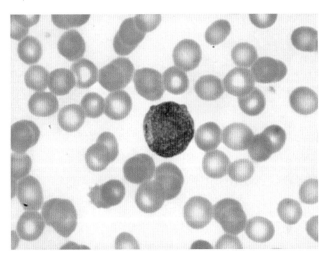

Figure 42-27 ■ Acute myeloid leukemia. Blast with Auer rod, abnormal, typically azurophilic, lysosomal granule, in cytoplasm.

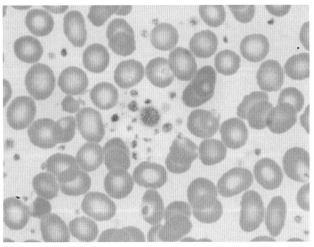

Figure 42-30 ■ Peripheral blood smear from a patient with essential thrombocythemia. Platelets are markedly increased in number. Large platelets are present.

PLATE 11

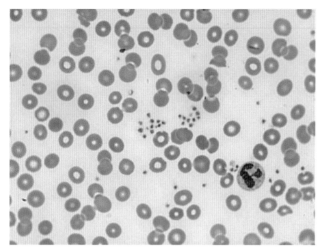

Figure 42-31 ■ Platelet clump.

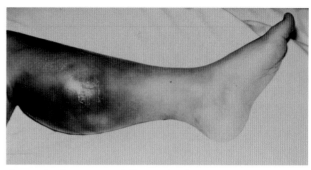

Figure 44-3 ■ Hemophilia A with intramuscular and sub-cutaneous hemorrhage.

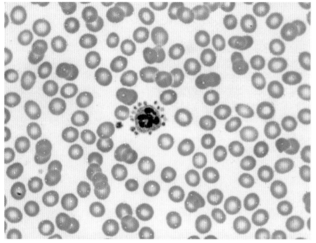

Figure 42-32 ■ EDTA-induced platelet satellitism. Platelets are adherent to the neutrophil.

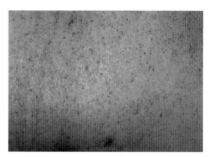

Figure 44-7 ■ Fabry disease. (From Hoffman R, Benz EJ Jr, Shattil SJ, Furie B, Cohen HJ, Silberstein LE, McGlave P [eds]: Hematology: Basic Principles and Practice, 3rd ed. Philadelphia: Churchill Livingstone, 2000.)

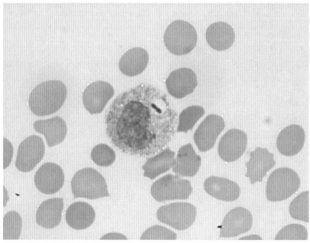

Figure 42-33 ■ Bacteria (E. coli) phagocytized in neutrophil.

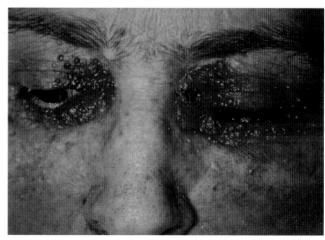

Figure 44-10 ■ Immunoglobulin related primary amyloidosis with extensive periorbital hemorrhagic cutaneous lesions.

PLATE 12

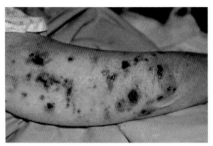

Figure 44-18 ■ Leukocytoclastic vasculitis. (From Hoffman R, Benz EJ Jr, Shattil SJ, Furie B, Cohen HJ, Silberstein LE, McGlave P [eds]: Hematology: Basic Principles and Practice, 3rd ed. Philadelphia: Churchill Livingstone, 2000.)

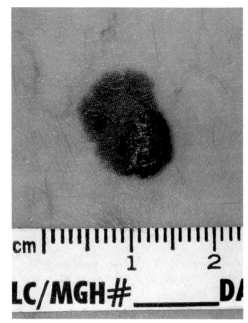

Figure 45-3 ■ Melanoma arising in association with a pre-existing compound nevus on the thigh of a woman in her 40s. Note elevation and irregularity of surface.

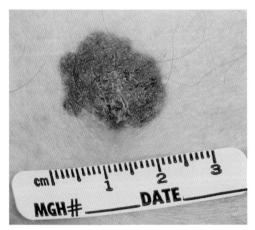

Figure 45-1 ■ Superficial spreading melanoma, level II, 0.43 mm in thickness on the arm of a male over age 60. Note asymmetry (A), irregularity of border (B), variation in color (C), and size: approximately 1.5 mm (D).

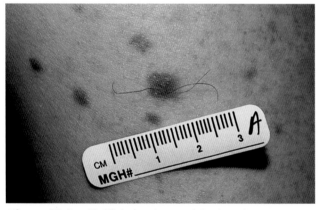

Figure 45-4 ■ Multiple benign nevi. Lesions have reasonably regular contours and uniform pigment patterns.

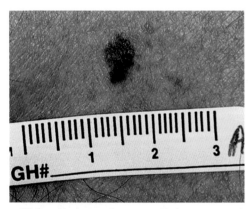

Figure 45-2 ■ Early melanoma. Note asymmetry (A), irregularity of border (B), and variation in pigment pattern (C). Lesion is 7 mm in greatest dimension (D).

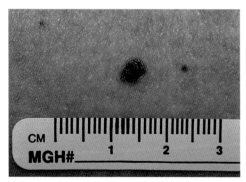

Figure 45-5 ■ Acquired compound nevus. Raised lesion, relatively uniform color, pigment pattern, and border. Onset, after birth.

PLATE 13

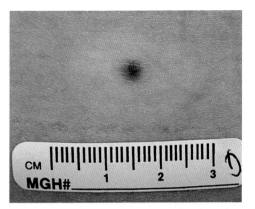

Figure 45-6 ■ Halo nevus. One mechanism by which the body rids itself of nevi is through an inflammatory response that destroys the mole and surrounding normal epidermal melanocytes. Halo nevi may be seen in patients who have a melanoma at some other location on their body. Note the hypopigmentation surrounding the central lesion.

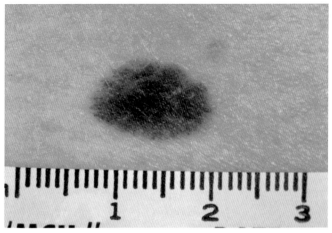

Figure 45-8 ■ Compound dysplastic nevus.

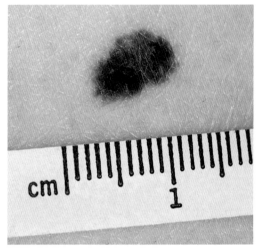

Figure 45-9 ■ Compound dysplastic nevus.

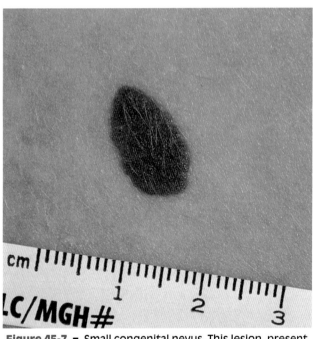

Figure 45-7 ■ Small congenital nevus. This lesion, present from birth, has uniform pigmentation, regular contours, and increased hair.

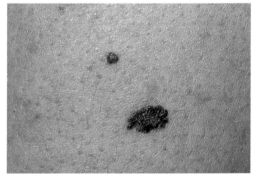

Figure 45-10 ■ Compound dysplastic nevus. Raised lesion, often >6 mm, may vary in size and shape from the patient's other nevi. Borders may be less distinct than those of benign acquired nevi.

PLATE 14

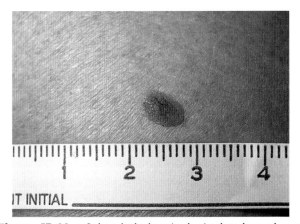

Figure 45-11 ■ Seborrheic keratosis. Lesion is a plaque with a waxy surface. Can be flesh colored to very dark.

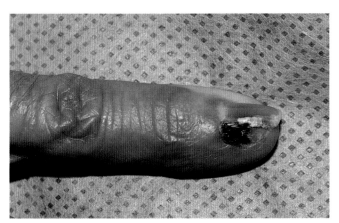

Figure 45-12 ■ Pseudo-Hutchinson sign in patient with hemorrhage and fungal infection of the nail plate. Note the pigmentation in the posterior nailfold.

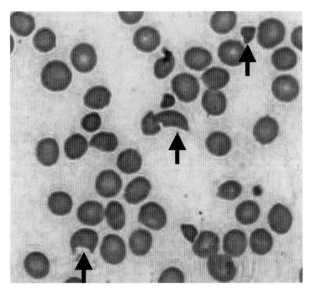

Figure 57-2 ■ Peripheral blood smear in thrombotic thrombocytopenic purpura. The peripheral blood smear in thrombotic thrombocytopenic purpura is characterized by schistocytes and red blood cell fragments (arrows). The number of schistocytes in thrombotic thrombocytopenic purpura can vary greatly and does not correlate well with severity, but they are the sine qua non of thrombotic thrombocytopenic purpura.

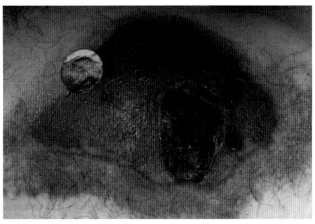

Figure 59-4 ■ Warfarin-induced skin necrosis. Central area of necrosis is surrounded by a well-circumscribed area of erythema. Circular defect at the margin is the biopsy site.

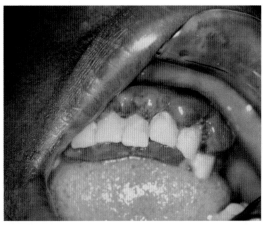

Figure 60-5 ■ Gingival hyperplasia in a 55-year-old patient presenting with monocytic acute myeloid leukemia, FAB type M5.

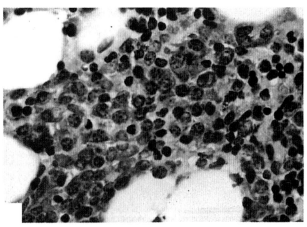

Figure 63-1 ■ Bone marrow biopsy section demonstrates clusters of immature, blast-like plasma cells (plasma blasts). (From Naeim F: Atlas of Bone Marrow and Blood Pathology. Philadelphia: WB Saunders, 2001.)

PLATE 15

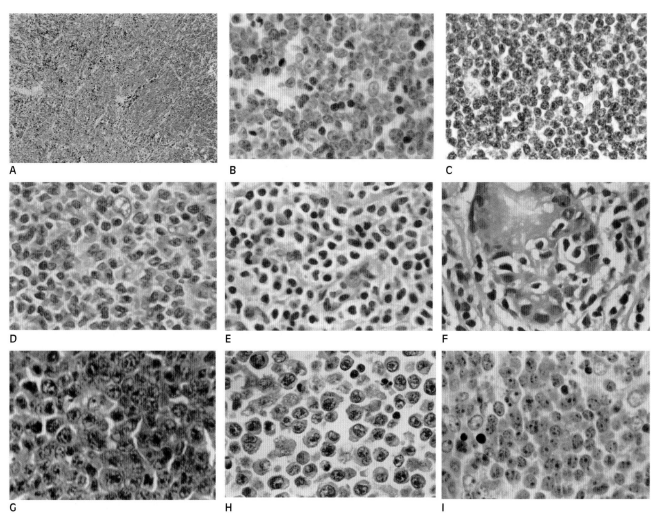

Figure 64-1 ■ *A*, Lymphoblastic lymphoma with diffuse pattern. *B*, Precursor T cell lymphoblastic lymphoma. *C*, B cell small lymphocytic lymphoma. *D*, Mantle cell lymphoma. *E*, Nodal marginal zone lymphoma (monocytoid cells). *F*, Lymphoepithelial lesion in extranodal marginal zone lymphoma of mucosal-associated lymphoid tissue type. *G*, Diffuse large B cell lymphoma. *H*, Diffuse large B cell lymphoma (plasma cell variant). *I*, Burkitt's lymphoma.

PLATE 16

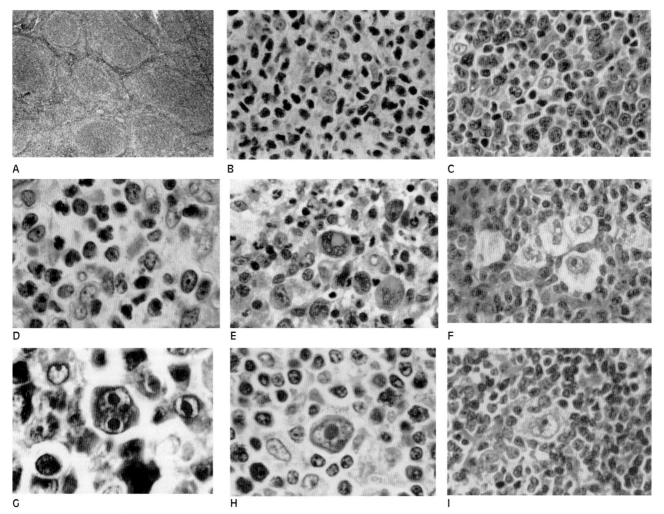

Figure 64-2 ■ *A*, Malignant lymphoma with follicular pattern. *B*, Follicular lymphoma, grade 1. *C*, Follicular lymphoma, grade 3. *D*, Peripheral T cell lymphoma. *E*, Anaplastic large cell lymphoma. *F*, Lacunar cell. *G*, Reed-Sternberg cell. *H*, Mononuclear Hodgkin's cell. *I*, L & H cell.

Figure 68-1 ■ Sites of primary extranodal lymphoma. (Adapted from Sutcliffe SB, Gospodarowicz MK: Localized extranodal lymphomas. In Keating A, Armitage J, Burnett A, et al [eds]: Haematological Oncology. Cambridge, Mass., Cambridge University Press, 1992, pp 189–222. Reprinted with the permission of Cambridge University Press.)

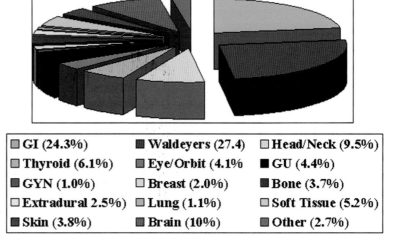

▢ GI (24.3%)	■ Waldeyers (27.4)	▢ Head/Neck (9.5%)
▢ Thyroid (6.1%)	▨ Eye/Orbit (4.1%	■ GU (4.4%)
■ GYN (1.0%)	▢ Breast (2.0%)	▨ Bone (3.7%)
▢ Extradural 2.5%)	▨ Lung (1.1%)	▨ Soft Tissue (5.2%)
■ Skin (3.8%)	▨ Brain (10%)	▨ Other (2.7%)

PLATE 17

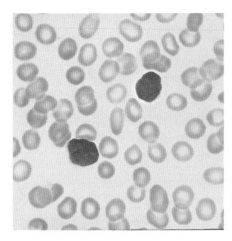

Figure 69-3 ■ Sézary cells in the peripheral blood.

Figure 73-1 ■ Teardrops (dacryocytes) in myelofibrosis.

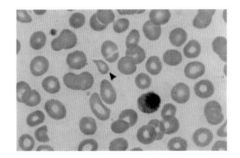

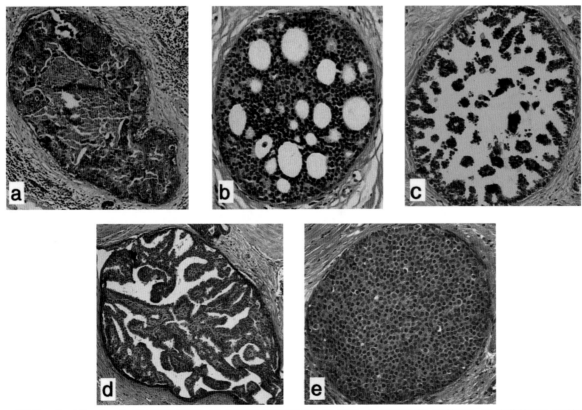

Figure 75-1 ■ Architectural classifications of ductal carcinoma in situ. *A*, Comedo pattern. *B*, Cribiform pattern. *C*, Micropapillary pattern. *D*, Papillary pattern. *E*, Solid pattern. (From Schnitt S: Pathology of Breast Cancer. In Hayes DF [ed]: Atlas of Breast Cancer, 2nd ed. St. Louis: Mosby, 2000.)

PLATE 18

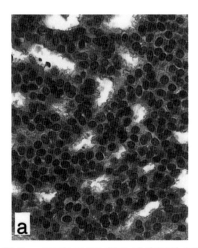
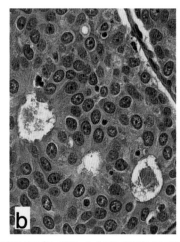
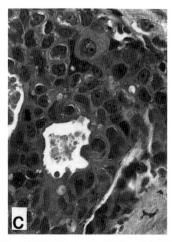

Figure 75-2 ■ Nuclear grading of ductal carcinoma in situ. *A*, Low nuclear grade. *B*, Intermediate grade. *C*, High nuclear grade. (From Schnitt S: Pathology of Breast Cancer. In Hayes DF [ed]: Atlas of Breast Cancer, 2nd ed. St. Louis: Mosby, 2000.)

Figure 81-1 ■ Intraoperative appearance of stage III epithelial ovarian cancer. Multiple implants are scattered throughout the peritoneal mesothelial surface of the upper abdomen.

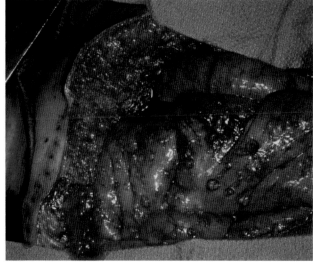

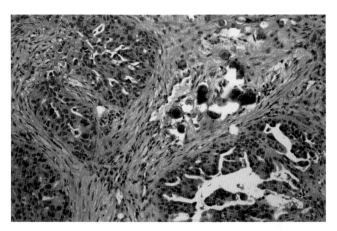

Figure 81-5 ■ Papillary serous ovarian cancer with psammoma bodies. Psammoma bodies are structures composed of concentric rings of calcification, often observed in papillary serous ovarian or primary peritoneal serous cancers. There are several psammoma bodies just to the right of center in this 40× (original magnification) photomicrograph (hematoxylin and eosin stain).

PLATE 19

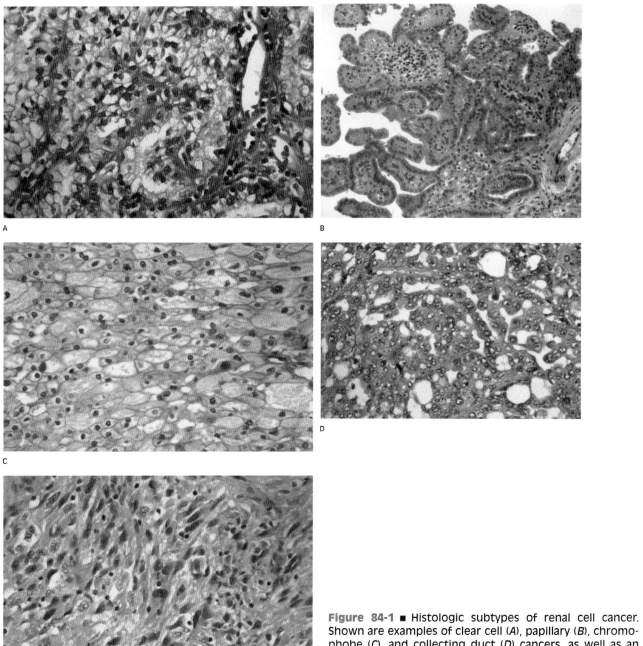

Figure 84-1 ■ Histologic subtypes of renal cell cancer. Shown are examples of clear cell (*A*), papillary (*B*), chromophobe (*C*), and collecting duct (*D*) cancers, as well as an example of a sarcomatoid renal cell carcinoma (*E*). (Photographs courtesy of Dr. Melissa Upton, Department of Pathology, Beth Israel Deaconess Medical Center.)

PLATE 20

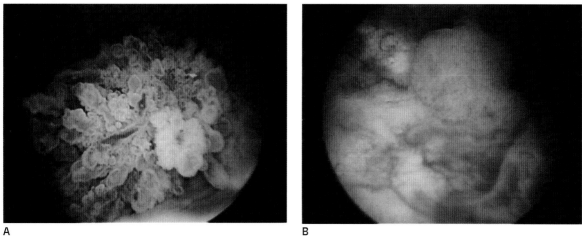

A   B

Figure 85-2 ■ Cystoscopic appearance of common superficial bladder cancers. *A*, Stage Ta grade 1–2. *B*, Stage T1 grade 3.

Figure 106-2B ■ Sentinel lymph node biopsy. *B*, Intraoperative lymphatic mapping with a vital blue dye in a patient with a right scapular melanoma. The dye was injected around the primary site. After 10 minutes, an axillary incision was made, and a blue-staining afferent lymphatic was identified (arrow) draining into a blue-staining node (the sentinel lymph node). This node contained a 5-mm focus of metastatic melanoma and was the only site of disease in the basin.

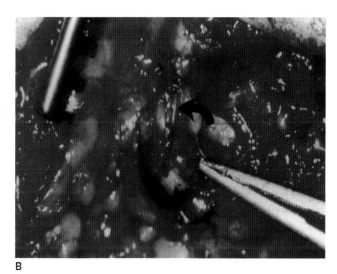

B

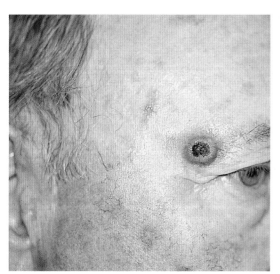

Figure 107-1 ■ Basal cell carcinoma that has become an ulcerating tumor. (From Callen JP, Paller AS, Greer KE, Swinyer LJ: Color Atlas of Dermatology, 2nd ed. Philadelphia: WB Saunders, 2000.)

PLATE 21

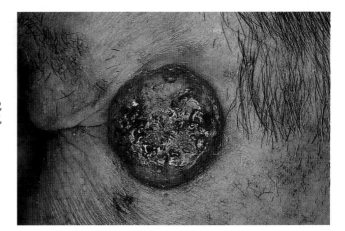

Figure 107-3 ■ Squamous cell carcinoma. (From Callen JP, Paller AS, Greer KE, Swinyer LJ: Color Atlas of Dermatology, 2nd ed. Philadelphia: WB Saunders, 2000.)

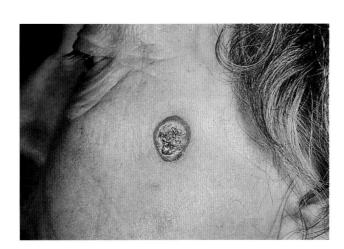

Figure 107-4 ■ Keratoacanthoma. (From Callen JP, Paller AS, Greer KE, Swinyer LJ: Color Atlas of Dermatology, 2nd ed. Philadelphia: WB Saunders, 2000.)

Figure 107-6 ■ Merkel cell carcinoma. (From Callen JP, Paller AS, Greer KE, Swinyer LJ: Color Atlas of Dermatology, 2nd ed. Philadelphia: WB Saunders, 2000.)

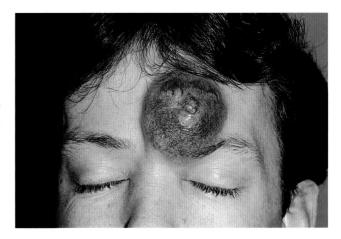

PLATE 22

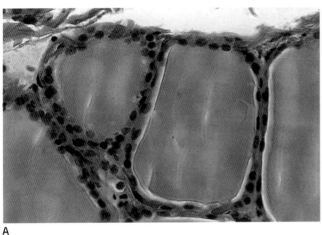
A

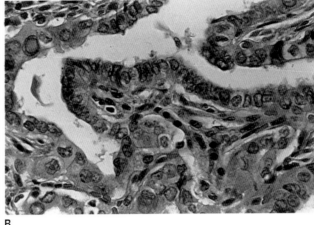
B

Figure 108-2 ■ Microscopic sections of normal thyroid tissue (*A*) and papillary carcinoma of the thyroid (*B*). In the normal thyroid, the follicular cells are arranged in follicles, and the cells have hyperchromatic nuclei. In the carcinoma, the cells are crowded together, and the nuclei overlap, are pale-staining, and have grooves and pseudo-inclusions.

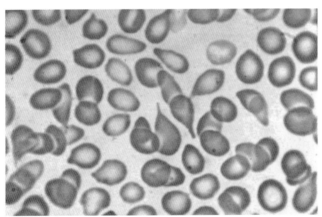

Figure 114-1 ■ Teardrop cells are seen most prominently in thalassemias and diseases involving bone marrow infiltration by fibrosis or malignancy. Erythrocytes are distorted as they travel through the vasculature of an abnormal bone marrow or spleen. Pointed ends may be sharp or blunt. (From Tkachuk DC, Hirschmann JV, McArthur JR: Atlas of Clinical Hematology. Philadelphia: WB Saunders, 2002.)

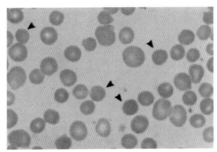

Figure 114-2 ■ Spherocytes in immune-mediated hemolytic anemia. (From Hoffman R, Benz EJ Jr, Shattil SJ, et al [eds]: Hematology: Basic Principles and Practice, 3rd ed. New York: Churchill Livingstone, 2000.)

PLATE 23

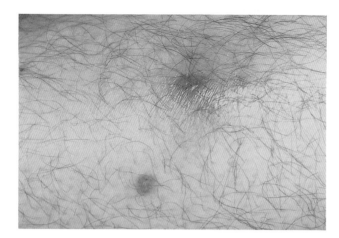

Figure 115-2 ■ Cutaneous manifestation of pseudomonals sepsis. A 28-year-old man with acute myeloid leukemia developed a fever and these palpable skin lesions on his arms and legs five days after receiving chemotherapy. Biopsy confirmed a necrotizing vasculitis with thrombosis, characteristic of ecthyma gangrenosum. Both skin biopsy and blood cultures grew *Pseudomonas aeruginosa*.

Figure 115-4B ■ Aspergillosis. A 48-year-old man with myelodysplastic syndrome developed fever, cough, and pleuritic chest pain 12 days after receiving chemotherapy. His neutrophil count was 0.02/mm^3. and chest radiograph showed a peripheral cavitary infiltrate. Video-assisted thoracoscopic biopsy revealed branching invasive hyphae characteristic of invasive pulmonary aspergillosis (*B*).

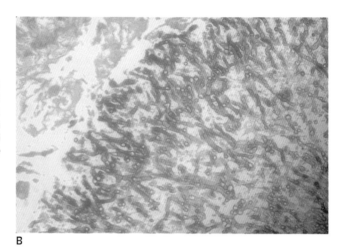

B

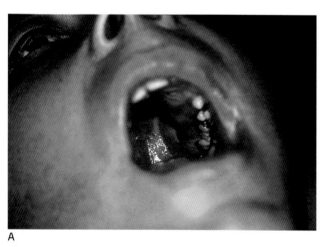

A

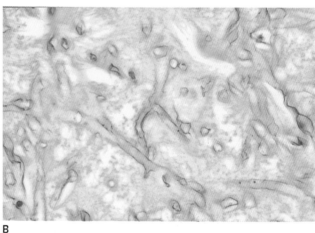

B

Figure 115-5 ■ Mucormycosis. This rapidly evolving oral lesion occurred in a patient with chronic lymphocytic leukemia in the setting of fever to 101.0°F and chemotherapy-induced neutropenia (*A*). Autopsy results (*B*) and postmortem cultures demonstrated mucormycosis, a largely fatal complication of advanced cancer. Prompt surgical evaluation is required in patients with suspected mucormycosis.

Preface

Hematology and oncology have become integrated disciplines. Combined divisions of hematology-oncology have been established in medical schools and hospitals across the United States; most major fellowship programs offer combined training programs in hematology and oncology; practitioners frequently hold dual memberships in the American Society of Hematology and the American Society for Clinical Oncology; and dual board certification in hematology and oncology is increasingly common. Because of this interdigitation, we thought that it would be helpful to assemble in a single textbook an approach to the clinical practice of this combined specialty. The intent is to provide a clinically useful, readily accessible guide to the diagnosis and management of patients with hematologic and neoplastic diseases. Rather than just joining two textbooks into a single volume, we have made a substantial effort to achieve a meaningful integration of these two fields. The result, we believe, is a source of information that fills the niche between the encyclopedic textbooks of hematology and of medical oncology and the broad textbooks of internal medicine by maintaining a clinical focus throughout. A wide audience, including hematologists/oncologists, family practitioners, general internists, oncology nurse practitioners, hematology-oncology trainees, medical students, and residents, should find this approach useful in clinical care and in preparation for Board examinations.

The book is organized differently from standard textbooks of hematology and oncology. The chapters in the first section (**Presentations**) focus on individual presenting symptoms and/or findings and describe the best approach to sort through the differential diagnosis, determine whether the problem is hematologic or oncologic, and to rapidly ascertain the definitive diagnosis. The chapters in the second section each describe a specific disease with a focus on evaluation and management. Authors of the individual chapters were selected for their clinical skills and experience and were encouraged to impart the thought processes

and decision-making that they themselves utilize in clinical practice. Each author was invited to include one or more brief discussions of particularly useful or insightful clinical "pearls of wisdom" regarding diagnosis and therapy. Chapters do not contain individual citation references; instead each chapter ends with a list of suggested relevant reading considered important by the author and generally recent in origin. Liberal use of figures, tables, images, photographs and diagrams of heuristic value are included in each chapter.

The major textbooks of hematology and of oncology, including *Hematology: Basic Principles and Practice* (Hoffman et al.) and *Clinical Oncology* (Abeloff et al.) by our publisher, Elsevier, typically are organized according to various diseases. Yet patients come to the attention of clinicians because of symptoms, physical signs, or abnormal laboratory and radiologic data. In order to make a diagnosis, one needs to distinguish among the multiple causes and whether the likely diagnosis lies in the realm of general medicine or in hematology or oncology. For example, when confronted with a specific clinical presentation, what is the constellation of symptoms and signs that make you lean toward one diagnosis or another? What are the clues that make you suspicious of an underlying hematologic or oncologic disorder as opposed to a general internal medicine problem? How do you distinguish potential nonmalignant from malignant disorders? What algorithms do you use for coming to the diagnosis—that is, laboratory studies, imaging, invasive procedures—and in what order? Since this is a hematology-oncology text, we focus on the hematologic and oncologic disorders that may present in this fashion. In some cases, 99% of patients presenting with a particular symptom complex may have a problem unrelated to hematology or oncology. We focus on the 1% of patients and provide the clues that you should use to separate them from the larger subset. For example, laboratory detection of hypercalcemia is not usually due to a hematologic or oncologic disorder. After outlining potential general medical causes, we indicate what components suggest an underlying neoplasm, such as the presence of hypercalcemic symptomatology. In sum, we describe rational approaches to establishing a definitive diagnosis, using a parsimonious, efficient, clinically intuitive approach based upon probabilities and presenting concomitant features. The second section, on principles of **Therapeutics**, provides an understanding of various treatment modalities, the biologic effects underlying their activity, and their appropriate application.

The third section, on **Evaluation and Treatment** of specific disorders, is a disease management section. Here, epidemiology, genetics, prognostic factors, and pathophysiology are discussed with a focus on their utility in enhancing clinical diagnosis and the determination of therapy. Differential diagnosis is discussed only briefly, since the **Presentations** section of the text provides a strategy for making diagnoses. The disease management chapters nevertheless describe the range of presenting signs and symptoms, laboratory findings, and radiographs typical of each disease. The chapters emphasize the varying histologic subtypes, staging procedures, and the implications for therapeutic strategies and outcomes. Rather than provide lengthy tables of the results of therapeutic clinical trials, the conclusions about the current standard single or combined modality therapy are given in instances where there is a consensus view. Ongoing general and supportive care management approaches, specific recommendations for appropriate follow-up evaluations, and the acute toxicities and late sequelae of treatment are also considered. We have intended that the recommendations emphasize one or more of the best available therapies and highlight persisting controversies in management. We have specifically avoided description of speculative or experimental therapies whose value is unproven.

Section four, on **Special Considerations in Treatment**, and section five, on **Supportive Care**, consider issues specific to subsets of patients with cancer, and they establish guidelines to anticipate and treat problems as they arise during the course of disease and therapy in patients with cancer.

The editors thank Marc Strauss for his efforts early on to get this book underway; Joanne Husovski, our developmental editor, whose diligent participation made this project feasible; and Dolores Meloni, who helped to oversee the timely completion of this book.

Bruce Furie
Peter A. Cassileth
Michael B. Atkins
Robert J. Mayer

Contents

Contributors   v

Preface   xvii

Contents   xix

SECTION I
Presentations   1

General

1 Weight Loss and Anorexia   3
Peter A. Cassileth

2 Fever of Unknown Origin   9
Robert W. Finberg

3 Pruritus   14
Peter A. Cassileth

Head

4 Headache   19
Eric Wong

5 Seizures   23
Steven C. Schachter

6 Cranial Neuropathy   27
Eric Wong and Subramanian Hariharan

7 Encephalopathy and Neuropathy   32
Patrick Y. Wen

Neck

8 Neck Mass   43
David S. Caradonna, Arthur M. Lauretano

9 Hoarseness   50
Elie E. Rebeiz and Stanley Shapshay

Breast

10 Palpable Breast Masses   59
Barbara L. Smith

11 The Abnormal Mammogram   65
Barbara L. Smith

12 Nipple Discharge   71
Barbara L. Smith

Pulmonary

13 Dyspnea   75
Corina Akerele and Joseph A. Sparano

14 The Solitary Pulmonary Nodule   81
Phillip M. Boiselle and Armin Ernst

15 Pleural Effusion   87
Scott Swanson and Hasan F. Batirel

16 Hilar and Mediastinal Adenopathy   94
Joseph LoCicero III

17 Superior Vena Cava Syndrome   98
Tracey Evans and Thomas J. Lynch Jr.

18 Hemoptysis   106
Armin Ernst and Robert L. Thurer

Abdomen

19 Bowel Obstruction   109
Monica M. Bertagnolli

20 Focal Liver Lesions   115
Gaston Morillo

21 Ascites   128
Kevin R. Fox

22 Splenomegaly   135
David P. Schenkein

23 Dysphagia   139
Stuart J. Spechler

24 Gastrointestinal Bleeding   144
Keith E. Stuart

Bone

25 Pathologic Fractures   149
Mohamed Anwar Hau and Henry J. Mankin

26 Back Pain   156
Eric Wong

Genitourinary

27 Renal and Adrenal Masses   165
Martina Morrin and Robert C. Eyre

28 Hematuria 173
Dinesh Singh and Aria F. Olumi

29 Testicular Mass   179
Pasquale Benedetto

30 Vaginal Bleeding   184
Kris Ghosh and Jonathan M. Niloff

Blood Chemistry Abnormalities

31 Hypercalcemia   191
Stephen Richman

32 Elevated Bilirubin   196
Peter A. Cassileth

33 Immunoglobulin Abnormalities   200
Philip R. Greipp

34 Iron Studies: Normal and Abnormal   207
Nancy C. Andrews

Hematological Abnormalities

35 Lymphadenopathy   213
Peter Kozuch and Michael L. Grossbard

36 Thrombocytopenia and Thrombocytosis   221
David J. Kuter

37 Anemia   232
William C. Aird

38 Quantitative Abnormalities of Leukocytes   241
Geraldine P. Schechter

39 Pancytopenia   251
Anne Moore

40 Erythrocytosis   256
Peter T. Curtin

41 Bleeding Disorders   265
Bruce Furie

42 Morphologic Abnormalities of the Peripheral Blood   272
Beria Cabello Inchausti and R. Judith Ratzan

43 Venous Thromboembolic Disease   283
Howard A. Liebman

Skin

44 Cutaneous Manifestations of Bleeding and Thrombotic Disorders   293
Donald Feinstein

45 Pigmented Skin Lesions   305
Arthur J. Sober

Difficult Diagnoses

46 Cancer of Unknown Primary   313
Richard M. Stone

Section II
Therapeutics   319

47 Radiation Oncology   321
Theodore S. Lawrence and George T. Henning

48 Cancer Chemotherapy   330
William N. Hait, Barton A. Kamen, Eric H. Rubin, and Susan Goodin

49 Surgical Oncology   362
Monica M. Bertagnolli

50 Biologic Therapy   376
Nancy L. Lewis and Louis M. Weiner

51 Hematopoietic Stem Cell Transplantation   391
Stephen J. Forman and Margaret R. O'Donnell

52 Growth Factors   419
Jacob M. Rowe

53 Transfusion Medicine   431
Steven R. Sloan and Leslie E. Silberstein

Section III
Evaluation and Treatment of Hematologic and Oncologic Disease   441

Hematologic Disorders

54 Bone Marrow Failure Syndromes   443
Elaine Sloand and Jaroslaw Maciejewski

55 Red Blood Cell Disorders   455
Peter W. Marks

56 White Cell Disorders   475
Laurence Alan Boxer

57 Platelet Disorders: Acquired and Congenital   485
Christopher L. Carpenter

58 Coagulation Disorders: Acquired and Congenital   498
Craig M. Kessler and Arafat Tfayli

59 Venous Thromboembolism 511
Jeffrey I. Weitz

Hematologic Malignancies

60 Acute Myeloid Leukemia 521
Larry D. Cripe and Martin S. Tallman

61 Acute Lymphoblastic Leukemia 549
Richard A. Larson

62 Myelodysplasia 566
Jeanne E. Anderson

63 Multiple Myeloma, Macroglobulinemia, and Amyloidosis 581
Mohamad A. Hussein and Martin M. Oken

64 Diagnosis of Malignant Lymphoma and Hodgkin's Disease 601
Gerald E. Byrne Jr. and Clarence C. Whitcomb

65 Hodgkin's Disease 615
Thomas M. Habermann and Joseph P. Colgan

66 Low-Grade Non-Hodgkin's Lymphoma 636
R. Gregory Bociek and James O. Armitage

67 Intermediate- and High-Grade Lymphoma 648
Ann Mellott and Leo I. Gordon

68 Extranodal Non-Hodgkin's Lymphoma 660
David P. Schenkein

69 Peripheral T Cell Lymphomas 664
Stephen M. Ansell

70 Adult T Cell Leukemia/Lymphoma 672
R. Judith Ratzan

71 Chronic Myeloid Leukemia 676
Richard T. Silver

72 Chronic Lymphocytic Leukemia and Hairy Cell Leukemia 688
Bruce D. Cheson

73 Polycythemia Vera, Idiopathic Myelofibrosis and Essential Thrombocythemia 701
Jerry L. Spivak

Breast Cancer

74 Breast Cancer—Staging and Prognosis 715
Craig A. Bunnell, Eric P. Winer, and Judy E. Garber

75 Noninvasive Breast Cancer 726
Virginia Borges and Steven E. Come

76 Locally Invasive Breast Cancer 737
Julie J. Olin and Hyman B. Muss

77 Metastatic Breast Cancer 750
Charles L. Shapiro

78 Breast Cancer: Supportive Measures and Follow-up Care 763
Harold J. Burstein

Gynecologic Cancer

79 Carcinoma of the Cervix, Vulva, and Vagina 769
Michael V. Seiden and AnneKathryn Goodman

80 Endometrial Cancer 782
Michael G. Muto

81 Ovarian Cancer 791
Stephen A. Cannistra

82 Trophoblastic Tumors 804
Donald P. Goldstein and Ross S. Berkowitz

Genitourinary Cancer

83 Testicular Germ Cell Cancer 813
Jacqueline Vuky and Robert J. Motzer

84 Renal Cancer 825
Jared A. Gollob

85 Superficial Bladder Cancer 842
Michael A. O'Donnell

86 Muscle-Invasive Bladder Cancer 850
Bruce J. Roth

87 Prostate Cancer 859
Yoo-Joung Ko and Glenn J. Bubley

Gastrointestinal Cancer

88 Esophageal Cancer 875
David Ilson

89 Gastric Cancer 887
Jeffrey A. Meyerhardt and Charles S. Fuchs

90 Hepatobiliary Cancers 899
Alan P. Venook

91 Pancreatic Cancer 908
Jeffrey W. Clark

92 Colorectal Cancer 921
Robert J. Mayer

93 Anal Carcinoma 938
David P. Ryan

Thoracic Cancer

94 Small Cell Lung Cancer 943
Joseph J. Merchant and Joan H. Schiller

95 Non–Small Cell Lung Cancer 958
Daniel D. Karp and Robert Thurer

96 Thymoma   983
Patrick J. Loehrer Sr.

97 Mesothelioma   991
Joseph Aisner

Head and Neck Cancer

98 Primary Head and Neck Cancer   999
Fadlo R. Khuri and Edward S. Kim

99 Second Primary Cancers of the Head and Neck   1012
Fadlo R. Khuri

100 Salivary Gland Carcinoma   1017
Roy B. Sessions and Douglas K. Frank

Sarcoma

101 Bone Sarcomas   1027
Shreyaskumar R. Patel and Robert S. Benjamin

102 Soft-Tissue Sarcomas   1038
Pasquale Benedetto

Neuro-Oncology

103 Primary Brain Tumors   1049
Stuart A. Grossman

104 Brain Metastases   1062
Minesh P. Mehta and Ivo Tremont-Lukats

105 Epidural Tumors and Spinal Cord Compression   1077
Fred Hochberg

Cutaneous Malignancies

106 Melanoma   1085
Lawrence E. Flaherty and Jared A. Gollob

107 Nonmelanoma Skin Cancer   1104
Reed E. Drews and Lara Kelley

Endocrine Cancer

108 Thyroid Cancer   1117
Robert D. Utiger

109 Adrenal Cancer   1129
William K. Oh

110 Neuroendocrine Cancer   1133
Matthew H. Kulke

111 Pituitary Cancer   1139
Robert D. Utiger

Section IV
Special Considerations in the Treatment of Patients with Cancer   1145

112 Cancer of Unknown Primary   1147
Melanie B. Thomas and James L. Abbruzzese

113 Cancer and the Immunocompromised Host   1155
David T. Scadden and Jonathan W. Friedberg

114 Hematologic Manifestations of Cancer   1166
John K. Erban

115 Febrile Neutropenia   1173
Joel T. Katz and Lindsey R. Baden

116 Thromboembolic Manifestations of Cancer   1179
James D. Levine

117 Tumor Lysis Syndrome   1187
Daniel J. De Angelo

Section V
Supportive Care of the Patient with Cancer   1191

118 Screening and Genetic Counseling for the Patient with Cancer   1193
Jeffrey N. Weitzel

119 Unorthodox Approaches to Cancer Therapy   1209
Brent Bauer and Charles L. Loprinzi

120 Psychosocial Issues   1224
Elizabeth M. Thomas, Carlos J. Sandoval, and Sharlene M. Weiss

121 Sexual Dysfunction   1235
Abraham Morgentaler

122 Symptom Management   1240
Janet L. Abrahm

Index   1261

Clinical Hematology
and Oncology

Section I
Presentations

General
Head
Neck
Breast
Pulmonary
Abdomen
Bone
Genitourinary
Lymphoid
Blood Chemistry Abnormalities
Hematologic Abnormalities
Skin
Cancer of Unknown Primary

Chapter 1
Weight Loss and Anorexia

Peter A. Cassileth

Cachexia (from the Greek *kakos* for "bad" + *hexis* "condition") is a syndrome involving loss of greater than 5% to 10% of the patient's weight associated with anorexia and weakness. Other manifestations include early satiety, fatigability, and poor performance status. In the absence of deliberate dieting, cachexia can be due to a vast array of medical problems. The potential etiologies include any severe chronic disease (inflammation, infection, and cancer), major organ function impairment (advanced cardiac, renal, pulmonary, or hepatic disease), endocrine (hyperthyroidism) or metabolic (diabetes mellitus) disorders, neurologic disease (impaired swallowing), medications (opiates, chemotherapy), malabsorption, or depression. In the great majority of patients presenting with the complaint of unexplained wasting, a careful history and physical examination, combined with routine laboratory studies, will usually point in the direction of the underlying diagnosis. This chapter focuses specifically on the cachexia that is associated with cancer.

The degree of cancer-associated cachexia (called *cachexia* or *cancer cachexia* hereafter in this chapter) correlates poorly with the extent of the tumor. It is the most common paraneoplastic syndrome, occurring in more than 50% of patients at some time in their disease course. Cachexia most frequently develops in patients with lung and gastrointestinal (GI) cancers and is only occasionally found in patients with breast cancer or the hematologic malignancies, even when these diseases are far advanced. Loss of weight in patients with cancer at the time of diagnosis is an adverse prognostic factor that is associated with a poorer response to therapy and shorter survival than occur in patients with equivalent-stage disease who are not wasting.

Pathogenesis

Anorexia, or loss of appetite, occurs in 80% of patients with advanced cancer. Many factors can be involved in the genesis of anorexia, including oral or esophageal mucositis, chemotherapy-induced alterations in taste and smell sensations, radiation-induced decreased salivary flow, obstructive lesions of the gastrointestinal tract, nausea and/or vomiting, neurologic damage, depression, and uncontrolled pain.

The syndrome of cachexia is itself a cause of anorexia. Some of the cytokines discussed below that are responsible for cachexia also act directly on the brain to cause centrally induced anorexia. Cancer-associated weight loss exhibits distinctive characteristics that distinguish it from the changes that occur in starvation (Table 1-1). The increase in basal energy expenditure is not simply from increased consumption of energy sources by the cancer, because it can occur in patients with early stage cancers. Simple lack of or reduction in food intake does not therefore explain the mechanism of cachexia. If, in fact, anorexia were the major factor in cachexia, then aggressive feeding by any of several routes would be able to correct the problem. The changes of cachexia, however, persist even after forced, increased calorie intake.

Other metabolic changes accompany the increase in basal body expenditure, such as increased gluconeogenesis and decreased synthesis and increased catabolism of both fats and proteins. Protein loss from

DIAGNOSIS

Differential Diagnosis of Weight Loss

A number of circumstances other than cancer cause weight loss, such as the following.

Decreased Food Intake

Anorexigenic drugs: Cancer chemotherapeutic agents and certain oral antibiotics, such as erythromycin

Neurologic impairment of swallowing or chewing: Parkinson's disease or after a cerebrovascular accident

Psychiatric disorders: Anorexia nervosa, depression, anxiety, dementia

Oral abnormalities: Poor dentition or gum disease

The elderly patient

Impaired Utilization of Nutrients

Diabetes mellitus, malabsorption disorders, other gastrointestinal disease

Increased Metabolic Activity

Hyperthyroidism, pheochromocytoma, increased exercise

Severe Chronic Disease

Impaired function of the heart, lungs, or kidneys

Inflammatory disorders such as rheumatoid arthritis

Chronic infection such as HIV infection or tuberculosis

Cancer

If symptoms or findings of cancer are not present, then the diagnosis of an occult cancer as the cause of weight loss involves the exclusion of other possibilities. Elderly patients can pose a major problem, as many of them not uncommonly experience weight loss without a specific explanation. Whether to embark in this setting on a search of the patient's entire body for cancer by means of endoscopy, X-ray studies, and CT and MRI scans is a matter of clinical judgment.

---

striated voluntary muscle leads to muscle weakness and debilitation. In starvation, protein is conserved in part by the generation of an alternate energy source, namely, ketone bodies derived from the breakdown of fat. This does not occur in cachexia. The failure of glucose uptake by muscle tissue contributes to the excessive proteolysis and the development of relative insulin resistance.

A number of cytokines, produced by the tumor or secondarily by monocytes and/or lymphocytes, partic-ipate in the development of cachexia (Table 1-2). Tumor necrosis factor is thought to be an important determinant of cachexia. But even when the effects of tumor necrosis factor are blocked, cachexia persists, supporting the role of the other mediators in producing metabolic derangement. Among its many deleterious effects, tumor necrosis factor suppresses the function of lipoprotein lipase, which is necessary for the storage of fat in tissues. Uncoupling proteins were originally identified in murine adipose tissue. A proton gradient across mitochondrial membranes is involved in the cells' ability to generate energy in the form of adenosine triphosphate from adenosine diphosphate during the breakdown of fat. Uncoupling proteins blocks the linkage between the oxidation of fat and adenosine triphosphate generation, forcing the body to use protein catabolism to generate energy, leading to the dramatic loss of skeletal muscle. Proteolysis-inducing factor is a tumor-derived proteoglycan found

Table 1-1 ■ Comparison of Features of Cachexia and Starvation

Cachexia	Starvation
Loss of fat and muscle protein, reduced lean body mass	Loss of fat, relative preservation of lean body mass
Increased resting energy expenditure	Decreased resting energy expenditure
Syndrome mediators, such as proteolysis inducing factor, not found in nonwasting patients with cancer	No specific mediators
Increased gluconeogenesis	Decreased glucose production

Table 1-2 ■ Mediators of Metabolic Changes in Cachexia

Tumor necrosis factor-α	Proteolysis-inducing factor
Interleukin-1	Uncoupling proteins
Interleukin-6	

in cancer patients who have cachexia but not in those patients with cancer who do not experience weight loss. Interleukin-1 may influence anorexia by increasing the levels of tryptophan, a precursor of serotonin, in the brain. Serotonin, as well as interleukin-1 itself, has anorexigenic effects on the hypothalamus. Interestingly, leptin, which is normally made in fat tissue and suppresses appetite by its effects on the hypothalamus, is not apparently involved in the cachexia of malignancy. Measured levels appear to be low rather than elevated.

Therapy

General Considerations

Because it is a paraneoplastic syndrome, cachexia is most effectively managed by successful treatment of the underlying cancer. If antitumor therapy is not feasible or fails to achieve a response, then the decision of whether to employ nutritional measures should be based on studies documenting objective benefit from such treatment and on an understanding of what one is trying to accomplish for the patient.

Eating food in response to a good appetite is a major source of pleasure in daily life. Such satisfaction is eliminated by cachexia, causing great distress for patients with advanced cancer, whose lives are compromised by other aspects of cancer and its treatment. At the same time, the general concept that good nutrition is essential to good health causes the patient's family great concern. The family believes that the patient's survival will be shortened because of malnutrition and that in the absence of good nutrition, the patient will be unable to "fight" the cancer. Pressing nutritional goals on the patient affords family members an opportunity to play a functional role in an area they think they understand, instead of being relegated to the position of a helpless observer. The treating clinician is not immune to similar feelings. The result is that all those concerned with the patient's well-being place great emphasis on oral, enteral, or parenteral nutrition. The perception that it is important to maintain good nutrition frequently leads caregivers to ignore the expenses involved, the lack of demonstrable benefit, and the discomfort this occasions for the patient. The problems are physical in the case of managing enteral tubes or intravenous lines for nonoral alimentation and psychological in the case of oral feedings. Because of the patient's anorexia and the struggle of family members to force oral intake, conflict develops between the patient's desire to satisfy the family and resentment because family members do not understand the difficulty of complying with their wishes.

Table 1-3 ■ Steps in Alleviating Anorexia

- Control pain.
- Treat oral infection.
- Use topical remedies for oral mucositis.
- Encourage smaller, more frequent meals.
- Allow the patient to select food items regardless of their nutritive value and macronutrient composition.
- If feasible, increase mobility, ambulation, and activities of daily living.
- Metaclopramide is useful in patients who have delayed gastric emptying or gastroparesis causing nausea, vomiting, early satiety, and anorexia.
- Recognize and treat underlying depression.

It is important to provide the family with information about the role and limitation of maintaining nutrition in far-advanced cancer. Families need to know that cachexia neither fosters nor inhibits the growth of the cancer. Studies have clearly shown that attempts by any route to force nutrition do not improve survival; do not restore positive nitrogen balance; do not improve the frequency, degree, or duration of response to therapy; and do not improve the quality of life. With this knowledge in mind, many families become less insistent that any and all nutritive measures be employed. Others cannot reconcile the data with what seems obvious to them, and the physician is then reluctantly obliged to try to increase caloric intake.

Like wasting, anorexia is troubling for patients and families. Therapy with specific orexigenic (antianorexia) agents is discussed in later sections. In some patients, factors other than cachexia contribute to, or are the principal causes of, anorexia. They should not be overlooked because many of these factors can be treated to the patient's benefit (Table 1-3). For patients who are in pain, pain relief may dramatically improve appetite and interest in food. Patients experience early satiety, and small, frequent feedings may be better tolerated than full meals. If they are consulted, nutritionists will create a dietary menu and employ nutritional supplements in an attempt to achieve nutritional goals. However, randomized studies show no benefit from nutritional counseling and construction of these diets. Moreover, these diets are less likely to be ingested than are food items that are selected for their appeal rather than their nutritional value. Given the absence of value from forced nutrition, allowing patient choice instead affords a better opportunity to reduce anorexia. A study of foods selected and eaten by cachectic patients with cancer showed that the percentage distribution of macronutrients, proteins, fats, and carbohydrates ingested did not differ from the distribution in control hospitalized patients without cancer. The concern that self-selection of foods is problematic because of aversion to specific nutrients—protein, for example— appears to be unwarranted. Depression is a major cause of anorexia even in the general population. It needs attention and therapy in patients with cancer as well. One should always be alert to the possibility in patients with previously or currently active cancer that weight loss may be secondary to depression-induced anorexia rather than cachexia.

Enteral Feedings

If increased caloric intake is necessary but cannot be accomplished orally, then enteral rather than parenteral feeding should be employed, provided that the gastrointestinal tract and its mucosal surface are intact. Percutaneous endoscopic gastrostomy is a useful means of establishing enteral nutrition. The major risk is the potential for fluids to back up from the stomach and cause aspiration pneumonia. Other side effects include diarrhea, constipation, nausea and vomiting, abdominal cramps, and bloating. Randomized studies of enteral feedings continued for more than three months in patients with advanced cancer showed no difference versus nonenterally fed control patients in the outcomes of weight gain, anthropometric measures, response to treatment, survival, and quality of life.

Total Parenteral Nutrition

Although total parenteral nutrition is advocated by many as therapy for the cachexia of patients with cancer, randomized studies have shown not only no benefit from total parenteral nutrition, but also increased morbidity and shortened survival, due largely to an increased risk of infection. In 1989, a consensus panel reviewed the clinical data on total parenteral nutrition for the American College of Physicians and concluded, "The routine use of parenteral nutrition for patients undergoing chemotherapy should be strongly discouraged, and, in deciding to use such therapy in malnourished patients whose malnutrition is judged to be life threatening, physicians should take into account the possible exposure to increased risk." To date, these conclusions remain unchanged.

Randomized studies previously suggested benefit from total parenteral nutrition in the following three circumstances: perioperatively for cancer resection if the patient is severely malnourished before surgery; prophylactically in autologous and allogeneic bone marrow transplantation, and in patients undergoing aggressive combined modality therapy for treatment of head and neck cancer. However, a large meta-analysis of total parenteral nutrition perioperatively or in critically ill patients failed to show any improvement in mortality or complication rates. Acute complications and duration of initial hospital stay after allogeneic and autologous transplantation have markedly decreased since the substitution of peripheral blood stem cells for bone marrow stem cells. The ensuing rapid reconstitution of the bone marrow largely obviates the need for prophylactic total parenteral nutrition in this circumstance. In patients with head and neck cancer, it is simpler, cheaper, and as effective to use enteral feedings (via percutaneous endoscopic gastrostomy) instead of total parenteral nutrition. The remaining potential uses for total parenteral nutrition are for patients who are or will be undergoing active anticancer treatment in whom malnutrition has or will occur and whose gastrointestinal tract does not permit enteral feeding. As was noted earlier, in the absence of gastrointestinal tract malfunction or injury, there are few confirmed indications for the application of total parenteral nutrition to treat the cachexia of malignancy.

Progesterone

Agents in this class include megestrol acetate (Megace) and medroxyprogesterone acetate (Depo-Provera); the former agent has been more extensively studied. Their orexigenic effects in a variety of cancers were first noted when patients under hormonal treatment for breast cancer were observed to gain weight. In vitro, medroxyprogesterone reduces the production of the cytokines, interleukin-1-β, interleukin-6, and tumor necrosis factor by peripheral blood mononuclear cells. The principal side effects of these progestational agents are peripheral edema, deep vein thromboses (the risk seems to increase if chemotherapy is administered simultaneously), and mild suppression of the pituitary-adrenal axis, leading in some patients to a diminished glucocorticoid response to stress. Impotence can occur in men and vaginal spotting in women.

Megestrol acetate is available as 20-mg and 40-mg tablets and in the form of an oral suspension. Whereas doses in excess of 160 mg/day do not improve the antitumor effects in breast cancer, dose escalation studies in patients with a wide variety of cancers indicate that increasing the total daily dose to 800 mg daily (but not beyond this level) increases the antianorexia effects. The dose-response data make it clear that the orexigenic effects are separate from its antitumor effects in patients with breast cancer. Medroxyprogesterone acetate can also be given orally, 500 mg bid, but it

Table 1-4 ■ Randomized Trial of Dexamethasone versus Megestrol Acetate in Cancer Cachexia

Feature	Dexamethasone	Megestrol Acetate	
Dose	0.75 mg QID PO	800 mg/day PO	
Discontinued Rx prematurely	36%	25%	$P = .03$
Myopathy	18%	6%	$P = .0006$
Infection	16%	11%	NS
Phlebothrombosis	1%	5%	$P = .06$
Cushingoid appearance	6%	1%	$P = .0008$
Insomnia	4%	1%	$P = .005$
Peptic ulcer	3%	0%	$P = .04$
Cost	$0.30/day (4-mg tablet)	$10.25/day (800-mg suspension)	

Adapted from Loprinzi CL, et al: Randomized comparison of megestrol acetate vs dexamethasone vs fluoxymestrone for the treatment of cancer anorexia/cachexia. J Clin Oncol 1999;17:3299-3306. This was a three-arm randomized trial, including fluoxymestrone. Increases in appetite enhancement, food intake, and nonfluid weight gain were equivalent with dexamethasone and megestrol acetate and inferior with fluoxymestrone (data not shown).
NS = not significantly different; PO = orally.

appears in some studies to be slightly less effective than megestrol acetate.

Although patients have improved appetite and gain weight, there is no evidence that these agents increase the frequency of response to chemotherapy or prolong survival. Moreover, most of the resulting weight gain occurs in fat and not in muscle protein (lean body mass).

Corticosteroids

Glucocorticoids, such as prednisone 10 to 20 mg/day or dexamethasone 3 to 6 mg/day, are as effective as megestrol in improving appetite and food intake, but their side effect profile is worse (Table 1-4). High-dose corticosteroids cause myopathy and muscle weakness, decreasing mobility in these already debilitated patients. Chronic administration also can cause dysphoria, insomnia, hypokalemia, immunosuppression and infections, edema, and glucose intolerance. Corticosteroids remain useful for the patient who is already bedridden or whose survival prognosis is too short for the side effects to develop materially while offering the advantage of their anti-inflammatory effects in relieving other tumor-related symptoms, such as pain.

Testosterone may offer some benefit in men with cancer cachexia who have low serum testosterone levels, but the effects are minimal.

Eicosapentaenoic Acid

Eicosapentaenoic acid (EPA) is derived from fish oil. It is an essential polyunsaturated fatty acid of the omega-3 (N-3) class. Eicosapentaenoic acid acts as a precursor to prostanoid synthesis that results in the production of prostaglandins, leukotrienes, and thromboxanes that are less inflammatory and prothrombotic than those usually derived from arachidonic acid. Dietary omega-3 fatty acids have been shown to reduce the production of interleukin-1 and tumor necrosis factor. Eicosapentaenoic acid also seems to block end organ responsiveness to proteolysis-inducing factor and lipid-mobilizing factors, thereby antagonizing some of the events contributing to cancer cachexia. Although preliminary results from clinical trials show activity, a randomized study is necessary to confirm eicosapentaenoic acid's apparent utility.

Thalidomide

Thalidomide shortens the half-life of tumor necrosis factor's messenger RNA, thereby potentially ameliorating some of its side effects. On the basis of studies of its effectiveness in the treatment of patients infected with HIV, thalidomide may help to improve nutrition and weight in patients with cancer.

Adenosine Triphosphate

Adenosine triphosphate infusions were given by intravenous infusion over 30 minutes every 2 to 4 weeks to patients with cancer cachexia and non-small-cell lung cancer. Improvement was demonstrated in comparison to a nontreated control, but the study was only single-blind, and the margin of improvement, although statistically significant, was not clinically meaningful. Additional studies are required.

Anti-Inflammatory Agents

Ibuprofen, by interfering with prostaglandin synthesis, blocks the cachectic effects of tumor necrosis factor and interleukin-1. Administration of ibuprofen, 400 mg tid orally, to patients with pancreatic cancer caused a reduction in the excessive resting energy expenditure. Nonsteroidal anti-inflammatory drugs may ease other manifestations, such as pain, adding to their value. Studies are evaluating the efficacy of combining nonsteroidal anti-inflammatory agents with megestrol acetate.

Agents with Borderline or No Efficacy

Pentoxyphylline inhibits the production of tumor necrosis factor by monocytes and T lymphocytes. It is not effective in cancer cachexia, indicating that tumor necrosis factor is only one of the causes of the syndrome.

Dronabinol is a cannabis derivative that can improve appetite, but it is less effective than megestrol acetate.

Cyproheptadine is a serotonin antagonist. Although serotonin effects on the brain play a role in the cachexia of malignancy, cyproheptadine has shown benefit only in patients with the carcinoid syndrome, whose cancers generate large amounts of serotonin.

Ondansetron blocks serotoninergic receptors in animals but has not been useful in treating the anorexia of malignancy in humans.

Melatonin reduces the synthesis of 5-hydroxy-tryptophan, a serotonin precursor. Its clinical utility has not yet been convincingly demonstrated, but it may prove ultimately to have a role in therapy.

Suggested Reading

American College of Physicians: Parenteral nutrition in patients receiving cancer chemotherapy. Ann Intern Med 1989;110:734–736.

Argiles JM, Lopez-Soriano FJ: Host metabolism: A target in clinical oncology. Med Hypotheses 1988;51:411–415.

Barber MD, McMillan DC, Preston T, et al: Metabolic response to feeding in weight-losing pancreatic cancer patients and its modulation by a fish-oil-enriched nutritional supplement. Clin Sci 2000;98:389–399.

Bing C, Brown M, King P, et al: Increased gene expression of brown fat uncoupling protein (UCP) 1 and skeletal muscle UCP2 and UCP3 in MAC16-induced cancer cachexia. Cancer Res 2000;60:2405–2410.

Body JJ: The syndrome of anorexia-cachexia. Curr Opinion Oncol 1999;11:255–259.

Edelman MJ, Gandara DR, Meyers FJ, et al: Serotoninergic blockade in the treatment of the cancer anorexia-cachexia syndrome. 1999;Cancer 86:684–689.

Gogos CA, Ginopoulos, Salsa B, et al: Dietary omega-3 polyunsaturated fatty acids plus vitamin E restore immunodeficiency and prolong survival for severely ill patients with generalized malignancy: A randomized trial. 1998;Cancer 82:395–402.

Hetland DK, MacDonald S, Keefe L, et al: Total parenteral nutrition in the critically ill patient. JAMA 1998;280:2013–2019.

Inui A: Cancer anorexia-cachexia syndrome: Are neuropeptides the key? 1999;Cancer Res 59:4493–4501.

Jatoi A, Kumar S, Sloan, Nguyen PL: On appetite and its loss. J Clin Oncol 2000;18:2930–2932.

Jatoi A, Loprinzi CL: Current management of cancer-associated anorexia and weight loss. Oncol 2001;15:497–509.

Jatoi A, Loprinzi CL, Sloan J, Goldberg RM: Is ATP (adenosine 5′-triphosphate), like STP, a performance-enhancing additive for the tanks of cancer patients? [Editorial]. J Natl Cancer Inst 2000;92:290–291.

Levine JA, Morgan MY: Preservation of macronutrient preferences in cancer anorexia. Br J Cancer 1998;78:579–581.

Loprinzi CL, Kugler KW, Sloan JA, et al: Randomized comparison of megestrol acetate vs dexamethasone vs fluoxymestrone for the treatment of cancer anorexia/cachexia. J Clin Oncol 1999;17:3299–3306.

Mantovani G, Maccio A, Esu S, et al: Medroxyprogesterone acetate reduces the in vitro production of cytokines and serotonin involved in anorexia/cachexia and emesis by peripheral blood mononuclear cells of cancer patients. Eur J Cancer 1997;33:602–607.

McMillan DC, Wigmore SJ, Fearon KC, et al: A prospective randomized study of megestrol acetate and ibuprofen in gastrointestinal cancer in patients with weight loss. Br J Cancer 1999;79:495–500.

Ovesen L, Allinsgstrup L, Hannibal J, et al: Effect of dietary counseling on food intake, body weight, response rate, survival, and quality of life in cancer patients undergoing chemotherapy: A prospective, randomized study. J Clin Oncol 1993;11:2043–2049.

Puccio M, Nathanson L: The cancer cachexia syndrome. Semin Oncol 1997;24:277–287.

Symposium on Cachexia of Cancer in Semin Oncol 1998; 25(Suppl 6), 1998.

Todorov P, Cariuk P, McDevitt T, et al: Characterization of a cancer cachectic factor. Nature 1996;79:739–742.

Veterans Affairs Total Parenteral Nutrition Cooperative Study Group: Perioperative total parenteral nutrition in surgical patients. N Engl J Med 1991;325:525–532.

Weisdorf SA, Lysne J, Wind D, et al: Positive effect of prophylactic total parenteral nutrition on long-term outcome of bone marrow transplantation. Transplant 1987;43:833–838.

Chapter 2
Fever of Unknown Origin

Robert W. Finberg

Fever in patients with hematologic or nonhematologic cancers can be either a feature of the underlying malignancy or a signal that urgent therapeutic intervention is needed. The challenge to the clinician is to determine which of these alternatives applies to a given patient. Fever is often a manifestation of malignancy and can be the presenting sign. The knowledge that elevations in body temperature in general are controlled by the release of cytokines provides insight into the mechanisms by which cancers can cause fever. Ultimately, one or more proteins produced by the host resets the hypothalamic temperature regulator. Atrial myxoma, a tumor that may present with sustained fever, is one example. In this setting, increased production of interleukin-6, a cytokine that induces fever, is in major part the responsible agent. In a similar fashion, in infection, the proteins, lipoproteins, or polysaccharides of the infecting microorganism, whether it is a bacteria, virus, or fungus, activate the host cells to produce cytokines. Successful diagnosis and treatment of fever in patients with cancer depend on recognition of the underlying predisposition to infection and the selection of the appropriate and timely therapeutic response.

Causes of Fever of Unknown Origin

Acute febrile episodes in normal hosts are most often due to infections, commonly viral illnesses. Fever of unknown origin is frequently a perplexing problem in clinical medicine, however, because of the broad array of diseases that may be responsible for this finding. For almost four decades, fever of unknown origin was defined by the criteria of Petersdorf and Beeson (1961). The definition focused on the population of apparently normal hosts with prolonged fever of more than 3 weeks' duration, temperature greater than 38.3°C (101°F), and no defined cause after 1 week of hospitalization. This definition was recently modified. The requirement for hospitalization was eliminated because of the availability of improved noninvasive diagnostic techniques and decreased use of hospitalization for diagnostic studies and empiric therapy. In patients without known prior disease, the most likely causes of a fever of unknown origin are infection, neoplasms, and collagen vascular diseases. Of the infections found in these patients, tuberculosis, intra-abdominal abscesses, chronic cholecystitis, culture-negative endocarditis, and other occult, chronic infections are common. Despite the high frequency of carcinomas of the breast, lung, and colon in the general population and the fact that these cancers, when metastatic (especially to the liver), occasionally cause fever, the most common tumors that cause fever of unknown origin are lymphomas, renal cell carcinomas, and atrial myxomas. This is presumably because these particular cancers more often than other cancers are associated with cytokine production. In recent years, the common causes of fever of unknown origin in chronically

DIAGNOSIS

Initial Approach to Fever in a Patient with Cancer

Infections are the cause of death in the majority of patients with hematologic malignancies and a major cause of morbidity and mortality in patients with other cancers. In evaluating febrile patients with cancer, the clinician should answer the following questions as a guide to the pace and selection of approaches to diagnosing and treating a potential infectious etiology:

- Is the patient neutropenic?
- Could the patient have an obstructed viscus (such as an obstructed ureter or bronchus)?
- Have other anatomic abnormalities occurred as a result of cancer or treatment?
- Has the patient received a bone marrow transplant or cytotoxic chemotherapy?

Table 2-1 ■ Infections in Cancer Patients

Type of Cancer	Site of Infection	Likely Organisms
Lung	Lung Postobstructive pneumonia	*Streptococcus pneumoniae* Aerobic gram-negative species, and oral anaerobes
Lung	Lung	Tuberculosis
Breast	Arm (impaired lymphatic drainage after axillary node dissection)	Recurrent bacterial infection with streptococci or staphylococci
Colon	Intra-abdominal abscess	Gram-negative aerobes, *S. bovis*
Prostate/Renal	Urine	Gram-negative aerobes
Chronic lymphocytic leukemia/ multiple myeloma	Lungs, ears, disseminated	*S. pneumoniae, Haemophilus influenzae,* *Neisseria meningitidis*
Leukemias	Skin, GI tract	Aerobic gram-positive and gram-negative bacteria

TREATMENT

Urgent Therapy in Patients with Fever

Immediate institution of appropriate antibiotics is required in a febrile patient not only in the setting of profound neutropenia or after autologous or allogeneic stem cell transplantation, but also when the patient has undergone splenectomy.

A splenectomized patient with a fever is a medical emergency. After splenectomy, the patient is not at increased risk of having an infection. However, if the patient contracts an infection by encapsulated organisms (such as *Streptococcus pneumoniae, Haemophilus influenzae,* or *Neisseria meningitidis*), the loss of the spleen's reticuloendothelial function as a filter of blood-borne pathogens enhances the risk of developing a devastating, uncontrolled bacteremia. In general, high doses of a third-generation cephalosporin (such as ceftriaxone) should cover most of these organisms. Where resistance to *H. influenzae* or *S. pneumoniae* is likely to be a problem, the addition of vancomycin (for resistant pneumococcus) or other agents (for resistant *H. influenzae*) should be considered. Because of the danger of these infections, some authorities recommend that splenectomized patients keep orally administered antibiotics available at home in case they are delayed in reaching an emergency room.

immunosuppressed, HIV-infected patients were found to be *Mycobacterium avium* infection, pneumocystis carinii, cytomegalovirus, disseminated histoplasmosis, and lymphoma.

These considerations of potential causes of fever in other populations do not apply to patients who have already been diagnosed with cancer and present with a fever. The approach necessarily varies depending on the type of underlying malignancy as well as the treatment the patient is receiving. Fevers in certain types of cancer are typically associated with infections by specific microorganisms and in specific locations, as outlined in Table 2-1.

General Considerations

It is essential that the managing clinician who is approaching a febrile patient with cancer first consider the patient's underlying risk for life-threatening infec-tion and rapidly determine whether the patient requires immediate antibiotics. Although in most cases the pace of the evaluation of patients with chronic fevers need not be hurried, speed is essential in certain groups of patients.

Life-Threatening Emergencies

Patients who are splenectomized, are severely neutropenic, or have status post stem cell transplantation are at high risk of rapidly progressive and overwhelming fatal infections because of their inability to contain bloodstream bacteremias. These patients should receive broad-spectrum antibiotic coverage immediately after appropriate cultures are obtained from blood and other potential sites of infection. Treatment should then be refined on the basis of the results of cultures and other studies.

Common Infections

Patients with organ-related cancers (especially lung, colon, and kidney) will often occlude normally patent structures such as ureters or bronchi, impairing drainage. The resulting pooling of the obstructed, ordinarily sterile, fluids becomes a site for ready infection by even a small number of invasive organisms. Infections of this nature are caused by commensal microorganisms that normally inhabit the skin surface or mucosa of the gastrointestinal tract.

Impairment of host response to infection is a common predisposing cause in patients with cancer. For example, granulocytopenia is a frequent consequence of cytotoxic chemotherapy, especially in patients who are treated with high doses, such as those with acute leukemia. Granulocytopenia, especially when the absolute granulocyte count is less than 500/μL, is a major risk factor for infections and for fatality from infection. Early empiric therapy with antibiotics can be life-saving in this setting. Patients who become neutropenic following cytotoxic chemotherapy are also subject to severe infection by skin, mouth, and gastrointestinal tract flora, owing to the concomitant damage and breakdown of protective mucosal linings. Because of the lack of circulating granulocytes, the infiltrating bacteria are not eliminated. They reach the bloodstream, bacteremia results, and other structures become infected. Usually, these bacteria are Gram-positive organisms such as staphylococci or streptococci from the skin surface or aerobic Gram-negative organisms found in the gastrointestinal tract.

As a result of high-dose cytotoxic chemotherapy and the development of neutropenia and immunosuppression, patients are subject to infections with intracellular organisms such as mycobacteria, *Nocardia*, fungi (especially cryptococcus, histoplasmosis, and coccidioidomycosis in the appropriate setting), and viruses (especially the herpesvirus group).

It is essential to recognize that the signs of infection, usually found in the intact host, are often not present in patients with granulocytopenia because pus formation and inflammatory responses are diminished or absent. For example, some redness and accompanying pain may be the only sign of cellulitis. Similarly, pneumonias can present without purulent sputum, findings of rales and rhonchi on physical examination, or even, at times, without chest X-ray abnormalities. Careful assessment of the patient's status is needed, since the clinician must rely on relatively subtle clues to diagnose infections.

The key to appropriate therapy is the understanding that as long as the underlying condition (granulocytopenia) persists, the patient remains at risk and antibiotics must be continued. Although conventionally, patients with cancer and febrile neutropenia are treated with intravenous antibiotics in the hospital setting, studies suggest that in a selected subset of "low-risk" patients, intravenous or oral therapy at home may be a safe alternative.

Fungal Infections

It is not surprising that patients who are treated with broad-spectrum antibacterial agents should develop fungal infections. The use of agents that eliminate the normal bacterial colonizers of the skin and gastrointestinal tract results in overgrowth in these areas by fungi, especially *Candida* species. In patients who are already colonized with *Aspergillus*, or when *Aspergillus* is found in the environment, *Aspergillus* species also become a therapeutic problem. The high fatality rate of patients who developed proven, culture- or biopsy-confirmed fungal infections has led to the use of antifungal therapy, given empirically when the setting and findings suggest a high risk of ongoing, albeit occult, fungal infection. Thus when fever continues in a culture-negative patient with persistent neutropenia after 4 to 7 days of antibacterial antibiotics, antifungal therapy is usually instituted. Although amphotericin B is usually used as the fungal antibiotic, liposomal amphotericin B appears to be as effective with lower toxicity, and trials with new broad-spectrum azoles (such as voriconazole) are underway.

In summary, the febrile neutropenic patient should receive antibacterial agents early on, followed by antifungals if fever persists, with careful attention to culture data and the clinical state of the patient.

Bone Marrow (Stem Cell) Transplantation

Patients undergoing bone marrow transplantation have nearly total abrogation of immune host response due to loss of lymphocytes as well as granulocytes. These patients are therefore subject to a wide variety of infections that are not seen in normal hosts or patients with cancer in general. These infections tend to occur in a predictable manner based on time after transplantation. Bacterial infections appear early as a consequence of neutropenia. As reconstitution of granulocytes occurs, lymphocyte number and function remain impaired, and after several weeks, increasing risk is observed for infections by higher bacteria (*Nocardia* and *Actinomyces*) and fungi (*Candida* and *Aspergillus*). Herpes simplex infection is most likely to occur in the immediate posttransplant period, whereas cytomegalovirus infection (a serious problem

TREATMENT

Treatment of Patients with Fever and Neutropenia

The choice of treatment for a febrile neutropenic patient must recognize the importance of errors of omission (failing to treat empirically with antibiotics that would be effective against all likely organisms) and commission (using too many antibiotics, which leads to drug toxicity and antibiotic resistance). General guidelines include the following:

- A careful history with particular attention to previous antibiotic use and prior history of infections and a careful physical examination with special attention to the skin and mucous membranes are essential. Assessment of liver function tests and a chest X-ray are indicated. Blood and urine cultures (and cultures of other potential sites if suggested by the clinical situation) should be obtained prior to starting antibiotics.
- The antibiotic regimen that is chosen should treat both Gram-positive cocci and Gram-negative rods. Early studies demonstrated the usefulness of two drugs (usually a semisynthetic penicillin and an aminoglycoside) to achieve broad-spectrum coverage. Recent studies of initial single-agent therapy with third-generation cephalosporins that are active against

Pseudomonas (such as ceftazidime) or carbipenems (such as imipenem) show equal efficacy.

- The choice of an antibiotic regimen should be based in part on the organisms and their antibiotic sensitivities that are known to be present in the environment in which the infection occurred.
- Once data from cultures are available, the antibiotic regimen may be refined, but the spectrum should not be narrowed as long as granulocytopenia persists.
- In general, antibiotics should be continued until the patient is no longer neutropenic.
- If the patient remains febrile and neutropenic after 4 to 7 days of treatment with antibacterial agents, an antifungal agent should be added.
- Avoid the tendency to switch antibiotics in patients with persisting fevers in the absence of guidance by culture data. Care is compromised by the confusion resulting from polypharmacy, as the patients are prone to drug rashes and other manifestations of drug toxicity.

Unless an underlying focus of infection has been identified, all antibiotics should be stopped once the granulocyte count is greater than 500/µL.

DIAGNOSIS

Approach to the Stem Cell Transplant Recipient with Fever

Stem cell transplant recipients develop different infections at different times following the transplant. Knowledge of when after the infusion of stem cells the fever developed is one of the most critical pieces of information in establishing a diagnosis, as indicated below for approximate periods of time:

Early (<30 days). Infections from bacteria on the skin and gastrointestinal tract and herpes simplex virus.

Middle (30 to 100 days). Infections by the higher bacteria (*Nocardia* and *Actinomyces*) and fungi (particularly *Candida* and *Aspergillus*). Cytomegalovirus (particularly in allogeneic trans-

plant patients) is a problem in this time period. Fever may also be caused by the development of graft-versus-host disease in allogeneic stem cell transplant recipients. Veno-occlusive disease of the liver may present with liver function abnormalities (primarily a rising serum bilirubin), ascites, fever, and abdominal pain at this time.

Late (3 to 12 months). Bacteremias with encapsulated organisms (*Streptococcus pneumoniae, Haemophilus influenzae*), varicella-zoster virus, and toxoplasmosis and pneumocystis carinii infection in patients who do not receive prophylactic antibiotics.

after allogeneic stem cell transplants that also occasionally supervenes after autologous stem cell transplants) occurs one to three months posttransplant and is rarely seen in the first few days or weeks following infusion of stem cells. Herpes zoster infection (either

disseminated or localized) usually does not occur for weeks to months following infection. The risk of its occurrence is approximately 50% after either autologous or allogeneic stem cell transplantation and does not subside for at least a year following transplant.

Therefore the differential diagnosis of fever in a bone marrow transplant should take into account not only the patient's signs and symptoms, but also the time following transplant.

Suggested Reading

Arbo MJ, Fine MJ, Hanusa BH, et al: Fever of nosocomial origin: Etiology, risk factors, and outcomes. Am J Med 1993;95:505–512.

Armstrong WS, Katz JT, Kazanjian PH: Human immunodeficiency virus–associated fever of unknown origin: A study of 70 patients in the United States and review. Clin Infect Dis 1999;28:341–345.

Arnow PM, Flaherty JP: Fever of unknown origin. Lancet 1997;350:575–580.

Bodey GP, et al: Quantitative relationships between circulating leukocytes and infection in patients with acute leukemia. Ann Intern Med 1966;64:328.

Finberg RW, Talcott JA: Fever and neutropenia: How to use a new treatment strategy [Editorial]. N Engl J Med 1999;34:362–363.

Gill FA, et al: The relationship of fever, granulocytopenia and antimicrobial therapy to bacteremia in cancer patients. Cancer 1977;39:1074–1079.

Mackowiak PA: Concepts of fever. Arch Intern Med 1998; 158:1870–1881.

Petersdorf RG, Beeson PB: Fever of unexplained origin: report on 100 cases. Medicine 1961;40:1–30.

Pizzo PA: Fever in immunocompromised patients [Review]. N Engl J Med 1999;341:893–900.

Pizzo PA, et al: A randomized trial comparing ceftazidime alone with combination therapy in cancer patients with fever and neutropenia. N Engl J Med 1986;315:552.

Schwartz PE, Sterioff S, Mucha P, et al: Postsplenectomy sepsis and mortality in adults. J Am Med Assoc 1982;248:2279.

Sickles EA, Greene WH, Wiernik PH: Clinical presentation of infection in granulocytopenic patients. Arch Intern Med 1975;135:715–719.

Van Dissel JT, van Langeveld P, Westendorp RG, et al: Anti-inflammatory cytokine profile and mortality in febrile patients. Lancet 1998;351:950–953.

Walsh TJ, Finberg RW, Arndt C, et al: Liposomal amphotericin B for empirical therapy in patients with persistent fever and neutropenia. N Engl J Med 1999;340:764–771.

Chapter 3
Pruritus

Peter A. Cassileth

Introduction

The word *pruritus* is a Latin noun derived from the verb "to itch" and does not mean inflammation, as its common misspelling, "pruritis," could lead one to infer. Itching is a troublesome symptom, most commonly associated with a variety of primary inflammatory dermatologic disorders, especially eczema and other acute and chronic dermatitides. When obvious skin lesions are present, their pattern and distribution frequently suggest the diagnosis and/or lead to punch biopsies of the skin and a histologic diagnosis. But itching can also be a manifestation of a number of systemic diseases and can provide a diagnostic clue to their presence. This chapter focuses on systemic causes of pruritus in the setting where there are no visible skin lesions. When a patient has generalized pruritus of unknown origin and no rash, a search for an underlying nondermatologic disease is required. One has to be aware, however, that intense scratching can itself induce a range of secondary dermatologic abnormalities, such as excoriation, lichenification, hyperpigmentation or hypopigmentation. To examine the untraumatized skin, one looks at the upper posterior thorax where, in a butterfly pattern, there is an area of skin out of reach of the hands.

Table 3-1 contains a list of systemic disorders associated with pruritus without skin rash. Dryness of the skin (xerosis), aquagenic pruritus (discussed under "Polycythemia Vera" below), and neurodermatitis (due to depression and/or anxiety) are common causes of pruritus in the general population, especially in the elderly. For this reason, isolated case reports and retrospective reviews claiming a relationship between pruritus and some diseases should be viewed skeptically. Examples are the associations reported between pruritus and multiple myeloma, essential thrombocythemia, acute leukemia, myelodysplasia, iron deficiency, or carcinomas of the breast, lung, and colon. They may be only chance associations.

Obstructive Hepatobiliary Disease

Extrahepatic or intrahepatic obstruction of the flow of bile causes itching. The etiology varies remarkably and includes intrahepatic cholestasis caused by tumors or drugs, cholangitis, primary biliary cirrhosis, and viral hepatitis or extrahepatic cholestasis due to common duct obstruction by stones, cancer, fibrosis, or enlarged lymph nodes. The itching is worse on the hands and feet and increases at night. It not uncommonly appears before substantial liver function test abnormalities or jaundice is apparent. Pruritus can thus be among the earliest symptoms, even being the dominant one at presentation. Pruritus has been attributed to bile acid accumulation, but the severity of pruritus does not correlate with the accumulation of bile salts. Treatment directed at reducing or altering the bile acid pool by administration of ursodeoxycholic acid, cholestyramine, or colestipol has not been very helpful. Each of these has troublesome side effects. Relief of cholestatic pruritus has been claimed with the use of rifampin, phototherapy, or plasmapheresis in some uncontrolled studies.

Opioidergic neurotransmitters in the brain play a role in pruritus. In biliary obstruction, endogenous opioids accumulate. Supporting the significance of this observation are the facts that the opioid antagonist naltrexone can cause an opioid withdrawal-like syndrome in some patients with biliary obstruction and that it relieved itching in these patients in a controlled randomized study.

Chronic Renal Disease

Correlating in severity with the extent of renal damage, pruritus is a frequent symptom in chronic, not acute, renal failure. In most patients, itching is paroxysmal and can be localized or generalized. It has been attributed to a dialyzable uremic product, such as increased bile acids (but dialysis provides only moderate relief), high calcium-phosphorus product

Table 3-1 ■ Systemic Diseases Causing Generalized Pruritus Without Skin Rash

Endocrine disorders:	Thyrotoxicosis, hypothyroidism (dry skin), diabetes mellitus, hyperparathyroidism
Hepatobiliary obstruction:	Intrahepatic or extrahepatic
Hematologic disorders:*	Polycythemia vera, Hodgkin's lymphoma, non-Hodgkin's lymphoma, mastocytosis, hypereosinophilic syndrome, mastocytosis, cutaneous T cell lymphomas (mycosis fungoides, Sézary syndrome)
Solid tumor neoplasms	
Chronic renal failure	
Idiopathic:	Aquagenic pruritus, neurodermatitic excoriation
Drug reactions:	Opioids and allergic drug reactions
Neurologic disorders:	Multiple sclerosis; brain infarct, abscess, or tumor; intramedullary tumors, neurofibromatosis, or postherpetic neuralgia

*Other hematologic disorders are associated with itching and a rash, such as cold urticaria produced by cryoglobulinemia, cryofibrinogenemia, and cold agglutinin disease or with the occurrence of angioedema in C1-esterase inhibitor deficiency (can be a congenital disorder or acquired in patients with lymphomas).

with calcium salt deposition in the skin (but parathyroidectomy is rarely effective and severity of the itch is not related to parathyroid levels), opioid retention, or neuropathy. Oral activated charcoal is a simple, nontoxic, and apparently effective therapy in this circumstance. What prurigenic substance or substances are bound to the charcoal as it passes through the intestine is unclear.

Opioids and Central Nervous System Effects

Administration of epidural morphine causes pruritus in the anatomically associated skin segments. Narcotics, including codeine and oxycodone, can cause generalized pruritus by a central nervous system, rather than an allergic, mechanism. It can occur after orally administered narcotics but is more often noted after parenteral administration. The itching tends to be localized to the face, neck, and upper chest. Substitution of a different morphine congener may allow continuation of analgesic therapy without recurrent pruritus. Accumulation of endogenous opioids, such as the encephalins and endorphins, can also cause itching. Stimulation of opioid receptors in the brain triggers itching. The neurologic disorders noted in Table 3-1 presumably can cause pruritus by direct or indirect (through pressure effects) stimulation of these centers.

Allergic Drug Reactions

Drug allergy usually induces some kind of skin eruption and itching, but it is well to remember that severe pruritus without skin rash can at times be an initial manifestation.

Polycythemia Vera and Aquagenic Pruritus

Aquagenic pruritus refers to the syndrome of itching after exposure to water. It is a not uncommon symptom in the general population of otherwise entirely healthy people. It usually starts before age 30 and can be evoked intermittently by fresh or salt water at any temperature or by sweating. The palms, soles, and scalp are usually spared. It is a bothersome but not very intense problem. A much more severe version of aquagenic pruritus occurs in patients with polycythemia vera (PCV). Itching after showering or bathing is a common and often the presenting symptom in polycythemia vera. The sensation of pruritus increases on exposure to hot water and or with vigorous toweling after water contact. Itching lasts for 15 to 60 minutes. Some patients are so desperate to avoid this symptom that they eschew bathing or showering entirely. With the exception of benign aquagenic pruritus, this symptom is virtually pathognomonic for polycythemia vera. Increased histamine release from basophils (and their tissue representatives, the mast cells) is not the cause, because antihistamines are ineffective therapy, and pruritus does not occur in the face of the basophilia associated with other myeloproliferative syndromes. Clinical responses in polycythemia vera can be obtained by administration of hydroxurea, alkylating agents, or phlebotomy, but they generally do not (or only minimally) relieve pruritus. Thus far, only interferon-α has been effective. Unfortunately, interferon is expensive and is associated with side effects, making it difficult to justify this therapy for most patients unless the itching is intolerable.

Lymphomas

Pruritus without skin infiltration occurs in approximately 25% of patients with Hodgkin's disease (HD) and is the only presenting symptom in 5% to 10% of patients. Pruritus is no longer recognized as an unfavorable prognostic finding in Hodgkin's disease. It can be localized over affected areas or generalized and can be quite severe. It is a useful clue to the diagnosis and its return after initial treatment indicates disease recurrence. The pruritus is totally resistant to all symptomatic therapy and responds only to control of the underlying Hodgkin's disease.

Pruritus less often affects patients with non-Hodgkin's lymphoma (NHL). It is noted in only 2% of patients at presentation and is more frequent in the well-differentiated histologic subtypes.

Other Hematologic Diseases

Unlike the subcutaneous nodules of Hodgkin's disease, the leukemia cutis of acute leukemias and infiltration of the skin by adult T-cell leukemia/lymphoma are nonpruritic. Although cutaneous T cell lymphoma usually causes skin lesions that mimic a wide variety of benign dermatoses, on occasion only itching is present and the skin appears normal. Biopsy of normal skin in this circumstance reveals the typical lesions of mycosis fungoides. Hypereosinophilic syndromes are occasionally associated with pruritus and are not relieved by histamine blockade. One or more visible and palpable intracutaneous masses that urticate on gentle stroking (Darier's sign) are usually present in mastocytosis and systemic mastocytosis (urticaria pigmentosa). Occasionally, the skin appears normal in these diseases, and biopsy is necessary to make the diagnosis.

Cancer

Pruritus occurs in metastatic carcinoid, but other symptoms from excess serotonin, such as wheezing and diarrhea, are more frequent and predominate. Almost every variety of cancer has been linked to pruritus. Given the low frequency of pruritus as a symptom in the common cancers, such as breast, lung, colon, and prostate, it is difficult to rule out a chance association, especially since in the elderly, idiopathic pruritus and cancer each occur independently with a substantial incidence. Moreover, the intensity of pruritus does not correlate with the extent of tumor, and the psychological stress of carrying the diagnosis of a malignancy may contribute to the sensation of pruritus in these patients. Many oncologists nevertheless believe that visceral abdominal spread of carcinoma can cause pruritus as a paraneoplastic symptom. Because this is at best a rare event, one should first exclude common causes of pruritus in cancer patients, such as drug reactions or biliary obstruction, before attributing pruritus to a distant effect of the tumor itself.

General Therapeutic Considerations

In both dermatologic and nondermatologic disease, the pathophysiology of itching (as well as why scratching provides relief) is unknown (Figure 3-1). It is probably multifactorial in etiology, but which of the many hypotheses proposed is/are correct and how much of a varying role they play in different clinical circumstances is uncertain. Consequently, treatment of pruritus is largely empiric and frequently limited in providing symptomatic relief. The best approach to alleviate pruritus due to underlying nondermatologic disease is by control or elimination of the disease, which is often difficult to accomplish. On the basis of purely theoretical considerations, a large number of agents have been prescribed in attempts to eliminate this symptom. Unfortunately, only a limited number of these therapies have been evaluated in randomized, double-blind, placebo-controlled trials. Usually, the results of carefully controlled studies have been negative. The placebo effect in patients with pruritus is particularly strong, inducing as much as a 30% to 50% response rate. Larger numbers of patients than are ordinarily entered on these studies are therefore required to be sure that no difference exists. Moreover, if, as suspected, pruritus is multifactorial, then single-agent therapy of any kind is likely to be only marginally effective. It is not surprising that no current therapy has been approved by the Food and Drug Administration (FDA) for the relief of pruritus as a primary symptom.

The fine unmyelinated nerve fibers that carry the sensation of itch from the epidermal/dermal junction have no specific receptors. Stimulation of these nerve endings by the release of factors alone or in combination can cause itching. These include histamine, interleukin-2, peptidases, eicosanoids such as prostaglandin E_2, serotonin, and substance P. Which, if any, are operative in a patient is unknown. Given the limited efficacy of available systemic agents, topical therapy often offers the best means of palliation. Such measures include cool compresses, emollients, oatmeal baths, exposure to ultraviolet light (with or without psoralens), topical anesthetics and steroids, and capsaicin (the active ingredient of chile pepper that depletes substance P). Oral antihistamines are ineffective except those congeners that cause sedation, since histamine is not the primary mediator of

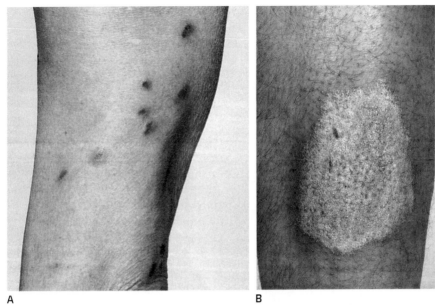

A   B

Figure 3-1 ■ Changes in the skin due to scratching from intense pruritus in a patient with biliary tract obstruction and jaundice. *A*, Excoriations from excavations of the skin by the patient's nails. *B*, Lichenification is thickening of the skin with exaggeration of the skin creases from rubbing the skin in the same site repetitively. (From du Vivier A: Atlas of Cinical Dermatology, 3rd ed. London, Churchill Livingstone, 2002.) (See Color Plate 1.)

DIAGNOSIS

Diagnostic Considerations in Pruritus

In general, one should suspect a diagnosis of polycythemia vera in patients who present with post-bathing pruritus. Routine blood counts provide confirmation.

The diagnosis of Hodgkin's or non-Hodgkin's lymphoma should be the first consideration in patients with nonaquagenic pruritus and no skin rash, provided that routine blood chemistries (liver and renal function and calcium levels) are in good order and no current medication appears to be the likely cause.

Given its rarity as a presenting symptom of solid organ cancers, a search for occult malignancy in a patient with otherwise unexplained pruritus is not warranted.

itching here as it is in urticarial diseases. In this regard, antidepressants and/or anxiolytics may ameliorate some aspects of this awful symptom in chronically afflicted patients.

Suggested Reading

Bernhard JD: Itch: Mechanisms and Management of Pruritus. New York: McGraw-Hill, 1994.

Greaves MW, Wall PD: Pathophysiology of itching. Lancet 1996;348:938–340.

Kam PCA, Tan KH: Pruritus: Itching for a cause and relief? Anaesthesia 1996;51:1133–1138.

Millikan LE: Pruritus: Unapproved treatments or indications. Clin Dermatol 2000;18:149–151.

Steinman HK, Greaves MW: Aquagenic pruritus. J Am Acad Dermatol 1985;13:91–96.

Yosipovitch G, David M: The diagnostic and therapeutic approach to idiopathic generalized pruritus. Int J Dermatol 1999;38:881–887.

Chapter 4
Headache

Eric Wong

Headache is common in the general population. Distinguishing between benign and malignant causes of headache is often difficult. This is particularly true for cancer patients, in whom the cause of headaches is often multifaceted; they can be related to brain metastasis, treatment effect, or other systemic disorders unrelated to cancer. While a busy clinician may decide to obtain neuroimaging for any patient with a persistent headache, this practice would clearly lead to considerable waste of resources and provoke unnecessary anxiety in patients. However, if the headache complaint is evaluated systematically and the appropriate diagnostic studies are performed, one can often determine a correct diagnosis with minimal excess resource utilization. The algorithm for evaluating headaches in the general population is shown in Figure 4-1. It includes a detailed history with particular attention to the patient's headache pattern, coexisting medical conditions, and neurologic examination. In the patient with known cancer, one must also take into consideration the primary malignancy, cancer staging, and neuroimaging findings.

Presentation and Evaluation of Headaches

Headaches are caused by irritation of the meninges, meningeal vasculature, scalp, or extracranial muscles and nerves. The brain parenchyma itself has no sensory fibers for pain. In fact, brain surgery can be done in fully awake patients under local anesthesia. In the general population, headaches are usually caused by migraine, muscle tension, or head pain related to cervical spine degenerative disease, but other causes such as temporal arteritis, bacterial meningitis, or temporomandibular joint dysfunction are possible. Primary brain tumors or brain metastases are rare causes, being responsible for well under 1% of the headaches in the general population. Clues for distinguishing headaches that are related to cancer from those related to other causes are listed in Table 4-1.

The intracranial processes associated with headaches are caused by raised intracranial pressure from mass effects, obstructive hydrocephalus, or both. Headaches can also occur as a result of meningeal irritations as tumor cells infiltrate the leptomeninges. Extracranial causes of headaches include metastasis to the calvarium or the upper cervical spine. It is also important to recognize that the potential causes of headaches may differ depending on the primary malignancy (Table 4-2). For example, intracranial metastasis from cancers of breast and lung typically cause mass effects, obstructive hydrocephalus, or both. In contrast, intracranial metastases are rare in patients with multiple myeloma, while headaches in such patients may be a symptom of blood hyperviscosity.

In taking a history, particular attention should be directed toward the cardinal features of headaches: quality, location, severity, duration, and temporal pattern. Additional information on the exacerbating or ameliorating factors and associated neurologic features is also helpful (see Table 4-1). According to one study of patients with known systemic cancer, 77% of the headaches are of tension type, 9% are migrainous, and 14% fall into other patterns. It is noteworthy that headaches from raised intracranial pressure can arise

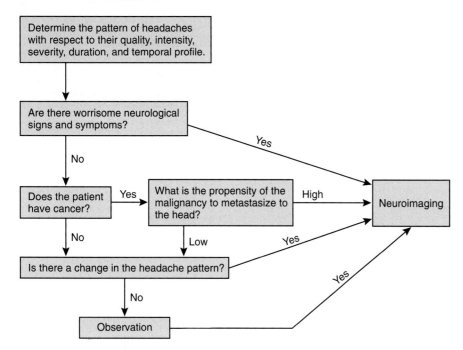

Figure 4-1 ■ Algorithm for evaluating headaches in the general population.

Table 4-1 ■ Distinguishing Features of Various Types of Headaches

Headache	Quality	Location	Severity	Duration	Temporal Pattern	Exacerbating Factors	Associated Deficits
Aneurysm bleed	Throbbing	Diffuse	The worst	Unremitting	Constant	Changes in body position, cough, sneeze, or Valsalva maneuver, neck movement	Coma, focal neurologic deficit
Brain tumor	Pressure	Diffuse	Can be severe	Unremitting	Constant	Changes in body position, cough, sneeze, or Valsalva maneuver	Papilledema or any focal neurologic deficit
Cervical neuritis	Sharp	Occiput	Mild/moderate	Days/weeks	Constant	Neck movement	Limitation in neck movement
Cluster	Throbbing	Unilateral	Severe	Days/weeks	Intermittent	Light, sound, alcohol	Rhinorrhea, conjunctival injection, miosis, ptosis
Hydrocephalus	Pressure	Diffuse	Can be severe	Unremitting	Constant	Changes in body position, cough	Papilledema or double vision
Meningitis	Pressure	Diffuse	Severe	Unremitting	Constant	Head motion	Papilledema, Kernig or Brudzinski signs, nausea, vomiting
Migraine	Throbbing	Unilateral	Usually severe	Hours	Intermittent	Light, sound, alcohol	Blurry vision, flashing light
Temporal arteritis	Ache	Temple	Mild/moderate	Unremitting	Constant	Local compression	Blindness

---

DIAGNOSIS

Headache: Who Needs Neuroimaging?

Headaches that worsen with raised intrathoracic pressure: These headaches are intensified by coughing, sneezing, or Valsalva maneuvers.

Nocturnal headaches: Headaches that awaken a patient at night should be taken seriously. Most benign headaches, such as migraines, tension headaches, or cluster headaches, actually improve with sleep. Nocturnal headaches are commonly associated with mass effect.

Headaches associated with worrisome neurologic signs: These signs include papilledema, nausea, projectile vomiting (the word *projectile* refers to the sudden nature of the vomiting, not the trajectory), syncope, a change in mental status, or seizure.

Headaches that worsen with changes in body position: This phenomenon usually indicates intracranial mass effect.

The worst headache of one's life: Although this type of headache is often related to an intracranial aneurysm bleed, an occasional cancer patient with a sudden tumor bleed may experience this phenomenon as well, particularly when blood seeps into the ventricles or subarachnoid space.

Changes in headache characteristics: When there is a change in headache quality, particularly with the associated neurologic signs and symptoms mentioned above, neuroimaging is indicated.

---

from a large brain tumor causing mass effect or from obstructive hydrocephalus caused by either tumor compression or leptomeningeal blockage of cerebrospinal fluid outflow. These patients quite often have the classic triad of increased intracranial pressure: headache, nausea, and papilledema. Such headaches can be exacerbated by activities that increase the intrathoracic pressure, such as coughing, sneezing, or Valsalva maneuvers. In addition, these headaches are often worse at night, frequently awakening the patient. These nocturnal headaches are a result of the transient increases in pCO_2, a potent cerebral vasodilator, during sleep. Other worrisome symptoms include increases in headache intensity with changes in body position, the onset of positional vertigo, the development of positional vertigo or vomiting, or the sudden loss of consciousness.

Management of Headaches

The symptomatic management of cancer-related headaches includes surgical interventions, radiation therapy, dexamethasone, and nonspecific drug treatments for pain (Table 4-3). Patients with mass effect from intracranial tumors, large calvarial masses invading the intracranial cavity and compressing the brain, or obstructive hydrocephalus usually need urgent neurosurgical evaluation for either resection of the mass or creation of a ventriculoperitoneal shunt. Dexamethasone can be a temporizing measure until definitive intervention is performed. If necessary, opioids may be used to alleviate headaches, but they can depress mental alertness, making an accurate assessment of neurologic function difficult. Fortunately, most patients do not need urgent neurosurgi-

---

Table 4-2 ■ Selected Cancer-Related Headaches and Their Mechanisms

Cancer	Brain Tumor	Hydrocephalus	Calvarial Metastasis	Hyperviscosity
Acute lymphocytic leukemia	–	+	–	+
Breast carcinoma	+	+	+	–
Germ cell tumor, non-seminoma	+	+	–	–
Glioma	+	+	–	–
Lung cancer, small-cell	+	+	–	–
Lung cancer, non-small-cell	+	+	–	–
Multiple myeloma	–	–	+	+
Non-Hodgkin's lymphoma	+	+	–	–
Prostate carcinoma	–	–	+	–
Renal cell carcinoma	+	–	+	–

Table 4-3 ■ Symptomatic Management of Cancer-Related Headaches

Etiology	Potential Interventions
Mass effect from tumor	Dexamethasone, neurosurgical resection, ventriculoperitoneal shunt, or opioids
Hydrocephalus	Ventriculoperitoneal shunt, dexamethasone, opioids
Calvarial metastasis	Radiation therapy, tricyclic antidepressant (amitriptyline, nortriptyline, or imipramine), anticonvulsants (carbamazepine or gabapentin), or opioids
Hyperviscosity	Plasmapheresis, phlebotomy, or leukopheresis

cal intervention. For headaches caused by calvarial metastases, radiation therapy may alleviate pain. An alternative is the use of both acute and chronic pain medications. Opioids are effective medications for acute pain, while drugs such as tricyclic antidepressants and anticonvulsants can suppress chronic pain by altering the neurochemical profile of the brain's perception of pain. As a result, they take longer to work than opioids or other narcotics. Finally, patients with hyperviscosity syndrome may need plasmapheresis to treat elevated levels of immunoglobulins, phlebotomy to alleviate increased red cell mass, or leukopheresis to reduce leukostasis related to leukemia.

Suggested Reading

Caraceni A: Clinicopathologic correlates of common cancer pain syndromes. Hemat Oncol Clin North Am 1996;10:57–78.

Chidel MA, Suh JH, Barnett GH: Brain metastases: Presentation, evaluation, and management. Cleve Clin J Med 2000; 67:120–127.

Clouston PD, DeAngelis LM, Posner JB: The spectrum of neurological disease in patients with systemic cancer. Ann Neurol 1992;31:268–273.

Forsyth PA, Posner JB. Headaches in patients with brain tumors: A study of 111 patients. Neurology 1993;43:1678–1683.

Manfredi PL, Shenoy S, Pavne R: Sumatriptan for headache caused by head and neck cancer. Headache 2000;40:758–760.

Victor M, Ropper AH: Adams and Victor's Principles of Neurology. New York: McGraw-Hill, 2001, pp 175–203.

Chapter 5
Seizures

Steven C. Schachter

Introduction

Recurrent seizures affect 2 to 4 million Americans. The prevalence is highest in people under the age of 20 years, though the incidence increases over the age of 70 years to more than 100 cases per 100,000. Although brain tumors are the most feared etiology, they are fortunately an infrequent cause. Fewer than 5% of children with epilepsy have brain tumors, though up to one half of children with tumors in the cerebral hemisphere have seizures as the initial presenting symptom. The likelihood of brain tumors among adults with new-onset epilepsy is approximately 12% and is highest among the elderly.

High-grade glial tumors and brain metastases are less likely to cause seizures than are low-grade, well-differentiated gliomas, including low-grade astrocytomas, oligodendrogliomas, dysembryopathic neuroepithelial tumors, gangliogliomas, and hamartomas. These lesions tend to be well circumscribed with minimal surrounding edema, may or may not enhance, and tend to be located in the temporal or frontal lobes. The most frequently encountered epileptogenic intra-axial tumors in children are astrocytomas and oligodendrogliomas. In adults, oligodendrogliomas are the most epileptogenic (and calcify in up to 40% of cases), followed by astrocytomas, glioblastoma multiforme, and metastases. Meningiomas, the most common extra-axial intracranial tumor (approximately 20% of all intracranial tumors), cause seizures as the initial presentation in up to 50% of cases.

The pathophysiologic mechanisms associated with tumor-associated epilepsy are not well understood but probably include focal hypoxia, mass effect, metabolic imbalance, pH abnormalities, amino acid and neuroreceptor disturbances, immunologic activity, and reduced inhibition from nearby cerebral regions.

This chapter reviews the clinical evaluation and management of seizures with particular emphasis on patients with intracranial neoplasms.

Clinical Evaluation of Seizures

History

Before initiating therapy, the clinician must obtain a thorough history from the patient and observers with particular attention to descriptions of actual seizures, including the circumstances leading up to the seizure, the ictal behaviors, and the postictal state. Partial seizures (seizures that arise from a focal area of cerebral cortex) are the most common type of seizure in patients with and without brain tumors. Simple partial seizures (also called auras) may take a variety of forms, including lateralized motor movements, affective sensations, and sensory illusions. During complex partial seizures (formerly called psychomotor seizures), patients appear to be awake but are not in contact with others in their environment and do not respond normally to instructions or questions. They often seem to stare into space and either remain motionless or engage in repetitive behaviors, called automatisms. If physically restrained, patients may become hostile or aggressive. The seizures typically last less than 3 minutes and may be immediately preceded by an unusual feeling or movement (aura). Afterward, the patient may be somnolent and confused and may have a headache for up to several hours (Figure 5-1).

A generalized tonic-clonic seizure (also called grand mal seizure, major motor seizure, or convulsion) may begin with an aura that is rapidly followed by loss of consciousness, often in association with a loud noise. Then the muscles of the extremities and the chest and back stiffen, and the patient may appear cyanotic. After approximately 1 minute, the muscles begin to jerk and twitch for an additional 1 to 2 minutes. During this clonic phase, the tongue may be bitten, and frothy, bloody sputum may appear, often mentioned by observers. Once the twitching movements end, the postictal phase begins. The patient is initially in a deep sleep, breathing deeply, and then gradually wakes up, often complaining of a headache.

There are no ictal characteristics that reliably distinguish seizures due to tumors from nontumoral causes; however, olfactory auras, if present, are most commonly due to tumors, typically in the temporal lobe.

Neurologic Examination and Diagnostic Studies

Cognitive disturbances or lateralizing findings on the neurologic examination, such as hyperreflexia or weakness, may be an indication of brain dysfunction. However, there are no neurologic signs that are specific for tumors, and the examination is often normal, particularly in patients with slow-growing tumors.

Laboratory evaluations are appropriate to rule out a metabolic cause for seizures, such as hyponatremia and hypoglycemia, and to obtain baseline screening before antiepileptic drugs are begun. An abnormal electroencephalogram (EEG) substantiates the diagnosis of seizures if epileptiform discharges are present, and marked unilateral slowing may be suggestive of a space-occupying lesion. However, a substantial proportion of patients with seizures and brain tumors have normal electroencephalograms; therefore a normal EEG rules out neither seizures nor an underlying tumor. Furthermore, a positive electroencephalogram may be nonspecific, because electroencephalogram abnormalities are associated with other conditions such as migraine headaches and vascular insufficiency.

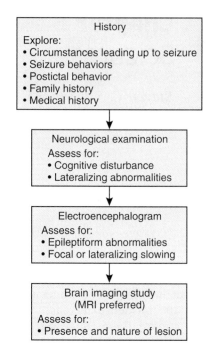

Figure 5-1 ■ Evaluation of seizure disorder.

A neuroimaging study should be obtained for all patients with partial seizures to look for a structural brain abnormality. Alerting the neuroradiologist to the possibility of a brain tumor is important. Brain magnetic resonance imaging is preferred over computed tomography (CT) for identifying tumors (Figure 5-2), because the computed tomography scan appearance

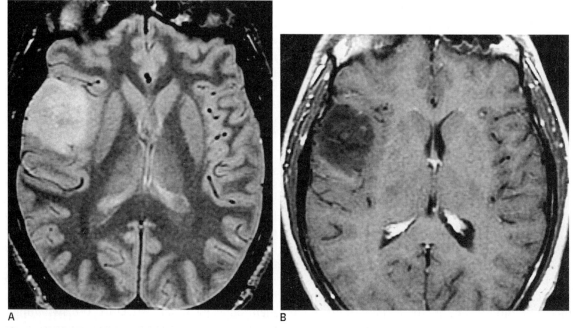

A   B

Figure 5-2 ■ T$_2$ and T$_1$ weighted magnetic resonance imaging images of a glioma. (From Chin CY, Chang S, Dillon WP: Brain and Spinal Cord Tumors. In Bragg DG, Rubin P, Hricak H [eds]: Oncologic Imaging. Philadelphia: WB Saunders, 2002, p. 141.)

of tumors may be nonspecific and therefore may be misinterpreted. If initially negative, magnetic resonance imaging scans should be repeated if (1) there is a suspicion of a tumor on the initial magnetic resonance imaging, (2) there is progressive worsening of a patient's neurologic examination or cognitive function, or (3) the frequency or severity of a patient's seizures increases. However, not all patients with epilepsy due to brain tumors have worsening of their seizure frequency over time, and some patients become seizure free. Therefore the clinician should not rely on seizure frequency alone in deciding when to repeat neuroimaging studies in patients without a known cause for their seizures.

Treatment

Pharmacologic Therapy

The goals of treatment are to prevent seizures without causing disabling side effects or worsening existing neurologic deficits. Unfortunately, drug therapy with a single agent does not provide adequate seizure relief for a substantial number of patients, particularly patients with seizures associated with brain tumors. However, before considering combination antiepileptic drug therapy because of lack of efficacy, the clinician should check serum concentrations to determine whether a patient has been noncompliant with the treatment regimen or the dose is inadequate (Table 5-1). Antiepileptic drug serum concentrations are also helpful to evaluate whether a patient's complaints are likely to be related to the patient's antiepileptic drugs

and to establish the therapeutic concentration for a patient whose seizures come under control. Serum concentrations that are associated with neurotoxicity vary from one patient to another and may occur within the so-called therapeutic range, especially in patients with brain tumors. Free (rather than total) concentrations are useful in managing antiepileptic drug dosages (particularly phenytoin and valproate) when patients have low albumin levels or take other tightly protein-bound medications.

There is no known "best" antiepileptic drug combination. The practical difficulty with combination therapy is that troublesome or disabling side effects are very common. Both pharmacokinetic and pharmacodynamic mechanisms account for most drug-drug interactions. Consequently, combinations of drugs with different side effect profiles and combinations that do not have a significant potential for drug-drug interactions are advisable.

Nonpharmacologic Therapy

Excision of epileptogenic tumors may be considered if pharmacologic therapy is ineffective, the overall prognosis is favorable, and the lesion is surgically accessible. For example, in one series of patients with seizures due to meningiomas who underwent surgery, nearly two thirds became seizure-free postoperatively. Lesions that are deep-seated or that are close to critical cerebral areas (such as the motor strip) may require a computer-assisted stereotactic approach. Low-dose gamma knife radiosurgery applied to a sufficient volume of brain tissue around the tumor has also been reported to be effective.

Prophylactic Therapy

Given the substantial risk of seizures, some clinicians use antiepileptic drugs as prophylaxis against seizures in nonepileptic patients diagnosed with brain tumors. This practice is somewhat controversial and not supported by the literature. For instance, a randomized, double-blind study of patients with at least one supratentorial brain lesion showed no difference in the incidence of first seizures between patients treated with valproate and those treated with placebo.

Psychosocial Issues

The diagnosis of epilepsy is associated with substantial psychosocial consequences. Memory disturbances, fatigue, and dizziness—often related to antiepileptic drugs—are frequent complaints and may limit activities of daily living. Coping with the unpredictability of seizures is challenging. Loss of independence due to inability to drive (see next paragraph) or work can be

Table 5-1 ■ Drugs Commonly Prescribed for Seizures and Their Usual Target Range for Plasma Levels

Drug	Brand Name	Target Range (μg/mL)
Carbamazepine	Tegretol, Carbatrol	4-12
Clonazepam	Klonopin	0.02-0.08
Clorazepate	Tranxene	Not established
Ethosuximide	Zarontin	50-100
Felbamate	Felbatol	Not established
Gabapentin	Neurontin	Not established
Lamotrigine	Lamictal	Not established
Levetiracetam	Keppra	Not established
Oxcarbazepine	Trileptal	Not established
Topiramate	Topamax	Not established
Tiagabine	Gabitril	Not established
Phenobarbital		15-40
Phenytoin	Dilantin	10-20
Valproate	Depakote, Depakene	50-150
Zonisamide	Zonegran	Not established

TREATMENT

Pharmacologic Anticonvulsant Therapy

No drugs have been shown to be superior to others for seizures secondary to brain tumors. Our practice is to start with oxcarbazepine, carbamazepine, phenytoin, or valproate. Of this group, oxcarbazepine is best tolerated and least likely to cause drug-drug interactions or be affected by hepatic dysfunction. Therefore oxcarbazepine is our drug of choice unless treatment must be started urgently, in which case intravenous phenytoin or fosphenytoin is our preference. Because oxcarbazepine is relatively new and more expensive than the other first-line drugs for partial seizures, some physicians prefer carbamazepine, phenytoin, or valproate.

We have found oxcarbazepine, the 10-keto analogue of carbamazepine, to be better tolerated than carbamazepine. The dose in adults can be initiated at 150 to 300 mg daily and titrated over 2 to 3 weeks to 900 to 1800 mg daily as needed. Rash occurs less frequently with oxcarbazepine than with carbamazepine, as do other side effects such as drowsiness, dizziness, headache, double vision, nausea, vomiting, and ataxia. Hyponatremia is more commonly seen with oxcarbazepine than with carbamazepine, although patients are rarely symptomatic.

Carbamazepine should be introduced in low doses (100 to 200 mg daily) with 100- to 200-mg increments every 3 to 14 days, depending on the urgency of the situation, to a target dose of 600 to 1200 mg daily. Side effects include double vision, headache, dizziness, nausea, and vomiting. Infrequent idiosyncratic reactions include a morbilliform rash in approximately 10% of patients, the syndrome of inappropriate antidiuretic hormone, and a reversible mild leukopenia. Rarely, Stevens-Johnson syndrome, aplastic anemia, and toxic hepatitis are seen. Drug interactions are common because carbamazepine accelerates the metabolism of many lipid-soluble drugs.

Phenytoin may be started at the maintenance dose, typically 300 mg/day in two divided doses in adults (5 to 8 mg/kg/day in children) or more rapidly by the intravenous route if necessary with parenteral phenytoin or fosphenytoin. Neurotoxic side effects include ataxia, nystagmus, dysarthria, asterixis, and somnolence. Phenytoin is associated with rash in approximately 5% of patients. Rare idiosyncratic reactions include Stevens-Johnson syndrome, hepatitis, bone marrow suppression, lymphadenopathy, and a lupuslike syndrome. Phenytoin induces hepatic enzyme function and may displace tightly protein-bound drugs.

Valproate should be started at 500 mg once or twice daily and titrated to 1000 to 1500 mg daily as needed. Side effects include dose-related tremor, weight gain, and hair thinning or loss. Rarely, stupor, encephalopathy, and hepatotoxicity can occur. Other sporadic problems include thrombocytopenia and pancreatitis. Valproate inhibits hepatic enzyme function.

Other antiepileptic drugs that may be beneficial as adjunctive therapy are gabapentin, lamotrigine, topiramate, tiagabine, levetiracetam, and zonisamide (see Table 5-1).

---

emotionally devastating. Consequently, comorbid psychiatric conditions are common, including depression, anxiety, and panic disorders. Depression generally presents with a chronic course interrupted by recurrent symptom-free periods of hours to several days. Selective serotonin reuptake inhibitors are unlikely to exacerbate seizures, whereas monoamine oxidase inhibitors and nontricyclic antidepressants are probably best avoided.

Driving regulations for patients with seizures vary from state to state, and clinicians should consult their state's motor vehicle authority to advise their patients about any applicable legal restrictions. In most states, 3- to 12-month seizure-free intervals are required before patients can legally drive. Some states still require mandatory reporting of patients with seizures by physicians; however, the majority of states rely on patients to self-report.

Suggested Reading

Balestrini MR, Zanette M, Micheli R, Fornari M, Solero CL, Broggi G: Hemispheric cerebral tumors in children: Long-term prognosis concerning survival rate and quality of life—considerations on a series of 64 cases operated upon.

Childs Nerv Syst 1990;6:143–147.

Beaumont A, Whittle IR: The pathogenesis of tumour associated epilepsy. Acta Neurochir (Wien) 2000;142:1–15.

Engel J: Surgery for seizures. N Engl J Med 1996;334:647–652.

Glantz MJ, Cole BF, Friedberg MH, et al: A randomized, blinded, placebo-controlled trial of divalproex sodium prophylaxis in adults with newly diagnosed brain tumors. Neurology 1996;46:985–991.

Moots PL, Maciunas RJ, Eisert DR, Parker RA, Laporte K, Abou-Khalil B: The course of seizure disorders in patients with malignant gliomas. Arch Neurol 1995;52:717–724.

Quesney LF: Clinical and EEG features of complex partial seizures of temporal lobe origin. Epilepsia 1986;27(Suppl 2):S27–S45.

Schachter SC: Antiepileptic drug therapy: General treatment principles and application for special patient populations. Epilepsia 1999;40(Suppl 9):S20–S25.

Schrottner O, Eder HG, Unger F, Feichtinger K, Pendl G: Radiosurgery in lesional epilepsy: Brain tumors. Stereotact Funct Neurosurg 1998;70(Suppl 1):50–56.

Sjors K, Blennow G, Lantz G: Seizures as the presenting symptom of brain tumors in children. Acta Paediatr 1993;82:66–70.

Villemure JG, de Tribolet N: Epilepsy in patients with central nervous system tumors. Curr Opin Neurol 1996;9:424–428.

Chapter 6
Cranial Neuropathy

Eric Wong and Subramanian Hariharan

Cranial neuropathies are uncommon cancer-related complications, but they can result in disabling deficits. According to one retrospective review, fewer than 10% of patients with systemic cancer present with this problem. As the cranial nerves project from the brain stem via the subarachnoid space and skull base to the cranial tissues, they can be damaged by a variety of malignant conditions either directly or indirectly. For example, tumor infiltration into the base of the skull or the leptomeningeal space can cause cranial nerve deficits. These deficits can also occur as a late sequela of radiation to the head and neck region. Equally important, cancer patients may have concomitant systemic diseases, such as diabetes, viral syndromes, or neuromuscular disorders, that can result in cranial neuropathies independent of the malignancy. The key to arriving at a correct diagnosis is twofold: (1) to localize the lesion in the cranial nerves versus the brain stem or brain and (2) to determine the potential causes on the basis of the temporal presentation of neurologic deficits, the primary malignancy, cancer staging, prior therapies, and concomitant illness. The spectrum of cranial neuropathies in cancer patients includes parenchymal metastasis to the brain, leptomeningeal metastasis, metastasis to the bones at the base of skull, treatment-related neuropathies, and other cranial neuropathies unrelated to cancer. The algorithm for evaluation of a patient presenting with a cranial neuropathy is depicted in Figure 6-1. The various components of this algorithm are elaborated in Tables 6-1 and 6-2.

Presentation of Cranial Neuropathies

The evaluation of cranial neuropathies in cancer patients should be considered within the context of the primary malignancy, if already known, and cancer staging. Different primary malignancies have different metastatic patterns to the brain and the surrounding structures such as the leptomeninges and the skull base (see Table 6-1). For example, patients with prostate cancer almost never have brain metastasis, but they frequently have cranial nerve deficits as a result of micrometastases to the clivus or sphenoid wing. In contrast, it is unusual for patients with renal cell carcinoma to have leptomeningeal spread. A solitary metastasis to the brain parenchyma is the usual metastatic pattern. Another important consideration is cancer staging. Patients with lung metastases from a systemic malignancy are particularly vulnerable to developing coexistent metastases to the brain, the leptomeninges, or the bones at the skull base, while patients with non-Hodgkin's lymphoma involving the paranasal sinuses and testes frequently have leptomeningeal spread.

Because each of the 12 cranial nerves has different motor and sensory functions, recognizing the pattern of cranial nerve deficits is important in narrowing the number of potential diagnoses. Table 6-2 lists the patterns of cranial nerve deficits and their respective cancer-related and non-cancer-related causes. As a rule of thumb, cancer-related cranial neuropathies usually evolve over weeks or months. In contrast, acute cranial nerve deficits occurring over minutes or hours are typically vascular in nature. For example, a patient having diabetic oculomotor nerve palsy would present with a sudden onset of double vision. Other deficits that take years to develop are usually, but not exclusively, caused by neurodegenerative diseases, as in the case of tongue weakness from amyotrophic lateral sclerosis.

In general, patients having multiple cranial nerve dysfunctions are more likely to have cancer as the underlying etiology than are those with only one deficit. The exact incidence of malignancy in patients presenting with multiple cranial neuropathies is unclear, because this phenomenon has not been adequately studied in the general population. The best data available are for patients with bilateral facial nerve palsies; about 20% of newly diagnosed patients are eventually found to have an underlying malignancy. In contrast, the incidence of cancer is probably

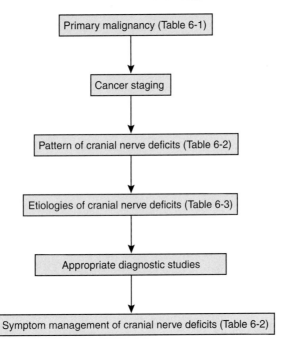

Figure 6-1 ■ Algorithm for evaluating cranial neuropathy in the cancer patient.

1% or less in the general population presenting with a unilateral facial palsy.

Evaluation of Cranial Neuropathies

Once the pattern of deficit has been determined, a differential diagnosis of the etiology can be generated. The diagnostic evaluations needed depend on the location of the suspected lesion in (1) the parenchyma of the brain, (2) the base of the skull, (3) the pituitary gland and the structures surrounding the sella, or (4) the leptomeningeal space (see Table 6-2). In general, MRI is far superior to CT in delineating intracranial structures. The only exception is in the evaluation of skull base lesions, for which CT can display the bony structures better than MRI. In patients with suspected leptomeningeal metastasis, a lumbar puncture may be necessary to find supportive evidence. However, a lumbar puncture would be contraindicated in most patients with raised intracranial pressure, noncommunicating obstructive hydrocephalus, or a spinal block. In these situations, a consultation with a neurosurgeon or a neuro-oncologist to expedite diagnostic and treatment decisions may be worthwhile. Approximately 30% of patients with leptomeningeal metastasis will have a negative MRI, despite their cerebrospinal fluid being positive for malignant cells, while another 30% of patients will have a positive MRI but a negative cerebrospinal fluid cytology. It is also important to recognize that treatment-related cranial neuropathies, such as those caused by radiation or chemotherapy, are diagnoses of exclusion.

Management of Cranial Neuropathies

Symptomatic management of cancer-related cranial nerve deficits is indicated to prevent potential complications. If the deficits are caused by tumor infiltration of the brain parenchyma, leptomeningeal space, or base of the skull, dexamethasone is indicated to lessen

Table 6-1 ■ **Common Metastatic Pattern of Selected Malignancies Causing Cranial Neuropathies**

Cancer	Brain Parenchyma	Leptomeninges	Base of Skull
Acute lymphoblastic leukemia	–	+	–
Acute myeloid leukemia	–	+	–
Breast carcinoma	+	+	+
Colon cancer	+	–	–
Germ cell tumors			
Seminoma	–	–	–
Non-seminoma	+	+	–
Lung cancer, small-cell	+	+	–
Lung cancer, non-small-cell	+	+	–
Melanoma	+	+	–
Non-Hodgkin's lymphoma			
Low-grade	–	–	–
Intermediate-grade	+	+	–
High-grade	+	+	–
Prostate carcinoma	–	–	+
Renal cell carcinoma	+	–	–

Table 6-2 ■ Some Common Cranial Nerve Deficits Seen in Cancer Patients

Cranial Nerves	Pattern of Deficit	Cancer-Related Causes	Non-Cancer-Related Causes	Symptomatic Management of Cancer-Related Causes
I, olfactory nerve	Loss of smell and taste	Unusual presentation	Head trauma or postsurgical	None
II, optic nerve	Homonymous hemianopsia	Brain metastasis	Stroke, abscess, demyelination	Dexamethasone
	Monocular blindness	Optic nerve glioma, ischemia from hypercoagulability	Demyelination, diabetes, sarcoidosis, orbital apex syndrome	Dexamethasone for tumor; aspirin or heparin for cancer-related hypercoagulability
	Bitemporal hemianopsia or monocular → binocular blindness	Pituitary tumors, craniopharyngioma	Unusual presentation	Dexamethasone
	Papilledema	Increased intracranial pressure from intracranial tumors	Increased intracranial pressure from pseudotumor cerebri, stroke, abscess, demyelination	Dexamethasone
III, IV, VI, oculomotor, trochlear, and abducent nerves	Double vision	Pituitary apoplexy, base of skull metastasis, sphenoid wing meningioma, increased intracranial pressure from intracranial tumors	Diabetes, sarcoidosis, spontaneous or postlumbar puncture intracranial hypotension	Dexamethasone, eye patch to cover one eye; prism glasses
	Unilateral dilated pupil	Uncal herniation caused by increased intracranial pressure from intracranial tumors	Uncal herniation from intracranial bleed, encephalitis, or demyelination	Mannitol, hyperventilation, and neurosurgical intervention for uncal herniation
V, trigeminal nerve	Chin numbness	Metastatic tumors to the lower jaw	Unusual presentation	No symptomatic treatment needed
	Cheek/gum numbness	Nasopharyngeal carcinoma	Nasal sinus abscess	No symptomatic treatment needed
	Facial numbness	Base of skull metastasis, sphenoid wing meningioma, leptomeningeal metastasis	Sarcoidosis, stroke	No symptomatic treatment needed
	Facial pain	Unusual presentation	Tic douloureux	Anticonvulsant therapy, tricyclic antidepressant

Table continues

Table 6-2 ■ Some Common Cranial Nerve Deficits Seen in Cancer Patients—cont'd

Cranial Nerves	Pattern of Deficit	Cancer-Related Causes	Non-Cancer-Related Causes	Symptomatic Management of Cancer-Related Causes
VII, facial nerve	Lower facial weakness only	Brain metastasis	Stroke, demyelination, abscess	Dexamethasone
	Upper and lower facial weakness	Leptomeningeal metastasis, base of skull metastasis	Bell's palsy, sarcoidosis, postsurgical	Dexamethasone; moisture chamber, lacrilube, and artificial tears for incomplete closure of the eye; tarsorrhaphy
VIII, cochlear and vestibular nerves	Hearing loss	Leptomeningeal metastasis, base of skull metastasis, vestibular schwannoma, meningioma, platinum-induced neurosensory hearing loss	Otitis media, age-related	Dexamethasone
	Vertigo	Leptomeningeal metastasis, base of skull metastasis	Benign positional vertigo, vestibular neuronitis, labyrinthitis brainstem stroke	Dexamethasone; vestibular exercises for desensitization; meclizine tablet or scopolamine patch
IX, X, glossopharyngeal and vagus nerves	Swallowing difficulty	Leptomeningeal metastasis, base of skull metastasis, nasopharyngeal carcinoma, radiation	Amyotrophic lateral sclerosis, stroke	Dexamethasone; saliva suction; gastroenterostomy tube feeding
	Carotid sinus syndrome	Base of skull metastasis	Idiopathic carotid sinus hypersensitivity	Dexamethasone; hydration
XI, accessory nerve	Neck and shoulder weakness	Base of skull metastasis, leptomeningeal metastasis	Torticollis (muscle hypertrophy), dystonia (muscle hypertrophy)	Dexamethasone; physical therapy to prevent shoulder joint contracture; sling to support weak shoulder and upper arm
XII, hypoglossal	Tongue weakness	Base of skull metastasis, glomus tumor, chordoma, radiation	Amyotrophic lateral sclerosis	Dexamethasone; gastroenterostomy tube feeding

---

DIAGNOSIS

Diagnostic study for evaluation of cranial neuropathies

Optimal diagnostic study for the evaluation of cranial neuropathies depends on the region of involvement as follows:

Brain: MRI with gadolinium
Pituitary: MRI of the sella with gadolinium
Base of skull metastasis: CT of the petrous temporal bone with bone windows
Leptomeningeal metastasis: MRI with gadolinium, lumbar puncture, or both

---

the degree of cranial nerve deficits. It is important to use dexamethasone to temporize cranial nerve deficits until definitive diagnostic studies are done and to wean it when the appropriate treatments are given. In cases of lymphoma and leukemia, a false negative diagnosis can result when there is a delay in performing a diagnostic evaluation after dexamethasone administration. This is because dexamethasone is oncolytic to lymphoma and leukemia cells, and it can also change the neuroimaging pattern by altering blood-brain barrier permeability. Furthermore, long-term dexamethasone use is associated with significant immune suppression, muscle weakness, weight gain, leg swelling, and infrequently gastritis and bowel perforation.

Special therapeutic interventions are available for specific cranial nerve deficits. For example, patients with double vision will need an eye patch to cover one eye. Most patients are particularly bothered by double vision, although they can still function with monocular vision even though they lack depth perception. When double vision is fixed and permanent, a neuro-ophthalmologic evaluation is indicated for prescription of prism glasses to realign vision. In addition, incomplete closure of one eye is often encountered in patients with peripheral facial nerve palsy. This leads to an impairment in blinking and in inadequate lubrication of the cornea. As a result, the cornea can be damaged by desiccation or external abrasion. To prevent corneal scarring and loss of eyesight, application of a moisture chamber, lubricant, and artificial tears is often needed. If none of the aforementioned interventions help, forced eyelid closure with a stitch, or tarsorrhaphy, is necessary. Also, vertigo can be caused by cancer infiltration or drug-related impairment of a vestibular nerve. When this symptom occurs, vestibular exercises, meclizine, or application of a scopolamine patch may lessen the discomfort. Patients with swallowing difficulty and tongue weakness are at risk of aspiration pneumonia. In severe cases, suctioning is needed to prevent aspiration of saliva and a gastroenterostomy is needed for tube feeding. Finally, chronic shoulder weakness from accessory nerve dysfunction can progress to frank contracture of the shoulder joint, setting off a chain of events leading to autonomic dysfunction in the upper extremity, osteoporosis, and pain. To prevent these secondary complications, regular physical therapy to improve joint mobility is indicated. When there is pain, treatment with a tricyclic antidepressant or anticonvulsant may help.

Suggested Reading

Clouston PD, DeAngelis LM, Posner JB: The spectrum of neurological disease in patients with systemic cancer. Ann Neurol 1992;31:268–273.

Haerer AF: DeJong's The Neurologic Examination, 5th ed. Philadelphia: JB Lippincott, 1992.

Keane JR: Bilateral seventh nerve palsy: Analysis of 43 cases and review of the literature. Neurology 1994;44:1198–1202.

Levin VA: Cancer of the Nervous System. New York: Churchill Livingstone, 1996.

Posner JB: Neurologic Complications of Cancer. Philadelphia: FA Davis, 1995.

Chapter 7
Encephalopathy and Neuropathy

Patrick Y. Wen

Two of the most common neurologic complaints in cancer patients are encephalopathy and peripheral neuropathy. This chapter reviews the evaluation of patients with these two problems.

Encephalopathy

Encephalopathy is a nonspecific term for diffuse cerebral dysfunction. It is most commonly used to refer to patients with an acute confusional state. This is a rapidly developing, reversible change in behavior characterized by clouding of consciousness, incoherent train of thought, and difficulty with attention and concentration.

Most patients who become encephalopathic will have one or more of the benign causes outlined in Table 7-1. However, in a minority of patients (fewer than 5%), the encephalopathy may be the first manifestation of an underlying cancer. The most common cause is a brain tumor. These tumors may cause encephalopathy by their mass effect or by provoking seizures. Another cause is metabolic encephalopathy produced by the underlying cancer, such as hypercalcemia in patients with myeloma or the syndrome of inappropriate antidiuretic hormone secretion (SIADH) in patients with small-cell lung cancer. Other less common cancer-related causes for patients presenting with encephalopathy include leptomeningeal metastases, strokes, and disseminated intravascular coagulation, opportunistic infections, and paraneoplastic limbic encephalitis (Table 7-2).

Encephalopathy is common in patients with a known cancer. Encephalopathy was the most common reason for neurologic consultation at Memorial Sloan Kettering Cancer Center, accounting for 17% of all consultations. It is present in 14% to 40% of patients hospitalized with cancer and is associated with an increased mortality rate. The etiology of encephalopathy is usually multifactorial. In addition to the usual causes of encephalopathy present in general medical patients, cancer patients have other causes that must also be considered (see Table 7-1), including cerebral dysfunction resulting from direct infiltration of the nervous system by cancer or indirect effects on the nervous system resulting from infection, chemotherapy, nutritional deficiency, and paraneoplastic disorders. The most common causes of encephalopathy in cancer patients in descending order of frequency are drug toxicity, infection, organ dysfunction, brain lesion, hypoxia, electrolyte imbalance, sensory or environmental factors (e.g., intensive care unit psychosis), radiotherapy to the brain, chemotherapy, and surgery. In most patients, a careful medical history and selective laboratory and radiographic evaluation (Table 7-3) will lead to a specific diagnosis.

Differential Diagnosis

Confusion must be differentiated from a variety of other disorders. Patients with Wernicke's aphasia have a disorder of language resulting from injury to the superior temporal gyrus in the dominant hemisphere. They have problems with comprehension and naming and make frequent paraphrasic errors that may be mistaken for confusion. Their level of consciousness is normal. Wernicke's aphasia is usually caused by a stroke or brain metastasis. Patients with transient global amnesia have a striking loss of short-term memory but a normal level of consciousness. This is usually a benign process that is not directly related to the patient's underlying cancer. Patients with psychosis frequently have incoherent thought processes that may resemble confusion, but their level of consciousness is normal and does not fluctuate with time. Patients with dementia have a problem with short-term memory and often other cognitive functions such as language, praxis, and executive function. However, the onset is usually subacute or chronic, and the level of consciousness is normal.

Clinical Evaluation

Special attention to the patient's presentation and history will often lead to the correct diagnosis. Factors

---

Table 7-1 ■ Causes of Encephalopathy

Nonmalignant Causes

Metabolic
Hypoxia
Hypercapnia
Electrolyte imbalance
Hypoglycemia
Uremia
Abnormal liver function
Drug toxicity or withdrawal
Nutritional deficiency, including Wernicke's encephalopathy
and B_{12} deficiency

Infectious
Sepsis
Meningitis and encephalitis

Endocrine
Hypothyroidism and hyperthyroidism

Cerebrovascular Disorders,
Avasculitis
Demyelination
Psychiatric Disorders
Including depression and psychosis

Causes Related to Direct Effects of the Cancer

Brain metastases
Leptomeningeal metastases
Seizures
Hydrocephalus

Causes Related to Indirect Effects of Cancer

Opportunistic infections
Cerebrovascular disorders
Toxic effects of chemotherapy and radiation therapy
Nutritional deficiency
Paraneoplastic disorders

---

that are of particular importance include the temporal onset of the encephalopathy, evidence of infection, or hypoxia; history of alcohol or drug use; medications; neurologic features such as headaches or focal deficits that may suggest brain or leptomeningeal metastases or cerebrovascular disorders; and loss of consciousness or clonic activity to suggest seizures. The patient's antineoplastic therapy is also important, as some agents, such as ifosfamide, high-dose methotrexate, and high-dose cytosine arabinoside, are associated with a higher incidence of encephalopathy. The extent of the patient's disease is also of importance. Patients with lung metastases may be hypoxic, while those with liver metastases may have hepatic encephalopathy. Patients with widely disseminated and uncontrolled systemic disease are more likely to have metastatic disease in the central nervous system. The patient's underlying cancer should also be taken into account. For example, while all types of lung cancer may be associated with brain metastases, patients with adenocarcinoma of the lung have a higher incidence of encephalopathy associated with disseminated intravascular coagulation, marantic endocarditis, and leptomeningeal metastases. Patients with small-cell lung cancer may have paraneoplastic limbic encephalitis associated with the anti-Hu antibody. In contrast, patients with squamous carcinoma of the lung are much less likely to have either disseminated intravascular coagulation, leptomeningeal metastases or paraneoplastic syndromes.

The general and neurologic examinations are important to determine the correct diagnosis. The general examination may help to exclude infection, dehydration, and hypoxia. The mental status examination is important in confirming that the patient has an acute confusional state and excluding the other conditions described above, which can be mistaken for confusion, such as Wernicke's aphasia, transient global amnesia, depression, psychosis, and dementia. The presence of asterixis usually indicates the presence of a metabolic encephalopathy. Focal deficits may suggest brain or leptomeningeal metastases or cerebrovascular disorders. The presence of visual field abnormalities may suggest that a parietal occipital lesion from either metastases or infarction is causing the confusion. The presence of intermittent eye deviation or hippus raises the possibility of nonconvulsive status epilepticus. Patients with confusion, cerebellar ataxia, sensory neuronopathy, or autonomic dysfunction may have paraneoplastic encephalomyelitis.

Laboratory Evaluation

The laboratory tests should be based on the diagnoses suggested by the history and examination (see Table 7-3). Most patients should have a complete blood count (CBC), electrolytes, glucose, calcium, renal and liver function tests, ammonia level, and oxygen saturation. Since infection is a common cause of encephalopathy, most patients should also have a urine culture, a chest X-ray, blood cultures if febrile, and possibly a lumbar puncture. Patients who are immunocompromised will require more extensive testing to exclude infection than will patients who are not immunocompromised. Other blood tests that are useful in certain encephalopathic patients include drug toxicity screen, thyroid function tests, HIV test, rapid plasmin reagent, antinuclear antibodies, and Lyme titer. Patients who are suspected of having a paraneoplastic syndrome should have measurement of serum anti-Hu antibody. Other autoantibodies that may be obtained include the anti-Ma (ataxia and encephalomyelitis), anti-Ta (encephalomyelitis in patients with testicular cancer), and anti-CV2

Table 7-2 ■ **Neoplastic Causes of Encephalopathy in Patients Without a Known Cancer: Diagnosis and Appropriate Laboratory Tests**

Cause	Laboratory or Imaging Studies
Tumors (primary brain tumors and metastases)	CT or MRI with contrast
Metabolic abnormalities (especially hypercalcemia and hyponatremia)	*Hypercalcemia* Albumin, phosphate, urinary calcium Parathyroid hormone, parathyroid hormone–related protein Search for underlying neoplasm, especially immunoelectrophoresis, urine Bence Jones proteins, chest X-ray, bone scan
	Hyponatremia Urine and serum osmolarities, TSH, A.M. cortisol Search for underlying neoplasm, especially chest X-ray
Leptomeningeal metastases	Lumbar puncture, MRI of brain or spine with contrast
Cerebrovascular disorders	MRI with diffusion imaging, MR angiography Hypercoagulable workup, echocardiogram, Holter monitor Search for underlying neoplasm
Disseminated intravascular coagulation	Search for underlying neoplasm
CNS infections	HIV test Possible search for underlying neoplasm
Paraneoplastic limbic encephalitis	EEG, CSF examination, serum autoantibodies Search for underlying neoplasm

---

Table 7-3 ■ **Laboratory and Radiologic Evaluation of an Encephalopathic Patient**

Blood Tests

In Most Patients
  Complete blood count
  Electrolytes
  Glucose
  BUN/creatinine
  Liver function tests
  Calcium
  Toxin screen
  Ammonia
  Thyroid function tests

In Selected Patients
  Autoantibodies for paraneoplastic disorders (anti-Hu, CRMP-3 and -5, Ma, Ta antibodies)
  Serologic test for syphilis
  ANA
  HIV
  Lyme titer

Oxygen Saturation and Arterial Blood Gases

Urine Culture and Blood Cultures (if Infection is suspected)

Radiology
  Chest X-ray
  MRI or CT scan of brain with contrast

Electroencephalography

Lumbar Puncture

(encephalomyelitis, usually in small-cell lung cancer patients) antibodies.

An electroencephalogram (EEG) is useful in excluding nonconvulsive status epilepticus. Encephalopathic patients usually have generalized slowing. Occasionally, this is more pronounced over a mass lesion or stroke.

All cancer patients who are encephalopathic should undergo neuroimaging. Computed tomography (CT) or preferably magnetic resonance imaging (MRI) is useful in excluding brain metastases, cerebral infarction or hemorrhages, abscesses, hydrocephalus, and frequently leptomeningeal metastases. They can also occasionally be helpful in diagnosing herpes encephalitis or paraneoplastic limbic encephalitis. Both of these conditions may be associated with abnormal T2 signal in the temporal lobes.

A lumbar puncture should be performed if central nervous system infection or leptomeningeal metastases are suspected. In both conditions, there may be cerebrospinal fluid pleocytosis, elevated protein, and occasionally hypoglycorrhea. The availability of herpes simplex and varicella-zoster virus polymerase chain reaction tests has enabled these causes to be excluded more rapidly. Patients who are suspected of paraneoplastic encephalomyelitis should also have a lumbar puncture, as their cerebrospinal fluid (CSF) often shows a mild lymphocytic pleocytosis, elevated protein, and the presence of oligoclonal bands. Specific autoantibodies may also be present in the cerebrospinal fluid.

Specific Causes of Encephalopathy in Cancer Patients

Direct Involvement of the Nervous System by Cancer

Brain Metastases

Brain metastases are present in approximately one third of patients with cancer. They can cause encephalopathy directly by infiltrating the brain (especially when there are multiple lesions) or bleeding or indirectly by producing seizures, SIADH, or cerebral infarction by occluding a venous sinus.

Leptomeningeal Metastases

Leptomeningeal metastases may produce encephalopathy in a minority of patients with cancer either by infiltration of the underlying cerebral cortex or by causing seizures, SIADH, hydrocephalus, or cerebral infarction.

Indirect Involvement of the Nervous System

Cerebral Infarction and Hemorrhage

Cerebral infarction can occur in patients who are hypercoagulable from either an underlying neoplasm or its therapy. These patients may develop cerebral infarction as a result of thrombosis of arteries and veins, emboli from nonbacterial thrombotic endocarditis, or disseminated intravascular coagulation and, rarely, thrombotic thrombocytopenic purpura. Cerebral hemorrhage may occur as a result of thrombocytopenia or bleeding into vascular brain metastases such as occurs with melanoma and choriocarcinoma.

Complications of Therapy

Certain antineoplastic agents are associated with an increased risk of encephalopathy. Chemotherapeutic agents such as ifosfamide or high-dose cytosine arabinoside or immunotherapeutic agents such as interferon-α and interleukin-2 are frequently associated with acute encephalopathies. Intrathecal or high-dose methotrexate, especially when administered after cranial irradiation, may result in a delayed leukoencephalopathy. Certain drugs are associated with vasculopathies. For example, asparaginase may lead to venous sinus thrombosis.

Paraneoplastic Syndromes

Cancer patients may present with an encephalopathy as a result of paraneoplastic limbic encephalitis. The pathogenesis is uncertain but probably results from an autoimmune response directed against tumor antigens but cross-reacting with neuronal antigens, resulting in inflammation of the temporal lobes. The best-characterized paraneoplastic syndrome causing encephalopathy is paraneoplastic encephalomyelitis. This is usually associated with the presence of the anti-Hu antibody in patients with small-cell lung cancer. In addition to the limbic encephalitis, these patients often have evidence of a more widespread encephalomyelitis and sensory neuronopathy. Encephalopathy has also been associated with the anti-CV2 (CRMP-3 and CRMP-5) antibodies (in small-cell lung cancer), the anti-Ma antibody (in a variety of cancers), and the anti-Ta antibody (in testicular cancer).

Opportunistic Infections

Most central nervous system infections can cause encephalopathy. Viral encephalitis is especially likely to produce encephalopathy, but severe meningitis and brain abscesses may also do so, especially if there are multiple lesions or significant mass effect.

TREATMENT

Management of Patients with Encephalopathy

The optimal management of patients with encephalopathy requires treatment of the underlying cause. Since several factors frequently contribute to the encephalopathy, it is important that all potential etiologic factors be corrected. Any medications that could contribute to the encephalopathy should be discontinued if they are not absolutely necessary. The patient's metabolic status should be optimized. Oxygen should be given if there is evidence of even mild hypoxia. Any intercurrent infections should be treated. Patients should empirically be given thiamine and multivitamins, as mild Wernicke's encephalopathy is often misdiagnosed. Even if the cause is recognized early and treated, the encephalopathy frequently takes time to resolve. In general, elderly patients with preexisting cognitive and neurologic deficits take longer to recover than younger patients with no prior neurologic problems. Patients are often agitated and difficult to manage. They should be placed in a bright, controlled environment with minimal distractions. The presence of a family member or a sitter may be helpful. Occasionally, patients will require sedation with medications such as lorazepam and haloperidol. Newer neuroleptics such as olanzepine, risperidone, and seroquel produce fewer extrapyramidal side effects and are increasingly being used in place of haloperidol. Soft physical restraints and posey vests may sometimes be necessary but should be used only as a last resort to ensure patient safety.

Table 7-4 ■ Clinical Features of Neuropathy

Type of Nerve Involved	Abnormalities
Motor	Wasting, weakness, unsteadiness, areflexia, fasiculation, cramps, deformities, e.g., pes cavus, hypotonia
Sensory	Sensory loss, clumsiness, ataxia, "tingling," "pins and needles," areflexia, hypotonia, "burning," allodynia or hyperpathia—perception of nonpainful stimuli as painful
Autonomic	Postural hypotension, impotence, hyperhidrosis, gustatory sweating, bowel or bladder dysfunction, anhidrosis
Trophic	Charcot joints, foot ulceration

Peripheral Neuropathy

Nerve injury has a limited repertoire of clinical expression (Table 7-4). The clinical features depend on which nerves are affected and whether sensory, motor, or autonomic fibers are involved. Involvement of the peripheral nerves usually results in numbness, burning, parasthesias, and weakness. The distribution of the numbness and weakness depends on the nerves affected. Patients with peripheral neuropathies usually experience symmetric distal sensory loss and weakness, while patients with mononeuropathy multiplex will have asymmetric numbness and weakness in the distribution of specific peripheral nerves. Involvement of autonomic nerves may result in bladder and bowel dysfunction, impotence, and postural hypotension.

Causes

The most common causes of neuropathies in the general population are diabetes, alcohol, and peripheral nerve entrapment. These and other etiologies are listed in Table 7-5.

A small minority of patients who present with neuropathies will have a previously undetected cancer as the underlying cause. Approximately 5% of patients with peripheral neuropathies have monoclonal gammopathies. Although most of these patients have monoclonal gammopathy of unknown significance, approximately 10% will have a neoplastic cause such as multiple myeloma or Waldenstrom's macroglobulinemia. Other neoplastic causes of neuropathies are extremely rare and account for fewer than 1% to 2% of all causes. Cancer should be considered especially in patients with rapidly progressive or severe neuropathies without an obvious etiology. A neoplastic cause should also be considered in patients with sensory neuronopathies, mononeuropathy multiplex, and painful, progressive plexopathies.

Table 7-5 ■ Causes of Neuropathies

Nonmalignant Causes

Diabetes
Peripheral nerve entrapment
Alcohol
Nutritional deficiency (e.g., B_{12} and thiamine)
Infections (leprosy, Lyme disease, HIV, syphilis)
Paraproteinemia
Guillain-Barré syndrome and chronic inflammatory
    demyelinating polyneuropathy
Hereditary disorders (e.g., Charcot-Marie-Tooth)
Metabolic disorders (e.g., uremia)
Connective tissue diseases
Toxins
Sarcoidosis
Vasculitis
Hypothyroidism
Amyloidosis

Causes Specific to Cancer Patients

Chemotherapy (e.g., vinca alkaloids, taxanes, cisplatin,
    thalidomide, suramin)
Radiation therapy injury
Paraneoplastic disorders (Guillain-Barré syndrome, brachial
    neuritis, vasculitis, sensory neuronopathy)
Paraproteinemia
Tumor infiltration of nerves

Patients with a known diagnosis of cancer may have additional causes of neuropathies. Approximately 20% of cancer patients have mild axonal neuropathies. The etiology is often unclear, but it may be partly nutritional, as many of these patients are cachectic. Compression neuropathies, especially peroneal palsies, are also fairly common for the same reason. Many chemotherapeutic agents are neurotoxic and result in neuropathies. Drugs that commonly produce neuropathies include the vinca alkaloids, taxanes, cisplatin, oxaliplatin, thalidomide, and suramin. Most of these are axonal neuropathies, although cisplatin affects predominantly the dorsal root ganglion and leads to profound sensory loss to all modalities. Peripheral nerves are relatively resistant to radiation therapy, but brachial or lumbosacral plexopathies may occasionally result from irradiation. Neuropathies associated with paraproteinemia may be caused by multiple myeloma and Waldenstrom's macroglobulinemia. Other paraneoplastic neuropathies are relatively uncommon. Guillain-Barré syndrome and brachial plexopathies have been described in patients with Hodgkin's lymphoma, while patients with the anti-Hu antibody frequently have a sensory neuronopathy (which closely resembles a peripheral neuropathy) or less commonly an autonomic neuropathy. A paraneoplastic vasculitic neuropathy has also been described. Direct infiltration of nerves is uncommon but may rarely occur in patients with lymphomas and carcinomas, producing a mononeuropathy multiplex.

Differential Diagnosis

Neuropathies must be distinguished from diseases of the central nervous system (especially the spinal cord), muscle disorders (myopathies), disorders of nerve roots (polyradiculopathies), and disorders of the neuromuscular junction. This can often be accomplished by performing a careful neurologic examination. Spinal cord disorders are associated with weakness in a pyramidal distribution, hyperreflexia, extensor plantar responses, and a sensory level. Myopathies are usually associated with proximal muscle weakness and normal sensation and reflexes. Neuromuscular junction disorders may be associated with fatigability, normal sensation, and normal reflexes (myasthenia gravis) or with variable weakness, normal sensation, and areflexia (Lambert-Eaton myasthenic syndrome). It is also important to localize the site of the neuropathy as accurately as possible, that is, to differentiate a peripheral neuropathy from a disorder of dorsal root ganglion (neuronopathy), brachial or lumbosacral plexus (plexopathy), or involvement of multiple peripheral nerves (mononeuropathy multiplex). Peripheral neuropathies will have symmetric distal loss of sensation and strength affecting the lower extremities more that the upper extremities and diminished or absent reflexes, neuronopathies may have intact reflexes, and plexopathies will have unilateral or asymmetric weakness and sensory loss in the distribution of the affected plexus. Mononeuropathies have asymmetric weakness and numbness in the distribution of specific peripheral nerves such as the ulnar or peroneal nerves. This differentiation can sometimes be difficult clinically, and electrodiagnostic testing may be necessary (Figure 7-1).

Clinical Evaluation of Patients

A careful history and physical examination and selective use of laboratory tests, including electrodiagnostic studies, will often allow the site of the neuropathy to be localized and the underlying etiology to be determined in the majority of patients. However, in approximately 20% of patients, the precise diagnosis may not be determined despite extensive evaluation.

Some considerations in the evaluation include the fiber type involved (i.e., motor, sensory, or autonomic), the location of the neuropathy (peripheral neuropathy, mononeuropathy multiplex, or plexopathy), how quickly the neuropathy has developed, whether it is predominantly axonal (e.g., vincristine neuropathy) or demyelination (e.g., monoclonal gammopathies), the presence of associated systemic conditions (e.g., diabetes), and whether there is a family history (e.g., hereditary sensorimotor neuropathies). In cancer patients, additional questions that may be useful include whether the tumor could be infiltrating adjacent nerves (e.g., brachial plexopathy in patients with breast cancer), whether the cancer can indirectly affect the nerve (e.g., paraneoplastic neuropathies), and what drugs the patient has been exposed to (e.g., vinca alkaloids, cisplatin, taxanes).

Laboratory Evaluation of Patients

Table 7-6 summarizes the laboratory evaluation of patients with neuropathies. The extent of evaluation will vary considerably among patients. Frequently, the cause of the neuropathy is clear from the history and examination (e.g., neuropathy following treatment with paclitaxel). However, even in these patients, other conditions may be contributing to the development of the neuropathy, and it is often useful to exclude these with blood tests (e.g., glucose, creatinine, B_{12}, TSH serum protein electrophoresis). Electrophysiologic examination (nerve conduction study and electromyography) has a limited role in some patients. These tests are helpful in confirming the presence of a neuropathy and differentiating it from related disorders. It helps to localize entrapment neuropathies and determine whether the neuropathy is primarily axonal or demyelinative. These tests can also provide objective data concerning the severity and chronicity of the neuropathy. A nerve biopsy is necessary only on rare occasions in patients with progressive neuropathies to exclude specific conditions such as tumor infiltration or vasculitis.

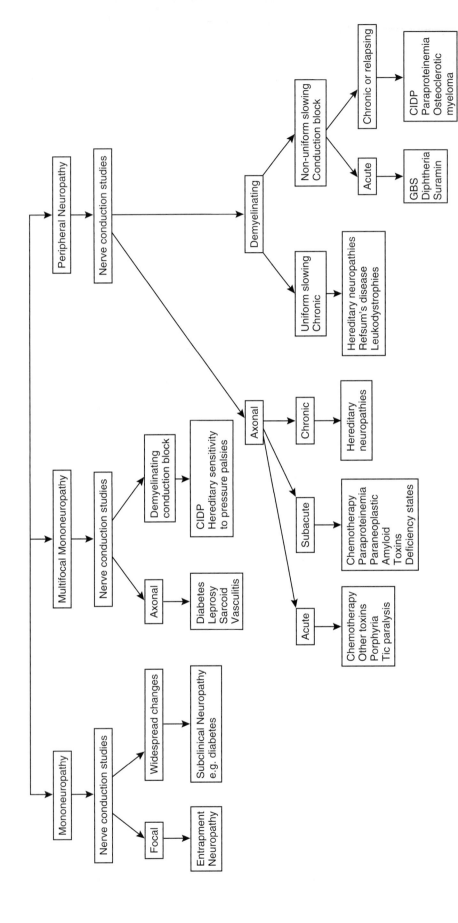

Figure 7-1 ■ Approach to the evaluation of a patient with peripheral neuropathy.

Considerations in the Evaluation of Neuropathies

What fiber types are involved?
(Motor, sensory, or autonomic)

What is the localization of the neuropathy?
(Peripheral neuropathy, mononeuritis multiplex, radiculopathy, or plexopathy)

How quickly is the neuropathy progressing?
(Acute neuropathies may be caused by Guillain-Barré syndrome, toxic neuropathy secondary to chemotherapy, vasculitis, and critical illness. Most other causes have a slower course.)

Is it a predominantly axonal or demyelinating neuropathy?
(Vincristine generally causes an axonal neuropathy, while most paraproteinemias cause a demyelinating neuropathy.)

What underlying systemic disorder is there?
(Diabetes, hypothyroidism, uremia, HIV, B_{12} deficiency, heavy alcohol use)

Is there a family history of neuropathy?
(Hereditary motor and sensory neuropathy [Charcot-Marie-Tooth disease], hereditary predisposition to pressure palsies)

Can the cancer directly infiltrate the nerve?
(For example, breast cancer invading the brachial plexus, intravascular lymphoma infiltrating peripheral nerves)

Can the cancer indirectly affect the nerve?
(Paraproteinemias, paraneoplastic neuropathies, and neuronopathies)

What neurotoxic agents has the patient been exposed to?
(Chemotherapeutic agents such as vinca alkaloids, taxanes, and cisplatin)

Table 7-6 ■ Diagnostic Tests for Patients with Neuropathies

Blood Tests

Screening Tests for Most Patients
Glucose, creatinine, B_{12}, TSH, serum protein electrophoresis

Screening Test for Some Patients
Lyme titer, RPR, ANA, cryoglobulins, anti-GM1 antibody, anti-MAG antibody, genetic tests for hereditary sensitivity to pressure palsy and hereditary sensorimotor neuropathies (Charcot-Marie-Tooth disease), anti-Hu antibody in patients with sensory neuronopathy (small-cell lung cancer)

Urine Tests

24-hour urine for porphyrins and Bence Jones protein

Lumbar Puncture

Paraneoplastic syndromes may have CSF pleocytosis and oligoclonal bands; CIDP may show elevated CSF protein; CSF cytology may be helpful in excluding leptomeningeal metastases, which can sometimes resemble polyneuropathies.

Electromyography and Nerve Conduction Studies

Confirms neuropathy, excludes other conditions, diagnoses entrapment neuropathies, differentiates axonal from demyelinating neuropathies, and provides objective data concerning severity.

Nerve Biopsy

Cancer-Related Causes	*Benign Causes*
Tumor infiltration	Sarcoidosis
Vasculitis	Vasculitis
Monoclonal gammopathy	Amyloidosis
Amyloidosis	Hereditary sensitivity to pressure palsy
	Metachromatic leukodystrophy
	Charcot-Marie-Tooth disease types 1 and 3
	Refsum disease
	Chronic inflammatory demyelinating polyradiculopathy (CIDP)
	Leprosy

Punch Skin Biopsy

Minimally invasive test that may be helpful in sensory neuropathies.

Management of Patients with Neuropathies

Despite optimal therapy, most neuropathies tend to improve slowly or not at all. As a result, an important aspect of the management of patients with neuropathies is to treat the symptoms. Regardless of the underlying etiology, many patients with neuropathies will experience paresthesia and pain. Topical capsaicin cream, which depletes the neurotransmitter substance P from the pain fibers, may be helpful in patients with mild symptoms. When the symptoms are more troublesome, tricyclic antidepressants such as amitriptyline and anticonvulsants such as gabapentin, carbamazepine, phenytoin, lamotrigine, and topiramate may be useful. Other medications that may occasionally be helpful include clonazepam, clonidine, and mexiletine. Non-steroidal anti-inflammatory medications, tramadol, and occasionally opiates may decrease the severity of pain in some patients. Corticosteroids may help with radiculopathies, compression neuropathies such as carpal tunnel syndrome, and plexopathies. Patients with weakness or sensory ataxia may benefit from physical and occupational therapy. Splints are useful in some patients with compression neuropathies.

Specific Causes of Neuropathy in Cancer Patients

Idiopathic Neuropathies

Cancer patients have a high incidence of neuropathies. Although these are often caused by chemotherapeutic agents or other identifiable causes, a large number of patients have mild axonal neuropathies of unclear etiology. It is likely that these neuropathies are caused by a combination of factors, including nutritional deficiencies, metabolic changes, and medications, although a paraneoplastic syndrome cannot be excluded.

Compression Neuropathies

Because cancer patients frequently experience profound weight loss and may be bed bound for prolonged periods, compression neuropathies such as peroneal palsies are common.

Chemotherapy

The most common cause of neuropathy in cancer patients is chemotherapy. Drugs that commonly produce neuropathies include the vinca alkaloids, taxanes, cisplatin, oxaliplatin, thalidomide, and suramin. Most of these drugs produce predominantly axonal neuropathies, although there can be both demyelinating and axonal features in severely affected patients. Cisplatin affects predominantly the dorsal root ganglion and leads to profound sensory loss to all modalities.

Radiation Therapy

Peripheral nerves are relatively radioresistant. Rarely, delayed radiation injury to the brachial or lumbosacral plexus may occur.

Paraneoplastic Syndromes

Monoclonal gammopathies associated with conditions such as multiple myeloma and Waldenstrom's macroglobulinemia may cause neuropathies. Hodgkin's disease has been associated with brachial neuritis and Guillain-Barré syndrome. Subacute sensory neuronopathies or autonomic neuropathies can occur in patients with the anti-Hu antibody (usually in patients with small-cell lung cancer). Very rarely, a paraneoplastic vasculitis can lead to mononeuropathy multiplex.

Tumor Infiltration of Nerves

Breast, lung, and head and neck cancers may infiltrate the brachial plexus, while tumors in the abdomen and pelvis may infiltrate the lumbosacral plexus. With both types of plexopathy, there is usually pain, weakness, and numbness in the extremities. Very rarely, tumor cells may actually infiltrate peripheral nerves.

Management of Patients with Neuropathies

The optimal management of neuropathies depends on treating the underlying cause. After careful clinical evaluation and laboratory testing, a diagnosis can usually be made in most patients. Frequently, several conditions may be contributing to the neuropathy.

Suggested Reading

Antoine JC: Paraneoplastic sensory neuropathy, demyelinating features, and response to immunotherapy. Muscle Nerve 1998;21:1811–1813.

Blaes F, Strittmatter M, Merkelbach S, et al: Intravenous immunoglobulins in the therapy of paraneoplastic neurological disorders. J Neurol 1999;246:299–303.

Bosch EP, Mitsumoto H: Disorders of peripheral nerves. In Bradley WG, Daroff R, Fenichel G, and Marsden CD (eds): Neurology in Clinical Practice, 3rd ed. Boston: Butterworth-Heineman, 2000, pp 2045–2130.

Breimberg HR, Amato AA: Neuromuscular complications of cancer neurologic clinics.

Clouston PD, DeAngelis LM: The spectrum of neurologic disease in patients with systemic cancer. Ann Neurol 1992; 31:268–273.

Corbo M, Balmaceda C: Peripheral neuropathy in cancer patients. Cancer Invest 2001;19:369–382.

Evoli A, Lo Monaco M, Marra R, et al: Multiple paraneoplastic diseases associated with thymoma. Neuromuscul Disord 1999;9:601–603.

Koehler PJ, Buscher M, Rozeman CA, et al: Peroneal nerve neuropathy in cancer patients: A paraneoplastic syndrome? J Neurol 1997;244:328–332.

Mendez Ashla MF: Delirium In Bradley WG, Daroff R, Fenichel G, and Marsden CD (eds): Neurology in Clinical Practice, 3rd ed. Boston: Butterworth-Heineman, 2000, pp 25–36.

Posner JB: Neurologic Complications of Cancer. Philadelphia: FA Davis, 1995.

Rubin DI, Kimmel DW, Cascino TL: Outcome of peroneal neuropathies in patients with systemic malignant disease. Cancer 1998;83:1602–1606.

Schiff D, Wen PY(eds): Cancer Neurology. Totowa, NJ: Humana Press 2002.

Strub RL, Black FW: Organic Brain Syndromes: An Introduction to Neurobehavioral Disorders. Philadelphia: FA Davis, 1981.

Stubgen JP: Neuromuscular disorders in systemic malignancy. Curr Opin Neurol 1997;10:371–375.

Thambisetty MR, Scherzer CR, Yu Z, et al: Paraneoplastic optic neuropathy and cerebellar ataxia with small cell carcinoma of the lung. J Neuroophthalmol 2001;21:164–167.

Tuma R, DeAngelis LM: Altered mental status in patients with cancer. Arch Neurol 57:1727–1731, 2000.

Chapter 8
Neck Mass

David S. Caradonna and Arthur M. Lauretano

Introduction

Patients presenting with a neck mass represent a diagnostic challenge owing to the multiple potential causes. The practitioner, whether generalist or specialist, must consider a wide array of differential diagnoses, which may be influenced by the patient's age group, risk factors, and concomitant medical conditions. Differential diagnoses may include congenital, inflammatory, infectious, and neoplastic causes. The etiology of the neck mass may best be defined by age groups. In patients younger than age 40 years, a neck mass most likely represents a benign disorder, most commonly an inflammatory process such as bacterial or viral lymphadenitis. The second most common cause in this age group is congenital or developmental lesions, followed finally by the neoplastic lesions. In contrast, in patients over age 40 years, neoplasms should be the primary consideration; inflammatory masses represent the second most common etiology, congenital masses being a distant third consideration in this older age group. In fact, some sources note a higher proportion of malignancy with increasing age, further supporting the importance of age in assessing a patient with a new neck mass.

Risk factors for neoplastic neck disease include a history of irradiation in childhood, a history of tobacco use, and a history of alcohol abuse. On the other hand, maternal hydramnios may be a risk factor for cystic hygroma. The location of the mass may be helpful in establishing both a diagnosis and a prognosis in that congenital/developmental masses usually occur in consistent locations, while inflammatory and metastatic disease generally follow an orderly pattern of lymphatic spread. In many respects, the clinician's ultimate goal is to separate the benign from the malignant and to ascertain whether surgical or nonsurgical therapy will be most appropriate.

Differential Diagnosis of the Neck Mass

Neck masses can be categorized as follows: benign primary neoplasms of the neck, congenital neck masses, inflammatory neck masses, malignant primary neoplasms of the neck, and metastatic neoplasms to the neck.

Benign primary neoplasms of the neck arise from normal structures found in the neck, which undergo neoplastic degeneration. These changes can range from neural crest tissue to adipose tissue (Table 8-1). Congenital neck masses are typically seen in the pediatric population and are usually identified prior to the age of 40 (Table 8-2). Inflammatory neck masses are certainly the most common and have a wide variety of sources (Table 8-3). Primary malignant neoplasms of the neck (Table 8-4) are far less common than is metastatic neck disease. The most common form of metastatic neck disease is squamous cell carcinoma.

Clinical Evaluation
History

Evaluation of the neck mass must begin with a careful and thorough history. The age of the patient should immediately allow the clinician to assess the relative likelihood of the entities within the differential

Table 8-1 ■ Benign Primary Neoplasms of the Neck

Paraganglioma	Neurofibroma
Carotid paraganglioma	Traumatic neuroma
Vagal paraganglioma	Lipoma
Schwannoma	

diagnosis: inflammatory > congenital > neoplastic for patients younger than 40; neoplastic > inflammatory > congenital for patients over 40. The physician should inquire about constitutional symptoms, including fever, night sweats, malaise, and weight loss. Symptoms of upper respiratory infection or tonsillitis/pharyngitis may indicate a viral or bacterial etiology for the neck mass such as a reactive lymphadenitis or possibly a secondary infection of a thyroglossal duct cyst, cystic hygroma, or branchial cleft cyst. Exposure to an infectious agent may also indicate a cause. For example, a history of exposure to a patient with streptococcal tonsillitis, viral upper respiratory infection, or tuberculosis may influence the physician's assessment of the mass. The presence of other head and neck pathology may also indicate the etiology of the neck mass. For example, infections of the ear, scalp, eyes/orbits, nose/sinuses, salivary glands, or tonsils/pharynx may lead to reactive lymphadenitis, and malignant neoplasms of these same regions may result in metastases to cervical nodes. The clinician should also assess for any recent trauma or exertion, as hematoma and laryngoceles may be associated with such precipitants. One should also carefully assess the patient's past medical history, medications, allergies, and social and family history. A careful review of systems should be performed, and information regarding weight loss, fever, malaise, and other constitutional symptoms should be obtained. Information such as the presence of dysphagia, odynophagia, otalgia, voice changes, stridor, nasal/sinus symptoms, and clots may indicate otolaryngologic pathology. In addition, the physician should inquire about smoking and alcohol use, foreign travel, and occupational and sexual history, as these

Table 8-2 ■ Congenital Neck Masses

Cystic hygroma	Thyroglossal duct cyst
Hemangioma	Thymic masses
Teratoma	Dermoid cyst
Muscular anomalies	Laryngocele
Branchial anomalies	

Table 8-3 ■ Inflammatory Neck Masses

Bacterial/viral cervical lymphadenitis
Neck space infections
Infectious mononucleosis
Myobacterial lymphadenitis
Cat scratch disease
Fungal/parasitic/spirochetal lymphadenitis
Sarcoidosis
Amyloidosis
HIV/AIDS

factors greatly influence the differential diagnosis (Figure 8-1).

Concomitant medical conditions may indicate the cause of the neck mass. For example, a history of lymphoma, AIDS, prior or current cancer (particularly a primary head and neck cancer), tuberculosis, sarcoidosis, or other systemic infection/inflammatory processes may provide a ready explanation for the new mass. Prior irradiation (especially low-dose) may be a risk factor for parotid carcinoma and parotid pleomorphic adenoma.

The duration of the mass and the rapidity of its growth may also be very helpful in evaluating its etiology, especially when considered in the context of the other information provided in the patient's history. For example, a rapidly developing, tender mass following a viral prodrome or bacterial tonsillitis will likely indicate a reactive node, while a slowly enlarging, nontender mass in a smoker will raise significant concern for metastatic cancer, even if a primary carcinoma is not obvious. However, reactive nodes may persist for a long period of time before regressing, may not always regress completely, and may not always be tender. Additionally, lymph nodes containing metastatic cancer may potentially grow rapidly and become painful as a consequence of central necrosis, secondary infection, or internal hemorrhage. Some metastatic nodes may even fluctuate in size, a characteristic that is more often associated with benign

Table 8-4 ■ Primary Malignant Neoplasms of the Neck

Salivary gland (parotid and submandibular)
Lymphoma
Thyroid/parathyroid gland
Cutaneous malignancy
Angiosarcoma
Hemangiopericytoma

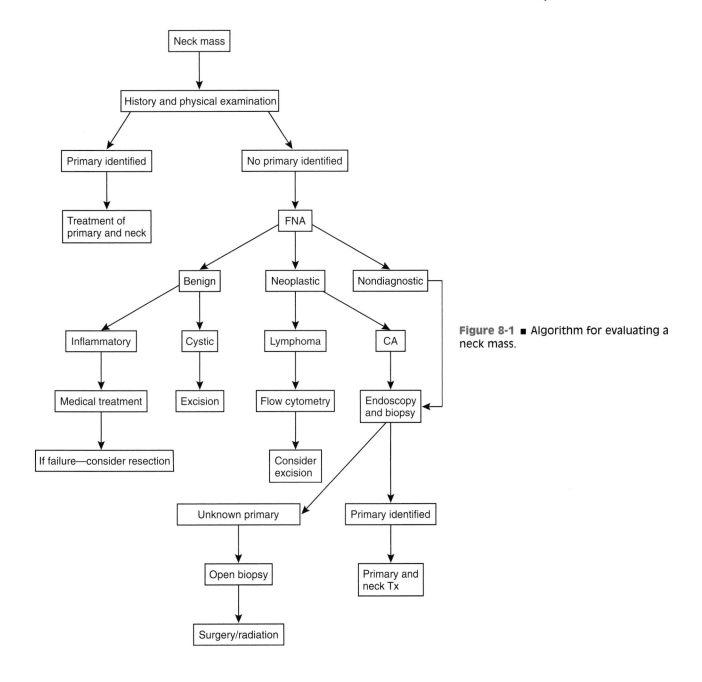

Figure 8-1 ■ Algorithm for evaluating a neck mass.

reactive adenopathy; however, such malignant nodes will generally grow over time. Consequently, any neck mass that has been present for one month, especially if it is increasing in size, should be carefully and thoroughly evaluated; in fact, one may wait even less time in a patient with significant risk factors for a malignant disease.

Physical Examination

A thorough and complete head and neck examination is mandatory for any patient presenting with a neck mass (Figure 8-2). The examiner must not overlook the skin, including the entire scalp. The skin should be assessed via both inspection and palpation for surface lesions. The ears, nose, nasopharynx, oral cavity, oral pharynx, larynx, and hypopharynx must also be examined. This examination should include bimanual palpation of the oral cavity and oral pharynx. The nasopharynx and larynx/hypopharynx may be visualized with the mirror or flexible endoscope; however, the examiner must be confident that complete visualization of all the structures of the upper aerodigestive tract (from nasal tip to cricopharyngeus and upper trachea) has been achieved. Radiologic evaluation is not a substitute for a

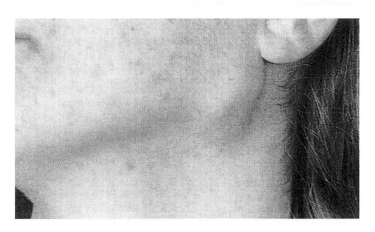

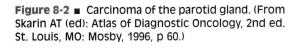

Figure 8-2 ■ Carcinoma of the parotid gland. (From Skarin AT (ed): Atlas of Diagnostic Oncology, 2nd ed. St. Louis, MO: Mosby, 1996, p 60.)

thorough physical examination of this region, particularly in uncovering small, superficial mucosal lesions. Although the paranasal sinuses cannot be directly visualized, inspection of the drainage areas within the nose and palpation of the sinuses themselves may yield important information about these structures. The examiner should evaluate for specific otolaryngologic signs such as trismus, stridor, neck stiffness, epiphora, loose teeth, cranial nerve deficit, or fetid breath; the presence of serous otitis media may indicate a nasopharyngeal primary as a potential source of the neck mass.

In assessing the neck mass itself, the clinician must first visually inspect the mass. The overlying skin should be inspected for color, ulceration, fistulous tracts, or cutaneous neoplasm. The mass should then be palpated, with assessment of mobility, tenderness, pulsation, fluctuance, and consistency. The presence of warmth may indicate infection but also could be from neovascularization in a neoplasm. Fixation of the mass to adjacent structures should be assessed to determine the extent of disease and, if possible, the structures that may be encountered and potentially jeopardized if surgical treatment is necessary.

The clinician should also examine the entire neck. Although most otolaryngologic pathology involving the neck lies anterior to the trapezius muscle, the true posterior neck should be fully evaluated as well. The examiner may choose to stand behind, beside, or in front of the patient to perform the neck examination with the patient in the sitting position. Many examiners will assess the patient from all of these vantage points. One must be careful not to overlook the supraclavicular nodes and the thyroid, as well as the body and tail of the parotid glands.

The clinician assessing the neck mass should be willing to broaden the scope of examination as indicated by the head and neck findings. One should auscultate the mass for bruits, particularly for a pulsatile mass. If a bruit is noted, it should be distinguished, if possible, from a carotid bruit or a transmitted cardiac murmur. The clinician should auscultate and percuss the chest if pulmonary disease is suspected and examine for axillary or inguinal adenopathy.

In patients presenting with supraclavicular adenopathy, one should think of infraclavicular pathology, including breast cancer, lung cancer, or intra-abdominal disease. The clinician should assess the patient for cachexia, fever, toxic appearance, or localized or diffuse stigmata of either trauma or inflammatory infectious or metastatic disease. Evidence of additional organ involvement should also be sought. For example, splenomegaly and hepatomegaly (infectious mononucleosis, portal hypertension); digital clubbing; and abnormal pulmonary findings such as wheezing, barrel chest, or distant lung sounds (chronic obstructive pulmonary disease) may be helpful not only in identifying the neck mass etiology, but also in determining how the patient will fare with proposed additional testing and ultimate treatment.

Diagnostic Tests

Although the history and physical examination remain the most essential parts of assessing the patient with a neck mass, various diagnostic tests may be helpful in further narrowing or confirming the diagnosis, delineating the extent of the neck mass, and assisting in the development of a treatment plan.

Radiographic Assessment

Computed tomography and magnetic resonance imaging scans can be helpful in defining the location and extent of the neck mass, its consistency (solid, cystic, or mixed), and its relationship to adjacent structures. Vascularity may be assessed via computed tomography or magnetic resonance imaging, and in some cases, magnetic resonance angiography may be employed. Computed tomography and magnetic resonance imaging/angiography should be performed with contrast. These studies may also be helpful in the evaluation of an ill-defined mass or the patient with a large neck. Ultrasound provides a rapid means to assess for cystic versus solid lesions and, consequently, has been particularly valuable for evaluation of thyroid lesions. Ultrasound is also valuable in the pediatric population or in pregnant women, for whom exposure to radiation may be undesirable.

Computed tomography and ultrasound may be used for image-guided fine needle aspiration. Plain films of the neck are of limited use but may be helpful in the neonate, in emergency evaluations, and in cases of trauma. Plain films of the chest or computed tomography scans of the chest may be essential in patients with suspected tuberculosis sarcoid or lung or distant neoplasm. Angiography may be necessary to further define a vascular mass or to enable preoperative embolization.

Laboratory Tests

Skin tests may be considered if mycobacterial disease is in the differential diagnosis. Thyroid function testing should be performed if there is suspicion of thyroid pathology; however, most patients with thyroid neoplasms are euthyroid. A complete blood count may be helpful, but the absence of an elevated white blood cell count does not rule out an infectious etiology for the neck mass. Liver function tests may be useful in patients who are suspected of having infectious mononucleosis or distant metastatic carcinoma. A sedimentation rate is nonspecific but may be elevated in infection, neoplasm, or granulomatous disease. Sjögren's antibodies (SS-A, SS-B) may be helpful in the evaluation of a neck mass that proves to be salivary gland enlargement. Cultures of the pharynx or sinuses may be helpful in identifying suspected infectious causes for the neck mass. Viral titers (acute and convalescent) and heterophile testing may detect evidence for Epstein-Barr virus, cytomegalovirus, and mumps infection.

Fine Needle Aspiration

Careful history and physical examination combined with appropriate testing will produce a diagnosis for the neck mass in 90% of patients. However, it may be necessary to obtain tissue to either confirm the diagnosis or identify an as yet undiagnosed cause. The standard initial means of obtaining tissue is via fine needle aspiration. This technique may easily be performed in the office setting. Excisional or incisional biopsies should be avoided. If the clinician feels that the mass is difficult to access, the fine needle aspiration may be performed under computed tomography or ultrasound guidance. Fine needle aspiration can be used to differentiate solid from cystic masses and benign from malignant lesions. Material may be obtained for cytology as well as the microbiology studies. For cystic masses, an attempt should be made to biopsy the wall of the cyst as well as aspirating the cyst contents. For some benign cysts, fine needle aspiration may actually be therapeutic.

Fine needle aspiration is typically indicated for the persistent mass when no obvious primary neoplasm has been identified or to confirm that the neck mass represents a metastasis from a previously identified primary tumor. Although fine needle aspiration can verify the solid or cystic nature of a neck mass, the presence of a cyst does not rule out malignancy. Similarly, the documentation of an infection does not rule out underlying neoplasm. Fine needle aspiration has both false-negative and false-positive rates in the 5% to 10% range. If the fine needle aspiration is nondiagnostic, it should be repeated. If it is still nondiagnostic, consideration should be given to an open biopsy. Of note, an open or excisional biopsy is frequently necessary to differentiate lymphoma from reactive adenopathy and to provide substantial tissue for phenotypic analysis of the lymphoma. By contrast, fine needle aspiration is very accurate in detecting squamous cell carcinoma.

Open Biopsy

If the fine needle aspiration is nondiagnostic or lymphoma is suspected clinically (and particularly after the fine needle aspiration yields lymphocytes), open biopsy may be necessary. Open biopsy should also be considered if the fine needle aspiration is repeatedly benign despite clinical disease progression. Open biopsy generally should be excisional. Exceptions include extremely large masses, particularly in situations in which the ultimate treatment would not involve full surgical excision of the lesion (e.g., lymphoma, tuberculosis). Excisional biopsies of neck masses, including resection of presumed benign lesions such as branchial cleft cysts, should include a frozen section. If the frozen section analysis shows squamous cell carcinoma (Figure 8-3), then it is generally recommended that the appropriate neck dissection be performed. Alternatively, some have proposed that excision of the node alone followed by radiation therapy may be equally effective (see Chapter 98).

Panendoscopy

Panendoscopy is a useful component of the evaluation for patients whose neck mass proves to be squamous cell carcinoma. The endoscopic assessment of the larynx, pharynx, esophagus, and bronchial tree

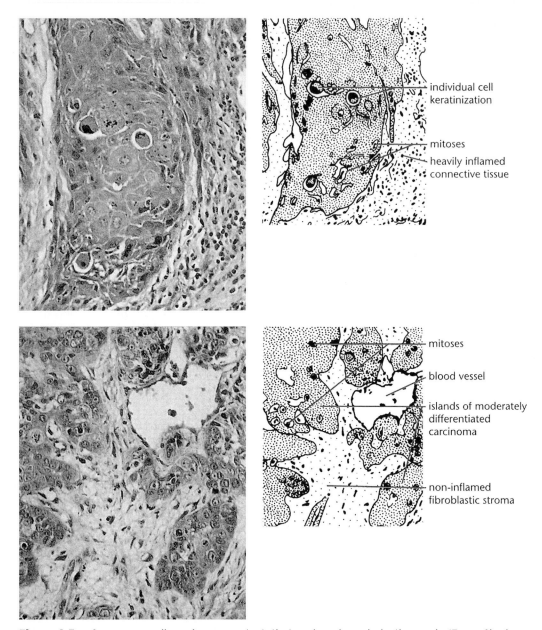

Figure 8-3 ▪ Squamous cell carcinoma metastatic to a lymph node in the neck. (From Skarin AT [ed]: Atlas of Diagnostic Oncology, 2nd ed. St. Louis, MO: Mosby, 1996, p 32.)

can identify a primary lesion (if previously unknown), assess the extent of the primary disease, and identify synchronous second primary cancers. It is important to note that even when a patient with a clearly defined primary squamous cell carcinoma identified within the upper aerodigestive tract presents with a neck mass, a panendoscopy still is appropriate to assess the extent of the disease and to rule out second primaries. One may perform the definitive biopsies of the primary site at the time of the endoscopy if an office biopsy was not possible. In such cases, fine needle aspiration of the neck mass should still be performed to confirm metastatic disease. In patients without a defined primary site, panendoscopy should include directed biopsies of likely primary sites, including tonsils, base of the tongue, hypopharynxpyriform sinuses, and nasopharynx. Many now advocate ipsilateral or bilateral tonsillectomy as part of the evaluation of such a patient. The course of treatment in such patients will likely be determined by both the panendoscopy results and the pathologic evaluation of the neck mass.

Suggested Reading

Jacobs C: The internist in the management of head and neck cancer. Ann Intern Med 1990;113:771–778.

McGuirt WF: The neck mass. Med Clin North Am 1999; 83(1):219–234.

Chapter 9
Hoarseness

Elie E. Rebeiz and Stanley Shapshay

Introduction

Hoarseness is a term that is commonly used to describe changes in the voice quality. It is a symptom of disease processes involving phonation, the production of speech. The specific causes of hoarseness are many and are best determined after obtaining a detailed medical history of the circumstances preceding the onset of hoarseness and performing a thorough physical examination.

The most common causes of hoarseness are benign processes; however, neoplastic growths can lead to hoarseness and should be considered carefully in certain situations. Table 9-1 lists the common causes of hoarseness. In the absence of an upper respiratory tract infection, any patient with hoarseness persisting for more than two weeks requires a complete evaluation. In particular, when the patient has a history of tobacco use, cancer of the head and neck must be considered. A number of different cancers can cause hoarseness by a variety of different mechanisms. Laryngeal cancer frequently presents with hoarseness due to a direct extension of the tumor to the vocal folds. Base of tongue and hypopharynx cancers can cause hoarseness by interfering with the airflow. Thyroid and other neck neoplasms, as well as lung cancer, can also lead to hoarseness, either by direct extension into the larynx or by involvement of the recurrent laryngeal nerves causing vocal fold paralysis.

Definition and Etiology of Hoarseness

Hoarseness and dysphonia are defined as an abnormal voice quality. There are three phases in speech production. The initial pulmonary phase entails air inhalation and lung inflation, followed by expulsion of air from the pulmonary tree into the trachea. As this column of air reaches the vocal folds, they vibrate at a frequency characterized by their proximity and tension; this is the laryngeal phase. The forced air then enters the pharynx. Hoarseness is due to processes involving the true vocal folds, including swelling of the mucosa overlying the vocal folds or a tumor arising on the surface of the vocal folds (Figure 9-1). These processes cause the vocal folds to vibrate at lower frequency, thus causing speech to have a hoarse quality. The patient's complaint of hoarseness may be different than the physician's perception. It is important that the physician consider the complaint of the patient and family members when evaluating hoarseness. Voice quality may be described as breathy, strained, rough, tremorous, or weak. Often, patients present with increased vocal effort or vocal fatigue, which may be perceived as hoarseness. Possible diagnoses based on voice quality are presented in Table 9-2.

Causes of Hoarseness

Voice abuse is one of the most common causes of hoarseness and can lead to other vocal pathologies such as vocal fold nodules. Other benign causes for hoarseness include viral infections that result in edema of the vocal fold mucosa, thus altering the vibratory frequency and producing a hoarse voice. This, however, is self-limiting and temporary. Good vocal hygiene can prevent and treat some pathologic conditions, and voice therapy plays an essential role in managing some cases of hoarseness. Gastroesophageal reflux disease is also known to cause hoarseness. This can usually be successfully treated with proton pump inhibitors and diet control. Gastroesophageal reflux disease has also been implicated as a potential causative agent for laryngeal carcinoma. Causes of hoarseness are summarized by broad category in Table 9-3.

Malignant tumors are most commonly seen in adults, and primary laryngeal cancer is by far the most common malignancy. The most common primary laryngeal cancer is squamous cell carcinoma. Other types include sarcoma, lymphoma, and metastatic

Table 9-1 ■ Common Causes of Hoarseness

Functional dysphonia	Abnormal use of the vocal mechanism despite normal anatomy. Related to stress, psychological disturbance, or acquired compensatory technique.
Laryngeal papilloma	Growths on the larynx caused by human papilloma viral infection.
Muscle tension dysphonia	A voice disorder resulting from excessive or unequal tension while speaking. This condition results from improper speaking technique and is commonly associated with reflux laryngitis.
Viral laryngitis	Edema of the vocal folds, usually following a cold.
Reflux laryngitis	Inflammation of the larynx caused by gastric acid irritation.
Reinke's edema	An accumulation of fluid in the vocal folds. Associated with smoking and vocal abuse. Occurs with reflux laryngitis.
Spasmodic dysphonia	Irregular voice breaks and interruptions of phonation. This is a focal dystonia of the laryngeal muscles.
Vocal fold paralysis	Weakness or immobility of the vocal fold(s).
Vocal nodules	Fibrotic formations on the vocal folds. Commonly referred to as "nodes."
Arytenoid dyslocation	Immobility of the vocal fold

tumors. Metastatic tumors include renal cell carcinoma, breast cancer, and melanoma. Sarcomas are rare in the larynx; however, Kaposi's sarcoma can occur in patients with AIDS.

Glottic lesions are the most common laryngeal cancers and usually present early with hoarseness (see Figure 9-1). As the disease progresses, symptoms will include throat irritation, pain, hemoptysis, dysphagia resulting in weight loss, stridor and referred pain to the ear.

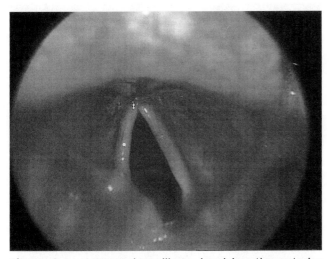

Figure 9-1 ■ Laryngeal papilloma involving the anterior commissure and both vocal folds. (See Color Plate 1.)

Other cancer-related causes of hoarseness include vocal fold paralysis. Causes of vocal fold paralysis and their relative frequencies are summarized in Table 9-4. Patients with vocal fold paralysis present with a breathy, weak voice, caused by incomplete adduction of the vocal folds. Vocal fold paralysis (Figure 9-2) is frequently due to compression of the vagus nerve or the recurrent laryngeal nerve in the neck or chest, most commonly secondary to lung or thyroid cancer. It can also be caused by injury of the recurrent laryngeal nerve during surgery (Table 9-5). In addition to hoarseness, patients will present with aspiration, most commonly with liquids but sometimes with solid food. Dysphagia can also be present. Aspiration results from incomplete closure of the true and false vocal folds as well as anesthesia of the supraglottic larynx from injury to the superior laryngeal nerve. Imaging from the base of the skull to the level of the arch of the aorta is required in the evaluation of this condition.

Evaluation of Patients with Hoarseness

The proper diagnostic workup for a patient with hoarseness begins with a thorough review of the history of the hoarseness, its duration, and any associated complaints. A comprehensive physical examination of the head and neck region is also required.

Table 9-2 ■ Diagnosis of Hoarseness Based on Voice Quality

Voice Quality	Differential Diagnosis
Breathy	Vocal fold paralysis, abductor spasmodic dysphonia, functional dysphonia
Hoarse	Vocal fold lesion, muscle tension dysphonia, reflux laryngitis
Low-pitched	Reinke's edema, vocal abuse, reflux laryngitis, vocal fold paralysis, muscle tension dysphonia
Strained	Adductor spasmodic dysphonia, muscle tension dysphonia, reflux laryngitis
Tremor	Parkinson's disease, essential tremor of the head and neck, spasmodic dysphonia, muscle tension dysphonia
Vocal fatigue	Muscle tension dysphonia, vocal fold paralysis, laryngitis, vocal abuse

Table 9-3 ■ Differential Diagnosis of Hoarseness

Neoplastic

Squamous cell cancer of the larynx
Vocal fold polyp/nodules
Vocal fold granulomas
Vocal fold cyst
Laryngeal papilloma
Lung cancer

Inflammatory

Gastroesophageal reflux laryngitis
Viral laryngitis
Bacterial laryngitis
Allergic laryngitis
Reinke's edema

Neurologic

Vocal fold paralysis (unilateral)
Spasmodic dysphonia
Movement disorder (Parkinson's disease)
Essential tremor
Cerebrovascular accident

Miscellaneous

Vocal abuse
Vocal fold atrophy
Vocal fold scarring
Hypothyroidism (myxedematous laryngitis)
Muscle tension dysphonia
Medications

In the absence of an upper respiratory tract infection, any patient with hoarseness persisting for more than two weeks requires evaluation. The history can yield important information and help to narrow the differential diagnosis. An essential part of a thorough history is elucidating the patient's voice use pattern. This process includes an evaluation of the patient's "vocal personality type" (amount and style of voice use), recent voice use (such as screaming at a baseball game), and vocal environment (where the patient uses his or her voice, such as talking while wearing earmuffs on an assembly line). A history of hearing loss in the patient or in a family member may be a contributing factor in voice abuse. This abuse is a common, often preventable, cause of dysphonia and may be underestimated by the patient, so it is impor-

tant to question the patient and family members specifically about patterns of voice misuse. In any patient with hoarseness and a history of tobacco use, head and neck cancer is the first diagnosis suspected, as hoarseness is often the only presenting symptom.

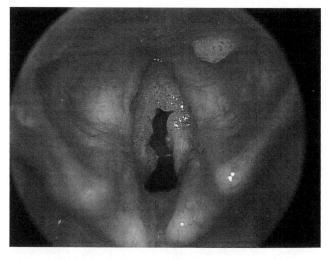

Figure 9-2 ■ Vocal fold paralysis. The folds do not meet properly during phonation. (See Color Plate 1.)

Table 9-4 ■ Etiologies of Vocal Fold Paralysis

Neoplasm: 35%	Inflammation: 12%
Surgical: 25%	Central: 7%
Idiopathic: 15%	Trauma: 6%

Table 9-5 ■ Surgical Procedures Associated with Risk of Injury to the Vagus and/or Recurrent Laryngeal Nerves

Cardiac/thoracic surgery	Neck surgery
Lung resection	Carotid artery surgery
— Ligation of patent ductus	— Neck dissection
— Valve repair	— Thyroid surgery
— Coronary artery bypass (rare)	— Anterior cervical disc surgery
— Thymectomy	— Tracheotomy (rare)
— Mediastinoscopy	Skull base surgery
— Esophagectomy	Tracheal intubation
— Tracheal surgery	

To obtain a complete history, the physician should be certain to cover several critical items in their patient interview.

Physical Examination

A thorough head and neck examination, including assessment of hearing acuity, upper airway mucosa, tongue mobility, and the function of other cranial nerves, is essential in the evaluation of dysphonia. Examination of the neck should also be performed, and the examiner should look for any scars from previous operations (carotid endarterectomy, cervical spine repair, or thyroidectomy) or any neck masses. Visualization of the larynx using indirect laryngoscopy or flexible nasolaryngoscopy is essential for the eval-

uation. The purpose of these procedures is to look for masses on the vocal folds, erythema, or edema of the mucosa and to assess vocal fold motion. It is essential to visualize the entire larynx. If clinical suspicion is high, the patient should also be examined for signs of systemic disease, such as hypothyroidism, or neurologic dysfunction, such as tremor, Parkinson's disease, or multiple sclerosis.

Ancillary Testing

If, after the examination, the definitive diagnosis is still in question or the working diagnosis prompts further evaluation, ancillary testing should be performed. If the patient describes symptoms of thyroid dysfunction, if the thyroid feels abnormal, or if there is diffuse

DIAGNOSIS

Hoarseness: The Critical Elements of the Clinical History

- Characteristics of the dysphonia. This includes both the physician's perceptions of the patient's voice (voice quality being wet or gurgly) and the patient's responses to the timing, duration, course, and description of their voice as well as a family member's assessment.
- Past medical and surgical history:
  - History of previous intubation, neck surgery, trauma, and types of medicines the patient is taking, in particular asthma inhalers.
  - History of previous head and neck carcinoma or family history of cancer.
- Tobacco use and alcohol consumption.
- Tendency for vocal abuse: Any voice abuse behavior at home and work or singing.
- History of allergies.
- Swallowing abnormalities: Weight loss, dysphagia, chronic cough, or aspiration symptoms or if there is a history of recurrent pneumonia.
- Gastroesophageal reflux disease: Dietary

history, symptoms of reflux disease, and history of treatment for these symptoms.
- Auditory acuity: History of hearing problems, previous audiometric evaluations if suspicious.
- Shortness of breath/stridor: History of difficulty breathing, stridor, and any history of asthma or emphysema.
- Emotional status of the patient: Evaluation of the patient's well-being and if there has been a large amount of stress or emotional anxiety in the recent past.
- Frequent throat clearing and coughing activities: History of excessive throat clearing or coughing, any postnasal drip or recent upper respiratory infection, and any throat clearing or coughing during the interview.
- Past history of voice difficulty: Any history of prior episodes of voice dysfunction and treatment rendered.

edema of the vocal fold mucosa, then it is appropriate to order a serum thyroid-stimulating hormone level. For patients with a suspected neoplastic process, lung imaging and liver function tests are ordered to screen for possible distant spread. Various other procedures may also be indicated and are described in the following sections.

Videostroboscopy

Videostroboscopy was popularized with the recent development of fiber-optic cables, powerful light sources, and video recording devices, which allow for better visualization of the larynx. It can be performed in the physician's office, without sedation, by simple local anesthesia of the nasal cavity. The devices are easy to use, and the visual data are easy to interpret. It has recently become an important addition to the practice of laryngology.

The concept of videostroboscopy is based on the fact that vocal fold vibration involves high-speed, minute vibrations; thus a subtle change in the mucosa or tension of the vocal fold that results in hoarseness may be observed and will be viewed in slow motion. Videostroboscopy is especially important in the evaluation of subtle lesions affecting the vibration of the cords and in submucosal pathology. The technique allows for the discovery of small lesions such as a vocal fold scar, hemorrhage, or cyst and can determine whether a malignant lesion is superficial or invasive.

Videostroboscopy provides still photos of the mucosa in rapid succession at various stages of phonation and has the ability to record and play back the video images synchronized with audio recordings of the patient's speech. This is therefore an invaluable tool for measuring patient response to treatment and to assess, in some instances, early cancer recurrence.

Videostroboscopy gives the clinician valuable data regarding glottic closure and gap; precise evaluation of vocal fold motion, supraglottic function, and vibratory portions of the fold; recorded information about laryngeal function during phonation, functional measures of the creation of the "mucosal wave." Stiffness of the mucosa is readily noted, and masses that are not easily diagnosed by routine physical examination may be easily seen and distinguished from invasive processes.

Imaging

Imaging is particularly important in the evaluation of laryngeal cancer and vocal fold paralysis. Plain films of the chest often yield valuable information and should be ordered as part of the workup of hoarseness of uncertain origin to screen for pulmonary masses. Computerized tomography (CT) scanning is better at identifying lung masses or evaluating the cause of a paralyzed vocal fold. Patients with laryngeal lesions that are likely to be cancerous should also have a computed tomography scan of both the neck and chest to evaluate for metastases and synchronous lung primaries. Neck computed tomography scans also help in determining the extent of laryngeal tumors. Lateral neck films should be reserved for patients who have a tenuous airway from an infectious process.

Computed tomography scanning of the neck is an important diagnostic tool in evaluating laryngeal pathology of unknown origin. When there is associated pain or the cause of the hoarseness is not ascertained from physical examination or videostroboscopy, it is appropriate to obtain a neck computed tomography scan. It is important for the computed tomography scan to cover the entire course of the recurrent laryngeal nerve, that is, from skull base to mediastinum. The scan should also be performed with contrast to better visualize a tumor. Neck computed tomography scans are also important in cases of idiopathic arytenoid dysfunction for the same reasons. Fine cuts (1 mm) through the larynx are helpful in distinguishing subtle abnormalities. The computed tomography scan should be reviewed by both the otolaryngologist, who has a better idea of the anatomy of the neck, and the radiologist, who can identify occult and incidental disease processes in areas that are unfamiliar to the otolaryngologist (such as the cervical vertebrae and the lungs). A head magnetic resonance imaging scan is also helpful in some instances. These include situations in which concomitant central nervous system pathology, such as a stroke, increased intracranial pressure, or brain infarct, is suspected. In addition, when multiple cranial neuropathies are associated with the hoarseness, a head magnetic resonance imaging may better identify tumors at the skull base and brain stem.

For patients with arytenoid dysfunction or vocal fold paralysis and suspected aspiration, a modified barium swallow study will identify the severity of aspiration. This may allow the speech therapist to identify aspiration and teach the patient basic compensatory measures to avoid it. For the patient with suspected reflux or the patient who complains of associated dysphagia, a barium swallow can identify gastroesophageal reflux disease and other pathology (dynamic and static) that may be indirectly affecting vocal fold function.

Electromyography/Electroglottography

Although not readily available in most medical care centers, electromyography or electroglottography may provide useful information in evaluating and treating the patient with hoarseness. Electroglottography determines when the vocal folds are open or closed and how rapidly they are closing. It is performed by placing recording electrodes over the thyroid cartilage. A low-current signal is conducted through the tissues to the recording electrodes. There is greater current flow when the folds are closed than when they are open. This study is limited, however, by the requirement for good contact of the vocal folds in order for the signal to be transmitted.

A neurologist usually performs electromyography, often with the assistance of an otolaryngologist. The test is performed by placing needle electrodes into the intrinsic laryngeal musculature and measuring the electric activity. The test is useful for further evaluating patients with vocal fold paralysis, especially within one year of the paralysis. The possibility of the vocal fold function returning can be evaluated by reviewing the electric potentials emitted. This technique can readily establish whether the cord has been permanently denervated (i.e., is iatrogenic) and allows for appropriate surgical planning in rehabilitating the paralyzed cord. Electromyography is also used to distinguish cricoarytenoid dislocation or fixation from vocal fold paralysis and to distinguish recurrent laryngeal nerve paralysis from complete vocal fold paralysis.

Diagnostic Rigid Endoscopy

With the current technology, the need for rigid endoscopy under general anesthesia has been greatly diminished. However, direct laryngoscopy, esophagoscopy, and bronchoscopy still have diagnostic value if the office flexible endoscopic exam is nondiagnostic and/or the suspicion of cancer is great.

The most frequent use for rigid endoscopy under general anesthesia in the evaluation of the hoarse patient is to enable biopsy of a suspicious lesion. Rigid endoscopy is performed in all patients with laryngeal cancer, if possible, to ascertain the extent of the tumor and to evaluate for synchronous primary lesions. It should also be performed in all patients with hoarseness in whom a diagnosis cannot be established by other methods. It is also reasonable to perform rigid endoscopy in any patient who has persistent or recurrent vocal symptoms or persistent pain in the head and neck region. If no diagnosis is found, it is wise to continue to follow the patient monthly, with repeated examinations, radiographs, and endoscopies until the cause of the patient's symptoms is determined.

Direct Laryngoscopy for Biopsy and Resection

Direct laryngoscopy under general anesthesia is the best way to evaluate a laryngeal mass and to rule out malignancy. If a patient has history of head and neck malignancy, a thorough endoscopic examination includes visualization of the larynx, hypopharynx, esophagus, and tracheobronchial tree.

Under direct visualization, a laser can be used to biopsy and excise early tumors of the true vocal folds. The lesions that are most suitable for transoral laser excisional biopsy are hyperkeratoses, dysplasia, carcinoma in situ, and early invasive squamous cell carcinoma (T1 tumors).

Endoscopic excision of T1 laryngeal carcinoma offers a 90% cure rate, which is comparable to the rate for radiotherapy. In addition, endoscopic excision offers a one-session treatment, in contrast to the many treatment sessions required with radiotherapy. In addition, endoscopic excision is associated with less morbidity, can be repeated in cases of failure, and permits examination of the pathology margins. In our practice, radiation therapy is reserved for treatment failures, recurrences, or second primary tumors, which frequently can occur in patients with head and neck cancers.

Endoscopic excision also offers some benefits when used for diagnosis and staging of laryngeal cancer. This technique helps to determine the degree of invasion of the vocal ligament and muscle. This has generated the concept of biologic staging. Endoscopic evaluation can upgrade the tumor from a T1 vocal fold carcinoma to a somewhat more aggressive T3 lesion. This greately affects the treatment plan, prognosis, and ultimate voice quality. If the tumor is found to invade the thyroid cartilage, the tumor can then be upstaged to a stage T4. Because computed tomography scanning does not accurately determine invasion of thyroid cartilage, particularly at the anterior commissure, endoscopic diagnosis is especially valuable.

Management

Hoarseness

An integral aspect of the management of hoarseness is the maintenance of good vocal hygiene. Patients should be advised to avoid straining their voices by shouting, whispering, or attempting to talk over excessive background noise. The importance of hydration should be emphasized. Certain medications, such as antihistamines and drugs that dry the mucosa through anticholinergic side effects (such as tricyclic antidepressants), may also create unfavorable voice changes, and these drugs should be avoided if possible. Irritants such as tobacco, alcohol, marijuana, and industrial chemicals should be avoided.

Voice therapy may be helpful in some situations. It is a behavior-based process in which maladaptive vocal habits and techniques are replaced with appropriate uses of the vocal mechanism. The treatment

TREATMENT

Criteria for Performing Endoscopic Laser Excision of a Laryngeal Lesion

Several criteria that need to be considered before performing endoscopic laser excision of a laryngeal lesion include the following: The lesion should be minimally invasive, should be localized to the midportion of the true vocal fold, and should not extend to the anterior commissure, the vocal process of the arytenoid cartilage, or the supraglottic or subglottic larynx. Minor involvement up to 1 to 2 mm along the floor of the ventricle may be managed endoscopically. Vocal fold mobility should be normal, which indicates superficial character of the lesion. A lesion involving the anterior commissure should not be excised, because the distance between the tumor and the thyroid perichondrium is small, and it is difficult to obtain good surgical margins. If the tumor extends into the anterior commissure region, recurrence is likely with any endoscopic technique.

Endoscopic management of laryngeal neoplasia presupposes adequate laryngoscopic exposure with a wide-bore laryngoscope. In approximately 10% to 15% of patients, in our experience, the larynx is difficult to expose because of a narrow dental arch, large tongue, previous neck surgery, or radiotherapy-induced tissue contracture.

Once the laryngoscope is in place, the entire table can be moved into various positions without changing the exposure. The advantage of using the laser is noncontact microprecision in a bloodless field. The potential disadvantage is the risk of thermal damage to the vocalis muscle.

Toluidine supravital staining is used to determine areas of dysplasia and to help, in cases of multicentricity, to guide to areas to be biopsied. It reduces the incidence of false-negative biopsies.

When areas of carcinoma in situ are identified, a deeper excision exposing the vocalis muscle is required, and a 2- to 3-mm margin around the tumor is obtained. This is important for proper assessement of the depth of invasion and for complete excision. If the lesion is found to violate the vocal ligament, then the diagnosis is changed to invasive carcinoma. Excision should be done in an even plane, respecting the vocal ligament. The specimen is oriented carefully for the pathologist for the evaluation of margins. A full-thickness specimen should be obtained, because the pathologist needs to determine any invasion of the basal epithelial membrane. A shallow specimen often results in a biopsy report in which invasion cannot be determined. The use of the CO_2 laser for endoscopic excision can be extended to a T1 invasive squamous cell carcinoma. Although these lesions can be successfully treated with radiotherapy, laser excision offers many benefits. A small exophytic lesion, limited to the midfold, not reaching the anterior commissure or the vocal process of the arytenoid, can be totally excised intraorally.

---

process incorporates auditory, visual, and proprioceptive feedback channels to produce a healthy and efficient voice. Voice therapy is typically administered 6 to 14 times (in 30- to 40-minute sessions) over a six- to eight-week period. Following therapy, examination of the larynx and documentation of improvement are done routinely.

Vocal Fold Paralysis

To correct the vocal fold paralysis, medialization of the vocal folds can be achieved by performing a thyroplasty technique. First described by Isshiki, this procedure involves displacing and stabilizing a rectangular, cartilaginous window at the level of the vocal fold, pushing the soft tissue medially. This is performed under local anesthesia to allow the patient to phonate during the procedure. The degree of medialization can be determined intraoperatively by the quality of the patient's voice. This procedure is typically performed in an outpatient setting and is reversible.

Other means for correcting the gap resulting from vocal fold paralysis is intracordal injection of autolo- gous fat or Gelfoam paste. This is a relatively safe outpatient procedure, with quick satisfactory results. Both procedures reestablish a satisfactory voice and, if done properly, prevent aspiration of liquid and food particles.

It is important to also involve a speech pathologist in the management of patients with complicated laryngeal symptoms including hoarseness. Speech pathologists are invaluable in teaching the patient compensatory mechanisms for speech, and swallowing function can be improved in many patients with aspiration, preventing pulmonary complications and allowing for oral feeding.

Suggested Reading

Mendenhall WM, Parsons JT, Stringer SP, Cassisi NJ: Management of Tis, T1, and T2 squamous cell carcinoma of the glottic larynx. Am J Otolaryngol 1994;15:250–257.

Miller RH, Duplechain JK: Hoarseness and vocal fold paralysis. In Bailey B (ed): Head and Neck Surgery: Otolaryngology, 3rd ed. Philadelphia: Lippincott-Raven, 2001.

Rebeiz EE, Shapshay SM: Benign lesions of the larynx. In Bailey B (ed): Head and Neck Surgery: Otolaryngology, 3rd ed. Philadelphia: Lippincott-Raven, 2001.

Ridley MB, Kelly JH, March BR, Roa RA: Office diagnostic techniques, the adult patient. In Fried MP (ed): The Larynx: A Multidisciplinary Approach, 2nd ed. St. Louis, MO: Mosby, 1996.

Shapshay SM, Rebeiz EE: Laser management of laryngeal cancer. In Silver C. (ed): Laryngeal Cancer. New York: Thieme Medical Publishers, 1991.

Chapter 10
Palpable Breast Masses

Barbara L. Smith

The discovery of a palpable breast mass can be a cause of great concern to a woman and her physician. Although the majority of breast masses will prove to be benign, many breast cancers present as a palpable mass. The strategy for evaluation of a palpable mass incorporates physical examination, imaging, and histologic features to distinguish between benign and malignant masses.

A variety of palpable abnormalities may be found in the breast, including discrete palpable masses and areas of vague thickening or nodularity. Palpable masses fall into several categories, which are listed in Table 10-1.

Evaluation of a Palpable Mass

History

In evaluating a patient with a palpable mass, a thorough history should include documentation of risk factors for breast cancer, including hormonal and reproductive risk factors, family history of breast and ovarian cancer, and any malignant or atypical histology on prior breast biopsies. The patient should be asked about prior cysts, palpable abnormalities, or pain that is suggestive of baseline fibrocystic disease.

The history of the presenting mass includes determining how long the mass has been present, whether it has changed in size since first noted, and, for premenopausal women, whether there is any variation in size or tenderness with the menstrual cycle.

Physical Examination

Physical examination of the breasts includes inspection of the skin, palpation of the breasts, examination of the nipples for discharge, and palpation of the axillary and supraclavicular lymph node areas. If an abnormal area is identified, its size, contour, texture, tenderness, and position are evaluated. The overlying skin is examined for dimpling or erythema, and mobility on the underlying chest wall is determined.

Palpable abnormalities may be discrete masses, distinct from surrounding normal tissue, or more vaguely defined areas of asymmetric nodularity or lumpiness. Diffuse, bilateral, symmetric nodularity is almost always benign, resulting from the variable texture of normal breast tissue. Tenderness of a breast abnormality suggests a benign cause, although some malignant lesions may also be tender.

The risk of malignancy is greater for a palpable mass arising in a woman who is older, has multiple risk factors for breast cancer, or presents with other suspicious physical findings such as palpable axillary nodes, fixation of the mass to skin or chest wall, skin dimpling, nipple discharge or erosion, or bloody nipple discharge. It is important to remember, however, that the majority of breast malignancies have no physical findings other than the palpable lesion. Most palpable breast cancers are mobile and do not present with enlarged axillary nodes.

Imaging Studies

It is critical to remember that as many as 10% to 15% of palpable breast cancers will not be visualized on mammography. Some of these cancers will also be

Table 10-1 ▪ Palpable Breast Masses

Discrete palpable masses

Cysts
Simple cysts
Complex cysts
Abscesses
Cystic malignancies

Solid masses

Fibroadenomas, lactating adenomas
Fibrocystic change, fibrosis
Lipomas
Fat necrosis
Sebaceous cysts
Duct ectasia/periductal mastitis
Phylloides tumors
Primary breast cancers
Tumors metastatic to the breast
Lymphoma

Vague thickening or nodularity

Fibrocystic change, fibrosis
Primary breast cancers
Fat necrosis
Duct ectasia/periductal mastitis
Primary breast cancer

DIAGNOSIS

Malpractice Litigation

Failure to diagnose breast cancer is one of the most frequent causes of malpractice litigation. Litigation is most likely when a patient reports a palpable mass but the examining clinician fails to fully evaluate and biopsy the lesion. Such delays in diagnosis may be avoided by careful workup of palpable masses and appropriate and timely tissue diagnosis.

mogram and/or ultrasound examination does not eliminate the need for biopsy of a palpable solid mass.

Management of Specific Palpable Masses

Discrete Palpable Masses

Discrete masses, that is, those that are clearly distinguishable from surrounding normal breast tissue, may be either solid or cystic. It is important to recognize that physical examination alone is not accurate in distinguishing a cyst from a solid mass.

Cysts

A palpable mass that is suspected to be a cyst should be confirmed as such by aspiration or by ultrasound (see Figure 10-1). If there is any concern that the palpable lesion does not correlate in size or location with the lesion visualized by ultrasound, the lesion should

missed by ultrasound examination. As a result, the role of mammography in evaluation of a palpable mass is to obtain additional information about the mass and to look for synchronous lesions in the ipsilateral and contralateral breast. A normal mam-

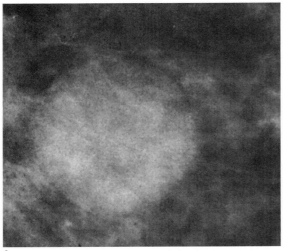
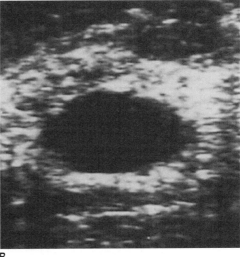

A   B

Figure 10-1 ▪ Comparison of mammogram and sonogram of a simple cyst. *A,* The mammogram shows a well-circumscribed mass with well-defined borders. *B,* The sonogram shows an absence of internal echoes, well-circumscribed margins, round contours, and a bright posterior wall. (From Grainger RG, Allison D [eds]: Diagnostic Radiology: A Textbook of Medical Imaging, 3rd edition. London: Churchill Livingstone, 1997, p 2005.)

be aspirated to confirm that it is cystic. For very large cysts, removal of the mass by aspiration also permits a more thorough examination of the surrounding breast tissue. A cyst that is complex on ultrasound examination requires aspiration to be sure that there is no solid component. Any solid component that remains should be biopsied. Bloody cyst fluid or a mass that persists after aspiration is worrisome for malignancy, and the aspirated fluid should be sent for cytologic analysis. Biopsy is generally indicated in this setting even if the cytologic analysis is negative for malignancy. If cyst fluid is not bloody and no mass remains after aspiration, there is little chance of malignancy, and the fluid need not be sent for cytology.

If a cyst is aspirated without prior ultrasound documentation that it was a simple cyst, the patient should be reexamined in four to eight weeks. Fewer than 10% of simple cysts will recur after aspiration. When the same cyst recurs rapidly after aspiration, it should be reaspirated, and the cyst contents should be sent for cytologic analysis. A biopsy should be performed if the cytology is suspicious or if the cyst recurs again. Appearance of a new cyst in a different area of breast tissue, however, does not require this additional workup and should be evaluated and aspirated as a new problem. Additional cysts may be expected over time in more than half of patients.

Solid Masses

Discrete masses within the breast that are solid, either by ultrasound criteria or by failing to yield fluid on appropriately guided aspiration attempts, require a tissue diagnosis to exclude malignancy (see Figure 10-2). Physical examination alone is inaccurate in identifying a mass as benign or malignant. Prior to biopsy, it is appropriate to order a mammogram in a woman over 35 years of age to look for synchronous lesions (see Figure 10-3). As was mentioned earlier, as many as 10% to 15% of palpable breast cancers will not be visualized on mammography. Therefore, negative imaging studies do not eliminate the need for obtaining a tissue diagnosis of a discrete solid mass.

Options for biopsy of palpable lesions include fine needle aspiration biopsy, core needle biopsy, and open surgical biopsy.

Vague Thickening or Nodularity

Normal breast texture is often heterogeneous, particularly in premenopausal women. These variations in texture may create areas that feel firmer to palpation than surrounding tissue and might or might not be tender. Such vague areas are of particular concern, as it may be difficult to rule out a malignancy such as lobular carcinoma, which produces only a vague mass.

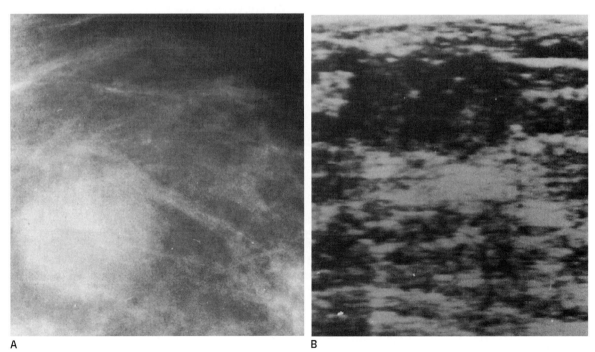

A   B

Figure 10-2 ■ Comparison of mammogram and sonogram of a fibroadenoma. *A*, The mammogram shows a well-circumscribed mass with well-defined borders. *B*, The sonogram shows a mass with internal echoes. (From: Grainger RG, Allison D [eds]: Diagnostic Radiology: A Textbook of Medical Imaging, 3rd edition. London: Churchill Livingstone, 1997, p 2004.)

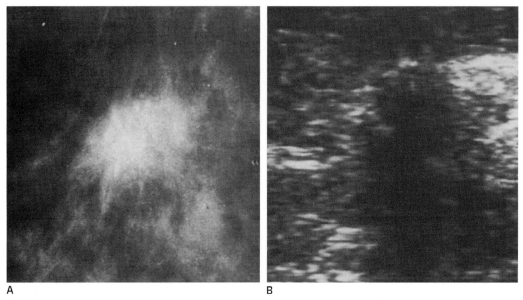

A   B

Figure 10-3 ■ Comparison of mammogram and sonogram of an infiltrating ductal carcinoma. *A,* The mammogram shows an irregular, speculated mass. *B,* The sonogram shows irregular borders and decreased internal echoes. (From Grainger RG, Allison D [eds]: Diagnostic Radiology: A Textbook of Medical Imaging, 3rd edition. London: Churchill Livingstone, 1997, p 2006.)

In evaluating a nodular area, it should first be compared with the corresponding area of the opposite breast for symmetry. Symmetric areas of thickening are rarely pathologic. Asymmetric areas, particularly those that are tender, often represent fibrocystic disease and often resolve spontaneously. To avoid unnecessary biopsies, vague areas of thickening in premenopausal women should be reexamined after one or two menstrual cycles. If the asymmetry resolves, the finding was most likely due to a benign process, and the patient may return to routine follow-up. Areas of asymmetry that persist, however, must be viewed with some suspicion. Such patients should be referred to a surgeon for evaluation and potential biopsy. It is appropriate to order a mammogram at this point to rule out synchronous lesions in a woman over age 35 who has not had a mammogram within the past six months.

Areas of vague asymmetry are of greater concern in postmenopausal women, as benign fibrocystic disease is less likely to be present and the risk of malignancy is higher. Postmenopausal women who are on hormone replacement therapy may be expected to have some cyclic changes in breast texture but are also at increased risk for development of breast cancer. Postmenopausal women with asymmetric nodularity should be evaluated with mammography and ultrasound, and biopsy should be considered.

Fine needle aspiration biopsy is generally not appropriate for areas of vague thickening, as tumors that produce only vague masses often have intermingled normal tissue, and sampling error can be high. Open surgical biopsy is generally required for adequate sampling to rule out malignancy.

Palpable Abnormalities in Pregnant or Lactating Women

Physical diagnosis of breast malignancy may be extremely difficult in the setting of pregnancy or lactation. While engorgement or diffuse thickening of the breasts may be expected during pregnancy and lactation, distinct masses, asymmetric tissue, or any area of persistent concern to the patient should be evaluated promptly, without waiting for delivery or the elective cessation of lactation. Such patients should be referred promptly to a surgeon for evaluation and possible biopsy.

The causes of breast masses during pregnancy include all the common breast lesions of premenopausal women, including fibroadenomas, fibrocystic change, fibrosis, and occasionally breast carcinoma. Lactating adenomas are benign lesions that grossly resemble fibroadenomas that may appear during pregnancy or lactation.

Mammography is generally not performed during pregnancy, as much because of the density of breast tissue and resulting low mammographic sensitivity as because of concern about radiation to the fetus. Mammographic sensitivity is also poor during lactation and for three or four months following cessation of breast feeding. Ultrasound may be useful in distinguishing cystic from solid palpable lesions and for evaluating contour and internal texture.

Biopsy can be performed safely during pregnancy and lactation, and diagnostic biopsy should not be postponed until the completion of pregnancy or lactation. Core needle biopsy or fine needle aspiration biopsy guided by palpation or core needle biopsy with ultrasound guidance is the preferred method for diagnosis. Open biopsy is reserved for atypical or nondiagnostic findings. Open biopsy during lactation may result in a milk fistula that requires weaning to heal. Despite this possibility, open biopsy should not be delayed if needle biopsy approaches do not provide a definitive diagnosis of a palpable mass.

Biopsy Options for Palpable Masses

Fine Needle Aspiration Biopsy

Fine needle aspiration using a 23- to 25-gauge needle may be performed with minimal patient discomfort at the time that a palpable mass is identified on physical examination. In interpreting results, it is important to recognize that the false-negative rate of fine needle biopsy is high. A diagnosis of normal or fibrocystic breast tissue raises the possibility that the lesion was not sampled, and open or core biopsy should be performed. Cytology diagnostic of a specific benign lesion such as a fibroadenoma or lactating adenoma may generally be relied on if it is in keeping with the clinical features of the lesion, and no further workup is required. It has been suggested that no further workup is required when "triple negative" criteria have been achieved, that is, a benign-feeling physical examination, benign mammogram, and benign fine needle aspiration result.

False-positive cytology readings on fine needle aspiration biopsies are rare, generally no more than 1% to 2%. As a result, a diagnosis of malignancy on a fine needle aspiration biopsy is reliable enough to proceed with lumpectomy and axillary staging but is generally not considered sufficient to proceed with mastectomy. Histologic confirmation of malignancy with core biopsy or open biopsy should be obtained before a breast is removed.

Core Needle Biopsy

A core needle biopsy removes an 11- or 14-gauge cylinder of tissue from the targeted lesion. The tissue that is obtained is analyzed by conventional pathology, and hormone receptor and other marker studies are readily performed.

Core needle biopsy may be performed by using mammographic or ultrasound guidance or without image guidance in the office setting using palpation to identify the target lesion. Palpation-guided core biopsy is most appropriate for larger lesions, when it is unlikely that the lesion will be missed. For small, mobile lesions, there can be a significant rate of false-negative results due to the technical difficulty of accurately placing and firing the core biopsy needle by palpation alone. Small lesions are best approached by core needle biopsy with image guidance.

Core needle biopsy has largely replaced incisional biopsy for making specific histologic diagnosis and obtaining hormone receptors and other markers for locally advanced breast cancers. Core biopsy also allows clip placement to identify the original location of the tumor to guide lumpectomy for the increasing percentage of patients with a clinical complete response to neoadjuvant chemotherapy. Core biopsy is ideal for large lesions or chest wall recurrences, in which the larger sample permits more detailed pathology and easy determination of hormone receptor assays than does fine needle aspiration biopsy.

Interpretation of Results

Core Biopsy

Atypical hyperplasia on a core biopsy reading is an indication for open biopsy, as there is a high frequency of ductal carcinoma in situ found when additional tissue is obtained. A finding of a cellular fibroadenoma on core biopsy requires open biopsy, as the lesion may actually be a phylloides tumor. The finding of extracellular mucin on core biopsy raises the possibility of an adjacent mucin-producing malignancy, and additional tissue should be obtained by open biopsy. Any core needle biopsy, especially a non-image-guided core biopsy, that yields benign or fibrocystic tissue should be viewed with some suspicion owing to the risk of technical or sampling error. Open biopsy should be considered if there is any discordance between such a benign reading and the clinical or mammographic features of the sampled lesion.

Open Biopsy

The decreased cost, time, and patient discomfort of core needle biopsy have led to increasingly selective use of the open surgical biopsy approach. Open biopsy is now generally reserved for patients whose lesions are not visualized on imaging studies, for areas of vague thickening, for atypical or nondiagnostic core needle biopsy results, or when the patient has a strong preference for complete excision of the lesion. Many breast surgeons prefer that the most suspicious lesions be approached by core biopsy rather than open biopsy. Lesions that are found to be malignant may then be excised widely on the first trip to the operating room, which gives a better cosmetic result than a diagnostic biopsy and a re-excision.

The vast majority of open breast biopsies are now performed under local anesthesia or local anesthesia with intravenous sedation. General anesthesia is reserved for the patient who requires excision of multiple lesions, for which the amount of local anesthetic required would exceed the maximum safe dose.

Suggested Reading

Cady B, Steele GD, Morrow M, Gardner B, Smith BL, Lee NC, Lawson HW, Winchester DP: Evaluation of common breast problems: Guidance for primary care Physicians. CA Cancer J Clin 1998;48:49–60.

Ciatto S, Cariaggi P, Bulgaresi P: The value of routine cytologic examination of breast cyst fluids. Acta Cytol 1987;31:301–304.

Smith BL, Souba WW: Breast procedures. In ACS Surgery: Principles and Practice. New York: WebMD, 2002.

Chapter 11
The Abnormal Mammogram

Barbara L. Smith

The widespread use of screening mammography has led to the identification of breast cancers at progressively smaller sizes and earlier stages. Mammography has the potential to identify a breast cancer years before it becomes a palpable mass. Identification of smaller tumors is associated with higher survival rates, increased rates of breast-conserving surgery as an alternative to mastectomy, and decreased likelihood that chemotherapy will be required.

On the other hand, the false-positive rate of screening mammography is significant. To avoid missing early, potentially curable cancers, the threshold for recommending biopsy is low, and in most series, only 10% to 30% of lesions for which biopsy is recommended will be malignant. Algorithms for managing an abnormal mammogram should recognize that the majority of lesions that are identified will be benign and strive to identify abnormalities that may be safely observed rather than biopsied. When biopsy is required, approaches should minimize the discomfort, anxiety, time, and cost of the process.

Mammographers have developed a series of criteria by which they grade their degree of suspicion that a given mammographic finding represents a malignancy. The American College of Radiology has developed the BI-RADS (Breast Imaging Reporting Data System) system for categorizing abnormalities identified on mammography and to guide clinicians in managing an abnormal mammogram (Table 11-1). Examples of mammograms reflecting various lesions are presented in Figure 11-1. In general, additional diagnostic imaging studies or biopsy procedures recommended by the mammographer should be performed.

Additional Diagnostic Imaging Studies

Abnormalities that are identified on an initial screening mammogram may be further characterized with additional imaging studies, including compression or magnification views, ultrasound, and magnetic resonance imaging (MRI).

Compression and Magnification Views

Additional mammographic views may be performed to investigate abnormalities found on standard views. Compression views may spread out superimposed normal tissues, and areas of vague density may resolve (Figure 11-2). Compression may also highlight a suspicious mass that was initially obscured by surrounding normal tissue. Magnification views can provide additional information about calcifications that increase or decrease suspicion of malignancy.

Ultrasound

Ultrasound is useful in determining whether a lesion identified by physical examination or mammography is cystic or solid (Figure 11-3) and to better define its size, contour, and internal texture (Figure 11-4).

MRI and Other Imaging Modalities

Magnetic resonance imaging is a promising addition to breast imaging options. With gadolinium contrast, many malignant lesions enhance relative to normal breast parenchyma. Although some benign lesions such as fibroadenomas also enhance with gadolinium, malignant lesions appear to enhance more rapidly and often to a greater extent (Figure 11-5).

The sensitivity and specificity of magnetic resonance imaging in distinguishing benign from malignant lesions is still being defined. Magnetic resonance imaging is proving useful in assessing the extent of vaguely defined tumors, in identifying unsuspected multifocal disease, and in helping to identify patients who are not eligible for breast-conserving surgery. It also appears that magnetic resonance imaging can distinguish locally recurrent tumor from surgical scarring and radiation change after lumpectomy and radiation, although it does not provide reliable readings until 18

Table 11-1 ■ The BI-RADS Classification

BI-RADS 0: Need additional imaging evaluation
BI-RADS 1: Negative
BI-RADS 2: Benign finding
BI-RADS 3: Probably benign, short interval follow-up
BI-RADS 4: Suspicious abnormality, biopsy should be considered
BI-RADS 5: Highly suggestive of malignancy

Source: From American College of Radiology. Breast Imaging Reporting and Data System (BI-RADS™). Reston, VA: American College of Radiology; 1995.

months or more after completion of surgery or radiation therapy.

Nuclear medicine studies such as sestimibi scintimammography and positron emission tomography (PET) scanning remain primarily investigational tools. There is currently no role for thermography or xerography in the evaluation of abnormalities identified on screening mammography.

Short-Interval Follow-Up for Probably Benign Lesions

In an effort to minimize the number of benign biopsies, short-interval follow-up rather than biopsy is recommended for lesions that are judged to be "probably benign" (BI-RADS 3). Biopsy is reserved for lesions that change and become more suspicious during follow-up. Sickles (1991) reported prospective follow-up of 3184 consecutive probably benign mammographic abnormalities with a protocol obtaining repeat mammograms at six months after the initial finding, 6 to 12 months later, and then annually for two more examinations. Only 17 (0.5%) of these 3184 probably benign lesions subsequently proved to be malignant on biopsy. Other series have confirmed the low risk of malignancy and safety of short-interval follow-up for these low suspicion mammographic findings.

At the present time, the "probably benign" mammography category is used for lesions for which the risk of malignancy is thought to be in the 1% range. Although there is some variation in the schedule used for short-interval follow-up, common schedules include the Sickles schedule or mammograms every six months on the affected side for two years, with annual films on the contralateral side. Routine screening is resumed when the follow-up interval has been completed.

Patients with probably benign readings of their mammograms should be reassured that this category carries a very low risk of malignancy and that biopsy is not likely to be required.

Abnormalities for Which Biopsy Is Recommended

When an abnormality that is seen on mammography is judged to be indeterminate or suspicious for malignancy (BI-RADS 4) or highly suggestive of malignancy (BI-RADS 5), biopsy is recommended. Core needle biopsy has become the preferred approach for diagnostic biopsy for the majority of lesions seen on mammography or ultrasound. Open surgical biopsy with wire localization is increasingly reserved for diagnosis of lesions not amenable to core biopsy.

Core Needle Biopsy

Core needle is a less invasive and less costly alternative to open surgical biopsy for diagnosis of nonpalpable breast lesions identified on mammography or by ultrasound (Parker 1991, Meyer 1996). A core needle biopsy removes several 11- or 14-gauge cylinders of tissue from a lesion using ultrasound or stereo mammography views to guide the needle. Suction may be applied via vacuum-assisted core biopsy devices to draw additional tissue into the biopsy needle.

The location and features of the lesion to be biopsied, for example, its size or whether it is a mass or faint calcifications, determine the feasibility and advisability of core needle biopsy. Most lesions that can be visualized on ultrasound examination are amenable to core biopsy. Abnormalities that are visualized only on mammography require a stereotactic biopsy approach in which the lesion is positioned within the device's biopsy window, stereo mammogram views are obtained, and the biopsy needle is advanced into breast tissue. Appropriate positioning might not be possible for certain peripheral locations within the breast or for women with severe arthritis or other conditions that preclude positioning on the biopsy table. Stereotactic core biopsy might not be possible in thin women, as the standard excursion of the spring-loaded biopsy needle requires a minimum thickness of the compressed breast tissue to avoid having the needle pierce the opposite side of the breast. Lesions that are very close to the chest wall or skin might not be amenable to core biopsy if there is concern that the excursion of the needle will pierce skin or chest wall muscle. If technical considerations make core biopsy impossible, open surgical biopsy with wire localization is required.

Tissue specimens obtained by core biopsy are analyzed by conventional pathology, and hormone receptor and tumor marker assays may be readily performed.

It is important for the ordering clinician to recognize the limitations of core biopsy to be able to cor-

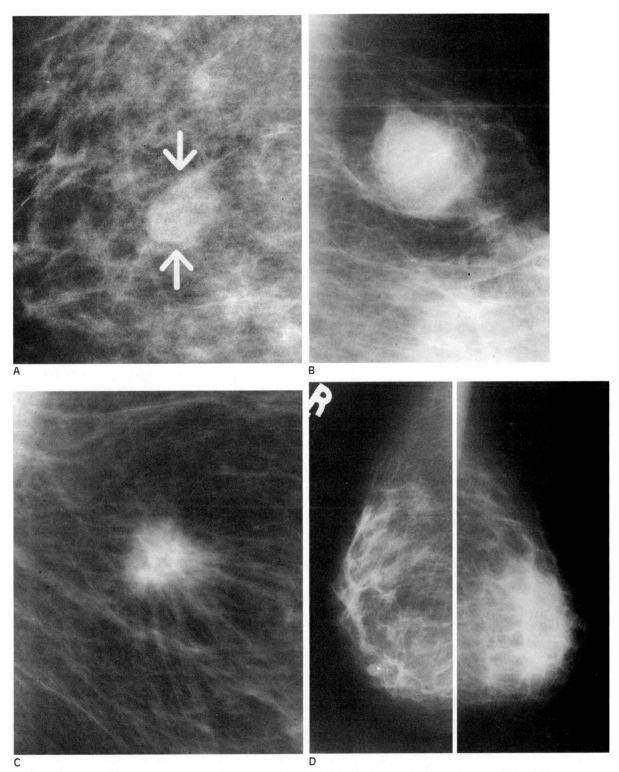

Figure 11-1 ■ Mammography of various breast lesions identified by biopsy. *A*, Fibroadenoma. *B*, Medullary carcinoma. *C*, Infiltrating ductal carcinoma. *D*, Inflammatory carcinoma.

Continued

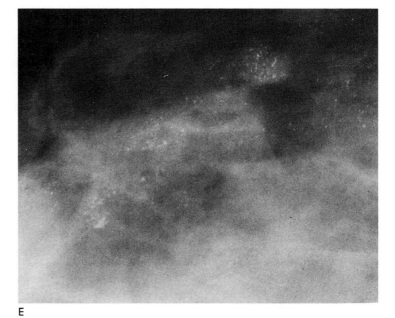

Figure 11-1 cont'd ■ *E*, Calcifications associated with a malignant ductal carcinoma. (From Griff SK, Dershaw DD: Breast cancer. In Bragg DG, Rubin P, Hricak H [eds]: Oncologic Imaging, 2nd ed. Philadelphia: WB Saunders, 2002, pp 265-294.)

E

rectly interpret its results. If the core biopsy pathology is discordant with the mammographic findings, for example, if only benign breast tissue is identified after core biopsy of a suspicious, spiculated mass, the biopsy should be repeated or the patient should be referred for open surgical biopsy. In addition, pathologic interpretation of certain lesions may be difficult on core biopsy. Distinguishing atypia from carcinoma in situ on core biopsy may be extremely difficult. The finding of atypical ductal hyperplasia requires open surgical biopsy to rule out malignancy, with up to half of subsequent open biopsies showing carcinoma in situ. The finding of a cellular fibroadenoma on core biopsy raises the possibility of a phylloides tumor, and

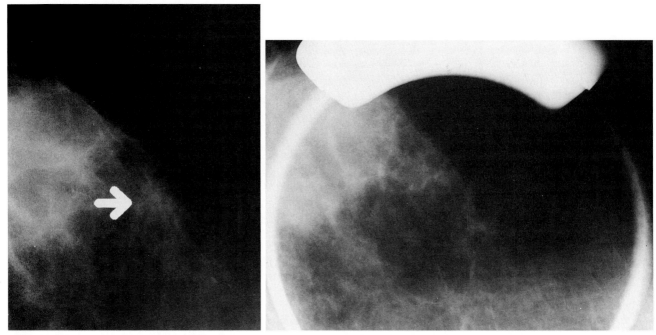

Figure 11-2 ■ Spot compression. The suspicious lesion on the left (arrow) dissipates on compression and closer magnification (right). (From Griff SK, Dershaw DD: Breast cancer. In Bragg DG, Rubin P, Hricak H [eds]: Oncologic Imaging, 2nd ed. Philadelphia: WB Saunders, 2002, pp 265-294.)

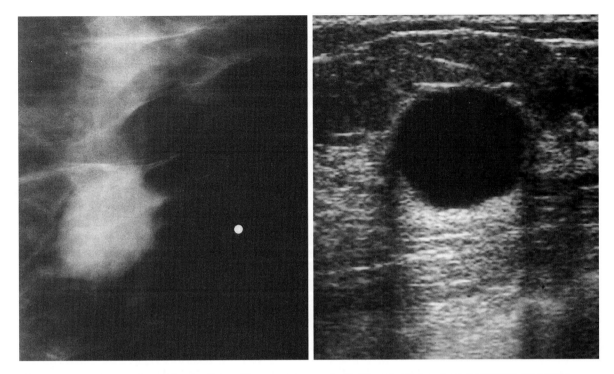

Figure 11-3 ■ Comparison of a simple cyst by mammography (left) and ultrasonography (right). The mass is partially defined in the mammogram, but its borders are obscured. The sonogram shows a smooth-walled lesion that is well defined, strongly suggesting a benign simple cyst. (From Griff SK, Dershaw DD: Breast cancer. In Bragg DG, Rubin P, Hricak H [eds]: Oncologic Imaging, 2nd ed. Philadelphia: WB Saunders, 2002, pp 265-294.)

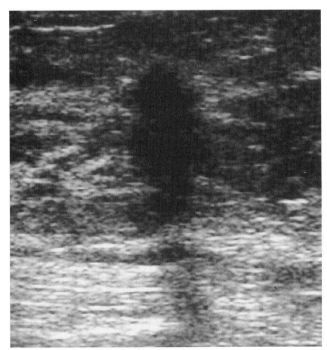

Figure 11-4 ■ Sonography of a malignant breast mass. Inhomogeneous echo pattern and irregular margins are prominent characteristics. (From Griff SK, Dershaw DD: Breast cancer. In Bragg DG, Rubin P, Hricak H [eds]: Oncologic Imaging, 2nd ed. Philadelphia: WB Saunders, 2002, pp 265-294.)

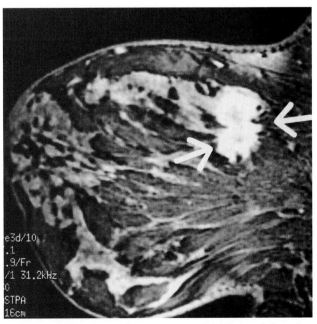

Figure 11-5 ■ Magnetic resonance imaging of invasive ductal carcinoma. Postgadolinium sagittal imaging. Arrows indicate mass. (From Griff SK, Dershaw DD: Breast cancer. In Bragg DG, Rubin P, Hricak H [eds]: Oncologic Imaging, 2nd ed. Philadelphia: WB Saunders, 2002, pp 265-294.)

excisional biopsy should be performed. Identification of necrosis or extravasated mucin in a core biopsy requires excisional biopsy to rule out malignancy.

The use of core needle biopsy for diagnosis of breast cancer can result in fewer surgical procedures and reduced cost in comparison with diagnosis by needle-localized open surgical biopsy. In one series, an average of 1.25 open surgical procedures were required for definitive treatment of a nonpalpable breast malignancy diagnosed by core needle biopsy, compared with an average of nearly two surgical procedures when open surgical biopsy was used for diagnosis (Smith 1997).

Open Surgical Biopsy with Needle Localization

For patients who choose or require diagnostic open surgical biopsy of a nonpalpable lesion or for patients with a nonpalpable malignancy diagnosed on core needle biopsy, preoperative wire localization of the lesion is required to direct the surgeon to the appropriate area. A localizing wire is placed adjacent to the target lesion using mammographic or ultrasound guidance. Wire localization for lesions visualized by magnetic resonance imaging can usually be performed with computed tomography (CT) guidance if the lesion is not identified on mammography or ultrasound. Systems for magnetic resonance imaging-guided localization of lesions are not yet widely available.

After the localizing wire is placed, the surgeon removes a piece of tissue around the wire so as to include the lesion with a rim of surrounding normal breast tissue. A specimen radiograph of the excised tissue is obtained before the patient leaves the operating room to be sure that the lesion is contained within the specimen. Diagnostic biopsies are generally performed under local anesthesia. Therapeutic wide excision of nonpalpable malignancies that were previously diagnosed as malignant by core biopsy is often performed under monitored or general anesthesia as an outpatient procedure.

The Missed Lesion

In 1% to 2% of wire-localized excisional biopsies, specimen radiography will show that the targeted lesion is not present in the excised tissue. Most often, this results from a change in the position of the localizing wire between placement and final excision. Other possibilities include inaccurate placement of the wire, failure of the surgeon to remove sufficient tissue around the wire, or a cystic lesion that ruptures during excision.

If the targeted lesion in not present in the specimen radiograph, the surgeon may consider immediately excising a limited amount of additional tissue if the likely location of the lesion can be deduced. Large amounts of tissue should not be removed blindly, however. It is often preferable to close the incision and perform a repeat mammogram in three or four weeks, as soon as the patient is able to tolerate compression. If the lesion remains, a repeat localization and excision may be performed.

Suggested Reading

American College of Radiology: Breast Imaging Reporting and Data System (BI-RADS™). Reston, VA: American College of Radiology, 1995.

Kopans DB, Smith BL: Preoperative, imaging guided needle localization, and biopsy of nonpalpable breast lesions. In Harris JR, Hellman S, Lippman M, Morrow M (eds): Diseases of the Breast. Philadelphia: JP Lippincott, 1996.

Meyer JE, Christian RL, Lester SC, et al: Evaluation of nonpalpable solid breast masses with stereotaxic large-needle core biopsy using a dedicated unit. Am J Roentgenol 1996;167:179–182.

Parker SH, Lovin JD, Jobe WE, et al: Nonpalpable breast lesions: Stereotactic automated large-core biopsies. Radiol 1991;180:403–407.

Sickles EA: Periodic mammographic follow-up of probably benign lesions: Results in 3,184 consecutive cases. Radiol 1991;179:463–468.

Smith DN, Christian R, Meyer JE: Large-core needle biopsy of nonpalpable breast cancers: The impact on subsequent surgical excisions. Arch Surg 1997;132:256–259.

Chapter 12
Nipple Discharge

Barbara L. Smith

Nipple discharge in most patients will have a benign etiology, but 1% to 2% of breast cancers present with nipple discharge and no other physical examination or mammographic findings. The aim of the evaluation of the symptom of nipple discharge is to sort out potentially malignant from benign causes.

Types of Discharge

Important features that are used in characterizing nipple discharge include the color of the discharge, the presence or absence of blood, whether the discharge is unilateral or bilateral, from a single duct or multiple ducts, and whether the discharge is spontaneous (spots the clothing), or appears only with active efforts to express it. Malignant discharge is usually unilateral, from a single duct, spontaneous, and bloody or watery. Benign discharge is bilateral, from multiple ducts, is not spontaneous, and does not contain blood. Galactorrhea is a spontaneous, milky discharge from multiple, bilateral ducts.

Physiologic Discharge

Small amounts of fluid may be expressed by pressure from the nipples of as many as 60% to 70% of healthy women. Physiologic nipple discharge is usually bilateral, appears from multiple ducts, and may be white, yellow, green, or dark blue in color. It is observed only with active manipulation of the nipple and does not occur spontaneously. A guaiac test on the fluid will be negative for occult blood. In the absence of a palpable mass or mammographic abnormality, this type of discharge requires no further evaluation or treatment, and only routine breast cancer screening is required.

Galactorrhea

Galactorrhea is a bilateral, often spontaneous, copious milky discharge, usually associated with elevated prolactin levels. Galactorrhea is almost never caused by a breast malignancy and may be distinguished from physiologic discharge under the microscope by the presence of fat in the secretions. As many as one third of women who have galactorrhea associated with amenorrhea will be found to have prolactin-secreting pituitary tumors. Conversely and of note, only 30% of patients with elevated serum prolactin levels will have a clinical picture of galactorrhea. Other causes of galactorrhea include hypothyroidism, chest wall trauma, and certain medications.

The evaluation of galactorrhea includes measurement of serum prolactin levels and thyroid function tests. Prolactin levels are measured in the morning, fasting, and in a nonstressed state. Levels greater than 150 ng/mL suggest a pituitary tumor, and a magnetic resonance imaging (MRI) scan of the head should be performed. The degree of prolactin elevation may correlate with tumor size. Prolactin levels in the 25 to 100 ng/mL range suggest hypothyroidism, renal disease, or medication-induced elevation. Medications that affect dopamine synthesis are the commonest causative agents in galactorrhea. Agents linked to galactorrhea include α-methyldopa, metoclopramide, cimetidine, phenothiazines, tricyclic antidepressants, opiates, and calcium channel blockers.

Treatment of galactorrhea is based on the underlying etiology. Medication-induced galactorrhea is corrected by discontinuing the offending agent. Galactorrhea associated with elevated prolactin with no evidence of a pituitary tumor is treated with bromocryptine when copious or when associated with infertility or menstrual abnormalities. Pituitary adenomas are managed on the basis of size. Microadenomas with no mass effect are followed with serial magnetic resonance imaging studies and with bromocryptine for infertility or menstrual abnormalities. Macroadenomas that are producing a mass effect in the pituitary are often treated with bromocryptine to shrink the lesion prior to surgical resection.

Pathologic Discharge

Nipple discharge that is unilateral and spontaneous increases the possibility that the discharge is due to malignancy. Bloody discharge is of greatest concern, although malignant discharge may be watery or of any color. Fewer than 10% of cases of bloody nipple discharge will be caused by a malignancy. A papilloma or other benign process is responsible for the discharge in the majority of cases. Postmenopausal women with nipple discharge are more likely to have an underlying malignancy than are premenopausal women.

Diagnostic Evaluation of the Patient

As is true in any woman presenting with a breast complaint, a thorough history and physical examination should be performed, and appropriate imaging studies should be obtained. A mammogram should be performed in the evaluation of pathologic nipple discharge for any woman more than 35 years of age. Any palpable or mammographic lesions identified should undergo biopsy.

Physical Examination Technique

Careful physical examination should be performed to identify any palpable masses present in the breast or any enlarged axillary nodes. In the absence of any other palpable abnormalities, the examination focuses on characterizing the discharge and identifying the area of the breast producing the discharge. The nipple is squeezed to elicit discharge. Manual pressure sweeping from the periphery of the breast toward the nipple may be helpful in bringing fluid toward the nipple. The patient herself may be able to efficiently elicit the discharge. The position of the duct from which discharge is obtained should be documented. A test for occult blood should be performed on any fluid that is obtained. The presence of occult blood increases the likelihood of malignancy, but a negative test does not rule it out.

The Role of Ductography and Cytology

Debate continues about the value of ductography (galactography) in the evaluation of single-duct nipple discharge. The majority of studies suggest that ductograms rarely provide data that change the need for surgery or the surgical procedure performed. Advocates of ductograms think that occasionally a ductogram will identify a peripheral lesion that would be missed on standard duct excision or will allow preoperative wire localization of a lesion, resulting in a smaller volume of excision.

False negative rates of ductography may be as high as 40% in patients with breast cancer presenting as nipple discharge. As a result, a negative ductogram does not eliminate the need for further evaluation and tissue diagnosis in a patient with pathologic nipple discharge.

There may be a role for ductography in young women with pathologic nipple discharge who hope to preserve the ability to breast-feed. If a peripheral cause of the discharge is identified, a more peripheral incision may be used. The finding of a focal lesion may potentially allow ductogram-guided wire localization and more limited tissue resection.

Cytologic analysis of nipple discharge is rarely useful. False-negative results of up to 35% have been reported, and false-positive results are also observed. A positive cytologic reading will still require duct excision to define the extent and histology of the malignancy, and given the risk of a false negative, surgery is still required for negative cytology.

The potential role of duct lavage and ductoscopy in evaluation of a patient with single-duct discharge is under investigation, as is the potential utility of magnetic resonance imaging.

Other Markers of Malignancy

Attempts to identify markers, such as carcinoembryonic antigen (CEA), prostate-specific antigen, p53, bFGF, or microsatellite DNA alterations, that exhibit good specificity and sensitivity for the presence of malignancy in nipple aspirate fluid have been largely unsuccessful.

Surgical Evaluation

Duct excision (microdochectomy) is the procedure of choice for determining the cause of single-duct nipple discharge. The surgeon's goal is to excise the duct from which the discharge arises, with as little additional tissue as possible. Local anesthesia, with or without sedation, is generally sufficient for this procedure. A circumareolar incision is made, and a nipple skin flap is raised. A fine lacrimal duct probe can usually be inserted into the discharging duct to allow palpation of the course of the duct to facilitate excision. The duct containing the probe is excised with a margin of surrounding tissue from just below the nipple dermis for 4 to 5 cm deep into breast tissue. The majority of ductal pathology will be within 5 cm of the nipple and will be contained in a specimen of this size.

If it is not possible to pass the lacrimal duct probe into the discharging duct, the skin incision is made and the nipple skin flap raised as above. A dark, secretion-filled pathologic duct can often be visualized and excised. If no single secretion-filled duct is identified, the entire subareolar duct complex must be excised from immediately beneath the nipple dermis to 4 to 5 cm deep into breast tissue.

Breast tissue is reapproximated beneath the nipple prior to skin closure to avoid nipple retraction or indentation of the areola. Nipple sensation is generally not affected by this procedure.

Results of Duct Excision

If a malignancy is found, the histology and size of the underlying lesion dictate management. In patients with cancer of the breast whose nipple discharge is unassociated with palpable or mammographic abnormalities, the histology is usually one of low-grade or intermediate-grade ductal carcinoma in situ (DCIS), with or without areas of invasion. The papillary histologic subtype is often seen. Surgical options include wide excision with radiation or mastectomy. Mastectomy is used when clean margins are not obtained on lumpectomy or if the patient prefers this option. The presence of nipple discharge in a patient with breast cancer does not require excision of the nipple and areola in patients undergoing lumpectomy.

If a single benign papilloma is found, no further treatment is required, and there is no increase in the risk of future breast cancer. Less commonly, pathology will identify multiple papillomas or juvenile papillomatosis. Often, one of the papillomas produces a palpable mass. These conditions may be associated with an increased risk of breast cancer, and careful screening is appropriate.

Other benign conditions such as duct ectasia (see below), a nipple adenoma, or fibrocystic disease may be found on duct excision. No further treatment is required. When no specific lesion is identified as the cause, patients should be followed closely with physical examinations and mammograms to be sure that a malignancy was not missed by the excision.

Other Clinical Situations Associated with Nipple Discharge

Nipple Irritation

A number of benign processes of the nipple may mimic discharge. Irritation of the nipple during exercise (jogger's nipple) may produce erosions and drainage. Eczema or other dermatitis may also produce erosion and drainage. Topical treatment results in prompt resolution of symptoms.

Bloody Discharge in Pregnancy

Bloody nipple discharge may occur in the second or third trimester of pregnancy. The discharge is usually bilateral and from multiple ducts. It is thought to arise as a result of the increased vascularity of breast duct tissue, which is part of duct development in preparation for lactation. In the absence of a palpable mass, the patient may be safely followed, and the discharge is likely to resolve spontaneously.

If an area of palpable concern is identified or if unilateral single duct discharge persists, further evaluation is warranted. Ultrasound may be helpful, but the density of breast tissue during pregnancy makes mammography of little value. Needle or open biopsy may be safely performed if a focal lesion is identified. Biopsy should not be delayed until after delivery or after completion of lactation.

Paget's Disease

Nipple discharge associated with erosion, itching, or chronic crusting of the nipple raises the possibility of Paget's disease of the nipple, a special form of breast cancer. The differential diagnosis of these nipple changes includes eczema, nipple adenoma, malignant melanoma, Bowen's disease (intraepidermal carcinoma), syphilitic chancre, and the inflammatory changes of duct ectasia/periductal mastitis. Biopsy is required to distinguish among these possibilities.

Clinical Features

Paget's disease accounts for 1% to 2% of presentations of breast cancer. The nipple changes of Paget's disease result from cancer cell proliferation within the epidermis of the nipple. Tumor cells may be present as small nests or as full-thickness replacement of the epidermis.

Nipple ulceration is present in as many as 90% of cases. Other common findings include itching or burning of the nipple, nipple discharge, erythema, crusting or scabbing of the nipple, vesicle formation, and nipple retraction. Patients with Paget's disease confined to the nipple itself are more likely to present with symptoms of itching, pain, and scaling without ulceration. Initially, the nipple changes may have a relapsing and remitting course with temporary healing of ulcerated areas. A breast mass is present in association with the nipple changes in approximately 30% to 40% of cases. The breast masses may be present in any part of the breast, although many are in a subareolar location.

Diagnosis

A brief course of topical steroids may be tried if a benign etiology for the observed nipple changes is suspected. Failure of the nipple changes to resolve completely or recurrence after cessation of therapy requires diagnostic biopsy. The diagnosis of Paget's disease is made by full-thickness biopsy of the nipple with biopsy of any associated palpable or mammographic abnormalities.

Treatment

The treatment of Paget's disease continues to be debated. In the past, mastectomy was recommended for all patients with Paget's disease owing to concerns about multifocal involvement of the breast. As with other breast cancer presentations, breast conservation is increasingly used in the initial therapy of Paget's disease, involving lumpectomy, with excision of the nipple and areola, and radiation. Systemic chemotherapy or hormone therapy is used as dictated by the underlying carcinoma.

The prognosis of patients with Paget's disease depends on the stage of the underlying breast carcinoma. The prognosis is not altered by the presence of clinically apparent nipple changes. For patients with Paget's disease confined to the nipple, with no underlying malignancy, the prognosis is similar to that of pure ductal carcinoma in situ, with long-term survival rates in the 90% to 100% range after mastectomy. Local recurrence rates after breast-conserving treatment are similar to those seen after breast conservation for ductal carcinoma in situ.

Duct Ectasia/Periductal Mastitis

Unilateral nipple discharge consisting of thick, pasty, white material may be caused by a chronic relapsing form of infection known as periductal mastitis or duct ectasia. The subareolar ducts become dilated, thin-walled, and filled with thick secretions. A sequence of mixed aerobic and anaerobic infections may occur, resulting in inflammatory changes and scarring of the subareolar ducts. Chronic discharge, retraction or inversion of the nipple, subareolar thickening, or a chronic fistula from the subareolar ducts to the periareolar skin may result. Palpable masses and mammographic changes that mimic carcinoma can occur. This condition appears to be more common among women who smoke or who have diabetes.

Duct ectasia/periductal mastitis is most often a clinical diagnosis. At the initial evaluation, physical examination and mammography are performed, and any suspicious lesions biopsied. Care should be taken to avoid open biopsy during periods of active infection, as wound infection, fistulas, and chronic abscesses may result. Antibiotic treatment prior to biopsy can prevent these complications, with the option of needle biopsy for suspicious areas in the setting of a refractory infection.

Duct ectasia in its early stages may occasionally be found on duct excision for unilateral single-duct discharge. If there is no associated infection, no further treatment is required. Such patients may or may not go on to develop chronic duct ectasia/periductal mastitis.

Episodes of infection present initially with subareolar pain and mild erythema. If they are treated at this stage, warm soaks and oral antibiotics can suffice. Antibiotic treatment should cover both aerobic and anaerobic skin flora, regardless of whether anaerobic species are identified on culture, because treatment is often unsuccessful unless anaerobic coverage is included. If an abscess develops, incision and drainage are required. Repeated infections are treated by excision of the entire affected subareolar duct complex after the acute infection has completely resolved, with intravenous antibiotic coverage during the perioperative period. Rare patients will have recurrent infections and persistent fistulas that require excision of the nipple and areola.

Suggested Reading

Ambrogetti D, Berni D, Catarzi S, Ciatto S: The role of ductal galactography in the differential diagnosis of breast carcinoma. Radiol Med (Torino) 1996;91:198–201.

Chaudary MA, Millis RR, Davies GC, Hayward JL: The diagnostic value of testing for occult blood. Ann Surg 1982;196:651–655.

Ciatto S, Bravetti P, Cariaggi P: Significance of nipple discharge clinical patterns in the selection of cases for cytologic examination. Acta Cytol 1986;30:17–20.

Das DK, Al-Ayadhy B, Ajrawi MT, et al: Cytodiagnosis of nipple discharge: A study of 602 samples from 484 cases. Diagn Cytopathol 2001;25:25–37.

Dinkel HP, Gassel AM, Muller T, et al: Galactography and exfoliative cytology in women with abnormal nipple discharge. Obstet Gynecol 2001;97:625–629.

Florio MG, Manganaro T, Pollicino A, et al: Surgical approach to nipple discharge: A ten-year experience. J Surg Oncol Suppl 1999;71:235–238.

Jardines L: Management of nipple discharge. Am Surg 1996;62:119–122.

King TA, Carter KM, Bolton JS, Furman GM: A simple approach to nipple discharge. Am Surg 2000;66:960–966.

Mitchell G, Trott PA, Morris L, et al: Cellular characteristics of nipple aspiration fluid during the menstrual cycle in healthy premenopausal women. Cytopathol 2001;12:184–196.

Morrison C: The significance of nipple discharge: Diagnosis and treatment regimes. Prim Care 1998;2:129–140.

Orel SG, Dougherty CS, Reynolds C, et al: MR imaging in patients with nipple discharge: Initial experience. Radiol 2000;216:248–254.

Sakafora GH: Nipple discharge: Current diagnostic and therapeutic approaches. Cancer Treat Rev 2001;27:275–282.

Shen KW, Wu L, Lu JS, et al: Fiberoptic ductoscopy for breast cancer patients with nipple discharge. Surg Endoscopy 2001;15:1340–1345.

Chapter 13
Dyspnea

Corina Akerele and Joseph A. Sparano

Dyspnea is a subjective feeling of breathlessness, an uncomfortable awareness of breathing. It is often associated with tachypnea. Interference with normal ventilation and oxygenation can be due either to direct organ involvement by cancer or indirect effects of cancer or its treatment. The principal causes of dyspnea in the patient with cancer are listed in Table 13-1; in some cancers, several mechanisms may be involved. For example, lung cancer can cause dyspnea by airway obstruction, pleural effusion, and/or pulmonary parenchymal disease.

In patients with advanced cancer, one needs to consider the possibility that a benign condition is causing dyspnea rather than assuming that it is must be due to the cancer. Examples of these nonmalignant complications include congestive heart failure due to arteriosclerotic cardiovascular disease, asthmatic bronchitis in patients with chronic obstructive pulmonary disease, anemia due to gastrointestinal (GI) tract bleeding, fluid retention from corticosteroid therapy or renal failure, and anxiety states. The search for a nonmalignant cause of dyspnea is particularly important in patients with metastatic cancer to avoid missing an opportunity for effective, nonantitumor therapy.

Dyspnea can therefore be a consequence of the disease, its treatment, associated complications, or comorbid medical conditions that are unrelated to the malignant disease. Pulmonary and/or pleural metastases are the most common cause of dyspnea in patients with solid tumors. These complications usually cause the gradual onset of dyspnea. An acute onset suggests either acute pulmonary infection, overwhelming sepsis, or a cardiovascular event such as a pulmonary embolus, myocardial ischemia, or cardiac tamponade. Pulmonary infections, sepsis, or drug reactions are most common in patients who have acute or chronic leukemias or other bone marrow malignancies and in those who receive high-dose chemotherapy plus radiation therapy followed by stem cell transplantation.

Because of the lung's reserve capacity, in patients who have normal intrinsic pulmonary function, numerous pulmonary metastatic deposits, even when large, might not cause dyspnea. More often, dyspnea develops in patients who have lymphangitic spread of cancer. Lymphangitic spread tends to be diffuse, and the extent of involvement is frequently greater than is appreciated on chest X-rays or scans. The dissemination throughout the lung causes dyspnea both by impairing gas exchange and by increasing the stiffness of the lung, reducing compliance, and increasing the work of breathing. Pulmonary function studies show a restrictive pattern and a diminished carbon monoxide–diffusing capacity (DLCO).

Pleural Effusion

Pleural fluid is normally rapidly formed and reabsorbed. Increasing the rate of formation and/or blocking reabsorption causes pleural fluid accumulation. Common nonmalignant causes include congestive heart failure and hypoalbuminema. Cancer-related pleural effusions are most commonly due to increased capillary permeability and/or impaired pleural lymphatic drainage. The most commonly associated malignancies are lung cancer, breast cancer, and lymphomas. Dyspnea results from lung compression; the

Table 13-1 ■ Common Causes of Dyspnea in Cancer Patients

Cause	Direct Effects of Invasive Cancer	Complications of Cancer or Its Treatment
PULMONARY:		
Obstructive airway disease	Airway obstruction Recurrent laryngeal nerve paralysis	Hypersensitivity reaction associated with chemotherapy
Parenchymal lung disease	Metastases	Pneumonia Chemotherapy-induced pneumonitis Radiation-induced pneumonitis
Pleural pathology	Metastases/malignant effusion	Pneumothorax (associated with catheter insertion) Chemotherapy-associated effusion (e.g., docetaxel)
Chest wall or respiratory muscles	Tumor involving chest wall Phrenic nerve paralysis Pathologic rib fracture	
CARDIAC:		
Heart disease	Myocardial/epicardial metastases Primary tumor (atrial myxoma)	Radiation-induced myocardial toxicity Cardiomyopathy (due to anthracyclines)
Pericardial disease	Metastases/malignant effusion	Chemotherapy-associated pericardial effusion (e.g., docetaxel) Radiation pericarditis
VASCULAR:		
Pulmonary vessels	Superior vena cava obstruction Carcinoid syndrome	Pulmonary embolus Drug-induced vasculopathy (e.g., busulfan)
OTHER CAUSES:		
	Metabolic (tumor lysis syndrome) Hyperviscosity Leukostasis	Progestational agents Anxiety Anemia Metabolic acidosis

severity of the symptom correlates with the rate and extent of fluid accumulation.

If lymphatic obstruction is the cause, as can occur with lymphomatous involvement of mediastinal and hilar lymph nodes, the fluid may have the characteristics of a transudate. If the thoracic duct is trapped by lymphoma, the transported fat seeps into the pleural space, resulting in a chylothorax due to the accumulation of lipid-laden milky-appearing fluid. More often, malignant effusions are due to invasion of the pleural surfaces by cancer. Deposits on these serosal surfaces cause capillary leakage of blood, impaired drainage, and shedding of malignant cells into the fluid. In the absence of chest trauma or pulmonary infarction, a bloody pleural effusion is virtually pathognomonic of a malignant effusion. Analysis of the fluid shows exudative features, including a specific gravity greater than 1.015, protein greater than 3 g/dL, pleural/serum protein ratio greater than 0.5, and pleural/serum lactate dehydrogenase (LDH) ratio greater than 0.6. A more detailed discussion of pleural effusions appears in Chapter 15.

Pericardial Effusion

Neoplastic pericardial effusions arise from impairment of pericardial lymphatic drainage and the stimulus of cancer deposits on the pericardial surface. This occurs most commonly in patients with lung cancer and metastatic breast cancer but can also develop from deposits of chloroma (collections of leukemia blast cells) or lymphomatous invasion.

Drug-Induced Pulmonary Toxicity

Pulmonary toxicity occurs as a complication of radiation therapy to the chest or after cytotoxic therapy. Drugs that have a 5% or greater risk of causing pulmonary toxicity include bleomycin, gemcitabine, methotrexate, carmustine, cytarabine, and mitomycin-C. Drugs that less frequently cause pulmonary damage include cyclophosphamide, busulfan, procarbazine, and vinorelbine. A number of other chemotherapeutic agents have only rarely been implicated as a cause of pulmonary abnormalities.

Pulmonary toxicity can be caused by oxidant injury of the phospholipid membranes of the alveolar and supporting cells of the lung. Such damage is mediated by reactive oxygen intermediates produced by bleomycin, cyclophosphamide, and nitrosoureas; hypersensitivity reactions to methotrexate or procarbazine; and cytokine release after mitomycin-C.

The clinical presentation and therapy of the pulmonary toxicity resulting from the most commonly associated agents are shown in Table 13-2. An acute presentation consistent with noncardiogenic pulmonary edema can occur within minutes or hours of administration in the case of bleomycin, cyclophosphamide, methotrexate, and cytarabine. In contrast, pulmonary fibrosis can develop gradually months or years after therapy had been discontinued in the case of ifosfamide, melphalan, busulfan, lomustine, and carmustine. The diagnosis is usually made based on exclusion of other potential causes, including lymphangitic metastatic spread, infection, hemorrhage, or pulmonary edema. Blood transfusions can, within 24 hours, cause noncardiogenic pulmonary edema due to leukoagglutinins. Acknowledgment of this possibility, which resolves within 24 to 48 hours, can spare the patient needless therapy and diagnostic procedures for pulmonary infection.

Evaluation

Dyspnea occurring at rest or with minimal exertion requires a prompt evaluation of the cause, starting with a directed history and physical examination. The past medical history should explore whether there is a history of pulmonary or pleural metastases; comorbid cardiac, pulmonary, or thromboembolic disease; current and prior anticancer therapies; and current medications. Critical elements of the symptom review include the acuity of onset; whether it occurs at rest, with minimal exertion, or with substantial exertion; and whether other symptoms, such as chest pain, hemoptysis, or leg swelling and pain, are present. Dull aching shoulder pain may provide a clue to the presence of diaphragmatic tumor implants, because the pain sensation from the diaphragm is referred to the same sensory level in the cervical cord as the shoulder region. Physical examination should determine the patient's cardiac, pulmonary, and mental status and whether cyanosis is present. Initial laboratory studies include a complete blood count, routine blood chemistries, pulse oximetry, and chest X-ray.

Additional studies are based on the suspected etiology of the dyspnea. These may well include arterial blood analysis of pH, pCO$_2$, and bicarbonate for metabolic acidosis; electrocardiogram for cardiac ischemia; pericardial effusion, or pericarditis; echocardiogram for congestive heart failure, pericardial effusion, intracardiac clot, or tumor; and spiral computerized tomography of the chest for pulmonary emboli, pleural metastatic deposits, parenchymal disease, or extent of lymphangitic carcinomatosis. Bronchoscopy and transbronchial biopsy may be necessary to rule out pulmonary drug toxicity. In this circumstance, the changes in the lung are nonspecific and nondiagnostic, but biopsy performs a useful service in ruling out other potential causes.

If a pleural effusion is present, then diagnostic thoracentesis should be performed to document the characteristics of the fluid and the presence of malignant cells. The cells in the fluid should be concentrated by cytospin and subjected to cytologic examination. In some cases, it may be difficult to identify with certainty that malignant cells are present, and additional studies such as special stains of indeterminate cells by anti-carcinoembryonic antigen (CEA) or antiepithelial membrane antigen, for example in the case of adenocarcinoma, may be diagnostic. Pleural biopsy is often successful in obtaining malignant cells. If this procedure is necessary, it should be performed in the presence of the pleural effusion so that the visceral pleura is displaced away from the biopsy needle and less subject to injury. Finally, if need be, in the case of suspected but undocumented malignancy in the chest, thoracoscopy can be employed.

Chest X-ray in patients with a pericardial effusion shows the typical globular, water bottle appearance of the cardiac silhouette. Echocardiogram provides definitive evaluation of the quantity of the pericardial effusion and the presence of pericardial tumor deposits. Computed tomography (CT) scan of the chest helps to define the extent of intrathoracic disease. Electrocardiograms show low QRS voltage and nonspecific ST-T wave changes. Percutaneous pericardiocentesis, carefully monitored in an intensive-care setting, is necessary to demonstrate that the effusion is neoplastic in origin, rather than due to an intercurrent illness.

Therapy

The choice of therapy depends on the cause of the dyspnea, the underlying diagnosis (solid tumor versus hematologic disease), the aims of overall therapy (palliation versus an attempt at cure or remission), whether the neoplasm remains responsive to anticancer treatment, a cost/benefit analysis of the likelihood of complications and of symptom resolution from treatment, and the patient's advance directives. Treatment should be directed to the underlying cause whenever feasible. For patients who are treated in the palliative care setting, treatment should be directed at the cause when there is a reasonable expectation that it may result in

Table 13-2 ■ Clinical Features and Management of Chemotherapy or Radiation-Induced Pulmonary Toxicity

Drug	Clinical Presentation	Management
Bleomycin	Pneumonitis (up to 10%) — Symptoms: Dyspnea, cough, fever, fatigue, malaise — Signs: Fine rales — Chest X-ray: Patchy infiltrates (usually lower lung fields) or nodular lesions mimicking metastases — Risk factors: cumulative dose >200IU, oxygen, age >70 years, prior pulmonary irradiation — Course: May progress to pulmonary fibrosis or result in death (1%) Acute chest pain syndrome (rare) Idiosyncratic anaphylactoid reaction (1% of lymphoma patients)	Prevention — Chest X-ray every 1–2 weeks; discontinue if infiltrates appear — Measure serial DLCO; discontinue if it decreases to <30% to 35% of pretreatment value — Use O_2 saturation <25% during/after surgery Treatment — Immediate drug withdrawal — Limit inhaled oxygen — Corticosteroids — Evaluate and consider rechallenge
Gemcitabine	Acute dyspnea syndrome (common: ~23%; severe 3%) — Symptoms: Dyspnea occurring within hours/days — Signs: None or bronchospasm (latter occurs in <2%) — Chest X-ray: No acute findings — Predisposing factors: Lung carcinoma/metastases Drug-induced pneumonitis or pulmonary edema (rare)	— Continue treatment — Obtain chest X-ray if occurs/persists beyond 24 hours — Discontinue treatment
Methotrexate	Pneumonitis (3% to 8%) — Symptoms: Dry cough, dyspnea, chest pain — Signs: None or rales — Chest X-ray: pleural effusion, adenopathy, infiltrates, or nodules Predisposing factors: None; may occur at very low doses and after oral, intravenous, or intrathecal administration	— Leucovorin rescue not protective — Consider corticosteroids
Cytarabine	Pneumonitis — Symptoms: Cough, fever, dyspnea, chest pain — Signs: None or rales — Chest X-ray: Infiltrates — Predisposing factors: High-dose (>1–3 gm/m² per dose), mucositis, streptococcal bacteremia	— Difficult to distinguish from infection — Commonly associated with diarrhea — Treat associated infections
Carmustine	Pneumonitis (associated with high-dose therapy) — Symptoms: Cough, fever, dyspnea — Signs: None or rales — Chest X-ray: Infiltrates — Predisposing factors: High dose (>600 mg/m²), advanced age, lung irradiation, lung disease, administration of other cytotoxic agents	Prevention — Restrict dose to <450 mg/m² if prior mediastinal irradiation Treatment — Corticosteroids
Radiation	Symptoms — Fever, dyspnea — Occurs 2–3 months post RT to lungs — Chest X-ray: Infiltrate with sharp border corresponding to radiation field — Predisposing factors: Cigarettes	Corticosteroids

relief of symptoms. Examples include drainage of a pleural or pericardial effusion or ascites, palliative irradiation, antibiotics, endoscopically guided laser therapy and/or stent insertion to open an occluded bronchus, and treatment of congestive heart failure.

If the cause is neoplastic invasion of the lungs, pleura, or pericardium, the use of chemotherapy requires that the neoplasm remain sensitive to treatment, as can occur in patients with lymphomas, breast cancer, or testicular cancer. In these settings, successful therapy can prolong life and relieve symptoms, including dyspnea. Direct antitumor therapy is not usually feasible in far-advanced disease in which either the disease is resistant or the patient is unable or unwilling to tolerate intervention other than symptomatic measures. In these circumstances, relief of dyspnea is best accomplished by oxygen therapy, given by nasal prongs or mask, and administration of morphine, which reduces the perception of dyspnea. Morphine should be given orally if feasible; otherwise, it should be given parenterally by an intravenous route. Severe dyspnea creates a sense of suffocation for patients. It is a terrifying and overwhelming symptom. Morphine should be given in whatever doses are necessary to secure the patient's comfort. Even though there is the potential for respiratory depression, this approach is not contraindicated in patients with far-advanced cancer.

Anemia that is severe (hemoglobin less than 8 g/dL) can of itself cause dyspnea or amplify the symptoms of patients with borderline cardiopulmonary function. Anemia is readily correctable by packed red blood cell transfusions but may be withheld in the terminal phases of disease if symptom relief can be achieved by other means. Congestive heart failure, whether secondary to drug toxicity—from adriamycin, for example—or from arteriosclerotic cardiovascular disease, will respond to the usual measures. Although the benefits of corticosteroids for drug- or radiation-induced pulmonary toxicity is unproven and the effective dose is unknown, some patients do appear to respond to prednisone. Shortness of breath is frightening, and the experience of dyspnea can be exacerbated by anxiety. A trial of anxiolytics may be warranted for some patients.

Malignant pleural effusions can be managed by sclerotherapy. This involves insertion of a thoracostomy tube, whose placement can be facilitated by thoracoscopy. The tube is connected to underwater sealed drainage to remove the pleural fluid and allow the visceral and parietal surfaces of the pleura to come into apposition. One of a number of agents can then be instilled to elicit an inflammatory reaction on the pleural surfaces. Drainage is continued, and the surfaces fibrose together, obliterating the pleural space in a process called pleurodesis. Agents that are commonly used for this purpose include tetracycline, bleomycin and other chemotherapeutic drugs, radioactive isotopes, and talc. Talc is effective if it is delivered over the entire pleural surface under visual guidance by thoracoscopy. Resolution of the pleural effusion occurs in 50% to 60% of cases. In cases that fail to respond, the pleural effusion becomes loculated, and the procedure cannot usually be repeated. External beam radiation may be of use in patients whose pleural effusion is due to lymphoma, primarily when the effusion is secondary to mediastinal lymph node replacement and lymphatic obstruction.

Percutaneous pericardiocentesis can provide transient relief of a malignant pericardial effusion and is useful if cardiac tamponade is present or threatened. Durable control can be obtained by other means. It is feasible to establish drainage through placement of a tube into the pericardial space, using a subxiphoid approach. It is then feasible to instill chemotherapy in an attempt to fuse the visceral and parietal pericardial linings together, in a fashion similar to that described for pleurodesis. Control of the pericardial effusion is more reliably accomplished by surgical resection of the pericardium. This allows drainage into the pleural space and prevents cardiac compression by continuing pericardial fluid formation. The success of this procedure correlates with the extent of pericardium that can be removed. The appropriateness of surgery depends on whether the patient's expected survival is long enough to justify the procedure.

Suggested Reading

Diagnosis

Boutin C, Astoul P: Diagnostic thoracoscopy. Clin Chest Med 1998;19:295-305.

Bruera E, Schmitz B, Pither J, et al: The frequency and occurrence of dyspnea in patients with advanced cancer. J Pain Symptom Manage 2000;19:357-362.

General

David CL: Palliation of breathlessness. Cancer Treat Res 1999;100:59–73.

DeCamp MM, Mentzer SJ, Swanson SJ, et al: Malignant effusive disease of the pleura and pericardium. Chest 1997;112:291S–295S.

Fenton KN, Richardson JD: Diagnosis and management of malignant pleural effusion. Am J Surg 1995;170:69–74.

Keefe DL: Cardiovascular emergencies in the cancer patient. Semin Oncol 2000;27:244–255.

Kreisman H, Wolkove N: Pulmonary toxicity of antineoplastic therapy. Semin Oncol 1992;19:508–520.

Petrakis I, Katsamouris A, Drossitis I, et al: Usefulness of thoracoscopic surgery in the diagnosis and management of thoracic diseases. J Cardiovasc Surg 2000;41:767–771.

Ripamonti C: Management of dyspnea in advanced cancer patients. Support Care Cancer 1999;7:233–243.

Tsang TS, Seward JB, Barnes ME, et al: Outcomes of primary and secondary treatment of pericardial effusion in patients with malignancy. Mayo Clin Proc 2000;75:248–253.

Wolkowicz J, Sturgeon J, Rawji M, et al: Bleomycin-induced pulmonary function abnormalities. Chest 1992;101:97–101.

Specific Treatment

Allard P, Lamontagne C, Bernard P, et al: How effective are supplementary doses of opioids for dyspnea in terminally ill cancer patients? A randomized continuous sequential clinical trial. J Pain Symptom Manage 1999;17:256–265.

Anderson TM, Ray CW, Nwogu CE, et al: Pericardial catheter sclerosis versus surgical procedures for pericardial effusions in cancer patients. J Cardiovasc Surg 2001;42:415–419.

Chan A, Rischin D, Clarke CP, et al: Subxiphoid partial pericardiostomy with or without sclerosant instillation in the treatment of symptomatic pericardial effusions in patients with malignancy. Cancer 1991;68:1021–1025.

Chen YM, Shih JF, Yang KY, et al: Usefulness of pig-tail catheter for palliative drainage of malignant pleural effusions in cancer patients. Supp Care Cancer 2000;8:423–426.

Colleoni M, Martinelli G, Beretta F, et al: Intracavitary chemotherapy with thiotepa in malignant pericardial effusions: an active and well-tolerated regimen. J Clin Oncol 1998;16:2371–2376.

Colt HG, Russack V, Chiu Y, et al: A comparison of thoracoscopic talc instillation: Slurry, and mechanical abrasion pleurodesis. Chest 1997;111:442–448.

Liu G, Crump M, Goss PE, et al: Prospective comparison of the sclerosing agents doxycycline and bleomycin for the primary management of malignant pericardial effusion and cardiac tamponade. J Clin Oncol 1996;14:3141–3147.

Milanez RC, Vargas FS, Filomeno LB, et al: Intrapleural talc for the treatment of malignant pleural effusions secondary to breast cancer. Cancer 1995;75:2688–2692.

Rodriguez-Panadero F: Current trends in pleurodesis. Curr Opinion Pulm Med 1997;3:319–325.

Von Hoff DD: Phase I trials of dexrazoxane and other potential applications for the agent. Semin Oncol 1998;25(4 Suppl 10):31–36.

Chapter 14
The Solitary Pulmonary Nodule

Phillip M. Boiselle and Armin Ernst

In the United States alone, it has been estimated that roughly 150,000 new solitary pulmonary nodules are detected by radiography and computed tomography (CT) each year. Considering recent advances in lung nodule detection, most notably the use of low-dose helical computed tomography for lung cancer screening, this number will likely increase significantly in the near future.

A solitary pulmonary nodule is defined as a focal area of increased lung opacity with a round or oval configuration that measures less than 3 cm in diameter (Figure 14-1). The distinction between a nodule and a mass is based on size criteria, a mass being defined as an opacity greater than 3 cm in diameter. This somewhat arbitrary size criterion is used for the following reasons: (1) The vast majority of lesions greater than 3 cm in diameter are malignant, whereas a slight majority of lesions less than this size are benign; (2) the presence of calcification is helpful in distinguishing benign from malignant lesions only if a nodule measures less than 3 cm in diameter; and (3) bronchogenic carcinomas less than 3 cm in diameter are less likely to be associated with lymph node metastases and have a better prognosis than larger lesions.

Once a nodule has been detected, the primary goal is to differentiate benign and potentially malignant (also referred to as "indeterminate") nodules as accurately as possible (Table 14-1). Specifically, one aims to detect and remove all solitary malignant lesions while avoiding unnecessary and costly workups (possibly including thoracotomies) for benign or nonisolated lesions. This is an important fact, as the five-year survival rate after removal of a malignant solitary pulmonary nodule is 40% to 80%, compared to the dismal outlook of lung cancer that is detected at later stages. This highlights the need for effective means of early lung cancer detection.

A variety of clinical data can be used to help determine the likelihood of malignancy, including patient age, smoking history, history of prior malignancy, and presenting symptoms. For example, a lung nodule detected in a 35-year-old nonsmoker with no history of prior malignancy is associated with a very low probability of malignancy, whereas the opposite is true for a lung nodule detected in a 70-year-old smoker.

Although indeterminate lung nodules have historically required invasive assessment such as biopsy or resection for definitive diagnosis, two new noninvasive methods of nodule assessment may help to reduce the number of unnecessary biopsies and thoracotomies. Unlike traditional imaging techniques, which rely on morphologic features to distinguish between malignant and benign nodules, these methods are based on more specific physiologic parameters. These emerging techniques include computed tomography nodule enhancement, which assesses nodule vascularity, and positron emission tomography (PET) imaging, which evaluates nodule glucose metabolism.

Traditional Imaging Techniques: Conventional Radiography and Computed Tomography

Conventional Radiography

Conventional radiography plays a limited role in distinguishing benign from malignant pulmonary nodules. In general, when a nodule is detected by chest radiography and does not meet the standard radiographic criteria (benign calcification pattern or stability for >2 years) for benignancy, computed tomography is the preferred initial method for further evaluation.

Computed Tomography

Computed tomography is extremely helpful for both confirming and characterizing solitary pulmonary nodules detected by chest radiography. Computed tomography is also more sensitive than radiography for detecting small pulmonary nodules.

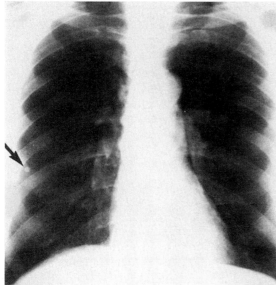

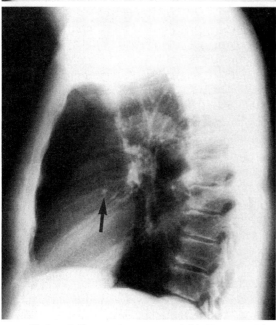

Figure 14-1 ■ Solitary pulmonary nodule. (From Mettler FA: Essentials of Radiology. Philadelphia: WB Saunders, p 89, 1996.)

Table 14-1 ■ **Differential Diagnosis of Solitary Pulmonary Nodules**

Neoplasm

Malignant
  Bronchogenic carcinoma*
  Carcinoid
  Pulmonary metastasis*
  Lymphoma
Benign
  Hamartoma*

Infection

  Granuloma (tuberculosis or fungal)*
  Rounded pneumonia
  Lung abscess
  Hydatid cyst

Inflammatory

  Rheumatoid arthritis
  Wegener's granulomatosis
  Lymphomatoid granulomatosis

Vascular/Embolic

  Arteriovenous malformation
  Venous varix
  Pulmonary infarction

Traumatic

  Hematoma

Miscellaneous

  Intrapulmonary lymph node
  Rounded atelectasis
  Bronchogenic cyst

*The most common causes of resected solitary pulmonary nodules.

With regard to computed tomography technique, one should initially perform a noncontrast scan with thin-section images through the nodule to allow an accurate determination of nodule density and margins. Specific features to assess on computed tomography images include size, contours and margins, relationship to vessels and bronchi, cavitation, and density.

1. *Size.* The size of a nodule is directly proportional to the likelihood of malignancy. In general, the smaller the size of a nodule, the more likely that it is benign. However, despite the well-established relationship between nodule size and malignancy, no size criterion allows exclusion of malignancy.

To date, the significance and management of very small nodules, defined as less than 5 mm in diameter, is somewhat controversial. Such small nodules are often managed by serial follow-up computed tomography scans to document two-year stability. Unfortunately, however, the detection of a malignant growth rate in such small nodules may be difficult to detect with traditional computed tomography measurement methods. Recently developed three-dimensional, volumetric methods of measurement using helical computed tomography data have been shown to be more accurate than conventional methods and will likely play an important role in nodule measurement in the future.

2. *Contours and margins.* Primary lung neoplasms typically have irregular contours and spiculated margins (Figure 14-2). Indeed, the presence of spiculated margins is highly predictive of malig-

DIAGNOSIS

Chest Radiography of Pulmonary Nodules

Conventional chest radiography has historically been the primary imaging tool for detecting pulmonary nodules. Importantly, there are only two accepted radiographic criteria for a benign solitary pulmonary nodule on conventional radiographs: lack of interval growth for at least two years and the identification of a benign calcification pattern within a smoothly marginated pulmonary nodule.

Comparison with prior studies is essential for determining two-year stability. If prior radiographs are unavailable at the time of initial interpretation, all possible attempts should be made to procure them to allow for assessment of interval growth. Comparison with prior studies also allows one to estimate the growth rate of a nodule. The majority of malignant nodules have a nodule volume doubling time between 30 and 400 days. When estimating nodule growth rates, it is important to be aware of the relationship between diameter and nodule volume. For example, an increase in nodule diameter of only 25% results in a doubling of nodule volume.

There are four recognized benign patterns of calcification: diffuse, central, popcorn, and laminar calcification. Importantly, stippled and eccentric calcification patterns can be seen in up to 15% of malignant lung carcinomas and therefore are not indicative of a benign process. The latter calcification patterns are seen more frequently at computed tomography than at radiography, owing to the higher sensitivity of computed tomography for detecting small foci of calcification.

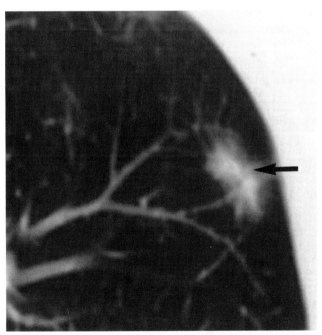

Figure 14-2 ■ Peripheral nodule on chest computed tomography. The presence of irregular and spiculated margins is highly predictive of a malignancy.

nancy. In contrast, benign nodules are usually characterized by smooth contours and well-defined margins; however, this appearance is not sufficient as a sole criterion for making a benign diagnosis. For example, pulmonary metastases are also often characterized by smooth contours and well-defined margins. Because lobulated contours can be seen in both benign and malignant conditions, this appearance should be considered indeterminate.

3. *Vascular and bronchial relationships.* The identification of a feeding artery and draining vein to a solitary nodular opacity is diagnostic of an arteriovenous malformation. In contrast, the identification of a systemic vascular supply from the aorta is diagnostic of a sequestration. Another important factor to consider is the relationship of a pulmonary nodule to the adjacent bronchi. The "positive bronchus" sign refers to the identification of a bronchus leading directly into a pulmonary nodule (Figure 14-3). The identification of air bronchograms within a lung nodule is more commonly associated with malignant nodules than with benign nodules, particularly if the observed bronchi are tortuous, ectatic, or abruptly cut off. The presence of focal bubblelike lucencies within a nodule has been referred to as *pseudocavitation* and is characteristic of bronchoalveolar cell carcinoma.

4. *Cavitation.* In general, cavitation is more frequently associated with malignant nodules than with benign nodules. The wall thickness of a cavity can be somewhat helpful in determining the likelihood of benignancy. Very thin-walled cavities (1- to 4-mm in diameter) are very often benign. Cavities with wall thickness between 5 mm and 15 mm should be considered indeterminate, and wall thickness greater than 15 mm is highly suggestive of malignancy.

5. *Density.* Computed tomography densitometry, which refers to computerized calculations of com-

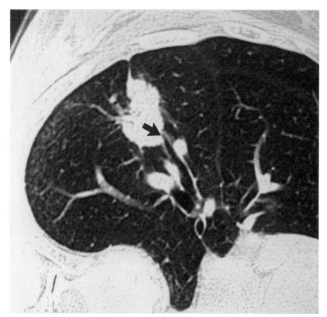

Figure 14-3 ■ A positive bronchus sign visualized on chest computed tomography.

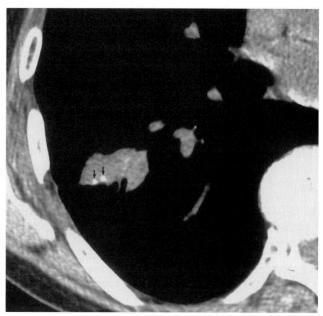

Figure 14-4 ■ Eccentric, stippled calcifications (arrows) within a lesion visualized on chest CT. This pattern does not rule out a malignant process.

puted tomography numbers within a nodule, can be quite helpful for confirming the presence of calcium and fat within a nodule (Figure 14-4). With regard to calcification, its presence or absence is considered the most important feature in distinguishing benign from malignant nodules. It is well recognized that computed tomography is more sensitive than conventional radiography for detecting calcification; moreover, thin-section computed tomography images are more sensitive than thick-section computed tomography images for this purpose. Although the presence of calcification is usually readily apparent by visual inspection of a thin-section computed tomography image, a pixelogram can be obtained for confirmation by placing a cursor over the lesion. Values greater than +200 Hounsfield units are indicative of the presence of calcification. The most reliable indicator of benignancy is the presence of diffuse calcification.

The identification of fat within a solitary pulmonary nodule is suggestive of a benign process such as hamartoma or lipoid pneumonia. With regard to hamartomas, they are the most common benign pulmonary neoplasms. Hamartomas can frequently be diagnosed with computed tomography by the identification of focal or diffuse fat attenuation, a combination of fat and calcification, or a diffuse "popcorn" pattern of calcification. The detection of fat by visual inspection can be con-

firmed with a pixelogram to allow for a confident diagnosis.

Specific Benign Diagnoses Using Traditional Imaging Methods

An assessment of the morphologic and densitometric features of a solitary pulmonary nodule may allow for a specific benign diagnosis to be made in a majority of cases of granuloma, hamartoma, round atelectasis, mucoid impaction, arteriovenous malformation, and pulmonary sequestration. All nodules that do not clearly meet the computed tomography criteria for a specific benign process should be considered indeterminate.

New Imaging Methods: Computed Tomography Enhancement and Positron Emission Tomography Imaging

Computed Tomography Enhancement

Computed tomography nodule enhancement relies on the principle that neoplastic nodules are more vascular than are benign nodules. In a study of 356 nodules, computed tomography nodule enhancement demonstrated a sensitivity of 98% and a specificity of 58%, and it was concluded that the absence of significant lung enhancement (less than 15 computed tomography number units) strongly predicts benignity.

DIAGNOSIS

Approach to a Patient with an Indeterminate Pulmonary Nodule

When one is faced with a patient with indeterminate pulmonary nodule on chest radiography or computed tomography scan, an attempt to review previous imaging studies is mandatory. If the lesion is stable over time, no further invasive workup is indicated. The criteria for benignity on chest computed tomography scan and individual risk factors as determined by patient history and physical examination should be taken into account in assessing the risk for the lesion's being malignant. If there is a high likelihood of cancer and the patient is a good surgical candidate, our preferred approach is surgical biopsy and, if indicated, resection. In the patient with increased surgical risk and lower likelihood of the lesion's being malignant, we usually perform additional imaging, such as positron emission tomography, or perform less invasive diagnostic maneuvers as dictated by the location of the lesion. This approach avoids unnecessary surgical procedures in this patient population.

The use of computed tomography nodule enhancement requires rigorous adherence to the study protocol, which employs the use of serial spiral computed tomography acquisitions before and after the intravenous administration of nonionic contrast. Postinjection scans are performed at one-minute intervals for four minutes following contrast administration, and nodule enhancement is determined by obtaining a region of interest within the nodule center.

It is important to be aware that there are specific nodule requirements for this protocol. Nodules should be relatively spherical in shape and homogeneous in appearance, without evidence of necrosis, calcification, cavitation, or fat. Moreover, patients should be able to perform reproducible breath-holds.

At present, the role of this technique is evolving. Although its strong negative predictive value is quite helpful in nodule management, the specificity of this test for malignancy is less than ideal.

Positron Emission Tomography Imaging

Positron emission tomography imaging employs the use of F-18 fluorodeoxyglucose, a radiolabeled D-glucose analog, to assess the metabolic activity of a pulmonary nodule (Figure 14-5). This technique relies on the well-known principle that neoplastic cells demonstrate increased glucose metabolism compared to normal tissues and most benign processes. Numerous investigators have shown that positron emission tomography–fluorodeoxyglucose (PET-FDG) imaging differentiates malignant and benign nodules with a high degree of accuracy. Although the reported sensitivity and specificity of positron emission tomography–fluorodeoxyglucose imaging of solitary pulmonary nodules have been uniformly high, this technique is not without limitations. For example, false-positive results may be encountered in cases of active granulomatous infections such as tuberculosis, and false-negative results may be encountered with bronchoalveolar cell carcinoma and carcinoid tumors.

State-of-the-art dedicated positron emission tomography scanners can reliably assess nodules as small as 7 mm in diameter. As positron emission tomography imaging becomes more widely accessible, its role in the assessment of solitary pulmonary nodules will likely increase in coming years.

Biopsy Methods

Definitive diagnosis can be established only by obtaining cytologic or histologic specimens. If a positive benign diagnosis is established, thoracotomy or thoracoscopy can be avoided. Biopsies are considered for indeterminate nodules. Nodules that are most likely

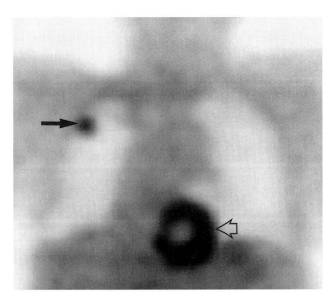

Figure 14-5 ■ Anterior-posterior positive positron emission tomography image of the chest in a patient with a right upper lobe nodule.

malignant should undergo surgical resection; nodules that have a very low likelihood of being malignant should be followed radiographically.

Transthoracic needle biopsy is usually performed under imaging (mainly computed tomography) guidance. The sensitivity for identifying a malignant nodule is higher than that for determining a benign diagnosis and may reach 95% for peripheral malignant nodules. False-negative results appear to depend on technique, and rates up to 30% have been described. The main complication of transthoracic needle biopsy is a pneumothorax. Risk factors for pneumothorax include more central lesions and the presence of emphysema, among others.

Larger nodules, especially if they exhibit a positive bronchus sign, may be amenable to bronchoscopy with transbronchial biopsy. The yield of this procedure depends on the location of the nodule and its size. Lesions less than 2 cm in diameter located in the outer third of the lung have the lowest yield. Conversely, central and large lesions are well accessed and the diagnosis is determined with a high sensitivity. This makes a bronchoscopic approach attractive for those lesions, as transthoracic needle biopsy and surgical resections are more difficult in more central regions of the lung. Complication rates are generally less than those that occur with transthoracic needle biopsy. Newer ultrathin bronchoscopes that reach airways beyond the ninth generation are being evaluated, and they may show promise in reaching, visualizing, and biopsying peripheral pulmonary nodules without the need for transbronchial biopsy or general anesthesia.

Thoracoscopy or thoracotomy is indicated for the resection of pulmonary nodules that are malignant or highly likely to be malignant, if there are no medical contraindications and the patient wishes to proceed. Video-assisted thoracoscopy is associated with a low morbidity and short hospital stay in selected patients.

Generally, the mortality rate for resection of malignant pulmonary nodules by thoracotomy is around 3%, and that for benign lesions is around 1%. A biopsy with frozen section may be performed and a resection as indicated and if possible can then be performed as dictated by the patients' clinical status. Persistent air leaks and incomplete lung reexpansion are the most common complications.

The treatment of patients with solitary pulmonary nodules following biopsy or resection is totally dependent on the histologic diagnosis. The management of patients who have been determined to have primary lung cancer is described in Chapters 94 and 95.

Suggested Reading

Al-Sugair A, Coleman RE: Applications of PET in lung cancer. Semin Nucl Med 1998;28:303–319.

Boiselle PM, Ernst A, Karp DD: Lung cancer detection in the 21st century: Potential contributions and challenges of emerging technologies. Am J Roentgenol 2000;175:1215–1221.

Coleman RE: PET in lung cancer. J Nucl Med 1999;40:814-820.

Erasmus JJ, Connolly JE, McAdams HP, Roggli VL: Solitary pulmonary nodules: Part I. Morphologic evaluation for differentiation of benign and malignant lesions. Radiographics 2000;20:43–58.

Erasmus JJ, McAdams HP, Connolly JE: Solitary pulmonary nodules: Part II. Evaluation of the indeterminate nodule. Radiographics 2000;20:59–66.

Henschke CI, McCauley DI, Yankelevitz DF, et al: Early lung cancer action project: Overall design and findings from baseline screening. Lancet 1999;354:99–105.

McLoud TC (ed): Thoracic Radiology: The Requisites. St. Louis: Mosby, 1998, 340–343.

Ost D, Fein A: Evaluation and management of the solitary pulmonary nodule. Am J Respir Crit Care Med 2000;162:782–787.

Swensen SJ, Viggiano RW, Midthun DE, et al: Lung nodule enhancement at CT: Multicenter study. Radiol 2000; 214:73–80.

Chapter 15
Pleural Effusion

Scott Swanson and Hasan F. Batirel

Introduction

Pleural effusion results from the imbalance between secretion and absorption of pleural fluid. Annually, more than one million patients are expected to present with a pleural effusion. A wide variety of diseases, both pulmonary and nonpulmonary in origin, manifest with pleural effusion.

Pleural fluid is generated from parietal pleura as well as interstitial spaces. The rate of pleural fluid entry into the pleural space has been calculated to be 0.01 mL/kg per hour in a 30-kg sheep, but this rate can increase by 20-fold with a change in physiologic conditions. Parietal pleural lymphatics will absorb the fluid at a rate of 0.20 mL/kg per hour. A very small amount of fluid is thought to circulate through the visceral pleura. A 70-kg man can absorb 500 mL of pleural fluid per day via lymphatic channels.

The pathophysiologic mechanism of fluid accumulation varies according to the primary etiology. An increase in pleural fluid formation or a decrease in lymphatic clearance will cause accumulation of fluid inside the pleural cavity. Increased pulmonary capillary wedge pressure as seen in congestive heart failure, increased systemic venous pressure as seen in superior vena cava syndrome, or decreased serum albumin as seen in cirrhosis cause an imbalance in hydrostatic and oncotic pressures in the pleural cavity, resulting in fluid accumulation. Abdominal diseases that cause ascites can also lead to fluid accumulation in the pleural cavity, the fluid passing through transdiaphragmatic channels. Malignant disease causes pleural effusion by increasing fluid production due to pleural tumor implants or by decreasing absorption due to lymphatic or bronchial obstruction. Malignant effusion can also result from other effects of a tumor, such as hypoalbuminemia or tumor embolus to the pulmonary artery. Radiation therapy and some of the chemotherapeutic agents (methotrexate, cyclophosphamide, and bleomycin) may cause pleuritis and associated effusion by inducing pleural fibrosis.

Differential Diagnosis

The causes of pleural effusion can be divided into two groups; they are due to either benign (Table 15-1) or malignant disease (Table 15-2) processes. Most of the patients complain of dyspnea and pleuritic pain. Cough is often reported, particularly when the effusion is sizable.

Overall, congestive heart failure is the most common cause of a pleural effusion. Forty percent of patients with congestive heart failure develop pleural effusion. The effusion tends to be bilateral and generally equal in size. It is due to left-sided heart failure, which causes an elevated pulmonary capillary wedge pressure and hence leakage of excessive fluid from lung interstitium. A second common cause of a benign pleural effusion is parapneumonic effusion, which may occur in 40% to 60% of all patients with pneumonia. Other causes of benign pleural effusion include nephrotic syndrome and hepatic hydrothorax. Hepatic hydrothorax is typically right-sided and may vary from small to massive in size. In 10% of benign pleural effusions, no definite cause can be identified.

Malignant tumors are often associated with a pleural effusion and must always be considered in the differential diagnosis. Every tumor that has the capability to metastasize or that arises from a structure adjacent to or involving the pleural space can cause a malignant effusion. Malignant effusions in general are more likely to be associated with symptoms than are benign effusions. Chest pain, weakness, and weight loss are common presenting complaints. Lung carcinoma is by far the most common cause of a malignant pleural effusion. The next most common is breast carcinoma, which accounts for 25% of malignant pleural effusions. Other malignancies include lymphomas, abdominal tumors such as gastric and ovarian carcinomas, and mesothelioma.

Table 15-1 ■ Causes of Benign Pleural Effusions

Cardiopulmonary Pathologies

Congestive heart failure
Pericardial disease (constrictive pericarditis)
Superior vena cava obstruction
Pulmonary emboli
Sarcoidosis
Pulmonary infections
Asbestos exposure

Abdominal Pathologies

Cirrhosis
Nephrotic syndrome
Peritoneal dialysis
Gastrointestinal diseases (esophageal perforation, pancreatic disease, intra-abdominal
    abscesses, diaphragmatic hernia)
Radiation therapy
Drug-induced pleural disease (nitrofurantoin, dantrolene, methysergide, bromocriptine,
    procarbazine, amiodarone, methotrexate, bleomycin)

Systemic Pathologies

Collagen vascular diseases:
    Rheumatoid arthritis
    Systemic lupus erythematosus
    Drug-induced lupus erythematosus
    Sjögren's syndrome
    Wegener's granulomatosis
    Churg-Strauss syndrome

Radiology

The first diagnostic tool for the workup of a malignant pleural effusion is a chest X-ray. Most cases of pleural effusion will be seen clearly on chest X-ray because only 200 to 300 mL of fluid is needed to cause blunting of the costophrenic angle. However, in cases in which the presence of an effusion is unclear (atelectasis, pneumonia, pleural scarring versus pleural effusion), a lateral decubitus chest X-ray and ultrasonogram can assist in the diagnosis by more precisely demonstrating the exact location and amount of the

pleural fluid. As little as 50 to 100 mL of pleural fluid can be seen on a lateral decubitus chest X-ray.

With the advent and widespread availability of computed tomography (CT), a chest computed tomography scan is often the next test obtained after a chest X-ray. A chest computed tomography scan will give precise, comprehensive, anatomic information about the effusion and the condition of the associated lung, mediastinal structures, and chest wall involvement in case of a tumor. It is difficult to evaluate loculated fluid collections adjacent to the mediastinal surface of the lung or those from chest wall disease without a computed tomography scan. Chest computed tomography is not operator dependent as is the case with an ultrasonographic evaluation.

Radiologic studies will not be able to distinguish the etiology of the effusion. If an obvious tumor is noted, then an associated malignant pleural effusion is likely.

Interventional Procedures

Where pleural effusion is found on the X-ray, invariably a diagnostic, or if the patient has severe dyspnea due to massive pleural effusion, therapeutic thoracen-

---

Table 15-2 ■ Most Common Causes of Malignant Pleural Effusions

Lung carcinoma	Pancreatic cancer
Breast cancer	Carcinoid
Ovarian carcinoma	Mesothelioma
Hodgkin's lymphoma	Esophageal carcinoma
Non-Hodgkin's lymphoma	Thymic carcinomas
Gastric cancer	Thoracic sarcomas
Hepatic cancer	Head and neck cancers

tesis is indicated. If the fluid is loculated, the site should be marked via ultrasonography or computed tomography scan to maximize the chances of a successful tap and minimize complications. Thoracentesis with a large-bore (17-gauge) needle is performed under local anesthesia. The most common site for a freely flowing moderate or large effusion is in the midscapular line in the sixth or seventh intercostal space. The procedure is usually performed with the patient seated on a bed or stretcher leaning slightly forward with his or her elbows resting on a pillow situated on a small table. If the patient is unable to sit up, then the patient may be positioned in the decubitus position with the side of the effusion down. For a therapeutic thoracentesis, a large amount (greater than 2 L) of fluid should be aspirated slowly, typically over 1 hour to prevent reexpansion pulmonary edema.

If the thoracentesis is nondiagnostic, closed pleural biopsies or surgical biopsy (either via pleuroscopy or video-assisted thoracic surgery) can establish an exact histologic diagnosis. The diagnostic accuracy of a closed pleural biopsy is 39% to 75%, thoracentesis is 40% to 87%, and accuracy with video-assisted thoracic surgery is close to 100%. If a surgical resection is contemplated, then a surgical biopsy should be done because it is the most dependable way to distinguish the exact etiology of the malignancy (i.e., adenocarcinoma versus mesothelioma).

Fluid Analysis

The analysis of the pleural fluid can classify an effusion as a transudate or an exudate. The combination of fluid characteristics will suggest either a benign or a malignant etiology (Table 15-3).

Initial thoracentesis fluid should be sent for glucose, amylase, protein, and lactate dehydrogenase (LDH) levels. In addition, pH, differential cell count, microbiologic cultures, Gram stain, and cytologic

analysis should be obtained. Further tests can be done to assess other pathologies such as tuberculosis, systemic vascular diseases, and chylothorax. At least 50 mL of fluid should be aspirated to have an adequate sample for these tests.

Malignant effusions are exudative in nature. The relative protein level is more than 0.5 (pleura/serum), and the lactic acid dehydrogenase ratio exceeds 0.6 (pleura/serum). Grossly bloody fluid is suggestive of a malignant effusion, though it is also seen with a pulmonary embolism. A serosanguinous fluid does not exclude malignancy, as in the case of mesothelioma that frequently causes a more uniformly serous-appearing fluid. In 20% of patients, the glucose level may be low, and this predicts poor patient prognosis, possibly due to increased tumor burden.

Management

Figure 15-1 shows a schematic approach to the diagnosis and treatment of pleural edema.

Benign Pleural Effusion

Benign pleural effusions (see Table 15-1) are generally secondary to systemic disease or thoracic infection, so treatment of the primary condition or disease typically resolves the effusion. In congestive heart failure, increasing left heart performance decreases the amount of fluid around the lungs. If the fluid is extensive and causes shortness of breath, a therapeutic thoracentesis is indicated. Parapneumonic effusions are reabsorbed after antibiotic treatment. Empyemas should be drained and treated with antibiotics as an initial step.

Malignant Pleural Effusion

Management of malignant pleural effusion can be a challenge (Figures 15-2, 15-3, and 15-4). Patients with malignant pleural effusion have a diminished life expectancy. In a series by Chernow and Sahn, the average life expectancy of these patients was 3.1 ± 0.5 months with a median survival of 2.2 months. The mortality rate was 54% within the first months and 84% at six months. Therefore there are two major concerns in the management of pleural effusion: to relieve the patient of his or her dyspnea and simultaneously to optimize the quality of the remaining life.

The histology and site of the tumor causing the pleural effusion affect treatment. Pleural effusions associated with lymphoma resolve very quickly with chemotherapy or mediastinal irradiation. Small-cell lung carcinomas respond well to chemotherapy, and the fluid resolves rapidly. Unfortunately, these malignancies are less common in patients with pleural

Table 15-3 ■ Pleural Fluid Characteristics in Benign and Malignant Pleural Effusion

	Benign[†]	Malignant
Cytology	Benign cells	Malignant cells
Color	Serous	Serosanguinous
Protein*	Low (<0.5)	High (≥0.5)
LDH*	Low (<0.6)	High (≥0.6)
Cells/μL	Low (<1000)	High (≥1000)
Glucose (mg/dL)	Normal/High (≥40)	Low (<40)

[†]Empyema can have fluid characteristics similar to those of a malignant effusion.
* Ratio of the concentrations in pleura/serum.

**PATIENT WITH SHORTNESS OF BREATH,
PLEURITIC PAIN AND/OR COUGH**

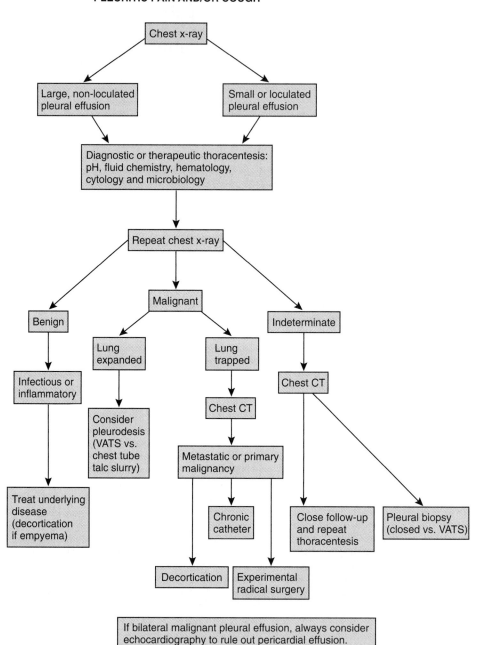

Figure 15-1 ■ Diagnostic and treatment approach to a patient with pleural effusion.

effusion than are non-small-cell lung and breast carcinomas, which often pose a management dilemma.

Different treatment modalities can be used in these more common etiologies with varying success rates:

1. Chest tube. Simple chest tube drainage is successful in preventing fluid reaccumulation in only 20% of malignant pleural effusion patients.

Therefore pleurodesis with a chemical agent such as talc is generally added to this treatment option. When placing a chest tube, one should be well aware of the status of the underlying lung. If the lung is trapped, chest tube drainage will not allow the lung to fully reexpand, which is the critical issue necessary for successful pleurodesis.

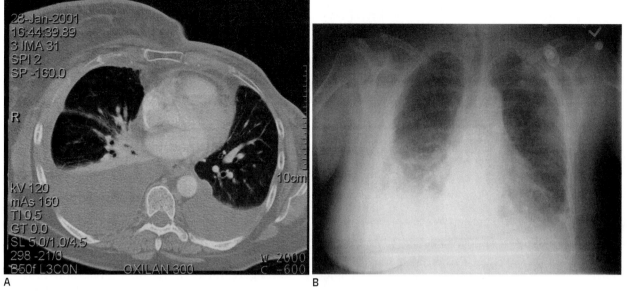

Figure 15-2 ■ A 54-year-old woman with a history of breast carcinoma. She now presents with shortness of breath. *A*, Chest computed tomography scan showed bilateral pleural effusion (right > left). *B*, Talc pleurodesis was performed via thoracoscopy, which resulted in mild postoperative interstitial edema.

2. Pleurodesis via chest tube or video-assisted thoracic surgery. If the repeat chest X-ray after an initial therapeutic thoracentesis demonstrates full lung expansion (see Figure 15-3), pleurodesis should be performed to achieve a long-term palliation due to the high rate (greater than 80%) of recurrent effusion. In case of bilateral malignant effusion (see Figure 15-2), the side with more fluid should be drained initially, and pleurodesis should rarely be performed simultaneously to

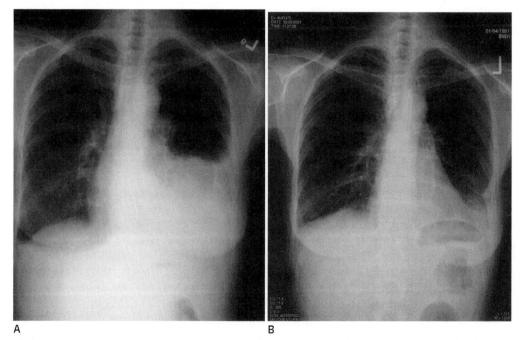

Figure 15-3 ■ A 50-year-old woman operated on two years ago due to cervical cancer was admitted with shortness of breath and dyspnea on exertion. *A*, An initial chest X-ray shows moderate-sized left pleural effusion. *B*, Therapeutic thoracentesis was performed to relieve her dyspnea. The lung was fully expanded after thoracentesis. Talc pleurodesis was performed one week later owing to recurrence of her effusion and was successful in obliterating pleural space.

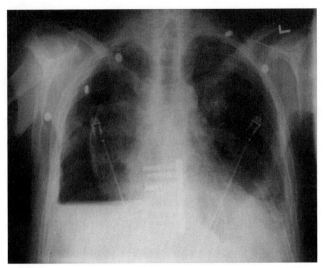

Figure 15-4 ■ A 36-year-old man with known stage IV non-small-cell lung cancer. Chest X-ray revealed trapped lung after thoracentesis. This patient was managed with a chronic pleural catheter.

avoid the possibility of bilateral adult respiratory distress syndrome (ARDS), which would be fatal. Pleurodesis can be performed via a bedside chest tube or in the operating room using video-assisted thoracic surgery. If the patient is concerned about pain, simple loculations need attention, or a biopsy is necessary, then the procedure should be performed in the operating room. A key factor in this decision is the patient's general condition and whether he or she will tolerate general anesthesia.

The aim of pleurodesis is to induce pleuritis and therefore obliterate any space in which fluid can reaccumulate. Pleurodesis was first discovered when nitrogen mustard was injected into the pleural cavity as a therapeutic drug in cases of malignant pleural effusion. Subsequently, new agents were introduced. Currently, talc, either insufflated or as slurry; tetracycline derivatives (doxycycline); and bleomycin are used with variable success. Talc is the most commonly used and the most effective. Insufflation of 3 to 6 g of talc via video-assisted thoracic surgery controls the malignant pleural effusions in 95% of patients. Talc slurry, 10 g of talc in 150 to 250 mL of saline, is also very effective, with a success rate of over 85%. In general, however, complications from talc are more common with doses over 4 g. We therefore limit talc to 4 g either in slurry form or when insufflated.

Talc slurry is done through a chest tube at the bedside with local anesthetic added to minimize discomfort. The chest tube is clamped for 2 hours while the patient is turned in different positions to achieve adequate distribution of the agent. Then the chest tube is drained and connected to 20-cm H_2O suction and maintained for 24 to 48 hours. The chest tube is generally removed at the end of 48 hours when the drainage is less than 200 mL per day.

Recently, a prospective trial through Cancer and Leukemia Group B (CALGB-9334) comparing these two techniques has been completed. The results comparing talc slurry at the bedside with video-assisted thoracic surgery talc insufflation are pending at this time but should be available in the near future.

Rarely, acute pneumonitis or adult respiratory distress syndrome (1% to 2%) may occur and can be difficult to treat, particularly if the contralateral lung is diseased. These complications are more likely to occur in patients with lymphangitic spread of the tumor. The blockage of lymphatic drainage by tumor may cause acute lung edema and injury if talc pleurodesis is attempted.

Other sclerosing agents are available in addition to talc. Doxycycline, an antibiotic, is effective in 60% to 70% of patients. Bleomycin, a chemotherapeutic agent, can be used with an overall success rate of 50% to 60%, but it is substantially more expensive than talc. A prospective study comparing talc, bleomycin, and tetracycline in malignant pleural effusions showed a successful pleurodesis rate of 97%, 64%, and 33% for these drugs, respectively. In the study mentioned above, talc was administered via thoracoscope, whereas bleomycin and tetracycline were given via chest tube.

3. Chronic indwelling pleural catheter. A chronic catheter should be considered for patients with a trapped lung due to visceral pleural thickening or extensive involvement of underlying lung tissue (see Figure 15-4). In these patients, simple chest tube insertion or pleurodesis via chest tube/video-assisted thoracic surgery is not successful because the lung does not reexpand to adhere to the parietal pleura. Options for this situation include decortication of the tumor rind that is trapping the lung (discussed in following sections) or a chronic drainage catheter. A Pleur-x (Denver Biomaterials, Golden, CO) catheter is inserted in the pleural space and tunneled through the subcutaneous tissue in a similar fashion to a chronic central intravenous line. The catheter is 8 French. Potential disadvantages are that it can become obstructed or infected, leading to an empyema. The patient is educated to drain the fluid every day or every other day. Early data suggest that it

is an effective, safe, and simple palliative option. In 100 patients recently reported by Putnam and colleagues from the MD Anderson Cancer Center, no mortality was seen due to the procedure. Morbidity was 19%, mainly the result of malfunction or infection (5% empyema rate). Sixty percent of the procedures were performed in an outpatient setting. The second type of catheter, the pleuroperitoneal shunt (Denver Biomaterials, Golden, CO), is placed subcutaneously and transfers fluid from the pleural to the peritoneal space. A button compression system is used to actively pump the fluid. This shunt requires significant patient education and, in addition, is not often used in the United States owing to its poor success rate. However, a group in London has reported 95% palliation with this catheter in 160 patients and recommends this method for cases of trapped lung.

4. Decortication and radical surgery. If the repeat chest X-ray shows partial lung expansion, decortication can also be considered in patients with relatively good medical condition and reasonable life expectancy. Decortication consists of surgical removal of the visceral and parietal pleura to free the trapped lung and achieve full lung expansion. Fry and Khandekar analyzed 24 patients with malignant pleural effusion who underwent partial pleurectomy. Successful pleurodesis was achieved in 21 patients (88%); the remaining three patients died owing to postoperative complications. Yim et al. reported a 100% success rate with partial thoracoscopic decortication in 16 patients; however, there was a 30% morbidity rate (bleeding and prolonged air leak). Decortication can be performed via a thoracotomy or video-assisted thoracic surgery in cases with a longer life expectancy and good general condition. Experimental surgical trials of radical extrapleural pneumonectomy for patients who have lung carcinoma with malignant pleural effusion are being carried out at centers in Japan and the United States. Preliminary information suggests that the technique is feasible and achieves excellent local control in a selected patient population.

In cases in which malignant mesothelioma is the cause of the malignant effusion, the treatment options in addition to those above include radical surgery with a more curative intent. In a series of 183 patients with malignant pleural mesothelioma by Sugarbaker et al., multimodality treatment including extrapleural pneumonectomy and adjuvant therapy resulted in 38% two-year and 15% five-year survival rates. The operative mortality was 3.8%. In a subgroup of patients with epithelial cell histology, negative resection margins and negative extrapleural lymph node status ($n = 31$), survival was 46% at five years, and median survival was fifty-one months. The poor prognostic factors were sarcomatoid cell type and extrapleural lymph node metastasis.

Suggested Reading

Chernow B, Sahn SA: Carcinomatous involvement of the pleura: An analysis of 96 patients. Am J Med 1977;63:695–702.

Fry WA, Khandekar JD: Partial pleurectomy for malignant pleural effusion. Ann Surg Oncol 1995;2(2):160–164.

Genc O, Petrou M, Ladas G, Goldstraw P: The long-term morbidity of pleuroperitoneal shunts in the management of recurrent malignant effusions. Eur J Cardiothorac Surg 2000;18:143–146.

Hartmann DL, Gaither JM, Kesler KA, et al: Comparison of insufflated talc under thoracoscopic guidance with standard tetracycline and bleomycin pleurodesis for control of malignant pleural effusions. J Thorac Cardiovasc Surg 1993;105:743–748.

Light RW: Malignant pleural effusions. In Pleural Diseases, 3rd ed. Baltimore: Williams and Wilkins, 1995, pp 94–116.

Putnam JB, Walsh GL, Swisher SG, Roth JA, Suell DM, Vaporciyan AA, Smythe WR, Merriman KW, DeFord LL: Outpatient management of malignant pleural effusion by a chronic indwelling pleural catheter. Ann Thorac Surg 2000;69(2):369–375.

Sahn SA: Diseases of the pleura and pleural space. In Baum GL, Crapo JD, Celli BR, Karlinsky JB: Textbook of Pulmonary Diseases, 6th ed. Philadelphia: Lippincott-Raven, 1998, pp 1483–1498.

Sugarbaker DJ, Flores RM, Jaklitsch MT, et al: Resection margins, extrapleural nodal status, and cell type determine postoperative long-term survival in trimodality therapy of malignant pleural mesothelioma: Results in 183 patients. J Thorac Cardiovasc Surg 1999;117(1):54–63.

Swanson SJ, Sugarbaker DJ: Surgery and pleural space: Fibrothorax, thoracoscopy and pleurectomy. In Baum GL, Crapo JD, Celli BR, Karlinsky JB: Textbook of Pulmonary Diseases, 6th ed. Philadelphia: Lippincott-Raven, 1998, pp 1499–1503.

Yim APC, Chung SS, Lee TW, et al: Thoracoscopic management of malignant pleural effusions. Chest 1996;109:1234–1238.

Chapter 16
Hilar and Mediastinal Adenopathy

Joseph LoCicero III

Enlarged lymph nodes in the mediastinum and the hilus of the lung are nonspecific findings that could represent anything from infection to cancer to a disease of unknown cause. Even with histopathologic evaluation of the enlarged nodes, the diagnosis may be elusive. Information gleaned from varied sources, including the patient's history and physical examination, the radiographic appearance and distribution of the nodes, and the pathologic and microbiologic evaluation, all combine to help the clinician arrive at a definitive diagnosis.

By standard convention, the hilar and mediastinal nodes are categorized by the American Joint Committee on Cancer (AJCC) classification of thoracic nodes. Figure 16-1 shows the location of the mediastinal and hilar nodes.

These include the upper and lower paratracheal nodes (stations 2 and 4), the subcarinal nodes (station 7), and the hilar nodes (station 10).

Clinical Presentation and Evaluation

Patients presenting with mediastinal adenopathy can display a variety of signs and/or symptoms. Symptoms typically relate directly to compression and/or impingement on adjacent structures. For example, compression of the airway by paratracheal lymph nodes may cause a chronic cough. Compression of the superior vena cava may lead to eyelid or facial edema, headaches, or plethora. Compression of the esophagus usually causes dysphagia but may mimic heartburn and reflux. Compression of the atria or pulmonary arteries may cause shortness of breath or dyspnea on exertion. Often, patients will have few if any symptoms relating to the enlargement of mediastinal nodes. Hilar adenopathy rarely causes symptoms but occasionally causes wheezing or dyspnea.

History remains the most important piece of information short of pathologic evaluation of the adenopathy. In addition to symptoms, obtaining travel history and potential exposure to granulomatous diseases is sometimes critical. Infectious diseases that commonly cause nodal enlargement leading to local problems are tuberculosis, histoplasmosis, and blastomycosis. A prior history of malignancy may be helpful, but few cause hilar or mediastinal adenopathy except for lymphoma, esophageal cancer, renal cell cancer, melanoma, and lung cancer.

Radiologic Evaluation

Clues to diagnosis can also be obtained from the radiologic appearance of these lesions. Computed tomography (CT) provides the most useful information in the evaluation of hilar and mediastinal adenopathy. To provide the most data and thus the best chance at diagnosis, the study should be performed with and without contrast. In a patient with a probable lung cancer, as in Figure 16-2, the presence of paratracheal nodes is highly suspicious for metastasis. Nodes larger than 1.2 mm in short axis, as seen on standard views of a computed tomography scan, probably contain cancer. However, in practice, any node larger than 8 mm should be evaluated.

Nodes in the mediastinum posterior to the airway may cause compression of the esophagus as in Figure 16-3. Such patients present with complaints of dysphagia. Although esophagram and esophagoscopy can be nondiagnostic in this scenario, computed tomography scans will demonstrate the mediastinal adenopathy.

When nodes are present in the paratracheal area and the hila of both lungs in an asymptomatic patient, as seen in Figure 16-4, the most common condition is sarcoidosis. This is particularly true if the nodes are not confluent but show some individual shape, even if they are contiguous. Much lower in the differential diagnosis for such a presentation is lymphoma. When mediastinal nodes are large and confluent without individual shape, as seen in Figure 16-5, one should have a much higher index of suspicion for lymphoma. Nodes in patients with lym-

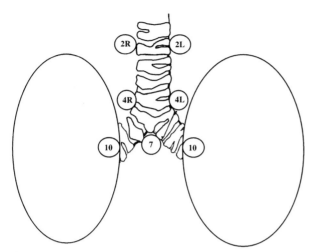

Figure 16-1 ■ Schematic drawing that demonstrates the nodal stations in the paratracheal (2 and 4), subcarinal (7), and hilar (10) regions.

phoma can reach considerable size without causing symptoms.

Often, the contrast phase of the computed tomography scan can be very helpful in evaluating mediastinal adenopathy. When mediastinal adenopathy reaches large proportions, the superior vena cava (SVC) may be compressed or obliterated. The contrast-enhanced computed tomography of the chest will often demonstrate the superior vena cava obstruction shown in Figure 16-6. Sometimes, benign conditions such as Castleman's disease may present with superior vena cava obstruction (Figure 16-7). In this situation,

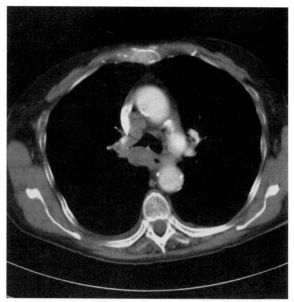

Figure 16-3 ■ This patient presented with dysphagia. The initial esophagram and esophagoscopy were nondiagnostic. The computed tomography demonstrated the mediastinal adenopathy both anterior and posterior to the airway and in proximity to the esophagus with no discernible lung lesion. In this case, the pathology was small-cell lung cancer.

the lymph nodes are highly vascular, and the contrast appears early in the nodes at about the same time as the aorta. This information is helpful not only in narrowing the differential diagnosis, but also in choosing the biopsy approach (see Chapter 17).

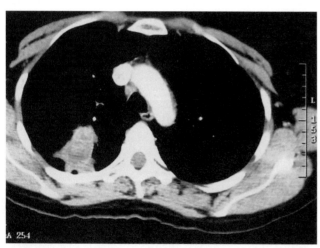

Figure 16-2 ■ Panel from the contrast phase of a standard computed tomography of the chest demonstrates a classic non-small-cell carcinoma with associated mediastinal adenopathy. The image clearly shows the cancer in the right upper lobe and shows an enlarged right paratracheal node (station 4R in Figure 16-1).

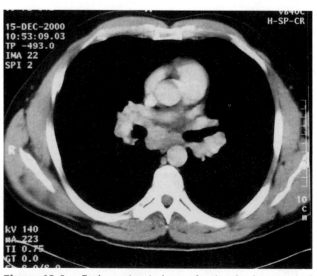

Figure 16-4 ■ Early contrast phase of a standard computed tomography of the chest demonstrating an abnormal number of enlarged hilar and mediastinal (subcarinal) lymph nodes in an asymptomatic patient. Biopsy by mediastinoscopy yielded a diagnosis of sarcoidosis.

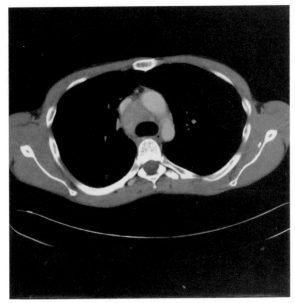

Figure 16-5 ■ Contrast phase of a standard computed tomography of the chest showing a homogeneous paratracheal mass. Biopsy demonstrated lymphoma.

Laboratory Evaluation

Laboratory investigations may make the diagnosis without resorting to invasive biopsies. In the case of suspicion for sarcoidosis, an elevated angiotensin-converting enzyme level may be sufficient for confirmation. In a young man with an unknown

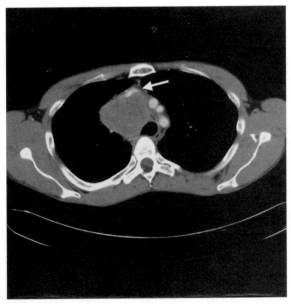

Figure 16-6 ■ Contrast phase of a standard computed tomography of the chest illustrating a large paratracheal mass compressing the superior vena cava (arrow). Biopsy yielded non-small-cell lung carcinoma.

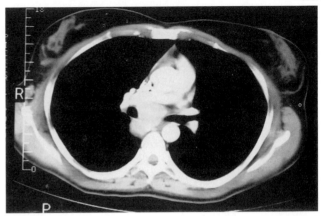

Figure 16-7 ■ Contrast phase of a standard computed tomography of the chest showing a mass, which has a similar density to the blood vessels. This suggests that the mass is highly vascular. The diagnosis confirmed at operation was Castleman's disease.

mediastinal mass, one should always obtain beta HCG and alpha-fetoprotein levels prior to biopsy or treatment, as elevated levels will point toward a diagnosis of a germ-cell tumor.

Diagnostic Procedures

The method for biopsy of hilar and mediastinal adenopathy should be tailored to the situation. It may be possible to arrive at a diagnosis with only minimal invasion and little added risk to the patient. Large masses in the anterior mediastinum are best approached by a radiologically guided needle biopsy. Large-bore needles are available for core biopsies so that histology as well as flow cytometry may be performed. Large nodes in proximity to the airway or the esophagus may be biopsied by using endoscopic methods. Diagnostic accuracy can be greatly enhanced through guidance with real-time computed tomography or ultrasound imaging, which ensures accurate needle placement in the mass. In many institutions, the cytologist will come to the endoscopy suite to perform the cytological evaluation immediately. This allows additional passes with the needle to ensure maximal yield. With a combination of these methods, it is much less common to need a surgical mediastinoscopy or a mediastinotomy to confirm the diagnosis.

Management

In addition to disease-specific therapy, urgent local treatment should be considered for alleviation of symptoms. The symptoms that require immediate attention are dyspnea and dysphagia. Venous obstruction may cause headaches, upper body edema, plethora, and dyspnea. Radiation will usually palliate

---

DIAGNOSIS

Biopsy of Hilar Mediastinal Adenopathy

Hilar adenopathy with no associated lung lesions is likely to be caused by benign disease. The most common disease identified in this setting is sarcoidosis.

Evaluation includes a careful history to identify constitutional symptoms of sarcoidosis, a computed tomography with contrast, pulmonary function tests (with diffusion capacity), and a determination of the serum level of angiotensin-converting enzyme.

Biopsy is not often needed but can be provided through minimally invasive tests such as bronchoscopy with transbronchial biopsy and/or transtracheal needle biopsy. Only under rare circumstances is it necessary to perform a mediastinoscopy.

DIAGNOSIS

Mediastinal Adenopathy

Mediastinal adenopathy with no associated lung lesions most often is due to a malignancy. The most common etiologies are lymphoma and small-cell lung cancer.

Evaluation includes a careful history to identify constitutional symptoms and a computed tomography with contrast.

Biopsy is needed to direct therapy. Depending on location, a radiologically directed needle biopsy with the help of cytopathology may make the diagnosis. Other tests include bronchoscopy with transtracheal needle biopsy and surgical mediastinal exploration.

---

these symptoms, but if dyspnea is very significant, immediate placement of an airway stent may be necessary. After radiation has taken effect, the stent can sometimes be removed. Of less immediate concern is esophageal obstruction, which can be managed with esophageal stent placement prior to completion of radiation therapy when causing significant symptoms.

Suggested Reading

Roth JA, Ruckdeschel JC, Weisenberger TH: Thoracic Oncology, 2nd ed. Philadelphia: WB Saunders, 1995.

Shields TW, LoCicero J, Ponn R: General Thoracic Surgery, 5th ed. Philadelphia: Lippincott Williams & Wilkins, 2000.

Chapter 17
Superior Vena Cava Syndrome

Tracey Evans and Thomas J. Lynch Jr.

When blood flow from the superior vena cava to the right atrium is obstructed, the result is a constellation of symptoms and signs known as superior vena cava syndrome. Over the course of the past century, the causes of superior vena cava syndrome obstruction have changed from primarily infectious to overwhelmingly malignant. Cancer causes 90% of the 15,000 estimated cases of superior vena cava in the United States per year. Often, superior vena cava syndrome is a patient's first sign or symptom of malignancy. Making a correct diagnosis and initiating therapy in a timely fashion are essential for optimal management of the superior vena cava syndrome.

Classically, the superior vena cava syndrome was considered to be an oncologic emergency requiring immediate radiation therapy, frequently before a firm diagnosis could be established. Clinicians feared that superior vena cava obstruction would rapidly lead to cerebral and laryngeal edema and would thereby cause irreversible neurologic damage and respiratory failure. Invasive procedures presented increased risk to the acutely ill patient with superior vena cava obstruction who could not tolerate the delay in treatment required for a diagnostic workup. Furthermore, radiation was the standard of care for the malignancies most likely to produce superior vena cava syndrome, and few alternatives were available.

We now know that superior vena cava obstruction is not rapidly fatal and that diagnostic procedures do not carry prohibitive risk. In addition, modern chemotherapy can improve outcomes in many patients with superior vena cava syndrome. For some, the appropriate chemotherapy can result in cure. Patients with the superior vena cava syndrome are typically in great physical distress and oftentimes are just learning that a malignancy is the cause of their discomforts. Compassion dictates a rapid and accurate diagnosis so that optimal treatment can proceed.

Anatomy

The superior vena cava is easily obstructed secondary to its anatomy. It is a large, low-pressure, compressible vessel within the middle mediastinum (Figure 17-1). The joining of the right and left brachiocephalic veins forms the beginning of the superior vena cava, which then extends for 6 to 8 cm before terminating in the right atrium. The distal 2 cm are located within the pericardial sac. The azygos vein opens into the superior vena cava posteriorly just above the pericardial reflection. Pathology in a number of strategic places can obstruct blood flow. The trachea, right bronchus, pulmonary artery, and aorta surround the superior vena cava. The thymus is located directly anterior to the superior vena cava, as is a goiter with substernal extension. The subcarinal, perihilar, and paratracheal lymph nodes abut the superior vena cava. These lymph nodes drain the right lung and the lower lobe of the left lung.

If a superior vena cava obstruction progresses sufficiently slowly for collateral systems to mature, symptoms may be minimal. The azygos system is the most important collateral circulation in superior vena cava obstruction, and the site of obstruction relative to the azygos vein also contributes to the severity of symptoms. If the obstruction occurs above the level where blood from the azygos vein enters the superior vena cava, venous drainage from the upper body can continue to flow into the distal superior vena cava and into the right atrium through the azygos vein. If the obstruction is located below the junction of the superior vena cava and azygos vein, blood flows retrograde through the azygos system and ultimately into the inferior vena cava. However, if, as in most cases, the azygos system is involved in the obstruction, blood flow from the upper body must find alternative pathways to the inferior vena cava. These pathways include the internal mammary veins, lateral thoracic veins, paraspinous veins, subcutaneous veins, and, rarely, esophageal varices.

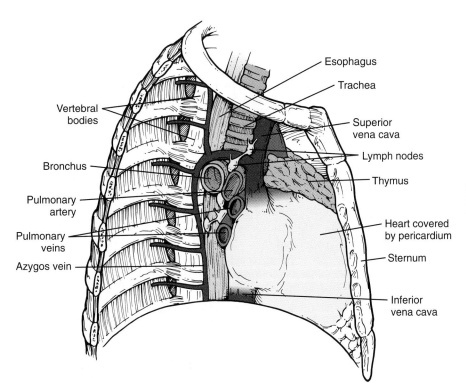

Figure 17-1 ■ The right side of the mediastinum with the right lung removed.

The Causes of Superior Vena Cava Syndrome

The shift from infectious to malignant causes for superior vena cava syndrome over the past 50 years is a result of better antibiotic therapy and the dramatic rise in the incidence of lung cancer. In a review of 250 cases in the literature from 1904 to 1946, primary intrathoracic tumors accounted for 36% of the cases, aortic aneurysms for 30%, and mediastinitis for 15%. Syphilis was the cause of superior vena cava syndrome via mediastinitis or aortic aneurysm in 35%. More recent series have found that malignancy causes superior vena cava obstruction in more than 90% of cases (Table 17-1). Lung cancer, either as a primary tumor or more often through mediastinal nodal spread, accounts for the great majority of all cases of superior vena cava syndrome. While only 20% of all cases of lung cancer are small cell, in some series, this histology accounts for up to 50% of cases of superior vena cava obstruction due to lung cancer. Approximately 8% of patients with small cell lung cancer and 4% of patients with non–small cell lung cancer (NSCLC) develop superior vena cava syndrome at some point in their disease. Lymphoma is the second most common cause of superior vena cava and most cases are due to large-cell and lymphoblastic subtypes. Hodgkin's disease and follicular lymphoma are rare causes. Approximately 4% of all cases of lymphoma result in superior vena cava syndrome.

Malignancies other than lung cancer and lymphoma account for about 10% of cases of superior vena cava syndrome. The most common of these is metastatic breast cancer. While thymomas are rare tumors, a significant proportion of patients with locally advanced thymomas present with superior vena cava syndrome. Other malignant causes of superior vena cava syndrome include germ-cell tumors, esophageal cancer, metastatic gastrointestinal and genitourinary tumors, and melanoma.

There are several important nonmalignant causes of superior vena cava syndrome. Superior vena cava

Table 17-1 ■ Etiologies of Superior Vena Cava Obstruction

Malignancy	95%
Lung cancer	65%
Lymphoma	15%
Breast cancer	5%
Germ-cell	2%
Thymic cancer	2%
Other cancer	4%
Benign	**5%**
Central venous device related	1%
Mediastinal fibrosis	3%

obstruction secondary to thrombosis or fibrosis in association with central venous catheters and pacemaker wires has been increasing in frequency over the past two decades. Given the frequency with which implantable catheters are used for administration of chemotherapy, catheter-related complications are an increasingly common cause of superior vena cava obstruction in patients with known active malignancies. Therefore cancer patients with catheters require confirmation that tumor is the cause of superior vena cava obstruction prior to undergoing antineoplastic treatment.

In pediatric cases, superior vena cava obstructions most commonly follow cardiovascular surgery to correct congenital heart defects. Mediastinal tumors, usually non-Hodgkin's lymphoma, are the second most frequent etiology. It is estimated that obstruction of the superior vena cava occurs in 5% of children with non-Hodgkin's lymphoma. Other tumors that can present with superior vena cava obstruction in the pediatric population are acute lymphoblastic leukemia, Hodgkin's disease, and neuroblastoma. Tracheal compression occurs with increased frequency in children with mediastinal tumors. The term "superior mediastinal syndrome" describes the clinical scenario in which a mediastinal tumor produces both superior vena cava obstruction and tracheal compression. Mediastinal fibrosis secondary to histoplasmosis is the third most common cause of superior vena cava syndrome in children.

Clinical Presentation

Patients with superior vena cava obstruction present with swelling of the head, face, and neck; a feeling of fullness (or suffusion); and dyspnea (Figure 17-2). Symptoms are frequently worse with lying down or bending over. Edema of the arms is also commonly seen. Less frequent symptoms include cough, chest pain, hemoptysis, and headache. Symptoms may be due to the underlying malignancy rather than to superior vena cava obstruction per se. Weight loss, for example, is also a common complaint of superior vena cava syndrome patients but is most certainly a result of the underlying malignancy. The duration of symptoms can be a clue to the underlying etiology. Benign causes can develop slowly over years, while sudden onset of symptoms most likely includes an element of thrombosis.

The most common physical findings in the patient with superior vena cava syndrome are dilated neck veins, facial edema, dilated chest wall veins, upper extremity swelling, and cyanosis secondary to venous engorgement. The striking change in appearance secondary to edema can be difficult to appreciate if the observer has not seen the patient prior to venous obstruction. Viewing an old photograph such as a driver's license can be helpful. The diagnosis is generally easy to make on history and physical exam alone. Superior vena cava syndrome can be distinguished from congestive heart failure and cardiac tamponade by the lack of any lower extremity edema. In subtle

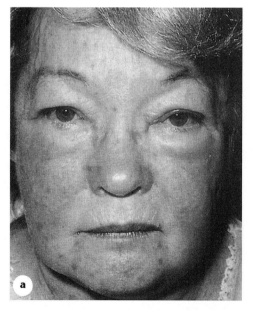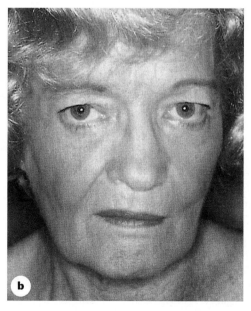

Figure 17-2 ■ Squamous cell carcinoma causing superior vena cava syndrome. *A,* Marked facial edema and plhethera. *B,* Postradiation therapy. (From Skarin AT [ed]: Atlas of Diagnostic Oncology, 2nd ed. St. Louis, MO: Mosby, 1996, p 88.)

cases of superior vena cava syndrome, Pemberton's sign (increased facial suffusion with elevation of the arms) can confirm the diagnosis. Signs and symptoms of respiratory obstruction or neurologic dysfunction such as stridor, wheezing, obtundation, or seizures are rare but important to assess. It is in these cases that superior vena cava syndrome becomes a true emergency requiring immediate therapy. While theoretically, the vascular obstruction itself can cause respiratory obstruction via laryngeal edema, more commonly, a mediastinal mass causes central airway compression in addition to superior vena cava syndrome. Similarly, neurologic symptoms can be a result of increased intracranial pressure from vascular obstruction, but the clinician must rule out other complications of malignancy such as brain metastases or hypercalcemia.

Diagnostic Evaluation

Chest X-rays in patients with superior vena cava syndrome are usually abnormal. A widened superior mediastinum is the most common abnormality (Figure 17-3). Pleural effusions, usually on the right side, occur in many cases of superior vena cava obstruction. However, up to 16% of chest X-rays can be normal in the setting of obstruction of the superior vena cava either because of a benign etiology for the syndrome or, more commonly, because a thoracic malignancy is not well visualized.

Computed tomography scan is now the most often used modality for confirming the diagnosis of superior vena cava syndrome (Figure 17-4). Prior to the widespread use of computed tomography scanning, venography had been used to confirm the obstruction of blood flow within the superior vena cava. This is now rarely necessary. In a patient with clinical superior vena cava syndrome, the finding of a mass lesion compressing the superior vena cava or the presence of a clot in the superior vena cava is sufficient to establish the diagnosis of superior vena cava obstruction.

Is Superior Vena Cava Syndrome a Life-Threatening Oncologic Emergency?

Lokich and Goodman stated in a 1975 *JAMA* review of superior vena cava syndrome, "In our experience, the pitfalls in the management of superior vena cava syndrome relate to overzealous efforts to establish the site of obstruction and to determine a specific histopathologic diagnosis. These efforts . . . may lead to life-threatening complications, such as respiratory obstruction, aspiration, and hemorrhage." Statements such as these led to a widespread perception that still persists that superior vena cava syndrome is an oncologic emergency. Many published series of patients since then have established that the patient with superior vena cava syndrome is not in immediate danger. In a review of 90 publications encompassing 1986 cases of superior vena cava syndrome, only one death was thought to be secondary to the superior vena cava syndrome itself: a case in which death resulted from aspiration of uncontrolled epistaxis.

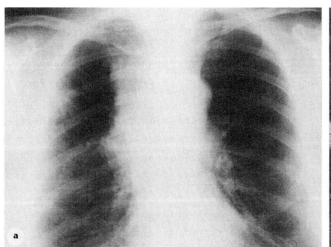 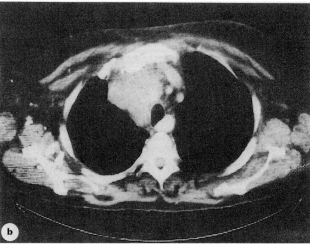

Figure 17-3 ■ Radiographs showing superior vena cava syndrome. *A,* Chest X-ray. *B,* CT scan. (From Skarin AT [ed]: Atlas of Diagnostic Oncology, 2nd ed. St. Louis, MO: Mosby, 1996, p 89.)

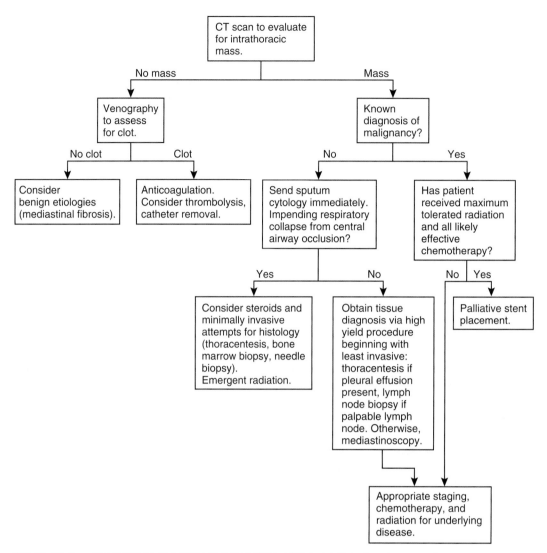

Figure 17-4 ■ Approach to the patient presenting with superior vena cava syndrome.

Managing Superior Vena Cava Syndrome in the Patient with Previously Known Malignancy

If the patient presenting with signs and symptoms of superior vena cava syndrome has a known diagnosis of an active malignancy as a likely etiology, appropriate therapy can proceed quickly without the need for obtaining additional tissue. In some instances in which a mediastinal mass is seen on computed tomography scan of a patient with a prior diagnosis of cancer, a positron emission tomography (PET) scan can confirm that the mass is active malignancy and not simply a residual posttherapy mass. For patients with responsive tumors such as small cell lung cancer or lym-

phoma, chemotherapy is a reasonable initial option. For patients in whom response to chemotherapy is unlikely, such as non–small cell lung cancer, radiation therapy is the standard of care. If the patient is unlikely to respond to chemotherapy and has received maximum radiation therapy, stent placement may be required to palliate symptoms. Patients with a known malignancy, however, may have superior vena cava secondary to thrombosis, especially if a central venous catheter is present. This may be particularly true if the computed tomography scan fails to show convincing evidence of tumor progression. For these patients, anticoagulation is essential. If symptoms fail to respond to anticoagulation, then catheter removal may be indicated.

Evaluating and Treating Superior Vena Cava Syndrome in a Patient without a Histologic Diagnosis

Two thirds of the patients who present with superior vena cava syndrome do not have a prior diagnosis of malignancy. These patients require a diagnostic workup with some urgency to establish a histologic diagnosis. It is critical to obtain adequate tissue prior to initiation of radiation therapy because radiation will frequently make interpretation of subsequent biopsy specimens impossible. This is less likely to be a problem for tumors such as non-small-cell lung cancer, since this tumor is less radiosensitive, and few patients with non-small-cell lung cancer who have this presentation will be cured. However, for germ-cell tumors, small-cell lung cancer, thymic carcinoma, and, most important, lymphomas, cure is possible, and it is critical to correctly diagnose the tumor. The chemotherapeutic strategies for a primary mediastinal germ-cell tumor are clearly different from those for a large-cell lymphoma. Furthermore, within the diagnosis of lymphoma, distinctions are significant: Burkitts-like lymphoma will have a different treatment approach than Hodgkin's disease.

There are multiple methods by which to make a histologic diagnosis in patients with superior vena cava obstruction, and the challenge lies in choosing the least invasive method that nonetheless has a high enough diagnostic yield that the patient may rapidly receive treatment (see Figure 17-4). Careful physical examination and review of radiographic images are essential in selecting the right approach. If the patient has a pleural effusion, thoracentesis can establish the diagnosis and ease dyspnea. Palpable lymph nodes or other easily accessible tissues are excellent sites for biopsy. Otherwise, it is our practice to proceed directly to mediastinoscopy.

Several recent series have established the safety and high diagnostic yield of mediastinoscopy in patients with superior vena cava obstruction. However, health care providers must pay careful attention to signs and symptoms of airway obstruction prior to the patient's receipt of general anesthesia. Partially obstructed airways can completely collapse when the negative intrathoracic pressure of spontaneous respiration keeping them open is replaced by positive pressure ventilation. Anesthetic relaxation of bronchial smooth muscle also contributes to airway obstruction. General anesthesia in the setting of airway obstruction can render ventilation impossible, and patients can die abruptly. High central venous pressures increase the risk of bleeding for patients with superior vena cava obstruction. For this reason, mediastinoscopy is often performed in the reverse Trendelenburg's position.

Masses causing superior vena cava obstruction are usually accessible high in the mediastinum, so distal dissection is unnecessary, and bleeding deep within the mediastinum is uncommon.

Given the simplicity of obtaining sputum for cytology, it is reasonable to send this test immediately while the patient is being readied for lymph node biopsy or mediastinoscopy. If sputum cytology provides a diagnosis, the more invasive procedures need take place only if required for appropriate staging. We would not recommend delaying higher-yield diagnostic procedures if sputum cytology cannot be obtained quickly or if the patient has any evidence of respiratory impairment or physical discomfort.

Treatment

Treatment of superior vena cava obstruction should be directed at the underlying cause. Symptomatic relief occurs within hours when a newly diagnosed lymphoma or small-cell lung cancer is treated with appropriate chemotherapy. For patients who experience rapid relief, often no additional therapy specific to the superior vena cava syndrome is necessary. If a patient is in significant discomfort or has evidence of respiratory compromise, it is often helpful to give two or three days of external beam radiation while initiating chemotherapy. Once symptoms are controlled, clinical considerations can determine whether to continue radiotherapy.

Radiation therapy is the standard of care for superior vena cava obstruction caused by relatively chemotherapy-resistant tumors such as non-small-cell lung cancer. Approximately 80% of patients with non-small-cell lung cancer will have improvement in symptoms with radiation therapy, most of these within two weeks. While there are reports of symptom resolution with chemotherapy alone in non-small-cell lung cancer, we do not recommend this approach as standard therapy, since response rates to modern chemotherapy regimens are at best 30%.

Between 10% and 20% of patients with superior vena cava syndrome due to lung cancer will have recurrence of superior vena cava obstruction symptoms following maximum radiation. Although survival in this setting is short, the symptoms are sufficiently distressing to warrant aggressive attempts at palliation.

Percutaneous stent placement is quite useful in this setting. It is technically successful in about 80% of cases, and relief of symptoms occurs promptly, usually within 72 hours. Venography is essential prior to stent placement. Oftentimes, if venography demonstrates a clot, stent placement follows thrombolysis. However, there are reports of successful procedures in which stents were placed across a clot, thereby wedging the clot against the wall of the superior vena cava. Tumor invasion of the superior vena cava and complete occlusion were once believed to be contraindications to stent placement, but stents have been successfully deployed in both settings. Possible complications of stent placement include stent migration, renal insufficiency from contrast dye, and perforation of the superior vena cava with resultant mediastinal hemorrhage and cardiac tamponade. Because stent placement is so rapidly effective, the increased venous return can lead to pulmonary edema. Stent reocclusion can occur by either tumor ingrowth or thrombosis. Our practice has been to anticoagulate patients long-term following stent placement with either coumadin or low-molecular-weight heparin. Others have advocated shorter periods (such as three months) of anticoagulation following stent placement.

Supportive Care

While the definitive treatments described above are the most important aspects of therapy for the patient with superior vena cava syndrome, there are some simple palliative maneuvers that can ease discomfort in the interim. If a patient presenting with superior vena cava syndrome is unstable from a respiratory or circulatory standpoint, hospital admission is appropriate. A comfortable, stable patient may be suitable for aggressive outpatient workup and therapy. Whether in the hospital or at home, simple bed rest with elevation of the head of the bed offers significant palliation for the patient with superior vena cava syndrome. This allows for mobilization of edema by reducing cardiac output and permitting gravity to assist in collateral drainage. Administration of oxygen can help to ease dyspnea for patients who are hypoxic and can further lower cardiac output. Diuretics and a low-salt diet can produce rapid resolution of upper body edema, but the effect is transient if the underlying obstruction persists. Steroids, though often used, have never been proven to improve symptoms or survival. Use of steroids in an animal model of superior vena cava syndrome had no clinical impact. Steroids may improve symptoms in patients with lymphoma or lymphoblastic leukemia due to their antineoplastic effect. However, they can make pathologic specimens difficult to interpret, so their use should be limited to patients who are in severe distress from airway obstruction or cerebral edema.

Role of Anticoagulation

In cases in which primary thrombosis results in the obstruction of the superior vena cava, anticoagulation with or without thrombolysis is the treatment of choice. The role of anticoagulation in the obstruction of the superior vena cava secondary to extrinsic compression is unclear. Autopsy studies in the first half of the twentieth century revealed thrombosis in 66% of patients with superior vena cava syndrome; however, anticoagulation in superior vena cava syndrome does not improve outcome. Nonetheless, many centers treat superior vena cava syndrome syndrome with anticoagulants as a matter of course. We do not anticoagulate patients with superior vena cava syndrome unless there is evidence on computed tomography of thrombosis of the superior vena cava or catheter-related thrombosis. For other patients, anticoagulation interferes with the diagnostic procedures that are the cornerstone of managing the patient with superior vena cava syndrome. Patients with advanced malignancies have a high likelihood of thrombotic complications regardless of superior vena cava obstruction. Clinicians should carefully evaluate patients for symptoms and signs of pulmonary embolism and treat accordingly.

Prognosis

The underlying disease is the primary determinant of prognosis for patients with superior vena cava syndrome. Patients with non-small-cell lung cancer usually have advanced disease with associated poor prognosis. Long-term survival is nonetheless possible, and for patients without evidence of distant metastases, we treat aggressively with multimodality therapy and curative intent. Limited-stage small-cell lung cancer can cause superior vena cava obstruction, given its tendency to form bulky nodal metastases. Patients with limited-stage small-cell lung cancer can achieve a five-year survival rate of approximately 10% regardless of superior vena cava obstruction. Patients with lymphoma causing superior vena cava have a more favorable prognosis, with a five-year survival rate of approximately 40%. Patients with germ-cell tumors causing superior vena cava are frequently cured, and patients with benign causes can survive decades without specific treatment and with substantial improvement in symptoms as collateral pathways mature.

Suggested Reading

Abner A: Approach to the patient who presents with superior vena cava obstruction. Chest 1993;103:394S–397S.

Ahmann F: A reassessment of the clinical implications of the superior caval syndrome. J Clin Oncol 1984;2:961–969.

Chen JC, Bongard F, Klein SR: A contemporary perspective on superior vena cava syndrome. Am J Surg 1990;160:107–211.

Lokich JJ, Goodman R: Superior vena cava syndrome. Clin Management JAMA 1975;231:58–61.

McIntire FT, Skyes EM Jr: Obstruction of the superior vena cava: A review of the literature and report of two personal cases. Ann Intern Med 1949;30:925–960.

Nieto AF, Doty DB: Superior vena cava obstruction: Clinical syndrome, etiology, and treatment. Curr Probl Cancer 1986;10:443–484.

Parish JM, Marschke RF Jr, Dines DE, Lee RE: Etiologic considerations in superior vena cava syndrome. Mayo Clin Proc 1981;56:407–413

Porte H, Metois D, Finzi L, et al: Superior vena cava syndrome of malignant origin: Which surgical procedure for which diagnosis? Eur J Cardiothorac Surg 2000;17:384–388.

Sculier JP, Feld R: Superior vena cava obstruction syndrome: Recommendations for management. Cancer Treat Rev 1985;12:209–218.

Yellen A, Rosen A, Reichert N, Lieberman Y: Superior vena cava syndrome: The myth—the facts. Am Rev Respir Dis 1990;141:1114–1118.

Yim CD, Sane SS, Bjarnason H: Superior vena cava stenting. Radiol Clin North Am 2000;38:409–424.

Chapter 18
Hemoptysis

Armin Ernst and Robert L. Thurer

Hemoptysis is the expectoration of blood or blood-stained sputum. The appearance of blood is frightening to patients, as it may herald serious underlying disease, and it often constitutes a diagnostic challenge. Hemoptysis is a common presenting symptom and may account for up to 5% of visits in a pulmonary practice. Owing to the mixture of blood with saliva, the amount and rate of bleeding are usually overestimated by both patients and health care providers.

Hemoptysis is commonly classified by the amount of expectorated blood. Scant hemoptysis describes flecks of blood in the sputum and does not exceed 20 mL of blood per day. This is the most common presentation of hemoptysis to an outpatient practice. Frank hemoptysis denotes expectoration of blood or blood clots (less than 300 mL per day), and massive hemoptysis is reserved for the patient with volumes higher than 300 mL per 24 hours and may be life threatening.

Differential Diagnosis

It is important to differentiate pseudohemoptysis from true hemoptysis. Clinical features assist in differentiating between hemoptysis and hematemesis.

Bleeding from the lung originates from one of two vascular systems: the high-pressure bronchial circulation or the low-pressure pulmonary circulation. These systems are interconnected, as the bronchial circulation supplying the pulmonary tissues drains into the pulmonary veins by means of intervascular connectors. This constitutes part of the physiological right-to-left shunt. Bleeding may originate from either but more than 90% of the time originates from the bronchial artery system.

The spectrum of underlying diseases leading to hemoptysis has changed over the years and varies with the geographic location. In developed countries, malignancies are the leading cause, closely followed by infectious disorders such as bronchitis. In developing countries, infectious disorders such as tuberculosis are more common. Table 18-1 lists the most common diagnoses associated with hemoptysis.

Clinical Evaluation

When patients present with scant or frank hemoptysis, the clinician must formulate a rational diagnostic workup. Massive hemoptysis, on the other hand, requires rapid stabilization and interventions first, before a workup can be pursued.

DIAGNOSIS

Differentiation of Hemoptysis from Pseudohemoptysis

It can be difficult to determine whether the blood that is coughed up originated from the tracheobronchial tree or pulmonary parenchyma. Other sources may be the nares, oropharynx, or gastrointestinal tract; evaluation by an otolaryngologist may be helpful. Another cause of pseudohemoptysis is infection with *Serratia marscecens*, which can cause sputum to stain red without blood being present. The following list addresses the clinical features in the differentiation between hemoptysis and hematemesis.

Hemoptysis (Pseudohemoptysis)	Hematemesis
Blood may be frothy	Blood is never frothy
Usually bright red blood	Usually dark red blood
No food particles	May be mixed with food particles
Usually followed by blood-tinged sputum	No blood-tinged sputum
Preceded by cough	Preceded by nausea/vomiting

Note: Hemoptysis can cause nausea and vomiting, and hematemesis may result in dyspnea.

Table 18-1 ■ Differential Diagnosis of Hemoptysis

Causes	Frequency
Malignant Diseases	40%
Non–small cell lung cancer	60%
Small cell lung cancer	20%
Metastatic, non-lung cancer	15%
Other	5%
Acute/chronic bronchitis	31%
Tuberculosis	12%
Pneumonia	6%
Lung abscess	4%
Pulmonary embolism and infarction	4%
Others	4%
Arteriovenous pulmonary malformation	
Mitral stenosis	
Foreign body	
Fungal infections	
Cystic fibrosis	
Bronchiectasis	
Goodpasture's syndrome	
Idiopathic hemosiderosis	
Catamenial hemoptysis	
Alveolar hemorrhage	

In the stable patient with scant or frank hemoptysis, a physical exam focused on the chest, neck, and oropharynx should be performed. Basic laboratory evaluation is aimed at detecting anemia or coagulopathies, and the patient should be asked about workplace, exposures, and smoking habits. This part of the evaluation guides in assessing probabilities for particular diseases but is usually not diagnostic. If the suspicion of bronchitis or similar infectious disorders is high, a short course of antibiotics and cough suppressant can be considered in the young patient (under age 40 years) without risk factors for malignancy.

Imaging

If the hemoptysis does not stop or recurs and the patient has significant risk factors such as age over 40 years or a smoking history, a chest X-ray should be performed. Although rarely diagnostic, a chest X-ray is quite valuable in localization of bleeding if an abnormality is present.

After this basic assessment, referral to a pulmonologist for further evaluation is appropriate. Frequently, a chest computed tomography will be performed, but as with the basic chest X-ray, it mainly serves as a guide to abnormalities without being in itself diagnostic.

Bronchoscopic Evaluation

It is generally accepted that bronchoscopy is appropriate for almost all patients with hemoptysis. Flexible bronchoscopy is a well-tolerated procedure performed on an outpatient basis that allows direct visualization of the central airways and frequently helps to establish a specific diagnosis. Bronchoscopy offers the highest diagnostic yield when performed as quickly as possible after the bleeding or, even better, during the episode. Waiting until hemoptysis has resolved decreases the chance of achieving a diagnosis. It is important to remember that a significant number of patients (up to 20%) with normal imaging studies have malignancies diagnosed by bronchoscopy only. Therefore a normal chest X-ray or chest computed tomography cannot be relied on as having excluded a serious disease, especially in the airways. If imaging abnormalities are present that could not be reached by bronchoscopy, surgical biopsy can be considered if dictated by the clinical situation.

Some patients will have both negative imaging and a negative bronchoscopic evaluation. In this instance, hemoptysis is described as cryptogenic. No guidelines exist as to how to follow these patients. Studies suggest that the incidence of cancer in this population is low but may reach 6% over several years. It seems that higher age and tobacco use may be associated with a higher incidence, and it appears prudent to follow these patients closely. For the most part, patients with one-time cryptogenic hemoptysis do well without appearing at risk for serious disease.

Other Diagnostic Tests

Newer diagnostic tools have recently been introduced. Autofluorescence bronchoscopy uses a blue-light source with the anticipated outcome of detecting occult malignant changes in the airways. Ultra-thin bronchoscopes designed to reach beyond the ninth generation of bronchial differentiation allow for more of the tracheobronchial tree to be visualized, and imaging methods such as positron emission tomography (PET) scanning may increase the yield of identifying malignancies. While potentially useful, the utility of these new tools in the workup of patients with hemoptysis has not yet been validated in clinical trials.

If hemoptysis occurs in patients with a known malignancy, there is frequently less of a diagnostic challenge. It is important to remember that patients with cancer still can develop pulmonary infections leading to hemoptysis. In general, bronchoscopy and imaging are aimed at identifying and localizing a presumed malignant focus in order to determine appropriate palliative therapy, as hemoptysis is distressing to the patient and, if left untreated, can progress to a life-threatening complication.

Management

If a patient presents with massive hemoptysis, immediate management takes priority over establishing the exact etiology. Patients should be admitted to an intensive care unit with urgent pulmonary and thoracic surgical consultation. Maintenance of a stable airway is of paramount importance. Mild sedation, cough suppression, and stool softeners may be helpful to decrease the rate of bleeding, but oversedation must be avoided, because it may lead to an inability to clear the airways. If the bleeding site is known, the patient is positioned with "the good side up" to avoid aspiration. Patients generally do not die from anemia, but rather from asphyxiation related to the tracheobronchial tree filling with blood.

If the patient is unstable, intubation is performed to secure the airway and allow for suctioning. Flexible and rigid bronchoscopy are performed not only to clear the airways and localize the bleeding source, but also to intervene therapeutically.

Therapeutic endoscopic options include tissue destructive therapy such as laser for endobronchial lesions, installation of iced saline or epinephrine, and placement of endobronchial obturators or occlusion catheters to stabilize a patient quickly.

Once a patient is stabilized or if bleeding continues, further steps must be considered. Because most bleeding arises from the bronchial circulation, angiographic embolization of feeding vessels with gel foam or coils or vascular stent placements should be attempted before resorting to emergent surgery. Embolization, when technically feasible and performed by an experienced interventional radiologist, is over 85% successful. Complications include backwash of occlusion material into the circulation and accidental occlusion of spinal arteries.

Surgical intervention in the acute phase is associated with a mortality of 10% to 50% as a result of difficult airway control in bleeding patients. If the bleeding is caused by a lesion requiring resection, the patient should be stabilized for an elective, rather than urgent, operation. If emergency resection is required, an anesthesia team that is familiar with difficult airway problems should be available. Early surgical consultation is essential to allow multidisciplinary decision making for these complex patients.

Radiation therapy may control bleeding from malignant airway or parenchymal lesions, but the effects may be delayed. It is better used once the bleeding source has been identified and stabilized. Radiation therapy directed at the identified lesion in the stabilized patient may significantly reduce the rate of recurrent bleeding.

The mortality for patients with massive hemoptysis depends on the underlying problem. Patients with end-stage malignant disease and tumor erosion into a major vessel may experience massive hemoptysis as a fatal event. On the other hand, patients may present with massive hemoptysis as a result of a primary tracheal tumor and can undergo curative surgical resection after stabilization. The life expectancy after massive hemoptysis due to benign diseases is usually quite good.

Suggested Reading

Boiselle PM, Ernst A, Karp DD: Lung cancer detection of the 21st century: Potential contributions and emerging technologies. Am J Roentgenol 2000;175:1215–1221.

Cahill BC, Ingbar DH: Massive hemoptysis: Assessment and management. Clin Chest Med 1994;15:147–167.

Colice GI: Detecting lung cancer as a cause of hemoptysis in patients with a normal chest radiograph. Chest 1997;111: 877–884.

Dweik RA, Stoller JK: Role of bronchoscopy in massive hemoptysis. Clin Chest Med 1999;20:89–105.

Haponik EF, Chin R: Hemoptysis: Clinicians' perspectives. Chest 1990;97:469–475.

Johnston H, Reisz G: Changing spectrum of hemoptysis: Underlying causes in 148 patients undergoing diagnostic flexible fiberoptic bronchoscopy. Arch Intern Med 1989;149:1666–1668.

Mapel DW: Hemoptysis season. Chest 2000;118:288–289.

Sharma OP: The problem of diffuse alveolar hemorrhage syndromes. Curr Opin Pulm Med 1998;4:247–250.

Stein PD, Afzal A, Henry JW, Villareal CG: Fever in acute pulmonary embolism. Chest 2000;117:39–42.

Tak S, Abluwalia G, Sharma SK, et al: Hemoptysis in patients with a normal chest radiograph: Bronchoscopy-CT correlation. Australas Radiol 1999;43:451–455.

Uflacker R, Kaemmerer A, Picon PD, et al: Bronchial artery embolization in the management of hemoptysis: Technical aspects and long-term results. Radiol 1985;157:637–644.

Chapter 19
Bowel Obstruction

Monica M. Bertagnolli

Introduction

Bowel obstruction is a common clinical problem that occurs in approximately 4% of patients with a history of abdominal or pelvic surgery for benign disease and is a presenting feature in 15% of large bowel malignancies. Nonneoplastic disorders can also produce symptoms of obstruction, including abdominal pain, nausea, and anorexia. These symptoms can also occur as a result of a wide variety of conditions, including viral infection, appendicitis, inflammatory bowel disease, diverticulitis, *Clostridium difficile* colitis, mesenteric adenitis, and chemotherapy toxicity.

Differential Diagnosis

The signs, symptoms, and differential diagnosis of intestinal obstruction vary according to the level of obstruction (Table 19-1).

Gastric Outlet Obstruction

A gastric outlet or duodenal obstruction is characterized by emesis of nonbilious material with minimal or no abdominal distension. Gastric outlet obstruction can be caused by severe peptic ulcer disease, a diagnosis that is suggested by a history of use of nonsteroidal anti-inflammatory medications and chronic epigastric pain relieved by meals. This type of obstruction is produced when acute inflammation causes edema and spasm of the pylorus. Gradual onset of gastric outlet or duodenal obstruction in the setting of weight loss and early satiety suggests a malignant etiology, such as locally advanced gastric, pancreatic, or periampullary cancer.

Small Bowel Obstruction

Small bowel obstruction often presents with the relatively sudden onset of colicky abdominal pain, obstipation, and abdominal distension. This diagnosis is confirmed by findings of dilated loops of fluid-filled small bowel with decompression of distal intestine on a plain film of the abdomen (Figure 19-1) or abdominal computed tomography (CT) scan. Most small bowel obstructions occur in patients with a history of abdominal or pelvic surgery and are caused by extrinsic compression of the bowel lumen by postoperative adhesions. Small bowel obstruction can also result from hernia incarceration or from inflammatory strictures related to Crohn's disease. Rare causes of small bowel obstruction include gallstone ileus, mesenteric volvulus, intra-abdominal abscess, and tumor.

Large Bowel Obstruction

Colonic obstruction is most often caused by a primary colorectal malignancy, although it may also be produced by volvulus or diverticulitis. When tumor is the cause, the point of obstruction is likely to reside in the left colon, as the liquid character of the stool in the proximal colon permits its passage until very late in the course of the disease. The development of symptoms of large bowel obstruction is generally more gradual than that of small bowel obstruction. Patients presenting with colonic obstruction usually report increasing constipation, decreased appetite, frequent laxative use, and eventually abdominal distension. Vomiting is an uncommon and late symptom of colonic obstruction. In large bowel obstruction, the degree of dilatation of the small bowel depends on the

Table 19-1 ■ Causes of Intestinal Obstruction in Adults

Gastric Outlet

Peptic ulcer disease
Gastric carcinoma
Pancreatic or distal bile duct tumors
Annular pancreas

Small Intestine

Postsurgical adhesions	75%
Incarcerated hernia	15%
Small bowel neoplasia (carcinoid, lymphoma, gastrointestinal stromal tumor (GIST), lipomas)	
Inflammatory bowel disease	
Mesenteric volvulus	
Extrinsic compression by tumor (advanced ovarian, colorectal, pancreatic, gastric tumors are most common):	Rare
Extrinsic abscesses and hematomas	
Radiation-associated strictures	
Gallstones	
Impactions: fecal, bezoar, barium	

Colon

Colon cancer	65%
Volvulus	15%
Diverticulitis	10%
Hernia	
Intussusception	
Inflammatory bowel disease	
Pelvic recurrence of rectal cancer	Rare
Carcinomatosis	
Ischemic stricture	
Foreign body/impaction	

Rectum

Rectal cancer
Epidermoid anal cancer
Infection (abscess)

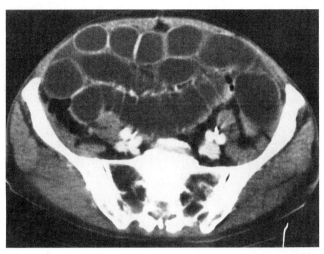

Figure 19-1 ■ Plain film of the abdomen in a patient with small bowel obstruction. (Source: From Herlinger H and Maglinte D: Clinical Radiation of the Small Intestine. WB Saunders, 1989, p 63.)

patients with occult malignancy elsewhere in the abdomen. The eponym Ogilvie's syndrome has since been broadened to include pseudo-obstruction of the colon from any cause. Ogilvie's syndrome is characterized by abdominal distention in the absence of pain in patients that are hospitalized for a related primary medical condition. The patient's abdomen is generally soft and nontender, and the course of the pseudo-obstruction is benign. In rare instances, however, pseudo-obstruction can result in cecal perforation. The patients who are most at risk for this complication are those who are immunosuppressed or who suffer hemodynamic collapse due to acute illness. The colonic dilatation produced by pseudo-obstruction can even cause respiratory difficulties in a patient with a tenuous ventilatory status.

Conditions associated with Ogilvie's syndrome include many that are common in cancer patients, such as narcotics use, diabetes mellitus, advanced age, chemotherapy or radiation therapy, surgery, sepsis, electrolyte abnormalities, or renal failure. The management of Ogilvie's syndrome includes discontinuing oral intake, instituting intravenous hydration, close observation with serial abdominal exams, avoidance of associated agents such as narcotics, correction of electrolytes, and periodic abdominal films to assess colon diameter. Endoscopic decompression of the colon is indicated for patients whose colonic diameter exceeds 10 to 12 cm. In the most extreme and persistent cases, tube cecostomy is performed to avoid cecal perforation. Urgent laparotomy is indicated for patients who show signs of deterioration, including abdominal tenderness or other evidence of perforation or sepsis.

competence of the ileocecal valve. Rarely, proximal colonic obstruction is misdiagnosed as a small bowel obstruction when the ileocecal valve is incompetent, and plain films of the abdomen show dilated, fluid-filled small bowel loops. In the setting of a competent ileocecal valve, colonic dilatation may become massive. Bowel diameter, measured on abdominal plain films, is used to predict the probability of imminent perforation, and a cecal diameter of 12 cm or greater is a cause for concern.

Ogilvie's Syndrome

In 1948, William Ogilvie reported two cases of massive dilatation of the colon without distal obstruction in

Bowel Obstruction in Patients with a History of Malignancy

Of patients who present with a bowel obstruction within five years of treatment for a primary gastrointestinal cancer, 30% to 50% will have a nonmalignant cause of their obstruction. Even for patients with a known recurrent gastrointestinal or ovarian malignancy, benign causes of small bowel obstruction are relatively common, comprising approximately 30% of these cases. All too often, however, patients with recurrent intestinal tumors and bowel obstruction have diffuse intraperitoneal disease in which attempted surgical treatment at best is ineffective and at worst may contribute substantially to disease morbidity. It is not surprising, therefore, that the hospital mortality of bowel obstruction from recurrent intra-abdominal tumor is 20% to 40%. The diagnostic goal is to distinguish patients who have a benign cause of obstruction from those who have localized recurrent obstructive cancer and those who have diffuse abdominal carcinomatosis. Preoperative imaging is essential for these complicated cases, as the presence of extensive tumor can make full surgical exploration difficult or impossible.

Initial Evaluation and Management

The evaluation of a patient with abdominal pain, nausea, and vomiting begins with the history and physical examination. The presence of obstipation associated with abdominal distention suggests a diagnosis of bowel obstruction, although these findings can be misleading, particularly in elderly or acutely ill patients or those with prolonged narcotics use. Plain films of the abdomen, including flat plate and upright or lateral decubitus views, are the next step in diagnosis. The patterns of gas may provide clues to the etiology of the obstruction, as shown in Figure 19-2. Free air seen on lateral decubitus or upright films is evidence of intestinal perforation and indicates the need for emergency surgery. In cases in which plain films are equivocal, spiral computed tomography scan with oral contrast is performed. These methods are generally sufficient to distinguish a mechanical bowel obstruction from a nonobstructing condition such as Ogilvie's syndrome, although on rare occasions a contrast study is required.

Once the level and likely cause of bowel obstruction have been determined, the clinical presentation dictates the immediate care of the patient. All patients require careful assessment of fluid and electrolyte status and monitoring of urine output. Fluid resuscitation should begin immediately and should proceed during the evaluation period along with judicious

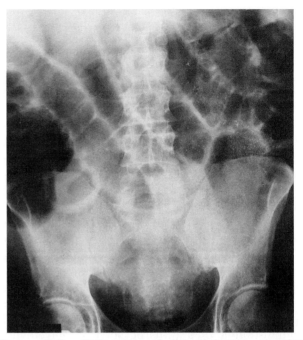

Figure 19-2 ■ Radiograph of the abdomen, showing dilated small and large bowel caused by partial obstruction of the descending colon by a colon cancer. (Source: From Bragg DG, Rubin P, and Hricak H: Oncologic Imaging, 2nd ed. WB Saunders, 2002, p 440.)

use of pain medications and serial abdominal examination. Patients with prolonged vomiting due to gastric outlet obstruction may present with a profound hypochloremic, hypokalemic metabolic alkalosis, requiring careful potassium replacement during fluid resuscitation. Small bowel obstruction may be associated with significant third-space fluid loss in addition to the dehydration produced by vomiting and lack of oral intake. The patient's cardiovascular status should be assessed and optimized, as cardiopulmonary complications are a common cause of morbidity and mortality in patients who require surgery for intestinal obstruction.

Gastric outlet obstruction is initially managed by nasogastric suction and intravenous hydration. When the patient's fluid and electrolyte status is stable, upper endoscopy is performed to determine or confirm the etiology, and appropriate intervention can then be planned. Complete small or large bowel obstruction is suggested by a lack of air in the intestine distal to the point of obstruction, by vomiting and by prolonged obstipation with significant abdominal distention. Treatment of complete bowel obstruction involves nasogastric suction, intravenous hydration, broad-spectrum antibiotics, and urgent laparotomy to relieve the obstruction and prevent further complications such as perforation or ischemic intestinal necrosis. In the early stages, no tests can definitively determine whether in fact a small bowel obstruction is complete.

The decision to proceed with emergency laparotomy relies on the surgeon's clinical judgment based on findings of abdominal tenderness or systemic signs of intestinal vascular compromise, perforation, or infection in association with tachycardia that is unresponsive to hydration, continuing fluid requirement, fever, or elevated white blood cell count.

For surgery involving the colon, it is clear that cleansing the bowel of stool reduces postoperative infection and anastomotic complications. It is therefore important to identify patients with partial large bowel obstruction for whom laparotomy can be delayed until after mechanical bowel preparation is accomplished. Such delay is reasonable in patients who do not have significant nausea or vomiting or abdominal tenderness and do have evidence of air or computed tomography contrast material in the intestine distal to the site of obstruction. These patients are treated with intravenous hydration and broad-spectrum antibiotics, with no oral intake other than administration of a cathartic such as polyethylene glycol or Phospho-soda. These agents are given gradually, generally over twice the time usually given for preoperative administration (12 to 24 hours). During bowel preparation, the patient is monitored by serial abdominal exams, and oral intake is discontinued if evidence of progression of the obstruction develops. This complication is unusual, however, and most patients who are prepared in this manner can undergo resection of their tumor with a primary anastomosis 24 to 48 hours after admission, in a setting that reduces postoperative morbidity and mortality.

Operative Management

The management of bowel obstruction is both site and disease specific. Care must be taken to preserve the physiologic reserves of patients who are potential surgical candidates, including the use of total parenteral nutrition if a trial of nonoperative management is attempted.

Gastric outlet obstruction caused by peptic ulcer disease generally resolves with nonoperative management, including nasogastric decompression, intravenous hydration, and proton pump inhibitor therapy. In rare instances, bypass surgery is required. If carcinoma is the cause of gastric outlet or duodenal obstruction, resection is attempted. Unfortunately, tumors that present in this manner are almost always too advanced for local resection, and the patient is therefore managed by bypass surgery. Patients with extremely bulky disease that prohibits bypass can benefit from decompressive gastrostomy.

Surgery is performed in patients who have small bowel obstruction caused by extrinsic compression of postsurgical adhesions or hernia incarceration when conservative management fails to resolve the obstruction. Surgery involves lysis of adhesions or hernia reduction and herniorrhaphy. Resection is required only when loss of intestinal blood supply by extrinsic compression causes bowel necrosis. In almost all of these cases, resection with primary reanastomosis can be performed. Foreign bodies or gallstones rarely are the cause of small bowel obstruction, usually at the ileocecal valve, which is the narrowest portion of the small intestine. These obstructions are treated by enterotomy to allow extraction of the foreign body. Intrinsic obstructing lesions of the small bowel, such as tumor, are managed by resection, with node dissection if indicated. Occasionally, small bowel obstruction occurs in the setting of diffuse involvement of the peritoneum with tumor. In this instance, it can be difficult to determine the exact location of obstruction, and the bowel lumen may be compromised in multiple locations. In addition, tumor encasement of the intra-abdominal contents can make the mobilization required for resection and reanastomosis difficult or impossible. Bypass of the obstructed segment successfully relieves the obstruction in some cases, but recurrent obstructive symptoms are common.

Approximately 15% of patients with colon cancer present with some degree of large bowel obstruction, and another 3% to 8% present with perforation of the colon. Patients with these complications are generally older and have more advanced disease at the time of surgery, resulting in a crude five-year survival rate of 25% to 35%. Although the presence of obstruction or perforation is generally associated with advanced disease, 30% to 50% of these colon cancers will prove to be stage II. The five-year survival for these high-risk stage II patients is less than for those presenting without complications. When adjusted for the increased mortality associated with emergency surgery in the setting of obstruction or perforation, however, the long-term survival rate of patients presenting with obstructing colon cancers is similar to that of stage-matched patients without obstruction.

The intraoperative management of patients presenting with complete large bowel obstruction depends on the location of the tumor and the condition of the patient. Lesions of the cecum, ascending, and transverse colon are resected by means of a right colectomy or extended right colectomy with a primary ileocolic anastomosis. Descending colon and sigmoid lesions are also resected, generally followed by a primary anastomosis. On-table lavage of the proximal colon may be performed prior to anastomosis if a large column of stool threatens to compromise the anastomosis during the early healing period. The prior practice of staged operations for obstructing left-sided lesions (resection and diverting colostomy followed by secondary surgery later to effect reanastomosis) has largely been replaced by immediate anastomosis. Using the preceding guidelines, this approach permits primary anastomosis to be accomplished safely and avoids the morbidity and mortality associated with a second operation for colostomy closure.

Sometimes, however, complete obstruction produces ischemia of the proximal intestine, and the surgeon may determine that primary anastomosis cannot safely be performed. This situation is best managed by creation of an end colostomy with mucus fistula or Hartmann's pouch, followed by colostomy closure once the proximal bowel has recovered. Similar precautions are sometimes required for patients with perforated cancers, particularly when intra-abdominal contamination is high and evidence of sepsis is present.

Patients with obstructing high rectal cancers are generally managed by resection in a manner similar to those with sigmoid tumors. Although uncommon, patients with cancers in the distal rectum can also present with obstruction. In this case, the advanced nature of the local disease invariably makes primary resection of the tumor difficult or impossible. These patients are best managed by diverting sigmoid colostomy and mucus fistula, followed by chemotherapy and radiation. For patients whose tumors respond to therapy, surgical resection is then considered and generally requires abdominoperineal resection.

It is unusual for a patient with diffuse carcinomatosis to present with an acute complete intestinal obstruction. Instead, these patients usually have a protracted course of nausea, vomiting, crampy abdominal pain, and abdominal films consistent with partial bowel obstruction. These patients are generally managed nonoperatively with nasogastric decompression, intravenous hydration or total parenteral nutrition, antiemetics, and judicious use of pain medications (see Chapter 122, "Symptom Management"). Nonoperative management is often only a temporary solution, as approximately 50% of these patients will eventually progress to complete obstruction. Moreover, after the bowel obstruction resolves following nonoperative management, patients often continue to have obstructive symptoms.

For patients with complete bowel obstruction due to diffuse intra-abdominal tumor spread, surgery to relieve the obstruction is rarely successful. In this case, surgery is generally reserved for the few patients who have maintained a good performance status. Survival in this patient population is extremely limited, particularly for patients whose nutritional status is compromised. Here, treatment is palliative. Anecdotal reports suggest that octreotide can alleviate the symptoms of malignant bowel obstruction, providing relief of nausea and pain in patients with advanced disease.

Suggested Reading

Baines M, Oliver DJ, Carter RL: Medical management of intestinal obstruction in patients with advanced malignant disease: A clinical and pathological study. Lancet 1985;2:990–993.

Burkhill GJ, Bell JR, Healy JC: The utility of computed tomography in acute small bowel obstruction. Clin Radiol 2001;56:350–359.

Ellis CN, Boggs HW, Slagle GW, Cole PA: Small bowel obstruction after colon resection for benign and malignant diseases. Dis Colon Rectum 1991;34:361–371.

Feuer DJ, Broadley KE, Shepherd JH, Barton DP: Systematic review of surgery in malignant bowel obstruction in advanced gynecological and gastrointestinal cancer: The Systematic Review Steering Committee. Gynecol Oncol 1999;75:313–322.

Fielding LP, Phillips RKS, Fry JS, Hittinger R: Prediction of outcome after curative resection for large bowel cancer. Lancet 1986;11:904–907.

Frank C: Medical management of intestinal obstruction in terminal care. Can Fam Physician 1997;43:259–265.

Furakawa A, Yamasaki M, Furuichi K, et al: Helical CT in the diagnosis of small bowel obstruction. Radiographics 2001;21:341–345.

Kelly WE Jr, Brown PW, Lawrence W Jr, Terz JJ: Penetrating, obstructing, and perforating carcinomas of the colon and rectum. Arch Surg 1981;116:381–384.

Lohn JW, Austin RC, Winslet MC: Unusual causes of small bowel obstruction. J R Soc Med 2000;93:365–368.

Longo WE, Virgo KS, Johnson FE, et al: Risk factors for morbidity and mortality after colectomy for colon cancer. Dis Colon Rectum 2000;43:83–91.

Macari M, Megibow A: Imaging of suspected acute small bowel obstruction. Semin Roentgenol 2001;36:108–117.

Maginte DD, Kelvin FM, Rowe MG, et al: Small bowel obstruction: Optimizing radiologic investigation and nonsurgical management. Radiology 2001;218:39–46.

Mercadante S, Ripamonti C, Casuccio A, et al: Comparison of octreotide and hyoscine butylbromide in controlling gastrointestinal symptoms due to malignant inoperable bowel obstruction. Support Care Cancer 2000;8:188–191.

Mulcahy HE, Skelly MM, Husain A, O'Donoghue DP: Long-term outcome following curative surgery for malignant large bowel obstruction. Br J Surg 1996;83:46–50.

Runkel NS, Hinz U, Lehnert T, Buhr HJ, Herfarth C: Improved outcome after emergency surgery for cancer of the large intestine. Br J Surg 1998;85:1260–1265.

Runkel NS, Schlag P, Schwarz V, Herfarth C: Outcome after emergency surgery for cancer of the large intestine. Br J Surg 1991;78:183–188.

Schnoll-Sussman F, Kurtz RC: Gastrointestinal emergencies in the critically ill cancer patient. Semin Oncol 2000;27:270–283.

Weiss SM, Skibber JM, Rosato FE: Bowel obstruction in cancer patients: Performance status as a predictor of survival. J Surg Oncol 1984;25:15–17.

Wilson MS, Ellis H, Menzies D, et al: A review of the management of small bowel obstruction: Members of the Surgical and Clinical Adhesions Research Study (SCAR). Ann R Coll Surg Engl 1999;81:320–328.

Woolfson RG, Jennings K, Whalen GF: Management of bowel obstruction in patients with abdominal cancer. Arch Surg 1997;132:1093–1097.

Chapter 20
Focal Liver Lesions

Gaston Morillo

This chapter presents an overview of the use of imaging methods in the evaluation of the liver in the oncologic patient. Only the most common liver tumors of the adult are discussed (Table 20-1). The objective of any imaging modality is to detect lesions, to determine their number and location in the liver, and, when possible, to establish their etiology. In other instances, only a differential diagnosis may be rendered. Imaging studies are also used as guidance for percutaneous procedures such as biopsies or tumor ablation and for planning surgical excision of lesions.

Imaging Modalities

Several imaging methods are available for the evaluation of focal liver lesions. The one that is most commonly used at present is spiral/helical computed tomography (spiral CT), which has supplanted traditional or conventional computed tomography scanning. With spiral/helical computed tomography, the entire abdomen can be examined in a few seconds, and, if necessary, the chest and the pelvis also can be included using the same bolus of intravenous contrast material. The speed of the examination is greatly appreciated by the cancer patient. Multiple thin slices can be obtained during a single breath-holding episode, avoiding motion artifacts and generating images of excellent quality. The resulting studies are highly reproducible and therefore allow relatively accurate comparison of serial examinations. The volumetric acquisition of data in a few seconds is also used for performing computed tomography angiography and to generate multiplanar and three-dimensional reconstructions of the images, providing additional information for diagnosis.

The spiral/helical computed tomography evaluation of most focal liver lesions requires intravenous administration of iodinated contrast agents. Some patients with a history of renal insufficiency, significant allergies, or previous severe reactions to the con-

trast material might not be suitable candidates for the procedure. Premedication may be required in selected cases. An appropriate venous access might not be readily available in some patients, precluding the use of contrast agents.

Magnetic resonance imaging (MRI) is becoming more widely used in the assessment of liver lesions. Magnetic resonance imaging has been used mostly as a problem-solving technique for patients whose previous ultrasound or computed tomography scans have been inconclusive or patients who could not be exposed to iodinated contrast agents. The inherent high-contrast resolution of magnetic resonance imaging allows reliable characterization of different soft tissues. Breath-holding techniques and the use of contrast agents have widened the indications for magnetic resonance imaging in the cancer patient. Gadolinium-based extracellular contrast agents, which behave in a manner similar to iodinated contrast agents, do not affect renal function significantly. The incidence of severe undesirable reactions is very low, making them appropriate for use in patients with allergic histories. Currently, the most important contraindications for magnetic resonance imaging are related to the presence of ferromagnetic materials implanted in the body, such as cerebral aneurysmal surgical clips, cochlear implants, neurostimulators, pacemakers, cardioverter defibrillators, and heart valve prostheses, among others.

Ultrasound is a readily available modality and is an expeditious way to characterize the ubiquitous liver cysts that may have been considered indeterminate by computed tomography or to confirm that a lesion is not a simple cyst and that further evaluation is needed. Ultrasound is most useful for the assessment of the hepatic vascular system, particularly in patients with hepatocellular carcinoma, to exclude portal vein tumor thrombosis. Ultrasound is also used as a guide for interventional procedures such as drainage of hepatic fluid collections, percutaneous biopsy, and/or ablation of accessible lesions. Intra-

Table 20-1 ▪ Focal Liver Lesions in the Adult

Benign Cystic Lesions

Abscess
Hematoma
Biloma
Simple cysts
Polycystic liver disease
Hemangioma
Biliary cystadenoma
Bile duct adenoma
Multiple bile duct hamartomas

Benign Solid Lesions

Focal nodular hyperplasia
Regenerative and dysplastic nodules
Hepatocellular adenoma
Focal fat infiltration
Lipoma, angiomyolipoma, myelolipoma
Inflammatory pseudotumor

Malignant Tumors

Metastases
Hepatocellular carcinoma
Fibrolamellar hepatocellular carcinoma
Cholangiocarcinoma
Biliary cystadenocarcinoma
Hepatic epithelioid hemangioendothelioma
Angiosarcoma
Malignant fibrous histiocytoma
Primary lymphoma

operatively, ultrasound is an excellent modality for the detection and localization of lesions that have not been visualized either preoperatively or by direct visual inspection.

There has been a resurgence of the applications of nuclear medicine in the evaluation of focal liver lesions due to the development of new imaging equipment and new imaging radiopharmaceuticals. Positron emission tomography (PET) is being used as a technique for functional imaging. It has the advantage of being able to evaluate not only the liver but the entire body when searching for tumor deposits. Positron emission tomography provides images of metabolic activity depending on the uptake of fluorine-18-labeled deoxyglucose (FDG) by the tumor, reflecting the use of glucose by different tissues. It has shown the capacity to identify or characterize tumor that is not visualized by other imaging modalities, and it appears to be able to differentiate between active tumor and residual fibrosis posttreatment. For the evaluation of neuroendocrine tumors, In-111 octreotide scintigraphy has been used with success.

Positron emission tomography has some limitations, since FDG also accumulates in inflammatory or infectious areas as well as in certain normal organs such as the liver, gastrointestinal tract, kidneys, and lymph nodes. Positron emission tomography images have relatively low spatial resolution, and the images might not provide anatomic landmarks for localization purposes. However, it is possible to combine the positron emission tomography images with computed tomography or MR images for anatomic localization.

Interventional radiologic procedures have specific indications such as embolization of the vascular supply of tumors, chemotherapy embolization, or percutaneous ablation of tumors using either ethanol injection, microwaves, laser radiofrequency waves, or cryoablation. Computed tomography hepatic angiography and computed tomography arterial portography using an intra-arterial catheter are very accurate for documenting liver tumors, particularly for the preoperative planning of surgical excision of metastases. However, with the development of spiral/helical computed tomography, their use has decreased.

Imaging Manifestations of Focal Liver Lesions

The following criteria are used to describe focal liver lesions: (a) morphology (size, shape, margins, and interface with the surrounding liver); (b) texture or internal architecture (liquid, solid, mixed, or complex); and (c) response to the administration of contrast material (lack of enhancement or pattern of enhancement).

The morphologic description of lesions is the same for all imaging modalities. The texture of a lesion is usually compared to the surrounding, presumably normal, liver. Contrast agents are used to evaluate the vascularity of a lesion and to increase conspicuity of the lesion by either enhancing the lesion itself more than the liver or enhancing the surrounding liver more than the lesion. Contrast agents increase detectability of lesions and allow a more reliable characterization of such lesions.

On ultrasound, the internal architecture of a lesion can be anechoic with good sound transmission in the case of fluid-containing lesions, hyperechogenic for solid lesions, or hypoechogenic or complex if there are both fluid and solid components. Computed tomography allows density measurements for water, fat, other soft tissues, calcium, and gas, expressed in Hounsfield units. On computed tomography, lesions are either hypodense, hyperdense, or isodense with the liver. Magnetic resonance imaging uses different techniques or pulse sequences to characterize tissues. Tissues have different magnetic relaxation times, represented by time constants T1 and T2. On T1-weighted images, the presence of fluid in cysts or in areas of necrosis usually appears hypointense in relation to the liver but may be slightly isointense. Blood and fat may appear hyperintense. Solid tissues usually appear isointense unless they contain fat or blood. On T2-weighted images, fluid is very hyperintense and very bright; solid tissue may be slightly to moderately hyperintense, and complex lesions show hypointense and hyperintense signal with a heterogeneous signal due to the presence of liquid and solid components.

Use of Contrast Materials

The liver receives approximately 75% of its blood supply through the portal vein and the remainder from the hepatic artery. Tumors are supplied mostly by the hepatic artery. Intravenous administration of contrast agents takes advantage of this blood supply to increase the difference in appearance between normal liver and suspected focal liver lesions. Contrast agents are used to assess the vascularity of lesions, to increase their conspicuity and detectability, and to display the vascular anatomy and the relationship between the lesions and the hepatic vessels.

Iodinated contrast agents and gadolinium chelates are administered intravenously as a bolus, and images are obtained immediately during the early arterial phase of enhancement of the liver, followed by acquisitions during the portal venous phase (biphasic technique). In some cases, particularly when using magnetic resonance imaging, nonenhanced images are obtained prior to the administration of the contrast material. Some lesions may require acquisition of delayed images for further characterization (multiphasic techniques). Nonenhanced images are useful for detecting changes that may be obscured by the contrast agent, such as calcifications, fat, or hemorrhage.

The degree of enhancement of the lesions is useful for their characterization as hypervascular or hypovascular, and the pattern of enhancement allows identification of certain lesions, such as hemangiomas.

In addition to gadolinium chelates, other substances can be used for magnetic resonance imaging images to improve detectability and characterization of lesions. Superparamagnetic iron oxide particles (ferumoxides) are selectively taken up by the reticuloendothelial system, decreasing the signal intensity of normal liver. Manganese-based agents (mangafodipir trisodium) are taken up by hepatocytes, increasing the signal intensity of the normal liver, and are eliminated through the biliary system, resulting in opacification of the bile ducts. Newer agents such as gadobenate

dimeglumine combine extracellular and hepatocytic functions, providing additional information for the diagnosis of liver lesions. These agents increase detectability of liver lesions, a feature that is particularly useful when surgical resection is planned. Some of these contrast materials provide a more confident histologic diagnosis in certain cases.

Imaging of Metastases

Metastases are the most common malignant liver tumors (Figure 20-1). Like all focal liver lesions, they are usually round or ovoid and may have either a solid, mixed, or pseudocystic texture, although occasionally they may appear completely cystic owing to extensive necrosis. The margins of the lesions are usually irregular and indistinct, although they may be smooth and well defined.

On nonenhanced computed tomography, metastases appear hypodense or isodense. Some may show calcific deposits, particularly those arising from mucinous carcinomas of the gastrointestinal tract or from the ovary. After administration of contrast material, most metastases appear hypovascular (Figure 20-2) and are best imaged during the portal venous phase of contrast enhancement (Table 20-2). Hypervascular metastases (Table 20-3) have a rich blood supply and become substantially hyperdense during the hepatic arterial phase of contrast enhancement, promptly becoming isodense with surrounding liver during the portal venous phase, rendering them either not detectable or less conspicuous in this stage (Figures 20-3 and 20-4). Larger complex lesions with solid and necrotic components show irregular margins with inhomogeneous and sometimes pseudoseptated appearance. The pseudocystic lesions can be properly characterized by the peripheral, halolike enhancement surrounding the nonenhancing center. This ring enhancement is continuous and usually of even thickness, in contrast to the peripheral nodular enhancement that is seen with hemangiomas. On delayed images, there may be a peripheral washout of the contrast agent with residual central enhancement.

On nonenhanced T1-weighted magnetic resonance imaging, metastases are either hypointense or isointense, and they may have either smooth or irregular margins. Lesions with evidence of bleeding as well as some melanoma metastases may show a hyperintense signal in this pulse sequence. On T2-weighted images, these lesions become hyperintense, frequently with inhomogeneous signal intensity (Figure 20-5). After the administration of gadolinium chelates, they behave in a manner similar to that of the enhanced computed tomography images. Some metastases, particularly from colon carcinoma, may

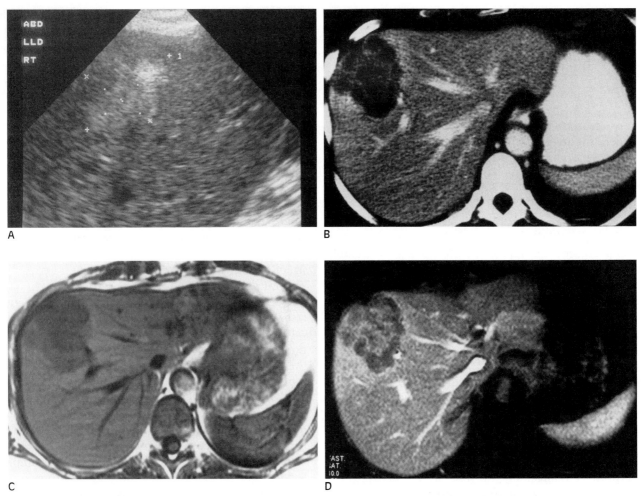

Figure 20-1 ■ Metastasis from colon carcinoma. *A,* Hyperechogenic lesion on ultrasound. *B,* Inhomogeneous lesion, predominately necrotic during portal venous phase computed tomography. *C,* Hypointense lesion on T1-weighted image. *D,* Inhomogeneous appearance of the lesion on the T2-weighted images using fat saturation. Clear visualization of hepatic veins.

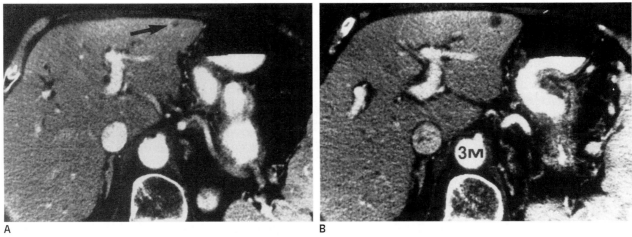

Figure 20-2 ■ Metastasis from pancreatic carcinoma. *A,* Portal venous phase computed tomography shows a 6-mm hypodense lesion (arrow) simulating a cyst. *B,* Three months later, the lesion has increased to 12 mm. Magnetic resonance imaging may help to differentiate a cyst from metastasis.

Table 20-2 ■ Hypodense Liver Lesions

Benign nonneoplastic cystic lesions
Biliary cystadenoma
Multiple bile duct hamartomas
Hemangioma
Lymphoma
Metastases from carcinoma of
    Colon
    Lung
    Breast
    Pancreas
    Stomach
    Head and neck tumors

Note: Some of the above lesions remain hypodense with and without intravenous contrast enhancement; others may show partial or complete enhancement.

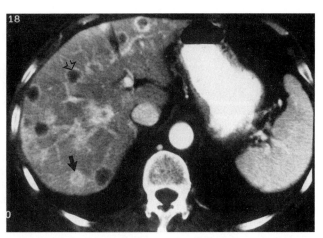

Figure 20-3 ■ Mixed hypervascular (black arrow) and hypovascular necrotic lesions (open arrow) with enhancing periphery during the arterial phase of computed tomography. Compare to the appearance of hemangiomas in Figure 20-11.

show a halo sign or a target pattern, which is highly characteristic of these lesions.

On ultrasound, metastases are usually hypoechogenic or complex in appearance, but some may be hyperechogenic (see Figure 20-1).

There are many variables in determining the size of a lesion, such as differences in the spatial and contrast resolution of different imaging methods. Measurements obtained during contrast enhancement may be smaller than those in the nonenhanced images

owing to accumulation of the contrast material in the periphery of the lesion, rendering this area isodense or isointense with the surrounding liver. Unidimensional or bidimensional measurements as well as intraobserver and interobserver discrepancies also introduce variables that must be taken in consideration. The capability of spiral/helical computed tomography and of magnetic resonance imaging for providing three-dimensional images allows measurements in three planes and volumetric determinations. The practical applications of such methods have not been demonstrated.

Table 20-3 ■ Hypervascular Liver Tumors

Primary Liver Tumors

Hemangioma
Hepatocellular carcinoma
Focal nodular hyperplasia
Hepatocellular adenoma
Sarcomas

Metastases From

Endocrine neoplasms:
    Carcinoid
    Islet cell tumors
    Pheochromocytoma
    Thyroid
    Nonendocrine neoplasms
    Melanoma
    Breast
    Renal cell carcinoma
    Sarcomas
    Choriocarcinoma

Note: Some of the above lesions do not always show intense enhancement following intravenous contrast material administration and may appear hypodense.

Hepatocellular Carcinoma

Hepatocellular carcinoma is the second most common malignant liver tumor, frequently developing in a cirrhotic liver caused by either viral hepatitis or alcohol abuse. The lesion may present as a single, multifocal, or disseminated tumor. It is highly vascular, it may have a capsule, and it may cause tumoral thrombosis of the portal vein. Metastases from the tumor can occur to abdominal lymph nodes and to distant sites.

Tumors less than 10 mm in size have variable appearances and may be difficult to differentiate from regenerating or dysplastic nodules, which are usually present in the cirrhotic liver. Hypervascular nodules, regardless of size, should be suspicious for tumor. Nonenhanced computed tomography images may show evidence of bleeding and occasionally calcifications in the lesion. The hepatic arterial phase shows substantial enhancement of the tumor with rapid washout of the contrast agent in the portal venous phase, the tumor becoming hypointense or isointense

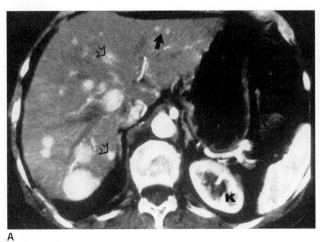
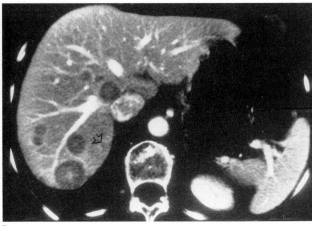

A   B

Figure 20-4 ■ Metastases from carcinoid tumor. *A,* Hypervascular metastases on arterial phase computed tomography becoming hypodense on portal venous phase. *B,* Some lesions (arrows) either are not demonstrated or appear less conspicuous during the venous phase.

in relation to the surrounding liver (Figure 20-6). A rim or capsule may be identified. Larger tumors appear inhomogeneous owing to central necrosis and hemorrhage.

Fibrolamellar hepatocellular carcinoma has been described as a tumor with better long-term prognosis than typical hepatocellular carcinoma. It usually occurs in young adults with no evidence of chronic liver disease and with normal tumor marker levels. The imaging manifestations are similar to those of the typical hepatocellular carcinoma, although a central scar, with calcification, is frequently seen.

On T1-weighted images, both tumors usually appear hypointense to liver, although some may be isointense (Figure 20-7). Both tumors may show high signal intensity due to bleeding, and the typical

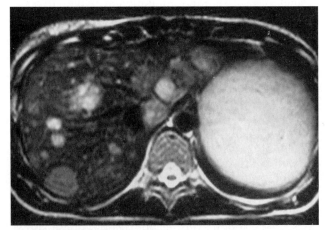

Figure 20-5 ■ Metastases from neuroendocrine pancreatic tumor. On T2-weighted images, some of the lesions appear very hyperintense while others are only moderately hyperintense. Compare to signal intensity of the cerebrospinal fluid.

hepatocellular carcinoma may show fat content (Table 20-4). On T2-weighted images, they show variable degrees of hyperintensity, frequently with an inhomogeneous appearance, particularly in the presence of necrosis and hemorrhage. Hepatocellular carcinoma shows contrast enhancement similar to that described with computed tomography, although fibrolamellar hepatocellular carcinoma appears to be less vascularized. Magnetic resonance imaging is believed to be more reliable than computed tomography in the detection and evaluation of hepatocellular carcinoma in the advanced cirrhotic liver.

Intrahepatic Cholangiocarcinoma

Intrahepatic cholangiocarcinoma is the second most common primary hepatic malignant tumor. It can be classified as either peripheral or hilar in location, the latter usually originating at the confluence of the right and left hepatic ducts. The peripheral type is manifested as a focal liver mass that is similar to other liver tumors, usually without associated dilatation of the bile ducts. It appears hypodense in the portal venous phase of computed tomography and shows partial enhancement in delayed images. It is hypointense on nonenhanced T1-weighted images and becomes

Table 20-4 ■ **Hyperintense Liver Lesions (MRI) (T-1 weighted images)**

Hepatocellular carcinoma	Fatty tumors
Hepatocellular adenoma	Blood
Focal fat infiltration	Abscess

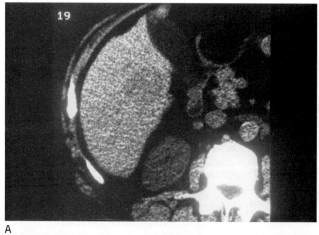

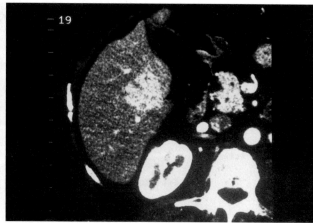

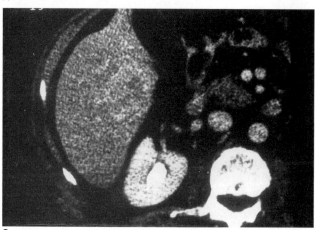

Figure 20-6 ■ Hepatocellular carcinoma. *A*, Faint hypodense lesion on nonenhanced computed tomography. *B*, Intense, slightly inhomogeneous enhancement of the tumor during the arterial phase computed tomography. *C*, On delayed image, there is rapid washout of the contrast material.

hyperintense on the T2-weighted pulse sequences. The tumor may show early peripheral enhancement with gadolinium chelates, becoming progressively inhomogeneous with central enhancement on delayed images (Figure 20-8).

The hilar type of intrahepatic cholangiocarcinoma, or Klatskin's tumor, is manifested by dilatation of the intrahepatic bile ducts and normal-appearing extrahepatic ducts. Since these patients present with jaundice, ultrasound of the liver is usually the initial

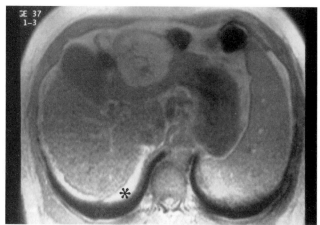

Figure 20-7 ■ Hepatocellular carcinoma. Gradient-echo MR image. Small liver with finely irregular surface and hypertrophy of the caudate lobe. Numerous small dark siderotic nodules in the liver, splenomegaly, and small amount of ascites (*) are indicative of cirrhosis. Tumor in the left hepatic lobe, medial to the gallbladder.

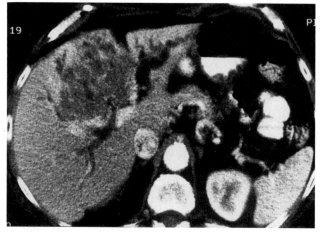

Figure 20-8 ■ Peripheral cholangiocarcinoma. Arterial phase computed tomography. Poorly enhancing predominately necrotic mass with irregular margins causing dilatation of the right and left hepatic ducts.

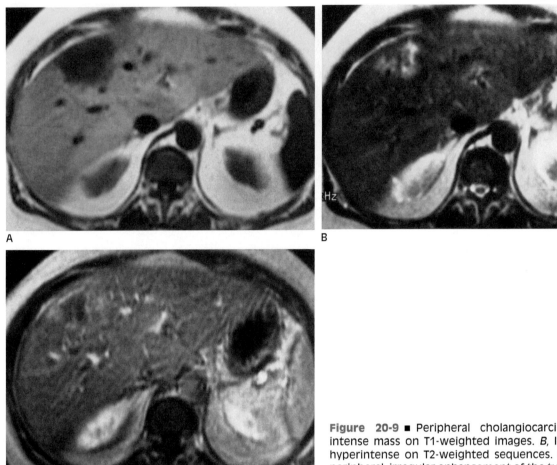

Figure 20-9 ▪ Peripheral cholangiocarcinoma. *A,* Hypointense mass on T1-weighted images. *B,* Inhomogeneously hyperintense on T2-weighted sequences. *C,* Predominately peripheral, irregular enhancement of the tumor. The findings are not specific for this diagnosis.

examination for evaluation of the bile ducts. On computed tomography, a hypodense or isodense mass may be seen in the hepatic hilum, showing enhancement on delayed images (Figure 20-9). Magnetic resonance imaging may show a hyperintense lesion on T2-weighted images. These lesions can be clearly demonstrated by MR cholangiography. Direct opacification of the bile ducts by either endoscopic retrograde cholangiography or percutaneous transhepatic cholangiography may be performed for diagnostic and decompression purposes.

Benign Focal Liver Lesions

Benign hepatic tumors (see Table 20-1) have been reported in over 50% of the general population. Most of them may not have any clinical significance. However, these lesions must be characterized in order to exclude either a primary malignant liver tumor or the presence of metastases in a cancer patient. Lesions less than 15 mm found in patients with known tumors more frequently are benign than malignant, but 11.6% of them have been reported to represent metastases. Abscesses, hematomas, and bilomas usually can be diagnosed on the basis of the clinical history. In this section, only some of the more common cystic and solid benign liver tumors are reviewed.

Liver Cysts

Liver cysts and hemangiomas are the most common focal liver lesions. Cysts may be solitary or multiple and include polycystic liver disease and bile duct hamartomas. Cysts may be unilocular or septated, varying in size from a few millimeters to several centimeters. They may be complicated by intracystic hemorrhage simulating a malignant tumor at imaging, but they rarely become infected. Simple cysts have smooth margins, sharp interface with the surrounding liver, and homogeneous internal architecture. They show total lack of enhancement with contrast material.

Simple cysts are completely anechoic by ultrasound, with good sound transmission, producing a bright reflective zone behind the posterior wall of the cyst (Figure 20-10). On computed tomography, the cysts are hypodense, with water density. On T1-

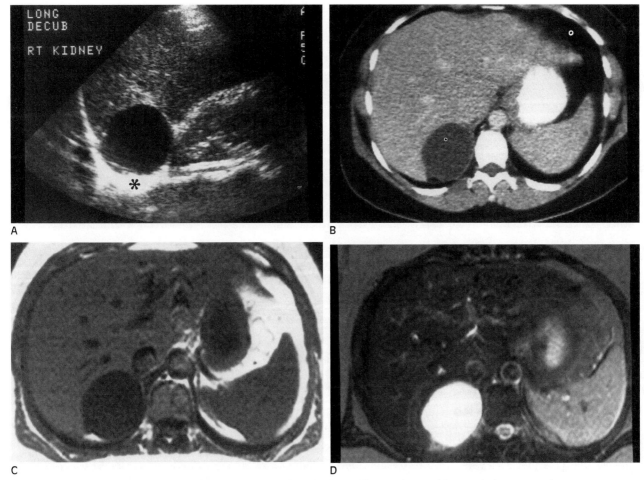

Figure 20-10 ■ Liver cyst. *A,* Ultrasound shows anechoic lesion with good sound transmission (*). *B,* The lesion appears hypodense on enhanced computed tomography images. *C,* Hypointense lesion on T1-weighted images. *D,* Hyperintense on the T2-weighted sequences.

weighted images, they appear hypointense, and on T2-weighted sequences, they become very hyperintense, with signal intensity similar to that of cerebrospinal fluid or bile.

Liver Hemangiomas

Hemangiomas are composed of cystic, blood-filled spaces lined with endothelium and separated by fibrous septa. They appear hyperechogenic on ultrasound, but some either may be hypoechogenic or may have a complex appearance. On unenhanced computed tomography, they are hypodense. During a multiphasic spiral/helical computed tomography examination, they have a characteristic appearance. In the arterial phase, they show intense, peripheral, and discontinuous nodular enhancement, similar in density to adjacent arteries. This phase is followed by progressive centripetal filling-in of the lesion, becoming homogeneously enhanced in delayed images with a density similar to that of portal veins. Small lesions may show complete early and persistent enhancement simulating hypervascular tumors, although the enhancement of hemangiomas may be more prolonged on delayed images. Large lesions may have central fibrosis or hyaline degeneration preventing complete opacification, giving the impression of a central scar. These larger lesions may simulate fibrolamellar hepatocellular carcinoma. On unenhanced magnetic resonance imaging, hemangiomas show changes similar to liver cysts. However, their pattern of enhancement with gadolinium chelates is the same as with enhanced computed tomography (Figure 20-11).

Biliary Cystadenoma

Biliary cystadenomas have an appearance similar to that of benign cysts except for the presence of internal septations and small calcifications in the septa and in the cyst walls (Figure 20-12). The septations may be thick and nodular. They have malignant potential; therefore surgical excision is usually indicated.

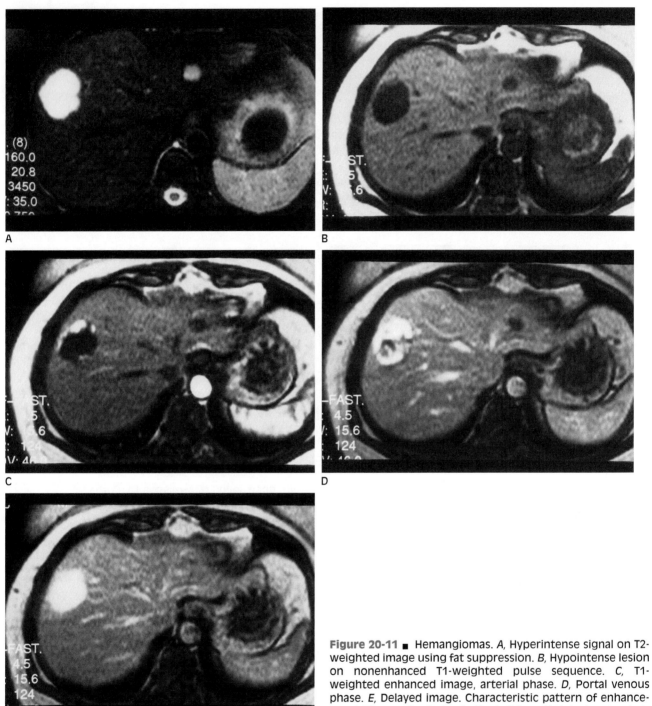

Figure 20-11 ■ Hemangiomas. *A*, Hyperintense signal on T2-weighted image using fat suppression. *B*, Hypointense lesion on nonenhanced T1-weighted pulse sequence. *C*, T1-weighted enhanced image, arterial phase. *D*, Portal venous phase. *E*, Delayed image. Characteristic pattern of enhancement. The smaller lesion in the left hepatic lobe has an atypical appearance that may simulate other lesions.

Focal Nodular Hyperplasia

Focal nodular hyperplasia is a benign lobulated, hypervascular tumor with histology similar to normal liver. It is composed of hepatocytes, Kupffer's cells, bile ductules, and blood vessels. The hyperplastic hepatocytes are arranged in lobules separated by fibrous septa radiating from a central scar that contains large arteries and nonfunctioning bile ductules. It is the

second most common benign liver tumor after hemangiomas.

Focal nodular hyperplasia (FNH) may appear isodense or hypodense on nonenhanced computed tomography but shows intense, brief enhancement during the arterial phase, becoming isodense with rapid washout of the contrast material in the portal venous phase, at which time it might not be detectable. The central scar is hypodense both on the

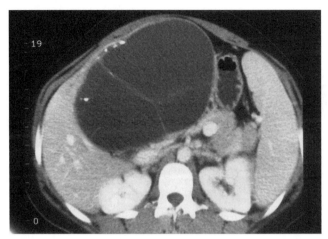

Figure 20-12 ■ Cystadenoma. Enhanced computed tomography. Benign-appearing cyst except for small calcifications in septa and in the cyst walls. Cannot exclude malignancy.

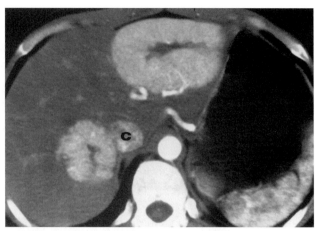

Figure 20-13 ■ Two examples of focal nodular hyperplasia. Arterial phase computed tomography. Hypervascular lesions with typical central scar (C = IVC).

unenhanced images and on the arterial and venous phases but shows increased density on delayed images (Figure 20-13). On magnetic resonance imaging, the lesion is isodense or hypointense on T1-weighted images and slightly hyperintense on T2-weighted sequences. The pattern of enhancement is similar to the one seen with computed tomography. The central scar is hypointense on T1-weighted images, becoming hyperintense on delayed, postcontrast enhanced, T1-weighted sequences. The scar is hyperintense on the T2-weighted images.

Hepatocellular Adenoma

Hepatocellular adenoma is a benign tumor composed of hepatocytes arranged in sheets and cords without an acinar architecture. No bile ductules and no portal venous tracts are present. The tumor is very vascular, with a tendency to bleed and to rupture, and may undergo malignant transformation. It is commonly found in women taking oral contraceptives and may occur in men using anabolic steroids as well as in patients with glycogen storage disease.

The tumor is isodense or hypodense on non-enhanced computed tomography, but areas of bleeding may appear hyperdense. The tumor appears hypervascular, with variable degrees of increased enhancement depending on its size. Large lesions have central areas of necrosis and hemorrhage (Figure 20-14). On T1-weighted images, the tumor is usually hypointense, although the presence of bleeding and/or fat content may cause areas of increased signal

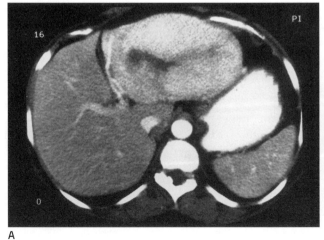

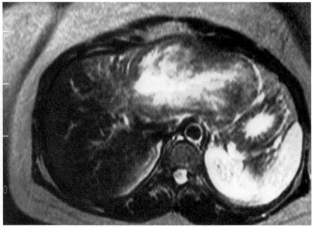

A   B

Figure 20-14 ■ Adenoma. *A*, Arterial phase computed tomography. *B*, T2-weighted MR image. Central necrosis simulating scar. Similar findings can be seen with other lesions.

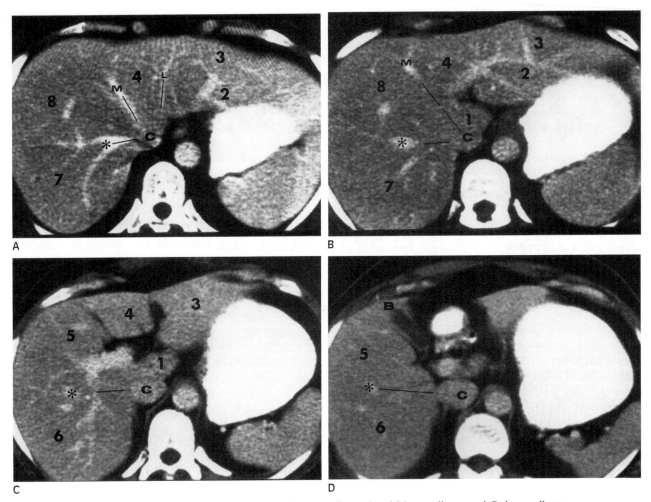

Figure 20-15 ■ Liver segments. *A*, Upper liver, *B*, mid-upper liver, *C*, mid-lower liver, and *D*, lower liver. These levels are usually well seen by computed tomography and magnetic resonance imaging.

intensity on this sequence. On T2-weighted images, the tumor is slightly hyperintense to liver with inhomogeneous areas of increased signal intensity owing to necrosis and hemorrhage. It is frequently impossible to distinguish between hepatocellular adenoma and hepatocellular carcinoma. Given the tendency of this type of lesion to bleed and because of its malignant potential, they are usually treated surgically.

Segmental Anatomy of the Liver

To identify the location of lesions within the liver, a segmental anatomic description is used (Figure 20-15). The right and left hepatic lobes are separated by a vertical oblique plane extending through the middle hepatic vein (M) and the fissure for the gallbladder. The right lobe is divided by the right hepatic vein (*) into anterior segments 8 and 5 and posterior segments 7 and 6. The right portal vein separates the superior and inferior segments of the right lobe. Segment 1 is the caudate lobe. The left lobe is divided into a medial and a lateral segment. The medial segment (4) is located between the middle (M) and the left (L) hepatic veins superiorly and between the fissure for the gallbladder and the fissure for the round ligament inferiorly. The lateral segment has two subsegments, 2 and 3, separated by the left portal vein (C = IVC, B = gallbladder).

DIAGNOSIS

Guidelines in Imaging Focal Liver Lesions

- Spiral/helical computed tomography has been shown to have 85% accuracy in the detection of colon metastases in the liver.
- Most liver lesions can be characterized by enhanced, single-phase spiral/helical computed tomography.
- Nonenhanced spiral/helical computed tomography should be combined with enhanced computed tomography whenever possible (dual-phase or biphasic computed tomography); otherwise, magnetic resonance imaging is preferred over unenhanced computed tomography.
- Hypervascular lesions are better evaluated by triple-phase spiral/helical computed tomography or magnetic resonance imaging.
- After the initial study, hypervascular lesions may be followed up by dual-phase spiral/helical computed tomography or magnetic resonance imaging.
- Lesions usually appear larger without contrast enhancement.
- Some lesions show a characteristic appearance that allows a confident diagnosis. Variants of these same lesions may present with atypical, nondiagnostic appearance.

- A solitary focal liver lesion with malignant features may represent either a primary liver tumor or a metastatic lesion.
- It may be impossible to characterize lesions that are very small or very large lesions that show necrosis and hemorrhage.
- Magnetic resonance imaging is an excellent alternative method for the evaluation of the liver, including diffuse liver disease such as increased iron deposition and fatty infiltration (hepatic steatosis).
- Magnetic resonance imaging can be used either as a primary diagnostic modality or whenever iodinated contrast agents may be contraindicated. It is also indicated when other examinations are inconclusive, in patients with advanced cirrhosis, and in the assessment of resectability of liver metastasis.
- The follow-up of liver lesions should be done using the same modality every time.
- Appropriate clinical information is critical for the adequate tailoring of the examination to the problem to be solved.

Suggested Reading

Craig JR, Peters RL, Edmonson HA: Tumors of the liver and intrahepatic bile ducts. In Atlas of Tumor Pathology, Second Series, Fascicle 26. Washington, DC: Armed Forces Institute of Pathology, 1989.

Hopper KD, Singapuri K, Finkel A: Body CT and oncologic imaging. Radiology 2000;215:27–40.

Horton KM, Bluemke DA, Hruban RH, et al: CT and MR imaging of benign hepatic and biliary tumors. Radio Graphics 1999;19:431–451.

Ito K, Honjo K, Fujita T, et al: Liver neoplasms: Diagnostic pitfalls in cross-sectional imaging. Radiographics 1996;16: 273–293.

Ros PR (guest ed): Hepatic imaging. Radiol Clin North Am 1998;36:237–365.

Sica GT, Ji H, Ros PR: CT and MR imaging of hepatic metastases. Am J Roentgenol 2000;174:691–698.

Chapter 21
Ascites

Kevin R. Fox

Introduction

Ascites is defined as the abnormal accumulation of fluid within the peritoneal cavity. In the clinical practice of oncology, most cases of ascites will occur as a result of progressive carcinoma within this cavity, resulting in diffuse involvement of all peritoneal surfaces by metastatic carcinoma. However, the practicing oncologist must not allow this fact to overshadow his or her obligation to consider the broader definition of ascites as it pertains to the adult population in general. Cancer patients can and will occasionally develop ascites for a variety of nonmalignant reasons, which might or might not be a direct result of the underlying neoplasm. A cursory summary of the various causes of ascites is shown in Table 21-1. This table is not intended to provide a comprehensive list of the possible causes of ascites in all patients but is rather a means of establishing a rational differential diagnosis in the cancer patient who presents with ascites either at the time of diagnosis or at some point during the course of his or her illness. This table divides ascites into nonmalignant and malignant types and assumes that most cases of nonmalignant ascites, with the exception of chylous ascites and infectious ascites, are the ultimate result of portal hypertension, a phenomenon that, in turn, may have a variety of causes.

The pathophysiology and pathogenesis of ascites are complex. In the practice of hepatology, nonmalignant ascites (ascites that is not caused by diffuse peritoneal carcinomatosis) is typically assumed to be a result of either portal hypertension, a general excess of total body sodium and water, or both. The patient with cardiac failure and ascites, for example, will have both processes at play simultaneously, while the patient with a thrombosed hepatic vein (Budd-Chiari syndrome) will have portal hypertension as their initial physiologic insult, with subsequent hepatic insufficiency contributing to both increasing derangements of salt and water metabolism, resulting in total body salt and water excess. A variety of theories exist as to why ascites should occur at all in the setting of liver disease; these theories are not germane to the practice of clinical oncology, except that they may dictate treatment strategies that depart from those used to treat malignant ascites.

However, the pathogenesis of malignant ascites has relatively little to do with sodium and water excess but rather is a consequence of direct tumor invasion of subdiaphragmatic lymphatic channels and consequent perversion of normal peritoneal lymphatic drainage. The tumor types that are most associated with ascites, listed in Table 21-2, are essentially those tumor types that have the greatest predilection for peritoneal dissemination. Thus ovarian (Figure 21-1) and gastrointestinal cancers account for most of the cases of malignant ascites encountered in clinical practice. Other factors may, of course, contribute to ascites formation in the cancer patient who has no involvement of the peritoneum, including obstruction of portal or hepatic veins by thrombus or progressive intrahepatic tumor, hypoalbuminemia, or coexisting renal or hepatic dysfunction. For purposes of management, it is essential to distinguish between "malignant" ascites, in which malignant tumor has gained access to the peritoneal cavity, and "nonmalignant" ascites, in which the accumulation of ascitic fluid stems from some other insult to the liver or peritoneum.

Bedside Diagnosis

The bedside approach to the patient with ascites will depend, of course, on the circumstances under which the ascites is discovered. In the clinical practice of oncology, we will assume that ascites is usually detected under one of two circumstances. First and most frequently, ascites will be discovered or suspected on the basis of the physical examination of the patient who complains of abdominal pain or fullness, obstipation, or dyspnea, the latter due to impairment of

Table 21-1 ▪ Causes of Ascites in the Cancer Patient

Nonmalignant Ascites
    Portal hypertension
      Heart failure
      Pericardial constriction
      Hepatic vein occlusion/obstruction
      Portal vein occlusion/obstruction
      Intrinsic liver disease
      Renal disease
    Chylous ascites
      Retroperitoneal injury or obstruction
    Infectious ascites

Malignant Ascites
    Metastatic carcinomatosis
    Primary peritoneal carcinomatosis
    Lymphoma
    Mesothelioma
    Primary intra-abdominal or metastatic sarcoma

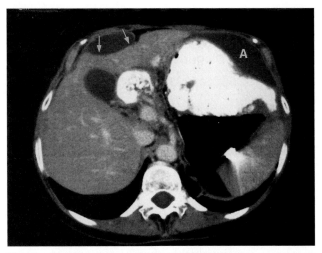

Figure 21-1 ▪ Ascites due to intraperitoneal metastasis from ovarian carcinoma. CT scan through the upper abdomen with the patient in the prone position shows intraperitoneal fluid collections anterior to the liver and splenic flexures (pericolonic ascites identified by A). The ascites indents the contour (arrows) of the medial segment of the left lobe of the liver. Nonmalignant ascites will not indent the liver contour. (Courtesy of Stephen E. Rubesin, M.D., Hospital of the University of Pennsylvania.)

diaphragmatic excursion. The physical examination in the symptomatic patient will usually demonstrate the abdomen to be at varying degrees of distention, relatively dull to percussion, and occasionally possessed of the "fluid wave" or "shifting dullness" that is so often described in medical texts. On many occasions, however, the examination will be equivocal, and the physical examination will be unable to distinguish readily among other causes of a distended abdomen, such as ileus, early bowel obstruction, massive hepatomegaly, or tumor mass. Under such circumstances, proper medical care demands the use of noninvasive strategies such as ultrasonographic imaging to identify the presence, location, and quantity of the ascitic fluid. Oncologists should have a low threshold for ultrasonographic testing if their confidence in the physical examination is anything but complete.

The second set of circumstances under which ascites may be discovered is the incidental finding of modest amounts of ascitic fluid on noninvasive abdominal imaging studies done for purposes of staging or otherwise evaluating for extent of disease. Medical texts state, with some variation, that ascites will not become clinically detectable until between 500 mL and 1500 mL of fluid has accumulated in the peritoneal cavity. The management of asymptomatic ascites in such patients should be approached differently from management of symptomatic patients, as is discussed below.

Diagnostic Approach: Symptomatic Ascites

When the cancer patient has accumulated enough ascitic fluid to become symptomatic, an efficient diagnostic strategy is mandatory. Although there will be an immediate temptation to proceed to paracentesis, the practitioner should pause and entertain the differential diagnosis of nonmalignant causes of ascites. Is there any reason to suspect severe underlying cardiac, renal, or hepatic dysfunction unrelated to the cancer itself? Could the patient be infected? If there are no elements in the medical history (congestive heart failure, preexisting chronic liver disease, renal failure, fever, acute abdominal pain) that make these other, nonmalignant causes patently obvious, then the diagnostic paracentesis should proceed straightaway.

When considering paracentesis, the use of ultrasound imaging for identification and localization of

Table 21-2 ▪ Tumor Types Associated with Malignant Ascites

Common	Uncommon
Ovary	Breast
Colon	Lymphoma
Stomach	Mesothelioma
Uterus	Biliary ducts
Pancreas	Plasmacytoma

Table 21-3 ■ Essential Elements of the Diagnostic Workup of Ascites, with Features Suggestive or Diagnostic of Malignant Ascites

Parameter	Feature
Gross inspection	Bloody or cloudy
Cytology	Positive for malignant cells
Protein level	Ascites/serum ratio >0.4
Lactate dehydrogenase	Ascites/serum ratio >1.0
Cell counts	Total count >1000 μL
Gram stain and culture	Negative for bacteria
Albumin	Serum/ascites albumin <1.1

ascites is an invaluable but sometimes overused device. If the practitioner is confident in the physical examination, then a small-volume paracentesis should be performed to yield enough fluid (minimum 200 mL) to complete a comprehensive diagnostic workup. This author prefers, for diagnostic taps, the use of plastic intravenous catheters (18-gauge or higher) placed in the lower abdominal quadrants midway between midline and axillary line. Other locations, including midline infraumbilical locations, may be selected and should depend on one's prior training, experience, and confidence in the physical findings.

The essential elements of a comprehensive diagnostic workup are included in Table 21-3. Measurement of albumin, protein, lactate dehydrogenase, and amylase, as well as samples for gram stain, bacterial culture, and, most important, cytology, should be sent. As the diagnosis of malignant ascites rests on the finding of malignant cells in the ascitic fluid, submission of fluid for cytology should take precedence if the amount of fluid obtained is unexpectedly meager. Gross inspection of the fluid usually provides a strong clue as to the origin of the ascites: Fluid that is grossly bloody or cloudy is usually malignant or infected, while fluid that is frankly serous may be due to portal hypertension, and fluid that is milky indicates a high lipid content (chylous ascites) and implies injury or obstruction to retroperitoneal lymphatics. Although we should always rely on the cytologic examination to clinch the diagnosis of true malignant ascites, the other parameters may provide valuable clues. An ascites/serum ratio greater than 1.0 for lactic acid dehydrogenase or greater than 0.4 for protein or a leukocyte count greater than 1000/mL is strongly suggestive of malignant ascites, provided that evidence of bacterial infection has been ruled out. The serum/albumin ascites gradient is an excellent means of identifying ascites due to portal hypertension and is able to distinguish ascites of this cause from other

causes. The serum albumin (g/dL) minus the ascitic albumin (g/dL) provides the formula for the gradient; if this number is greater than 1.1, the ascites is probably due to portal hypertension rather than a malignant exudate.

If the cancer patient proves to have nonmalignant ascites, with no cytologic evidence of cancer, low cell counts, low protein, albumin, and lactic acid dehydrogenase content, then the oncologist must consider further diagnostic evaluation to establish treatable causes of nonmalignant ascites (see Table 21-1). Some form of liver imaging should be obtained to rule out cancer-related causes of nonmalignant ascites, such as hepatic or portal vein thrombosis or obstruction of the portal triad by tumor. Magnetic resonance imaging is the diagnostic study of choice under these circumstances. The therapeutic management of malignant and nonmalignant ascites is discussed in following sections.

Diagnostic Approach: Asymptomatic Ascites

The diagnostic strategy for the patient whose ascites is found incidentally during investigations of the peritoneal cavity for other reasons should follow the same logic as that for the symptomatic patient with one obvious question interposed: Will a diagnostic workup matter? Will it make any difference in the treatment, well-being, or outcome for the patient? The lymphoma patient with limited supradiaphragmatic disease in whom locoregional radiation therapy is being contemplated after an abbreviated course of systemic chemotherapy and who has even a modest amount of ascitic fluid on routine abdominal CT scan staging should have every effort made to establish the origin of the ascites, as this will markedly alter treatment strategy if the ascites is caused by lymphoma. Conversely, the patient with metastatic breast cancer who is being restaged after a failure of systemic therapy will not necessarily have her treatment altered because of the incidental finding of ascites on abdominal CT scan, and therefore an aggressive diagnostic workup is not indicated. The cancer patient with unexplained fever, who has no symptoms referable to the abdomen and who is found to have ascites incidentally on the abdominal CT scan performed as part of the "fever of unknown origin" workup, is deserving of an aggressive diagnostic approach, as not all cases of early infectious peritonitis will produce dominant abdominal symptoms.

In considering the diagnostic approach in the asymptomatic patient, blind paracentesis into a normal or marginally abnormal abdomen is not warranted. Here again, ultrasound guidance to establish location, quantity, and accessibility is mandatory before a bedside procedure is considered. If the bedside tap fails to yield adequate fluid for all components of the diagnostic workup and if obtaining adequate peritoneal fluid is essential to establishing a rational overall treatment strategy, then surgical consultation for laparoscopic evaluation under general anesthesia will be necessary. The workup of ascitic fluid so obtained should be identical to the workup in the symptomatic patient.

Treatment: Symptomatic Nonmalignant Ascites

Patients with a known diagnosis of cancer will have nonmalignant ascites in up to one third of cases. Fluid retention due to congestive heart failure, hepatic insufficiency of malignant or nonmalignant origin, or renal failure can be assumed to be secondary to generalized salt and water excess and can be managed with some combination of bed rest, salt restriction (less than 500 mg of sodium intake per day), potassium-sparing diuretics (spironolactone up to 400 mg per day), and loop diuretics (furosemide or ethacrynic acid). If these measures are applied patiently in sequence, most patients with ascites of such origin can diurese 1 to 2 L of ascitic fluid per day. The use of more aggressive diuretic regimens to achieve greater daily volumes of fluid loss is potentially harmful by producing volume contraction, potentially precipitating hepatic encephalopathy, worsening renal failure, and hypokalemia. For the patient whose ascites is accompanied by hypoalbuminemia due to impaired hepatic synthetic function and/or nutritional compromise, regular infusions of albumin are of no proven value and cannot be recommended.

Patients whose ascites is "nonmalignant" but are directly related to the presence of intra-abdominal carcinoma and resulting lymphatic or venous obstruction provide much greater challenges. Malignant tumors in the liver or porta hepatis, which cause portal hypertension and ascites, can be ameliorated by the use of systemic chemotherapy (particularly in the case of malignant lymphoma of the porta hepatis) or occasionally by the use of external beam radiation therapy, using the latter only if the treatment field and dose do not threaten normal liver parenchyma. Tumors of the hepatic parenchyma proper may cause occlusion or thrombosis of the hepatic veins (Budd-Chiari syndrome) or inferior vena cava, resulting in significant hepatic dysfunction and ascites. The value of systemic anticoagulation in relieving thrombosis-related hepatic dysfunction and ascites is doubtful, and

anticoagulants should be used cautiously if systemic antitumor therapy is not an option.

The treatment of ascites secondary to infectious peritonitis is relatively straightforward. The patient who has nonmalignant ascites (cytologically negative) and an ascitic fluid white blood cell count containing more than 250 neutrophils/μL should be presumed to have bacterial peritonitis until proven otherwise and treated empirically with antibiotics. Spontaneous bacterial peritonitis rarely develops in truly malignant ascites and usually occurs when the ascites is due to portal hypertension. The most likely offending microbes are typically enteric gram-negative bacteria such as *Escherichia coli* and *Klebsiella* species, but *Streptococcus pneumoniae* is a frequent offender as well. Therefore presumptive antibacterial therapy should include either ampicillin/sulbactam, a quinolone, or a second-generation cephalosporin, with the choice of antibiotic dependent on the hospital's current antibiotic susceptibility patterns for these organisms.

The treatment of chylous ascites is a substantial, but thankfully uncommon, challenge. Chylous ascites must be assumed to be secondary to lymphatic obstruction in the retroperitoneal space. Antitumor therapy against relatively chemotherapy-sensitive malignancies such as lymphoma might bring about prompt resolution of chylous ascites, but in the setting of chemotherapy-refractory disease, treatment options are much less clear. External beam radiation therapy to a defined retroperitoneal tumor mass can be considered. Consultation with the interventional radiology service to cannulate the cisterna chylae is an option that is reserved for the most desperate of circumstances.

The practice of repeated paracenteses for symptomatic relief should be approached cautiously in the patient with nonmalignant ascites. When ascites results from generalized salt and water excess with concurrent portal hypertension, repeated large-volume paracentesis should be reserved for patients in whom all other approaches have failed. Overzealous removal of such ascites may result in hypotension, volume contraction, and may precipitate hepatic encephalopathy and renal insufficiency in the fashion of overzealous diuresis. No more than 1 or 2 L of ascitic fluid should be removed during any one procedure. Patients with infectious ascites should undergo repeat paracentesis only for the relief of intractable symptoms.

The use of peritoneovenous shunting devices (Denver or LeVeen shunts) in patients with nonmalignant ascites is debatable, as such shunts are prone to substantial failure and complication rates, and should be reserved only for the most refractory cases (see below).

Table 21-4 ■ Treatment Options in Malignant Ascites Management

Hemodynamic
 Bed rest
 Salt restriction
 Diuresis

Chemotherapeutic
 Systemic
 Intracavitary

Mechanical
 Debulking surgery
 Repeat paracentesis
 Peritoneovenous shunts

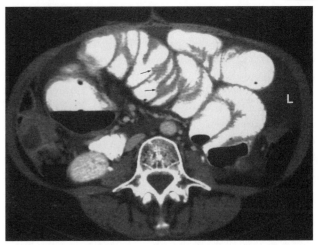

Figure 21-2 ■ Ascites due to intraperitoneal metastasis from ovarian carcinoma. CT scan through the lower abdomen obtained with the patient in the prone position shows ascitic fluid in the right and left paracolic gutters (left paracolic gutter ascites identified by L). Small intestinal loops are mildly dilated and tethered by metastases. Focal thickening of the wall of the small intestine is due to intraperitoneal implants (representative implants indicated by arrows). (Courtesy of Stephen E. Rubesin, M.D., Hospital of the University of Pennsylvania.)

Treatment: Symptomatic Malignant Ascites

Treatment strategies for patients whose ascites is malignant in origin (cytologically positive) are relatively straightforward and can be divided roughly into four categories: hemodynamic, chemotherapeutic (both systemic and intracavitary), and mechanical (Table 21-4). The first two categories require little discussion. The use of salt restriction and diuresis is of little value in treating ascites that is truly malignant. Patients with accompanying portal hypertension from coexisting hepatic involvement by tumor can be considered such candidates for such intervention, but expectations for significant long-term success should be guarded. As in the case of nonmalignant ascites, the use of albumin infusions is not encouraged for the hypoalbuminemic patient. The use of systemic chemotherapy as the primary treatment modality for malignant ascites requires that the malignancy be reasonably chemotherapy sensitive and that the patient's abdominal symptoms be modest. The severely symptomatic patient should have some mechanical effort made to remove ascites for comfort reasons before systemic chemotherapy is contemplated. The newly diagnosed lymphoma patient has an excellent chance of rapid palliation and potential cure with systemic chemotherapy alone but should not be required to remain uncomfortable while awaiting chemotherapy's benefits. Repeated paracentesis until the chemotherapy-induced reduction of ascites is realized constitutes the most humane approach to care. A similar juxtaposition of chemotherapy and intermittent paracentesis can be applied to any patient who stands a reasonable chance of response to chemotherapy in the first place: Metastatic cancers of breast, ovarian, colonic, pancreatic, or gastric origin will fall under this heading, but under no circumstances should such a patient be denied the symptomatic benefits of paracentesis while awaiting an uncertain response to chemotherapy. The use of methotrexate, while no longer a major consideration in the treatment of most chemotherapy-sensitive malignancies, is discouraged in the patient with ascites, as methotrexate can accumulate in ascites, with resulting slow release into the systemic circulation and potential augmentation of clinical toxicity.

Most of the available information regarding the use of intraperitoneal drug therapy (intracavitary therapy) is derived from the ovarian cancer literature and involves the use of intraperitoneal cisplatinum, alone or in combination with other agents. In this literature, intraperitoneal cisplatinum was not intended to treat ascites per se, but rather was given as part of the overall treatment strategy for the patient with newly diagnosed or recurrent ovarian cancer. Only one clinical trial randomized patients to receive purely intracavitary versus purely systemic chemotherapy at the time of diagnosis, and it did not show a difference in overall survival or response rates in a small number of patients. While intraperitoneal cisplatinum clearly has some palliative benefit in patients with recurrent ovarian carcinoma or peritoneal carcinomatosis (Figure 21-2), insufficient data exist to support the routine use of intraperitoneal chemotherapy for the treatment of ascites due to other tumor types.

Mechanical approaches to the treatment of malignant ascites include surgical evacuation of the peritoneal space, repeat paracentesis, and shunting procedures. Radical surgical approaches to the treatment of ascites are encouraged only when an aggressive surgical approach is part of the overall treatment strategy of a particular patient. The newly diagnosed patient with ovarian cancer and ascites will undergo aggressive debulking surgery as part of her long-term treatment plan; such an approach is not necessarily appropriate for patients with refractory or recurrent carcinomas of other origins. An aggressive surgical approach in some patients with sarcoma or mesothelioma of the peritoneum has been advocated as a prelude to intracavitary chemotherapy, but such an approach is not appropriate except in qualified institutions.

The use of repeat paracentesis is probably the most frequently used palliative approach to ascites treatment in general oncology practice. Large volumes of ascitic fluid can be removed in a single procedure, generally without regard to the hemodynamic consequences of overzealous paracentesis in patients whose ascites is secondary to portal hypertension. This author prefers to use 3-inch metal thoracentesis needles (18-gauge or higher) for palliative therapeutic taps in order to avoid the premature collapse of plastic catheters. With or without ultrasound guidance, volumes of fluid in excess of 5 L can be removed on repeated occasions. With each procedure, however, the risk of infection, visceral injury, leaking, or electrolyte imbalance increases. For this reason, a variety of implantable shunting devices have been developed for long-term palliation of malignant ascites.

The standard shunting devices (known as the LeVeen or Denver shunt) are essentially single lengths of flexible plastic tubing. One end of the tube has numerous side-perforations, and it is this end that is placed in the peritoneal cavity. The tube exits the peritoneal cavity through a subcostal incision and is tunneled subcutaneously along the anterolateral thorax until it enters the circulation via the subclavian or jugular vein. The constant pressure gradient between the abdomen and thorax, a gradient that increases with each inhalation and subsequent drop in intrathoracic pressure, favors spontaneous flow from peritoneum to general circulation. All shunting devices contain a one-way valve, which maintains flow in a cephalad direction, and in the case of the Denver shunt, the valve can be pumped manually by the patient or caretaker to encourage cephalad flow.

Peritoneovenous shunts neither prolong survival nor necessarily enhance quality of life; they should be considered to spare patients the logistic inconvenience and discomfort of repeat paracentesis. Peritoneovenous shunts have a high failure rate, typically due to shunt occlusion. Disseminated intravascular coagula-

Table 21-5 ▪ Considerations in Placing a Peritoneovenous Shunt (after Souter et al., 1983)

Rapid reaccumulation of ascites after paracentesis
No evidence of loculation of fluid on abdominal imaging
Nonviscous ascites
Survival anticipated to be more than three months

tion is a complication of shunt placement but may occur much less frequently in the patient with malignant ascites than in the patient whose ascites is secondary to portal hypertension. Patients undergoing peritoneovenous shunting do so as an overall palliative strategy and generally survive for up to six months, with a few patients surviving for more than a year; these poor survival times are reflective of the patient's underlying disease process. Guidelines for patient selection for shunting procedures are shown in Table 21-5.

Malignant Ascites as a Presenting Sign of Disease

On occasion, patients with no known cancer history will present with symptomatic ascites, which, on diagnostic paracentesis, reveals carcinoma. The workup that ensues should depend primarily on the sex of the patient. As more than three fourths of women presenting with malignant ascites will have gynecologic malignancies, the workup should proceed accordingly, with ultrasound evaluation of the ovaries and a careful gynecologic examination. Failure to disclose a primary tumor by these means should lead to either laparoscopy (which will successfully identify the primary tumor in the majority of cases) or exploratory laparotomy, with plans to perform a debulking procedure if an ovarian or peritoneal primary tumor is found. Because male patients are likely to have gastrointestinal primary tumors when presenting with malignant ascites, endoscopic evaluation of the gastrointestinal tract is the most sensible diagnostic undertaking. The yield of laparoscopy in disclosing a primary tumor in men has been evaluated less extensively but should be considered when a thorough evaluation of the gastrointestinal tract has failed.

Overview of Care

The grim reality of ascites management in general oncologic practice is that the patient with ascites will develop this complication as a late event during the phase of progressive decline from his or her underlying malignancy. For this reason, aggressive means to palliate ascites are often not indicated. A sensible mechanical approach to management should be conducted in the context of an overall palliative treatment strategy. The greatest challenge to the oncologist is the identification of the patient who develops ascites that can be managed for extended periods of time because the ascites stems from some unrelated, nonmalignant cause. Every patient deserves at least a comprehensive workup to rule out such treatable causes of ascites.

Suggested Reading

Alexander HR, Fraker DI: Shunting procedures for malignant ascites and pleural effusions. In Lotze MT, Rubin JB (eds): Regional Therapy for Malignant Ascites and Pleural Effusions. Philadelphia: Lippincott-Raven, 1997, p 271.

Chu CM, Lin SM, Peng SM, et al: The role of laparoscopy in the evaluation of ascites of unknown origin. Gastrointest Endosc 1994;40:285.

Parsons SL, Watson SA, Steele RJ: Malignant ascites. Br J Surg 1996;83:6–14.

Runyon BA: Care of patients with ascites. N Eng J Med 1994;330:337.

Souter RG, Tarin D, Kettlewell MG: Peritoneovenous shunts in the management of malignant ascites. Br J Surg 1983; 70:478.

Tempero MA, Davis RB, Reed E, Edney J: Thrombocytopenia and laboratory evidence of disseminated intravascular coagulation after shunts for ascites in malignant disease. Cancer 1985;55:2718.

Chapter 22
Splenomegaly

David P. Schenkein

Introduction

Splenic enlargement occurs in a number of hematologic disorders and is not an issue when the underlying cause is known. Patients who present with splenomegaly as their principal and/or sole abnormality do pose diagnostic challenges. Distinguishing a malignant from a benign cause in these patients is paramount to undertaking their care. As Table 22-1 shows, the list of potential causes is lengthy. Splenomegaly can result from the following problems: infiltration by granulomas, cancer, parasitic and infectious organisms, deposition of proteins or lipids, elevated splenic venous pressure due to increased portal venous pressure or splenic vein thrombosis, extramedullary hematopoiesis in myeloproliferative syndromes and severe hemolytic anemias, splenic hyperplasia due to increased activity in clearing red blood cells in hemolytic anemias or secondary to lymphoid proliferation in response to viral infections and inflammatory, and immunologic disease.

Clinical Presentation

The underlying condition and the rapidity of the enlargement often dictate the clinical presentation. The majority of patients with moderate splenomegaly are asymptomatic. Symptoms, when they occur, are generally related to splenic size such as early satiety (due to compromise of stomach volume by splenic enlargement), loss of lean body mass, abdominal fullness and distention, or pain from splenic infarction. Splenic infarction usually causes left upper quadrant pain that is referred to the left shoulder due to diaphragmatic irritation. Physical examination may disclose a splenic friction rub. Unlike the splenic infarcts that occur in children with sickle-cell disease, these most often occur in adult patients with sickle-cell variants or with massive splenomegaly from myeloproliferative disorders. The clinical diagnosis can often be confirmed by observing a wedge-shaped hypodense defect in the spleen on computed tomography (CT) scan. These usually resolve spontaneously over seven to ten days; splenic rupture very rarely occurs. Splenic rupture can occur in patients with infectious mononucleosis during the initial two weeks of illness, when the spleen expands rapidly owing to T-lymphocyte proliferation.

Clinical Evaluation

Up to 50% of moderately enlarged spleens are not palpable. Physical examination will detect splenomegaly only after the spleen has tripled in volume. Once the spleen, which lies posteriorly, has increased from its normal weight in the adult of 150 to 175 mg to approximately 450 mg, it can be palpated anteriorly on abdominal examination. In contrast, a common error is not palpating low enough in the abdomen to feel the edge of a massively enlarged spleen that can extend into the pelvis. The pathognomonic friction rub that can be heard in the setting of a splenic infarct is another often overlooked clinical finding. It is best to examine the abdomen for splenomegaly from the right side of the patient both in the fully supine position and with the patient in the right lateral position using both palpation and percussion techniques. Imaging modalities such as the computed tomography scan (Figure 22-1), ultrasound, and nuclear isotopic scans are often used to supplement the physical examination. Imaging of the spleen can detect filling defects (Figure 22-2), determine the size of an impalpable but enlarged spleen, and alert one to other findings that help to establish the diagnosis.

Differential Diagnosis

The differential diagnosis of splenomegaly encompasses most disciplines within internal medicine. Despite the broad scope of potential diagnoses, the number of possible explanations for an enlarged spleen markedly decreases after a full history is

Table 22-1 ■ Differential Diagnosis of Splenomegaly

Infections

Infectious mononucleosis due to Epstein-Barr virus or cytomegalovirus
Acute and chronic bacterial infections
Disseminated mycobacterial or fungal infection
Parasitic red blood cell infestations, such as malaria and babesiosis
HIV disease
Viral hepatitis
Acute viral infections
Rickettsial infections
Toxoplasmosis
Splenic abscess
Other: histoplasmosis, leishmaniasis, trypanosomiasis, Lyme disease, syphilis

Infiltrative Diseases

Benign: Gaucher's disease or other glycogen storage disease
Malignant: Hodgkin's disease, non-Hodgkin's lymphoma, leukemias, splenic metastases, systemic mastocytosis, amyloidosis
Extramedullary hematopoiesis in myeloproliferative syndromes or severe hemolytic anemia

Immunologic Disorders

Felty's syndrome: rheumatoid arthritis, splenomegaly, and neutropenia
Systemic lupus erythematosus
Immune hemolytic anemias
Congenital or acquired hypogammaglobulinemia, secondary to splenic hyperplasia
Serum sickness
Graft versus host disease
Sarcoidosis
Sjögrens syndrome
Large granular lymphocytosis and neutropenia
Drug hypersensitivity reactions, especially phenytoin

Nonimmunologic Hemolytic Anemias

Sickle-cell disease: in children until autoinfarction occurs
Sickle-cell variants, such as sickle-cell disease
Congenital spherocytosis or elliptocytosis
Thalassemia

Elevated Splenic Vein Pressure

Cirrhosis
Hepatic vein obstruction
Portal vein obstruction
Chronic congestive heart failure
Splenic vein thrombosis

Anatomic Splenic Abnormalities

Cysts, hamartomas

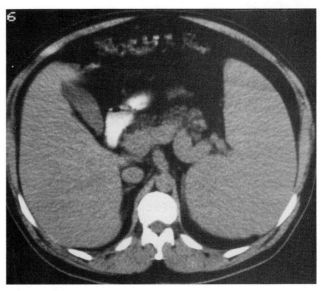

Figure 22-1 ■ Splenomegaly. (From Grainger RG, Allison DJ: Diagnostic Radiology, 3rd ed. Churchill Livingstone 1999, p 2580.)

obtained, a careful physical examination is performed looking for other manifestations of disease, and the blood counts and peripheral blood smear are analyzed. For example, it should become clear whether an underlying infectious or immunologic inflammatory disorder is the likely cause. Appropriate tests then help to make the specific diagnosis.

The complete blood count, peripheral blood smear, reticulocyte count, and bilirubin frequently provide clues to a hematologic disorder and allow assessment of whether hemolysis is present. The information then guides the choice of additional investigative studies.

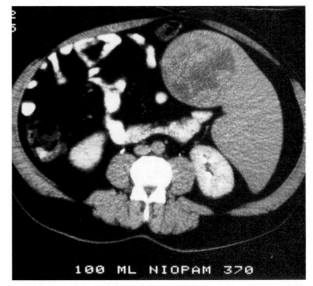

Figure 22-2 ■ Splenomegaly with filling defects. (From Grainger RG, Allison DJ: Diagnostic Radiology, 3rd ed. Churchill Livingstone, 1999, p 2580.)

DIAGNOSIS

Considerations in the Evaluation of Splenomegaly

- Patients with idiopathic immune thrombocytopenia (ITP) do not have an enlarged spleen, despite the increased destruction of antibody-coated platelets in the spleen. If splenomegaly is present in a patient with thrombocytopenia, then the low platelet count is due to one of the disorders listed in Table 22-1. For example, the thrombocytopenia could be a secondary immunologic manifestation in a patient with systemic lupus erythematosus or lymphoma or could be due to a nonimmune cause such as hypersplenism.
- If the platelet count is less than 50,000/μL, then hypersplenism, although it might be present, is not usually the sole cause of the lowered platelet count.
- In non-Hodgkin's lymphomas, splenomegaly is almost always due to diffuse lymphomatous infiltration of the spleen. This can be confirmed on CT scan, but splenic defects are rare. In contrast, in Hodgkin's disease, splenic enlargement is usually secondary to nonspecific lymphoid hyperplasia, a secondary manifestation of Hodgkin's disease. In Hodgkin's disease, direct involvement of the spleen is focal and nodular. The nodules are very rarely numerous or large enough to cause splenomegaly. As a result, computed tomography scanning in Hodgkin's disease does not detect deposits in the spleen, and enlargement does not necessarily reflect that splenic disease is present.
- In very aggressive non-Hodgkin's lymphomas, splenic involvement can be substantial, revealing space-occupying lesions and tumor necrosis on computed tomography scan.
- The largest spleens occur in patients with a myeloproliferative disorder, such as in the advanced stages of chronic myeloid leukemia, polycythemia vera, essential thrombocythemia, and myelofibrosis. These spleens limit gastric intake, causing weight loss, which can be masked by the contribution of increasing splenic weight.
- In patients with splenomegaly, a reticulocyte count should be obtained even if the hemoglobin and hematocrit are normal. An elevated reticulocyte count may disclose an unanticipated compensated hemolytic anemia.
- In a small number of otherwise normal individuals (15% of children, 3% of young adults), the spleen may be palpable 2 cm below the left costal margin. This represents residual, slowly resolving splenic hyperplasia due to a prior viral infection, such as infectious mononucleosis. If the patient is asymptomatic and routine blood counts, platelet count, and reticulocyte count are normal, further investigation is unnecessary.
- In apparently normal individuals one must be wary of occult liver disease. For example, hepatic schistosomiasis can lead to cirrhosis and portal hypertension while routine liver function tests remain entirely normal. A study of portal blood flow can verify the presence of congestive splenomegaly.

Hypersplenism

Although cytopenias may be manifestations of a primary hematologic disorder, reductions in the number of red blood cells, platelets, and/or white blood cells can occur as a manifestation of hypersplenism. Hypersplenism can develop in patients who have splenomegaly due to splenic hyperplasia or infiltrative disease of the spleen, but it is more likely to appear in circumstances in which splenic venous pressure is increased, most commonly by cirrhosis of the liver. The cytopenia(s) caused by splenomegaly due to elevated portal venous pressure do not result from increased destruction of red blood cells, platelets, or white blood cells. Usually, the total body mass of these cells is normal. The fraction of these cells in the circulation is reduced because of increased, transient sequestration in the spleen. Under stress, the spleen releases these elements. As much as 60% of the total platelet population may be in the spleen in the patient with hypersplenism. The net effect is that the platelet count generally does not fall lower than 50,000/μL on the basis of hypersplenism alone. Moreover, reduced blood counts due to hypersplenism do not require therapy because the reductions are modest, the cells are still available if needed, and the patient is not at risk for infection from leukopenia, bleeding from thrombocytopenia, or symptoms from anemia.

Bone Marrow Aspiration and Biopsy

A bone marrow examination should be performed whenever the potential for a malignant (e.g., leukemia, lymphoma) or infiltrative (Gaucher's) disease exists that is not otherwise apparent from the preceding evaluation. On occasion, some infections, such as systemic mycobacterium tuberculosis, and other granulomatous disorders associated with splenomegaly may be diagnosed after bone marrow aspiration/biopsy, with or without cultures being obtained. In immunologic disorders, such as autoimmune warm antibody hemolytic anemia or immune thrombocytopenia, bone marrow evaluation may be warranted because these can be secondary manifestations of Hodgkin's or non-Hodgkin's lymphomas.

Splenic Aspiration/Biopsy

Although occasionally used at some centers, splenic biopsies are generally avoided because of the high risk of bleeding complications. The rare splenic biopsy is performed today under computed tomography scan or ultrasonic guidance. This procedure is reserved for drainage of an abscess or fluid collection rather than to obtain a tissue diagnosis. If splenic tissue is required to make a diagnosis, then splenectomy is usually performed.

Splenectomy is rarely necessary for diagnostic purposes because ancillary studies such as imaging, blood counts, blood chemistries, and flow cytometry of the peripheral blood and/or bone marrow reveal the diagnosis in most circumstances.

Suggested Reading

Bora P, Gomber S, Agarwal V, Jain M: Splenic tuberculosis presenting as hypersplenism. Ann Trop Paediatr 2001;21:86–87.

Calvo-Romero JM: Magnetic resonance imaging in primary lymphoma of the spleen. Arch Intern Med 2000;160:1706–1707.

Cleary JE, Burke WM, Baxi LV: Pregnancy after avascular necrosis of the femur complicating Gaucher's disease. Am J Obstet Gynecol 2001;184:233–234.

Klopfenstein KJ, Grossman NJ, Fishbein M, Ruymann FB: Cavernous transformation of the portal vein: A cause of thrombocytopenia and splenomegaly. Clin Pediatr 2000;39:727–730.

Liu DC, Meyers MO, Hill CB, Loe WA Jr: Laparoscopic splenectomy in children with hematological disorders: Preliminary experience at the Children's Hospital of New Orleans. Am Surg 2000;66:1168–1170.

Mazonakis M, Damilakis J, Maris T, et al: Estimation of spleen volume using MR imaging and a random marking technique. Eur Radiol 2000;10:1899–1903.

Messinezy M, MacDonald LM, Nunan TO, et al: Spleen sizing by ultrasound in polycythemia and thrombocythaemia: Comparison with SPECT. Br J Haematol 1997;98:103–107.

Neudorfer O, Hadas-Halpern J, Elstein D, et al: Abdominal ultrasound findings mimicking hematological malignancies in a study of 218 Gaucher patients. Am J Hematol 1997;55:28–34.

Secil M, Goktay A, Dicle O, Pirnar T: Splenic vascular malformations and portal hypertension in hereditary hemorrhagic telangiectasia: Sonographic findings. J Clin Ultrasound 2001;29:56–59.

Sheth SG, Amarapurkar DN, Chopra KB, et al: Evaluation of splenomegaly in portal hypertension. J Clin Gastroenterol 1996;22:28–30.

Shurin, SB: The spleen and its disorders. In Hoffman R, Benz E, Shattil SJ, Furie B, Cohen HJ, Silberstein LE (eds): Hematology. New York: Churchill Livingstone, 1999, pp 821–829.

Swaroop J, O'Reilly RA: Splenomegaly at a university hospital compared to a nearby count hospital in 317 patients. Acta Haematol 1999;102:83–88.

Tincani E, Cioni G, D'Alimonte P, et al: Value of the measurement of portal blood flow velocity in the differential diagnosis of asymptomatic splenomegaly. Clin Radiol 1997;52:220–223.

Wenzel JS, Donohoe A, Ford KL, et al: Primary biliary cirrhosis: MR imaging findings and description of MR imaging periportal halo sign. Am J Roentgenol 2001;176:885–889.

Chapter 23
Dysphagia

Stuart J. Spechler

Dysphagia is the perception that there is an impediment to the normal passage of swallowed material. Patients with dysphagia frequently relate that swallowed food "gets stuck" or "just won't go down right." Dysphagia can be caused by benign or malignant disorders that either obstruct the esophagus or interfere with its motor function. When cancers cause dysphagia, they generally do so through one of three mechanisms:

1. Primary tumors of the esophagus or proximal stomach grow to cause intrinsic, mechanical obstruction of the esophageal lumen.
2. Cancers involving structures adjacent to the esophagus (e.g., mediastinal lymph nodes) grow to encircle or invade the organ and cause extrinsic, mechanical narrowing of the esophagus.
3. Uncommonly, malignancies affect the esophageal muscle and its innervation to disrupt peristalsis, interfere with lower esophageal sphincter relaxation, or both. Such motor dysfunction can be caused by local tumors that invade the esophageal neural plexuses or by remote tumors that presumably release humoral factors that disrupt esophageal motility as part of a paraneoplastic syndrome.

Initial Assessment of the Patient with Dysphagia

On the basis of a careful history alone, the clinician can predict, with an accuracy of approximately 80%, whether dysphagia is caused by a benign or malignant disorder. The physical examination is important for assessing the patient's performance status and ability to tolerate any contemplated therapies, but only infrequently does the physical examination provide specific clues to the etiology of dysphagia (e.g., a palpable left supraclavicular (Virchow's) lymph node may suggest dysphagia due to a malignancy within the abdomen).

Some key elements of the history are highlighted in the following paragraphs.

Is the dysphagia for solid foods, liquids, or both? Tumors that cause dysphagia by narrowing the esophageal lumen usually pose little barrier to the passage of liquids until very late in the course of the disease when the obstruction becomes complete. Consequently, patients with dysphagia caused by partially obstructing tumors characteristically experience swallowing difficulty only when they ingest solid foods. In contrast, diseases that disrupt esophageal motility may cause dysphagia for liquids as well as solids. Although malignancies rarely can cause motility disorders manifested by dysphagia for liquids (e.g., pseudoachalasia), the vast majority of patients with dysphagia due to cancer complain of dysphagia for solids alone.

Where does the patient perceive that ingested material sticks? Patients with esophageal obstruction usually perceive that swallowed material sticks at a point that is either above or at the level of the lesion that is causing the obstruction. It is uncommon for patients to perceive that swallowed material sticks at a level substantially below that of the obstructing lesion. The perception that a swallowed bolus sticks above the suprasternal notch is of little value in localizing the obstruction, because this sensation could be caused by a lesion located anywhere from the pharynx to the gastroesophageal junction. If the patient localizes the obstruction to a point below the suprasternal notch, however, the chances are excellent that the dysphagia is caused by a disorder that involves the esophagus.

Are there symptoms of oropharyngeal dysfunction? Oropharyngeal dysphagia usually results from diseases that affect the striated muscles of the oropharynx or their innervation (e.g., muscular dystrophies, cerebrovascular accidents). Patients with these neuromuscular diseases may experience difficulty in initiating a swallow, and swallowing may be accompanied by nasopharyngeal regurgitation, pulmonary aspiration, and a sensation that residual material remains in the pharynx. If any of these symptoms are prominent, evaluation for oropharyngeal dysfunction may precede tests for esophageal disorders. Large tumors of the head and neck can cause dysphagia by obstructing the oropharynx, but such large tumors seldom cause major diagnostic difficulties.

Is the dysphagia rapidly progressive? Rapid progression of dysphagia (over a period of weeks to months) associated with profound weight loss strongly suggests malignancy. In contrast, patients with benign esophageal disorders typically complain of dysphagia that progresses either slowly (over a period of months to years) or not at all, and the dysphagia usually does not result in substantial weight loss. It is decidedly unusual for patients with dysphagia due to cancer to describe symptoms that have persisted for more than one year.

Are there risk factors for esophageal cancer? Cigarette smoking and alcohol abuse are strong risk factors for squamous cell carcinomas of the head and neck and esophagus. For this reason, presumably, head and neck cancer is strongly associated with esophageal cancer and vice versa. Barrett's esophagus, the condition in which the squamous lining of the distal esophagus is replaced by a metaplastic intestinal-type epithelium, is a strong risk factor for esophageal adenocarcinoma. The new onset of dysphagia in a patient who is known to have Barrett's esophagus suggests the possibility of this cancer. Heartburn, the cardinal symptom of gastroesophageal reflux disease (GERD), is also an established risk factor for esophageal adenocarcinoma, presumably because gastroesophageal reflux disease causes Barrett's esophagus. However, most patients with dysphagia due to benign peptic strictures also have a history of long-standing heartburn. Consequently, conclusions regarding the etiology of dysphagia should not be based primarily on the presence or absence of heartburn.

Is the patient immunosuppressed? Infectious esophagitis occurs frequently in patients whose immune system has been compromised severely by advanced malignancy, by infection with the human immunodeficiency virus, or by organ transplantation with the administration of potent immunosuppressive drugs. Most esophageal infections are caused by one or a combination of only three organisms: candida, cytomegalovirus, and herpes simplex virus. Odynophagia (pain on swallowing) is usually the predominant symptom for patients with infectious esophagitis, but many patients experience some dysphagia as well.

Diagnostic Tests

Physicians continue to debate whether to perform a barium swallow early in the evaluation of dysphagia or whether it is more cost-effective to bypass the radiographic study and to proceed directly to endoscopic evaluation of the esophagus. Those who advocate early radiology contend that the barium swallow provides valuable anatomic information that may help to prevent procedural complications and to direct therapy. For example, a barium swallow can identify lesions that might pose potential hazards such as a large Zenker's diverticulum that could be perforated by the unwary endoscopist. For patients with malignant esophageal strictures so tight that they cannot be traversed by the endoscope, a barium esophagogram can provide information on the extent of the tumor that may be helpful in staging and in directing the appropriate therapy. Also, an initial barium swallow provides an objective baseline record of the esophagus that can be useful in assessing the response to therapy or progression of disease. Proponents of early endoscopy argue that this procedure is virtually always required in the evaluation of dysphagia, regardless of the radiographic findings, and that a barium swallow usually does not provide sufficient additional information to justify its added expense and inconvenience. Despite all the proposed advantages for early radiographic evaluation, no study yet has shown that performance of a barium swallow prior to endoscopy decreases complications or improves outcomes for patients with dysphagia. In the absence of meaningful studies validating the cost-efficacy of either approach, this debate will continue.

When a barium swallow demonstrates an esophageal stricture, features that suggest malignancy include irregular borders and sharp angles (in contrast to the smooth, gradual tapering that is typical of benign peptic strictures) (Figure 23-1). Most benign peptic strictures are located in the distal esophagus, and cancer becomes more likely for strictures that involve the middle and proximal esophagus. Cancers in mediastinal lymph nodes that cause dysphagia by encasing the esophagus also typically involve the middle and proximal esophagus. Unless contraindicated by serious comorbidity, endoscopic evaluation is recommended for virtually all patients with dysphagia either to establish or to confirm a diagnosis. Unlike the radiologist, the endoscopist can obtain biopsy and brush cytology specimens of esophageal lesions that can establish the diagnosis of specific neoplasms or infections. Endoscopy also is more sensitive than radiology for identifying small mucosal lesions of the esophagus. Endoscopically, primary esophageal malignancies typically appear as nodular lesions that protrude into the lumen of the esophagus (Figure 23-2). Extrinsic and submucosal lesions that cause dysphagia appear endoscopically as areas of narrowing that are lined by normal-appearing mucosa.

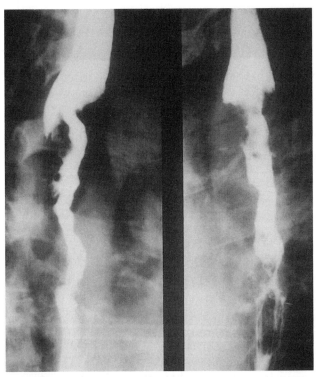

Figure 23-1 ■ Barium swallow of an advanced cancer of the esophagus. The proximal edge of the ulcerated tumor forms an abrupt shelf that gives the lesion the appearance of an apple core. (Reprinted, with permission, from the Clinical Teaching Project of the American Gastroenterological Association.)

Most malignant causes of dysphagia will be identified by barium swallow and/or endoscopy. Endoscopic biopsy specimens can establish the diagnosis of the specific tumor that is causing the dysphagia for primary epithelial malignancies of the esophagus and stomach, for tumors that invade the wall of the esophagus to involve the mucosa, and for submucosal tumors that are exposed by overlying ulceration. When the barium swallow or endoscopic examination identifies an extrinsic lesion causing dysphagia by esophageal compression, computed tomography (CT) of the chest may be helpful to suggest a specific diagnosis (e.g., enlarged mediastinal lymph nodes, primary lung tumor). Sometimes, a primary tumor of the esophagus or stomach causes dysphagia by infiltrating the wall of the esophagus without breaking through the mucosa. Such tumors may be located deep in the submucosa, beyond the reach of standard, endoscopic mucosal biopsy forceps. In these cases, CT may help to define the extent of submucosal tumor involvement. Needle biopsy sampling of such lesions may be accomplished using guidance provided by CT or by endoscopic ultrasonography.

As was mentioned previously, some tumors cause dysphagia by disturbing esophageal motor function through either local or systemic effects. When such tumors cause motility abnormalities similar to those of primary, idiopathic achalasia (e.g., incomplete relaxation of the lower esophageal sphincter, absent peristalsis), the condition is called secondary achalasia or pseudoachalasia. If the clinical history strongly suggests pseudoachalasia due to malignancy (e.g., onset in old age, rapid progression of symptoms, profound weight loss), tests such as computed tomography or endosonography might be necessary to demonstrate the neoplasm. Esophageal manometry can establish the type of motility disorder, but no manometric feature is specific for dysmotility due to malignancy.

Management

An approach to the management of patients with dysphagia due to cancer is outlined in Figure 23-3. When a barium swallow or endoscopic examination has established that dysphagia is due to a tumor that involves the esophagus, either primarily or by invasion, the next step is an evaluation of the patient's fitness to undergo treatment. Tumor staging (often involving CT and endosonography for primary esophageal tumors) may be performed to assess the appropriate treatment options, which are often dependent on the tumor stage. These data are used to determine whether treatment directed at the primary tumor is feasible. Such treatments usually involve a choice among surgery, radiation therapy, chemother-

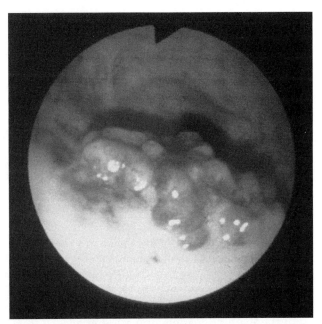

Figure 23-2 ■ Endoscopic photograph showing a nodular carcinoma of the esophagus. (Reprinted, with permission, from the Clinical Teaching Project of the American Gastroenterological Association.) (See Color Plate 2.)

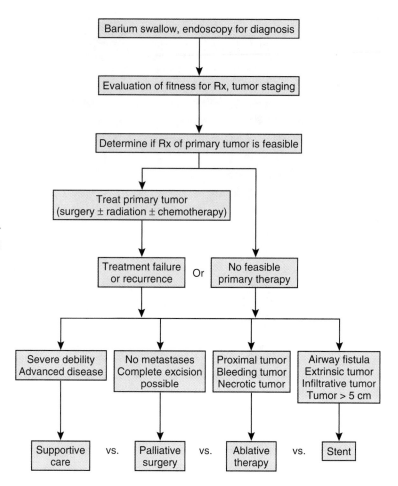

Figure 23-3 ■ Management algorithm for patients with dysphagia due to cancer involving the esophagus.

apy, or some combination of these three modalities. The use of research protocols is recommended to direct this choice for patients with tumors whose treatment is disputed.

If treatment of the primary tumor is feasible and the patient is able to maintain adequate oral intake, then initial treatment is directed only at the primary tumor. Palliative therapies designed to open the obstructed esophagus such as tumor dilation, endoscopic ablative treatments, and stent placement generally are not used at this point unless the patient cannot maintain adequate oral intake and palliation by the primary therapy is likely to be delayed. For example, it might take weeks for chemoradiation therapy to provide relief of dysphagia in patients with advanced esophageal malignancies. For such patients who have severe dysphagia, a dysphagia-palliating therapy may be combined with treatment of the primary tumor.

If there are no feasible primary therapies, if treatments directed at the primary tumor fail or if the tumor recurs, then there are a number of palliative treatment options to manage the dysphagia. Tumor

dilation with mercury-filled rubber bougies, wire-guided dilators (e.g., Savary-Gilliard), or balloons can be helpful occasionally, but such dilation often is ineffective and at best provides only very short-lived results. For patients who are severely debilitated and who have advanced disease, the most humane option may be only supportive care with careful attention to pain control. If there are no apparent metastases and complete excision of the tumor is possible, then surgery sometimes can provide excellent palliation for primary esophageal tumors. Other options include ablative therapies (e.g., photodynamic therapy, Nd:YAG laser, chemical ablation) or stents. Patients often cannot tolerate stents that are positioned in the cervical esophagus, and so other palliative modalities should be chosen for patients with very proximal esophageal tumors. Stents might not provide good palliation for patients who have tumors that are necrotic or bleeding; ablative therapy may be preferable in these circumstances. Gastroesophageal reflux can be a problem for stents that cross the gastroesophageal junction, but symptoms usually can be controlled with antisecretory therapy such as proton pump inhibitors. Esophagobronchial fistulae generally are best managed with a stent that occludes the connection between the esophagus and airway. Also, stents are preferable to ablative therapy for tumors that are extrinsic or infiltrative. Ablative therapy may be difficult and time-consuming for patients with very long tumors, and stenting may be preferable in these circumstances.

Proprietary esophageal stents are available in a variety of models and sizes. Fixed-diameter stents are made of plastic and often are reinforced with a metallic core to resist kinking and compression. Placement of a fixed-diameter stent requires that the lumen first must be dilated to a diameter slightly larger than that of the stent, a procedure that is associated with substantial morbidity and mortality due to perforation and bleeding. Subsequent dislocation of the plastic stent is a complication that affects 5% to 10% of patients. Most modern endoscopists prefer to use expandable metal stents. These prostheses are introduced in a compressed form, constrained in a sheath. When the stent is positioned within the narrowed area, the sheath is removed, and the stent expands. This obviates the practice of esophageal dilation prior to stent placement. If the stent does not have an internal plastic lining, the tumor can grow between the wire mesh and eventually obstruct the lumen. Incomplete expansion of the stent within the tumor also is

a potential problem, and these stents can be difficult to remove safely if they do not function adequately. Finally, expandable stents are far more expensive than the plastic prostheses.

Suggested Reading

Boyce HW: Palliation of dysphagia of esophageal cancer by endoscopic lumen restoration techniques. Cancer Control 1999;6:73–83.

Castell DO, Donner MW: Evaluation of dysphagia: A careful history is crucial. Dysphagia 1987;2:65–71.

Castell DO, Knuff TE, Brown FC, et al: Dysphagia. Gastroenterology 1979;76:1015–1024.

Cook IJ, Kahrilas PJ: AGA technical review on management of oropharyngeal dysphagia. Gastroenterology 1999;116:455–478.

Ott DJ, Gelfand DW, Wu WC, Chen YM: Radiologic evaluation of dysphagia. JAMA 1986;256:2718–2721.

Ponec RJ, Kimmey MB: Endoscopic therapy of esophageal cancer. Surg Clin North Am 1997;77:1197–1217.

Saidi RF, Marcon NE: Nonthermal ablation of malignant esophageal strictures: Photodynamic therapy, endoscopic intratumoral injections, and novel modalities. Gastrointest Endosc Clin N Am 1998;8:465–491.

Spechler SJ: AGA technical review on treatment of patients with dysphagia caused by benign disorders of the distal esophagus. Gastroenterology 1999;117:233–254.

Chapter 24
Gastrointestinal Bleeding

Keith E. Stuart

Gastrointestinal (GI) bleeding is a common medical problem that is more often due to benign than malignant causes. Gastrointestinal bleeding can, however, be the presenting sign of an unsuspected cancer, can complicate the course of a known tumor, or can develop as a complication of antineoplastic therapy. Gastrointestinal bleeding may be an acute event, giving immediacy to the clinical evaluation, or it may be a chronic problem that is identified only on discovery of an anemia or by routine screening. This chapter discusses a rational approach to the evaluation of gastrointestinal bleeding, with emphasis on the clinical context in which it appears. The mode of presentation—acute hemorrhage, chronic bleeding and anemia, or on cancer screening—determines the likelihood of finding a cancer and the direction of investigation. Iron deficiency anemia in the absence of an obvious explanation, such as menses in women, is most often due to occult gastrointestinal bleeding.

Acute Upper Gastrointestinal Bleeding

Hematemesis is the most dramatic manifestation of upper gastrointestinal bleeding, which has an incidence of about 100/100,000 population annually. The overall mortality rate from acute hemorrhage may be as high as 10%. Chronic blood loss in the stools may also be a result of upper gastrointestinal blood loss. A number of potential causes are listed in Table 24-1. Patients who are on oral anticoagulants, have other coagulation factor deficiencies, congenital or acquired, or are thrombocytopenic, do not usually have acute gastrointestinal bleeding without an underlying upper gastrointestinal tract lesion.

Approximately 50% of upper gastrointestinal bleeding is caused by peptic ulcer disease, and a substantial proportion is either caused or exacerbated by the use of aspirin or other nonsteroidal anti-inflammatory medications. Bleeding from varices usually occurs in patients with chronic liver disease, but even in this group of patients, peptic ulcer is the most common cause. Angiodysplasia is another common source of bleeding. It occurs more frequently in patients with chronic renal failure, aortic stenosis, and cirrhosis. Less common causes include Mallory-Weiss tears, esophagitis, and Dieulafoy's lesions (bleeding submucosal vessels without ulceration). Upper gastrointestinal tract malignancies account for only 1% to 5% of major episodes of upper gastrointestinal bleeding.

Variceal hemorrhage is the most life-threatening cause of upper gastrointestinal bleeding. Recent management techniques have reduced the once fearsome mortality rate from an acute episode from 50% to 20%. Patients with cirrhosis have a 40% risk of bleeding from either esophageal or gastric varices, which result from portal hypertension. Immediate endoscopic evaluation and treatment are vital, and the high mortality rate, likelihood of rebleeding, and presence of hepatic insufficiency generally mandate intensive-care monitoring

Most bleeding gastric or duodenal malignancies are adenocarcinomas, primarily involving the stomach. Approximately 1% of gastric neoplasms are gastrointestinal lymphomas, including mucosial associated lymphoid tumors (MALT) lesions. Gastric carcinoids are infrequent sources of gastrointestinal bleeding. Biopsy is generally definitive in differentiating the histology of the tumor, and further systemic workup is tailored to the specific tumor type.

Cancer can also lead to the development of occult portal hypertension and bleeding from varices or portal gastropathy. Portal vein occlusion can be caused by direct invasion of the vein or tumor-mediated thrombosis. It occurs in hepatocellular carcinomas, in cancers such as pancreatic adenocarcinoma that are metastatic to the liver, and in invasive renal carcinoma. Hepatocellular carcinoma is increasing in incidence as a cause of upper gastrointestinal bleeding, due to the increasing incidence of hepatitis C–induced cirrhosis. Ten percent of cirrhotic patients develop hepatocellular carcinoma. The risk increases, ironi-

Table 24-1 ■ Causes of Upper Gastrointestinal Bleeding

Benign Disease
Peptic ulcer disease
Variceal bleeding from portal hypertension
Angiodysplasia of the stomach
Mallory-Weiss tears of the esophagus
Dieulafoy's lesion

Malignancy
Adenocarcinoma of the stomach
Lymphoma of the stomach (mucosal-associated lymphoid tumors or other non-Hodgkin's lymphomas)
Gastric carcinoid
Variceal bleeding from portal hypertension due to:
  Large hepatomas
  Portal vein thrombosis by cancer
  Myeloproliferative disease: polycythemia vera, myelofibrosis
Chemotherapy-induced mucosal erosion and ulceration

Table 24-2 ■ Causes of Acute Lower Gastrointestinal Bleeding

Benign Disease
Colonic diverticulosis
Colitis: ischemic, ulcerative, or granulomatous
Colonic angiodysplasia
Hemorrhoids
Colonic polyps
Colonic endometriosis in women

Malignancies
Colonic adenocarcinoma
Anal squamous cell carcinoma
Radiation-induced colitis

cally, in alcohol-induced cirrhosis when patients manage to abstain, because they survive decades longer than individuals who remain chronic alcoholics.

In polycythemia vera, hepatic vein thrombosis results in Budd-Chiari syndrome and portal hypertension. In myelofibrosis, increased blood flow from the spleen to the liver and extramedullary hematopoiesis obstructing intrahepatic blood flow are causes of portal hypertension.

Evaluation of Acute Upper Gastrointestinal Bleeding

Endoscopy is the modality that is most widely employed in the evaluation of upper gastrointestinal bleeding. Endoscopy is more sensitive in uncovering the source of the blood loss than are radiographic imaging techniques, which successfully identify the source less than half the time. Endoscopy also allows a biopsy to be obtained during the investigative procedure. Endoscopy offers a further advantage over radiologic imaging studies in the setting of active bleeding. Hemostasis can be established in 90% of cases by endoscopic intervention, using injection therapy (with materials such as epinephrine, saline, ethanol, sclerosants, fibrin glue, or thrombin), thermal or laser coagulation, clipping, or banding. Although most upper gastrointestinal bleeding stops spontaneously, prompt endoscopic intervention within 24 hours may significantly reduce the risk of rebleeding and mortality. Failing this, radiographic embolization or surgery may be necessary in severe situations.

Acute Lower Gastrointestinal Bleeding

Acute gastrointestinal bleeding from the lower gastrointestinal tract is approximately one fifth as common as bleeding from the upper gastrointestinal tract, although 80% of patients with any source of gastrointestinal blood loss will have evidence of it in their stools. The incidence is somewhat higher in men and rises with advancing age. The mortality rate is generally less than 5%. The exact character of the stools helps to indicate the location of the bleeding lesion. Bright red or dark red stools generally point to a colonic or rectal source, while melena (black stools) suggests an upper gastrointestinal source. Of course, patients with a particularly brisk upper gastrointestinal bleed may present with red stools, but the presence of hemodynamic compromise usually will help to sort this out. Alternatively, black, tarry stools may develop from a small intestinal or right colonic source in the setting of slow colonic transit time. The great majority of lower gastrointestinal bleed episodes will stop spontaneously, but many rebleed intermittently.

The potential causes of acute lower gastrointestinal bleeding (Table 24-2) are numerous and include diverticulosis, angiodysplasia, various forms of colitis, and hemorrhoids. These benign disorders are much more often the cause of overt lower gastrointestinal bleeding than are gastrointestinal cancers and polyps. Colorectal tumors (both cancer and polyps) account for a minority of such events, because bleeding in these circumstances tends to be low-grade and chronic. Hyperplastic polyps are less likely to bleed than adenomas, and polyps less than 1 cm in diameter are unlikely to bleed. Rectal cancers and cancers of the left hemicolon are more likely to cause overt bleeding than are lesions of the right colon. Mucosal erosions caused by squamous cell cancers of the anus commonly present with acute, albeit not usually massive, bleeding.

Colonoscopy for overt rectal bleeding shows that approximately 10% of episodes are due to cancer and 20% to polyps. Fifty percent of patients with positive tests for occult blood in the stool have colonic lesions, and 12% of these are cancers. But 30% of colorectal cancers are associated with false-negative stool testing for blood.

Evaluation of Acute Lower Gastrointestinal Bleeding

The diagnostic approach to acute lower gastrointestinal bleeding is determined by whether or not the bleeding has stopped and by the hemodynamic urgency of the situation. In acute bleeding, surgical intervention is always a possibility, and the rapid determination of the source is necessary. Radionuclide scans using technetium 99m–labeled red blood cells can detect bleeding that is at a rate as slow as 0.1 mL/min, whereas angiography is less sensitive, requiring blood loss of more than 0.5 mL/min. Either test has variable sensitivity, ranging from 26% to 78% in identifying a bleeding source. Both studies can demonstrate extravasation and luminal pooling. Angiography has the advantage of occasionally diagnosing the cause as well as the location of the bleeding, for example, by detecting a characteristic tumor blush of neoplastic vessels. Intra-arterial vasopressin, or rarely embolization, offers potential therapeutic possibilities with angiography as well. Moreover, radionuclide localization frequently requires the use of a subsequent test, such as angiography or colonoscopy.

Colonoscopy in the setting of acute bleeding may be problematic in that patients may be hemodynamically unstable and will require a full bowel preparation for adequate visualization of the colonic lumen. Visibility may be poor owing to retained fecal matter or rapid bleeding. Nevertheless, colonoscopy identifies the acute bleeding site in 48% to 90% of patients. The use of this test is almost inevitable sooner or later in cases of lower gastrointestinal bleeding because of the need for direct visualization, biopsy, and occasionally therapeutic intervention.

Intra-Abdominal Catastrophe

Although it is not an example of luminal blood loss, hemoperitoneum may still be classified as a type of gastrointestinal bleeding that can be the presenting sign of an abdominal malignancy. Five percent of cirrhotic patients with ascites have bloody ascites, and about 25% of these are due to hepatoma. In sub-

Saharan Africa, where hepatocellular carcinoma secondary to aflatoxin ingestion or hepatitis B infection has a more virulent course than it does in Asia or the West, up to 25% of new diagnoses may present with signs of abdominal catastrophe. The tumor ruptures through the liver capsule, spilling tumor cells and blood into the peritoneal cavity. Urgent surgical intervention is required, but where it is available, arterial embolization can be useful in halting the bleeding. The use of chemoembolization in this setting is hazardous, owing to the possible delivery of the chemotherapeutic agent directly to the peritoneum.

Hemoperitoneum or bloody ascites can also be seen in malignancies involving the peritoneal surface. Malignant ascites is most frequently due to gynecologic tumors in women, although 10% (and the majority in men) result from gastrointestinal malignancies. Even so, malignant ascites is rarely significantly bloody. Perforations from luminal cancer lesions generally present with peritonitis, but slowly erosive tumors may cause blood loss into the peritoneum.

Hemobilia

Bleeding originating in the biliary tract is rarely a cause of occult or overt gastrointestinal bleeding. Trauma to the biliary tract may cause hemorrhage and may present with the triad of biliary colic, jaundice, and gastrointestinal bleeding. Although most commonly a result of instrumentation or direct hepatic damage, invasive cholangiocarcinoma and hepatocellular carcinoma are neoplastic considerations in the evaluation and differential diagnosis.

Chronic Gastrointestinal Bleeding

Chronic gastrointestinal tract blood loss frequently presents as iron-deficiency anemia or is detected in nonanemic patients by screening tests for occult bleeding. The site may be in the upper or lower gastrointestinal tracts.

Evaluation of Chronic Gastrointestinal Bleeding

Barium or air-contrast enemas may miss about 20% of lesions but are less expensive and slightly less invasive than colonoscopy. The utility of colonoscopy may be limited by poor bowel preparation or, rarely, by an obstructive lesion. In the latter case, virtual colonoscopy can be useful. This is a relatively new technique using high-resolution computed tomography scanning (after an adequate bowel preparation) to reproduce the entire lumen of the colon. The diagnostic accuracy of this modality is similar to that of colonoscopy, but the imaging study does not provide an opportunity to biopsy suspicious lesions.

Upper gastrointestinal radiographic series are useful in patients with symptoms of obstructive pathology but have limited success in diagnosing sources of bleeding. Only 80% of lesions causing bleeding in the stomach can be identified, compared with more than 95% when endoscopy is performed.

In approximately 5% to 10% of gastrointestinal bleeding episodes, the source remains unknown even after upper and lower endoscopy. In some cases, the bleeding is coming from the small intestine, where angiodysplasia, ulcers, diverticula, and tumors can arise. Workup is frequently difficult and frustrating for the patient (and the physician). Barium enteroclysis has a yield of less than 10%, but recent advances in endoscopic technology (longer and more maneuverable scopes) enable experienced gastroenterologists to visualize and intervene, if necessary, in much of the small intestine beyond the ligament of Treitz.

Gastrointestinal Bleeding as a Complication in Patients with a Known Cancer

It is important to avoid the temptation to assume that all problems in the cancer patient are due to the cancer itself. The same principles of common disorders and sequence of investigation and intervention detailed previously hold as well for patients with known malignancy. For instance, endoscopic studies have shown that less than 20% of upper gastrointestinal bleeding in patients with malignancy is due to actual involvement by tumor. Gastritis, ulcers, and varices are still the most likely culprits, while diverticulosis and angiodysplasia cause the majority of colonic bleeding.

Nevertheless, a number of possible tumor-specific sources of bleeding can be discovered endoscopically. Known mucosal lesions may rebleed, or tumors that are not thought to involve the intestinal lumen (such as adjacent pancreatic or hepatocellular cancers) may have eroded into the duodenal lumen. New primary cancers may arise and bleed in patients who are at risk because of their current tumors. For instance, a known colon cancer confers a threefold risk of developing a new colorectal malignancy. Shared risk factors may lead to the development of an esophageal cancer in a patient with a hepatoma. Melanoma has a predilection for metastases to the small intestine, which can cause gastrointestinal bleeding. Any potential cause of gastrointestinal bleeding in the cancer patient may be enhanced by concurrent therapy with nonsteroidal anti-inflammatory agents, anticoagulation, or thrombocytopenia.

Thrombocytopenia is generally treatment-related but occasionally may be seen as a result of extensive marrow infiltration by cancer of the breast, prostate, or lung. Hematologic malignancies usually also cause this problem by direct bone marrow involvement, but lymphoid neoplasms in particular may be associated with secondary immune-mediated thrombocytopenic purpura.

Bleeding from mucosal tumor involvement is usually self-limited but can make further treatment decisions difficult because of the need to avoid nonsteroidal anti-inflammatory drugs and anticoagulation. Surgery is generally inappropriate for these very ill patients and/or technically impossible due to tumor extension. Discrete lesions may be treatable with local radiation therapy, depending on location. Endoscopic cautery is often feasible, and occasionally an intraluminal stent may be able to tamponade the bleeding lesion.

Gastrointestinal Bleeding as a Complication of Cancer Treatment

While many chemotherapeutic agents are associated with nausea and vomiting, this is commonly due to a central nervous system effect, rather than direct gastrointestinal toxicity. However, several endoscopic studies of cancer patients receiving different chemotherapeutic regimens, such as cyclophosphamide, methotrexate, and 5-fluorouracil for breast cancer, 5-fluorouracil for colon cancer, and etoposide and cisplatin for lung cancer, demonstrate a significant increase in gastric and duodenal bleeding from direct chemotherapy-induced mucosal toxicity. These include erosions, diffuse gastritis, and frank ulcerations. Intra-arterial chemotherapy using floxuridine delivered via the hepatic arteries can also cause gastritis, erosions, gastric ulcers, and chemical necrosis. Chemoembolization of hepatic lesions may lead to gastritis and gastrointestinal blood loss as well.

Few studies of prophylaxis have been reported, but a group from Ferrara, Italy, has conducted several interventional studies of oral medication during chemotherapy. Omeprazole was significantly better than either misoprostol or placebo in preventing gastroduodenal damage. Moreover, in another study, omeprazole and ranitidine were better than placebo in preventing ulcers and epigastric discomfort. The omeprazole-treated group of patients was less likely than the ranitidine group or the placebo group to show global endoscopic deterioration.

Many patients develop iatrogenic thrombocytopenia from marrow-suppressive chemotherapy, but few of these experience spontaneous bleeding unless there is a preexisting source of gastrointestinal blood loss. Radiation colitis is associated with the development of mucosal telangiectasias, which can result in acute gastrointestinal bleeding occurring as late as three years after pelvic, rectal, or prostatic irradiation treatments.

Suggested Reading

Bryant TH, Jackson JE: The radiographic appearance of non-specific small intestinal ulceration. Clin Radiol 2002;57: 117–122.

Elting LS, Rubenstein EB, Martin CG, et al: Incidence, cost, and outcomes of bleeding and chemotherapy dose modifications among solid tumor patients with chemotherapy-induced thrombocytopenia. J Clin Oncol 2000;19:1137–1146.

Enns R: Acute lower gastrointestinal bleeding: Part 1. Can J Gastroenterol 2001;15:509–516.

Enns R: Acute lower gastrointestinal bleeding: Part 2. Can J Gastroenterol 2001;15:517–521.

Fallah MA, Prakash C, Edmundowicz S: Acute gastrointestinal bleeding. Med Clin North Am 2000;84:1183–1208.

Helms JF, Sandler RS: Colorectal cancer screening. Med Clin North Am 1999;83:1403–1422.

Lambert R: Diagnosis of esophagogastric tumors. Endoscopy 2002;34:129–138.

Mulcahy HE, Patel RS, Postic G, et al: Yield of colonoscopy in patients with nonacute rectal bleeding: A multicenter database study of 1,766 patients. Am J Gastroenterol 2002;97: 328–333.

Podiula PV, Ben-Menachem T, Batra SK, et al: Managing patients with acute, nonvariceal gastrointestinal hemorrhage: Development and effectiveness of a clinical care pathway. Am J Gastroenterol 2001;96:208–219.

Rollhauser C, Fleischer DE: Nonvariceal upper gastrointestinal bleeding. Endoscopy 2002;34:111–118.

Sartori S, Trevisani L, Nielsen I, et al: Randomized trial of omeprazole or ranitidine versus placebo in the prevention of chemotherapy-induced gastroduodenal injury. J Clin Oncol 2000;18:463–467.

Schnoll-Sussman F, Kurtz RC: Gastrointestinal emergencies in the critically ill patient. Semin Oncol 2000;27:270–283.

Schuetz A, Lauch KW: Lower gastrointestinal bleeding: Therapeutic strategies, surgical techniques and results. Langenbecks Arch Surg 2001;386:17–25.

Wu JC, Sung JJ: Ulcer and gastritis. Endoscopy 2002;34:104–110.

Chapter 25
Pathologic Fractures

Mohamed Anwar Hau and Henry J. Mankin

Pathologic fractures represent a major medical challenge. A pathologic fracture may represent the first sign of cancer, of cancer recurrence, or of disease progression. Pathologic fracture through a metastatic focus represents a major threat to the patient's functional status and is often a cause of profound disability.

In dealing with patients with pathologic fractures, several issues must be explored:

1. *Establishing the diagnosis.* Although the diagnosis is often quite clear on the basis of physical findings and imaging studies, sometimes considerable effort must be made to be certain that one is dealing with a pathologic fracture.
2. *Identifying and staging the underlying disease.* One must first define the nature of the primary disease and then define the extent of that disease.
3. *Determining the extent of the damage to the bone and*

DIAGNOSIS

Considerations in the Evaluation of Pathologic Fractures

- Primary tumors that may cause a pathologic fracture include not only the malignant ones, such as osteosarcoma, chondrosarcoma, lymphoma of bone, myeloma, and Ewing's tumor, but also benign or low-grade lesions, such as giant-cell tumor, nonossifying fibroma, hemangioma, unicameral bone cyst, adamantinoma, aneurysmal bone cyst, and osteoblastoma.
- For the most part, secondary cancers that affect the skeleton include carcinomas of the breast, prostate, lung, kidney, and, less commonly, thyroid, bowel, and bladder. All except lung cancers metastasize, as a rule, to the bones above the knees and elbows. Because of Batson's plexus, prostatic carcinoma almost always affects the pelvis and spine.
- Approximately 20% of metastatic tumors from the lung, 60% of those from breast, and 90% of those from prostate demonstrate extraordinary

bone production at the site. Myeloma, thyroid, and renal cell metastases are almost always purely lytic.
- Pathologic fractures involving the pelvic bone have a much higher mortality rate than those that occur in other sites.
- In general, a solitary primary site (without metastasis) or a solitary metastatic deposit has a better outcome than those in multiple sites and, for the most part, should have more aggressive treatment.
- Metastatic deposits with a prolonged disease-free interval appear to have a better prognosis than those that are present at the time the primary is discovered.
- Tumors, especially primary ones that develop a pathologic fracture, have a poorer prognosis for survival and are much more difficult to treat with limb-sparing surgery.

the effect of the injury on the patient. Occasionally, emergency treatment may be necessary, such as a patient with a pathologic fracture of the femur causing injury to the femoral artery or sciatic nerve.

4. *Immediate treatment.* Stabilization of the patient and relief of pain are important aspects of early therapy.

5. *Definitive treatment.* Treatment varies widely depending on the nature and extent of the primary tumor, the number and location of additional metastatic sites, the extent of the bone and soft tissue damage at the local site, and the projected efficacy and morbidity of the various treatment approaches. In addition, other factors, such as the family constellation and living conditions and the threat to the patient's ability to care for him or herself, must be taken into account.

Presenting Features

Pathologic fracture should be suspected when patients present with the following symptoms and signs:

1. *Bone pain without traumatic injury.* The pain of pathologic fracture may be subtle if the initial event is a stress-type fracture (Figure 25-1). Typically, such pain is often related to weight bearing. Although pain is sometimes relieved by rest, it is frequently more intense at night. Pain from undiagnosed pathologic fracture will usually increase to the point at which function is impaired (e.g., the patient's arm is held immobile, or the patient develops a limp or is even unable to walk).

2. *Sudden giving way of an arm or a leg.* This may occur without warning and with minimal trauma. Such fractures are often painful and grossly disabling. Classically, a fracture of the proximal femur or humerus with displacement of the fragments may be preceded by only minor discomfort; but at the time of the event, it may be associated with severe pain, deformity, and functional disability. If a nerve or blood vessel is compromised, decreased sensation, motor function, or vascular perfusion of the distal extremity may be evident.

3. *A deformity or mass at the site of the fracture.* Some patients who do not present with acute pain will develop a mass at the site of the injury related to partial healing. The mass may be variably tender, and the bone may be deformed, producing a varus or valgus position of the structures below the fracture site (Figure 25-2).

4. *Special circumstances related to spine fractures.* A fracture of one or several vertebrae may cause acute neurologic deficits. These include quadriplegia or

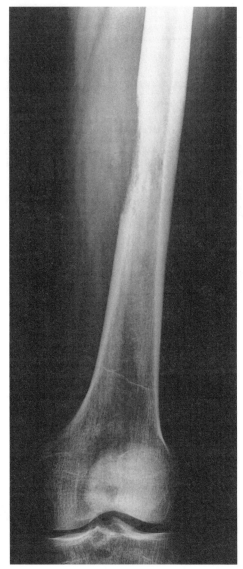

Figure 25-1 ■ An anteroposterior radiograph of the left femur of a 53-year-old man with renal cell carcinoma. At the level of the midshaft, there is a destructive lesion that has undergone a linear stress fracture. The bone is not deformed, but the patient's pain was excessive.

upper extremity nerve functional loss for lesions in the cervical spine; paraplegia, Brown-Sequard syndrome, or sensory nerve deficits for lesions in the thoracic spine; or urinary retention or bowel incontinence for the lesions in the lumbar or sacral spine (Figure 25-3).

Differential Diagnosis of the Underlying Disease

The various underlying causes of pathologic fracture and their approximate frequencies are presented in Table 25-1. Patients with osteopenia may develop frac-

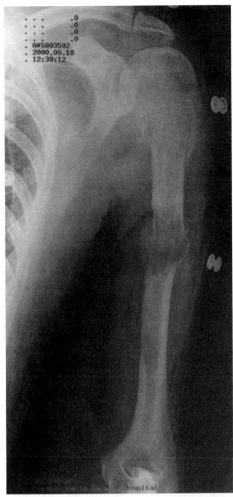

Figure 25-2 ■ The patient shown in Figure 25-1 complained of a tender mass in the arm. The radiograph shows multiple pathologic fractures representing renal cell metastases.

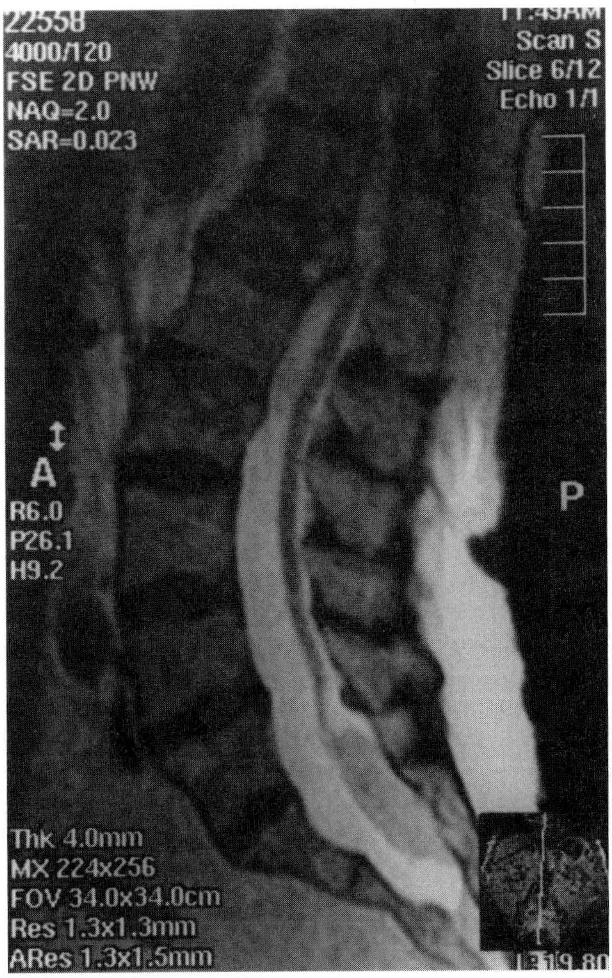

Figure 25-3 ■ A sagittal magnetic resonance imaging of the lumbar spine in a 76-year-old woman with breast cancer demonstrating pathologic fractures of the lumbar spine.

Table 25-1 ■ Approximate Frequency of Causes of Pathologic Fractures in Adults

Metastatic carcinoma	70%
Myeloma/lymphoma	10%
Osteosarcoma	2%
Chondrosarcoma	1%
Benign disorders including unicameral bone cyst, nonossifying fibroma, fibrous dysplasia, giant-cell tumor, and eosinophilic granuloma.	17%

Note that the frequencies will vary considerably with the age of patients seen and with the type of practice. For example, the rates for osteosarcoma and Ewing's sarcoma will be considerably higher in a pediatric oncology practice.

tures with minimal trauma; hence entities other than malignancy must be considered in the differential diagnosis of patients who present with pathologic fractures. These include osteoporosis, osteomalacia, hyperparathyroidism, osteomyelitis, tuberculosis, sarcoid, hyperthyroidism, fibrous dysplasia, Paget's disease, Hand-Schüller-Christian disease, Sudeck's atrophy, and such rare genetic entities as neurofibromatosis, osteogenesis imperfecta, Gaucher's disease, and a host of others. Many of these can be ruled out by a careful history and physical examination, laboratory studies, and often quite characteristic findings on imaging studies. If the patient has known primary malignant disease, parsimony of diagnosis (Occam's razor) predicts that cancer is the cause of a pathologic fracture even if the patient has been treated effectively and is without known recurrence. However, even in the face of a history of primary cancer, one must consider these other entities if clinical evaluation does not establish metastatic cancer as the etiology.

Clinical Evaluation

The simplest way to assess the presence of the fracture is by physical examination and biplanar radiographic imaging of the site. The former often demonstrates tenderness, deformity, limb shortening, and abnormal mobility. The X-rays, computed tomography (CT), or magnetic resonance imaging (MRI) will show not only the fracture, but almost always additional bone pathology. Radiologic changes may include edema, a soft tissue mass, cortical erosion, trabecular disruption, and sometimes increased density usually in close juxtaposition to the bone fragments (Figure 25-4).

The evaluation of a patient with a documented pathologic fracture should include the following:

1. A careful history and physical examination, including a rectal and pelvic examination and palpation of the breasts, abdomen, and thyroid gland.
2. A ^{99M}technetium bone scan to detect other sites of bony involvement.
3. If the spine is involved, an X-ray and magnetic resonance imaging of the affected segmental region.
4. A computed tomography study of the chest with extension below the diaphragm to see the liver, spleen, and kidneys and, if suspected as the primary site, the abdominal and pelvic viscera.
5. A mammogram for women.
6. A laboratory screen including a complete blood count, immunoelectrophoresis, sedimentation rate, blood urea nitrogen (BUN), creatinine, alkaline phosphatase, calcium, phosphorus, and, in males, a prostatic specific antigen (PSA).

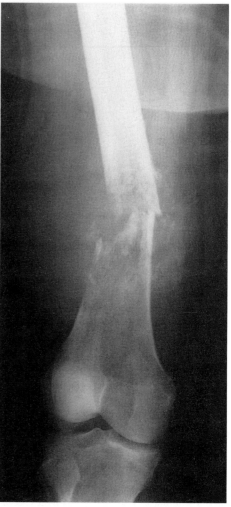

Figure 25-4 ■ An anteroposterior radiograph of the right femur of a 53-year-old woman with a primary osteosarcoma. Note the pathologic fracture, the severe deformity, the soft tissue mass, the cortical erosion, and the trabecular disruption.

DIAGNOSIS

Patient Evaluation

1. A careful history and physical is essential.
2. In people over age 45 years, studies should be done to rule out breast, lung, kidney, and prostate carcinomas and lymphoma and myeloma. In people under age 40, suspect primary tumors, chiefly osteosarcoma, giant-cell tumor, chondrosarcoma, and so on.
3. Imaging screens and especially bone scans and computed tomography scans of chest and abdomen as well as computed tomography scans and magnetic resonance imagings of the fracture site are helpful in assessing the extent of the problem and the primary site.
4. Laboratory tests must include, in addition to the usual studies, a prostatic specific antigen for prostate cancer in men and an immunoelectrophoresis for multiple myeloma.
5. A needle biopsy is sometimes necessary to determine the nature of the lesion, especially in young people with no known primary tumor.

7. If myeloma, lymphoma, or leukemia is suspected, a skeletal survey and bone marrow biopsy should be done.
8. A thyroid scan should be done if a thyroid mass is felt, and a gallium scan if lymphoma is suspected. Magnetic resonance imaging of the brain may be helpful if the patient has neurologic deficits.
9. If necessary, a computed tomography–guided or open biopsy of either the fracture site and/or another more readily accessible site often provides the proper diagnosis.

Following the aforementioned studies, it should be possible to establish the primary site and the extent of the metastatic spread. One must be able to define whether the fracture is at the site of a primary tumor (osteosarcoma, as seen in Figure 25-4, chondrosarcoma, or Ewing's tumor) or is a metastasis from lung, breast, prostate, kidney, or other less frequent sites, such as thyroid, bowel, bladder, uterus, or esophagus. In both groups, it is essential to establish whether the tumor at the pathologic fracture site is the only site of disease or one of many.

Primary Management of Pathologic Fractures

The immediate management of pathologic fractures is similar to management of other fractures. An attempt should be made to define the extent and nature of the injury, the effect on adjacent neurovascular structures, and the degree of deformity present. Such an analysis is usually performed by using a careful physical examination and initial biplanar imaging studies. This may be particularly difficult with lesions of the spine, and at times more extensive studies such as magnetic resonance imagings or electromyograms (EMGs) are required. If a vascular compromise is suspected in an extremity or the pelvis, an angiogram may be very useful in further defining the problem. If no acute neurovascular problem exists, the usual course to follow is to temporarily immobilize the patient using a sling and swathe, brace, or cast for the upper extremity and traction, pillow-splinting, or bracing for a lower-extremity fracture. Injuries to nerves such as the radial, ulnar, or peroneal may respond promptly to such treatment. Spinal cord or nerve root compression may require immediate treatment with immobilization and intravenous corticosteroids to reduce the degree of inflammation. Urgent or emergent surgery is rarely necessary, and generally surgical management should be delayed until the extent and nature of the primary or metastatic neoplastic process is clearly defined.

If the fracture is determined to be caused by a primary tumor of bone or a solitary metastatic neoplasm, then subsequent treatment should be aimed at eliminating the disease. If, on the other hand, the patient is discovered to have cancer involving multiple bony and/or visceral sites, it is more appropriate in most cases to provide a palliative treatment. The period of delay prior to definitive treatment may be used for establishing the diagnosis and stage of disease and, if necessary, obtaining appropriate consultation (radiology, pathology, radiation and medical oncology, and, if necessary, neurology and neurosurgery) to provide a multidisciplinary approach to the overall management.

Definitive Treatment

Patient management can be divided into four categories:

1. *Patients with primary neoplasms of bone that, although aggressive, are unlikely to metastasize.* These include chiefly giant-cell tumor of bone, unicameral and aneurysmal bone cysts, nonossifying fibroma, ossifying fibroma, osteoblastoma, and adamantinoma. Although the ultimate treatment approach may vary considerably for each of these, it seems logical to reduce the fracture if it is displaced and allow it to partially heal and then treat the underlying lesion according to its potential to recur. Giant-cell tumors are now best treated by curettage, phenolization, and cementation (Figure 25-5); bone cysts by injection or addition of allograft

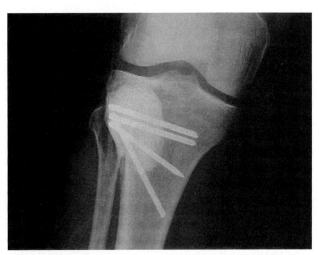

Figure 25-5 ■ A 39-year-old male with a giant-cell tumor of the proximal tibia treated with curettage, phenolization, and cement packing.

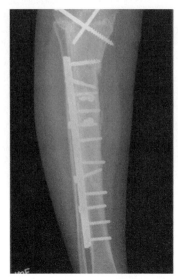

Figure 25-6 ■ Treatment of a recurrent adamantinoma of the tibia with resection and allograft replacement.

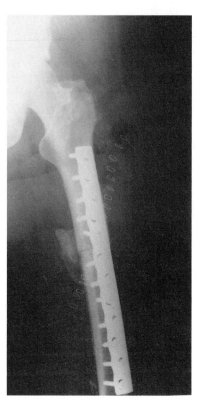

Figure 25-7 ■ A 40-year-old male with a chondrosarcoma of the proximal femur was treated with an osteoarticular allograft

chips; nonossifying fibroma, ossifying fibroma, and osteoblastoma by curettage and insertion of bone chips or struts; and adamantinoma (which may metastasize) by resection and allograft replacement (Figure 25-6). Hardware should be added where needed to increase the stability of the repair.

2. *Patients with primary high-grade malignant tumors that have not yet metastasized.* These include chiefly osteosarcoma, malignant fibrous histiocytoma, Ewing's sarcoma, lymphoma, and, at times, chondrosarcoma and plasmacytoma. This group is best treated by appropriate chemotherapy and at times radiation prior to surgical management. Radiation may be all that is needed for patients with plasmacytoma and lymphoma. In addition, chondrosarcomas are less sensitive to either radiation or chemotherapy and therefore are usually treated by primary resection after a short time period for healing of the fracture. As to the type of surgery, wide margins are ideal, and after resection, an osteoarticular or intercalary allograft or a modular prosthetic implant provides the best functional result (Figure 25-7). It should be noted that amputation may be an appropriate treatment for pathologic fractures that have resulted in a large soft tissue extension that would make a wide margin more difficult to achieve.

3. *Patients with metastatic disease.* If the lesion is solitary, it is appropriate to treat the patient in a fashion similar to those with primary lesions, with the hope that there will be no other metastases or that they will be controllable by techniques such

as radiation and chemotherapy. This approach is certainly appropriate for breast, thyroid, and sometimes renal cell metastases but is less likely to be of any value in the management of patients with lung cancer.

4. *Patients with widespread metastases from either a primary bone tumor or a carcinoma.* These patients are best treated palliatively. If the fracture is a problem, it may be treated with prosthetic implants, plates, and screws or by insertion of a rod with or without the addition of cement and or bone graft (Figure 25-8). Radiation or bisphosphonates may be used alone or may be added to the surgical management system, particularly for patients with lytic bony metastases. The objectives are to relieve pain and improve function and, if possible, to restore ambulation. A special note should be added for patients with spinal tumors, for whom palliation may consist of decompressing the canal and fusing the spine from both the front and the back. In these cases, interoperative radiation is often the best approach to relieving pain and slowing the progress of the disease. Such patients are discussed in more detail in Chapter 26.

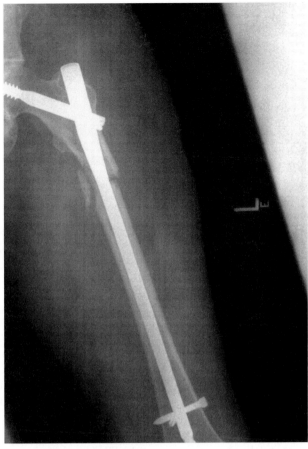

Figure 25-8 ■ A 60-year-old woman with widespread metastases and a pathologic fracture of her proximal left femur secondary to breast carcinoma. She was treated by stabilization with a reconstruction intramedullary nail and subsequent radiation therapy.

Suggested Reading

Algan SM, Horowitz SM: Surgical treatment of pathologic hip lesions in patients with metastatic disease. Clin Orthop 1996;332:223–231.

Coleman RE: Skeletal complications of malignancy. Cancer 1997;80:1588–1594.

Frassica FJ, Frassica DA, McCarthy EF, Riley LH 3rd: Metastatic bone disease: Evaluation, clinicopathologic features, biopsy, fracture risk, nonsurgical treatment and supportive management. Instr Course Lect 2000;49:453–459.

Harrington KD: Orthopedic surgical management of skeletal complications of malignancy. Cancer 1997;80:1614–1627.

Weinstein JN: Differential diagnosis and surgical treatment of pathologic spine fractures. Instr Course Lect 1992;41:301–315.

Chapter 26
Back Pain

Eric Wong

Back pain is a common problem in the general population. The potential etiologies range in severity from benign conditions such as chronic degenerative disease of the spine to those that require urgent intervention, such as epidural spinal cord compression from a vertebral metastasis. Although magnetic resonance imaging has revolutionized the neuroimaging of the spine and its adjacent neuroanatomy by offering detailed structural resolution, the proper diagnosis of back pain still depends on a physician's clinical acumen. The diagnostic neuroimaging study, for the most part, is just for confirmatory purposes or to exclude certain diagnoses in the original differential. In patients with a known history of cancer, the natural history of the primary malignancy and the presenting features of the back pain are important; this information will help to distinguish between cancer-related back pain and back pain from other causes. An algorithm for the evaluation of back pain is described in Figure 26-1.

Evaluation of Back Pain

The Location of Back Pain

The location of back pain is an important feature to recognize during an initial evaluation. Cervical and lumbar back pains are common in degenerative diseases of the spine, such as osteoarthritis and rheumatoid arthritis. This is a result of repetitive flexion and extension movements over years or decades at the cervical and lumbar levels. Although many patients have degenerative spine disease, thoracic back pain, especially in a cancer patient, should arouse concern for spinal metastasis. The thoracic level is the most stable part of the spine, as the ribs and sternum help to stabilize the thoracic spine from any flexion and extension motions; therefore degenerative spine disease developing at the thoracic level is distinctly uncommon. Consequently, plain films of the spine should be performed on patients presenting with persistent

thoracic back pain, and magnetic resonance imaging or computed tomography spine imaging should be performed on cancer patients with new onset of thoracic back pain.

The Quality of Back Pain

The quality of back pain can offer a clue to the underlying etiology. A sharp, shooting pain in a dermatomal distribution often indicates radicular nerve involvement, as in nerve compression at a neuroforamen by hypertrophied bone in osteoarthritis or a laterally situated intervertebral disk. Back pain that has a burning quality quite often suggests herpes zoster neuralgia; in this case, a search for vesicles and a detailed neurosensory examination of the affected dermatome are helpful. A dull, aching pain is less specific, since it may arise from a vertebral body, epidural space, or subarachnoid space or from within the spinal cord itself when the spinothalamic tract is involved. Spasms of the spine often arise from the longitudinal paraspinal muscles, and this feature is not very helpful for localizing the affected spinal level. In these situations, the presence of associated neurologic signs and symptoms could help to narrow the number of diagnostic possibilities.

The Temporal Pattern of Back Pain

The time course of onset of back pain provides another clue to the etiology. Acute back pain, occurring in seconds or minutes, is usually traumatic in nature. A compression fracture of an osteoporotic vertebral body for example, can present with acute back pain. By contrast, metastatic spine tumors typically cause a subacute onset of back pain over days or weeks. An important feature of this type of pain is its escalating tempo. Patients frequently complain of crescendo pain needing increasing amount of analgesics. This tempo of pain escalation frequently signals an ominous underlying cause of the back pain. Nevertheless, crescendo back pain can occur in other settings, such

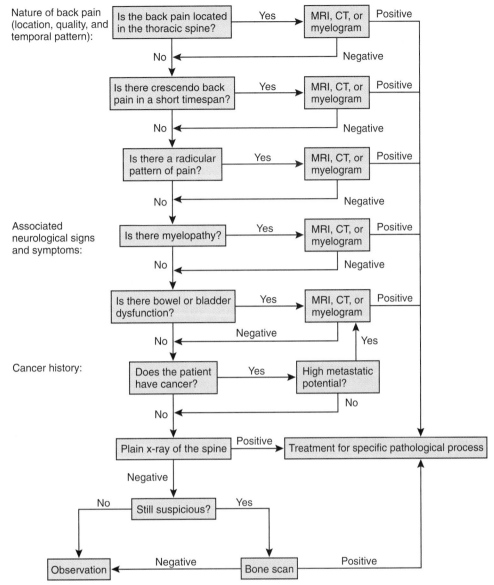

Figure 26-1 ■ Algorithm for the evaluation of back pain in cancer patients.

as an epidural abscess or an epidural hematoma. Finally, chronic back pain that evolves over years is most likely to be degenerative in nature.

Associated Neurologic Signs and Symptoms

The associated neurologic signs and symptoms offer important clues to a correct diagnosis, and they should be an important component of the evaluation of patients with back pain. For example, coughing, sneezing, or Valsalva maneuvers increase cerebrospinal fluid (CSF) pressure and thereby cause increased back pain in an area of spinal canal narrowing. This is frequently noted in cancer patients

with epidural spinal cord compression by metastatic tumors, but it can be seen in patients with intervertebral disk herniation, fracture of the spine, epidural abscess, or epidural hematoma resulting in compromise of the spinal canal. Although neurologic signs and symptoms do not indicate a specific etiology for the back pain, they can direct the clinician to the site of spine disease. Similarly, meningismus of the spine usually arises from an irritating process in the subarachnoid space of inflammatory, infectious, or hemorrhagic nature. The inciting agent can be intrathecal chemotherapy causing arachnoiditis or bacteria causing bacterial meningitis. Subarachnoid bleeding can be a result of hemorrhage from a leptomeningeal tumor located in the subarachnoid space, from a traumatic spinal tap in a patient with a low platelet count or coagulopathy, or as a result of spontaneous bleeding from a spinal arteriovenous malformation. Because the entire paraspinal musculature can go into spasm, it is hard to localize the spinal level where this process originates.

It is also important to recognize myelopathy in patients with back pain. Patients who present with myelopathy should undergo an urgent diagnostic investigation so that the appropriate treatment can be quickly instituted to prevent irreversible neurologic sequelae. In obvious cases, patients experience motor or sensory dysfunction below the level of spinal cord compromise. The motor problems may include hyperreflexia or spasticity, while sensory deficits may include a sensory level below which sensation to pinprick or temperature is lost. Depending on the severity of spinal cord impairment, loss of proprioception, ataxia, or autonomic dysfunction (such as changes in sweating pattern at a given spinal level) may occur. In addition, a spastic bladder, manifesting as a complaint of urinary urgency and a small postvoid residual of urine on catheterization, is an upper motor neuron equivalent of bladder dysfunction, suggesting spinal cord compromise above the conus medullaris. In contrast, a flaccid bladder, with large post-void residual and infrequent overflow incontinence, is a typical result of conus medullaris and cauda equina dysfunction.

The Natural History of the Primary Malignancy

For patients with a history of malignancy, it is important to take into consideration the likelihood of recurrence, specifically spinal metastasis, in the evaluation of new onset of back pain. Lung carcinoma, breast cancer, and prostate cancer commonly recur in bone, and epidural compression can result from a vertebral metastasis. Other cancers that are less commonly associated with epidural metastasis include melanoma, renal cell carcinoma, colorectal cancers, and lymphoma. In contrast, epidural metastasis from leukemia is distinctly unusual. By recognizing the natural pattern of metastasis based on the primary malignancy, one can make an estimate of the likelihood that the back pain may arise from epidural spinal cord compression, leptomeningeal metastasis, dural metastasis, or other nonmalignant causes.

Diagnostic Neuroimaging

The selection of the appropriate diagnostic neuroimaging test has to be individualized on the basis of the suspected etiologies. First, magnetic resonance imaging scan of the spine is the diagnostic modality of choice to look for any spinal pathology. For example, epidural compression of the spinal cord by vertebral metastasis can be easily recognized on a sagittal magnetic resonance imaging image of the spine, along with the degree of spinal cord compression, intramedullary signal changes, and associated neuroforaminal compression. The magnetic resonance imaging is also helpful in detecting concurrent intramedullary metastasis and leptomeningeal metastasis, as 16% of these patients have simultaneous leptomeningeal disease metastasis. This additional information is often helpful in selecting patients for surgical intervention and in planning of the radiation field. In nonmalignant cases, magnetic resonance imaging is useful in detecting epidural infection, such

DIAGNOSIS

Back Pain Can Be a Medical Emergency

Back pain in patients who have or have had cancer requires prompt clinical evaluation. As in patients without cancer, benign lesions such as osteoarthritis or disk disease can be the cause. In this case, rapid reassurance allays the patient of anxiety about the possibility that cancer is causing the symptom. But back pain may also be caused by metastases to the vertebral bodies, epidural space, and leptomeninges. Back pain can also herald encroachment of the spinal cord by vertebral metastasis with potentially devastating consequences. One should therefore ask the patient about associated symptoms of spinal cord compromise, such as increased back pain with cough, sneeze, or Valsalva,

motor weakness, or sensory deficit. For example, vertebral compression of the conus in the lower thoracic level can cause lower extremity weakness, as well as urinary retention and constipation due to bladder and bowel dysfunction. Spinal cord injury by metastatic cancer can become irreversible if it is not treated promptly. For this reason, cancer patients complaining of back pain should be considered for magnetic resonance neuroimaging of the spine or consultation by a neuro-oncologist. Inevitably, these additional evaluations may lead to higher medical cost, but the prevention of devastating spinal cord deficits would warrant this approach.

as an epidural abscess. This condition usually starts in a disk, and a notable diskitis, manifesting as irregular disk border in the adjacent vertebral bodies, can be seen on magnetic resonance imaging. Spinal stenosis, intervertebral disk protrusion, and foraminal stenosis are common pathologies that can be seen on the magnetic resonance imaging of the spine as well. Finally, the uncommon spinal subarachnoid hemorrhage can be detected on magnetic resonance imaging. This type of hemorrhage can occur in patients with melanoma or choriocarcinoma or those with coagulopathy, particularly after a lumbar puncture, or in patients suffering a bleed emanating from a spinal arteriovenous malformation.

Plain myelography and computed tomography myelogram are useful alternatives for patients who cannot tolerate magnetic resonance imaging owing to metallic artifacts from spinal instrumentation, magnetic resonance imaging incompatible aneurysm clips, claustrophobia, cardiac pacemaker, or recent surgery. A major drawback of these procedures, however, is the need to inject a contrast agent into the subarachnoid space in the lumbar thecal sac or the cisterna magna, depending on the site and etiology of back pain. Although a plain myelography can demonstrate epidural block of contrast flow along the spinal canal or flow defects around the nerve roots, it does not offer direct visualization of the pathological process as with magnetic resonance imaging. In contrast, the axial images of a computed tomography myelogram offer some structural information about neural elements inside the spinal canal; however, these images can be degraded by metallic artifacts seen in patients who have had prior spinal instrumentation.

A bone scan can be a helpful adjunct to magnetic resonance imaging, plain myelography, or computed tomography myelogram studies. The radionuclide is sequestered in areas of increased blood flow or areas with new bone formation. When it is difficult to distinguish degenerative from metastatic disease to the spine, a bone scan can demonstrate other areas of radionuclide uptake that are more typical of either metastasis or degenerative spine disease. Likewise, a plain X-ray of the spine can detect poor mineralization in patients with osteoporosis that may have resulted from menopause, prior irradiation, or chronic corticosteroid use.

Differential Diagnosis

The various etiologies of back pain and their differential presentations are described in Table 26-1 and in

Table 26-1 ■ Common Etiologies of Back Pain in Cancer Patients

Etiology	Location	Quality	Time Pattern	Neurological Deficits	Neuroimaging Features
Epidural compression by metastasis	Anywhere	Ache	Subacute	Myelopathy, sensory level, point tenderness, worse with reclining	MRI with epidural compression or myelogram shows flow block
Vertebral compression fracture	Thoracic and lumbar	Sharp pain or ache	Acute	Point tenderness, worse with reclining	MRI with vertebra compression, X-ray shows osteoporosis or both
Degenerative disease of the spine	Cervical and lumbar	Ache	Chronic	Worse with movement, sitting, or standing; better with reclining	MRI with disk, spondylosis, spinal stenosis or neuroforaminal stenosis
Meningismus	Anywhere	Ache or spasm	Subacute	Neck stiffness, Kernig's or Brudzinski's sign	MRI with subarachnoid enhancement or blood
Herpes zoster	Anywhere	Burning or stabbing	Acute	Radiculopathy (motor or sensory), transverse myelitis	MRI with enhancement in a nerve root or spinal cord
Bacterial infection	Thoracic and lumbar	Ache	Subacute	Myelopathy, sensory level, point tenderness, worse with reclining	MRI with epidural compression or Myelogram shows flow block

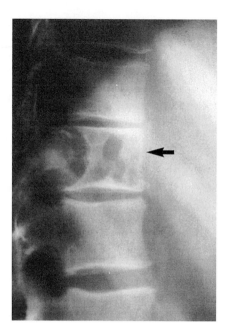

Figure 26-2 ■ Lytic lesions of T12 associated with multiple myeloma. (From Skarin AT [ed]: Atlas of Diagnostic Oncology, 2nd ed. St. Louis, MO: Mosby, 1996, p. 537.)

more detail in following sections. Even patients with known cancer can have benign causes of back pain, so it is important to know the clinical features of these entities as well.

Epidural Spinal Cord Compression by Metastatic Tumor

Epidural spinal cord compression is the most likely condition to be associated with cancer. It is a serious condition and deserves immediate attention. The pain is typically a dull, aching pain located at the affected level of the spine. At times, there is focal tenderness at a particular level on palpation, particularly when there is tumor infiltration into the posterior elements. The pain can also worsen with reclining but improves with standing or sitting. When there is obvious myelopathy, the diagnosis is often certain. However, varying signs may occur depending on the location of the spinal cord compression. For example, in a patient with a laterally situated spine metastasis, radiculopathy or ataxia can result. The diagnosis can be confirmed by magnetic resonance imaging demonstrating an epidural mass causing compression of the spinal cord and compromising the cerebrospinal fluid space. Both lytic lesions (Figure 26-2) and blastic lesions can be associated with significant back pain. A detailed dis-

cussion of epidural spinal cord compression is provided in Chapter 105 of this book.

Compression Fracture of Osteoporotic Vertebral Body

Because osteoporosis is prevalent in the elderly, compression of a vertebral body can occur secondary to osteoporotic changes in the spine. Although this phenomenon is by far most common in postmenopausal woman, it can also occur in cancer patients who have had remote irradiation to the spine or who are using corticosteroids chronically. The vertebral compression often occurs at the level of the thoracic or lumbar spine, primarily because these levels are responsible for weight bearing. Magnetic resonance imaging of the spine often detects compression of a vertebral body without adjacent disk space changes. A plain X-ray of the spine would help to detect the loss of bone mineralization that is typical of osteoporosis.

Degenerative Disease of the Spine

Intervertebral disk herniation, spondylosis of the spine, spinal stenosis, and neuroforaminal stenosis are common manifestations of the degenerative process of the spine. An intervertebral disk herniation usually occurs at the most mobile portions of the spine, as in the C5-6, C6-7, L4-5, and L5-S1 intervertebral spaces, resulting in nerve root compression, spinal cord compression (if this is a cervical disk), or both. Disk herniation at other levels of cervical and lumbar spines is less common, and a thoracic disk herniation is rare. The pain is usually aggravated by movement, sitting, or Valsalva maneuver and improves with reclining. The pain is typically in a radicular distribution with associated reflex changes, such as diminution of an Achilles tendon reflex or a triceps jerk. There may be numbness in the associated dermatomal distribution. Likewise, spondylosis of the spine occurs at the cervical and lumbar levels because these sections of the spine have high mobility and are subjected to chronic flexion and extension. Degenerative disease of the thoracic spine is rare because the thoracic spine is stabilized by the ribs and sternum. Patients with cervical spondylosis, depending on the location of spondylitic compression, can have myelopathy, dermatomal sensation loss, or motor radiculopathy. Spinal stenosis and neuroforaminal stenosis are caused by hypertrophy of the facet joints in the spinal column. Severe spinal stenosis in the lumbar region can cause a syndrome of spinal claudication resulting in back pain, leg numbness, and leg weakness and simulating vascular claudication of the lower extremities. Neuroforaminal stenosis can cause focal motor weakness, dermatomal sensory loss, or both.

Magnetic resonance imaging scans of the affected area can easily demonstrate an intervertebral disk, spondylitic bone spur, stenotic spinal canal, or neuroforaminal stenosis. However, in patients who cannot undergo magnetic resonance imaging, plain myelography and computed tomography myelogram can demonstrate the defects.

Herpes Zoster Spinal Radiculopathy or Myelopathy

Herpes zoster eruptions can result in radicular back pain and, in severe cases, transverse myelitis. Frequently, the pain is burning and stabbing. This unpleasant sensation typically precedes the development of a rash or vesicles. However, changes in the affected dermatome, such as abnormal touch sensation (paresthesia), unpleasant sensation when touched (dysesthesia), or lingering pain after stimulation (hyperpathia), can be detected when a detailed neurosensory examination is performed. In severe cases, a transverse myelitis, with signs of spinal cord dysfunction, can result owing to the spread of the zoster causing inflammation of the spinal arteries. The magnetic resonance imaging may show enhancement along a nerve root or on the pial surface of the spinal cord. The cerebrospinal fluid may show pleocytosis and elevated protein.

Meningismus

Meningismus is spinal spasms caused by subarachnoid irritation by an inflammatory process, infection, or blood. The spasms involve the entire paraspinal region from the base of the neck to the sacrum, and therefore it has poor localizing value. It is these spasms that give rise to stiff neck as well as Kernig's and Brudzinski's signs. Cancer patients may experience arachnoiditis from chemotherapy administered to the subarachnoid space, spinal meningitis from immune compromise, or bleeding in the subarachnoid space from metastatic tumors, spinal arteriovenous malformation, coagulopathy, or lumbar puncture. Magnetic resonance imaging of the entire spine is necessary to detect the location of a bleed or to locate areas of tumor infiltration or arteriovenous malformation. A spinal tap is needed to obtain cell counts as well as culture and sensitivity. Empiric antibiotics may be necessary until the final culture results come out.

Epidural Back Pain from Bacterial Infections

Diskitis, epidural abscess, and vertebral osteomyelitis are potential infectious causes of back pain located in the epidural space. These processes can be seen in patients with diabetes mellitus, intravenous drug abuse, or compromised immune system, as well as patients with cancer. The process can spread to the spine by arterial or venous routes. The infectious organism often causes a diskitis initially, as the penetrating arteries to the spine first enter the intervertebral disk space. When left untreated, the infection spreads to the adjacent vertebral body and epidural space, resulting in vertebral myelitis and epidural abscess. The infectious organism can also spread to the spinal epidural space via the Batson's venous plexus. This plexus is more extensive in the lumbar and lower thoracic spine, and patients with chronic urinary tract infections are particularly predisposed to the development of epidural abscess at these sites. These patients describe back pain near the site of the epidural abscess. The pain typically has an aching quality, and patients often have associated point tenderness and worsening pain with reclining. Although patients might not have a fever, their sedimentation rate is usually elevated. The diagnosis is confirmed on magnetic resonance imaging scan by detecting an epidural fluid collection with associated changes in the disk space and vertebral body. A plain X-ray of the spine may be helpful,

Table 26-2 ■ **Management of Back Pain**

Etiology	Management
Epidural compression by metastasis	Surgery, radiation, chemotherapy, or any combination
Vertebral compression fracture	Symptomatic treatment with NSAID, antidepressants, anticonvulsants, opioids, calcium, or vitamin D
Degenerative disease of the spine	Surgery or symptomatic treatment with NSAID or opioids
Meningismus	Treat underlying cause; symptomatic treatment with NSAID or opioids
Herpes zoster neuralgia	Anti-viral medication, antidepressants, anticonvulsants, NSAID, or opioids
Bacterial infection	Antibiotics and surgical drainage; symptomatic treatment with NSAID or opioids

as it can show the irregular disk borders of the adjacent vertebral bodies at the site of diskitis. At times, there may be vertebral body collapse as well. The treatment is surgical drainage and a prolonged course of antibiotics.

Management of Back Pain

There are three general considerations in the management of back pain: (1) treatment of the underlying pathology, (2) symptomatic management of back pain, and (3) prevention of future disabling neurologic sequelae. The underlying pathology causing back pain dictates the type of treatment that is needed (Table 26-2). For example, surgery, radiation, and, in some cases, chemotherapy would be appropriate treatments for epidural spinal cord compression from metastatic tumor to the spine. Although symptomatic management is a primary consideration in patients with osteoporosis and degenerative disease of the spine, in severe cases, as in spinal claudication caused by compression of the cauda equina, spine instability from osteoporosis, or myelopathy from cervical spondylosis, surgical decompression by laminectomy can relieve pain, neurologic deficits, and progression of neurologic signs. For patients with herpes zoster neuropathy, particularly those with a compromised immune system, early treatment with antiviral medication is needed.

The symptomatic treatment of back pain typically involves the use of medications for the abortive and preventive control of pain. This strategy typically includes nonopioid analgesics and, if necessary, opioid analgesics. Commonly used nonopioid analgesics include antidepressants (e.g., amitriptyline, nortriptyline, and imipramine), anticonvulsants (e.g., gabapentin, carbamazepine, lamotrigine, and valproic acid), nonsteroidal anti-inflammatory drugs, and muscle relaxants; but other drugs such as α_2-adrenergic agonist (e.g., clonidine), local anesthetics (e.g., lidocaine or mexiletine), neuroleptics, and corticosteroids also may have efficacy in controlling back pain. A good example of the use of these drugs is the treatment of postherpetic neuropathic pain. If it is left untreated, adjacent dermatomes may develop a heightened sensation to pain (hyperalgesia) as a result of molecular changes in the spinal cord from chronic pain sensitization. Early treatment with an anticonvulsant such as gabapentin or a tricyclic antidepressant such as nortriptyline can help to prevent such pain progression.

Opioid analgesics are usually reserved for moderate to severe back pain, particularly for cancer-related malignant pain. A typical strategy involves the use of nonopioid analgesics as initial treatment for back pain, such as nonsteroidal anti-inflammatory drugs or tramadol. When the pain escalates, nonopioid analgesics could be used in combination with a low-potency opioid analgesic, such as codeine, hydrocodone, or oxycodone. When the pain escalates further and becomes severe, opioid analgesics with high potency (such as hydromorphone or morphine) and those in long-acting forms (such as fentanyl patch or sustained-release morphine) become the primary analgesic agents, with nonopioid analgesics used to augment pain control. Sustained-release forms of opioids avoid variations in drug level and pain associated with intermittent opioid dosing, thus reducing the occurrence of rebound pain. Another important method of opioid delivery is via a PCA pump. This allows for both basal and command dosing of opioid, thus providing optimal pain relief while minimizing the sedating side effect of the opioid. In patients with intractable chronic back pain, surgical interventions such as intrathecal opioids or baclofen, nerve block, neurectomy, dorsal rhizotomy, thalamectomy, or cingulotomy may be considered. But these procedures should be performed only after careful neurologic, neurosurgical, and psychiatric evaluations.

The prevention of neurologic sequelae is a paramount concern in the management of patients with back pain. This requires the recognition of potentially serious causes of back pain that may result in irreversible myelopathy and/or other neurologic dysfunctions. The long-term neurologic sequelae that may result include paralysis, bowel or bladder incontinence, and myelopathic pain. For example, early recognition of epidural compression of the spinal cord by metastatic spinal tumors, prompt administration of corticosteroids, and definitive treatment for the metastatic spinal tumor can prevent paralysis and/or irreversible bowel and bladder dysfunction. Likewise, patients with early signs of myelopathy from compression fracture of the vertebral body require urgent neurosurgical evaluation for possible decompression and spine stabilization. Those with an epidural abscess require immediate broad-spectrum antibiotics and an early and neurosurgical evaluation for potential drainage.

Suggested Reading

Clouston PD, DeAngelis LM, Posner JB: The spectrum of neurological disease in patients with systemic cancer. Neurol 1992;31:268–273.

Herkowitz HN, Garfin SR, Balderston RA, et al: Rothman-Simeone: The Spine, 4th Edition. Philadelphia: WB Saunders, 1998.

Portenoy RK, Kanner RM (eds): Pain Management: Theory and Practice. Philadelphia: FA Davis, 1996.

Portenoy RK, Lipton RB, Foley KM: Back pain in the cancer patient: An algorithm for evaluation and management. Neurol 1987;37:134–138.

Posner JB: Spinal metastases. In Neurologic Complications of Cancer. Philadelphia: FA Davis, 1995, pp 111–142.

Wasserstrom WR, Glass JP, Posner JB: Diagnosis and treatment of leptomeningeal metastases from solid tumors: Experience with 90 patients. Cancer 1982;49:759–772.

Chapter 27
Renal and Adrenal Masses

Martina Morrin and Robert C. Eyre

Advances in radiologic imaging and more widespread use of sophisticated scanning techniques in the past decade have dramatically improved our ability to detect and evaluate renal and adrenal masses. Biologically important solid and cystic lesions can now be detected at very early stages by ultrasonography, computed tomography, or magnetic resonance imaging and can be characterized with a high degree of accuracy in the majority of cases. Moreover, the availability of new, minimally invasive treatment modalities, such as radiofrequency ablation and ultrasonic and cryosurgical ablation, and the current enthusiasm for nephron-sparing surgery have increased the options for clinical management of small lesions.

Hematuria, flank pain, or a palpable abdominal mass is an obvious presenting symptom or physical finding that focuses attention on urinary tract pathology. However, renal or adrenal masses produce a wide spectrum of symptoms ranging from sudden, life-threatening retroperitoneal hemorrhage to subtle or nonspecific complaints such as early satiety, unexplained weight loss, myalgia, flushing, and lethargy. Physical findings such as new onset of hypertension or a right varicocele or laboratory abnormalities such as anemia, polycythemia, elevated erythrocyte sedimentation rate, or elevation in liver enzymes may be the only clues that point to possible renal or adrenal pathology.

Incidence of Renal and Adrenal Masses

Abdominal computed tomography (CT) scans, often performed for an increasing number of nonurologic indications, demonstrate renal cystic lesions in at least 25% to 33% of patients. It is estimated that 0.1% to 0.3% of the population undergoing abdominal computed tomography or ultrasound have a detectable solid renal mass, of which about 80% will be renal cell carcinoma. Incidentally discovered adrenal masses are found by computed tomography or magnetic resonance imaging (MRI) in 0.6% to 1.3% of patients. Almost all are benign and asymptomatic. Autopsy series show an incidence of unsuspected adrenal masses of 1.3% to 8.7%. Incidentally discovered adrenal malignancies at autopsy are extremely rare.

Renal Masses

Cystic Renal Lesions

Simple renal cysts are found in approximately 50% of the population over the age of 50. They are usually cortical in position and asymptomatic unless they are large enough (10 to 20 cm) to cause symptoms of vague flank or upper abdominal pain or fullness, a noticeable change in abdominal girth, or early satiety (usually left-sided cysts). Cysts of this size are often palpable on abdominal examination. They should not be considered a cause of microscopic or gross hematuria.

Renal cysts can usually be fully evaluated by either ultrasound or a combination of ultrasound and computed tomography. Essential ultrasound criteria of a simple cyst include (a) a smooth, sharply marginated wall, (b) no internal echoes, and (c) posterior acoustic enhancement. If these criteria are fulfilled, no further investigation is required. Complex cysts may contain

Table 27-1 ▪ Bosniak Classification of Renal Cysts

Category 1: Simple Cyst

Anechoic with sharply marginated smooth walls on US.*
Well-marginated, nonenhancing, low-attenuation (0–20 HU),
    thin, smooth walls.

Category 2: Mildly Complicated Cysts

May contain thin septae or a small amount of calcification in an
    otherwise thin outer wall
Hyperdense cysts 3 cm or less in diameter, nonenhancing,
    homogeneous, 40–90 HU, smooth wall

Category 3: Indeterminate Cysts

Irregular wall, many septae, heavier calcification
Includes multilocular cysts, multilocular cystic nephroma, cystic
    renal cell carcinoma

Category 4: Cysts Containing Solid Features†

Irregular, thick margins, thick septae, nodularity in wall,
    calcification, enhancement

HU: Hounsfield units; US: Ultrasound.
*If any portion of the lesion measures >20 HU, perform a contrast study.
†These lesions should be considered malignant until proven otherwise.

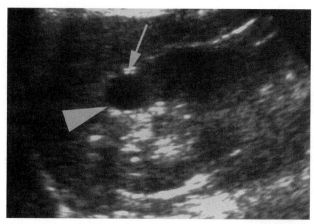

Figure 27-1 ▪ Renal ultrasound examination showing a simple cyst with a smooth, sharply marginated wall (arrow), no internal echoes (arrowhead), and posterior acoustic enhancement.

a variety of elements such as a solid component, irregularity of the wall, internal septation, high attenuation, or calcification that necessitate further evaluation with either computed tomography or magnetic resonance imaging. Cysts containing thin septations or minimal calcifications confined to the wall but no other abnormality are usually benign. Computed tomography evaluation of simple cysts requires both contrast-enhanced and noncontrast scans. Essential computed tomography criteria of simple cysts include a smooth, thin, sharply marginated wall; a uniform density of 0 to 20 Hounsfield units; and no enhancement with contrast medium. Benign cysts can sometimes be hyperdense on unenhanced computed tomography, with attenuation values of 20 to 100 Hounsfield units. The increased attenuation is often due to calcium carbonate, proteinaceous fluid, or high iron content within the cyst following hemorrhage.

The Bosniak classification system uses computed tomography criteria to divide cystic masses into four categories in order of increasing malignant potential (Table 27-1). Category 1 lesions are reliably benign and can be observed; category 2 and 3 cysts are associated with intermediate risks of malignancy (up to 50% for category 3); and category 4 cysts are associated with a 96% risk of cancer. An irregular or thick cyst wall has been considered one of the most worrisome features of indeterminate cystic lesions, although this feature may also be seen in

infected cysts. Other associated features, such as the presence of mural nodules or intense enhancement of the wall, increase the likelihood of malignancy. Cystic lesions less than 1.5 cm in diameter may occasionally mimic solid lesions because of partial volume averaging.

Magnetic resonance imaging is being used with increasing frequency to further characterize indeterminate cysts. Although it cannot detect calcification, gadolinium contrast can accurately evaluate soft tissue thickening, wall irregularity, and wall enhancement. Since renal cell carcinomas may exhibit cystic growth patterns (Figure 27-1) (five different types are described: multilocular, cystic, unilocular, cystic necrotic, and tumor arising from a cyst wall), detailed radiologic analysis of complex cysts and an appropriately aggressive surgical approach to Bosniak category 3 and 4 lesions are of importance.

Solid Renal Masses

All solid renal masses, regardless of size, should be considered malignant unless they fulfill specific criteria associated with benign lesions. Computed tomography can detect 47% of renal masses below 5 mm in diameter and 75% of masses between 10 and 15 mm in diameter. Imaging during the nephrographic phase best demonstrates lesion enhancement and arterial and venous structures (for preoperative staging), while imaging in the corticomedullary phase is most helpful in differentiating pseudotumors such as a column of Bertin from malignant masses. Given the accuracy of current imaging capabilities, it is only rarely necessary for patients to undergo a diagnostic biopsy of a solid renal mass prior to therapy. Indications for a biopsy include differentiating lymphoma or metastatic disease from primary renal cell carcinoma. Computed tomography and magnetic resonance imaging have virtually replaced angiography or vena cavography for preoperative staging of the lymph nodes, adrenal glands, renal vein, and inferior vena cava and establishing a vascular "road map" for planning partial nephrectomies.

Approximately 85% of all solid renal masses that are detected incidentally on computed tomography scan are malignant, and about 85% of these malignant masses are renal cell carcinomas. Calcification can occur in about 10% of renal cancers, although cancers less than 3 cm in diameter are not usually calcified. Most masses have attenuation values of greater than 20 Hounsfield units on unenhanced scans. Scans before and after contrast medium are essential, with enhancement greater than 20 Hounsfield units suggesting malignancy. Renal cell cancers, which are very vascular, may enhance to the same degree as the renal cortex. If small, they may be missed on corticomedullary phase images but be seen as hypodense lesions on nephrographic images. The overall accuracy of computed tomography for staging renal cell carcinoma is 72% to 90%. While conventional computed tomography has an accuracy for detecting renal vein involvement of 50% to 80%, spiral computed tomography increases the sensitivity of detecting renal vein and lymph node involvement to 88% to 95%, with a specificity of 99% to 100%.

Magnetic resonance imaging may be used in patients who cannot be assessed by contrast-enhanced computed tomography because of either an allergy to iodinated contrast media or renal insufficiency. On T1-weighted images, renal cell carcinomas are typically lower in signal intensity than normal parenchyma but may have high signal intensity due to foci of hemorrhage. On T2-weighted images, renal cell carcinomas are generally hyperintense compared to the normal kidney, although hemorrhage within the tumor can have a lower signal. Tumor detection is improved by intravenous administration of gadolinium contrast medium and fat suppression. After contrast, most but not all renal cell carcinomas enhance greatly. Peripheral enhancement is characteristic of predominantly cystic necrotic renal cell carcinoma lesions, while homogeneous enhancement is encountered in small, solid masses. A breath-hold flow-sensitive sequence should be used to evaluate flow in renal veins and inferior vena cava. With this technique, images are obtained axially from the right atrium to the bifurcation of the inferior vena cava. MR angiography and venography may be performed with a bolus of intravenous contrast. This approach gives information about the tumor, its vascular supply, the status of nodes and adjacent organ involvement, venous

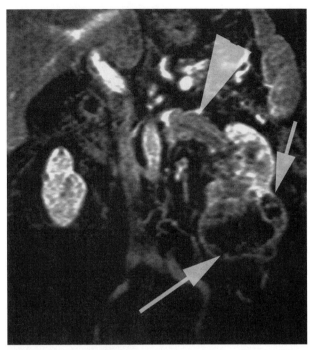

Figure 27-2 ■ Magnetic resonance image illustrating a large renal cell carcinoma with tumor thrombus. T1-weighted image postadministration of intravenous gadolinium illustrating a large, complex renal cell carcinoma in the lower pole of the left kidney (arrows). Enhancing tumor thrombus is seen within the left renal vein (arrowhead).

thrombus (Figure 27-2), and the presence or absence of liver metastases. While computed tomography and ultrasound allow accurate preoperative staging in over 90% of patients with renal cell carcinoma, the perirenal extent of surrounding vessel, nodal, and organ involvement is often overstated by these imaging modalities in comparison to magnetic resonance imaging.

Renal cell carcinoma can usually be differentiated from benign renal masses and other malignant lesions by utilizing the specific capabilities of computed tomography and magnetic resonance imaging; however, one should never lose sight of other valuable clinical details. The most common benign lesions include focal nephritis (a "pseudotumor" created by localized edema seen as a hypodense lobar mass in a patient with clinical pyelonephritis), angiomyolipoma (distinguished by identifying fat density in the lesion on computed tomography) (Figure 27-3), or oncocytoma. Less frequently seen are hemangiomas, lymphangiomas, leiomyomas, and lipomas. No reliable radiologic criteria currently exist to differentiate renal cell carcinoma from oncocytoma, and since oncocytomas tend to gradually enlarge and may coexist with renal cell carcinoma, resection is appropriate.

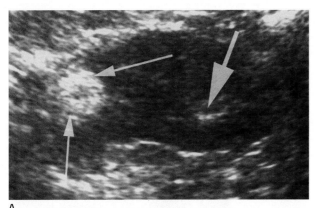

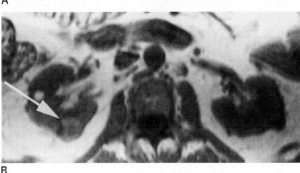

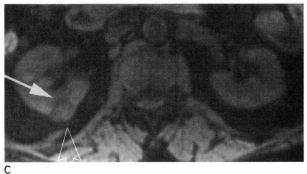

Figure 27-3 ■ Angiomyolipoma. *A,* Sonogram shows a 3-cm, homogeneously echogenic mass at the upper pole of the right kidney (small arrows). The echogenicity of this mass is similar to that of the fat in the renal medulla (large arrow). *B,* T1-weighted image without fat saturation shows the 3-cm mass right kidney with a peripheral bright signal rim (arrow). *C,* T1-weighted with fat saturation shows a drop in signal in the periphery of the lesion relative to the non-fat-saturated image in *B,* indicating the presence of fat within the lesion.

In addition to renal cell carcinoma, other malignant lesions that must be considered in the differential diagnosis of renal masses include transitional cell tumors of the renal pelvis (larger lesions often invade the parenchyma), lymphoma, and metastatic lesions. Primary neoplasms of the renal pelvis comprise almost 10% of malignant renal masses, of which transitional cell carcinoma is the most common. Incidental radiologic diagnosis of these tumors is more unusual,

generally because they may only have a papillary growth pattern, and may not be suspected unless focal calyceal or ureteral obstruction are noted on computed tomography or there is an obvious mass or filling defect in the renal pelvis. Patients usually present with hematuria (see Chapter 28), at which time a more focused computed tomography evaluation using 5-mm cuts may disclose the mass. However, cystoscopy, retrograde ureteropyelography, and ureteroscopy remain essential parts of evaluating possible renal pelvic and other ureteral lesions.

Metastatic tumors to the kidney are the most common multifocal malignant renal neoplasm and most occur as a result of hematogenous spread. Fewer than 10% arise from direct growth from adjacent organs such as the adrenals or pancreas or from lymphatic spread. The most common primary sites to metastasize to the kidney include lung, colon, and breast. Typically, the lesions are peripheral, multifocal, bilateral, hypovascular, and asymptomatic. If a patient with a known history of another cancer presents with a suspicious renal lesion, biopsy is appropriate, since management of the lesion may be determined by the primary tumor type.

Primary lymphoma of the kidney is very rare because there is no intrarenal lymphoid tissue. Secondary renal involvement may be caused either by direct infiltration with contiguous growth or by hematogenous spread. Lymphoma of the kidney can present as solitary or multiple masses, as direct infiltration from retroperitoneal lymph nodes, or as diffuse infiltration resulting in enlargement of one or both kidneys. The most common pattern of involvement is multiple masses ranging from 1 to 3 cm in diameter. On computed tomography, masses are typically bilateral and homogeneous and exhibit minimal enhancement after intravenous contrast. A cystic appearance is rarely seen and usually reflects necrosis in patients undergoing chemotherapy. Many patients initially present with renal failure from either parenchymal replacement, bilateral ureteral obstruction from bulky retroperitoneal adenopathy, or both. In most circumstances, when renal lymphoma is suspected, a percutaneous biopsy of the kidney or, preferably, an involved periaortic lymph node will establish the diagnosis.

Adrenal Masses

Most adrenal masses are incidentally found by computed tomography or magnetic resonance imaging. The vast majority are nonfunctioning and asymptomatic and require no further evaluation or treatment. Primary malignant lesions of the adrenal gland are rare, accounting for 0.02% of cancers and 0.2% of all

Table 27-2 ■ Classification of Functioning Adrenal Carcinoma

Cushing's syndrome
Virilization in females
    Increased DHEA 17-ketosteroids
    Increased testosterone
Feminizing syndromes in men
Hyperaldosteronism
Mixed combination of above

cancer deaths. Since up to 79% of adrenal tumors secrete a variety of hormones that produce clinical symptoms or signs and over 90% are greater than 6 cm in diameter, a practical approach to evaluation of adrenal masses focuses on both their size and their functionality (Table 27-2).

Of note, many tumors secrete multiple products, and some metabolites may be nonfunctional or secreted in such low amounts that physiologic changes are not evident. A selective, cost-effective biochemical assessment of an adrenal mass should include tests to rule out a pheochromocytoma (e.g., serum or urine catecholamine level), potassium levels in hypertensive cases, and glucocorticoid evaluation when clinical stigmata of Cushing's syndrome or virilization are present.

The ability of computed tomography and magnetic resonance imaging to localize and characterize adrenal lesions has reduced the need for extensive biochemical evaluation. All functional masses and those over 5 cm in diameter should be evaluated and surgically removed (Figure 27-4).

Benign adrenal masses that may require surgical evaluation include adenomas, myelolipomas, or metastases. Adenomas are usually less than 5 cm in diameter, solitary, and often associated with atrophy of the opposite gland. They are usually nonfunctional but may rarely present with Cushing's syndrome or hyperaldosteronism. Adrenal hyperplasia, however, is a more common cause of hyperaldosteronism. Most adrenal adenomas appear slightly hypointense to the liver on T1-weighted images and either slightly hyperintense or isointense to liver on T2-weighted images. Chemical-shift MR imaging takes advantage of the fact

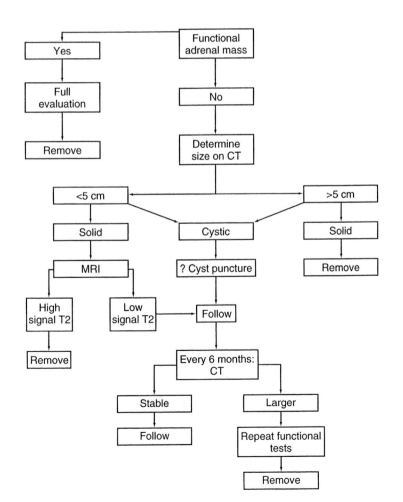

Figure 27-4 ■ Algorithm for evaluation of incidentally found adrenal mass. (From Walsh PC, et al [eds]: Campbell's Urology, 7th edition, Philadelphia, WB Saunders, 1998, p. 2933.)

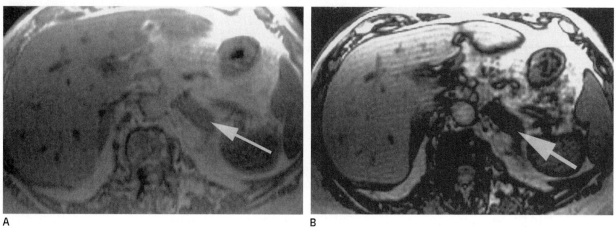

A   B

Figure 27-5 ■ Chemical-shift magnetic resonance image showing fractional intravoxel lipid confirming the presence of an adrenal adenoma. *A*, T1-weighted gradient echo in-phase image showing intermediate signal in the left adrenal mass (arrow). *B*, T1-weighted gradient echo opposed-phase image showing a drop-off in signal within the left adrenal mass consistent with an adrenal adenoma.

that many adenomas contain "fractional intravoxel lipid," which contributes to a drop-off in signal when opposed-phase imaging is performed. An adrenal-spleen signal ratio (ASR) threshold of 70 indicates a benign lesion, and no further workup is required in these patients. Lesions with an adrenal-spleen signal ratio greater than 70 should have a biopsy performed, depending on the clinical situation (Figure 27-5). Myelolipomas are also usually less than 5 cm in diameter and nonfunctional and may occasionally cause pain. Since they are composed of hematopoietic and adipose tissue, they will have a characteristic appearance on computed tomography or magnetic resonance imaging that should differentiate them from other lesions (Figure 27-6). Observation of lesions with this appearance is appropriate.

Many different primary tumors have a high propensity to metastasize to the adrenal glands, including melanoma, breast, lung, and renal carcinomas. In fact, primary adrenocortical carcinoma (Figure 27-7) is much less common than metastatic tumors to the adrenal. Consequently, the incidental finding of a suspicious, asymptomatic adrenal lesion should always prompt a search for an occult primary tumor. Computed tomography-guided fine needle aspiration of indeterminate adrenal lesion can provide a diagnosis in over 90% of cases. Treatment depends on the underlying primary disease. Bilateral adrenal metastasis may produce adrenal insufficiency. Special attention should be given to evaluating the adrenal gland in any patient who is found to have a renal carcinoma because of the current trend to spare the adrenal gland in many instances when performing a radical or partial nephrectomy (see Chapter 84, "Renal Cell Carcinoma").

Pheochromocytoma

Although pheochromocytoma is the causative factor for hypertension in less than 1% of the population and

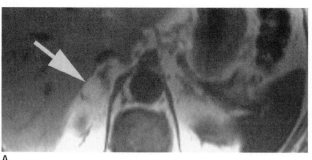
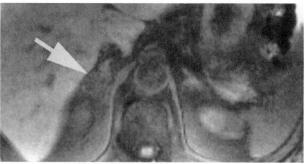

A   B

Figure 27-6 ■ Magnetic resonance image showing fat suppression within an adrenal myelolipoma. *A*, T1-weighted gradient echo in-phase image showing a high signal mass within the right adrenal gland. *B*, Fat-suppressed T1-weighted in-phase image showing marked drop in signal within this mass consistent with an adrenal myelolipoma.

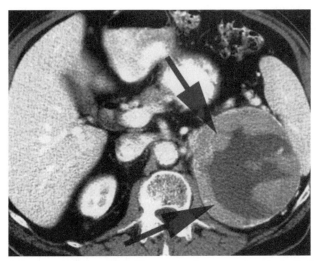

Figure 27-7 ■ Computed tomography scan showing a left adrenal carcinoma. Enhanced computed tomography scan shows a 7-cm mass within the left adrenal gland with nodular enhancement of the wall and central low-density area due to necrosis. This mass displaces the spleen laterally and left kidney inferiorly.

is a rare underlying etiology for an adrenal mass, its recognition is critical because of the potentially lethal effects from sustained or paroxysmal hypertension. Clues to the diagnosis of pheochromocytoma include new onset and often widely fluctuating hypertension, severe headache, excessive generalized sweating, palpitations with or without tachycardia, anxiety, and tremulousness. Rarely, patients who are found to have a pheochromocytoma are normotensive. The diagnosis is confirmed by demonstrating elevated levels of catecholamines, metanephrine, or vanillylmandelic

acid (VMA) in the urine or serum. Several drugs or food substances can affect these levels.

Pheochromocytoma can occur bilaterally, or in an ectopic location such as the organ of Zuckerkandl, and may rarely be malignant. Typically, a pheochromocytoma is very bright on T2 magnetic resonance imaging images. Sagittal and coronal images are particularly helpful to demonstrate the anatomic relationships of the tumor to surrounding tissue (Figure 27-8).

When a pheochromocytoma is clinically suspected but not confirmed by laboratory data, it may be helpful to perform a ^{131}I metaiodobenzylguanidine imaging study. This has been found to be particularly helpful in the diagnosis of multiple lesions, extra-adrenal locations, residual masses, and malignant pheochromocytomas.

Suggested Reading

Renal Masses

Bosniak MA: Diagnosis and management of patients with complicated cystic lesions of the kidney. Am J Roentgenol 1997;169:819–821.

Kallman DA, King BF, Hattery RR, et al: Renal vein and inferior vena cava tumor thrombus in renal cell carcinoma: Computed tomography, ultrasound, magnetic resonance imaging and venacavography. J Comput Assist Tomogr 1992;16:240–247.

Marotti M, Hricak H, Fritzche P, et al: Complex and simple renal cysts: Comparative evaluation with MR imaging. Radiology 1987;162:679–684.

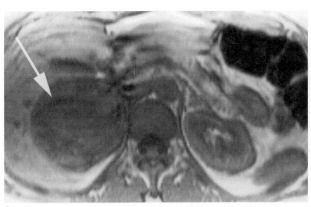

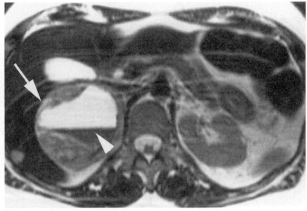

A   B

Figure 27-8 ■ Magnetic resonance image showing a right adrenal pheochromocytoma. *A*, Axial T1-weighted gradient echo image showing a 6-cm inhomogeneously low-signal mass within the right adrenal gland. The left adrenal gland is normal. *B*, T2-weighted image shows layering of low- and high-signal areas within the pheochromocytoma consistent with areas of necrosis. This layering effect is not due to hemorrhage because of the lack of signal consistent with blood degradation products on the T1-weighted images.

McNicholas MM, Raptopoulos VD, Schwartz RK, et al: Excretory phase computed tomography urography for opacification of the urinary collecting system. Am J Roentgenol 1998;170:1261–1267.

Schlicter A, Schubert R, Werner W, et al: How accurate is diagnostic imaging in determination of size and multifocality of renal cell carcinoma as a prerequisite for nephron-sparing surgery? Urol Int 2000;64:192–197.

Adrenal Masses

Belldegrun A, deKernion J: What to do about the incidentally discovered adrenal mass. World J Urol 1989;7:117–120.

McNicholas MM, Lee MJ, Mayo-Smith WW, et al: An imaging algorithm for the differential diagnosis of adrenal adenomas and metastases. Am J Roentgenol 1995;165:1453–1459.

Chapter 28
Hematuria

Dinesh Singh and Aria F. Olumi

Introduction

Hematuria, or blood in the urine, either gross (visible) or microscopic, is a common symptom. The prevalence estimates for microscopic hematuria in screened populations range from 3% to 20%. This broad range reflects differences in the composition of the populations studied and the number of screening studies performed. Since hematuria is frequently a harbinger of serious underlying pathology, including cancer, it is essential for the clinician to be aware of the screening tests, the workup, the differential diagnosis (Table 28-1), and management of hematuria.

General Considerations

The finding of hematuria often causes patients great distress. The commonest causes of transient hematuria are cystitis and menstrual blood contamination of the urine. When hematuria is persistent, no etiology will be found in the majority of patients, but the incidence of renal or urologic tumors is approximately 15%. Bladder carcinoma accounts for more than 90% of the malignancies identified, and renal cancer

for approximately 2% to 5% of these. Approximately 80% of patients with bladder cancer will exhibit either gross or microscopic hematuria, whereas gross hematuria is distinctly uncommon in renal cancer. Hematuria can result from therapy. Radiation-induced cystitis and hemorrhagic cystitis from cyclophosphamide may occur more than 20 years after treatment. Because a substantial percentage of patients with hematuria are found to have genitourinary tumors, a complete urologic evaluation is warranted.

Several substances may color the urine red in the absence of red blood cells in the urine. These include (1) medicines such as the antibiotics rifampin, nitrofurantoin, sulfamethoxazole, pyridium, and phenytoin; (2) phenolphthalein (a component of some laxatives); (3) artificial food coloring; and (4) anthocyanins in beets (most often in children with iron deficiency anemia) and berries.

Urine Dipstick Testing

The urine dipstick is a useful initial screening test because it is highly sensitive to the presence of hemoglobin in the urine. When the test is positive, evalua-

DIAGNOSIS

Renal Carcinoma

One should be wary of the possibility that microscopic hematuria is caused by a urologic neoplasm. This is especially true when a patient carries another diagnosis, of a neoplasm or a nonneoplastic medical problem. In this circumstance, there is a tendency to believe that the hematuria is related to the known condition. This can lead to failure to recognize that a renal cancer coexists.

A number of symptoms and findings can provide useful clues to the presence of renal cancer. For example, patients with renal cancer can have constitutional symptoms of fever and weight loss and may

manifest peripheral neuropathy. Abnormal laboratory studies also appear as paraneoplastic manifestations, not due to dissemination of the cancer. These include abnormal liver function tests, anemia, erythrocytosis (in approximately 5% of affected patients), hypercalcemia, and marked elevation of the sedimentation rate (to more than 90 mm/hour). The latter is due to increased levels of the acute phase reactant, haptoglobin. This increase can be so high that the alpha-2 protein fraction, most of which is haptoglobin, is increased on serum protein electrophoresis.

Table 28-1 ■ Differential Diagnosis of Hematuria

Urologic Malignancy

Bladder cancer
Renal cell carcinoma
Prostate cancer
Ureteral transitional cell carcinoma
Metastatic carcinoma
Urethral cancer
Penile cancer
Renal or prostatic lymphoma

Nonmalignant Renal Disease

Pyelonephritis
Immunologic glomerulonephritides
Calculus
Polycystic kidney disease
Papillary necrosis: diabetes, sickle-cell disease
Anemia

Renal Trauma

Benign prostatic hyperplasia
Prostatitis
Prostate or bladder trauma from indwelling catheter

Cystitis

Infection
Radiation
Cyclophosphamide

Urethritis or Urethral Polyps

Renal Vascular Disease

Abdominal aortic aneurysm
Renal artery embolism, thrombosis, or stenosis
Renal vein thrombosis

Strenuous Exercise

Table 28-2 ■ Risk Factors for Harboring Significant Urologic Disease

Smoking history
Occupational exposure to chemicals or dyes (benzenes or aromatic amines)
History of gross hematuria
History of pelvic irradiation
Prior treatment with cyclophosphamide

Adopted from Grossfeld GD, et al: Evaluation of asymptomatic microscopic hematuria in adults: The American Urological Association best practice policy. II: Patient evaluation, cytology, voided markers, imaging, cystoscopy, nephrology evaluation, and follow-up. Urology 2001;57: 604-610.

cell casts suggests glomerular pathology and the possibility of an underlying glomerulonephritis.

Normally, 1 to 2 million red blood cells are excreted in the urine daily. Therefore what degree of microscopic hematuria constitutes clinically meaningful hematuria requiring investigation is not well defined. The Best Practice Policy Panel on Asymptomatic Microscopic Hematuria published guidelines, which state that the presence of more than three red blood cells per high power field in a patient who has any of the risk factors for urologic disease noted in Table 28-2 warrants a complete urologic workup.

One needs to be aware, however, that there is no completely "safe" lower limit for the number of red blood cells per high power field, because patients with fewer than three red blood cells per high power field may harbor urologic tumors. The clinician should maintain a high index of suspicion and must use his or her judgment in determining whether a complete workup is warranted in patients with minimal microscopic hematuria.

History

A thorough history is part of the initial evaluation of a patient presenting with hematuria. The history should assess the degree of hematuria, its timing ("hematuria" concomitant with menses may be normal urine contaminated by vaginal blood or could be related to urinary tract endometriosis), history of previous hematuria, related risk factors (see Table 28-2), urologic instrumentation or catheterization, recent trauma, previous episodes of hematuria, presence of clots, shapes of any clots (vermiform clots indicate the upper urinary tract as the source), and/or relationship to strenuous exercise (strenuous exercise can cause a brief, less than 48-hour, "runner's hematuria").

Microscopic hematuria does not cause dysuria unless it is due to cystitis or urethritis. Flank pain asso-

tion should proceed to urinary sediment analysis. The urine dipstick screening test may be falsely positive for hematuria secondary to the presence of myoglobinuria, hemoglobinuria (from intravascular hemolysis), or povidone/iodine contamination. In contrast, a patient with very hypotonic urine can have a true positive urinalysis and a falsely negative examination of the urinary sediment. In this case, the hypotonicity lyses the red blood cells, and none may be seen under light microscopy.

Other dipstick analyses or the results of microscopic examination of the urinary sediment may suggest an etiology for the hematuria. For example, the presence of leukocyte esterase and nitrites suggests a urinary tract infection. The presence of ≥2+ protein and/or dysmorphic red blood cells and/or red blood ciated with hematuria usually results from a focus of bleeding in the upper urinary tract, such as a blood clot or a calculus. Gross hematuria indicates that the lesion is postglomerular. The timing of gross hematuria is also informative. Initial hematuria, or hematuria at the initiation of micturition, indicates a source in the urethra. Total hematuria, or hematuria throughout the urine stream, suggests that the bladder is the site of the bleeding. Terminal hematuria, or blood seen at the end of the voided stream, indicates pathology arising near the bladder neck or from the prostate (prostatic contraction occurs at the end of urination).

A careful history and physical examination combined with the results of the urinalysis and urinary sediment usually serve to focus attention on the likely locus, if not the etiology, of the blood in the urine.

Evaluation

Assessment of the lower and upper urinary tracts is necessary to evaluate any patient who has either gross hematuria or clinically significant microscopic hematuria. In an adult, the working presumption must be that the hematuria is due to cancer until proven otherwise. After dipstick and microscopic urine analysis, the three cardinal components of a full hematuria evaluation include urine cytology, cystoscopy, and upper urinary tract imaging.

Urine cytology for the possibility of a transitional cell carcinoma of some urothelial site is best obtained from a midstream voided specimen. Its sensitivity varies greatly with the degree of differentiation of the tumor. For instance, urine cytology has a greater than 90% sensitivity for detecting high-grade (grade III)

cancer or carcinoma in situ of the bladder. However, for lower-grade transitional cell carcinoma, the sensitivity falls to approximately 70% for grade II lesions and to less than 30% for grade I lesions. Despite its low sensitivity in the detection of a well-differentiated transitional cell carcinoma, urine cytology is clearly useful in identifying patients who have early-stage cancers. Molecular markers of urothelial cancer, such as NMP22, BTA, telomerase, and P53, can be assayed in the urine, but their diagnostic utility is not well defined.

Upper-tract imaging approaches vary at different clinical centers. The study of choice in the past was an intravenous pyelogram (IVP). Although good visualization of the urinary tract is obtained, the renal parenchyma is not evaluable, small lesions (less than 3 cm in diameter) within the kidney may not be seen, and the technique does not distinguish between large renal masses and renal cysts. By contrast, an ultrasound can assess the renal parenchyma and distinguish masses from cysts; however, its ability to assess the ureters in fine detail is limited.

For these reasons, an abdominal and pelvic computed tomography scan with and without contrast has become the standard mode for imaging the urinary tract. Figure 28-1 demonstrates a precontrast and postcontrast computed tomography scan of a patient with a left renal mass consistent with renal cell carcinoma. As shown, the computed tomography scan images the renal parenchyma and readily differentiates renal cysts from renal masses. A precontrast computed tomography scan is the study of choice for a patient who is suspected of having a kidney stone. A postcontrast computed tomography scan helps to evaluate solid parenchymal lesions because contrast-

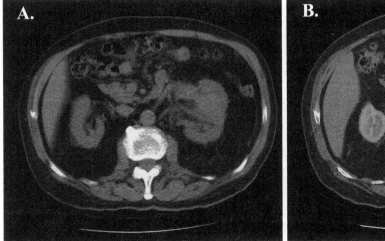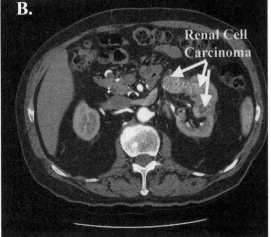

Figure 28-1 ■ Precontrast (*A*) and postcontrast (*B*) abdominal computed tomography demonstrating a large left renal mass in a patient who presented with microscopic hematuria.

DIAGNOSIS

Caveats About Urine Cytology

Urine cytology should be deferred:

- In the setting of gross hematuria because the results will not be informative.
- After instrumentation or Foley catheter placement because these interventions can introduce sloughed cells from the urethral lining into the urinary sample, leading to their interpretation as atypical cells.

- After the administration of radiocontrast material either during a cystoscopic procedure or from an intravenous pyelogram, because the radiopaque dye can alter cytologic morphology.
- For at least three months after a patient has received intravesical Bacillus Calmette-Guerin treatment for bladder cancer, because the resulting urothelial reaction can lead to a false-positive diagnosis of cancer.

enhancing renal masses are usually malignant. The computed tomography scan also shows areas of calcification, which can be informative beyond the detection of urolithiasis. Up to 90% of centrally calcified masses are malignant, whereas only 20% of peripherally calcified masses are malignant, and only 1% of simple cysts are calcified. The collecting system including the ureters can be well visualized, and the bladder mucosa can be evaluated for large filling defects on the excretory phase of the computed tomography scan. If a bladder or renal tumor is identified, the size of the corresponding draining lymph nodes can be evaluated for staging purposes. Invasion of the renal vein or inferior vena cava by tumor thrombosis from a renal carcinoma can be seen as well. For smaller renal tumors, the size and location of the mass are useful in the consideration of a partial versus a total nephrectomy. The findings on the computed tomography scan may influence the approach to subsequent cytoscopy if it is required. For instance, computed tomography imaging of a ureteral mass will guide the urologist to include ureteroscopy and possibly a biopsy in the same procedure as cytoscopy.

Cystoscopy allows direct visualization of the lower urinary tract, namely, the urethra and the bladder (Figure 28-2). When a computed tomography scan of the abdomen cannot be performed with contrast because of a history of a severe allergic reaction to contrast material or compromised renal function, cystoscopy affords an opportunity to study the upper tracts via a retrograde pyelogram, by injecting radiocontrast dye up the ureteral orifice into the renal pelvis without systemic administration (Figure 28-3).

Management of Gross Hematuria

Hematologist/oncologists do encounter patients with substantial gross hematuria, most commonly caused by bladder tumors, prostate cancer, benign prostatic hyperplasia, and cystitis secondary to radiation treatment (radiation cystitis) or as a complication of cyclophosphamide treatment (hemorrhagic cystitis). When the hematuria is not profuse, the patient should be kept well hydrated to minimize clot formation.

Gross hematuria leading to blood clot formation and acute urinary retention is more difficult to control. Continuous copious bladder irrigation with saline delivered through a three-way indwelling Foley catheter is necessary to wash out clots and prevent their reformation. In most cases, the continuous bladder irrigation can be titrated in volume and

TREATMENT

Pitfalls in the Management of Gross Hematuria

Many clinicians misguidedly place a three-way urinary catheter to treat a patient with gross hematuria and clot retention. The caliber of a catheter represents a measure of the diameter of the total catheter. Therefore the diameter of the outflow port, through which clots are evacuated, is much smaller in a three-way catheter than in a comparably sized two-way catheter. One should first place a large-caliber two-way catheter to facilitate evacuation of the clot. Then one can substitute a three-way catheter for continued irrigation to prevent clot reformation.

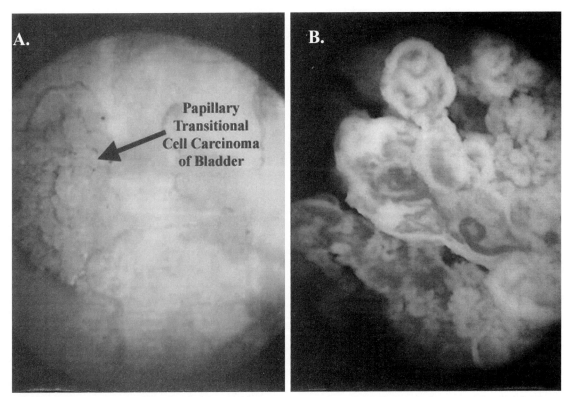

Figure 28-2 ■ Cystoscopic image of a bladder tumor at low (*A*) and high (*B*) magnifications from a patient who presented with gross hematuria.

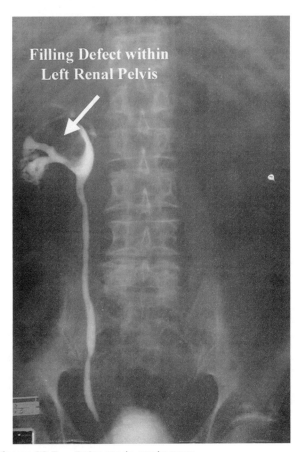

Figure 28-3 ■ Retrograde pyelogram.

discontinued within several days, and the catheter can be removed. After initiating the continuous bladder irrigation, any offending irritant agent must be stopped, and any existing coagulopathy must be corrected.

If the bleeding still persists and its origin is the bladder, especially in cases of nonfocal, diffuse bladder hemorrhage such as occurs in radiation cystitis or hemorrhagic cystitis, additional measures administered by means of cystoscopy become necessary. Alum is a substance that promotes clot formation and can be instilled as a continuous drip through an indwelling catheter. This requires no anesthesia and does not cause any great degree of bladder scarring. Since alum is supplied as an aluminum potassium sulfate or aluminum ammonium sulfate salt, toxic levels of aluminum, potassium, or ammonia may accumulate in the serum.

Formalin and silver nitrate are more caustic than alum but may more readily induce cessation of bleeding by precipitation of protein at the bleeding sites. A cystogram must be done first to rule out the presence of vesicoureteral reflux, because both agents are harmful to the upper urinary tracts. General or spinal anesthesia is also required because their instillation is painful. The result of this therapy can be a scarred, contracted, dysfunctional or nonfunctional bladder.

These measures should therefore be reserved for patients who fail less toxic approaches.

Suggested Reading

Alishahi S, Byrne D, Goodman CM, Baxby K: Haematuria investigation based on a standard protocol: Emphasis on the diagnosis of urologic malignancy, J R Coll Surg Edinb 2002;47:422–427.

Avidor Y, Nadu A, Matzkin H: Clinical significance of gross hematuria and its evaluation in patients receiving anticoagulant and aspirin treatment. Urology 2000;55:22–24.

Froom P, Froom J, Ribak J: Asymptomatic microscopic hematuria: Is investigation necessary? J Clin Epidemiol 1997;50:1197–1200.

Grossfeld GD, Litwin MS, Wolf JS, et al: Evaluation of asymptomatic microscopic hematuria in adults: The American Urological Association best practice policy. I: Definition, detection, prevalence, and etiology. Urology 2001;57:599–603.

Grossfeld GD, Litwin MS, Wolf JS, et al: Evaluation of asymptomatic microscopic hematuria in adults: The American Urological Association best practice policy. II: Patient evaluation, cytology, voided markers, imaging, cystoscopy, nephrology evaluation, and follow-up. Urology 2001;57:604–610.

Hall CL: The patient with hematuria. Practitioner 1999;243:564–568.

Jaffe JS, Ginsberg PC, Gill R, Harkaway RC: A new diagnostic algorithm for the evaluation of microscopic hematuria. Urology 2001;57:889–894.

Khadra MH, Pickard RS, Charlton M, et al: A prospective analysis of 1,930 patients with hematuria to evaluate current diagnostic practice. J Urol 2000;163:524–527.

Lammerer RL, Gibson S, Kovacs D, et al: Comparison of urine dipstick and urinalysis at various test cutoff points. Ann Emerg Med 2001;38:505–512.

Lang EK, Macchia RJ, Thomas R, et al: Computerized tomography tailored for the assessment of microscopic hematuria. J Urol 2002;167:547–554.

Newhouse JH, Amis ES Jr, Bigongiari LR, et al: Radiologic investigation of patients with hematuria: American College of Radiology Appropriateness Criteria. Radiology 2000;215(Suppl):687–691.

Sokolsky MC: Hematuria. Emerg Med Clin North Am 2001;19:621–631.

Chapter 29
Testicular Mass

Pasquale Benedetto

Numerous benign conditions may present as scrotal swelling, including hydrocele, spermatocele, epididymal cysts, simple or complex testicular cysts, varicocele, epididymitis, orchitis, abscess, rare infections such as tuberculosis or syphilis, sarcoidosis, infarction, vasculitis, or hematoma. These conditions occur with much greater frequency than neoplastic diseases. Although malignant diseases of the testicle are uncommon relative to benign testicular disorders, such conditions are important because they include malignancies that are highly curable. Therefore prompt diagnosis is important to facilitate treatment and optimize chances for prolonged survival.

General Considerations

Important factors to consider in evaluating a patient who presents with a "testicular" mass include whether the mass is intratesticular or extratesticular, the age of the patient, and the presence or absence of symptoms.

The location of the lesion as testicular versus extratesticular can usually be made on the basis of the physical exam (see the following sections). In situations in which the results of a physical examination are unclear, ultrasound is invariably definitive. Extratesticular masses in the adult are usually cystic and benign, while intratesticular lesions are more commonly due to malignant conditions. Malignant extratesticular lesions are frequently solid on ultrasound. A large percentage of such lesions are paratesticular sarcomas. These typically occur in the younger, prepubertal patient population. Tumors arising from spermatic cord structures are less common and are distinguished by their paratesticular rather than intratesticular location on exam and ultrasound.

Most clinically apparent intratesticular masses are malignant. The type of lesion varies with the age at presentation. Intratesticular neoplasms most often present in young adults, generally between the ages of 15 and 40, with a median age in the third decade. Germ-cell tumors predominate in this age group, lymphoma or stromal tumors being much less common. Such tumors, particularly germ-cell neoplasms, must be suspected in any young adult who presents with an enlargement of the testicle documented by ultrasound to be an intratesticular solid mass.

While children more commonly present with paratesticular neoplasms, intratesticular lesions do occur in this age group. The differential diagnosis for an intratesticular mass in a child includes germ-cell tumors, lymphoma, and testicular presentation of acute lymphoblastic leukemia. Within the germ-cell category, embryonal-cell carcinoma, yolk sac (endodermal sinus) tumors, or teratomas predominate. Seminomas are rare in the pediatric age group. In contrast, seminoma represents the most common germ-cell neoplasm in men over age 50. However, testicular masses in this age group more commonly result from other neoplastic diseases, most notably non-Hodgkin's lymphomas. Fewer than 1% of all germ-cell neoplasms occur in Blacks; hence some of the diagnostic considerations mentioned above may be different in this ethnic group.

History

The patient's history and presenting symptoms can provide important diagnostic clues as to the etiology of a testicular mass. The rapidity of the enlargement, the presence or absence of pain, a prior history of trauma, a history of testicular maldescent, fever, back pain, breast tenderness, and fatigue are all potentially relevant to the diagnosis. Pain, tenderness, and fever are more likely associated with infectious etiologies. Prior trauma suggests the possibility of hematoma, although it is not unusual to obtain a history of trauma in a patient with an apparent tumor. In these instances, the trauma appears to call attention to the presence of a testicular abnormality rather than to be a causative factor in the malignant differentiation. Maldescent of the testicle (cryptorchidism) is associated with a considerable increase in the incidence of testicular cancer; therefore in patients with such a history, the suspicion for testicular cancer should be heightened. Curiously, 20% of patients with testicular cancer and a history of cryptorchidism will present with tumor in the normally descended testis. Breast tenderness is an important clue to possible ectopic hormone production by tumor, usually the beta subunit of human chorionic gonadotropin (beta-hCG) produced by a nonseminomatous germ-cell tumor. Gynecomastia or hirsutism, on the other hand, may indicate the presence of other endocrine syndromes that are typically associated with stromal tumors. Finally, back pain may signify retroperitoneal nodal metastases.

Physical Examination

On physical examination, one can usually identify the scrotal mass as either intratesticular or extratesticular, smooth or irregular, hard or fluctuant, and/or tender. All of these descriptors lend information to the examiner regarding the differential diagnosis (Figure 29-1). In general, physical examination including transillumination will usually identify a hydrocele or spermatocele. These conditions are usually associated with a smooth contoured mass that transilluminates. Varicoceles and epididymal cysts are common extratesticular lesions. The former are usually irregular, wormlike, but soft; the latter are usually smooth. The hallmark of malignant tumors is the presence of an irregularly contoured, firm or hard mass, although occasionally, the only finding is an enlargement of the testicle relative to the contralateral gland.

Acute infectious etiologies, such as epididymitis, usually are tender to palpation, although this might not be the case with chronic conditions. Most tumors of the testicle are not painful; therefore pain as a presenting symptom leads one to consider conditions such as torsion, infarct, hemorrhage, trauma, or infection. Torsion is an emergency situation that requires prompt attention to avoid testicular damage. Doppler ultrasonography or radionuclide scanning may be most helpful in distinguishing torsion from epididymitis, an alternative consideration in a patient who presents with acute testicular pain.

Fever often implies an infectious etiology. This diagnosis is further supported by an elevation of the white blood cell count, positive urethral or urine culture, or white cells on urethral smear or urine Gram stain.

Other physical exam findings that are helpful include the presence of cervical adenopathy, an indicator of an advanced malignancy; breast tenderness, suggesting a germ-cell neoplasm; or feminization in an adult male or masculinization in a child, suggesting the possibility of functioning stromal tumor such as a Sertoli-Leydig cell tumor.

DIAGNOSIS

Evaluation of Testicular Masses

- Intratesticular solid masses in adults should raise the suspicion of neoplasm and initiate early evaluation. While ancillary laboratory studies may be helpful, they should not dissuade from surgery.
- Extratesticular lesions are more commonly benign in adults and can frequently be observed.
- In children, scrotal pathology is unusual, and the possibility of malignant disease should always be suspected, occasioning prompt evaluation and intervention.

Laboratory Evaluation

The evaluation of a patient who is suspected of having a testicular tumor should include serum assays for the tumor markers, alpha-fetoprotein and beta-hCG. These oncofetal proteins are expressed in most nonseminomatous tumors and in a small percentage of seminomas (beta-hCG only). Elevation of these markers is highly correlated with the presence of a germ-cell tumor. Elevations in the serum lactate dehydrogenase (LDH) is useful but not diagnostic of malignancy, as it is commonly elevated in infectious or inflammatory states. However, in the patient with an obvious neoplastic condition, an elevation of the lactate dehydrogenase implies rapid cell turnover and high tumor burden, usually indicative of tumor outside of the confines of the testis itself.

Abnormalities of the blood counts are most likely seen with acute and chronic infectious etiologies. Tumors, in general, are not associated with abnormalities in routine blood tests except for the testicular presentation of acute lymphoblastic leukemia, in which the hemogram will demonstrate circulating blasts. Testicular relapse of acute lymphoblastic leukemia might not be associated with an abnormal peripheral smear, but the antecedent history will provide a clue to the diagnosis.

Imaging

Ultrasound should be the initial diagnostic study in a patient presenting with a scrotal mass. Ultrasound has

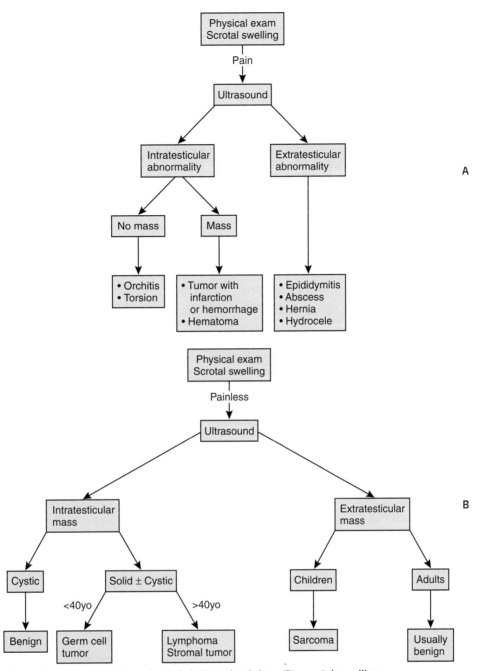

Figure 29-1 ■ Evaluation of painful (A) and painless (B) scrotal swelling.

a very high degree of sensitivity. The study should be able to identify the location of the lesion as intratesticular versus extratesticular or paratesticular and to distinguish a solid, cystic, or complex mass from other inflammatory findings. As was mentioned previously, the identification of an intratesticular solid mass places malignancy at the top of the differential diagnosis.

An ultrasound of the normal testis demonstrates homogeneous echogenicity with well-defined borders. Generally, germ-cell tumors are hypoechoic, but they may have areas of hyperechogenicity. It should be noted that the ultrasound does not always identify a solid mass. Embryonal-cell carcinomas are only slightly hypoechoic in comparison to normal testis and therefore may initially be missed until there is distortion of the contour of the normal testis. Other descriptors, including "heteroechogenic," "hypervascular," and "inhomogeneous" should alert the clinician to the possibility of a neoplasm. Other clues to the diagnosis of a germ-cell neoplasm include the presence of microlithiasis, cystic spaces with solid components, and calcifications.

Stromal tumors appear as hypoechoic lesions and are essentially indistinguishable from other neoplasms. Although hyperechoic, homogeneous lesions are generally benign, lymphoma usually has this appearance.

Benign lesions within the testis include cysts. These are easily identified and require no further intervention as long as there are no solid components. The presence of a solid component within a cyst necessitates further investigation, since teratocarcinomas typically present with cystic spaces. Mumps orchitis has a fairly characteristic appearance on ultrasound, typically presenting as a uniform, hypoechoic testicular enlargement without focality or irregularity of the testicular contour. In contrast to testicular neoplasms, there is frequently no "normal"-appearing testis. Hematomas likewise usually create an abnormal appearance to the entire testis. While testicular torsion has a typical ultrasound appearance, this diagnosis is usually made by the clinical history, specifically the sudden onset of severe testicular pain. Doppler studies may be helpful in this situation by documenting decreased or absent blood flow.

Other imaging modalities rarely provide useful additional information. While magnetic resonance imaging (MRI) scan can provide more detail of an intratesticular mass, this is rarely important.

Approach to the Patient with a Testicular Mass

A patient presenting with a scrotal swelling should undergo a good physical examination, including scrotal transillumination, to determine whether the swelling is intratesticular or extratesticular. If this distinction cannot be made on the basis of examination alone, then one should proceed to ultrasound. An extratesticular mass that is smooth and transilluminates points to the diagnosis of hydrocele.

In general, a patient presenting with an intratesticular solid mass should be considered to have a neoplasm until proven otherwise. These lesions usually are asymptomatic or minimally painful at presentation. The young adult with a documented intratesticular mass should proceed to surgical intervention. On the basis of the presumptive diagnosis of a germ-cell neoplasm, an inguinal orchiectomy should be performed. A biopsy of the testis is rarely indicated in a patient who is suspected of having a tumor. Perhaps the only indication would be the patient with a presumptive tumor diagnosis who has only one testis. In less clear situations, more information may be required before proceeding to a procedure as definitive as orchiectomy. Tumor markers can be helpful. An elevated alpha-fetoprotein and beta-hCG is essentially incontrovertible evidence of a malignant germ-cell neoplasm, nonseminomatous type, since no other disease state is associated with an elevation of both proteins. Elevation of either tumor marker is strongly supportive of the diagnosis. However, the absence of a marker does not mitigate against the diagnosis of a germ-cell tumor, since at least 10% of patients with nonseminomatous disease and more than 90% of patients with seminoma do not express markers. Therefore only a positive value is helpful in deciding to explore the patient if there is some hesitancy. While tumor markers should be obtained preoperatively, the need for surgical therapy should not be based on the value of the markers, since cancer may exist in the absence of an elevated marker.

In clinical practice, it is not uncommon for the diagnosis of cancer to be delayed while the patient is treated for possible epididymitis. The pathogenesis of epididymitis requires a sexually active individual or a patient with a structural abnormality. Therefore inquiries into prior urinary tract infections and sexual activity are important. Lack of pain, pyuria, or bacteria on a urethral Gram stain should call into question the diagnosis of epididymitis. In any event, if antibiotic treatment does not result in prompt resolution of the swelling (one to two weeks), alternative diagnoses should be entertained. In particular, the diagnosis of tumor must be considered, and orchiectomy performed.

If the patient is older than 40 years, an intratesticular mass still carries a high likelihood of malignancy, but the differential is expanded to include lymphoma and stromal tumors.

In an asymptomatic patient, the demonstration of a testicular mass implies the presence of tumor until proven otherwise. If ultrasound evaluation confirms a solid intratesticular mass, the study should be followed by surgical intervention without delay. However, if the imaging study confirms a purely cystic lesion, the patient can be followed, given the essentially benign nature of this finding. As was mentioned previously, it is important to be sure the cystic lesion has no solid component.

The presence of pain at diagnosis renders the possibility of a number of other acute illnesses. Of prime importance is the diagnosis of testicular torsion, as a delay in diagnosis of this entity may result in testicular infarction. The presentation of torsion is usually cataclysmic, with uncontrollable pain prompting emergency intervention. Doppler ultrasound may help to establish a low-flow state consistent with the presumptive diagnosis. Other etiologies that produce rapid onset of pain include hemorrhage secondary to trauma that should be obvious by history or infection that should be supported by laboratory data. Occasionally, a patient with a tumor will present with pain secondary to hemorrhage. The diagnosis will usually be established on the basis of the history and ultrasound.

Extratesticular lesions in the adult are usually benign, but the presence of a solid mass warrants consideration of the rare tumors that occur in the area. In the child, testicular abnormalities are uncommon, and genitourinary sites for sarcomas are frequent. Therefore a higher index of suspicion of tumor exists in this context, and earlier surgical intervention is necessary.

Suggested Reading

Bosl GJ, Bajorin DF, Sheinfeld J, Motzer RJ: Cancer of the testis. In DeVita VT Jr, Hellman S, Rosenberg SA (eds): Cancer: Principles and Practice of Oncology, 5th ed. Philadelphia: Lippincott-Raven, pp 1397–1425.

Lau MWM, Taylor PM, Payne SR: The indications for scrotal ultrasound. Br J Radiol 1999;72:833–837.

Micallef M, Torreggiani WC, Hurley M, et al: The ultrasound investigation of scrotal swelling. Int J STD AIDS 2000; 11:297–302.

The Scrotum. In Cochlin D, Dubbins P, Goldberg B, Alexander A (eds): Urogenital Ultrasound: A Text Atlas. Philadelphia: Lippincott, 1994, pp 196–224.

Walsh PC, Retik AB, Wein AJ, Vaughan ED (eds): Campbell's Urology, 8th ed. Philadelphia: WB Saunders, 2002.

Chapter 30
Vaginal Bleeding

Kris Ghosh and Jonathan M. Niloff

Introduction

Vaginal bleeding is one of the most common symptoms affecting women. The term *vaginal bleeding* implies that the origin of the bleeding is the reproductive tract, including the uterus, cervix, vagina, or vulva. Other sources of bleeding should always be excluded, such as bleeding from the rectum or urinary tract. Patients often confuse bleeding from hemorrhoids and urinary infections with vaginal bleeding.

Vaginal bleeding in an abnormal pattern may be dysfunctional (hormonal) in nature or may reflect organic pathology. The major causes of vaginal bleeding are not hematologic or oncologic. Only 15% of cases of vaginal bleeding are related to cancer. Vaginal bleeding is considered abnormal when there is excessive menstrual flow (greater than 80 cc), prolonged duration of menses (more than 7 days), menses occurring too frequently (less than 21 days apart), intermenstrual bleeding, bleeding occurring prior to menarche, and bleeding after sexual intercourse. The most worrisome bleeding is that which occurs after menopause. It should be considered indicative of cancer until proven otherwise.

Differential Diagnosis

Abnormal vaginal bleeding can be divided into four categories: systemic disease, dysfunctional causes, complications of pregnancy, and reproductive tract disease (Table 30-1).

Blood dyscrasias such as von Willebrand disease can present as vaginal bleeding. Other disorders that affect platelet function, including idiopathic thrombocytopenia, hypersplenism, sepsis, and leukemia, can cause abnormal vaginal bleeding. These coagulopathies typically present at the time of menarche. Coagulation disorders are diagnosed in 20% of adolescent females who require hospitalization for abnormal vaginal bleeding. Routine screening for coagulation defects should be reserved for women with suggestive clinical signs such as petechiae or bruising. Other systemic causes of vaginal bleeding include anticoagulation therapy, cirrhosis, and hypothyroidism.

Dysfunctional bleeding is the predominant cause of abnormal vaginal bleeding in the reproductive years. Dysfunctional bleeding results from alterations in neuroendocrine function, most commonly anovulation. Examples include eating disorders such as anorexia nervosa, excessive physical exercise, thyroid disease, excess androgen syndromes, and diabetes mellitus. Oral contraceptives and menopausal estrogen replacement therapy are two common forms of exogenous hormone treatment that are often complicated by vaginal bleeding.

Pregnancy and its complications should always be considered in the differential diagnosis of vaginal bleeding during the reproductive years. A pregnancy test should therefore be included in the initial evaluation of abnormal vaginal bleeding in this age group. If the pregnancy test is positive, ultrasound will establish the presence or absence of an intrauterine gestation. Common complications of pregnancy that result in bleeding include a threatened, missed, or incomplete abortion and ectopic pregnancies (see Table 30-1). Gestational trophoblastic disease, a neoplasm characterized by the abnormal proliferation of trophoblastic tissue, may present with bleeding (Figure 30-1). High serum human chorionic gonadotropin (HCG) levels are observed among women with gestational trophoblastic disease and can be helpful in differentiating this entity from other sources of bleeding. A human chorionic gonadotropin titer greater than 100,000 mIU/mL is suggestive of trophoblastic disease. Other manifestations of gestational trophoblastic disease are hypertension prior to 24 weeks' gestation, nausea and vomiting, abdominal pain, and uterine size greater than expected for the gestational age. If trophoblastic disease is suspected, the best diagnostic test is a pelvic ultrasound. Gestational trophoblastic disease has a characteristic sonographic appearance

Table 30-1 ■ Differential Diagnosis of Vaginal Bleeding

Systemic Disease

Von Willebrand disease
Hypersplenism
Thrombocytopenia
Leukemia
Anticoagulation therapy
Cirrhosis

Dysfunctional Bleeding

Hypothyroidism
Excess androgen syndromes
Diabetes mellitus
Exogenous hormones (e.g., oral contraceptives)
Anorexia nervosa
Excessive physical exercise
Polycystic ovary syndrome
Chronic anovulation

Complications of Pregnancy

Threatened abortion
Incomplete abortion
Gestational trophoblastic disease
Missed abortion
Ectopic pregnancy

Reproductive Tract Disease

Vulva/perineum
  Trauma
  Foreign body
  Hypoestrogenism
  Vulvar dystrophy
  Vulvar/vaginal cancer
Cervix
  Cervicitis
  Cervical polyp
  Cervical cancer
Uterus
  Endometritis
  Leiomyomata
  Endometrial polyps
  Endometrial hyperplasia
  Uterine cancer

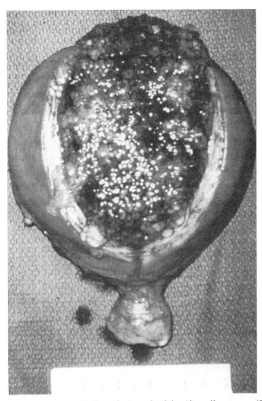

Figure 30-1 ■ Gestational trophoblastic disease. (From Morrow CP, Curtin JP: Synopsis of Gynecologic Oncology, 5th ed. New York: Churchill-Livingstone, 1998, p 319.)

usually described as a "snowstorm." A fetus is usually not present.

Evaluation: General

The evaluation of vaginal bleeding from the reproductive tract should follow an orderly progression based on anatomy. The vulva and the perineum should be examined first. In prepubertal girls, vulvitis with excoriation or trauma may be a cause of bleeding. In the elderly, common diagnoses are vulvar atrophy due to hypoestrogenism and vulvar dystrophy. Most important, any suspicious lesion or area of abnormal pigmentation should be biopsied to rule out malignancy.

The entire vagina should be visualized with a speculum, and any suspicious areas should be biopsied. Vaginal atrophy due to hypoestrogenism or prior radiation therapy is a common problem and often presents with postcoital bleeding. In the prepubertal patient, vaginitis, a foreign body, or trauma should be suspected with the complaint of vaginal bleeding. In examining the reproductive tract in an adolescent female, congenital abnormalities should always be looked for.

The cervix is a common source of vaginal bleeding. Its evaluation includes inspection and palpation. The Pap smear is a good screening test for cervical neoplasia. However, if a lesion is observed on the cervix, it should be biopsied to establish a histologic diagnosis. A Pap smear should not be relied on in the face of a gross lesion. Also included in the differential diagnosis are cervicitis, particularly chlamydial cervicitis, which can present with irregular or postcoital spotting; cervical polyps; and cervical leiomyomata.

DIAGNOSIS

Disorders of Hemostasis Associated with Vaginal Bleeding

Thrombocytopenia, particularly when the platelet count is below 40,000 to 50,000/μL and especially when the platelet count is below 10,000/μL, is associated with excessive menstrual bleeding. Therefore a platelet count should be performed with a complete blood count to rule out thrombocytopenia when vaginal bleeding may be a presentation of idiopathic thrombocytopenic purpura, acute leukemia, or drug-induced thrombocytopenia, for example. Although medications such as aspirin can aggravate an existing bleeding tendency, it is unusual for aspirin alone in an otherwise healthy woman to cause excessive vaginal bleeding.

Patients with hereditary disorders of hemostasis have a lifelong history of bleeding and bruising from multiple sites, and prolonged duration or excessive bleeding during menses is just a single manifestation. These patients should be evaluated for von Willebrand's disease or a congenital thrombocytopathy. In the former, von Willebrand factor activity is decreased; in the latter, platelet function is abnormal. To rule out von Willebrand disease, the plasma von Willebrand factor antigen, Ristocetin cofactor activity, and Factor VIII are measured. Unless these values are less than 50% of normal, von Willebrand's disease does not explain the excessive bleeding. However, the level of von Willebrand factor does fluctuate, and patients with low normal values should have these tests repeated on a separate occasion. Patients with hereditary thrombocytopathies also have a lifelong history of easy bruising, which may be aggravated by specific medications, including those that contain aspirin or nonsteroidal anti-inflammatory agents. An abnormal bleeding time and perhaps abnormal platelet aggregation studies may assist in making the proper diagnosis; however, the diagnosis of hereditary thrombocytopathy is often a diagnosis of exclusion.

The uterus is the most common source of bleeding from the genital tract. In prepubertal girls, the most frequent diagnosis is precocious puberty. Among postmenarchal women, the differential diagnosis of uterine bleeding includes endometritis (infection), endometrial polyps, submucosal leiomyomata, endometrial hyperplasia, and invasive endometrial cancer. Endometrial biopsy or dilation and curettage (D&C) is the procedure used to diagnose endometrial hyperplasia and invasive endometrial cancer. Histologic evaluation of the endometrium by one of these techniques is mandatory in women with abnormal uterine bleeding who are older than age 35 years, are obese, or have a history of anovulation. The dilatation and curettage has now largely been replaced by the office endometrial biopsy, when technically feasible, as the initial test of choice. Dilatation and curettage, with or without visual inspection of the endometrial cavity (hysteroscopy), is generally reserved for patients who are not able to tolerate an office biopsy or have cervical stenosis. Pelvic ultrasound is the best test for evaluating the endometrial thickness and the uterine contour. A thickened endometrium may suggest endometrial neoplasia but may also be observed with endometrial polyps and tamoxifen therapy in the absence of neoplasia. Despite improvements in the sensitivity of ultrasound, with newer technologies such as Doppler flow and sonohysterography, endometrial tissue is still required to differentiate endometrial neoplasia from benign entities. The Pap smear is not a useful test for evaluating the endometrium; however, the presence of endometrial cells on a Pap smear from a postmenopausal woman requires further evaluation to exclude an endometrial cancer.

Evaluation: Specific

It is important to consider the entire differential diagnosis in every patient with abnormal vaginal bleeding. All women of childbearing age with abnormal bleeding should have a careful history and physical examination, a Pap smear (if one has not been performed in the previous 12 months), and a pregnancy test if clinically appropriate. Thyroid function tests, liver function tests, complete blood count, clotting studies, a Gram stain/wet prep of the vaginal fluid, and endometrial biopsy are performed when indicated by the history and physical examination. Ultrasound using a vaginal probe transducer allows a better assessment of the endometrium and adnexa, particularly in obese women. Endometrial sampling should be performed to evaluate abnormal bleeding in women who are at risk for endometrial polyps, hyperplasia, or carcinoma.

Among women with postmenopausal bleeding, transvaginal ultrasound may be used to evaluate the uterine lining. It has been suggested that an endometrial thickness of less than 5 mm indicates a low probability of endometrial cancer.

In children with vaginal bleeding, if no obvious cause of bleeding is visible externally or in the distal

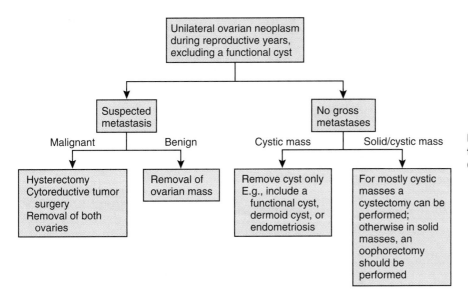

Figure 30-2 ■ Treatment algorithm for ovarian neoplasm during reproductive years.

vagina, an examination under anesthesia with an endoscope may be necessary to completely visualize the vagina and cervix. A pelvic ultrasound may also provide helpful information in this age group.

In the adolescent females, a pregnancy test and coagulation studies should be performed.

Management

In the prepubertal age group, management of bleeding is directed to the specific cause of bleeding. For example, in bleeding due to nonspecific vulvovaginitis, further evaluation of a foreign body is needed. In cases of vulvar dystrophy, a short course of steroid cream may be helpful. Vaginal and ovarian tumors should be managed in consultation with a gynecologic oncologist (Figure 30-2).

In the adolescent group, management of bleeding abnormalities related to thyroid disease, androgen excess, hematologic abnormalities, and pregnancy should be directed to the underlying condition. In cases of mild or moderate anovulatory bleeding, oral contraceptives can be utilized. In cases of severe acute bleeding, management includes stabilization of the patient including correction of any coagulopathy, treatment with intravenous conjugated estrogens in cases of anovulation, and, at times, a dilatation and curettage for immediate control of blood loss.

In women of reproductive and postmenopausal age, bleeding is managed with either progesterone or combined oral contraceptives. The surgical management of abnormal bleeding should be reserved for situations in which medical therapy has been unsuccessful or is contraindicated. Surgical management includes dilatation and curettage or hysterectomy. In cases of cervical, uterine, or vaginal cancer, consulta-

tion should again include the expertise of a gynecologic oncologist.

Pelvic Mass

A pelvic mass may be gynecologic in origin or may arise from other pelvic structures, most commonly the urinary tract or bowel. Gynecologic pelvic masses most frequently arise from the uterus and ovaries (Figure 30-3).

Differential Diagnosis

The differential diagnosis of a pelvic mass found on physical examination or an imaging study is vastly different in a prepubertal child, in an adolescent, during the reproductive years, or during the postmenopausal period.

In premenarchal girls, small pelvic masses are rarely detected, as pelvic examinations are not routinely performed. Large pelvic-abdominal masses commonly present with symptoms such as abdominal enlargement, pain, and the perception of a mass. The differential diagnosis includes gynecologic tumors as well as adrenal masses and Wilms' tumor. Physiologic causes of ovarian enlargement are rare prior to menarche, but anatomic variants such as ectopic pelvic kidney and sacral meningocele occur with some frequency (Table 30-2). All pelvic or abdominal masses in premenarchal patients must be presumed to be neoplastic and usually require prompt surgical exploration after appropriate imaging.

Approximately 60% of ovarian neoplasms in this age group are germ-cell tumors including dysgerminomas, endodermal sinus tumors, embryonal carcinomas, immature teratomas, and choriocarcinomas.

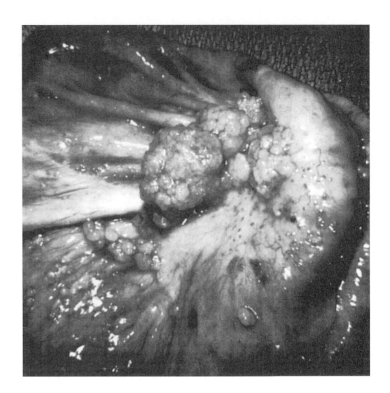

Figure 30-3 ■ Obvious ovarian malignancy. (From Morrow CP, Curtin JP: Synopsis of Gynecologic Oncology, 5th ed. New York: Churchill-Livingstone, 1998, p 230.)

Benign dermoid cysts and the gonadal stromal tumors (granulosa cell tumors, arrhenoblastoma, and thecoma) are the next most common ovarian masses and occur with roughly equal frequency.

Malignant germ-cell tumors may secrete glycoproteins, which may exert hormonal effects. They can also serve as tumor markers. Classically, human chorionic gonadotropin is produced by choriocarcinoma or embryonal carcinoma elements. Cases of precocious puberty have been associated with increased serum levels of human chorionic gonadotropin produced by these neoplasms. Alpha-fetoprotein is secreted by endodermal sinus and embryonal carcinoma elements. The gonadal stromal tumors can also, at times, secrete hormonal substances. The production of estrogens or androgens may result in clinically obvious manifestations in this age group and can be confirmed with serum estradiol or testosterone assays. As many of these germ-cell tumors arise in dysgenetic gonads, karotyping should be obtained. The presence of the Y chromosome can lead to malignant transformation of gonadal tissue.

In the reproductive years, physiologic pelvic masses are common. An early intrauterine pregnancy can enlarge the uterus and soften the lower uterine segment to create the false impression of a mass distinct from the uterus (Hegar sign). Physiologic cystic enlargement of the ovaries is common among ovulatory women. These follicular or corpus luteal cysts are usually unilateral and can grow to 10 to 12 cm in diameter. On occasion, they cause pain secondary to rupture, hemorrhage, or torsion. Because these cysts are much more common than pathologic cysts and usually resolve without intervention, a conservative approach is recommended.

Malignant germ-cell tumors peak in the teenage years and are rare after the age of 30. Gonadal stromal neoplasms are uncommon throughout the reproductive years. Most ovarian neoplasms diagnosed during the reproductive era are benign (80% to 85%). The most common are dermoid cysts and serous and mucinous cystadenomas (see Table 30-2). Ovarian adenocarcinomas account for most of the ovarian malignancies in this age group with a frequency that increases as menopause approaches. They may present at a relatively earlier age among women with hereditary ovarian cancer syndromes.

Ectopic pregnancy may present as an adnexal mass and requires immediate attention. The diagnosis is suggested by the presence of an adnexal mass, the absence of an intrauterine pregnancy on ultrasound examination, and an elevated serum human chorionic gonadotropin level.

The most common pelvic masses that do not originate from the ovary are uterine leiomyomata. These benign, smooth muscle tumors occur in at least 20% of women during their reproductive years. One half of these women have symptoms that are directly related attributable to the leiomyomata. Symptoms include pelvic pain or pressure, urinary frequency, and

Table 30-2 ■ Differential Diagnosis of a Pelvic Mass

Nonpathologic

Full bladder
Stool in the colon
Pelvic kidney
Intrauterine pregnancy
Functional ovarian cyst

Pathologic

Nongynecologic
Diverticulosis-diverticulitis
Appendiceal abscess
Colon cancer

Bladder diverticulum
Bladder cancer
Peritoneal inclusion cysts

Mesenteric cysts

Anterior sacral meningocele

Gynecologic, benign
Salpingo-oophoritis
Tubo-ovarian abscess
Endometriosis
Leiomyomata (uterine/ovarian)
Ectopic pregnancy
Tumorlike conditions of the ovary
    Polycystic ovaries
    Pregnancy luteoma
    Hyperplasia of ovarian stroma and hyperthecosis
    Surface epithelial inclusion cysts
    Paraovarian cysts

Gynecologic, malignant

Ovarian neoplasms including ovarian cancer
Fallopian tube neoplasms

---

excessive vaginal bleeding. Uterine sarcomas are rare and are characterized by rapid growth and bleeding.

With the onset of menopause, the ovaries become progressively smaller over a period of several months. Because physiologic cysts do not develop in these atrophic ovaries, an adnexal mass in a postmenopausal woman is presumed to be neoplastic. The diagnosis of ovarian carcinoma must be excluded. Because ovaries in postmenopausal women become atrophic, any palpable postmenopausal ovary should raise the suspicion of a neoplasm.

Evaluation

Physical examination is the first step in the evaluation of a pelvic mass. Proper preparation of the patient is important. A full urinary bladder or a rectum replete with stool may compromise an examination or masquerade as pathology itself. Other factors that can impede a proper examination include pain, lack of psychological preparation, inadequate relaxation, and obesity. The best clinical evaluation of the adnexa is accomplished with a bimanual abdominal-rectovaginal examination. In prepubertal girls in whom the hymeneal ring is intact, a digital rectal examination may be substituted for a vaginal examination. In the adolescent age group, a history and a physical examination including a sexual history are critical to making the proper diagnosis.

Laboratory tests may include a complete blood count and a pregnancy test. Tumor markers (human chorionic gonadotropin, AFP, and lactate dehydrogenase) should be attained if a germ-cell tumor is suspected. Tumor markers such as CA125 have little utility in a premenopausal woman, as many benign conditions such as uterine leiomyomata, pelvic inflammatory disease, pregnancy, and endometriosis can cause an elevation of the CA125. The most common diagnosis among premenopausal women with an adnexal mass and an elevated CA125 is endometriosis.

Ultrasound continues to be the best imaging test to evaluate a pelvic mass. Solid adnexal masses, bilateral cystic masses, and cysts greater than 10 cm in diameter are presumed to be pelvic neoplasms, and surgery should be performed to establish a diagnosis. Magnetic resonance imaging has been demonstrated to be helpful in evaluating congenital uterine malformations. It should be obtained only selectively. Percutaneous guided aspiration of pelvic cysts should be avoided owing to the risk of dissemination of cancer cells.

In the postmenopausal woman, the pelvic examination, CA125 level, and ultrasound are helpful in discriminating benign from malignant masses (Figure 30-4). Simple ovarian cysts less than 5 cm in diameter associated with normal CA125 levels have a low risk for malignancy and can be followed. Larger masses and complex masses require evaluation. An elevated CA125 in postmenopausal women is highly suggestive of malignancy. On the other hand, a normal CA125 in the presence of a suspicious mass cannot be relied on to exclude malignancy, as it has only modest sensitivity for early-stage ovarian cancer. Ovarian cancer rarely presents with parenchymal liver metastases. If such lesions are present, an alternative primary should be searched for. An ultrasound and CA125 level constitute a sufficient preoperative evaluation in most postmenopausal women with pelvic masses. Computed tomography (CT), magnetic resonance imaging (MRI), cystoscopy, or sigmoidoscopy may be used selectively if the origin of the mass is unclear.

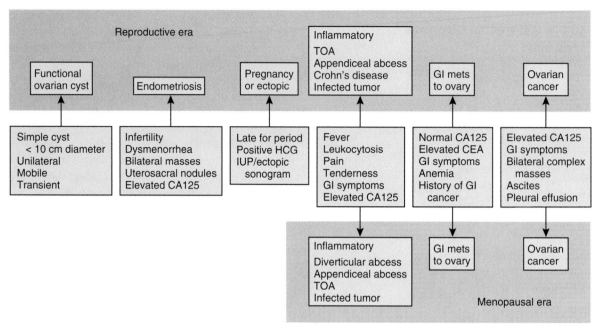

Figure 30-4 ■ Diagnosis of a pelvic mass.

Management

In prepubertal girls, most unilocular cysts are benign and will regress in three to six months, thus requiring only close observation. In adolescent girls, most unilocular cysts can be followed conservatively; however, in cases in which there is uncertainty of diagnosis, issues of future fertility must be recognized, and management may include a unilateral procedure rather than a more radical approach. Thus a unilateral cystic adnexal mass smaller than 8 to 10 cm in an asymptomatic ovulating woman should be followed for four to eight weeks, anticipating spontaneous regression. If the mass has not disappeared at the end of the observation period, surgical intervention is recommended.

In reproductive-age and postmenopausal women, management is based on the likeliness of malignancy. In cases of small (less than 5 cm), unilocular, asymptomatic cysts, one may feel comfortable with close observation as a mode of management. In cases

of obvious malignancy, resection of both ovaries is indicated. In cases of other benign pelvic masses such as uterine leiomyomata, surgical management is reserved for cases in which symptoms such as pain and bleeding are refractory to conservative modalities.

Suggested Reading

Barber HRK, Graber EA: The PMPO (postmenopausal palpable ovary syndrome). Obstet Gynecol 1971;38:921–930.

Claessens AE, Cowell CA: Acute adolescent menorrhagia. Am J Obstet Gynecol 1981;139:277–280.

Norris HJ, Jensen RD: Relative frequency of ovarian neoplasms in children and adolescents. Cancer 1972;30:713–719.

Schutter EM, Kenemans P, Sohn C, et al: Diagnostic value of the pelvic examination, ultrasound, and serum CA125 in postmenopausal women with a pelvic mass: An international multicenter study. Cancer 1994;74:1398–1406.

Van den Bosch T, Vanendael A, Van Schoubroeck D, et al: Combining vaginal ultrasonography and office endometrial sampling in the diagnosis of endometrial disease in postmenopausal women. Obstet Gynecol 1995;85:349–352.

Blood Chemistry Abnormalities

Chapter 31
Hypercalcemia

Stephen Richman

Hypercalcemia occurs in approximately 18 per 100,000 population and is therefore a not infrequent finding when routine blood chemistries are obtained in asymptomatic patients. Although hypercalcemia can occur in cancer as a paraneoplastic syndrome, with or without bone involvement, it rarely occurs in the absence of symptoms from the hypercalcemia itself or from the underlying malignancy. Usually, therefore, the differential diagnosis between a benign or malignant etiology of hypercalcemia can be accomplished on the basis of history, symptoms, clinical findings, and/or the presence of other accompanying blood test abnormalities.

Of the etiologies listed in Table 31-1, primary hyperparathyroidism is the most likely diagnosis in asymptomatic patients, and hypercalcemia of malignancy is the most likely diagnosis in symptomatic patients. In primary hyperparathyroidism, parathormone levels by immunoassay will be elevated, whereas they will be low (or within the normal range) in the hypercalcemia of malignancy. The other diagnoses in Table 31-1 account for fewer than 10% of cases. Although it is an infrequent cause of hypercalcemia, the proclivity for self-medication with herbal remedies and vitamins makes it necessary to question the possibility of known or unrecognized (in complex preparations) vitamin D intake.

Hypercalcemia occurs in 10% of cancers overall, at some time in the course of disease, primarily concentrated at two time points: at initial diagnosis and, more often, in the later, advanced stages of disease. If hypercalcemia of malignancy is part of the initial presentation, it resolves with initial successful therapy and then reappears if and when the tumor recurs. Hypercalcemia occurring as a late manifestation of disseminated cancer that is resistant to therapy can often be controlled by hypocalcemic therapy administered in the context of the overall goals of palliative care and the patient's general status. The three malignancies most frequently associated with hypercalcemia are, in order of decreasing frequency, multiple myeloma, breast cancer, and non-small-cell lung cancer. Hypercalcemia is much less common in other neoplastic diseases. Reflecting the frequency of associated symptomatic disease, malignancy is the most common cause of hypercalcemia in hospitalized patients. Unusually, in breast cancer that is metastatic to bone, the initiation of therapy with tamoxifen, an antiestrogen, can be associated with increased bone pain and hypercalcemia. This tamoxifen flare is caused by a transient stimulus of the breast cancer. The flare starts within several days or two weeks of the institution of therapy and then resolves in most, but not all, patients. This reaction in patients whose acute symptoms subside despite continuation of tamoxifen seems to be predictive of a good ultimate antitumor response. On occasion, until the flare subsides, hypocalcemic therapy may be required.

It is important to recognize that hypercalcemia in cancer patients can develop from nonmalignant causes, especially coincidental primary hyperparathyroidism, and that other problems, such as immobilization, or medications, such as thiazides, can contribute to the hypercalcemia of malignancy.

Table 31-1 ■ Differential Diagnosis of Hypercalcemia

Noncancer Etiology
Primary hyperparathyroidism (parathyroid adenoma)
Excess vitamin D ingestion
Prolonged immobilization
Familial benign hypercalcemia (defective calcium sensor)
Lithium therapy
Sarcoidosis (increased 1,25 dihydroxyvitamin D)
Hyperthyroidism

Cancer-Related Etiology
Multiple myeloma
Metastatic breast cancer (from disease or tamoxifen-induced flare)
Non-small-cell lung cancer (primarily squamous cell carcinoma)
Parathyroid carcinoma
Multiple endocrine neoplasia
Other malignancies

Mechanisms of Hypercalcemia

Calcium homeostasis is maintained by a balance of competing activities, namely, calcium adsorption to and resorption from bone, urinary calcium excretion and reabsorption by the kidney, and calcium absorption and loss from the gastrointestinal (GI) tract. The (1,25) dihydroxylated form of vitamin D enhances calcium absorption from the gastrointestinal tract, fosters conversion of monocytes to osteoclasts, and induces osteoclast differentiation. Parathormone, released by the parathyroid glands, stimulates osteoclast-mediated bone resorption, calcium reabsorption (normally 85% of filtered calcium is reabsorbed) from the renal tubules, and hydroxylation of (25) hydroxylated vitamin D to the (1,25) dihydroxylated form. Parathormone's effects on bone are antagonized by calcitonin. Renal reabsorption of calcium is reduced by sodium in the proximal tubules. In the plasma, the majority of calcium is bound to protein or complexed with ions such as bicarbonate and citrate. Approximately 40% of circulating calcium in the plasma is in the ionized, metabolically active form. The ionized form controls the feedback loop of humoral (parathormone) response to changes in plasma calcium levels.

Plasma Calcium Determinations

Total calcium levels in the plasma normally range from 8.8 to 10.4 mg/dL; more than 50% is bound to protein, principally to albumin. When these proteins are reduced in the circumstances of malnutrition, an uncorrected total calcium level may be misleading.

The following is a simple but useful formula to correct the measured calcium level to reflect the alterations in the level of albumin:

$$\text{Calcium (corrected) mg/dL} = \text{Calcium (measured) mg/dL} - \text{Albumin g/dL} + 4.0$$

Direct measurement of ionized calcium (average value 4.6 to 5.0 mg/dL) is a better means of assessing the functional activity of calcium than is the level of total calcium. In multiple myeloma, for example, the total calcium level may be normal in circumstances where the paraprotein is acting as a calcium-binding protein, reducing the level of ionized calcium available to the tissues. In general, however, in hypercalcemia due to other malignancies ionized calcium determinations are not necessary.

Hypercalcemia of Malignancy

The hypercalcemia of malignancy can develop owing to either local or systemic (humoral) factors. In malignancies that are metastatic to bone, bone resorption occurs, but only a fraction of cases are associated with hypercalcemia. There is thus no direct relationship between the extent of malignant osteolysis and the likelihood of hypercalcemia. Other factors must contribute to the cause of hypercalcemia in this circumstance. In most cases of hypercalcemia of malignancy, the cause is secretion of a humoral factor, called parathormone-related protein (PTHrP), by the neoplastic cells. This protein, although larger than parathormone, exhibits substantial homology to parathormone in the sequence of the first 30 amino acids. Both parathormone and parathormone-related protein bind to the same receptor. The effects of parathormone-related protein therefore mimic those of parathormone.

Local secretion of a variety of biologically active factors by osteolytic metastases to bone also can contribute to hypercalcemia. These factors include cytokines such as the interleukins 1, 6, and 11; tumor necrosis factor; transforming growth factor beta; interferon gamma; and prostaglandins. They also stimulate osteoclast activity.

Production of parathormone-related protein (Table 31-2) is usually the cause of hypercalcemia associated with squamous cell carcinomas of the lung, head, and neck and renal carcinomas. Multiple myeloma is a cancer that causes hypercalcemia due to secretion of local osteolytic factors. Hypercalcemia occurring in breast cancer may be produced by either or both mechanisms.

Rarely, in lymphomas and leukemias, excessive production of 1,25 dihydroxyvitamin D causes hypercalcemia. In contrast, the hypercalcemia often present

Table 31-2 ■ Etiologic Factors in the Hypercalcemia of Malignancy

	Squamous Carcinomas	Breast Carcinoma	Myeloma	Lymphoma
Parathormone-related protein	+	+	−	−*
Local osteolytic factors	−	+	+	−
Increased vitamin D	−	−	−	+

*Increased PTHrP (parathormone-related protein) can occur in HTLV-1 associated lymphomas.

in the adult T-cell leukemia/lymphoma associated with HTLV-1 infection is due to production of parathormone-related protein.

Signs and Symptoms

The signs and symptoms of hypercalcemia of malignancy are nonspecific and can develop acutely, presenting as a medical emergency or as a subacute, symptomatic or chronic, asymptomatic disorder. Demonstrable signs and symptoms depend not only on the level of free ionized calcium in the circulation, but also on the rate of rise in plasma calcium and the patient's medical condition.

Symptoms of hypercalcemia occur singly or variably in combination. These include anorexia, nausea, vomiting, constipation, dehydration, and neurologic symptoms such as weakness, depression, apathy, stupor, or coma. Great care must be given to avoid automatically ascribing these symptoms to the disease itself or side effects of therapy, thereby failing to check a calcium level and missing an opportunity to successfully intervene. For example, in a stuporous patient with cancer, hypercalcemia of malignancy should be part of the differential diagnosis, which includes brain or meningeal metastases, sepsis, hypoglycemia, or central nervous system hemorrhage. As a general rule, hypercalcemia must be considered whenever a patient who has an active malignancy experiences unexplained deterioration in mobility, activity, appetite, affect, or mentation. This is essential because hypercalcemia of malignancy so often occurs in patients with an advanced malignancy, when calcium determinations may not be regularly obtained.

Hypercalcemia causes renal tubular damage resulting in impairment of renal concentrating ability and natriuresis leading to polyuria, dehydration, and rising blood urea nitrogen and creatinine levels. These renal events and consequent dehydration further elevate the calcium level. Electrocardiograms may reveal a shortened Q-T interval as another manifestation of hypercalcemia, and the patient may develop cardiac arrhythmias.

Laboratory evaluation includes calcium, phosphorous, electrolytes, magnesium, blood urea nitrogen, creatinine, and, of course, albumin levels. If the patient is newly diagnosed with cancer, then initial staging evaluation may be required. If the patient carries a previous diagnosis of cancer, then the advent of hypercalcemia may signal disease relapse/progression, requiring documentation of disease status.

Therapy

Since hypercalcemia of malignancy, by definition, is due to tumor, treatment should ideally proceed on two fronts. If feasible, therapy to reduce the tumor burden should be initiated as soon as possible. Unfortunately, in many patients, hypercalcemia of malignancy occurs or recurs after many antitumor treatment options have been exhausted, and treatment must be directed solely at the hypercalcemia itself.

1. Fluid volume expansion with saline is the first step in treatment. This restores blood volume, increases the glomerular filtration rate, and induces a natriuresis and simultaneous calciuresis. A high flow rate of intravenous fluid volume replacement with saline is employed (Table 31-3), and the patient's cardiovascular reserve needs to be considered. This hydration-natriuresis process plays an important role in facilitating additional therapy but should not be used as the sole treatment. Used alone, it repletes the contracted extracellular volume, improves renal function, and enhances calciuresis, but its calcium-lowering effects are modest. Moreover, it does not deal with the issue of increased calcium mobilization. Therefore specific pharmacologic measures should be undertaken soon after diagnosis. Loop diuretics, such as furosemide, which were previously advocated to promote calciuresis during hydration, are best employed only as needed to prevent volume overload in patients receiving large volumes of fluids intravenously.

2. Bisphosphonate (analogues of pyrophosphate) therapy is the most frequently used specific anti-

Table 31-3 ■ Summary of Treatment for Hypercalcemia of Malignancy

Agent	Dose	Comment
Saline	250–500 mL/h IV	First maneuver to correct dehydration and correct/maintain renal function
Loop diuretics	40–80 mg IV (furosemide)	As needed to maintain fluid balance
Bisphosphonates	60–90 mg IV (pamidronate) 4–8 mg IV (zoledronic acid)	Cornerstone of current therapy
Calcitonin	2–8 IU/kg/q6-12 hr SQ or IM	Emergency therapy
Corticosteroids	40–100 mg/day (prednisone)	Only in corticosteroid-sensitive tumors
Plicamycin	25 µg/kg IV (restrict total dose to 1 mg)	Backup therapy

hypercalcemic agent. Approximately half of an administered dose is excreted by the kidneys, and the other half is adsorbed to bone. In bone, bisphosphonates interfere with osteoclast activity. Until recently, of a number of bisphosphonates, pamidronate in doses of 60 mg or 90 mg intravenously over 2 to 4 hours was the treatment of choice. Side effects consist of fever, which may be significant, and malaise. Decrease in calcium levels occurs in 24 to 48 hours, and normalization requires four days or more. Another bisphosphonate, zoledronic acid, was recently shown to be more effective than pamidronate in a randomized clinical trial. Response rates (88%), time to normalization of calcium levels, and duration of response (30 to 40 days) were significantly better after zoledronic acid, with a similar profile of side effects. Ease of administration (zoledronic acid in a 4-mg or 8-mg dose can be given via 5-minute infusion) is also a substantial advantage over the lengthy time required to administer pamidronate.

In the presence of bone metastases, especially in breast cancer and multiple myeloma, continued administration of bisphosphonate therapy can reduce the risk of bony events, such as pathologic fractures, vertebral body collapse, and pain, that come from continued resorption of bone. However, continuing therapy has not been shown to improve overall survival or increase objective evidence of bone response. Suggestions that bisphosphonates have some antitumor effects and can retard the development of bone metastases have not yet been confirmed.

3. Calcitonin reduces calcium levels by inhibiting bone resorption and increasing renal excretion. It is not useful for chronic therapy because resistance develops to repeated doses, but it is the most rapidly acting of the hypocalcemic agents (onset of effect in 2 to 4 hours) and is the initial agent of choice in patients with severe hypercalcemia. The duration of effect is brief, and it is ineffective in

the hypercalcemia of malignancy when administered by nasal insufflation. It can be given subcutaneously but acts more quickly if given intramuscularly, provided that the patient's platelet count is not low and the patient's coagulation status is otherwise not compromised.

4. Corticosteroids decrease osteoclast-mediated bone resorption and gastrointestinal tract calcium absorption. Against the hypercalcemia of malignancy, corticosteroids are most useful in those cancers in which they can induce an antitumor response, such as in the hematologic malignancies and, in some cases, breast cancer. It is not useful for other cancers associated with hypercalcemia.

5. Plicamycin (formerly called mithramycin) was developed as an antitumor antibiotic, but it was abandoned because of excessive toxicity, principally to platelets and the kidneys. The recommended dose of 25 µg/kg can result in toxicity. If the dose is held to a total of 1 mg, toxicity is rarely seen, even if the drug is administered two to three times weekly to control hypercalcemia. It is generally reserved for use in patients when bisphosphonate therapy has failed.

Gallium nitrate, an agent that was originally developed for its antitumor properties, was discovered to have calcium-lowering effects. Although approved for use as an antihypercalcemic agent, it was recently withdrawn from the market. Oral phosphorous administration lowers calcium levels but causes diarrhea and nausea, metastatic calcification, and renal insufficiency. Its toxicity generally precludes its role in therapy.

Suggested Reading

Burtis WJ, Brady TG, Orloff JJ, et al: Immunochemical characterization of circulating parathyroid hormone-related protein in patients with humoral hypercalcemia of cancer. N Engl J Med 1990;322:1106–1112.

Coleman RE: Metastatic bone disease: Clinical features, pathophysiology and treatment strategies. Cancer Treat Rev 2001;27:165–176.

Kim SJ, Shiba E, Maeda I, et al: Screening for primary hyperparathyroidism (PHPT) in clinic patients: Differential diagnosis between PHPT and malignancy-associated hypercalcemia by routine blood tests. Clin Chem Acta 2001;305:35–40.

Major P, Lortholary A, Hon J, et al: Zoledronic acid is superior to pamidronate in the treatment of hypercalcemia of malignancy: A pooled analysis of two randomized, controlled trials. J Clin Oncol 2001;19:558–567.

Martin TJ, Moseley JM: Mechanisms in the skeletal complications of breast cancer (Review). Endocrine-Related Cancer 2000;7:271–284.

Marx SJ: Hyperparathyroid and hypoparathyroid disorders. N Engl J Med 2000;343:1863–1875.

Niesvizsky R, Warrell RP Jr: Pathophysiology and management of bone disease in multiple myeloma. Cancer Invest 1997;15:85–90.

Oyajobi BO, Anderson DM, Traianedes K, et al: Therapeutic efficacy of a soluble receptor activator of nuclear factor kappaB-IgG Fc fusion protein in suppressing bone resorption and hypercalcemia in a model of humoral hypercalcemia of malignancy. Cancer Res 2001;61:2572–2578.

Pecherstorfer M, Schilling T, Blind E, et al: Parathyroid hormone-related protein and life expectancy in hypercalcemic cancer patients. J Clin Endocrinol Metab 1994;78:1268–1270.

Potts JT Jr: Hyperparathyroidism and other hypercalcemic disorders (Review). Adv Intern Med 1996;41:165–212.

Syed MA, Horwitz MJ, Tedesco MB, et al: Parathyroid hormone-related protein-(1—36) stimulates renal tubular calcium reabsorption in normal human volunteers: Implications for the pathogenesis of humoral hypercalcemia of malignancy. J Clin Endocrinol Metab 2001;86:1525–1531.

Theriault RL, Hortobagyi GN: The evolving role of bisphosphonates (Review). Semin Oncol 2001;28:284–290.

Chapter 32
Elevated Bilirubin

Peter A. Cassileth

Introduction

Approximately 85% of bilirubin production is derived from the breakdown of old red blood cells. The balance comes from the normally small fraction of ineffective erythropoiesis in the marrow and from the metabolism of heme-containing proteins such as the hepatic cytochromes, muscle myoglobin, and enzymes such as catalase. Since red blood cells normally have a life span of 120 days, somewhat less than 1% of the red blood cell mass is removed daily and replaced by newly formed cells. As red blood cells are removed from the circulation, hemoglobin is released and in turn degraded into heme and globin moieties. The globin undergoes protein catabolism, and the heme component is oxidized to biliverdin and then reduced to bilirubin. Bilirubin circulates in the blood in an unconjugated form at a concentration of 0.8 to 1.2 mg/dL. It is a polar, water-insoluble compound that circulates firmly bound to albumin as a transport protein. Measurement of this form of bilirubin by a colorimetric method requires the addition of another solute to accelerate the reaction. Since the determination requires an extra procedural step, the reaction is called an "indirect" one, and the bilirubin so quantified is called indirect bilirubin. The terms *unconjugated bilirubin* and *indirect bilirubin* identify the same substance. Liver cells extract bilirubin from its albumin binding. Once in the cell, bilirubin is conjugated in a series of steps to a monoglucuronide and diglucuronide catalyzed by glucuronyl transferase, which transfers glucuronides from uridine diphosphoglucuronic acid (UDPG). Conjugated bilirubin is water soluble and measurable "directly" by the colorimetric method. Direct bilirubin is transported across the cell membrane into the biliary radicals, passing through the biliary ducts into the duodenum, where it colors the stool. The small amount of direct reacting bilirubin in the serum of normal individuals reported by the chemistry laboratory overstates its actual amount. Essentially, all bilirubin in the serum is indirect in normal patients, and direct bilirubin appears in the blood in significant amounts only when there is obstruction of bile flow or hepatic cell damage. Because of its albumin binding, indirect bilirubin is not filtered through the kidney, and therefore bilirubin is not in the urine in normal patients or even those with substantial elevations of serum levels. In contrast, direct reacting bilirubin usually only loosely binds to albumin. Direct bilirubin easily dissociates from albumin and is cleared (filtered at the glomerulus and incompletely reabsorbed at the renal tubules) into the urine, where it is detectable as bilirubinuria on dipstick testing. Its presence in the urine is a useful clue to the presence of an elevated serum direct bilirubin.

Elevation of the serum bilirubin can occur either because of excess production of bilirubin or because of abnormalities in its clearance by means of hepatic uptake and transport through the biliary ducts to the small intestine. Defects in bilirubin processing can be analyzed in part on the basis of the accumulation and relative proportions of direct and indirect bilirubin that accumulate in the blood. If more than half of the total bilirubin is in the direct fraction, then for the purposes of differential diagnosis, the jaundice is due to conjugated bilirubin. In contrast, in hemolytic states, indirect bilirubin rises predominantly. An outline of the causes of hyperbilirubinemia appears in Figure 32-1.

The yellowing of the tissues that occurs due to bile pigment accumulation is difficult to detect until total bilirubin levels reach 2 to 2.5 mg/dL. Jaundice is most readily detectable by examination of the sclera, where elastin is present and is highly bilirubin-avid. The liver has an enormous reserve capacity to handle a bilirubin load. For example, tying off one of the two main hepatic ducts does not increase the serum bilirubin. It is estimated that a loss of more than 75% of hepatocytes is necessary before the bilirubin rises. Jaundice is rare even with extensive metastases (unless there is biliary obstruction) because usually an adequate

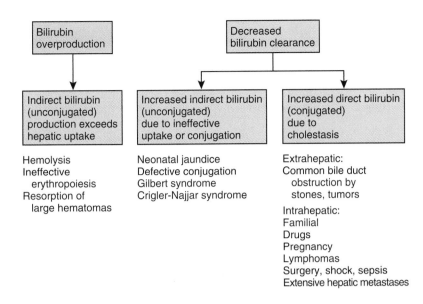

Figure 32-1 ■ Causes of hyperbilirubinemia.

Note: Hepatocellular diseases, such as hepatitis, cirrhosis, veno-occlusive disease, and graft-versus-host disease raise both direct and indirect serum bilirubin levels in varying proportions.

DIAGNOSIS

Protracted Hyperbilirubinemia

Prolonged obstructive jaundice causes the development of a nonenzymatic covalent bond between direct (conjugated) bilirubin and albumin. When the obstruction is relieved, an elevated direct bilirubin can persist for weeks, long after other liver function tests become normal. This bilirubin is only slowly cleared as the albumin itself is metabolized, with a $T_{1/2}$ of 15 days.

---

number of functional hepatocytes persist to metabolize the bilirubin load. Yet less overt but diffuse obstruction of the biliary radicals by a variety of infiltrative processes can cause jaundice.

Increased Indirect Bilirubin

Hemolysis

Both intravascular and intravascular hemolysis lead to increased production of bilirubin from the accelerated destruction of red blood cells. In severe chronic hemolytic anemias, such as sickle-cell anemia or warm antibody autoimmune hemolytic anemia, bone marrow red blood cell production, even under intense stimulus by erythropoietin, can achieve a maximum rate of approximately 7 to 8 times normal. At this turnover rate, the increased bilirubin production raises

serum levels relatively modestly because of the reserve capacity of liver clearance mechanisms. The maximum indirect bilirubin level in this circumstance does not exceed 4 to 5 mg/dL. Higher levels than these suggest the presence of concomitant liver disease. Indeed, in less severe hemolytic anemias, such as hereditary spherocytosis or cold agglutinin hemolytic anemia, the bilirubin will be within the normal range in half of the affected patients. A small rise in direct bilirubin can accompany the increase in indirect bilirubin because of increased efflux back into plasma of bilirubin after conjugation in the liver. During hemolysis, other blood chemistry abnormalities result from the release of transaminases and lactic dehydrogenase from the red blood cells. Because the alkaline phosphatase (not a red blood cell component) does not increase, it helps to clarify that liver disease is not the cause of the elevated serum enzymes. Other diagnostic abnormalities in hemolytic anemia are discussed in Chapter 55.

Ineffective Erythropoiesis

Ineffective erythopoiesis refers to premature red blood cell death in the bone marrow before their release into the circulation. In conditions such as myelodysplasia or megaloblastic anemias, the indirect bilirubin can rise owing to increased ineffective erythropoiesis and/or an associated slightly shortened red blood cell survival. Indirect bilirubin levels increase only slightly, staying within the normal range in more than half of the patients. In myelodysplasia, however, the lactic dehydrogenase (LDH) levels rise only slightly in a small percentage of patients owing to release of the lactic dehydrogenase from red blood cells, whereas in megaloblastic anemias, the lactic dehydrogenase is markedly elevated (many times normal) owing in part to its release from white blood cell precursors (ineffective leukopoiesis).

Neonatal Jaundice

The capacity for hepatic uptake and glucuronidation of bilirubin is impaired in early neonatal life compared to that of an adult. Physiologic jaundice thus commonly occurs in the first days of life. It usually spontaneously declines by the end of the first week and returns to normal levels by the end of the second week. Its frequency and severity are inversely related to the maturity of the neonate. The increase in indirect bilirubin results from a shortened red blood cell survival of the fetal red blood cells, insufficient activity of the urinary uridine diphosphoglucuronic acid glucuronyl transferase enzyme necessary for glucuronidation, and some reabsorption of bilirubin from the intestinal tract. The average elevation is approximately 5 to 6 mg/dL, although the bilirubin level occasionally rises to 10 to 15 mg/dL. Ordinarily, there are no adverse effects, and kernicterus, brain damage from diffusion of indirect bilirubin into the central nervous system, does not occur. Phototherapy (exposure to ultraviolet light) in these children is rarely needed. Phototherapy lowers bilirubin levels by creating water-soluble isomers that can be excreted without glucuronidation.

Defective Glucuronide Conjugation

Three congenital disorders caused by deficient activity of uridine diphosphoglucuronic acid glucuronyl transferase lead to chronically elevated indirect bilirubin levels. These are, in order of increasing severity of the defect, Gilbert syndrome and Crigler-Najjar syndrome, types II and I. Gilbert syndrome is probably inherited as an autosomal dominant gene, whereas the Crigler-Najjar syndromes appear to be autosomal recessive. Crigler-Najjar syndrome type I is fortunately a very rare disorder. It is associated with sustained high levels (greater than 20 mg/dL) of indirect bilirubin (and total inability to conjugate bilirubin to the direct form) that resist various modes of therapy. There is a high frequency of severe brain damage from kernicterus and early mortality. Although superficially similar, Crigler-Najjar syndrome type II retains partial ability to conjugate bilirubin and readily corrects the elevated bilirubin after the administration of phenobarbital or other drugs that induce uridine diphosphoglucuronic acid glucuronyl transferase activity. Type II carries a

---

DIAGNOSIS

Low-Grade Hyperbilirubinemia

The most common causes of an elevated indirect bilirubin in adults are Gilbert syndrome and hemolysis.

---

risk of kernicterus in the newborn period, but thereafter, apart from jaundice, health is normal.

Gilbert syndrome is the most common and mildest of these three syndromes. Its frequency in the population is variously estimated at 3% to 10%. A male preponderance is observed even though this is not a sex-linked trait. This has been attributed to the lower level of bilirubin production in women, whose red blood cell mass is smaller than men's. The increased indirect bilirubin is usually less than 3 mg/dL, but its level can rise under the stimulus of stress, fever, fasting, exertion, surgery, alcohol intake, or infection. This is an entirely benign condition. It is nevertheless an important one because it is so frequently detected on blood chemistry screening studies and may be inadvertently attributed to disease. It is easily recognized by the isolated increase of indirect bilirubin in liver function tests and the absence of findings of hemolysis such as anemia, increased lactic dehydrogenase, or reticulocytosis.

Increased Direct Dilirubin

Biliary Tract Obstruction

Biliary obstruction causes predominantly the elevation of serum direct (conjugated) bilirubin with some secondary increase in indirect bilirubin. Depending on the degree and duration of the obstruction, secondary damage to hepatocytes may cause an increase in serum transaminases and elevate the lactic dehydrogenase. The elevation of direct bilirubin in the circulation is virtually always accompanied by a substantial increase in the serum alkaline phosphatase. This is not due only to increased transfer of alkaline phophatase from the liver; rather, it is due to the fact that cholestasis triggers a markedly increased rate of hepatic synthesis of alkaline phosphatase. No single blood test or pattern of abnormal blood chemistries allows one to distinguish between intrahepatic and extrahepatic sites of obstruction to biliary flow.

Extrahepatic Cholestasis

Extrahepatic obstruction is due to blockage of the common bile duct by gallstones, cholangiocarcinomas (arising from the duct itself), carcinoma of the head of the pancreas (ampullary or periampullary cancer), strictures (postoperative scarring), or external compression of the common duct by tumor masses caused by or secondary to metastases to periportal lymph nodes. Computed tomography (CT) scan of the abdomen and/or ultrasound readily reveals dilated bile ducts and helps to define the potential cause. The elevation of bilirubin in total obstruction reaches a maximum of approximately 35 mg/dL because renal excretion of direct bilirubin modulates the final achievable level.

Intrahepatic Cholestasis

When obstruction and dilatation of the biliary tree are not the cause of an elevated direct bilirubin, then causes of intrahepatic cholestasis need to be considered. As is noted in Figure 32-1, the third trimester of pregnancy can be associated with cholestasis, and at times Hodgkin's and non-Hodgkin's lymphomas can induce intrahepatic cholestasis as a paraneoplastic finding without direct or substantial involvement of the liver. In contrast, carcinomas must diffusely and extensively involve the liver before jaundice results. Dubin-Johnson syndrome and Rotor's syndrome are congenital disorders; the former exhibits impaired excretion of conjugated bilirubin and a darkly stained liver, and the latter shows impaired hepatic storage of conjugated bilirubin and no liver pigmentation. Both are benign diseases.

After extensive surgery and substantial blood replacement, intrahepatic cholestasis may develop and persist for more than one week. The cause is unknown, but it probably requires hypotensive shock for its genesis, since similar events occur occasionally after sepsis and/or shock without surgery.

The most common cause of intrahepatic cholestasis is drug administration, notably tricyclic antidepressants, testosterone or anabolic steroids, general anesthetics, oral contraceptives, and various antibiotics and chemotherapy agents.

Suggested Reading

Deiss A: Destruction of erythrocytes: In Lee GR, Foerster J, Lukens J, Paraskevas F, Greer JP, and Rodgers GM (eds): Wintrobe's Clinical Hematology, Baltimore: Williams & Wilkins, 1999, pp 280–299.

Isselbacher KJ: Bilirubin metabolism and hyperbilirubinemia. In Fauci AS, Braunwald E, Isselbacher KJ, Wilson J, Martin JB, Kasper DL, Hauser SL, Longo DL (eds): Harrison's Principles of Internal Medicine, New York: McGraw-Hill, 1998, pp 1672–1677.

Kaplan LM, Isselbacher KJ: Jaundice. In Fauci AS, Braunwald E, Isselbacher KJ, Wilson J, Martin JB, Kasper DL, Hauser SL, Longo DL (eds): Harrison's Principles of Internal Medicine, New York: McGraw-Hill, 1998, pp 249–254.

Sassa S, Kappas A: Disorders of heme production and catabolism: In Handin RI, Lux SE, Stossel TP (eds): Blood: Principles and Practice of Hematology, Philadelphia: JP Lippincott, 1995, pp 1496–1523.

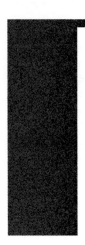

Chapter 33
Immunoglobulin Abnormalities

Philip R. Greipp

During an annual clinical evaluation in an asymptomatic individual, the finding of an elevated sedimentation rate or of an increased or decreased total globulin level on the report of blood chemistries can lead to further evaluation for an immunoglobulin abnormality. Immunoglobulin abnormalities, or gammopathies, are also commonly detected when a serum protein electrophoresis or test for quantitative immunoglobulins is ordered during the evaluation for a medical problem. Any increase or decrease in immunoglobulin levels necessitates a consideration of the underlying diagnosis.

Immunoglobulins are antibodies of several different classes, namely, IgG, IgA, IgM, IgD, and IgE. Each antibody is composed of four amino acid chains: two identical heavy chains and two identical light chains. The heavy chains and the light chains have constant and variable regions. The variable regions are part of the immunoglobulin's Fab fraction and account for that antibody's antigenic specificity. The constant regions of the heavy chains (called γ, α, μ, δ, and ε) constitute the Fc fraction of the immunoglobulin molecule. These constant regions establish the specific class of the antibody molecule. The light chains are only of two types, κ or λ, for all classes of immunoglobulins. The IgG fraction represents 75% of the total of immunoglobulins, and IgA represents 20%. The kappa:lambda light chain ratio is normally approximately 2:1.

Antibody output is increased in response to antigenic inflammatory or infectious antigenic stimuli or as a result of autonomous proliferation of the cells that produce antibodies. In the normal sequence of events, antigenic stimuli result in a lymphoproliferative response with production of IgM and IgD antibodies. With the passage of time, 2 to 3 weeks, populations of plasma cells are derived from these cells and durably secrete IgG, IgA, and IgE. This explains why the presence of IgM antibodies to an infectious organism identifies that the infection is recent rather than old. IgD and IgE exist in such minute concentrations that special studies are required to determine their level. Table 33-1 displays the normal adult ranges of immunoglobulin concentration in the serum.

A serum protein electrophoresis provides preliminary evaluation of immunoglobulin abnormalities. This test is performed on an agarose gel or cellulose acetate backing. Serum proteins migrate at different rates in the electrical field, and the proteins appear as bands when they are suitably stained. A densitometer reading of a cellulose acetate strip provides a graphic display, such as that shown for a normal individual in Figure 33-1A. If immunoglobulins are increased, one must first determine whether the increase is polyclonal, arising from multiple clones or monoclonal, arising from a single clone of plasma cells. In a polyclonal gammopathy caused by an infectious or inflammatory condition, the gamma globulin fraction is diffusely increased, resulting in a broad band in the gamma globulin fraction. If the increase

DIAGNOSIS

Initial Considerations in the Evaluation of an Immunoglobulin Abnormality

If hypogammaglobulinemia is present, is it hereditary or acquired? If hypergammaglobulinemia is present,

Is it polyclonal? If so:
Is there an underlying infectious, inflammatory, or neoplastic disorder?
Is it monoclonal? If so:
What is the concentration of the monoclonal protein?
Is there evidence to suggest multiple myeloma, solitary plasmacytoma, Waldenström's macroglobulinemia, amyloidosis, or another plasma cell disorder?

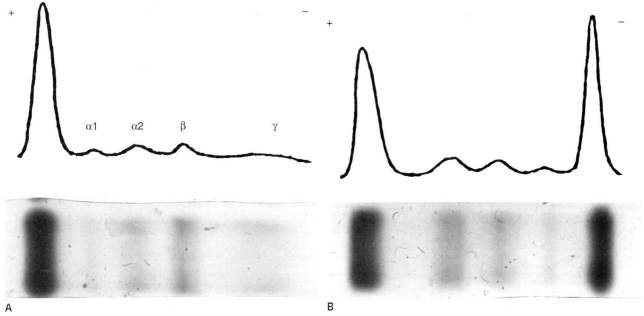

Figure 33-1 ▪ Zone electrophoresis on cellulose acetate with densitometric scans. *A,* Normal human serum. The large left peak is serum albumin. Most of the alpha-1 protein fraction consists of alpha-1 antitrypsin, whereas haptoglobin makes up most of the alpha-2 fraction. Immunoglobulins are largely contained in the gamma globulin fraction but extend into the range of beta globulins. *B,* Serum with a large monoclonal spike in the mid gamma globulin fraction. Note that the background of normal polyclonal gamma globulin on either side of the spike is markedly reduced in comparison with Figure 33-1A. (From Leddy JP: Electrophoretic and immunochemical analysis of human immunoglobins. In Hoffman R, Benz EJ Jr, Shattil SJ, Furie B, Cohen HJ, Silberstein LE, McGlave P [eds]: Hematology: Basic Principles and Practice, 3rd ed. New York: Churchill Livingstone, 2000, p 2505.)

is monoclonal, the increased antibody is all of one type, resulting in a narrow heightened band on electrophoresis as shown in Figure 33-1B, the so-called M-protein, protein spike, or paraprotein. The finding of a monoclonal gammopathy raises the question of a lymphoid or plasma cell malignancy.

Differential Diagnosis

Immunoglobulin disorders can be considered in three categories: polyclonal gammopathy, hypogammaglobulinemia, and monoclonal gammopathy. By working within this framework (see Table 33-1), the cause of each patient's immunoglobulin abnormality can be diagnosed.

Polyclonal Gammopathy

Polyclonal gammopathy is a heterogeneous increase in globulins. By definition, it represents an increased output of gamma globulins by nonneoplastic plasma cells. A polyclonal increase in immunoglobulins may be due to an increase in any one class or several classes of immunoglobulins, such as IgG, IgA, or IgM. Several tests, such as a serum protein electrophoresis and determination of quantitative immunoglobulin levels, can confirm that the increase in gamma globulins is polyclonal rather than monoclonal. In polyclonal gammopathy, one observes not only the typical broad-based increase in the gamma region of the electrophoretic tracing, but also an increase in immunoglobulins with no evidence to suggest a monoclonal gammopathy on immunofixation. At times, a

Table 33-1 ▪ Normal Range of Immunoglobulin Concentrations in Adults

IgG	IgA	IgM
560–1,800 mg/dL	85–380 mg/dL	45–250 mg/dL

monoclonal gammopathy may be found in association with a background polyclonal increase in gamma globulin. Quantitation of the increase in immunoglobulins might not suffice to rule out a monoclonal protein, which requires a study of the plasma proteins by immunofixation.

Uncovering the cause of a polyclonal gammopathy is not usually difficult. One of the causes listed in Table 33-2 should be readily identifiable from the history, physical examination, blood counts, and

Table 33-2 ■ Differential Diagnosis of Immunoglobulin Abnormalities

Polyclonal Gammopathy
Chronic or acute infections, including AIDS
Inflammatory diseases
  Collagen vascular disease, such as systemic lupus
    erythematosus
  Rheumatoid arthritis
  Temporal arteritis (polymyalgia rheumatica)
Liver disease
  Acute and chronic hepatitis
  Cirrhosis
Sarcoidosis
Cancer
  Metastatic cancer
  Renal cell carcinoma
  Hodgkin's disease

Hypogammaglobulinemia
Congenital disorders in childhood, such as Bruton's X-linked
  form
Acquired common variable immunodeficiency in adults
Cancer
  Multiple myeloma
  Non-Hodgkin's lymphoma
  Hodgkin's disease
  Chronic lymphocytic leukemia
  Thymoma
Amyloidosis

Monoclonal Gammopathy
Monoclonal gammopathy of undetermined significance
  IgG or IgA monoclonal immunoglobulins
  Monoclonal IgM (macroglobulin) immunoglobulin
Asymptomatic (smoldering) multiple myeloma
Multiple myeloma
  POEMS syndrome (peripheral neuropathy, osteosclerosis,
    endocrinopathy, monoclonal M-protein, sclerodactyly)
Solitary plasmacytoma
Amyloidosis, light chain type
Monoclonal macroglobulin (IgM) increase
  Waldenström's macroglobulinemia
  Non-Hodgkin's lymphoma
  Chronic lymphocytic leukemia

routine blood chemistries. In patients who are asymptomatic or who have minimal and/or nonspecific symptoms, the presence of polyclonal gammopathy can lead to the diagnosis of a previously unsuspected illness. For example, polyclonal gammopathy and anemia with shoulder girdle stiffness can be salient features leading to a diagnosis of polymyalgia rheumatica (temporal arteritis). But elderly patients with polymyalgia may be asymptomatic. The presence of a mild anemia and polyclonal gammopathy (reflected in a markedly elevated red blood cell sedimentation rate of more than 100 mm/hour) may be the only clues that trigger the temporal artery biopsy necessary to make the diagnosis. Similarly, liver disease can be occult, with minimal or no abnormalities in liver enzymes, bilirubin, or serum albumin. Imaging of the liver by computed tomography (CT) scan and ultrasound may show enlargement and the echogenic heterogeneity characteristic of chronic liver disease. In a patient with polyclonal gammopathy, the presence of lymphadenopathy and/or splenomegaly on physical examination or on computed tomography scan can suggest a diagnosis of lymphoma or sarcoid. Castleman's syndrome is one lymphoproliferative disorder in which a monoclonal gammopathy is often found superimposed on a polyclonal gammopathy. The T-cell lymphoma, formerly called angioimmunoblastic lymphadenopathy with dysproteinemia (AILD), often shows a small monoclonal protein in the setting of a polyclonal gammopathy as well.

Hypogammaglobulinemia

Recurrent pyogenic infections, such as pneumonia, otitis, and sinusitis, due to encapsulated bacteria such as pneumococcus, streptococcus, staphylococcus, or *Haemophilus influenzae* are a common presentation of patients with hypogammaglobulinemia. In infancy and childhood, this history suggests a congenital, X-linked recessive form of hypogammaglobulinemia, called Bruton's. In adolescents or young adults, this presentation, associated with low levels of IgG, IgA, and IgM, suggests an acquired hypogammaglobulinemia, called common variable immunodeficiency. This is the most common cause of hypogammaglobulinemia. Treatment consists of intravenous immunoglobulin replacement therapy and appropriate antibiotics. The family history may disclose that other members of the family have immunologic disorders such as autoimmune disease and lymphoma.

In common variable immunodeficiency, the spleen is enlarged in one third of patients. The benign lymphoid proliferation in the spleen probably represents a response to the repeated infections these patients experience. The risk of developing a lymphoma is markedly increased. The splenic hyperplasia and the hypogammaglobulinemia may be markers that the patient has an underlying immunologic dyscrasia that predisposes to lymphoma, as is true in the immunodeficient patient with AIDS. Similarly, thymoma is often associated not only with hypogammaglobulinemia, but also with a variety of autoimmune diseases, including myasthenia gravis, warm antibody hemolytic anemia, and pure red cell aplasia.

Studies of a patient's immunoglobulins are usually directed at determining whether a monoclonal gammopathy is present. The level of normal immunoglobulins is frequently reduced in the presence of a monoclonal gammopathy. The reduced immunoglobulins are another risk factor for infection in these patients. It is well to bear in mind, however, that hypogammaglobulinemia may be the only detectable immunoglobulin abnormality in disorders that are commonly associated with a monoclonal gammopathy, such as multiple myeloma, non-Hodgkin's lymphoma, Hodgkin's disease, chronic lymphocytic leukemia, amyloidosis, and other gammopathy-related diseases. One would especially want to exclude the diagnosis of multiple myeloma as a cause of hypogammaglobulinemia in elderly patients by obtaining a serum protein electrophoresis and immunofixation. Urinary protein electrophoresis and immunofixation may also be useful in this circumstance to detect monoclonal light chain protein. Patients with light chain myeloma (producing only the light chain moiety of the immunoglobulin molecule) commonly present with hypogammaglobulinemia without evidence of a serum monoclonal protein because the kidneys readily excrete the light chain.

Monoclonal Gammopathy

Monoclonal Gammopathy of Undetermined Significance

Most patients with a monoclonal gammopathy do not have multiple myeloma. They have a benign neoplastic proliferation of plasma cells; the plasma cells, by definition, comprise less than 10% of the marrow cellularity. The increased plasma cells in the bone marrow are scattered throughout, rather than appearing in focal collections or clusters. Monoclonal gammopathy of undetermined significance (MGUS) can be found on serum protein electrophoresis in 2% of the population who are more than 50 years old and 3% to 5% of the population who are more than age 60 years and are otherwise healthy. Progression is nonexistent or very slow, analogous to what occurs in a benign colonic polyp.

DIAGNOSIS

Studies in the Evaluation of a Monoclonal Gammopathy*

Hemoglobin, hematocrit, white blood cell count, platelet count
Serum calcium and creatinine
Lactic acid dehydrogenase (LDH)
Liver function tests (alkaline phosphatase is usually low in multiple myeloma)
Urinalysis
Serum and urinary protein electrophoresis and immunofixation
Quantitative immunoglobulins
Metastatic bone survey
Bone marrow aspiration/biopsy
Magnetic resonance imaging or computerized tomographic scanning of the lumbar spine or suspected areas of involvement

* The extent of studies actually obtained depends on the level of suspicion for a given cause, as outlined in the text.

Given the frequency of monoclonal gammopathy of undetermined significance in healthy individuals, the chance occurrence of osteoporosis and a monoclonal gammopathy in the elderly population is not infrequent. Careful evaluation is required to avoid the erroneous diagnosis of multiple myeloma in such patients. At the same time, a patient with monoclonal gammopathy of undetermined significance needs close monitoring to be sure that the level of monoclonal protein is not increasing over time. Similarly, a patient with metastatic cancer and lytic bone lesions may have an incidental monoclonal gammopathy. In this case, a bone marrow aspiration/biopsy is necessary to clarify the diagnosis.

The monoclonal protein, also called the M-protein or paraprotein, in monoclonal gammopathy of undetermined significance is most commonly of the IgG immunoglobulin subtype and less often of the IgA type. In patients with monoclonal gammopathy of undetermined significance, the level of the monoclonal protein is less than 3 g/dL in the case of IgG and less than 2 g/dL in the case of IgA. Since the process is benign, these individuals do not suffer end organ damage such as anemia, renal failure, hypercalcemia, bone lesions, or extramedullary growth in tissues. Practically speaking, a patient with an IgG M-protein that is less than 3 g/dL (or an IgA M-protein less than 2 g/dL) who has normal hemoglobin, calcium, and creatinine can be diagnosed with reasonable certainty as having monoclonal gammopathy of undetermined significance. Generally, one does not have to obtain bone X-rays or a bone marrow examination unless the IgG or IgA M-protein is at a higher level or there are symptoms such as bone pain. At the same time, one needs to be aware that the diagnosis of monoclonal gammopathy of undetermined significance implies that the outcome is uncertain. The need for long-term follow-up is implicit in the uncertainty of the diagnosis and the 1% annual risk that a patient IgG or IgA monoclonal gammopathy of undetermined significance will manifest multiple myeloma or amyloidosis.

A minority of patients with an IgM monoclonal gammopathy of undetermined significance will have an IgM monoclonal protein, measuring less than 1 g/dL. IgM monoclonal gammopathy is usually associated with lymphoma and chronic lymphocytic leukemia and not with multiple myeloma. Unless these patients are completely asymptomatic, blood counts and physical examination are normal, and the IgM M-protein level is less than 1 g/dL, a search for an underlying lymphoma should be initiated. Evaluation should include computed tomography scan of the abdomen and a bone marrow aspirate/biopsy. With continued follow-up, many of these patients will ultimately manifest a lymphoproliferative disorder. Very rarely, an IgM type of amyloidosis supervenes. The likelihood of developing an overt lymphoma in IgM monoclonal gammopathy of undetermined significance is greater than the risk of conversion of an IgG or IgA type of monoclonal gammopathy of undetermined significance to multiple myeloma.

A monoclonal gammopathy of undetermined significance of IgD or IgE types is rarely diagnosed because the small increments in M-protein result in minimal increase in their normally low concentrations in the serum. The resulting protein band on serum protein electrophoresis would be so indistinct that it would go undetected. By the time a monoclonal IgD and IgE M-protein is increased enough to be appreciated, the patient usually already has a well-established malignant plasma cell disorder, and the bone marrow may be heavily infiltrated with plasma cells. An IgD monoclonal protein generally indicates a diagnosis of multiple myeloma, and an IgE M-protein is commonly associated with plasma cell leukemia.

If a free monoclonal light chain is found in the serum or in the urine, the likely diagnosis include myeloma, amyloidosis, or light chain deposition disease. In some instances, even when the urine free monoclonal light chain measures more than 300 mg/24 hours, no malignancy can be detected, and the patient is then diagnosed as having idiopathic Bence-Jones proteinuria.

Asymptomatic (Smoldering) Multiple Myeloma

The most common malignant disorder of plasma cells is multiple myeloma. A substantial subset of patients, perhaps 10% to 20%, whose findings meet the criteria for the diagnosis of multiple myeloma do not have symptoms of bone pain or evidence of disease progression. These patients are diagnosed as having asymptomatic (smoldering) multiple myeloma. In contrast to monoclonal gammopathy of undetermined significance, the bone marrow contains more than 10% plasma cells, and the level of IgG protein or of IgA protein is more than 3 g/dL and 2 g/dL, respectively. The hemoglobin is at normal or near-normal levels, and the calcium and creatinine levels are normal as well. These patients can be safely followed without treatment. The data thus far do not show a survival advantage if treatment is begun before the patient becomes symptomatic (from anemia or bone pain) or shows progressive worsening of peripheral blood counts or abnormal blood chemistries (e.g., rising calcium and creatinine). Like patients with monoclonal gammopathy of undetermined significance, these patients should be followed every three to four months. Follow-up studies include complete blood and platelet counts, serum calcium, creatinine, serum protein electrophoresis with measurement of the M-protein, and quantitative measurement of the involved immunoglobulin, for example, IgG levels in patients with IgG monoclonal gammopathy. Sometimes such patients will have small asymptomatic lytic lesions of bone on magnetic resonance imaging (MRI) scans reflecting abnormal patterns of activity in the bone marrow. Despite the presence of documented bone disease and/or bone marrow plasma cells that can be more than 30%, these patients can remain clinically well for years with any specific intervention. Bisphosphonates such as pamidronate or zoledronic acid should be used to prevent progressive osteoporosis.

Multiple Myeloma

Multiple myeloma usually presents with a monoclonal gammopathy associated with renal insufficiency, hypercalcemia, unexplained anemia, or bone pain. An important aspect of the history is the characteristic movement-related bone pain, most often the result of involvement of the axial skeleton. Bone lesions occur in two thirds of patients with myeloma. Percussion tenderness of the spine and tenderness of the sternum are typical of myeloma, especially of the IgA subtype, which more often than the IgG subtype is associated with extramedullary extension. Characteristic thoracic or lumbar nerve root pain suggests destructive involvement of a vertebral body or posterior elements with extramedullary extension and nerve root impingement. Left unchecked, such involvement can lead to spinal cord compression with symptoms of extremity weakness or numbness, positive cough-sneeze effect or interference with bowel or bladder control, and ultimately paralysis. During a review of systems, one may encounter the classic symptoms of hypercalcemia: lassitude, somnolence, nausea, loss of appetite, constipation, polydipsia, and polyuria. Hypercalcemia is caused by lysis of bone and requires prompt therapy to correct or prevent its symptoms and complications, particularly renal failure.

Solitary Plasmacytoma

Sometimes, myeloma forms a localized growth of plasma cells as an isolated tumor mass, called a solitary plasmacytoma. The growth usually occurs in bone but may also occur in extramedullary tissues. A common presentation is back pain with a vertebral mass and a monoclonal gammopathy. If bone marrow aspiration/biopsy is negative for multiple myeloma, a site-directed biopsy of the lesion must be done to make the diagnosis. Computed tomography–guided biopsy may be recommended in certain instances; in other cases, an orthopedic or neurosurgical approach is needed.

Amyloidosis

A history of other affected family members may lead to consideration of familial forms of amyloidosis. Amyloidosis can also develop secondary to long-standing chronic infections, such as osteomyelitis, and/or inflammatory disorders, such as familial Mediterranean fever.

Amyloidosis of the primary systemic or light chain type is most often recognized when an elderly patient who has symptoms and/or findings of either nephrotic syndrome, heart failure, neuropathy, or hepatomegaly presents with a monoclonal gammopathy. The monoclonal gammopathy in systemic primary amyloidosis is usually of the lambda light chain type. Amyloid can infiltrate the tongue, causing macroglossia. Orthostatic hypotension due to an autonomic neuropathy is a marker of cardiac involvement by amyloid. Angina, jaw, or buttock claudication due to ischemia may signal microvascular amyloidosis. Joint pain due to synovial infiltration by amyloid causes tenderness and apparent hypertrophy of the muscles about the shoulder, the so-called shoulder pad syndrome. A burning sensation in the skin due to a characteristically painful small fiber peripheral neuropathy and carpal tunnel syndrome are often seen.

DIAGNOSIS

Diagnosing Amyloidosis

Amyloidosis should be considered when a patient has otherwise unexplained:

Nephrotic syndrome
Congestive heart failure
Peripheral neuropathy
Carpal tunnel syndrome
Orthostatic hypotension
Hepatomegaly
Malabsorption
Mucosal and cutaneous bleeding
Macroglossia

Mucosal bleeding and a prolonged prothrombin time in a patient with amyloidosis suggest the possibility of factor X clotting factor deficiency. This occurs in rare patients due to adherence of factor X to the amyloid fibrils, thereby reducing its serum concentration. Isolated acquired factor X deficiency is virtually diagnostic of amyloidosis. However, mucosal and cutaneous bleeding is more often caused by vascular amyloid deposits and associated brittle blood vessels. Ecchymoses, called *amyloid purpura,* are frequently periorbital and can be extensive at times. These may be elicited by Valsalva maneuvers, when straining to defecate, for example. The peripheral blood smear usually contains Howell-Jolly bodies and other evidence of hyposplenism when splenomegaly due to amyloid deposition occurs.

Diagnosis is accomplished by biopsy of appropriate tissue (subcutaneous fat) and demonstrating positive Congo red staining on light microscopy of suspicious deposits.

Waldenström's Macroglobulinemia

An IgM monoclonal gammopathy is rarely a presenting sign of myeloma. An IgM M-protein is most often encountered in patients with the Waldenström's macroglobulinemia, chronic lymphocytic leukemia, or non-Hodgkin's lymphoma. Lymphadenopathy, hepatomegaly, and/or splenomegaly are common in these patients and are rarely seen to any substantial degree in patients with multiple myeloma. The diagnosis of lymphoma or chronic lymphocytic leukemia is easily made. In Waldenström's macroglobulinemia, the bone marrow is infiltrated with lymphocytoid plasma cells, variably admixed with lymphocytes and plasma cells.

Suggested Reading

Dimopoulos MA, Galani E, et al: Waldenstrom's macroglobulinemia. Hematol Oncol Clin North Am 2001;13:1351–1366.

Fonseca R, Greipp P: Multiple myeloma. In Rakel RE, Bope ET (eds), Conn's Current Therapy, Philadelphia, WB Saunders, 2001, pp 466–469.

Kyle RA, Therneau TM, Rajkumar SV, et al: A long-term study of prognosis in monoclonal gammopathy of undetermined significance. N Engl J Med 2002;346:564–569.

Kyle RA, Rajkumar SV: Monoclonal gammopathies of undetermined significance. Hematol Oncol Clin North Am 1999; 13:1181–1202.

Gertz MA, Lacy MQ, et al: Amyloidosis. Hematol Oncol Clin North Am 1999;13:1211–1233.

Chapter 34
Iron Studies: Normal and Abnormal

Nancy C. Andrews

Clinical disorders of iron metabolism result from perturbation of normal iron balance. The manifestations are best understood by considering how the metal is distributed in the body. More than 60% of iron in normal individuals is incorporated into the functional heme group in red blood cell hemoglobin. Consequently, anemia is the most prominent finding in iron deficiency. Erythroid iron is recycled by reticuloendothelial macrophages found in the liver and spleen. This recycling process is disrupted in the setting of chronic inflammation, resulting in the anemia of chronic disease, which is characterized by increased macrophage iron content but decreased availability of iron for erythropoiesis. Iron in excess of the body's needs is deposited in storage, primarily in hepatocytes. The liver therefore is a primary target organ affected in iron overload, along with the heart and the pancreas.

Morphologic Evidence of Iron Deficient Erythropoiesis

When the body's iron stores are depleted, iron becomes limiting for erythropoiesis, and newly made erythrocytes are poorly hemoglobinized. Since erythrocytes normally live for about four months, it takes some time for iron-restricted erythropoiesis to become apparent in the bulk population of red blood cells. The first morphologic finding is a decrease in the hemoglobin content of reticulocytes (CHr). Although the hemoglobin content of reticulocytes measurement is not widely available yet, a recent study of pediatric patients concluded that it is a highly sensitive marker of iron deficiency. As the iron-deficient erythrocyte population becomes a larger fraction of the total, the hemoglobin and hematocrit levels decrease. This is due to decreases in both erythrocyte hemoglobin content (mean corpuscular hemoglobin, MCH) and cell volume (mean corpuscular volume, MCV). Marked anemia that is not accompanied by decreased mean corpuscular hemoglobin and mean corpuscular

volume does not result from iron deficiency alone. Either it is a combination of two etiologies (e.g., folate deficiency and iron deficiency, mild iron deficiency and acute blood loss) or the diagnosis of iron deficiency is incorrect. Conversely, decreased mean corpuscular hemoglobin and mean corpuscular volume values in individuals with normal hematocrit and hemoglobin levels are unlikely to signify iron deficiency. Iron deficiency leads to variability in erythrocyte size, reflected in an increased red cell distribution width (RDW). A red cell distribution width greater than 15% is highly sensitive but not specific for iron deficiency.

The blood smear is useful when iron deficiency is longstanding, though it may be normal early on. Erythrocytes appear hypochromic and microcytic, consistent with the decreased mean corpuscular hemoglobin and mean corpuscular volume values. Wide variation in erythrocyte size (anisocytosis, explaining the increased red cell distribution width) and shape (poikilocytosis) occurs. Elongated pencil cells and target cells may be seen, particularly when iron deficiency is profound. Typically, the reticulocyte count is low. However, intermittent use of iron supplements may stimulate bursts of accelerated erythropoiesis, resulting in transient reticulocytosis. An increased platelet count frequently accompanies iron deficiency and may be evident on the blood smear. White blood cell numbers and morphology are usually normal.

Routine Wright-Giemsa staining of iron-deficient bone marrow aspirates may show nonspecific changes, such as normoblasts with minimal amounts of cytoplasm and ragged borders; however, neither of these morphologic findings is invariably present or specific for iron deficiency. The iron that is available for erythropoiesis can be examined by staining with Perls' Prussian blue, which makes iron appear blue-green against a light background. Small iron granules may be present in some normoblasts, but round iron granules in macrophages give the best indication of iron available to red cell precursors. Decreased macrophage iron is highly suggestive and the earliest sign of iron deficiency, occurring even before the hemoglobin decreases or red blood cell indices are altered. One must be wary of interpreting iron deficiency on the basis of absent iron on staining of a bone marrow *biopsy* because decalcification with acidic fixatives or nonbuffered formalin may solubilize iron from the sample and allow it to leach away. At least two slides should be examined from the patient, in parallel with a similarly treated control slide.

Biochemical Indicators of Iron Deficiency and Iron Overload

Iron, Iron-Binding Capacity, and Transferrin Saturation

In normal individuals, nearly all serum iron is carried by the abundant plasma glycoprotein transferrin, which has two high-affinity iron-binding sites. The total serum iron-binding capacity (TIBC) is primarily a measure of transferrin-binding sites unless an exogenous iron chelator (e.g., desferrioxamine) is present. The amount of transferrin tends to be elevated in iron deficiency and decreased in iron overload. Serum iron is measured by acidification of serum in the presence of a reducing agent to release iron from transferrin. It shows circadian variability and sensitivity to recent dietary or medicinal intake of iron. For that reason, it is best to perform this test early in the morning in a fasting state. It is rarely useful to measure either the serum iron or total serum iron-binding capacity alone because these results are best interpreted in combination. The transferrin saturation is the ratio of serum iron to total iron-binding capacity. It is expressed as a percentage that describes the occupancy of transferrin-binding sites with iron.

Transferrin saturation less than 10% is considered diagnostic of iron deficiency, and less than 16% is suggestive. Iron-deficient patients often have elevated serum transferrin (and TIBC). Under some circumstances, it is useful to examine intestinal iron absorption by giving a 1- to 2-mg/kg oral dose of elemental iron in the form of an iron salt (e.g., ferrous sulfate) and measuring serum iron just before and 1 to 2 hours after the dose is taken. Iron-deficient patients with normal intestinal absorptive capacity show a significant increase in serum iron after the test dose. A blunted response indicates a problem with enteral iron uptake. Some clinicians have attempted to use this test to make the diagnosis of iron deficiency, relying on the fact that intestinal iron absorption is increased when iron stores are depleted; however, more reliable tests are available for that purpose.

Serum iron and transferrin saturation may also be low in patients who have anemia of chronic disease due to inflammation or malignancy. These patients have an impairment of macrophage iron release that results in decreased loading of iron onto transferrin. It is useful to note that anemia of chronic disease is typically associated with low serum transferrin and abundant iron in macrophages. Measurements of serum ferritin and serum transferrin receptor may also be useful in distinguishing iron deficiency from anemia of chronic disease (see the following sections).

In normal individuals, serum transferrin saturation ranges from 20% to 40%. However, in the setting of iron overload, iron values may equal or even exceed the number of transferrin iron-binding sites. Patients with hereditary hemochromatosis characteristically have elevated serum transferrin saturation. In adults, repeated values greater than 45% are highly suggestive of hemochromatosis. Patients with other iron overload disorders, particularly those with a distinct disorder found in sub-Saharan Africa, may have tissue iron overload associated with less extreme increases in transferrin saturation. Similarly, African-Americans with iron overload do not typically have transferrin saturations as high as those seen in patients with hereditary hemochromatosis.

Serum Ferritin

Ferritin is the major storage molecule for iron within cells. It can be released by tissue damage. It is also present in the serum of normal individuals, though the source of normal serum ferritin has not been definitively identified. Nonetheless, it is a useful marker of iron status. Serum ferritin contains little iron and is measured by an immunoassay. Low values (less than 10 μg/L) invariably indicate iron deficiency, as there are no known conditions that artifactually lower the serum ferritin level. Borderline low values (less than 20 μg/L) indicate that iron stores are low and may indicate frank iron deficiency, particularly in patients who are anemic.

There are several possible explanations for a high serum ferritin level. It may indicate increased iron stores due to genetic iron overload disorders or transfusional iron loading. However, serum ferritin should not be considered a quantitative assessment of iron stores; measurement of liver iron (see the following sections) is far more accurate. Ferritin levels can rise severalfold as part of an acute-phase response to inflammation and to an even greater extent if there is significant tissue destruction. Tissue ferritin concentrations are several orders of magnitude greater than serum ferritin concentrations. Hence relatively minor tissue damage may have a marked effect on serum fer-

DIAGNOSIS

Iron Studies in Disease

Serum Iron	Total Iron-Binding Capacity	Percent Saturation	Ferritin	Etiology
Decreased	Increased	Decreased (≤15%)	Decreased	Iron-deficiency anemia Estrogen Rx Oral anticontraceptives
Decreased	Decreased	Decreased (≤15%)	Normal or increased	Anemia of chronic disease
Decreased	Decreased	Decreased (≤15%)	Normal or decreased	Anemia of chronic disease + iron-deficiency anemia
Normal or increased	Normal or decreased	Increased	Increased	Hemochromatosis Aplastic anemia Myelodysplasia Megaloblastic anemia Alcoholism Chronic hepatitis

Notes:

- Patients on estrogens may have iron-binding capacity and percent saturation consistent with iron-deficiency anemia, even when they are not iron deficient.
- Iron studies are abnormal in the anemia of chronic disease regardless of whether iron deficiency is present. In the anemia of chronic disease, if the ferritin level is ≤12 μg/L, then the patient is iron deficient; if the ferritin level is >100 μg/L, then iron deficiency is not present. Between these two values, the only certain means of determining the iron status is by iron stain of the bone marrow aspirate.
- Circumstances of ineffective erythropoiesis, red cell hypoplasia, and liver disease can alter iron studies in the direction of those found in

hemochromatosis. Although the increased iron saturation and ferritin levels are usually substantially higher in hemochromatosis, the values may be indeterminate (especially in alcoholics with liver disease), requiring liver biopsy and quantitative iron assay to make the diagnosis.
- Iron studies can vary and are most accurate when obtained in the fasting state in the morning.
- An isolated serum iron determination is useless as a diagnostic tool.
- The anemia of chronic disease regularly lowers the serum iron and iron-binding capacity, rendering these studies less helpful in the presence of infection, inflammation, or malignancy.

ritin levels. Neoplastic conditions, including neuroblastoma, hepatocellular carcinoma, germ-cell tumors, and malignant histiocytosis, are characteristically associated with hyperferritinemia. Any of these conditions can confound the use of ferritin levels in assessment of iron status. Finally, there is a rare syndrome in which hyperferritinemia is associated with autosomal-dominant congenital cataracts. This is not a disorder of iron metabolism; rather, it results from dysregulated overexpression of ferritin protein in the absence of iron overload.

Serum ferritin levels are age dependent, as are levels of body iron stores. Serum ferritin is elevated in term newborns, reflecting the iron accumulated during the third trimester. Levels drop during the first six months of life as iron is used to support growth and expansion of the red blood cell mass. Ferritin

levels remain relatively low throughout childhood because little iron is stored while body size is rapidly increasing. Ferritin levels begin to rise after adolescence. However, menstrual blood losses limit iron storage in female patients; at any given age, average ferritin values are greater in men than in menstruating women. Ferritin levels increase in women after they reach menopause. Despite these caveats, serum ferritin values can be helpful in monitoring iron stores during treatment for iron deficiency or overload, as long as they are considered in context.

Serum Transferrin Receptor

Serum transferrin receptor is a normal proteolytic cleavage product of the cell surface receptor for transferrin. Cell-bound transferrin receptor is abundant on developing erythroid precursors but absent from mature erythrocytes. It is shed into the plasma during late erythroid differentiation. Levels of serum transferrin receptor are increased in patients with iron deficiency and in patients with disorders associated with ineffective erythropoiesis (e.g., thalassemia syndromes, sideroblastic anemia, congenital dyserythropoietic anemias). When ineffective erythropoiesis can be ruled out, serum transferrin receptor is a useful marker for iron deficiency. It can be particularly helpful in distinguishing anemia of chronic disease from iron deficiency when the diagnosis is uncertain. The ratio of serum transferrin receptor to the log of ferritin (TfR-F index) is particularly helpful for making this distinction. Values greater than 1.5 indicate iron deficiency alone or in combination with an inflammatory condition; values less than 1.5 are characteristic of anemia of chronic disease. The TfR-F index also appears to be sensitive enough to detect iron deficiency before anemia is apparent.

Protoporphyrin Levels

Protoporphyrin IX is the precursor molecule that incorporates iron to form heme. In iron deficiency, the lack of iron leads to production of free protoporphyrin and protoporphyrin in which zinc is substituted for iron. Lead poisoning also impairs incorporation of iron into protoporphyrin. Free erythrocyte protoporphyrin (FEP) and zinc protoporphyrin (ZPP) levels are frequently used in children to detect lead poisoning. The zinc protoporphyrin assay is simple to perform: It involves placement of a drop of blood on a coverslip and measurement of the absorbance at 420 nm in a hematofluorometer. The assay requires oxygenated blood, but it is not dependent upon hematocrit. It is easily performed in an office setting. In contrast, the free erythrocyte protoporphyrin test requires a more complex assay procedure, but it is more sensitive. Both levels are elevated in iron deficiency; levels are very high when iron deficiency is complicated by lead poisoning and in erythropoietic protoporphyria. However, these tests are not specific; protoporphyrin measurements and the protoporphyrin/heme ratio may also be elevated in the anemia of chronic inflammation. Levels are low when there is a defect in hemoglobin synthesis that does not limit iron acquisition or incorporation—for example, in thalassemia syndromes.

Detection of Blood Loss

Abnormal blood loss is the most common cause of iron deficiency. Each milliliter of whole blood contains approximately 0.4 mg of iron. Therefore chronic blood loss may deplete iron stores even if the amount lost is small. Aside from menstrual losses, the gastrointestinal tract is the most common site of occult and apparent bleeding. Two tests for occult stool blood are in common use. The Hemoccult test involves the application of a small stool sample to paper impregnated with guaiac, a plant resin that serves as an indicator substance. Guaiac is oxidized to a blue color if blood is present when the sample is treated with hydrogen peroxide. The test is less sensitive if the sample has dried out; in that situation, saline should be applied first. The test should be repeated on multiple occasions because bleeding may be intermittent. Upper gastrointestinal bleeding may be harder to detect because the test is most sensitive for hemoglobin, which is digested as it passes through the gut. Hemoglobin and myoglobin from meat do not cause the test to be positive unless they are consumed in very large amounts. However, peroxidase activities present in red meats and induced by administration of some drugs (e.g., aspirin) can occasionally result in false positives. Medicinal iron does not give a false positive test in spite of the fact that it darkens the stools.

Evaluation of Tissue Iron Content

When clinically significant iron overload is suspected, on the basis of iron studies, a magnetic resonance imaging (MRI) study of the liver may produce a distinctive, virtually diagnostic scan. This has reduced the necessity for liver biopsy to directly measure the extent of iron overload, although liver biopsy is still considered by many to be the gold standard for determining body iron burden. Hepatic iron concentration (in micrograms of iron per 100 mg dry weight of liver tissue) is measured by atomic absorption spectroscopy. When necessary, this can be done on deparaffinized tissue blocks. Values less than 140 μg/100 mg are considered normal, whereas values greater than 240 μg/100 mg are diagnostic of iron overload. In parallel, histologic sections should be stained with Perls' Prussian blue to determine whether excess iron is present in Kupffer cells or liver parenchymal cells. Liver iron is most prominent in hepatocytes in hereditary hemochromatosis. When liver biopsy cannot be performed, repeated phlebotomy (the weekly removal of one unit of blood) offers an alternative method to quantify and confirm the presence of excess iron load.

Genetic Testing for Iron Overload Disorders

Twenty-five years ago, it was discovered that most patients with hemochromatosis show genetic linkage

DIAGNOSIS

Diagnosing Genetic Iron Overload

The clinical diagnosis of genetic iron overload is evolving rapidly, and it is now clear that hemochromatosis, once thought to be a single disorder, has multiple distinct etiologies. However, several simple principles continue to apply. Clinically significant iron overload is invariably associated with elevated serum ferritin and usually associated with elevated serum transferrin saturation. While ferritin may be increased for other reasons (inflammation, malignancy, and hyperferritinemia/cataract syndrome), the combination of elevated ferritin and clinical signs of iron overload and/or elevated transferrin saturation demands further investigation. The next step depends on available data and clinical judgment. In patients with a known *HFE* C282Y homozygous relative or a high prior probability based on their ancestry, it may be sufficient to send a blood sample for *HFE* gene analysis. Most C282Y homozygotes with serum evidence of iron overload do not need a liver biopsy prior to starting phlebotomy.

Increasingly, asymptomatic patients are referred for evaluation because they have a family member who is a known C282Y homozygote. Under these circumstances, the *HFE* gene test can provide some indication of the likelihood that the patient will develop hemochromatosis. However, it is important to remember that iron overload rarely presents before adolescence, because children have increased iron needs to support their growth. Furthermore, not all C282Y homozygotes will develop iron overload as adults. For these reasons, patients who are discovered to be asymptomatic C282Y homozygotes must have liver biopsies and/or periodic serum chemistries performed to monitor for the development of iron overload.

It is now clear that some patients with inherited hemochromatosis syndromes may have other *HFE* mutations or defects in other genes, because *HFE*-associated hemochromatosis accounts for only approximately two thirds of the cases of genetic iron overload. There are at least four other, non-*HFE* iron-loading disorders, including a form with juvenile onset. At least one appears to be inherited in an autosomal dominant manner, while others appear to be autosomal recessive, complicating the task of genetic counseling. The gene has been identified for only one of these non-*HFE* disorders. The genes that are responsible for the other inherited iron overload disorders are likely to be identified over the next few years, adding to the roster of gene tests for this disorder.

Finally, it is important to bear in mind that there are other clinically significant iron overload disorders that do not resemble hemochromatosis. Rare patients may have congenital atransferrinemia or congenital aceruloplasminemia, each of which leads to increased intestinal iron absorption and pathologic distribution of iron in the body. When suspected, these are easily identified by measurement of serum transferrin and ceruloplasmin, respectively.

---

of the disease to the human major histocompatibility (HLA) complex on chromosome 6p. Recently, this information led to positional cloning of the defective gene *HFE* and the development of a gene-based test. A large majority of patients with histocompatibility leukocyte antigen–associated hemochromatosis carry a unique missense (C282Y) mutation that converts amino acid 282 of the HFE preprotein (amino acid 260 of the mature protein) from cysteine to tyrosine. This mutation appears to have arisen in a single individual of Celtic origin, and it has spread throughout the world in a pattern consistent with Celtic migration. This mutation has never been found in individuals without European ancestry (e.g., Asians and Black Africans). Patients who are homozygous for the C282Y mutation are at risk for developing clinically significant hemochromatosis. Patients with one C282Y allele and one other allele are generally not at risk, though some may develop iron overload when their slight genetic susceptibility is combined with environmental factors such as viral hepatitis or alcoholism.

The clinical significance of most of the other alleles is still uncertain.

Suggested Reading

Iron Deficiency

Brugnara C, Zurakowski D, DiCanzio J, et al: Reticulocyte hemoglobin content to diagnose iron deficiency in children. JAMA 1999;281:2225.

Punnonen K, Irjala K, Rajamaki A: Serum transferrin receptor and its ratio to ferritin in the diagnosis of iron deficiency. Blood 1997;89:1052.

Suominen P, Punnonen K, Rajamaki A, et al: Serum transferrin receptor and transferrin receptor-ferritin index identify healthy subjects with subclinical iron deficits. Blood 1998;92:2934.

Iron Metabolism and Laboratory Studies

Andrews NC: Medical progress: Disorders of iron metabolism. N Engl J Med 1999;341:1986.

Cook JD: The measurement of serum transferrin receptor. Am J Med Sci 1999;318:269.

Gottschalk R, Wigand R, Dietrich CF, et al: Total iron-binding capacity and serum transferrin determination under the influence of several clinical conditions. Clin Chim Acta 2000;293:127.

Labbe R, Vreman H, Stevenson D: Zinc protoporphyrin: A metabolite with a mission. Clin Chem 1999;45:2060.

Iron Overload States

Cazzola M, Skoda R: Translational pathophysiology: A novel molecular mechanism of human disease. Blood 2000; 95:3280.

Cullen LM, Anderson GJ, Ramm GA, et al: Genetics of hemochromatosis. Annu Rev Med 1999;50:87.

Feder JN, Gnirke A, Thomas W, et al: A novel MHC class I-like gene is mutated in patients with hereditary haemochromatosis. Nat Genet 1996;13:399.

Gordeuk V, Mukiibi J, Hasstedt SJ, et al: Iron overload in Africa: Interaction between a gene and dietary iron content. N Engl J Med 1992;326:95.

Olynyk JK, Cullen DJ, Aquilia S, et al: A population-based study of the clinical expression of the hemochromatosis gene. N Engl J Med 1999;341:718.

Pietrangelo A, Montosi G, Totaro A, et al: Hereditary hemochromatosis in adults without pathogenic mutations in the hemochromatosis gene. N Engl J Med 1999;341: 725.

Piperno A, Sampietro M, Pietrangelo A, et al: Heterogeneity of hemochromatosis in Italy. Gastroenterology 1998;114: 996.

Powell LW, George DK, McDonnell SM, et al: Diagnosis of hemochromatosis. Ann Intern Med 1998;129:925.

Simon M, Bourel M, Fauchet R, et al: Association of HLA-A3 and HLA-B14 antigens with idiopathic haemochromatosis. Gut 1976;17:332.

Hematologic Abnormalities

Chapter 35
Lymphadenopathy

Peter Kozuch and Michael L. Grossbard

Introduction

Lymphadenopathy is encountered by physicians in all medical specialties and requires comprehensive assessment and timely management. Specific algorithms, described below, to assess abnormal lymph nodes can be helpful in designing an orderly evaluation of the patient presenting with lymphadenopathy. Lymph nodes can enlarge owing to polyclonal expansion of lymphocytes in response to the stimuli of infection or antigen exposure or as a component of autoimmune diseases. In contrast, in lymphomas and leukemias, nodal enlargement is due to a monoclonal expansion of lymphocytes. Tumors of epithelial cell origin, melanomas, and germ-cell tumors may infiltrate lymph nodes. Rarely, lymphadenopathy can be caused by abnormal lipid deposition in the setting of lipid storage diseases. Table 35-1 outlines the numerous disorders associated with lymphadenopathy.

Definitions

Lymphadenopathy refers to nodes that are abnormal in size, number, or consistency. Normal lymph nodes are nontender and mobile within the surrounding tissue, soft but slightly rubbery, with well-defined borders. The normal limits of lymph node size vary by anatomic location. In the inguinal chain, lymph nodes may occasionally be as large as 2 cm in diameter in healthy adults. Submandibular and axillary lymph nodes may be palpable in an otherwise healthy individual. It is difficult therefore to define with certainty the upper size limit of a normal lymph node. Among a selected group of patients who were referred to a lymphoma/leukemia unit for further work-up of unexplained adenopathy, nonspecific adenopathy was the final diagnosis in 89%, 50%, and 22% of patients with nodes less than 1×1 cm, less than 1×1 to 1.5×1.5 cm, and greater than 1.5×1.5 cm, respectively. In the patients whose lymph nodes measured greater than 1.5×1.5 cm, 40% had tuberculosis, toxoplasmosis, or mononucleosis; 31% had non-Hodgkin's lymphoma or Hodgkin's disease; and 7% were diagnosed with metastatic cancer. The nearly 80% incidence of malignancy or infectious disease in this report from a referral hematologic malignancy clinic is not generalizable to other practice settings. Nevertheless, the relationship of lymph node size to the likelihood of involvement by malignant or infectious disease is well established. It is rare for a lymph node less than 1 cm in diameter to be clinically significant. Concern about the etiology of lymph node enlargement increases as it exceeds 1.5 cm in diameter. As with all abnormal clinical and laboratory findings, the significance of an enlarged lymph node must be viewed in the broad context of other factors, including location, acuity/chronicity, patient age, gender, and associated symptoms. Any lymph node measuring 2 cm or greater in diameter that persists for more than four weeks, even if present as an isolated finding, must be viewed with suspicion. In this setting, further evaluation is mandatory, including lymph node biopsy (and cultures of the biopsy, where appropriate) for possible malignant or infectious etiologies irrespective of patient age or gender, presence or absence of symptoms, or location of the lymph node.

Localized adenopathy is defined as abnormal lymph nodes in one region (e.g., anterior cervical

213

Table 35-1 ▪ Causes of Lymphadenopathy

Infectious diseases:

1. Viral: mononucleosis syndromes (Epstein-Barr virus, cytomegalovirus), hepatitis, HIV
2. Bacterial: streptococci, staphylococci, cat-scratch disease, chancroid, Lyme disease, tuberculosis, atypical mycobacteria, primary and secondary syphilis
3. Fungal: histoplasmosis, coccidioidomycosis
4. Chlamydial: lymphogranuloma venereum, trachoma
5. Parasitic: toxoplasmosis
6. Rickettsial: rickettsialpox

Immune-mediated diseases:

1. Autoimmune disorders: rheumatoid arthritis, systemic lupus erythematosus
2. Drug hypersensitivity: diphenylhydantoin, allopurinol, carbamazepine, captopril, quinidine
3. Other hypersensitivity reactions: serum sickness
4. Graft-versus-host disease

Hematologic malignancies: Non-Hodgkin's lymphoma, leukemias, and Hodgkin's disease

Metastatic cancer

Disorders of unknown etiology associated with lymphadenopathy as a prominent feature: Angioimmunoblastic lymphadenopathy, Castleman's disease, sarcoidosis, inflammatory pseudotumor of lymph nodes
Other: Hyperthyroidism, hyperlipidemia

---

chain), generalized adenopathy is enlarged nodes in two or more noncontiguous areas (e.g., bilateral axillary adenopathy), and regional adenopathy consists of involvement of two or more contiguous areas. These distinctions are of limited utility in the differential diagnosis because many of the conditions listed in Table 35-1 can manifest either local, regional, or generalized lymphadenopathy.

General Concepts in the Evaluation of Lymphadenopathy

History

The history and physical examination allow the practitioner to reach the first decision point in the evaluation of a patient's lymphadenopathy. Critical historical information includes the presence of constitutional symptoms, past medical history, medications, and social history. Localizing symptoms can be coupled to physical examination findings to help define a differential diagnosis (Table 35-2). Constitutional symptoms include persistent unexplained weight loss of at least 10% from the patient's baseline, fever greater than 38°C, fatigue, and drenching night sweats. Constitutional symptoms are classically associated with Hodgkin's disease but also suggest other serious diseases such as non-Hodgkin's lymphomas, leukemia, some metastatic solid tumors, inflammatory disease, and chronic infections such as HIV and tuberculosis.

The patient's past medical history should be reviewed for possible associations with the presenting complaint. A prior cancer history should prompt the consideration of locoregional or distant recurrence of virtually any malignancy. Breast cancer, melanoma, and low-grade lymphomas may relapse many years after primary therapy. A history of prior radiation therapy to the chest should raise the suspicion of a secondary malignancy, particularly breast cancer, which can presenting with adenopathy (cervical, supraclavicular, or axillary). Adenopathy in sexually active adults and those with a history of blood product transfusion or intravenous drug use prompts consideration of a diagnosis of HIV or hepatitis infection. Opportunistic infections and lymphomas should be considered in patients who are immunocompromised due to advanced HIV infection or who are receiving chronic immunosuppressive therapy for autoimmune disorders or after organ or bone marrow transplantation.

Patient age must be considered in the assessment of lymphadenopathy. In young adults, lymphadenopathy is usually due to infections, including viral or bacterial upper respiratory tract infections, mononucleosis, toxoplasmosis, or tuberculosis in endemic areas. Adenopathy in patients age 50 years or older, however, is more likely due to malignancy. A review of the patient's medication list may reveal use of a drug that is associated with hypersensitivity reactions that include adenopathy as a prominent feature. Aspects of the social history may offer important clues to the diagnosis (Table 35-3).

Physical Examination

The physical examination starts with examination of the region that is the focus of the patient's complaint but must also include careful palpation of the other major nodal basins. The anterior and posterior cervical node areas; preauricular lymph nodes; submandibular and submental lymph nodes; supraclavicular, infraclavicular, axillary, epitrochlear, inguinal, and femoral lymph node areas; and the spleen should be examined. The bidimensional size of lymph nodes, their mobility in relation to surrounding tissue and overlying skin, and their consistency should be documented. The pads of the fingertips should be used to palpate the skin and soft tissue of each nodal basin. The anterior cervical and supraclavicular lymph nodes

Table 35-2 ■ Lymph Node Groups and Their Drainage Areas

Lymph Node Group	Drainage Areas	Differential Diagnosis	Evaluation and Follow-up
Suboccipital nodes	Scalp	Local infections, tick bites Systemic infections: EBV, cytomegalovirus, toxoplasmosis, HIV Melanoma	Treatment of local infection, serologic evaluation for systemic infection Biopsy atypical nevus or suspicious nodules
Submental lymph nodes	Tongue, conjunctivae, lower lip, floor of mouth, anterior tongue	Local infections: head and neck, sinuses, eyes, pharynx, ears Head and neck carcinomas Low-grade lymphoma	Treat local infections Suspected carcinoma: refer to head and neck surgeon for evaluation and biopsy
Anterior cervical lymph nodes (one of the most frequent areas of adenopathy)	Pharnyx, tongue, pinna, parotid	Local infection: ear, pharynx, dental Systemic diseases: HIV, tuberculosis, cytomegalovirus, mononucleosis, sarcoidosis, and lymphomas	Treat local infections Serologic evaluation for systemic infections
Posterior cervical lymph nodes	Scalp, neck, skin of arms, thorax	Advanced head and neck, breast, thyroid, and lung cancer	Suspected carcinoma: refer to head and neck surgeon Many cases of isolated anterior cervical adenopathy are attributed to nonspecific etiologies; posterior cervical adenopathy is more often associated with diagnosable pathology
Preauricular adenopathy	Eyelids and conjunctivae, pinna	Local infections	Treat local infection
Supraclavicular adenopathy (almost always pathologic)	Mediastinum, lungs, esophagus, stomach, breast	Malignancy: lung, gastrointestinal tumors (the so-called Virchow's node if a gastrointestinal tumor has metastasized to the left supraclavicular lymph node); breast, germ-cell, and lymphomas Nonmalignant: tuberculosis, sarcoidosis, toxoplasmosis	Definitive diagnosis: biopsy of largest or most rapidly growing accessible lymph node
Axillary adenopathy	Upper extremities, breast, thorax	Local infections or injury of the hands and arms, cat-scratch disease Malignancy: breast cancer in men and women, melanoma, lymphoma	Treat the local infection or injury Breast exam, mammography, biopsy suspicious findings
Epitrochlear adenopathy	Ulnar aspect of forearm and hand	Local infections, secondary syphilis, sarcoid Lymphoma	Serological evaluation of syphilis Treat local infection Biopsy of largest or most rapidly growing accessible lymph node
Inguinal adenopathy	Penis, scrotum, vulva, vagina, perineum, lower abdominal wall, lower anal canal, lower extremity	Infections or trauma of the lower extremity Sexually transmitted diseases: lymphogranuloma venereum, primary syphilis, genital herpes, chancroid Malignancy: metastatic cancer from primary rectal or genital cancers, lower extremity melanomas Lymphoma	Evaluation and therapy of sexually transmitted disease Biopsy suspicious lesions

Table 35-3 ■ Social History and Associated Etiologies of Lymphadenopathy

High-risk behavior
- Sexual: HIV, cytomegalovirus, hepatitis, syphilis, herpes simplex I and II, chancroid (*Haemophilus ducreyi*), chlamydia (lymphogranuloma venereum)
- Intravenous drug use: HIV

Occupational history/hobbies
- Hunters, trappers: tularemia
- Fishermen, slaughterhouse workers: erysipeloid (*Erysipelothrix rhusiopathiae*)
- Domestic cat exposure: cat-scratch disease, toxoplasmosis
- Tick bites: tularemia, Lyme disease

Demographic clues: poverty-stricken, homeless, medical worker or relief worker: tuberculosis

Travel history
- Southwestern United States (Arizona, Southern California, New Mexico, western Texas): coccidioidomycosis, bubonic plague
- Southeastern and central United States: histoplasmosis
- Southeast Asia, India, Northern Australia, Central or West Africa: African trypanosomiasis (sleeping sickness)
- Central and South America: American trypanosomiasis (Chagas' disease)
- East Africa, Mediterranean, China, Latin America: leishmaniasis (kala-azar)
- Mexico, Peru, Chile, India, Pakistan, Egypt, Indonesia: typhoid fever

Undercooked meat: toxoplasmosis

are best examined when the clinician is positioned first behind and then in front of the patient. Increased opportunity to palpate supraclavicular lymph nodes occurs when the patient's shoulders are rotated inward. Asking the patient to breathe deeply and then perform a Valsalva maneuver facilitates examination of the supraclavicular lymph nodes by elevating the soft tissue behind the clavicle.

The axillary lymph node exam should include palpation of the axillary apex and continue inferiorly along the midaxillary line over the rib cage to the level of the inferior border of the pectoralis major. The anterior border of the axillary lymph node chain extends to the tissue just deep to the lateral border of the pectoralis muscles, the lateral border extends along the upper inner aspect of the humerus, and the posterior border extends to the lateral border of the latissimus dorsi. The area that is drained by an enlarged lymph node should be carefully inspected for evidence of inflammation, infection, or tumor.

Several findings suggest the presence of carcinoma metastatic to lymph nodes, such as a rock-hard texture due to dense replacement of nodal tissue or secondary to the reactive fibrosis (desmoplasia) that the carcinoma elicits. Such nodes may become immobile and fixed in place owing to extracapsular tumor extension into the adjacent tissues. The clumping together of otherwise distinct, separate lymph nodes is referred to as matting and can be a sign of metastatic carcinoma extending beyond lymph node capsules, binding neighbor lymph nodes to one another. These changes are not specific for carcinoma; they are also seen in lymph nodes involved by tuberculosis, sarcoidosis, and lymphogranuloma venereum. Conversely, the absence of these features does not rule out the possibility of metastatic cancer.

Lymph nodes that are enlarged, nontender, and of a soft, rubbery, or fleshy consistency are classic for lymphoma but are also observed in carcinomas, notably small-cell lung and breast cancers. The lymph nodes in low-grade lymphomas can wax and wane spontaneously without treatment and do not necessarily show the inexorable progression in size of other cancers. Although tender lymph nodes are more often associated with inflammatory or infectious processes, they also appear in some patients with Hodgkin's disease. In general, any kind of malignancy that is undergoing rapid proliferation and expansion stretches the lymph node capsule and/or exerts pressure on nearby structures, causing pain. Small (usually less than 1 cm), localized, firm, fibrotic lymph nodes can persist for long periods of time after an episode of infection in the region the nodes drain.

Evaluation of Local or Regional Adenopathies

Cervical adenopathy is the most frequent site of local or regional adenopathy. Abnormal lymph nodes here usually are due to benign processes such as upper respiratory tract infections, dental infections, or viral illnesses such as mononucleosis. Infectious etiologies are suggested by a history of recent symptoms of upper respiratory tract, odontogenic, or generalized infection. The physical findings may include inflammation localized to the region of symptomatology and tender, enlarged nodes in the draining lymphatic basins (see Table 35-2). Patients should be instructed to see the physician if signs or symptoms persist for more than four weeks after initial evaluation and therapy.

The principal malignant causes of cervical adenopathy are metastatic spread of head and neck, lung, and thyroid cancers and lymphomas. Persistent adenopathy, associated with general constitutional symptoms, and/or localizing symptoms such as pain, dyspnea, hoarseness, or dysphagia are suspicious for

metastatic carcinoma. Particularly in patients age 50 years or older and in current or former smokers, fine needle aspiration (FNA) of the lymph nodes should be obtained.

Supraclavicular adenopathy is usually caused by malignancy or infection. The thorax and retroperitoneum drain into the supraclavicular lymph node basins. Malignant causes of supraclavicular adenopathy include germ-cell, gastrointestinal, lung, breast, head, and neck carcinomas and lymphomas, whereas infectious etiologies include sarcoidosis, tuberculosis, and toxoplasmosis. Symptoms and signs that are suggestive of these tumors help to direct subsequent radiographic and/or endoscopic evaluations. Fine needle aspiration by an experienced operator is again an attractive diagnostic option in these readily accessible nodes.

The approach to axillary adenopathy should include an evaluation for associated injury or infection of the ipsilateral upper extremity. If carcinoma is found in the lymph node, then even if it is an isolated finding in a woman or a man, both breasts need to be evaluated for breast cancer, by physical examination, mammography, and/or breast ultrasonography.

Inguinal lymphadenopathy is usually secondary to nonmalignant causes such as sexually transmitted diseases and infection or trauma of the lower extremities; however, enlarged inguinal lymph nodes may be the first presentation of a lymphoma or an occult lower extremity melanoma. Cancers of the lower genital tract, anus, and perineum may also metastasize to the inguinal lymphatic chain. Evaluation should therefore include inspection and palpation of the skin of the lower extremities, including the soles of the feet, subungual areas, intertriginous areas, perineum, and lower genital tract, with particular attention to the possibility of cutaneous melanoma, other carcinomas, and infections. A digital rectal examination should also be part of the evaluation of inguinal adenopathy.

Mediastinal or hilar adenopathy discovered on chest X-ray or chest computed tomography (CT) may be due to nonmalignant disease such as sarcoidosis (especially if it is symmetrical and bilateral), particularly when encountered in young adults. Unilateral hilar adenopathy can occur in tuberculosis and histoplasmosis or lung and esophageal cancers. It is rare in non-Hodgkin's lymphomas unless pulmonary involvement is present. Bilateral hilar adenopathy is most commonly due to Hodgkin's disease or sarcoid. Lymphomas, lung and esophageal cancer, germ-cell tumors, and thymomas may enlarge mediastinal lymph nodes.

Abdominal or retroperitoneal adenopathy incidentally encountered on computed tomography scanning is usually a manifestation of cancer. Germ-cell tumors, distal colorectal cancer, prostate cancer, and lymphomas often involve the retroperitoneal lymph nodes. Further workup such as endoscopy and laparoscopic or percutaneous needle biopsy of the lymph nodes resolves the issue if the diagnosis is not already apparent elsewhere. In carcinoma of unknown origin that presents in men as central masses in the mediastinum or retroperitoneum, the germ-cell tumor markers α-fetoprotein and β-hCG and a testicular ultrasound should be obtained.

Enlarged lymph nodes in the chest or abdomen can present with ascites. Aspiration and, if appropriate, culture of the ascitic fluid usually assist in the diagnosis. In general, the more fluid sent for cytopathology and cell block analysis, the better the diagnostic yield. The optimal approach to obtaining a biopsy of enlarged internal lymph nodes is based on patient preference, available surgical or interventional radiology expertise, and anatomic considerations.

Generalized adenopathy, including splenomegaly, is suggestive of systemic illness and may be due to autoimmune disorders, sarcoidosis, or infections such as mononucleosis, toxoplasmosis, tuberculosis, or Lyme disease. Lymphoproliferative disorders are the malignant diseases that are most commonly associated with generalized lymphadenopathy.

Decision Points

The history and physical exam may be diagnostic, suggestive, or nondiagnostic regarding the cause of a patient's lymphadenopathy (Figure 35-1). Diagnoses that can be made on the basis of the history and physical alone include pharyngitis, conjunctivititis, upper respiratory tract infections, and other focal infections such as cellulitis, cat-scratch disease, and tinea. Empiric treatment is appropriate.

A suggestive or nondiagnostic history and physical requires confirmatory testing. For example, a patient with malaise, fever, and generalized adenopathy may have any one or a combination of infectious or neoplastic diseases, for example, HIV infection and lymphoma. A complete blood count can help to diagnose benign and malignant causes of lymphadenopathy, including hematologic disorders and carcinoma invading the bone marrow. Additional testing can include HIV, hepatitis serologies, heterophile antibody, IgM cytomegalovirus (CMV) antibody, IgM toxoplasmosis antibody, and PPD (tuberculin skin test) placement. If arthritic, dermatologic, renal, or neurologic symptomatology suggests autoimmune disease, then appropriate serologic studies are needed.

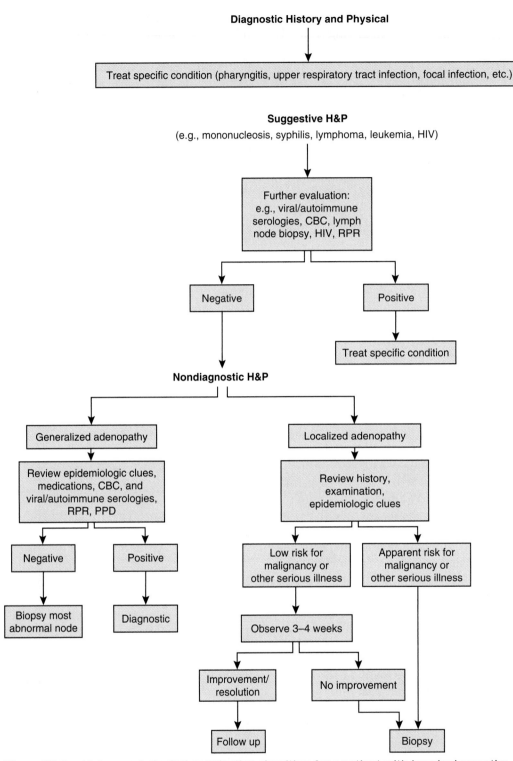

Figure 35-1 ■ History and physical examination algorithm for a patient with lymphadenopathy.

Pitfalls in Lymph Node Sampling

Empiric therapy with corticosteroids can create problems in the evaluation of unexplained adenopathy. Only rarely is adenopathy life-threatening so that anti-inflammatory therapy is warranted, as can occur in superior vena cava syndrome or when the upper airway is compromised by enlarged and/or infiltrating lymph nodes. Empiric corticosteroid therapy in patients with rapidly proliferating lymphoid malig-

---

DIAGNOSIS

Lymph Node Biopsy Considerations

Conditions that always warrant a lymph node biopsy:

- Adenopathy that develops over weeks to months
- A lymph node (other than an inguinal lymph node) larger than 2 cm in diameter
- A lymph node that is rock hard or matted in texture
- Lymphadenopathy associated with unexplained weight loss, fatigue, or cytopenias

Minimal additional evaluation to assess common causes of lymphadenopathy:

- HIV, hepatitis serologies
- Medication review
- Complete blood count

Potential pitfalls of lymph node biopsies:

- Do not interpret a negative biopsy as anything more than nondiagnostic. Ensure appropriate follow-up of patients with negative biopsy results.
- Avoid corticosteroid administration prior to a lymph node biopsy. (It reduces the accuracy of histologic diagnosis because of lymphocyte depleting effects.)

---

nancies such as high-grade lymphomas or acute lymphoblastic leukemia can initiate unexpected and hazardous tumor lysis syndrome. Equally important, corticosteroid-induced lympholysis can make histologic classification of lymphoproliferative diseases difficult or impossible. One should avoid, if possible, performing a biopsy of the inguinal lymph nodes, which are frequently nonspecifically enlarged from local irritation and infection. The largest and/or most rapidly changing nodes should be targeted to increase the diagnostic yield of lymph node fine needle aspiration or biopsy. Lymph node biopsy should also be avoided during suspected mononucleosis (due to either Epstein-Barr virus or cytomegalovirus) or toxoplasmosis, as these infections can result in histologic changes in the enlarged lymph nodes that mimic lymphoma.

A final diagnosis of negative for malignancy from the pathologist on a fine needle or lymph node biopsy should be considered neither final nor negative from a clinical perspective. If the suspicion of a cancer diagnosis was high enough to prompt the biopsy, then a negative result should be viewed instead as being nondiagnostic. For example, in some studies, up to one quarter of patients with nonspecific findings on lymph node biopsy proved to have a specific diagnosis, usually a lymphoma, shortly after the first biopsy. The appropriate next step is to either repeat a fine needle aspiration of the same or a different lymph node or to excise a different node. With an experienced operator, fine needle aspiration or core needle biopsy usually yields enough tissue for definitive histologic diagnosis and allows for additional immunostaining for diagnostic markers of malignancy such as cytokeratins, estrogen/progesterone receptors, S-100, and HER-2-neu expression. When a hematologic malignancy is suspected, a touch preparation for Wright-Giemsa staining can be helpful, and some of the biopsy should be conserved for flow cytometry. In some circumstances, flow cytometry remarkably facilitates the histologic diagnosis and subclassification and, in the case of suspected lymphomas, offers an opportunity to document whether the cellular abnormalities are clonal (malignant).

Suggested Reading

Ferrer R: Lymphadenopathy: Differential diagnosis and evaluation. Am Fam Physician 1998;58:1313–1320.

Pangalis G, Vassilakopoulos T, Boussiotis V, Fessas P: Clinical approach to lymphadenopathy. Semin Oncol 1993;20:570–582.

Saltzstein SL: The fate of patients with non-diagnostic lymph node biopsies. Surgery 1965;58:659–662.

Sinclair S, Beckman E, Ellman L: Biopsy of enlarged superficial lymph nodes. JAMA 1974;228:602–603.

Storm FK, Mahvi D, Hafez GR: Retroperitoneal masses, adenopathy, and adrenal glands. Surg Oncol Clin N Am 1995;4:75–84.

Tarantino DR, McHenry CR, Strickland T, Khiyami A: The role of fine needle aspiration biopsy and flow cytometry in the evaluation of persistent neck adenopathy. Am J Surg1998;76:413–417.

Chapter 36
Thrombocytopenia and Thrombocytosis

David J. Kuter

Introduction

With the routine use of automated blood counting devices, a complete blood count (CBC) including the platelet count is obtained on virtually all patients entering the medical arena. Abnormalities in platelet number are commonly observed in these routine blood counts. The finding of an elevated or decreased platelet count may indicate a primary bone marrow process or may reflect other underlying medical problems. The key to the evaluation of patients with platelet counts above or below the normal level is (1) the extent of increase or decrease of the platelet count, (2) associated changes in red and white blood cells, (3) the presence of related symptoms, (4) the duration of the platelet count abnormality, and (5) patient and physician concern.

Thrombocytopenia

Platelet Counts and Bleeding Risks

Bleeding risks associated with low platelet counts are difficult to quantify given that bleeding is a complex response not just to platelet count but also to platelet function, vascular integrity, comorbid medical conditions, and surgical procedures. In general, platelet counts above 100,000/μL are associated with normal hemostasis in virtually all circumstances, and platelet counts as low as 50,000/μL are adequate for most surgical procedures. Between 50,000/μL and 10,000/μL, the bleeding risk with procedures or trauma is increased; however, spontaneous bleeding is relatively rare in the absence of platelet dysfunction.

Most individuals with spontaneous bleeding due solely to thrombocytopenia have platelet counts under 10,000/μL.

Most prior studies assessing the bleeding risk of thrombocytopenia have been performed in leukemic patients who had a wide variety of comorbid medical conditions and concomitant antiplatelet medications. These studies suggest that below 100,000/μL, there is a greatly increased risk of spontaneous bleeding. In contrast, most patients with immune thrombocytopenic purpura (ITP) have considerably less bleeding at comparable platelet counts. Although it is difficult to judge the exact risk of bleeding for any particular thrombocytopenic patient, given the inability to quantify the extent of concomitant platelet dysfunction, the following general guidelines seem to be adequate:

1. Platelet counts above 100,000/μL are associated with normal hemostasis.
2. Platelet counts between 10,000/μL and 50,000/μL should have no increased risk of spontaneous or surgical bleeding.
3. Platelet counts between 10,000/μL and 50,000/μL have an increased risk of surgical bleeding and a minimal risk of spontaneous bleeding.
4. Platelet counts below 10,000/μL, depending on the cause, are associated with an increased risk of spontaneous bleeding and significant hemorrhage with procedures.

Presenting Symptoms

Most thrombocytopenic patients are devoid of symptoms. If symptoms are present, they may range from minor to severe bleeding. Epistaxis, ecchymoses, petechiae, increased menstrual bleeding, and microscopic hematuria are common; melena and gross hematuria are far less frequent. Hemarthroses are uncommon. The risk of central nervous system bleeding is low. Symptoms vary not only with the platelet count, but also with the cause of the thrombocytopenia and the extent of platelet dysfunction. For example, immune thrombocytopenic purpura patients at 10,000/μL may have no bleeding whatsoever, whereas myelodysplastic syndrome patients at that level commonly bleed. Renal insufficiency or neurologic problems ranging from headache to coma should prompt a rapid evaluation of such individuals for thrombotic microangiopathy (thrombotic thrombocytopenic purpura [TTP]/hemolytic uremic syndrome (HUB)) or internal bleeding. Finally, the presence of thrombosis in the presence of thrombocytopenia should raise concern about thrombotic thrombocytopenic purpura/hemolytic uremic syndrome, disseminated intravascular coagulation (DIC), or heparin-induced thrombocytopenia with thrombosis.

Patient History

Patients should be questioned about bleeding or thrombotic presenting symptoms. A complete review of patient medications used within the past three to six months is key. Many medications that are associated with drug-induced thrombocytopenia may linger in adipose tissues or may be complexed to blood cells for weeks or months after the last administration of the drug. Equally important is the use of illicit drugs ranging from heroin to cocaine; many of these illicit drugs are "cut" with other compounds such as quinine or talc that may themselves precipitate thrombocytopenia. Vaccinations, particularly atypical vaccinations such as those for anthrax or yellow fever, should be questioned. Potential exposures to HIV, including blood transfusions, sexual contacts, and drug abuse, are important to discern. A history of recent viral or bacterial infection is relevant.

The presence of liver disease with the potential for splenomegaly should be sought. Autoimmune disorders ranging from Hashimoto's thyroiditis to systemic lupus erythematosus are specific items to be questioned. Other comorbid diseases such as clotting disorders and certainly current symptoms of bleeding, bruising, melena, hematuria, and heavy menses need to be discerned. A family history of thrombocytopenia or a history in the patient of chronically low platelet counts should be elicited. Prior medical records documenting the duration of the thrombocytopenia are of great value. Finally, there have been suggestions of ethnic variations in platelet counts. In hospitalized patients, a precipitous drop in platelets to fewer than 10,000/μL within several hours or days of a blood transfusion might suggest posttransfusion purpura. Other causes of such abrupt drops in platelet count are disseminated intravascular coagulation, sepsis, and drug-induced immune thrombocytopenic purpura.

Pregnancy is commonly associated with multiple types of thrombocytopenia.

Physical Examination

Most patients with a thrombocytopenia lack specific symptoms and physical findings. Nonetheless, the most common associations with thrombocytopenia on the physical examination are those that indicate bleeding: ecchymoses, petechiae, and hematomas on the skin, conjunctiva, and oral mucosa. Funduscopic examination for retinal hemorrhage and rectal examination for occult blood in the stool may reveal abnormalities due to thrombocytopenia. Finally, an examination of the abdomen will assess hepatosplenomegaly. Patients should be assessed for the stigmata of chronic liver disease. In pediatric patients, the absence of the radius bone may be associated with the thrombocytopenia with absent radius (TAR) syndrome. The presence of neurologic findings such as headache, seizure, coma, confusion, or simply an altered mental status should heighten the awareness for thrombotic microangiopathy, as should findings of renal insufficiency. Ischemia or infarction of digits or limbs may indicate thrombotic thrombocytopenic purpura/hemolytic uremic syndrome but can also be seen with disseminated intravascular coagulation and heparin-induced thrombocytopenia and thrombosis.

In evaluating patients with thrombocytopenia, reliance on the concept of "wet" versus "dry" purpura appears to be helpful. The presence of a few petechiae and bruises often goes along with an indolent clinical course and rare major bleeding complications. Patients who have significant petechiae, ecchymoses, and hematomas as well as occult blood in the stool often have a severe thrombocytopenia and a major risk for additional bleeding.

Evaluation of Thrombocytopenia

Whether to evaluate for thrombocytopenia and how to evaluate for thrombocytopenia depend on the symptoms and the platelet count. Most symptomatic patients, those with moderate-to-severe thrombocytopenia (platelets less than 50,000/μL), and those with concomitant anemia and/or leukopenia will usually require a complete evaluation. The extent of evaluation of mild decreases in platelet counts (50,000/μL) in asymptomatic individuals remains one of physician preference, patient concern, and plan for surgical procedures.

DIAGNOSIS

Thrombocytopenia: Who Needs Evaluation?

Patients with hemorrhagic or thrombotic symptoms. Symptomatic patients have platelet counts well below 50,000/μL, often less than 10,000/μL, and lack primary hemostasis. The presence of concomitant platelet dysfunction often exacerbates the bleeding problem. Paradoxically, thrombotic symptoms also occur in thrombocytopenic patients and warrant immediate evaluation for thrombotic microangiopathy, disseminated intravascular coagulation, and heparin-induced thrombocytopenia. **Asymptomatic patients with platelet counts < 50,000/μL.** These patients have a variable risk of spontaneous bleeding but probably have an increased risk of hemorrhage with surgery or procedures. Most have a diagnosable cause for the thrombocytopenia.

Asymptomatic patients with platelet counts < 100,000/μL requiring surgery. For patients with normal platelet function, a platelet count of 50,000/μL provides adequate hemostasis but a value over 100,000/μL may provide an additional margin of safety. A diagnosable cause of the thrombocytopenia is usually uncovered in this group.
Patients who also have red cell or white blood cell abnormalities. Although anemia and/or leukopenia may accompany thrombocytopenia due to autoantibody formation, serious bone marrow processes such as leukemia, aplastic anemia, and myelodysplasia are the major concern here and need to be evaluated.

Platelet Count Less Than 100,000/μL with Central Nervous System, Renal, or Thrombotic/Hemorrhagic Symptoms

A first principle in evaluating thrombocytopenic patients is to rule out thrombotic microangiopathy, acute disseminated intravascular coagulation, heparin-induced thrombocytopenia, and acute bleeding. Patients with renal dysfunction and/or CNS symptoms require an immediate emergency evaluation of the blood smear, bilirubin, lactate dehydrogenase (LDH), haptoglobin, D-dimer/fibrin degradation products, PT, PTT, and reticulocyte count to assess for thrombotic thrombocytopenic purpura/hemolytic uremic syndrome and acute disseminated intravascular coagulation. If on heparin, a platelet factor 4-heparin antibody test should be performed if available. A computed tomography (CT) scan will determine whether acute central nervous system or retroperitoneal bleeding is occurring.

Platelet Counts 150,000/μL to 100,000/μL, Normal Red and White Blood Cell Counts, Asymptomatic, More Than 1 Year Duration

Patients with a long history of mild thrombocytopenia and prior stable platelet counts probably require no specific evaluation except for review of medications, physical examination to assess spleen size, an analysis of the smear, review of the platelet histogram, and a mean platelet volume (MPV). Autoimmune testing (anticardiolipin antibody, antinuclear antibody, rheumatoid factor, antithyroid antibodies, direct antiglobulin test) and erythrocyte sedimentation rate may be done in those with a family history or symptoms of such disorders. Many of these patients have no firm diagnosis or

will have mild splenomegaly or mild autoimmune disease or be considered a normal variant. On review of these findings, reassurance is usually given and a recommendation that platelet counts be followed every six months for two years, then annually.

Platelet Counts 100,000/μL to 50,000/μL, Normal Red and White Blood Cell Counts, Asymptomatic

Most patients will be asymptomatic and will have adequate hemostasis for most surgical procedures. Evaluation in this group is quite variable but usually includes a physical examination assessing spleen size, review of the peripheral blood smear, and review of the platelet histogram and mean platelet volume as well as blood tests looking for the presence of autoimmune processes and occasionally a toxic screen in those in whom a drug abuse history cannot be conclusively ruled out. HIV testing in those with risk factors is recommended. Renal function tests, lactate dehydrogenase, bilirubin direct/total, and urinalysis are done to exclude mild chronic thrombotic microangiopathy and a fibrinogen, PT and PTT, and D-dimer test are done to exclude chronic disseminated intravascular coagulation. If these tests are unremarkable, patients are followed every three to six months for approximately two years to assess stability of counts. If any of the aforementioned autoimmune tests are positive, such as antinuclear antibody and/or antithyroid antibody test, the presumption is that these patients have mild immune-based thrombocytopenia and, in the absence of symptoms, warrant no therapy at these platelet counts but do deserve frequent follow-up.

Platelet Counts Less Than 50,000/μL and/or Abnormalities of Red or White Blood Cell Counts

The extent of symptoms in this patient group varies enormously. The evaluation of these patients includes all the studies done for those with thrombocytopenia ranging from 100,000/μL to 50,000/μL but in addition includes a stool guaiac test to assess for blood loss and a bone marrow examination to assess the adequacy of megakaryocyte production.

The Role of Bone Marrow Analysis and Antiplatelet Antibodies

Bone Marrow Analysis

When to perform a bone marrow analysis is always an issue. Most thrombocytopenic patients do not require a bone marrow biopsy and aspirate for diagnosis. However, this procedure is indicated in all patients with severe thrombocytopenia when diagnosis and therapy will be affected by bone marrow findings. A common concern is that bone marrow biopsy in the thrombocytopenic patient presents a significant bleeding risk; however, significant bleeding is uncommon and does not mandate prophylactic platelet transfusions. The rationale for performing a bone marrow analysis is to assess the adequacy of bone marrow stores of megakaryocytes as well as to observe any associated red cell or white cell disorder. Not until the platelet count declines below approximately 50,000/μL can changes in megakaryocyte number be assessed histologically (Figure 36-1). The linear decline in platelet count is related to a logarithmic rise in megakaryocyte number and ploidy. In patients with thrombocytopenia as the only presenting hematologic

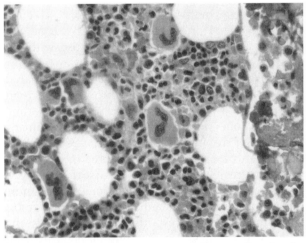

Figure 36-1 ■ Bone marrow megakaryocytes in immune thrombocytopenic purpura. Bone marrow biopsy of patient with chronic immune thrombocytopenic purpura showing a four-fold to five-fold increase in megakaryocyte number. (See Color Plate 2.)

finding, a bone marrow performed in patients whose platelet counts are above 50,000/μL is usually not informative about the megakaryocyte content.

A bone marrow aspirate and usually a biopsy should be performed in the following situations:

1. Two or more lineages are abnormal except in clear cases of thrombotic thrombocytopenic purpura/hemolytic uremic syndrome or Evans syndrome.
2. There is no clear explanation for the moderate or severe thrombocytopenia.
3. Symptoms demand a rapid answer.
4. Platelet count is less than 50,000/μL and especially if it is less than 20,000/μL.

Antiplatelet Antibody Testing

In most cases of thrombocytopenia, antiplatelet antibody tests are of little help. The sensitivity and specificity of these antibody tests appear poor, and these tests have little predictive value with regard to the diagnosis of thrombocytopenia. In their current formats, such antiplatelet antibody testing cannot be recommended.

Diagnosis of the Cause of Thrombocytopenia

Table 36-1 summarizes the relevant causes of thrombocytopenia.

Artifactual and Cell Counter Abnormalities

During the collection and processing of blood for routine complete blood count, temperature or antibody-mediated phenomenon can cause platelet clumping as can an inadequate amount of anticoagulant. These result in platelet clumps that yield a low platelet count when blood cells are counted by automated instrumentation. An example of such clumped platelets is provided in Figure 36-2 in which an asymptomatic patient was found to have a platelet count of 2,000/μL. However, on evaluation of the smear, the patient had a normal number of platelets, most of which had been clumped. If clumping recurs, the problem can usually be resolved by drawing the sample into an acid-citrate-dextrose or heparin tube at 37° and performing the analysis immediately. Another problem with automated platelet counts is the fact that the cell counter "gates" for the platelet "window" may be too narrow to count all of the larger platelets. This problem is best assessed by analyzing the platelet size histogram or by reviewing the blood smear. A hint of the presence of large platelets is an increased mean platelet volume.

Dilutional Thrombocytopenia

Thrombocytopenia in hospitalized patients occurs following the transfusion of large amounts of red blood cells after major trauma or major surgery complicated

Table 36-1 ▪ Causes of Thrombocytopenia

Artifact or cell counter problem
Dilution
Splenic sequestration
Decreased production
    Primary bone marrow disorders
        Aplastic anemia
        Myelodysplasia
        Acute leukemia
        Familial thrombocytopenia
        Thrombocytopenia with absent radius syndrome
    Infection
        HIV
    Toxins/drugs
    Radiation
    Vitamin/nutritional deficiencies
        Vitamin B_{12}
        Iron deficiency, severe
    Metabolic disorders
        Hypothyroidism
        Adrenal insufficiency
        Gaucher's disease
    Thrombopoietin deficiency
    Thrombopoietin receptor defect
Increased destruction
    Nonimmune
        Disseminated intravascular coagulation
        Thrombotic thrombocytopenic purpura
        Hemolytic uremic syndrome
        Giant cavernous hemangiomas
        Burns
        Sepsis
        Continuous venovenous hemofiltration
        Renal transplant rejection
        Intra-aortic balloon pump
        Cyclosporin A therapy
        Von Willebrand disease, type 2b
    Immune
        Fab-mediated
            Immune thrombocytopenic purpura
                Drug-associated
                Idiopathic
            Posttransfusion purpura
            Neonatal, isoimmune thrombocytopenia
        Fc-mediated
            Heparin
                Immune complex

by a bleeding. Since packed red blood cells are mostly used in this situation, there is a decline in the platelet count in these bleeding patients.

Splenomegaly

The platelet count declines inversely and proportionally to increasing spleen size owing to splenic sequestration. The platelet mass, not the platelet count, is regulated in normal physiology, and approximately one third of the total platelet mass is normally sequestered in the spleen. Commonly, platelet counts of 50,000/μL to 70,000/μL have been found in individuals with cirrhosis and associated splenomegaly and have been presumed to be due to splenic sequestration. More recent data suggest a more complicated mechanism of thrombocytopenia in liver disease. Since the liver is the primary site of production of the major regulator of platelet production, thrombopoietin, recent studies suggest that some if not all of the thrombocytopenia associated with liver disease might be due to diminished thrombopoietin production.

Decreased Platelet Production

As listed in Table 36-1, a large number of disorders ranging from metabolic disorders to toxin/drug exposure to inherited or acquired problems of marrow function is associated with thrombocytopenia. The thrombocytopenia is associated with a decrease in megakaryocyte number, size, and ploidy; however, there are exceptions to this concept of decreased platelet production being associated with decreased bone marrow megakaryocytes. "Ineffective thrombopoiesis" (decreased platelet production from a normal or often increased megakaryocyte mass) accounts for the thrombocytopenia associated with HIV infection, B_{12} deficiency, and some patients with myelodysplastic syndrome.

Increased Destruction

Normal platelet survival ranges from 7 to 10 days. This normal clearance mechanism of the platelet may be augmented in thrombocytopenic disorders by nonimmune or immune mechanisms. Nonimmune causes of increased platelet consumption include acute and chronic disseminated intravascular coagulation, thrombotic thrombocytopenic purpura, and hemolytic uremic syndrome as well as the rare vascular abnormalities such as giant cavernous hemangiomas or von Willebrand disease, type IIB. Burns, rejection of transplanted kidney, use of cyclosporin A, continuous venovenous hemofiltration (CVVH), and intra-aortic balloon pump (IABP) counterpulsation are all commonly associated with thrombocytopenia. Sepsis can also induce thrombocytopenia in the absence of disseminated intravascular coagulation. Immune consumption of platelets depends on the presence of antibody binding either directly to platelet antigens via its Fab region or to the platelet Fc receptor by the antibody Fc portion in antigen-antibody complexes; both lead to removal of platelets by the spleen and liver. In addition, the presence of antibody directed against platelet antigens may lead to platelet dysfunction, whereas the binding of antigen-antibody com-

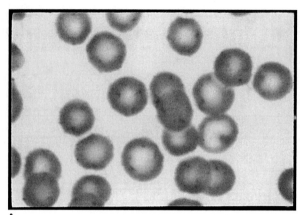
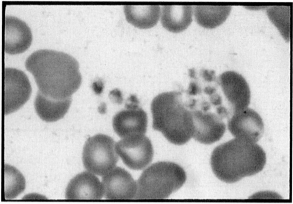

A   B

Figure 36-2 ■ Platelet clumping. Peripheral blood smear of patient showing no platelets in one field (*A*) but large platelet clumps in another field (*B*). (See Color Plate 2.)

DIAGNOSIS

Thrombocytopenia: The Complete Evaluation

History. Assess for bleeding/thrombotic symptoms, duration of thrombocytopenia, exposure to drugs and toxins, recent vaccinations, family history, and ethnic origin. Review old medical records to assess prior blood counts and abnormalities in red and white blood cells.

Physical examination. Look for signs of hemorrhage (petechiae, ecchymoses, and occult blood in stool), thrombosis, adenopathy, hepatosplenomegaly, and liver disease.

Review complete blood count, peripheral blood smear, and platelet histogram. This will exclude artifactual causes of thrombocytopenia and provide information about platelet size and granularity as well as red and white blood cell morphology. The presence of schistocytes, spherocytes, polychromatophilic red blood cells, or atypical white blood cells (i.e., Pelger-Huet cells) should be specifically noted.

Exclude disseminated intravascular coagulation/ thrombotic thrombocytopenic purpura/ hemolytic uremic syndrome/heparin-induced thrombocytopenia. Chronic and acute disseminated intravascular coagulation can be assessed with prothrombin time, partial thromboplastin time, fibrinogen, and D-dimer (or fibrin degradation products). Check blood urea nitrogen, creatinine, lactate dehydrogenase, bilirubin (direct and total), urinalysis, and haptoglobin to assess for thrombotic thrombocytopenic purpura/hemolytic uremic syndrome. If the patient is on heparin, check PF4-heparin antibody test.

Exclude HIV infection. Both early and late disease can be associated with thrombocytopenia.

Assess for autoimmune disorders. Since thrombocytopenia accompanies so many autoimmune processes, direct antiglobulin test, antinuclear antibody, antithyroid antibody, antiphospholipid antibody, and erythrocyte sedimentation rate should identify these.

Consider metabolic disorders and von Willebrand disease. Cortisol, thyroid-stimulating hormone, glucocerebrosidase activity, and von Willebrand's panel will assess these possibilities.

Perform bone marrow examination. An aspirate and biopsy will distinguish decreased platelet production from increased platelet destruction as well as provide important information about marrow cellularity and the red and white blood cell precursors.

plexes to the Fc receptor may cause platelet aggregation, such as occurs in heparin-induced thrombocytopenia. The Fab-mediated processes include neonatal isoimmune thrombocytopenia, the rare but probably underdiagnosed posttransfusion purpura, and immune thrombocytopenic purpura. Fc-mediated responses depend on the presence of a drug such as heparin or the presence of immune complexes such as in HIV disease.

Thrombocytosis/Thrombocythemia

Disorders of elevated platelet counts are divided into benign reactive causes and malignant causes due usually to myeloproliferative disorders and, occasionally, myelodysplastic syndromes. The benign causes have been historically called "thrombocytosis" and are not associated with clotting risks; the platelet count elevation here is usually an acute phase reaction. The

DIAGNOSIS

Elevated Platelet Count: Who Needs Evaluation?

Patients with thrombosis and/or hemorrhage. Although most patients have reactive thrombocytosis and no related symptoms, the presence of symptoms heightens the concern for myeloproliferative or myelodysplastic disorders. These symptomatic patients may have platelets with either increased or decreased function.

Asymptomatic patients with persistent (>3 month) platelet count elevations over 450,000/μL. These patients will have either myeloproliferative disorder of myelodysplastic syndrome, splenectomy, or a reactive thrombocytosis due to iron deficiency, infection/inflammation, or malignancy. **Patients with associated abnormalities in red or white blood cells.** Thrombocythemia is seen in all of the myeloproliferative disorders, and elevated red or white blood cell values help to confirm the diagnosis of polycythemia vera, chronic myeloid leukemia, or agnogenic myeloid metaplasia. Patients with thrombocythemia and unexplained anemia or leukopenia should be evaluated for myelodysplasia (the 5q⁻ syndrome).

malignant causes have been referred to as "thrombocythemia" and are considered to have an increased thrombotic or bleeding risk. Most cases of elevated platelet counts are "reactive."

Relationship of Platelet Count to Thrombosis Risk

There is little to suggest that an elevated platelet count is an independent thrombotic risk factor in patients with reactive thrombocytosis. A possible exception to this may be in patients with malignant solid tumors with venous thrombosis. In contrast, 75% of patients with thrombocythemia due to myeloproliferative disorders do have an increased thrombosis risk. These thrombi are often arterial, involving digits, the central nervous system, and fundi; less common are venous clots, although hepatic vein thrombosis (Budd-Chiari syndrome) occurs with increased frequency in this patient group. The exact relationship of this increased risk to the platelet count rise and the type of myeloproliferative disorder is unclear. Some patients with essential thrombocythemia and platelet counts of 350,000/μL on treatment may have thrombosis, whereas some untreated essential thrombocythemia patients with platelet counts over 1 million/μL may have no problems for decades. Variations in the platelet function may account for these differences. Age may also be a relevant variable, since several studies have showed increased thrombosis in essential thrombocythemia patients over age 60 years. Thrombocythemia associated with polycythemia vera may be more thrombogenic than that in patients with essential thrombocythemia. Paradoxically, about 25% of patients with thrombocythemia due to myeloproliferative disorders (and many with elevated platelet counts due to myelodysplasia) have bleeding problems. The elevated platelet count in these bleeding patients is usually accompanied by a significant decrease in platelet function.

Presenting Symptoms

Most patients undergoing evaluation for an elevated platelet count are referred solely because of a numeric elevation and are asymptomatic. Those with reactive thrombocytosis will rarely have thrombotic or bleeding symptoms; almost all of their symptoms are attributable to the underlying associated conditions. In those with thrombocythemia, arterial thrombotic symptoms predominate and include stroke, transient ischemic attacks, visual field losses/blindness, digital ischemia/infarction/necrosis, myocardial infarction/ischemia, and bowel infarction. Erythromelalgia (transient painful erythema of the hands and feet) is associated with myeloproliferative disorders. Less common events in thrombocythemia are hepatic vein obstruction with abdominal pain, ascites, and jaundice or mesenteric or splenic artery thrombosis. Bleeding is found in a minority of thrombocythemic patients.

Patient History

The goal of the history is to elicit thrombotic symptoms and to distinguish reactive causes of platelet elevation from those due to myeloproliferative disorders or myelodysplastic syndromes. Since reactive thrombocytosis is the more common, close attention should be paid to infectious or inflammatory symptoms. A personal or family history of systemic lupus erythematosus, rheumatoid arthritis, thyroiditis, and inflammatory bowel disease should specifically be queried, as should recent bacterial infections such as pneumonia or cellulitis. Joint pain, joint stiffness, and the presence of skin rashes are symptoms of special importance. A history of iron deficiency or surgical splenectomy should be elicited. A history of elevated hemoglobin or white blood cells, pruritus, and splenomegaly with or without splenic infarction may be found in patients with myeloproliferative disorder; anemia or leukopenia suggests myelodysplastic syndrome. Bone pain and nights sweats are common in chronic myeloid leukemia and myeloid metaplasia. A history of arterial or venous thrombosis should be determined. Patients should be questioned about prior cerebrovascular accident, myocardial infarction, retinal infarctions, retinal "blind spots," and digital ischemia as well as the presence of erythromelalgia.

In evaluating both thrombocytosis and thrombocythemia, medical records documenting the duration and extent of the elevated platelet count are helpful.

Physical Examination

The goal in the physical examination is to distinguish thrombocythemia from reactive thrombocytosis and to uncover evidence of prior thrombosis. Splenomegaly and hepatomegaly are found in myeloproliferative disease. Pallor may indicate myelofibrosis or myelodysplastic syndrome, whereas plethora and conjunctival suffusion would suggest polycythemia vera. Evidence of digital ischemia or the presence of erythromelalgia favor thrombocythemia. Joint pain, stiffness, effusion, or skin rash would be consistent with reactive thrombocytosis, as would the absence of hepatomegaly or splenomegaly. Temperature elevation, skin rash, and signs of chronic infection should be assessed. More subtle findings of chronic infection such as dental abscesses, infected sebaceous cysts, chronic prostatitis, and chronic urinary tract infections are often missed.

Evaluation of the Elevated Platelet Count

Physicians are called to evaluate a platelet count elevation in two general situations. The first is the hospitalized medical or surgical patient with a de novo documented platelet count elevation. These are usually reactive and transient and require minimal evaluation. The second is usually in the outpatient setting of a patient who has had a persistent platelet count elevation over 450,000/μL for over several months. In both circumstances, the physician is called on to answer four general questions: Why is the platelet count elevated? What is the thrombosis risk? Can any of the patient's symptoms be ascribed to the elevated platelet count? What is the appropriate therapy?

Hospitalized Medical/Surgical Patients

Except in the rather uncommon situation of a patient with previously undiagnosed myeloproliferative disorder presenting with arterial thrombosis, the elevated platelet count in this patient group is usually a reactive thrombocytosis and has no thrombosis risk. The elevated platelet count should be documented by reviewing the smear, platelet histogram, and mean platelet volume. Review of the medical record to demonstrate a recently normal platelet count should suffice to exclude thrombocythemia and should also allow one to uncover recent surgical procedures, infections, gastrointestinal bleeding, inflammatory problems, or recent thrombocytopenia that have incited the increased platelet count. Serum iron, total iron-binding capacity, ferritin, erythrocyte sedimentation rate, and C-reactive protein as well as an antinuclear antibody and rheumatoid factor help to document iron deficiency and inflammatory causes of reactive thrombocytosis. Platelet counts over 1 million/μL can be observed in patients with multiple reactive causes, such as inflammatory bowel disease with concomitant iron deficiency. Bone marrow biopsy is rarely revealing, and the reactive thrombocytosis usually resolves with treatment of the underlying disease.

Outpatients with Persistent Platelet Counts Greater Than 450,000/μL

Platelet counts persistently elevated above 450,000/μL warrant evaluation to distinguish reactive thrombocytosis from thrombocythemia. Although the median platelet count in reactive thrombocytosis is less than that of patients with thrombocythemia, the use of a platelet count of 1 million/μL to distinguish between these two types of disorders is untested and unreliable. Most patients are asymptomatic and have a reactive thrombocytosis. History, lack of thrombotic events, and absence of splenomegaly often point to one of the causes of reactive thrombocytosis. The peripheral blood smear, platelet histogram, mean platelet volume, serum iron, total iron-binding capacity, ferritin, erythrocyte sedimentation rate, C-reactive protein, antinuclear antibody, and rheumatoid factor may help to confirm this impression. Chronic urinary tract infections, dental abscesses, chronic prostatitis, and osteomyelitis may be associated with thrombocytosis.

In the absence of iron deficiency, inflammation, or infection, the likelihood of a thrombocythemic disorder increases. An elevated hemoglobin and red blood cell mass help to diagnose polycythemia vera, whereas an increased white blood cell count and presence of the bcr/abl translocation will diagnose chronic myeloid leukemia. Anemia and a leukoerythroblastic blood smear with teardrop erythrocytes should prompt evaluation by bone marrow biopsy of agnogenic myeloid metaplasia; skeletal radiographs may also show osteosclerosis. Many patients will present with a several-year history of elevated platelet count, modest leukocytosis, and normal hemoglobin. If the mean cell volume is normal and iron saturation is normal (to exclude patients with polycythemia vera who are iron deficient), most such individuals probably do not need a bone marrow examination to exclude polycythemia vera, chronic myeloid leukemia, or agnogenic myeloid metaplasia. If the platelet count is greater than 600,000/μL, the patient can be presumed to have essential thrombocythemia (or early polycythemia vera with thrombocytosis). If the platelet count is 450,000 to 600,000/μL, no clear diagnosis of essential thrombocythemia can be made. Many patients probably have an early myeloproliferative disease, and this can sometimes be supported by a bone marrow examination that demonstrates features of myeloproliferative disease, specifically hypercellularity and increased megakaryocytes. Patients with anemia or leukopenia accompanying the elevated platelet count usually either have the "spent phase" of myeloproliferative disease or have myelodysplastic syndrome. A bone marrow examination with chromosome analysis is helpful to distinguish between these disorders. Patients with the spent phase of myeloproliferative disease usually have splenomegaly.

Diagnosis of the Cause of Elevated Platelet Count

Table 36-2 lists the common causes of elevated platelet counts.

Table 36-2 ▪ Causes of Thrombocytosis

Artifact or cell counter problem
Postsplenectomy
Reactive thrombocytosis
  Acute hemorrhage
  Iron deficiency
  Infection/inflammation
  Rebound thrombocytosis
  Malignancy
Familial thrombocytosis
Thrombocythemia
  Myeloproliferative disorders
    Essential thrombocythemia
    Polycythemia vera
    Chronic myeloid leukemia
    Agnogenic myeloid metaplasia with myelofibrosis
  Myelodysplastic syndromes
    5q- syndrome
    3q21q26 syndrome

Artifactual or Cell Counter Problem

Small circulating blood particles may be mistakenly counted as platelets. The typical situation is in patients with severe autoimmune hemolytic anemia, in whom small red cell fragments may be erroneously counted as platelets. The presence of Howell-Jolly bodies in red cells can also lead to reports of high platelet counts. A manual count or review of the smear assesses for this possibility; a manual check of the blood smear is a part of most laboratory procedures.

Postsplenectomy

Approximately one third of the body's platelet mass is sequestered in the spleen, where it is readily exchangeable with the circulating platelets. Since the body regulates the entire body platelet mass, when the spleen is removed, the platelet count three to four months later assumes a new steady state value that is about 40% to 50% higher than the preoperative value. If a patient has a preoperative platelet count of 400,000/μL, near the upper limit of normal, then several months later the postoperative platelet count can be 600,000/μL. It should also be noted that many patients immediately postsplenectomy have a characteristic transient platelet count rise to well over 1 million/μL that is due to perioperative inflammation and possibly some indirect early effect of splenic removal on thrombopoiesis.

Reactive Thrombocytosis

Acute Hemorrhage
The platelet count acutely rises within 24 hours of major hemorrhage.

Iron Deficiency
Thrombocytosis occurs in moderate-to-severe iron deficiency by a nonthrombopoietin mechanism. With very severe iron deficiency, hematopoiesis declines, and thrombocytopenia occurs.

Infection/Inflammation
The platelet count behaves as an acute phase reactant. In situations in which the fibrinogen and sedimentation rate are elevated, the platelet count is commonly increased. This is probably mediated by interleukin-6 (IL-6), a potent stimulator of platelet production.

Rebound Thrombocytosis
After any severe thrombocytopenia, the normal physiological response mechanisms produce a rebound thrombocytosis that peaks four to ten days later and then resolves. The extent of the rebound is inversely proportional to the extent and duration of the preceding thrombocytopenia. A common example

DIAGNOSIS

Elevated Platelet Count: The Complete Evaluation

History. Assess for prior thrombosis, erythromelalgia, and hemorrhage. Inquire about iron deficiency (pica, prior iron therapy, and blood loss). Review old blood counts to determine the duration of platelet findings and concomitant red and white blood cell values.

Physical examination. The presence of hepatosplenomegaly, plethora, erythromelalgia, or digital ischemia/infarction would suggest myeloproliferative disease or, rarely, myelodysplasia. Abdominal ultrasound or computed tomography may be needed to assess spleen size in some patients. Signs of inflammation (malar rash, joint stiffness/erythema/swelling), infection (cutaneous ulcer, fistulae), or iron deficiency (angular stomatitis, nail changes, pica) would indicate a reactive process. The presence of adenopathy would suggest an infectious or malignant etiology.

Review complete blood count, peripheral blood smear and platelet histogram. These tests confirm the platelet count elevation and provide information about platelet size and granularity. Rouleauxed or hypochromic/microcytic red cells would suggest reactive thrombocytosis, whereas teardrop red cells, elevated white blood cell count, leukoerythroblastic findings, or Pelger-Huet cells would suggest myelodysplasia or myeloproliferative syndrome. Howell-Jolly bodies and nucleated red blood cells suggest asplenia.

Evaluate for causes of reactive thrombocytosis. Send Fe, total iron-binding capacity, ferritin, urine culture, sedimentation rate, C-reactive protein, antinuclear antibody, and rheumatoid factor to evaluate for iron deficiency, infection, and inflammation. Panorex films of teeth are considered in those with dental symptoms.

If no reactive etiology is found, evaluate for myeloproliferative disease/myelodysplastic syndrome. Elevated hemoglobin or white blood count should prompt direct assessment for polycythemia vera or chronic myeloid leukemia. A bone marrow evaluation is often indicated to distinguish agnogenic myeloid metaplasia and myelodysplastic syndrome from essential thrombocythemia.

---

of this is the rebound thrombocytosis that occurs after resolution of an acute drug-induced thrombocytopenia.

Malignancy

Thrombocytosis is seen in less than 10% of malignancies at diagnosis. The elevation in platelet count is probably due to inflammation and inflammatory cytokines. Thrombocytosis is associated with an increased risk of thrombosis, but whether this is a risk factor independent of other tumor procoagulants is unclear.

Familial Thrombocytosis

Four families have been described that have a defect in the regulatory sequences of the thrombopoietin gene that result in increased production of thrombopoietin and platelet counts up to 1 million/μL.

Thrombocythemia

Myeloproliferative Disorders

All of the myeloproliferative disorders may be associated with thrombocythemia and an increased risk of thrombosis or bleeding. The platelets that are synthesized in these disorders are dysplastic and are characterized by either increased or decreased function.

Essential thrombocythemia is defined as a platelet count over 600,000/μL in the absence of causes for reactive thrombocytosis and not associated with an elevated red blood cell mass, Philadelphia chromosome, or significant marrow fibrosis. The thrombocythemia associated with polycythemia vera may precede the elevated red cell mass by years. The thrombocythemia associated with chronic myeloid leukemia is usually seen simultaneously with the elevated white blood cell count. In agnogenic myeloid metaplasia with myelofibrosis, massive splenomegaly and a leukoerythroblastic blood smear accompany mild thrombocytosis.

Myelodysplastic Syndromes

Although most patients with myelodysplastic syndrome have thrombocytopenia, a small group with the 5q- syndrome or the 3q21q26 syndrome has elevated platelet counts.

Suggested Reading

Harker LA: Kinetics of thrombopoiesis. J Clin Invest 1968; 47:458–465.

Harker LA: Regulation of thrombopoiesis. Am J Physiol 1970;218(5):1376–1380.

Harker LA, Finch CA: Thrombokinetics in man. J Clin Invest 1969;48:963–974.

Kuter DJ: The physiology of platelet production. Stem Cells 1996;14(Suppl 1):88–101.

Kuter D: The regulation of platelet production. In Kuter DJ, Hunt P, Sheridan W, and Zucker-Franklin D (eds): Thrombopoiesis and Thrombopoietins: Molecular, Cellular, Preclinical and Clinical Biology, Totowa, NJ, Humana Press, 1997, pp 377–395.

Kuter DJ. Megakarypoiesis and thrombopoiesis. In Beutler E, Lichtman MA, Coller BS, Kipps TJ, and Seligsohn U (eds): Williams' Hematology, 6th ed., New York: McGraw-Hill, 2001, pp 1339–1356.

Chapter 37
Anemia

William C. Aird

An operational definition of anemia is a hemoglobin or hematocrit value lower than two standard deviations below the mean. The normal range for the hemoglobin and hematocrit varies according to age, sex, and altitude of residence. At sea level, normal adult men have a hemoglobin value between 14 and 16 g/dL, while normal menstruating women have a hemoglobin value between 12 and 15.5 g/dL. The higher values in men are due to the androgenic red blood cell stimulus.

A decrease in hemoglobin level reduces the oxygen-carrying capacity of the blood; this can result in a variety of symptoms and physical findings. A number of mechanisms act to reduce the impact of lowered oxygen-carrying capacity in the blood. Increased plasma volume compensates for the loss in total blood volume. The cardiovascular system compensates for the reduced oxygen-carrying capacity of blood by increasing the heart rate and stroke volume. The respiratory rate and tidal volume increase. In the red blood cell, 2,3-diphosphoglycerate derived from the glycolytic pathway, accumulates. The increasing concentration of this normal metabolite shifts the hemoglobin-oxygen dissociation curve so that more oxygen is unloaded to the tissues. When anemia develops gradually over time, the compensatory mechanisms come into play, diminishing potential symptomatology when the patient is at rest. Symptoms of weakness, fatigue, and shortness of breath still may develop on exertion or when underlying cardiac or pulmonary disease impairs the compensatory physiologic responses to anemia. In the absence of substantial organ dysfunction and with the slow onset of anemia, even elderly patients can tolerate hemoglobin levels as low as 7 g/dL. One should bear this in mind in approaching patients with chronic anemia to avoid iron overload from unnecessary transfusions and to minimize the risk of infection from blood products. Red blood cell transfusion in chronic anemia should be administered on the basis of the presence and degree of resulting symptoms and not solely on the hemoglobin and/or hematocrit levels.

History and Physical Examination

A comprehensive medical history may elicit data and/or symptoms that provide useful clues to the cause of anemia (Table 37-1). The ethnic background of the patient and/or a family history of anemia may suggest a congenital cause for the disease, such as an underlying hemoglobinopathy or enzyme deficiency state. The social history, including alcohol use, eating habits, and prior treatment with iron, vitamin B_{12}, or folate, may provide important clues about nutritional deficiencies. Finally, a history of blood transfusion and/or the availability of previously documented blood counts can help to determine whether the anemia is of recent onset or chronic.

On physical examination, the patient with acute bleeding may present with signs of intravascular volume depletion, such as postural changes in blood pressure and heart rate. Nonspecific findings of anemia include pallor of the skin, mucous membranes, nailbeds, palmar creases, and/or conjunctiva. Manifestations of cardiac hyperkinesis may be present, including a bounding pulse, tachycardia, systolic bruits over the carotid arteries, venous hums, or systolic ejection murmurs. Patients with profound anemia or with concomitant medical conditions may show mental status changes and signs of high output cardiac failure. Apart from these general findings, some abnormalities on physical examination may suggest specific types of anemia (Table 37-2). For example, jaundice in the absence of liver disease may be due to hemolysis. Splenomegaly can cause hypersplenism (with reduction in platelets, red blood cells, and/or white blood cells). or can result from splenic hyperplasia due to increased red blood cell clearance in hemolytic anemias. Splenomegaly also raises the question of an underlying lymphoma or myeloproliferative disease. Cutaneous changes can reflect iron deficiency. Angular cheilitis (fissures at the angles of the mouth) and glossitis are observed in patients with nutritional deficiencies. Nail changes, including brittleness and spooning,

Table 37-1 ■ Symptoms or History Associated with Causes of Anemia

Thalassemia

Family history
Mediterranean ethnic background (β-thalassemia)
Asian ethnic background (α-thalassemia)
Prior transfusions
Growth retardation (thalassemia major)
Aplastic crisis
Cholelithiasis with bilirubin gallstones
Leg ulcers

Sickle Cell Disease

Family history
African ethnic background
Vaso-occlusive crises
Recurrent bacterial infections
Growth retardation
Leg ulcers
Priapism
Hematuria
Cerebrovascular accident
Aplastic crises

Iron Deficiency

Pica (craving for and ingestion of ice, starch, clay)
Burning tongue
Chapped lips
Dry skin
Dysphagia: esophageal web formation
Menorrhagia
GI tract blood loss: melena, peptic ulcer disease, hemorrhoids
Hemoptysis
Multiple prior pregnancies
Lead exposure (children)

Vitamin B$_{12}$/Folate Deficiency

Nutritional deficit (either)
Soreness of tongue (either)
Weight loss (either)
Inflammatory small bowel disease of resection (either)
Gastrectomy (vitamin B$_{12}$ deficiency)
Tropical or celiac sprue (folate deficiency)
Alcoholism (folate deficiency)
Paresthesias, unsteady gait, mental status changes (vitamin B$_{12}$ deficiency)

Immune Hemolytic Anemia

Lymphoproliferative disease, connective tissue disease, or HIV infection

Anemia of Chronic Disease

Symptoms of underlying cancer, infection or connective tissue disease

Presence of Liver Disease, Renal Disease, or Hypothyroidism

Table 37-2 ■ Specific Signs in Patients with Anemia

Jaundice

Liver disease
Congenital and acquired hemolytic anemias of diverse causes

Cutaneous Changes in Iron Deficiency

Cheilitis, or fissuring of the angles of the mouth
Glossitis
Dry skin
Nails: brittleness, longitudinal ridging, spooning (koilonychia)

Splenomegaly

Thalassemia
Sickle-cell variants such as sickle-cell disease or sickle thalassemia
Lymphoma
Chronic myeloid or lymphocytic leukemia
Myeloproliferative syndromes

Abnormalities in Vitamin B$_{12}$ Deficiency (Pernicious Anemia)

Glossitis
Vitiligo
Prematurely gray hair
Dorsal column findings

are associated with iron deficiency. Leg ulcers occur in patients with congenital hemolytic anemia, primarily in sickle-cell anemia. The presence of ecchymoses or petechiae raises the possibility of concomitant thrombocytopenia. Findings of chronic liver disease, rheumatoid arthritis, myxedema, or uremia may provide clues about the underlying cause of anemia. Similarly, the presence of abdominal scars from gastrectomy, terminal ileal resection, or splenectomy may help to narrow the differential diagnosis. Changes in gait or loss of position/vibration senses may indicate underlying pernicious anemia (vitamin B$_{12}$ deficiency).

Laboratory Diagnosis

Routine tests in the evaluation of an anemia should include a complete blood count, red blood cell indices, platelet count, examination of a peripheral blood smear, a reticulocyte count, and a bilirubin determination. In conjunction with the clinical presentation and physical findings, the results of these initial studies guide the choice of additional tests. In most cases the history, physical examination, and the following analysis of laboratory studies will obviate the need for a bone marrow aspirate or biopsy in the

DIAGNOSIS

Indications for a Bone Marrow Aspirate and Biopsy in Isolated Anemias

Most cases of isolated anemia can be diagnosed without the need for a bone marrow aspirate or biopsy. This is particularly true for patients with appropriate reticulocyte response (e.g., acute blood loss or hemolysis). In patients with inappropriately low reticulocyte counts, a bone marrow aspirate or biopsy may be helpful in the following situations:

Microcytic anemia. In some patients, suspected iron deficiency may be masked by underlying chronic disease. For example, patients with rheumatoid arthritis and iron deficiency secondary to NSAID-induced gastrointestinal blood loss may have a ferritin within the "normal" range. In these individuals, iron deficiency can be diagnosed by an iron stain of the bone marrow.

Macrocytic anemia. The most common causes of macrocytosis are diagnosed by a combination of history, physical examination, complete blood count, and ancillary blood tests. When the diagnosis is still in doubt, a bone marrow aspirate and biopsy may help to rule out an underlying myelodysplastic syndrome or early aplastic anemia.

Normocytic anemia. The differential diagnosis of normocytic anemia with inappropriate bone marrow response may be divided into systemic diseases and primary bone marrow disorders. If there is no evidence for a nonhematologic disorder (endocrine, liver, renal, chronic inflammatory disease), a bone marrow aspirate and biopsy should be performed to rule out pure red cell aplasia, aplastic anemia, myelodysplastic syndrome, or other infiltrative diseases.

evaluation of anemia, except when infiltration of the bone marrow by a malignant disorder may be the underlying etiology.

Red Blood Cell Indices

Hemoglobin values are expressed as grams of hemoglobin per liter of whole blood. The hematocrit represents the proportion of whole blood that is occupied by red blood cells and is expressed as a percentage. The hemoglobin, hematocrit, and red blood cell count can be used to calculate the red blood cell indices. The indices include the mean corpuscular volume (MCV), which measures red blood cell size, mean corpuscular hemoglobin (MCH), which measures the absolute amount of hemoglobin, and mean corpuscular hemoglobin concentration (MCHC), which measures the concentration of hemoglobin within the red blood cell:

Mean corpuscular volume (fL) = Hematocrit × 10/Red blood cell count ($10^6/\mu L$) resulting in a normal value of 90 fL ± 8 (i.e., 45 × 10/(5 x $10^6/\mu L$))

Mean corpuscular hemoglobin (pg) = Hemoglobin (g/dL) × 10/Red blood cell count ($10^6/\mu L$) resulting in a normal value of 30 pg ± 3 (i.e., 15 × 10/(5 × $10^6/\mu L$))

Mean corpuscular hemoglobin concentration (g/L) = Hemoglobin (g/dL) × 10/Hematocrit or mean corpuscular hemoglobin/mean corpuscular volume resulting in a normal value of 33 g/dL ± 2 (i.e., 15 × 10 /45)

One needs to be aware not only of the range of normal values contained within two standard deviations from the mean of these values, but also of the fact that various changes in red blood cell shape or aggregation can lead to artifactual abnormalities in the indices, which are determined by automated cell counters.

Although all of these indices are of value in the differential diagnosis of anemia, a satisfactory morphologic classification of three subsets of anemias can be based solely on the value of the mean corpuscular volume. Thus anemias can consist of small red blood cells (microcytic) (Figure 37-1), normal size red blood cells (normocytic), or large red blood cells (macrocytic). The red blood cells in microcytic anemias contain reduced amounts of hemoglobin, the mean corpuscular hemoglobin is low, and the cells usually appear hypochromic. The mean corpuscular hemoglobin concentration is usually within the normal range in macrocytic and normocytic anemias, and the cells appear normochromic. The mean corpuscular hemoglobin concentration is helpful in distinguishing among microcytic anemias and is increased in the spherocytic red blood cells of patients who have hereditary spherocytosis or acquired warm antibody-mediated hemolytic anemia, because the cell water content is reduced in these disorders. Table 37-3 lists the common disorders associated with either hypochromic, microcytic indices, macrocytosis, or normocytic red blood cells. This preliminary classification provides a basis for the further investigation of the underlying cause of the anemia.

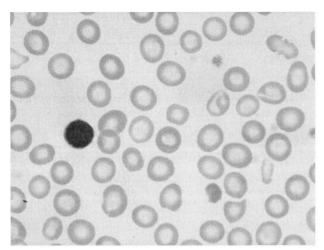

Figure 37-1 ■ Hypochromic red blood cells. Many are also microcytic (original magnification ×100, oil). (See Color Plate 6, same as Fig. 42-5. Courtesy of Cabello Inchausti B: Chapter 42 of this book.)

Table 37-3 ■ Classification of Anemias on the Basis of the Mean Corpuscular Volume

Microcytic Hypochromic Anemia	Normocytic Anemia
Iron deficiency	Renal disease
Thalassemia	Liver disease
Lead intoxication	Anemia of chronic disease
Anemia of chronic disease	Hematologic malignancies
	Hemolytic anemias
Macrocytic Anemia	Aplastic anemia
Megaloblastic anemia due to:	Pure red cell aplasia
Folate deficiency	Bone marrow infiltration by
Vitamin B$_{12}$ deficiency	fibrosis, metastases
Chemotherapy	Endocrine disorders:
Myelodysplasia	Hypothyroidism
Reticulocytosis > 10%	Hyperthyroidism
Liver disease	Hypogonadism
Postsplenectomy	Hypopituitarism
Alcoholism	

Bear in mind that in patients with a megaloblastic anemia (macrocytic) and simultaneous iron deficiency (microcytic), the mean corpuscular volume may be normal. In myelodysplasia, macrocytosis is a common finding, but a second population of hypochromic microcytic cells is present in some patients (more often in the congenital rather than acquired form), leading to a normal mean corpuscular volume. In this circumstance the variation in cell size (anisocytosis) results in an elevated value for the red cell distribution width (RDW), a measure of the coefficient of variation of red cell volume. The red cell distribution width adds a dimension of information to the mean corpuscular volume. For example, both thalassemia and iron deficiency are microcytic, hypochromic anemias, but the red cell distribution width is elevated in iron deficiency and generally normal in thalassemias, with some exceptions.

Peripheral Smear

Examination of the peripheral blood smear is an essential component in the evaluation of a patient with anemia (see Chapter 42, Morphologic Abnormalities in the Peripheral Blood). Clues to the differential diagnosis are found in studying red cell size, color, and shape and the presence or absence of inclusions (Table 37-4, Figure 37-2). The quantity and morphology of platelets and/or white blood cells may also help to define the problem.

Reticulocytes

As red cell precursors differentiate in the bone marrow, they eventually discard their nucleus (Figure 37-3). The early anucleate cell contains residual RNA and can be detected in the peripheral blood using standard Giemsa stains (polychromatophilic or bluish-red red blood cells), a supravital stain (such as methylene blue showing black clumps of precipitated RNA) (Figure 37-4), or flow cytometry (RNA-containing red blood cells). The reticulocyte count provides important information about whether the bone marrow is appropriately responding to anemia by increasing the bone marrow red blood cell activity, which should result in an increase in reticulocytes. The reticulocyte count is usually reported as a percentage of the total red cell count, but this value may be misleading. For example, a 1% reticulocyte count is normal, representing an absolute count of approximately 50,000/μL, that is, 1% of an average red blood cell count of 5,000,000/μL. If anemia reduces the red blood cell count to half-normal, or 2,500,000/μL, a 1% reticulocyte count would not be normal. It would represent a failure of an appropriate response to the anemia because the absolute reticulocyte count of 25,000/μL indicates half-normal production of red blood cells. To effectively assess the significance of a reticulocyte count, it is well to consider the absolute, rather than the relative, reticulocyte count.

The Diagnostic Approach to Anemia

The red blood cell indices provide a helpful starting point in evaluating an anemia. As shown in Table 37-3, finding a microcytic, hypochromic (decreased mean corpuscular volume), or macrocytic (increased mean corpuscular volume) anemia substantially narrows down the possible etiologies. The next step is to assess the pathophysiology underlying the anemia. Is the

Table 37-4 ■ Evaluation of the Peripheral Blood Smear

Red Blood Cells

Agglutination: in cold antibody autoimmune hemolytic anemia (cold agglutinin disease)
Rouleaux formation: elevated erythrocyte sedimentation rate
Increased central pallor: hypochromic (anemia)
Decreased (absent) central pallor: spherocytic anemia
Increased blue-staining (polychromatophilic) cells: reticulocytosis in hemolytic anemias or acute blood loss

Shape Changes

Pencil- or cigar-shaped cells: iron deficiency anemia
Elliptocytes: hereditary elliptocytosis
Spherocytes: hereditary spherocytosis, warm antibody autoimmune hemolytic anemia
Microspherocytes: microangiopathic hemolytic anemias such as thrombotic thrombocytopenic purpura
Sickle cells: sickle-cell anemia
Teardrop cells: myelofibrosis
Target cells: liver disease, thalassemia, Hb C, iron deficiency anemia
Cell fragments (schistocytes): microangiopathic hemolytic anemia
Burr cells (echinocytes): renal failure
Spur cells (acanthocytes): severe liver disease
"Bite" cells: glucose-6-phosphate dehydrogenase deficiency
Oval macrocytes: megaloblastic anemia
Acanthocytes: postsplenectomy

Inclusions

Basophilic stippling: disordered red blood cell production
Howell-Jolly bodies: asplenia or hyposplenia
Nucleated red blood cells: hyperproliferative marrow or marrow infiltration

White Blood Cells

Increased number: infection, myeloproliferative or lymphoproliferative disorder
Decreased number: decreased bone marrow production
Inclusions such as toxic granulation or Dohle bodies: infection
White blood cell precursors in the circulation: marrow infiltration of diverse causes, bacterial infection, leukemias, myeloproliferative disease
Hypersegmented granulocytes: megaloblastic anemia (vitamin B_{12} or folate (deficiency)
Pelger-Huet cells (binucleate, mature granulocytes): myelodysplasia, myeloproliferative disease, myeloid leukemias

Platelets

Increased number: inflammatory disease, myeloproliferative syndromes, iron deficiency, postsplenectomy
Large platelets: increased bone marrow production in response to peripheral destruction, myeloproliferative syndromes, marrow infiltration

marrow responding adequately or inadequately to the stimulus of anemia and are the red blood cells surviving normally or being destroyed prematurely (or lost because of hemorrhage)? The reticulocyte count provides a simple means of measuring bone marrow erythroid activity. The level of serum bilirubin is a helpful but relatively insensitive indicator of hemolysis. The level of the serum lactate dehydrogenase correlates well with the intensity of hemolysis, whether intravascular or extravascular (e.g., intramedullary). In all cases, the laboratory determinations of blood counts, red blood cell indices, reticulocyte count, and bilirubin are complementary to and not a substitute for careful examination of the peripheral blood smear.

Light microscopic examination offers additional information of great importance about the morphology of the red blood cells, white blood cells, and platelets.

Microcytic, Hypochromic Anemia

Microcytic anemias (mean corpuscular volume less than 80 fL) usually arise from a defect in hemoglobin synthesis and are often associated with hypochromia. The most common causes of microcytic anemia are thalassemia, iron deficiency, and the anemia of chronic disease.

The quantitative abnormalities of globin synthesis, or thalassemias, vary in their severity depending

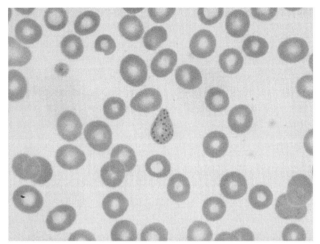

Figure 37-2 ■ Basophilic stippling. Punctate, bluish inclusions throughout the red cell (original magnification ×100 oil). (See Color Plate 8, same as Fig. 42-17. Courtesy of Cabello Inchausti B: Chapter 42 of this book.)

on the number of genes affected and the absence or presence of coinherited hemoglobinopathies. β-thalassemia major is diagnosed in childhood and is associated with severe transfusion-dependent anemia and marked abnormalities on the peripheral smear, while β-thalassemia minor is associated with a milder degree of anemia, less striking morphologic changes, and an elevated hemoglobin A₂ (± increased hemoglobin F) on hemoglobin electrophoresis. In

α-thalassemia, which is also associated with hypochromic, microcytic anemia, the hemoglobin electrophoresis is normal, and the diagnosis is confirmed by more advanced molecular studies. The reticulocyte count is elevated in α- or β-thalassemia and less than normal in iron deficiency and the anemia of chronic disease. However, in patients with thalassemia who develop an aplastic crisis secondary to parvovirus infection or megaloblastic crisis secondary to folate deficiency, the reticulocyte count will be reduced.

In uncomplicated cases of iron deficiency, the serum iron and ferritin are low, and the total iron-binding capacity is elevated. In the presence of systemic illness such as inflammation, infection, or cancer, both the serum iron and the iron-binding capacity fall regardless of the presence or absence of iron deficiency, rendering these iron studies uninterpretable. The serum ferritin is a more reliable determination of the extent of iron stores, even though it can on occasion be mildly falsely elevated (see Chapter 34, Iron Studies) in the setting of inflammatory or infectious disease. Even in these circumstances, one can use an adjusted threshold for the ferritin level in diagnosing iron deficiency. For example, in rheumatoid arthritis a ferritin level less than 40 mg/L (which is in the normal range) indicates that iron deficiency is present. The sine qua non for the diagnosis of iron deficiency anemia is by iron stain of a bone marrow aspirate. This is rarely necessary. Iron deficiency

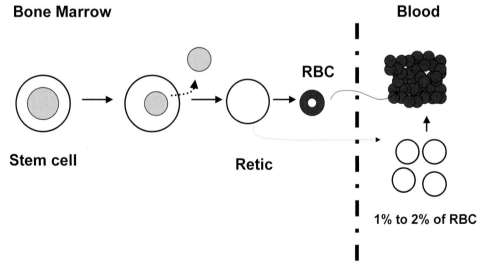

Figure 37-3 ■ Reticulocytes. Red blood cells are derived from erythroid precursor cells in the bone marrow. During differentiation, red blood cells begin to synthesize hemoglobin and lose their nucleus. At this stage, the red blood cell has residual RNA in its cytoplasm. In Giemsa stains, the RNA lends a bluish color to the red of the hemoglobin, resulting in mixing of colors, called polychromatophilia. Supravital stains renders the RNA as blue-black clumps in the reticulocyte. An alternative method for identifying and counting these young red blood cells is by flow cytometry, in which the cells are marked by an RNA-specific fluorophore. In the absence of anemia, reticulocytes normally make up 1% to 2% of the total red blood cell count. Retic = reticulocyte; RBC = red blood cell count.

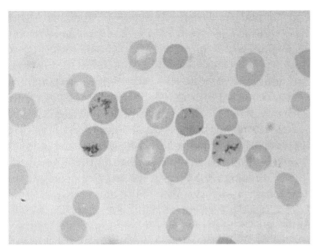

Figure 37-4 ■ Reticulocytes. The structures inside red cells represent precipitated ribonucleoprotein by new methylene blue. On air-dried smears stained with Wright stain, they are polychromatophilic cells (original magnification ×100, oil). (See Color Plate 8, same as Fig. 42–18. Courtesy of Cabello Inchausti B: Chapter 42 of this book.)

anemia always arises from increased demand (childhood or pregnancy) or blood loss. Indeed, in the absence of a history of multiparity or heavy menses in women or at any time in men, the diagnosis of iron deficiency should always trigger an investigation for a source of blood loss. If microcytic hypochromic indices are present and the hemoglobin is 9 g/dL or greater, the anemia is not due to iron deficiency because the indices in iron deficiency anemia remain normochromic and normocytic until the hemoglobin falls below this level.

Microcytic indices occur in 20% to 30% of patients with the anemia of chronic disease. However, in contrast to iron deficiency, the hemoglobin is rarely less than 9 g/dL, and, unlike severe iron deficiency or thalassemia, the mean corpuscular volume is rarely less than 70 fL. A serum ferritin level is helpful in evaluating patients with the anemia of chronic disease for the presence of concurrent iron deficiency. Less common causes of microcytic anemia include the rare congenital sideroblastic anemias, lead poisoning, hemoglobin D, and congenital fragmentation syndromes.

Macrocytic Anemia

The differential diagnosis of macrocytic anemia (mean corpuscular volume greater than 100 fL) includes folate or B_{12} deficiency, drug-induced disorders of DNA synthesis (as occurs after cancer chemotherapy), myelodysplastic syndrome, alcoholism, liver disease, and hypothyroidism (Table 37-3). In all of these cases, the reticulocyte count is reduced, either because of ineffective erythropoiesis in the bone marrow (mega-loblastic anemia and myelodysplasia) or because of increased peripheral destruction (liver disease). As a general rule, a mean corpuscular volume greater than 120 fL is most often associated with a diagnosis of vitamin B_{12} or folate deficiency, whereas a mean corpuscular volume of 100 to 120 fL may arise from any of the aforementioned disorders. One needs to be aware that because reticulocytes are larger than mature red blood cells, an increased reticulocyte count can also cause macrocytosis. The clinical presentation and peripheral smear provide important clues to the diagnosis. The presence of macro-ovalocytes and hypersegmented neutrophils is virtually pathognomonic of folate or vitamin B_{12} deficiency, the finding of target cells and/or acanthocytes is consistent with liver disease, and the presence of Pelger-Huet cells (hyposegmented neutrophils) (Figure 37-5) raises the possibility of myelodysplasia. Concomitant leukopenia and/or thrombocytopenia may be seen in megaloblastic anemias or myelodysplasia.

Normocytic Normochromic Anemia

The differential diagnosis of normocytic anemias includes a myriad of possible causes, including the anemia of chronic disease. The potential causes can be considered in two groups based on the reticulocyte count.

Increased Reticulocyte Count

When anemia is associated with an increased reticulocyte count, the bone marrow is responding appropriately to either blood loss, sequestration in the spleen, or increased red cell destruction (hemolysis). Acute blood loss (Figure 37-6), which can be internal or external, and hypersplenism are usually obvious from the clinical presentation. Intravascular or extravascular hemolysis is supported by the findings of an increased lactate dehydrogenase (LDH) and bilirubin and decreased haptoglobin.

An outline of potential causes of hemolytic anemias appears in Figure 37-7, dividing the causes into immune-mediated and nonimmune-mediated illnesses. Immune-mediated hemolytic anemias are detected by the direct and indirect antiglobulin (Coombs') test or a cold agglutinin screen. Nonimmune-mediated hemolytic anemias may arise from extracorpuscular or intracorpuscular defects. Microangiopathic hemolytic anemias are the most common causes of extracorpuscular hemolysis; the diagnosis requires documentation of red blood cell fragmentation on peripheral smear. In this circumstance, red blood cells are sheared and fragmented into schistocytes due to traumatic injury as they pass through fibrin strands forming in the blood vessels (e.g., in

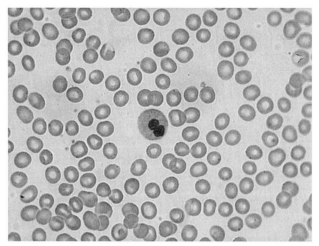

Figure 37-5 ■ Bilobed Pelger-Huet cell (original magnification ×60). (See Color Plate 9, same as Fig. 42-22. Courtesy of Cabello Inchausti B: Chapter 42 of this book.)

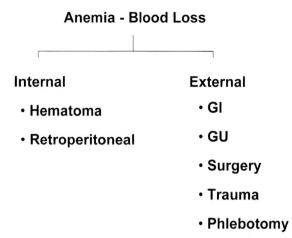

Figure 37-6 ■ Acute blood loss anemia. GI = gastrointestinal; GU = genitourinary.

thrombotic thrombocytopenic purpura and disseminated intravascular coagulation) (Figure 37-8) or are pushed through areas of high-velocity turbulence (e.g., in leaks around heart valves). Microangiopathic hemolytic anemias are frequently accompanied by varying degrees of thrombocytopenia. Thrombotic thrombocytopenic purpura (TTP) and hemolytic

uremic syndrome (HUS) often present with other features, including fever, mental status changes, and/or renal failure. Disseminated intravascular coagulation (DIC) may occur as a complication of sepsis or cancer, while microangiopathies associated with artificial heart valves, drugs, transplantation, pregnancy, or malignant hypertension are diagnosed in the appro-

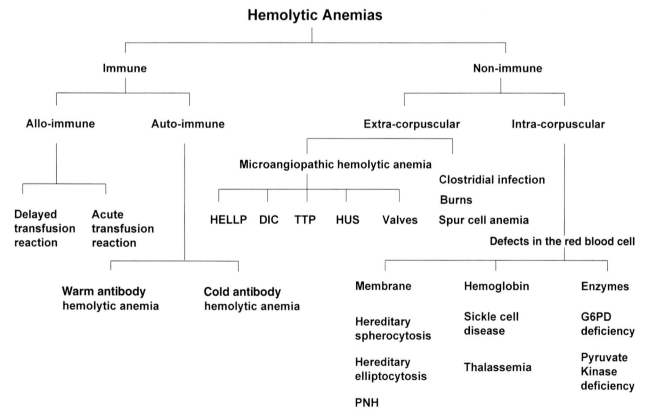

Figure 37-7 ■ Hemolytic anemia. HELLP = hemolytic anemia, elevated liver enzymes and low platelets occurring during pregnancy; DIC = disseminated intravascular coagulation; TTP = thrombotic thrombocytopenic purpura; HUS = hemolytic uremic syndrome; Valves = defective heart valves, PNH = paroxysmal nocturnal hemoglobinuria.

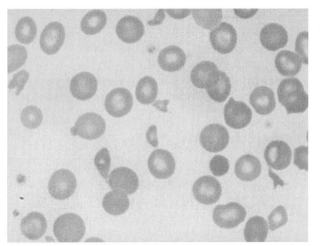

Figure 37-8 ■ Fragmented red cells in a patient with microangiographic hemolytic anemia (original magnification ×100, oil). (See Color Plate 7, same as Fig. 42-7. Courtesy of Cabello Inchausti B: Chapter 42 of this book.)

priate clinical context. The intracorpuscular causes of hemolytic anemia may be divided into those that involve the red cell membrane, hemoglobin mutations, or intracellular enzymes. Acquired red cell membrane abnormalities include spur cell anemia, a rare complication of end-stage liver disease that is associated with the presence of spur cells (also termed acanthocytes) in the peripheral smear.

Paroxysmal nocturnal hemoglobinuria (PNH) is an acquired membrane abnormality that renders the red cell at increased risk for complement-mediated hemolysis. Patients with paroxysmal nocturnal hemoglobinuria may present with a history of nocturnal hematuria and/or thrombosis and may have other cytopenias. While the leukocyte alkaline phosphatase (LAP) score is typically decreased, the diagnosis is confirmed by flow cytometric analyses confirming loss of glycosylphosphatidyl-inositol-anchored proteins, such as CD55 and/or CD59, on the surface of circulating blood cells. Congenital membrane disorders such as hereditary spherocytosis and elliptocytosis are associated with a history of mild anemia and gallstones and the finding of mild splenomegaly. The diagnosis is based on characteristic red cell morphology on the peripheral smear. Sickle-cell anemia is the most common qualitative hemoglobinopathy associated with anemia. The diagnosis is based on the history and the finding of sickled red cells on the peripheral smear and of hemoglobin S on hemoglobin electrophoresis. Enzyme deficiency states (glucose-6-phosphate dehydrogenase or pyruvate kinase deficiency) are commonly associated with a compensated hemolytic anemia and are diagnosed by enzyme assays.

Reduced Reticulocyte Count

An inappropriately low reticulocyte count in the face of an anemia indicates a problem with bone marrow production of red cells. In normochromic normocytic anemias, a low reticulocyte count can be due to the anemia of chronic disease developing iron deficiency anemia (before it becomes hypochromic and microcytic), aplastic anemia, or pure red blood cell aplasia. In the latter two diseases, the reticulocyte count is severely reduced, frequently to less than 0.5%.

DIAGNOSIS

Evaluating a Patient with Anemia

Anemia may gradually appear over 24 to 48 hours after a patient is hospitalized. At bed rest, extravascular fluid reenters the circulation, diluting the concentration of red blood cells reflected in the hemoglobin and hematocrit. This can suggest the presence of a previously unrecognized anemia and does not represent a new development. Similarly, after an acute bleed, the hemoglobin and hematocrit does not fall immediately. The decline is delayed until plasma volume increases in an attempt to maintain euvolemia.

Minimal decrements or increments in hemoglobin and hematocrit outside the normal range may not require further investigation. It is well to remember that 2.5% of the normal population will have values more than two standard deviations from the mean.

An elevated serum bilirubin is frequently sought to document that hemolysis is occurring. A markedly low total bilirubin of 0.1 to 0.3 mg/dL is also a helpful clue to diminished heme production occurring in otherwise uncomplicated iron deficiency anemia, aplastic anemia, or pure red cell aplasia.

A clue to the presence of either red cell aplasia or aplastic anemia is the presence of an extremely low reticulocyte count of 0.1% to 0.4%. The reticulocyte count usually remains normal on a percentage basis in other causes of inadequate erythroid response to anemia such as occurs in the anemia of chronic disease, iron deficiency, or megaloblastic anemia.

Schistocytes characterize all of the microangiopathic hemolytic anemias, but the additional findings on peripheral blood smear of circulating nucleated red blood cells and the presence of microspherocytes (smaller than those generally seen in congenital and acquired spherocytic anemias) are peculiar to thrombotic thrombocytopenic purpura.

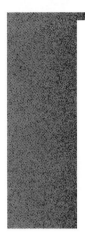

Chapter 38
Quantitative Abnormalities of Leukocytes

Geraldine P. Schechter

Abnormalities in the relative and absolute concentrations of peripheral blood leukocytes frequently provide clues to an underlying diagnosis. The patient's history and physical examination also offer important leads to pursue. Of paramount importance in directing the evaluation of these disorders, and not yet displaced by the advances in flow cytometry, polymerase chain reaction (PCR), or cytogenetic analysis, is the microscopic examination of the peripheral blood smear by an experienced hematologist.

Neutrophilia

Reactive Neutrophilic Leukocytosis

Microbial infection, inflammatory disorders, ischemia with tissue necrosis, and trauma are the most common causes of neutrophilia (absolute concentration of neutrophils greater than 7500/µL) (Table 38-1). Hematologists are usually called in to explain neutrophilia when the referring physician has not identified one of these disorders and therefore entertains a diagnosis of chronic myeloid leukemia or other myeloproliferative disorder. Since infection is so common a cause of neutrophilic leukocytosis, the possibility of occult bacterial infection such as chronic osteomyelitis, endocarditis, intra-abdominal infection, and urinary tract infections must always remain an important consideration. Viral and mycobacterial infections are usually associated with normal leukocyte counts but, when severe, may exhibit marked leukocytosis. Modest neutrophilia is frequently found in patients with inflammatory and autoimmune disorders, such as polyarteritis, Crohn disease, Wegener's granulomatosis, and adult-onset Still disease. Patients with severe alcoholic hepatitis may have marked leukocytosis to levels of 20,000/µL in the absence of infection.

The leukocytosis that is found in certain patients with solid tumor malignancies, particularly lung, epidermoid, gastric, and renal cancers, is associated with endogenous production of granulocyte colony-stimulating factors (G-CSF). These malignancies may not be overt; therefore a screening evaluation for cancer including computed tomography (CT) of the chest and abdomen is indicated in selected patients.

Most patients with serious infection or inflammation will mount a leukocytosis between 10,000/µL and 20,000/µL. White blood cell counts greater than 25,000/µL suggest abscess formation or overwhelming infection. The peripheral blood smear will show a predominance of segmented neutrophils and band neutrophils, usually less than 20% of the latter, but few circulating eosinophils and basophils, presumably owing to stress hormone release. The neutrophils will frequently exhibit enhanced granular staining ("toxic

---

Table 38-1 ■ Causes of Neutrophilia

Infection
Inflammatory disorders
Tissue necrosis, traumatic injury, stress
  Major surgery, burns, myocardial infarction, alcoholic hepatitis
  Seizures, exercise, unipolar depression
Hormones and medications
  Corticosteroids, lithium, granulocyte colony-stimulating factors, GM-CSF, G-ESF
  Pregnancy
Nonhematopoietic malignancies
  Lung, epidermoid, renal, bladder, and many others
    Endogenous tumor CSF or other cytokine production
    Tumor necrosis, undefined stimuli
Clonal myeloproliferative disorders
  Philadelphia chromosome-positive and -negative chronic myeloid leukemia
  Chronic myelomonocytic leukemia
  Polycythemia vera
  Myeloid metaplasia and myelofibrosis
  Chronic neutrophilic leukemia
Hyposplenism and asplenia
Smoking-related
Idiopathic (? hereditary)

granulation," Figure 38-1) and occasionally the pale blue Döhle bodies (Figure 38-2) in the cytoplasm. Immature leukocytes such as metamyelocytes or myelocytes are uncommon and, if present, suggest poor bone marrow reserve or overwhelming infection. Most patients with reactive neutrophilic leukocytosis are easily distinguished from patients with chronic myeloid leukemia in that the numbers of immature myeloid cells are limited and they lack the eosinophils and basophils that make up the "colorful" leukocytosis exhibited by the patients with chronic myeloid leukemia. Bone marrow aspirates and biopsies are usually not necessary; they will simply display a hypercellular marrow without dysplasia and normal percentages of blasts and promyelocytes. The relative frequency of leukemia versus reactive leukocytosis and leukemoid reactions at various levels of neutrophilia is illustrated in Table 38-2.

Leukemoid Reactions

Occasionally, patients with solid tumors or severe infections may have striking elevations in leukocyte counts to greater than 50,000/μL or even 100,000/μL with increased numbers of immature myeloid cells ("shift to the left") mimicking chronic myeloid leukemia sufficiently to be called leukemoid reactions. The diagnostic challenge is to determine whether the neutrophilia is entirely reactive or whether there is a coexisting myeloproliferative disorder. The inexpensive cytochemical stain for leukocyte alkaline phosphatase (LAP) can be useful here; it is elevated in reactive leukocytosis (Figure 38-3) and low in Philadelphia-positive chronic myeloid leukemia. However, an increased leukocyte alkaline phosphatase score is not specific for reactive neutrophilia, since it

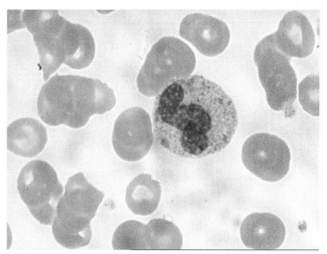

Figure 38-2 ■ Döhle bodies in stress leukocytosis (original magnification ×100, oil). (See Color Plate 3.)

can be found in other myeloproliferative disorders such as polycythemia vera, some cases of myeloid metaplasia, and the rare chronic neutrophilic leukemia.

The presence of nucleated red cell precursors in combination with immature myeloid cells in the peripheral blood defines a leukoerythroblastic reaction and suggests marrow infiltration with metastatic tumor, a clonal myeloproliferation, or myelofibrosis. Therefore for a patient whose peripheral smear shows considerable immaturity or a leukoerythroblastic picture, examination of the bone marrow aspirate and biopsy is an important diagnostic step to confirm metastatic tumor infiltration or a hematopoietic clonal disorder. Breast and prostate cancers metastasizing to the marrow commonly exhibit a leukoerythroblastic picture. Finding marked myeloid immaturity or fibrosis in the marrow is consistent with chronic myeloid leukemia or other myeloproliferative disorders. Patients with an exuberant "leukemoid" but nonleukemic reaction show normal differentiation with predominantly mature myeloid cells and few blasts

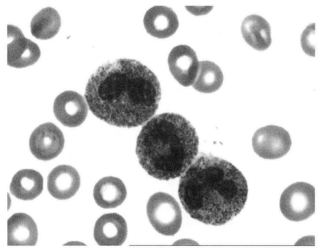

Figure 38-1 ■ Toxic granulation in a patient with neutrophilic leukocytosis (original magnification ×100, oil). (See Color Plate 3.)

Table 38-2 ■ Levels of Neutrophilic Leukocytosis and Likely Diagnosis

WBC	Likely Etiology
<20,000/μL	Reactive leukocytosis >> leukemia
20,000–30,000/μL	Severe infection > leukemia
30,000–50,000/μL	Leukemia > leukemoid reaction (granulocyte colony-stimulating factor related)
50,000–100,000/μL	Leukemia >>> leukemoid reaction
>100,000/μL	Leukemia

WBC (white blood cell count); > (more likely), >> (much more likely); >>> (very much more likely).

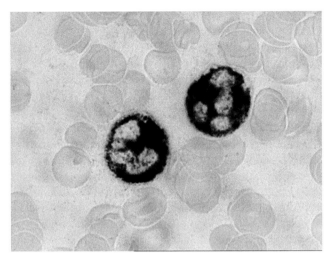

Figure 38-3 ■ Increased leukocyte alkaline phosphatase in a patient with reactive leukocytosis (original magnification ×100, oil). (See Color Plate 3.)

and promyelocytes. Cytogenetic analysis can be useful in distinguishing leukemoid reactions from clonal leukemias when an abnormal karyotype is detected; however, a normal karyotype does not eliminate the possibility of leukemia.

Postsplenectomy Neutrophilia

A portion of the circulating neutrophils is normally sequestered in the splenic circulation. Splenic dysfunction or asplenia is associated with a moderate rise in neutrophils, as is found for example in adult patients with sickle-cell anemia whose spleen has undergone autoinfarction. Splenic dysfunction or asplenia can be recognized by the presence of nuclear fragments (Howell-Jolly bodies; see Figure 42-16 in Chapter 42) in circulating red cells. In the early postoperative period following splenectomy, the rise in white blood cell count is more pronounced, presumably because of the surgical trauma and inflammation in conjunction with the elimination of the sequestration site. With recovery from surgery, the white blood cell count usually decreases to the upper level of the normal range, 10,000 to 12,000/μL.

Other Mild Chronic Neutrophilias

Occasionally, patients are seen who have a chronic mild to moderate neutrophilic leukocytosis, usually less than 16,000/μL, in whom no etiology or associated illness is found after years of follow-up. These outliers may represent a familial neutrophilia. Another possibility to consider is smoking-related leukocytosis. Cigarette smokers as a group have higher average leukocyte counts than do nonsmokers, and some may exceed the normal range. Patients with

unipolar depression may exhibit leukocytosis; however, it is often not clear whether the neutrophilia is drug-induced or secondary to the mood disorder. Lithium increases neutrophil concentrations by stimulating granulocyte colony-stimulating factor production. Since the neutrophilia appears to have little clinical consequence, no intervention is necessary. Systemic corticosteroids, either iatrogenic or endogenous (Cushing disease or adrenal tumors), predictably cause neutrophilia due to marrow stimulation and decreased egress of leukocytes into the tissues.

Rare patients, usually children or adolescents with recurrent infections and leukocytosis, need to be evaluated for congenital leukocyte defects that impair neutrophil function. These entities, including leukocyte adhesion deficiency, Chédiak-Higashi syndrome, and chronic granulomatous disease, are discussed in Chapter 56.

Neutrophilia with Splenomegaly or Peripheral Blood Myeloid Immaturity

The combination of neutrophilia and palpable splenomegaly should immediately suggest a hematopoietic malignancy. Occasionally, lymphomas present with a minor leukocytosis, but more likely, these are the presenting features of clonal myeloproliferative disorders. A patient who exhibits immature leukocytes, including myelocytes, promyelocytes, and blasts in the peripheral blood smear (Figures 38-4 and 38-5) with or without splenomegaly, requires a prompt bone marrow examination with chromosomal analysis. The most common of these disorders is Philadelphia chromosome-positive (Ph-positive) chronic myeloid leukemia, which is easily recognized by the left-shifted myeloid population recapitulating

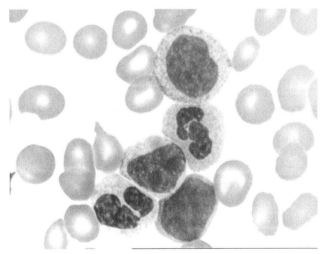

Figure 38-4 ■ Left-shifted myeloid cells in the peripheral blood in a patient with chronic myeloid leukemia (original magnification ×100, oil). (See Color Plate 3.)

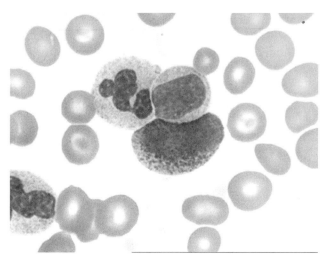

Figure 38-5 ■ Immature myeloid cells in the peripheral blood, including a promyelocyte (original magnification ×100, oil). (See Color Plate 3.)

the cellular distribution of the bone marrow in the peripheral blood accompanied by eosinophils and basophils. The percentage of blasts and promyelocytes in the blood will be less than 10%; if it is higher, a diagnosis of blast crisis of chronic myeloid leukemia or acute leukemia should be considered. Chronic myeloid leukemia patients are commonly anemic and exhibit thrombocytosis, but normal hemoglobin and platelet levels may be seen early in the course, particularly in those diagnosed from a routine complete blood count.

Other myeloproliferative disorders that present similarly include Philadelphia chromosome-negative (Ph-negative) leukemia, polycythemia vera with progression into the so-called spent or burnt-out phase when anemia and leukocytosis become prominent, and myeloid metaplasia with myelofibrosis. Philadelphia chromosome-negative chronic myeloid leukemia may be indistinguishable morphologically from Philadelphia chromosome-positive chronic myeloid leukemia or exhibit an excess of monocytes, making the label of chronic myelomonocytic leukemia more appropriate. A history of previous erythrocytosis is helpful in diagnosing a transformation of polycythemia vera, or abnormal chromosomal abnormalities such as del 20q may suggest it. Marrow fibrosis in a patient with splenomegaly and Philadelphia chromosome-negative chronic myeloid leukemia points to agnogenic myeloid metaplasia with myelofibrosis. The importance of specifically defining these disorders by chromosomal analysis relates to treatment and prognosis, particularly now that targeted therapy against the chronic myeloid leukemia is available. If traditional karyotyping is unrevealing, then fluorescence in situ hybridization (FISH) or polymerase chain reaction should be pursued to identify the bcr-abl translocation. If the bone marrow aspirate is unsuccessful (a "dry tap"), then chromosomal analysis or fluorescence in situ hybridization should be attempted on peripheral blood leukocytes to detect the bcr-abl translocation.

A rare myeloproliferative disorder, chronic neutrophilic leukemia, can mimic a reactive neutrophilic leukocytosis in that very high concentrations of neutrophils are unaccompanied by significant immaturity in the peripheral blood or bone marrow. Del 20q or del 11q23 is occasionally detected in such patients, or polymerase chain reaction may show an atypical bcr-abl translocation (p230 bcr-abl). Often the diagnosis is made after prolonged follow-up when no other etiology emerges. Serum electrophoresis in these patients frequently reveals a monoclonal gammopathy.

Patients with chronic myeloid leukemia or other myeloproliferative disorders with leukocyte counts greater than 100,000/μL usually do not exhibit the effects of leukostasis that are seen in patients with acute leukemia with similar levels of white blood cells. Leukapheresis is rarely necessary in patients who have mainly mature neutrophils circulating, whereas it is essential to prevent hypoxia and central nervous system dysfunction in acute leukemia patients with blast counts greater than 50,000 to 100,000/μL.

Neutropenia

Absolute neutrophil counts between 1000 and 1500/μL are considered mild neutropenia and are only occasionally associated with significant infection. Patients with an absolute neutrophil count between 500 and 1000/μL have a moderate risk of infection. Levels less than 500/μL indicate severe neutropenia, which carries a high risk of bacterial infection and fungal superinfection. The severity and duration of the neutropenia and the history and type of prior infections are important considerations in evaluating the patient. Clues to the etiology include the presence of splenomegaly and abnormalities of the hemoglobin and platelet levels. A careful medication history, both prescribed and over-the-counter, is a critical part of the evaluation. Table 38-3 lists the causes of neutropenia.

Neutropenia Resulting from Infection

A number of acute and chronic infections are characterized by the presence of neutropenia. Viral infections, including measles, varicella, and acute hepatitis, are not infrequently accompanied by transient leukopenia and neutropenia that are not associated with significant clinical consequences. Certain bacterial

Table 38-3 ■ Causes of Neutropenia

Infections
 Viral
  Childhood exanthems
  Acute hepatitis
  Infectious mononucleosis
  Acute and chronic HIV infection
  Bacterial, fungal, mycobacterial, protozoan
  Overwhelming sepsis
  Salmonella
  Malaria
Ethnic or familial neutropenia
Cytotoxic chemotherapy
Radiation therapy
Idiosyncratic medication-induced neutropenia
 Semisynthetic penicillins, phenothiazines, gold salts
  Sulfa drugs, antithyroid medications, procaine amide
  Anti-convulsants, captopril, clozapine
Alcohol neutropenia
Splenomegaly with sequestration
 Cirrhosis
Lymphoproliferative disorders with or without splenomegaly
 Hairy cell leukemia
 T cell large granular lymphocytosis
Autoimmune disease
 Systemic lupus erythematosus
 Felty's syndrome
 Autoimmune neutropenia
Cyclic neutropenia
Myelodysplasia or acute leukemia

infections are regularly associated with neutropenia such as salmonellosis (typhoid fever). Falling neutrophil counts in the face of bacterial infections that are usually associated with leukocytosis ominously predict overwhelming sepsis, poor marrow reserve, or both.

Transient neutropenia and leukopenia may occur in the acute phase of human immunodeficiency (HIV) infection. In the late stages, when CD4 levels fall below 50/μL, chronic neutropenia is a frequent finding and often a diagnostic challenge. The role of drug toxicity, particularly due to sulfamethoxazole–trimethoprim, and opportunistic infections need to be considered in the evaluation. In the febrile HIV-positive patient with worsening neutropenia, bone marrow examination and culture should be performed. The bone marrow biopsy should be stained for tuberculosis and fungal organisms. In these severely immunosuppressed patients, bone marrow examination is frequently useful in demonstrating systemic infection caused by *Mycobacterium avium intracellulare*, *Mycobacterium tuberculosis*, *Histoplasma capsulatum*, or *Cryptococcus neoformans*. Non-Hodgkin's

lymphoma or Hodgkin's disease may also be diagnosed in the bone marrow biopsy. Most often, the default diagnosis for the neutropenia is HIV marrow dysplasia, particularly when associated with a hypocellular marrow and peripheral blood neutrophils exhibiting the Pelger-Huet anomaly (bilobed nuclei, Figure 42-22 in Chapter 42). The frequent response to granulocyte colony-stimulating factors suggests that HIV neutropenia relates in part to a deficiency in the endogenous production of these factors by T cells. In HIV patients with a history of frequent bacterial infections, it may be necessary to resort to chronic granulocyte colony-stimulating factor therapy sufficient to maintain the neutrophil count at 1000/μL.

Acute and Febrile Neutropenia

Severe isolated neutropenia with an absolute neutrophil count below 500/μL, called agranulocytosis when the count is less than 200/μL, is usually the result of a drug reaction. Therefore a careful drug history is mandatory. Drugs that are well known for causing neutropenia on an idiosyncratic basis include phenothiazine, gold salts, antithyroid medications, carbamazepine, clozapine, captopril, and semisynthetic penicillins (Table 38-3). Chemotherapeutic drugs (particularly alkylating agents, nucleoside analogues, and anthracyclines) and radiation therapy regularly cause dose-dependent myelosuppression and will usually cause other cytopenias as well as neutropenia. Chemotherapy- or radiation-induced neutropenia usually does not present a diagnostic dilemma. However, prolonged delays in recovery beyond the usual three to four weeks after a cycle of treatment may raise concerns about other diagnoses, such as myelodysplasia or marrow involvement with tumor, but most often reflect a decline in bone marrow reserve following multiple cycles of chemotherapy. Other, more unusual causes of severe isolated neutropenia include cyclic neutropenia, autoimmune neutropenia, and T cell large granular lymphocytosis.

Fever in patients with an absolute neutrophil count below 1000/μL, particularly those with levels below 500/μL, requires prompt institution of broad-spectrum antibiotic coverage, which, depending on the circumstances, patient status, and expected duration of neutropenia, can be given orally or intravenously. For example, febrile solid tumor and lymphoma patients who have received only moderately myelosuppressive therapy and who are expected to have a more transient neutropenia may safely receive outpatient treatment with antibiotics and granulocyte colony-stimulating factors, particularly if absolute neutrophil counts are greater than 500/μL.

Isolated Mild Neutropenia

The diagnosis of so-called "ethnic" neutropenia frequently seen in African Americans and other groups reflects the use of a reference range of normal neutrophil levels derived from individuals of European origin. An absolute neutrophil count of 1200 to 1800/μL is found in a sizeable number of otherwise healthy African Americans, usually men, and has also been reported in various groups in the Middle East. Levels of 900 to 1200/μL may also be noted in these individuals. Because similar levels of neutropenia are seen in serious hematologic disorders, consideration of other causes is necessary before concluding that ethnic neutropenia is present. Benign ethnic neutropenia is the likely explanation in the patient who reports long-standing mild neutropenia without a history of bacterial infections and who has a normal red blood cell and platelet count. A normal physical examination with no evidence of splenomegaly and a normal peripheral blood smear on microscopic examination gives added confidence in the diagnosis. In patients without knowledge of previous blood counts and particularly patients who have had documented "normal" blood counts in the past, the problem can be somewhat more challenging. However, the clinician should be aware that these individuals elevate their neutrophil counts into the "normal" range in response to infection, corticosteroids, and intense exercise. The etiology of ethnic neutropenia in individuals of African origin appears to be a lower bone marrow reserve compared to that of individuals of European origin; this is of apparently no clinical consequence. Bone marrow examination is not necessary to confirm this diagnosis. In situations in which an absolute concentration of neutrophils below 1000/μL raises concern, a hydrocortisone stimulation test can confirm the presence of an adequate bone marrow reserve indicated by an increment of more than 1600/μL bands and segmented neutrophils three to five hours after an intravenous bolus of 200 mg of hydrocortisone.

Other Chronic Neutropenias

Mild neutropenia and leukopenia due to splenic sequestration is frequently associated with the presence of splenomegaly. These patients generally do not have frequent infections. The need for a bone marrow examination will depend on the recognition of the underlying systemic illness. Bone marrow aspiration will not usually reveal any new information in patients with cirrhosis, chronic hepatitis, systemic lupus erythematosus, or human immunodeficiency, all of whom have uncomplicated mild neutropenia. On the other hand, a patient with splenomegaly

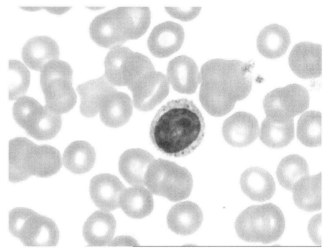

Figure 38-6 ■ Large granular lymphocyte (original magnification ×100, oil). (See Color Plate 3.)

and/or other cytopenias without clinical or laboratory evidence of the aforementioned entities requires an examination of the bone marrow to rule out marrow infiltrative disorders such as hairy cell leukemia, lymphoma, myelofibrosis, and myelodysplasia. Flow cytometry of the marrow and peripheral blood may be useful to identify a clonal lymphoid population, particularly when abnormal lymphoid cells are noted on microscopic examination. Excess granular lymphocytes (greater than 700/μL) in the peripheral blood smear (Figure 38-6) accompanying a mild lymphocytosis should raise suspicion of T cell large granular lymphocytosis, which can be confirmed by flow cytometry. Bone marrow examination with chromosomal analysis is indicated if macrocytosis, bilobed neutrophils (Pelger-Huet cells), or poorly granulated neutrophils suggestive of myelodysplasia are seen. In an effort to control the costs of these evaluations, it is useful to view the stained smear of the bone marrow aspirate to help decide the need for these additional studies.

Lymphocytosis: Absolute, Relative, and Atypical

The initial evaluation of lymphocyte count abnormalities depends on the answer to two questions: Is the lymphocytosis absolute or relative, and are atypical lymphocytes seen in the peripheral blood smear? A relative lymphocytosis occurs when neutropenia develops, because the percentage of lymphocytes in the peripheral smear automatically increases. The absolute lymphocyte concentration, however, remains less than 5000/μL. When increased numbers of "reactive" or "atypical" lymphocytes accompany the neutropenia, the differential diagnosis should include a viral or other nonbacterial infection, such as viral hepatitis, cytomegalovirus infection, acute HIV infection, measles, or toxoplasmosis. Infectious mononucleosis and immune drug reactions may present in this fashion as well, but not infrequently an absolute lymphocytosis occurs, raising the absolute lymphocyte count to more than 4000/µL.

Absolute Lymphocytosis

The differential diagnosis of an absolute lymphocytosis (Table 38-4) is highly dependent on age and geography. In adolescents, infectious mononucleosis (Figure 38-7) is the most common cause. In most cases it is the result of Epstein-Barr infection of B cells with an exuberant reactive response by T cells that results in the remarkable pleomorphic lymphocyte morphology. In severely ill patients with this disorder, particularly when presenting at an older age than the usual adolescent, the markedly abnormal lymphocyte morphology may suggest a diagnosis of acute lymphoblastic leukemia or lymphoma. Concerns about an underlying lymphoid malignancy can be heightened further by complications such as autoimmune thrombocytopenia and/or hemolytic anemia. Generally, however, review of the peripheral smear by an experienced hematologist and the confirmatory serologic tests for heterophil antibodies or specific antibodies to the Epstein-Barr virus will lead to the correct diagno-

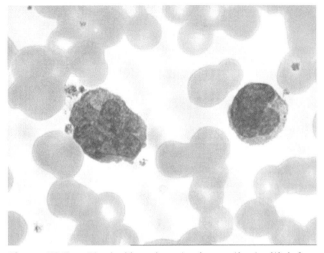

Figure 38-7 ■ Atypical lymphocytes in a patient with infectious mononucleosis (original magnification ×100, oil). (See Color Plate 4.)

sis. If Epstein-Barr viral titers are negative, tests for antibodies to cytomegalovirus and toxoplasma should be obtained.

Immunologic drug reactions are another common cause for reactive lymphocytosis that can mimic lymphoma; phenytoin and sulfa drugs are frequent offenders. The reactions are frequently accompanied by rash, adenopathy, fever, and striking atypical T cell lymphocytosis.

Diagnosing Clonal Lymphocyte Disorders

In adults, an absolute lymphocytosis should raise concerns about clonal lymphoproliferative disorders. The presence of splenomegaly and peripheral lymphadenopathy will reinforce that concern. In their absence, immunophenotyping by flow cytometry or immunocytochemistry may be the simplest initial approach. Patients presenting with 5000 to 10,000 lymphocytes/µL not infrequently are found to have T cells, which show no evidence of aberrance in their antigen profile and therefore are presumed to be reactive. Approximately one half of the patients with mild lymphocytosis will be discovered to have a clonal B cell disorder. Most of these patients will have early, stage 0, B cell chronic lymphocytic leukemia (B-CLL). Flow cytometry findings of dim surface immunoglobulin with expression of only one light chain, either kappa or lambda, plus positivity for CD5 and CD23 will confirm a diagnosis of chronic lymphocytic leukemia. The morphology of the lymphocytes in B cell chronic lymphocytic leukemia is usually fairly uniform and very similar to normal lymphocytes (Figure 38-8), but increased cell fragility results in many "smudge" cells when the blood smear is made

---

Table 38-4 ■ Causes of Lymphocytosis

Reactive lymphocytosis with atypical lymphocytes
Viral infections
Mononucleosis syndromes
  Epstein-Barr virus, cytomegalovirus, toxoplasmosis
Hypersensitivity reactions to drugs
  Phenytoin, sulfa drugs
Clonal lymphocytic disorders
  B cell disorders
    Chronic lymphocytic leukemia
    Prolymphocytic leukemia
    Mantle cell lymphoma
    Follicular lymphoma
    Hairy cell leukemia and variant
    Marginal zone lymphoma (splenomegaly with circulating villous lymphocytes)
  T cell disorders
    Cutaneous T cell lymphoma (Sézary syndrome)
    Adult T cell leukemia-lymphoma
    T cell large granular lymphocytosis
    Prolymphocytic leukemia
    Peripheral T cell lymphoma

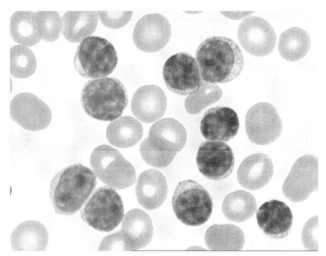

Figure 38-8 ■ Lymphocytosis due to chronic lymphocytic leukemia (original magnification ×100, oil). (See Color Plate 4.)

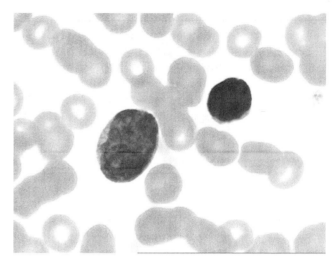

Figure 38-9 ■ Circulating lymphoma cells from a patient with follicular lymphoma (original magnification ×100, oil). (See Color Plate 4.)

for microscopic examination. If the physical examination and the hemoglobin and platelet level are normal, further evaluation in these typical early-stage patients is unnecessary. In patients with higher white blood cell counts and evidence of progression in the form of adenopathy and splenomegaly, bone marrow examination and computed tomography scans are appropriate to assess the patient's tumor burden and need for therapy.

The overwhelming majority of patients with lymphocyte concentrations above 10,000/μL have B cell chronic lymphocytic leukemia. Lymphocyte counts in these patients commonly range from 20,000 to 120,000/μL and occasionally reach levels greater than 200,000/μL.

Other Clonal Lymphoid Disorders

Lymphoid morphology or flow cytometry findings atypical for B cell chronic lymphocytic leukemia alert the clinician to the likelihood of less frequent lymphoproliferative states. For example, plasmacytoid lymphocytes in the smear will point to a diagnosis of Waldenström's macroglobulinemia that will be confirmed by finding an IgM paraprotein in the serum. Lymphocytes with cleaved or irregular nuclei (Figure 38-9), particularly when found in patients with prominent adenopathy and a minor lymphocytosis, suggest follicular lymphoma or mantle cell lymphoma. Flow cytometry of these patients' tumor cells will show bright surface immunoglobulin and different antigen profiles than are found in chronic lymphocytic leukemia.

Patients presenting with lymphocytosis and prominent splenomegaly but without adenopathy suggest other diagnoses. When immature prolympho-

cytes make up more than one half of the peripheral lymphocytosis, the diagnosis is most likely T or B prolymphocytic leukemia. If the lymphocytes have prominent villi or appear "hairy" (Figure 38-10), splenic lymphoma with villous lymphocytes, marginal zone lymphoma, or hairy cell leukemia and its variants should be considered.

Convoluted T lymphocytes should immediately raise suspicion of cutaneous T cell lymphoma or Sézary syndrome in the patient with a long-standing rash or adult T cell leukemia-lymphoma (ATLL) in patients who originated from the Caribbean or Southern Japan and have a brief history of skin involvement or hypercalcemia.

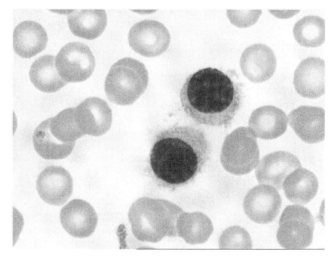

Figure 38-10 ■ Circulating hairy cells from a patient with hairy cell leukemia (original magnification ×100, oil). (See Color Plate 4.)

Monocytosis and Monocytopenia

A relative (greater than 10%) or absolute monocytosis (greater than 800/µL) is rarely the most important clue leading to an underlying diagnosis. The most frequent causes, chronic infections and inflammatory disorders, will raise the monocyte count only modestly, rarely more than 20% of the leukocytes or more than 2000/µL, and are frequently also associated with lymphopenia. Patients with severe neutropenia may announce their imminent recovery by the appearance of monocytes in the peripheral blood. Patients with Hodgkin's disease and other lymphomas may exhibit a reactive monocytosis. The monocytosis noted in acute and chronic myeloid leukemias and myelodysplasia are most likely due to monocytic differentiation of the malignant clone.

Monocytopenia (less than 300/µL) occurs regularly in patients with agranulocytosis and aplastic anemia and other neutropenic disorders, reflecting the origin of the monocyte from the myeloid stem cell. Monocytopenia also occurs in patients on chronic corticosteroid therapy. Profound monocytopenia is a useful diagnostic clue to the presence of hairy cell leukemia. It unvaryingly accompanies this disorder and probably accounts for the resulting propensity to develop opportunistic infections such as atypical mycobacterial infection and cryptococcosis.

Eosinophilia

Diagnostic Evaluation

The differential diagnosis of eosinophilia has been described by an anonymous wit as "wheezes, worms, and weird diseases," reflecting its association with atypical immunologic responses, unusual antigens, and poorly understood syndromes and malignancies. Fortunately, the most common causes for peripheral blood eosinophilia (more than 300/µL) are responses to immunologic stimuli, which are usually readily apparent from the patient's history or physical examination. For patients with mild eosinophilia (less than 1500/µL), a history of asthma, allergic rhinitis, chronic eczema, or a newly instituted drug, particularly when accompanied by a rash, quickly solves the problem. In patients with more severe and chronic eosinophilia, the evaluation often requires more detective work if there is no clinical evidence of cancer and the routine serial stool examinations for ova and parasites do not reveal invasive roundworm parasitic infestations such as by strongyloides or ascaris. For a patient with the clinical picture of myalgias, periorbital edema, and cardiomyopathy, a muscle biopsy may reveal trichina. Hodgkin's disease, cutaneous T cell lymphoma, and occasionally other non-Hodgkin's lymphoma can be associated with eosinophilia. Computerized tomographic examination of the chest and abdomen for evidence of lymphoma may be helpful when these disorders are suspected. If the peripheral smear reveals eosinophilic myelocytes or more immature myeloid cells or if splenomegaly is found, a bone marrow examination with chromosome analysis is important to confirm a diagnosis of eosinophilic leukemia or Philadelphia chromosome-positive chronic myeloid leukemia.

Eosinophilic Syndromes

Unusual syndromes of unknown etiology that are associated with eosinophilic accumulation in specific organs and tissues include evanescent pulmonary eosinophilic infiltrates (Löffler's syndrome), eosinophilic fasciitis (which may be associated with aplastic anemia), eosinophilic granulomatous cellulitis (Well's syndrome), and allergic granulomatosis (pulmonary vasculitis with neuropathy and asthma, Churg-Strauss syndrome).

The term *idiopathic hypereosinophilic syndrome* is reserved for patients with severe hypereosinophilia (greater than 1500/µL but often more than 5000/µL) sustained for over six months who have no other identified cause of eosinophilia. These patients, usually men, have multiorgan involvement, including any combination of thromboembolic events, due to myocardial necrosis and endocardial fibrosis, central and peripheral neuropathies, pulmonary infiltrates, angioedema and other cutaneous lesions, and splenomegaly. The cardiac damage and thromboembolic events are believed to be due to toxicity induced by the eosinophil granular proteins and can also be seen in patients with documented reactive eosinophilia secondary to parasitic infestation. In some patients with idiopathic hypereosinophilia abnormal expansions of T helper-2 type lymphocytes have been found. These expansions often appear to be monoclonal, suggesting that an occult T cell lymphoproliferative disorder is stimulating interleukin-5 (IL-5) or other cytokines to increase eosinophilic proliferation.

Hypereosinophilic patients presenting with evidence of end organ damage should have prompt treatment with corticosteroids. In those who do not respond, hydroxyurea or other chemotherapy agents or interferon may be useful in controlling the eosinophilia and clinical manifestations. Occasional patients may have sustained eosinophilia of unknown etiology for years without clinical evidence of end organ damage and do not require treatment. It may be prudent in this circumstance to recommend periodic echocardiographic monitoring in these patients to look for early evidence of endocardial damage and thrombosis.

Suggested Reading

Chang R, Wong GY: Prognostic significance of marked leukocytosis in hospitalized patients. J Gen Intern Med 1991;6: 199–203.

Darko DF, Fose J, Gillin JC, et al: Neutrophilia and lymphopenia in major mood disorders. Psychiatry Res 1988;25: 243–251.

Elliott MA, Dewald GW, Tefferi A, Hanson CA: Chronic neutrophilic leukocytosis (CNL): A clinical, pathologic and cytogenetic study. Leukemia 2001;15:35–40.

Evans RH, Scadden DT: Haematological aspects of HIV infection. Clin Haematol 2000;13:215–230.

Faderl S, Talpaz M, Estrov Z, Kantarjian HM: Chronic myelogenous leukemia: Biology and therapy. Ann Intern Med 1999;131:207–219.

Haddy TB, Rana SH, Castro O: Benign ethnic neutropenia: What is a normal absolute neutrophil count? J Lab Clin Med 1999;133:15–22.

Jaffe ES, Harris NL, Stein H, Vardiman JW (eds): WHO Classification of Tumors: Pathology and Genetics of Tumors of Haematopoietic and Lymphoid Tissues. IARC Press, 2001.

Loughran TP: Clonal diseases of large granular lymphocytes. 1993;Blood 82:1–14.

Mason BA, Lessin L, Schechter GP: Marrow granulocyte reserves in healthy American Blacks. Am J Med 1979;67:201–205.

Parry H, Cohen S, Schlarb JE, Tyrell DA, et al: Smoking, alcohol consumption and leukocyte counts. Am J Clin Pathol 1997;107:64–67.

Rothenberg ME: Eosinophilia. N Engl J Med 1998;338: 1592–1600.

Roufosse F, Schandene L, Sibille C, et al: Clonal Th2 lymphocytes in patients with the idiopathic hypereosinophilic syndrome. Brit J Haematol 2000;109:540–548.

Schechter GP: Chronic lymphocytic leukemia. In Rich R, Fleisher TA, Schwartz BA, Shearer WT, Strober W (eds): Clinical Immunology, 2nd ed. St. Louis: Mosby-Yearbook, 2001.

Van der Klauw MM, Goudsmit R, Halie MR, et al: A population-based cohort study of drug-associated agranulocytosis. Arch Intern Med 1999;22:369–376.

Weller PF, Bubley GJ: The idiopathic hypereosinophilic syndrome. Blood 1994;83:2759–2779.

Chapter 39
Pancytopenia

Anne Moore

Pancytopenia describes simultaneous low peripheral blood counts in all three cell lines: red cells, white cells, and platelets. It is not a diagnosis but a presentation of some underlying general medical or primary hematologic disorder. Pancytopenia is due to one of two processes: decreased production of peripheral blood cells, for example, aplastic anemia, or increased destruction or sequestration as in hypersplenism. The challenge to the physician is to understand why the patient is pancytopenic and to treat the underlying condition.

Pancytopenia, if it is mild (Table 39-1), may cause no symptoms and may be found at the time of a routine medical examination. By contrast, severe pancytopenia may be life-threatening and require emergency attention to make an accurate diagnosis and to treat the patient. Most patients with moderate pancytopenia come to the physician with a symptom related to the low blood counts. The most common presenting symptom is fatigue and shortness of breath on exertion as a result of anemia. A patient may also seek medical attention because of easy bruising and bleeding associated with a low platelet count. Since mild to moderate levels of leukopenia are generally well tolerated, infection is not the usual presenting complaint. However, a previously healthy patient with a high fever and severe sore throat or other infection such as a perirectal abscess should be assessed for possible leukopenia.

When the physician discovers that a patient has pancytopenia, the most helpful information is the prior blood count. For example, if the blood count was normal at an earlier time and the patient now has moderate pancytopenia, the physician will search for a recent event such as a new medication to explain the change in blood counts. On the other hand, if the low blood counts have been unchanged for the past five years, the physician considers a chronic condition such as hypersplenism (splenomegaly with cytopenia and a hypercellular bone marrow), perhaps caused by a prior splenic vein thrombosis.

History and Physical Examination

At the time of initial evaluation of the pancytopenic patient, a careful history and physical examination may lead to the most likely diagnosis (Table 39-2). The history of the present illness should allow the physician to establish a time line for the development of the pancytopenia. Most important, is this a sick patient or a "well" patient? An acutely ill patient with pancytopenia should be considered a medical emergency. Most patients will not be acutely ill when they present with low blood counts, although they may be chronically unwell. For the symptomatic patient, when did he or she notice the symptoms of anemia? Has the patient noticed shortness of breath on climbing the stairs? When did that start? How fast has it progressed? If the patient complains of bleeding due to thrombocytopenia, when did he or she first notice problems? Has the patient had dental work or any surgery that would have tested the hemostatic process? For example, if the patient had a tooth extracted with no difficulty six weeks ago and now has a platelet count of 25,000/μL, the very low blood counts can be assumed to be of recent origin. Previous physical examinations are important. A history of an enlarging spleen over many years might be a clue to hypersplenism or to Gaucher disease as an explanation for the pancytopenia.

Table 39-1 ▪ Pancytopenia : A Working Definition

	White Blood Cell Count (/μL)	Hemoglobin (g/dL)	Platelets (/μL)
Mild	2500–3500	9.0–11.0	75,000–100,000
Moderate	1500–2500	7.5–9.0	45,000–75,000
Severe	<1500	<7.5	<45,000

Table 39-2 ■ Causes of Pancytopenia

Primary disease of bone marrow elements
  Inherited
    Fanconi's anemia
    Schwachman-Diamond syndrome
  Acquired
    Myelodysplasia
    Myelofibrosis
    Acute myeloid or lymphoblastic leukemia
    Hairy cell leukemia
    Non-Hodgkin's lymphoma
    Paroxysmal nocturnal hemoglobinuria
    Irradiation of the bone marrow

Hypersplenism
  Hairy cell leukemia
  Portal hypertension
  Non-Hodgkin's lymphoma involving the spleen
  Sarcoidosis
  Chronic infection of the spleen, such as brucellosis
  Collagen vascular disease—systemic lupus erythematosus
  Rheumatoid arthritis—Felty's syndrome
  Glycogen storage disease—Gaucher's syndrome

Myelophthisis, involvement of the bone marrow by an infiltrative process
  Carcinoma metastatic to the bone marrow
  Lymphomatous marrow involvement
  Glycogen storage disease—Gaucher's syndrome

Immune-mediated disorders against bone marrow precursors
  Aplastic anemia
  Graft-versus-host disease after blood transfusion in an immunosuppressed patient
  Collagen vascular disorder—systemic vasculitis
  Rheumatoid arthritis—Felty's syndrome

Other causes
  Panyhypopituitary states
  Hypothyroidism
  Legionnaire's disease
  Q fever
  Anorexia nervosa

The social history of the pancytopenic patient is very important. Medication, both prescribed and over-the-counter, is a common cause of a patient presenting with new pancytopenia. All medications are suspect, and patients should be carefully questioned about recreational drugs as well as alternative therapies such as vitamins and herbs, which they may forget to report. All medications should be discontinued if possible in a patient with the new onset of pancytopenia. Although dietary deficiencies of vitamin B_{12} (such as in the vegan diet) and folic acid are associated primarily with megaloblastic anemia, leukopenia and thrombocytopenia may also occur and may confuse the diagnosis. Chronic alcoholism is associated with liver disease and hypersplenism. Alcohol can also suppress the bone marrow directly and lead to pancytopenia. Anorexia nervosa may be associated with pancytopenia, with "gelatinous transformation" of the bone marrow. A travel history should also be elicited. Malaria is associated with pancytopenia, primarily because of hypersplenism. Risk factors for AIDS should also be explored, although pancytopenia is usually not seen until late in the disease. Occupational history and toxin exposures may reveal links to pancytopenia, benzene exposure being the most frequently cited as a cause for aplastic anemia.

The majority of patients presenting with pancytopenia have no family history of blood disorders. However, a careful family history is still warranted. The patient should be asked not only if there is a family history of blood disease, but also if there are family members who have had splenectomy or cholecystectomy suggesting a chronic hereditary hemolytic anemia. For example, patients with sickle-cell disease and hereditary spherocytosis are prone to transient aplastic crisis, a serious complication of parvovirus

TREATMENT

Emergency Management of the Patient with Severe Pancytopenia

- Stop all medication, including over-the-counter products.
- Obtain serum vitamin B_{12} and folic acid levels, and administer vitamin B_{12}, 1000 µg IM and folic acid 1 mg PO.
- Treat with broad-spectrum antibiotics for fever and/or infection. Granulocyte colony-stimulating factors may be considered in this setting.
- Transfuse with irradiated red blood cells if hemoglobin is less than 6.0 to 7.0 g/dL or for symptom relief.

- Consider platelet transfusion with irradiated platelets if platelets are less than 5000/µL or if the patient is bleeding.
- Perform bone marrow aspirate and biopsy with appropriate ancillary studies (Table 39-3).
- If aplastic anemia is confirmed on bone marrow biopsy, begin evaluation of the patient and siblings for possible bone marrow transplant. It is wise to initiate tissue typing and to contact a bone marrow transplant center early in the course of the disease. Use only irradiated blood products.

infection. Fanconi's anemia is an inherited aplastic anemia that usually presents in childhood. However, there are variants of Fanconi's anemia that present with pancytopenia in adulthood, and chromosomal analysis demonstrating increased sensitivity to DNA-damaging agents may be necessary to make this diagnosis.

The review of systems and the physical examination offer many clues. History of a prior malignancy should alert the clinician to the possibility of metastases to the bone marrow. Common solid tumors that metastasize to the bone marrow are breast cancer, prostate cancer, small-cell carcinoma of the lung, and malignant melanoma. Lymphoma may cause pancytopenia based on hypersplenism or on direct bone marrow involvement. In addition, prior chemotherapy and radiation therapy may lead to myelodysplasia presenting as pancytopenia. A patient with AIDS may develop pancytopenia as part of the clinical spectrum of the disease, independent of drug therapy. Dermatologic disorders are important. A rash, particularly a recent rash, is an important clue and may lead to the diagnosis of a vasculitis, which may be associated with an autoimmune pancytopenia. Respiratory symptoms such as shortness of breath due to a pleural effusion should lead the clinician to suspect tuberculosis with myelophthisis or systemic lupus erythematosus with autoimmune pancytopenia as a cause of the low blood counts. A patient reporting easy satiety or left upper quadrant discomfort should lead to a search for an enlarged spleen, which may not be readily appreciated on physical examination. Splenomegaly may be associated with hypersplenism in patients with nonmalignant disorders such as cirrhosis of the liver, splenic vein thrombosis, and Gaucher's disease. Gaucher's disease also causes pancytopenia by infiltrating the bone marrow with the characteristic Gaucher's cell, a macrophage that is rich in glucosylceramide. A patient with agnogenic myeloid metaplasia with myelofibrosis characteristically has an enlarged spleen at diagnosis but only occasionally presents with pancytopenia. A history of hepatitis, usually non-A, non-B, non-C, within the six months prior to the development of pancytopenia may point to the diagnosis of aplastic anemia, a rare but potentially fatal complication of this disease. A history of rheumatoid arthritis in a patient with splenomegaly and pancytopenia suggests Felty's syndrome.

Laboratory Testing

When a patient is found to be pancytopenic, the blood count should always be repeated before alarming the patient. The next step is the examination of the peripheral blood smear. Because of the low white blood count, examination of the white blood cell distribution and morphology may benefit from a smear made from a buffy coat. The white cell differential count reveals the distribution of white cells, the percentage of mature granulocytes being most important for the patient. The absence of mature granulocytes places the patient at severe risk for infection and should be considered a medical emergency. Abnormal white blood cells, for example, myeloblasts, promyelocytes, or myelocytes, suggest an infiltrative process in the bone marrow such as acute leukemia or metastatic cancer. Cells extrinsic to the normal hematopoietic system such as hairy cells may be seen on a peripheral blood smear. Hairy cell leukemia typically presents with pancytopenia, and only a few hairy cells may be seen in the peripheral blood.

The morphology of the white blood cells is important. Hypersegmentation of the granulocytes and the presence of "giant bands" may lead to a clinical diagnosis of pernicious anemia. Hypogranulation and hyposegmentation of the granulocytes may be the first clue to a diagnosis of myelodysplastic syndrome in an elderly patient. Myelodysplastic syndrome is a clonal disorder of the hematopoietic stem cell that presents clinically with cytopenias of one or more cell lines associated with an abnormal bone marrow.

Red cell indices and morphology are also important in the evaluation of the pancytopenic patient. Macrocytosis (with an elevated mean corpuscular volume [MCV]) in a pancytopenic patient should raise the question of severe vitamin B_{12} or folic acid deficiency. A mildly elevated mean corpuscular volume and the presence of target cells should alert the clinician to the possibility of pancytopenia on the basis of liver disease, usually alcoholic cirrhosis with hypersplenism. An unexplained mild elevation of the mean corpuscular volume in a patient with pancytopenia may be a clue to myelodysplastic syndrome. Refractory anemia (with or without sideroblasts) and refractory anemia with excess blasts are the most common categories of myelodysplastic syndrome. The red cell population in these disorders may be both microcytic and macrocytic; poikilocytosis with various abnormal forms may be seen on a peripheral blood smear. Nucleated red cells (which may falsely elevate an automated white blood cell count) are never seen in a normal blood smear. Their presence indicates extramedullary hematopoiesis or myelophthisis and may be a clue to myelofibrosis or to metastatic cancer in the bone marrow.

The reticulocyte count is usually low in the patient with pancytopenia, indicating inadequate bone marrow response to anemia. Occasionally, the reticulocyte count is elevated, suggesting increased peripheral red blood cell destruction as part of the clinical

---

Table 39-3 ■ Bone Marrow Studies in the Pancytopenic Patient

Bone Marrow Aspirate

Cellularity, maturation, and morphology of all three cell lines, myeloid/erythroid ratio, presence of extrinsic cells, iron stores and presence of ringed sideroblasts

Biopsy

Architecture and cellularity, presence of extrinsic cells, presence of fibrosis using reticulin stain

Culture

Bacteria, mycobacteria, fungus

Histochemistry

Peroxidase (acute myelocytic leukemia), tartrate-resistant acid phosphatase (hairy cell leukemia)

Cytogenetics

Chromosomal abnormalities such as 5q- (myelodysplasia) or t(15;17) associated with acute promyelocytic leukemia

Immunophenotype

Lymphocyte subsets (for lymphoma or leukemia in the marrow)

Immunogenotype

Immunoglobulin and T cell receptor rearrangement (e.g., large granular lymphocyte syndrome)

---

picture, as in a patient with autoimmune disease. Paroxysmal nocturnal hemoglobinuria (PNH), a clonal disorder of the hematopoietic stem cell, may present with a low white blood cell and platelet count as well as a hemolytic anemia with an elevated reticulocyte count.

Platelet morphology may be helpful. For example, giant, bizarre platelets may indicate a myelodysplastic syndrome.

Bone marrow examination should be considered early in the evaluation of all pancytopenic patients and should be performed without delay in the patient with severe pancytopenia. It may be reasonable to observe the asymptomatic patient with mild or moderate pancytopenia to see whether the pancytopenia resolves before doing a bone marrow examination. This is particularly true, for example, if the physician suspects drug-induced pancytopenia and the drug has been stopped. To spare the patient unnecessary discomfort from repeated marrow examinations, the hematologist should be prepared to perform aspiration and biopsy with special studies (see Table 39-3) at the time of the initial marrow examination. Samples should be placed in the appropriate media, and arrangements should be made in advance with the laboratory. If the initial morphologic examination of the stained bone marrow aspirate is diagnostic, the

special studies may not need to be sent. For example, if the bone marrow aspirate reveals acute promyelocytic leukemia, the immunophenotype studies are not necessary. The hematologist should be prepared to make the most of a scanty specimen when performing a bone marrow on a pancytopenic patient. If the hematologist encounters a "dry tap," which is common in aplastic anemia, hairy cell leukemia, and myelofibrosis and in some cases of myelodysplastic syndrome, he or she should make a "touch prep" of the biopsy for morphologic analysis before placing the biopsy core in the fixative for pathology. If a second site also yields a dry tap, the biopsy itself can be divided and placed in the various media for the additional studies required, for example, cytogenetics or culture for bacteria or mycobacteria. The biopsy can be gently teased with a small-gauge needle after it is placed in the medium.

If an aspirate is obtained, the smears can be prepared and stained immediately. A marrow aspirate is examined for the degree of cellularity, for the presence of normal megakaryocytes, and for full maturation of myeloid and erythroid cell lines with normal morphology. Extrinsic cells are sought, both malignant and nonmalignant, for example, Gaucher's cells. A hypercellular, monotonous marrow is typical of acute leukemia or, more rarely, lymphoma involving the

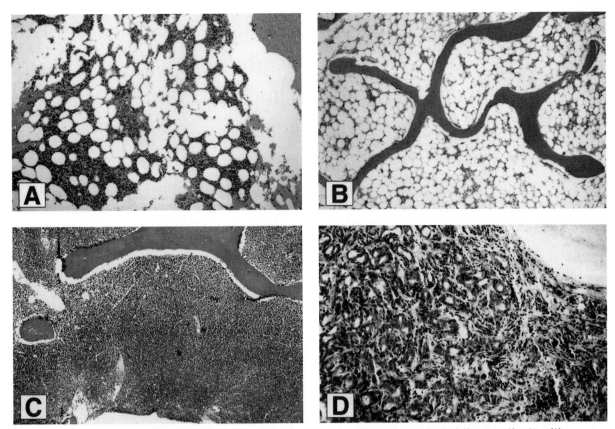

Figure 39-1 ■ Bone marrow biopsies from a patient with normal blood counts and three patients with severe pancytopenia, stained with hematoxylin and eosin. *A*, Normal cellularity, approximately 50% fat and 50% cells (×40 [original magnification]); higher power (not shown) reveals heterogeneity of the cell population with normal maturation and morphology of megakaryocytes, myeloid and erythroid precursors. *B*, Aplastic anemia, with replacement of most of the marrow space with fat (×40 [original magnification]). *C*, Lymphoma replacing the marrow with homogeneous infiltration and obliteration of the fat (×40 [original magnification]). *D*, Metastatic breast cancer replacing marrow with glandular pattern seen at high power (×200 [original magnification]).

marrow. A hypercellular marrow with some variety in cell type but morphologic abnormalities of the erythroid and myeloid cell lines is typical of myelodysplastic syndrome (MDS). An extremely hypocellular aspirate suggests a hypoplastic or aplastic marrow, but a biopsy is essential to confirm this. Occasionally, a marrow packed with extrinsic cells or with leukemia is too dense to yield an aspirate, and the hematologist is deceived about the true cellularity. Special stains for iron stores also allow the hematologist to look for ringed sideroblasts that may be present in myelodysplastic syndrome. The bone marrow biopsy requires 24 to 48 hours for processing. The biopsy is most valuable for the architecture of the marrow. A hypocellular aspirate with an extremely hypocellular biopsy is diagnostic of aplastic anemia. A marrow biopsy is also helpful for diagnosing malignant conditions such as leukemia, metastatic cancer, or lymphoma to explain pancytopenia. Figure 39-1 shows bone marrow results for three different patients with pancytopenia, along with normal results. Results of the ancillary bone

marrow studies may be necessary to establish a definite cause for pancytopenia.

Suggested Reading

Ball SE: The modern management of severe aplastic anemia. Br J Haematol 2000;110:41–53.

Barrett J, Saunthararajah Y, Molldren J: Myelodysplastic syndromes and aplastic anemia: Distinct entities or diseases linked by a common pathophysiology? Semin Hematol 2000;37:15–29.

Bennett JM, Catovsky D, Daniel MT, et al: Proposed revised criteria for the classification of acute myeloid leukemia: A report of the French-American-British Cooperative Group. Ann Intern Med 1985;103:620–625.

Buckley PJ: Examination and interpretation of bone marrow biopsies and aspirate smears. In Hoffman R, Benz EJ, Shattil SJ, et al (eds): Hematology: Basic Principles and Practice, New York: Churchill Livingstone, 1995, pp 2214–2222.

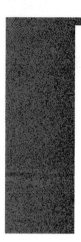

Chapter 40
Erythrocytosis

Peter T. Curtin

Introduction

An increase in the concentration of red blood cells, whether measured as number of cells, hemoglobin or hematocrit, is designated erythrocytosis. Polycythemia describes an increase in total mass of red cells in the body. Erythrocytosis can result from an increase in red cell mass (polycythemia or absolute erythrocytosis) or can result from a reduced plasma volume (apparent erythrocytosis). When a patient presents with an elevated hematocrit, the critical diagnostic objectives are first to determine whether absolute erythrocytosis is present and second to distinguish polycythemia vera from other causes of absolute erythrocytosis. Identification of patients with polycythemia vera is particularly important given the significant morbidity and mortality associated with this disorder.

The starting point of evaluation of erythrocytosis is a complete blood count (CBC). It is generally more useful to define erythrocytosis in terms of the hematocrit rather than the hemoglobin, since coexisting iron deficiency can occur and typically lowers the hemoglobin level more than the hematocrit. By definition, individuals with a hematocrit or hemoglobin level above the upper limit of the normal ranges for males and females can be said to have an erythrocytosis. It is important to obtain more than a single complete blood count before determining that an individual has erythrocytosis. Individuals with a stable elevated hematocrit or hemoglobin should generally be investigated further by measurement of their red cell mass. Examination of normal reference values for hematocrit indicates that the 99 percentile values for males and females are 52% and 48%, respectively. Thus, individuals with repeated hematocrit values above these levels should undergo red cell mass measurement. However, males and females with hematocrit values above 60% and 56%, respectively, can be assumed to have an absolute erythrocytosis and do not need to have red cell mass measurement. Individuals with a high normal hematocrit level and unexplained splenomegaly should have red cell mass measurement to exclude an absolute erythrocytosis.

Erythrocytosis: Absolute Versus Apparent

The initial step in the diagnostic evaluation of the patient with documented erythrocytosis is to determine whether the erythrocytosis is absolute or apparent. In most patients, this involves the measurement of red cell mass by dilution in blood of radiolabeled autologous red cells. This test is of value because the hematocrit, particularly when modestly elevated, does not reliably correlate with increased red cell mass. Demonstration of an elevated red cell mass in patients without a clear cause of erythrocytosis identifies a group deserving of close follow-up and additional, subsequent investigation. Using a standardized method of red cell measurement produces very reproducible results. Expressing results of red cell mass studies in terms of body weight leads to inaccuracy in the obese individual, as fatty tissue is relatively avascular. The International Council for Standardization in Hematology currently recommends expressing results in terms of body surface area, as results for 98% of males and 98% of females fall within plus or minus 25% of the mean value at any give body surface area. These limits were chosen as the normal range. Thus, a diagnosis of absolute erythrocytosis is made when the measured red cell mass is more than 25% above the mean predicted value for an individual's body surface area, while apparent erythrocytosis is present when the measured red cell mass falls within the normal range. This measurement therefore provides a good separation of individuals with a raised hematocrit value. In centers where red cell mass measurements are not available, all patients must undergo comprehensive evaluation as if they had absolute erythrocytosis.

Table 40-1 ■ The Classification of Absolute Erythrocytosis

Primary Erythrocytosis
  Congenital
    Erythropoietin receptor truncation
  Acquired
    Polycythemia vera

Secondary Erythrocytosis
  Congenital
    High-oxygen-affinity hemoglobin
    Autonomous high erythropoietin production
  Acquired
    Hypoxemia
    Renal disease
    Tumor

Idiopathic Erythrocytosis

Classification of Absolute Erythrocytosis

The absolute erythrocytoses can be classified into three general groups as shown in Table 40-1. The first is primary erythrocytosis, in which the abnormality is intrinsic to the erythroid progenitor compartment. Congenital primary erythrocytosis is due to truncation of the cytoplasmic portion of the erythropoietin receptor leading to excessive signaling in response to erythropoietin binding. A family history may be elicited in individuals with this rare disorder. The serum erythropoietin level is low in congenital primary erythrocytosis. Acquired primary erythrocytosis is due to the clonal, myeloproliferative disorder polycythemia vera. Secondary erythrocytosis is the result of an intrinsically normal erythroid progenitor compartment responding to increased erythropoietin secretion. A large number of disorders that can result in congenital and acquired secondary erythrocytosis are shown in Table 40-2. Idiopathic erythrocytosis is used for individuals who, at initial investigation, cannot be assigned to have either primary or secondary erythrocytosis.

Medical History and Physical Examination

The medical history should attempt to document the time of onset of erythrocytosis and whether erythrocytosis has been progressive. The discovery of prior normal hematocrit values can effectively eliminate congenital disorders. In the absence of prior complete blood counts, the duration of plethora may be esti-

mated by questioning the patient or family members. Inquiry should be made regarding the presence, duration, and severity of headache, dizziness, or visual changes, which may reflect cerebral vascular engorgement or hyperviscosity-induced reductions in cerebral blood flow. The patient should be asked about itching after bathing, which is characteristic of polycythemia vera. Early satiety or left upper quadrant pain can reflect splenomegaly. Signs and symptoms that are suggestive of polycythemia vera are listed in Table 40-3. A history of prior thrombotic, cardiovascular, or pulmonary disease should be sought. The duration and magnitude of smoking and alcohol consumption should be determined. Inquiry into symptoms that are suggestive of sleep apnea, such as snoring, awaking unrefreshed, and daytime somnolence, should be made, particularly in obese individuals. A family

Table 40-2 ■ Causes of Secondary Erythrocytosis

Congenital

  High-oxygen-affinity hemoglobin
  Methemoglobinemia
  Decreased 2,3-diphosphoglycerate
  Autonomous high erythropoietin production (Chuvash polycythemia)

Acquired

  Arterial hypoxemia
    High altitude
    Chronic mountain sickness
    Cyanotic heart disease
    Chronic lung disease
    Hypoventilation (Pickwickian syndrome, sleep apnea)
  Impaired oxygen delivery
    Smoking
    Carbon monoxide poisoning
  Renal disease
    Renal artery stenosis
    Renal transplantation
    Cystic lesions
    Hydronephrosis
  Hepatic disease
    Cirrhosis
    Hepatitis
  Neoplastic
    Renal cell carcinoma
      Hepatoma
      Other carcinomas
      Adrenal tumors
      Cerebellar hemangioblastoma
      Uterine fibroids
    Pharmacologic
      Erythropoietin
      Androgens

Table 40-3 ▪ Signs and Symptoms of Polycythemia Vera

Headache
Dizziness
Visual changes
Mental clouding
Facial plethora
Pruritus (particularly after bathing)
Early satiety or left upper quadrant discomfort
Gout
Abnormal bleeding (particularly gastrointestinal tract)
Digital ischemia
Stroke or transient ischemic attack

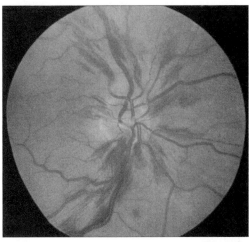

Figure 40-2 ▪ Retinal changes in a patient with polycythemia vera. Note distension of retinal vessels and hemorrhage and mild swelling of the optic disc in a patient with a hemoglobin level of 23.5 g/dL, blurred vision, headache, and confusion. (From Hoffbrand AV, Pettit JE: Color Atlas of Clinical Hematology, 3rd ed. St. Louis: Mosby, 2000, p 248.) (See Color Plate 5.)

history of erythrocytosis may suggest the presence of high-oxygen-affinity hemoglobin or one of the rare familial erythrocytosis syndromes.

Patients with absolute erythrocytosis, regardless of the etiology, may have signs of vascular distension, including plethora (Figure 40-1), dilated retinal veins (Figure 40-2), and conjunctival injection. The abdomen should be carefully examined for the presence of splenomegaly (Figure 40-3), a finding that is suggestive of polycythemia vera. Examination findings of cardiopulmonary disease may suggest the cause of a secondary erythrocytosis due to hypoxia.

Diagnostic Studies Performed in All Patients

A careful approach to the evaluation of absolute erythrocytosis must take into account both the causes of secondary erythrocytosis (see Table 40-2) and the

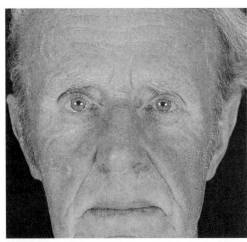

Figure 40-1 ▪ Facial plethora in a man with polycythemia vera. (From Hoffbrand AV, Pettit JE: Color Atlas of Clinical Hematology, 3rd ed. St. Louis: Mosby, 2000, p 247.) (See Color Plate 5.)

diagnostic criteria for polycythemia vera (Table 40-4). A number of diagnostic studies should be considered in all patients (Table 40-5). The results of these initial tests are used to determine which additional tests should be undertaken in individual patients.

Complete Blood Count

The red blood cell indices should be examined for evidence of iron deficiency, given its frequency in patients with polycythemia vera. This is particularly important in the setting of a modestly elevated hematocrit or in individuals with a normal hematocrit and other clinical features that are suggestive of polycythemia vera. In the absence of infection or other apparent causes of reactive leukocytosis, an elevated neutrophil count supports a diagnosis of polycythemia vera. A modest neutrophilic leukocytosis also occurs in smokers, particularly heavy smokers. In the absence of a reactive cause, thrombocytosis is also a minor criterion for polycythemia vera.

Oxygen Saturation

Determination of oxygen saturation is useful to exclude some forms of secondary erythrocytosis. Pulse oximetry is useful in determining the arterial oxygen saturation. It is important to stress, however, that pulse oximetry will not detect an elevated carboxyhemoglobin level. Particularly in cigarette smokers, the carboxyhemoglobin level must be determined directly and subtracted to give an adequate value for the oxygen saturation. Oxygen saturation below 92% has

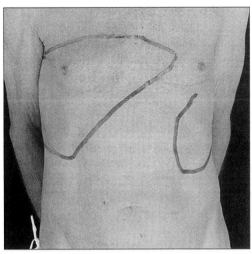

Figure 40-3 ■ Enlargement of liver and spleen in a patient with polycythemia vera. (From Hoffbrand AV, Pettit JE: Color Atlas of Clinical Hematology, 3rd ed. St. Louis: Mosby, 2000, p 248.)

been used to suggest a potential causal relationship with erythrocytosis. Oxygen saturation can vary throughout the day in given individuals, and intermittent reductions can result in erythrocytosis. Nocturnal desaturation can explain erythrocytosis in individuals who otherwise would be classified as having idiopathic erythrocytosis. Inquiry should be made into symptoms suggesting the sleep apnea syndrome, such as snoring, waking unrefreshed, and somnolence during the daytime, particularly in the obese patient. Smokers often have increased values of carboxyhemoglobin, but typically their hematocrits are only minimally higher than those of nonsmokers. While smoking is rarely the cause of absolute erythrocytosis, the elevated carboxyhemoglobin level in heavy smokers may contribute to the erythropoietic drive in those with underlying hypoxic lung disease.

Ferritin and Vitamin B$_{12}$

Determination of serum ferritin and vitamin B$_{12}$ levels may be helpful in suggesting the presence of polycythemia vera. Low ferritin values are more commonly seen in polycythemia vera than in secondary erythrocytoses, and absence of stainable iron in the marrow has been regarded as a hallmark of polycythemia vera. Vitamin B$_{12}$ levels may be elevated in polycythemia vera due to transcobalamin release from an increased granulocyte mass. Folate deficiency has been reported in polycythemia vera.

Renal and Liver Function Tests

Examination of renal and liver function tests may be useful. Mild renal impairment has been associated with a moderate absolute erythrocytosis in some individuals. Renal ultrasound is an important investigation in all patients to identify polycystic kidneys or other anatomic abnormalities given the various renal lesions associated with erythrocytosis. Cirrhosis of the liver and excessive alcohol intake with impaired liver function may occasionally cause absolute erythrocytosis due to associated hypoxemia, decreased erythropoietin catabolism, or increased hepatic production. Uric acid is frequently elevated in individuals with polycythemia vera and may be associated with gout.

Abdominal Ultrasound

An abdominal ultrasound is indicated in all patients. Simple renal cysts are commonly found but, unlike polycystic kidneys, are rarely associated with erythrocytosis. On occasion, very large renal cysts or hydronephrosis may cause sufficient renal ischemia to cause erythrocytosis. Renal cell carcinoma is occasionally (fewer than 5% of cases) associated with erythrocytosis (Figure 40-4). Ultrasound can be useful

---

Table 40-4 ■ Proposed Diagnostic Criteria for Polycythemia Vera

A1	Raised red cell mass (>25% above mean normal predicted value) or Hct ≥ 60% in males or 56% in females
A2	Absence of cause of secondary erythrocytosis
A3	Palpable splenomegaly
A4	Clonality marker (abnormal marrow karyotype)
B1	Thrombocytosis (platelet count: >400,000/μL)
B2	Neutrophilic leukocytosis (neutrophil count: >10,000/μL, >12,500/μL in smokers)
B3	Splenomegaly demonstrated by scan
B4	Characteristic BFU-E growth or decreased serum erythropoietin level
A1+A2+A3 or A4	Establishes diagnosis of polycythemia vera
A1+A2+two of B	Establishes diagnosis of polycythemia vera

Table 40-5 ■ Evaluation of Absolute Erythrocytosis

Tests Performed in All Patients

Complete blood count
Blood urea nitrogen and creatinine
Liver function tests
Uric acid
Ferritin
Vitamin B_{12}
Serum erythropoietin
Arterial oxygen saturation
Abdominal ultrasound

Tests Performed in Selected Patients

Bone marrow aspiration and biopsy
Marrow karyotype
Burst-forming unit erythroid culture
Immunohistochemical staining for megakaryocyte *c-mpl*
Quantitation of PRV-1 expression in granulocytes
Oxygen dissociation curve (P_{50})
Erythropoetin receptor analysis
Chest X-ray
Pulmonary function tests
Echocardiogram
Sleep study

in assessing both liver disease and splenic size. Hepatocellular carcinoma is associated with erythrocytosis in fewer than 10% of cases (Figure 40-5). Splenic enlargement can be detected by scanning before it is palpable (Figure 40-6). In the absence of liver disease, splenic enlargement, whether palpable or documented by ultrasound, supports a diagnosis of poly-

cythemia vera. There is, however, some variability in ultrasound spleen sizing among radiologists along with variation in splenic size according to the age and size of the individual. In light of this, splenic enlargement established by scanning is only a minor criterion for the diagnosis of polycythemia vera.

Computed Tomography

Computed tomography images of the abdomen can reveal malignant processes associated with polycythemia. Images of the kidney (see Figure 40-4*B*) can reveal renal cell carcinoma. Images of the liver (see Figure 40-5*B*) can reveal primary hepatocellular carcinoma. Both diseases can be associated with erythropoietin or an erythropoietin-like substance production.

Serum Erythropoietin

In polycythemia vera, serum erythropoietin levels are low or low normal at presentation and remain low despite normalization of hematocrit by phlebotomy. However, low serum erythropoietin levels can also occur in other causes of erythrocytosis at times when hematocrit levels are elevated. This limits the specificity of a low erythropoietin level for polycythemia vera in the setting of an elevated hematocrit, but it remains useful as a minor criterion. An elevated serum erythropoietin level is strong evidence against polycythemia vera. In secondary erythrocytosis due to arterial hypoxemia, erythropoietin levels are usually elevated. In other forms of secondary erythrocytosis, results are variable, and a normal value does not exclude secondary erythrocytosis.

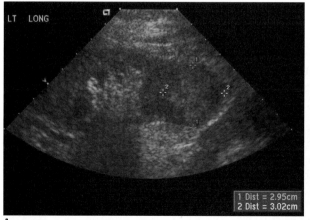

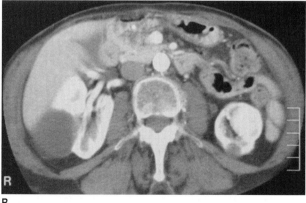

Figure 40-4 ■ Renal cell carcinoma and erythrocytosis. *A*, Ultrasound of left kidney in a woman with erythrocytosis shows a 3 × 3 cm mass (indicated by cursors); *B*, Computed tomography scan shows an enhancing mass in the left kidney that was found to be a renal cell carcinoma. A small left kidney cyst and a large right kidney cyst are also present.

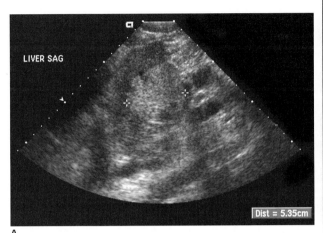

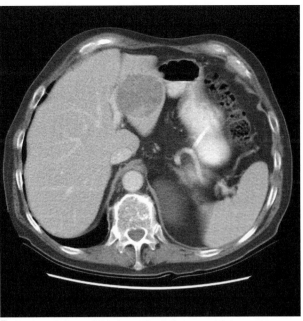

Figure 40-5 ■ Hepatocellular carcinoma and erythrocytosis. *A*, Ultrasound of liver in a man with erythrocytosis shows a 5 × 5 cm mass (indicated by cursors); *B*, Computed tomography scan shows a mass in the left lobe of the liver that was found to be a hepatocellular carcinoma.

Diagnostic Studies Performed in Selected Patients

Bone Marrow Aspiration and Biopsy

Bone marrow aspirate and biopsy should be performed in patients with absolute erythrocytosis unless a clear causative diagnosis has been established. The characteristic marrow appearance in polycythemia vera includes hypercellularity with trilineage hyperplasia, pleomorphic megakaryocytes with giant forms, and increased ploidy and clustering of megakaryocytes (Figure 40-7). The reticulum may be normal or moderately increased in polycythemia vera, and often iron stores are decreased or absent. Quantitative and qualitative megakaryocyte abnormalities and decreased iron stores are not commonly seen in secondary erythrocytosis. Owing to interobserver variation, these findings are most useful in supporting a diagnosis of polycythemia vera. Marrow studies may identify early myelofibrotic changes or findings that are suggestive of leukemic transformation. Marrow examination should be performed before undertaking cytoreductive therapy.

Marrow Karyotype

Marrow karyotype studies should be performed on all marrow samples obtained to evaluate erythrocytosis. The identification of an acquired, karyotypic abnor-mality indicates the presence of a clonal disorder and is a major criterion for the diagnosis of polycythemia vera. From 10% to 20% of patients with polycythemia vera have karyotypic abnormalities, including 20q-, trisomy 8, trisomy 9, 13q-, and deletions of chromosome 5 or 7.

Burst-Forming Unit Erythroid Assays

Marrow progenitors from polycythemia vera patients have burst-forming unit erythroid (BFU-E) that are

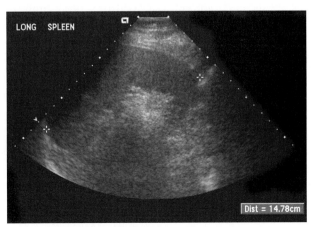

Figure 40-6 ■ Ultrasound demonstration of mild splenomegaly in a patient with polycythemia vera.

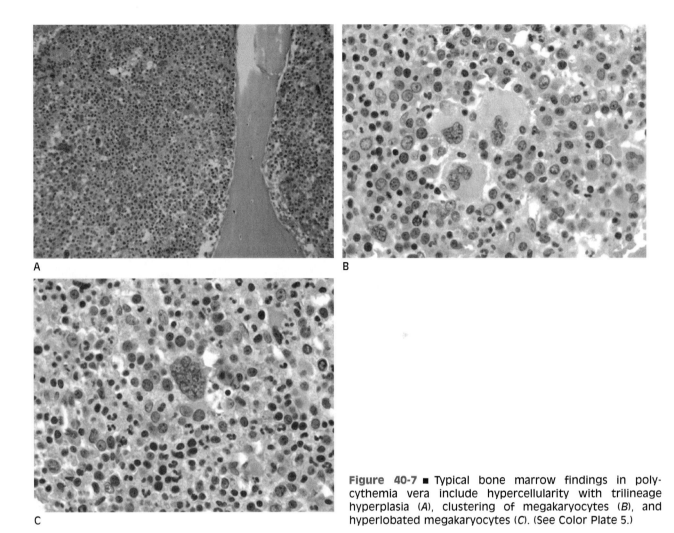

Figure 40-7 ▪ Typical bone marrow findings in polycythemia vera include hypercellularity with trilineage hyperplasia (*A*), clustering of megakaryocytes (*B*), and hyperlobated megakaryocytes (*C*). (See Color Plate 5.)

more sensitive than normal to several different growth factors, including erythropoietin, interleukin-3, stem cell factor, and insulin-like growth factor. Burst-forming unit erythroid will develop in the absence of exogenous erythropoietin in cultures of peripheral blood or marrow cells from patients with polycythemia vera. Growth of these endogenous erythroid colonies is not generally seen in patients with secondary erythrocytosis, and this assay has been proposed as a reliable diagnostic marker of polycythemia vera. Unfortunately, the number of burst-forming unit erythroids that grow in this assay varies considerably among patients with polycythemia vera, and the colonies tend to be poorly hemoglobinized and therefore difficult to score. A more reliable approach is to measure a dose-response curve of burst-forming unit erythroid and erythropoietin. This assay yields similar results in patients with erythropoietin receptor truncation. These culture-based techniques are laborious,

expensive, and often not readily available. They have more utility in the research setting than in the routine diagnosis of polycythemia vera.

Immunohistochemical Staining for Megakaryocyte *c-mpl*

Recent studies have shown decreased megakaryocyte expression of the thrombopoietin receptor (*c-mpl*) in patients with polycythemia vera but not in secondary erythrocytosis. These studies suggest that *c-mpl* staining may complement marrow histology in supporting a diagnosis of polycythemia vera.

Quantitation of PRV-1 Expression in Granulocytes

Subtractive hybridization was used to search for genes that are differentially expressed in granulocytes from patients with polycythemia vera versus normal controls. This led to the identification of the PRV-1 gene, a novel member of the urokinase plasminogen activator receptor (uPAR) superfamily, which is expressed at high levels in granulocytes from patients with polycythemia vera but not in granulocytes from normal controls. Expression was observed in normal controls that had been treated with granulocyte colony stimulating factor. PRV-1 expression was not observed in a limited number of patients with secondary erythrocytosis, chronic myeloid leukemia, or acute myeloid leukemia.

Oxygen Dissociation Curve (P_{50})

The partial pressure of oxygen at which hemoglobin is 50% saturated with oxygen is a convenient measure of the affinity of hemoglobin for oxygen. A reduced P_{50} indicates hemoglobin with an increased affinity for oxygen. This results in impaired oxygen release in tissues and a compensatory erythrocytosis. Measurement of the P_{50} is essential in individuals with unexplained erythrocytosis to identify those with high-oxygen-affinity hemoglobin, congenital methemoglobinemia, or the rare patient with congenital deficiency of 2,3-diphosphoglycerate. Many of the high-oxygen-affinity hemoglobin mutants are not detected by routine electrophoresis. Therefore, measurement of P_{50} is the appropriate first step in evaluating these individuals. Once a hemoglobin mutant has been excluded by using electrophoresis at both alkaline and acid pH and isoelectric focusing, an assay of erythrocyte 2,3-diphosphoglycerate should be performed. Hemoglobin oxygen dissociation studies are available in only a few research laboratories.

Truncation of the Erythropoietin Receptor

The rare individual with truncation of the erythropoietin receptor will present with unexplained erythrocytosis and, typically, a low serum erythropoietin level. Erythroid progenitor bone marrow cells from these individuals grow in culture independent of erythropoietin, similar to those from patients with polycythemia vera. Unlike in polycythemia vera, however, erythropoiesis is polyclonal. The truncation of the erythropoietin receptor results in loss of a C-terminal, intracytoplasmic negative regulatory domain. This domain plays an important role in down-modulation of the signal after ligand-induced signaling through the erythropoietin receptor. Inquiry into the presence of additional affected family members and genetic studies are appropriate in these rare individuals with primary erythrocytosis in the absence of other diagnostic criteria for polycythemia vera. Both autosomal dominant inheritance and sporadic occurrence have been reported.

Idiopathic Erythrocytosis

A heterogeneous group of patients with absolute erythrocytosis cannot be classified as having a clear cause. In approximately 5% to 10% of these patients, features that are definitive for polycythemia vera will emerge over a few years. In other patients, a cause of secondary erythrocytosis, such as nocturnal arterial hypoxemia, will be recognized ultimately. It is most important to not incorrectly ascribe a cause of erythrocytosis in a given patient. When there is doubt as to the diagnosis, it is best to follow the patient closely and to reevaluate the patient periodically.

Apparent Erythrocytosis

Apparent erythrocytosis has previously been known by a number of names including relative, stress, spurious, and pseudo-polycythemia. Approximately one third of these individuals have a reduced plasma volume below the normal range, but the majority have an increase in the red cell mass and a reduction in plasma volume. A number of possible underlying mechanisms have been identified, including hypertension, renal disease, fluid loss, alcohol, obesity, smoking, arterial hypoxemia, and an early stage of development of absolute erythrocytosis.

It is particularly important to exclude renal disease and arterial hypoxemia. A sleep study should be performed if there are symptoms to suggest nocturnal arterial oxygen desaturation. Previously, it was found that erythropoietin levels were normal in apparent erythrocytosis, but a recent study has shown that some of these patients have serum erythropoietin levels below the normal range.

Over a follow-up period of several months, in approximately one third of patients the hematocrit will fall into the normal range. In another third, the hematocrit is variably in the normal range or just slightly elevated. This leaves one third of these patients with a consistently raised hematocrit. These patients warrant extended follow-up.

Suggested Reading

Michiels JJ, Barbui T, Finazzi G, Fuchtman SM, Kutti J, Rain JD, Silver RT, Tefferi A, Thiele J: Diagnosis and treatment of polycythemia vera and possible future study designs of the PVSG. Leuk Lymphoma 2000;36:239–253.

Pearson TC: Diagnosis and classification of erythrocytoses and thrombocytoses. Baillieres Clin Haematol 1998;11:695–720.

Pearson TC: Evaluation of diagnostic criteria in polycythemia vera. Semin Hematol 2001;38(1 Suppl 2):21–24.

Prchal JT: Pathogenetic mechanisms of polycythemia vera and congenital polycythemic disorders. Semin Hematol 2001; 38(1 Suppl 2):10–20.

Tefferi A: Diagnosing polycythemia vera: A paradigm shift. Mayo Clin Proc 1999;74:159–162.

Temerinac S, Klippel S, Strunck E, Roder S, Lubbert M, Lange W, Azemar M, Meinhardt G, Schaefer H-E, Pahl HL: Cloning of PRV-1, a novel member of the uPAR receptor superfamily, which is overexpressed in polycythemia rubra vera. Blood 2000;95:2569–2576.

Chapter 41
Presentation of Bleeding Disorders

Bruce Furie

Hereditary and acquired bleeding disorders present to medical attention following episodes of spontaneous bleeding or bruising or after serious bleeding complications following trauma or a surgical procedure. A careful medical history and laboratory evaluation will usually lead to a specific diagnosis. With a diagnosis in hand, the bleeding risk of a specific surgical procedure can be estimated, and a rational plan can be developed for taking patients safely through surgery or to manage intermittent episodes of spontaneous or traumatic bleeding.

The Spectrum of Bleeding Disorders

Bleeding disorders can be classified in four separate categories: (1) coagulation disorders, (2) von Willebrand disease, (3) fibrinolytic disorders, and (4) platelet function abnormalities. Within this framework, each patient can be examined, and his or her bleeding abnormality can be diagnosed. Although the medical history may provide some important clues to a specific diagnosis and guide the laboratory evaluation, a complete and systematic laboratory evaluation is the most reliable method to confirm a suspected diagnosis.

Special attention to the patient presentation and history facilitates arriving rapidly at the correct diagnosis. Issues on which to focus include the nature and site of bleeding, the temporal relationship of this bleeding episode to other medical problems or medications, a family history of similar bleeding disorders, and the distinction between congenital and acquired disorders. Presentation of intermittent, chronic bleeding from mucosa, including epistaxis or lower gastrointestinal bleeding, hints of either a platelet defect or von Willebrand's disease. Delayed bleeding following surgery may be the result of excessive fibrinolysis. Hemarthrosis is often associated with hemophilia. Easy bruisability is a very common complaint, and the yield on its evaluation may be low; it can be associated with platelet defects or medications that interfere

with platelet function. Excessive bleeding following tooth extraction is a common presentation of a congenital bleeding disorder but can be associated with all hemostatic disorders. Usually, patients with congenital bleeding disorders have a lifelong history of clinical problems. However, some congenital disorders may be mild and express themselves only following surgery or serious injury. A lifelong bleeding problem that manifests itself during the rigors of childhood is likely to be congenital. A patient who is currently under evaluation for a bleeding disorder and who underwent major surgery uneventfully 10 years earlier is likely to have an acquired abnormality.

Concurrent disease may be associated with a bleeding disorder. For example, a coagulopathy and severe liver disease are likely to be causally related owing to impaired synthetic function. Acquired disorders are often associated with the use of certain medications, particularly medications that are known to interfere with platelet function or to be associated with the lupus anticoagulant. Aspirin and aspirin-containing compounds are famously associated with a bleeding tendency owing to their interference with prostaglandin synthesis in platelets; alcohol use can aggravate this effect. However, many other drugs interfere with platelet function, including nonsteroidal anti-inflammatory drugs. Accidental or surreptitious ingestion of warfarin may be suspected in a patient who is deficient in the vitamin K–dependent blood-clotting proteins but otherwise free of any causes of vitamin K deficiency. This coagulopathy in its most serious form can be a manifestation of psychiatric disease and is seen in subjects with access to warfarin and who may be associated with the health professions. Superwarfarins, such as brodifacoum, are rodenticides that can cause severe deficiency of the vitamin K–dependent proteins. A family bleeding disorder is always suggestive of a hereditary disorder, and it can include any of the four categories. A coagulopathy that is hereditary and afflicts male members of the family is suggestive of the X-linked diseases hemophilia A (Factor VIII deficiency) and hemophilia B (Factor IX deficiency). However, the absence of a family history does not preclude a congenital coagulopathy, since about one third of patients with hemophilia do not have a history of this disease in their family.

From the initial interview and examination of the patient, it should be possible to address the following questions:

1. Should this patient undergo a limited or extensive laboratory workup of hemorrhagic disorders?
2. Is this bleeding disorder more likely to be acquired or more likely to be hereditary?
3. Is this likely to be a disorder of clotting proteins, platelets, fibrinolysis, or von Willebrand factor?
4. Does the gender of the patient assist in eliminating certain diagnoses?
5. Do medications or intercurrent illness play a role?
6. Is this evaluation for an immediate acute bleeding problem that requires treatment, or is the evaluation to understand the nature of the disorder for pending or future surgery or potential trauma-induced emergency?

Once the answers to these questions have been established, the primary effort is to combine this information with that obtained from a laboratory evaluation to place the disorder within one of the following four categories: coagulation disorders, von Willebrand disease, fibrinolytic disorders, and platelet disorders.

Coagulation Disorders

Abnormalities of blood coagulation are reflected in the prolongation of the partial thromboplastin time (PTT) or the prothrombin time (PT; see Table 41-1). Because the PTT and PT are widely available and highly reliable, these tests should be used to screen for coagulation abnormalities (Figure 41-1). A clinically significant coagulation disorder caused by a deficiency of the activity of one or more blood-clotting proteins is not possible if the PTT and PT are within the normal range. In general, the PTT or PT is prolonged when a coagulation protein activity is at least below 40% to 60% of the normal value. Unless the PTT or PT is prolonged, the deficiency in itself is not sufficient to cause a clinically relevant bleeding disorder. Prolongation of the PTT or PT usually warrants determination of the proteins that are biologically deficient by measurement of the level of specific clotting factors. The pattern of this deficiency leads to a specific diagnosis. For example, deficiency of the vitamin K–dependent

DIAGNOSIS

Bleeding Presentations: Who Needs Evaluation?

Epistaxis: This is a common complaint among otherwise healthy children and a common complication of medical disorders of adults. Epistaxis does not necessarily indicate a hemostatic abnormality. Evaluation should be reserved for patients with an unusual frequency of epistaxis or unusual quantity of blood loss. Environmental conditions (e.g., low humidity), anatomic lesions such as vascular abnormalities, and other local defects must be distinguished from abnormalities of hemostasis. Bleeding from both nares hints of a systemic abnormality.

Heavy menses: Heavy menses may be associated with von Willebrand disease. More commonly, there is no hemostatic abnormality, and an endocrine evaluation is of higher yield.

Easy bruisability: A very common problem, especially among women, this complaint does not warrant workup unless the symptoms and signs are extreme.

Bleeding following tooth extraction: Significant bleeding following tooth extraction, particularly when transfusion is necessary, is a critical historic feature indicating the likelihood of a hemostatic abnormality.

Hematomas: Hematoma formation following injury is not uncommon and does not warrant evaluation unless the hematoma is unusually large (out of proportion to the injury). Hematomas that are recurrent and multiple require evaluation.

Excessive bleeding following surgery: Postoperative bleeding almost always requires evaluation.
Family history of bleeding tendency
Incidental prolonged PTT or prothrombin time

Hemarthrosis: Spontaneous hemarthrosis is almost always associated with hemophilia.

Table 41-1 ■ Coagulation Disorders That Can Cause Bleeding

Combined Prolongation of the PTT and PT

Vitamin K deficiency
Liver disease
Factitious purpura
Warfarin
Acquired inhibitor to factor V
Factor X deficiency and amyloidosis
Disseminated intravascular coagulation
Deficiency of factors X or V or prothrombin

Prolongation of the PT Only

Factor VII deficiency

Prolongation of the PTT Only

Hemophilia A (factor VIII deficiency)
Hemophilia B (factor IX deficiency)
Factor XI deficiency
Factor VIII inhibitor

blood coagulation proteins suggests vitamin K deficiency, pharmacologic inhibition of synthesis of the vitamin K–dependent proteins, or a hereditary defect in vitamin K–dependent carboxylation. An isolated hereditary deficiency of factor VIII or factor IX suggests hemophilia. Factor XI deficiency is most likely hereditary. Liver disease is associated with general synthetic defects in the blood coagulation proteins, whereas DIC is associated with consumption of these proteins. A circulating anticoagulant can be diagnosed with the PTT obtained from a mix of patient plasma and normal plasma.

Von Willebrand Disease

Von Willebrand disease is the most common hereditary bleeding disorder. It is easily diagnosed by two, or ideally three, blood tests: the Ristocetin cofactor assay, a measure of the biological activity of von Willebrand factor; factor VIII activity; and von Willebrand factor antigen. Care must be taken to obtain these results from a reliable laboratory, since misdiagnoses (false positives) are common. In the most common forms of von Willebrand disease, von Willebrand factor antigen is decreased in plasma (Type I) or von Willebrand factor antigen is normal but the activity is decreased (Type IIa). The bleeding time is prolonged in von Willebrand disease.

Fibrinolytic Disorders

After clot formation and wound healing, the fibrin clot is dissolved enzymatically by plasmin via the fibrinolytic pathway. Excess fibrinolysis can be associated with a bleeding disorder. A simple albeit old-fashioned method of screening for excessive fibrinolytic activity employs the euglobulin clot lysis time. Abnormalities of the euglobulin clot lysis time can also be due to α2-antiplasmin deficiency, levels of which can be monitored as well.

Platelet Function Abnormalities

Most platelet function abnormalities, both acquired and congenital, are difficult to measure using the available laboratory assays. The bleeding time has been shown to be an inadequate screening test to predict bleeding and is now reserved for confirmation of bleeding disorders such as von Willebrand's disease. Platelet aggregation studies, the only platelet function tests that are routinely available, are limited to the demonstration of the expression of a functional fibrinogen receptor (glycoprotein IIb-IIIa), the presence of fibrinogen and granule secretion. No other methods are currently available for the routine monitoring of platelet function in the clinical laboratory. Platelet adhesiveness, measured as the percentage of platelets in platelet-rich plasma that bind to a glass bead column, is no longer routinely available in most laboratories.

Diagnosis

Acquired Bleeding Disorders

The clinical manifestations of vitamin K deficiency are usually excessive bleeding following surgery or spontaneous ecchymoses in the face of an elevated prothrombin time and partial thromboplastin time. There is a deficiency of the four vitamin K–dependent blood clotting proteins, factor VII, factor X, factor IX, and prothrombin, in the absence of deficiency of one or more of the blood-clotting proteins that do not require vitamin K for their synthesis. Vitamin K deficiency is usually due to malabsorption of fat-soluble vitamins or, following complicated surgery, can be typically observed in hospitalized patients with no food intake who are treated with antibiotics. Also, malabsorption syndromes, specifically intestinal malabsorption due to inflammatory bowel disease or diseases of the biliary tree, can be complicated by vitamin K deficiency. It is not possible for a normal healthy individual to become vitamin K deficient on the basis of diet alone. Rarely, vitamin K deficiency is observed with certain medications. For example, ingestion of excessive amounts of aspirin leads to oxidation of vitamin K and subsequent severe vitamin K deficiency.

Factitious purpura, historically associated with surreptitious warfarin ingestion but more recently also associated with ingestion of "superwarfarins," such as the rodenticide brodifacoum, reflects the consequences of exposure to inhibitors of vitamin K. Patients may have no manifestations other than a prolonged PT and PTT, or they may have severe spontaneous bleeding into soft tissue, mucosal bleeding including epistaxis, or extreme menstrual bleeding. There is a deficiency of the four vitamin K–dependent blood clotting proteins, factor VII, factor X, factor IX, and prothrombin, thus causing elevation of the PTT and PT. This occurs in the absence of deficiency of the blood-clotting proteins that do not require vitamin K for their synthesis. Warfarin intoxication can be proven by demonstration of warfarin in the serum in a typical "tox" screen. When superwarfarin ingestion is suspected, specific serum assays (e.g., brodifacoum)

can be obtained from commercial laboratories to confirm the diagnosis.

Disseminated intravascular coagulation (DIC) can occur in two forms. In its fulminate form, it is associated with an acute hemorrhagic syndrome characterized by ecchymoses, epistaxis, gastrointestinal (GI) bleeding, hematuria, hematomas, and bleeding from venapuncture sites. In its chronic form, it is associated with thrombosis, including purpura fulminans, gangrene of the distal portions of digits, and tissue necrosis. Disseminated intravascular coagulation is caused by pathologic activation of the blood coagulation system, resulting in overwhelming of the natural anticoagulant mechanisms and the consumption of the coagulation proteins, including fibrinogen. Acute disseminated intravascular coagulation is characterized by a prolonged PT or PTT, low platelet count, and evidence of fibrinolysis, as manifested by an elevated D-dimer and fibrin split products. This syndrome is most commonly associated with septicemia but is also observed in obstetrical complications, including reten-

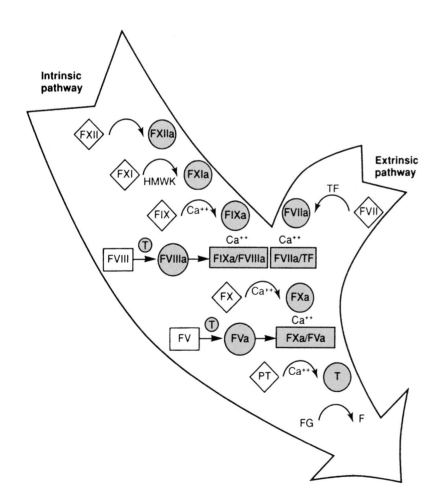

Figure 41-1 ■ Pathways of blood coagulation. The extrinsic pathway is measured by the prothrombin time. The intrinsic pathway is measured by the PTT. (From Furie B, Furie BC: Molecular basis of blood coagulation. In Hoffman R, Benz EJ Jr, Shattil SJ, Furie B, Cohen HJ, Silberstein LE, McGlare P [eds]: Hematology: Basic Principles and Practice, 3rd ed. New York: Churchill Livingstone, 2000, p 1784.)

TREATMENT

Relapsing Thrombotic Thrombocytopenia Purpura

Some patients with thrombotic thrombocytopenic purpura relapse episodically and re-present regularly with fulminant thrombotic thrombocytopenic purpura. Such cases require careful and watchful monitoring to identify the relapse prior to the development of the full clinical syndrome. Since thrombocytopenia and microangiopathic hemolytic anemia are the hallmarks of this disease, regular monitoring of the platelet count and the serum lactate dehydrogenase can provide adequate warning. Red cell fragmentation is associated with the release of lactate dehydrogenase in the plasma, so lactate dehydrogenase is a direct measure of hemolysis.

---

tion of a dead fetus, placental abruption, and amniotic fluid emboli. Chronic disseminated intravascular coagulation may be more indolent. Chronic disseminated intravascular coagulation is characterized by a minimal prolongation of the PT and PTT, a low platelet count, and evidence of significant fibrinolysis, including a low fibrinogen and elevated D-dimer assay. Microangiopathy may or may not be present.

Thrombotic thrombocytopenic purpura (TTP) is characterized by severe thrombocytopenia, microangiopathic hemolytic anemia, hematuria, transient neurologic signs, and gastrointestinal bleeding. The pathogenesis of thrombotic thrombocytopenic purpura appears to be due to absence or inhibition of a plasma protease that cleaves von Willebrand factor high molecular weight multimers. Episodes of thrombotic thrombocytopenic purpura may occur following viral infection. Significant microangiopathy is observed on the peripheral blood smear by the presence of schistocytes, which are markedly deformed red blood cells. The smear also is characterized by few platelets, consistent with the low platelet count. The extremely elevated lactate dehydrogenase (LDH) is due to hemolysis. Few conditions other than thrombotic thrombocytopenic purpura are associated with such high levels of the lactate dehydrogenase. The partial thromboplastin time and prothrombin time are always normal. Very high molecular weight multimers of von Willebrand's factor characterize the analysis of plasma from these patients. Both the platelet count and the lactate dehydrogenase are useful monitors of thrombotic thrombocytopenic purpura activity.

Liver disease in its severe form is associated with a clinically important coagulopathy. The PT and PTT are prolonged owing to deficiency of most of the blood coagulation proteins. All blood-clotting proteins are synthesized in the liver, with the exception of factor VIII, which is also synthesized in other tissues. The coagulopathy of liver disease is often associated with the sequelae of severe liver disease: jaundice, hepatomegaly, splenomegaly, hypoalbuminemia, and low blood urea nitrogen (BUN). Diagnostic difficulties arise when patients with severe liver disease present with a coagulopathy that might be caused by both liver disease and an additional disease process, such as disseminated intravascular coagulation.

Inhibitors of blood coagulation can manifest themselves with severe spontaneous bleeding or can be entirely silent. The lupus anticoagulant is associated with thrombosis, not bleeding. The PTT is usually prolonged and is not corrected in mixing studies. The specific lupus anticoagulant assay and the hexagonal phase phospholipid assay are important for documenting the presence of a lupus anticoagulant. The most common bleeding syndrome associated with an inhibitor is due to a factor VIII inhibitor. This may be observed during the postpartum period, in elderly patients, and in patients who are exposed to certain medications. The partial thromboplastin time is prolonged and is not corrected in mixing studies. A deficiency of factor VIII can be documented. It is essential to quantify the factor VIII inhibitor concentration using the Bethesda assay, since the titer of the inhibitor dictates appropriate therapy. Treatment of actively bleeding patients with factor VIII inhibitors is challenging and should be the domain of a specialist in coagulation. Acquired inhibitors of von Willebrand factor lead to accelerated clearance of von Willebrand factor and a bleeding syndrome similar to the hereditary form of von Willebrand disease. This syndrome is most commonly associated with dysproteinemias, including patients with lymphoproliferative disorders and Waldenström's macroglobulinemia.

The von Willebrand factor antigen, Ristocetin cofactor activity, and factor VIII activity are usually low, in parallel, in a situation in which the PTT, now prolonged, was documented to be previously normal. Often these patients have a serum monoclonal gammopathy documented.

Factor X deficiency associated with primary amyloidosis is a rare disorder that is caused by rapid clearance of newly synthesized factor X. Isolated factor X deficiency in the absence of evidence of a congenital deficiency is suggestive of this syndrome. Although some patients may already carry a diagnosis of amyloidosis when the factor X deficiency is discovered, factor X deficiency and bleeding may be the presenting sign and symptom for a subset of patients with primary AL-type amyloid.

Acquired disorders of platelet function are often associated with certain medications. This can be associated with frank bleeding, although, more commonly, medications are associated with ecchymoses and purpura. Aspirin inhibits prostaglandin synthetase irreversibly, whereas ibuprofen inhibits prostaglandin synthetase reversibly. Abnormalities in the platelet aggregation studies indicate the absence of a secondary wave of aggregation due to the inhibition of granule release.

Congenital Bleeding Disorders

Hemophilia is the hereditary deficiency of the activity of factor VIII (hemophilia A) or factor IX (hemophilia B). Hemophilia A and hemophilia B are clinically indistinguishable, and both are associated with a prolonged PTT. The diagnosis is made by specific factor assay. In its mild form (factor VIII or factor IX levels greater than 4%), hemophilia may be latent until trauma, postoperative bleeding following surgery, or a prolonged PTT brings it to medical attention. In contrast, severe hemophilia (factor VIII or factor IX levels less than 1%) is associated with spontaneous hemarthrosis, hematomas, and internal bleeding.

Factor VII deficiency is a rare autosomal hereditary disorder. It is characterized by a normal PTT and a prolonged PT. Diagnosis is made with a factor VII assay.

Factor X deficiency, prothrombin deficiency, and factor V deficiency are rare autosomal hereditary disorders. Each is characterized by a prolonged PTT and PT. Diagnosis is documented by specific factor assay.

Von Willebrand disease, the most common hereditary bleeding disorder, is due to a deficiency in the activity of von Willebrand factor. This activity is assayed in the laboratory as Ristocetin cofactor activity. Levels below 50% of normal are consistent with von Willebrand disease. In general, the activity level correlates with the bleeding tendency. This bleeding is most often manifested by epistaxis and gastrointestinal bleeding. Often, the von Willebrand factor antigen is about the same level as the Ristocetin cofactor, as in Type I von Willebrand disease. However, Type IIa von Willebrand disease is characterized by low activity and normal antigen levels. Type IIb von Willebrand disease is associated with a gain-of-function mutation such that there is tighter binding between von Willebrand factor and platelets. Elevation of the von Willebrand factor level is associated with thrombocytopenia. Type III von Willebrand disease, which is very severe and associated with spontaneously bleeding, involves abnormalities at both alleles. Since von Willebrand factor is the carrier protein for factor VIII, low levels of von Willebrand factor lead to correspondingly low levels of factor VIII. In one form of von Willebrand disease in which there is a mutation in the site that interacts with factor VIII, patients have the phenotype of hemophiliacs with factor VIII deficiency, although the mutation is within the von Willebrand factor gene.

Factor XI deficiency is a common hereditary disorder observed mainly in populations derived from Ashkenazi Jews. The disorder is characterized by a prolonged PTT and a low concentration of factor XI. Unlike hemophilia A and hemophilia B, factor XI deficiency is an autosomal disease. In its heterozygous form, the factor XI concentration is between 30% and 50%, causing a prolongation of the PTT. In the homozygous form, the factor XI level can range from 0% to 30%.

Congenital thrombocytopathies, that is, platelets with abnormal function, are relatively common and can be associated with easy bruising and mucocutaneous bleeding. In most cases, the platelet count is normal. Glanzmann's thrombasthenia, characterized by a deficiency or functional defect in glycoprotein IIb-IIIa, is associated with abnormal platelet aggregation. There is a bleeding tendency, although serious bleeding is not common. Bernard-Soulier syndrome is caused by a deficiency or functional defect in glycoprotein Ib. The platelets are large and morphologically abnormal. The syndrome is characterized by a defect in platelet adhesion. May-Hegglin anomaly, with the presence of Pelger-Huet cells and a low platelet count, also includes a defect in platelet function. A number of other rare disorders, some characterized at the molecular level and others poorly described, include Gray platelet syndrome (with a deficiency of alpha granules), storage pool disease (with defective granules), Scott syndrome (abnormal membrane architecture), and release disease (abnormal granule release), combine to partially define patients with congenitally abnormal platelet function. There are no specific laboratory tests to demonstrate that patients are at risk for intraoperative bleeding. The patient's medical history, especially the response to prior surgery, is predictive of potential bleeding problems.

Hyperfibrinolysis syndrome is a hereditary disorder associated with increased risk of delayed postsurgical bleeding. Usually, the hemostatic evaluation is normal except for a shortened euglobulin clot lysis time.

Factor XII, high-molecular-weight kininogen, and prekallekrein deficiencies are of interest because they are characterized by a prolonged PTT but are not associated with a bleeding disorder.

Suggested Reading

Furie B, Bouchard B, Furie BC: Vitamin K–dependent carboxylation. Blood 1999;93:1798–1808.

Furie B, Limentani SA, Rosenfield CG: A practical guide to the evaluation and treatment of hemophilia. Blood 1994;84:3–9.

George JN, Shattil SJ: The clinical importance of acquired abnormalities of platelet function. N Engl J Med 1991; 324:27–39.

Weitzel JN, Sadowski JA, Furie BC, Maroose R, Mount ME, Murphy MJ, Furie B: Hemorrhagic disorder caused by surreptitious ingestion of a long-acting vitamin K antagonist/rodenticide, brodifacoum. Blood 1990;76:2555–2559.

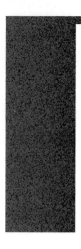

Chapter 42
Morphologic Abnormalities of the Peripheral Blood

Beria Cabello Inchausti and R. Judith Ratzan

Few physicians today make peripheral blood smears, stain the slides, or personally review them; slide preparation and interpretation are routinely performed by automated cell counters. The new hematology analyzers not only report red blood cell, white blood cell, and platelet counts as well as red blood cell indices, but also prepare the slides and provide white blood cell differential counts and morphologic assessments. Despite this impressive technology, microscopic examination of the machine-stained blood slide by the concerned clinician still adds an important dimension to patient care. This approach yields clues that enable one to immediately make the definitive diagnosis or to develop a focused, parsimonious investigation of the patient's problems by further studies. This chapter reviews the specific morphologic abnormalities that can be usefully identified on inspection of the peripheral blood smear.

General Approach

A systematic approach to the examination of the smears should be used to ensure that all cellular elements are carefully evaluated. Prior to microscopic examination, the appearance of the slide to the eye can be useful. A bluish tinge to the coloring of the slide suggests staining due to increased and/or abnormal plasma proteins or marked leukocytosis.

Examination at low-power magnification (Figure 42-1) is used initially to assess the overall number and distribution of leukocytes, search for platelet clumps, and identify red blood cell rouleaux formation or agglutination. In rouleaux formation, the red blood cells align one on the other so that they resemble stacks of coins (Figure 42-2). This is especially marked in the presence of monoclonal gammopathies but also occurs in any circumstance that elevates the sedimentation rate due to polyclonal increase in gammaglobulins and/or fibrinogen. In agglutination, the red blood cells stick to each other, usually because an antibody is coating the red cell surface, blocking the normally repulsive interaction of the negatively charged red blood cell membrane. Such clumping of the red blood cells appears as irregular or rounded clusters, resembling bunches of grapes (Figure 42-3). The shape of the red blood cells, characteristics of white blood

DIAGNOSIS

Morphology Presentations

- Macrocytosis commonly occurs in myelodysplasia and multiple myeloma. It also occurs in B_{12} and folate deficiency, but in those conditions, the macrocytes are macro-ovalocytic, and hypersegmentation of the granulocytes occurs.
- Anemia from blood loss may first present as a normochromic, normocytic anemia. It is only with continued iron loss that the cells undergo morphologic changes, first to microcytic cells and finally to microcytic and hypochromic cells.
- Toxic granulation of the neutrophils in a patient who is suspected of bacterial infection indicates that bacteremia is present.

- The red cell distribution width is increased in iron deficiency anemia (variable red cell size) and normal in thalassemias (fairly uniform red blood cell size), helping to distinguish between these two hypochromic, microcytic anemias. The red blood cell (RBC) count is also helpful, as it is normal in thalassemia and decreased in iron deficiency.
- The presence of Howell-Jolly bodies (nuclear remnants) in the red blood cells postsplenectomy rules out residual functioning splenic tissue.

Figure 42-1 ■ Peripheral blood smear. Low-power appearance. Well spread smear with even distribution of cells (original magnification ×10). (See Color Plate 6.)

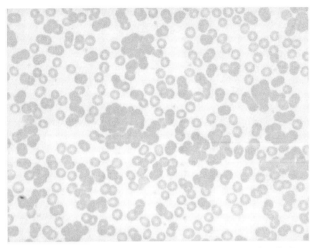

Figure 42-3 ■ Blood smear. Agglutination of red cells in a patient with cold agglutinins (original magnification ×40). (See Color Plate 6.)

cells, and platelet morphology are best evaluated by using the oil immersion lens. This may also be achieved with a "dry" 60× objective. The best area for evaluation is where the red blood cells are just touching, without overlapping (Figure 42-4).

Red Cell Abnormalities

In reviewing the smear, it is important to assess the size and shape of the red blood cells, the extent of hemoglobinization, and whether red blood cell inclusions are present. The average red blood cell is 6 to 8 μm in diameter, approximately the size of the nucleus of a well-differentiated lymphocyte. One can therefore use the lymphocyte to determine whether the red cell size is normal (normocytic), larger than normal (macrocytic), or smaller than normal (micro-

cytic). The red cell indices are helpful to confirm these visual findings. Because of its biconcave shape (like a dumbbell), the normal (normochromic) red blood cell is round with a small area of central pallor that is about one third of the cell diameter and fades gradually toward the more deeply stained periphery of the cell (see Figure 42-4). When the amount of hemoglobin per red blood cell decreases, the central area becomes larger and paler, and the cells are described as hypochromic (Figure 42-5). Hypochromic cells are characteristic of congenital sideroblastic anemia. A dimorphic population of red cells (normochromic and hypochromic in the same film) is present in the female carriers of congenital sideroblastic anemia as well as in the acquired sideroblastic anemias, especially idiopathic (subtype of myelodysplasia syndrome). A dimorphic population is also found after transfusion

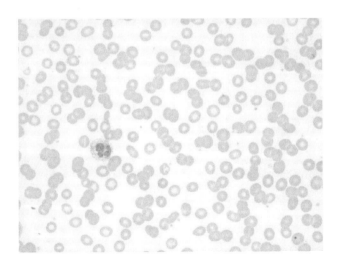

Figure 42-2 ■ Blood smear showing rouleaux formation (original magnification ×40). (See Color Plate 6.)

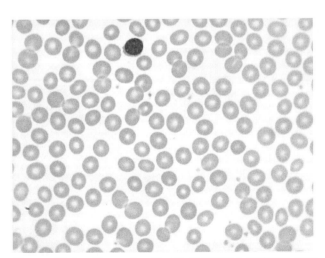

Figure 42-4 ■ The red cells are separated without overlapping. Normal red blood cells with little variation in size and small area of central pallor (original magnification ×60). (See Color Plate 6.)

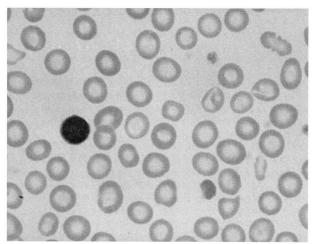

Figure 42-5 ■ Hypochromic red blood cells. Many are also microcytic (original magnification ×100, oil). (See Color Plate 6.)

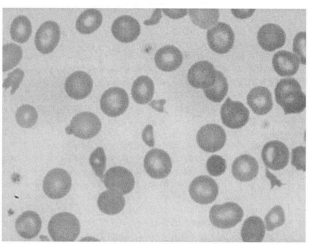

Figure 42-7 ■ Fragmented red cells in a patient with microangiopathic hemolytic anemia (original magnification ×100, oil). (See Color Plate 7.)

with normal red cells into a patient with a hypochromic anemia. This same picture may be seen for several weeks after initiation of iron replacement therapy for iron deficiency.

Inherited and acquired hematologic disorders produce widely variable changes in the shape of red blood cells. Normally, erythrocytes are fairly uniform circular discs, with only slight variation in size. Anisocytosis refers to the finding of a marked degree of difference in cell size, whereas poikilocytosis refers to abnormalities in cell shape. These variations in red blood cell shape are described by their appearance, for example, as crenated cells (burr cells, echinocytes), teardrop cells, schistocytes, stomatocytes, target cells, bite cells, acanthocytes or spur cells, and sickle cells. Crenated cells are red cells with spicules that are evenly distributed over the cell surface. They are usually an artifact of slide preparation and must be

distinguished from true abnormalities. Teardrop cells are typical of agnogenic myeloid metaplasia (myelofibrosis) (Figure 42-6). In this disorder, nucleated red blood cells, megakaryocytic fragments, large platelets, and white blood cell precursors are commonly seen.

Schistocytes are fragmented cells found in microangiopathic anemias where red blood cells are traumatized within the circulation, culminating in intravascular hemolysis. Causes include heart valve hemolysis, disseminated intravascular coagulation (DIC), thrombotic thrombocytopenic purpura (TTP), and hemolytic uremic syndrome (HUS) (Figure 42-7). The thrombocytopenic purpura/hemolytic uremic syndrome combination can be triggered by some medications such as mitomycin, ticlopidine, and clopidogrel; by diseases such as HIV; or after gastrointestinal infection with some strains of *Escherichia coli*. Because treatment of thrombocytopenic purpura/hemolytic

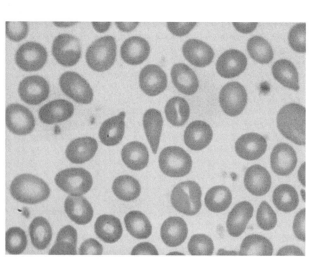

Figure 42-6 ■ Abnormally shaped cell in the form of a teardrop (original magnification ×100, oil). (See Color Plate 6.)

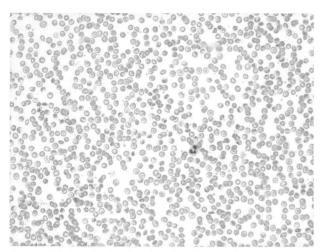

Figure 42-8 ■ Red cells showing hemoglobin in greater concentration at the rim of the cell and at the center producing a "target" appearance (original magnification ×20). (See Color Plate 7.)

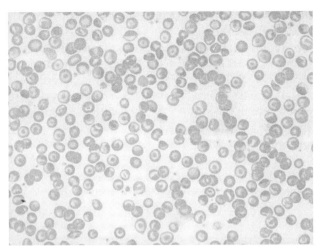

Figure 42-9 ■ Peripheral smear of a patient with hemoglobin C disease. Note elongated structure of hemoglobin crystals within a hypochromic red blood cell and many target cells (original magnification ×40). (See Color Plate 7.)

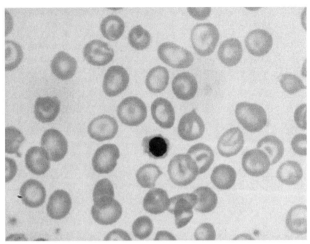

Figure 42-10 ■ Smear of a patient with thalassemia intermedia showing target cells and hypochromia with a nucleated red blood cell (original magnification ×100, oil). (See Color Plate 7.)

uremic syndrome must be initiated rapidly, it is important to examine the smear if there is any question of this diagnosis. The peripheral blood smear is virtually pathognomonic, exhibiting schistocytes of several types, including small cell fragments, helmet cells, or bite cells plus microspherocytes and nucleated red blood cells. Stomatocytes have a peculiar slit in the area of central pallor. These cells are generally seen in alcoholic liver disease. Target cells (Figure 42-8) are a result of increased red blood cell surface area and may be seen in liver disease, homozygous hemoglobin C disease (Figure 42-9), hemoglobin S/C disease, and the thalassemias (Figure 42-10). Inherited abnormalities in either qualitative or quantitative hemoglobin production can produce red blood cells with specific morphologic findings. Sickle-cell disorders are associated with production of hemoglobin S (Figure 42-11). This

abnormal hemoglobin causes sickling of the red blood cells on deoxygenation. Most of these cells are reversibly sickled, reassuming a normal red blood cell shape on oxygenation, whereas other cells are irreversibly sickled and unable to revert to normal. Sickling increases in areas of blood flow stasis, leading to tissue infarction and painful crises. Hemolysis, the destruction of red blood cells at an increased rate, is often accompanied by an increase in the number of young red blood cells; these are the reticulocytes. On routine Wright-stained smears, the reticulocyte appears slightly blue-pink (polychromatophilic cell) and somewhat larger than the mature red blood cells (Figure 42-12). The bluish color is due to residual RNA, which precipitates after exposure to supravital stains, forming dark inclusions in the cell that permit the enumeration of the reticulocytes as a percentage of the

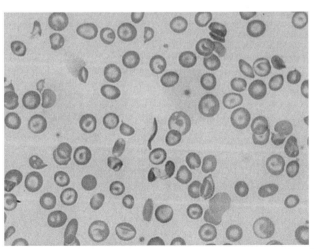

Figure 42-11 ■ Sickle cell in a patient with sickle-cell disease. Target cells and two red cells showing condensation of hemoglobin toward one side of the cell (original magnification ×60). (See Color Plate 7.)

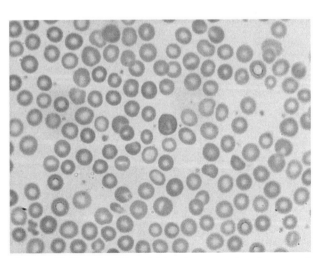

Figure 42-12 ■ Peripheral blood smear showing a polychromatophilic cell in the center of the field. These cells are large and usually lack central pallor (original magnification ×60). (See Color Plate 7.)

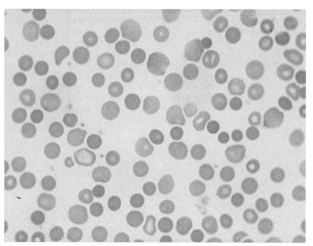

Figure 42-13 ■ Blood smear from a patient with autoimmune hemolytic anemia showing spherocytes, dense staining cells that tend to be microcytic (original magnification ×60). (See Color Plate 8.)

total red blood cell count. Spherocytes are red blood cells that have lost surface membrane. They round up, lose their biconcave shape, and assume a spherical appearance with loss of central pallor. They are extremely rare in normal persons, in whom they represent senescent cells. They are seen in patients with hereditary spherocytosis or warm antibody-induced autoimmune hemolytic anemia (AIHA) (Figure 42-13). In contrast, spherocytes are absent in cold agglutinin hemolytic anemias. In considering an immune-mediated hemolytic anemia, clues to cold agglutinin disease are usually also provided by a spurious elevation of the red blood cell mean corpuscular volume (MCV), in association with disparate readings on determination of the hemoglobin and hematocrit. These changes are caused by clumping of the red blood

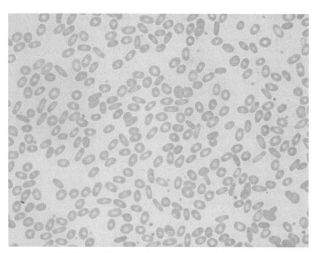

Figure 42-14 ■ Elliptocytes. The red blood cells are pencil- or cigar-shaped in a typical case of congenital elliptocytosis (original magnification ×40) (See Color Plate 8.)

cells at room temperature as they pass through automated cell counters. Elliptocytes (Figure 42-14) are seen as an inherited disorder, similar to hereditary spherocytosis. Elliptocytosis can occur without any significant hematologic disorder, but in some patients, it is associated with a mild hemolytic state. Bite cells are formed when individuals with G-6PD deficiency are exposed to drugs such as sulfonamides. Their appearance is that of a cell missing a small area. Burr or crenated cells are notably seen in uremia and represent cells with numerous evenly spaced projections. Spur (acanthocytes) cells seen in terminal liver disease are similar but with fewer and irregular projections.

Categories of Red Blood Cell Abnormalities in Anemias

Red blood cells in anemia may be either (1) normochromic, normocytic; (2) hypochromic, microcytic; or (3) macrocytic. The category of normochromic, normocytic anemia does not distinguish among a number of causes of reduced hemoglobin caused by a wide range of disorders such as metastatic cancer, inflammatory disease, or infection. The latter two categories are, however, extremely helpful in pinpointing the cause of anemia.

In the hypochromic, microcytic anemias, small, poorly hemoglobinized red blood cells are produced. This results from abnormalities in heme synthesis (iron insertion into heme), globin production (thalassemias), or both (lead poisoning). Iron deficiency should always be considered as indicative of blood loss, through either the gastrointestinal tract in men and postmenopausal women or vaginally due to menstruation in the premenopausal woman. The importance of making this diagnosis is in pursuing the etiology of the source of blood loss. In addition to the hypochromic/microcytic red blood cells, helpful clues to the presence of severe iron deficiency include cigar-shaped cells, marked anisocytosis, and an increase in platelet count. Hypochromic/microcytic anemia can also occur even when iron stores are normal because of defects in iron metabolism. The anemia of chronic disease and congenital sideroblastic anemias represent examples of this mechanism. Despite adequate iron stores in the reticuloendothelial cells of the bone marrow, iron transfer into heme in the developing red blood cell precursors is impaired. In the sideroblastic anemias (related to myelodysplasia), this problem can be quite pronounced, leading to the accumulation in red blood cell precursors of large amounts of iron within mitochondria that are peculiarly positioned in a perinuclear distribution. Visualized on iron stains of the bone marrow, these are called ringed sideroblasts.

In the peripheral blood, one can observe mixed red cell populations, including microcytic/hypochromic cells, normal cells, and some macrocytosis.

Hereditary defects in globin synthesis in the thalassemias lead to a decrease in the formation of hemoglobin even though iron is available. The resulting erythrocytes are markedly hypochromic and microcytic, similar to the changes in severe iron deficiency. An increased reticulocyte count, increased iron stores, normal red cell distribution width (RDW), and normal or actually increased red blood cell count distinguish thalassemia from iron deficiency.

Lead poisoning induces hypochromic/microcytic changes because lead interferes with both globin chain and heme synthesis pathways.

Macrocytic anemias are generally normochromic. Deficiency of B_{12} or folate leading to a megaloblastic bone marrow and macrocytic red blood cells in the peripheral blood are treatable causes of macrocytic anemia. The typical red cell in this condition has a macro-ovalocytic shape (Figure 42-15). Nucleated red blood cells (megaloblastic appearing) and red cells with Howell-Jolly bodies (nuclear remnants) may appear in the circulation. White blood cell abnormalities occur as well. In fact, the pathognomonic finding for the diagnosis of B_{12} or folic acid deficiency is the presence of hypersegmented granulocytes. Normal granulocytes generally do not have more than three or four lobes. An increase in the average lobe count above this number or the finding of even a single six-lobed granulocyte is highly suggestive of a diagnosis of megaloblastic anemia. It is worth remembering that other causes of macrocytosis exist, including myelodysplasia, increased reticulocyte count (because they are larger than normal red blood cells), red cell agglutination, and antineoplastic drugs that interfere with DNA synthesis such as hydroxyurea, methotrexate, or 6-mercaptopurine. These latter antimetabolites can also cause megaloblastic changes in the bone marrow despite normal folic acid and B_{12} levels.

Red Cell Inclusions

Erythrocyte inclusions develop as a manifestation of functional hyposplenia (as in sickle-cell anemia or splenic infarctions) or asplenia (postsplenectomy), an abnormality in red blood cell production, or instability of the hemoglobin molecule. Adequate splenic function serves to remove inclusions that can occur normally such as Howell-Jolly bodies (Figure 42-16) in circulating red blood cells (residual DNA) or the occasional nucleated red blood cell. Splenic hypofunction results in Pappenheimer bodies, which are complexes of ferric iron and protein that occur in disorders of hemoglobin production. In similar circumstances, red blood cells may demonstrate iron granules (siderocytes). Basophilic stippling (aggregated ribosomes) is a common finding in lead poisoning, thalassemia, or myeloproliferative disorders (Figure 42-17). It is a nonspecific finding, however, and can be found in a number of other hematologic disturbances. Special stains with supravital dyes are needed to see the residual RNA in reticulocytes (Figure 42-18) or the Heinz bodies (precipitated hemoglobin attached to the inner membrane surface) that occur in inherited mutant unstable hemoglobins or after severe oxidative injury (as happens in G-6PD deficiency) (Figure 42-19).

White Blood Cell Abnormalities

Careful evaluation of the white blood cells (WBCs) provides useful information regarding the patient's

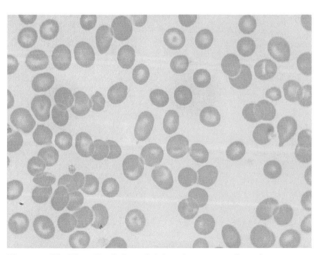

Figure 42-15 ■ Peripheral blood smear showing macro-ovalocytes (egg-shaped cells). These cells are different from elliptocytes (original magnification ×60). (See Color Plate 8.)

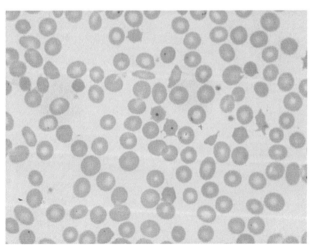

Figure 42-16 ■ Howell-Jolly bodies. Round nuclear remnants in the red cells. There are also acanthocytes (spur cells) (original magnification ×60). (See Color Plate 8.)

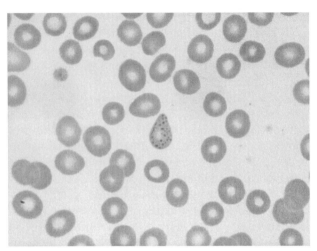

Figure 42-17 ■ Basophilic stippling. Punctate, bluish inclusions throughout the red cell (original magnification ×100, oil). (See Color Plate 8.)

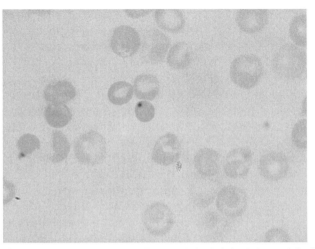

Figure 42-19 ■ Heinz body. Crystal violet stain (original magnification ×100, oil). (See Color Plate 9.)

status and/or underlying illness. Increase in the white blood cell count occurs in infection, leukemic disorders, and nonhematologic malignancies that infiltrate the bone marrow. The latter is termed myelophthisis, and the result is a leukoerythroblastic blood picture with circulating early white blood cell and red blood cell precursors. A decreased white blood cell count is noted in hypersplenism, collagen vascular disease, some viral infections, aplastic anemia, drug toxicity (due to direct marrow damage or immunologic injury), and immune neutropenias (such as in Felty's syndrome) or after chemotherapy. In considering the white blood cell differential count, one should be sure to convert the percentages of white blood cell subsets into absolute counts by multiplying by the total white blood cell count. For example, by percentage, a 35% neutrophil count is low, but if the total

white blood cell count is 10,000/μL, then the absolute number of granulocytes is normal. Toxic granulation of the neutrophils is present in severe infections (Figure 42-20), and a left shift in the granulocytes may be seen, with the appearance of white blood cell precursors, including metamyelocytes and myelocytes. Hyposegmentation of the granulocytes is called the Pelger-Huet anomaly. In these cells, the appearance of the cytoplasm and chromatin is normal, but the nucleus is either monolobed or bilobed (rather than the usual three to four lobes) with a thin bridge of chromatin connecting them. This anomaly, which is due to failure of the normal lobe development, is a not uncommon congenital disorder that is of no clinical significance (provided that it is not misinterpreted as an increase in band forms suggesting a shift in the granuloctyes), but it also can occur as part of myelo-

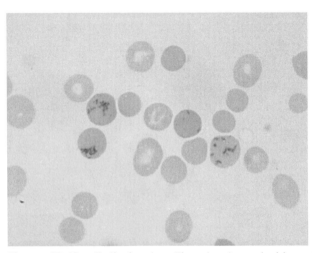

Figure 42-18 ■ Reticulocytes. The structures inside red cells represent precipitated ribonucleoprotein by new methylene blue. On air-dried smears stained with Wright stain, they are polychromatophilic cells (original magnification ×100, oil). (See Color Plate 8.)

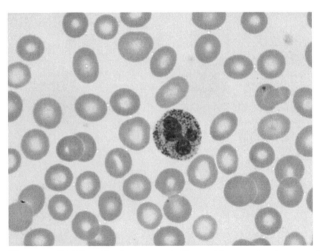

Figure 42-20 ■ Toxic granulation. The cytoplasm of this band neutrophil shows granules diffusely scattered throughout the cytoplasm (original magnification ×100, oil). (See Color Plate 9.)

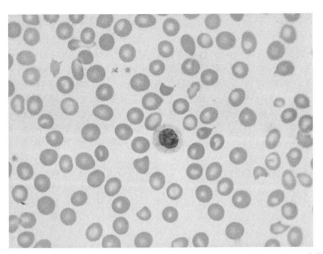

Figure 42-21 ■ Monolobed Pelger-Huet cell. Neutrophil with mature (clumped) chromatin. The nucleus failed to develop lobes (original magnification ×60). (See Color Plate 9.)

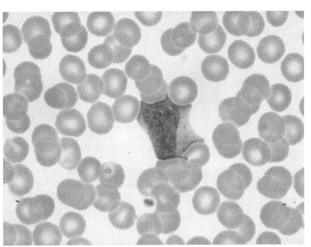

Figure 42-23 ■ Atypical lymphocyte. The morphology of atypical lymphocytes is variable. This one is large with abundant cytoplasm. Young man with infectious mononucleosis (original magnification ×100, oil). (See Color Plate 9.)

proliferative or myelodysplastic disorders (Figures 42-21 and 42-22). Rare disorders such as Chédiak-Higashi syndrome show a decreased white blood cell count, but the granulocytes, eosinophils, and monocytes have abnormal giant dark inclusions (large, coalesced lysosomal granules). Atypical lymphocytes are seen in viral infections, toxoplasmosis, or severe inflammatory disease. In these circumstances, the cells are large and the cytoplasm is a deep blue (RNA-rich), frequently with immature nuclear chromatin, but the absolute lymphocyte count is not increased. The atypical lymphocytes that appear in mononucleosis, whether caused by Epstein-Barr virus (EBV) or cytomegalovirus (CMV), are increased in number and striking in appearance. Many of the cells may appear similar to the lymphoblasts of acute lymphoid leukemia, whereas others are increased in size owing

to much increased but pale cytoplasm, which frequently contains vacuoles. The atypical lymphocytes are, in fact, activated T lymphocytes that develop as a cytocidal response to the Epstein-Barr virus– or cytomegalovirus-infected B lymphocytes (Figure 42-23).

The leukemias are usually readily identified on the peripheral smear. Chronic lymphocytic leukemia (CLL) presents with increased numbers of well-differentiated small lymphocytes (Figure 42-24). Characteristically, these cells are mechanically fragile, and when they are pushed along on a slide, some tend to disrupt, resulting in multistranded unidentifiable cell remainders called basket or smudge cells. It is important to examine the smear of patients with chronic lymphocytic leukemia and anemia for the

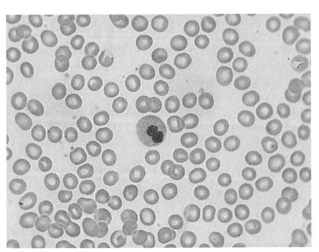

Figure 42-22 ■ Bilobed Pelger-Huet cell (original magnification ×60). (See Color Plate 9.)

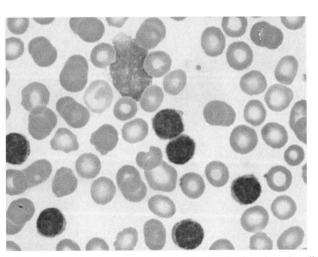

Figure 42-24 ■ Chronic lymphocytic leukemia. Small lymphocytes with dense nuclear chromatin and a very thin rim of cytoplasm. Note smudge cell at top of figure (original magnification ×100, oil). (See Color Plate 9.)

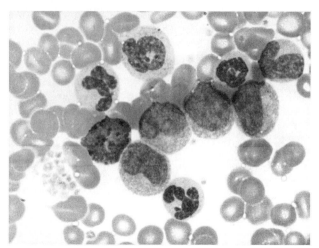

Figure 42-25 ▪ Peripheral blood smear. Chronic myeloid leukemia. Spectrum of granulocytic precursors with a basophil (cell with prominent, dark-stained granules) (original magnification ×100, oil). (See Color Plate 10.)

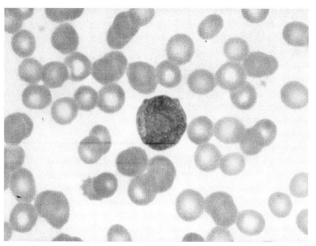

Figure 42-27 ▪ Acute myeloid leukemia. Blast with Auer rod, abnormal, typically azurophilic, lysosomal granule, in cytoplasm (original magnification ×100, oil). (See Color Plate 10.)

presence of spherocytes, because a direct antiglobulin-positive warm antibody hemolytic anemia not infrequently supervenes in these patients.

The white blood cells in peripheral smear in patients with chronic myeloid leukemia (CML) appear similar to the array of white blood cell precursors that are normally seen in the bone marrow, including a spectrum of myeloblasts, promyelocytes, myelocytes, metamyelocytes, and bands forms (Figure 42-25). Similarly, white blood cell abnormalities may be present in the other myeloproliferative disorders such as myelofibrosis with myeloid metaplasia. In this last disorder, these changes are accompanied by nucleated red blood cells, schistocytes, and large atypical platelets (megakaryocytic fragments).

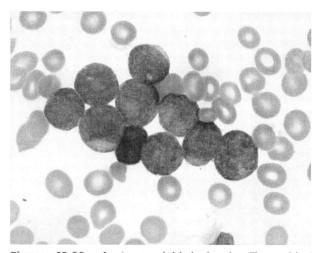

Figure 42-26 ▪ Acute myeloid leukemia. These blasts have fine chromatin, prominent nucleolus, and very little cytoplasm (original magnification ×100, oil). (See Color Plate 10.)

Acute leukemias generate blast forms, which are either myeloid or lymphoid, in the peripheral blood. Distinguishing between these two major types on Wright-Giemsa stain is sometimes difficult, but the appearance of Auer rods (red, sharply outlined, rod-shaped structures in the cytoplasm) indicates myeloid differentiation (Figures 42-26 and 42-27). Precise classification of the different types requires integration of data from immunophenotyping, cytochemical stains, and morphologic evaluation. The FAB classification of acute myeloid leukemia includes types M0 to M7, depending on the degree of differentiation and the type of blast. The first three types, M0, M1, and M2, vary from undifferentiated to more differentiated forms. M3 to M7 subtypes are categorized on the basis of type of the predominant blast cell produced. These include acute promyelocytic leukemia (M3), mixed myelo-monocytic differentiation (M4), monoblastic (M5), erythroblastic (M6), and megakaryoblastic (M7).

The FAB classification identifies three subtypes of acute lymphocytic leukemia: L1 (small lymphoblasts with minimum cytoplasm and inconspicuous nucleoli, L2 (large lymphoblasts with prominent nucleoli), and L3 (cells that are identical to those found in Burkitt's lymphomas) (Figures 42-28 and 42-29).

Platelet Abnormalities

Abnormal platelet forms appear in the myeloproliferative disorders, including essential thrombocythemia, chronic myeloid leukemia, myelofibrosis, and polycythemia vera. These platelets are the products of the defective stem cell clones in these diseases. They are associated in the bone marrow with atypical megakaryocytes and in the peripheral blood with giant

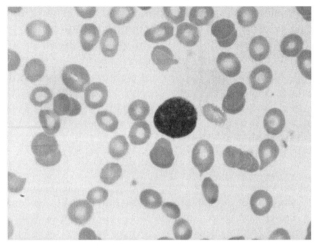

Figure 42-28 ■ Acute lymphocytic leukemia, L1 morphology (original magnification ×100, oil). (See Color Plate 10.)

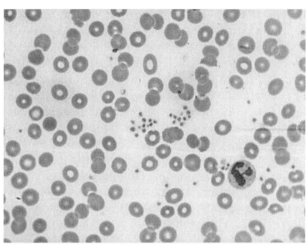

Figure 42-31 ■ Platelet clumps (original magnification ×60). (See Color Plate 11.)

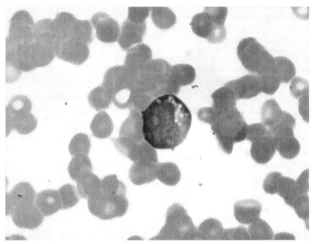

Figure 42-29 ■ Acute lymphocytic leukemia, L3 morphology. This lymphoblast shows a prominent nucleolus and fairly abundant cytoplasm with vacuoles (original magnification ×100, oil). (See Color Plate 10.)

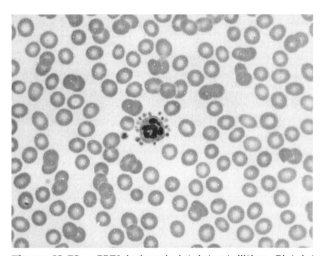

Figure 42-32 ■ EDTA-induced platelet satellitism. Platelets are adherent to the neutrophil (original magnification ×60). (See Color Plate 11.)

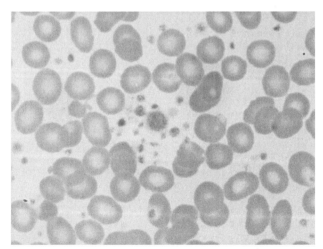

Figure 42-30 ■ Peripheral blood smear from a patient with essential thrombocythemia. Platelets are markedly increased in number. Large platelets are present (original magnification ×100, oil). (See Color Plate 10.)

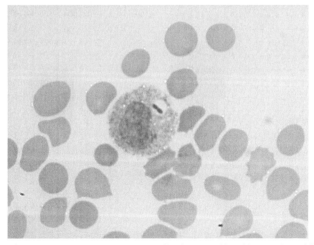

Figure 42-33 ■ Bacteria (*E. coli*) phagocytized in neutrophil (original magnification ×100, oil). (See Color Plate 11.)

platelets from abnormal fracturing of large amounts of the megakaryocyte cytoplasm. The platelet counts in myeloproliferative disorders can be normal, reduced, or increased (Figure 42-30). If they are increased in number, one has to consider alternative explanations, such as iron deficiency, chronic blood loss, inflammatory disease, solid malignancy, Hodgkin's disease, or postsplenectomy status.

The peripheral smear must be examined microscopically whenever the laboratory reports a low platelet count. Occasionally, clumping of platelets or platelet "satellitism" occurs when a patient's blood is drawn into a tube with ethylenediaminetetraacetic acid (EDTA) as the anticoagulant. A spuriously low platelet count results because the automated cell counters are gated on platelet size and do not include these clumps in the count (Figures 42-31 and 42-32). If blood is drawn in a tube with citrate as the anticoagulant, the automated counter will determine the true platelet count.

Infections as a Cause of Abnormalities in the Peripheral Smear

In rare circumstances, and usually associated with overwhelming bacteremia, careful inspection reveals bacterial inclusions in the white blood cells (Figure 42-33). These are most readily recognized at the feathery, tail end of the blood smear. In endemic areas, or in patients from endemic areas, careful perusal of the red cells will allow identification of a patient infected with malaria or babesia.

Suggested Reading

Dacie JV, Lewis SM: Practical Haematology, 7th ed. London: Churchill Livingstone, 1991.

Hall R, Malia RG: Preparation, staining, and examination of blood films. In Medical Laboratory Haematology. London: Butterworths, 1984, pp 130–171.

Henry JB: Clinical Diagnosis and Management by Laboratory Methods, 19th ed. Philadelphia: WB Saunders, 1996.

Schumacher HR, Garvin DF, Triplett DA: Introduction to Laboratory Hematology and Hematopathology. New York: Alan R. Liss, 1984.

Van Assendelft OW: Interpretation of the quantitative blood cell count, in Koepke JA (ed): Practical Laboratory Hematology. New York: Churchill Livingstone, New York, 1991, 61–97.

Williams WJ, Beutler E, Lichtman MA, et al (eds.): Hematology, 5th ed. New York, McGraw-Hill, 1995.

Chapter 43
Venous Thromboembolic Disease

Howard A. Liebman

Clinical Assessment

The patient presenting with a painful swollen leg from a deep vein thrombosis (DVT) is a common clinical scenario. This painful and disabling medical condition has added significance when there is extension of thrombosis into the proximal popliteal and/or common femoral veins, since this may be associated with the potentially fatal complication of pulmonary embolus. Numerous studies have shown that clinical examination alone is inadequate in making a valid diagnosis. Only 20% to 30% of patients with clinically suspected deep vein thrombosis have documented thrombosis after objective testing. Even in the presence of leg pain, tenderness, and/or swelling and excluding other obvious causes of leg swelling, only 42% of patients in one study were confirmed to have a deep vein thrombosis by venography. Frequently observed alternative diagnoses include superficial phlebitis of varicose veins, musculoskeletal injuries, chronic edema, and inflammatory arthritis. In the cancer patient, many of the classic clinical findings of deep vein thrombosis such as leg swelling, pain, and increased warmth with erythema can also result from lymphatic obstruction by tumor, external tumor compression of veins, superficial or deep infection, and metastatic disease to bone or soft tissue.

A carefully structured patient history and physical examination, when combined with assays for plasma D-dimer, can speed diagnosis and reduce the number of objective diagnostic studies. Clinical features that can predict a pretest probability of deep vein thrombosis have been validated in a series of well-designed studies and are listed in Table 43-1. The clinician should consider each of these clinical features in the evaluation of the patient. Nearly 80% of patients with a high pretest probability of deep vein thrombosis will have evidence of proximal deep vein thrombosis on compression ultrasound compared to fewer than 5% of patients with a low pretest probability. A moderate or intermediate pretest probability is associated with

an objectively documented deep vein thrombosis in 30% of patients. The significance of this clinical exercise is that patients with a high pretest probability and a negative compression ultrasound should have further evaluation with either contrast venography or a repeat ultrasound within five to seven days. Patients with a moderate pretest probability and a negative ultrasound should also undergo a repeat study within seven days. If the repeat study is negative, no further evaluation is indicated. Patients with low pretest probability and a negative ultrasound need no further studies or follow-up to rule out a deep vein thrombosis. A diagnostic algorithm for the evaluation of patients with a suspected deep vein thrombosis is presented in Figure 43-1.

Several other historical and clinical features, although less well validated, can provide important information regarding the probability of deep vein thrombosis and the risk of an underlying prothrombotic state. Superficial thrombophlebitis of calf vein varicosities is rarely associated with deep vein thrombosis. In contrast, superficial thrombophlebitis of the greater saphenous vein can be associated with deep venous involvement and even pulmonary embolism. There are also reported associations between the development of spontaneous superficial thrombophlebitis and prothrombotic states resulting from underlying cancer or the antiphospholipid syndrome. Therefore, the development of idiopathic superficial phlebitis alone in patients without obvious varicosities should alert the clinician to the possibility of these underlying prothrombotic disorders. Clinical probability models have concluded that a family history of thromboembolic disease is not predictive of a deep vein thrombosis and does not contribute to a determination of pretest probability. However, a history of venous thrombosis in first-degree relatives does increase the probability of detecting an underlying inherited prothrombotic defect in patients with an objectively documented idiopathic deep vein thrombosis.

Table 43-1 ■ Clinical Features Predicting Pretest Probability of Deep Vein Thrombosis

History

Active cancer within the last 6 months

Paralysis, paresis, or recent plaster immobilization of the lower extremities

Recently bedridden for more than 3 days or major surgery within 4 weeks

Postpartum within 4 weeks

Symptoms and Signs

Localized tenderness along the distribution of the deep venous system

Entire leg swollen

Calf swelling by more than 3 cm when compared with the asymptomatic leg* (measured 10 cm below tibial tuberosity)

Pitting edema (greater in the symptomatic leg)

Collateral superficial veins (nonvaricose)

Source: Adapted from Wells et al. (1997). A high pretest probability is defined as three or more of the features listed above. Moderate pretest probability is one to two features, and a low pretest probability is none of the above or the presence of an alternative diagnosis. The presence of an alternative diagnosis as likely or greater than a deep vein thrombosis is considered as a negative feature (×2).

*In patients with symptoms in both legs, the more symptomatic leg is used.

Pulmonary embolism is the most devastating manifestation of venous thromboembolic disease. Autopsy studies have found evidence of lower extremity thrombosis in approximately 80% of patients with pulmonary embolism. However, at presentation, only 15% to 20% of patients with objectively documented pulmonary embolism have clinically apparent lower extremity deep vein thrombosis. The clinical manifestations of pulmonary embolism can vary greatly. Patients can present with circulatory collapse associated with shock and cardiac arrest. A more common presentation is the acute onset of shortness of breath with pleuritic chest pain and occasional hemoptysis. Other patients will manifest only increased shortness of breath aggravated by exercise.

Dyspnea is the most common symptom of pulmonary embolism, and in patients with objectively documented embolus, dyspnea is reported by over 70%. Circulatory collapse occurs in approximately 10% of patients, and pulmonary embolism with chest pain and pulmonary infarction may occur in 50% to 60% of patients. Tachypnea (respiratory rate of 20 per minute or greater) and tachycardia are the most frequent signs of pulmonary embolism and, when combined with dyspnea, are observed in over 90% of patients with objectively documented pulmonary

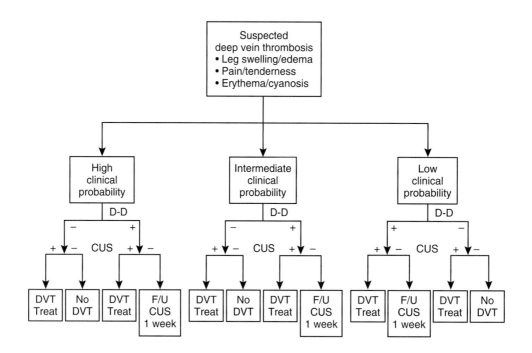

D-D: D-dimer assay
CUS: Compression ultrasound

Figure 43-1 ■ Algorithm for the diagnosis of suspected deep vein thrombosis.

Table 43-2 ▪ Clinical Features Predicting Pretest Probability of Pulmonary Embolism

History

Historical risk factors as listed in Table 43-1

Previous or new objective diagnosis of deep vein thrombosis or pulmonary embolism

Symptoms and Signs

Respiratory features:*
  Dyspnea at rest or with exertion
  Tachypnea (respiratory rate ≥ 20/min)
  Pleuritic chest pain or nonretrosternal chest pain
  Hemoptysis
  Pleural rub
  Arterial saturation of less than 92% on room air
Supporting diagnostic features:
  Low-grade temperature
  Tachycardia (>100/min)
  Chest radiograph consistent with pulmonary embolism

Source: Adapted from Wells et al. (1998). Patients with historical risk factors, at least two respiratory features, and all supporting diagnostic features without an alternative diagnosis as or more likely than pulmonary embolism are considered high probability of pulmonary embolism. Without historical risk factors but with appropriate signs and symptoms, patients are considered to have a moderate probability. In the presence of no risk factors and an alternative diagnosis as likely or more likely than pulmonary embolism, patients are considered to be low probability. Patients with fewer than two respiratory symptoms and atypical respiratory or cardiac symptoms but historical risk factors and no alternative diagnosis have a moderate pretest probability.
*Patients with typical respiratory features with the additional complicating clinical features such as syncope, blood pressure <90 mm Hg with a pulse of >100 beat/min, needing oxygen supplementation or respiratory assistance or new onset of right heart failure are considered high probability and even in the presence of an alternative diagnosis should be considered moderate probability.

embolism. Rales or wheezing can be heard in patients with pulmonary infarction, and an accentuated second pulmonary sound may be heard on cardiac auscultation. A low-grade fever has been reported to occur in up to 20% of patients, predominantly in patients with pulmonary infarction. Electrocardiogram abnormalities can be found in 5% to 10% of patients and may be more frequently observed in patients with underlying cardiopulmonary disease.

Most of the clinical symptoms and signs of pulmonary embolism are also found in other common cardiac and pulmonary disorders such as myocardial infarction, congestive heart failure, chronic obstructive pulmonary disease, and/or pneumonia. Therefore, the clinical symptoms and signs in patients with suspected pulmonary embolism should be considered in conjunction with the historical features listed in Table 43-1 that have been shown to predict for deep vein thrombosis. Additional pulmonary symptoms

and signs that will increase the pretest probability of a pulmonary embolism are listed in Table 43-2. However, even with the use of objective tests, the diagnosis of pulmonary embolism remains one of the most difficult diagnostic challenges. A schematic algorithm for the diagnosis of a pulmonary embolism is presented in Figure 43-2.

Laboratory Assessment and Diagnosis of Deep Vein Thrombosis

Tests that document in vivo hemostatic activation can provide helpful additional information in the evaluation of patients with suspected deep vein thrombosis and/or pulmonary embolism. Of the laboratory tests that are currently available, only assays for D-dimers have shown value in clinical assessment of patients with suspected deep vein thrombosis and pulmonary embolism. D-Dimers are the fibrinolytic breakdown product of Factor XIIIa-mediated cross-linked fibrin monomer and therefore document recent generation of thrombin. The prolonged blood half-life of the D-dimer makes it the preferred hemostatic marker for the evaluation of deep vein thrombosis when compared to other hemostatic activation markers such as prothrombin fragment 1·2, thrombin-antithrombin complexes, or fibrinopeptide A.

A number of D-dimer assay systems of different sensitivities have been studied. These include bedside whole blood assays, latex bead agglutination assays performed on plasma, and highly sensitive ELISA systems that can measure D-dimer levels accurately down to 10 ng/mL. In patients with objectively documented deep vein thrombosis, the commonly used latex agglutination assay has a reported sensitivity of 50% to 80% and specificity of 60% to 90%. Although the positive predictive value of the latex agglutination system is only 50% to 80% in most studies, its negative predictive value is reported to be 80% to 95%. Studies evaluating D-dimer ELISA systems in the diagnosis of deep vein thrombosis have uniformly reported greater sensitivities but lower specificity than the latex agglutination assay. Therefore the determination of D-dimer levels by ELISA have a greater negative predictive value. A typical clinical example of the use of the D-dimer assay is a negative D-dimer in a patient with suspected deep vein thrombosis who had a low clinical pretest probability. The combined negative predictive value for deep vein thrombosis of both tests would be nearly 100%. The measurement of plasma D-dimer by the ELISA method may be particularly helpful in the evaluation of patients with suspected pulmonary embolism and inconclusive ventilation-perfusion lung scans. A positive D-dimer ELISA without obvious other causes of D-dimer elevations would support

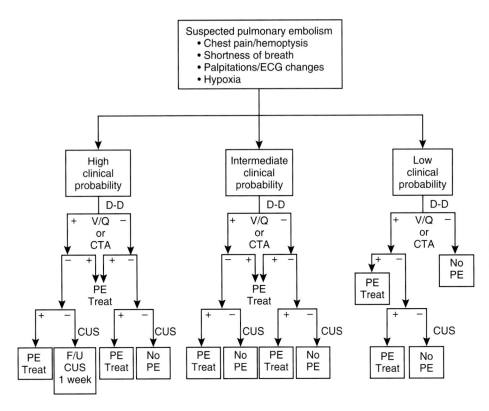

Figure 43-2 ■ Algorithm for the diagnosis of suspected pulmonary embolism.

V/Q = Ventilation perfusion scan
CTA = Computerized tomographic angiogram
D-D = D-dimer assay
CUS = Compression ultrasound

further evaluation with pulmonary angiography. A negative assay would effectively rule out a pulmonary embolus. The use of the D-dimer assay in the evaluation of patients with suspected deep vein thrombosis and/or pulmonary embolism is presented in the diagnostic algorithms (see Figures 43-1 and 43-2).

A number of commonly observed clinical conditions can reduce the specificity and the negative predictive value of the D-dimer assays. Significant elevations of D-dimers have been reported in patients with soft tissue bleeding, rheumatologic disorders, active inflammatory bowel disease, acute and chronic infections, and malignancy. Many of these disorders are associated with increased risk of deep vein thrombosis and therefore will lower the clinical utility of the D-dimer assay in patients who are suspected of having a deep vein thrombosis and/or pulmonary embolism.

Cancer patients presenting with a new thromboembolic episode should have a careful hemostatic evaluation prior to the initiation of therapy. Laboratory studies to be performed should include screening tests for hemostatic function such as a prothrombin time, partial thromboplastin time, thrombin time,

quantitative fibrinogen, and platelet count. These studies are important in determining whether a thrombotic event is the clinical manifestation of chronic disseminated intravascular coagulation (DIC) and providing a baseline for monitoring subsequent therapy.

While abnormalities in these screening assays may provide important corroborative evidence of underlying chronic disseminated intravascular coagulation, care must be given in assessing patients with underlying liver disease or extensive hepatic metastasis. The platelet count may be depressed secondary to extensive bone marrow involvement with tumor or due to the marrow suppressive effects of radiation therapy or chemotherapy. Therefore, a diagnosis of chronic disseminated intravascular coagulation should not be made without studies that indicate excess thrombin generation. When a D-dimer assay is used as the only test for thrombin generation, caution must be exercised in interpreting results in patients who have had recent surgery, bleeding into tissues, effusions, cirrhotic liver disease, and renal failure. However, markedly elevated D-dimers combined with abnormalities in the screening assays in a cancer patient who presents with a thrombotic episode is almost always diagnostic of chronic disseminated intravascular coagulation. The need for follow-up laboratory studies will be determined by the specific therapies that are chosen for the treatment of the thrombotic event and the primary malignancy.

Objective Tests for the Diagnosis of Deep Vein Thrombosis and Pulmonary Embolism

Contrast venography is the reference objective diagnostic imaging procedure for the diagnosis of lower extremity deep vein thrombosis; however, in clinical practice, venography is rarely performed, and noninvasive imaging techniques have replaced this more invasive diagnostic procedure. Impedance plethysmography and duplex ultrasound with compression have been validated as procedures for the diagnosis of proximal lower extremity deep vein thrombosis. Of the two diagnostic procedures, compression ultrasound venous imaging has proven to be the more sensitive and specific noninvasive test. Appropriate scans will examine the leg in two areas: the common femoral vein at the inguinal ligament and the popliteal vein at the knee joint line traced down to the point of trifurcation of the calf veins. The veins are scanned in the transverse plane with lack of full venous compressibility as the sole criterion for an abnormal study (Figure 43-3). However, the validity of a positive or negative study will depend on the techniques that are used and the experience of the ultrasound technician and radiologist.

Occasionally, problems unique to the cancer patient, such as tumor compression of iliac or lower extremity veins, may result in an inaccurate or nondiagnostic study. However, these diagnostic complications are rare, and compression venous ultrasonography remains the most commonly used objective diagnostic procedure for the determination of lower extremity deep vein thrombosis. When combined with pretest probability testing and sensitive D-dimer testing, compression ultrasound can diagnose proximal deep vein thrombosis in over 98% of patients.

Patients with distal (calf veins) and superficial venous thrombosis are at significantly lower risk of pulmonary embolism. However, in the cancer patient, these lower-risk thrombotic complications can be a harbinger of a more serious prothrombotic state: Trousseau's syndrome. These patients should have laboratory evaluations looking for evidence of the chronic disseminated intravascular coagulation associ-

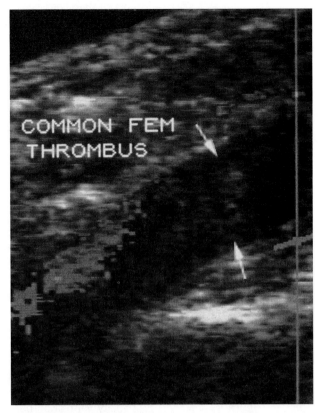

Figure 43-3 ■ A compression colored ultrasound demonstrating a noncompressible common femoral vein (white arrows) documenting the presence of a deep venous thrombosis.

ated with Trousseau's syndrome. However, even cancer patients without laboratory evidence of chronic disseminated intravascular coagulation should be followed closely and have follow-up compression ultrasound to exclude propagation into the proximal deep venous system.

Like contrast venography, pulmonary contrast angiography remains the diagnostic gold standard for the objective diagnosis of pulmonary embolism. The invasive nature of this procedure has limited its use, and less definitive noninvasive objective tests are more often utilized. Ventilation-perfusion lung scintigraphic scans have been demonstrated to have high specificity and sensitivity. Ventilation-perfusion lung scans are usually interpreted as (1) high probability with one or more segmental or two or more large (greater than 75%) subsegmental perfusion defects with normal ventilation (Figure 43-4), (2) a normal study with no perfusion defects or (3) a nondiagnostic or indeterminate scan that is neither normal nor high probability. In consideration of these three potential imaging interpretations, the addition of the pretest probability evaluation and D-dimer assay can greatly assist in determining the likelihood of an accurate

Ventilation Scan

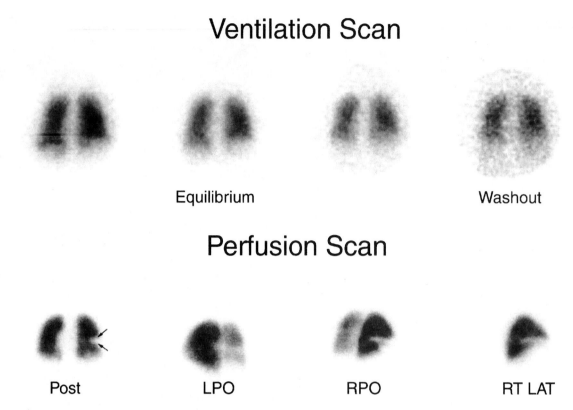

Equilibrium   Washout

Perfusion Scan

Post   LPO   RPO   RT LAT

Figure 43-4 ■ High probability ventilation-perfusion lung scan in a patient with a suspected pulmonary embolism. The black arrows indicate segmental perfusion defect. The patient is a 51-year-old female receiving adjuvant chemotherapy for stage II breast cancer. She had sudden onset of right-side pleuritic chest pain and moderate dyspnea worse with exertion. She was afebrile and had a normal chest X-ray.

diagnosis. Also, studies using compression ultrasound or contrast venography of the lower extremities in patients with documented pulmonary embolism have found evidence of deep vein thrombosis in 30% to 60%. Therefore, in patients in whom clinical suspicion for pulmonary embolism remains high despite indeterminate or low-probability imaging studies, a lower-extremity compression ultrasound should be performed.

Examples of this combined approach to pulmonary embolism diagnosis could include the following: A patient with a low pretest probability, a negative D-dimer assay, and an indeterminate scan would most likely (less than 5%) not have a pulmonary embolism. In contrast, a patient with a high or moderate pretest probability, a positive D-dimer assay, and an indeterminate scan would very likely have a pulmonary embolism. This patient should have lower-extremity compression ultrasound and, if this study is negative, undergo a pulmonary angiogram. A diagnostic algorithm for the investigation of a patient with suspected pulmonary embolism is presented in Figure 43-2.

Computed chest tomography (CT) angiogram, also termed spiral computed tomography, has been shown to be reliably specific in the diagnosis of pulmonary embolism involving central (main pulmonary artery) and first-order pulmonary arteries (lobar arteries) (Figure 43-5). It is much less sensitive in the evaluation of embolus to the segmental and subsegmental vessels. In a recent prospective study, the sensitivity of spiral computed tomography was only 70%, and the specificity was 91%. If spiral computed tomography is combined with pretest probability testing, D-dimer assays, and compression ultrasound of the lower extremities, the false negative results are greatly reduced. Cancer patients can have a number of pulmonary complications that complicate the diagnosis of embolism. Among these are included primary lung tumors, pulmonary metastasis, pulmonary infections, and pulmonary reactions to radiation and chemotherapeutic drugs. Therefore, spiral computed tomography can have certain advantages over the ventilation-perfusion scan in the cancer patient and most specifically in the patient with an abnormal chest X-ray. It

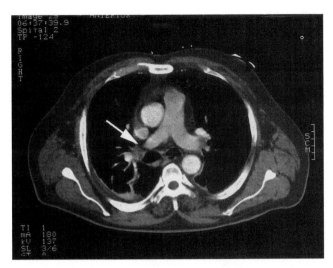

Figure 43-5 ■ A computed tomography pulmonary angiogram showing a clot in the right superior branch of the pulmonary artery (white arrow). The patient is a 63-year-old male with metastatic bladder cancer. The patient had the sudden onset of nonpleuritic chest pain and dyspnea. Chest X-ray showed a widened mediastinum and several pulmonary nodules consistent with metastases.

can differentiate among pulmonary metastasis, tumor compression, and invasion of pulmonary arteries and pulmonary embolus. However, in the patient with a normal chest X-ray, ventilation-perfusion lung scanning remains the diagnostic imaging procedure of choice.

Evaluation of the Prothrombotic Risk Factors in Patients with an Idiopathic Deep Vein Thrombosis

There is increasing evidence that acquired and genetic risk factors alone or in combination with transient risks such as pregnancy, oral contraceptive use, or immobilization can predispose patients to thromboembolism. A great deal of controversy remains regarding which patients should be studied and the clinical significance of these risk factors in the individual patient with a history of deep vein thrombosis or pulmonary embolism. Even more controversial is the issue of screening family members without a history of deep vein thrombosis for genetic defects. However, evaluating a patient for an acquired or inherited thrombophilic risk factor may be less controversial when the tests are performed in the context of the risks associated with recurrent venous thrombosis. Recurrent thrombosis may be fatal in 5% of patients, and 30% of patients with recurrence will develop the postphlebitic syndrome. Retrospective studies have shown that thrombotic recurrence is most common in patients with the antiphospholipid syndrome (lupus anticoagulant), homozygous Factor V Leiden, or deficiencies of antithrombin or protein C and in patients with combined risk factors. In individuals with these prothrombotic factors, the risk of recurrent thrombosis may outweigh the 2% to 3% annual risk of major bleeding associated with long-term oral anticoagulation.

DIAGNOSIS

Screening Laboratory Evaluation for the Thrombophilic Patient

1. *Coagulation-based assay for activated protein C resistance.* First-generation assays cannot be performed on patients who are receiving heparin or warfarin or have the lupus anticoagulant. Second-generation assays using Factor V–deficient plasma can be performed on anticoagulated patients. A positive result should be confirmed for the Factor V Leiden mutation. Assays for activated protein C resistance and Factor V Leiden is unnecessary in individuals of Asian (China, Japan, or Korea), native African, or Native American descent.

2. *Genetic screen for the prothrombin G20210A mutation.* Unnecessary in individuals of Asian (China, Japan, or Korea), native African, or Native American descent.

3. *Functional assays for antithrombin, protein C, and protein S.* Functional assays for protein C and S cannot be performed in patients receiving vitamin K antagonists (warfarin). An abnormal functional assay should be followed by immunologic assays for the deficient factor.

4. *Functional assay for Factor VIII activity.* Should be performed with concomitant measurement of C-reactive protein (CRP) or sedimentation rate. Elevated levels should be confirmed with a second specimen.

5. *Coagulation assay for the lupus anticoagulant and an ELISA for antiphospholipid (anticardiolipin) antibodies.* A positive lupus anticoagulant assay should be repeated to confirm.

6. *Measurement of fasting plasma homocysteine levels.* Patients with elevated homocysteine levels should have a repeat sample drawn for simultaneous measurement of serum folate and B_{12} levels.

Therefore, without clear guidelines from well-designed prospective clinical trials, the decision regarding screening of patients for inherited or acquired thrombophilia can be made only with a consideration of a high risk of recurrent thrombosis. Screening is appropriate in patients with a documented idiopathic deep vein thrombosis and/or pulmonary embolism under the age of 40 years, older patients with a strong family history of venous thromboembolism in first-degree relatives, women under the age of 30 years who develop thrombosis on oral contraceptives, and women who develop antepartum thrombosis. Also, the severity of the initial thrombotic event is an important consideration in patient screening, since a recurrent thrombotic event in such patients may have a greater risk of morbidity and mortality. In selecting which screening assays to perform, consideration should also be given to the patient's racial and ethnic background. A list of thrombophilic risk factors that should be evaluated in selected patients with idiopathic deep vein thrombosis is given in Table 43-3.

Thromboembolic events have been reported to occur before the diagnosis of cancer. Several studies have suggested that there is an increased risk of cancer in patients with idiopathic and recurrent thromboembolism. Two large registry studies support this premise, finding a three to five times increased incidence of cancer in patients with primary or idiopathic deep vein thrombosis and pulmonary embolism when compared to the general population. However, this increased risk was primarily observed during the first 6 to 12 months of follow-up. The risk rapidly declined to that of the general population after one year. In addition, a follow-up report by one registry found that an initial clinical presentation with thrombosis predicted a poorer prognosis and shorter survival.

A prospective randomized trial evaluated the efficacy of an aggressive cancer evaluation in patients who present with an initial idiopathic venous thrombosis. Patients with recurrent thrombosis or with documented inherited prothrombotic defects were excluded. In the patients who underwent the aggressive cancer screening protocol, an underlying malignancy was found in 13%. In the control group, who underwent a routine examination on presentation with deep vein thrombosis/pulmonary embolism, a cancer was diagnosed in 10% during the following two years. Patients who were diagnosed by the aggressive cancer screen had earlier stages of disease than were the control patients. However, it is unknown whether this earlier diagnosis significantly improves survival. At present, a routine aggressive cancer evaluation cannot be recommended for patients presenting with idiopathic thrombosis. An appropriate

examination should include a careful history and physical examination, chest radiograph, stool for occult blood, pelvic examination in females, and a serum prostate acid phosphatase (PSA) in males who present over the age of 50. Symptomatic patients should have a computed tomography scan or abdominal pelvic ultrasound examinations when indicated. In the prospective cancer screening trial, computed tomography scanning of the chest, abdomen, and pelvis proved to be the most productive in detecting an occult malignancy.

Suggested Reading

Baron JA, Gridley G, Weiderpass E, et al: Venous thromboembolism and cancer. Lancet 1998;351:1077–1080.

Table 43-3 ■ Inherited and Acquired Causes of Venous Thrombosis

Common Inherited

Factor V Leiden (G1691 Factor V mutation)*
Prothrombin G20210A mutation*
Factor VIII activity (150%)†
Homocysteinemia‡

Rare Inherited

Protein C deficiency
Protein S deficiency
Antithrombin deficiency
Dysfibrinogenemia

Common Acquired

Cancer
Antiphospholipid antibodies (lupus anticoagulant and anticardiolipin antibodies)
Myeloproliferative disorders
Autoimmune hemolytic anemias

Rare Acquired

Paroxysmal nocturnal hemoglobinuria
Elevated homocysteine levels, due to folate or B_{12} deficiency

---

*Factor V Leiden and prothrombin G20210A mutations are not found in persons of Far Asian (Chinese, Korean or Japanese), African, or Native American descent.
†Factor VIII is an acute phase reactant. Levels should be obtained with simultaneous measurement of other acute phase reactants, such as the sedimentation rate or C reactive protein. Levels should be repeated at least once.
‡Homocyteine levels should be drawn with simultaneous folate and B_{12} levels. Should be repeated at least twice with fasting sample. The most common inherited cause of elevated levels is homozygous C677T mutation of the methyltetrahydrofolate reductase gene. However, thrombotic risk correlates with homocysteine levels and not presence of mutation. This discrepancy may be due to the variations in an individual's dietary folate intake.

Cranley J, Canos AJ, Sull WJ: The diagnosis of deep venous thrombosis: Fallibility of clinical symptoms and signs. Arch Surg 1976;111:34–36.

Heijboer H, Buller HR, Lensing AWA, et al: A comparison of real-time compression ultrasound with impedance plethysmography for the diagnosis of deep-vein thrombosis in symptomatic outpatients. N Engl J Med 1993;329:1365–1369.

Hull R, Hirsh J, Sackett DL: Replacement of venography in suspected venous thrombosis by impedance plethysmography and ^{125}I-fibrinogen leg scanning. Ann Intern Med 1981;94:12–15.

Hull RD, Hirsh J, Carter CJ, et al: Pulmonary angiography, ventilation lung scanning and venography for clinically suspected pulmonaary embolism with abnormal perfusion lung scan. Ann Intern Med 1983;98:891–899.

Kearon C, Ginsberg JS, Douketis J, et al: Management of suspected deep venous thrombosis in outpatients by using clinical assessment and D-dimer testing. Ann Intern Med 2001;135:108–111.

Lee AYY, Julian JA, Levine MN, et al: Clinical utility of a rapid whole-blood D-dimer assay in patients with cancer who present with suspected acute deep venous thrombosis. Ann Intern Med 1999;131:417–423.

Lensing AWA, Hirsh J, Ginsberg JS, Buller HR: Diagnosis of venous thrombosis. In Colman RW, Hirsh J, Marder VJ, et al (eds): Hemostasis and Thrombosis: Basic Principles and Clinical Practice, 4th ed. Philadelphia: Lippincott Williams & Wilkins, 2000, pp 1277–1301.

Perrier A, Howarth N, Didier D, et al: Performance of helical computed tomography in unselected outpatients with suspected pulmonary embolisms. Ann Intern Med 2001;135: 88–97.

Seligsohn U, Lubetsky A: Genetic susceptibility to venous thrombosis. N Engl J Med 2001;344:1222–1231.

Sorensen HT, Mellemkjaer L, Steffensen FH, et al: The risk of a diagnosis of cancer after primary deep venous thrombosis or pulmonary embolism. N Engl J Med 1998;338:1169–1173.

The PIOPED Investigators: Value of the ventilation/perfusion scan in acute pulmonary embolism: Results of the Prospective Investigation of Pulmonary Embolism Diagnosis. JAMA 1990;263:2753–2759.

Wells PS, Anderson DR, Bormanis J, et al: Value of assessment of pretest probability of deep-vein thrombosis in clinical management. Lancet 1997;350:1795–1798.

Wells PS, Ginsberg JS, Anderson DR, et al: Use of a clinical model for safe management of patients with suspected pulmonary embolism. Ann Intern Med 1998;129:997–1005.

Chapter 44
Cutaneous Manifestations of Bleeding and Thrombotic Disorders

Donald Feinstein

Hereditary and acquired hemorrhagic disorders may frequently present with bleeding into the skin or subcutaneous tissues that is visible on physical examination. However, since many hereditary and acquired vascular disorders without systemic hemostatic defects may also present in the skin, a major problem is to be able to differentiate the lesions of primary vascular disorders from those seen in patients with a systemic hemostatic defect. Moreover, there are many normal individuals who occasionally may bleed into their skin for unknown reasons. In addition to bleeding disorders that may present in the skin, thrombotic disorders may also, initially, be present with a skin lesion, which is frequently hemorrhagic. In evaluating cutaneous lesions, the history is extremely important in formulating a differential diagnosis of cutaneous lesions.

History

Besides a careful physical examination, the history is extremely important in evaluation of patients with bleeding and thrombotic disorders. The major problems encountered in this situation are the following:

1. Many normal individuals without a bleeding disorder will complain of excessive bleeding into the skin as well as from other sites.
2. Many normal individuals with bleeding disorders may not complain of excessive bleeding into the skin and/or from other sites.

Therefore the history must be much more extensive in evaluating these patients, and it should be supplemented by screening laboratory studies of the hemostatic system.

Besides the manifestations of skin bleeding, it is important to determine the following:

1. The incidence and extent of spontaneous mucous membrane bleeding from the nose, throat, gingiva, and gastrointestinal tract.
2. The amount and extent of bleeding after any trauma or invasive procedure.
3. The amount of bleeding after dental extractions (particularly wisdom teeth) or tonsillectomy and adenoidectomy.
4. Whether transfusion of blood products, packing, or extra suturing was ever required.
5. The amount and severity of menstrual flow and whether there ever was excessive postpartum bleeding.
6. Whether excessive bruising or bleeding occurred with the use of certain medications such as aspirin, NSAIDs, and warfarin.
7. Whether there is concurrent disease, particularly renal or hepatic disease.

The identification of severe hereditary and acquired disorders is usually not a problem. In contrast, mild to moderate hereditary bleeding disorders may be difficult to differentiate from acquired disorders, particularly if the individual has not suffered significant trauma or undergone an invasive procedure. Family history may also be helpful in differentiating a hereditary from an acquired disorder if there is excessive bleeding in first-degree relatives. In taking a family history, it is also extremely important to inquire about invasive procedures that first-degree relatives may have undergone and whether or not they have any knowledge or evidence of excessive bleeding (such as requiring blood transfusions or reoperation).

Physical Examination of the Skin

Although a complete physical examination is important in evaluating patients with a possible bleeding disorder, a careful examination of the skin can provide important information. Although cutaneous bleeding may provide an important clue to an underlying bleeding disorder, recurrent bleeding that is confined only to the skin may be a manifestation of a primary vascular or dermatologic disorder. Frequently, primary vascular and dermatologic lesions are somewhat raised (i.e., palpable), in contrast to the flat cutaneous lesions that are associated with a primary bleeding disorder. The lesions that are classically seen as a reflection of a systemic hemostatic disorder are petechiae, purpura, and ecchymoses.

Petechiae are small (<3 mm) round, red spots that are small hemorrhages and thus are nonblanchable (Figure 44-1). They usually appear as multiple lesions in areas of increased venous pressure (on the lower extremities; below bra straps, belts, or stockings; and on the neck, face, and upper chest after coughing, vomiting, or straining at stool). They may also occur on mucous membranes (i.e., mouth, nasopharynx, and gastrointestinal tract). Petechiae stem from extravasation of blood from very small vessels and result from a loss of integrity of the microvascular endothelium. The loss of integrity of the endothelium

may be secondary to increased venous pressure alone, thrombocytopenia, primary vascular defect, or, less commonly, a qualitative platelet defect. When petechiae are seen, the most important initial laboratory study is a platelet count, and if that is normal, then the most likely cause is a primary vascular defect.

Purpura is another form of cutaneous bleeding that is frequently not confined to areas of increased venous pressure, and thus it may coalesce anywhere in the body, including the mucous membranes. They are red to purple in color, are round, and usually vary from 3 mm to 1 cm in diameter (Figure 44-2). Multiple lesions may occur and thus appear to be much larger than usually seen with a single lesion. Therefore the larger lesions are not perfectly round and have irregular borders. Purpuric lesions are seen in patients with severe thrombocytopenia and in patients with primary vascular defects. The former can frequently (but not always) be differentiated from the latter because they are flat and nonpalpable. Primary vascular lesions may either be raised (palpable) or flat. Thus when purpuric lesions are seen, the only differential diagnosis is whether there is severe thrombocytopenia or not. If severe thrombocytopenia is ruled out, then the purpura must be ascribed to a primary endothelial cell defect. The endothelial cell defects may result from a variety of different conditions, which will be discussed below, in patients with primary vascular disorders without any systemic hemostatic abnormality.

Ecchymoses are bruises that are larger than 3 mm and have a reddish to bluish color when first formed and then become yellow to green with age. Ecchy-

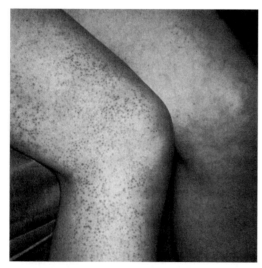

Figure 44-1 ■ Petechiae in a patient with severe thrombocytopenia.

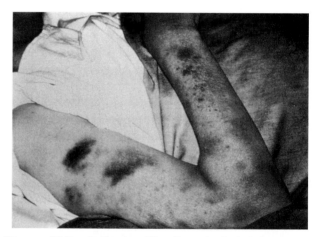

Figure 44-2 ■ Patient with disseminated intravascular coagulation secondary to adenocarcinoma of the stomach metastatic to bone marrow. Patient had both severe thrombocytopenia and a low fibrinogen. Note petechiae and purpura on forearm and ecchymoses on arm.

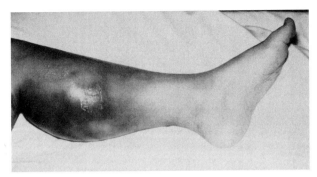

Figure 44-3 ■ Hemophilia A with intramuscular and subcutaneous hemorrhage. (See Color Plate 11.)

moses may appear spontaneously or with trauma and may be mildly painful and tender. When ecchymoses are found in greater than normal number and with no history of trauma, the condition is usually called easy bruisability. This condition is found in approximately 25% of normal men and 50% of normal women who have no identifiable systemic bleeding problem. In contrast, ecchymoses may be a manifestation of any systemic hemostatic disorder, including thrombocytopenia, coagulation factor deficiencies, qualitative platelet defects, and primary vascular defects. When ecchymoses are associated with thrombocytopenia, they usually accompany petechiae and purpura. When subcutaneous bleeding is massive and particularly when it is associated with intramuscular or intra-articular bleeding, it usually is secondary to a severe coagulation factor deficiency (Figure 44-3).

Hereditary Primary Vascular Disorders

Hereditary hemorrhagic telangiectasia or Rendu-Osler-Weber syndrome is an autosomal-dominant disorder characterized by multiple telangiectatic lesions involving the skin and mucous membrane associated with mucous membrane bleeding from the nose and gastrointestinal tract. This appears to result from various mutations in the endoglin gene, which is an integral membrane glycoprotein expressed on endothelial cells in blood vessels that serves as a binding protein for transforming factor beta. Like many other hereditary diseases, it probably arises from many different types of mutations. The actual pathophysiologic mechanism by which the genetic defects result in telangiectatic lesions is unknown. The bleeding from mucous membranes is secondary to very fragile vessels, although occasional hemostatic defects have been reported. The cutaneous lesions usually appear sometime between 20 and 40, and they usually measure 1 to 3 mm in diameter. They are found mostly on the face, lips, ears, nailbeds, and finger pads (Figures 44-4 and 44-5). The number of lesions varies from a few to many. Although bleeding from the nose and gastrointestinal tract is common, easy bruisability is rare. Besides bleeding phenomena, these patients may develop arteriovenous malformations, particularly involving the pulmonary arteriovenous system, and thus they may develop significant right-to-left shunts with paradoxic arterial emboli. Arteriovenous shunts may also occur in the brain or in other organs.

Kasabach-Merritt syndrome

These patients usually have very large cavernous hemangiomas (Figure 44-6). Bleeding may occur, not

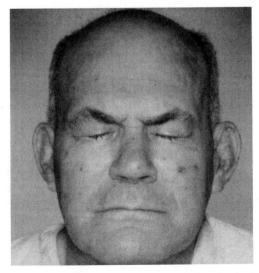

Figure 44-4 ■ Hereditary hemorrhagic telangiectasia.

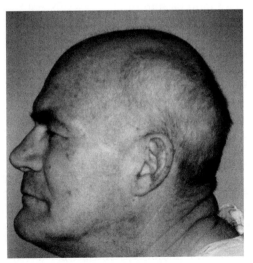

Figure 44-5 ■ Hereditary hemorrhagic telangiectasia.

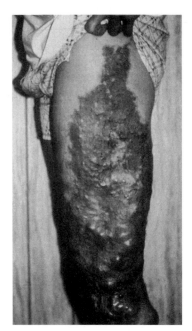

Figure 44-6 ■ Kasabach-Merritt syndrome.

Figure 44-7 ■ Fabry disease. (From Hoffman R, Benz EJ Jr, Shattil SJ, Furie B, Cohen HJ, Silberstein LE, McGlave P [eds]: Hematology: Basic Principles and Practice, 3rd ed. Philadelphia: Churchill Livingstone, 2000.) (See Color Plate 11.)

only because of the hemangioma, but also because there is significant localized intravascular coagulation, and therefore the patient may present with easy bruising in other uninvolved areas of skin.

Hereditary Disorders of Connective Tissue

Ehlers-Danlos disease, osteogenous imperfecta, pseudoxanthoma elasticum, and Marfan syndrome are all hereditary disorders of connective tissue that have a variety of different manifestations. All of them are characterized by easy bruisability, but the bruisability is more frequent and more significant in patients with Ehlers-Danlos disease and pseudoxanthoma elasticum than in patients with osteogenous imperfecta and Marfan syndrome. Moreover, the patients with Ehlers-Danlos disease and its various subtypes and patients with pseudoxanthoma elasticum also have fairly significant mucous membrane bleeding.

Fabry's Disease

Fabry's disease (angiokeratoma corporis diffusum) is a hereditary X-linked disorder of glycolipid metabolism that leads to accumulation of glycolipid, leading to multisystem disease. The skin lesions are variable in numbers and distribution but are usually found on the trunk, extremities, and genitalia. They consist of nonblanchable 1- to 4-mm red, blue, or black macules or papules (Figure 44-7). These patients usually have no evidence of excessive mucocutaneous bleeding.

Ataxia Telangectasia

Ataxia telangectasia is an autosomal-recessive disorder that is characterized by telangiectasia, cerebellar ataxia, recurrent sinopulmonary infections, immunodeficiency, and an increased incidence of malignancies. The most common initial presentation is cerebellar ataxia. Telangiectatic lesions appear later in childhood and are located in exposed areas of the skin, including eyelids, ears, face, dorsum of hands, and bulbar conjunctivae. There is no increased tendency for mucocutaneous bleeding from these lesions.

Acquired Primary Vascular Disorders Without Vasculitis

In the absence of thrombocytopenia, purpura must be ascribed to a primary endothelial cell defect. These defects may result from a variety of different conditions, including the following:

1. Senile purpura results from loss or supporting subcutaneous connective tissue and results in purple to red patches, which frequently have irregular borders (Figure 44-8). They usually involve the forearms and dorsum of the hands but may also involve the lower extremities. The skin is usually very thin and fragile, and the purpura may remain for long periods of time before resolution.
2. Corticosteroid excess, whether due to medication or to Cushing's syndrome, results in purpura that are almost identical in appearance and distribution to those of senile purpura. It also probably stems from the loss of subcutanenous supporting tissue.
3. Scurvy results in perifollicular purpura or petechiae (Figure 44-9). In more severe cases, large ecchymoses of the lower extremities and hemorrhagic gingivitis may also occur.

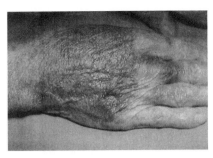

Figure 44-8 ■ Senile purpura. (From Hoffman R, Benz EJ Jr, Shattil SJ, Furie B, Cohen HJ, Silberstein LE, McGlave P [eds]: Hematology: Basic Principles and Practice, 3rd ed. Philadelphia: Churchill Livingstone, 2000.)

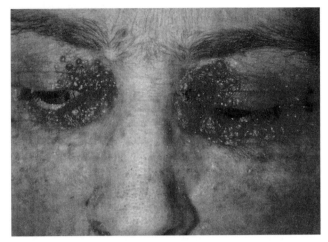

Figure 44-10 ■ Immunoglobulin-related primary amyloidosis with extensive periorbital hemorrhagic cutaneous lesions. (See Color Plate 11.)

4. Amyloidosis frequently involves blood vessels and causes increased vascular fragility, and bleeding from minimal trauma. Moreover, many different amyloidotic cutaneous lesions may occur with secondary bleeding (Figure 44-10). There are usually other clinical (cardiomyopathy, nephrotic syndrome, hepatomegaly) and laboratory abnormalities (monoclonal immunoglobulin in serum and/or urine) that suggest the diagnosis. In addition, patients with amyloidosis may develop excessive bleeding because of acquired Factor X-deficiency or increased fibrinolysis.
5. Type I cryoglobulinemia (see the discussion below).
6. Infection (bacterial, viral, rickettsial, fungal, or parasitic) may produce purpuric and/or petechial lesions as the major presenting problem (Figures 44-11 through 44-13). This may result from thrombocytopenia, a primary vascular defect, or a combination of both. The thrombocytopenia can be caused by disseminated intravascular coagulation (DIC), sepsis syndrome without DIC, splenomegaly, decreased thrombopoiesis, or a combination of these mechanisms.
7. Telangiectasias similar to those seen in hereditary hemorrhagic telangectasia (see below) are seen in the CREST syndrome but, like other telangiectatic lesions, are blanchable (Figure 44-14).
8. Spider angiomata are seen in normal women and in patients with chronic liver disease. They are blanchable and are distinguished by a central feeding vessel with smaller vessels extending from it.

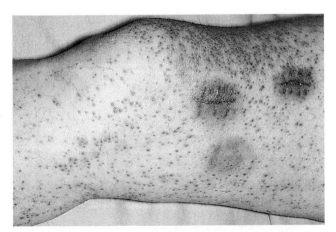

Figure 44-9 ■ Scurvy. Vitamin C deficiency results in perifollicular purpura, corkscrew hairs, and ecchymoses. (From Callen JP, Paller AS, Greer KE, Swinyer LJ [eds]: Color Atlas of Dermatology, 2nd ed. Philadelphia: WB Saunders, 2000.)

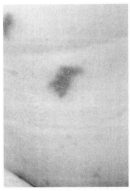

Figure 44-11 ■ Meningococcemia. (From Hoffman R, Benz EJ Jr, Shattil SJ, Furie B, Cohen HJ, Silberstein LE, McGlave P [eds]: Hematology: Basic Principles and Practice, 3rd ed. Philadelphia: Churchill Livingstone, 2000.)

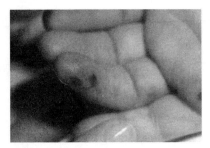

Figure 44-12 ■ Acute bacterial endocarditis. (From Hoffman R, Benz EJ Jr, Shattil SJ, Furie B, Cohen HJ, Silberstein LE, McGlave P [eds]: Hematology: Basic Principles and Practice, 3rd ed. Philadelphia: Churchill Livingstone, 2000.)

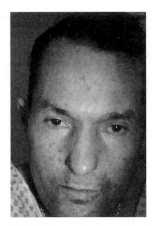

Figure 44-14 ■ CREST. (From Hoffman R, Benz EJ Jr, Shattil SJ, Furie B, Cohen HJ, Silberstein LE, McGlave P [eds]: Hematology: Basic Principles and Practice, 3rd ed. Philadelphia: Churchill Livingstone, 2000.)

Acquired Primary Vascular Disorders with Vasculitis

Patients with a variety of vasculitides may present with different hemorrhagic cutaneous lesions. However, the majority of the lesions are purpuric and are palpable. These patients may also develop petechiae, nonpalpable purpura, and ecchymosis as well as microvascular ischemic lesions. These disorders include not only the primary vasculitic disorders, such as Schönlein-Henoch purpura, but also those associated with mixed cryoglobulinemia, particularly the one associated with chronic hepatitis C.

Mixed cryoglobulinemia and Schönlein-Henoch purpura should always be considered when a patient is seen with extensive predominantly lower extremity palpable purpura, arthralgias, and renal involvement (Figure 44-15). They can be easily differentiated from one another by the presence of IgA immune complexes in Schönlein-Henoch vasculitic skin lesions in contrast to cryoglobulinemia and hepatitis C antibody in patients with chronic hepatitis C. Mixed

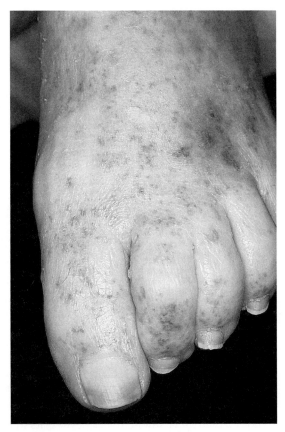

Figure 44-15 ■ Cryoglobulinemia. (From Callen JP, Paller AS, Greer KE, Swinyer LJ [eds]: Color Atlas of Dermatology, 2nd ed. Philadelphia: WB Saunders, 2000.)

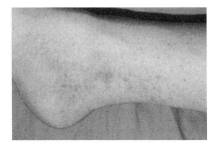

Figure 44-13 ■ Rocky Mountain spotted fever. (From Hoffman R, Benz EJ Jr, Shattil SJ, Furie B, Cohen HJ, Silberstein LE, McGlave P [eds]: Hematology: Basic Principles and Practice, 3rd ed. Philadelphia: Churchill Livingstone, 2000.)

cryoglobulinemia consists of a monoclonal IgM and polyclonal IgG (type II cryoglobulinemia) or polyclonal IgM and polyclonal IgG (type III cryoglobulinemia). In contrast, type I cryoglobulinemia consists of pure monoclonal IgM or IgG. Type I patients may develop ischemia or necrotic skin lesions or acral ischemia (fingers, toes, nose, ears, etc.) when exposed to cold environmental temperatures because of intravascular precipitation of protein. The skin lesions differ from those seen in patients with mixed cryoglobulinemia in that there is no evidence of vasculitis on biopsy and crops of purpuric lesions of the lower extremities are unusual. The patient's monoclonal immunoglobulin may be in low concentration, and thus associated with monoclonal gammopathy of undetermined significance, or in high concentration, and thus associated with multiple myeloma or macroglobulinemia of Waldenström. In testing for cryoglobulinemia, it is important to maintain the blood at 37°C until the serum is removed. Once the presence of cryoglobulin is detected, the serum should be studied by serum protein electrophoresis and immunofixation to determine whether it is mixed (type II or III) or pure monoclonal (type I). Patients with idiopathic cold hemagglutinin have a monoclonal kappa IgM antibody that is usually directed to the I antigen on the red cell surface, which results in hemolytic anemia. The agglutinated red cells may cause acral microvascular obstruction, which may or may not be reversible with warning. The monoclonal IgM is usually not a precipitating protein (cryoglobulin), and the vascular lesions do not show any evidence of vasculitis.

Patients with systemic autoimmune disorders (SLE, scleroderma, etc.) and patients with either small- or large-vessel vasculitis may develop a variety of different cutaneous lesions. These include palpable purpuric lesions, petechiae, ecchymosis, subungual splinter hemorrhages, livedo reticularis, telangec-

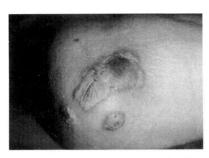

Figure 44-17 ■ Wegener's granulomatosis. (From Hoffman R, Benz EJ Jr, Shattil SJ, Furie B, Cohen HJ, Silberstein LE, McGlave P [eds]: Hematology: Basic Principles and Practice, 3rd ed. Philadelphia: Churchill Livingstone, 2000.)

tasias, chronic skin ulcers, digital ischemia, and areas of skin necrosis (Figures 44-16 through 44-18).

Hypergammaglobulinemic purpura is a syndrome first described by Waldenström that differs from the other disease that he first described, macroglobulinemia of Waldenström. It is characterized by polyclonal hyperimmunoglobulinemia, an elevated erythrocyte sedimentation rate, and frequently a mild anemia and leukopenia. It has marked predilection for young women, and the purpura usually involves the lower extremities and is palpable in the great majority of cases (Figure 44-19). Patients may have arthralgias and low-grade fever. The episodes of purpura usually resolve after a few days, and recurrences are fairly common but unpredictable. Cryoglobulins are not present. The syndrome may also occur as a secondary phenomenon in patients with systemic autoimmune disease such as systemic lupus erythematosus and Sjögren's syndrome. Skin biopsies usually show evidence of vasculitis, and the vessels are frequently positive for both IgM and IgG. Circulating immune complexes can also be found.

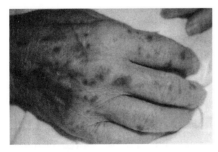

Figure 44-16 ■ Rheumatoid vasculitis. (From Hoffman R, Benz EJ Jr, Shattil SJ, Furie B, Cohen HJ, Silberstein LE, McGlave P [eds]: Hematology: Basic Principles and Practice, 3rd ed. Philadelphia: Churchill Livingstone, 2000.)

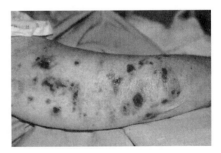

Figure 44-18 ■ Leukocytoclastic vasculitis. (From Hoffman R, Benz EJ Jr, Shattil SJ, Furie B, Cohen HJ, Silberstein LE, McGlave P [eds]: Hematology: Basic Principles and Practice, 3rd ed. Philadelphia: Churchill Livingstone, 2000.) (See Color Plate 12.)

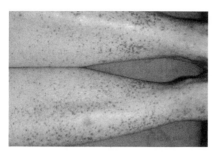

Figure 44-19 ■ Hyperglobulinemic purpura. (From Hoffman R, Benz EJ Jr, Shattil SJ, Furie B, Cohen HJ, Silberstein LE, McGlave P [eds]: Hematology: Basic Principles and Practice, 3rd ed. Philadelphia: Churchill Livingstone, 2000.)

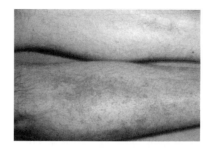

Figure 44-21 ■ Schamberg's pigmented purpuric eruption. (From Hoffman R, Benz EJ Jr, Shattil SJ, Furie B, Cohen HJ, Silberstein LE, McGlave P [eds]: Hematology: Basic Principles and Practice, 3rd ed. Philadelphia: Churchill Livingstone, 2000.)

Miscellaneous Disorders Without Hemostatic Defects

Autoerythrocyte sensitization (psychogenic purpura) is an extremely rare disorder characterized by recurrent, spontaneous ecchymotic lesions in patients with no evidence of any systemic hemostatic defect. The cutaneous lesions are always preceded and accompanied by pain in the involved area. The area then becomes erythematous, raised, and warm, and this is followed by the development of an ecchymosis (Figure 44-20). The erythema and swelling usually subside within 24 to 72 hours of the development of the bruise. These symptoms are frequently recurrent. This disorder usually affects young women who have significant underlying psychological problems. The lesions can be reproduced by injection of 0.1 mL of autologous red cells.

There is a group of miscellaneous primary dermatologic disorders (with a variety of eponyms such as Schamberg's progressive pigmentary dermatosis, Majocchi's purpura annularis, Lichen aureus, and Gaugerot-Blum purpura) that are usually associated with a purpura and petechial eruption that evolve into brown pigmented lesions (Figures 44-21 through 44-23). The latter is due to hemosiderin deposits. Acutely, there is an upper dermal infiltrate with extravasation of red blood cells around capillaries. Other common skin disorders such as contact dermatitis and drug eruptions may also be complicated by the formation of petechiae and purpura.

Patients with "gloves and socks" papular purpura syndrome present with pruritic edema and erythema of hands and feet followed by the development of petechiae and purpura in the same distribution. In addition, the oral mucosa may be involved. This syndrome most commonly occurs with parvovirus B_{19} infection, and the patients frequently have systemic findings including fever, cytopenias, abnormal hepatic tests, and an exanthem.

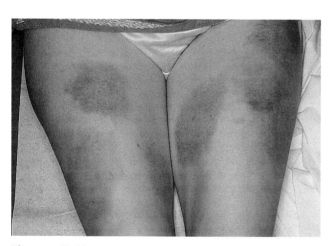

Figure 44-20 ■ Gardner-Diamond syndrome or autoerythrocyte sensitization syndrome. Trauma initiates the purpuric lesion. (From Callen JP, Paller AS, Greer KE, Swinyer LJ [eds]: Color Atlas of Dermatology, 2nd ed. Philadelphia: WB Saunders, 2000.)

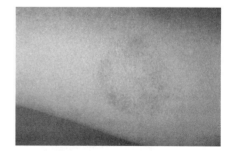

Figure 44-22 ■ Majocchi's pigmented purpuric eruption. (From Hoffman R, Benz EJ Jr, Shattil SJ, Furie B, Cohen HJ, Silberstein LE, McGlave P [eds]: Hematology: Basic Principles and Practice, 3rd ed. Philadelphia: Churchill Livingstone, 2000.)

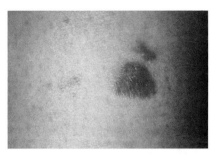

Figure 44-23 ■ Lichen aureus. (From Hoffman R, Benz EJ Jr, Shattil SJ, Furie B, Cohen HJ, Silberstein LE, McGlave P [eds]: Hematology: Basic Principles and Practice, 3rd ed. Philadelphia: Churchill Livingstone, 2000.)

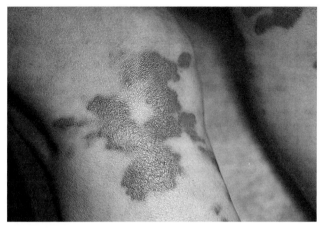

Figure 44-25 ■ Kaposi's sarcoma. (From Callen JP, Paller AS, Greer KE, Swinyer LJ [eds]: Color Atlas of Dermatology, 2nd ed. Philadelphia: WB Saunders, 2000.)

Chronic venous stasis of the lower extremities or chronic edema of any cause (CHF, liver disease, nephrotic syndrome, etc.) may be associated with extravasation of blood in the form of petechiae and purpura with evolution into persistent brownish pigmentation of the lower extremities due to hemosiderin deposits (Figure 44-24).

Skin and mucous membrane lesions due to Kaposi's sarcoma are frequently confused with hemorrhagic lesions. They may be found anywhere on the skin and mucous membrane. They may be as small as a few millimeters or as large as a few centimeters. They may be flat or palpable and brown to red in color (Figure 44-25).

Cutaneous Findings in Patients with Thromboembolic Disorders

A variety of thromboembolic problems secondary to a variety of pathophysiologic mechanisms may present with cutaneous findings:

1. Not only is disseminated intravascular coagulation (DIC) associated with petechiae, purpura, and ecchymoses due to the hemostatic consumption,

but the generation of excess thrombin with downregulation of the fibrinolytic system can result in ischemic hemorrhagic necrosis of skin and subcutaneous tissue, acral ischemia, and gangrene of distal extremities. This picture is usually seen in patients with DIC and hypotension associated with severe infection (so-called secondary purpura fulminans) (Figure 44-26; see also Figure 44-2).

Primary purpura fulminans is associated with single or scattered very large ecchymoses, some of which may become gangrenous and are usually located in the lower extremities or the buttocks (Figure 44-27). It frequently (but not always) is preceded (by one to two weeks) by a viral or strep-

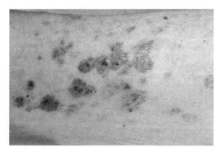

Figure 44-24 ■ Stasis purpura (palpable). (From Hoffman R, Benz EJ Jr, Shattil SJ, Furie B, Cohen HJ, Silberstein LE, McGlave P [eds]: Hematology: Basic Principles and Practice, 3rd ed. Philadelphia: Churchill Livingstone, 2000.)

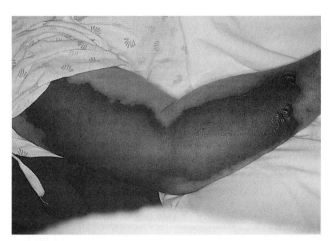

Figure 44-26 ■ Disseminated intravascular coagulopathy in a patient with gram-negative sepsis. (From Callen JP, Paller AS, Greer KE, Swinyer LJ [eds]: Color Atlas of Dermatology, 2nd ed. Philadelphia: WB Saunders, 2000.)

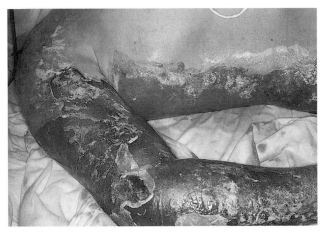

Figure 44-27 ▪ Primary purpura fulminans. (From Callen JP, Paller AS, Greer KE, Swinyer LJ [eds]: Color Atlas of Dermatology, 2nd ed. Philadelphia: WB Saunders, 2000.)

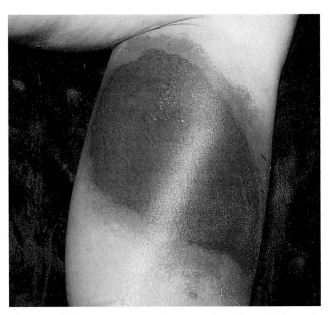

Figure 44-28 ▪ Warfarin skin necrosis. (From Callen JP, Paller AS, Greer KE, Swinyer LJ [eds]: Color Atlas of Dermatology, 2nd ed. Philadelphia: WB Saunders, 2000.)

tococcal infection, which appears to trigger an episode of DIC resulting in hemorrhagic infarction of the skin and subcutaneous tissue. A similar syndrome occurs in neonates with homozygous protein C deficiency.

2. Warfarin skin necrosis occurs in a rare patient (women more than men) who was started on warfarin, usually three to six days previously. The lesions begin with painful, sometimes erythematous patches, which rapidly involve into ecchymotic plaques followed by gangrene (Figures 44-28 and 44-29). The lesions frequently develop in skin overlying fatty areas such as the thighs, buttocks, and breasts but may involve other parts, including the penis. Pain in an ecchymotic fatty area in patients recently started on oral anticoagulants (particularly high initial doses) is an important clue to the diagnosis. Pathologically, the lesion consists of widespread microvascular thrombi. It is frequently associated with heterozygosity for a protein C defect wherein the heterozygote state is converted to the homozygous state because of the short half-life of protein C, making the thrombophilic state more dominant because of the long half-life of Factors II and X. The lesions may also occur in patients with protein S deficiency and in patients with Factor V Leiden. However, it may also occur in patients without any definite evidence of thrombophilia.

3. Venous limb gangrene resembles secondary purpura fulminans in that it results in distal limb ischemic tissue necrosis in the presence of palpable arterial pulses. The limb that is affected is the one affected by a deep vein thrombosis and therefore the reason that heparin was initially given. It occurs in the setting of heparin-induced thrombocytopenia after the heparin is discontinued and warfarin is initiated. The patients who develop venous limb gangrene usually have a higher International Normalized Ratio (INR) than other individuals receiving warfarin for a deep venous thrombosis who did not develop venous limb gangrene. The pathophysiologic mechanism that is thought to be operative in these patients is the generation of excess thrombin in the presence of inadequate levels of protein C due to increased

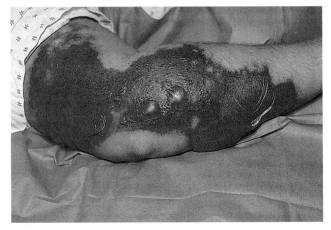

Figure 44-29 ▪ Warfarin skin necrosis. (From Callen JP, Paller AS, Greer KE, Swinyer LJ [eds]: Color Atlas of Dermatology, 2nd ed. Philadelphia: WB Saunders, 2000.)

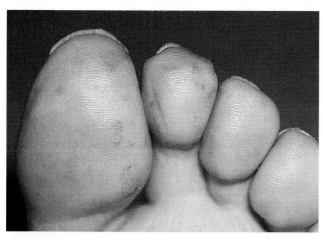

Figure 44-30 ■ Cholesterol emboli. (From Callen JP, Paller AS, Greer KE, Swinyer LJ [eds]: Color Atlas of Dermatology, 2nd ed. Philadelphia: WB Saunders, 2000.)

consumption and warfarin-induced deficiency. It differs from warfarin skin necrosis in that only a minority of patients with warfarin necrosis develop ischemia of distal limbs.

4. Heparin-induced thrombocytopenia may also be associated with arterial ischemia secondary to platelet-rich thrombi (white-clot syndrome), but the ischemia stems from arterial obstruction rather than small-vessel venous thrombi as seen with venous limb gangrene.

5. Antiphospholipid antibody syndrome is characterized by an elevated level of anticardiolipin antibody and/or the presence of lupus anticoagulant activity in phospholipid-dependent coagulation assays plus the clinical findings of arterial or venous thrombosis, fetal loss, and thrombocytopenia. Patients may develop livedo reticularis, digital ischemia, or central skin necrosis.

6. Fat embolism may occur immediately after hip or knee replacement or one to three days after severe trauma. Cutaneous findings include widespread petechiae frequently involving upper extremity, truncal, and conjuctival vessels.

7. Atheroemboli usually stem from atherosclerotic lesions in the aorta and result in a variety of skin lesions, including petechiae, purpura, livedo reticularis, and spotty digital ischemia. Pulses are usually preserved. The syndrome is difficult to diagnose but should be considered whenever the above findings are seen in older males who have undergone vascular intervention or who are receiving anticoagulants.

8. Emboli to cutaneous vessels resulting in a purpuric and/or petechial lesion may result from cho-lesterol embolism from atherosclerotic plaques, from fat embolism after trauma or bone marrow necrosis, or from fibrin platelet aggregates from infected cardiac valves in patients with endocarditis (Figure 44-30).

9. Vasculitic lesions may result in microvascular obstruction and ischemic skin lesions (see the preceding discussion).

10. Cryoglobulinemia (with or without vasculitis) or idiopathic cold hemagglutinin disease can also occasionally cause digital ischemia and/or necrotic skin lesions due to microvascular obstruction.

Suggested Reading

Breathnach S: Amyloidosis of the skin. In Freidberg IM, Eisen AZ, Wolff K, Goldsmith LA, Katz SI, Fitzpatrick TB (eds): Fitzpatrick's Dermatology in General Medicine, 5th ed. New York: McGraw-Hill, 1999, p 1756.

Cocoub P, Fabiani FL, Musset L, et al: Mixed cryoglobulinemia and hepatitis C virus. Am J Med 1994;96:124.

Cohen SJ, Pittelkow MR, Su WPD: Cutaneous manifestations of cryoglobulinemia: Clinical and histopathologic study of seventy-two patients. J Am Acad Dermatol 1991;25:21.

Coller BS, Schneiderman PI: Clinical evaluation of hemorrhagic disorders: The bleeding history and differential diagnosis of purpura. In Hoffman R, Benz EJ Jr, Shattil SJ, Furie B, Cohen HJ, Silberstein LE, McGlave P (eds): Hematology: Basic Principles and Practice, 3rd ed. Philadelphia: Churchill Livingstone, 2000, p 1824.

Desnick RJ, Eng CM: Fabry disease. In Freidberg IM, Eisen AZ, Wolff K, Goldsmith LA, Katz SI, Fitzpatrick TB (eds): Fitzpatrick's Dermatology in General Medicine, 5th ed. New York: McGraw-Hill, 1999, p 1812.

Eby CS: Warfarin-induced skin necrosis. Hematol Oncol Clin North Am 1993;7:1291.

Falk RH, Comenzo RL, Skinner M: The systemic amyloidoses. N Engl J Med 1997;337:898.

Feinstein DI, Marder VJ, Colman RW: Consumptive thrombohemorrhagic disorders. In Colman RW, Hirsh J, Marder VJ, Clowes AW, George JN (eds): Hemostasis and Thrombosis: Basic Principles and Clinical Practice, 4th ed. Philadelphia: Lippincott, Williams & Wilkins, 2000, p 1197.

Guttmacher AE, Marchuk DA, White RI: Hereditary hemorrhagic telangiectasia. N Engl J Med 1995;333:918.

Haitjema T, Westermann CJJ, Overtoom TTC, et al: Hereditary haemorrhagic telangiectasia (Osler-Weber-Rendu syndrome): New insights into pathogenesis, complications, and treatment. Arch Intern Med 1996;156:714.

McCrae KR, Feinstein DI, Cines DB: Antiphospholipid antibodies and the antiphospholipid syndrome. In Colman RW, Hirsh J, Marder VJ, Clowes AW, George JN (eds): Hemostasis and Thrombosis: Basic Principles and Clinical Practice, 4th ed. Philadelphia: Lippincott, Williams & Wilkins, 2000, p 1339.

McGehee WG, Klotz TA, Epstein DJ, Rapaport SI: Coumadin necrosis associated with hereditary protein C deficiency. Ann Intern Med 1984;101:59.

Mulliken JB, Virnelli-Grevelink S: Vascular anomalies. In Freidberg IM, Eisen AZ, Wolff K, Goldsmith LA, Katz SI, Fitzpatrick TB (eds): Fitzpatrick's Dermatology in General Medicine, 5th ed. New York: McGraw-Hill, 1999, p 1175.

Patrignelli R, Sheikh SH, Shaw-Stiffel TA: Henoch-Schönlein purpura: A multisystem disease also seen in adults. Postgrad Med 1995;97(5):123.

Piette WW: Hematologic diseases. In Freidberg IM, Eisen AZ, Wolff K, Goldsmith LA, Katz SI, Fitzpatrick TB (eds): Fitzpatrick's Dermatology in General Medicine, 5th ed. New York: McGraw-Hill, 1999, p 1867.

Rappersberger K, Stingl G, Wolff K: Karposi's sarcoma. In Freidberg IM, Eisen AZ, Wolff K, Goldsmith LA, Katz SI, Fitzpatrick TB (eds): Fitzpatrick's Dermatology in General Medicine, 5th ed. New York: McGraw-Hill, 1999, p 1195.

Rees MM, Rodgers GM: Bleeding disorders caused by vascular abnormalities. In Lee GR, Foerster J, Lukens J, Paraskeva F, Greer JP, Rodgers GE (eds): Wintrobe's Clinical Hematology, 10th ed. Baltimore: Williams & Wilkins, 1999, p 1633.

Sontheimer RD, Tu JH, Mandell B, Soter NA, Cornelius LA, Katz SI, Sutej P, Provost T, Klippel JH, Winchester R, Holubar K, et al: Skin manifestations of rheumatologic diseases. In Freidberg IM, Eisen AZ, Wolff K, Goldsmith LA, Katz SI, Fitzpatrick TB (eds): Fitzpatrick's Dermatology in General Medicine, 5th ed. New York: McGraw-Hill, 1999, pp 1993–2098.

Warkentin TE, Elavathil LJ, Hayward CPM, Johnston MA, Russett JL, Kelton JG: The pathogenesis of venous limb gangrene associated with heparin-induced thrombocytopenia. Ann Intern Med 1997;127:804.

Warkentin TE, Kelton GJ: A 14-year study of heparin-induced thrombocytopenia. Am J Med 1996;101:502.

Wenstrup RJ: Heritable disorders of connective tissue with skin changes. In Freidberg IM, Eisen AZ, Wolff K, Goldsmith LA, Katz SI, Fitzpatrick TB (eds): Fitzpatrick's Dermatology in General Medicine, 5th ed. New York: McGraw-Hill, 1999, p 1835.

Chapter 45
Pigmented Skin Lesions

Arthur J. Sober

The evaluation of pigmented skin lesions is a common concern for health care providers in many disciplines. All clinicians who have the opportunity to examine the skin should be able to distinguish those pigmented lesions that are suspicious (primarily melanoma and its precursors) from the myriad of banal pigmented lesions of skin (benign nevi, seborrheic keratoses, ephelides, and certain vascular lesions).

Faced with the frequency of common pigmented lesions, the clinician has only two questions to answer: (1) Is this person likely to develop a melanoma? (2) Is this lesion likely a melanoma?

Who is at risk? Current risk factor models can separate individuals whose risk for melanoma may differ by several hundredfold. Table 45-1 lists the features that are associated with an increased risk for melanoma. Overall lifetime risk for melanoma in the United States for a Caucasian is about 1 in 75. The evaluation of a given pigmented lesion may be more or less suspicious depending on the patient's other risk factors.

What are the factors that raise suspicion that a pigmented lesion might be a melanoma? For almost two decades, the ABCDs of melanoma have been a useful tool to assist in recognizing a pigmented lesion of potential concern. Table 45-2 defines the ABCDs for recognition of potentially suspicious pigmented lesions. Occasionally, an E has been added to the list for "enlargement" or "elevation" (Figures 45-1 through 45-3). Increase in size and change in color are the most frequently observed changes in thin (curable) melanoma (Table 45-3). Itching of a lesion is nonspecific but was observed on direct query in about one fifth of patients with thin primary tumors (see Table 45-3). Elevation was more associated with thicker melanomas, as were bleeding, tenderness, and ulceration (see Table 45-3).

In addition to the ABCDs of diagnosis, several algorithms assist in evaluating patients with pigmented lesions. Weinstock proposed a nine-step model with these action items: ACT, IGNORE, and WATCH (Table 45-4). ACT suggests evaluation by a dermatologist and possible biopsy. IGNORE indicates reassurance of the patient. WATCH suggests reexamination at two months and at six months. Table 45-5 indicates the range of potential actions that are available following the evaluation of patients for melanoma. Robinson proposed a six-step model for the evaluation of pigmented lesions based on the Weinstock model (Table 45-6).

Evaluation of Specific Pigmented Lesions

Lesions to be differentiated from melanoma include benign melanocytic lesions, such as lentigines, blue nevi, junctional, dermal, compound, and dysplastic nevi; vascular lesions (hemangiomas, hematomas) and pigmented nonmelanocytic malignancies (pigmented basal cell carcinoma, pigmented squamous cell carcinoma, in situ or Bowen disease); pigmented fibrotic lesions (pigmented dermatofibromas); and pigmented benign keratinocytic lesions (seborrheic keratoses, epidermal nevi) and exogenous pigment (tattoo) (Table 45-7 and Figures 45-4 through 45-12). Examination with oil, magnification, and tangential illumination can be helpful in the diagnostic evaluation. This process is called epiluminescence microscopy (ELM). The presence of a pigmented network pattern establishes the presence of a melanocytic lesion.

The lack of a network usually implies a nonmelanocytic growth. The algorithm in Figure 45-13 describes the approach to distinguishing benign from malignant lesions using epiluminescence microscopy. Three epiluminescence microscopy findings have a high degree of specificity for melanoma: (1) "radial streaming," linear streaks of pigmentation at the edge of the lesion perpendicular to the border and (2) "pseudopods," thickened branching pigment pattern at lesional edge, both representing the radial growth phase of the tumor; and (3) "blue-gray veil," bluish-

Table 45-1 ■ Factors Associated with Increased Individual Risk for Melanoma

Greatly Elevated Risk

More than 100 nevi
Two or more close family members with melanoma
Prior melanoma
Xeroderma pigmentosum
A changing pigmented lesion

Moderately Elevated Risk

A few dysplastic nevi
Giant congenital nevus
Family history of melanoma
Chronic Psoralen plus ultraviolet A radiation exposure as
    therapy

Modest Elevation of Risk

Easy burn, poor tan
Freckles
Small congenital nevus
Blue or gray eyes
Blond or red hair
Immunosuppression
History of severe sunburns

Table 45-2 ■ Suspicious Features: The ABCDs of Melanoma

A = lesional asymmetry
B = border irregularity
C = color variation
D = diameter >6 mm
E = enlargement or elevation

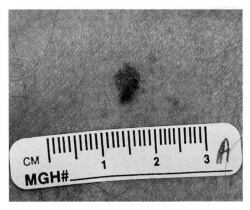

Figure 45-2 ■ Early melanoma. Note asymmetry (A), irregularity of border (B), and variation in pigment pattern (C). Lesion is 7 mm in greatest dimension (D). (See Color Plate 12.)

gray or white areas within the lesion representing partial tumor regression.

Figure 45-14 describes an overall approach to individuals with pigmented lesions. It is important to examine the complete skin surface, including the scalp. A good source of illumination and magnifying lens can greatly assist in the evaluation. If melanoma is suspected, palpation of the regional lymph nodes and the cutaneous surface between the possible primary site and the regional nodes is worthwhile to detect possible satellite, in-transit, or nodal metastases. A review of systems may also be of help in identifying the presence of distant disease.

Not all melanomas are pigmented; perhaps 5% are amelanotic. In these cases, the diagnosis is made by the pathologist after biopsy of a new, changing, or otherwise suspicious lesion (bleeding, ulceration, pain, etc).

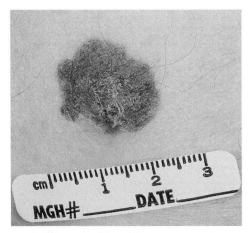

Figure 45-1 ■ Superficial spreading melanoma, level II, 0.43 mm in thickness on the arm of a male over age 60. Note asymmetry (A), irregularity of border (B), variation in color (C), and size: approximately 1.5 mm (D). (See Color Plate 12.)

Table 45-3 ■ Percentage of Patients with Melanoma Presenting with the Following Signs and Symptoms by Primary Tumor Thickness

| | Thickness (mm) | | | |
	<0.85	0.85–1.69	1.70–3.64	≥3.65
Size	55	49	51	72
Color change	49	47	45	58
Elevation	36	51	59	82
Bleeding	13	25	48	63
Ulcer	5	15	33	50
Tenderness	8	7	14	19
Itching	20	30	29	46

Values represent percentage of patients who noted that sign or symptom at presentation.

Table 45-4 ■ Algorithm for the Evaluation of Pigmented Lesions

1.	ACT	Patients who are at "very high risk"; annual exam by a dermatologist
2.	IGNORE	Clearly benign pigmented lesions (see Table 45-7)
3.	IGNORE	Lesions of less than 3 weeks' duration
4.	ACT	Ulcerated, eroded, bleeding, or crusted lesions of greater than 3 weeks' duration
5.	IGNORE	Flat, unchanging lesions less than 3 mm in diameter
6.	ACT	Lesions meeting ABCD criteria or change in color, size, surface, or shape
7.	ACT	Black lesions in fair complexioned individuals
8.	IGNORE	Nonchanging lesions, less than 6 mm, lacking the features of ACT
9.	WATCH	All lesions not classified as "ACT" or "IGNORE"

Table 45-5 ■ Potential Actions Available in the Management of Patients with Pigmented Lesions

1. Reassure patient that lesion is benign
2. Follow lesion for change:
   By patient only (at 2-month intervals)
   By patient and care provider (at 6- to 12-month intervals)
3. Biopsy lesion if suspicious
4. Refer to dermatology, surgery, or plastic surgery

Table 45-6 ■ Screening Patients with Pigmented Lesions

1. Annual skin exam by a dermatologist for patients at greatly or moderately increased risk
2. Reassure and educate patients for the signs and symptoms of melanoma if none of their pigmented lesions meet the criteria for biopsy
3. Reassure and educate patients for lesions of less than 3 weeks' duration
4. Reassure and educate patients with flat unchanging pigmented lesions less than 3 mm in diameter
5. Biopsy or refer for further evaluation and potential biopsy lesions that demonstrate three or four markedly abnormal features of the ABCDs or rapid change in a single feature
6. Reevaluate at 2 to 6 months all lesions that are not classified under items 2–5

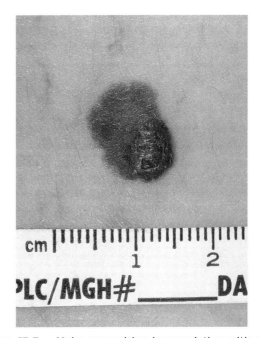

Figure 45-3 ■ Melanoma arising in association with a pre-existing compound nevus on the thigh of a woman in her 40s. Note elevation and irregularity of surface. (See Color Plate 12.)

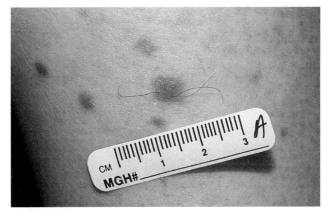

Figure 45-4 ■ Multiple benign nevi. Lesions have reasonably regular contours and uniform pigment patterns. (See Color Plate 12.)

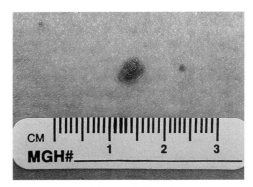

Figure 45-5 ■ Acquired compound nevus. Raised lesion, relatively uniform color, pigment pattern, and border. Onset, after birth. (See Color Plate 12.)

Table 45-7 ■ **Differential Diagnosis of Cutaneous Melanoma** (See Figures 45-4 through 45-12)

Benign nevus	
Compound	Round or oval shape, well-demarcated. Smooth bordered. May be dome-shaped or papillomatous: colors range from flesh colored to very dark brown, with individual nevi being relatively homogenous in color.
Junctional	Flat to barely raised brown lesion. Sharp border. Fine pigmentary stippling visible especially upon magnification.
Blue	Gunmetal or cerulean blue, blue-gray. Stable over time. One half occur on dorsa of hands and feet. Lesions are usually single, small 3 mm to <1 cm. Must be distinguished from nodular melanoma.
Lentigo	Flat, uniformly medium or dark brown lesion with sharp border. Solar lentigines are acquired lesions on sites of chronic solar exposure (face and backs of hands). Lesions are 2 mm to >1 cm. Solar lentigines have reticulate pigmentation upon magnification.
Pigmented dermatofibroma	Lesion is not well demarcated visually, is firm, and dimples downward when compressed laterally. Usually <6 mm.
Tattoo (traumatic, medical, or cosmetic)	In medical tattoo, lesions are small pigmentary dots, often blue or green, that make a regular pattern (rectangle). Traumatic tattoos are irregular, and pigmentation may appear black.
Seborrheic keratosis	Rough, sharp-bordered lesions that feel waxy and "stuck on"; range in color from flesh to tan, to dark brown. Presence of keratin plugs in surface is helpful for discriminating especially dark lesions from melanoma.
Pigmented basal cell carcinoma	Papular border. May have central ulceration. Usually on a sun-exposed surface in an older patient. Patient usually has dark brown eyes and dark brown or black hair.
Pigmented squamous cell, carcinoma, in situ (Bowen disease)	Variably pigmented plaque with slightly scaly or rough surface. Usually in individuals who tan well and who have brown eyes and dark brown or black hair.
Hemangioma	Dome-shaped reddish, purple, blue nodule. Compression with a glass microscope slide may result in blanching. Saccular pattern on epiluminescence microscopy. Must be distinguished from nodular melanoma.
Subungual hematoma	Maroon (red-brown) coloration. As lesion grows out from nail fold, a curving clear area is seen.
Café-au-lait macule	Flat, uniformly pigmented light chocolate colored lesion may be single or multiple.

Source: Adapted from Sober AJ, et al: Harrison's Principles of Internal Medicine, 14th ed. New York: McGraw-Hill, 1998, pp 543–549.

In individuals with large numbers of pigmented lesions, select for biopsy one or more lesions that is (are) out of phase with the rest, for example, a black lesion among brown ones or a red lesion among brown ones. Brown or tan lesions with a hint of pink or red may also be worth considering for diagnostic evaluation. Photographs of nevi may be of value in monitoring a patient's lesions for change. Photography tends to be one of two types: (1) total body photography with serial 35-mm slides, prints, or digital imaging to monitor for new or changing lesions in a patient with a large number of nevi or (2) individual lesional photography 1:1 or 2:1 with 35-mm slides, prints, digital images, or Polaroid images in a patient in whom one or up to several nevi are to be monitored more closely than the rest for change. In general,

photography is more helpful in revealing changes in size, shape, or pigment pattern than in determining color change. The latter is especially true for Polaroid photography. At present, in most settings, the obtaining of images is not reimbursable by health insurance. Nonetheless, it can prove quite helpful in recognizing possible early melanoma in patients with large numbers of atypical nevi. New or changing lesions tend to be scrutinized more avidly for malignancy than do stable established lesions.

Evaluation of Pigmented Lesions in Unusual Locations

In blacks and Asians, the palms, soles, nailbeds, and mucous membranes are the most common locations

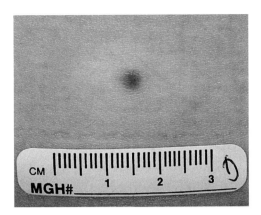

Figure 45-6 ■ Halo nevus. One mechanism by which the body rids itself of nevi is through an inflammatory response that destroys the mole and surrounding normal epidermal melanocytes. Halo nevi may be seen in patients who have a melanoma at some other location on their body. Note the hypopigmentation surrounding the central lesion. (See Color Plate 13.)

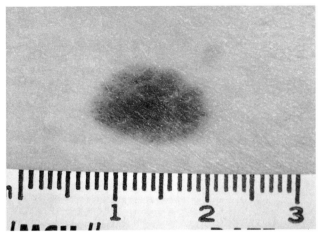

Figure 45-8 ■ Compound dysplastic nevus. (See Color Plate 13.)

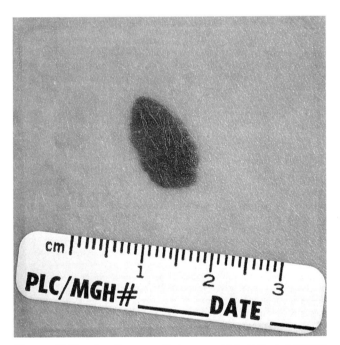

Figure 45-7 ■ Small congenital nevus. This lesion, present from birth, has uniform pigmentation, regular contours, and increased hair. (See Color Plate 13.)

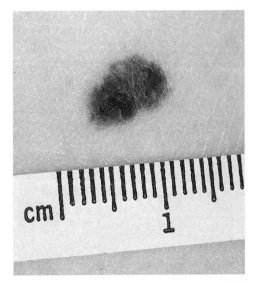

Figure 45-9 ■ Compound dysplastic nevus. (See Color Plate 13.)

for melanoma. The subungual location presents a special challenge since the site of origin of melanoma is in the nail matrix, a location that requires special skill in obtaining a diagnostic biopsy. Subungual melanoma needs to be distinguished from more common benign nevi of the nailfold and the even more common subungual hematoma. Benign nevi are usually thinner streaks of long duration and often involve multiple nails, while subungual hematomas occur following a clear history of trauma, are red-

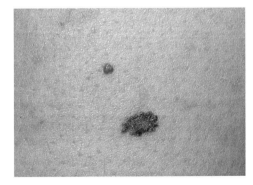

Figure 45-10 ■ Compound dysplastic nevus. Raised lesion, often >6 mm, may vary in size and shape from the patient's other nevi. Borders may be less distinct than those of benign acquired nevi. (See Color Plate 13.)

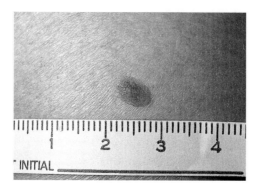

Figure 45-11 ■ Seborrheic keratosis. Lesion is a plaque with a waxy surface. Can be flesh colored to very dark. (See Color Plate 14.)

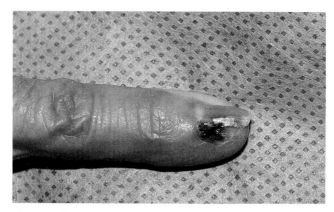

Figure 45-12 ■ Pseudo-Hutchinson sign in patient with hemorrhage and fungal infection of the nail plate. Note the pigmentation in the posterior nailfold. (See Color Plate 14.)

brown or maroon in color, and often lack posterior nailfold involvement. Subungual hematoma of acute onset can be diagnosed and treated by penetrating the nail plate with a heated paper clip and releasing the hemorrhage. Subungual hematomas "grow out" with follow-up and show progressive clearing of the proximal nail region. Pigmentation of the posterior nailfold (Hutchinson sign) is an ominous finding that may be observed with subungual melanoma (see Figure 45-12).

Acral plantar lesions present problems of early

recognition, as some have a tendency to be relatively amelanotic and thus may be confused with plantar warts. In addition, flat lesions may have appreciable thickness (downward growth). Finally, benign acral nevi can be confused histopathologically with acral melanoma because of the tendency of acral nevi to have benign nevus cells ascending in the epidermis. Nonetheless, the ABCD rule can usually be applied to the diagnosis of acral melanoma.

Conjunctival melanoma must be distinguished from benign conjunctival melanosis, which clinically

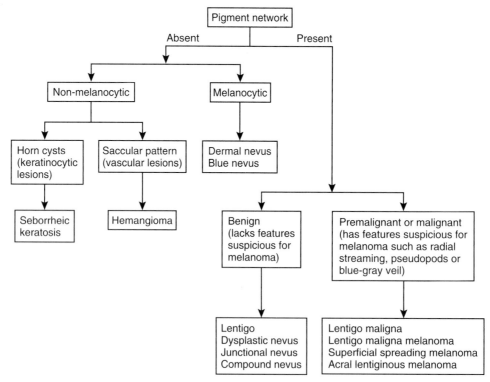

Figure 45-13 ■ Distinguishing benign from malignant lesions using epiluminescence microscopy.

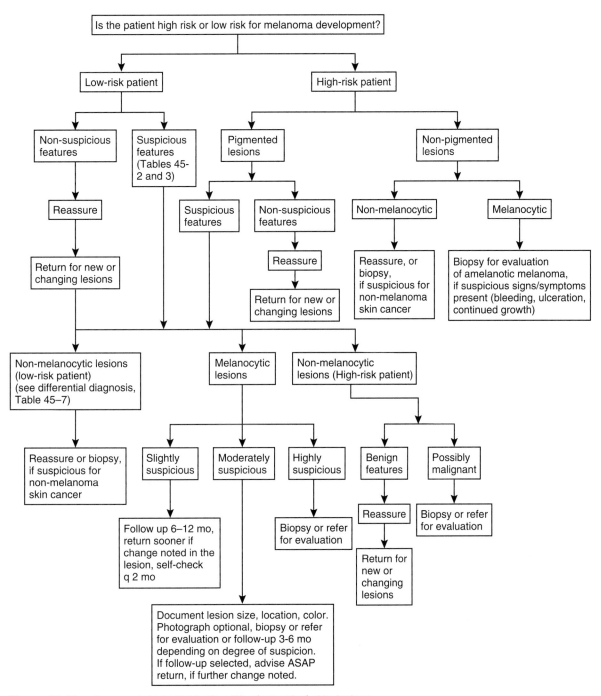

Figure 45-14 ■ Approach to individuals with pigmented skin lesions

may be similar. The distinction is based on histopathologic exam.

Oral mucosal melanoma must be distinguished from vascular lesions and blue-gray dental amalgam tattoos.

In evaluating irregular bordered and variably pigmented macular lesions of the genitalia (penis and vulva), one needs to be aware of conditions termed benign penile or vulvar lentiginosis. In these conditions, a rather alarming clinical appearance is associated microscopically with benign melanocytic proliferation. These lesions appear to behave in a stable manner, but follow-up for change is a reasonable course of action with rebiopsy as necessary.

Biopsy of Lesions of Concern

The optimal biopsy is an excisional biopsy under local anesthesia with narrow (1 to 2 mm) margins. This type of biopsy provides the entire specimen for the

DIAGNOSIS

Evaluation of Nailbed Lesions

Early diagnosis of subungual melanoma is challenging in part because of the rarity of diagnosis and in part because of the higher degree of technical skill needed to perform a nailbed matrix biopsy and the risk of permanent nail plate dystrophy resulting.

Features that would raise suspicion include the following:

- A new pigmented streak
- A solitary pigmented streak
- A broad pigmented streak
- Older individuals
- Pigmentation on posterior nailfold (Hutchinson sign)
- Deformity of nail plate
- African American or East Asian lineage

Factors that would lower suspicion include the following:

- Streak of long duration
- Narrow streak
- Streaks on multiple nails

- Young individuals
- Maroon color and history of trauma (subungual hematoma)
- History of pharmacologic drug use where medication has been associated with pigmentation of nails
- Pigmentation does not involve the posterior nailfold

Unfortunately, a history of trauma may be misleadingly present in patients with subungual melanoma.

Lesions that are considered suspicious by the above criteria should be considered for biopsy or close follow-up (photography may be helpful).

Biopsy needs to include nail matrix and must be evaluated by a pathologist who is familiar with the characteristics of subungual melanoma.

Once the diagnosis has been established, definitive management (surgical removal ± sentinel node identification) will depend on the extent of the lesion, tumor thickness, and the presence of any other adverse risk factors.

---

pathologist's review. Partial biopsy (punch or incisional) is not thought to increase risk of metastasis and is preferable to a further delay in diagnosis. It is important that sufficient representative tissue be provided to the pathologist in order to reach an accurate diagnosis. If partial biopsy is performed, biopsy of the most raised or thickest portion of the growth will usually establish the diagnosis. In a flat lesion, biopsy of the darkest area is suggested. Deep shave biopsies of thin primary melanomas may prove adequate, but superficial shave biopsies often transect deeper tumors, precluding accurate assessment of thickness. The caregiver who biopsies a lesion needs to be able to interpret the response from the pathologist. If the clinical impression does not fit with the histopathologic diagnosis, further action is needed, including dialogue with the pathologist regarding the adequacy of biopsy specimen (if the entire lesion was not removed), reexamination of the histopathologic material, deeper sections, and a possible second opinion from a pathologist who is more experienced in the diagnosis of difficult pigmented lesions.

Not all melanomas can be detected clinically even by the most knowledgeable and expert clinicians. Being aware of individuals who are at increased risk and the features that raise concern in a given pigmented lesion leads to the detection of most cutaneous melanomas. Since the overall survival rate of melanoma is in the 85% range, the majority of melanomas are detected and removed prior to the establishment of viable metastatic disease.

Suggested Reading

Fitzpatrick TB, Johnson RA, Wolff K, Suurmond D: Clinical Atlas and Synopsis of Clinical Dermatology, 4th ed. New York: McGraw-Hill, 2001, pp 270–311.

Friedman RJ, Rigel DS, Kopf AW: Early detection of malignant melanoma: The role of physician examination and self-examination of the skin. CA Cancer J Clin 1985;35: 130–151.

Rhodes AR: Public education and cancer of the skin: What do people need to know about melanoma and non-melanoma skin cancer? Cancer 1995;75:613–636.

Rhodes AR, Weinstock MA, Fitzpatrick TB, et al: Risk factors for cutaneous melanoma: A practical method of recognizing predisposed individuals. JAMA 1987;258:3146–3154.

Robinson JK: A 28-year-old fair-skinned woman with multiple moles. JAMA 1997;278:1693–1699.

Sober AJ, Day CL, Kopf AW, et al: Detection of "thin" primary melanomas. CA Cancer J Clin 1983;33:160–163.

Weinstock MA, Goldstein MG, Dube CE, et al: Basic skin cancer triage for teaching melanoma detection. J Am Acad Dermatol 1996;34:1063–1066.

Chapter 46
Cancer of Unknown Primary

Richard M. Stone

Introduction

On the basis of clinical and histologic findings, the organ of origin of a given neoplasm is usually readily apparent. However, about 1% of patients with cancer present with a syndrome in which the primary site is unknown. Such patients present a therapeutic dilemma because treatment is nonstandard and most such individuals fare poorly. Because of recent advances in diagnostic strategies, the incidence of metastatic cancer of unknown primary is declining. Nonetheless, owing to nonspecific presentations and confusing results on examination of biopsy specimens, it is likely that these challenging cases will persist at low frequency. In general, the strategy for patients with whom an initial evaluation does not reveal a primary site rests on two principles: detailed analysis of the pathology and special consideration of metastatic cancers that are responsive to therapy.

A reasonable definition for metastatic cancer of unknown primary site includes the following: (1) malignancy confirmed by a biopsy; (2) no obvious primary site despite careful history, physical examination, chest X-ray, computed tomogram of the abdomen and pelvis, complete blood count, and serum chemistry (including beta human chorionic gonadotropin, alpha fetoprotein, and prostate-specific antigen in men); (3) negative mammography in women; (4) a careful histologic examination that does not establish a definitive primary site; and (5) failure of additional directed diagnostic studies to reveal the organ of origin. Numerous investigations have shown that "blind endoscopy" (i.e., colonoscopy in the absence of abdominal symptoms or occult blood in the stool) is an unnecessary use of resources. On the other hand, symptoms and findings should be followed up carefully, such as cystoscopy for patients with microscopic hematuria.

The patient and family will exert great pressure on the physician to spare no expense and to use every available diagnostic tool in the search for the primary site of origin of the cancer. Substantial time and effort are required to educate the patient and family about the goals and limitations of the clinical evaluation. The diagnostic search should focus on those metastatic malignancies for which effective therapy exists. The patient and family will need considerable persuasion to understand that such therapy, where available, can be applied to the patient's benefit even when the primary site is undetectable and not surgically removed. (See also Chapter 112.)

Clinical Evaluation

Despite the availability of multiple invasive and costly diagnostic procedures, one of the key features of the workup is a thorough history and physical examination. One important but often overlooked feature is a history of a prior biopsy of any suspected lesion, even in the distant past. Such a lesion could have been mistakenly diagnosed as benign. Alternatively, the patient who is thought to have been cured of a localized cancer many years ago could be experiencing a late recurrence of the original neoplasm. Therefore any histologic specimens that were obtained in the past should be sought and reviewed. A thorough review of systems might yield clues such as abdominal pain, change in stool caliber, cough, or genitourinary bleeding that could indicate the direction for subsequent workup. The physical examination should include a thorough inspection of the oral cavity and possible indirect laryngoscopic exam, thorough inspection of the skin for visible or palpable lesions, a rectal exam with palpation of the prostate in men, and breast examination and pelvic exam and Pap smear in females. The increasingly widespread use of positron emission tomography (PET) scanning may diminish even further the incidence of cancers whose primary site remains unknown; however, at the moment, there are no data to support the routine use of this expensive diagnostic modality in patients with this entity. Moreover, positron emission tomography scans also yield false-positive findings, which could serve to broaden the cost and discomfort of an expanded diagnostic workup.

The pattern of the clinical presentation and findings may provide clues to the underlying diagnosis. Patients presenting with a neck mass with squamous histology (especially with a node located in a high or midcervical area) should be considered to have a tumor of the upper aerodigestive tract (head and neck cancer) unless proven otherwise. Such patients should undergo a detailed examination of the head and neck, including direct laryngoscopy, nasopharyngoscopy, and random blind biopsies. The most common location for an occult primary when a metastatic lesion with squamous histology is found in the neck is in the base of the tongue or tonsillar fossa. Primary thyroid cancer should also be considered, particularly in the absence of definitive squamous histology. Liver metastases from an adenocarcinoma without a clear primary may represent an occult cancer of the lung or gastrointestinal tract.

Pathology

Evaluation of a suspected metastatic cancer of unknown primary site requires consultation from a pathologist who is skilled in evaluating difficult-to-classify lesions. Histologic and pathologic review, especially in the current era when a battery of sophisticated immunohistochemical stains and molecular studies are available, can often be helpful in directing specific therapy. The pathologist will first attempt to classify, on morphologic grounds alone, whether the neoplastic tissue is of hematopoietic, connective tissue, or epithelial (be it glandular, squamous, or transitional) origin. Certain specific findings on histologic review will suggest a primary site. For example, psammoma bodies suggest ovarian or thyroid derivation, and signet ring cells suggest a gastric origin. The initial review leads to a diagnosis of moderately or well-differentiated adenocarcinomas in 60% of cases and poorly differentiated carcinomas/adenocarcinomas in 30%. The remainder consists of poorly differentiated malignant neoplasms that are not further classifiable as carcinomas, lymphomas, or sarcomas.

Immunohistochemical studies of biopsy specimens are often helpful in determining the cell of origin. For example, a positive leukocyte common antigen stain can indicate that a poorly differentiated neoplasm is of lymphoid origin. Such a finding could have a critical impact on therapy and prognosis, since even poorly differentiated neoplasms that stain for lymphoid antigens or specific B or T cell markers tend to respond as well to antilymphoma therapy as those cases which are more readily identifiable. The presence of epithelial membrane antigen or cytokeratin staining can confirm that the neoplasm is a carcinoma as opposed to HMB45, which is typical of melanoma, desmin in sarcoma, or a myoglobin in rhabdomyosarcoma. Within the category of adenocarcinomas, other immunohistochemical stains can direct the oncologist to the organ of origin, such as prostate-specific acid phosphatase or the cytokeratin pattern. For example, ovarian cancers are cytokeratin 20 negative but cytokeratin 7 positive; colorectal cancers tend to be cytokeratin 20 positive but cytokeratin 7 negative, and pancreatic cancers are positive for both these cytokeratin subtypes. Positive immunostaining for both p63 and cytokeratin 5/6 suggests a squamous cell origin. Table 46-1 lists a number of studies that could help to define the cell or origin. However, it is important to note that none of these tests are completely specific. For example, while sarcomas are desmin positive, certain sarcomas such as mesotheliomas are also cytokeratin positive. S-100 positivity, typically associated with melanomas, even amelanotic subtypes, may also be found in other tumors of neuroendocrine origin, such as small-cell lung cancer, carcinoid, or neuroepithelioma. Moreover, many routine laboratories are not equipped to provide all of these studies. Whether it is worthwhile to send specimens for analysis to a reference pathology laboratory depends on the need for this sophisticated level of discrimination.

Cytogenetic and molecular analysis can also help lead to a specific diagnosis. These studies require special handling of tumor biopsies. Therefore the clinician must have either a suspicion for metastatic cancer of unknown primary or perform these studies on a repeat biopsy. Ultrastructural studies require fixation in glutaraldehyde, and cytogenetic studies require fresh tissue. Electron microscopic evaluation can reveal the actin-myosin filaments that are typically seen in rhabdomyosarcoma, the secretory

Table 46-1 ■ Histologic/Cytologic Review of Biopsies from Patients with Metastatic Cancer of Unknown Primary Site

	Specific Tumor
Histology	
Psammomma bodies	Ovarian cancer, thyroid cancer
Signet ring morphology	Gastric or breast cancer
Immunocytochemistry	
Cytokeratin 7/20 pattern	CK7+/CK20–: lung cancer
	CK7+/CK20+: transitional cell carcinoma
Cytokeratin 5/6	Squamous cell carcinoma
Prostate specific antigen	Prostatic adenocarcinoma
HMB45	Melanoma
CA19-9	Pancreatic carcinoma
CA-125	Ovarian cancer
Thyroglobulin	Thyroid cancer
Gross-cystic disease protein	Breast cancer
S-100	Melanoma, neuroendocrine tumors
myoglobin	Rhabdomyosarcoma
calcitonin	Medullary carcinoma of the thyroid
leukocyte common antigen	Lymphoma
leu-M1	Hodgkin's disease
epithelial membrane antigen	Carcinoma
desmin	Sarcoma
alpha fetoprotein	Liver, stomach, germ cell
placental alkaline phosphatase	Germ cell
factor VIII	Kaposi's sarcoma, angiosarcoma
Cytogenetics	
Iso 12p; 12p–	Germ cell
t(11;22)	Ewing's sarcoma, primitive neuroectodermal tumor
3p–	Small cell, renal, mesothelioma
t(X;18)	Synovial sarcoma
t(12;16)	Myxoid liposarcoma
t(12;22)	Clear cell sarcoma (melanoma of small parts)
t(2;13)	Alveolar rhabdomyosarcoma
1p–	Neuroblastoma
Molecular studies	
BRCA1 mutation	Breast cancer
c-kit mutation	Gastrointestinal stromal cell tumor
Ig, TCR, bcl-2 rearrangement	Lymphoma

Source: Modified from Stone, RM: Metastatic cancer of unknown primary site. In Braunwald E, Fauci A, Kasper D, Hauser S, Longo D, Jameson L (eds): Harrison's Principles of Internal Medicine, 15th ed. New York: McGraw Hill, 2001, with permission.

granules found in neuroendocrine tumors, and/or the cell-cell junctions in carcinomas. Particularly in the evaluation of suspected sarcomas, cytogenetic evaluation provides a way to potentially identify a specific neoplasm. One of the best examples of this type of approach is the translocation between chromosome 11 and 22 seen in Ewing's sarcoma and in the related group of neoplasms, the primitive neuroepidermal tumors (see Table 46-1).

Particularly with the advent of molecularly targeted therapies, molecular biologic studies are becoming increasingly important in the evaluation of suspected neoplasms. For example, gastrointestinal stromal cell tumors tend to overexpress the c-kit membrane-associated tyrosine kinase proto-oncogene (CD117 on flow cytometric analysis). Moreover, most patients with gastrointestinal stromal cell tumors have been found to harbor an activating mutation in the c-kit gene. The protein resulting from this mutated gene is sensitive to the tyrosine kinase inhibitor imatinib mesylate (Gleevec). The impressive clinical responses that are noted with this drug in a gastrointestinal malignancy that is completely resistant to chemotherapy highlight the value of molecular studies.

Biological Behavior

Tumors that "don't follow the rules" by presenting in an unusual fashion or with difficult-to-classify histology may be considered to manifest intrinsically adverse biological behavior. One can intuit how biologically aggressive a cancer is that exhibits early dissemination from a minimal, inapparent primary lesion. One cytogenetic correlate of this aggressive behavior is a deletion of the long arm of chromosome 1. A group of patients presenting with nodal metastases from a squamous cell carcinoma that were presumed, but not identified, to have arisen from a head and neck cancer site were evaluated with cytogenetic studies. In one half of the patients, normal areas of the aerodigestive tract were found on biopsy to harbor the same microsatellite DNA pattern as was found in the nodal metastases. This raises the question of whether the genetically abnormal cells gave rise to metastases without first forming a focal tumor collection. At the moment, however, the heterogeneity of this category of neoplasms defies construction of a unifying biologically based hypothesis. The biologic variability in these patients with cancer of unknown primary is reflected in their median survival rate, which can range from 40 months for those with non-adenocarcinoma histology, limited metastatic sites, and no liver/bone/adrenal/pleural metastases to five months for those with liver metastases, age greater than 60 years, and nonneuroendocrine histology.

TREATMENT

Metastatic Cancer of Unknown Primary

1. Search for primary:
   No invasive diagnostic procedures unless indicated by other findings
   Thorough history and physical:
   Attention to prior biopsies
   Stool for occult blood
   Rectal and genital exam in men
   Breast, pelvic, and Pap smear in women
   Routine laboratory studies:
   Chest X-ray, mammogram (women), prostate-specific antigen (men), urinalysis
   Tumor marker studies (if indicated)
2. Pathology review:
   Selected histologic, immunocytochemical, cytogenetic, and molecular studies

   Exclude lymphoma, sarcoma, melanoma, neuroendocrine origin
3. Treatment:
   Define treatable entity (if possible)
   If LCA (CD45) positive, treat for non-Hodgkin's lymphoma
   If extragonadal germ-cell primary is likely, platinum-based chemotherapy
   If squamous-cell carcinoma in cervical lymph node, search for head and neck primary
   If axillary lymph node with adenocarcinoma, treat for stage II breast cancer
   If peritoneal carcinomatosis in a woman, treat for ovarian cancer

Treatment Considerations

Though metastatic cancer of unknown primary in general carries a poor prognosis, it is possible to define subgroups of patients who may do well or even be curable. Occult extragonadal germ-cell cancer represents one such subset of patients with metastatic cancer of unknown primary. They usually display one or more of the following features: age less than 50 years, tumor involving midline structures (organs or lymph nodes), an elevated serum alpha fetoprotein and/or beta human chorionic gonadotropin, or evidence of rapid tumor growth. Cytogenetic features are similar to those identified in highly chemotherapy-responsive germ-cell tumors of the testes. Approximately 15% to 20% of patients with this form of cancer of unknown primary experience prolonged disease-free survival after treatment with an intensive platinum-based chemotherapy program.

Some women present with disseminated cancer in the peritoneum but without an obvious ovarian primary. These patients may respond as do those with locally advanced ovarian cancer to platinum-based combination therapy with paclitaxel. This presentation has been termed the primary peritoneal papillary serous carcinoma or multifocal extra ovarian serous carcinoma syndrome. Gastrointestinal cancer, however, can also present with disseminated peritoneal carcinomatosis and would not be expected to respond to platinum-based chemotherapy. It is often possible to differentiate the likelihood of a colonic versus ovarian cancer if psammoma bodies or an elevated serum CA125 level, which are more consistent with ovarian cancer, are noted.

Women who present with an axillary mass that is proved on biopsy to be adenocarcinoma may be considered to have stage II breast cancer whether or not a breast primary is found and whether or not the tumor cells express estrogen or progesterone receptors. This presentation, if untreated, will demonstrate recurrent disease in the breast in one half of patients. In this situation, treatment with surgery and/or radiation therapy and adjuvant chemotherapy/hormonal therapy is administered as for women presenting with a proven primary cancer in the breast. Frequently, the mastectomy specimen fails to demonstrate the putative breast cancer primary despite meticulous review of the specimens by the pathologist.

Patients presenting with brain metastases without an obvious primary may fare better than was previously realized, especially if radiation and/or resection can successfully control the intracranial disease. Osteoblastic bone metastasis in males, particularly in the setting of an elevated serum prostate-specific antigen, should be considered to indicate metastatic prostate cancer, and therapy should be directed accordingly. Patients who present with this syndrome or are suspected of having primary head and neck cancer should receive definitive local therapy, including surgery and/or radiation therapy. Neoadjuvant therapy with a platinum-based chemotherapy regimen may also be beneficial.

Suggested Reading

Abruzzesse JL, et al: Analysis of a diagnostic strategy for patients with suspected tumors of unknown origin. J Clin Oncol 1995;13:2094.

Briasoulis E, Kalofonos H, Bafaloukas D, et al: Carboplatin plus pacitaxel in unknown primary carcinoma: A phase II Hellenic Cooperative Oncology Group Study. J Clin Oncol 2000;18:3101–3107.

Califaro J, et al: Unknown primary head and neck squamous cell carcinoma: Molecular identification of the site of origin. J Natl Cancer Inst 1999;91:599–604.

Ettinger DS, et al: NCCN practice guidelines for occult primary tumors. Oncology 1998;12:226–309.

Greco FA, Gray J, Burris HA, et al: Taxane-based chemotherapy for patients with carcinoma of unknown primary site. Can J Cancer 2001;7:203–212.

Hainsworth JD, Greco FA: Treatment of patients with cancer of an unknown primary site. N Engl J Med 1993;329: 275–263.

Hainsworth JD, Greco FA: Management of patients with cancer of unknown primary site. Oncology 2000;14:563–574.

Hess KR, Abruzzesse MC, et al: Classification and regression tree analysis of 1,000 consecutive patients with unknown primary carcinoma. Clin Cancer Res 1999;5:3403–3410.

Hillen HF: Unknown primary tumours. Postgrad Med J 2000;76:690–693.

Lassen U, Daugaard G, et al: 18F-FDG whole body positron emission tomography (PET) in patients with unknown primary tumours (UPT). Eur J Cancer 1999;35:1076–1082.

Moetzer RJ, Rodriguez E, Reuter VE, et al: Molecular and cytogenetic studies in the diagnosis of patients with poorly differentiated carcinomas of unknown primary site. J Clin Oncol 1995;13:274–282.

Muggia FM, Baranda J: Management of peritoneal carcinomatosis of unknown primary tumor site. Semin Oncol 1993;20:268.

Nguyen LN, Maor MH, Oswald MJ: Brain metastases as the only manifestation of an undetected primary tumor. Cancer 1998;83:2181–2184.

Shapiro DV, Jarrett AR: The need to consider survival, outcome, and expense when evaluating and treating patients with unknown primary carcinoma. Arch Intern Med 1995;155: 2050–2054.

Vlastos G, Jean ME, Mirza AN, et al: Feasibility of breast preservation in the treatment of occult primary carcinoma presenting with axillary metastases. Ann Surg Oncol 2001;8: 425–431.

Section II
Therapeutics

Chapter 47
Radiation Oncology

Theodore S. Lawrence and George T. Henning

Radiation oncology is a specialty that combines the fields of radiation biology, medical physics, and clinical medicine. In this chapter, we review how ionizing radiation interacts with tissue, both physically and biologically, and then focus on how to apply these concepts to treat cancer patients.

Ionizing radiation is measured in terms of gray (Gy) which is a joule of energy deposited in a kilogram of tissue. This term replaces the rad, which might be more familiar; however, because 100 rads is equal to 1 Gy, many radiation oncologists have attempted to preserve the status quo by expressing doses in terms of centigray (cGy), so 1 cGy equals 1 rad. Another old term that might be familiar is the rem (standing for "Roentgen equivalent in man"), which has been replaced by the Sievert. This term was created to reflect the fact that different forms of radiation have a different biological effect for the same physical dose. For instance, 1 Gy of neutrons has a much greater biological effect than does 1 Gy of photons. The rem was defined as a physical dose times a "quality factor" reflecting the biologic effect of a unit of dose. The rem (or a thousandth of a rem, mrem) comes up frequently in discussions of radiation protection in the context of maximum allowable exposure.

The interaction of ionizing radiation with biologic tissues depends on the energy of the radiation. At the lowest energies (50 to 250 KeV), the dominant interaction is via the photoelectric effect. An incoming photon of the right energy knocks out an orbital electron of the same energy. In the photoelectric effect, the absorption of photons depends strongly on the atomic number of the irradiated substance. Thus, these photons are very useful in diagnostic radiology to image bones compared to soft tissues and air. Higher-energy photons (in the range of 2 to 25 MeV) are the chief form of ionizing radiation used to treat patients. These penetrate deeply into tissue (Figure 47-1), as a function of energy, producing a phenomenon called skin sparing. This means that the deep tumor receives more dose than does the overlying

skin. These higher-energy photons interact with tissue chiefly through what is known as the Compton effect, in which the incident photon can eject orbital electrons by passing nearby. In this energy range, the chief determinant of energy deposition is the density of the tissue rather than the atomic number. This means that because bones are only slightly denser than soft tissue, these differ only modestly in absorption, whereas soft tissue and lung (which has a markedly lower electron density) differ dramatically.

Most radiation oncology departments treat patients with two forms of radiation: photons and electrons. Electrons interact directly with tissue, in contrast to photons, which affect tissues by the electrons that they eject. Thus, electrons tend to deliver a higher skin dose than photons, and their depth of penetration is highly dependent on their energy. They are useful in treating tumors that are within approximately 6 cm from the surface of the body. A few centers use protons, charged nuclei (such as He or Ne), or neutrons for radiation treatments. These particles offer certain theoretical benefits, but clinically, they are still largely investigational.

Radiation is administered by two methods: an external machine (teletherapy) or the implantation of radioactive sources in or around the tumor (brachytherapy). Although chiefly of historic interest in the United States, radiation can be delivered by using cobalt 60, a radioisotope that has been activated in a nuclear reactor. Although cobalt machines are very reliable, the relatively low energy (limited penetration for deep tumors) and greater difficulty in achieving sharp beam edges (which limits dose to normal tissues) have relegated cobalt machines to, at most, a palliative role. More commonly, external radiation is administered by using a linear accelerator. In this device, electrons are accelerated to high energies and either used directly or collided with a tungsten target that produces photons. The beams can be individually shaped to match that of the tumor using either a custom fabricated metal block or, more

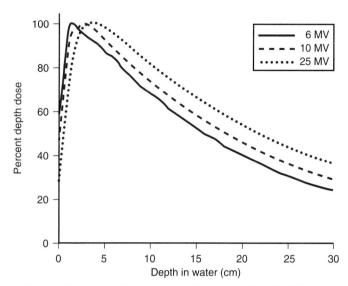

Figure 47-1 ■ Depth dose profiles for 6 MV, 10 MV, and 25 MV photon beams. The higher-energy beams exhibit a skin-sparing effect with a lower dose at the skin surface (depth = 0), and they penetrate deeper into the tissue.

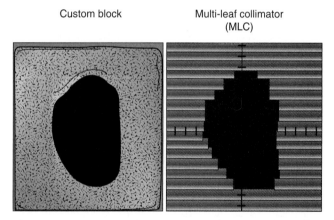

Figure 47-2 ■ Beam-shaping devices include the Cerrobend block on the left and the MLC collimator to define the same field shape on the right.

recently, a multileaf collimator (Figure 47-2). The latter has the advantage that it can be placed under computer control, permitting the efficient delivery of many complex fields for a single patient treatment (see the section entitled "Radiation Treatment Planning" later in this chapter).

Brachytherapy involves the placement of radioactive sources into or next to the tumor. It takes advantage of the fact that radiation dose falls off as the square of the distance from the source. Thus, if radioactive sources can be placed so that the tumor is within 1 cm of the sources, the dose that is received by normal tissues just 2 cm distant from the source and 1 cm distant from the tumor would be one quarter of the dose received by the tumor. Thus, it is sometimes possible to deliver a high dose to the tumor with only a modest dose to normal tissue. Disadvantages to brachytherapy are that it is hard to deliver a uniformly high dose to the tumor and that this form of treatment usually involves a surgical procedure. Placements can be permanent (giving very low-dose radiation over a long time period, often used for prostate cancer), or they can be temporary (as in cervix cancer). Traditional temporary brachytherapy involves delivering radiation over several days (low dose rate: in the range of 0.5 to 1 Gy/hour). A more recently developed form of temporary brachytherapy uses a high dose rate (HDR) applicator. In this approach, a highly radioactive source is placed near the tumor for only a few minutes. Radiation is delivered at dose rates resembling those used in teletherapy (in the range of 1 Gy/minute), and the procedure is repeated on a weekly basis three or more times. The use of high dose rate avoids the overnight hospital stay associated with low dose rate, radiation exposure to medical staff, and the potential for applicator movement. For these reasons, the use of high dose radiation brachytherapy has increased significantly over the last several years, particularly for the treatment of gynecologic malignancies. A wide variety of isotopes with differing depths of penetration can be used, which gives a great deal of flexibility to brachytherapy techniques.

The Interaction of Radiation with Cells

The chief targets of radiation in the cell appear to be DNA and the cell membrane. When ionizing radiation encounters biologic tissues, it can cause the ejection of electrons that interact directly with a target. A more common occurrence, however, is that the electron interacts with water to produce free radicals, which then can damage DNA breaks or the cell membrane. Radiation can produce both single- and double-strand DNA breaks. Single-strand DNA are usually efficiently repaired, as there is an intact template on which to replicate a repair patch, but occasionally, errors of repair are made. These and improperly repaired DNA double-strand breaks are probably the cause of the second malignancies that are caused in about 0.1% of patients undergoing a course of radiation therapy.

The most studied lesion induced by radiation that produces cell death is the DNA double-strand break. This damage can lead to cell death during a subsequent mitosis. Cells have elaborate mechanisms for repairing DNA damage, and even large amounts of damage are typically repaired within four to six hours. However, a single unrepaired DNA double-strand break can be sufficient to kill a cell. The presence of oxygen significantly increases the fixation of damage in DNA. This finding at least partly underlies the observation that hypoxic tumors tend to be more resistant to radiation than are well-oxygenated tumors and has led to research efforts to develop radiation sensitizers that can substitute for or increase oxygen during a course of radiation treatments.

It is possible that the DNA double-strand break repair process underlies the phenomenon known as sublethal damage repair. This term refers to the observation that splitting a single dose of radiation (for instance 8 Gy) into two 4-Gy doses separated by time decreases cell killing as the time between the fraction increases. A split of six hours is enough to lose any additivity of the fractions. This laboratory observation might explain the clinical finding that increasing fractionation improves normal tissue tolerance. It is also likely that this repair process explains the influence of dose rate on the radiation effectiveness. Radiation delivered at the low dose rates (such as 0.1 to 1 Gy/hour) of standard brachytherapy produces significantly less cell killing than the same dose of radiation delivered at typically external beam rates (1 to 3 Gy/minute) because of continuous repair during irradiation.

An alternative form of cell death produced by radiation is apoptosis, or programmed cell death, in which radiation initiates a series of steps leading to the activation of an enzyme that cleaves DNA. Other than in lymphocytes and spermatocytes, in which apoptosis dominates, apoptosis typically accounts for a minor fraction of the cell death resulting from ionizing radiation. The clinical significance of radiation-induced apoptosis in tumors is an active area of study.

Radiation can affect other parts of the cell, in particular the cell membrane. Radiation can stimulate signal transduction pathways originating in the membrane causing activation of growth factors (such as epidermal growth factor receptors) as well as death signals (such as tumor necrosis factor). The former may be analogous to a wound-healing response. It also may be responsible for the stimulation of regrowth of certain cancer cells that occurs during a course of radiation and is the basis for accelerated fractionation (see below).

Interaction of Radiation with Tissues and Organs

Although an enormous amount of progress has been made at the molecular and cellular levels, much of our knowledge of the effect of radiation at the levels of tissues and organs is still descriptive. This area remains important because concepts derived from experimental work at the organ level have led to important clinical trials involving the role of fractionation. On the basis of laboratory studies of radiation toxicity, side effects are classified as acute (such as mucositis and diarrhea) and chronic (such as fibrosis or radiation myelitis). Similarly, tissues are considered acutely responding (such as the pharynx or intestine) or late responding (such as the spinal cord). Acutely responding tissues tend to be composed of rapidly proliferating cells, whereas late-responding tissues tend to proliferate slowly, if at all. Experimental studies have suggested that fraction size has a much stronger influence on the toxicity of acutely responding tissues than on late responding tissues. For example, it has been shown experimentally that, in comparison to standard fractionation, giving multiple small fractions to the oral mucosa produces less long-term toxicity for the same acute toxicity, whereas fraction size appears to have little influence on radiation myelitis. Most tumors tend to respond as acutely responding tissues. These concepts have formed the basis for the hyperfractionation trials for head and neck cancer described below.

Why Does Radiation Therapy Work?

Before leaving the subject of how radiation interacts with cells, it is important to ask the simple question: Why does radiation therapy work? Perhaps the simplest explanation is that unirradiated cells can migrate into the treated zone to permit repair at the organ level after a tumor has been eliminated. Another possibility is that radiation turns on proliferation in normal cells (as alluded to above) that permits the normal tissues to regenerate more effectively than the tumor. (However, there is evidence that some tumors retain this ability of normal tissues and can also be stimulated to proliferate during therapy. This potential may be addressed by accelerated fractionation described below.) An additional possibility is that tumors have absent or disordered cell cycle checkpoints, so they progress inappropriately through the cell cycle after damage, whereas normal cells pause to repair damage prior to entering S phase or mitosis. The molecular, cellular, and organ basis for a therapeutic index is an area of great research interest to modern radiation biologists.

Radiation Treatment Planning

After a patient has been evaluated and a course of radiation is deemed to be of use, planning is initiated. This process involves six steps:

1. Determining the region that requires treatment. This process begins by defining the gross tumor volume (GTV), which is the gross tumor defined by the relevant modality: physical examination,

chest X-ray, computed tomography (CT), magnetic resonance imaging (MRI), positron emission tomography (PET), and so on. We then expand the gross tumor volume into the clinical target volume (CTV), which includes not only the gross tumor, but also regions that are at risk on the basis of our knowledge of the natural history of the illness. For instance, in the case of treating an advanced base of tongue cancer, we might wish to include the cervical neck nodes even though they are not grossly involved, as we might suspect that they harbor occult disease. Finally, we define a planning target volume (PTV) that includes the clinical target volume plus a margin for our uncertainty in aligning the patient each day (usually in the range of 5 mm) and for internal organ motion due to breathing or other processes. The purpose of radiation treatment planning, defined below, is to deposit sufficient radiation to the clinical target volume (which means treating the planning target volume) to control the tumor without producing unacceptable side effects to the surrounding normal tissue.

2. Localizing the patient and the involved region in three-dimensional space (in a manner that can be referenced to the linear accelerator). This step is traditionally performed by using an X-ray simulator (Figure 47-3). This device is configured similarly to a treatment unit, except that its purpose is to make diagnostic-quality X-rays that show the region to be treated. Simulators typically have fluoroscopic capabilities, permitting rapid determination of the relevant region based on bony anatomy. The head of the simulator can be rotated around the patient to take simulation films from almost any treatment angle. These films are compared to films obtained on the treatment machine on the first day and on a regular basis thereafter to verify the accuracy of treatment. More recently, the computed tomography simulator has been introduced. This device performs precisely the same functions, but the accuracy of localization is, of course, greatly increased by soft tissue information (see below). At the end of this session, reference marks are placed on the patient (or on an immobilization device such as a mask that fits tightly to the patient) to permit accurate alignment for treatment.

3. Registering the information from step 1 with the patient localization data from step 2. If the simulation process used an X-ray simulator, then only a tumor involving the bone can be registered directly. Otherwise, the radiation oncologist must reference the region to be treated with bony landmarks seen on the simulation film. In the case of computed tomography simulation, the tumor is visualized directly, although information from other modalities (for instance, magnetic resonance imaging for brain tumors) must also be registered with the computed tomography data set to define the region at risk. In addition to indicating the tumor, an equally important part of this process involves delineating the normal organs (that must be avoided).

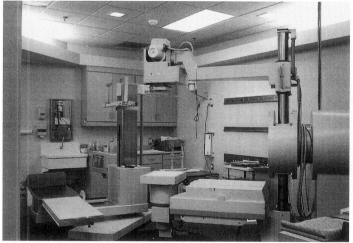
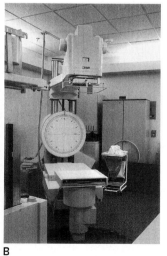

A   B

Figure 47-3 ■ Treatment simulator. The gantry rotates 365°, as does the treatment machine gantry, and it has delineator wires that allow definition of the treatment field. The table can be moved in three dimensions. An image intensifier is attached that allows fluoroscopy.

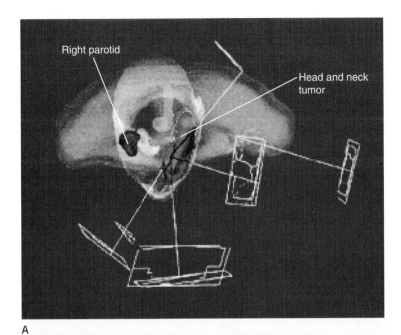

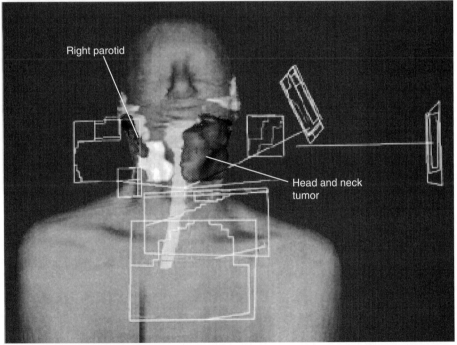

Figure 47-4 ■ The beam arrangement to treat a head and neck tumor while sparing the right parotid.

4. Determining beam arrangement. The complexity of this step varies tremendously depending on the clinical setting. In some cases, such as a proposed treatment of a bone metastasis to the upper thoracic spine, a single posterior field might be sufficient to treat the tumor. In other cases, such as head and neck cancer, in which an effort is being made to treat the tumor but spare the parotid glands, it might be necessary to use six to ten fields, each of which is subdivided (Figure 47-4). In traditional (forward) radiation planning, the expected dose distribution produced by a beam arrangement is calculated, and the physician decides whether the goals of planning have been achieved. If not, another beam arrangement is attempted. Plans can be displayed by using isodose lines or surfaces that indicate the region receiving more than a particular dose (Figure 47-5). Treat-

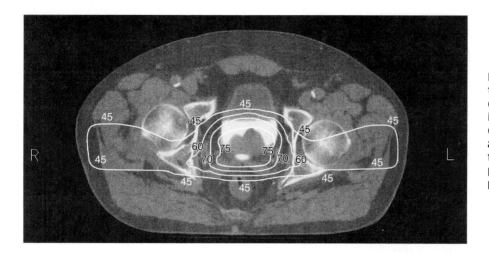

Figure 47-5 ■ The dose distribution for treatment of a prostate cancer is displayed on an axial image. Multiple axial, sagittal, and coronal images can be created, and each can be displayed with the isodose distribution for that plane to evaluate a treatment plan.

ment planning tools, such as dose volume histograms, yield additional information to help evaluate potential plans (Figure 47-6). An exciting area of research is to develop automated dose optimization (also called inverse planning), in which the physician defines a set of objectives that are to be met in treating the tumor and avoiding normal tissue and a computer determines the beam arrangement that would produce a satisfactory dose distribution.

5. Verification of beam arrangement. After an acceptable plan is found, the patient is aligned to

reference markers on the linear accelerator couch, and the beam arrangement is evaluated. Diagnostic images (and/or portal images, which are analogous to fluoroscopy images for the treatment unit) are obtained to verify that the planned beams treat the regions predicted by the treatment planning process.

6. Treatment. Radiation is typically delivered in daily fractions, from as few as 1 to over 40. Traditionally, the radiation therapist manually aligns the patient and manipulates the machine position and configuration to administer therapy. More recently, this process can be computer controlled, permitting complex multifield plans to be delivered accurately and efficiently. Each treatment typically takes less than 15 minutes, and the radiation beam is on for only a minute or two. An individual treatment typically produces no symptoms at the time that radiation is delivered (i.e., each treatment is much like undergoing a diagnostic X-ray). In addition, patients are not made radioactive by a treatment and can often return immediately to work or other routine activities.

Clinical Applications of Radiation Therapy

Although the use of radiation will be detailed in each of the organ-specific chapters, it is useful to give an overview of how radiation is applied in the treatment of cancer patients. It has been estimated that approximately half of all cancer patients will receive radiation at some point in their illness and that radiation will aid in the cure of 90,000 to 100,000 patients each year. This section begins with a discussion of fractionation, followed by some general comments about the use of radiation as curative, adjuvant, and palliative treatment.

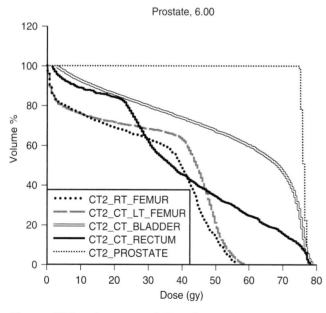

Prostate, 6.00

..... CT2_RT_FEMUR
– – – CT2_CT_LT_FEMUR
——— CT2_CT_BLADDER
——— CT2_CT_RECTUM
.... CT2_PROSTATE

Figure 47-6 ■ On a cumulative dose volume histogram (DVH), the percentage of an organ treated above a corresponding dose is displayed for each organ of interest. On this prostate plan, about 20% of the rectum is treated to greater than 70 Gy, and the dose to both the femoral heads is less than 60 Gy.

Fractionation

Standard fractionation for radiation therapy is defined as the delivery of one treatment of 1.7 to 2.25 Gy per day. This approach has a well characterized chance of tumor control and risk of normal tissue damage (as a function of volume). Altered fractionation schemes based on laboratory concepts have been proposed to improve the outcome for patients undergoing curative treatment and simplify the treatment for patients receiving palliative therapy. Two forms of altered fractionation have been tested for patients undergoing curative treatment: hyperfractionation and accelerated fractionation. Hyperfractionation is defined as the use of more than one fraction per day that delivers less radiation than a standard fraction. Compared to standard fractionation, hyperfractionation permits the delivery of a higher dose for the same extent of late toxicity. Thus, this approach would make the most sense in an attempt to escalate the dose to a tumor surrounded by acutely responding tissues in which the dose-limiting toxicity is expected to be chronic. Because tumors tend to behave as acutely responding tissues, the greater dose would also produce a greater cure rate. Because the acute toxicity is transient, the greater cure rate would be safely achieved. Randomized trials of standard radiation versus hyperfractionated radiation in the treatment of head and neck cancer support the hyperfractionation strategy.

The second approach is called accelerated fractionation. Here, the goal is to deliver more radiation in a shorter time period than can be achieved by using standard fractionation by administering more than one treatment a day in which each treatment is approximately equal to a standard fraction. Accelerated fractionation attempts to address the issue of accelerated repopulation alluded to above, in which tumors may increase their rate of proliferation during a course of fractionated radiation. A recent randomized trial comparing standard fractionation, hyperfractionation, and accelerated fractionation for patients with locally advanced head and neck cancer suggests that the altered fractionation schemes produce superior local control, validating these laboratory-based concepts.

Radiation Treatment Strategies

One of the most important uses of radiation is with curative intent. This includes using radiation to treat gross disease or as adjuvant therapy. In the case of gross disease, radiation is used as a curative treatment for patients with basal and squamous skin cancers, brain tumors, head and neck cancers, non–small cell and small cell lung cancer, esophageal cancer, cervix cancer, prostate cancer, anal cancer, and lymphoma. Although traditionally radiation was given alone, the addition of hormonal therapy and/or chemotherapy has improved the cure rate for patients with locally advanced stage of all of the above diseases (except skin cancer), representing a major advance in oncology.

Radiation therapy also plays a crucial role in adjuvant therapy. Adjuvant therapy is considered when gross resection of the tumor has been achieved, but there is a high risk of residual microscopic disease. Adjuvant therapy might not be indicated if the chance of recurrence is low (less than 10% to 15%) or if a local recurrence can be easily dealt with by a second surgical resection. However, in many circumstances, the chance of recurrence is higher, and local recurrence is morbid. Therefore, adjuvant therapy is recommended for many patients who have undergone resection of cancers of the brain, head and neck, lung, breast, stomach, pancreas, rectum, and soft tissue sarcoma. In the case of breast, stomach, pancreas, and rectal cancer, it appears that chemoradiation prolongs survival and local control, whereas in head and neck cancer, lung cancer, and soft tissue sarcoma, it decreases the risk of morbid local recurrence.

An important related treatment concept concerns the use of radiation (with or without chemotherapy) in organ preservation. An excellent example of a method of achieving organ preservation in the face of gross disease involves the use of chemotherapy and radiation to replace laryngectomy in the treatment of advanced larynx cancer. In contrast to some of the examples given in the preceding paragraph, the combination of radiation and chemotherapy does not improve overall survival compared to radical surgery. However, the organ conservation approach permits voice preservation in approximately two thirds of patients (see Chapter 98). The use of chemotherapy and radiotherapy to treat anal cancer can also be viewed in this light, with chemoradiotherapy producing organ conservation and cure rates that are superior to those of the radical surgery used decades ago.

There is even stronger evidence that the use of limited surgery with radiation can permit organ preservation compared to radical surgery alone. The best example here is surely the treatment of early-stage breast cancer, in which no fewer than seven randomized trials have demonstrated that lumpectomy plus radiation produces survival rates equal to those of modified radical mastectomy. Another important example is in the treatment of soft tissue sarcoma, in which limb-sparing surgery plus radiation produces survival rates equal to those resulting from amputation. Some patients with low-lying rectal cancers can avoid an abdominal perineal resection (and

Table 47-1 ■ A Comparison of Preoperative Versus Postoperative Adjuvant Irradiation with or without Chemotherapy

	Postoperative Treatment	Preoperative Treatment
Disadvantages	■ Treatment of larger fields is sometimes necessary to cover the entire surgical bed. ■ Disruption of the normal anatomy can complicate treatment. Disruption of the peritoneum can allow small bowel into the pelvis and limit the dose that can be given following pelvic resections.	■ Detailed pathologic staging information is lost. ■ Fibrosis from treatment can make surgery more complicated and difficult. There is the potential for increased postoperative morbidity and complications.
Advantages	■ Allows pathologic staging. Patients with early disease or metastatic disease might not need adjuvant treatment. ■ No delay in surgery. ■ Reported to make resection easier in cases such as sarcomas. Possibly better tolerated than when treating a patient shortly after major surgery. ■ Possibly smaller radiation therapy portals. Preoperatively often only the tumor plus margin will be treated, whereas postoperatively the entire surgical bed is treated.	■ Offers potential to reduce the tumor size and allow a surgery that might not otherwise be possible. ■ Offers the opportunity for organ sparing. By reducing tumor size, it might be possible to do a smaller resection.

colostomy) through radiation or chemoradiation, which can produce sufficient tumor regression to permit a wide local excision.

An issue that frequently arises is whether radiation therapy should be given preoperatively or postoperatively when surgery is planned. The relative advantages of preoperative versus postoperative treatment are summarized in Table 47-1. In general, as nonsurgical staging techniques improve, it appears that preoperative (chemo)radiation will ultimately displace postoperative treatment as it permits more patients to undergo organ conserving procedures and it appears to be less toxic.

Radiation is also important in palliation of symptoms produced by cancers even when cure is not possible. Treatment is highly effective in relieving the pain resulting from bony metastases. The combination of systemic treatment with narcotics and adjuvant medications (antidepressants, antiepileptic, and anti-inflammatory) with localized radiation to sites of severe pain can manage pain in the great majority of patients.

A special category that does not fit neatly into the above discussion concerns the role of radiation in oncologic emergencies. These include superior vena cava syndrome (typically resulting from either lymphoma or lung cancer) and spinal cord compression. In both of these cases, radiation (typically in combination with steroids) can produce detectable shrinkage within hours.

Summary and Future Directions

Radiation oncology has made enormous advances in the last 10 to 15 years based chiefly on the development of high-speed computers and sophisticated treatment-planning software. These improvements permit far better visualization of the target region in three-dimensional space as well as the ability to conform dose to the target with greater sparing of normal tissue. In addition to minimizing the treatment of normal tissues, this advanced treatment-planning software has permitted quantification. This had led to a much greater understanding of the relationships between volume of tissue treated and risk of complication. Taken together, these advances have permitted both the safe delivery of far higher doses of radiation than would have been considered possible just a few years ago (producing an improved cure rate for some cancers) and delivery of the same dose of radiation with decreased normal tissue toxicity (improving the quality of life) in other cases. These technical gains have been amplified by the recognition that multi-modality therapy (chemoradiation ± minimal surgery) is superior to radiation alone for many tumor types.

References

Bentel G: Radiation Therapy Planning, 2nd ed. New York: McGraw-Hill, 1995.

Bernhard EJ, McKenna WG, Muschel RJ: Radiosensitivity and the cell cycle. Cancer J Sci Am 1999;5:194–204.

Blank KR, Rudoltz MS, Kao GD, et al: The molecular regulation of apoptosis and implications for radiation oncology. Int J Radiat Biol 1997;71:455–466.

Bolla M, Gonzalez D, Warde P, et al: Improved survival in patients with locally advanced prostate cancer treated with radiotherapy and goserelin. N Engl J Med 1997;337:295–300.

Brizel DM, Albers ME, Fisher SR, et al: Hyperfractionated irradiation with or without concurrent chemotherapy for locally advanced head and neck cancer. N Engl J Med 1998;338:1798–1804.

Coia L, Moylan D: Introduction to Clinical Radiation Oncology, 3rd ed. Madison, WI: Medical Physics Publishing, 1998.

Cooper JS, Guo MD, Herskovic A, et al: Chemotherapy of locally advanced esophageal cancer: long-term follow-up of a prospective randomized trial (RTOG 85-01). JAMA 1992;281:1623–1627.

Dillman R, Herndon J, Seagren S, et al: Improved survival of stage III non-small-cell lung cancer: Seven-year follow-up of cancer and leukemia group B (CALGB) 8433 trial. J Natl Cancer Inst 1996;88:1210–1215.

Fisher B, Anderson S, Redmond CK, et al: Reanalysis and results after 12 years of follow-up in a randomized clinical trial comparing total mastectomy with lumpectomy with or without irradiation in the treatment of breast cancer. N Engl J Med 1995;333:1456–1461.

Flam M, John M, Pajak TF, et al: Role of mitomycin in combination with fluorouracil and radiotherapy, and to salvage chemoradiation in the definitive nonsurgical treatment of epidermoid carcinoma of the anal canal: Results of a phase III randomized intergroup study. J Clin Oncol 1996;14:2527–2539.

Fraas BA, Kessler ML, McShan DL, et al: Optimization and clinical use of multisegment intensity-modulated radiation therapy for high-dose conformal therapy. Semin Radiat Oncol 1999;9:60–77.

Fu KF, Pajak TF, Trotti A, et al: A Radiation Therapy Oncology Group (RTOG) phase III randomized study to compare hyperfractionation and two variants of accelerated fractionation to standard fractionation radiotherapy for head and neck squamous cell carcinomas: First report of RTOG 9003. Int J Radiat Oncol Biol Phys 2000;48:7–16.

Gunderson LL, Tepper JE: Clinical Radiation Oncology, 1st ed. New York: Churchill Livingstone, 2000.

Hall EJ: Radiobiology for the Radiologist, 5th ed. Philadelphia: Lippincott, 2000.

Khan F: The Physics of Radiation Therapy, 2nd ed. Baltimore: Williams and Wilkins, 1997.

Loeffler JS, Smith AR, Suit HD: The potential role of proton beams in radiation oncology. Semin Oncol 1997;24:686–695.

Miller TP, Dahlberg S, Cassady JR, et al: Chemotherapy alone compared with chemotherapy plus radiotherapy for localized intermediate- and high-grade non-Hodgkin's lymphoma. N Engl J Med 1998;339:21–326.

Morris M, Eifel PJ, Lu J, et al: Pelvic radiation with concurrent chemotherapy compared with pelvic and para-aortic radiation for high-risk cervical cancer. N Engl J Med 1999;340:1137–1143.

Nag S, Erickson B, Thomadsen B, et al: The American Brachytherapy Society recommendations for high-dose rate brachytherapy for carcinoma of the cervix. Int J Radiat Oncol Biol Phys 2000;48:201–211.

Perez CA, Brady LW: Principles and Practice of Radiation Oncology, 3rd ed. Philadelphia: Lippincott-Raven, 1998.

Pignon J, Arriagada R, Ihde DC, et al: A meta-analysis of thoracic radiotherapy for small-cell lung cancer. N Engl J Med 1992;327:1618–1624.

Ragde H, Elgamal AA, Snow PB, et al: Ten-year disease free survival after transperineal sonography-guided iodine-125 brachytherapy with or without 45-gray external beam irradiation in the treatment of patients with clinically localized, low to high Gleason grade prostate carcinoma. Cancer 1998;83:989–1001.

Rosen EM, Fan S, Rockwell S, et al: The molecular and cellular basis of radiosensitivity: Implications for understanding how normal tissues and tumors respond to therapeutic radiation. Cancer Invest 1999;17:56–72.

Rosenberg SA, Tepper J, Glatstein E, et al: The treatment of soft-tissue sarcomas of the extremities. Ann Surg 1982;196:305–315.

Rowinsky EK: Novel radiation sensitizers targeting tissue hypoxia. Oncology 1999;13:61–70.

The Department of Veterans Affairs Laryngeal Cancer Study Group: Induction chemotherapy plus radiation in patients with advanced laryngeal cancer. N Engl J Med 1991;324:1685–1690.

UKCCR Anal Cancer Trial Working Party: Epidermoid anal cancer: results from the UKCCR randomized trial of radiotherapy alone versus radiotherapy, 5-fluorouracil, and mitomycin. Lancet 1996;348:1049–1054.

Withers HR: Radiation biology and treatment options in radiation oncology. Cancer Res 1999;59:1676s–1684s.

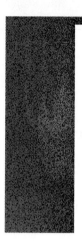

Chapter 48
Cancer Chemotherapy

William N. Hait, Barton A. Kamen, Eric H. Rubin, and Susan Goodin

The Biologic Basis of Cancer Therapeutics

In years past, a discussion of the principles of cancer chemotherapy would focus on the kinetics of cell kill by traditional cytotoxic agents and a variety of theoretical constructs designed to optimize the use of individual drugs and drug combinations. We now appreciate that anticancer drugs interfere with cellular processes that are altered in malignancy and that it is the interference with this pathophysiology that explains the pharmacology of both older and many newer agents. In this chapter, we attempt to place cancer therapeutic agents in the context of a modern understanding of cancer biology while highlighting recent advances in cancer treatment.

The origins of cancer involve complex interactions between the environment and genome that are affected by behavior and aging. The fundamental lesion is probably genetic; that is, changes occurring in DNA lead to functional alterations in proteins, which in turn result in cellular transformation. More than one genetic defect is usually required, and it is the accumulation of these changes over time that leads to malignant transformation. Cancer cells acquire the ability to proliferate through growth factor–growth factor receptor stimulation, loss of regulated cellular proliferation through abrogation of normal cell-cycle check points, and blocking the potentially lethal shortening of telomeric ends of the chromosome. These changes are attributable to mutations in oncogenes, tumor suppressor genes, and acquisition of enhanced cell viability through activation of genes that prevent cell death.

Traditionally, chemotherapeutic drug targets included DNA (nucleotide bases, enzymes of DNA synthesis, degradation, and repair), microtubules, and growth factor receptors. New targets include the protein products of mutated or overexpressed oncogenes (Her-2/neu, ras, bcr/abl), tumor suppressor genes (p53), cell surface antigens (CD33, CD20, IL2-R), antiapoptotic proteins (bcl-2), cell-cycle regulators (cyclin-dependent kinases), and telomerase, a reverse transcriptase that allows continuous cell replication.

Cancer cells also gain the capacity to invade locally and metastasize distantly. This process involves detachment of the malignant cell from the primary site, invasion through the basement membrane, access to the blood or lymphatic vessels, entry to distant organs through adherence to visceral capillaries, evasion of a variety of immunologic mechanisms designed to protect the host from "foreign invasion," and establishment of a new blood supply through angiogenesis. Agents in development that target these steps in the generation of a viable malignancy include angiogenesis inhibitors such as endostatins, angiostatins, thalidomide, and metalloproteinase inhibitors, such as marimastat. Figure 48-1 depicts the interactions of drugs that target pathways that are essential to malignant transformation.

Growth Factors, Receptors, and Signal Transduction

Normal cell division results from the interaction of growth factors with specific receptors, located in the plasma membrane, cytoplasm, or nucleus. Ligand/receptor interactions occurring at the cell surface initiate signal transduction cascades, culminating in uncoiling of DNA and activation of nuclear transcription factors that produce cell-proliferation molecules. Growth factor interactions with cytoplasmic and nuclear receptors lead to direct transcriptional activation of genes that contain specific response elements that are recognized by the occupied receptor. These pathways are usurped during the transformation of a normal cell to a malignant one.

The following discussion of current chemotherapeutic agents is based on the biologic classification of the agents (Table 48-1) as opposed to the more traditional classification of chemotherapeutic agents (Table 48-2).

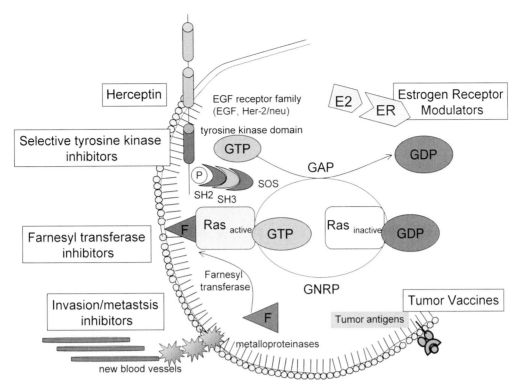

Figure 48-1 ■ Oncogenic pathways targeted by anticancer drugs.

Drugs That Affect Growth Factor/Receptor Interactions

Intracellular Receptors

The superfamily of intracellular receptors (or steroid-hormone superfamily) includes receptors for steroid hormones, thyroid hormones, retinoids, and vitamin D. The small hydrophobic ligands differ from one another but appear to act by a similar mechanism. Following diffusion across the plasma membrane, they bind to their cognate intracellular receptor protein. The binding of ligand to receptor creates a conformational change in the protein that releases it from its inhibitory chaperone (for example, a heat-shock protein, such as Hsp90), activating the receptor by exposing its DNA-binding domain. The specificity of the response in a given tissue or cell depends not only on the presence of the receptor, but also on additional regulatory proteins that cooperate with the ligand-bound receptor to activate gene transcription. Therefore drugs that affect intracellular receptors will have different effects on different tissues based not only on the presence of the receptor, but also on the cellular context in which the receptor resides.

Estrogen Receptor Modulators (ERMs)

The interaction of estrogen with the estrogen receptor localizes the complex to the nucleus, where in the presence of an appropriate array of corepressors and coactivators it binds to estrogen response elements through its DNA-binding domain and initiates transcription. It is these estrogen response genes that account for the normal actions of this hormone, including cellular viability, proliferation, and differentiation, as well as a variety of salutary effects on cognition. There are at least two types of estrogen receptors, ER-α and ER-β, which share significant homology within their DNA-binding domains. In contrast, there is significantly less homology in the carboxyl terminal hormone-binding domain, suggesting a mechanism for selective hormone action. The complex interaction between hormone, estrogen receptors, corepressors, and coactivators is believed to account for the potential for agonistic and antagonistic effects of drugs that bind to the estrogen receptor and alter its function.

Tamoxifen (Nolvadex)

Tamoxifen is the classic example of a drug that works by interfering with a growth factor–receptor interaction. Breast cancers that express estrogen and/or progesterone receptors appear to require estrogen-induced activation of gene transcription to maintain proliferation and viability. Disruption of this signaling leads to inhibition of cell growth and death of the cell. Tamoxifen is generally considered to be a cytostatic drug, because in vitro it causes rapidly cycling breast

Text continued on p. 343

Table 48-1 ■ Biologic Classification of Chemotherapy Agents

1. Growth Factor Receptor Interactions
   A. Estrogen receptor modulators
      i. Tamoxifen citrate (Nolvadex)
      ii. Toremifene (Fareston)
      iii. Raloxifene (Evista)
      iv. Fuluestrante (Faslodex)
   B. Antiandrogens
      i. Bicalutamide (Casodex)
      ii. Flutamide (Eulexin)
      iii. Nilutamide (Nilandron)
   C. Retinoic receptor modulators
      i. Tretinoin (Vesanoid)
      ii. Bexarotene (Targretin)
   D. Growth factor receptor family antagonists
      i. Trastuzumab (Herceptin)
   E. Miscellaneous
      i. Rituximab (Rituxan)
      ii. Gemtuzumab ozogomicin (Mylotarg)
      iii. Denileukin difitox (Ontak)

2. Agents That Decrease Circulating Growth Factors
   A. Aromatase inhibitors
      i. Aminoglutethimide (Cytadren)
      ii. Anastrozole (Arimidex)
      iii. Letrozole (Femara)
      iv. Exemestane (Aromasin)
   B. Luteinizing hormone–releasing hormone (LHRH)
      i. Goserelin (Zoladex)
      ii. Leuprolide (Lupron)

3. Drugs Affecting Nucleic Acid Synthesis: Alkylating Agents
   A. Nitrogen mustards
      i. Mechlorethamine hydrochloride (HN_2, Mustargen)
      ii. Cyclophosphamide (Cytoxan)
      iii. Ifosfamide (Ifex)
      iv. Melphalan (L-pam, L-phenylalanine, Alkeran)
      v. Chlorambucil (Leukeran)
   B. Nitrosoureas
      i. Carmustine (BCNU, BiCNU)
      ii. Lomustine (CCNU, CeeNU)
      iii. Semustine (methyl-CCNU)
      iv. Streptozocin (Zanosar)
   C. Alkyl sulfonates
      i. Busulfan (Myleran)
   D. Ethylenimines
      i. Thiotepa (Thioplex)
      ii. Hexamethylmelamine (Altretamine)
   E. Triazenes
      i. Dacarbazine (DTIC-DOME)
      ii. Temozolomide (Teniodar)
   F. Platinum analogues
      i. Cisplatin (Platinol)
      ii. Carboplatin (Paraplatin)

4. Inhibitors of Nucleic Acid Synthesis: Antimetabolites
   A. Folate antagonists
      i. Methotrexate (Folex)
      ii. Trimetrexate
   B. Purine analogues
      i. Mercaptopurine (6-MP, Purinethol)
      ii. Thioguanine (6-TG)
      iii. Cladribine (2-cda, 2-chloro-deoxyadenosine, Leustatin)
      iv. Fludarabine (Fludara)
      v. Pentostatin (Nipent)
   C. Pyrimidine analogues
      i. Cytarabine (ara-C, Cytosar-U)
      ii. Fluorouracil (5-FU, Adrucil)
      iii. Floxuridine (FUDR)
      iv. Gemcitabine (Gemzar)
      v. Capecitabine (Xeloda)
   D. Miscellaneous hormonal agents
      i. Estramustine (Emcyt)

5. Topoisomerase Inhibitors
   Topoisomerase II Inhibitors
   A. Anthracyclines
      i. Daunorubicin hydrochloride (Cerubidine)
      ii. Doxorubicin hydrochloride (Adriamycin)
      iii. Idarubicin (Idamycin)
      iv. Epirubicin (Ellence)
      v. Valrubicin (Valstar)
   B. Epipodophyllotoxins
      i. Etoposide (VP-16, Vepesid)
      ii. Tenoposide (VM-26, Vumon)
   C. Anthracendiones
      i. Mitoxantrone (Novantrone)
   Topoisomerase I Inhibitors
   A. Camptothecins
      i. Topotecan (Hycamtin)
      ii. Irinotecan (Camptosar)

6. Drugs Affecting the Mitotic Apparatus
   A. Vinca alkaloids
      i. Vinblastine (Velban)
      ii. Vincristine (Oncovin)
      iii. Vinorelbine (Navelbine)
   B. Imidazotetrazines
      i. Temozolomide (Temodar)
   C. Taxanes
      i. Paclitaxel (Taxol)
      ii. Docetaxel (Taxotere)

7. Drugs Affecting Oncogene Activity
      i. Imatinib mesylate (Gleevec)

Table 48-2 ■ Traditional Classification of Chemotherapeutic Agents

Class	Structure	Route	Target	Cancer Use	Toxicities
Alkylating Agents					
Nitrogen Mustards					
Mechlorethamine	(structure)	IV	Alkylation of N-7 of guanine	Hodgkin's disease, non-Hodgkin lymphoma	Nausea, vomiting, lacrimation, myelosuppression, mucositis, alopecia, vesicant
Cyclophosphamide; ifosfamide	(structure)	IV; PO		Acute and chronic lymphocytic leukemia, lymphomas, myeloma; neuroblastoma, breast, ovary, lung, Wilms' tumor, cervix, testis, sarcoma	Myelosuppression, mucositis, alopecia, emesis, dizziness, hemorrhagic cystitis, skin pigmentation, cardiac, renal, CNS (particularly ifosfamide, including seizures, altered mental status, coma, and paralysis at high doses), SIADH
Melphalan	(structure)	PO		Myeloma, breast, ovary, sarcoma	Myelosuppression
Chlorambucil	(structure)	PO		CLL, primary macroglobulinemia, Hodgkin's disease, non-Hodgkin lymphoma	Myelosuppression, secondary leukemias, and other tumors.
Ethylenimines and Methylmelamines					
Hexamethylmelamine	(structure)	IV		Ovary	Nausea and vomiting, diarrhea, myelosuppression
Thiotepa	(structure)	IV		Bladder, breast, ovary	Myelosuppression, mucositis, nausea, vomiting
Alkyl Sulfonates					
Busulfan	(structure)	PO		Chronic myelogenous leukemia	Myelosuppression, prolonged thrombocytopenia
Nitrosoureas					
Carmustine (BCNU)	(structure)	IV	O^6 of guanine, carbamoylation of ε-amino-lysines	Hodgkin's disease, non-Hodgkin lymphoma, astrocytomas, myeloma, melanoma	Delayed myelosuppression (nadir at 4–6 weeks); hepatic necrosis at high doses, nausea and vomiting, flushing; interstitial pulmonary fibrosis and renal failure at doses >1000 mg/m²

Continued

Table 48-2 ■ Traditional Classification of Chemotherapeutic Agents—Cont'd

Class	Structure	Route	Target	Cancer Use	Toxicities
Lomustine (CCNU)		PO		Hodgkin's disease, non-Hodgkin's lymphoma, astrocytomas, small cell lung cancer	Myelosuppression
Semustine (methyl-CCNU)		PO		Colon	Myelosuppression
Streptozotocin		IV		Insulinoma, carcinoid	Nausea, renal (proximal tubule effects), hepatic, mild to moderate myelosuppression
Triazenes					
Dacarbazine (DTIC)		IV	O^6 of guanine; N^7 of guanine	Melanoma, Hodgkin's disease, sarcomas	Myelosuppression, nausea, vomiting, flulike syndrome
Temozolomide		PO		Astrocytoma, melanoma	Lymphocytopenia, hepatic toxicity, nausea and vomiting, hyperglycemia, anemia, and thrombocytopenia
Bioreductive Alkylating Agents					
Mitomycin-C		IV	N^6 of adenine, N^7 and O^6 of guanine	Colon, rectum, breast, gastric, head and neck, lung, cervix	Myelosuppression with delayed recovery (6–8 weeks), nausea, vomiting, diarrhea, mucositis, dermatitis, asthenia, interstitial fibrosis, hemolytic-uremic syndrome, congestive heart failure

Platinating Agents

Drug	Route	Mechanism	Clinical uses	Toxicity
Cisplatin	IV	Inter- and intra-strand cross linking of DNA	Testis, ovary, bladder, head and neck, lung, thyroid, cervix, endometrium, neuroblastoma, osteogenic sarcoma	Renal toxicity, nausea and vomiting, peripheral neuropathy, ototoxicity, myelosuppression, electrolyte abnormalities (hypomagnesemia, hypocalcemia, hypophosphatemia), anaphylactoid reactions
Carboplatin	IV	→		Myelosuppression (thrombocytopenia)
Oxaliplatin	PO		Colon	Peripheral neuropathy, nausea and vomiting, myelosuppression

Nucleic Acid Synthesis Inhibitors

Folate Analogues

Drug	Route	Mechanism	Clinical uses	Toxicity
Methotrexate	IV, PO	Inhibition of dihydrofolate reductase, inhibits folate-dependent synthesis of purines and thymidylate	ALL, choriocarcinoma, non-Hodgkin's lymphoma, breast, head and neck, lung, osteogenic sarcoma	Myelosuppression, mucositis, renal failure, reversible pneumonitis, hepatic fibrosis (low-dose oral administration)

Pyrimidine Analogues

Drug	Route	Mechanism	Clinical uses	Toxicity
Fluorouracil (5-Fluorouracil); floxuridine (fluorodeoxyuridine, FUDR), capecitabine	IV, PO	Inhibition of thymidylate synthase; inhibition of RNA processing, incorporation into DNA	Breast, colon, stomach, pancreas, ovary, hepatoma head and neck, bladder, cervix, prostate	Myelosuppression, mucositis, nausea, diarrhea, hair loss, nail changes, pigmentation, chest pain, hand-foot syndrome
Cytarabine (cytosine arabinoside)	IV	Analogue of 2'-deoxycytidine; inhibition of DNA chain elongation	AML and ALL, non-Hodgkin's lymphoma	Myelosuppression, mucositis, conjunctivitis, reversible hepatic dysfunction
Gemcitabine	IV	Analogue of 2'-deoxycytidine; inhibits DNA synthesis; incorporated into DNA; inhibits ribonucleotide reductase	Pancreas, bladder, breast, lung	Myelosuppression, flulike syndrome, nausea

Continued

Table 48-2 ■ Traditional Classification of Chemotherapeutic Agents—Cont'd

Purine Analogues

Class	Structure	Route	Target	Cancer Use	Toxicities
Mercaptopurine		PO	Inhibits de novo purine production; incorporates into DNA	ALL, AML, CML	Myelosuppression, anorexia, nausea, vomiting, jaundice
Thioguanine		PO	Inhibits de novo purine production; incorporates into DNA	ALL, AML, CML	Myelosuppression, anorexia, nausea, vomiting
Fludarabine		IV	Inhibits DNA polymerase, primase, ribonucleotide reductase DNA and RNA	CLL, low-grade NHL	Myelosuppression, fever chills, asthenia, anorexia; depletion of CD4 cells can lead to opportunistic infections; peripheral neuropathy, altered mental status, seizure, optic neuritis, and coma at higher doses
Pentostatin (2-deoxycoformycin)		IV	Inhibits adenosine deaminase and blocks DNA synthesis	Hairy cell leukemia, cutaneous T cell lymphoma, CLL	Myelosuppression, nausea, vomiting, skin rashes, abnormal liver function; depletion of T cells can lead to opportunistic infections
Cladribine (2-chlorodeoxyadenosine)		IV	Incorporated into DNA and leads to strand breakage	Hairy cell leukemia, CLL, cutaneous T cell lymphoma, low grade lymphoma, Waldenström's macroglobulinemia	Myelosuppression, nausea, infections, fever, headache asthenia, skin rashes, tumor lysis syndrome.
Hydroxyurea		PO	Blocks conversion of ribonucleotides to deoxyribonucleotides; inhibits DNA synthesis	CML, polycythemia vera, essential thrombocytosis, melanoma	Myelosuppression, dermatologic changes

DNA Topoisomerase Inhibitors

Anthracyclines

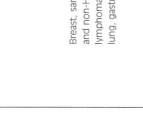

Drug	Structure	Route	Mechanism	Indications	Toxicity
Doxorubicin		PO	DNA intercalation; free radical generation after metabolism by cytochrome P450 reductase and NADPH, peroxidation of cell membrane lipids	Breast, sarcomas; Hodgkin's and non-Hodgkin's lymphoma, ALL, bladder, thyroid, lung, gastric, neuroblastoma	Cardiomyopathy, myelosuppression, mucositis, radiation recall, local flare reactions, vesicant
Daunomycin		PO		AML, ALL	
Idarubicin		PO		AML, ALL	
Epirubicin		IV		Breast, sarcomas, Hodgkin's and non-Hodgkin's lymphoma, ALL, bladder, lung, gastric	Less cardiac toxicity, alopecia, phlebitis, myelosuppression is dose-limiting

Continued

Table 48-2 ■ Traditional Classification of Chemotherapeutic Agents—Cont'd

Class	Structure	Route	Target	Cancer Use	Toxicities
Anthracenediones					
Mitoxantrone		IV	Less ability to form free radicals	AML, breast, prostate	Myelosuppression, nausea, vomiting, mucositis
Epipodophyllotoxins					
Etoposide		IV, PO	Form ternary complexes with topoisomerase II and DNA	Testis, lung, breast, Hodgkin's and non-Hodgkin's lymphoma, AML, Kaposi's sarcoma	Myelosuppression, nausea, vomiting, mucositis
Teniposide		IV, PO	Form ternary complexes with topoisomerase II and DNA	Pediatric ALL and AML	Myelosuppression, nausea, vomiting, hypotension
Dactinomycin (actinomycin-D)		IV	DNA intercalation, forms ternary complexes with DNA and topoisomerase II	Wilms' tumor, rhabdomyosarcoma, testis, choriocarcinoma, Kaposi's and Ewing's sarcoma	Nausea, vomiting, anorexia, myelosuppression, mucositis, alopecia, erythema and desquamation of skin, radiation recall, vesicant

Camptothecins

Irinotecan

IV — Form ternary complexes with topoisomerase I and DNA — Colon, ovary — Myelosuppression, diarrhea, alopecia

Topotecan

IV — Form ternary complexes with topoisomerase I and DNA — Ovary, lung — Myelosuppression, diarrhea, alopecia

Other DNA-Damaging Agents

Bleomycin

IV — DNA cleavage due to generation of reactive oxygen — Testis, non-Hodgkin's lymphoma, Hodgkin's disease, head and neck — Hypersensitivity reactions most prominent in patients with lymphomas, skin pigmentation and ulceration, interstitial pulmonary fibrosis

Continued

Table 48-2 ■ Traditional Classification of Chemotherapeutic Agents—Cont'd

Class	Structure	Route	Target	Cancer Use	Toxicities
Antimicrotubule Agents					
Vinca Alkaloids					
Vinblastine $R_1 = CH_3$		IV	Inhibit tubulin polymerization	Hodgkin's disease, non-Hodgkin's lymphoma, breast, testis	Myelosuppression, peripheral neuropathy, obstipation
Vincristine $R_1 = CHO$				ALL, neuroblastoma, Wilms' tumor, rhabdomyosarcoma, Hodgkin's disease, non-Hodgkin's lymphoma, small-cell lung	Peripheral neuropathy, myelosuppression, constipation, abdominal cramps, SIADH, vesicant
Vinorelbine (structure not shown)				Breast, lung	Myelosuppression, peripheral neuropathy, pain
Taxanes					
Paclitaxel R =		IV	Inhibit tubulin depolymerization	Ovary, breast, lung, bladder	Myelosuppression, alopecia totalis, peripheral neuropathy, pain, hypersensitivity reactions
Docetaxel R = OC(CH$_3$)$_3$				Ovary, breast, lung, bladder	Myelosuppression, alopecia totalis, peripheral neuropathy, pain, capillary leakage, cardiac arrhythmias, hypersensitivity reactions
Signal Transduction Modulators					
Antiestrogens					
Tamoxifen		PO	Block activation of estrogen receptor by estrogens (produce TGB-β; inhibit signal transduction enzymes)	Breast	Amenorrhea, hot flashes, nausea, weight gain, hypercalcemia, venous thrombosis, endometrial cancer
Toremifene (structure not shown)		PO		Breast, melanoma	Hot flashes, nausea, venous thrombosis

Drug	Route	Mechanism	Site	Toxicities
Raloxifene (structure not shown)	PO		Breast	Hot flushes, nausea, venous thrombosis
Antiandrogens				
Flutamide	PO	Block activation of the androgen receptor by dihydrotestosterone	Prostate cancer	Nausea, diarrhea, constipation, mastodynia, gynecomastia, galactorrhea, hot flashes, loss of facial hair
Bicalutamide (structure not shown)	PO	→		Similar to flutamide
Nilutamide (structure not shown)	PO	→		Similar to flutamide, also visual disturbances (delayed adaptation to dark)
Aromatase Inhibitors				
Aminoglutethimide	PO	Aromatase	Breast cancer	Glucocorticoid deficiency, skin rash, lethargy, orthostatic hypotension
Anastrazole	PO	→		Nausea, diarrhea, asthenia, headache, hot flashes, pain
Letrozole	PO	→		Headache, nausea, vomiting, constipation, heartburn
Exemestane	PO	Aromatase inactivator (irreversible)	Breast	Fatigue, hot flashes, pain, nausea, depression, and insomnia
Gonadotropin-Releasing Agents				
Leuprolide Buserelin (structure not shown) — pyro-Glu-His-Trp-Ser-Tyr-D-Leu-Leu-Arg-Pro-ethylamide	IM	Activate gonadotropin releasing hormone receptor and block subsequent activation by receptor desensitization	Prostate, breast	Loss of libido, impotence, hot flashes, diarrhea; increased pain at sites of bony metastases ("tumor flare") due to initial gonadotropin stimulation

Continued

341

Table 48-2 ■ Traditional Classification of Chemotherapeutic Agents—Cont'd

Class	Structure	Route	Target	Cancer Use	Toxicities
Progestins					
Megestrol acetate	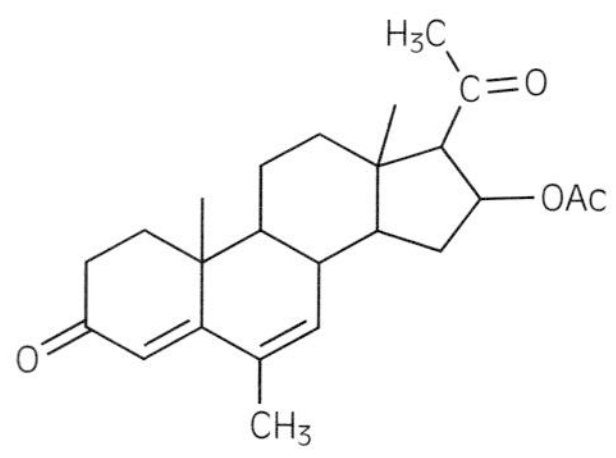 (structure shown)	PO		Breast, endometrial	Weight gain
Monoclonal Antibodies					
Rituximab (structure not shown)		IV	Binds to CD20 and activates humoral and cellular immunity	B-cell non-Hodgkin's lymphomas, CLL	Infusion-related: fever, chills, vomiting, urticaria, rash, rigors; non-infusion-related (uncommon): arrhythmias, pain, myalgias, angioedema, bronchospasm; myelosuppression; major toxicities associated with high numbers of circulating CD20-positive cells
Trastuzumab (structure not shown)		IV	Binds to HER-2/neu receptor, blocks cell proliferation; elicits immune response	Breast cancer	Fever, chills, pain at tumor site, diarrhea
Gemtuzumab ozogamicin, (monoclonal antibody linked with the chemotherapy agent calicheamicin) (structure not shown)		IV	The antibody portion binds to the CD33 antigen resulting in a complex that is internalized. On internalization, the calicheamicin derivative is released inside the lysosomes of the myeloid cell.	CD33 positive AML	Infusion-related (fever, nausea, chills, hypotension, shortness of breath), severe neutropenia and thrombocytopenia. Reports of hyperbilirubinemia or increased aminotransferase activity
Denileukin diftitox, DAB389IL-2 (Ontak) (Structure not shown.)		IV	Recombinant fusion protein consisting of peptide sequences for the enzymatically active and membrane translocation domains of diphtheria toxin and human IL-2	Persistent or recurrent cutaneous T cell lymphoma that express CD25 component of the IL-2 receptor	Infusion-related (hypotension, back pain, dyspnea, vasodilation, rash, chest pain), vascular leak syndrome (edema, hypoalbuminemia)

cancer cells to shift to a slower cycling state, increasing overall cell cycle transit times. Clinicians recognize, however, that patients receiving tamoxifen often experience partial or complete remissions, that is, the disappearance of half or all of the visible cancer cells, making cell death the ultimate result of tamoxifen's action.

Tamoxifen is a nonsteroidal antiestrogenic analog of clomiphene, the *trans*-isomer of triphenylethylene that was originally developed as a "morning-after" contraceptive. It is a nonselective estrogen receptor modulator that binds to estrogen receptors in normal and malignant tissues. Tamoxifen binds to α- and β-estrogen receptors and disrupts estradiol/estrogen receptor-mediated transcriptional activation in some but not all estrogen-responsive tissues. The estrogen receptor resides in the cytosol; on occupation by estradiol, it is transported to the nucleus, where it activates genes (including those encoding proliferation molecules) containing estrogen response elements. Tamoxifen is antiestrogenic in the breast and estrogenic in the uterus, liver, and bone. Other effects of tamoxifen that may contribute to its antiproliferative actions include the ability to decrease insulinlike growth factor 1 (IGF-1) and increase transforming growth factor-beta (TGF-β) in surrounding breast stroma.

Tamoxifen is active in several settings. In metastatic breast cancer, the response rate is directly proportional to the expression of hormone receptors, and activity is seen in both postmenopausal and premenopausal patients. Activity in premenopausal patients is approximately equal to that of ovarian ablation. In tumors that are strongly hormone-receptor positive, the response rate is greater than 60%; tamoxifen is of little benefit to women whose tumors do not express hormone receptors. Tamoxifen is also effective as adjuvant treatment of hormone-receptor-positive breast cancer, producing a greater than 30% reduction in the absolute annual odds of recurrence. For example, a patient with node-negative breast cancer carries a 10-year risk of recurrence of approximately 30%. In this patient, tamoxifen would decrease the risk of recurrence by 30%. Thus the absolute reduction would be 9% ($0.3 \times 0.3 = 0.09$), bringing the estimated risk of recurrence to 21%. Finally, tamoxifen may also be useful in the prevention of breast cancer. In the National Surgical Adjuvant Breast Program (NSABP) P-01 study, tamoxifen reduced the appearance of breast cancer over a three- to five-year period by approximately 50% in women without breast cancer who were at high risk for developing the disease.

Tamoxifen has been safely used by hundreds of thousands of women throughout the world who enjoy the benefits of treatment with few side effects.

However, tamoxifen does cause both bothersome and even life-threatening side effects in a small percentage of patients. These include hot flushes, menstrual irregularities, vaginal discharge, nausea, weight gain, venous thrombosis, and potentially serious effects on the uterus, including endometrial proliferation and rarely (in less than 0.3% of treated women) endometrial cancer.

Although discussion continues regarding the benefits of tamoxifen in patients whose tumors do not express readily measurable estrogen or progesterone receptors, it is our experience that few hormone-receptor-negative tumors respond. In fact, we use a few general guidelines when thinking about responsiveness to hormonal therapy in the treatment of breast cancer. First, the greater the expression of both estrogen receptor (ER) and progesterone receptor (PgR), the better the response in terms of magnitude and duration. Second, the duration of first response to a hormonal manipulation is a fairly accurate guide to subsequent treatment. For example, second-line hormonal therapy is likely to work half as well as first-line therapy in terms of both response and duration. Thus a patient who has enjoyed two years of good response to tamoxifen is likely to experience a 12-month duration of response to second-line therapy and a six-month duration to third-line hormonal treatment.

Selective Estrogen Receptor Modulators (SERMs)

Selective estrogen receptor modulators (SERMs) are antiestrogens with greater selectivity for one tissue over others by virtue of high-affinity interactions with the estrogen receptor or its subsets (α or β). We now appreciate that tissue selectivity may also depend on the relative expression of corepressor and coactivator molecules (see above).

Toremifene (Fareston)

Toremifene is a triphenylethylene selective estrogen receptor modulator that differs from tamoxifen by a single chlorine addition at position 4. Toremifene has the same affinity for the estrogen receptor as tamoxifen and has the potential for fewer estrogenic side effects. Moreover, preclinical data suggest that toremifene can maintain activity even in tamoxifen-refractory patients. In a phase III trial comparing toremifene 60 mg to tamoxifen 20 mg in 640 patients, Hayes et al. found toremifene to be as effective as tamoxifen in terms of response rate, median duration of response, median time to progression, and median survival. Toremifene side effects were, however, similar to those of tamoxifen and included vaginal discharge, bleeding, nausea, vomiting, and thromboses.

The incidence of endometrial cancer with long-term use of toremifene has not been determined.

Raloxifene (Evista)

Raloxifene is a nonsteroidal benzothiophene-derived estrogen receptor antagonist in the breast and uterus and an estrogen receptor agonist in bone and liver. The recent description of a raloxifene-response element in the promoter region of certain genes could account for some of its functional differences from tamoxifen and other selective estrogen receptor modulators. Raloxifene is currently under study as a chemopreventive agent based on results of the Multiple Outcomes of Raloxifene Evaluation (MORE) trial. Postmenopausal women with osteoporosis randomly received raloxifene (60 mg qd or bid) or placebo. After a median follow-up of 33 months, 27 of 2576 (1%) patients receiving placebo and 13 of 5129 (0.25%) patients receiving raloxifene developed breast cancer. Although the incidence of osteoporosis was reduced, four cases of endometrial cancer occurred in each group, and the incidence of thromboses was increased in the raloxifene group. These results led to a randomized study by the National Surgical Adjuvant Breast Program comparing the effectiveness of raloxifene to tamoxifen in reducing the risk of breast cancer. Pending these results, raloxifene is not currently FDA approved by the Food and Drug Administration (FDA) for the prevention or treatment of breast cancer, nor is its use currently recommended in these settings.

Androgen Receptor Antagonists

Antiandrogens, like antiestrogens, exert their effects by interrupting growth factor–growth factor receptor interactions that are essential for the viability of androgen-dependent cancers, most notably prostate cancer. Like the estrogen receptors described above, the transcriptional activity of the occupied androgen receptor is dependent on a transcription complex of coactivators and corepressors.

Bicalutamide (Casodex), Flutamide (Eulexin), Nilutamide (Nilandron)

Antiandrogens are competitive antagonists of the interaction between androgens and the androgen receptor, which normally leads to transcriptional activation of genes containing androgen-response elements in their promoter regions. Antiandrogens are effective treatment for prostate cancer when used in combination with a luteinizing hormone-releasing factor (LHRH) receptor agonist or orchiectomy. Although the three nonsteroidal antiandrogens that are currently approved by the Food and Drug

Administration for the treatment of prostate cancer have similar efficacy, their side effects may differ. Relatively common side effects include nausea, diarrhea, and constipation. Androgenic blockade results in predictable feminizing side effects in men, including mastodynia, gynecomastia, galactorrhea, hot flashes, and loss of facial hair. Nilutamide is associated with idiosyncratic reactions including visual disturbances manifesting as delayed adaptation to dark in up to 50% of patients. Interstitial pneumonitis and alcohol intolerance have also been reported.

Retinoic Acid Receptor Modulators

Retinoic acid receptors are transcription factors that allow normal maturation of a variety of tissues, including those of myeloid and lymphoid lineage. In acute promyelocytic leukemia, a characteristic translocation involving chromosomes 15 and 17 [t(15: 17)(q22;q12)] creates a fusion between the intron of the retinoic acid receptor alpha (RAR-α) gene and PML, a second protein with DNA-binding capacity. The fusion protein functions in a dominant fashion blocking the transcription of genes controlled by RAR-α by recruiting nuclear corepressors. It is believed that all-*trans* retinoic acid (Tretinoin, Vesanoid) releases the corepression activity, allowing transcription of genes involved in cellular differentiation.

All-*trans* Retinoic Acid (Tretinoin, Vesanoid)

All-*trans* retinoic acid has unique activity in the treatment of acute promyelocytic leukemia due to the t(15 :17) translocation. In both previously treated and untreated patients who receive a 30- to 90-day course of orally administered treatment, responses occur in more than 80% of patients. All-*trans* retinoic acid appears to be superior to treatment with chemotherapy alone, and the optimum initial therapy appears to be the concurrent use of both all-*trans* retinoic acid and anthracycline-based chemotherapy regimens. Side effects of all-*trans* retinoic acid include the retinoic acid syndrome (fever, pulmonary infiltrates and pulmonary insufficiency, pericarditis, and pleuritis), nausea, dry skin, and headache.

Bexarotene (Targretin)

Bexarotene is a retinoic acid analog that was given accelerated Food and Drug Administration approval for the treatment of cutaneous T cell lymphoma (CTCL). It is a highly selective antagonist of the retinoid "X" receptor and thereby interferes with the response of cells to derivatives of vitamin A. Bexarotene has activity in patients with cutaneous T cell lymphoma who have failed prior systemic chemotherapy. The most frequent side effects are reversible, asymptomatic increases in liver function tests, leukopenia, hypertriglyceridemia, and hypercalcemia.

Membrane Receptors

Epidermal Growth Factor (EGF)/EGF Receptor (EGFR)-Family Antagonists

Many growth factor–receptor interactions occur at the cell surface and are therefore amenable to different types of pharmaceutical agents such as antibodies and peptides. Several of these new agents are discussed below.

Trastuzumab (Herceptin)

HER-2/neu is a member of the epidermal growth factor receptor (EGFR) family of tyrosine kinases and is involved in the growth, invasion, and metastasis of breast cancer. The demonstration that overexpression of HER-2/neu in breast and ovarian cancer was associated with a poor prognosis led to a search for effective therapies aimed at this target, culminating in the approval of trastuzumab for the treatment of breast cancers that overexpress HER-2/neu.

Trastuzumab is an anti-HER-2/neu murine monoclonal antibody that contains a human IgG1 Fc region. It recognizes an extracellular epitope (amino acids 529–567) in the cysteine-rich II domain of HER-2/neu, an oncogene that is overexpressed in approximately 25% of breast cancers. Trastuzumab inhibits cell growth and induces CDK2 kinase inhibitor (p27^{KIP1}) and Rb (retinoblastoma gene) expression. It also restores sensitivity to TNF-α, upregulates E-cadherin and α-2 integrin, decreases vascular endothelial growth factor, fixes complement, activates antibody-dependent cell-mediated cytotoxicity, and downregulates inactive HER-2 homodimers.

In preclinical studies, trastuzumab was found to enhance sensitivity to cisplatin by decreasing DNA repair. Its effects were synergistic with cisplatin, thiotepa, docetaxel, and etoposide; additive with doxorubicin, paclitaxel, methotrexate, and vinblastine; and antagonistic with 5-fluorouracil.

In the clinic, the response rate to trastuzumab plus chemotherapy appears to be superior to the response rate to either alone. In a series of Phase II trials, the response rate to trastuzumab alone was 12% to 23% in patients who had previously been treated for metastatic breast cancer. Slamon and colleagues demonstrated in a randomized trial that the combination of trastuzumab plus paclitaxel was superior to trastuzumab plus an anthracycline owing to the cumulative cardiac toxicity of the trastuzumab-anthracycline combination. In this study, patients received either doxorubicin 80 mg/m^2 with cyclophosphamide (650 mg/m^2) or epirubicin (75 mg/m^2) plus cyclophosphamide or paclitaxel (175 mg/m^2 over 3 hours) with or without trastuzumab (4 mg/kg loading dose followed by 2 mg/kg weekly maintenance dose). The addition of trastuzumab improved median time to progression (7.4 months versus 4.6 months), response rate (50% versus 32%), duration of response (9.1 months versus 6.1 months), mortality rate at one year (22% versus 33%), and median survival rate (25.1 months versus 20.3 months) compared to chemotherapy alone. The frequency of cardiac toxicity increased when trastuzumab was combined with anthracycline plus cyclophosphamide (27% versus 8% with chemotherapy alone) or with paclitaxel (13% versus 1% with paclitaxel alone).

Trastuzumab is generally well tolerated. Fever and chills, pain at the tumor site, diarrhea, nausea, and vomiting were noted only 11 times in 768 administrations. With increasingly widespread use, rare deaths have occurred during drug administration.

Responses to trastuzumab may be long-lived, even in patients presenting with far advanced, heavily pretreated disease. In patients who are treated initially with trastuzumab and paclitaxel, after approximately nine months of paclitaxel, despite a good response, the toxicities (especially the neurotoxicity) from the taxane begin to become unbearable. In such cases, we have been able to maintain the response for one year or more by continuing the trastuzumab and decreased the dose and scheduling of paclitaxel to 75 mg/m^2 weekly, biweekly, and then monthly. One such patient relapsed in the central nervous system (CNS) despite a continuing systemic response. Following resection of the brain metastasis and radiation therapy, the patient was maintained successfully on trastuzumab alone for six additional months before disease progressed outside of the brain. This case highlights the inability of antibodies to cross the blood-brain barrier and serves as a reminder to be wary of the significance of central nervous system symptoms in a patient who is responding well to antibody therapy.

Rituximab (Rituxan)

The presence of the CD20 antigen on the surface of many B-cell lymphomas and in B-cell chronic lymphocytic leukemia was originally reported by Nadler and colleagues and by Almasri, respectively. The observation that antibodies to CD20 block cell cycle progression and differentiation supports the putative role of CD20 as a growth factor receptor. Rituximab is an antibody that is raised against CD20. It contains a human IgG1 Fc region, heavy-chain variable region sequences and human IgG1 heavy-chain and κ light-chain constant regions. The human Fc domain induces immune mediated B-cell lysis by complement-dependent and antibody-dependent cellular cytotoxicity and can induce apoptosis.

Rituximab is active against both indolent and intermediate-grade non-Hodgkin's lymphoma. In previously treated patients with low-grade lymphomas, response rates approach 50%, with a median time to response of seven weeks and a median time to progression of 10 months. In previously untreated low-grade non-Hodgkin's lymphoma, a dose of 375 mg/m^2 by intravenous infusion each week for four consecutive weeks resulted in responses in 21 of 39 patients (54%), and another 14 of 39 (36%) experienced disease stabilization. Thirteen patients were retreated at six months, and four additional responses were seen; four patients went from partial responses to complete responses after the second course of therapy. Rituximab has also been tested in combination with chemotherapy. For example, when rituximab was combined with cyclophosphamide, doxorubicin, vincristine, and prednisone (CHOP) in the treatment of low-grade B-cell lymphomas, the overall response rate was 95% (38 of 40); there were 22 complete responses (55%), 16 partial responses, and two nonresponders. The median duration of response was greater than 29 months. In addition, seven of eight patients who overexpressed bcl-2, t(14;18) translocations became bcl-2 negative (by the highly sensitive polymerase chain reaction test) with treatment. There was no added toxicity from combining rituximab with CHOP. In newly diagnosed patients with intermediate or high-grade non-Hodgkin's lymphoma, rituximab plus CHOP induced 63% complete responses and 33% partial responses with no noticeable increase in toxicity.

Rituximab is currently approved for a single course of therapy. However, despite a marked prolongation of half-life with a second course of treatment, retreatment within 12 months appears to be safe and beneficial. Zevalin (ibritumomab, Y-90) and Bexxar (I^{131} labeled tositumomab), which are radioactive congeners of rituximab, both target the CD20 antigen. They provide an opportunity to deliver relatively targeted radiation therapy to the lymphomatous deposits. Initial studies show that they can induce responses even in patients who have failed therapy with non-radioisotope-linked monoclonal antibodies such as rituximab.

Most side effects from rituximab are infusion-related (probably cytokine-mediated) and resolve completely within hours. These include fever, chills, vomiting, urticaria, rash, and rigors in 65% to 80% of patients during the first infusion. With each subsequent infusion, the frequency and severity of side effects diminish. In contrast, non-infusion-related toxicities are uncommon and include arrhythmias, pain, myalgias, fatigue, angioedema, and bronchospasm. Hematologic toxicity is mild and reversible. Despite the fact that normal B-cells are also destroyed with this therapy and immunoglobulin production is reduced, no substantial increase in infections has been noted. With the radioactive congeners of these antibodies, suppression of hematopoiesis does occur, requiring careful attention to the dose of radiation administered.

Gemtuzumab Ozogomicin (Mylotarg)

CD33 antigen expression is almost exclusively limited to the hematopoietic system and is present on the surface of acute myelogenous leukemia (AML) cells in greater than 80% of patients. Gemtuzumab is approved for the treatment of patients age 60 years or older who have CD33-positive acute myelogenous leukemia in first relapse and who are not candidates for cytotoxic chemotherapy. Gemtuzumab is a humanized recombinant IgG4κ monoclonal antibody against CD33 and is linked to calicheamicin, an anticancer antibiotic isolated from a bacterium that is found in caliche clay in Texas. Gemtuzumab selectively delivers calicheamicin to immature normal and leukemic cells of myelomonocytic origin.

Gemtuzumab showed activity in phase II trials in patients with CD33-positive acute myelogenous leukemia in first relapse (FAB type M3 [promyelocytic] and secondary leukemias were excluded). Good-risk patients were defined by a duration of first remission greater than one year and/or age less than 60 years. In these patients, the overall response rates with gemtuzumab were lower than those reported for similar patients treated with other drugs in first relapse: 30% versus 33% to 54%. In poor-risk patients, defined by a first remission duration less than one year and/or age over 60 years, the overall response rates were similar to those reported with chemotherapy (28% versus 14% to 44%).

Toxicities with gemtuzumab include alopecia, mucositis, and infections, but these are generally less severe than with chemotherapy. Myelotoxicity is similar or decreased in comparison with chemotherapy. Acute symptoms associated with the infusion are generally mild and self-limiting. Calicheamicin-related hepatotoxicity including grade 3 to 4 elevations of transaminases and bilirubin were seen in 14% and 24% of patients, respectively. Four patients developed veno-occlusive disease, and one subsequently died of liver failure.

Denileukin, Diftitox, DAB389IL-2 (Ontak)

Proliferation of helper T-cells occurs when they are stimulated to secrete interleukin-2 (IL-2), which then interacts with surface interleukin-2 receptors.

Denileukin is the first drug to target the interleukin-2 receptor. The expression of interleukin-2 receptors is normally dependent on the exposure of T-cells to specific antigens. Therefore under normal conditions, interleukin-2 causes the proliferation of only those T-cells that have encountered their specific antigen. The interleukin-2 receptors are composed of alpha and beta chains either as homodimers or heterodimers. The interleukin-2 receptor is constituitively expressed in the majority of cutaneous T-cell lymphomas, a malignancy of CD4+ helper T-cells. Cyclosporin, a drug that can inhibit generation of interleukin-2 receptors through suppression of interleukin-2 production, has been reported to have activity against cutaneous T-cell lymphomas. Other malignancies that overexpress the interleukin-2 receptor include hairy cell leukemia and T-cell acute lymphoblastic leukemia.

Denileukin is approved by the Food and Drug Administration for the treatment of persistent or recurrent cutaneous T-cell lymphomas that express the CD25 component of the interleukin-2 receptor. Denileukin is a fusion protein consisting of the cytotoxic A chain fragment of diphtheria toxin fused to interleukin-2. Therefore denileukin delivers a potent exotoxin to cutaneous T-cell lymphoma cells (and others) expressing the interleukin-2 receptor. A phase I study reported five complete and eight partial responses in 35 patients with cutaneous T-cell lymphoma. The median time to response was two months, and the duration of response was 2 to 39+ months. In subsequent studies, the overall response rate was 30% to 37%, including 10% to 14% complete responses.

The majority of side effects include flulike symptoms, acute hypersensitivity reactions, nausea and vomiting, infections, and transient elevation of liver function tests. The presence of antidiphtheria antibodies does not preclude a clinical response.

Drugs That Decrease Circulating Growth Factors

Drugs that decrease circulating growth factors interfere with growth factor–receptor interactions by decreasing available ligand. This is a characteristic of drugs that produce a medical adrenalectomy or hypophysectomy (luteinizing hormone-releasing factor agonists) or inhibit the peripheral conversion of hormones to their active forms through inhibition of aromatase. Aromatase is an enzyme complex made up of two proteins: aromatase cytochrome P450 (CYP19) and NADPH-cytochrome P450 reductase; inhibition of aromatase blocks the conversion of androgens to estrone in peripheral tissues including fat, liver, muscle, and breast. Inhibition of aromatase is an effective treatment for postmenopausal women with breast cancer, in whom the greatest source of estrogen comes from the conversion of androstenedione (produced in the adrenal) to estrone in liver, muscle, and fat. Recent comparisons of the newer aromatase inhibitors to tamoxifen suggest that they may have a therapeutic index as good as or better than tamoxifen when used as front-line therapy against breast cancer.

Aminoglutethimide was originally developed as an anticonvulsant. It is an inhibitor of cholesterol conversion to pregnenolone, and combined with dexamethasone, it suppresses adrenal function. This medical adrenalectomy produced responses in breast cancer due to inhibition of peripheral aromatization of androstenedione to estrone. Anastrazole, letrozole, and exemestane are more selective aromatase inhibitors than aminoglutethimide.

Aromatase inhibitors are approved for use in the treatment of postmenopausal women with hormone-responsive metastatic breast cancer. They also have activity as second-line hormonal agents in patients who have relapsed after responding to tamoxifen. In this setting, they are as effective as megestrol acetate but have fewer side effects. Aminoglutethimide produces glucocorticoid deficiency, mineralocorticoid deficiency, skin rash, lethargy, and orthostatic hypotension and therefore should no longer be used. Anastrazole and letrozole have greater affinity for the CYP19 aromatase than aminoglutethimide. They are therefore more selective and less toxic and do not require glucocorticoid replacement. Exemestane is an irreversible, aromatase inactivator that is structurally related to androstenedione, the natural substrate. It is a pseudosubstrate for aromatase that binds irreversibly to the active site of the enzyme causing its destruction, thereby lowering circulating estrogen concentrations. Exemestane has no detectable effect on adrenal synthesis of corticosteroids or aldosterone. Side effects include nausea, vomiting, and diarrhea (less than 30%). Preliminary studies suggest that these third-generation aromatase inhibitors may have activity equal to or greater than that of tamoxifen as well as fewer side effects.

Drugs That Alter Nucleic Acid Replication and Transcription

Growth factor–receptor interactions activate signal transduction cascades that culminate in DNA synthesis through transcriptional activation of cell proliferation genes. A good example is the signaling cascades that are mediated by the retinoblastoma protein (Rb); when phosphorylated by cyclinD1/cdk4, Rb releases bound transcription factors, E2F, which activate a series of genes involved in cell proliferation (e.g., thymidylate synthase, ribonucleotide reductase, and dihydrofolate reductase). Therefore it is not surprising that some of our most effective chemotherapeutic drugs interfere with downstream signal transduction events by inhibiting thymidylate synthase (fluoropyrimidines), ribonucleotide reductase (gemcitabine and hydroxyurea), and dihydrofolate reductase (methotrexate). Furthermore, transcriptional activation requires the unwinding of compacted DNA through the action of topoisomerases and histone deacetylases. These steps can be inhibited by alkylating and platinating agents and topoisomerase poisons, whereas drugs that target the function of histones are under intense investigation.

Alkylating Agents

The alkylating agents were the first compounds demonstrated to have anticancer activity. Louis Goodman, Alfred Gilman, and their colleagues at Yale University demonstrated that nitrogen mustard could abolish lymphomas in experimental animals and had chemotherapeutic effects in humans. The classes of alkylating agents are shown in Tables 48-1 and 48-2. Their mechanism of action is exemplified by the prototype, mechlorethamine, which forms a covalent bond between nucleotides on adjacent strands of DNA. Thus bifunctional alkylating agents disrupt DNA replication and transcription and lead to cell death.

Temozolomide is an oral alkylating agent approved for the treatment of brain tumors. It is the 3-methyl derivative of mitozolomide and is both less active and less toxic than the parent compound. The mechanism of action of temozolomide is similar to that of dacarbazine. Both drugs methylate N-7 and 0'6 positions on guanines (the latter is believed to produce the cytotoxic lesion). Temozolomide has a large volume of distribution that includes penetration into the central nervous system. Following ingestion and absorption, the triazene ring opens and generates monomethyl triazene (MTIC), the same metabolite that is formed by metabolic dealkylation of dacarbazine.

Temozolomide has activity against high-grade astrocytomas and melanoma. The most common untoward side effects from temozolomide are lymphocytopenia, increased transaminases, nausea and vomiting, hyperglycemia, anemia, and thrombocytopenia.

Platinating Agents

The therapeutic properties of cisplatin were deduced from studies of bacterial motility in electric currents, in which bacterial cell death was observed adjacent to platinum electrodes. Platinating agents kill cancer cells by creating irreversible intrastrand links in DNA that disrupt the normal process of gene transcription. Currently approved platinating agents are shown in Table 48-1. Cisplatin is part of a curative regimen for germ-cell tumors and has activity against a variety of carcinomas including those of lung, gastric, bladder, and head and neck. It is far less active against the hematopoietic malignancies. Carboplatin has an activity spectrum similar to that of cisplatin but differs in that its major toxicity is myelosuppression rather than nephrotoxicity. Oxaliplatin is approved for the treatment of colorectal cancer.

Inhibitors of Nucleic Acid Synthesis

Activation of growth factor receptors leads to phosphorylation of the retinoblastoma gene product, Rb. Once phosphorylated, Rb protein disassociates from a family of transcription factors, resulting in the activation of several genes that are critical to cell division. Therefore drugs that inhibit these enzymes such as 5-fluorouracil (thymidylate synthase), hydroxyurea (ribonucleotide reductase), and methotrexate (dihydrofolate reductase) are some of the most effective anticancer agents. Several new inhibitors of nucleic acid synthesis are discussed below.

Capecitabine (Xeloda)

Capecitabine is orally administered and is approved for metastatic breast cancer that is resistant to anthracyclines and taxanes. Capecitabine is the carbamate derivative of 5'-deoxy-5-fluorouridine, a prodrug that must be metabolically activated following ingestion. It is converted to 5'-deoxy-5-fluorocytidine by carboxylesterases in the liver, followed by conversion to 5'-deoxy-5-fluorouridine (DFUR) by cytidine deaminase in the liver and tumor tissue. 5'-Deoxy-5-fluorouridine is then converted to 5-fluorouracil by thymidine phosphorylase. The increased activity of thymidine phosphorylase in certain tumors compared to normal tissues may give capecitabine a potential advantage in terms of selectivity and activity over 5-fluorouracil.

Capecitabine is active against breast and colorectal cancer. In breast cancer patients who were refractory to paclitaxel, capecitabine produced a 20% response rate, an 8.1-month median duration of response, a 12.8-month median survival, and a decrease in cancer-related pain. In colorectal cancer patients, capecitabine produced responses in 20% to 28% of patients when given either on a continuous or intermittent schedule and regardless of whether leucovorin was added to the treatment regimen. The median time to progression was 30 weeks using the intermittent schedule, 17 weeks with the continuous schedule, and 24 weeks in the group receiving leucovorin. However, increased toxicity was seen with the combination of capecitabine plus leucovorin, particularly diarrhea and hand-foot syndrome.

Gemcitabine (Gemzar)

Gemcitabine, a deoxycytidine analogue (2'-deoxy-2',2'-difluorocytidine), was selected for development because of its activity against murine solid tumors. Gemcitabine inhibits DNA synthesis through several mechanisms that require activation of the drug by intracellular enzymes. First, the parent drug is metabolized by deoxycytidine kinases to the active diphosphate and triphosphate nucleosides, metabolites that inhibit DNA polymerase. Gemcitabine diphosphate also inhibits ribonucleotide reductase, the enzyme that generates the deoxynucleoside triphosphates required for DNA synthesis. Gemcitabine triphosphate competes with deoxycytidine triphosphate for incorporation into DNA. The reduction in the intracellular concentration of deoxycytidine triphosphate (by the action of the gemcitabine diphosphate) enhances the incorporation of gemcitabine triphosphate into DNA (self-potentiation).

Gemcitabine is approved for treatment of pancreatic cancer and is active against lung, breast, and bladder cancer. In pancreatic cancer, patients receiving gemcitabine compared to 5-fluorouracil demonstrated increases in survival, time to disease progression, and clinical benefit response (decreased analgesic consumption, reduced pain intensity, improved performance status, and weight gain). No confirmed objective tumor responses were observed, however, with either treatment. The primary endpoint was a prospectively defined clinical benefit response, a measure of clinical improvement based on change.

Data from two randomized clinical studies also support the use of gemcitabine with cisplatin as first-line treatment of patients with locally advanced or metastatic non-small-cell lung cancer. In one study, gemcitabine plus cisplatin showed improved median survival and time to disease progression compared to cisplatin alone in previously untreated patients with advanced inoperable non-small-cell lung cancer. The objective response rate on the gemcitabine plus cisplatin arm was 26% versus 10%, but the duration of response was similar. A randomized comparison of a similar group of patients receiving gemcitabine plus cisplatin versus etoposide plus cisplatin showed no significant difference in survival, although the objective response rate and median time to disease progression were better in patients receiving the gemcitabine combination therapy. Myelosuppression is the dose-limiting toxicity. Other side effects are generally mild and include mild nausea and vomiting, liver function abnormalities, and fever during drug infusion.

Inhibitors of DNA Topoisomerase

Replication of DNA and transcription of DNA to mRNA requires the unwinding of compacted DNA into a form that is more accessible to replication and transcription complexes. This alteration in DNA structure involves changes in DNA topology that are mediated by topoisomerases, which produce transient single-strand (topoisomerase I) or double-strand (topoisomerase II) breaks in DNA. Several natural-product antineoplastic drugs covalently bind to either topoisomerase I or to topoisomerase II and markedly alter the function of these critical enzymes.

The effect of topoisomerase-targeting drugs are different from those of most other anticancer enzyme inhibitors; topoisomerase-targeting drugs "poison" the enzymes by inhibiting religation of the DNA nicks produced during topoisomerase catalysis, that is, the drugs lock the enzyme in an "on" conformation. As replication or transcription complexes encounter drug/topoisomerase/DNA complexes, the resulting collisions produce DNA double-strand breaks that lead to cell death (Figure 48-2). Cancer cells have greater topoisomerase activity than normal cells, resulting in more drug-induced DNA damage and cell death. Differences in the processing of topoisomerase-mediated

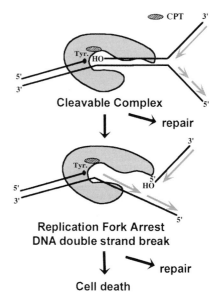

Figure 48-2 ■ Model of the collision of a replication fork with a camptothecin-topoisomerase I-DNA ternary complex. Repair of drug-induced, topoisomerase I-mediated DNA damage is possible either before or after the collision.

DNA damage by malignant versus normal cells may also be important in the selectivity of these drugs.

Drugs That Target Topoisomerase II

Currently approved topoisomerase II inhibitors such as doxorubicin, daunorubicin, etoposide, and teniposide are part of many combination chemotherapy regimens. Newly approved topoisomerase II drugs include liposomal doxorubicin (Doxil) and epirubicin (Ellence). Liposomal doxorubicin was originally approved in 1995 for Kaposi's sarcoma and is now approved for ovarian cancer. Epirubicin is approved as a component of adjuvant therapy for node-positive breast cancer.

The anthracyclines were isolated from *Streptomyces peucetius* var. *caesius*, and the antitumor activity of daunorubicin and doxorubicin was observed in the 1960s. The structures of the clinically used anthracyclines (see Table 48-2) explain their pharmacologic actions. For example, the planar, hydrophobic tetracycline ring linked to a daunosamine sugar through a glycosidic linkage and the positive charge at physiological pH allows intercalation into DNA. The adjacent quinone moieties encourage electron transfer reactions that generate oxygen free radicals.

Daunorubicin and doxorubicin differ only by a single hydroxyl at position C14, yet they have distinct spectra of antitumor activity. Idarubicin is a semisynthetic derivative of daunomycin (4-demothoxy-daunorubicin) that lacks the 4-methoxy group present on the parent compound. Epirubicin is an epimer of doxorubicin; the C4'-hydroxyl group on the amino sugar is in the equatorial rather than the axial position. This increases lipophilicity compared to doxorubicin. The liposome-encapsulated formulation of doxorubicin (Doxil) displays altered pharmacokinetics (e.g., a lower volume of distribution and greater AUC) but no major differences in activity (with the possible exception of epithelial ovarian cancer).

The anthracyclines are highly reactive and produce a variety of effects on biological systems. In addition to their effects on topoisomerase II (see above), anthracyclines intercalate into double-stranded DNA and produce structural changes that interfere with DNA and RNA synthesis. Anthracyclines generate reactive oxygen species, including oxygen free radicals, hydroxyl radicals, and hydrogen peroxide, that damage DNA, mRNA, proteins, and lipids; the peroxidation of lipids may account for much of the cardiac toxicity characteristic of these drugs.

The anthracyclines are active against solid and hematological malignancies. Doxorubicin has the broadest spectrum of activity. Its introduction in the 1960s and incorporation into combination regimens led to curative treatments for intermediate/high-grade non-Hodgkin's lymphoma with CHOP and less toxic treatment for Hodgkin's disease with ABVD (adriamycin, bleomycin, vinblastine, and DTIC). It is also active against Ewing's, osteogenic, and other soft tissue sarcomas. Doxorubicin is one of the most active drugs against breast cancer. Single-agent activity is similar to that of paclitaxel and is comparable to combination chemotherapy in patients with metastatic disease.

Daunorubicin is active against acute lymphocytic and myeloid leukemias. Although it has some activity against pediatric solid tumors, it has little activity against adult solid malignancies. Idarubicin is used predominantly in the treatment of adult acute myelogenous leukemia. Epirubicin has activity against breast, melanoma, colorectal, renal, gastric, pancreatic, ovarian, and lung cancer and hepatocellular soft tissue sarcoma. In addition, it is part of active regimens against Hodgkin's disease and non-Hodgkin's lymphoma. In the treatment of breast cancer, epirubicin has activity similar to that of doxorubicin.

Anthracyclines produce myelosuppression, mucositis, alopecia, nausea, vomiting, and increased skin pigmentation. Erythema at the injection site ("flare reaction") is benign, but extravasation into the surrounding tissues can lead to serious local complications, including full-thickness necrosis. Inflammation at sites of previous radiation ("radiation recall") can lead to unanticipated complications including pericarditis, pleural effusion, and skin rash.

All anthracyclines produce potentially serious cardiac effects. Acute effects include arrhythmias and ST-T wave changes, which are not usually life-threatening. A rare syndrome resembling acute pericarditis-myocarditis can occur that is characterized by a fall in cardiac ejection fraction, conduction abnormalities, pericardial effusion, and congestive heart failure. Congestive cardiomyopathy is more common and of greater clinical significance than the acute cardiac effects. Congestive cardiomyopathy is associated with mortality rates of approximately 30%. Myocardial damage occurs through several mechanisms including the generation of reactive oxygen species from the electron transfer from the semiquinone to quinone moieties of the anthracycline ring. The generation of hydrogen peroxide and the peroxidation of myocardial lipids contribute to myocardial damage.

Both cumulative dose and schedule of administration affect the incidence of cardiomyopathy. Cardiac toxicity correlates best to peak plasma concentration of the parent drug. Accordingly, more total drug can be given safely at low-dose weekly intervals or by continuous infusion than higher doses given every three to four weeks. A history of heart disease,

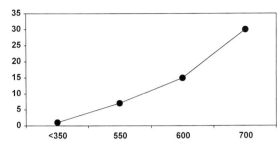

Figure 48-3 ■ The incidence of clinically detectable congestive heart failure as a function of cumulative doxorubicin dosing when doxorubicin is given at doses of 40 to 75 mg/m² as a bolus injection every three to four weeks.

hypertension, radiation to the mediastinum, age less than 4 years, or prior use of anthracyclines or other cardiac toxins may predispose patients to cardiac damage.

The incidence of clinically detectable congestive heart failure when doxorubicin is given at doses of 40 to 75 mg/m² as a bolus injection every three to four weeks is shown in Figure 48-3. When doxorubicin is given by a low-dose weekly regimen (10 to 20 mg/m² per week) or by slow continuous infusion over 96 hours, cumulative doses of greater than 500 mg/m² can be given. However, careful monitoring of cardiac function is still required and should increase in frequency at these cumulative doses. Doses of daunorubicin less than 1000 mg/m² (equivalent to 550/m² doxorubicin) are considered to be safe. Doses of idarubicin less than 290 mg/m² did not produce clinical congestive heart failure despite changes in cardiac ejection fraction. Epirubicin appears as active as doxorubicin and may have less cardiac toxicity.

Cardiac function can be monitored during treatment with anthracyclines using electrocardiography, echocardiography, or radionuclide ejection fractions. Anthracyclines should be avoided in patients with underlying cardiac disease (e.g., a baseline left ventricular ejection fraction of less than 50%) and should be discontinued after a documented decrease in ejection fraction of greater than 10% if this results in a value below the lower limit of normal, or a 20% decrease, regardless of the absolute value. It appears that each dose of anthracycline results in some muscle damage. With prolonged dosing, clinical congestive heart failure develops. Although routine monitoring of the ECG and cardiac ejection fraction are frequently advised and performed, there is no evidence that these tests provide early warning that the next dose will result in clinical manifestations of heart failure. Indeed, in a number of patients, unexpected congestive heart failure has developed one to two months after anthracyclines have been discontinued. Dexrazoxane (ADR-529) is a metal chelator approved

to decrease the myocardial toxicity of doxorubicin. Similar protective effects have been suggested for amifostine, an organic thiophosphate that is dephosphorylated to form a reactive thiol (N-2mercaptoethyl-1,3,-diaminopropane), which acts as a free radical scavenger.

Anthracenediones

Mitoxantrone

Anthracenediones lack the glycoside substituents of the anthracyclines (see Table 48-2). Mitoxantrone, the most active anthracenedione, was identified in the 1970s through a search for anthracycline analogs with less cardiac toxicity. The spectrum of antitumor activity is narrower than is true for doxorubicin. Its decreased cardiac toxicity may be because of mitoxantrone's diminished ability to generate oxygen free radicals. Mitoxantrone produces single- and double-stranded DNA breaks through poisoning of topoisomerase II.

Mitoxantrone has activity against acute leukemias and breast cancer. Response rates range from 50% to 70% when used in combination with cytosine arabinoside for the treatment of acute myelogenous leukemia. In breast cancer, mitoxantrone is as active as doxorubicin, but mitoxantrone is less often associated with cardiac toxicity.

Drugs That Target Topoisomerase I

Topotecan (Hycamtin)

Topotecan is a camptothecin derivative from the *Camptotheca acuminata* (Chinese yew) tree identified in the 1960s by Wani and Wahl. The original sodium salt formulation of camptothecin caused severe and unpredictable toxicity. The appreciation of the importance of pH-dependent lactone ring cleavage and drug inactivation led to the development of safer, more stable derivatives. Topotecan is a semisynthetic analog of camptothecin, created by adding a basic side chain at the 9-position of the A-ring of 10-hydroxycamptothecin (see Table 48-2). These substitutions increase solubility without requiring hydrolysis of the lactone (E-ring). The mechanism of action of topotecan is the poisoning of topoisomerase I leading to single- and double-stranded DNA breaks. The lactone ring is susceptible to pH-dependent reversible hydrolysis to carboxylic acid. The drug is active when in the lactone form.

Topotecan is approved for treatment of refractory ovarian cancer and relapsed small cell lung cancer. The major untoward side effect with topotecan is myelosuppression and fatigue. Diarrhea occurs in 15% of patients and is more severe when the drug is given by continuous infusion rather than in intermittent pulses. Alopecia occurs in 40% to 100% of patients.

Irinotecan (Camptosar, CPT-11)

Irinotecan is active in the treatment of colorectal cancer that is refractory to 5-fluorouracil. It is a semi-synthetic analog of camptothecin whose mechanism of action is similar to that of topotecan. Irinotecan is also approved for first-line therapy in combination with 5-fluorouracil and leucovorin for patients with metastatic colorectal cancer based on two large studies. A European study compared two 5-fluorouracil infusion schedules given with or without irinotecan, whereas a U.S. study compared irinotecan (125 mg/m²) alone to weekly irinotecan with 5-fluorouracil/leucovorin (weekly for four consecutive weeks every six weeks) and to leucovorin and 5-fluorouracil given as a daily bolus for five consecutive days every four weeks. Irinotecan alone was no better than 5-fluorouracil/leucovorin, but the combinations of therapy with irinotecan demonstrated a statistically significant improvement in median survival, time to tumor progression, and response rates for patients.

The major untoward side effects from irinotecan are myelosuppression and diarrhea. Irinotecan produces both early and late onset diarrhea. Early onset occurs during infusion or within 24 hours and is associated with other cholinergic side effects, including flushing, diaphoresis, lacrimation, salivation, and abdominal cramping. Late-onset diarrhea develops 24 hours after administration, most commonly after the second or third weekly dose.

In considering treatment of a patient with irinotecan, it is important to remember that diarrhea is a prominent side effect. Diarrhea that occurs within the first 24 hours can be treated with 0.25 to 1 mg of atropine intravenously. Diarrhea that occurs later results from the cytotoxic effects of the drug on the intestinal mucosa and can be life-threatening. Patients should be instructed to have loperamide available at home and at the onset of diarrhea should begin high-dose loperamide immediately. This consists of 4 mg initially then 2 mg every 2 hours until there are no further bowel movements for 12 hours. Patents with hepatic dysfunction or inherited hepatic metabolic abnormalities, such as Gilbert syndrome (see Chapter 32), are at increased risk for severe diarrhea while receiving irinotecan; the drug should be used with caution in these patients.

Drugs That Affect the Mitotic Apparatus

Following a growth-promoting signal either from the cell surface or through the interaction of intracellular receptors with specific genes, the cancer cell must replicate its DNA and undergo successive cellular divisions to create viable progeny. This requires the transition from interphase to metaphase, events that are mediated by microtubules. Microtubules form the mitotic spindle, maintain cell shape, organize the location of organelles, mediate intracellular transport, participate in secretion and neurotransmission, and promote cell motility required for invasion, metastases, and angiogenesis. Microtubules consist of α- and β-tubulin dimers that create 13 protofilaments that form hollow cylinders. The protofilaments are aligned with the same polarity. The (+) or fast-growing end extends from the nucleus to the plasma membrane, whereas the (−) or slow-growing end identifies a site of origin or nucleation of the microtubule, which often begins in the centrosome. Microtubules grow in spurts or may disappear completely. This process, called dynamic equilibrium, is an essential feature of microtubule physiology. Elongation of microtubules requires the addition of both α- and β-tubulin bound to GTP. GTP-bound β-tubulin forms a GTP cap at the elongating end. The GTP cap increases the affinity for other tubulin molecules and is a characteristic of rapid microtubule growth. During depolymerization, GTP is hydrolyzed more rapidly than it can be added, resulting in weakening of the bonds that hold the tubulin molecules together.

Oncogenes can affect the function of microtubules. For example, several microtubule-associated proteins are under the transcriptional control of the tumor suppressor oncogene, p53. In most instances reported to date, wild-type p53 represses the synthesis of these proteins; as a result, when p53 is functionally disabled through mutation or deletion, there is a transcriptional release of microtubule-associated proteins, such as MAP4 and stathmin.

Antimitotic drugs interfere with the physiology of microtubules and disable the normal mitotic apparatus. Moreover, by affecting microtubules in interphase cells, these drugs may also inhibit cell motility and normal subcellular organization. Finally, the sensitivity to our most useful antimitotic drugs (taxanes and vinca alkaloids) is influenced by the relative expression of microtubule-associated proteins; estramustine, an active drug against prostate cancer, may target microtubule proteins directly.

Drugs That Stabilize Polymerized Microtubules

The taxane paclitaxel was initially isolated from the Pacific yew tree, *Taxus brevifolius*. Taxanes interfere with the function of microtubules and thereby disrupt normal mitosis. Taxanes preferentially bind to the N-terminal 31 amino acids of the β-subunit of tubulin oligomers or polymers and inhibit microtubule depolymerization. At nanomolar concentrations, taxanes create a mitotic block without increasing the mass of microtubule polymers. At higher concentrations (1 mol drug per 1 mol tubulin dimer), taxanes stabilize microtubules independent of its effects on GTP or microtubule associated proteins. Taxanes are large alkaloid esters consisting of a taxane ring linked to a four-member oxetan ring at positions C-4 and C-5 (see Table 48-2). Docetaxel is a semisynthetic derivative that exhibits enhanced solubility in water and increased potency in vitro.

Paclitaxel and docetaxel are the two taxanes that are currently approved for clinical use. They share broad-spectrum antitumor activity against breast, lung, ovarian, and bladder cancers. Both drugs also have activity against lymphoid malignancies. Paclitaxel and docetaxel produce peripheral neuropathy, dose-limiting bone marrow suppression, and alopecia. Nausea, vomiting, and diarrhea are rarely severe. Docetaxel can cause vascular permeability (peripheral edema, pleural effusion, and ascites). Both paclitaxel and, less commonly, docetaxel can cause type I hypersensitivity reactions characterized by flushing, bronchospasm, dyspnea, and hypotension.

Vinca alkaloids were originally isolated from the pink periwinkle plant (catharanthys roseus, formerly *vinca rosea* Linn). The mechanism of action of the vincas is concentration related. At substochiometric concentrations, they bind to high-affinity sites at the ends of microtubules (Ka 5.3×10^{-5} M) and prevent microtubule polymerization. At higher concentrations, vincas bind to low-affinity, high-capacity sites (Ka $3-4 \times 10^{-3}$ M), leading to microtubule disintegration. The alkaloids are large symmetrical molecules consisting of a dihydroindole nucleus (vindoline) connected to an indole nucleus (catharanthine) by a methylene bridge (see Table 48-2). Vincristine and vinblastine differ by a single R1 substituent, whereas vinblastine and vindosine differ in the R2 and R3 positions; vinorelbine has a modification of the catharine ring.

The spectrum of activity and toxicities of the vincas are somewhat different. Vincristine is effective against non-Hodgkin's lymphoma, Hodgkin's disease, and pediatric solid tumors but plays less of a role in the treatment of adult solid tumors. Vinorelbine is active against breast and lung cancer. Vinblastine is most frequently used in the treatment of testicular cancer and Hodgkin's lymphoma and is a third-line agent in the treatment of breast cancer.

Major toxicities include dose-limiting myelosuppression and neurotoxicity. The most frequent neurotoxicities include constipation, numbness and tingling of the extremities, loss of deep tendon reflexes, and distal muscle weakness. Sensory changes often resolve with time and do not mandate discontinuation of the drug. In contrast, loss of motor function is a later and more serious side effect, requiring discontinuation of the medication and/or a search for contributing causes. The high frequency of severe constipation in patients receiving the vinca alkaloids requires that these patients be placed on prophylaxis with stool softeners and at times on laxatives as well.

Principles of Drug Dosing

For an anticancer drug to destroy a cancer cell, several things must occur: (1) the drug must enter the bloodstream and be activated or escape inactivation by drug metabolizing enzymes; (2) the drug must be at a therapeutic concentration when it reaches its target; (3) the drug-target interaction must result in the desired pharmacologic effect (e.g., receptor inactivation, enzyme inhibition, interference with microtubule function); and (4) these interactions must eventually produce cell death or a reversal of the malignant phenotype.

The ability of a drug to destroy a cancer cell grown in a flask far exceeds its ability to eradicate cancer in a patient. On the basis of in vitro studies, a mathematical model predicts that cell kill will increase exponentially based on the concentration of the drug and the duration of exposure. This model is based on a homogenous cancer cell population growing synchronously in log phase in vitro and therefore does not take into account the highly variable features in humans with cancer. Enormous heterogeneity exists in the frequency of cells undergoing spontaneous mutation, the percentage of cells in cell cycle at any one time, drug pharmacokinetics from patient to patient, interactions with other drugs, cancer cells in the same patient and between patients, and tumor vascularity. Tumor cell heterogeneity alone can produce significant differences in drug sensitivity. Heppner and colleagues treated three subpopulations of Balb/CfC3H mammary adenocarcinoma with cyclophosphamide, methotrexate, and 5-fluorouracil and found that the effects varied markedly, ranging from tumor regression to the actual promotion of metastases. Finally, although the model predicts that for any given time of exposure, increasing the drug concentration will increase cell kill, recent data from clinical trials challenge the notion that higher doses of drug are necessarily more effective.

The number of cellular mutations increases as a function of cell number. Nearly 50 years ago, cancer pharmacologists noted that the outcome of treatment was dependent on the stage of the disease and the health of the host. When an animal was treated shortly after inoculation of a small number of cancer cells, a single large dose of drug was more effective than fractionated smaller doses. However, once the tumor was established and the animal was symptomatic, the type of therapy that was curative for minimal disease actually worsened the outcome when used to treat advanced disease. Furthermore, treatment of animals with advanced-stage ascites tumors with smaller total doses of the same drug given in a multidose scheme achieved significant disease control and extended the life span of the animal. These results form the scientific basis for the current use of low-dose, weekly regimens being used successfully in the treatment of solid tumors.

The oxygenation of a tumor is a major determinant of drug sensitivity. The seminal work of Sartorelli and colleagues demonstrated that most chemotherapeutic drugs were significantly less active in the hypoxic environments produced in regions of poorly vascularized tumors. The exception was the mitomycins, which were actually more active under hypoxic conditions. Folkman's work on tumor angiogenesis led to the realization that tumors can attract their own blood supply and that the tumor vasculature was therefore an attractive therapeutic target.

The observation that tumor blood vessels grow more rapidly than those of endothelium of normal tissue has resulted in a new application of the relationship of time and dose of chemotherapy. So-called metronomic therapy, that is, the use of more frequent, smaller doses of conventional drugs such as cyclophosphamide and vinca alkaloids, may control tumor growth more effectively than conventional dosing schemes. Moreover, these regimens may be less toxic to the patient and may also be synergistic with more specifically designed antiangiogenic drugs. The principle of metronomic therapy is supported by empiric success in the clinic. For example, highly effective treatment for children with acute lymphoblastic leukemia relies heavily on a continuation phase of therapeutic cycles of outpatient therapy having a backbone of daily or even twice-daily 6-mercaptopurine and weekly methotrexate for up to three years. Both of these drugs (or metabolites) are antiangiogenic and bone marrows of treated children have an antiangiogenic appearance. The use of high doses of intravenous ifosfamide and etoposide over five days for treatment of patients with Ewing's sarcoma in the late 1980s resulted in a 60% (complete + partial responses) response rate and substantial toxicity. In contrast, oral cyclophosphamide for seven days followed on day 8 by a single dose of doxorubicin was at least as effective (19 of 23 complete responses) but far less toxic. More recently, weekly taxanes seem to have an equal or even better therapeutic index than higher doses given at less frequent intervals.

Once a cytotoxic concentration of drug is attained, another important variable is the duration of exposure. Experimental models of cytotoxicity with methotrexate showed that a one-log increase in duration of exposure produced a two-log increase in cell kill. In contrast, a one-log increase in concentration resulted only in a 0.3-log increase in cell kill. The duration of time that a drug can be present at an effective dose has been traditionally limited by toxicity to normal tissues. However, the development of newer agents that are highly selective for abnormalities present in the cancer cell or tumor vasculature may allow chronic, more effective, dosing. Alternatively, selectivity may be obtained by taking advantage of selective uptake or metabolism of the drug by tumor cells as compared to normal cells.

Drug schedule changes, by affecting mesenchymal support elements in the host, can influence the outcome of therapy. For example, stromal and tumor-associated macrophages contribute to the angiogenic proclivity of a tumor. Destruction of stromal components may explain the synergistic effect of low-dose, continuous chemotherapy regimens combined with endothelial specific drugs. Since vascular endothelial growth factor (VEGF) secretion by stromal cells may protect tumor cells from doxorubicin, the effect of drugs on the stromal elements is a consideration in the phenomenon of drug resistance. It may be necessary to inhibit this paracrine loop of cell growth stimulation with specific inhibitors against not only vascular endothelial growth factor, but also other angiogenic molecules. Finally, high-dose chemotherapy regimens can impair the host's immune response. Destruction of macrophages, dendritic cells, and T- and B-lymphocytes could allow tumor growth in the absence of an appropriate immune response from an otherwise immunocompetent host. In contrast, low doses of cyclophosphamide may actually enhance immune function.

Dose Modification Guidelines

Doses of chemotherapy are typically modified for changes in organ function as well as for alterations in blood counts. Tables 48-3 and 48-4 outline commonly utilized guidelines for dose reductions based on compromised renal or hepatic function. The occurrence of other toxicities such as myelosuppression, thrombocytopenia, neurotoxicity, and mucositis also require modification of therapy.

Rational Drug Selection Based on Pharmacogenomics

In years past, the selection of drugs for patients with cancer was based on empiric trials emanating from hints of activity in phase I clinical trials. Combination

Table 48-3 ■ Recommended Dose Modifications for Renal Dysfunction

Agent	Organ Dysfunction	Dose Modification
Bleomycin	CrCl = 30–60 mL/min	25–50% decrease
	CrCl = 10–30 mL/min	25–50% decrease
	CrCl<10 mL/min	50% decrease
Carboplatin	Renal insufficiency	Total dose = AUC X (CrCl +25)
Cisplatin	Use with caution in patients with CrCl <50 mL/min	
Cyclophosphamide	Renal failure	Decrease dose 50–75%
Etoposide	Decrease in proportion to CrCl: 15–50 mL/min	Decrease dose 25%
Fludarabine	Use with caution in patients with CrCl <60 mL/min	Decrease dose in proportion to CrCl
Hydroxyurea	Use with caution in patients with CrCl <60 mL/min	Decrease dose in proportion to CrCl
Ifosfamide	Renal failure	Decrease dose 50–75%
Methotrexate	Decrease in proportion to CrCl <60 mL/min Monitor levels closely	
Pentostatin	Dose in proportion to CrCl	
Streptozocin	Renal failure	Decrease dose 50–75%
Topotecan	CrCl 20–39 mL/min	Decrease dose 50%

Renal failure: creatinine clearance <25 mL/min.
CrCl: creatinine clearance.
AUC: Area under the concentration × time curve.
Note: For most drugs, only approximate guidelines can be offered with varying recommendations from multiple sources.

chemotherapy was based on a variety of useful preclinical models that in reality were often usurped by the necessity to combine drugs lacking similar toxicities. These approaches, although time consuming and fraught with errors along the way, nonetheless led to the cure of over 70% of children and many adults with malignant disease.

The future selection of drugs in the treatment of cancer will be based on our current understanding of molecular biology and pharmacology and determinants of drug sensitivity, coupled with our ability to decipher the expression of entire sets of genes in small clinical samples. By using DNA or tissue microarray, an individual's tumor can be phenotyped and a prediction made regarding drug sensitivity. Such predictions could then be converted into hypotheses to be tested in rational, well-designed clinical trials.

Just as the measurement of estrogen and progesterone receptors in breast cancer specimens identified the patients who were likely to respond to hormonal therapies, the measurement of newer drug targets in individual patients will undoubtedly lead to higher chances of response. Early approaches include quan-

tifying the expression of target receptors such as her-2/neu, which is present in approximately 30% of breast cancer, and the ability to detect the Ph chromosome in patients with leukemia to predict for response to trastuzumab and STI 571, respectively (see below).

This approach should also yield more precise predictions of which patients will respond to more traditional cytotoxic drugs. For example, several early studies suggest that the overexpression of thymidylate synthase and dihydropyrimidine dehydrogenase in a tumor specimen predict a poor response to fluoropyrimidines.

Rational selection of patients for treatment with antitubulin drugs is also under investigation. At the Cancer Institute of New Jersey, phenotyping includes several gene products that are critical determinants of sensitivity to tubulin-binding agents, including P-glycoprotein, p53, MRP, microtubule-associated protein 4 (MAP-4), and bcl-2. For example, patients whose tumors harbor wild-type p53 are invited to participate in protocols designed to determine whether induction of DNA damage with an anthracycline

Table 48-4 ■ Recommended Dose Modifications for Hepatic Dysfunction

Agent	Organ Dysfunction	Dose Modification
Anthracyclines	Hepatic Dysfunction*	
	Bilirubin 1.2–3.0 mg/dL	Decrease dose 50%
	Bilirubin 3.1–5.0 mg/dL	Decrease dose 75%
	Bilirubin >5.0 mg/dL	Omit
Docetaxel	Bilirubin >ULN	Do not give
	AST or ALT >1.5 ULN and	Do not give
	Alk Phos >2.5 ULN	
Etoposide	Bilirubin 1.5–3.0 mg/dL	Decrease dose 50%
	Bilirubin 3.1–5.0 mg/dL	Omit
Paclitaxel	Use with caution in hepatic failure	
Thiotepa	Use with caution in hepatic failure	
Vinblastine		
Vincristine	Bilirubin 1.5–3.0 mg/dL	Decrease dose 50%
Vinorelbine	Bilirubin 3.1–5.0 mg/dL	Omit

* No clear correlation of toxicity or pharmacokinetics has been proven.
ULN: upper limit of normal.
Note: For most drugs, only approximate guidelines can be offered with varying recommendations from multiple sources.

(doxorubicin) can induce p53 and repress MAP-4. This sequence is designed to then sensitize cells to the vinca alkaloid, vinorelbine. Preliminary data obtained from both peripheral blood mononuclear cells and patient samples confirm the feasibility of this approach.

In instances in which tumors overexpress bcl-2 and harbor mutant p53, patients are invited to participate in protocols designed to determine whether or not the combination of interferon α- and cis-retinoic acid can downregulate bcl-2 and sensitize cells to paclitaxel, as was shown in preclinical and phase I clinical trials.

Future Directions: Imatinib Mesylate (Gleevec)

Imatinib mesylate was designed to target the intracellular tyrosine kinase domain of a unique growth factor receptor. The drug inhibits the enzyme activity of BCR-ABL, the fusion product of a reciprocal chromosomal translocation involving the long arms of chromosomes 9 and 22. This chromosomal fusion, t(9:22) (q34.1;q11.21), creates an oncogenic tyrosine protein kinase that mediates signaling through its cytoplasmic tyrosine kinase domain. Imatinib mesylate competes for the binding of ATP at the ATP-binding domain of the kinase. It is the uniqueness of the fusion protein, the ability of the drug to bind to the nonphosphorylated ATP activation loop of the kinase, and the unusual ATP-binding motif that accounts for the relative specificity of this inhibitor.

Imatinib mesylate has shown exciting results in the treatment of chronic myelogenous leukemia (see Chapter 71). In patients in chronic phase of the disease, complete hematologic remissions were observed in 53 of 54 patients once therapeutic doses were achieved. Prolonged therapy produced cytogenetic remissions in 29 of these patients, with 13% experiencing complete disappearance of the Ph chromosome. Complete hematologic remissions were maintained with a median follow-up of 265 days. There was no dose-limiting toxicity. The drug also showed activity in patients with chronic myeloid leukemia in blast crisis and Ph+ acute lymphoblastic leukemia. Fifty-five percent of myeloid phenotype patients and 70% of lymphoid phenotype patients experienced partial or complete responses of two- to three-month duration. Finally, imatinib mesylate is also active against the rare gastrointestinal stromal cancer and may prove to be effective against other cancers driven by the c-kit oncogene, another tyrosine kinase.

These responses highlight the ability of drugs to destroy cancer cells by interrupting a critical cell viability signal rather than by directly damaging DNA or microtubules. Thus imatinib mesylate is a cytotoxic drug that works through a unique mechanism of action. Increasing knowledge of tumor cell genetics and their resulting role in malignant transformation should lead to further development of anticancer therapies targeted at specific biochemical reactions. Such drugs, developed by design rather than empirically, should provide agents that are not only highly effective, but also very selective in their attack, leading to reduced toxicity to normal tissues.

References

General Considerations and Dosing Strategies

Berd D, Maguire HC, Mastrangelo MJ: Potentiation of human cell-mediated and humoral immunity by low dose cyclophosphamide. Cancer Res 1984;44:5439–5443.

Fidler J, Ellis M: Chemotherapeutic drugs: More really is not better. Nature Med 2000;6:500–502.

Goldie JH, Coldman AJ: The genetic origin of drug resistance in neoplasms: Implications for systemic therapy. Cancer Res 1984;44:3643–3653.

Goldin A, Venditti JM, Humphreys SR, Mantel N: Modification of treatment schedules in the management of advanced mouse leukemia with amethopterin. J Natl Cancer Inst 1956;17:203–212.

Hainsworth JD, Burris HA, Erland JB, et al: Phase I trial of docetaxel administered by weekly infusion in patients with advanced refractory cancer. J Clin Oncol 1998;16:2164–2168.

Hanahan D, Bergers G, Bergsland E: Less is more, regularly: Metronomic dosing of cytotoxic drugs can target angiogenesis in mice. J Clin Invest 2000;105:1045–1047.

Hayes FA, Thompson EI, Hustu HO, et al: The response of Ewing's sarcoma to sequential cyclophosphamide and doxorubicin induction therapy. J Clin Oncol 1983;1:45–51.

Hensley ML, Schuchter LM, Lindley C, et al: American society of clinical oncology clinical practice guidelines for the use of chemotherapy and radiotherapy protectants. J Clin Oncol 1999;17:3333–3355.

Heppner GH, Miller BE: Tumor heterogeneity: Biological implications and therapeutic consequences. Cancer Metastasis Rev 1983;2:5–23.

Heppner GH, Dexter DL, DeNucci T, et al: Heterogeneity in drug sensitivity among tumor cell subpopulations of a single mammary tumor. Cancer Res 1997;38:3758–3763.

Keef DA, Capizzi RL, Rudnick SA: Methotrexate cytotoxicity for L5178Y asn⁻ lymphoblasts: Relationship of dose and duration of exposure to tumor cell viability. Cancer Res 1982;42:1641–1645.

Kennedy KA, Rockwell S, Sartorelli AC: Selective metabolic activation of mitomycin C by hypoxic tumor cells in vitro. Proc Am Assoc Cancer Res 1979;20:278 (abst #1129).

Meikle SR, Matthewes JC, Brock CS, et al: Pharmacokinetic assessment of nover anti-cancer drugs using spectral analysis and positron emission tomography: A feasibility study. Cancer Chemother Pharmacol 1998;42:183–193.

Poste GR, Greig R: On the genesis and regulation of cellular heterogeneity in malignant tumors. Invasion Metastasis 1982;2:137–176.

Rocca A, Colleoni M, Nole F, et al: Low dose oral methotrexate (MTX) and cyclophosphamide (CTX) in metastatic breast cancer (MBC): Antitumor activity and correlation with serum vascular endothelial growth factor (VEGF) levels. Proc Am Soc Clin Oncol 1999;18:121a.

Seidman AD, Hudis CA, McCaffrey J, et al: Dose-dense therapy with paclitaxel via weekly 1-hour infusion: Preliminary experience in the treatment of metastatic breast cancer. Semin Oncol 1997;24:S17–S17.

Wall ME, Wani MC: Camptothecin and taxol: Discovery to clinic—Thirteenth Bruce F. Cain Memorial Award lecture. Cancer Res 1995;55:753.

Growth Factor Receptor Interactions: Hormones

Bonneterre J, Thurlimann B, Tobertson JFR, et al: Anastrozole versus tamoxifen as first-line therapy for advanced breast cancer in 668 postmenopausal women: Results of the tamoxifen or arimidex randomized group efficacy and tolerability study. J Clin Oncol 2000;18:3748–3757.

Buchanan RB, Blamey RW, Duvert KR, et al: A randomized comparison of tamoxifen with surgical oophorectomy in premenopausal patients with advanced breast cancer. J Clin Oncol 1986;4:1326–1330.

Colletti RB, Roberts JD, Devlin JT, Copeland KC: Effect of tamoxifen on plasma insulin-like growth factor I in patients with breast cancer. Cancer Res 1989;49:1882–1888.

Crawford ED, Eisenberger MA, McLeod DG, et al: A controlled trial of leuprolide with and without flutamide in prostatic carcinoma. N Engl J Med 1989;321:419–424.

Cummings SR, Exkert S, Krueger KA, et al: The effect of raloxifene on risk of breast cancer in postmenopausal women. JAMA 1999;281:2189–2197.

Delmas PD, Bjarnason MH, Mitlak BH, et al: Effects of raloxifene on bone mineral density, serum cholesterol concentrations, and uterine endometrium in postmenopausal women. N Engl J Med 1997;337:1641–1647.

Evans RM: The steroid and thyroid hormone receptor superfamily. Science 1988;240:889–895.

Fisher B, Constantino J, Redmond C, et al: A randomized clinical trial evaluating tamoxifen in the treatment of patients with node-negative breast cancer who have estrogen-receptor positive tumors. N Engl J Med 1989;320:479–484.

Fisher B, Constantino JP, Wicherham DL, et al: Tamoxifen for prevention of breast cancer: Report of the National Surgical Adjuvant Breast and Bowel Project P-1 Study. J Natl Cancer Inst 1998;90:1371–1388.

Griffiths CT, Hall TC, Saba Z, et al: Preliminary trial of aminoglutethimide in breast cancer. Cancer 1973;32:31–37.

Hayes DF, Van Zyl JA, Goedhals L, et al: Randomized comparison of tamoxifen and two separate doses of toremifene in postmenopausal patients with metastatic breast cancer. J Clin Oncol 1995;13:2556–2566.

Hirsimaki P, Hirsimaki Y, Nieminen L, et al: Tamoxifen induces hepatocellular carcinoma in rat liver: A 1 year study with 2 antiestrogens. Arch Toxicol 1993;67:49–59.

Ingle JN, Krook JE, Green SJ, et al: Randomized trial of bilateral oophorectomy versus tamoxifen in premenopausal women with metastatic breast cancer. J Clin Oncol 1986;4:178–185.

Knabbe C, Lippman ME, Wakefield L, et al: Evidence that TGFβ is a hormonally regulated negative growth factor in human breast cancer. Cell 1987;48:417–428.

Klotz L: Hormone therapy for patients with prostate carcinoma. Cancer 2000;88(Suppl):3009–3014.

Legha SS: Tamoxifen in the treatment of breast cancer. Ann Int Med 1988;109:219–228.

Nabholtz JM, Buzdar A, Pollak M, et al: Anastrozole is superior to tamoxifen as first-line therapy for advanced breast cancer in postmenopausal women: Results of a North American Multicenter randomized trial. J Clin Oncol 2000;18:3758–3767.

Santen RJ, Lipton A, Kendall J: Successful medical adrenalectomy with aminoglutethimide: Role of altered drug metabolism. JAMA 1974;230:1661–1665.

Stearns V, Gelmann EP: Does tamoxifen cause cancer in humans? J Clin Oncol 1998;16:779–792.

Yang NN, Benugopalan M, Hardikar S, et al: Identification of an estrogen response element activated by metabolites of 17β-estradiol and raloxifene. Science 1996;273:1222–1225.

Retinoic Receptor Modulators

Fenaux P, Chastang C, Chevret S, et al: A randomized comparison of all-*trans* retinoic acid (ATRA) followed by chemotherapy and ATRA plus chemotherapy and the role of maintenance therapy in newly diagnosed acute promye-locytic leukemia. The European APL Group. Blood 1999;94:1192–1200.

Fenaux P, Chomienne C, Degos L: All-*trans* retinoic acid and chemotherapy in the treatment of acute promyelocytic leukemia. Semin Hematol 2001;38L13–38L25.

Frankel SR, Eardley A, Lauwers G, et al: The "retinoic acid syndrome" in acute promyelocytic leukemia. Ann Intern Med 1992;117:292–296.

Grignani F, De Matteis S, Nervi C, et al: Fusion proteins of the retinoic acid receptor-alpha recruit histone deacetylase in promyelocytic leukemia. Nature 1998;391:815–818.

Huang ME, Ye YYC, Chen SR, et al: Use of all-*trans* retinoic acid in the treatment of acute promyelocytic leukemia. Blood 1988;72:567–572.

Mangelsdorf DJ, Umesono K, Evans RM: The retinoid receptors. In Sporn MD, Roberts AB, Goodman DS (eds): The Retinoids: Biology, Chemistry, and Medicine, 2nd ed. New York: Raven Press, 1994, pp 319–349.

Melnick A, Licht JD: Deconstructing a disease: RARalpha, its fusion partners, and their roles in the pathogenesis of acute promyelocytic leukemia. Blood 1999;93:3167–3215.

Miller VA, Benedetti FM, Rigas JR, et al: Initial clinical trial of a selective retinoid X receptor ligand, LGD 1069. J Clin Oncol 1997;15:790–795.

Warrell RP Jr, Frankel SR, Miller WH Jr, et al: Differentiation therapy of acute promyelocytic leukemia with tretinoin (all-*trans* retinoic acid). N Engl J Med 1991;324:1385–1393.

Epidermal Growth Factor Response Family Receptors

Trastuzumab (Herceptin)

Baselga J: Current and planned clinical trials with trastuzumab. Sem Oncol 1999;26:78–83.

Baselga J, Tripathy D, Mendelsohn J, et al: Phase II study of weekly intravenous recombinant humanized anti-p-185HER2 monoclonal antibody in patients with HER2/neu overexpressing metastatic breast cancer. J Clin Oncol 1996;14:737–744.

Cobleigh MA, Vogel CL, Tripathy D, et al: Multinational study of the efficacy and safety of humanized anti-HER2 mono-clonal antibody in women who have HER2-overexpressing metastatic breast cancer that progressed after chemother-apy for metastatic disease. J Clin Oncol 1999;17:2639–2648.

Coussens L, Yang-Feng TL, Liao Y-C, et al: Tyrosine kinase receptor with extensive homology to EGF receptor shares chromosomal location with *neu* oncogene. Science 1985;230:1132–1139.

Hancock MC, Langton BC, Chan T, et al: A monoclonal anti-body against the c-erbB-2 protein enhances the cytotoxic-ity of cis-diamminedichloroplatinum against human breast and ovarian tumor cell lines. Cancer Res 1991;51:4575–4580.

Pegram M, Hsu S, Lewis G, et al: Inhibitory effects of combina-tions of HER-2/neu antibody and chemotherapeutic agents used for treatment of human breast cancers. Oncogene 1999;18:2241–2251.

Rizvi NA, Marshall JL, Dahut W, et al: A phase I study of

LGD1069 in adults with advanced cancer. Clin Cancer Res 1999;5:1658–1664.

Slamon DJ, Godolphin W, Jones LA, et al: Studies of the HER2/neu proto-oncogene in human breast and ovarian cancer. Science 1989;244:707–712.

Slamon DJ, Clark GM, Wong SG, et al: Human breast cancer: Correlation of relapse and survival with amplification of the HER-2/neu oncogene. Science 1987;235:177–182.

Slamon DJ, Godolphin W, Jones LA, et al: Studies of the HER2/neu proto-oncogene in human breast and ovarian cancer. Science 1989;244:707–712.

Slamon DJ, Leyland-Jones B, Shak S, et al: Addition of Herceptin (humanized anti-HER2 antibody) to first line chemotherapy for HER2 overexpressing metastatic breast cancer (HER2+/MBC) markedly increases anticancer activ-ity: A randomized, multinational controlled Phase III trial. Proc Amer Soc Clin Oncol 1998;17:98a.

Sliwkowski MX, Lofgreen JA, Lewis GD, et al: Nonclinical studies addressing the mechanism of action of trastuzumab. Sem Oncol 1999;26:60–70.

Vogel CL, Cobleigh MA, Tripathy D, et al: Efficacy and safety of Herceptin (trastuzumab, humanized anti-HER2 antibody) as a single agent in first-line treatment of HER2 overex-pressing metastatic breast cancer. Breast Cancer Res Treat 1998;50:232 (abstract).

Rituximab (Rituxan)

Almasri NM, Duque RE, Iturraspe J, et al: Reduced expression of CD20 antigen as a characteristic marker for chronic lymphocytic leukemia. Am J Hematol 1992;40:259.

Czuczman MS, Grillo-Lopez AJ, White CA, et al: Treatment of patients with low-grade B-cell lymphoma with the combination of chimeric anti-CD20 monoclonal antibody and CHOP chemotherapy. J Clin Oncol 1999;17:268–276.

Davis TA, White CA, Grillo-Lopez AJ, et al: Rituximab anti-CD20 monoclonal antibody therapy in non-Hodgkin's lymphoma: Safety and efficacy of re-treatment. J Clin Oncol 2000;18:3135–3143.

Golay JT, Clark EA, Beverly PC: The CD20 antigen is involved in activation of B cells from the G0 to the G1 phase of the cell cycle. J Immunol 1985;135:3795–3801.

Hainsworth JD, Burris HA, Morrissey LH, et al: Rituximab monoclonal antibody as initial systemic therapy for patients with low-grade non-Hodgkin's lymphoma. Blood 2000;95:3052–3056.

Link BK, Grossbard ML, Fisher RI, et al: Phase II pilot study of the safety and efficacy of rituximab in combination with CHOP chemotherapy in patients with previously untreated intermediate- or high-grade NHL Proc Am Soc Clin Oncol 1998;17:7.

Maloney DG, Smith B, Applebaum FR: The anti-tumor effect of monoclonal anti-CD2 antibody therapy includes direct anti-proliferative activity and induction of apoptosis in CD20 positive non-Hodgkin's lymphoma cell lines. Blood 1996;88:637a.

Nadler LM, Ritz J, Hardy R, et al: A unique cell surface antigen identifying lymphoid malignancies of B-cell origin. J Clin Invest 1981;67:134.

Reff ME, Carner K, Chambers KS, et al: Depletion of B-cells in vivo by a chimeric mouse human monoclonal antibody to CD20. Blood 1994;83:435–445.

Tedder TF, Aboyd AW, Freedman AS, et al: The B-cell surface molecule B1 is funtionally linked with B-cell activation and differentiation. J Immunol 1985;135:973–979.

Gemtuzumab (Mylotarg)

Sievers EL, Appelbaum FR, Spielberger RT, et al: Selective ablation of acute myelogenous leukemia using antibody-targeted chemotherapy: A phase I study of an anti-CD33 calicheamicin immunoconjugate. Blood 1999;93:3678–3684.

Sievers EL, Larson RA, Estey E, et al: Interim analysis of the efficacy and the safey of CMA-676 in patients at first relapse. Blood 1998;92:2527a.

Interleukin-2 Receptors

Colamonici OR, Rosolen A, Cole D, et al: Stimulation of the beta-subunit of the IL-2 receptor induces MHC-unrestricted cytotoxicity in T acute lymphoblastic leukemia cells and normal thymocytes. J Immunol 1988;141:1200–1205.

Cooper DL, Braverman IM, Sarris AH, et al: Cyclosporin treatment of refractory T-cell lymphomas. Cancer 1993;71:2335–2341.

Erber WN, Mason DY: Expression of the interleukin-2 receptor (Tac antigen/CD25) in hematologic neoplasms. Am J Clin Path 1988;89:645–648.

LeMaister CF, Saleh MN, Kuzel TM, et al: Phase I trial of ligand fusion-protein (DAB$_{389}$IL-2) in lymphomas expressing the receptor for interleukin 2. Blood 1998;91:399–405.

Olsen EL, Duvic M, Frankel A, et al: Pivotal phase III trial of two dose levels of denileukin diftitox for the treatment of cutaneous T-cell lymphoma. J Clin Oncol 2001;19:376–388.

Saleh MN, LeMaister CF, Kuzel TM, et al: Antitumor activity of DAB$_{389}$ IL-2 fusion toxin in mycosis fungoides. J Am Acad Dermatol 1998;39:63–73.

Alkylating Agents

Temozolomide

Bleehen NM, Newlands ES, Lee SM, et al: Cancer research campaign phase II trial of temozolomide in metastatic melanoma. J Clin Oncol 1995;13:910–913.

Middleton MR, Johnson JR, Middleton MR: Temozolomide for advanced, metastatic melanoma. J Clin Oncol 2000;18:158–166.

Newlands ES, Blackledge GR, Slack JA, et al: Phase I trial of temozolomide. Br J Cancer 1992;65:287–291.

Rosenberg B, Van Camp L, Krigas T: Inhibition of cell division in *Escherichia coli* by electrolysis products from a platinum electrode. Nature 1965;205:698–699.

Yung WK, Prados MD, Yaya-Tur R, et al: Multicenter phase II trial of temozolomide in patients with anaplastic astrocytoma or anaplastic oligoastrocytoma at first relapse. J Clin Oncol 1999;17:2762–2771.

Antimetabolites

Blum JL, Jones SE, Buzdar AU, et al: Multicenter phase II study of capecitabine in paclitaxel-refractory metastatic breast cancer. J Clin Oncol 1999;17:485–493.

Budman DR, Meropol NJ, Reigner B, et al: Preliminary studies of a novel oral fluoropyrimidine carbamate: Capecitabine. J Clin Oncol 1998;16:1795–1802.

Burris HA, Moore MJ, Andersen J, et al: Improvements in survival and clinical benefit with gemcitabine as first-line therapy for patients with advanced pancreas cancer: A randomized trial. J Clin Oncol 1997;15:2403–2413.

Cardenal F, Cabrezio PL, Anton A, et al: Randomized phase III study of gemcitabine-cisplatin versus etoposide-cisplatin in the treatment of locally advanced or metastatic non-small cell lung cancer. J Clin Oncol 1999;17:12–18.

Hertel LW, Boder GB, Kroin JS, et al: Evaluation of the antitumor activity of gemcitabine (difluoro-2'-deoxycytidine). Cancer Res 1990;50:4417–4423.

Huang P, Chubb S, Hertel L, et al: Action of 2', 2'-difluorodeoxycytidine on DNA synthesis. Cancer Res 1991;51:6110–6117.

Ishikawa T, Sekiguchi F, Fukase Y, et al: Positive correlation between the efficacy of capecitabine and deoxyfluridine and the ratio of thymidine phosphorylase to dihydropyrimidine dehydrogenase activities in tumors in human cancer xenografts. Cancer Res 1998;58:685–690.

Sandler AB, Nemunaitis J, Denham C, et al: Phase III trial of gemcitabine plus cisplatin vs cisplatin alone in patients with locally advanced or metastatic non–small-cell lung cancer. J Clin Oncol 2000;18:122–130.

Van Cutsem E, Findlay M, Osterwalder B, et al: Capecitabine, an oral fluoropyrimidine carbamate with substantial activity in advanced colorectal cancer: results of a randomized phase II study. J Clin Oncol 2000;18:1337–1345.

Topoisomerase Inhibitors

Bash-Babula JE, Alli EL, Toppmeyer D, Hait WN: Effect of doxorubicin treatment on p53 and microtubule-associated protein 4 (MAP-4) expression in patients with breast cancer. Am Assoc Cancer Res 2000;41:a2124.

Chen AY, Liu LF: DNA topoisomerases: Essential enzymes and lethal targets. Annu Rev Pharmacol Toxicol 1994;34:191–218.

Froelich-Ammon SJ, Osheroff N: Topoisomerase poisons: Harnessing the dark side of enzyme mechanism. J Biol Chem 1995;270:21429–21432.

Giovanella BP, Stehlin JS, Wall ME, et al: DNA topoisomerase I-targeted chemotherapy of human colon cancer in xenografts. Science 1989;246:1046–1048.

Wang JC: DNA topoisomerases. Annu Rev Biochem 1996;65:635–692.

Anthracyclines

Ahmann DL, Schaid DJ, Bisel HF, et al: The effect on survival of initial chemotherapy in advanced breast cancer: Polychemotherapy versus single drug. J Clin Oncol 1987;5:1928.

Alexander JN, Dainiak N, et al: Serial assessment of doxorubicin cardiotoxicity with quantitative radionuclide angiocardiography. N Engl J Med 1979;300:278–283.

Arcamone F, Cassinelli G, Fantini G, et al: Adriamycin, 14-hydroxy-daunomycin, a new antitumor antibiotic from *S. peucetius var. caesius*. Biotechnol Bioeng 1969;11:1101.

Bontenbal M, Andersson M, Wildiers J, et al: Doxorubicin vs epirubicin, report of a second-line randomized phase II/III study in advanced breast cancer. EORTC Breast Cancer Cooperative Group. Br J Cancer 1998;77:2257.

Cortes EP, Lutman G, Wanka J, et al: Adriamycin (NSC-123127) cardiotoxicity: A clinicopathologic correlation. Cancer Chemother Rep 1975;6:215.

Di Marco A, Gaetani M, Orezzi P, et al: Daunomycin, a new antibiotic of the rhodomycin group. Nature 1964;201:706.

Doroshow JH: Role of hydrogen peroxide and hydroxyl radical formation in the killing of Ehrlich tumor cells by anticancer quinones. Proc Natl Acad Sci USA 1986;83:4514.

Jones RB, Holland JF, Bhardwaj S, et al: A phase I–II study of intensive-dose adriamycin for advanced breast cancer. J Clin Oncol 1987;5:172.

Launchbury AP, Habboubi N: Epirubicin and doxorubicin: A comparison of their characteristics, therapeutic activity and toxicity. Cancer Treat Rev 1993;19:197.

Lefrak EA, Pitha J, Rosenheim S, et al: Clinicopathologic analysis of adriamycin cardiotoxicity. Cancer 1973;32:302.

Legha SS, Benjamin RS, Mackay B, et al: Reduction of doxorubicin cardiotoxicity by prolonged continuous intravenous infusion. Ann Intern Med 1982;96:133.

Sinha BK, Katki AG, Batist G, et al: Differential formation of hydroxyl radical by adriamycin in sensitive and resistant MCF-7 human breast tumor cells: Implication for the mechanism of action. Biochemistry 1987;26:3776.

Sledge GW, Neuberg D, Ingle J, et al: Phase III trial of doxorubicin (A) vs. paclitaxel (T) vs. doxorubicin + paclitaxel (A + T) as first-line therapy for metastatic breast cancer (MBC): An intergroup trial. Proc Am Soc Clin Oncol 1997;16:1a.

VonHoff DD, Layard MW, Basa P, et al: Risk factors for doxorubicin-induced congestive heart failure. Ann Intern Med 1979;91:710.

Mitoxantrone

Arlin Z, Feldman E, Mittelman A, et al: High dose short course mitoxantrone with high dose cytarabine is safe and effective therapy for acute lymphoblastic leukemia (ALL). Proc Am Soc Clin Oncol 1991;10:223.

Crepsi JD, Ivanier SE, Genovese J, Baldi A: Mitoxantrone affects topoisomerase activities in human breast cancer cells. Biochem Biophys Res Commun 1986;136:521–528.

Dutcher JP, Wiernik PH, Strauman JJ, et al: Mitoxantrone (MITOX) and cytosine arabinoside (ARA-C) in acute non-lymphocytic leukemia (ANLL) and blast crisis of chronic myelogenous leukemia (CML-B). Proc Am Soc Clin Oncol 1985;4:170.

Murdock KC, Child RG, Fabio PF, et al: Antitumor agents. I. 1,4-Bis[(aminoalkyl)amino]-9,10-anthracenedions. J Med Chem 1979;22:1024–1033.

Paciucci PA, Ohnuma T, Cuttner J, et al: Mitoxantrone in patients with acute leukemia in relapse. Cancer Res 1983;43:3919.

Shenkenberg TD, Von Hoff DD: Mitoxantrone: A new anticancer drug with significant clinical activity. Ann Intern Med 1986;105:67.

Antimetabolites

Douillard JY, Cunningham D, Roth AD, et al: A randomized phase III trial comparing inrinotecan (IRI) + 5FU/folinic acid (FA) to the same schedule of 5FU/FA in patients with metastatic colorectal cancer (MCRC) as front line chemotherapy. Proc Am Soc Clin Oncol 1999;18:233a;899.

Saltz LB, Locker PK, Priotta N, et al: Irinotecan plus fluorouracil and leucovorin for metastatic colorectal cancer. Irinotecan Study Group. N Engl J Med 2000;343:905–914.

Wilson L, Jordan MA: Microtubule dynamics: Taking aim at a moving target. Chem Biol 1995;2:569.

Drugs Affecting Mitotic Apparatus (Vinca Alkaloids and Taxanes)

Ahn J, Murphy M, Kratowicz S, et al: Down-regulation of the stathmin/Op 18 and FKBP25 genes following p53 induction. Oncogene 1999;18:5954–5958.

Himes RH: Interactions of the catharanthus [Vinca] alkaloids with tubulin and microtubules. Pharmacol Ther 1991;51:257.

Mitchison T, Kirschner M: Dynamic instability of microtubule growth. Nature 1984;312:237–242.

Murphy M, Hinman A, Levine A: Wild-type p53 negatively regulates the expression of a microtubule-associated protein. Genes Dev 1996;10:2971–2980.

Schiff PB, Fant J, Horwitz SB: Promotion of microtubule assembly in vitro by taxol. Nature 1979;277:665.

Skipper HE, Schabel FM, Mellet LB, et al: Implications of biochemical, cytokinetic, pharmacologic and toxicologic relationships in the design and optimal therapeutic schedules. Cancer Chemother Rep 1970;54:431–450.

Stearns ME, Tew KD: Antimicrotubule effects of estramustine, an antiprostatic tumor drug. Cancer Res 1985;45:3891–3897.

Angiogenesis Inhibitors

Browder T, Butterfield CE, Kraling BM, et al: Antiangiogenic scheduling of chemotherapy improves efficacy against experimental drug-resistant cancer. Cancer Res 2000;60:1878–1886.

Carmeliet P, Jain RK: Angiogenesis in cancer and other diseases. Nature 2000;407:249–257.

Folkman J: Fighting cancer by attacking its blood supply. Sci Am 1996;275:150–154.

Klement G, Baruchel S, Rak J, et al: Continuous low-dose therapy with vinblastine and VEGF receptor-2 antibody induces sustained tumor regression without overt toxicity. J Clin Invest 2000;105:R15–R24.

Perez-Atayde AR, Sallan SE, Tedrow U, et al: Spectrum of tumor angiogenesis in the bone marrow of children with acute lymphoblastic leukemia. Am J Pathol 1997;150:815–820.

Pettersson A, Nagy JA, Brown LF, et al: Heterogeneity of the angiogenic response induced in different normal adult tissues by vascular permeability factor/vascular endothelial growth factor. Lab Invest 2000;80:99–115.

Presta M, Rusnati M, Belleri M, et al: Purine analogue 6-methylmercaptopurine riboside inhibits early and late phases of the angiogenesis process. Cancer Res 1999;59:2417–2424.

Tyrosine Kinase Inhibition

DiPaola RS, Rafi MM, Vyas V, Toppmeyer D, et al: Phase I clinical and pharmacologic study of 13-cis-retinoic acid, interferon alfa, and paclitaxel in patients with prostate cancer and other advanced malignancies. J Clin Oncol 1999; 17:2213–2218.

Druker BJ, Lydon NB: Lessons learned from the development of an abl tyrosine kinase inhibitor for chronic myelogenous leukemia. J Clin Invest 2000;105:3–7.

Druker BJ, Sawyers CL, Kantarjian H, et al: Activity of a specific inhibitor of the bcr-abl tyrosine kinase in the blast crisis of chronic myeloid leukemia and acute lymphoblastic leukemia with the philadelphia chromosome. N Engl J Med 2001;344:1038–1042.

Druker BJ, Talpaz M, Riesta DJ, et al: Efficacy and safety of a specific inhibitor of the bcr-abl tyrosine kinase in chronic myeloid leukemia. N Engl J Med 2001;344:1031–1037.

Lugo TG, Pendergast AM, Muller AJ, Witte ON: Tyrosine kinase activity and transformation potency of bcr-abl ongene products. Science 1990;247:1079–1082.

Chapter 49
Surgical Oncology

Monica M. Bertagnolli

Introduction

The earliest successful surgical treatment of a gastrointestinal cancer was probably accomplished by Pillore of Rouen, who performed a cecostomy for an obstructing colon cancer in 1776. In 1844, Reybard reported a survival after resection and anastomosis for cancer of the colon. This is a remarkable accomplishment, considering that it antedates general anesthesia. In 1879, Billroth resected a sigmoid cancer and exteriorized the proximal bowel as a permanent colostomy. The first successful surgery for gastric carcinoma is attributed to Billroth in 1881. During this procedure, the antrum and pylorus were removed and the duodenum was sutured to the gastric cardia, an operation that later became known as a Billroth I gastrectomy. The first cancer operation to meet present-day standards of adequate primary tumor resection and complete lymphadenectomy was performed by Miles, who developed the combined abdominoperineal resection in 1926. In 1938, Whipple successfully resected a tumor in the region of the pancreatic head, a complex procedure involving removal of the distal stomach, duodenum, and pancreatic head, and requiring reanastomosis of the pancreatic duct, distal common bile duct, and stomach to the proximal jejunum. After World War II, advances in blood transfusion, antibiotics, metabolic support, and anesthesia substantially reduced the mortality from radical cancer resections such as these.

During the 1970s, the distinct natural histories of different tumors were recognized. For most solid tissue cancers, it became clear that tumor involvement of regional lymph nodes is an indicator of systemic disease and that a poor prognosis is unlikely to be improved by increasing the scope of aggressive local extirpation. In the latter part of the twentieth century, contributions from radiation therapy and chemotherapy produced modest improvements in survival when used as adjuvant therapy for patients with stage III colorectal cancer. Comparable gains are still lacking

for the other primary gastrointestinal cancers. This chapter reviews some of the general principles guiding surgical oncology for cancers involving the gastrointestinal tract.

Preoperative Risk Assessment

Although minimal-access surgery and early postoperative feeding have decreased the adverse physiologic impact of intestinal surgery, these operations still require general anesthesia. Cancer surgery is frequently performed on patients in their sixties and beyond, who are likely to have comorbid conditions and nutritional compromise by their tumors. Decision making in major cancer surgery requires balancing surgical risks and benefits, and the first step in this process involves assessing the patient's physiologic reserves. This is particularly important in cancer patients who are of advanced age, as age alone is not an accurate predictor of surgical risk. Physical classification systems to identify patients with increased risk of adverse outcomes following major surgery include those developed by the American Society of Anesthesiologists and by Goldman et al. (Table 49-1).

Because more than 50% of all major perioperative complications or deaths are related to cardiovascular disease, identifying cardiac risk factors present prior to surgery is critically important. Optimal perioperative physiologic support can decrease surgical morbidity and mortality in patients with cardiac disease. The most commonly used method of assigning cardiac risk for patients undergoing major surgery appears in Tables 49-2 and 49-3. On the basis of this classification, patients whose preoperative state places them in risk category III or IV should be considered for invasive perioperative monitoring. Patients with evidence of potentially treatable cardiovascular disease, such as unstable angina or transient ischemic attacks, should undergo complete evaluation and treatment of these conditions prior to tumor resection. For patients with good functional status and no signs

Table 49-1 ■ Functional Classification of Physical Status

Risk Category	American Society of Anesthesiologists	Goldman Classification
Class I	No physiologic, biochemical, or psychiatric disturbance; the pathologic process for which surgery is to be performed is localized and not conducive to systemic disturbance	Ordinary physical activity, such as walking and climbing stairs, does not cause angina. Angina occurs with strenuous or rapid or prolonged exertion at work or recreation.
Class II	Mild to moderate systemic disturbance caused either by the condition to be treated surgically or by other pathophysiologic processes	Slight limitation of ordinary activity. Angina occurs with walking or climbing stairs rapidly, walking uphill, walking or stair climbing after meals or in cold, in wind, under emotional stress, or only during the few hours after awakening. Angina occurs when walking more than two blocks on the level or climbing more than one flight of ordinary stairs at a normal pace and in normal conditions.
Class III	Severe systemic disturbance or pathology	Marked limitation of ordinary physical activity. Angina occurs when walking one to two blocks on the level and climbing one flight of stairs in normal conditions and at a normal pace.
Class IV	Severe systemic disorder that is immediately life-threatening and not always correctable by the operative procedure	Inability to carry on any physical activity without discomfort. Angina may be present at rest.
Class V	Moribund condition; little chance of surviving surgery	
Emergency (E)	Any patient in one of the classes listed above operated on in an emergency situation	

Table 49-2 ■ Goldman's Cardiac Risk Index

Risk Factor	Points
Jugular venous distension/S3 gallop	11
Myocardial infarction in the previous 6 months	10
Any rhythm other than sinus or premature atrial contractions on preoperative electrocardiogram	7
More than 5 premature ventricular contractions per minute on preoperative electrocardiogram	7
Age more than 70 years	5
Emergency procedure	4
Intrathoracic, intraperitoneal, or aortic operation	3
Poor general medical condition (arterial $PO_2 < 60$ mmHg or $>PCO_2$ 50 mmHg; $K^+ < 3$ mEq/L or BUN >50 mg/dL; abnormal serum glutamic-oxaloacetic transaminase; signs of chronic liver disease)	3
Hemodynamically significant aortic stenosis	3

Class	Point Total	Minor Complications	Life-Threatening Complications	Cardiac Deaths
I (N = 537)	0–5	532 (99%)	4 (0.7%)	1 (0.2%)
II (N = 316)	6–12	295 (93%)	12 (5%)	5 (2%)
III (N = 130)	13–25	112 (86%)	15 (11%)	3 (2%)
IV (N = 18)	≥26	4 (22%)	4 (22%)	10 (56%)

Table 49-3 ■ Reduction of Perioperative Cardiac Risk

Risk	Recommended Preoperative Cardiac Evaluation	Recommended Action
Low: Class I and <12 points	None	Proceed with surgery with usual monitoring
Medium: Class II or III, 12–26 points or cannot assess by history	Exercise testing or, if unable to exercise, dipyridamole thallium or stress echo	Consider invasive perioperative monitoring
High: Class IV or >26 points	Cardiac catheterization	Coronary artery revascularization, if possible, before surgery

of cardiovascular disease, the risk and cost of noninvasive preoperative cardiac evaluation are not warranted. These individuals have a very low risk of perioperative myocardial infarction or death from cardiac causes.

Nutrition

Most patients undergoing cancer surgery withstand the associated brief period of nutritional deficit and catabolism after surgery without difficulty. It is not unusual, however, to encounter patients whose nutrition is compromised. The degree of compromise can range from mild, with no adverse effect on treatment outcome, to cancer cachexia (see Chapter 1, "Weight Loss"), a paraneoplastic syndrome characterized by anorexia, and progression to multiple organ dysfunction. For many patients with intestinal tumors, anorexia and the resulting malnutrition are exacerbated by tumor-associated changes in gastrointestinal function and by the surgery, chemotherapy, and radiation therapy used to treat the tumor.

Nutritional assessment for patients with cancer includes a dietary history, with documentation of recent weight change, anorexia, early satiety, or dysphagia. Findings on physical examination that suggest malnutrition include evidence of muscle wasting; dry, flaky skin texture; brittle hair or unusual hair loss; and ridging or spooning of the nails. Important laboratory tests for nutritional evaluation include serum albumin and transferrin levels. These assessments allow patients to be classified into clinically relevant categories that indicate the extent of their nutritional reserves (Table 49-4).

Maintenance of adequate preoperative oral nutrition should be a high priority for all patients undergoing major surgery. This imperative is sometimes overlooked when gastrointestinal cancer patients receive multiple preoperative endoscopic or radiologic evaluations requiring fasting or have tumor-associated

Table 49-4 ■ Preoperative Nutritional Assessment

	Normal Nutritional Reserves	Mild-to-Moderate Nutritional Deficit	Severe Malnutrition
Weight	Normal, or recent loss <6% of body weight	Recent loss 6% to 12% of body weight	Recent loss ≥12% of body weight
Physical exam	Normal	Normal	Muscle wasting, skin, hair or nail changes
Serum albumin level	≥3.5 g/dL	2.6–3.4 g/dL	≤2.5 g/dL
Serum transferrin level	≥200 mg/dL	151–199 mg/dL	≤150 mg/dL

anorexia or nausea. Controversy remains over the clinical benefits of nutritional intervention in cancer patients. In the most extreme case of patients with severe malnutrition, most studies support the use of perioperative total parenteral nutrition (TPN). Aggressive nutritional support is also necessary for patients whose treatment will result in prolonged periods (10 to 14 days) of inadequate nutritional intake. The benefits to these patients, including decreased operative morbidity and mortality and improved wound healing, exceed the increased risk due to total parenteral nutrition-related infections. Patients with severe nutrition should receive a minimum of seven days of nutritional therapy before a major surgical procedure and should continue to receive adequate nutrition, via total parenteral nutrition or feeding jejunostomy if necessary, as soon as possible after surgery. For all other patients, the risks of total parenteral nutrition–related complications are probably greater than the benefits of decreased recovery time and marginally improved outcome. It is clear, however, that maximizing enteral nutrition by early postoperative feeding or nasogastric or jejunostomy feedings when necessary and feasible is an effective, safe, and sometimes overlooked way to speed patient recovery. Enteral nutrition should be given precedence over parenteral nutrition whenever possible.

Staging

Accurate staging enhances the care of gastrointestinal cancer patients and becomes even more important as new therapeutic modalities emerge. Patients who are known to have localized disease can avoid extensive surgery or toxic adjuvant therapies, and identification of clinically significant micrometastatic disease selects a group of patients who are likely to benefit from adjuvant therapy. The wide range of treatment responses that are observed within the present staging categories for gastrointestinal cancers suggest that these categories are too encompassing and that, particularly for stage II disease, more precise delineation is needed. Approaches to improve gastrointestinal cancer staging include surgical methods, such as staging laparoscopy and sentinel node excision, as well as new techniques for examining tissue employing immunohistochemical and molecular markers.

Staging Laparoscopy

The application of minimally invasive technology has decreased staging and treatment morbidity for gastrointestinal cancer patients. In many patients, for example, staging laparoscopy makes it possible to avoid a laparotomy, especially for cancers of the gas-

troesophageal junction, stomach, liver, and pancreas. Because laparoscopy is best used to examine the visible surfaces of the peritoneum and the abdominal organs, the sensitivity of laparoscopy for detection of unresectable disease is significantly increased by the application of endoscopic or laparoscopic ultrasound.

In a study of patients with upper gastrointestinal malignancies, including lower esophageal, gastric, and pancreatic cancers, laparoscopy alone provided additional staging information compared to conventional imaging in one half of the patients. The added information contributed to advancing the clinical stage of most of these patients, but some were downstaged after the procedure. The value of laparoscopy was enhanced by the addition of ultrasonography, which changed the clinical management in one half of the patients by supplying more detailed information than that obtained with conventional imaging, including undisclosed portal vein invasion and liver metastases. In a prospective study of 103 consecutive patients with gastric adenocarcinoma, laparoscopy was the most sensitive of several staging studies in the detection of hepatic, nodal, and peritoneal metastases. Its accuracy rate was 99%, compared to 76% for ultrasound and 79% for computed tomography (CT) of the abdomen. In another group of patients with pancreatic cancer who had no evidence of distant disease by computed tomography, laparoscopy confirmed intra-abdominal disease extension in one quarter of the patients. In the remaining three quarters of patients, angiography documented vascular invasion in half of those without apparent metastatic disease. As a measure of the improved staging precision, 30 of 40 patients proceeding to laparotomy were found to be resectable.

In 50 patients with liver metastases, laparoscopy with laparoscopic ultrasound detected disease that precluded curative hepatic resection in 23 patients (46%). These included new lesions not seen on magnetic resonance imaging (MRI) or computed tomography scans in 14 patients (28%). Laparoscopy with laparoscopic ultrasound is highly useful in determining unresectability in patients with hepatic metastases, without the need for open laparotomy. This technique is most useful for upper gastrointestinal malignancies that exhibit peritoneal spread missed by noninvasive imaging techniques.

Laparoscopy also provides the opportunity to perform peritoneal lavage for peritoneal cytology. The use of peritoneal cytology for staging of gastrointestinal malignancies is controversial, however. For example, in a large series of patients, which included 87 esophageal cancers, 72 proximal bile duct tumors, 236 periampullary pancreatic cancers, 17 cancers of the pancreatic body or tail, and 7 primary and 32 metastatic liver cancers, peritoneal lavage altered the assessment of stage and accurately predicted unresectable disease in only 6 (1.3%) patients. Moreover, of 28 patients with positive cytology, 3 proved to be falsely positive, and those 3 cancers were resected at laparotomy. The contribution of peritoneal lavage cytology to staging remains uncertain.

Sentinel Nodes in Gastrointestinal Cancer

The clinical importance of individual tumor cells from solid tissue malignancies discovered in lymph nodes, bone marrow, or circulating blood is unclear. Tumors readily shed individual cells into the circulation, and these can be detected in tissue samples by polymerase chain reaction (PCR)-based methods. The clinical importance of circulating tumor cells resides in their ability to lodge in host tissues and form independently proliferating metastatic colonies. Such "micrometastases" likely represent a small fraction of the cells shed from a tumor. To date, numerous studies have failed to correlate the presence of small numbers of tumor cells in lymph nodes, bone marrow, or circulating blood with the clinical behavior of tumors. This distinction is obviously most important for tumors that are responsive to adjuvant therapies, such as colorectal or gastric cancers.

Conventional staging of gastrointestinal tumors involves inspection of a single section from each identified lymph node by light microscopy after hematoxylin and eosin (H&E) staining. One way to improve the sensitivity of detection of nodal metastases is to examine multiple sections from multiple levels in each mesenteric lymph node. Clearance of the mesenteric fat with solvents can be used to increase the total number of lymph nodes sampled from a colectomy specimen. Both of these processes are prohibited by the time and expense involved in their execution. The sentinel lymph node sampling technique offers a potential means to obviate these laborious methods. It is routinely used for the staging of malignant melanoma and breast cancer. A tracer, consisting of dye or radioactive colloid, is injected near the tumor. This tracer is taken up by the lymphatics adjacent to the tumor and transported to the nearest draining lymph node. The node is identified by the surgeon and removed for extensive histopathologic examination. Cancer cells entering the tumor site's lymphatic drainage colonize the lymph nodes in a sequential fashion. Thus, the first draining node, or "sentinel" node, should be positive if any of the nodes beyond that level are positive. This has been confirmed clinically and histologically in approximately 96% of melanoma cases and 95% of breast cancers.

In a prospective study of 76 consecutive colorectal cancer patients, a sentinel node was identified successfully in 99% of patients using an injection of isosulfan blue at the tumor site. All of the mesenteric lymph nodes from patients in this study were then examined by a multilevel sectioning technique. In 96% of patients whose sentinel lymph nodes were free of metastases, all other draining lymph nodes were negative as well. Of patients who had demonstrable metastases in their sentinel nodes, 17% had no other regional draining nodes involved on complete lymph node dissection and examination.

Although effective in increasing the detection of nodal metastases in melanoma, examining sections at multiple levels in the sentinel node in gastrointestinal cancer does not improve staging. All of the 542 lymph nodes that were extracted from colon cancer primary resection specimens that were negative on the basis of standard single-level hematoxylin and eosin examination remained negative after multiple-level sectioning. Occult metastases were not identified even after immunohistochemistry using monoclonal anticytokeratin antibody against cytokeratin-18, CAM 5.2. Multilevel sectioning seems unnecessary in evaluating the regional lymph nodes from patients with gastrointestinal cancer. Whether sentinel node localization and analysis can be used to guide therapy in stage II colon cancer requires evaluation in a multi-institutional clinical trial.

Radioimmune-Guided Surgery

Radioimmune-guided surgery provides intraoperative localization of tumor in tissues that would not ordinarily be identified and removed as part of a standard cancer resection. The opportunity exists not only for extended resection, but also for the use of intraoperative radiation therapy or for adjuvant postoperative chemotherapy and/or radiation therapy. The technique involves injecting a radiolabeled monoclonal antibody into the patient three to four weeks prior to surgery. A monoclonal antibody directed against the epithelial tumor antigen, tumor-associated glycoprotein-72, is used most often for defining the extent of gastrointestinal cancers. The antibody is labeled with ^{125}I and therefore must be administered with a thyroid-blocking agent such as potassium iodide. During exploratory laparotomy, in addition to the usual inspection and palpation, the abdomen is scanned with a handheld gamma probe, taking as background the count corresponding to circulating blood, obtained at the bifurcation of the aorta. The local tumor field and associated nodal basins are then scanned for increased signal, which indicates residual disease. Complete survey of the abdomen with the gamma probe also includes the liver, stomach, duodenum, and posterior retroperitoneum, including kidneys and pelvis. Problems with the technique include low specificity in lymph node tissue, possibly due to clearance of the antibody by the reticuloendothelial system.

Radioimmune-guided surgery may have prognostic value. In a multicenter phase III trial for recurrent or metastatic intra-abdominal cancer, surgical decision making was altered by radioimmune guided surgery 20% of the time, by extending the resection to adjacent tissues. In patients with liver metastases, radioimmune-guided surgery located identified occult metastases in the periportal lymph nodes of 29% of patients and identified those who were not likely to be cured by liver resection. Radioimmune-guided surgery has not yet demonstrated an impact on patient treatment morbidity or survival, and this technique is costly and fairly cumbersome.

Molecular Characterization of Tumors

Tumor-associated genotypic or phenotypic markers add to conventional assessment of histologic grade or degree of invasion by measuring cell cycle control, angiogenic potential, or genomic stability, to name a few functional categories (Table 49-5).

Measurement of thymidylate synthase is one example of how a tumor-associated marker can provide useful clinical information. Thymidylate synthase is an enzyme required for DNA synthesis, as it converts 2'-deoxyuridine 5'-monophosphate (dUMP) to thymidine 5'-monophosphate (dTMP). Thymidylate synthase is a critical target for 5-fluorouracil, the most commonly used chemotherapeutic agent for gastrointestinal malignancies. DNA synthesis is inhibited by 5-FU through formation of a ternary complex between thymidylate synthase, a metabolite of 5-fluorouracil called fluorodeoxyuridine monophosphate (FdUMP), and a tetrahydrofolic folic acid derivative. Increased expression of thymidylate synthase predicts a poor response to chemotherapy regimens using 5-fluorouracil.

Most reports linking genotypic or phenotypic characteristics of tumors to clinical outcome are single-marker studies, performed either retrospectively or prospectively with a small number of patients. Although some of these markers, such as thymidylate synthase, appear to have independent prognostic value, their clinical utility remains in question because of variability in laboratory methods, differences in treatment within the study cohort, and insufficient clinical follow-up.

Extent of Resection of Primary Tumor

As understanding of tumor biology has progressed, the surgical techniques used to remove cancers have evolved. Advances in endoscopy, radiology, and perioperative support have led to earlier diagnosis and an increase in the number of long-term survivors of cancer. Cancer surgery techniques include sharp, rather than blunt, dissection of the tissue planes, en bloc tumor resection with avoidance of tumor cell spillage, complete regional lymphadenectomy, and as wide a tumor margin as possible without undue morbidity to the patient. Apart from the recognition of the importance of tumor-free excision margins, however, it has been extremely difficult to objectively measure the impact of differences in surgical technique on treatment outcome. Moreover, the value of the "more is better" approach to cancer surgery was challenged by the observation that in many cancers at the time of surgery, the disease is already systemic and not localized.

Accurate measurement of the extent of surgical resection may be one of the most important pieces of clinical information for a gastrointestinal cancer patient. The importance of proper handling of operative specimens prior to and during examination by the surgical pathologist cannot be overestimated. Complicated specimens demand a substantial amount of experience and knowledge to be properly examined, and a microscopic diagnosis is of limited value unless it is interpreted in the context of essential clinical data. Only the operative surgeon understands fully the relationship of the tumor to the remaining tissues and the method or thoroughness of the resection. The addition of complementary molecular and micrometastatic tumor analyses to standard histopathology makes collaboration between the surgical pathologist and the cancer surgeon all the more critical to optimal cancer treatment.

Table 49-5 ■ Markers of Prognosis or Treatment Response

Carcinoembryonic antigen	PCNA	p53
Thymidylate synthase	Ki67	p21
Thymidylate phosphorylase	Cyclin D1	p27
Matrix metalloproteinases	Ploidy	Myc
Cathepsin D	Apoptotic index	Bcl2/Bax
Si LeA/Si LeX	Microvascular density	17pLOH
CD44 v6, v8–10	VEGF	18qLOH
Plasminogen activator	Sucrase-isomaltase	DCC
UPA receptor	Prolactin receptor	Ki-ras
Her/2-neu	Vitamin D receptor	Microsatellite instability

Laparoscopic Cancer Resections

Minimally invasive surgical techniques have gained widespread application in general surgery over the past 10 years. Laparoscopic resections of the gallbladder and spleen have become preferred operations because they provide a significant reduction in patient morbidity compared to open procedures. The laparoscopic approach is also frequently used to treat benign diseases of the stomach and large bowel such as gastroesophageal reflux, diverticulitis, or inflammatory bowel disease. The use of laparoscopy for potentially curative resection of gastrointestinal cancers, however, has been approached with caution by the surgical oncology community. The overriding concern is that the short-term benefits of decreased hospital stay and earlier return to activities compared to laparotomy might not be worthwhile if the result is a decreased cure rate, an endpoint that takes many years to determine. Many surgeons also question whether laparoscopic techniques allow for an adequate regional lymphadenectomy and whether laparoscopic excision is associated with an increased rate of local or distant recurrence. As instruments and operative techniques have improved, adequate extent of surgical resection, including lymphadenectomy, no longer appears to be a significant issue. Early data from series of laparoscopic colon cancer resections suggested a small but increased risk of incisional (port-site) recurrence. A review of clinical data for the past 10 years, however, suggests that the incidence of incisional tumor recurrences following laparoscopic colectomy is comparable to that of open colectomy. Full acceptance of laparoscopic colectomy as standard treatment for potentially curable malignant gastrointestinal tumor awaits the results of the NIH's ongoing randomized clinical trial.

Intraoperative Radiation Therapy

Another promising addition to the surgical management of gastrointestinal tumors is the delivery of radiation to the tissues at the time of surgery, or intraoperative radiation therapy. The combination of intraoperative radiation therapy with preoperative or postoperative external beam radiation and chemotherapy theoretically allows delivery of a maximal dose of radiation therapy, as dose-limiting structures such as the small bowel or bladder can be excluded from the intraoperative radiation therapy field. The currently available methods of delivering intraoperative radiation therapy include electron beam and high-dose brachytherapy. This latter method involves the application of radiation through a flexible catheter system that can conform to complicated areas of anatomy such as the deep pelvis. Single-dose electron beam intraoperative radiation therapy is equivalent to two to three times the equivalent dose of external beam radiation in terms of antitumor effect. This treatment is best applied in cases in which the risk of local recurrence without systemic metastases is relatively high. For this reason, intraoperative radiation therapy has been used for management of locally advanced rectal cancer, for which from 15% to 30% of patients develop isolated locoregional recurrence. Intraoperative radiation therapy may also be appropriate when dose-limiting structures permit limited delivery of external beam radiation, even though the chance of systemic recurrence is high, as occurs in selected patients with gastric, esophageal, pancreatic, or bile duct malignancies.

Results from randomized, controlled trials comparing intraoperative radiation therapy to external beam radiation alone are not yet available; however, comparison of intraoperative radiation therapy with historical controls suggest a benefit in locoregional disease control and prevention of local recurrence. Although the results are promising, the reported series are small, the patients differ in many respects from the historical controls, and the patient populations are heterogeneous with regard to operative and radiation therapy techniques. Comparisons of morbidity are also lacking.

Intraoperative Radiation Therapy and Peritoneal Chemotherapy

A small number of patients with gastrointestinal malignancies develop involvement of the peritoneal surfaces without evidence of disease in other organs such as liver or lungs. Primary tumors that classically give rise to this condition are mucinous adenocarcinoma of the colorectum or adenocarcinoma of the stomach, small bowel, or appendix. In some cases, particularly for low-grade malignancies such as grade I mucinous adenocarcinoma or pseudomyxoma peritonei, significant local disease control can be achieved by cytoreductive surgery, often with the addition of intraperitoneal chemotherapy. Cytoreductive surgery involves stripping the peritoneum from the surfaces of the diaphragm, anterior abdominal wall, and pelvis, in addition to an omentectomy and perhaps a splenectomy, cholecystectomy, or antrectomy as well. The extent of tumor reduction achieved by cytoreductive surgery is the most important prognostic indicator for patients treated with intraperitoneal chemotherapy. In a group of 86 patients with peritoneal carcinomatosis treated with cytoreductive surgery and intraperitoneal chemotherapy with mitomycin C and 5-fluorouracil, 64% of patients were alive at three years if no visible tumor remained or implants were less than 2.5 mm in diameter. None of the patients with tumor implants greater than 2.5 mm following the cytoreductive procedure were alive at three years.

Intraperitoneal chemotherapy is administered via catheters positioned in the abdominal cavity at the time of cytoreductive surgery. The theoretical advantage of intraperitoneal chemotherapy is that maximal doses can be delivered to the tumor-bearing peritoneal surface by this approach, as a tenfold higher concentration is tolerated by intraperitoneal administration than can be administered systemically. Recent studies suggest that for patients with resected gastric and colon cancer, the intraperitoneal fluid distribution remains adequate in 94% of patients at six months, and combined intravenous and intraperitoneal dosing of 5-fluorouracil produces a peritoneal fluid to plasma drug concentration ratio of 100:1.

Intraperitoneal administration concentrates chemotherapeutic agents in the hepatic parenchyma. Because local and hepatic metastases are the most common pattern of recurrence for patients with stage II and III colorectal cancer, the effectiveness of adjuvant intraperitoneal chemotherapy was assessed. In a randomized trial of 241 patients with resected stage III colon cancer, Scheithauer et al. demonstrated a significant improvement in disease-free and overall survival following six months (six courses) of 5-fluorouracil + leucovorin given both systemically and intraperitoneally, compared to the same agents given only systemically. Recently, Vaillant et al. extended this observation to stage II colon cancer. The role of intraperitoneal chemotherapy for routine adjuvant therapy of colorectal and other intra-abdominal malignancies, such as gastric or pancreatic tumors, has yet to be defined but appears promising.

The cytostatic effect of some chemotherapeutic agents is potentiated by hyperthermia, perhaps through improved tissue penetration. In addition, application of chemotherapy to the abdominal cavity at the time of surgery offers the theoretical advantages of access of the chemotherapeutic agent to all tissue surfaces before the tumor cells are isolated by the healing process. Residual tumor cells that are freely mobile in the abdominal cavity at the completion of the cytoreductive surgery are also potentially treated before closure of the operative field. Intraperitoneal hyperthermic chemotherapy entails aggressive surgical debulking followed by heated intraperitoneal perfusion of chemotherapy, generally with agents such as mitomycin C or cisplatin. Single-arm as well as some randomized clinical studies suggest that this treatment reduces local recurrence of gastric cancer and may increase disease-free survival of patients with disseminated spread of appendiceal, colorectal, and pancreatic cancers. Responding patients are generally limited to those with minimal peritoneal spread or those at high risk owing to bulky locoregional disease. In a series of 200 patients treated with this modality, complications, including pancreatitis, fistula formation, bleeding, and hematological toxicity, occurred in approximately 27% of patients, and the treatment-related mortality rate was 1.5%. In the absence of other effective but less morbid treatments, intraperitoneal chemotherapy alone or with intraoperative hyperthermia remains an option for management of this patient population with an otherwise dismal prognosis.

Hepatic Artery Infusion

Over one half of all patients with metastatic colorectal cancer develop liver metastases, and in many of these, the liver is the only or the predominant site of disease. Resection of limited disease in the liver clearly increases survival and offers the possibility of cure. Cryotherapy can also successfully ablate limited liver disease, and this technique has been added to the options that are available both in the operating room and via percutaneous access. Other nonoperative ablative techniques include percutaneous injection of lesions with ethanol and application of radiofrequency energy via probes. These procedures are useful for patients with impaired physical reserves but are limited to those with small lesions that are relatively few in number. Unfortunately, many patients with colorectal cancer present with liver-only disease that is not amenable to resection or ablation. Because tumor metastases derive their blood supply from the hepatic artery, whereas hepatocytes are supplied by the hepatic vein, intra-arterial administration of the 5-fluorouracil metabolite (FUDR) produces significant intratumoral drug levels while theoretically limiting hepatic toxicity. A high first-pass extraction of 5-fluorouracil metabolite (approximately 95%) limits the systemic effect of hepatic artery infusion. Despite the favorable drug ratio between tumor and hepatocytes, hepatic artery infusion is associated with the potentially fatal complications of drug-induced hepatitis and sclerosing cholangitis.

For unresectable hepatic metastases, the effects of hepatic artery infusion added to standard intravenous chemotherapy have been difficult to assess. The available studies include small patient numbers and are problematic because of crossover between treatment arms and inability to establish adequate hepatic artery perfusion in some patients who are randomized to receive this treatment. Meta-analyses of the randomized trials reported to date, however, suggest that hepatic artery infusional therapy increases the short-term survival rate by 10% to 15%.

Patients who undergo successful resection of a hepatic colorectal metastasis have a 70% to 80% incidence of disease recurrence, and in approximately 50% of these recurrences, the liver will be the only site of disease. In one study, coordinated by the Eastern Cooperative Oncology Group, 109 patients with liver-only colorectal cancer metastases were preoperatively randomized to either surgery alone or surgery plus hepatic artery infusional chemotherapy with 5-fluorouracil metabolite, followed by infusional 5-fluorouracil. With a median follow-up of four years, the three-year recurrence free survival rate in the surgery alone group was 34%, compared to 58% in patients receiving combined modality therapy ($P = .039$). A second randomized study compared hepatic artery infusion of 5-fluorouracil metabolite and dexamethasone combined with systemic 5-fluorouracil and leucovorin to treatment with systemic 5-fluorouracil and leukovorin alone in this same patient population. The two-year disease-free survival rate was 85% in the group receiving hepatic artery infusional chemotherapy compared to 69% in the systemic-treatment-only arm. These two studies suggest that chemotherapy, including hepatic artery infusional chemotherapy, may increase survival following resection of isolated hepatic metastases from colorectal cancer.

Management of Malignant Bowel Obstruction

Bowel obstruction is relatively common in gastrointestinal cancer patients, whether it is the initial presentation of an intestinal malignancy, produced by recurrent or metastatic disease, or associated with benign causes such as postoperative adhesion formation (see Chapter 19, "Bowel Obstruction"). Approximately 15% of patients with intestinal cancer exhibit some degree of obstruction on presentation, and another 3% to 8% present with perforation of the carcinoma. Patients with these complications are generally elderly and have advanced disease at the time of surgery, resulting in a crude five-year survival rate of 25% to 34%. Prompt surgical intervention is essential for patients with acute intestinal obstruction or perforation. Even for distal colonic lesions, most patients with good physiologic status and a relatively brief duration of preoperative symptoms can be treated by resection of the tumor with primary anastomosis, avoiding a temporary diverting ileostomy or colostomy. For colorectal tumors, although the presence of obstruction or perforation is generally associated with advanced disease, 30% to 50% of these cases will prove to be limited to stage II disease. The five-year survival rate for these "high-risk" stage II patients is less than that for those presenting without complications, particularly for perforated tumors, for which the five-year survival rate approaches that of patients with stage III disease.

One of the more difficult problems faced by a surgeon is the management of bowel obstruction in a patient with a past history of abdominal cancer. The cause of intestinal obstruction is benign in one third of patients who present within five years of treatment for a primary gastrointestinal cancer. Of the remaining two thirds, approximately one half have carcinomatosis that can be identified by computed tomography or by physical examination. The goal is to identify patients with benign or localized disease whose obstruction can be treated or palliated surgically. All too often, however, patients with recurrent intestinal tumors and bowel obstruction have diffuse intraperitoneal disease. In this setting, attempted surgical treatment is at best ineffective and at worst may contribute substantially to disease morbidity. It is not surprising, therefore, that the hospital mortality rate of bowel obstruction from recurrent intra-abdominal tumor is 20% to 40%.

The operative approach to intestinal obstruction in patients with a history of intra-abdominal malignancy is dictated by the extent of tumor and the location of the obstruction. Preoperative imaging is essential for these complicated cases, as the presence of extensive tumor can make full surgical exploration difficult or impossible. Spiral computed tomography scanning is an excellent method for determining the extent of disease and frequently the point of obstruction. Care must be taken to preserve the physiologic reserves of patients who are potential surgical candidates, including the use of total parenteral nutrition if a trial of nonoperative management is attempted. Surgical exploration is clearly indicated for patients with a history of intra-abdominal malignancy whose physical examination and imaging studies suggest localized intestinal obstruction. Not only will a significant proportion of these patients have benign disease as the etiology of their obstruction, but for patients with good performance status, surgery to relieve localized malignant obstructions can improve the patient's quality of life by relieving nausea, vomiting, and abdominal pain. Palliative procedures consist of lysis of adhesions, small bowel bypass, decompressive colostomy, and gastrostomy. Complete resection of recurrent disease is possible only in rare instances.

It is unusual for a patient with diffuse carcinomatosis to present with an acute complete intestinal obstruction. Instead, these patients usually have a protracted course of nausea, vomiting, crampy abdominal pain, and abdominal films that are consistent with partial bowel obstruction. These patients are generally managed nonoperatively with nasogastric decompression, intravenous hydration or total parenteral nutrition, antiemetics, and judicious use of pain medications. Nonoperative management is often only a temporary solution, as approximately 50% of these patients will eventually progress to complete obstruction. In addition, patients whose obstructions resolve following nonoperative management often continue to have obstructive symptoms after discharge. Unfortunately, for those with a significant disease burden, these symptoms also persist in patients receiving palliative surgery for gastrointestinal cancer.

For patients with complete bowel obstruction due to diffuse intra-abdominal tumor spread, surgery to relieve the obstruction is rarely successful. In this case, surgery is generally reserved for patients with good performance status, as those with widespread visceral metastases whose activities are limited are particularly unlikely to benefit from surgery.

Surgical Management of Complications of Radiation Therapy

Radiation-induced bowel injury can be manifest as an acute or chronic problem. Acute radiation enteritis is experienced by almost all patients receiving pelvic or abdominal radiation therapy. This complication is due to radiation-induced injury to the actively dividing cells of the intestinal mucosa, which causes nausea, vomiting, abdominal pain, diarrhea, or tenesmus. The symptoms generally resolve within a few weeks of completion of therapy. The treatment of acute radiation enteritis includes antiemetics, pain medication, and maintenance of hydration.

Chronic radiation injury to the intestine is a progressive condition characterized histologically by chronic inflammation, fibrosis, and obliterative endarteritis. The period between radiation exposure and clinical manifestations of a chronic radiation-associated injury averages two years but can occur within months or not for many years. Chronic radiation-associated destruction of the intestine can progress to become a transmural injury leading to obstruction, bleeding, perforation, and fistula and stricture formation. In one large series of patients undergoing radiation therapy with or without chemotherapy for rectal cancer, the incidence of chronic proctitis was 12.5%, and 5% of patients developed chronic enteritis. Operation for therapy of complications of chronic enteritis was required in 5% of the patients.

Optimal operative intervention in these patients consists of resection of the involved intestine with reanastomosis. For friable segments of strictured small intestine that are adherent deep in the pelvis or cannot be resected for other reasons, an intestinal bypass procedure is the treatment of choice, with diversion or exclusion reserved for the most recalcitrant cases. If necessarily left in place, the diseased segment is subject to additional complications, such as ulceration, bleeding, and fistula formation; secondary surgery may therefore be needed in up to one half of patients. Perioperative mortality rates from severe complications of radiation enteritis may be as high as 40% to 50%.

The practice of preoperative radiation and chemotherapy for rectal cancer may decrease the incidence of chronic radiation enteritis. The preoperative pelvis is free of adhesions, allowing techniques such as prone positioning, maintenance of a full bladder, and use of a "belly board" to move the small intestine out of the radiation field more effectively. In addition, improved general mobility of the intestine prevents repeated delivery of radiation to the same area of intestine. Treatment-related toxicity appears to be the same as for patients receiving postoperatively adjuvant therapy.

Prophylactic Gastrointestinal Cancer Surgery

For the lower gastrointestinal tract, cancer prevention is effectively achieved by endoscopic surveillance with removal of premalignant adenomas from the intestinal tract. There are three clinical disorders, however, in which colorectal cancer develops either with high frequency or by acceleration of the adenoma-carcinoma sequence to the extent that prophylactic colectomy or proctocolectomy becomes an appropriate option for consideration. These conditions include familial adenomatous polyposis, hereditary nonpolyposis colorectal cancer, and chronic ulcerative colitis (see Chapter 92, "Colorectal Cancer").

Familial Adenomatous Polyposis

Familial adenomatous polyposis is an autosomal-dominant cancer predisposition syndrome characterized by the development of hundreds to thousands of colorectal adenomas and the inevitable progression to colorectal cancer by the third to fourth decade of life. Familial adenomatous polyposis is now recognized as a systemic disease caused by a germline mutation of the *APC* gene, and the phenotype can include desmoid tumors, duodenal adenomas and carcinomas, mandibular osteomas, congenital hypertrophy of the retinal pigmented epithelium, and cutaneous epidermoid tumors. Although treatment with nonsteroidal anti-inflammatory medications (NSAIDs) such as sulindac or celecoxib reduces the number and size of the polyps, total proctocolectomy is the most successful method of cancer prevention. Since 8% to 12% of these patients also develop duodenal carcinomas, lifetime surveillance of the upper gastrointestinal tract is also crucial.

Prophylactic surgery for patients with familial adenomatous polyposis involves either total proctocolectomy, generally with J-pouch ileoanal reconstruction, or total colectomy with ileorectal anastomosis, followed by lifetime surveillance of the remaining rectal segment. The choice of operation requires balancing the higher rate of complications of total proctocolectomy against ileorectal anastomosis, which carries the long-term risk of cancer developing in the retained rectal segment. Before age 50, the cumulative risk of rectal carcinoma in patients receiving an ileorectal anastomosis is 10%, but the risk increases markedly in patients more than 50 years old. The absence of a rectum in patients undergoing ileoanal anastomosis produces tolerable symptomatology when the procedure is performed in young adulthood. After the procedure, teenagers experienced a mean daytime and nighttime stool frequencies of 4 ± 1.5 and 1 ± 1, respectively; daytime incontinence was exceedingly rare; and impotence or retrograde ejaculation did not occur. These outcomes, plus elimination of the risk of cancer, lead most patients with familial adenomatous polyposis to opt for total proctocolectomy.

Hereditary Nonpolyposis Colorectal Cancer

Hereditary nonpolyposis colorectal cancer is transmitted as an autosomal-dominant familial syndrome with a high risk of development of colorectal cancer, but precursor colonic adenomas are not abundant as in familial adenomatous polyposis. These families also have a high incidence of endometrial, gastric, and urothelial carcinomas. Hereditary nonpolyposis colorectal cancer is caused by germline defects in genes encoding DNA mismatch repair enzymes. Faulty mismatch repair creates an enhanced potential for malignant transformation in the intestinal epithelium, a finding that is also present in 12% to 16% of "sporadic" colorectal cancers. Because of the associated DNA repair defects, the time to progression from adenoma to carcinoma may be accelerated in these patients. In contrast to patients with familial adenomatous polyposis, fewer individuals with hereditary nonpolyposis colorectal cancer develop colorectal cancer, and the natural history of the illness is difficult to predict. Because of this uncertainty, the practice of prophylactic subtotal colectomy for germline carriers of mismatch repair mutations is controversial. However, if a patient with hereditary nonpolyposis colorectal cancer develops a colorectal at a young age, particularly those with multiple colonic adenomas,

most surgeons agree that subtotal colectomy is appropriate.

Chronic Ulcerative Colitis

Chronic ulcerative colitis is an autoimmune disorder of the large intestine characterized by abdominal pain, bleeding, and persistent inflammation, ulceration, and stricture formation that carries a substantial risk of subsequent colorectal cancer. Approximately 10% to 25% of patients with active chronic ulcerative colitis for 25 or more years develop colorectal cancer, and colorectal cancer is the cause of death in up to 15% of these patients. The management of patients with chronic ulcerative colitis must include lifelong frequent surveillance colonoscopy with biopsy to detect precancerous dysplasia. In some cases, depending on the age at onset, the severity of the disease, and the patient's wishes, prophylactic total proctocolectomy is performed.

References

Chemotherapy

Bozzetti F, Vaglini M, Deraco M: Intraperitoneal hyperthermic chemotherapy in gastric cancer: Rationale for a new approach. Tumori 1998;84:483–488.

Drake JC, Voeller DM, Allegra CJ, Johnston PG: The effect of dose and interval between 5-fluorouracil and leucovorin on the formation of thymidylate synthase ternary complex in human cancer cells. Br J Cancer 1995;71:1145–1150.

Hirose K, Katayama K, Iida A, et al: Efficacy of continuous hyperthermic peritoneal perfusion for the prophylaxis and treatment of peritoneal metastasis of advanced gastric cancer: Evaluation by multivariate regression analysis. Oncology 1999;57:106–114.

Johnston PG, Lenz HJ, Leichman CG, et al: Thymidylate synthase gene and protein expression correlate and are associated with response to 5-fluorouracil in human colorectal and gastric tumors. Cancer Res 1995;55:1407–1412.

Leichman CG, Lenz HJ, Leichman L, et al: Quantitation of intratumoral thymidylate synthase expression predicts for disseminated colorectal cancer response and resistance to protracted-infusion fluorouracil and weekly leucovorin. J Clin Oncol 1997;15:3223–3229.

Lenz HJ, Danenberg KD, Leichman CG, et al: p53 and thymidylate synthase expression in untreated stage II colon cancer: Associations with recurrence, survival, and site. Clin Cancer Res 1998;4:1227–1234.

Loggie BW, Fleming RA, McQuellon RP, et al: Cytoreductive surgery with intraperitoneal hyperthermic chemotherapy for disseminated peritoneal cancer of gastrointestinal origin. Am Surg 2000;66:561–568.

Paradiso A, Simone G, Petroni S, et al: Thymidylate synthase and p53 primary tumor expression as predictive factors for advanced colorectal cancer patients. Br J Cancer 2000;82:560–567.

Portilla AG, Martinez de Lecea D, Stevens M, Sugarbaker PH: Relevant points to consider for selection of patients with peritoneal carcinomatosis for cytoreductive surgery and IP chemotherapy. Br J Surg 1998;85(s):21–22.

Salonga D, Danenberg KD, Johnson M, et al: Colorectal tumors responding to 5-fluorouracil have low gene expression levels of dihydropyrimidine dehydrogenase, thymidylate synthase, and thymidine phosphorylase. Clin Cancer Res 2000;6:1322–1327.

Scheithauer W, Kornek GV, Marczell A, et al: Combined intravenous and intraperitoneal chemotherapy with fluorouracil + leucovorin vs. fluorouracil + levamisole for adjuvant therapy of resected colon carcinoma. Br J Cancer 1998;77:1349–1354.

Speyer JL, Collins JM, Dedrick RL, et al: Phase I and pharmacologic studies of 5-fluorouracil administered intraperitoneally. Cancer Res 1980;40:567–572.

Stephens AD, Alderman R, Chang D, et al: Morbidity and mortality analysis of 200 treatments with cytoreductive surgery and hyperthermic intraoperative intraperitoneal chemotherapy using the coliseum technique. Ann Surg Oncol 1999;6:790–796.

Vaillant J-C, Nordlinger B, Deuffic S, et al: Adjuvant intraperitoneal 5-fluorouracil in high-risk colon cancer: A multicenter phase III trial. Ann Surg 2000;231:449–456.

Yeh KH, Shun CT, Chen CL, et al: High expression of thymidylate synthase is associated with the drug resistance of gastric carcinoma to high dose 5-fluorouracil-based systemic chemotherapy. Cancer 1998;82:1626–1631.

Familial Gastrointestinal Cancer Syndromes: Prophylactic Surgery

Giardiello FM, Hamilton SR, Krush AJ, et al: Treatment of colonic and rectal adenomas with sulindac in familial adenomatous polyposis. N Engl J Med 1993;328:1313–1316.

Groden J, Thliveris A, Samowitz W, et al: Identification and characterization of the familial adenomatous polyposis coli gene. Cell 1991;66:589–600.

Heiskanen I, Jarvinen H: Fate of the rectal stump after colectomy and ileorectal anastomosis for familial adenomatous polyposis. Int J Colorectal Dis 1997;12:9–16.

Kinzler KW, Nilbert MC, Su L-K, et al: Identification of FAP locus genes from chromosome 5q21. Science 1991; 253:661–665.

Lasher BA: Recommendations for colorectal cancer screening in ulcerative colitis: A review of research from a single university-based surveillance program. Am J Gastroenterol 1992;87:168–175.

Lennard-Jones JE, Melville DM, Morson BC, et al: Precancer and cancer in extensive ulcerative colitis: Findings among 401 patients over 22 years. Gut 1990;31:800–806.

Lynch HT, Smyrk T: Hereditary nonpolyposis colorectal cancer (Lynch syndrome): An updated review. Cancer 1996;78:1149–1167.

Nugent KP, Phillips RK: Rectal cancer risk in older patients with familial adenomatous polyposis. Br J Surg 1992; 79:1204–1206.

Parc YR, Moslein G, Dozois RR, et al: Familial adenomatous polyposis: Results after ileal pouch-anal anastomosis in teenagers. Dis Colon Rectum 2000;43:893–898.

Penna D, Karthueser A, Parc R, et al: Secondary proctectomy and ileal pouch-anal anastomosis after ileorectal anastomosis for familial adenomatous polyposis. Br J Surg 1993;80:1621–1623.

Rodriguez-Bigas MA: Prophylactic colectomy for gene carriers in hereditary nonpolyposis colorectal cancer: Has the time come? Cancer 1996;78:199–201.

Steinbach G, Lynch PM, Phillips RK, et al: The effect of celecoxib, a cyclooxygenase-2 inhibitor, in familial adenomatous polyposis. N Engl J Med 2000;342:1946–1952.

Winawer SJ, Zauber AG, Ho MN, et al: Prevention of colorectal cancer by colonoscopic polypectomy. New Engl J Med 1993;329:1977–1981.

Intestinal Obstruction

Baines M, Oliver DJ, Carter RL: Medical management of intestinal obstruction in patients with advanced malignant disease: A clinical and pathological study. Lancet 1985;2:990–993.

Mercadante S, Ripamonti C, Casuccio A, et al: Comparison of octreotide and hyoscine butylbromide in controlling gastrointestinal symptoms due to malignant inoperable bowel obstruction. Support Care Cancer 2000;8:188–191.

Mulcahy HE, Skelly MM, Hussain A, O'Donoghue DP: Long-term outcome following curative surgery for malignant large bowel obstruction. Br J Surg 1996;83:46–50.

Turnbull ADM, Guerra J, Starnes HF: Results of surgery for obstructing carcinomatosis of GI, pancreatic, or biliary origin. J Clin Oncol 1989;7:381–386.

Woolfson RG, Jennings K, Whalen GF: Management of bowel obstruction in patients with abdominal cancer. Arch Surg 1997;132:1093–1097.

Laparoscopy

Abbasakoor F, Senapati PSP, Brown TH, Manson J: Laparoscopy and laparoscopic ultrasonography in upper gastrointestinal cancer: Do they improve staging? Br J Surg 1998;85:412 (abstract).

Fernandez-del Castillo C, Rattner DW, Warshaw AL: Further experience with laparoscopy and peritoneal cytology in the staging of pancreatic cancer. Br J Surg 1995;82:1127–1129.

Fusco MA, Paluzzi MW: Abdominal wall recurrence after laparoscopic assisted colectomy for colon cancer: Report of a case. Dis Colon Rectum 1993;36:858–861.

John TG, Greig JD, Crosbie JL, et al: Superior staging of liver tumors with laparoscopy and laparoscopic ultrasonography. Ann Surg 1994;220:711–719.

Stell DA, Carter CR, Stewart I, Anderson JR: Prospective comparison of laparoscopy, ultrasonography, and computed tomography in the staging of gastric cancer. Br J Surg 1996;83:1260–1262.

Stocchi L, Nelson H: Laparoscopic colectomy for colon cancer: Trial update. J Surg Oncol 1998;68:255–267.

Stocchi L, Nelson H: Wound recurrences following laparoscopic-assisted colectomy for cancer. Arch Surg 2000; 135:948–958.

Tate JJT, Kwok S, Dawson JW, et al: Prospective comparison of laparoscopic and conventional anterior resection. Br J Surg 1993;80:1396–1398.

Wexner SD, Cohen SM: Port site metastases after laparoscopic colorectal surgery for cure of malignancy. Br J Surg 1995;82:295–298.

Wexner SD, Cohen SM, Johansen OB, et al: Laparoscopic colorectal surgery: A prospective assessment and current perspective. Br J Surg 1993;80:1602–1605.

Liver Metastases and Intra-arterial Infusion Therapy

Goldberg RM, Fleming TR, Tangen CM, et al: Surgery for recurrent colon cancer: Strategies for identifying resectable recurrence and success rates after resection. Ann Intern Med 1998;129:27–35.

Harmantas A, Rotstein LE, Langer B: Regional versus systemic chemotherapy in the treatment of colorectal carcinoma metastatic to the liver. Cancer 1996;78:1639–1645.

Kemeny MM, Adak S, Lipsitz S, et al: Results of the intergroup Eastern Cooperative Oncology (ECOG) and Southwest Oncology Group (SWOG) prospective randomized study of surgery alone versus continuous hepatic artery infusion of FUDR and continuous systemic infusion of 5-FU after hepatic resection for colorectal liver metastases. Proc Am Soc Clin Oncol 1999;18:264a.

Kemeny N, Cohen A, Huang Y, et al: Randomized study of hepatic arterial infusion (HAI) and systemic chemotherapy (SYS) versus SYS alone as adjuvant therapy after resection of hepatic metastases from colorectal cancer. Proc Am Soc Clin Oncol 1999;18:263a.

Meta-Analysis Group in Cancer: Reappraisal of hepatic arterial infusion in the treatment of nonresectable liver metastases from colorectal cancer. J Natl Cancer Inst 1996;88:252–258.

Solbiati L, Goldberg SN, Ierace T, et al: Hepatic metastases: Percutaneous radio-frequency ablation with cooled-tip electrodes. Radiology 1997;205:367–373.

Preoperative Assessment

Buzby GB: The Veterans Affairs TPN Cooperative Study Group: Perioperative TPN in surgical patients. N Engl J Med 1991;325:525–532.

Goldman L, Caldera DL, Nussbaum SR, et al: Multifactorial index of cardiac risk in non-cardiac surgical procedures. N Engl J Med 1977;297:845–850.

Radiation Enteritis

Deitel M, To TB: Major intestinal complications of radiotherapy. Arch Surg 1987;122:1421–1424.

Galland RB, Spencer J: The natural history of clinically established radiation enteritis. Lancet 1985;8440:1257–1258.

Mann WJ: Surgical management of radiation enteropathy. Surg Clin North Am 1991;71:977–990.

Miller AR, Martenson JA, Nelson H, et al: The incidence and clinical consequences of treatment-related bowel injury. Int J Radiat Oncol Biol Phys 1999;43:817–825.

Waddell BE, Rodriguez-Bigas MA, Lee RJ, et al: Prevention of chronic radiation enteritis. J Am Coll Surg 1999;189:611–624.

Radiation Therapy and Combined Modality Therapy

Bodner WR, Hilaris BS, Mastoras DA: Radiation therapy in pancreatic cancer: Current practice and future trends. J Clin Gastroenterol 2000;30:230–233.

Farouk R, Nelson H, Gunderson LL: Aggressive multimodality treatment for locally advanced unresectable rectal cancer. Br J Surg 1997;84:741–749.

Gunderson LL, Martin JK, Beart RW, et al: Intraoperative and external beam irradiation for locally advanced colorectal cancer. Ann Surg 1988;207:52–60.

Gunderson LL, Nelson H, Martenson J, et al: Locally advanced primary and recurrent colorectal cancer: Disease control and survival with IOERT containing regimens. Int J Radiat Oncol Biol Phys 1995;32(Suppl 1):267.

Harrison LB, Enker WE, Anderson LL: High-dose-rate intraoperative radiation therapy for colorectal cancer. Oncology 1995;9:737–741.

Henning GT, Schild SE, Stafford SL, et al: Results of irradiation or chemoirradiation for primary unresectable, locally recurrent, or grossly incomplete resection of gastric adenocarcinoma. Int J Radiat Oncol Biol Phys 2000;46:109–118.

Hyams DM, Mamounas EP, Petrelli N, et al: A clinical trial to evaluate the worth of preoperative multimodality therapy in patients with operable carcinoma of the rectum: A progress report of National Surgical Breast and Bowel Project Protocol R-03. Dis Colon Rectum 1997;40:131–139.

Swedish Rectal Cancer Trial: Improved survival with preoperative radiotherapy in resectable rectal cancer. N Engl J Med 1997;336:980–987.

Willett CG: Intraoperative radiation therapy in resected bile duct cancer. Int J Radiat Oncol Biol Phys 2000;46:523–524.

Willett CG, Shellito PC, Tepper JE, et al: Intraoperative electron beam therapy for primary locally advanced rectal and rectosigmoid carcinoma. J Clin Oncol 1991;9:843–849.

Wilson LD, Chung JY, Haffty BG, et al: Intraoperative brachytherapy, laryngopharyngoesophagectomy, and gastric transposition for patients with recurrent hypopharyngeal and cervical esophageal carcinoma. Laryngoscope 1998;108:1504–1508.

Sentinel Lymph Node Biopsies

Gershenwald JE, Colome MI, Lee JE, et al: Patterns of recurrence following a negative sentinel lymph node biopsy in 243 patients with stage I or II melanoma. J Clin Oncol 1998;16:2253–2260.

Reintgen D: Lymphatic mapping and sentinel node harvest for malignant melanoma. J Surg Oncol 1997;66:277–281.

Turner RR, Ollila DW, Krasne DL, Giuliano AE: Histopathologic validation of the sentinel lymph node hypothesis for breast carcinoma. Ann Surg 1997;226:271–276.

Veronesi U, Paganelli G, Galimberti V, et al: Sentinel-node biopsy to avoid axillary dissection in breast cancer with clinically negative lymph-nodes. Lancet 1997;349:1864–1867.

Staging

Arnold MW, Young DC, Hitchcock CL, et al: Radioimmunoguided surgery in primary colorectal carcinoma: An intraoperative prognostic tool and adjuvant to traditional staging. Am J Surg 1995;170:315–318.

Calaluce R, Miedema BW, Yesus YW: Micrometastasis in colorectal carcinoma: A review. J Surg Oncol 1998;67:194–202.

Clarke MP, Kane RA, Steele G Jr, et al: Prospective comparison of preoperative imaging and intraoperative ultrasonography in the detection of liver tumors. Surgery 1989; 106:849–855.

Fong Y, Cohen AM, Fortner JG, et al: Liver resection for colorectal metastases J Clin Oncol 1997;15:938–946.

Little AR, Warren RS, Moore D, Pallavincini MG: Molecular cytogenetic analysis of cytokeratin 20-labeled cells in primary tumors and bone marrow aspirates from colorectal carcinoma patients. Cancer 1997;79:1664–1670.

Makary MA, Warshaw AL, Centeno BA, et al: Implications of peritoneal cytology for pancreatic cancer management. Arch Surg 1998;133:361–365.

Nicholson AG, Marks CG, Cook MG: Effect of lymph node status of triple leveling and immunohistochemistry with CAM 5.2 on node negative colorectal carcinomas. Gut 1994;35:1447–1448.

O'Sullivan GC, Collins JK, Kelly J, et al: Micrometastases: Marker of metastatic potential or evidence of residual disease? Gut 1997;40:512–515.

O'Sullivan GC, Collins JK, O'Brien F, et al: Micrometastases in bone marrow of patients undergoing "curative" surgery for gastrointestinal cancer. Gastroenterology 1995;109: 1535–1540.

Ragaelson SR, Kronborg O, Larsen C, Fenger C: Intraoperative ultrasonography in the detection of hepatic metastases from colorectal carcinoma. Dis Col Rectum 1995; 38:355–360.

Soeth E, Vogel I, Roder C, et al: Comparative analysis of bone marrow and venous blood isolates from gastrointestinal cancer patients for the detection of disseminated tumor cells using reverse transcription PCR. Cancer Res 1997;57:3106–3110.

van Dijkum N, Els JM, Sturm PD, et al: Cytology of peritoneal lavage performed during staging laparoscopy for gastrointestinal malignancies: Is it useful? Ann Surg 1998; 228:728–733.

Chapter 50
Biologic Therapy

Nancy L. Lewis and Louis M. Weiner

Introduction

Surgery, radiotherapy, and cytotoxic agents have long been the mainstays of cancer treatment. While these approaches have been effective to a considerable extent, cancer remains a leading cause of morbidity and mortality worldwide. There is a continued need for the development of more effective, more selective, and less toxic therapeutic strategies.

Biologic therapy is a rapidly emerging area of antineoplastic treatment. Advances in the fields of molecular and cell biology have furthered our understanding of the mechanisms of carcinogenesis, metastasis, and host immune response. As the details of cell signaling pathways, angiogenesis, genetic alterations, and cellular immune dysfunction are elucidated, researchers and clinicians are discovering novel targets for therapeutic intervention. This chapter provides a broad overview of our current understanding of cancer biology and some of the advances being made in the area of biologically directed cancer therapeutics.

Cytokines

Cytokines comprise a very large group of soluble proteins produced by cells of the immune system and function as autocrine and paracrine cellular signals. Cytokines are a diverse group of proteins ranging from 15 to 40 kDa in size. They include the families of interferons, interleukins, hematopoietic growth factors, tumor necrosis factor, and insulinlike growth factor. While each cytokine has somewhat unique and specialized roles, all serve to modulate cell growth, activation, differentiation, and cell death via receptor binding and ultimately signal transduction. Table 50-1 is a partial list of cytokines that have active roles in the treatment of cancer patients.

Interferons are naturally occurring glycoproteins that are produced in response to viral infections, antigen or mitogen exposure, and other cytokines. Interferon-α (IFN-α) is leukocyte-derived, and two

recombinant forms of interferon are available for clinical use: interferon-α2a and interferon-α2b. Interferon-β is produced largely by fibroblasts, and interferon-γ, the most potent immunomodulator in this group, is derived from T lymphocytes. Although the exact mechanism of action remains incompletely understood, interferons have a variety of effects that include well-documented antitumor and antiviral activity (Table 50-2).

The term *interleukins* literally means "between leukocytes." This family of cytokines is composed of at least 18 members, and new members continue to be identified. The specific functions of each cytokine have been determined with knockout mouse models. Most of the interleukins serve as stimulators of lymphocyte activation, growth, differentiation, and/or mediators of inflammation (Table 50-3). Some have demonstrated clinical use. For example, interleukin-11 (IL-11) has been shown to alleviate chemotherapy-induced thrombocytopenia. Interleukin-2, perhaps the most widely studied interleukin, has shown modest therapeutic efficacy in both renal cell cancer and melanoma and received FDA approval in 1992 and 1998, respectively.

There are two broad classes of cytokine receptors. Type I receptors are composed of two subunits, α and β, and depending on the particular ligand, the subunits can be interchangeable. Ligands for type I receptors include interleukin-1 through interleukin-9, interleukin-13, interleukin-18, granulocyte-macrophage colony-stimulating factor (GM-CSF), granulocyte colony-stimulating factor (G-CSF), and erythropoietin (EPO). The association of the two subunits of the type I receptor results in effective signal transduction. Three subclasses of type I receptors have cytoplasmic tyrosine kinase domains. Subclass 1 includes growth factor receptors for HER-2/*neu* and epidermal growth factor receptor (EGFR). Subclass 2 is bound by insulin and insulinlike growth factor (IGF-1). Platelet-derived growth factor (PDGF) and Flt-3 ligand bind to subclass 3.

Table 50-1 ▪ Cytokines

Interferons	IFN-α, IFN-β, IFN-γ
Interleukins	IL-2, IL-4, IL-11
Tumor necrosis factor	TNF α, TNF β
Hematopoietic growth factors	EPO, GM-CSF, G-CSF, TPO, IL-11, SCF

Type II cytokine receptors also have α and β subunits. Tumor necrosis factors, interleukin-10 and interferons bind to these cell surface receptors, inducing the oligomerization of the α and β chains. These subunits are associated with Janus kinases (Jak-1 and Jak-2) or, alternatively, tyrosine kinase 2 (depending upon the interferon). The Janus kinase complex phosphorylates tyrosine residues, which serve as docking sites for signal transducers and activators of transcription (STAT) molecules. Once signal transducers and activators of transcription are phosphorylated, they are transported to the nucleus and promote transcription. Examples of ligands that bind to the tumor necrosis factor (TNF) receptor family include tumor necrosis factor, nerve growth factor (NGF), CD30, and fas ligand. Tumor necrosis factor and fas ligand binding to this receptor triggers apoptosis via the caspase cascade, which results in proteolysis of cellular structural proteins such as polyadenosine diphosphate ribose polymerase.

Both interferon-α2a and interleukin-2 have demonstrated activity against metastatic renal cancer and melanoma and remain a component of standard therapies for these diseases. In addition, treatment with interferon-α has resulted in significant responses in patients with hairy cell leukemia, chronic myelogenous leukemia (CML), Kaposi's sarcoma, and non-Hodgkin's lymphoma and has been approved by

Table 50-2 ▪ Antitumor Activity of Interferons

Immunomodulation
- Activation of natural killer cells, T$_c$ cells
- Induction of major histocompatibility class I antigens
- Induction of gp96, a heat shock protein associated with antigen presentation

Antiproliferative activity
Inhibition of angiogenesis
Regulation of cell differentiation and growth
Modulation of gene expression
Signal transduction
Proapoptotic effects
Antiviral effects

Table 50-3 ▪ Key Functions of Selected Interleukins

Interleukin	Produced By	Function
IL-2	Activated T cells	Activated T cell proliferation Antitumor effects on melanoma and renal cell carcinoma
IL-4	Activated T cells	B lymphocyte activation, especially IgE Stimulates eosinophils
IL-6	Many cell types	Key inflammatory mediator
IL-8	Macrophages, endothelial cells	Chemotaxis and activation of neutrophils Stimulates angiogenesis
IL-11	Mesenchymal cells	Promotes hematopoiesis, especially platelets
IL-18	Macrophages	Induces interferon-γ synthesis

the FDA for these uses. Interferon-α is also commonly used for intravesical therapy of recurrent transitional cell carcinoma of the bladder. Neither interferon-α nor interleukin-2 is without significant toxicity, however. Side effects of cytokine treatment can include fever, chills, nausea, vomiting, diarrhea, anorexia, myalgias, arthralgias, neuropsychiatric changes such as somnolence and depression, and, in the case of interleukin-2, vascular leak syndrome leading to hemodynamic instability, interstitial pulmonary edema, and renal insufficiency. We are only beginning to understand the complicated network of intercellular and intracellular signaling and how it influences cell growth, differentiation, and death. Clearly, these cytokines do play a significant role in the control of the immune system, and some have demonstrated antitumor activity, although the mechanisms are still poorly understood.

Monoclonal Antibodies

The advent of hybridoma technology, pioneered by Kohler and Milstein, allows for the production of large quantities of highly purified specific antibodies directed against single antigenic epitopes. Monoclonal antibodies, which have gained widespread use for diagnostic testing, are now being used with therapeutic intent in the treatment of a variety of malignancies.

Immunoglobulins are naturally produced by B lymphocytes as a result of foreign antigen stimulation. There exist a variety of isotopes: IgG, IgM, IgA, IgE, and IgD. The basic IgG structure is a relatively large 150-kDa protein composed of two light and two heavy

Table 50-4 ■ Therapeutic Uses of Monoclonal Antibodies

Therapeutic targeting vehicles
Perturbation of cell signaling
Promote tumor lysis
Induce apoptosis
Immunization against tumor antigens
Depletion of cells from allogeneic transplant grafts

Table 50-5 ■ Tumor-Associated Targets for Monoclonal Antibodies

Tissue-specific differentiation antigens	CD20, CD33, CD52
Growth factor receptors	HER2/*neu*, epidermal growth factor receptor
Oncofetal proteins	Carcinoembryonic antigen, CD17 1-A
Tumor-specific antigens	PSA, L6
Soluble growth factor ligands	Vascular endothelial growth factor

chains that can be cleaved enzymatically by pepsin and papain to the Fc and (Fab)₂ fragments. The Fab domain provides the antigen-binding site that is complementary to a single antigen epitope. This domain confers a high degree of specificity for each antibody. The Fc domain is the segment of the antibody molecule that interacts with effector cells of the immune system and can activate the complement cascade. This portion of the antibody also dictates the half-life of the molecule.

Monoclonal antibodies have numerous potentially therapeutic effects; these are listed in Table 50-4. Once bound to a target cell, antibodies result in cellular death by direct and indirect mechanisms of action. Most commonly, tumor cell lysis occurs via complement-mediated or antibody-dependent cellular cytotoxicity (ADCC). Antibody binding has been shown to lead to cellular apoptosis. Cell signaling pathways can be perturbed by antibody-mediated inhibition of receptor-ligand interaction by either binding to the ligand or blocking the receptor. Antibodies that are conjugated to radionuclides and chemotherapeutic agents have been administered as "magic bullets," serving as vehicles to transport these cytotoxic agents to specific cellular targets. Anti-idiotypic antibodies have been used to immunize patients against tumor antigens (see the section "Vaccine Therapy" for more detail). Finally, antibodies that are targeted against T cell surface markers have been used to deplete T cells from allogeneic transplant grafts.

Ideally, antigenic targets for monoclonal antibody development should be expressed on malignant cells only, should be present in abundance on the cell surface, and should not be shed into the vasculature or surrounding interstitium. Targets for which antibodies have been developed are listed in Table 50-5. Tissue-specific cell surface markers CD20, CD33, and CD52 are found on B cells, leukemic blasts, and T and B lymphocytes, respectively. Growth factor receptors such as HER2/*neu*, which is overexpressed in approximately 20% of breast cancers, and the epidermal growth factor receptor, found on many malignant

tumors including head and neck, lung, colorectal, and renal tumors, are also excellent targets for monoclonal antibody-directed therapy.

Oncofetal proteins, which may be expressed in fetal tissues, are expressed almost exclusively on malignant cells in the adult. Carcinoembryonic antigen is commonly followed as a tumor marker in gastrointestinal malignancies and has been used extensively as an antigenic target for both monoclonal antibody and vaccine development.

Unconjugated antibodies are thought to exert their antitumor effects through complement-mediated and antibody-dependent cellular cytotoxicity mechanisms. Two unconjugated antibodies have gained FDA approval in the United States. Rituximab (Rituxan, IDEC Pharmaceuticals, San Diego, California), a chimeric anti-CD20 antibody, has been shown to have a very high response rate when administered with standard CHOP chemotherapy for patients with low-grade follicular non-Hodgkin's lymphoma. The addition of rituximab to CHOP chemotherapy increases complete response rates from 60% to 75% and significantly improved the event-free and overall survival rates in elderly patients with diffuse large-cell lymphoma. Trastuzumab (Herceptin, Genentech, San Francisco, California), the second FDA-approved antibody, is a recombinant humanized antibody against HER2/*neu*. It binds to the extracellular domain of this growth factor receptor and has demonstrated significant antitumor activity in patients with chemotherapy-refractory breast cancer whose tumors overexpress the HER2/*neu* receptor. In phase II studies, response rates ranged from 11.6% to 24%. In phase III trials, patients were randomized to receive chemotherapy alone versus chemotherapy + trastuzumab. The overall response rate in the trastuzumab arm was 62% compared with 36.2% in the chemotherapy-alone arm.

Other unconjugated antibodies are being investigated in patients with T cell lymphoma, melanoma, colon cancer, and neuroblastoma. One of the newer humanized antibodies against the epidermal growth factor receptor, cetuximab, has shown a 22.5% response rate when administered with irinotecan in patients with metastatic colorectal cancer who previously failed irinotecan therapy.

Bispecific antibodies are monoclonal antibodies that are designed not only to recognize tumor antigens, but also to increase the immune response by simultaneously binding to cell surface molecules on a variety of effector leukocytes. Antibody binding to these leukocytes will presumably lead to activation of the immune system at the target tissue site. Bispecific molecules have been prepared to bind to tumor antigens and to the FcγRI receptor on neutrophils, monocytes, and macrophages and the FcγRIII receptor on macrophages, natural killer cells, and CD3/TCR on T cells and CD44 on natural killer (NK) cells.

Anti-idiotypic antibodies are discussed in greater detail in the vaccine section. Briefly, anti-idiotype antibodies that contain a surrogate tumor epitope can be used to immunize patients. This results in the production of an anti-anti-idiotype antibody that recognizes and binds to the original tumor epitope. This approach may be advantageous in that it results in the development of an antibody that is relatively selective for a single tumor epitope and is less likely to cross-react with other shared antigens that are commonly found in normal tissue.

The antitumor activity of monoclonal antibodies can be enhanced by conjugating the antibody to a toxic moiety. Antibodies have been conjugated to chemotherapeutic agents, plant and bacterial toxins, and radionuclides. Chemotherapeutic agents that have been linked to monoclonal antibodies include adriamycin and, more recently, calicheamicin; the latter conjugate has been tested in leukemia. Plant toxins include ricin, which is derived from castor beans and inhibits protein synthesis through binding to ribosomal elongation factor-2. Similarly, antibodies coupled to *Pseudomonas* exotoxin A kill targeted cells by inhibiting protein synthesis. All of these immunoconjugates require internalization of the antibody/conjugate complex for cytotoxic effects. Radionuclides that have been coupled to monoclonal antibodies include yttrium-90 and iodine-131. The advantage of radioimmunoconjugates is that internalization of the antibody is not required. In addition, radioimmunoconjugates can kill even malignant cells within a tumor population that underexpress the target antigen through the bystander effect, as high-energy β emissions can travel a distance of several millimeters (e.g., more than one cell diameter).

Several preexisting or potential hurdles must be overcome to enable the extended applicability of monoclonal antibody therapy. Antibodies are relatively large molecules compared with standard chemotherapeutic agents. Accordingly, they have slower distribution kinetics and demonstrate poor tissue penetration. Coupled with a heterogeneous blood supply within tumors and high intratumoral interstitial pressures, antibodies frequently fail to penetrate the tumor to an optimal extent. To circumvent this problem, alterations in antibody structures that minimize or completely remove the Fc portion have been investigated. Single-chain variable fragments, diabodies, and minibodies are all smaller than IgG but retain antigen recognition sites with the same binding affinity while exhibiting improved diffusion and distribution capacities.

Initially, monoclonal antibodies were generated in mice. Unfortunately, the development of human anti-mouse antibodies (HAMA) precluded multiple dosing administration of such murine antibodies. With the advent of recombinant technology, chimeric, "humanized" antibody production circumvented this problem. Chimeric antibodies are formed by fusing the DNA coding for the mouse variable region with the human constant region of IgG, resulting in smaller amounts of foreign protein. Antibodies can now be essentially fully "humanized" by incorporating the murine protein sequence region of the antibody that interacts directly with the antigen into a completely human Ig framework. Not only is the formation of human anti-mouse antibodies eliminated, but humanized Fc regions can be engineered to enhance interactions with effector cells.

Other potential resistance mechanisms that may lead to ineffective antibody therapy include down-modulation of tumor antigens by tumor cells, release of antigens into the microvasculature resulting in the binding of antibodies before they reach their targets, and cross-reactivity of normal tissues leading to toxicity and insufficient tumor binding. The identification of additional genetic changes that occur during tumorigenesis may enable better targeting of gene products that are unique to malignant cells and, eventually, the surmounting of these barriers.

Vaccine Therapy

The observation made by William Coley that some tumors regressed as a result of immune activation in response to bacterial toxins has made the concept of immunotherapy for cancer an attractive one. Much of the work that has been done in the development of cancer vaccines began in the melanoma model, as these tumor cells demonstrate naturally high immunogenicity. The identification of tumor-reactive lymphocytes, the presence of autoimmune-mediated destruction of melanocytes in patients with vitiligo, and reports of spontaneous melanoma regressions have fueled interest in developing ways to channel an immunologic response directed against tumors.

Understanding the cellular interactions that result in a specific antitumor immune response has improved markedly over the past few decades. Activation of the immune response by specific antigens occurs via the humoral antibody mediated pathway (B cell activation) or direct cellular mechanisms (T cell activation). Antibodies recognize antigens that are in their native protein state, usually on the surface of cell targets. Binding results in complement-mediated or antibody-dependent target cell death. T cells, on the other hand, can recognize cytoplasmic or membrane-bound protein fragments that are presented in the context of class I or II major histocompatibility (MHC) antigens. There are two types of T lymphocytes, cytotoxic and helper cells, which recognize antigens via the T cell receptor. The T cell receptor closely interacts with the CD3 molecule, which in turn triggers intracellular signaling pathways. Activation of CD8+ "cytotoxic" T lymphocytes occurs when antigen-presenting cells process peptide fragments and transport them to the cell surface in association with class I major histocompatibility molecules. CD4+ T helper T cells are activated when similar peptides are presented in association with class II major histocompatibility molecules. Activation of CD4+ cells results in the secretion of cytokines and lymphokines that in turn induce B cells to secrete immunoglobulin and activate CD8+ cells. The processing and presenting of exogenous antigen can be carried by a number of different antigen-presenting cells, such as B cells, macrophages, and monocytes. Bone marrow–derived dendritic cells are the most efficient antigen-presenting cells and express high levels of both class I and II major histocompatibility molecules. These cells are capable of migrating to distant sites, including lymph nodes, where the bulk of antigen processing and presentation occurs.

Several types of cellular proteins within malignant cells can give rise to smaller peptides that are recognized by cytotoxic T lymphocytes. These include oncogenes, mutated cellular proteins, nonmutated tissue-specific proteins, families of proteins that are unique to cancer and testis, and viral proteins. Oncogenes may be overexpressed, as in the case of HER2/*neu* in approximately 20% of breast cancers, or mutated like the mutated ras p21 family of proto-oncogenes (K-ras, H-ras, N-ras). These affected genes are vital for cell signaling and growth. Point mutations in the *ras* gene are seen in a variety of cancers and have been reported to occur in approximately 90% of

pancreatic tumors and 50% of colorectal cancers. These mutations lead to the constitutive transduction of growth-promoting signals. Given their prevalence and function in cell growth, overexpressed or mutated oncogenes are not only potentially useful targets for vaccine development, but also promising targets for cell cycle inhibitory agents (see the section entitled "Cell Signaling").

Tissue-specific proteins, particularly those expressed by normal and malignant melanocytes, have been studied. These include tyrosinase, gp100, MART-1, and tyrosine-related proteins 1 and 2 (TRP-1, TRP-2). These proteins are involved in tissue differentiation pathways and the synthesis of melanin.

A group of antigens is encoded by large families of genes that are expressed only in malignant cells or the normal testis. These genes are located on the X chromosome and code for a variety of antigens expressed in melanoma (MAGE), gastrointestinal tumors (GAGE), breast (BAGE), and renal (RAGE) cancers.

Mutated cellular proteins with or without carbohydrate residues can serve as tumor-associated antigens (see Table 50-6). Examples include ras, p53, β-catenin, and p16 protein products. Finally, a number of viruses have been shown to play a role in the malignant transformation of normal cells. These include human papillomavirus (HPV) (types 16, 18, 31, 33, and 45), human herpes virus-8, and hepatitis B, which have been linked to cervical cancer, Kaposi's sarcoma, and hepatoma, respectively. The viral proteins expressed by these cancer cells can be recognized by cytotoxic T lymphocytes. One human papillomavirus viral oncoprotein, E6 protein, has been shown to bind the tumor suppressor p53 and target its degradation through the ubiquitin pathway. Another oncoprotein, E7, binds to pRB, resulting in unchecked entry into the cell cycle. Both of these antigenic viral proteins serve as excellent potential targets for vaccine strategies.

Autologous tumor proteins that have been shown to elicit cytotoxic T lymphocyte responses include the

Table 50-6 ■ Tumor-Associated Antigens

Tumor-Associated Antigens	Examples
Oncogenes	p21
Mutated cellular protein	p53
Nonmutated tissue-specific protein	gp100, TRP-1, TRP-2
Cancer testis	MAGE
Viral	Human papillomavirus, E6, E7

family of heat shock proteins (HSPs). These chaperone proteins are associated with almost all proteins generated within a cell and serve to promote survival under adverse conditions. The expression of heat shock proteins is thought to confer resistance to chemotherapy and radiation-induced apoptosis. Members of this family include Mcl-1, Bcl-2, Bcl-x, and glutathione S-transferase.

In addition to cellular proteins, many tumor-associated carbohydrate moieties are present on the surface of tumor cells. Examples include Lewis Y, Globo H, Tn, TF, sTn, and the gangliosides GM2, GD2, and GD3 that are expressed on melanoma cells. Although these antigens are often prominently expressed, they tend to be weakly immunogenic, and adjuvant immunogens may be required to elicit significant immune responses.

Tumor-associated antigens that serve as targets for therapeutic vaccines fall into two broad categories: shared antigens and unique antigens. Shared antigens are present on tumors from many different patients, while unique antigens are expressed only by one patient's tumor. Distinct vaccine approaches have been tried in an effort to enhance immune reactivity to either shared or unique antigens. Autologous tumor cell–based vaccines have the advantage of presenting all tumor-associated antigens, including potentially unique antigens, to the patient's immune system; however, this approach is labor-intensive, is not widely applicable to larger populations, and may be limited by the availability of tumor cells. On the other hand, purified molecules that are shared by most melanoma cells, such as whole tumor antigens, heavily glycosylated proteins (mucins) or tumor-associated carbohydrate antigens, can be synthesized for widespread use. While they might not be highly immunogenic themselves, these molecules can be administered in the presence of adjuvants to increase their immunogenicity. One disadvantage of this approach is that these highly purified vaccines may contain antigens that can be expressed only in the context of a particular human leukocyte antigen (HLA) molecule, limiting the general applicability of this approach.

With the advent of genetic engineering, recombinant vaccines have emerged. For example, the genetic modification of tumor cells has been widely explored. Genes that encode cytokines (GM-CSF, IL-2, IL-4, IL-6, IL-12 or IFN-γ), immunogenic peptides, costimulatory molecules, or major histocompatibility proteins may increase the immune recognition of and response to either autologous or allogeneic tumor cells. Alternatively, tumor-associated antigens such as carcinoembryonic antigen (CEA) have been incorporated into viral vectors, such as vaccinia, and shown to trigger both humoral and cell-mediated pathways of immune response. Anti-idiotypic antibodies that mimic protein and nonprotein antigenic epitopes represent a novel and interesting approach to eliciting tumor antigen-specific immune responses. The antigen-combining site of each antibody, the idiotype, is a unique, clonally derived structure that stimulates the production of a series of host antibodies. Accordingly, an idiotype-containing antibody (i.e., AB1) that binds to a tumor antigen induces the production of anti-idiotype antibodies (i.e., AB2). AB2, a portion of which contains a surrogate tumor epitope recognized by the AB1, can immunize patients, leading to the production of anti-anti-idiotype antibodies (i.e., AB3), some of which bind to the original tumor epitope. Anti-idiotype strategies that mimic tumor antigens are under investigation as cancer vaccines. These vaccines can be thought of as highly purified antigen epitopes that stimulate immune responses against defined tumor antigen epitopes. In contrast, immunization with tumor antigens may be problematic, since the immune response to the whole antigen may induce reactivity to epitopes that are shared by unrelated, normal cellular antigens. One example of an anti-idiotypic vaccine is CeaVAC, which contains an anti-idiotypic internal image of carcinoembryonic antigen, a tumor-associated antigen that is frequently overexpressed in colon cancers. Other anti-idiotypic antibodies are designed to stimulate immune responses to disialoganglioside GD2 on melanoma cells or ACA-125 on ovarian cancer cells.

Finally, dendritic cell vaccines have emerged as exciting new strategies for inducing tumor-protective immune responses. Dendritic cells can be expanded in vitro after isolation from the peripheral blood or bone marrow in the presence of GM-CSF and IL-4 and can be pulsed with relevant tumor antigens (or transfected with cDNA encoding such antigens) and reinfused as primed antigen presenters.

Many tumor vaccines have completed phase I clinical trial evaluations. In general, vaccines have produced minimal adverse effects. Several vaccines have induced peptide-specific T cell responses as measured by in vitro assays such as the enzyme-linked immunospot (ELISPOT) assay, lymphocyte proliferation studies, limiting dilution analysis, and human leukocyte antigen–tetramer staining. Despite such documented immune responses, the antitumor effects of vaccine-based therapies have been disappointing.

Several potential mechanisms of resistance to vaccine-based therapies have been identified. As tumor cells become more poorly differentiated, they may lose expression of antigens, costimulatory molecules, or downregulate major histocompatibility expression. They may produce immunosuppressive cytokines such as transforming growth factor-β (TGF-β) and interleukin-10 or may upregulate heat shock proteins or Fas ligand. In addition, selective pressures exerted by an activated immune system may result in a population of highly resistant and poorly immunogenic cells. Immune tolerance or anergy to the antigen may occur via alterations in the T cell receptor signal transduction, T cell clonal exhaustion, and replicative senescence. Despite these potential pitfalls, vaccine therapy remains an attractive adjunct to standard treatment with surgery, chemotherapy, and cytokine therapy and may ultimately find its niche in the adjuvant or preventative settings.

Gene Therapy

Gene therapy is defined as the transfer of genetic material with therapeutic intent. More specifically, it entails the insertion of genetic sequences into the genome of a target cell (be it a malignant cell, a normal functional cell, or a nonfunctional nonmalignant cell) to produce a new cellular function. Traditionally, such therapy has been developed for diseases for which a given gene product is notably absent or abnormal, such as cystic fibrosis, adenosine deaminase deficiency, severe combined immunodeficiencies, or hemoglobinopathies. As understanding of the genetic alterations that occur during tumorigenesis and subsequent development of chemotherapeutic drug resistance increases, gene therapy may become a rational therapeutic approach for cancer treatment as well.

Proto-oncogenes are normal counterparts of oncogenes, which usually function to promote signal transduction and gene transcription. Mutations in these proto-oncogenes, such as point mutations, amplifications, translocations, or rearrangements, may activate these genes. Tumor suppressor genes, such as p53 and retinoblastoma (Rb), play integral roles in cell cycle regulation and are required to inhibit cell growth. Cells are normally maintained in G_0/G_1 of the cell cycle. Normal Rb regulates release from G_1, and normal p53 determines the cell's response to stress or DNA damage, that is, cell cycle arrest versus apoptosis. Usually, a cell needs only one normal copy of a tumor suppressor gene to function normally. The functional loss of both alleles due to mutation and/or deletion causes growth dysregulation. Frequently, a mutation in one allele leads to the production of a mutant protein that binds to and inactivates the structurally normal protein encoded by the other allele. This is termed a dominant negative mutation.

As was noted above, cell growth is tightly regulated through a complex network in which the Rb protein plays a central role. Phosphorylation of the Rb protein results in increased transcription of other genes, increased protein synthesis, and subsequently increased cell growth. This phosphorylation step is controlled by cyclins, cyclin-dependent kinases (CDKs), and p21, a potent inhibitor of CDKs. p53 exerts its DNA checkpoint activities by regulating p21 function and therefore indirectly affects Rb function. p53 is mutated in more than 50% of human cancers, making this mutation one of the most common genetic events found in malignancy. Replacement of a normal p53 protein is therefore one of the many attractive goals that could be accomplished through gene therapy.

In the setting of malignancy, the goals of genetic manipulations fall into several categories (Table 50-7). Gene therapy can be used to boost the immune system by enabling immunomodulation and inflammatory cytokine production at the tumor site, or by stimulating an antitumor response through overexpression of class I major histocompatibility antigens or costimulatory molecules on tumor cells. Alternatively, tumor cells might be influenced to undergo apoptosis via the insertion of a "suicide gene" or insertion of a wild-type p53 tumor suppressor gene. In addition, the sensitivity of tumor cells to chemotherapy or radiation might be augmented via genetic modification. Alternatively, normal hematopoietic stem cells could be protected from chemotherapy and radiation by inserting genes that confer chemoresistance such as MDR-1 or a mutated dihydrofolate reductase (DHFR). Finally, gene therapy could be used in the development of tumor vaccines by increasing the expression of tumor antigens such as gp100, MART-1, and carcinoembryonic antigen (see the section entitled "Vaccine Therapy").

For gene therapy to be effective, the genetic material must be delivered to the target cells. This can be accomplished via one of several delivery systems, including the use of viral and nonviral vectors (Table 50-8). Both RNA and DNA viral vectors are in widespread use in clinical trials. Although viruses are highly efficient at cell entry and genomic integration,

Table 50-7 ■ Potential Applications of Gene Therapy in Malignancy

Immunomodulation of host tissues
Programmed cell death
Replacement of a mutated gene with wild-type functional counterpart
Augmentation of chemotherapy sensitivity
Tumor vaccine development
Protection of host tissues
Alteration of tumor biology

Table 50-8 ■ Vector Delivery Systems

Viral

RNA: retroviruses
DNA: Adenovirus
- Papova virus
- Papilloma virus
- Pox virus (vaccinia, fowl pox, canary pox)
- Herpes virus (Epstein-Barr virus)

Chemical

Calcium-phosphate precipitation
Diethylaminodiethyl dextran precipitation

Physical

Microinjection
Electroporation
Receptor mediated
Centrifugation
Osmotic lysis

Fusion

Liposomal fusion
Red blood cell fusion

they may also be highly immunogenic, leading to eradication by the immune system. Commonly used viral vectors include retroviruses, adenoviruses, pox viruses, and herpes viruses. Retroviral vectors have a very high degree of infectivity and integrate efficiently into the target cell genome, resulting in high-level and relatively stable gene expression; however, retroviruses can infect only dividing cells. Adenoviruses, on the other hand, can infect both resting and dividing cells, can be rendered replication-defective if need be, and can be genetically modified to delete all adenoviral gene products, making it less likely that these viruses will be rapidly eliminated by host immune mechanisms. Nonetheless, adenoviral vectors still induce potent host antiviral responses that attenuate viral activity on subsequent exposure. Other methods of delivering genetic material to intended target cells include direct introduction of naked DNA and chemical, physical, or cell fusion methods.

As was noted previously, systemic administration of various cytokines results in significant toxicity (see the section entitled "Cytokines"). Insertion of genes encoding for various cytokines into tumor cells may allow for localized expression at the tumor site, thereby decreasing systemic toxicity. As was discussed previously, these cytokines play a potential role in regulating apoptosis, differentiation of antigen presenting cells, including dendritic cells, and enhancing immune effector cell chemotaxis and survival. Numerous

clinical trials of cytokine-gene modified tumor cells have been completed or are ongoing, particularly in patients with melanoma and renal cell carcinoma, albeit with limited benefit to date.

Several attempts to insert "suicide genes" into tumor cells are underway and have demonstrated promising results. For example, inserting the gene for herpes simplex virus–thymidine kinase (HSV-TK) into tumor cells renders them sensitive to the antiviral agent ganciclovir. Ganciclovir is taken up by cells and phosphorylated by thymidine kinase and, once phosphorylated, is incorporated into the DNA, terminating DNA elongation. In addition to this direct effect, phosphorylated ganciclovir can be transported across the cell membrane from thymidine kinase$^+$ cells to thymidine kinase$^-$ cells, resulting in a bystander effect. Another potential benefit to this approach is that herpes simplex virus proteins can generate a cytotoxic T lymphocyte response at the site of the tumor.

An emerging field of gene therapy involves the use of reverse complementary or "antisense" oligonucleotides, which are molecules 13 to 30 nucleotides in length that target specific mRNA. Antisense oligonucleotides bind and inhibit translation into the corresponding protein and therefore block expression of target genes. Antisense oligonucleotides accomplish this in two ways. Oligonucleotide-mRNA is a substrate for endogenous ribonuclease, which cleaves the mRNA part of the complex. In addition, the oligonucleotide-mRNA inhibits sliding of the 40S ribosomal subunit during protein synthesis. Antisense oligonucleotides have been generated against several oncogenes (c-myc, c-myb, ras), antiapoptotic proteins (bcl-2), tumor suppressor genes (p53), tyrosine kinase receptors (c-kit), angiogenic molecules (bFGF), and abnormal fusion genes (bcr-abl) and are currently in clinical trials.

A novel use of gene therapy is to target normal host tissues and confer resistance to more conventional therapies such as chemotherapy or radiation, so that higher doses of the therapeutic agents can be administered safely. Several such applications have been used in an attempt to protect hematopoietic stem cells. One example is to insert the multidrug resistance gene (MDR-1) into bone marrow cells. This gene codes for P glycoprotein, an adenosine triphosphate (ATP)—dependent transmembrane efflux pump that confers resistance to a number of widely used chemotherapeutic agents such as anthracyclines, taxol, vincristine, and etoposide. Resistance to methotrexate has been accomplished by inserting a mutated dihydrofolate reductase gene that confers this property. The dihydrofolate reductase enzyme, which converts dihydrofolate to tetrahydrofolate, a necessary step in purine synthesis, is normally bound by methotrexate, thus inactivating it. The mutated dihydrofolate reductase enzyme has less affinity for methotrexate and is therefore able to maintain its enzymatic function.

Several impediments to the development of gene therapy of stem cells have been identified. First, stem cells have very low levels of retroviral receptor expression. Receptor levels are increased after cytokine stimulation and are present in greater numbers on mobilized peripheral blood stem cells as well as fresh cord blood. Second, stem cells tend to have low levels of proliferation. As was noted previously, certain vectors, particularly retroviral vectors, require replicating cells for infection. It has been shown that proliferation rates can be increased by incubating cells with growth factors (interleukin-3, interleukin-6, stem cell factor (SCF), and Flt-3) and/or cell substrates such as mesenchymal and stromal cells. Perhaps the greatest obstacle is that many proliferating stem cells differentiate, thereby losing their replicative capacity, and no longer pass on their newly acquired chemo-protective mechanisms to daughter cells.

Although gene therapy has therapeutic potential, several major obstacles to its application remain. Given the large number of tumor cells, the lack of vector specificity, and the degree of heterogeneity within a given tumor, a paramount concern is to determine how vector-mediated therapy can be selectively delivered to every tumor cell. With this in mind, there is ongoing research into developing vectors with conditional replicative competency. For example, a viral vector is being developed that is replication deficient in cells with normal p53 function. As a consequence, the virus is taken up by all cells but replicates only in cells with p53 mutations. Vectors that require tumor-specific promoters that are not present in normal cells may also be able to overcome such specificity obstacles. For example, bispecific antibodies (discussed in the Monoclonal Antibody section) that bind to adenoviral vectors as well as tumor-specific targets may facilitate the selective localization of the viruses to tumor sites. Such approaches may eventually overcome the selectivity concern and enable more widespread clinical application of gene therapy in many different hematologic and oncologic disorders.

Antiangiogenic Therapy

It has long been known that tumors require a vascular supply for growth, invasion, and distant spread. Only recently, however, has it been shown the tumors themselves produce substances that induce new blood vessel formation. Dr. Folkman and colleagues have identified several tumor angiogenic factors. These factors promote angiogenesis, which is needed for

Table 50-9 ■ Stimulators and Inhibitors of Angiogenesis

Angiogenic Agents	Antiangiogenic Agents
Vascular endothelial growth factor	Angiostatin
Basic fibroblast growth factor	Endostatin
Acidic fibroblast growth factor	Platelet factor 4
Interleukin-8	Thrombospondin
Placental growth factor	Thalidomide
Angiopoietin-1	Paclitaxel
Transforming growth factor-β	Interferons

delivery of oxygen and nutrients to tumors as well as for removal of catabolites. In addition, new vessel formation is a prerequisite for blood-borne metastasis to distant sites. These angiogenic molecules belong to the vascular endothelial growth factor and fibroblast growth factor families and include vascular endothelial growth factor (VEGF), plasminogen activators, angiopoietin-1, acidic and basic fibroblast growth factor (aFGF and bFGF), and transforming growth factor-β (Table 50-9). Angiogenesis is delicately regulated by stimulators as well as inhibitors of this process. More than 40 endogenous inhibitors of human angiogenesis have been identified. These fall into five main categories: antiangiogenic proteolytic fragments, interleukins, interferons, matrix metalloproteinase inhibitors, and others. Antiangiogenic proteolytic fragments are naturally occurring fragments of larger proteins. Examples include angiostatin and endostatin. Angiostatin is a 38-kDa fragment of plasminogen, and endostatin is a 20-kDA fragment from the C terminal domain of type XXVIII collagen. Interleukins and interferons are leukocyte-derived cytokines that can be proangiogenic (interleukin-8) or antiangiogenic (interleukin-4, interleukin-10, and interleukin-12). Interleukin-12, which stimulates natural killer cells as well as cytotoxic T lymphocytes, exerts its antiangiogenic effects by inducing interferon-γ expression, which in turn induces inducible protein 10 (IP-10) and MIG-1. Interferon-α and -β inhibit angiogenesis by downregulating the expression of bFGF. Matrix metalloproteinases (MMPs) are enzymes secreted by tumors that digest the basement membrane and extracellular matrix, thereby enabling tumor cells to invade local tissues. Endothelial cells utilize matrix metalloproteinases to develop microvasculature. Examples of tissue inhibitors of MMPs include troponin-1 and marimastat. These agents have been shown in preclinical experiments to inhibit vascular smooth muscle cell migration and prevent tumor cell invasion and distant metastases. Other agents that demonstrate antiangiogenic properties include thrombospondin-1 (TSP-1), a 450-kDa adhesive glycoprotein found in platelet α-granules that helps to stabilize platelet aggregates, and platelet factor 4, which is also released from platelet α-granules. Endothelial monocyte activating polypeptide-2 (EMAP-II) demonstrates antiangiogenic properties by upregulating tumor necrosis factor. The tumor suppressor genes p53 and p16 inhibit angiogenesis by upregulating TSP-1 and downregulating vascular endothelial growth factor. Fumagillin, a naturally occurring product of *Aspergillus fumigatus*, inhibits blood vessel formation as well.

While angiogenesis is a normal part of wound healing, tissue repair, reproduction, growth, and development, uncontrolled angiogenesis can be pathologic. This is evident in patients who have diabetic retinopathy, macular degeneration, and other inflammatory disorders. In addition, once tumor cells make the "angiogenic switch" and begin releasing angiogenic factors, they demonstrate the ability for growth, invasion, and metastasis. Inhibiting this angiogenic switch is therefore an attractive goal for antineoplastic therapy.

Several preclinical assays have been developed to screen and compare agents for their antiangiogenic properties. In vitro assays include culturing endothelial cells from a variety of sources. Internalization of magnetic microbeads by capillary endothelial cells, chemotactic assays, and growing cells in collagen and fibrin gels that serve as an artificial extracellular matrix offer methods to quantitate antiangiogenic activity. A more labor-intensive aortic ring model can be used. In vivo assays include the chicken chorioallantoic membrane assay that has been used to screen new agents.

Issues to consider in clinical trial development include how best to administer these agents (by oral, subcutaneous, or intravenous routes) and measurement of clinical as well as biologic endpoints. Given the cytostatic nature of most antiangiogenic agents, which do not demonstrate direct tumor lytic effects, stable disease, freedom from progression, or survival rather than tumor response may be the appropriate endpoint in clinical trials. Commonly, time to tumor progression, tumor response, and overall survival are used. In the setting of antiangiogenic therapy, functional imaging can be utilized to measure the effect of a particular treatment on tumor metabolism, oxygen consumption, blood flow, and receptor expression. In addition, the measurement of biologic markers such as circulating vascular endothelial growth factor and basic fibroblast growth factors may serve as biologically important endpoints. The measurement of microvessel density on tumor pathology specimens and endothelial cell proliferation and migration assays may also be surrogate endpoints. Finally, with the advent of microarray technology, differential gene expression may produce valuable information.

Antiangiogenic agents that are currently in clinical trials include TNP-470, a fumagillin analog. This agent has been in phase I clinical trials on three different regimens, including a one-hour intravenous infusion thrice weekly, a four-hour weekly intravenous infusion, and a continuous five-day infusion administered every 21 days. Dose-limiting toxicities have largely been neurocerebellar. This agent is now in phase II study in several cancers, including glioblastoma multiforme, pancreas, cervical, and renal cell cancers. A recombinant humanized mouse monoclonal antibody against vascular endothelial growth factor has been shown to bind circulating vascular endothelial growth factor and to decrease tumor-derived angiogenesis. This antibody has completed phase I clinical trials and is being examined in patients with breast, hormone refractory prostate, renal cell, colon, or lung cancers. Matrix metalloproteinase inhibitors such as marimastat, AG3340, COL-3, and Bay 12-9566 are all in clinical trials. In addition to blocking the binding of growth factors such as vascular endothelial growth factor to their target receptors, an alternative is to block the signaling of the growth factor receptor. A novel group of small molecules that inhibit tyrosine kinase function in the signaling pathway have been developed and are discussed in more detail in the section entitled "Cell Signaling." Finally, thalidomide, an agent that was used in the 1950s as a sedative but was removed from the market after it was demonstrated to be teratogenic (infants born to mothers using this drug were born without limb formation), is now being revisited as a treatment for several cancers. It is thought to exert antiangiogenic effects by modulating vascular endothelial growth factor levels and by downregulating tumor necrosis factor expression. Thalidomide has shown activity in patients with myeloma or renal cell carcinoma and is currently being studied in patients with melanoma, breast, colon, or prostate cancer, mesothelioma, or glioblastoma multiforme. Toxicities have included somnolence, headache, dry mouth, and peripheral neuropathy.

Cell Signaling

A cell receives multiple external stimuli from its surrounding environment that dictate its growth, differentiation, activation, and eventually planned senescence and death. These signals may be produced by specialized endocrine cells at distant sites (hormonal), by neighboring cells (paracrine), or by the cell itself (autocrine). These molecules may be small and hydrophilic and readily diffuse across the cell membrane or large, hydrophobic molecules that send their message via binding to a cell surface receptor.

There are three types of cell membrane receptors: ion channels, G-protein receptors, and enzyme-linked receptors. Most of the cell growth and differentiation signaling occurs through the latter two. G-protein receptors are large, single-chain polypeptides with an extracellular N-terminus. The protein traverses the cell membrane seven times and ends with its C-terminus on the cytoplasmic side. Ligand binding occurs on the extracellular domain, and G-protein activation occurs on the intracellular side. G-proteins are made up of α, β, and γ subunits, with a guanosine diphosphate (GDP) molecule linked to the α subunit. With ligand binding, guanosine triphosphate (GTP) replaces the guanosine diphosphate, and the α-guanosine triphosphate complex dissociates from the β and γ subunits, leaving the membrane and entering the cytosol. This leaves both the β-γ complex and the α-guanosine triphosphate complex to interact with effectors, initiating cell activation. Alpha-guanosine triphosphate interacts with adenylyl cyclase, which converts adenosine triphosphate to cAMP. In addition, protein kinases that phosphorylate tyrosine, serine, and threonine residues are activated as is phospholipase C. The cell activation signal stays on until GTPase hydrolyses guanosine triphosphate to guanosine diphosphate. Guanosine diphosphate-α returns to the membrane, joins the β and γ subunits and returns to the resting position. Enzyme-linked cell-surface receptors are either cytokine receptors or members of the receptor tyrosine kinase family. Cytokine docking results in a conformational change that induces phosphorylation and activation of members of the Janus kinase family of kinases. Ligands for the receptor tyrosine kinases include growth factors such as epidermal growth factor and platelet-derived growth factor. Docking of the ligand induces receptor dimerization. The cytoplasmic tail of the tyrosine kinase receptors have intrinsic kinase activity resulting in an autophosphorylation, which triggers a cascade of protein kinase activation and ultimately cell activation via phospholipase C. Activation of phospholipase C cleaves the membrane-bound phosphatidylinositol diphosphate to inositol triphosphate and diacylglycerol. As a result, calcium is released from the endoplasmic reticulum, activating a protein kinase cascade. Similarly, diacylglycerol activates protein kinase C. Signals generated at the membrane via protein kinase activity reach the nucleus via mitogen-activated protein (MAP) kinases. Once activated, mitogen-activated proteins enter the nucleus and induce early-response gene transcription, causing the cell to enter the cell cycle.

The cell cycle is tightly regulated by a series of protein kinases called cyclin-dependent kinases (CDKs). They are activated by binding with their cyclin protein and are present and functioning at specific points in the cell cycle. There are checkpoints throughout the cycle that result in cell cycle arrest or delay in response to stress or DNA damage. The first occurs at G_1/S, and this is regulated by the p53/Rb pathways described previously. When Rb is in its dephosphorylated state, it binds to E2F, a transcription factor, and suppresses further induction of genes involved in DNA synthesis. Once phosphorylated, Rb dissociates from E2F and the cell enters S phase.

In the event that p53 or the Rb gene is mutated, as occurs in over 50% of cancers, cells can enter the cycle unchecked, despite possessing DNA damage. In addition, certain tumors such as mantle cell lymphoma have a chromosomal translocation t(11;14) that results in increased expression of cyclin D1. Knowledge of the cyclin-dependent kinase/cyclin complexes makes these rational targets for anticancer therapy. Indeed, several cyclin-dependent kinase modulators are currently in early-stage clinical trials.

Although there are several known signal transduction pathways, three require special mention: the Ras, PTEN-Akt, and epidermal growth factor pathways. The Ras family is a group of more than 50 small guanosine triphosphate–binding proteins, which relay signals from the Ras tyrosine kinase. Ras associated with guanosine diphosphate is anchored to the inner cell membrane. Like G-proteins, when the extracellular ligand binding occurs, guanosine triphosphate replaces guanosine diphosphate with the help of an effector protein, Sos. Ras-guanosine triphosphate induces intracellular phosphorylation events that result in cell activation, differentiation, and division. In the presence of GTPase-activating proteins (GAPs), guanosine triphosphate is converted to guanosine diphosphate, the Ras signaling cascade is halted, and the cell returns to its resting state. For Ras to function, it must be bound to the cytoplasmic cell membrane. After being synthesized in the cytoplasm, posttranslational modification enables transport of ras to the cell membrane. Farnesylation (addition of a 15-C farnesyl group to the C-terminal cystine residue of ras) is accomplished by a farnesyl transferase enzyme. Alternatively, addition of a 20-C group occurs via geranyl geranyl protein-transferase. Three members of the Ras family (H-, K-, and N-) are cellular proto-oncogenes. Point mutations have been well documented. Tumor-associated Ras mutants are resistant to GTPase-activating protein–mediated GTPase amplification, and the resulting Ras signal is stuck in the "on" position. Mutated Ras occurs in approximately 20% to 30% of all cancers, including up to 90% of all pancreatic cancers. In cancer cells, ras preferentially undergoes farnesylation, whereas in normal cells, geranyl geranyl transport is more common. Thus inhibition of the farnesyl transferase protein represents a rational anticancer strategy. Three types of farnesyl transferase inhibitors exist: monoterpenes (molecules that compete for the farnesyl moiety), peptidomimetics that mimic the Ras C-terminal CAAX box, and bisubstrate analogs that do both. While these drugs were specifically designed to target Ras farnesylation, preclinical and early clinical data reveal a lack of correlation between inhibition of tumor cell growth and Ras mutations. It has been more recently discovered that a critical target protein, Rho-B, demonstrated sensitivity to farnesyl transferase inhibition by blocking tumor growth. Although most of the Rho proteins undergo geranyl protein transferase, Rho-B, which is involved in regulating cytoskeletal formation, undergoes farnesylation. Certain cancers, such as inflammatory breast cancers, express Rho-B linking this protein to cellular growth functions as well.

Irrespective of mechanism, farnesyl transferase inhibitors have shown preclinical antitumor effects and are now in phase I/II clinical trials with and without standard chemotherapeutic agents. Side effects include gastrointestinal toxicity and myelosuppression. At this point, it remains unclear whether these agents work synergistically with chemotherapy and whether they should be given on a long-term basis.

Other new drugs are being designed with the aim of inhibiting alternative signaling pathways that are involved in cell proliferation. The mammalian target of rapamycin (mTOR) (also known as FRAP, RAFT1, or RAPT1) is a member of the phosphoinositide 3 kinase–related kinases. It is a 290-kDa kinase that is triggered by activation of the PI3 kinase/Akt signal transduction pathway. PI3-kinase is a lipid kinase that phosphorylates phosphatidylinositol. Downstream, Akt, a serine-threonine kinase, is involved in regulating proapoptotic pathways as well as mRNA translation via mammalian target of rapamycin. Phosphorylation of mammalian target of rapamycin turns on $p70^{s6kinase}$, which phosphorylates the 40S ribosomal protein S6 leading to protein production. In addition, mammalian target of rapamycin phosphorylates 4E-BP1, which ultimately leads to the production of proteins involved in cell cycling. This pathway is regulated by the tumor suppressor pentaerythritol tetranitrate (PTEN), which inhibits the early activity of PI3-kinase. Cell lines with pentaerythritol tetranitrate mutations have constitutive activation of this pathway resulting in cell proliferation, dysregulation, and resistance to apoptosis. The fungicide rapamycin and its ester, CCI-779, have been shown to inhibit mammalian targets of rapamycin,

resulting in decreased mRNA translation and cell cycle arrest in tumor cell lines. CCI-779 is currently in phase I/II studies in a number of tumors, including renal, prostate, small-cell lung cancer, and melanoma.

A whole class of new agents has arisen from increased understanding of the functions of the epidermal growth factor receptor. Ligand binding to the epidermal growth factor receptor results in cell proliferation as well as promotion of angiogenesis. This receptor is overexpressed on a number of epithelial cancers, most notably non-small-cell lung, colorectal, breast, prostate, and head and neck cancer.

Several novel therapeutic agents have been developed to interfere with signaling through the epidermal growth factor receptor pathway. Preclinically, two monoclonal antibodies that target the epidermal growth factor receptor, ABX-EGF and C225, have been shown to block epidermal growth factor and transforming growth factor-α binding to that receptor. As a result, ligand-induced activation is averted, resulting in inhibition of cell cycle progression, decreased angiogenesis, decreased rates of metastasis, and increased sensitivity to chemotherapy- and radiation-induced apoptosis. These antibodies are now being studied in a variety of disease settings, with C225 showing evidence of some efficacy. Although these agents are relatively well tolerated, toxicities include an acneiform rash that on biopsy reveals a subepidermal neutrophilic infiltration and epidermal hyperproliferation. In addition, several oral tyrosine kinase inhibitors have been developed (e.g., OSI-774 and ZD1839) to selectively and directly inhibit the epidermal growth factor receptor tyrosine kinase activity, decreasing epidermal growth factor receptor autophosphorylation on ligand binding. Tyrosine kinase inhibition results in cell cycle arrest and apoptosis. These epidermal growth factor receptor tyrosine kinase inhibitor agents are showing promising single-agent antitumor activity in non-small-cell lung and other cancers.

In summary, there are strong preclinical data to support the idea that targeted therapies represent a promising new era in cancer treatment. Biologically active doses of these agents have been given to patients with chemotherapy-refractory tumors, and tumor responses and stabilization of disease have been reported. However, the ultimate role of these agents as cancer therapeutics remains to be determined.

Conclusion

Recent advances in the areas of genetics, immunology, and molecular and cell biology have begun to alter our approach to the treatment of malignancy. New drugs, aimed specifically at targets unique to malignant cells, are being developed. Several have completed clinical investigation and are available for widespread use. Many others are in the early stages of their development. Clinical endpoints that have traditionally been used to determine dosing of chemotherapeutic agents may no longer be applicable to these novel drugs. In particular, the linear dose response curves seen with conventional cytotoxic agents may no longer apply. While time to tumor progression and overall survival will continue to be important endpoints, surrogate and biologic measurements such as apoptosis, inhibition of angiogenesis, induction of specific immune response, production or reduction of signaling molecules, and gene expression will need to be measured and correlated with clinical outcomes to determine optimal dosing and scheduling of the novel agents. Ultimately, these agents may enable truly tumor-specific antineoplastic therapy.

References

General

Bi WL, Parysek LM, Warnick R, et al: In vitro evidence that metabolic cooperation is responsible for the bystander effect observed with HSV-TK retroviral gene therapy. Hum Gene Ther 1993;4:725–731.

Bunting KD, Galipeau J, Topham D, et al: Effects of retroviral-mediated MDR1 expression on hematopoietic stem cell self-renewal and differentiation in culture. Ann N Y Acad Sci 1999;872:125–140.

Dianzani F: Interferon treatments: How to use an endogenous system as a therapeutic agent. J Interferon Res 1992; (Special Issue):109–118.

Gibbons JJ, Discafani C, Peterson R, et al: The effect of CCI-779, a novel macrolide anti-tumor agent, on the growth of human tumor cells in vitro and in nude mouse xenograft in vivo. Proc Am Assoc Cancer Res 2000;40: 301.

Gibbons NB, Watson RW, Coffey RN, et al: Heat-shock proteins inhibit induction of prostate cancer cell apoptosis. Prostate 2000;45:58–65.

Jackson JH, Cochrane CG, Courne JR, et al: Farnesol modification of Kirsten-ras exon 4B protein is essential for transformation. Proc Natl Acad Sci U S A 1990;87:3042–3046.

Nauts HC, Swift WE, Coley BL: Treatment of malignant tumors by bacterial toxins as developed by the late William B. Coley, M.D., reviewed in the light of modern research. Cancer Res 1946;6:205.

Webb A, Cunningham D, Cotter F, et al: BCL-2 antisense therapy in patients with non-Hodgkin's lymphoma. Lancet 1997;349:1137–1141.

Wu X, Senechal K, Neshat MS, et al: The PTEN/MMAC1 tumor suppressor phosphatase functions as a negative regulator of the phosphoinositide 3-kinase/Akt pathway. Proc Natl Acad Sci U S A 1998;95:15,587–15,591.

Angiogenesis

Hanahan D, Folkman J: Patterns and emerging mechanisms of the angiogenic switch during tumorigenesis. Cell 1996;86:353–364.

Kerbel RS, Viloria-Petit AM, Okada F, et al: Establishing a link between oncogenes and tumor angiogenesis. Mol Med 1998;4:286–295.

Moore BB, Arenberg DA, Addison CL, et al: Tumor angiogenesis is regulated by CXC chemokines. J Lab Clin Med 1998;132:97–103.

Cancer Immunology

Ishii T, Udono H, Yamano T, et al: Isolation of MHC class I-restricted tumor antigen peptide and its precursors associated with heat shock proteins hsp70, hsp90, and gp96. J Immunol 1999;162:1303–1309.

Jain RK: Transport of molecules across tumor vasculature. Cancer Metastasis Rev 1987;6:559–593.

James SP: Current Protocols in Immunology, 1991;7.

Jerne NK: Towards a network theory of the immune system. Ann Immunol 1974;125:373–389.

Pittet MJ, Valmori D, Dunbar PR, et al: High frequencies of naïve Melan-A/MART-1-specific CD8(+) T cells in a large proportion of human histocompatibility leukocyte antigen (HLA)-A2 individuals. J Exp Med 1999;190:705–715.

Slansky JE, Rattis FM, Boyd, et al: Enhanced antigen-specific antitumor immunity with altered peptide ligands that stabilize the MHC-peptide-TCR complex. Immunity 2000;13:529–538.

Steinman RM: The dendritic cell system and its role in immunogenicity. Annu Rev Immunol 1991;9:271–296.

Steplewski Z, Lubeck M, Koprowski H: Human macrophages armed with murine immunoglobulin G2a antibodies to tumors destroy human cancer cells. Science 1983; 221:865–868.

Traversari C, van der Bruggen P, Van den Eynde B, et al: Transfection and expression of a gene coding for a human melanoma antigen recognized by autologous cytolytic T lymphocytes. Immunogenetics 1992;35:145–152.

Tsang KY, Zaremba S, Nieroda CA, et al: Generation of human cytotoxic T-cells specific for human carcinoembryonic antigen (CEA) epitopes from patients immunized with recombinant vaccinia-CEA (rV-CEA) vaccine. J Natl Cancer Inst 1995;87:982–990.

van Oers MH, Pinkster J, Zeijlemaker WP: Quantification of antigen-reactive cells among human T lymphocytes. Eur J Immunol 1978;8:477–484.

Vegh Z, Wang P, Vanky F, Klein E: Selectively down-regulated expression of major histocompatibility complex class I alleles in human solid tumors. Cancer Res 1993;53(10 Suppl):2416–2420.

Cytokines

Czerkinsky C, Andersson G, Ekre HP, et al: Reverse ELISPOT assay for clonal analysis of cytokine production: I. Enumeration of gamma-interferon-secreting cells. J Immunol Methods 1988;110:29–36.

Wu PC, Alexander HR, Huang J, et al: In vivo sensitivity of human melanoma to tumor necrosis factor (TNF)-alpha is determined by tumor production of the novel cytokine endothelial-monocyte activating polypeptide II (EMAII). Cancer Res 1999;59:205–212.

Genes and Cancer

Almoguera C, Shibata D, Forrester K, et al: Most human carcinomas of the exocrine pancreas contain mutant c-K-ras genes. Cell 1988;53:549–554.

Bos JL, Fearon ER, Hamilton SR, et al: Prevalence of ras gene mutations in colorectal cancer. Nature 1987;327:293.

Fritz G, Just I, Kaina B: Rho GTPases are overexpressed in human tumors. Int J Cancer 1999;81:682–687.

Ganly I, Kirn D, Eckhardt SG, et al: A phase I study of Onyx-015, an E1B attenuated adenovirus, administered intratumorally to patients with recurrent head and neck cancer. Clin Cancer Res 2000;6:798–806.

Hollstein M, Sidransky D, Vogelstein B, et al: p53 mutations in human cancers. Science 1991;253:49–53.

Scheffner M, Werness BA, Huibregtse JM, et al: The E6 oncoprotein encoded by human papillomavirus types 16 and 18 promotes the degradation of p53. 1990;Cell 63:1129–1136.

Smit VT, Boot AJ, Smits AM, et al: KRAS codon 12 mutations occur very frequently in pancreatic adenocarcinomas. Nucleic Acids Res 1988;16:7773–7782.

Gene Therapy

Munger K, Werness BA, Dyson N, et al: Complex formation of human papillomavirus E7 proteins with the retinoblastoma tumor suppressor gene product. EMBO J 1989; 8:4099–4105.

Reese JS, Koc ON, Gerson SL: Human mesenchymal stem cells provide stromal support for efficient CD34+ transduction. J Hematother Stem Cell Res 1999;8:515–523.

Growth Factor Receptors

Baselga J, Mendelsohn J: Receptor blockade with monoclonal antibodies as anti-cancer therapy. Pharmacol Ther 1994;64:127–154.

Dinney CPN, Bielenberg DR, Reich R, et al: Inhibition of basic fibroblast growth factor expression, angiogenesis, and growth of human bladder carcinoma in mice by systemic interferon-alpha administration. Cancer Res 1998;58:808–814.

Saltz L, Rubin M, Hochster H, et al: Cetuximab (IMC-C225) plus irinotecan (CPT-11) is active in CPT-11 refractory colorectal cancer (CRC) that expresses epidermal growth factor receptor (EGFR). Proc Am Soc Clin Oncol 2001;20:3a, abst 7.

van Golen KL, Davies S, Wu X et al: A novel putative low-affinity insulin-like growth factor-binding protein, LIBC (lost in inflammatory breast cancer) and RhoC GTPase correlate with the infflammatory breast cancer phenotype. Clin Cancer Res 1999;5:2511–2519.

Interferon

Golomb HM, Jacobs A, Fefer A, et al: α-2 IFN therapy of hairy-cell leukemia: A multicenter study of 64 patients. J Clin Oncol 1986;4:900–905.

Huang S, Hendriks W, Althage A, et al: Immune response in mice that lack the interferon-gamma receptor. Science 1993;259:1742–1745.

The Italian Cooperative Study Group of Chronic Myeloid Leukemia: Interferon α-2a as compared with conventional chemotherapy for the treatment of chronic myeloid leukemia. N Engl J Med 1994;330:820–825.

Kirkwood JM, Strawderman MH, Ernstoff MS, et al: Interferon α-2b adjuvant therapy of high risk resected cutaneous melanoma: The Eastern Cooperative Oncology Group trial est. 1684. J Clin Oncol 1996;14:7–176.

Medical Research Council Renal Cancer Collaborators: Interferon-α and survival in metastatic renal carcinoma: Early results of a randomized controlled trial. Lancet 1999; 353:14–17.

Pestka S, Langer JA, Zoon KC, et al: Interferons and their actions. Annu Rev Biochem 1997;56:727–777.

Quesada JR, Reuben J, Manning JT, et al: Alpha interferon for induction of remission in hairy-cell leukemia. N Engl J Med 1984;310:15–18.

Sen GC, Ransohoff RM: Adv Virus Res 1993;42:57–102.

Singh RK, Gutman M, Bucana CD, et al: Interferons alpha and beta downregulate the expression of basic fibroblast growth factor in human carcinoma. Proc Natl Acad Sci U S A 1995;92:4562–4566.

Interleukins

Kanegane C, Sgadari C, Kanegane H, et al: Contribution of the CXC chemokines IP-10 and Mig to the antitumor effects of IL-12. J Leukoc Biol 1998;64:384–392.

Parkinson D, Abrams J, Wiernik P, et al: Interleukin-2 therapy in patients with metastatic malignant melanoma: A phase II study. J Clin Oncol 1990;8:1650–1656.

Rosenberg SA, Yang JC, Topalian SL, et al: Treatment of 283 consecutive patients with metastatic melanoma or renal cell cancer using high-dose bolus interleukin-2. JAMA 1994;271:907–913.

Monoclonal Antibodies

Ballare C, Barrio M, Portela P, et al: Functional properties of FC-2.15, a monoclonal antibody that mediates human complement cytotoxicity against breast cancer cells. Cancer Immunol Immunother 1995;41:15–22.

Baselga J, Tripathy T, Mendelsohn J, et al: Phase II study of weekly intravenous recombinant humanized anti-p185HER2 monoclonal antibody in patients with HER2/neu overexpressing metastatic breast cancer. J Clin Oncol 1996;14:737–744.

Cobleigh MA, Vogel CL, Tripathy D, et al: Efficacy and safety of Herceptin (humanized anti-HER2 antibody) as a single agent in 222 women with HER2 overexpression who had relapsed following chemotherapy for metastatic breast cancer. Proc Am Soc Clin Oncol 1998;17:97a, abst 376.

Czuczman MS, Grillo-Lopez AJ, White CA, et al: Treatment of patients with low grade B-cell lymphoma with the combination of chimeric anti-CD20 monoclonal antibody and CHOP chemotherapy. J Clin Oncol 1999;17:268–276.

Kohler G, Milstein C: Continuous cultures of fused cells secreting antibody of predefined specificity. Nature 1975; 256:495–497.

Ortaldo JR, Woodhouse C, Morgan AC, et al: Analysis of effector cells in human antibody dependent cellular cytotoxicity with murine monoclonal antibodies. J Immunol 1987;138:3566–3572.

Pegram MD, Lipton A, Hayes DF, et al: Phase II study of receptor-enhanced chemosensitivity using recombinant humanized anti-p185 HER2/neu monoclonal antibody plus cisplatin in patients with HER2/neu-overexpressing metastatic breast cancer refractory to chemotherapy treatment. J Clin Oncol 1998;8:2659–2671.

Slamon D, Leyland-Jones B, Shak S, et al: Addition of Herceptin (humanized anti-HER2 antibody) to first line chemotherapy for HER2 overexpressing metastatic breast cancer (HER2+/MBC) markedly increases anticancer activity: A randomized, multinational controlled phase III trial. Proc Am Soc Clin Oncol 1998;17:98a, abstr 377.

Slamon DJ, Clark GM, Wong SG, et al: Human breast cancer correlation of relapse and survival with amplification of the HER2/neu oncogene. Science 1987;253:177–181.

Trauth B, Klas C, Peters A, et al: Monoclonal antibody-mediated tumor regression by induction of apoptosis. Science 1989;245:301–304.

Weiner LM: Bispecific antibodies in cancer therapy. Cancer J Sci Am 2000;6(Suppl 3):S265–S271.

Vaccines

Caspar CB, Levy S, Levy R: Idiotype vaccines for non-Hodgkin's lymphoma induce polyclonal immune responses that cover mutated tumor idiotypes: Comparison of different vaccine formulations. Blood 1997;90:3699–3706.

Foon KA, John WJ, Chakraborty M, et al: Clinical and immune responses in resected colon cancer patients treated with anti-idiotype monoclonal antibody vaccine that mimics the carcinoembryonic antigen. J Clin Oncol 1999;17:2889–2895.

Foon KA, Sen G, Hutchins L, et al: Antibody responses in melanoma patients immunized with an anti-idiotype antibody mimicking disialoganglioside GD2. Clin Cancer Res 1998;4:1117–1124.

Hsu FJ, Caspar CB, Czerwinski D, et al: Tumor-specific idiotype vaccines in the treatment of patients with B-cell lymphoma: Long term results of a clinical trial. Blood 1997;89:3129–3135.

Lindenmann J: Speculations on idiotypes and homobodies. Ann Immunol 1973;124:171–184.

Wagner U, Schlebusch H, Kohler S, et al: Immunological responses to the tumor-associated antigen CA 125 in patients with advanced ovarian cancer induced by the murine monoclonal anti-idiotype vaccine ACA125. Hybridoma 1997;16:33–40.

Chapter 51
Hematopoietic Stem Cell Transplantation

Stephen J. Forman and Margaret R. O'Donnell

Introduction

Hematopoietic cell transplantation has been used to establish marrow and immune function following high-dose chemotherapy or chemotherapy and radiation to treat a variety of acquired and inherited malignant and nonmalignant disorders. These include hematologic malignancies such as acute and chronic leukemia, lymphoma, multiple myeloma, and myelodysplasia as well as nonmalignant acquired bone marrow disorders such as aplastic anemia. In addition, genetic diseases, including thalassemia, sickle cell anemia, and various syndromes of combined immune deficiency, have all been cured by this approach. Autologous hematopoietic cell transplantation is used in the support of patients with lymphoid malignancies, myeloma, acute myelogenous leukemia, and selected solid tumors who are undergoing high-dose therapy for which hematologic toxicity would be the limiting factor.

Types of Transplantation

Three different types of hematopoietic stem cell transplantation are used in therapy:

1. Allogeneic hematopoietic stem cell transplantation involves infusion of stem cells that are derived from a donor other than the patient. This type of transplantation requires some degree of tissue compatibility between the donor and the recipient. Immunosuppressive agents are needed both to prevent rejection of the graft by the recipient and to prevent the potentially lethal reaction of the donor immune system against the patient, a phenomenon known as graft-versus-host disease (GVHD). Allogeneic hematopoietic stem cell transplantation is used to reestablish bone marrow and immunologic function after myeloablative treatment with high-dose chemotherapy with or without radiation therapy that is given for the treatment of certain acquired and inherited malignant and nonmalignant disorders. These include hematologic malignancies such as acute and chronic leukemia, lymphoma, multiple myeloma, and myelodysplasia as well as nonmalignant acquired bone marrow disorders such as aplastic anemia. Moreover, genetic diseases including thalassemia, sickle cell anemia, and various syndromes of combined immune deficiency have been cured by this approach.

2. Autologous hematopoietic stem cell transplantation involves the collection of stem cells from the patients themselves. These cells are cryopreserved prior to dose-intensive therapy. This presupposes that the disease process does not significantly involve the patient's bone marrow and/or peripheral blood and that the stem cell pool has not been so depleted in heavily pretreated patients that one cannot obtain an adequate number of stem cells to allow prompt marrow reconstitution. Autologous hematopoietic stem cell transplantation is used in the support of patients with lymphoid malignancies, myeloma, acute myeloid leukemia, and selected solid tumors undergoing high-dose therapy for which hematologic toxicity would be the limiting factor.

3. Syngeneic hematopoietic stem cell transplantation uses an identical twin as the stem cell donor.

Source of Hematopoietic Stem Cells

The early studies of hematopoietic stem cell transplantation used bone marrow stem cells harvested from the iliac crest of the patient or donor by multiple aspirates obtained in the operating room under general anesthesia. In the late 1980s, the availability of marrow-stimulating cytokines such as granulocyte colony-stimulating factor (G-CSF) and granulocyte-monocyte colony-stimulating factor (GM-CSF) made it feasible for hematopoietic stem cells to be collected via a leukopheresis technique from peripheral blood by mobilizing marrow precursor stem cells into the peripheral blood circulation. These cytokine-primed stem cells were used initially in autologous hematopoietic stem cell transplantation. Compared to stem cells obtained from the bone marrow; peripheral blood stem cells shortened the time to blood count recovery following high-dose therapy and dramatically decreased procedure-related morbidity and mortality rates in both autologous and allogeneic hematopoietic stem cell transplantation. Despite a substantially greater quantity of donor lymphocytes in peripheral blood versus bone marrow-derived stem cells, acute graft-versus-host disease was not increased in frequency or severity in allogeneic transplantation. Although the findings have been controversial, recent studies suggest that the extent and severity of chronic graft-versus-host disease may be somewhat increased.

As immunosuppressive medications improved and human leukocyte antigen (HLA) typing was refined, it became possible to use nonfamily donors who were phenotypically tissue matched. A number of potential sources for stem cells for allogeneic transplantation are listed in Table 51-1.

Allogeneic Hematopoietic Stem Cell Transplantation

Human Leukocyte Antigen–Typing to Identify a Donor

Matched related allogeneic hematopoietic stem cell transplantation involves a donor who is human leukocyte antigen matched to the recipient. Historically, human leukocyte antigen typing was performed on

Table 51-1 ■ Stem Cell Sources for Allogeneic BMT

Donor	Advantages	Disadvantages
Identical Twin		
(Syngeneic)	No need for immunosuppression No graft-versus-host disease	No graft-versus-tumor effect
Sibling Donor		
(6/6 or 5/6 HLA-A, HLA-B, and HLA-DR antigen match)	Rapid donor identification (2 weeks)	Graft-versus-host disease (25% to 40%) for non-T cell-depleted grafts Low graft rejection rate (2% to 5%) Only 30% of patients will have a histocompatible sibling donor
Matched Unrelated Donor		
	Extends donor availability (60% to 70% of patients will have a potential match) Increased graft-versus-tumor effect	Takes time to find donor: average of 3 to 4 months (range, 1.5 to greater than 6 months) Increased graft failure rate (5% to 10%) Increased graft-versus-host disease rate (50% to 60%)
Umbilical Cord Blood		
	Precise human leukocyte antigen matching not required Low graft-versus-host disease rate (10% to 20%) despite 1 or 2 human leukocyte antigen mismatch	Cell number is limited (reduced applicability to large recipient) Marrow engraftment is delayed No chance for second infusion for graft failure or donor lymphocyte infusion for relapse High graft failure rate (10%)
Haploidentical Family Member		
	Almost all patients have a sibling, parent, or child who is haploidentical These donors can be used if patient has relapsed or refractory disease and no other donor is available	Needs intensive immunosuppression (including T cell depletion of donor product) to achieve engraftment High risk of infectious complications Very high graft failure rate (10% to 15%)

blood samples obtained from the patient and potential donors utilizing serologic methods to identify the Class I (HLA A, B, and C) and Class II (DQ, DR) antigens. A match within a family is noted when the major Class I and Class II antigens (A, B, and DR) of the recipient and potential donor are identical. Phenotypic identity can be confirmed by testing the parents to determine the alleles of each set of antigens or molecular characterization of the alleles. Because a person receives one set of human leukocyte antigen antigens from each parent, the patient is haploidentical with each parent, and there is a 25% chance that any sibling will be histocompatible. Given the average family size in the United States and Europe, only 30% of patients who are in need of a donor will have a family match. For patients who do not have a donor in their immediate family, it is sometimes useful to perform an extended family search, particularly when there are close familial interrelationships. Approximately 5% of patients will have a relative that is matched for five of the six HLA A, B, and DR serologically defined antigens. Although the use of these individuals as donors in transplantation is associated with a greater risk of both graft rejection and graft-versus-host disease than when sibling donors are used, the survival rate appears to be comparable. Matched nonsibling relatives thus can be used, particularly for patients who cannot wait until a matched unrelated donor is located.

For patients who lack a family donor, finding a matched unrelated donor involves a search of the computer files of the National Marrow Donor Program and other registries around the world. Because there are multiple alleles at any given human leukocyte antigen locus, serologic identity does not necessarily imply genotypic identity as is the case among sibling pairs, in whom the molecular inheritance patterns are defined by the parents. The development of oligonucleotide probes has greatly increased the precision of human leukocyte antigen typing and has allowed for more precise selection of hematopoietic stem cell donors by matching molecular alleles in the Class I and Class II antigens. In general, the closer the molecular match of the donor and recipient, the better is the outcome from transplantation and the more likely it is that the result will approximate what can be achieved by utilizing a matched family donor. The distribution of human leukocyte antigen phenotypes is not random. Because of linkage disequilibrium, a number of the common HLA-A, B, and DR haplotypes found in human populations vary in frequency among racial and ethnic groups. Common haplotypes have been identified for the major ethnic groups; distinct and less common human leukocyte antigen types are seen in native Americans, African blacks, Japanese,

Ashkenazi Jews, and Asians. Patients of mixed racial origin with uncommon haplotypes are the most difficult to match. For these patients, the potential donor sources may be limited to either stem cells from family members who are only haploidentical or umbilical cord stem cells. The former causes frequent and severe graft-versus-host disease because of the degree of human leukocyte antigen mismatch. These haploidentical stem cells have to be T cell-depleted to moderate graft-versus-host disease effects, but T cell depletion increases the risk of disease relapse and failure of engraftment. Umbilical cord cells are perforce immunologically naive and, as donor cells, even if one or two antigens are mismatched with the host, do not cause excessive graft-versus-host disease. Although useful in the treatment of children, umbilical cord blood stem cells are infrequently used in adult hematopoietic transplantation. The small volume of blood obtainable from the umbilical cord blood usually does not contain an adequate number of stem cells to provide speedy bone marrow recovery in a full-sized adult.

The time constraints that are involved in the identification of a nonfamily donor means that the interval between initiating the donor search and setting up a transplantation requires a minimum of two months (including obtaining insurance authorization). However, for most patients the process takes between two and six months. This lengthy delay compromises the utility of matched unrelated donors transplantation for those patients with leukemia or bone marrow failure whose disease does not remain clinically stable. For this reason, patients should be human leukocyte antigen typed at diagnosis so that a donor search can be initiated, when indicated, without delay.

Principles Underlying Allogeneic Hematopoietic Stem Cell Transplantation

The conditioning or preparative regimen that is used for an allogeneic hematopoietic stem cell transplantation contains a therapeutic component that is intended to eliminate tumor cells in the recipient and an immunosuppressive component that is intended to prevent a host immune response that would reject the donor graft. The object is to obtain complete donor type hematopoietic and immunologic reconstitution, a state that is known as complete chimerism. Traditionally, the doses of radiation and chemotherapy that are employed take advantage of the steep dose-response curve that exists for many hematologic malignancies, but the maximally tolerated doses of the various regimens are limited by toxicity to non-hematopoietic organs, such as the liver, gastrointestinal (GI) tract, and lung.

Advantages of an allogeneic graft include (1) no contamination of the graft with tumor cells, (2) the potential for an immunologically based graft-versus-tumor effect, and (3) the ability to treat malignant and nonmalignant diseases in which the bone marrow is abnormal. The disadvantages of an allogeneic hematopoietic stem cell transplantation include (1) the time and difficulty in finding an appropriate human leukocyte antigen–matched donor if a family donor is not available and (2) the development of graft-versus-host disease after transplantation. Graft-versus-host disease contributes to the morbidity and mortality of the procedure. Delayed immunologic recovery results from the effects that graft-versus-host disease induces and from the use of immunosuppressive drugs to diminish graft-versus-host disease. Immune dysfunction after allogeneic hematopoietic stem cell transplantation increases the risk of infectious complications.

Graft-Versus-Tumor Effect

The risk of recurrent disease in patients undergoing transplantation for a hematologic malignancy is influenced by the donor source and the development of a graft-versus-host reaction. Relapse rates are highest in syngeneic hematopoietic stem cell transplantation and lowest in patients with mild to moderate graft-versus-host disease. Graft-versus-host disease is in fact the most significant independent prognostic factor associated with a decreased relapse rate after allogeneic hematopoietic stem cell transplantation. Both acute and chronic graft-versus-host disease are associated with a graft-versus-tumor effect even in patients with only minimal graft-versus-host disease when compared to patients with syngeneic donors who develop no graft-versus-host disease. Another measure of this effect is the observation that withdrawal of immunosuppressive therapy can cause disease regression in patients whose chronic myeloid leukemia, acute myeloid leukemia, or low-grade lymphoid malignancy relapses after allogeneic hematopoietic stem cell transplantation. The results in patients who receive T cell-depleted marrow during allogeneic hematopoietic stem cell transplantation for chronic myeloid leukemia make a circumstantial but compelling case for T cell mediation of graft-versus-host tumor effect. These patients have a far greater relapse rate (40% to 60%) than recipients of unmodified allogeneic marrow (10% to 15%). This phenomenon has found application in the infusion of donor lymphocytes (DLI) in patients who relapse. Donor T lymphocyte infusion in the absence of immunosuppressive medication reinduces remission in 60% of patients with chronic-phase chronic myeloid leukemia who relapse after

allogeneic hematopoietic stem cell transplantation, albeit at the price of generating a substantial degree of graft-versus-host disease.

Nonmyeloablative Hematopoietic Stem Cell Transplant

The recognition that malignant hematopoietic disease may respond to donor leukocyte infusion without requiring high-dose chemoradiotherapy raised the question of whether one could harness the graft-versus-tumor effect itself as the primary treatment of the disease. Treatments of varyingly reduced intensity and toxicity have been used to establish donor-derived hematopoiesis and harness the donor antitumor immune effect. The reduced doses of chemotherapeutic agents with or without total body irradiation are intended primarily for their immunosuppressive effects rather than for tumoricidal activity. After transplantation, immunosuppression is used to inhibit the host's immunologic response, facilitating engraftment of the donor stem cells. This technique was developed to provide allogeneic hematopoietic stem cell transplantation for patients whose advanced age or concomitant medical conditions would not permit the use of the usual intensive preparative regimens. Remissions have been achieved in some hematologic malignancies by this technique.

Preparative Treatment Regimens for Allogeneic Hematopoietic Stem Cell Transplantation

The initial treatment that is used to prepare a patient to accept an allograft should combine agents that are highly active against the underlying malignancy with agents that provide a degree of immunosuppression that is adequate to prevent the recipient from rejecting the donor's stem cells. Conditioning regimens usually employ drugs that exhibit steep dose-response curves against hematopoietic malignancies. Commonly used regimens are listed in Table 51-2. For high-dose therapy and allogeneic hematopoietic stem cell transplantation, two frequently used regimens are (1) total body irradiation (TBI) combined with either cyclophosphamide (CY) or etoposide (VP-16) and (2) cyclophosphamide (CY) combined with busulfan (BU).

Targeted therapeutic strategies are under investigation. For example, busulfan taken orally exhibits widely varying absorption rates, and the actual received dose is uncertain. An intravenous formulation of busulfan now allows for precise pharmacologic dose targeting, which appears to decrease both hepatic toxicity and relapse. Radiolabeled (^{131}I or ^{90}Y) antibodies that are targeted to myeloid (CD33) or lym-

Table 51-2 ■ Common Allogeneic Transplantation Conditioning Regimens for Malignancies

Radiation-Based

	Fractionated total body irradiation (FTBI) 1200 to 1320 (cGy) delivered in 6 to 11 dose fractions to whole body over 3 to 4 days, usually with lung shielding at 50% dose followed by either
FTBI/CY	Cyclophosphamide (CY) 60 mg/kg ideal body weight/day × 2 on days –3 and –2
	or
FTBI/VP-16	Etoposide (VP-16) 60 mg/kg IV adjusted ideal weight/on day –2

Chemotherapy Regimens

BU/CY	Busulfan (BU) 1 mg/kg/PO qid × 4 days or 0.8 mg/kg IV qid × 4 days on days –8 to –4 (dose targeted to achieve an AUC of 800 to 1200 ng/mL)
	Cyclophosphamide (CY) 60 mg/kg ideal body weight IV/day on days –3 and –2

Nonmyeloablative Therapy

Total body irradiation	200 cGy in 1 dose
+	
Fludarabine	25 mg/m^2 IV/day × 5 on days –6 to –2
or	
Fludarabine combined with melphalan	150 mg/m^2 IV on day –1

For Aplastic Anemia

CY/ATG	Cyclophosphamide (CY) 50 mg/kg ideal body weight IV × 4 days on days –5 to –2 as a single agent or combined with Anti-thymocyte globulin (ATG) 40 mg/kg IV day –4 to –2 (3 doses)

Minus days refer to days prior to stem cell reinfusion, which is day 0.
AUC = Area under the curve if a pharmacokinetic measurement of drug delivery (dose and time)

phoid (CD19 or CD45) antigens represent another approach. They offer the potential to increase the effective radiation dose delivered to the tumor while preventing injury to normal tissues.

The nonmyeloablative conditioning regimens are focused primarily on the immunosuppression of the host rejection mechanism, relying on the donor cells' graft-versus-tumor effect to be tumoricidal. The regimens combine a single dose of limited whole-body radiation (200 cGy) with fludarabine or fludarabine plus melphalan. These regimens allow engraftment of donor cells; complete chimerism (allogeneic hematopoietic stem cell fully functional in a non-identical host) is usually established within 30 to 60 days after infusion of stem cells.

For patients with aplastic anemia, the host immune status is the target of the conditioning regimen. Cyclophosphamide either alone or combined with antithymocyte globulin (ATG) currently represents the conditioning regimen for sibling donor hematopoietic stem cell transplantations. Additional immunosuppression is required in this circumstance if the stem cell source is an unrelated donor.

Common acute toxicities associated with these regimens are listed in Table 51-3. All recipients of dose-intensive regimens exhibit gastrointestinal side effects, including severe oral mucositis, which often requires narcotic analgesics and nutritional supplementation to provide adequate caloric intake. The oral mucositis may be exacerbated by reactivation of oral herpes simplex infection and in allogeneic hematopoietic stem cell recipients by methotrexate, which is a frequent component of graft-versus-host disease prophylaxis.

Veno-occlusive disease (VOD) results from injury to the endothelium in liver (and occasionally lung) caused by cytotoxic agents. The clinical manifestations are fluid retention, jaundice, hepatomegaly, right upper quadrant pain from distension of the liver capsule, and, in severe cases, ascites and hepatorenal syndrome. It is distinguished from other forms of liver injury by the relatively modest elevations of the blood levels of the liver enzymes, the transaminases, and alkaline phosphatase. The syndrome occurs in 5% to 20% of both allogeneic and autologous hematopoietic stem cell transplantation recipients. Factors that pre-

Table 51-3 ▪ Common Nonhematologic Toxicities of Agents Used in Transplantation Regimens

Agent	Early Toxicity	Late Toxicity
Total body irradiation	Mucositis, enteritis, nausea, vomiting	Sterility, leukemia (following autologous transplant), secondary cancers, cataracts, cardiomyopathy, interstitial pneumonitis
Cyclophosphamide	Nausea, vomiting, hemorrhagic cystitis, cardiomyopathy	Sterility, secondary leukemia (following autologous transplants), interstitial pneumonitis
Etoposide	Nausea, vomiting, mucositis, blisters, skin rash, enteritis, hypotension	Secondary leukemia (from autologous transplants)
Busulfan	Seizure, nausea, veno-occlusive disease	Secondary leukemia (following autologous transplants), alopecia, pulmonary fibrosis
Melphalan	Nausea	Peripheral neuropathy
Fludarabine	Hemolytic anemia	Prolonged immunosuppression, EBV related lymphoproliferative disease
Carmustine (BCNU)	Nausea, vomiting, seizure	Interstitial pneumonia, pulmonary fibrosis

dispose to veno-occlusive disease include prior hepatic injury from viral or chemical hepatitis, prior hepatic radiation therapy, iron overload from multiple blood transfusions, prior dose-intensive chemotherapy, particularly within the preceding year, and busulfan-based treatment regimens. Treatment is usually supportive and, except in severe cases, resolves within weeks. No specific therapy is available.

Graft-Versus-Host Disease and Its Prophylaxis and Treatment

Graft-versus-host disease is analogous, in reverse, to organ rejection (host-versus-graft) in solid organ transplants. The cytotoxic T cells from the donor recognize and react to differences in minor histocompatibility antigens on recipient tissues. In the acute phase, which usually occurs within 100 days of transplantation, the primary targets are usually the skin, liver, and gastrointestinal tract, resulting in skin rash, jaundice, nausea, vomiting, and diarrhea. Late or chronic graft-versus-host disease occurs in 30% to 75% of patients. It is more insidious and resembles aspects of collagen vascular disorders such as scleroderma, Sjögren's syndrome, or systemic lupus erythematosus. Malabsorption, chronic weight loss, and recurrent infections may supervene. Bronchiolitis obliterans occasionally occurs as a manifestation of chronic and can lead to respiratory insufficiency. Factors that reduce the risk of severe graft-versus-host disease are (1) complete (versus partial) human leukocyte antigen matching of donor and recipient, (2) matched related (versus unrelated) donor, (3) younger (versus older) age of donor and recipient, and (4) no or few (versus many)

pregnancies in the donor. The incidence of moderate to severe acute graft-versus-host disease ranges from 10% to 30% for patients with a family donor to 50% to 60% in recipients with a matched unrelated or partially matched family donor.

There are two strategies for graft-versus-host disease prophylaxis: One can either partially deplete the donor graft of T cells prior to infusion or administer drugs to inactivate the donor T cells. T cell depletion can be done mechanically by elutriation techniques or by immunologic means such as CD34 selection using immunomagnetic beads, e-rosetting, or exposure of the stem cell product to selected T cell antibodies such as Campath. T cell depletion successfully abrogates acute graft-versus-host disease but at the cost of both higher rates of graft failure and disease relapse. Drugs for prophylaxis include cyclosporine or its analog, tacrolimus, which is usually paired with a short course of methotrexate given on days 1, 3, 6, and 11 after transplantation. In situations in which the risk of graft rejection is high, such as aplastic anemia or mismatched grafts, antithymocyte globulin (ATG) is added to the preparative regimen prior to stem cell infusion, which inactivates host T cells and generates some early antigraft-versus-host disease effects. High doses of methylprednisolone are added to cyclosporine (or tacrolimus) to treat acute graft-versus-host disease. As the reaction subsides, these medications are slowly tapered. In patients with corticosteroid refractory acute graft-versus-host disease, agents such as mycophenolate, antithymocyte globulin, or monoclonal anti-T cell antibodies such as decluzimab are added sequentially to gain control of the syndrome. Although most patients do respond to corticosteroids, the mortality rate in corticosteroid-refractory patients is high and is often associated with intercurrent bacterial or fungal infections.

Chronic graft-versus-host disease may evolve directly from acute graft-versus-host disease or emerge later, 3 to 12 months after transplantation, as immunosuppression is tapered. Because the manifestations often develop slowly over time, end organ damage in connective tissue and lung may be relatively advanced before clinical symptoms are recognized. Cyclosporine or tacrolimus plus corticosteroids is the mainstay of chronic graft-versus-host disease therapy. For resistant graft-versus-host disease, psoralen-activated ultraviolet light irradiation administered by means of extracorporeal photopheresis may be effective. This involves establishing efferent and afferent intravenous lines to circulate the patient's blood through an external grid, where it is irradiated by ultraviolet light. This technique works by inactivating circulating T cells and dendritic cells. Other agents that are sometimes useful in the treatment of late chronic graft-versus-host disease include thalidomide, rapamycin, and mycophenolate. Patients with chronic graft-versus-host disease often have significant T cell immune deficiency and are prone to recurrent bacterial and fungal infection of lungs and sinuses. While there is significant morbidity and mortality associated with graft-versus-host disease, the heightened immune reactivity of donor T cells also conveys some protection against relapse of the primary malignancy.

Autologous Hematopoietic Stem Cell Transplantation

Principles Underlying Autologous Hematopoietic Stem Cell Transplantation

Autologous hematopoietic stem cell transplantation involves the reinfusion of the patient's stem cells to support the recovery of hematopoiesis after high-dose antitumor chemotherapy ± radiation therapy. The autologous grafted cells' sole contribution to the outcome is rapid reestablishment of hematopoiesis, which mitigates the toxicity of the regimen. The success of autologous hematopoietic stem cell transplantation ultimately depends on the sensitivity of the tumor to the high-dose preparative regimen. High-dose therapy is not uniformly tumor-ablative, in either the autologous or allogeneic transplantation setting, because many cancers contain small populations of tumor cells that are resistant to treatment, either intrinsically or acquired over the course of therapy and time. The treatment regimens may also be ineffective because the incremental increase in dose might

not be high enough to provide the intended tumor cell kill.

The probability that a tumor contains treatment-resistant cells, according to the Goldie-Coleman model, correlates with the size of the tumor and the spontaneous mutation rate of the cancer cells. This suggests that the optimal timing of high-dose therapy is early in the natural history of a tumor, when it is chemosensitive. Consistent with this hypothesis is the observation that patients undergoing transplantation after multiple relapses have an inferior disease-free survival rate compared with those who undergo transplantation early in their therapy. The development of resistant disease that leads to relapse is the major determinant of the difference in outcome. A disadvantage of autologous hematopoietic stem cell transplantation is the possibility of occult tumor cell contamination of the stem cell collection. Because of the concern that these tumor cells have the potential to repopulate and cause relapse, autologous hematopoietic stem cell transplantation is limited to patients who lack significant marrow or peripheral blood involvement at the time of stem cell harvesting. The relative merits and disadvantages of allogeneic versus autologous hematopoietic stem cell transplantation are outlined in Table 51-4. The choice of either an allogeneic or an autologous approach is influenced by the patient's condition, age, and disease status and the availability of a donor. Detailed discussion of the type of transplantation and its role in therapy follows in the sections on indications for transplantation in specific hematologic disorders.

Treatment Regimens for Autologous Hematopoietic Stem Cell Transplantation

The efficacy of autologous hematopoietic stem cell transplantation relies solely on the conditioning regimen. Because there is no need to incorporate immunosuppressive agents to allow engraftment in the autologous setting, the preparative regimens usually focus on combining drugs that are efficacious against a particular tumor. Their utility depends on whether tumor response rates improve with increased doses and the presence of nonoverlapping toxicities among the drugs combined in therapy. Whereas most allogeneic regimens combine two agents (fractionated total body irradiation plus etoposide or cyclophosphamide or busulfan plus cyclophosphamide), autologous transplantation preparative regimens may employ three or even four agents. Because many patients with lymphomas, including Hodgkin's disease, myeloma, and breast cancer, have had prior radiation therapy, the commonly used regimens (Table 51-5) do not contain radiation therapy. In patients

Table 51-4 ■ Comparison of Allogeneic Versus Autologous Stem Cell Transplantation

Allogeneic

Advantages

1. No tumor contamination of graft and no prior donor stem cell injury from chemotherapy decreases risk of subsequent myelodysplasia/acute leukemia
2. Graft-versus-tumor effect
3. Can be used for patients with marrow involvement by tumor or with bone marrow dysfunction such as aplastic anemia, hemoglobinopathies, or prior pelvic radiation

Disadvantages

1. Regimen-related toxicity limits use in older patients, usually only employed in patients less than age 55 years
2. Time to identify donor if no sibling donor is available; limited availability of matched unrelated donor for some ethnic groups
3. Early and late treatment-related mortality from graft-versus-host disease and infectious complications (20% to 40% depending on age and donor source)

Autologous

Advantages

1. No need to identify donor if peripheral blood stem cells uninvolved by tumor at time of collection
2. No immunosuppression = less risk of infections
3. No GVHD
4. Dose intensive therapy can be used for older patients (usually up to age 70)
5. Low early treatment-related mortality (2% to 5%)

Disadvantages

1. Not feasible if overt tumor cell contamination of peripheral blood or marrow stem cells
2. Stem cell damage from either prior chemotherapy and/or transplant regimen creates risk of subsequent myelodysplasia/acute leukemia (up to 10%)
3. No graft-versus-tumor effect
4. Diminished stem cell number from prior treatment may make it impossible to mobilize an adequate stem cell dose to permit rapid marrow reconstitution

who have received no prior radiation therapy, primarily patients with lymphoma or acute myeloid leukemia, fractionated total body irradiation can substitute for the carmustine (BCNU) in the treatment programs.

General Considerations In Hematopoietic Stem Cell Transplantation

Evaluating the Patient

Patients who are potential candidates for either autologous or allogeneic hematopoietic stem cell transplantation require a careful clinical evaluation as well as in-depth counseling by physicians, nurses, and social workers who are experienced in the procedure. The patients and their caregivers should be informed about the complications of the procedure and issues related to the preparative regimen, bone marrow hypoplasia, immunologic impairment, graft-versus-host disease, and other short- and long-term complications. These sessions deal with significant and sensitive issues, such as infertility, morbidity, mortality, and management of end-of-life issues, should they be required. Patients who are being evaluated for transplantation need to undergo repeated staging procedures to document the current extent of the disease, since this can influence the type of transplantation as well as the specific conditioning regimen to be utilized.

Cytogenetic studies of the patient's stem cells should be obtained before autologous hematopoietic stem cell transplantation. When allogeneic hematopoietic stem cell transplantation is indicated but a suitable sibling donor is unavailable, the search for a matched unrelated donor should proceed while efforts are made to stabilize the patient's disease until a histocompatible donor can be identified.

The patient's age and performance status are important factors in considering a patient for high-dose therapy. Allogeneic hematopoietic stem cell transplantation are generally restricted to patients younger than age 56 years, whereas autologous hematopoietic stem cell transplantation, because of lower toxicity, can be attempted in patients 60 years or older if their organ systems are physiologically sound. Studies that are required to assess the risk of morbidity and mortality from the transplantation procedure include assessment of the patient's cardiac, respiratory, hepatic, and renal function. For instance, a patient older than age 50 years who has a history of exposure to anthracycline drugs or radiation to the chest may be at increased risk for cardiac or pulmonary complications if high-dose cyclophosphamide is a component of the conditioning regimen. Significantly reduced diffusion capacity might be predictive of pulmonary complications, particularly for radiation-based conditioning regimens. Liver function test abnormalities need investigation, because liver disease can increase the risk of potentially fatal veno-

Table 51-5 ▪ Common Autologous Transplantation Conditioning Regimens

Radiation-Based Regimens

For leukemia and lymphoma	Fractionated total body irradiation (FTBI) 1200 cGy in 6 to 10 fractions over 3 to 4 days on days −8 to −5 (radiolabeled ^{131}I or ^{90}Y anti-CD20 is substituted in some clinical trials) + Etoposide (VP-16): 60 mg/kg IV on day −4 + Cyclophosphamide (CY): 100 mg/kg ideal weight IV on day −2

Chemotherapy Regimens

For Non-Hodgkin's Lymphoma and Hodgkin's Disease

BCV	Carmustine (BCNU): 150 mg/m^2 IV/day × 3 on days −6 to −4 + Etoposide (VP-16): 60 mg/kg actual weight IV on day −4 + Cyclophosphamide (CY): 100 mg/kg ideal body weight IV day −2
BEAM	Carmustine (BCNU): 300 mg/m^2 IV on day −6 + Etoposide (VP-16): 100 mg/m^2 q 12 hrs IV × 6 on days −5 to −2 + Cytarabine (ARA-C): 200 mg/m^2 q 12 hrs IV × 6 on days −5 to −2 + Melphalan: 140 mg/m^2 IV on day −1

For Acute Leukemias

BU/CY	Busulfan (BU) 1 mg/kg/PO qid × 4 days or 0.8 mg/kg IV qid × 4 days (dose is targeted to achieve an AUC of 800 to 1200 ng/mL) on days −8 to −4 + Cyclophosphamide (CY): 60 mg/kg ideal body weight IV/day on days −3 and −2

For Myeloma

Melphalan	140 to 200 mg/m^2 IV, 1 or 2 cycles 1 + BU/CY cycle 2
High-dose melphalan	140 to 200 mg/m^2 IV cycle 1 + BU/CY cycle 2
High-dose melphalan + total body irradiation	As a single cycle or tandem (2 sequential transplants)

Minus days refer to days prior to stem cell reinfusion, which is day 0.

occlusive disease. A liver biopsy might be necessary to exclude hepatic cirrhosis, which is a contraindication for any type of dose-intensive hematopoietic transplantation. Renal function is particularly important for allogeneic recipients, since the primary immunosuppressive medications, cyclosporine or tacrolimus, are both cleared by the kidneys and are nephrotoxic.

A history of previous infections, especially of invasive fungal diseases, should be sought. These may reactivate during the period of severe pancytopenia and immunosuppression that occurs after autologous and allogeneic hematopoietic stem cell transplantation. Some patients need antifungal prophylaxis as part of their treatment plan.

Psychosocial assessment of the patient is an important component of the evaluation not only to evaluate whether the patient should proceed to transplantation, but also to establish what will be required of the patient and family during the arduous process of transplantation and recovery. The transplantation team needs to understand the family's support structure and the capacity of the patient and family to adhere to instructions regarding the patient's medications and lifestyle restrictions, for example, restrictions on alcohol use, cigarette smoking, and exposure to others with infections. The patient's compliance with previous therapy and insight into diagnosis and prognosis require exploration. Given the multicultural nature of the society in which we live, obtaining a grasp of the patient's unique culture, religious convictions, literacy, and language skills is a component of the assessment.

All of these issues are even more important in the

pediatric population, in which there are special considerations. Although the rationale for the procedure as well as specific side effects and outcome issues are very similar, the most obvious difference in the evaluation is that the person for whom the procedure is intended is not the one who will give consent. The parents or the legal guardian of the minor child have a responsibility for decision making and therefore must have access to all the information to evaluate risk and benefits for any transplantation procedure. Nevertheless, the child is still the patient, the one who will have to endure the side effects of the procedure. The physicians and the pediatric staff must be sure to meet the needs of both the child and the parents.

Prevention and Treatment of Bacterial Infection in Transplantation Recipients

The neutropenia that follows a dose-intensive conditioning regimen places the patient at risk for bacterial infections. Endogenous bacteria, residing in the patient's gastrointestinal tract and mouth, are the principal source of infection. Exogenous sources of infection can be introduced, most commonly, during manipulation of venous access devices by the patient or health care providers. Many treatment regimens disrupt natural barriers to infection by desquamation of the skin and breakdown of the mucosal lining of the oropharynx and intestine.

In the autologous transplantation setting, using stem cells derived from the peripheral blood, this breach of natural defenses is transient, because recovery of blood counts is rapid. The risk of bacterial infection largely disappears once granulocyte recovery is established. A very small fraction of patients do, however, have decreased recovery of immunoglobulin production and are functionally asplenic. These patients may benefit from immunoglobulin replacement and penicillin prophylaxis.

In the allogeneic transplantation setting, the duration of neutropenia is similarly brief, but the opportunity for bacterial infection is greatly prolonged beyond the time of granulocyte recovery. Active graft-versus-host disease prolongs the period at risk by (1) continuing to damage mucosal surfaces, (2) necessitating immunosuppressive agents such as corticosteroids, and (3) creating the need for central venous access devices. In recipients of hematopoietic stem cells from histocompatible siblings or matched unrelated donors who develop graft-versus-host disease, acute bacterial infection accounts for 25% to 30% of treatment-related deaths within the first six months of transplantation. For patients who remain at high risk, immunoglobulin levels are monitored, and monthly replacement therapy is instituted for those who have continued hypogammaglobulinemia. Low-

dose penicillin prophylaxis is also recommended in those who are asplenic or who have functional asplenia.

Strategies for dealing with bacterial infection during neutropenia depend on the patient's history of infections, prior infecting organisms' antibiotic susceptibility, and institution-specific nosocomial infections. In centers where antibiotic-resistant organisms such as methicillin-resistant *Staphylococcus aureus* are prevalent, routine pretransplantation screening may identify patients who are colonized with these organisms. This knowledge will influence antibiotic choices during neutropenia and will affect contact isolation procedures to prevent spread of these organisms to other patients. Venous access devices may need to be replaced in patients who have previously documented bacteremia or fungemia with an organism that is difficult to eradicate from prosthetic devices.

Some studies have shown that the use of oral antibiotics during the conditioning regimen will decrease aerobic gastrointestinal tract flora, leading to fewer episodes of gram-negative sepsis. Empiric antibiotic therapy during febrile neutropenia should provide coverage for aerobic gram-positive and gram-negative organisms. Agents that are active against anaerobes and fungal infections are empirically added subsequently for patients who remain persistently febrile. Clinical trials are now evaluating whether keratinocyte growth factor may minimize oropharyngeal mucosal breakdown. The use of granulocyte colony-stimulating factor–primed stem cells as the source of hematopoietic reconstitution in both the autologous and the allogeneic transplantation setting has markedly decreased the morbidity and mortality risk of bacterial infection by shortening the duration of neutropenia by five to seven days.

Prevention and Treatment of Fungal Infections Post Transplantation

Mycotic infections in transplantation recipients are most often caused by *Candida* and *Aspergillus* species, and less often by mucor species. *Candida* overgrowth in the gastrointestinal tract occurs in neutropenic patients. The *Candida* then spreads via the bloodstream to other tissues. Fungal spores are ubiquitous in nature. Individuals such as ranch or construction workers are colonized during occupational exposure, or colonization may occur from hobbies such as gardening and dirt biking. The spores may remain dormant for decades, but in a patient receiving long-term immunosuppression, these agents can become active and invade tissues. Since the primary route of colonization is inhalation, the major sites of infection for *Aspergillus* species and mucormycoses are the nose, lung, and sinuses initially with later spread to the central nervous system (CNS). Because these organisms may be difficult to eradicate, prophylaxis and early detection are of the utmost importance. As part of pretransplantation screening, computed tomography (CT) scans of lung, liver, and spleen should be obtained to look for evidence of granulomas from prior fungal infections.

The incidence of fungal infection is less than 5% in autologous hematopoietic stem cell transplantation recipients and 5% to 15% in most allogeneic hematopoietic stem cell transplantation centers. The mortality rate is high (up to 80% in the systemic mycoses), and fungal infections represent the major cause of infectious deaths beyond 100 days after allogeneic hematopoietic stem cell transplantation.

Candida Infections

Candida overgrowth in the aerodigestive tract and female genitalia is commonly seen in patients who are treated with broad-spectrum antibiotics. In patients with profound neutropenia and mucosal breakdown due to dose-intensive chemoradiotherapy, the organism can gain access to the systemic circulation. *Candida* has a predilection for prosthetic devices and, once established, is almost impossible to eradicate with antifungal agents unless the prosthesis (usually a venous access device) is removed. From the colonized catheter, septic emboli are shed to the liver, spleen, and, less commonly, retina. The prophylactic use of fluconazole during conditioning and the subsequent neutropenia can significantly decrease colonization and fungemia, although fluconazole-resistant strains are now appearing.

Aspergillus Infections

Agents such as amphotericin or itraconazole are used to eradicate systemic, tissue-invasive fungal infections. In patients with nasal mucosal invasion or fungal sinusitis, surgical debridement of the tissues destroyed by hemorrhagic necrosis may be needed in addition to antifungal agents. *Aspergillus* infection of the lung can appear as an infiltrate on chest X-ray during neutropenia. As granulocytes reappear, tissue breakdown occurs, the almost pathognomonic fungus "ball" appears on chest X-ray, and the patient is at risk of serious pulmonary hemorrhage. Patients undergoing hematopoietic stem cell transplantation have difficulty resolving these infiltrates with antibiotic therapy alone due to immunologic function and often need pulmonary resection of the lesion.

Strategies for prophylaxis against *Aspergillus* species vary widely from institution to institution. In the absence of a reliable screening test for radiographically occult fungal infection, most investigators

choose to treat high-risk patients empirically with amphotericin (usually in a lipid formulation) or itraconazole or newer agents such as voriconazole and caspofungin. Patients who experience profound immunosuppression due to active graft-versus-host disease and the requirement for corticosteroid therapy or those who have a prior history of *Aspergillus* are at highest risk. The major drawback to universal prophylaxis is nephrotoxicity associated with long-term amphotericin use and liver function abnormalities associated with the azole-derived drugs.

Prevention and Treatment of Viral Infections After Hematopoietic Stem Cell Transplantation

Herpes viruses, including herpes simplex, cytomegalovirus (CMV), and varicella-zoster virus, are the most common cause of viral infection after transplantation. These infections usually represent reactivation of a preexisting latent virus in the adult patient, although primary varicella infections can occur in children. Reactivation is a consequence of the temporary immunoparalysis that accompanies allogeneic and autologous hematopoietic stem cell transplantation.

Herpes Simplex Infection

There are two subtypes of herpes simplex virus. Type 1 generally infects the oropharynx and typically establishes a latent infection in the trigeminal ganglia. Type 2 typically involves the genital or perineal area and establishes latency in the sensory ganglia of the lumbosacral plexus. In the absence of antiviral prophylaxis, 70% to 80% of autologous or allogeneic transplantation recipients who are seropositive for herpes simplex will reactivate virus within the first two to three weeks. Most of the infections involve the oropharynx, causing pain and decreased oral intake. Herpes simplex viral esophagitis and severe herpes simplex pneumonia can also occur. Randomized trials demonstrated that this reactivation can be prevented or minimized by prophylactic use of the antiviral acyclovir. The latent virus, however, is not eliminated by such treatment. Most recipients on immunosuppression are likely to reactivate once the acyclovir is stopped. Acyclovir has no substantial adverse effect on marrow recovery after transplantation. Therefore, patients who have a clinical history of vaginal or oral herpes simplex or antibody titers consistent with prior infection receive acyclovir prophylaxis to minimize this complication.

Cytomegalovirus

Cytomegalovirus is the most important herpetic infection that can affect long-term disease-free survival after allogeneic hematopoietic stem cell transplantation. As with herpes simplex virus, most patients who are seropositive for cytomegalovirus have latent infection, maintained in a dormant state by the host's intact immune system. In allogeneic hematopoietic stem cell transplantation, if approaches to control this potential infection are not part of the treatment plan, cytomegalovirus interstitial pneumonia develops in 20% to 40% of patients who either are seropositive for cytomegalovirus or receive stem cells from a seropositive donor. Mortality rates from respiratory failure were as high as 80% in the past. In the late 1980s, clinical studies showed that the combination of ganciclovir and intravenous immunoglobulin successfully treated 40% to 50% of allogeneic hematopoietic stem cell transplantation recipients who had established cytomegalovirus pneumonia. The median time to clinical infection with cytomegalovirus gastroenteritis, pneumonitis, or iritis is approximately 50-70 days after transplantation. Of particular note, although infection rates, determined by laboratory studies, are very similar in autologous stem cell recipients, the incidence of clinical cytomegalovirus disease is very low, suggesting that alloreactivity is a component of the pathogenesis of this disease.

The most important strategy for controlling cytomegalovirus infection after allogeneic hematopoietic stem cell transplantation is prevention. In seronegative recipients who have a seronegative donor, seronegative blood support should be used from the time of the original diagnosis and therapy to prevent primary infection. For the majority (more than 60%) of patients who are seropositive at diagnosis or who have a seropositive donor, other steps are necessary to forestall clinical expression of cytomegalovirus reactivation after transplantation. At present, two approaches are available for these patients: early detection of impending clinical activation or prophylaxis.

Early detection involves careful monitoring after transplantation for evidence of cytomegalovirus reactivation using blood cultures, detection of cytomegalovirus antigenemia, or polymerase chain reaction technology. Blood cultures are obtained twice weekly; they generally become positive two to three weeks before the development of pneumonia. Patients with documented blood infections should be treated preemptively with oral or intravenous ganciclovir for a minimum of five to six weeks. After completion of therapy, patients should continue to be screened for evidence of a secondary reactivation.

An alternative approach is the use of prophylactic ganciclovir in all patients who are seropositive. This is an effective strategy, but benefit from this approach has not been unequivocally demonstrated. While not all cytomegalovirus-seropositive transplant recipients will develop reactivation with positive blood cultures

during the course of transplantation, all recipients are at risk for the side effects of the prophylactic medication. These include marrow suppression and renal dysfunction. This places patients at risk for secondary infections and increases the costs of transplantation. Therefore, one can use either a risk-adapted technique, namely, administering antivirals during high-risk periods, such as when acute graft-versus-host disease is present, or monitor for reactivation during the first 100 days after transplantation and promptly initiate treatment at that time. Foscarnet is another antiviral that can be used effectively if cytomegalovirus resistance to ganciclovir develops.

Studies show that generation of a donor-derived immune response is the most important factor in preventing cytomegalovirus reactivation. Building on this information, clinical trials of the infusion of donor-derived cytomegalovirus-specific T cells are under investigation. These can alter the natural history of infection and protect most patients from clinical cytomegalovirus disease, eliminating the need for antiviral drugs. Other studies use donor immunization with cytomegalovirus-specific proteins or peptides to augment the immunologic response to reactivation of cytomegalovirus in the early months after transplantation.

Varicella-Zoster Infection

As is true of herpes simplex virus and cytomegalovirus, varicella-zoster infections can be primary infections, occurring from exposure during or after transplantation or recurrent infections or secondary, due to reactivation of latent virus. Primary infection produces the same clinical manifestations as chickenpox. After primary infection, the virus establishes latency in cells of the dorsal sensory ganglia of the spinal cord. Serum IgG antibodies provide evidence of past primary infection. When the endogenous latent virus reactivates, it causes herpes zoster, a painful vesicular eruption that is usually localized to one side and a single dermatome. In localized herpes zoster, the rash is usually preceded by pain and paresthesias in the involved dermatome that may antedate the eruption by several days to one week. The antecedent pain is often misdiagnosed as pleurisy, myocardial ischemia, cholecystitis or pancreatitis, renal colic, disc disease, or neuropathy, until the typical rash in a dermatomal distribution appears, leading to the correct diagnosis. In contrast to healthy subjects, patients after transplantation may develop widespread cutaneous dissemination with complications of pneumonia, hepatitis, encephalitis, and disseminated intravascular coagulation. Mortality in patients with visceral zoster is almost always due to viral pneumonia. Because more than 85% of individuals in the United States have had primary varicella-zoster infection, reactivation is the usual cause of the disease after transplantation. Prior to the availability of antiviral drugs, approximately 20% of patients had visceral dissemination, and 12% died from complications.

In the allogeneic hematopoietic stem cell transplantation setting, intravenous acyclovir is the drug of choice for treatment of primary and recurrent varicella-zoster infection. In the autologous hematopoietic stem cell transplantation setting with localized zoster, oral administration of famciclovir may suffice. Therapy is given for a minimum of seven days or for two days after cessation of new lesion formation and will lead to improvement in symptoms within 24 hours with decrease in the formation or elimination of new skin lesions. Either oral acyclovir or famciclovir is given prophylactically at some centers to prevent varicella-zoster infection after transplantation. Treatment is expensive and must be given for prolonged periods, because viral reactivation often occurs after prophylaxis is discontinued. For this reason, most centers eschew prophylaxis and instead instruct patients to report promptly the early signs and symptoms of infection so that treatment can be rapidly instituted.

Pneumocystis Infection

Pneumocystis carinii is a protozoal organism (recently reclassified as a fungus on the basis of molecular studies). It can cause pneumonitis in severely immunosuppressed patients, particularly those on corticosteroid therapy. Because patients are immunologically deficient after hematopoietic stem cell transplantation, all such patients receive antibiotic prophylaxis to prevent this infection. Trimethoprim-sulfamethoxazole, in a dose of one double-strength tablet twice daily, two days each week, is most commonly employed. It is used for all patients receiving corticosteroid therapy, patients with lymphoid malignancies after autologous hematopoietic stem cell transplantation, and all allogeneic recipients within the first six months after transplantation. It is continued beyond this time point in patients with active graft-versus-host disease. For patients who are allergic to this medication or develop neutropenia from it, aerosolized pentamidine, 300 mg inhaled monthly, can be substituted. Because of its variable distribution to different sites in the lung, aerosolized pentamidine is not as effective in prophylaxis as is trimethoprim-sulfamethoxazole.

Delayed Complications Following Hematopoietic Cell Transplantation

Successful application of techniques to reduce or eliminate the early complications of hematopoietic stem cell transplantation has increased the number of individuals who are at risk for the development of late complications. The etiology of these delayed events relates to a number of factors, including (1) the toxicity of the high-dose preparative regimen, (2) immunologic dysfunction developing in the recovering immune system after transplantation, and (3) the side effects of the immunosuppressive therapy that is required after allogeneic hematopoietic stem cell transplantation. Multiple organ systems can be affected. In the allogeneic setting, chronic graft-versus-host disease has a further deleterious effect. Both allogeneic and autologous hematopoietic stem cell recipients require long-term follow-up care to anticipate, prevent, and/or treat these events in patients whose initial illness has been cured by transplantation.

Respiratory Complications

Apart from pulmonary infections, the lung can be directly affected by toxicity from radiation therapy and chemotherapy, such as cyclophosphamide and carmustine. Occult lung injury during treatment can lead later to pulmonary fibrosis or reactive airway disease. In most patients, the loss of lung volume does not produce significant impairment in function. After allogeneic hematopoietic stem cell transplantation, the most serious respiratory problem is the development of bronchiolitis obliterans. It affects approximately 10% of all patients who have chronic graft-versus-host disease and usually appears within 3 to 24 months of transplantation. Clinically, patients experience cough, shortness of breath, and asthmatic symptoms. The histologic changes in the lungs are consistent with a graft-versus-host reaction, possibly aggravated by the recurrent bacterial pneumonias that are a prominent feature of this entity. The clinical course of bronchiolitis varies from a slowly progressive deterioration to a rapidly fatal necrotizing inflammation of the small airways. Administration of immunoglobulin as a component of chronic graft-versus-host disease therapy may decrease the incidence of obliterative bronchiolitis. Treatment is usually unavailing.

Autoimmune Disease

Patients who have chronic graft-versus-host disease often develop clinical disease manifestations that are similar to those observed in a number of autoimmune disorders, including scleroderma, primary biliary cirrhosis, polymyositis, and keratoconjunctivitis/sicca syndrome. Autoantibodies are frequently present. These include rheumatoid factor, antinuclear antibody and antimitochrondrial antibodies. Some patients develop antiacetylcholine receptor antibodies and clinical manifestations of myasthenia gravis. In the context of chronic graft-versus-host disease, a number of immunologically mediated hematologic problems can occur, such as immune thrombocytopenia, anemia, and neutropenia. The marrow itself may be a target, resulting in persistent thrombocytopenia, which is a poor prognostic factor in patients after allogeneic hematopoietic stem cell transplantation.

Thyroid Function Abnormalities

Endocrine abnormalities are the most frequent long-term complications of both autologous and allogeneic hematopoietic stem cell transplantation. Hypothyroidism is very common in patients who have received radiation therapy as part of their initial treatment for Hodgkin's disease. In addition to the functional abnormalities, these patients are at increased risk for benign or malignant tumors of the thyroid gland, related to prior radiation exposure to the neck. Patients who received radiation therapy to the neck area before or during transplantation should be monitored at least annually with thyroid function studies. A thyroid-stimulating hormone assay allows early, preclinical detection of impending hypothyroidism.

Adrenal Function Abnormalities

Many patients receive glucocorticoid therapy after allogeneic hematopoietic stem cell transplantation, and some patients require lengthy treatment for persistent chronic graft-versus-host disease. These patients develop the classic corticosteroid side effects, including cushingoid features, myopathy, bone loss, and iatrogenic suppression of endogenous cortisol production, resulting in relative adrenal insufficiency. A small subset of patients, particularly those who have had cranial irradiation followed by total body irradiation, may have severe effects on the pituitary gland.

Gonadal and Sexual Function Abnormalities

The effects of dose-intensive preparative regimens on gonadal function play an important role in any discussion before transplantation about the consequences of therapy. This is a particularly disturbing problem for young patients who wish to preserve fertility. The vast majority of patients who undergo transplantation will become sterile, and where possible, the potential for future biologic parenting should be preserved in men by sperm banking and in women by fertilized egg cryopreservation.

Gonadal function and fertility are highly influenced by the patient's age, antecedent therapy, and the regimen that is utilized for transplantation. Young patients who are conditioned with a cyclophosphamide-containing regimen may show only transient impairment of gonadal function, particularly patients with aplastic anemia. However, patients who are prepared with total body irradiation-containing regimens generally have lasting impairment, which is more likely to occur with advancing age. After transplantation, all patients should be evaluated for sexual dysfunction. In men, this can be treated with testosterone and Viagra. Premenopausal women who have undergone a chemical menopause should, unless there are contraindications, receive estrogen and progesterone replacement therapy. Low dose androgen therapy may have beneficial effects in women for improving libido and sexual satisfaction.

Ophthalmologic Problems

Cataracts are a frequent late complication in patients who receive total body irradiation or who require long-term corticosteroid use. Chronic graft-versus-host disease can cause keratoconjunctivitis sicca. Artificial tears may provide symptomatic relief in mild cases. Ligation of the canaliculi, which normally drain lacrimal fluid, may be necessary in severe cases to maintain surface moisture and prevent corneal ulceration and blindness.

Orthopedic Problems

Osteoporosis in patients after hematopoietic stem cell transplantation is related to several factors, including radiation therapy, glucocorticoid therapy, inactivity, and, most important in women, the development of premature menopause. Accelerated bone loss begins within the first 100 days after transplantation in both sexes. Therefore, it is important, where appropriate, to use hormone replacement therapy with estrogens and progesterone to increase bone mass in women along with calcium and vitamin D supplements. Testosterone replacement therapy in men will likely accomplish a similar effect. Serial bone density examinations should be part of the follow-up in all long-term survivors of transplantation, particularly those who continue to require corticosteroids for graft-versus-host disease therapy. Patients with decreased bone density should receive therapy with agents such as diphosphonates to stabilize or increase bone mass.

Avascular necrosis is another significant bony complication, related to corticosteroid administration. It can occur after either short-term or long-term therapy. The femoral head is most frequently involved, followed by the humerus. Pain is usually the first manifestation. Avascular necrosis can be documented by magnetic resonance imaging (MRI) examination. An orthopedic surgeon should evaluate the patient to determine the necessity for and timing of joint replacement.

Second Malignancies

A posttransplantation lymphoproliferative disorder, usually related to Epstein-Barr virus, can develop early (within 12 months) in the course of an allogeneic hematopoietic stem cell transplantation. This is most likely to occur in patients who undergo allogeneic hematopoietic stem cell transplantation using T cell-depleted or mismatched donor stem cells or after treatment of graft-versus-host disease with antithymocyte globulin.

Solid tumors occur not only after allogeneic stem cell transplantation, but also after syngeneic and autologous hematopoietic stem cell transplantation and generally arise in host cells. They are usually late manifestations. Because these cancers may appear many years after hematopoietic cell transplantation is performed, some caution is needed in determining whether they are in fact secondary, rather than primary, malignancies. An analysis of a large number of patients indicated the risk of developing second cancers to be approximately 2% at 10 years and 7% at 15 years after transplantation. The incidence of head and neck cancer, skin cancer, melanoma, thyroid cancer, and soft tissue sarcoma is increased. Prior radiation therapy in the autologous setting and radiation therapy and chronic graft-versus-host disease in the allogeneic setting are factors that contribute to the genesis of secondary cancers.

Myelodysplasia can develop as a consequence of autologous hematopoietic stem cell transplantation. The risk of its occurrence, one to seven years after hematopoietic stem cell transplantation, correlates with a variety of factors, principally antecedent therapy with alkylating agents and topoisomerase-2 inhibitors. Most studies indicate that the genetic damage to the stem cell that later causes a clonal malignancy is incurred prior to the transplantation procedure, from preceding chemotherapy exposure. Thus, extensive treatment prior to transplantation increases the risk of myelodysplasia, documented by the detection of genetic mutations in precursor cells harvested before transplantation. Patients who are candidates for autologous stem cell transplantation should have cytogenetic analysis of the marrow before stem cell collection, particularly those with extensive prior treatment. Patients should be counseled about this long-term risk.

Psychosocial Issues

The use of allogeneic and autologous hematopoietic stem cell transplantation places substantial emotional stress on patients and families and their relationships. A commitment to a positive outlook and the mustering of personal and familial strength are needed to cope with the rigors of therapy and the recovery phase, which may be lengthy and complicated. There-fore, it should not be surprising that there are long-term adjustments and rehabilitation requirements for patients after hematopoietic stem cell transplantation. Patients with chronic graft-versus-host disease have the most difficulties. These patients may suffer from reduced attention span, short-term memory deficit, depression, inability to attain sexual satisfaction, and low self-esteem. The psychosocial stresses before, during, and after transplantation require as much attention as the physical complications. Support, understanding, and focused discussions by the physician and other health care workers are necessary over the long term to minimize the difficulties and help patients deal successfully with problems as they arise.

Hematopoietic Stem Cell Transplantation in Specific Disorders

Acute Myeloid Leukemia

The role of hematopoietic stem cell transplantation in the treatment of acute myeloid leukemia (see Chapter 60) has evolved from one of a strategy of last resort to a treatment approach that is an integral part of postremission therapy. The change in perspective has been influenced in part by refinements in transplantation techniques, which have decreased the morbidity and mortality associated with the procedure. These include (1) improved infection prophylaxis, (2) the use of cytokines to mobilize both autologous and allogeneic hematopoietic stem cell products, reducing the duration of neutropenia, and (3) improved immunosuppressive measures that allow successful matched unrelated donor transplantation, thereby increasing access to allogeneic hematopoietic stem cell transplantation.

Moreover, increasingly, consideration of favorable and unfavorable prognostic factors is used to guide the choice of therapy (Figure 51-1). Cytogenetic studies have defined different risk groups, and these subsets now form the backbone of the therapeutic decision tree. Whether to consider allogeneic hematopoietic stem cell transplantation in therapy depends on the availability of a human leukocyte antigen–matched sibling or matched unrelated donor. Human leukocyte antigen typing should be routinely obtained in the initial evaluation of patients with newly diagnosed acute myeloid leukemia whose age and/or comorbid medical problems do not preclude transplantation.

Patients with acute promyelocytic leukemia enjoy a high disease-free survival rate with conventional-dose chemotherapy combined with all-trans retinoic acid in induction and maintenance. The patient's remission status can be monitored by following the level of the fusion protein (PML/RARα) produced by the t(15;17) translocation. Patients who show reemer-

1. Acute promyelocytic leukemia

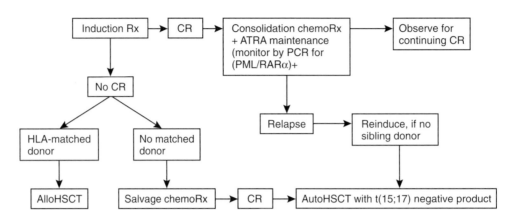

2. Good risk cytogenetics in acute myeloid leukemia (other than promyelocytic)

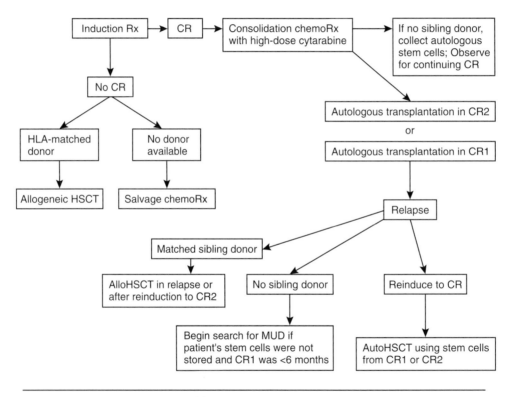

Allo = allogeneic; Auto = autologous; HSCT = hematopoietic stem cell transplantation;
CR = complete remission; ChemoRx = chemotherapy; ATRA = all-trans retinoic acid;
MUD = matched unrelated donor

Figure 51-1 ■ Treatment algorithm for acute myeloid leukemia in patients younger than age 60 years.

gence and/or a rising level of the fusion protein are likely to relapse. Transplantation, using either an allogeneic donor or an autologous product that demonstrably lacks the fusion protein, is reserved for patients with acute promyelocytic leukemia who relapse.

Patients with good risk cytogenetics [t(8;21), inv(16), t(16;16)] may achieve long-term remission with incorporation of cycles of high-dose cytarabine in postremission therapy. Autologous hematopoietic stem cell transplantation after one or more intensive chemotherapy courses in this group resulted in a somewhat better three-year disease-free survival rate (70% to 85%) than chemotherapy alone in randomized studies. Several treatment strategies are available for

3. Intermediate risk cytogenetics (type sib at diagnosis)

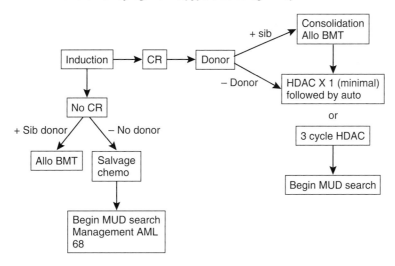

4. Poor risk cytogenetics

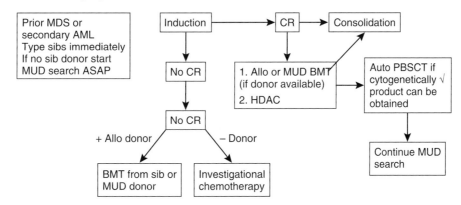

Figure 51-1 ■ Continued

this favorable prognosis group. These include (1) postremission courses of high-dose cytarabine, reserving allogeneic hematopoietic stem cell transplantation for treatment of relapse in patients who possess a human leukocyte antigen–matched sibling donor; (2) one or two cycles of high-dose cytarabine followed by autologous hematopoietic stem cell transplantation in first complete remission; or (3) postremission courses of high-dose cytarabine and the collection of autologous stem cells during initial remission that are held in reserve for autologous transplantation in second remission in patients who lack a histocompatible sibling.

Approximately half of adults with de novo acute myeloid leukemia are in the intermediate risk cytogenetics group; of these, approximately 90% appear to have a normal karyotype. Unfortunately, the three-year disease-free survival rate for this group is only 35% to 40% when high-dose cytarabine is used for postremission therapy. In this group of patients, both autologous and allogeneic (sibling) hematopoietic stem cell transplantation in initial complete remission appears to offer an improved disease-free survival rate of 50% to 55%. The patient's age, tumor burden at diagnosis, and infectious complications during induction or postremission therapy are factors that influence the choice of therapy after initial remission. In patients who are age 30 years or younger, the risk of graft-versus-host disease is relatively low. Allogeneic hematopoietic stem cell transplantation may be an attractive option because of its low relapse rate (15% to 20%). In older patients, allogeneic hematopoietic stem cell transplantation has a high treatment-related mortality rate (30% to 40%) and long-term morbidity. If transplantation is thought to be appropriate for this age group, then autologous hematopoietic stem cell transplantation offers an equivalent chance of long-term survival with a lower risk of short-term and long-term toxicity.

Patients whose leukemia cells show loss of part or all of chromosomes 5 or 7 or complex karyotypic abnormalities, as well as those patients with antecedent myelodysplasia or therapy-related leukemia have a very poor outcome when treated with conventional postremission therapy; the three-year disease-free survival rate is approximately 10%. Autologous hematopoietic stem cell transplantation has failed to improve on these results. Allogeneic hematopoietic stem cell transplantations can cure approximately 25% to 30% of patients in this group. If such patients lack a sibling donor, a search for a matched unrelated donor should be initiated early on, during induction therapy.

The use of a non-dose-intensive conditioning regimen coupled with allogeneic (matched sibling or matched unrelated volunteer) stem cell transplantation is under study as a means to extend the potential benefit of the graft-versus-tumor effect to patients who are either too old or too frail to tolerate high-dose preparative treatment regimens. This nonmyeloablative allogeneic hematopoietic stem cell transplantation approach may also prove to be useful as salvage therapy for patients who relapse after autologous hematopoietic stem cell transplantation. However, the procedure is associated with the risk of morbidity and mortality from graft-versus-host disease.

Myelodysplastic Syndromes

The myelodysplastic syndromes (see Chapter 62) encompass a spectrum of marrow disorders with variable degrees of ineffective hematopoiesis and predisposition to leukemic transformation. Survival ranges from months to a decade after diagnosis. Factors influencing outcome are the number of cytopenias, cytogenetic abnormalities, and the presence and percentage or quantity of myeloblasts in the bone marrow. The overwhelming majority of patients who have myelodysplasia are more than 60 years of age and are therefore ineligible for fully oblative allogeneic hematopoietic stem cell transplantation. There are, however, an increasing number of young patients who develop myelodysplasia as a sequela of chemotherapy or radiation therapy for lymphomas, germ cell tumors, or breast cancer. These secondary myelodysplasias have a very poor prognosis with conventional chemotherapy.

Decisions to utilize transplantation to replace the defective stem cells are influenced by the patient's age, prognosis, and comorbid conditions. Using the International Prognostic Index (see Chapter 62), patients with low-risk disease are usually not recommended for hematopoietic stem cell transplantation until they progress unless they have treatment-related myelodysplasia. For patients with intermediate-risk disease, allogeneic hematopoietic stem cell transplantation from a sibling or volunteer unrelated donor should be considered as primary therapy for patients younger than age 55 years. In this group, allogeneic hematopoietic stem cell transplantation can successfully restore normal hematopoiesis in 40% to 50% of patients. For patients with high-risk disease (more than 15% blasts in the marrow) or secondary acute myeloid leukemia, controversy exists as to whether induction chemotherapy should be employed before hematopoietic stem cell transplantation to reduce the "leukemic burden." Those patients who respond to initial chemotherapy have a lower risk of relapse following transplantation, but often in the attempt to improve the disease burden the patient becomes too debilitated. Those patients who fail induction have a very poor outcome. In patients who do not have a sibling donor, induction chemotherapy might be necessary as a temporizing measure while a matched unrelated donor is sought.

Acute Lymphoblastic Leukemia

Although acute lymphoblastic leukemia (see Chapter 61) is a highly curable malignancy in children between the ages of 2 and 12 years, the disease is much more difficult to eradicate in adolescents and adults. Conventional chemotherapy regimens in adult acute lymphoblastic leukemia provide an overall five-year disease-free survival rate of 20% or less. This is partially explained by the fact that a higher percentage (up to 50%) of adults carry unfavorable cytogenetic markers, such as the Philadelphia chromosome resulting from the t(9;22) translocation, t(4;11), t(1;19), and t(8;14).

Allogeneic stem cell hematopoietic stem cell transplantation in first complete remission is the treatment of choice for adults with high-risk acute lymphoblastic leukemia who have a histocompatible sibling donor. At the City of Hope, more than 100 such patients have undergone transplantation using fractionated total body irradiation and etoposide as the conditioning regimen and cyclosporine and methotrexate ± prednisone for graft-versus-host disease prophylaxis. The three-year disease-free survival rate is 63% with a relapse rate of only 8% but a 29% nonrelapse mortality rate due to graft-versus-host disease and infection. The results in patients with advanced disease are less favorable (Figure 51-2). For adults with high risk, such as those with Philadelphia chromosome–positive acute lymphoblastic leukemia who lack a histocompatible sibling, a matched unrelated donor search

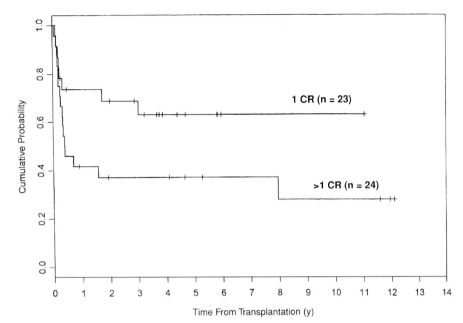

Figure 51-2 ■ Probability of disease-free survival in patients with Philadelphia chromosome–positive acute lymphoblastic leukemia transplanted in first remission (1 CR) or in more advanced stages (greater than 1 CR) using fractionated total body irradiation and high-dose etoposide as the conditioning regimen, $P = 0.02$ (see Table 51-2). Combines the data from the City of Hope and Stanford University. (Reprinted with permission from Snyder DS: Allogeneic stem cell transplantation for Philadelphia chromosome–positive acute lymphoblastic leukemia. Biol Blood Marrow Transplant 2000;6:597–603.)

should be instituted as soon as the diagnosis is made.

For patients who relapse following conventional chemotherapy, allogeneic hematopoietic stem cell transplantation represents the only potentially curative option. For patients who are fortunate enough to achieve a second remission, a 35% to 40% long-term disease-free survival rate is attainable after either a matched sibling or matched unrelated donor hematopoietic stem cell transplantation. Patients who undergo allogeneic hematopoietic stem cell transplantation for refractory acute lymphoblastic leukemia have a very poor outcome; the three-year disease-free survival rate is 10%.

Unfortunately, the graft-versus-leukemia effects of allogeneic hematopoietic stem cell transplantation in acute lymphoblastic leukemia are less than in acute or chronic myeloid leukemia. Thus, discontinuation of immunosuppression or the administration of donor lymphocyte infusions yields only transient responses in patients who relapse after transplantation. Because of the minimal response to donor lymphocyte infusions, there is less interest in exploring alternative nonmyeloablative hematopoietic stem cell transplantations in patients with acute lymphoblastic leukemia.

Autologous hematopoietic stem cell transplantation has only minimal value in patients with acute lymphoblastic leukemia, whether employed in first remission or at relapse. A French study compared multiple cycles of non-cross-resistant chemotherapy followed by maintenance therapy against an attenuated postremission chemotherapy course concluding in autologous hematopoietic stem cell transplantation. The three-year disease-free survival rate was 20% with either treatment approach.

Chronic Myeloid Leukemia (See Chapter 71)

Chronic myeloid leukemia is a myeloproliferative disorder characterized by a t(9;22) chromosomal translocation with a predictable natural history involving a chronic phase, an accelerated phase, and a terminal blast crisis. Therapeutic studies have focused on agents that could delay or block the progression of the disease. Considerable progress with new agents has occurred, but allogeneic hematopoietic stem cell transplantation remains the only curative therapy.

Disease status, age, and time from diagnosis to transplantation are the most important predictors of long-term survival. Approximately 70% to 75% of patients who are younger than age 40 years and undergo sibling donor allogeneic hematopoietic stem cell transplantation while they are in the chronic phase of the disease within the first year after diagnosis achieve long-term, disease-free survival. The combination of cyclophosphamide and busulfan is the most commonly used preparative regimen for chronic-phase chronic myeloid leukemia. The patients for whom an unrelated donor molecularly matched at the human leukocyte antigen Class I and Class II antigens can be identified have results that are very similar to those of matched sibling allografts. For disease that progresses beyond the chronic phase, cure is still possible but is less frequently achieved than in the chronic phase. Allogeneic hematopoietic stem cell transplantation provides a long-term disease-free survival rate of up to 40% in patients with accelerated or second chronic phase and 10% to 15% in patients in blast crisis.

Prior to the development of Gleevec for the treatment of chronic myeloid leukemia, the major question was whether a trial of interferon was appropriate before embarking on transplantation using a matched unrelated donor, particularly for young patients. Because of the high cure rate, physicians at transplantation centers believe that for patients younger than age 45 years who have a matched sibling or a matched unrelated donor, allogeneic hematopoietic stem cell transplantation within the first year after diagnosis is the treatment of choice. In patients older than age 45 years, many investigators recommend a trial of interferon prior to considering transplantation. For patients who have a major or complete cytogenetic response (reduction in the frequency or elimination of the Philadelphia chromosome) after six to nine months of interferon therapy, transplantation may be delayed until there is evidence of interferon resistance. This approach affords time to assess the response, identify a donor, and proceed to transplantation if the response to interferon is inadequate.

Gleevec, a specific tyrosine kinase inhibitor, is a remarkably effective and minimally toxic orally administered agent. It can induce complete cytogenetic remissions in some patients who are refractory to interferon. However, remissions induced by Gleevec in the accelerated phase or blast crisis of chronic myeloid leukemia are generally of short duration. Gleevec is easier to use (orally versus subcutaneous injection) and less toxic than interferon, and it can delay blast crisis, induce cytogenetic remissions, and prolong survival, more effectively than does interferon in newly diagnosed patients. Randomized trials using Gleevec ± cytarabine will assess the role and timing of allogeneic hematopoietic stem cell transplantation. The use of Gleevec to achieve a molecularly negative stem cell product, combined with high-dose chemotherapy and autologous stem cell rescue, might, in the future, prove to be an alternative to allogeneic hematopoietic stem cell transplantation for those who lack a suitable donor.

Nonmyeloablative transplantation may be another treatment option for elderly patients and those with compromised organ function. Donor lymphocyte infusions represent an effective salvage approach in patients who relapse after an allogeneic hematopoietic stem cell transplantation with a high-dose conditioning regimen. A reduced-intensity conditioning regimen that would still permit the establishment of donor-derived hematopoiesis could allow donor T cells to produce an effective graft-versus-tumor response.

Hodgkin's Disease

Approximately 85% to 90% of patients with limited-stage Hodgkin's disease (see Chapter 65) can be cured with extended field radiation or combined modality therapy. A high proportion of patients with advanced-stage Hodgkin's disease can also be cured with chemotherapy. Nevertheless, the disease progresses in 20% to 30% of patients during their initial treatment, and 30% of patients relapse after achieving an initial remission. Autologous hematopoietic stem cell transplantation offers an opportunity for cure in these patients. A consensus exists that patients who relapse after a chemotherapy-based regimen will have better overall survival, event-free survival, and freedom from progression after autologous hematopoietic stem cell transplantation than after salvage by conventional chemotherapy. The conditioning regimens that are commonly used are included in Table 51-5. Most patients who have been treated for Hodgkin's disease have had prior mediastinal or extensive bleomycin and adriamycin treatment, thus limiting the use of total body radiation.

Autologous hematopoietic stem cell transplantation is very effective in patients who have Hodgkin's disease at the time of initial relapse, when the disease is usually still too chemotherapy sensitive. The duration of first remission correlates strongly with the likelihood of a favorable outcome in these patients. Patients who received more than two prior chemotherapy regimens have an inferior outcome after autologous transplantation than do patients who have received less extensive prior therapy. Multiple salvage attempts increase the immediate and long-term toxicity from high-dose therapy and may select for chemoresistance. Nevertheless, although chemoresponsiveness to conventional therapy is routinely used to select patients for high-dose therapy with non-Hodgkin's lymphoma, it is not clear whether this principle applies to Hodgkin's disease. It may well be that low tumor burden, rather than chemosensitivity, is the important predictive factor for successful autologous transplantation. Patients with primary refractory Hodgkin's disease, defined as either minimal response or progression on standard induction chemotherapy, have a 30% to 40% progression-free survival after autologous stem cell hematopoietic stem cell transplantation. Although it has not been formally assessed in a randomized study, autologous hematopoietic stem cell transplantation appears to be more effective than

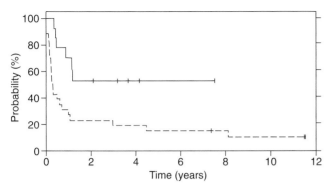

Figure 51-3 ■ Kaplan-Meier estimate of disease-free survival in patients with Hodgkin's disease failing induction therapy or in relapse who received high-dose therapy and autologous hematopoietic stem cell transplantation (solid line) compared to historical controls treated with conventional therapy (dashed line), *P* = <0.01. (Reprinted with permission from Yuen A, Rosenberg S, Hoppe R, et al: Comparison between conventional salvage therapy and high dose therapy with autografting for recurrent or refractory Hodgkin's disease. Blood 1997;89:814–822.)

conventional chemotherapy in relapsed disease or in those who fail to achieve a complete remission with initial therapy (Figure 51-3). The tendency for patients with Hodgkin's disease to relapse in previous sites of bulky disease has led to the practice of treating those areas with radiation therapy after recovery from autologous hematopoietic stem cell transplantation.

Whether to use autologous stem cell hematopoietic stem cell transplantation as therapy for patients with high-risk disease in first remission remains controversial. The recently developed International Prognostic Factor scoring system for Hodgkin's disease allows the identification of the small fraction (10% to 15%) of patients at presentation whose risk of treatment failure and short survival would justify early autologous hematopoietic stem cell transplantation; a progression-free survival rate of up to 75% to 100% in this circumstance has been reported from single-institution studies. An international trial is in process which randomizes high-risk patients in first remission to receive autologous stem cell transplantation either in initial remission or at relapse. This will determine whether early or delayed autologous transplantation is the most effective strategy.

Allogeneic hematopoietic stem cell transplantation has a limited role in the treatment of Hodgkin's disease, primarily owing to the high treatment-related mortality rate, which is 40% to 55% within the first year. The role of graft-versus-tumor effect is also not as well defined in Hodgkin's disease as it is in chronic myeloid leukemia and non-Hodgkin's lymphoma.

Therapy-related myelodysplasia and secondary acute myeloid leukemia are the most significant long-term complications of autologous stem cell hematopoietic stem cell transplantation for Hodgkin's disease. As is true of conventional chemotherapy for Hodgkin's disease, the incidence of secondary solid cancers is also increased.

Non-Hodgkin's Lymphoma

Autologous stem cell rescue has long been used to cure patients with chemosensitive diffuse aggressive non-Hodgkin's lymphoma (see Chapters 66, 67, 68, and 69) in relapse. In a randomized trial of autologous hematopoietic stem cell transplantation versus conventional chemotherapy in patients younger than age 60 years who had relapsed and then responded to a second-line therapy, autologous stem cell transplantation showed a significant benefit (Figure 51-4). The cure rates after autologous hematopoietic stem cell transplantation are influenced by the patient's age and the lymphoma's continuing sensitivity to chemotherapy. For example, the long-term disease-free survival rate is 40% to 50% in patients who have chemosensitive disease versus only 10% to 15% in patients whose disease fails to respond well to conventional salvage chemotherapy regimens prior to transplantation.

On the basis of these data, clinical trials examined the role of high-dose therapy and autologous stem cell hematopoietic stem cell transplantation in intermediate- and high-grade lymphomas in first

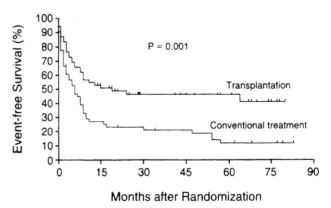

Figure 51-4 ■ Kaplan-Meier estimate of event-free survival of patients with chemosensitive relapsed non-Hodgkin's lymphoma randomized to receive additional salvage chemotherapy (conventional treatment) or autologous hematopoietic stem cell transplantation (dashed line). Five-year event-free survival rate 12% versus 46% for transplantation. (From Philip T, Guglielmi C, Hagenbeek A, et al: Autologous bone marrow transplantation as compared with salvage chemotherapy in relapses of chemotherapy-sensitive non-Hodgkin's lymphoma. N Engl J Med 1995;333:1540–1545. Copyright © 1995 Massachusetts Medical Society. All rights reserved.)

remission. The majority of patients did not benefit from early transplantation. The International Prognostic Index has identified a group of patients (intermediate-2 and high) whose relapse-free survival rate is less than 50%, and this subset of patients might nevertheless benefit from early autologous hematopoietic stem cell transplantation. Patients with delayed or incomplete responses to initial chemotherapy may be candidates for autologous stem cell hematopoietic stem cell transplantation.

The favorable results of autologous stem cell hematopoietic stem cell transplantation in patients with intermediate- or high-grade lymphoma led to its use in low-grade lymphomas. Even if autologous transplantation does not cure the disease or prolong survival, autologous hematopoietic stem cell transplantation might be deemed advantageous if a substantial proportion of patients achieved prolonged remission. The long and variable natural history for follicular lymphoma and the myriad therapeutic options make it difficult to interpret the results of hematopoietic cell transplantation. Patients who have a minimal disease burden and continued sensitivity to standard drug therapy do best after autologous hematopoietic stem cell transplantation. No plateau in the incidence of relapse over time occurs after autologous transplantation. Thus, there is no evidence that autologous hematopoietic stem cell transplantation is curative in the low-grade lymphomas.

Mantle cell lymphoma (see Chapter 67) appears to combine the worst aspects of both large cell and low-grade lymphoma in that, despite a high degree of chemosensitivity, the complete remission rate and overall survival rate are low, with a shorter time to progression than is seen in low-grade lymphomas. The data on the efficacy of autologous stem cell hematopoietic stem cell transplantation in the management of this lymphoma are conflicting. Some studies show an apparent increase in progression-free survival rates, whereas others show no effect. Because the natural history of disease in the great majority of these patients is so short, many physicians continue to use autologous stem cell hematopoietic stem cell transplantation despite the absence of data confirming its value.

Patients receiving allogeneic hematopoietic stem cell transplantation are usually those for whom autologous hematopoietic stem cell transplantation was not feasible because of overt persistent marrow or peripheral blood involvement. Some degree of a graft-versus-lymphoma effect is demonstrable clinically, particularly in the follicular lymphomas, similar to that observed in acute leukemia. Toxicity in this frequently elderly population is substantial, but the incidence of relapse among surviving patients is very low. For this reason, less intensive, nonmyeloablative chemotherapy regimens have been used to allow engraftment and establish a graft-versus-lymphoma effect. The early results have been very encouraging, confirming the role of the allograft in mediating an antitumor response in patients with low-grade lymphoma. This approach to allogeneic hematopoietic stem cell transplantation has several advantages. It can be applied to patients who have blood and marrow involvement, which commonly occurs in low-grade lymphoma. The use of stem cells from a normal donor also obviates the risk of myelodysplasia after transplantation. Reports from the National Bone Marrow Transplantation Registry compared the results of autologous and allogeneic hematopoietic stem cell transplantation in low-grade lymphomas and showed improved disease-free survival with allogeneic transplantation.

Multiple Myeloma

The malignant plasma cells in multiple myeloma (see Chapter 63) are inherently resistant to chemotherapy. Although the response rate to chemotherapy such as vincristine, adriamycin, and dexamethasone (VAD) or melphalan and prednisone is greater than 70%, complete remissions are very rare. Therefore, the disease is considered to be incurable by conventional chemotherapy.

Interest in the use of high-dose cytotoxic therapy developed from observations that patients undergoing syngeneic hematopoietic stem cell transplantation could have prolonged remissions. Historically, allogeneic hematopoietic stem cell transplantation for multiple myeloma had been limited by the high median age of the patient population, toxicity of the regimen, and high relapse rate. However, the systematic evaluation of high-dose melphalan, both with and without autologous stem cell support, demonstrated that patients could achieve a complete remission of the disease with intensified chemotherapy. Randomized trials determined the value of autologous stem cell hematopoietic stem cell transplantation (single or tandem, sequential) after initial chemotherapy for newly diagnosed multiple myeloma. These studies demonstrated that the progression-free and overall survival improved. Autologous stem cell transplantation early in treatment has become the standard approach for patients responsive to chemotherapy (Figure 51-5). Sequential, double (tandem) transplants appear to improve results further. Despite the improvement in survival, patients continue to have evidence of persistence of myeloma and will ultimately relapse. Strategies involving treatment with interferon, thalidomide, or antiangiogenesis factors

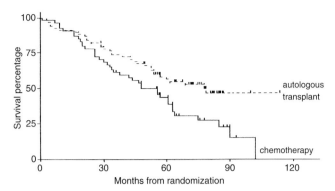

Figure 51-5 ■ Probability of survival in patients who are newly diagnosed with myeloma and who are younger than age 60 years after randomization to receive either conventional treatment (chemotherapy) or transplantation (conventional treatment followed by autologous hematopoietic stem cell transplantation). Vertical axis is probability, and horizontal axis is time in months. (Reprinted with permission from Attal M, Harousseau JL: Randomized trial experience of the Intergroupe Francophone du Myelome. Semin Hematol 2001;38:226-230 [The IFM 90 Trial].)

after hematopoietic stem cell transplantation are under investigation as a means to decrease the relapse rate.

The demonstration of a graft-versus-myeloma effect following allogeneic hematopoietic stem cell transplantation has renewed interest in the use of nonmyeloablative treatment regimens. These would appear to be ideal for patients with multiple myeloma, because these patients are often elderly and have concomitant medical problems that increase the hazards of a fully myeloablative regimen. Phase II studies show that a substantial proportion of patients receiving a nonmyeloablative regimen in allogeneic transplantation can achieve a complete remission of their disease. Determination of long-term outcome requires lengthier follow-up.

Clinical trials are in progress evaluating the combination of an autologous stem cell transplantation to cytoreduce the disease followed by nonmyeloablative therapy and allogeneic hematopoietic stem cell transplantation to provide immunotherapy, mediated by the allograft.

Aplastic Anemia

Severe aplastic anemia (see Chapter 54) in the majority of cases is thought to be mediated by an autoimmune reaction of host T cells against early hematopoietic precursors, producing severe pancytopenia. Treatment strategies other than supportive care focus on the use of immunosuppressive agents to (1) suppress the autoreactive T cells or (2) allow engraftment of normal hematopoietic stem cells from a human leukocyte antigen–matched sibling or unre-

lated donor. Patients older than age 40 years are treated initially with immunosuppressive therapy (cyclosporine, antithymocyte globulin, and prednisone). In selected cases, patients who fail this therapy can be considered for allogeneic hematopoietic stem cell transplantation.

For patients younger than age 40 years, an allogeneic marrow transplantation from a human leukocyte antigen–matched sibling can completely correct the abnormal hematopoiesis in 85% to 90% of recipients using a preparative regimen of cyclophosphamide (CY) alone or in combination with antithymocyte globulin (ATG) (Figure 51-6). These powerful immunosuppressive agents act to paralyze the cytotoxic T cells of the recipient prior to infusion of donor marrow, allowing successful primary engraftment in 95% of sibling recipients. The medications that are used for graft-versus-host disease prophylaxis also provide long-term suppression of host cytotoxic T cells. These medications (primarily cyclosporine) are tapered more slowly, over one year, than in patients with malignancies for two reasons: to prevent late graft failure from inadequately suppressed residual host T cells and to minimize the risks of graft-versus-host disease, since these patients do not require any antitumor benefit. Approximately 30% to 40% of patients who receive a sibling donor's marrow develop chronic graft-versus-host disease and require ongoing treatment. However, 85% of patients return to productive activities within one to two years after transplantation.

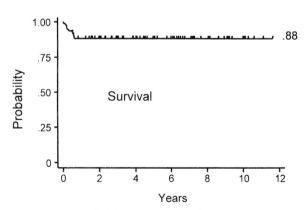

Figure 51-6 ■ Kaplan-Meier estimate of the probability of survival of 94 patients with aplastic anemia who underwent allogeneic hematopoietic stem cell transplantation from a *human leukocyte antigen*–matched sibling after a preparative regimen consisting of cyclophosphamide and antithymocyte globulin. (Reprinted with permission from Storb R, Blume KG, O'Donnell MR, et al: Cyclophosphamide and antithymocyte globulin to condition patients with aplastic anemia for allogeneic marrow transplantations: The experience in four centers. Biol Blood Marrow Transplant 2001;7: 39–44.)

Factors that adversely affect the outcome are (1) prolonged time to transplantation, because the long duration of neutropenia and attempts at immunotherapy to treat the disease predispose to fungal colonization and infection, and (2) multiple transfusions prior to transplantation, because increasing exposure to human leukocyte antigen antigens on blood leukocytes increases the risk of graft rejection. Therefore, for all newly diagnosed patients with severe aplastic anemia, the following guidelines are recommended: Human leukocyte antigen typing of the family should be done as quickly as possible, blood transfusions should be minimized, all blood products should be filtered to remove leukocytes and radiated (to kill lymphocytes that could engraft and initiate graft-versus-host disease), and all platelet products should be single nonrelated donor in origin (to avoid exposing and sensitizing the patient to minor histocompatibility antigens in the family, which would increase the risk and/or severity of both graft rejection and graft-versus-host disease after transplantation). Testing for chromosomal fragility should also be considered to exclude Fanconi's anemia. It is important to identify patients with increased chromosomal fragility, as they do not tolerate high-dose chemotherapy. They require substantial dose reduction of the drugs used in the preparative regimen to avoid unacceptable morbidity and mortality rates.

Patients who are younger than age 40 years who lack a human leukocyte antigen–matched sibling donor are initially treated with immunosuppressive therapy. If they fail to respond or later relapse, they should be considered for allogeneic transplantation using a matched unrelated donor. The risk of graft failure is higher (greater than 10%) than in early transplantation using a human leukocyte antigen–matched sibling donor because prior transfusions will have sensitized host T cells to human leukocyte antigens. Additional immunosuppression is therefore necessary to achieve engraftment. Current clinical trials combine radiation therapy given as either total body radiation or total lymphoid radiation plus cyclophosphamide ± antithymocyte globulin. The addition of radiation therapy increases the risk for late pulmonary toxicity and late second malignancies. The risk of extensive, chronic graft-versus-host disease is increased, but matched unrelated donor marrow transplantation can cure a substantial fraction of patients with severe aplastic anemia who fail to respond to immunosuppressive therapy.

For the small proportion of patients who do sustain late graft failure, a second transplantation using cyclophosphamide and antithymocyte globulin as the preparative regimen can successfully reestablish marrow function in approximately 50% of patients.

Transplantation for Breast Cancer

Breast cancer (see Chapters 76 and 77) is sensitive to a variety of chemotherapeutic agents, including alkylating drugs. The success of autologous stem cell hematopoietic stem cell transplantation in the hematologic malignancies led to attempts to use transplantation in the treatment of breast cancer as well. Autologous hematopoietic stem cell transplantation was used in women with metastatic breast cancer or as adjuvant therapy in women with high-risk disease (advanced stage II, stage III, and inflammatory carcinoma). Phase II trials reported high response rates and apparent improvement in disease-free survival. After high-dose chemotherapy, a proportion of women with metastatic breast cancer achieved complete remission, which rarely occurs after conventional-dose chemotherapy. In the adjuvant setting, patients with extensive nodal involvement or an aggressive primary tumor appeared to have longer, recurrence-free survival compared to historical controls. However, a large randomized trial of transplantation in the adjuvant setting conducted in the United States showed no significant improvement in overall and disease-free survival rates. In randomized trials of women with metastatic breast cancer, autologous transplantation did improve survival.

Currently, autologous hematopoietic stem cell transplantation in breast cancer is an investigational procedure. The development of new agents and the increasing application of biologic studies to distinguish among different patient subgroups (e.g., HER-2/neu positive or negative breast cancer) and guide the selection of appropriate therapy will affect the design of future trials of high-dose therapy in breast cancer.

References

Allogeneic Stem Cell Hematopoietic Stem Cell Transplantation

General Considerations
Beatty PG, Mori M, Milford E: Impact of racial genetic polymorphism on the probability of finding an HLA-matched donor. Transplantation 1995;60:778–783.

Bensinger WI, Martin PJ, Storer B, et al: Transplantation of bone marrow as compared with peripheral-blood cells from HLA-identical relatives in patients with hematologic cancers. N Engl J Med 2001;344:175–181.

Giralt S, Thall PF, Khouri I, et al: Melphalan and purine analog containing preparative regimens: Reduced-intensity conditioning for patients with hematologic malignancies undergoing allogeneic progenitor cell transplantation. Blood 2001;97:631–637.

Henslee-Downey PJ, Abhyankar SH, Parrish RS, et al: Use of

partially mismatched related donors extends access to allogeneic marrow transplant. Blood 1997;89:3864–3872.

McSweeney PA, Niederwieser D, Shizuru JA, et al: Hematopoietic cell transplantation in older patients with hematologous malignancies: Replacing high-dose cytotoxic therapy with graft-versus-tumor effects. Blood 2001;97: 3390–3400, 2001.

Michallet M, Bilger K, Garban F, et al: Allogeneic hematopoietic stem cell transplantation after nonmyeloablative preparative regimens: Impact of pretransplantation and post transplantation factors on outcome. J Clin Oncol 2001; 19:3340–3349.

Slavin S: Immunotherapy of cancer with alloreactive lymphocytes. N Engl J Med 2000;343:802–803.

Slavin S, Nagler A, Naparstek E, et al: Nonmyeloablative stem cell transplantation and cell therapy as an alternative to conventional bone marrow transplantation with lethal cytoreduction for the treatment of malignant and nonmalignant diseases. Blood 1998;91:756–763.

Socie G, Veum Stone J, Wingard JR, et al: Long-term survival and late deaths after allogeneic bone marrow transplantation. N Engl J Med 1999;341:14–21.

Acute Lymphoblastic Leukemia

Chao NJ, Forman SJ, Schmidt GM, et al: Allogeneic bone marrow transplantation for high-risk acute lymphoblastic leukemia during first complete remission. Blood 1991;78: 1923–1927.

Snyder DS: Allogeneic stem cell transplantation for Philadelphia chromosome-positive acute lymphoblastic leukemia. Biol Blood Marrow Transplant 2000;6:597–603.

Verhagen OJHM, Willemse MJ, Breunis WB, et al: Application of germline IGH probes in real-time quantitative PCR for the detection of minimal residual disease in acute lymphoblastic leukemia. Leukemia 2000;14:1426–1435.

Acute Myeloid Leukemia/Myelodysplasia

Anderson JE, Gooley TA, Schoch G, et al: Stem cell transplantation for secondary acute myeloid leukemia: Evaluation of transplantation as initial therapy or following induction chemotherapy. Blood 1997;89:2578–2585.

Andersson BS, Gajewski J, Donato M, et al: Allogeneic stem cell transplantation (BMT) for AML and MDS following i.v. busulfan and cyclophosphamide. Bone Marrow Transplant 2000;25:35–38.

Appelbaum FR, Anderson J: Allogeneic bone marrow transplantation for myelodysplastic syndrome: Outcomes analysis according to IPSS score. Leukemia 1998;12:25–29.

Arnold R, de Witte T, van Biezen A, et al: Unrelated bone marrow transplantation in patients with myelodysplastic syndromes and secondary acute myeloid leukemia: An EBMT survey. European Blood and Marrow Transplantation Group. Bone Marrow Transplant 1998;21: 1213–1216.

Aversa F, Terenzi A, Carotti A, et al: Improved outcome with T cell-depleted bone marrow transplantation for acute leukemia. J Clin Oncol 1999;17:1545–1550.

Bosi A, Laszlo D, Labopin M, et al: Second allogeneic bone marrow transplantation in acute leukemia: results of a survey by the European Cooperative Group for Blood and Marrow Transplantation. J Clin Oncol 2001;16:3675–3684.

Deeg HJ, Appelbaum FR: Hematopoietic stem cell transplantation in patients with myelodysplastic syndrome. Leuk Res 2000;24:653–663.

O'Donnell MR, Long GD, Parker PM, et al: Busulfan/cyclophosphamide as conditioning regimen for allogeneic bone marrow transplantation for myelodysplasia. J Clin Oncol 1995;13:2973–2979.

Sierra J, Storer B, Hansen JA, et al: Unrelated donor marrow transplantation for acute myeloid leukemia: An update of the Seattle experience. Bone Marrow Transplant 2000;26: 397–404.

Aplastic Anemia

Deeg HJ, Amylon MD, Harris RE, et al: Marrow transplants from unrelated donors for patients with aplastic anemia: Minimum effective dose of total body irradiation. Biol Blood Marrow Transplant 2001;7:208–215.

Socié G, Henry-Amar M, Bacigalupo A, et al: Malignant tumors occurring after treatment of aplastic anemia. N Engl J Med 1993;329:1152–1157.

Storb R, Blume KG, O'Donnell MR, et al: Cyclophosphamide and antithymocyte globulin to condition patients with aplastic anemia for allogeneic marrow transplantations: The experience in four centers. Biol Blood Marrow Transplant 2001;7:39–44.

Chronic Myeloid Leukemia

Elmaagacli AH, Beelen DW, Opalka B, et al: The risk of residual molecular and cytogenetic disease in patients with Philadelphia-chromosome positive first chronic phase chronic myelogenous leukemia is reduced after transplantation of allogeneic peripheral blood stem cells compared with bone marrow. Blood 1999;94:384–389.

Hansen JA, Gooley TA, Martin PJ, et al: Bone marrow transplants from unrelated donors for patients with chronic myeloid leukemia. N Engl J Med 1998;338:961–968.

McGlave PB, Shu XO, Wen W, et al: Unrelated donor transplantation for chronic myelogenous leukemia: 9 years' experience of the National Marrow Donor Program. Blood 2000;95:2219–2225.

Radich JP, Gehly G, Gooley T, et al: Polymerase chain reaction detection of the BCR-ABL fusion transcript after allogeneic marrow transplantation for chronic myeloid leukemia: Results and implications in 346 patients. Blood 1995;85: 2632–2638.

Sehn LH, Alyea EP, Weller E, et al: Comparative outcomes of T cell-depleted and non-T cell-depleted allogeneic bone marrow transplantation for chronic myelogenous leukemia: Impact of donor lymphocyte infusion. J Clin Oncol 1999;17:561–568.

Sierra J, Radich J, Hansen JA, et al: Marrow transplants from unrelated donors for treatment of Philadelphia chromosome-positive acute lymphoblastic leukemia. Blood 1997;90:1410–1414.

Slattery JT, Clift RA, Buckner CD, et al: Marrow transplantation for chronic myeloid leukemia: The influence of plasma busulfan levels on the outcome of transplantation. Blood 1997;89:3055–3060.

Graft-Versus-Host Disease

Cutler C, Giri S, Jeyapalan S, et al: Acute and chronic graft-versus-host disease after allogeneic peripheral-blood stem cell and bone marrow transplantation: A meta-analysis. J Clin Oncol 2001;19:3685–3691.

Przepiorka D, Anderlini P, Saliba R, et al: Chronic graft-versus-host disease after allogeneic blood stem cell transplantation. Blood 2001;98:1695–1709.

Speiser DE, Tiercy JM, Rufer N, et al: High resolution HLA matching associated with decreased mortality after unrelated bone marrow transplantation. Blood 1996;87:4455–4462.

Storek J, Gooley T, Siadak M, et al: Allogeneic peripheral blood stem cell transplantation may be associated with a high risk of chronic graft-versus-host disease. Blood 1997;90:4705–4709.

Sullivan KM, Storek J, Kopecky KJ, et al: A controlled trial of long-term administration of intravenous immunoglobulin to prevent late infection and chronic graft-vs-host disease after marrow transplantation: Clinical outcome and effect on subsequent immune recovery. Biol Blood Marrow Transplant 1996;2:44–53.

Wagner JL, Seidel K, Boeckh M, et al: De novo chronic graft-versus-host disease in marrow graft recipients given methotrexate and cyclosporine: Risk factors and survival. Biol Blood Marrow Transplant 2000;6:633–639.

Weiden PL, Flournoy N, Thomas ED, et al: Antileukemic effect of graft-versus-host disease in human recipients of allogeneic marrow grafts. N Engl J Med 1979;300:1068–1073.

Infections

Arvin AM: Varicella-zoster virus: Pathogenesis, immunity, and clinical management in hematopoietic cell transplant recipients. Biol Blood Marrow Transplant 2000;6:219–230.

Avery RK, Adal KA, Longworth DL, Bolwell BJ: A survey of allogeneic bone marrow transplant programs in the United States regarding cytomegalovirus prophylaxis and preemptive therapy. Bone Marrow Transplant 2000;26:763–767.

Boekh M, Gooley TA, Myerson D, et al: Cytomegalovirus pp65 antigenemia-guided early treatment with ganciclovir versus ganciclovir at engraftment after allogeneic marrow transplantation: A randomized double-blind study. Blood 1996;88:4063–4071.

Bowden RA, Slichter SJ, Sayers M, et al: A comparison of filtered leukocyte-reduced and cytomegalovirus seronegative blood products for the prevention of transfusion-associated CMV infection after marrow transplant. Blood 1995;86:3598–3603.

Ochs L, Shu XO, Miller J, et al: Late infections after allogeneic bone marrow transplantations: Comparison of incidence in related and unrelated donor transplant recipients. Blood 1995;86:3979–3986.

Prentice HG, Kibbler CC, Prentice AG: Towards a targeted, risk-based, antifungal strategy in neutropenic patients. Br J Haematol 2000;110:273–284.

Reed EC, Bowden RA, Dandliker PS, et al: Treatment of cytomegalovirus pneumonia with ganciclovir and intravenous cytomegalovirus immunoglobulin in patients with bone marrow transplants. Ann Intern Med 1988;109:783–788.

Van Burik J-A, Leisenring W, Myerson D, et al: The effect of prophylactic fluconazole on the clinical spectrum of fungal diseases in bone marrow transplant recipients with special attention to hepatic candidiasis: An autopsy study of 355 patients. Medicine 1998;77:246–254.

Walter EA, Greenberg PD, Gilbert MJ, et al: Reconstitution of cellular immunity against cytomegalovirus in recipients of allogeneic bone marrow by transfer of T cell clones from the donor. N Engl J Med 1995;333:1038–1044.

Wingard JR: Fungal infections after bone marrow transplant. Biol Blood Marrow Transplant 1999;5:55–68.

Non-Hodgkin's Lymphoma/Hodgkin's Disease

Gajewski JL, Phillips GL, Sobocinski KA, et al: Bone marrow transplants from HLA-identical siblings in advanced Hodgkin's disease. J Clin Oncol 1996;14:572–578, 1996.

Khouri IF, Keating M, Korbling M, et al: Transplant-lite: Induction of graft-versus-malignancy using fludarabine-based nonablative chemotherapy and allogeneic blood progenitor cell transplantation as treatment for lymphoid malignancies. J Clin Oncol 1998;16:2817–2824.

Molina A, Parker P, Stein A, et al: Allogeneic bone marrow transplantation for patients with incurable low-grade lymphoproliferative disorders. Blood 1996;88(Suppl 1):619a.

van Besien K, Sobocinski KA, Rowlings PA, et al: Allogeneic bone marrow transplantation for low-grade lymphomas. Blood 1998;92:1832–1836.

Multiple Myeloma

Bensinger WI, Buckner CD, Anasetti C, et al: Allogeneic marrow transplantation for multiple myeloma: An analysis of risk factors on outcome. Blood 1996;88:2787–2793.

Corradini P, Voena C, Tarella C, et al: Molecular and clinical remission in multiple myeloma: Role of autologous and allogeneic transplantation of hematopoietic cells. J Clin Oncol 1999;17:208–215.

Martinelli G, Terragna C, Zamagni E, et al: Molecular remission after allogeneic or autologous transplantation of hematopoietic stem cells for multiple myeloma. J Clin Oncol 18:2273–2281.

Umbilical Cord Hematopoietic Stem Cells

Gluckman E, Rocha V, Boyer-Chammard A, et al: Outcome of cord-blood transplantation from related and unrelated donors. N Engl J Med 1997;337:373–381.

Laughlin MJ, Barker J, Bambach B, et al: Hematopoietic engraftment and survival in adult recipients of umbilical-cord blood from unrelated donors. N Engl J Med 2001;344:1815–1822.

Rubinstein P, Carrier C, Scaradavou A, et al: Outcomes among 562 recipients of placental-blood transplants from unrelated donors. N Engl J Med 1998;339:1565–1577.

Wagner JE, Rosenthal J, Sweetman R, et al: Successful transplantation of HLA matched and HLA mismatched umbilical cord blood from unrelated donors: Analysis of engraftment and acute graft versus host disease. Blood 1996;88:795–802.

Autologous Stem Cell Transplantation

General Considerations

Bhatia R, Verfaillie CM, Miller JS, et al: Autologous transplantation therapy for chronic myelogenous leukemia. Blood 1997;89:2623–2634.

Schimmer AS, Qauermain M, Imrie K, et al: Ovarian function after autologous bone marrow transplantation. J Clin Oncol 1998;16:2359–2363.

Acute Myeloid Leukemia

Burnett AK, Goldstone AH, Stevens RMF, et al: Randomized comparison of addition of autologous bone-marrow transplantation to intensive chemotherapy for acute myeloid leukemia in first remission: Results of MRC AML 10 trial. Lancet 1998;351:700–708.

Cassileth PA, Harrington D, Appelbaum FR, et al: Chemotherapy compared with autologous or allogeneic bone marrow transplantation in the management of acute myeloid leukemia in first remission. N Engl J Med 1998;339:1649–1656.

Gorin NC: Autologous stem cell transplantation in acute myelocytic leukemia. Blood 1998;92:1073–1090.

Grimwade D, Walker H, Oliver F, et al: The importance of diagnostic cytogenetics on outcome in AML: Analysis of 1,612 patients entered into the MRC AML 10 trial. Blood 1998;92:2322–2333.

Krishnan A, Bhatia S, Slovak ML, et al: Predictors of therapy-related leukemia and myelodysplasia following autologous transplantation for lymphoma: An assessment of risk factors. Blood 2000;95:1588–1593.

Meloni G, Diverio D, Vignetti M, et al: Autologous bone marrow transplantation for acute promyelocytic leukemia in second remission: Prognostic relevance of pretransplant minimal residual disease assessment by reverse-transcription polymerase chain reaction of the PML/RARa fusion gene. Blood 1997;90:1321–1325.

Rohatiner AZS, Bassan R, Raimondi R, et al: High-dose treatment with autologous bone marrow support as consolidation of first remission in younger patients with acute myelogenous leukaemia. Ann Oncol 11:1007–1015.

Stein AS, O'Donnell MR, Chai A, et al: In vivo purging with high-dose cytarabine followed by high-dose chemoradiotherapy and reinfusion of unpurged bone marrow for adult acute myelogenous leukemia in first complete remission. J Clin Oncol 1996;14:2206–2216.

Zittoun RA, Mandelli F, Willemze R, et al: Autologous or allogeneic bone marrow transplantation compared with intensive chemotherapy in acute myeloid leukemia. N Engl J Med 1995;323:217–223.

Breast Cancer

Nieto Y, Champlin RE, Wingard JR, et al: Status of high-dose chemotherapy for breast cancer: A review. Biol Blood Marrow Transplant 2000;6:476–495.

Stadtmauer EA, O'Neill A, Goldstein LJ, et al: Conventional dose chemotherapy compared with high-dose chemotherapy plus autologous hematopoietic stem cell transplantation for metastatic breast cancer. N Engl J Med 2000;342:1069–1076.

Multiple Myeloma

Attal M, Harousseau J-L, Stoppa A-M, et al: A prospective, randomized trial of autologous bone marrow transplantation and chemotherapy in multiple myeloma. N Engl J Med 1996;335:91–97.

Barlogie B, Jagannath S, Vesole DH, et al: Superiority of tandem autologous transplantation over standard therapy for previously untreated multiple myeloma. Blood 1997;89:789–793.

Fermand J-P, Ravaud P, Chevret S, et al: High-dose therapy and autologous peripheral blood stem cell transplantation in multiple myeloma: Up-front or rescue treatment? Results of a multicenter sequential randomized clinical trial. Blood 1998;92:3131–3136.

Lokhorst HM, Schattenberg A, Cornelissen JJ, et al: Donor lymphocyte infusions for relapsed multiple myeloma after allogeneic stem cell transplantation: predictive factors for response and long-term outcome. J Clin Oncol 2000;18:3031–3037.

Non-Hodgkin's Lymphoma/Hodgkin's Disease

Andre M, Henry-Amar M, Pico J-L, et al: Comparison of high-dose therapy and autologous stem cell transplantation with conventional therapy for Hodgkin's disease induction failure: A case-control study. J Clin Oncol 1999;17:222–229.

Apostolidis J, Gupta RK, Grenzelias D, et al: High-dose therapy with autologous bone marrow support as consolidation of remission in follicular lymphoma: Long-term clinical and molecular follow-up. J Clin Oncol 18:527–536.

Blay J-Y, Gomez F, Sebban C, et al: The International Prognostic Index correlates to survival in patients with aggressive lymphoma in relapse: Analysis of the PARMA trial. Blood 1998;92:3562–3568.

Cao TM, Horning SJ, Negrin RS, et al: High-dose therapy and autologous hematopoietic cell transplantation for follicular lymphoma beyond first remission: The Stanford University experience. Biol Blood Marrow Transplant 2001;7:294–301.

Freedman AS, Gribben JG, Nadler LM: High-dose therapy and autologous stem cell transplantation in follicular non-Hodgkin's lymphoma. Leuk Lymphoma 1998;28:219–230.

Friedberg JW, Neuberg D, Stone RM, et al: Outcome in patients with myelodysplastic syndrome after autologous bone marrow transplantation for non-Hodgkin's lymphoma. J Clin Oncol 1999;17:3128–3135.

Gribben JG, Freedman AS, Neuberg D, et al: Immunologic purging of marrow assessed by PCR before autologous bone marrow transplantation for B cell lymphoma. N Engl J Med 1991;325:1525–1533.

Hahn T, Wolff SN, Czuczman M, et al: The role of cytotoxic therapy with hematopoietic stem cell transplantation in the therapy of diffuse large cell B cell non-Hodgkin's lymphoma: An evidence-based review. Biol Blood Marrow Transplant 2001;7:308–331.

Lillington DM, Micallef INM, Carpenter E, et al: Detection of chromosome abnormalities pre-high-dose treatment in patients developing therapy-related myelodysplasia and secondary acute myelogenous leukemia after treatment for non-Hodgkin's lymphoma. J Clin Oncol 2001;19: 2472–2481.

Mills W, Chopra R, McMillan A, et al: BEAM chemotherapy and autologous bone marrow transplantation for patients with relapsed or refractory non-Hodgkin's lymphoma. J Clin Oncol 1995;13:588–595.

Milpied N, Fielding AK, Pearce RM, et al: Allogeneic bone marrow transplant is not better than autologous transplant for patients with relapsed Hodgkin's disease. J Clin Oncol 1996;14:1291–1296.

Nademanee A, Molina A, Fung H, et al: High-dose chemo/radiotherapy and autologous bone marrow or stem cell transplantation for poor-risk advanced-stage Hodgkin's disease during first partial or complete remission. Biol Blood Marrow Transplant 1999;5:292–298.

Nademanee A, Molina A, O'Donnell MR, et al: Results of high-dose therapy and autologous bone marrow/stem cell transplantation during remission in poor-risk intermediate- and high-grade lymphoma: international index high and high-intermediate risk group. Blood 1997;90:3844–3852.

Philip T, Guglielmi C, Hagenbeek A, et al: Autologous bone marrow transplantation as compared with salvage chemotherapy in relapses of chemotherapy-sensitive non-Hodgkin's lymphoma. N Engl J Med 1995;333:1540–1545.

Press OW, Eary JF, Gooley T, et al: A phase I/II trial of iodine-131-tositumomab (anti-CD20), etoposide, cyclophosphamide, and autologous stem cell transplantation for relapsed B cell lymphomas. Blood 2000;96:2934–2942.

Sureda A, Arranz R, Iriondo A, et al: Autologous stem cell transplantation for Hodgkin's disease: Results and prognostic factors in 494 patients from the Grupo Espanol de Linfomas/Transplante Autologo de Medula Osea Spanish Cooperative Group. J Clin Oncol 2001;19:1395–1404.

Sweetenham JW, Carella AM, Taghipour G, et al: High-dose therapy and autologous stem cell transplantation for adult patients with Hodgkin's disease who do not enter remission after induction chemotherapy: Results in 175 patients reported to the European Group for Blood and Bone Marrow Transplantation. Lymphoma Working Party. J Clin Oncol 1999;17:3101–3109.

Sweetenham JW, Santini G, Qian W, et al: High-dose therapy and autologous stem cell transplantation versus conventional-dose consolidation/maintenance therapy as postremission therapy for adult patients with lymphoblastic lymphoma: Results of a randomized trial of the European Group for Blood and Bone Marrow Transplantation and the United Kingdom Lymphoma Group. J Clin Oncol 2001;19:2927–2936.

Verdonck LF, van Putten WLJ, Hagenbeek A, et al: Comparison of CHOP chemotherapy with autologous bone marrow transplantation for slowly responding patients with aggressive non-Hodgkin's lymphoma. N Engl J Med 1995;332:1045–1051.

Vose JM, Zhang M-J, Rowlings PA, et al: Autologous transplantation for diffuse aggressive non-Hodgkin's lymphoma in patients never achieving remission: a report from the autologous blood and marrow transplant registry. J Clin Oncol 2001;19:406–413.

Chapter 52
Growth Factors

Jacob M. Rowe

Introduction

Hematopoietic growth factors are glycoproteins that can be produced for pharmacologic use by recombinant DNA technology. They have many potential clinical uses in malignant and nonmalignant hematology. Several areas have been explored extensively, and much data are available from clinical trials. Other areas are of potential interest but have a paucity of clinical information.

Over the past two decades, the development of in vitro marrow clonogenic culture systems has led to the discovery of a family of interacting hematopoietic growth factors that have been demonstrated to have critical physiologic roles for controlling hematopoiesis in vivo. Of the many hematopoietic growth factors that have been cloned, only erythropoietin (EPO), granulocyte colony-stimulating factor (G-CSF), and granulocyte-macrophage colony-stimulating factor (GM-CSF) have seen widespread clinical use. Thrombopoietins have a limited clinical role, and several trials over the past decade have involved interleukin-2 (IL-2), interleukin-3, interleukin-11, macrophage colony-stimulating factor (M-CSF), stem cell factor (SCF), interleukin-6, and interleukin-1. Most of these have a limited, if any, therapeutic role at the present time, although they may be critical biologic factors in normal cell functioning.

Erythropoietic Growth Factors

Recombinant human erythropoietin is a purified glycoprotein that stimulates erythropoiesis. It is produced from mammalian cells into which the gene coding for human erythropoietin has been inserted and is indistinguishable from human urinary erythropoietin by biologic activity and immunologic reactivity. Endogenous erythropoietin is the only hematopoietic growth factor that behaves like a hormone. Produced mostly in the kidneys but also in the liver, erythropoietin interacts with the erythroid progenitor cells in the bone marrow to promote their proliferation and maintain their viability. Production of erythropoietin in humans is regulated by tissue oxygenation such that hypoxia or anemia stimulates erythropoietin production and erythrocytosis suppresses it. In general, plasma erythropoietin concentrations reflect erythropoietin production and can be used to define deficient states in which anemia may be amenable to correction by administration of recombinant erythropoetin (Table 52-1).

Of all hematopoietic growth factors, none has been as important clinically as erythropoietin. The use of erythropoietin over the past 15 years represents one of the most important advances in the management of patients with advanced renal disease with or without dialysis. Not only has this resulted in freedom from transfusion dependency and elimination of many of the risks associated with this, but it has also led to a significant improvement in quality of life for these patients. As a result of the development of erythropoietin, many patients with chronic renal failure are able to lead relatively normal lives. Over 95% of hemodialysis patients respond to erythropoietin and are able to achieve a hematocrit of 35% within three months of initiation of such therapy. Although erythropoietin is not dialyzable, it is commonly administered intravenously at the end of each dialysis at a dose of 75 to 150 units/kg. The variability in the required dose of erythropoietin is related to the enormous variation in the steady-state plasma erythropoietin level at any given level of anemia.

Initially, on the basis of theoretical considerations, there was serious concern that erythropoietin treatment might accelerate the progression of renal failure; therefore, erythropoietin was often withheld from predialysis patients with renal failure. The results of several prospective studies have been published, and it is now standard practice to offer erythropoietin to all patients with chronic renal failure if they have significant anemia and are symptomatic. Erythropoietin treatment in predialysis patients may affect the blood

Table 52-1 ■ Clinical Use of Recombinant Erythropoietin (EPO)

Absolute Indication	Often Useful	Possibly Useful
1. Anemia of chronic renal failure	1. Anemia of multiple myeloma	1. Perisurgical
2. Anemia of prematurity	2. Anemia of cancer	2. Anemia of chronic disease
3. Anemia secondary to platinum-based chemotherapy	3. Potentiation of preoperative autologous blood donation	3. Post-allogeneic bone marrow transplantation
	4. Myelodysplasia	
	5. Anemia of HIV infection	
	6. Chemotherapy-induced anemia	

pressure; therefore, close monitoring and possible adjustment of antihypertensive treatment are sometimes necessary. An increased incidence of seizures has been reported in renal failure patients who receive erythropoietin. However, recent studies have not confirmed this increase in incidence over renal failure patients who do not receive erythropoietin. Therefore, at the present time, erythropoietin is not contraindicated for patients with a previous history of seizures. Although higher hematocrits could lead to thrombosis of arteriovenous fistulas, the incidence among erythropoietin-treated patients is 5% to 10%, similar to the incidence in patients undergoing dialysis who do not receive erythropoietin.

During treatment with erythropoietin, it is essential to maintain adequate iron stores. Hemodialysis patients often receive this intravenously, as recommended by the National Kidney Foundation; however, the use of an oral iron preparation is perfectly acceptable. Inadequate iron supply is the commonest cause of a poor response to erythropoietin. Other, less common causes of a poor response to erythropoietin are intercurrent infections and excessive splenic hemolysis.

For patients with renal failure who are not transfusion-dependent, erythropoietin should nevertheless be given if the patient is symptomatic. In this instance, the recommended starting dose is 25 units/kg subcutaneously three times per week for the first month. If there has been no response, the dose can be escalated to 50 units/kg. Other clinical indications for the use of erythropoietin are summarized in Table 52-1. These include patients who have a prolonged anemia following treatment with platinum derivatives (cisplatin or carboplatin). These chemotherapeutic agents are associated with defective endogenous erythropoietin production, and randomized trials have demonstrated that patients benefit significantly from therapy with erythropoietin. Patients receiving other chemotherapeutic agents who have prolonged anemia and are transfusion-dependent are also likely to respond to erythropoietin. In all cases of chemotherapy-induced anemia, the patients who are most likely to benefit are those who are either anemic prior to initiation of therapy or those who became severely anemic after the first cycle.

In general, patients should only be treated with erythropoietin if a low level of endogenous erythropoietin has been demonstrated (Table 52-2). Myelodysplasia may be an exception to this rule.

Anemia of prematurity, although multifactorial, usually responds to erythropoietin at the dose of 250 units/kg subcutaneously three times a week. As with anemia of renal failure, iron supplementation must be given.

Myelodysplastic syndromes (MDS) comprise a heterogeneous group of clonal myeloid stem cell

Table 52-2 ■ General Recommendations for Therapy with EPO

1. EPO should be given only to patients who have a symptomatic anemia or are transfusion-dependent. This category also includes patients who are candidates for blood transfusions.
2. The cause of anemia must be clearly established prior to initiation of EPO. Even if EPO deficiency has been demonstrated, other factors such as iron deficiency or B_{12} or folate deficiency must be corrected.
3. In general, EPO therapy should be given only in those conditions in which data from clinical trials (preferably phase III), have demonstrated its efficacy.
4. It is not necessary to demonstrate a low level of EPO in patients with renal failure or in premature infants. In all other patients, with the exception of myelodysplasia, inadequate erythropoietin production should be documented.
5. In general, begin with a dose at the lower level known to be effective. Escalate after one month if this has been inadequate.
6. The target hematocrit is not always a "normal hematocrit." A level on the order of 35% to 37% will usually suffice and may prevent complications of EPO therapy.

disorders characterized by peripheral cytopenias and dysplasia of bone marrow progenitor cells (see Chapter 62). Myelodysplastic syndromes occur primarily among older adults with a median age of 70 years. The most important clinical problems arise from chronic anemia and from red cell transfusion-induced iron overload, bleeding due to low platelet counts, and infections as a consequence of neutropenia. A significant number of patients succumb to these complications of cytopenia prior to the onset of overt acute myelogenous leukemia. There is no effective therapy for myelodysplasia in older adults; the mainstay of therapy is supportive care. Younger adults who have a histocompatible sibling may be cured with allogeneic transplantation. Approximately 30% to 50% of transfusion-dependent patients with myelodysplastic syndromes respond to high doses of erythropoietin ($\geq$3 $\times$ 10,000 units/week). Of interest, synergy between granulocyte colony-stimulating factor and erythropoietin has been demonstrated for the production of normal and myelodysplastic erythroid precursors. Thus, approximately 40% of patients with myelodysplasia who are treated with a combination of granulocyte colony-stimulating factor and erythropoietin have an erythroid response. It has also been shown that patients responding to erythropoietin and granulocyte colony-stimulating factor had significantly lower serum erythropoietin level (<500 U/L), higher absolute reticulocyte counts, and normal cytogenetics. However, these criteria are not exclusive, and patients with higher erythropoietin levels are also known to respond. Because of the major cost involved in erythropoietin therapy and the difficulty in deciding which patients will respond, ongoing randomized trials are attempting to evaluate prospectively the role of erythropoietin, with or without granulocyte colony-stimulating factor, versus supportive care that does not include erythropoietin.

Myeloid Growth Factors

Myeloid growth factors, mainly granulocyte colony-stimulating factor and granulocyte-macrophage colony-stimulating factor, have enormous potential in the therapy of patients with hematologic malignancies. Guidelines for their use were published by the American Society of Clinical Oncology in 1996 and since then have been updated on two occasions. Table 52-3 outlines the circumstances where they are commonly used.

Acute Myeloid Leukemia

Many potential applications exist for the use of colony-stimulating factors in the treatment of acute myeloid leukemia (Table 52-4).

Table 52-3 ■ Use of Myeloid Growth Factors

1. Acute myeloid leukemia
2. Acute lymphoblastic leukemia
3. Stem cell transplantation
4. Myelodysplasia
5. Chemotherapy-induced neutropenia

Reducing Period of Neutropenia

Over the past decade, 14 major controlled trials of growth factors used after induction therapy in the acute myeloid leukemia have been reported (Table 52-5). Studies have been grouped according to the product used. Most important, the concern for safety has been laid to rest. The preponderance of the data from all of these clinical trials shows that the administration of growth factors at any time after induction therapy for acute leukemia is safe. Not only has this safety been demonstrated by the published results of induction therapy, but also the follow-up of these studies have failed to show any increase in the relapse rate among patients who went into complete remission with growth factors when compared with patients who did not receive growth factors. Virtually all of these studies demonstrated a significant reduction in the time required to reach an absolute neutrophil count of 500/μL or 1000/μL. Several studies reported varying degrees of reduction in morbidity, and one study showed a significant reduction in mortality. Despite these 14 well-controlled clinical investigations comprising over 3500 patients, controversy still abounds over the use of growth factors in acute myeloid leukemia. The results that have been obtained are not consistent, and the conclusions of the various authors differ. A meta-analysis cannot be performed owing to differences in the design and conduct of these clinical trials (Table 52-6). Particularly important may be differences in patient age, induction regimen, and disease state, whether de novo acute

---

Table 52-4 ■ Potential Uses of Growth Factors in Acute Myeloid Leukemia

- Reducing period of neutropenia
- Recruitment of cells into S-phase of the cell cycle (priming)
- Enhancement of antimicrobial function
- Induction of differentiation of leukemic cells
- Direct antileukemic effects
- Interruption of autocrine-paracrine loops
- Stem cell protection

Table 52-5 ■ Controlled Trials of Growth Factors After Induction Therapy in Acute Myeloid Leukemia

Study	N	Reduction in Days to ANC 1000/μL	Documented Reduced Morbidity	Leukemia Stimulation
GM-CSF (Sargramostin)				
Büchner et al., 1992	86	6–9*	+	No
Rowe et al., 1995	117	6*	+	No
GM-CSF (Molgrastim)				
Link et al., 1996	187	6*		No
Goldstone et al., 1997	803	5*		No
G-CSF (Lenograstin)				
Estey et al., 1994	197	13*		No
Heil et al., 1997	521	5*	+	No
Godwin et al., 1998	234	3–4*	+	No
G-CSF (Filgrastim)				
Stone et al., 1995	379	2*		No
Löwenberg et al., 1997	316	5*		No
Witz et al., 1998	209	6*		No

* $P = \leq .05$.

myeloid leukemia or more advanced disease. Also important is the timing of the growth factor administration, particularly in relation to the documentation of marrow hypoplasia. Differences in study product may exist, even among different cellular preparations of the same cytokine. Finally, the statistical endpoints that are used in these studies need to be considered carefully. Some of the studies were designed and sized to show differences in hematopoietic recovery, for example, but not to show differences in complete response rate or survival. It is also possible that at least in some of the studies, patient selection might have affected interpretation of the data.

Among studies investigating the use of growth factors in consolidation therapy, very few have shown benefit. Since patient numbers in these trials were small and the studies were not sized to show differences in neutrophil recovery during consolidation, failure to demonstrate such a difference does not imply that cytokines do not work in consolidation. In fact, the largest trial of growth factors in acute myeloid leukemia, which had an adequate sample size to assess reduction in neutropenia, demonstrated a statistically significant shortening of neutropenia among patients receiving growth factors during consolidation. Similar results were also reported by the Cancer and Leukemia Group B (CALGB) when cytokines were given after consolidation with diaziquone and mitoxantrone and in a recently published Groupe Ouest-Est Leucemies Aigues Myeloblastiques (GOELAM) study.

Several studies have evaluated the cost-effectiveness of cytokines when used during induction therapy. Table 52-7 outlines these clinical studies and their correlative cost analyses. Most studies in adults demonstrated a cost benefit for growth factors, although a cost-effectiveness study using the more toxic *Escherichia coli*—derived granulocyte-macrophage colony-stimulating factor was an exception. Therefore, one of the major considerations for withholding the use of cytokines in acute myeloid leukemia may no longer be compelling.

There are few areas in clinical medicine in which so many prospective clinical trials have been designed to answer a single question at the end of which the data remain equivocal. Considering that the major

Table 52-6 ■ Variability in the Design and Conduct of Clinical Studies of Cytokines in Acute Myeloid Leukemia

■ Patient age
■ Induction regimen used
■ Disease state
■ Timing of growth factor administration
■ Documentation of marrow hypoplasia
■ Differences in study product
■ Statistical endpoints
■ Patient selection

Table 52-7 ■ Clinical Results of Induction Chemotherapy from Cooperative Group Studies

Clinical Study	Growth Factor	Patients	Reduction in Neutropenia (days)	CSF Versus Control		
				Percent of Documented Infections	Days of Hospitalization	Incremental Cost of CSF Use
Laver et al., POG, 1998	G-CSF	88	Same	N.A.	9 versus 9	+$ 2497
Heil et al., International AML study, 1997	G-CSF	521	5	37 versus 36	20 versus 25*	–$ 2230
Godwin et al., SWOG, 1998	G-CSF	211	3	163 versus 141	29 versus 29	+$ 120
Rowe et al., ECOG, 1995	GM-CSF, yeast	117	4	52 versus 70 10 versus 36* Grade 4, 5	36 versus 38	–$ 2310

*P < 0.01.

reason for the reluctance to initiate clinical trials of cytokines in acute myeloid leukemia had been a concern for safety, it can now be stated unequivocally that this concern is unwarranted. With the apparent benefit that has been demonstrated in so many studies and the uniform finding of an improved neutrophil recovery time, it is not clear why hesitation to use cytokines in acute myeloid leukemia persists. The probability of infection and the risk of increased morbidity and mortality correlate directly with severity of neutropenia, although these observations may, at times, not be easy to demonstrate objectively. It is therefore difficult not to acknowledge the benefit to a patient undergoing induction therapy as a consequence of an improved neutrophil recovery time of approximately one week. The sense of well-being among patients (and physicians) at the early evidence of neutrophil recovery cannot be ignored, and therefore, it would seem that cytokines (granulocyte-macrophage colony-stimulating factor or granulocyte colony-stimulating factor) should be administered to all patients undergoing induction therapy for acute myeloid leukemia who are at high risk for therapy-related morbidity and mortality. The earlier published data were analyzed on the basis of an expectation of major differences in response rate or survival rate. This is clearly not the issue or the reason for the use of growth factors. Rather, cytokines should be considered important supportive care measures, much like central venous catheters. These indwelling catheters are not cost-effective, and they increase rather than decrease infections; nevertheless, virtually all physicians use them for the comfort and well-being of the patient.

These same considerations need to be employed regarding the use of cytokines.

Enhancement of Antimicrobial Function

Considerable speculation in preclinical investigations has focused on the potential for enhancing antimicrobial therapy with cytokines. In vitro, granulocyte-macrophage colony-stimulating factor increases phagocytic and fungicidal activity of neutrophils against *Candida albicans* and *Torulopsis glabrata*. Similarly, in vitro exposure of peripheral blood mononuclear cells to granulocyte-macrophage colony-stimulating factor increases phagocytosis of *Cryptococus neoformans*, and exposure of monocytes to granulocyte-macrophage colony-stimulating factor results in increased killing of *Candida albicans* and *Aspergillus fumigatus*. The mechanism of increased activity against *Candida* and *Aspergillus* appears to be unrelated to increased phagocytosis; rather, it is due to increased oxidative metabolism and production of toxic superoxide anions by monocytes.

Clinical data that support the use of cytokines in fungal infections have been limited to a few early phase I and II data. A hint of effectiveness was suggested by the Eastern Cooperative Oncology Group (ECOG) phase III study of cytokines in acute myeloid leukemia. In this study, 20 of 117 patients had unequivocally documented fungal infections, and the overall mortality rate in the granulocyte-macrophage colony-stimulating factor group was 13% compared with 75% in the placebo group (Table 52-8). Most of these patients, as expected, had *Aspergillus* or *Candida* infections, and there was no difference in fungal prophylaxis between the two groups. Basically, most patients receiving granulocyte-macrophage colony-stimulating factor survived their fungal infections, while most of those receiving placebo died. Clearly, caution is mandatory in dealing with relatively small numbers, but these data are intriguing. It is not known whether these results are due to direct stimulation of monocyte activity by granulocyte-macrophage colony-stimulating factor or to earlier neutrophil recovery, as was initially hypothesized during the design of the study.

Recruitment of Cells into S-Phase of the Cell Cycle (Priming)

Over the past decade, several groups have attempted to determine whether hematopoietic growth factors can be used to prime leukemic blasts by increasing the proportion in the active phase of the cell cycle, thereby, theoretically, increasing their susceptibility to S-phase-active agents such as cytosine arabinoside. In vitro studies have shown that growth factors such as granulocyte-macrophage colony-stimulating factor, granulocyte colony-stimulating factor, stem cell factor (c-kit ligand), interleukin-3, and others can increase the fraction of leukemic blasts in the S-phase. The effect that in vivo priming might have on leukemic blasts in their ultimate response to chemotherapy is unclear, despite a multitude of phase II and phase III studies. Detailed analysis of these studies shows that the clinical data remain conflicting and confusing. The finding of an increased number of blasts or recruitment into the S-phase of the cell cycle following the administration of a cytokine must be compared carefully with control patients, because untreated patients with acute myeloid leukemia often change their cell cycle kinetics and increase their blast cell counts. Table 52-9 outlines the controlled studies that have evaluated the role of cytokines as priming agents for acute myeloid leukemia. This clearly shows the variability in patient selection, cytokine used, type of therapy administered, and, of course, results. Just as was seen with the multiple studies on enhancement of neutrophil recovery, despite the vast number of clinical trials examining the use of cytokines as priming agents for acute myeloid leukemia, the results remain confusing. Only one study demonstrated stimulation of leukemia and a lower response rate among patients receiving priming therapy with E. coli—derived granulocyte-macrophage colony-stimulating factor, but it was not prospectively controlled, and the control group consisted of a historical cohort of patients who were treated on several different studies.

Thus, the preponderance of the evidence has established the safety of cytokines when used as priming agents. The only study to show a major positive effect of priming in patients with acute myeloid leukemia was the GOELAM study. This well-designed prospective placebo-controlled study showed no difference in complete response rate in granulocyte-macrophage colony-stimulating factor or placebo, but the two-year disease-free survival was significantly improved in the granulocyte-macrophage colony-stimulating factor group. The granulocyte-macrophage colony-stimulating factor group also showed a trend toward a longer overall survival rate. The fundamental difference with this study and all others is that the priming with the cytokine was not administered prior to the administration of chemotherapy, leading to the suggestion that some detrimental effect might occur following one or more days of blast cell stimulation without simultaneous cytotoxic therapy. However, this hypothesis remains unproven. Thus, in contrast to the established role of growth factors following induction therapy to ameliorate morbidity, no clear role of hematopoietic growth factors as priming agents as yet has been defined, and the use of cytokines as priming agents in the AML cannot be recommended outside of well-designed clinical studies.

Acute Lymphoblastic Leukemia

The use of growth factors for acute lymphoblastic leukemia (ALL) has largely bypassed the controversy that was described for acute myeloid leukemia. The data suggest that the use of cytokines in acute lym-

Table 52-8 ■ Incidence of Infection with GM-CSF Versus Placebo

	GM-CSF (n = 52)	Placebo (n = 47)	P value
Therapy-related mortality	3/52 (6%)	7/47 (15%)	0.18
Infection			
Grade 3, 4, 5	27/52 (52%)	33/47 (70%)	0.068
Grade 4, 5	5/52 (10%)	17/47 (36%)	0.002
Pneumonia			
Death/grade 3, 4	2/14 (14%)	7/13 (54%)	0.046
Fungal infection			
Death/grade 3, 4	1/8 (13%)	9/12 (75%)	0.02

From Rowe JM, Rubin A, Mazza JJ, et al: Incidence of infections in adult patients (>55 years) with acute myeloid leukemia treated with yeast-derived GM-CSF (sargramostim): Results of a double-blind prospective study by the Eastern Cooperative Oncology Group. In Hiddeman W, Büchner T, Worrman B (eds): Acute Leukemias V: Experimental Approaches and Management of Refractory Diseases. Berlin-Heidelberg: Springer-Verlag, 1996, pp 178–184.

Table 52-9 ■ Controlled Trials of Growth Factors as Priming Therapy for AML

Study	N	Cytokine	Day of Administration	Leukemia Stimulation	Cytokine Versus Control CR (%)	Survival (%)
Rowe et al., 1998	245	GM-CSF (yeast) versus placebo	−2	No	38/40	Same
Estey et al., 1994	197	G-CSF versus control	−1	No	63/53	Same
Estey et al., 1992	232	GM-CSF (*E. coli*) versus control	−8	Yes	48/65*	Worse with GM-CSF
Witz et al., 1998	229	GM-CSF (*E. coli*) versus placebo	+1	No	62/61	44/19* (24 months)
Peterson et al., 1996	174	GM-CSF (*E. coli*) versus placebo	−5	No	56/55	Same

*$P \leq 0.05$.

phoblastic leukemia, either during induction or in subsequent intensification, reduces the period of neutropenia and in several studies affects the morbidity and even mortality rates (Table 52-10). Thus, it has become established to recommend the use of growth factors, granulocyte colony-stimulating factor or granulocyte-macrophage colony-stimulating factor, at any stage of the long therapy for acute lymphoblastic leukemia where profound life-threatening neutropenia is expected as part of the therapeutic course.

Stem Cell Transplantation

There are three predominant uses of growth factors in bone marrow transplantation: enhancement of neutrophil recovery, prevention or therapy of graft failure, and mobilization of stem cells.

Enhancement of Neutrophil Recovery

Growth factors given after autologous or allogeneic bone marrow transplantation significantly shorten the period of neutropenia and reduce the hospital stay (Table 52-11). Various published randomized studies show reduction in significant neutropenia of anywhere from four to seven days with a similar short-

ening in the overall hospital stay. There are differences in Table 52-11 between the recovery after granulocyte-macrophage colony-stimulating factor and granulocyte colony-stimulating factor that do not reflect differences in study product; rather, they reflect evolving clinical practice. Most of the early studies with granulocyte-macrophage colony-stimulating factor were conducted using bone marrow as the source of stem cells, whereas most of the published randomized studies with granulocyte colony-stimulating factor used mobilized peripheral blood stem cells. The available data on growth factors after allogeneic bone marrow transplantation, based on several phase II and phase III studies, confirm that in this setting, there is also a more rapid neutrophil recovery and reduced hospital stay.

In general, the efficacy of enhanced neutrophil recovery is similar whether glycosylated or nonglycosylated granulocyte colony-stimulating factor is used (lenograstim or filgrastim) or glycosylated granulocyte-macrophage colony-stimulating factor (sargramostim). The nonglycosylated granulocyte-macrophage colony-stimulating factor (molgramostim) is more toxic and should probably not be used. During the last decade, multiple trials attempted

Table 52-10 ■ Randomized Studies of Growth Factors in Acute Lymphoblastic Leukemia

Study	N G-CSF Versus Control	Days to ANC >500 or 1000/μL G-CSF Versus Control	Incidence of Infections G-CSF Versus Control	Early Death G-CSF Versus Control	Leukemia Stimulation
Ottman, 1995	37/39	8/12.5	43%/56%	3%/6%	No
Geissler, 1997	25/26	16/26	40%/77%	4%/9%	No
Larson, 1998	102/96	16/22	Same	5%/11%	No

Growth Factors for Acute Myeloid Leukemia

Prospective clinical trials have demonstrated that growth factors are safe when given at any time during induction therapy for acute myeloid leukemia.

Growth factors given after induction therapy shorten the period of neutropenia by anywhere from two to seven days.

Five of the 14 major randomized studies have shown a significant reduction in morbidity if growth factors are administered during induction.

No major study has shown a detrimental effect from growth factors.

Studies of cost-effectiveness, although limited in scope, have also, in most instances, demonstrated a benefit for growth factors.

While glycosylation may confer important biological properties, the glycosylated and nonglycosylated granulocyte colony-stimulating factor preparations and granulocyte-macrophage colony-stimulating factor seem to be equally efficacious in reducing the period of neutropenia. However, nonglycosylated *E. coli*-derived granulocyte-macrophage colony-stimulating factor is more toxic than all other growth factors for acute myeloid leukemia and should not be used.

Granulocyte-macrophage colony-stimulating factor has a potential advantage when neutropenia is accompanied by fungal infection, and consideration should be given to the preferential use of granulocyte-macrophage colony-stimulating factor in such instances.

The data suggest that the best time to administer growth factors is after marrow aplasia has been demonstrated on day 10 to 14 of bone marrow. Thus, growth factors are recommended, as a supportive care measure, both following induction and consolidation therapy for acute myeloid leukemia.

In contrast to the role of growth factors following induction therapy to ameliorate morbidity, no clear role for growth factors as priming agent has yet been defined, and the use of cytokines for priming cannot be recommended outside of well-designed clinical trials.

to use other cytokines after stem cell transplantation. These involved predominantly the combination of granulocyte-macrophage colony-stimulating factor and granulocyte colony-stimulating factor, concurrently or sequentially, or combinations involving interleukin-3. Although various combinations of interleukin-3 with granulocyte-macrophage colony-stimulating factor or granulocyte colony-stimulating factor appeared to confer accelerated hematopoietic recovery, the toxicity of interleukin-3 does not seem to warrant routine use of interleukin-3 alone, in combination, or as a hybrid (PIXY 321) in routine clinical practice. In any event, the evolving clinical practice of mobilized peripheral blood stem cells has made use of growth factors after autologous transplantation less of a critical issue.

Graft Failure

Graft failure as well as poor graft function with prolonged cytopenias increases the hazards of bone marrow transplantation and affects patient survival. Graft failure, either primary or secondary, was more common in the early days of bone marrow transplantation, when the constitution of cells in the graft was

Table 52-11 ■ Randomized Trials of Growth Factors Following Autologous BMT

	ANC > 500 or 1000/μL (days)		Days of Hospitalization	
GM-CSF	**Cytokine or Placebo**		**Cytokine Versus Placebo**	
Nemunaitis et al., 1991	19	26	27	33
Rabinowe et al., 1991	14	21	23	28
Greenberg et al., 1996	18	27	29	32
G-CSF				
Spitzer et al., 1997	10	16	19	21
Klumpp et al., 1995	10.5	16	18	24
Linch et al., 1997	9	12	13	16
McQuaker et al., 1997	10	14	13	16

somewhat empiric. With current technologies and measurement of precise numbers of CD34-positive cells in the donor pool, graft failure is a lot less common. Nevertheless, a small proportion of patients undergoing allogeneic transplantation or, less commonly, autologous transplantation fail to engraft. Studies with granulocyte-macrophage colony-stimulating factor showed that growth factors significantly reduce the rate of graft failure, primary or secondary, and that sequential administration of different growth factors, that is, granulocyte-macrophage colony-stimulating factor followed by granulocyte colony-stimulating factor, offered no advantage over granulocyte-macrophage colony-stimulating factor alone in accelerating hematopoiesis or preventing lethal complications in patients with poor graft function after transplantation.

Because of the potential for enhancing antimicrobial function with granulocyte-macrophage colony-stimulating factor, it is not known whether the routine use of small doses of granulocyte-macrophage colony-stimulating factor after bone marrow transplantation is indicated. On the basis of theoretic considerations, in situations in which the neutrophils have recovered but the patient remains infected and severely immune-compromised, owing to graft-versus-host-disease (GVHD) or the therapy thereof, the use of granulocyte-macrophage colony-stimulating factor may help to prevent, or be an adjunct to the treatment of, fungal or other opportunistic infection. However, there are no prospective studies, to date, that have been performed confirming such a benefit.

Mobilization of Peripheral Blood Progenitor Cells

For the successful mobilization of progenitor cells of peripheral blood for clinical use, several approaches have been used:

1. Collecting cells during the recovery following intensive myelosuppressive chemotherapy;
2. Following the administration of growth factors, granulocyte colony-stimulating factor or granulocyte-macrophage colony-stimulating factor;
3. Using the combination of hematopoietic growth factors and myelosuppressive chemotherapy.

In practice, progenitor cells are most efficiently collected following the combination of chemotherapy and growth factors, although there is a significant proportion of patients in whom an adequate number of progenitor cells can be collected following the use of growth factors alone for mobilization. Table 52-12 outlines the current understanding of peripheral blood stem cell mobilization.

While the rate of engraftment using mobilized peripheral blood stem cells is more rapid than that following the use of unmobilized bone marrow stem cells, there is no fundamental difference in the rate of engraftment between mobilized peripheral blood stem cells and mobilized cells obtained from the bone marrow. In practice, mobilization of peripheral blood stem cells has become commonplace and is easily performed in the outpatient setting. The vast majority of autologous transplants are performed in this manner, and an increasing number of allogeneic stem cells are collected this way. Some countries prohibit the use of growth factors to healthy children who act as donors; however, the emerging data suggest that the risks, if any, are minimal.

Myelodysplasia

The myeloid growth factors, granulocyte-macrophage colony-stimulating factor and granulocyte colony-stimulating factor, are reported to be occasionally beneficial in increasing the neutrophil count and function in patients with myelodysplasia. The initial concerns about the safety of using glycoproteins known to stim-

---

Table 52-12 ■ General Guidelines for Mobilization of Peripheral Blood Stem Cells

- Both G-CSF and GM-CSF mobilize peripheral blood stem cells.
- There is a dose-response effect for both G-CSF and GM-CSF in peripheral blood stem cells mobilization.
- Combinations of cytokines and chemotherapy mobilize more peripheral blood stem cells than do cytokines alone.
- Patients who have received no or minimal prior chemotherapy have a greater than 90% likelihood of achieving an adequate collection of peripheral blood stem cells with cytokine/chemotherapy combinations.
- Patients who have received more than six months of alkylating agent therapy, fludarabine, or radiation therapy have only a 70% chance of obtaining adequate number of peripheral blood stem cells ($>1.5 \times 10^6$ CD34 cells/kg) using standard technique.
- For heavily pretreated patients, in whom there is a significant risk of nonmobilization using standard techniques, use of an early-acting cytokine such as stem cell factor (SCF) or flt3 ligand (Flt3 L) together with a late-acting cytokine (G-CSF or GM-CSF) is likely to significantly enhance the rate of peripheral blood stem cells mobilization and enable the transplant to take place.

Modified from Stiff PJ: Peripheral blood stem cell mobilization: Contemporary issues and early studies using Flt3 ligand. In Rowe JM, Lazarus HM, Carella AM (eds): Bone Marrow Transplantation. London: Martin Dunitz, 2000, pp 21–40.

ulate leukemic blast cell proliferation have been similar to those that were described in the earlier discussion of acute myeloid leukemia. Clinical data, however, have demonstrated that stimulation of leukemia does not appear to be of major clinical concern in myelodysplasia. Most studies have not shown an uncontrolled proliferation of leukemic blasts or significant negative effects on survival beyond the expected rate of transformation to frank acute myeloid leukemia. While most studies have shown a small but often significant effect on neutrophil proliferation, the biologic significance of this is not always clear.

Myelodysplasia is a disease of older adults, and conventional therapy is usually unsatisfactory. There is evidence that over 90% of patients have an increase in their neutrophil count.

Thus, it appears that granulocyte-macrophage colony-stimulating factor and granulocyte colony-stimulating factor have the capacity to affect a modest increase in mature myeloid elements. However, the clinical effects of these cytokines are limited, but in a palliative clinical setting, they may be important adjuncts to the supportive care of patients with myelodysplasia.

Chemotherapy-Induced Neutropenia

The routine use of growth factors for the primary prophylaxis of neutropenia following chemotherapy for solid tumors or lymphoma is not supported by data. Guidelines published by the American Society of Clinical Oncology suggest that this should be offered only when a therapeutic regimen has an expected rate of febrile neutropenia of at least 40%.

Once a patient has developed febrile neutropenia following a course of chemotherapy, it is common practice to administer this in future cycles as secondary prophylaxis. There are clear advantages in maintaining dose intensity, and thus, although convincing prospective data are lacking, such a practice seems reasonable. Growth factors are also used routinely as an adjunct to the therapy of febrile neutropenia following chemotherapy for solid tumors or lymphomas. In most cases, no more than a few days of growth factor administration are required.

TREATMENT

Anemia in Patients with Myelodysplasia

There is no role for prophylactic therapy using erythropoietin, with or without granulocyte colony-stimulating factor, among myelodysplasia patients who do not have symptomatic anemia.

For patients who are symptomatic and/or transfusion-dependent, the baseline erythropoietin levels should be obtained.

Patients who have an erythropoietin level <500 U/L should be started on erythropoietin at a dose of 150 units/kg daily, subcutaneously. This therapy should continue for at least four months.

If the response has not been adequate, then granulocyte colony-stimulating factor at a dose of 1 μg/kg/day subcutaneously should be added.

If there is no response to this combination after four to six weeks, the dose of erythropoietin may escalate to 300 units/kg/day.

If no response is demonstrated after two months, then erythropoietin should be discontinued. There is no point in attempting this therapy again at a future point.

Patients who have responded to any dose of erythropoietin or to a combination of erythropoietin and granulocyte colony-stimulating factor should be maintained on this dose for three months.

If the hematocrit is maintained on this dose, then a judicious attempt at gradual reduction of the erythropoietin dose may be attempted.

Most responses to erythropoietin, with or without granulocyte colony-stimulating factor, are not maintained for more than 12 months.

Most patients with an endogenous level of erythropoietin >500 U/L do not respond to erythropoietin, with or without granulocyte colony-stimulating factor. However, because there is a small subgroup of patients who respond to erythropoietin, it is reasonable to begin with a trial of erythropoietin at a dose of 300 units/kg/day with G-CSF for three months. Among this group, erythropoietin should be offered to patients who are transfusion-dependent and symptomatic.

If no response is seen, then the therapy with these growth factors should be discontinued.

During the initial therapy with erythropoietin, if the hematocrit increases to >40 mL/dL without transfusion support erythropoietin should be held and restarted when the hematocrit is ≤32 mL/dL. Furthermore, if the platelet count decreases more than 50% or falls to <20,000/μL, the erythropoietin should be held and restarted when the platelet count is >40,000/μL. If the platelet count has not increased to >40,000/μL, a repeat bone marrow should be performed to evaluate the disease status. If there is no evidence of disease progression, the treatment may restart at the same erythropoietin dose if the platelet count is >20,000/μL.

Thrombopoietic Growth Factor

Two recombinant thrombopoietins have been extensively studied and demonstrate some clinical activity. One is the full thrombopoietin molecule (TPO), and the other is the erythropoietin-like domain coupled with polyethylene glycol (PEG) to provide stability in vivo. This latter agent is known as polyethylene glycol-megakaryocyte growth and development factor (MGDF). To date, neither of these recombinant thrombopoietin products has received approval for clinical use. Both of these thrombopoietins have demonstrated in clinical trials some benefit in the prophylaxis of thrombocytopenia associated with chemotherapy by reducing the duration of thrombocytopenia. However, the data that have been obtained in clinical trials for acute myeloid leukemia or following stem cell transplantation have not shown a convincing benefit. However, both agents can be administered to normal platelet apheresis donors to increase the level of circulating platelets, thus increasing the yield following platelet apheresis.

Interleukin-3, interleukin-6, and interleukin-11 are potent stimulators of platelet production. However, interleukin-3 and interleukin-6 are too toxic for routine clinical use. On the other hand, interleukin-11 has a far less toxic profile and, in fact, has been approved by the Food and Drug Administration for the prevention of chemotherapy-induced thrombocytopenia. Interleukin-11 is a thrombopoietic growth factor directly stimulating the proliferation of the hematopoietic stem cells and megakaryocyte progenitor cells and induces megakaryocyte maturation resulting in increased platelet production.

On the basis of two randomized double-blind placebo-controlled trials, the current indication for interleukin-11 is for the prevention of severe thrombocytopenia and the reduction of platelet transfusions following myelosuppressive chemotherapy in patients with nonmyeloid malignancies who are at high risk for severe thrombocytopenia. At the current time, there are insufficient data to support the use of interleukin-11 after intensive chemotherapy for acute myeloid leukemia or bone marrow transplantation. Although these thrombopoietic growth factors are of great potential theoretic value, a clinical role similar to that of the myeloid growth factors or erythropoietin has not been established for them.

References

Büchner T, Hiddemann W, Koenigsmann M, et al: Recombinant human granulocyte-macrophage colony-stimulating factor after chemotherapy in patients with acute myeloid leukemia at higher age or after relapse. Blood 1992; 78:1190–1197

Estey E, Thall P, Kantarjian H: Treatment of newly-diagnosed acute myelogenous leukemia with granulocyte-macrophage colony-stimulating factor (GM-CSF) before and during continuous-infusion high-dose Ara-C plus daunorubicin: Comparison to patients treated without GM-CSF. Blood 1992;79:2246–2255.

Estey E, Thall P, Andreeff M, et al: Colony-stimulating factor before, during, and after fludarabine plus cytarabine induction therapy of newly diagnosed acute myelogenous leukemia or myeloid dysplastic syndromes: Comparison with fludarabine plus cytarabine without granulocyte colony-stimulating factor. J. Clin Oncol 1994; 12:671.

Geissler K, Koller E, Hubmann E, et al: Granulocyte colony-stimulating factor as an adjunct to induction chemotherapy for adult acute lymphoblastic leukemia: A randomized phase-III study. Blood 1997;90:590–596.

Godwin JE, Kopecky KJ, Head DR, et al: A double-blind placebo-controlled trial of granulocyte colony-stimulating factor in elderly patients with previously untreated acute myeloid leukemia: A Southwest Oncology Group Study (9031). Blood 1998;91:3605–3615.

Goldstone AH, Burnett AK, Wheatley K, et al: Attempts to improve treatment outcomes in acute myeloid leukemia (AML) in older patients: The results of the United Kingdom Medical Research Council AML11 trial. Blood 2001; 98:1302–1311.

Greenberg P, Advani R, Keating A, et al: GM-CSF accelerates neutrophil recovery after autologous hematopoietic stem cell transplantation. Bone Marrow Transplant 1996; 18:1057–1064.

Heil G, Hoelzer D, Sanz MA, et al: A randomized, double-blind, placebo-controlled, phase III study of filgrastim in remission induction and consolidation therapy for adults with *de novo* acute myeloid leukemia: The International Acute Myeloid Leukemia Study Group. Blood 1997;90:4710–4718.

Kaushansky K: Use of thrombopoietic growth factors in acute leukemia. Leukemia 2000;14:505–508.

Klumpp TR, Mangan KF, Goldberg SL, et al: Granulocyte colony-stimulating factor accelerates neutrophil engraftment following peripheral-blood stem cell transplantation: A prospective, randomized trial. J Clin Oncol 1995; 13:1323–1327.

Larson RA, Dodge RK, Linker CA, et al: A randomized controlled trial of filgrastim during remission, induction and consolidation chemotherapy for adults with acute lymphoblastic leukemia: CALGB study 9111. Blood 1998; 92:1556–1564.

Laver J, Amylon M, Desai S, et al: Randomized trial of r-metHu granulocyte colony-stimulating factor in an intensive treatment for T cell leukemia and advanced-stage lymphoblastic lymphoma of childhood: A Pediatric Oncology Group pilot study. J Clin Oncol 1998;16:522–526.

Linch DC, Milligan DW, Winfield DA, et al: G-CSF after peripheral blood stem cell transplantation in lymphoma patients significantly accelerated neutrophil recovery and shortened time in hospital: Results of a randomized BNLI trial. Br J Haematol 1997;99:933–938.

Link H, Wandt H, Schönrock-Nabulei, et al: G-CSF (lenograstim) after chemotherapy for acute myeloid leukemia: A placebo controlled trial. Blood 1996;88(suppl 1):2654a.

McQuaker IG, Hunter AE, Pacey S, et al: Low-dose filgrastim significantly enhances neutrophil recovery following autologous peripheral-blood stem cell transplantation in patients with lymphoproliferative disorders: Evidence for clinical and economic benefit. J Clin Oncol 1997; 15:451–457.

Nemunaitis J, Rabinowe SN, Singer JW, et al: Recombinant granulocyte-macrophage colony-stimulating factor after autologous bone marrow transplantation for lymphoid cancer. N Engl J Med 1991;324:1773.

NKF-DOA: Anemia Work Group: Guidelines. Am J Kid Dis 1997;80:8196.

Ottmann OG, Hoelzer D, Gracien E, et al: Concomitant granulocyte colony-stimulating factor and induction chemoradiotherapy in adult acute lymphoblastic leukemia: A randomized phase III trial. Blood 1995;86:444.

Ozer H, Miller LL, Schiffer CA, et al: American Society of Clinical Oncology. Recommendations for the use of hematopoietic colony-stimulating factors: Evidence-based, clinical practice guidelines. J Clin Oncol 1996;14:1957–1960.

Peterson B, George K, Bhalla K, Schiffer C: A phase III trial with or without GM-CSF administered before and during high dose cytarabine in patients with relapsed or refractory acute myelogenous leukemia (CALGB 9021). Proc Am Soc Clin Oncol 1996;15:3a.

Rabinowe SN, Nemunaitis J, Armitage J, Nadler LM: The impact of myeloid growth factors on engraftment following autologous bone marrow transplantation for malignant lymphoma. Semin Hematol 1991;28:6–16.

Rowe JM: The concurrent use of growth factors and chemotherapy in acute leukemia. Curr Opin Hematol 2000;7:197–200.

Rowe JM, Andersen JW, Mazza JJ, et al: Randomized placebo-controlled phase III study of granulocyte-macrophage colony stimulating factor in adult patients (>55–70 years) with acute myelogenous leukemia: A study of the Eastern Cooperative Oncology Group (E1490). Blood 1995;86:457–462.

Spitzer G, Adkins D, Mathews M, et al: Randomized comparison of G-CSF + GM-CSF vs G-CSF alone for mobilization of peripheral blood stem cells: Effects on hematopoietic recovery after high-dose chemotherapy. Bone Marrow Transplant 1997;20:921–930.

Stone RM, Berg DT, George SL, et al: Granulocyte-macrophage colony-stimulating factor after initial chemotherapy for elderly patients with primary acute myelogenous leukemia. Cancer and Leukemia Group B. N Engl J Med 1995;332:1671–1677.

Witz F, Sadoun A, Perrin MC, et al: A placebo-controlled study of recombinant human granulocyte-macrophage colony-stimulating factor administered during and after induction therapy for de novo acute myelogenous leukemia in elderly patients. Group Ouest Est Leucemies Aigues Myeloblastiques (GOELAM). Blood 1998;91:2722–2730.

Chapter 53
Transfusion Medicine

Steven R. Sloan and Leslie E. Silberstein

Introduction

Most blood transfusions consist of blood components such as red blood cells, platelets, plasma, or cryoprecipitate rather than whole blood. Several blood products can be prepared from one whole blood collection, and each component can be stored at optimal conditions that are specific for that component. Using apheresis technology, it is also feasible to collect cellular products enriched in lymphocytes, neutrophils, and hematopoietic progenitor/stem cells. In this chapter, we first discuss issues that pertain to all blood transfusions and then discuss issues pertinent to products that are used for hematology and oncology patients.

Blood Collection

Allogeneic Blood Donations

Most blood transfusions are collected from random volunteer donors who are unknown to the patient who is receiving the blood. Prior to donating, these donors must pass a screening process that involves a detailed questionnaire and a brief physical exam that usually involves checking the donor's vital signs. The questionnaire is designed to exclude donors who are at risk for transmitting blood-borne illnesses such as HIV, hepatitis B, hepatitis C, and malaria. In addition, donor blood is tested for HIV, hepatitis B, hepatitis C, human T-cell leukemia/lymphoma virus (HTLV), and syphilis. Only blood that tests negative for these diseases can be transfused. Blood donor centers keep track of which of their donors are ineligible to donate on the basis of history or test results and defer those people from donating. Many blood donations come from donors who repeatedly donate, and this has proven to be the safest blood.

Directed Blood Donations

Some patients might wish to receive blood from friends or relatives. Studies indicate that this blood can

be very slightly more risky than random banked blood because most of these donors are first-time donors. Additionally, some of these donors might not be completely honest when answering the questionnaire because the patient might wonder why they were unable to receive blood from their relative or friend. Individual blood bank policies vary on whether or not they allow directed blood donations.

Autologous Blood Donations

Patients who are expecting to need blood for a scheduled procedure may choose to donate blood for themselves. This is most frequently appropriate for orthopedic patients who have a high likelihood of requiring blood and usually have normal hematocrits. Autologous blood donations are not appropriate for hematology patients with red cell disorders such as sickle-cell disease. Oncology patients are often not candidates for autologous blood donations because they may develop anemia following blood donations.

Blood Components

Table 53-1 lists the blood products that are commonly available. Note that some blood banks stock only platelet concentrates prepared from whole blood collections, some stock only apheresis platelets,[1] and some stock both.

Red Blood Cells

Indications
Red blood cell transfusions increase the oxygen-carrying capacity of the blood for patients suffering from symptomatic anemia. Few patients with a hemoglobin level greater than 10 g/dL need a red

---

[1]Apheresis platelets are collected on apheresis machines that collect platelet-rich plasma with minimal contamination by erythrocytes or leukocytes. One unit of apheresis platelets provides a dose that is equivalent to six units of platelet concentrates.

Table 53-1 ■ Indication for Blood Products

Product	Volume (mL)	Indications
Packed red blood cells	225–300	Symptomatic anemia
Thawed plasma or fresh frozen plasma	180–300	Coagulopathy secondary to multiple factor deficiencies or thrombotic thrombocytopenic pupura
Platelet concentrate	~50	1. Prophylaxis: thrombocytopenia (Plt < 10,000/μL) or 2. Bleeding due to thrombocytopenia or dysfunctional platelets
Platelet apheresis	~170–300	Same as for platelet concentrates
Cryoprecipitate	~20	Hypofibrinogenemia, or factor XIII deficiency, von Willebrand's disease, hemophilia A

blood cell transfusion, while those with a hemoglobin level less than 8 g/dL may require a red blood cell transfusion. However, the oxygen-carrying requirements depend on the clinical situation, patients with a chronic anemia being able to tolerate lower hemoglobin concentrations than patients with anemia of acute onset. Neonates and older patients with atherosclerotic disease are at higher risk from anemia than are other patients.

Transfusion indications for patients with some hemoglobinopathies vary from the indications that are used for most patients. In general, patients with sickle-cell disease are chronically anemic and tolerate baseline hemoglobin levels that are often around 6 g/dL. In contrast, multiple secondary complications of thalassemia can be prevented by transfusing children with thalassemia to hemoglobin concentrations of 9 to 10 g/dL or greater. It is unclear whether adults with thalassemia also benefit from hemoglobin levels in this range.

Expected Response

One unit of red blood cells should increase the hemoglobin concentration by 1 g/dL in an average-size adult who is not actively bleeding.

Red Cell Immunology

A variety of antigens are present on red cell membranes. There is significant diversity in expression of these antigens between people. Many people's immune systems can make alloantibodies against antigens that are not present on their own red blood cells. Most but not all of these alloantibodies develop in response to exposure to foreign blood during a transfusion or exposure to fetal blood during pregnancy

and parturition. The ABO type, antibody screen, and cross-match are designed to minimize reactions associated with alloantibodies.

The presence or absence of the A and B antigens determines a person's blood type. These antigens are oligosaccharides that are present in plasma and on membrane glycosphingolipids of red cells, epithelial cells, and endothelial cells. During the first year of life, people who lack A or B oligosaccharides make antibodies to the A or B antigens, respectively. These antibodies develop in response to cross-reactive epitopes present on bacteria that colonize the gastrointestinal tract in the first few months of life. A person's blood group is determined by testing for the presence or absence of antigen on the red blood cells, the front type, and the presence or absence of antibodies in the serum, the back type.

A major incompatibility occurs when a person (blood recipient) has anti-A or anti-B antibodies that react with A and/or B antigens on transfused cells. This should occur only if there has been a clerical error during the blood-typing process. A minor incompatibility occurs when transfused plasma has anti-A or anti-B antibodies that react with the patient's red cells. The latter is not usually clinically significant but can be in pediatric patients or in adults who are transfused with large amounts of plasma or possibly with plasma with high-titer isohemaglutinins.

The Rh system is composed of several epitopes present on integral membrane proteins. Of these, the Rh D-antigen is the best known and most immunogenic. People who express the D-antigen are known as Rh-positive. While Rh-negative individuals can be transfused with Rh-positive blood, approximately 80% of Rh-negative people will develop an anti-D antibody.

If an individual makes an anti-D antibody, future red cell transfusions must be Rh-negative, and there is a significant risk of hemolytic disease of the newborn in future pregnancies. Other antigens such as c, C, e, and E are also part of the Rh system, and the absence or presence of the various Rh antigens constitutes a person's extended Rh phenotype. The extended Rh phenotype of transfused red blood cells is not routinely matched with the patient. If a patient makes an antibody to an Rh antigen, subsequent transfusions of red cells need to lack that antigen to prevent a hemolytic transfusion reaction.

There are several other red cell antigen systems to which patients may make antibodies. Not all antibodies are usually clinically significant. Antibodies to some of these, such as Kell (K), Kidd, and Duffy can cause hemolytic transfusion reactions and hemolytic disease of the newborn, while antibodies to others, such as Lewis group antigens, are usually clinically insignificant.

The Direct Antiglobulin Test

The direct antiglobulin test (DAT), also known as direct Coombs' test, detects antibody attached to the red blood cells in the patient's circulation (Figure 53-1). A positive direct antiglobulin test occurs in about 6% to 8% of hospitalized patients and may be due to a medication or underlying disease. In most of these cases, the positive direct antiglobulin test has no clinical consequences. In many cases, the cause of a positive direct antiglobulin test cannot be determined. The direct antiglobulin test is clinically important in two situations:

1. A positive direct antiglobulin test in a patient with a hemolytic anemia is consistent with an immune-mediated hemolytic anemia.

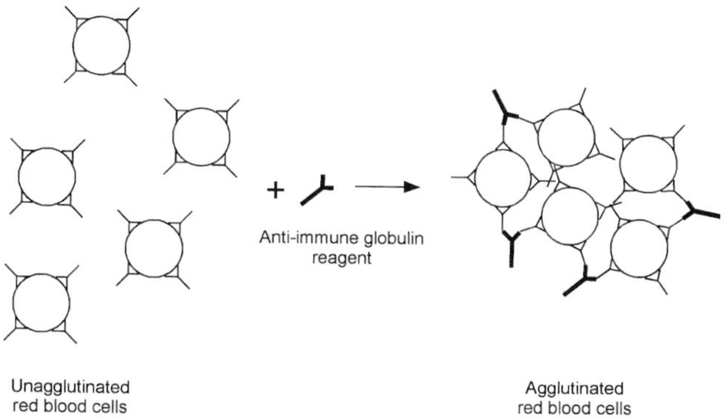

Figure 53-1 ■ The direct antiglobulin test. Unagglutinated red blood cells coated with immunoglobulin are incubated with anti-immune globulin reagent. The anti-immune globulin reagent binds to antibody coating the red blood cells, causing them to agglutinate.

2. A positive direct antiglobulin test that develops during a red blood cell transfusion or immediately following a transfusion strongly suggests that the patient has an antibody directed against the transfused red blood cells. This is consistent with a hemolytic transfusion reaction and requires a thorough investigation.

Identification of Compatible Red Cell Units

A flowchart depicting the steps in pretransfusion testing is shown in Figure 53-2.

Step 1. A patient's ABO and Rh(D) type are determined.

Step 2. An antibody screen is performed. This identifies unexpected alloantibodies to red cell antigens other than those directed to the A or B antigens. First, the patient's serum is mixed with different red cells of known phenotypes to determine whether the serum causes the cells to agglutinate. This part of the antibody screen is more likely to detect IgM antibodies that react at room temperature (cold reactive antibodies), since pentameric IgM can agglutinate red cells. Many IgM antibodies agglutinate red cells at cold temperatures but do not agglutinate red cells at 37°C. These antibodies are usually not clinically significant.

In the next step of the antibody screen, antihuman immune globulin (also known as Coombs' reagent) is added to the red cell/serum suspension. Some antihuman immune globulin detects complement (C3) that is usually fixed to the cells by IgM, some antihuman immune globulin detects IgG only, and some preparations are polyspecific. Usually, the antihuman immune globulin that is used for the antibody screen specifically recognizes IgG. The cells are incubated, centrifuged, and inspected for agglutination.

If any of the screening cells are positive, the serum is subsequently tested with a panel of cells of known phenotypes. The pattern of reactivity is used to determine the specificity of the alloantibodies in the patient's serum.

Step 3. The cross-match. A type specific unit is selected. If the patient has clinically significant alloantibodies, then the phenotype of the cells in the red cell unit is determined to ensure that the donor unit lacks the corresponding antigens. The patient's serum is cross-matched with red cells from the potential donor unit by mixing the patient's serum with the red cells and inspecting for agglutination. If the patient's serum has red cell alloantibodies, then the sensitivity of the cross-match is enhanced by determining whether agglutination occurs in the presence of anti-human immune globulin.

TREATMENT

Transfusion Support of Patients with Warm Autoimmune Hemolytic Anemia

Fatalities and severe morbidity due to warm autoimmune hemolytic anemia (WAIHA) can usually be prevented with proper management. Patients with warm autoimmune hemolytic anemia have the following:

- Anemia
- Increased lactate dehydrogenase, bilirubin, and plasma hemoglobin and decreased haptoglobin.
- A positive direct antibody test. While there are reports of patients with warm autoimmune hemolytic anemia having a negative direct antibody test, every effort should be made to find an alternative cause of hemolysis if the direct antibody test is negative.
- An antibody that reacts with all or most allogeneic red blood cells (a pan-reactive antibody) is typically present.

Because most patients have a panreactive antibody, transfused red blood cells are likely to have a short circulating half-life owing to extravascular clearance. In severe cases, a portion of the cells may undergo intravascular hemolysis. In addition to detecting the autoantibody, extensive serologic testing in the blood bank may detect underlying alloantibodies that may be present. These alloantibodies should be identified, since specific alloantibodies (e.g., anti-Kell antibodies) that recognize transfused red blood cells may accelerate hemolysis of the transfused red blood cells.

Blood bank testing may also reveal that the autoantibody has a relative specificity toward a particular antigen, usually an Rh antigen. For most cases, selecting red cell units on the basis of the relative specificity of the autoantibody will not help. However, in a few cases, the autoantibody specifically reacts with a particular Rh antigen and does not react with cells lacking that antigen. In these cases, cross-match compatible blood can be identified if the red cells lack the antigen recognized by the antibody.

Transfusions of these patients is riskier than most transfusions but must not be delayed if clinically necessary. Because the blood is most often cross-match incompatible and underlying alloantibodies may be present, there is a risk of a hemolytic transfusion reaction and blood transfusions should be minimized. If transfusions are necessary, the patient should be closely monitored for signs of a reaction. However, failing to transfuse may be more dangerous than the transfusion itself. Some patients urgently need a transfusion and should receive blood prior to the completion of laboratory testing.

Platelets

Indications

Platelet transfusions are used to control or prevent bleeding in a patient with thrombocytopenia or dysfunctional platelets. Most hematology or oncology patients who receive platelets have malignancies with treatment-induced thrombocytopenia. Platelet transfusions are usually ineffective and unnecessary in idiopathic thrombocytopenic purpura (ITP) and are contraindicated in thrombotic thrombocytopenic purpura (TTP).

Patients who have received cancer chemotherapy, especially those who received myeloablative therapy for a hematopoietic stem cell transplant, often become severely thrombocytopenic and require platelet transfusions. Most outpatients and stable inpatients do not require a platelet transfusion unless their platelet count drops below 10,000/μL. In contrast, some unstable inpatients may benefit from prophylactic platelet transfusions when the platelet count drops below 20,000/μL.

Expected Response

The count increment (CCI) is used to assess the effectiveness of the platelet transfusion.

$$CCI = \frac{[\text{posttransfusion platelet count (platelets/μL)} - \text{pretransfusion platelet count (platelets/μL)}] \times [\text{body surface area (m}^2\text{)}] \times 10^{11}}{[\text{number of platelets transfused}]}$$

In general, the count increment should be greater than 7500/μL within one hour of the transfusion. This corresponds to an increase in the platelet count by 13,000/μL in an average-size adult, and platelet count increases of 10,000 to 40,000/μL are commonly seen.

Immunology

While platelet membranes are coated with antigens, antibody screens and cross-matches are not usually necessary for platelet transfusions. However, patients may develop antibodies to antigens on platelet membranes, and these patients may require specially selected platelet products. Two groups of patients with antiplatelet antibodies may benefit from specially selected platelet products. One group consists of patients who have had multiple exposures to foreign antigens from pregnancies and blood transfusions. Another group includes fetuses and neonates whose plasma contains maternal antiplatelet antibodies

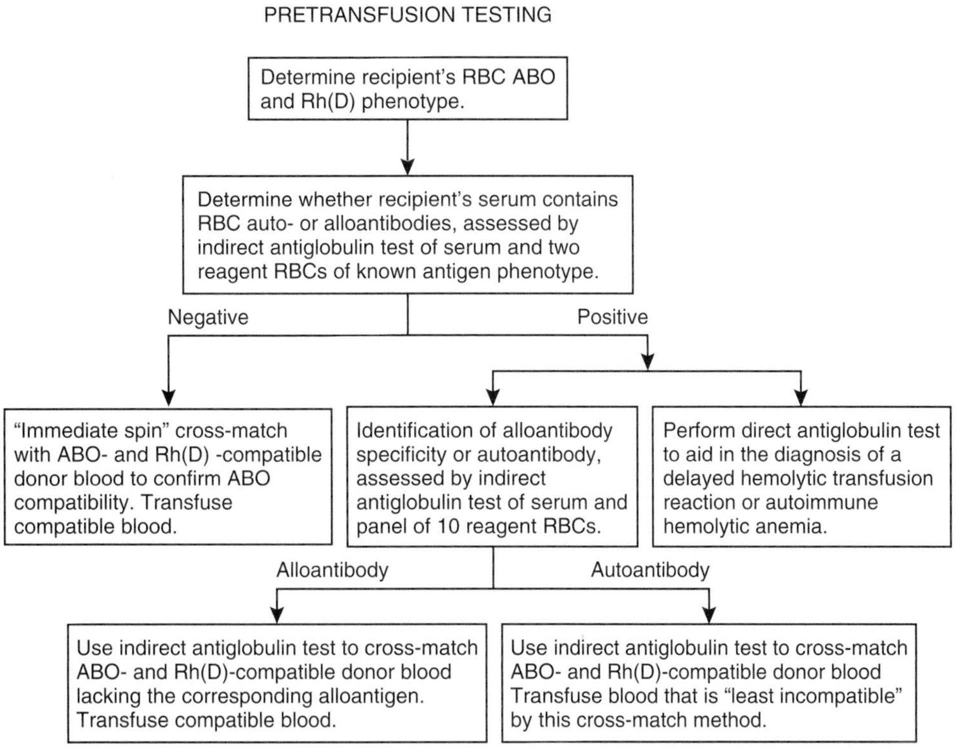

PRETRANSFUSION TESTING

Figure 53-2 ■ Laboratory algorithm for pretransfusion testing. Using this algorithm, almost all patients that don't have autoantibodies should receive compatible red blood cells. (From Tenen, MJ: In Hoffman, R., Benz, EJ Jr, Shattil, SJ, et al [eds]: Hematology Basic Principles and Practice, 3rd edition. Philadelphia: Churchill Livingstone, 2000, with permission.)

directed against antigens that are present on the fetal platelets.

Platelet Refractoriness

Approximately 10% to 15% of patients who require multiple platelet transfusions become refractory to the transfusions. This refractoriness is usually secondary to antibodies directed against epitopes on foreign platelets. In many cases, these antibodies are directed against foreign human leukocyte antigen (HLA) types. Nonresponsiveness to platelet transfusions can be associated with hemorrhagic events secondary to thrombocytopenia.

Some neonates may also be refractory to platelet transfusions. This occurs when pregnant women develop antibodies directed against fetal platelet antigens. Unlike antibodies to red cell antigens, this often occurs in the first pregnancy and can cause thrombocytopenia in the fetus and neonate. These antibodies are often directed against platelet proteins that are present on most donor platelets as well as the fetus's own platelets. HPA-1a is the antigen that is most frequently involved. In serious cases, a platelet donor who lacks the targeted antigen—often the mother—might need to be recruited.

Reducing the Incidence of Platelet Refractoriness

The incidence of platelet refractoriness following multiple transfusions can be reduced by leukoreducing transfused red blood cells and platelets. While leukocytes can provide a stimulus for primary immunization against foreign human leukocyte antigens, platelets do not usually provide such a stimulus. However, platelets appear to provide sufficient stimulus to provoke an anamnestic response. This is one reason for recommending that all patients with leukemia and all patients that are potential bone marrow transplant candidates receive leukoreduced blood components. However, this does not prevent refractoriness to platelet transfusions in all patients. Some patients may develop refractoriness to platelet transfusions despite the fact that blood transfusions were leukoreduced because they might respond to antigens that are still present in leukoreduced blood components or they might have been immunized to foreign antigens during pregnancies or from prior transfusions of non-leukoreduced blood.

Evaluation of Platelet Refractoriness

Patients who do not appear to respond to platelet transfusions need careful evaluation. First, posttransfusion platelet counts taken within two hours of the completion of the platelet transfusion help in differentiating refractoriness from alloimmunization from refractoriness due to other causes. Patients with splenomegaly, sepsis, disseminated intravascular coagulation (DIC), fevers, and ongoing hemorrhage may fail to respond to platelet transfusions. If these posttransfusion counts reveal that the patient consistently fails to respond to platelet transfusions, then alloimmunization is a likely cause.

Human Leukocyte Antigen–Matched and Cross-Matched Platelets

If posttransfusion platelet counts suggest that the patient is alloimmunized, there are two strategies the transfusion service may use to identify platelets to which the patient will respond. Some blood centers use platelets from donors who have a human leukocyte antigen type similar to that of the patient (human leukocyte antigen-matched platelets). The specificity of anti-human leukocyte antigen antibodies in the patient's serum can be determined, and this can also help to guide the selection of platelet products.

Some blood centers prefer to cross-match platelets. Platelet cross-matches are performed by a limited number of blood centers and can detect antibodies in a patient's serum that react with platelets in potential donor units. The cross-match may detect a variety of antibodies that can react with platelets. These include but are not limited to anti-human leukocyte antigen antibodies. Either of these approaches may identify platelets products that provide good responses for the patient. The particular approach used often depends on logistical aspects of the blood provider. Recently, many blood centers have found it easier to provide cross-matched rather than human leukocyte antigen-matched platelets.

A reasonable first approach is to use human leukocyte antigen-matched platelets for refractory patients. If the patient fails to respond to human leukocyte antigen-matched platelets, determination of the specificity of antibodies in the patient's sera helps to guide the selection of human leukocyte antigen-matched platelets. Occasionally, cross-matched platelets are used.

Fresh Platelets, Single-Donor Platelets, and Continuous Platelet Infusions

Several other strategies have been attempted to increase the response to platelet transfusions, but these have not been useful. Some studies suggest that some patients may respond better to transfusions of fresh platelets. However, the advantage is small, and platelets that are stored for their maximal shelf life retain enough of their function for clinical use, and fresh platelets do not provide significant benefit for patients who are refractory to platelet transfusions. Some physicians prefer to use single-donor platelets rather than pooled platelet concentrates. However, studies show that this does not generally improve the response to platelet transfusions.

In an attempt to overcome platelet refractoriness, some physicians have attempted to transfuse platelets as a continuous drip. There is little evidence to support the efficacy of this method of administration, and it has a potential disadvantage. As compared to platelets that are undergoing continuous agitation, platelets in suspension in a stationary bag during a continuous slow infusion are susceptible to storage lesions.

ABO Groups and Platelet Transfusions

Although platelet components contain plasma that contains ABO isohemaglutinins and platelet membranes have ABO antigens, these are usually of little clinical consequence. However, hemolysis from these transfused antibodies has been seen if the platelet unit contains a high-titer isohemagglutinin or if the patient is a young child. Some studies suggest better responses to platelets that do not express an ABO antigen recognized by antibodies present in the patient's serum. While ABO incompatibility is not usually the cause of severe platelet refractoriness, it might be worthwhile to use ABO-compatible platelets for patients who do not respond well to platelet transfusions from a donor of an incompatible ABO group.

Plasma (Thawed Plasma or Fresh Frozen Plasma)

Indications

Plasma transfusions provide multiple coagulation proteins. Patients who might need multiple coagulation factors include patients with severe liver disease and patients with massive hemorrhage or patients with congenital deficiency of blood coagulation proteins. Factor replacement may be indicated when the prothrombin time (PT) or partial thromboplastin time (PTT) exceeds 1.5 times the normal value but is often not needed until there is a more pronounced coagulopathy. Plasma is also used to treat thrombotic thrombocytopenic purpura by apheresis with plasma as a replacement fluid.

Purified factor preparations are usually more appropriate if the patient is deficient in only one coagulation protein, such as patients with hemophilia A (factor VIII) or hemophilia B (factor IX). These purified clotting factors may be of human or porcine origin and may be prepared from plasma or may be produced in cell culture using recombinant DNA technology.

Expected Response

Diffuse bleeding due to multiple coagulation factor deficiencies should be controlled when the clotting factor levels reach 20% to 50% of normal levels. These concentrations can be obtained with infusion of 2–6 units of plasma in a 70-kg adult.

Immunologic Considerations

Plasma can have red cell alloantibodies and should be compatible with the patient's red cells (Table 53-2).

Cryoprecipitate

Indications

Cryoprecipitate is composed of proteins that precipitated from plasma at cold temperatures. While cryoprecipitate contains fibrinogen, factor VIII, factor XIII, and von Willebrand factor, it is usually used for hypofibrinogenemia or dysfibrinogenemia and occassionally for factor XIII deficiencies. In the absence of high-purity concentrations of factor VIII or von Willebrand factor, cryoprecipitate can be used in emergent situations. Cryoprecipitate does not contain factor IX and should not be used to treat hemophilia B.

Expected Response

One unit of cryoprecipitate contains, on average, 250 mg of fibrinogen. The fibrinogen level should rise by ~8.5 mg/dL in a nonbleeding 70-kg patient per unit of infused cryoprecipitate.

Immunologic Considerations

Only clinically insignificant amounts of antibodies such as red cell isohemagglutinins are present in cryoprecipitate.

Hematopoietic Progenitor Cells

Indications

Hematopoietic progenitor cells, also referred to as stem cells, are the cells administered to patients requiring a bone marrow transplant. The hematopoietic progenitor cells may be harvested directly from the bone marrow or may be collected from the peripheral circulation by apheresis. The harvested cellular product may be purified by one of a number of different techniques and subsequently may be frozen by using a cryopreservative such as dimethylsulfoxide.

Autologous hematopoietic progenitor cells are collected from the patient. The patient, usually with malignant disease, is then treated with chemotherapy and/or radiation targeted to his disease. This treatment also damages the patient's bone marrow, and the patient is given hematopoietic progenitor cells to replace the damaged marrow.

Allogenetic hematopoietic progenitor cells are collected from a healthy donor. Patients receiving allogeneic hematopoietic progenitor cells are also usually cancer patients who receive toxic therapy targeted at their disease. Following the therapy, the patient receives the allogeneic hematopoietic progenitor cells to engraft a marrow that has been damaged previously by toxic therapy.

Increasingly, allogeneic hematopoietic progenitor cell transplants are being used to treat genetic diseases of the hematopoietic lineage such as sickle-cell anemia. In sickle-cell anemia, for example, the purpose of the transplant is to replace the patient's own hematopoietic cells that produce defective red cells with hematopoietic cells from a healthy donor.

Expected Response

A successfully engrafted marrow should produce mature hematopoietic cells that circulate in the peripheral arteries and veins. The myeloid lineage usually engrafts first; the neutrophil count rises to 500/μL between 11 and 17 days posttransplant. The platelet lineage usually engrafts next with the platelet count rising to 20,000/μL between 9 and 31 days posttransplant. Because of the relatively long life span of red blood cells, these patients do not usually become anemic. Hence, the hemoglobin and hematocrit are not usually used to measure the response to the transplanted hematopoietic progenitor cells.

Immunologic Considerations

The most frequent serious immunologic consequence of an allogeneic hematopoietic progenitor cell trans-

Table 53-2 ■ Compatibility of Transfused Plasma

Plasma Blood Type	Anti-Red Cell Antibodies Present	Use for Patients with Blood Type(s)
O	anti-A, anti-B	O
A	anti-B	A, O
B	anti-A	B, O
AB	None	AB, A, B, O

plant is graft-versus-host disease (GVHD). Graft-versus-host disease occurs when the donor's immune system reacts against the patient's cells that are recognized as "foreign." Human leukocyte antigen proteins are the most important antigens that mediate the development of graft-versus-host disease, but minor antigens can also contribute to the development of graft-versus-host disease. Perfectly human leukocyte antigen-matched allogeneic hematopoietic progenitor cell transplants from relatives are least likely to result in the development of graft-versus-host disease. Transplants from unrelated donors and transplants that are not perfect human leukocyte antigen matches are more likely to result in graft-versus-host disease.

Conversely, an immunologic benefit of an allogeneic hematopoietic progenitor cell transplant is a graft-versus-tumor effect in which the donor's immune system attacks the patient's tumor. This effect can be substantial and can lead to long-term remissions in some patients.

Hemolysis from ABO isohemaglutinins can also develop during or immediately after an infusion of an allogeneic hematopoietic progenitor cell product. Hematopoietic progenitor cell collections normally contain donor plasma and red blood cells. If the donor's red cells are incompatible with the patient's plasma, then red cells should be depleted from the hematopoietic progenitor cell product prior to transplant. Conversely, if the patient's red cells are incompatible with the donor's plasma, then donor plasma should be depleted from the hematopoietic progenitor cell product prior to the transplant. In some cases, the donor plasma may be substituted with plasma that is compatible with the patient's erythrocytes. Hemolysis can also occur during engraftment of an allogeneic bone marrow that is incompatible with the patient's original blood type. Donor lymphocytes can make antibodies that react with the patient's red blood cells, or the patient's lymphocytes can make antibodies that attack the donor's red blood cells. These complications are unusual but may be more common if the patient's own marrow has not been ablated for the transplant.

While allogeneic hematopoietic progenitor cells are engrafting, the patient will have red cells and antibodies derived from two different hematopoietic systems. These may be of different ABO types. In this event, blood products are chosen to be compatible with both the donor and recipient blood groups. Appropriate blood products are listed in Table 53-3.

Autologous hematopoietic progenitor cell transplants are not subject to the same immunologic complications as allogeneic transplants.

Table 53-3 ■ Blood Products for Bone Marrow Transplant Patients

Recipient	Donor	Red Cells	Plasma
A	O	O	A or AB
A	B	O	AB
A	AB	A or O	AB
B	O	O	B or AB
B	A	O	AB
B	AB	B or O	AB
AB	O	O	AB
AB	B	B or O	AB
AB	A	A or O	AB
O	A	O	A or AB
O	B	O	B or AB
O	AB	O	AB

Adverse Consequences of Blood Transfusions

Hemolytic Transfusion Reactions

Patients can develop acute or delayed hemolytic transfusion reactions. Acute hemolytic reactions can initially present with mild symptoms or can present as severe shock. Symptoms associated with an acute hemolytic reaction include flank pain, chest pain, dyspnea, a "sense of impending doom," chills, fever, and hematuria. Laboratory testing usually reveals hemoglobinemia, a positive direct antibody test, and increased plasma levels of lactate dehydrogenase (LDH), hemoglobin, and bilirubin. These reactions occur when transfused red blood cells are incompatible with the patient. This usually is due to an error in labeling the specimen sent to the blood bank or incorrectly matching the patient with the cross-matched unit of blood. Hence, a clerical check is a critical part of transfusion reaction investigations.

Acute hemolysis can occur if red blood cells are transfused with a nonisotonic solution. In addition, antibodies present in plasma have been reported to cause hemolysis of the patient's own red cells. Normally, significant quantities of incompatible plasma are transfused only during some platelet transfusions, and the vast majority do not cause hemolysis. However, hemolysis may occur in some pediatric patients or if the plasma in the platelet component has an exceptionally high titer of isohemaglutinin. Additionally, hemolysis can occur in patients who are undergoing an allogeneic hematopoietic progenitor cell transplant. This can be an acute event that occurs during or immediately after the transplant, or it can develop weeks after the administration of donor hematopoietic progenitor cells.

Allergic transfusion reactions are one of the most common types of transfusion reactions and are caused by allergies to proteins in the plasma contained in all blood products. Urticaria is usually the main symptom of a mild allergic transfusion reaction. Mild allergic reactions can be treated with an antihistamine and will often resolve. Mild allergic reactions rarely if ever develop into severe allergic transfusion reactions that are manifested by anaphylaxis and may need treatment with epinephrine and corticosteroids.

Febrile Nonhemolytic Transfusion Reactions

Cytokines released from damaged leukocytes can cause fever. These leukocytes may be damaged during storage of blood components or may be damaged after entering the patient in patients that have antibodies that recognize antigens on foreign white blood cells. Leukoreduction of blood components reduces the risk of these reactions, prestorage leukoreduction being more effective than poststorage leukoreduction. Antipyretics can help prevent or symptomatically treat these reactions. Although these reactions are not dangerous, fever may be a sign of a more serious reaction such as a hemolytic transfusion reaction or a septic transfusion reaction. Thus, a febrile reaction needs to be investigated carefully.

Volume overload can occur with transfusion of any blood component. All blood products have a high oncotic pressure, and patients who are susceptible to sudden changes in volume, such as patients with congestive heart failure, are especially prone to this adverse event. For this reason, patients who are susceptible to the effects of increased intravascular volume need to be transfused slowly.

Infectious disease transmission can occur with any blood component. In addition to viruses such as HIV, hepatitis B, hepatitis C, and human T-cell leukemia/lymphoma virus that can be transmitted in any blood component, bacteria and parasites can also infect some blood components. Bacteria can grow in platelets that are stored rocking at room temperature and some bacteria such as *Yersinia enterocolitica* can grow in packed red blood cells stored at 4° C. Bacteria do not grow in frozen products such as frozen plasma or cryoprecipitate.

Graft-Versus-Host Disease

Transfusions of cellular blood products, including red blood cells, platelets, and granulocytes, that contain leukocytes can result in graft-versus-host disease (Table 53-4). Graft-versus-host disease occurs when donor lymphocytes react with the patient's human antigen antigens and these lymphocytes proliferate.

Table 53-4 ■ Risk Groups for Transfusion-Associated Graft-Versus-Host Disease

Risk Well Defined

Bone marrow transplant recipients
Congenital immunodeficiency syndromes
Intrauterine transfusion
Transfusion from first-degree blood relatives
Hodgkin's disease

Risks Under Review

Premature newborns
Hematologic malignancies other than Hodgkin's disease
Solid tumors
Organ transplant recipients

No Risks Defined

Term newborns
AIDS

From Anderson KC, Goodnough LT, Sayers M, et al: Variation in blood component irradiation practice: Implications for prevention of transfusion-associated graft-versus-host disease. Blood 1991;77:2096, with permission.

Most transfusions do not result in graft-versus-host disease because the patient's own immune system usually recognizes the donor lymphocytes as foreign and prevents proliferation of the donor cells. Patients whose own immune systems fail to react to donor lymphocytes are susceptible to graft-versus-host disease. This can occur when the human leukocyte antigen types of the donor and patient are similar, which is often true when the blood donor is related to the patient. Leukoreduction of blood components by filtration does not prevent graft-versus-host disease. For this reason, cellular blood components from directed donors are usually irradiated with γ-rays to prevent proliferation of lymphocytes in the blood component. In addition, patients with compromised immune systems, such as fetuses, neonates, bone marrow transplant patients, patients with some types of leukemia or lymphoma, and patients on some forms of immunosuppressive therapy for solid organ transplants are at risk for graft-versus-host disease because their immune systems may fail to suppress transfused lymphocytes. For this reason, cellular blood products that are transfused to patients who are known to be immunocompromised and at risk for graft-versus-host disease are also irradiated. Unfortunately, identification of all patients at risk for graft-versus-host disease is increasingly difficult in an era with continuing development of new immunosuppressive drugs and increasing numbers of patients on immunosuppressive therapy.

Alloimmunization

Transfusion can stimulate antibodies to human leukocyte antigens or antigens on foreign red blood cells. The incidence of anti-human leukocyte antigen antibodies can be significantly reduced by using leukoreduced blood products. Currently, the only means to reduce the development of antibodies to red cell antigens is to minimize donor exposures or to transfuse only red cells that have a phenotype similar to that of the patient. This is frequently done for sickle-cell patients.

References

American Society of Anesthesiologists Task Force on Blood Component Therapy: Practice guidelines for blood component therapy: A report by the American Society of Anesthesiologists Task Force on Blood Component Therapy. Anesthesiology 1996;84:732–747.

Avent ND, Reid ME: The Rh blood group system: A review. Blood 2000;95:375–387.

Federowicz I, Barrett BB, Andersen JW, et al: Characterization of reactions after transfusion of cellular blood components that are white cell reduced before storage. Transfusion 1996;36:21–28.

Friedberg RC, Donnelly SF, Mintz PD: Independent roles for platelet crossmatching and HLA in the selection of platelets for alloimmunized patients. Transfusion 1994;34:215–220.

Garratty G (ed): Immunobiology of Transfusion Medicine. New York: Marcel Dekker, 1994.

Gelb AB, Leavitt AD: Crossmatch-compatible platelets improve count increments in patients who are refractory to randomly selected platelets. Transfusion 1997;37:624–630.

Gmur J, Burger J, Schanz U, et al: Safety of stringent prophylactic platelet transfusion policy for patients with acute leukaemia. Lancet 1991;338:1223–1226.

Heckman KD, Weiner GJ, Davis CS, et al: Randomized study of prophylactic platelet transfusion threshold during induction therapy for adult acute leukemia: 10,000/microL versus 20,000/microL. J Clin Oncol 1997;15:1143–1149.

Hoffman R, Benz EJ Jr, Shattil SJ, et al (eds): Hematology: Basic Principles and Practice, 3rd edition. Philadelphia: Churchill Livingstone, 2000.

Judd WJ, Barnes BA, Steiner EA, et al: The evaluation of a positive direct antiglobulin test (autocontrol) in pretransfusion testing revisited. Transfusion 1986;26:220–224.

Kattamis C, Touliatos N, Haidas S, Matsaniotis N: Growth of children with thalassaemia: Effect of different transfusion regimens. Arch Dis Child 1970;45:502–509.

Krishnan LA, Brecher ME: Transfusion-transmitted bacterial infection. Hematol Oncol Clin North Am 1995;9:167–185.

Larsson LG, Welsh VJ, Ladd DJ: Acute intravascular hemolysis secondary to out-of-group platelet transfusion. Transfusion 2000;40:902–906.

McCullough JJ: Transfusion Medicine. New York: McGraw-Hill, 1998.

Mollison PL, Engelfriet CP, Contreras M: Blood Transfusion in Clinical Medicine, 10th edition. Malden, MA: Blackwell Science, 1997.

Muller-Steinhardt M, Schlenke P, Wagner T, Kluter H: Transfusion of platelet concentrates from pooled buffy-coats: Comparison of bedside vs. prestorage leukofiltration. Transfus Med 2000;10:59–65.

Myhre BA, Figueroa PI: Infectious disease markers in various groups of donors. Ann Clin Lab Sci 1995;25:39–43.

Panzer S, Auerbach L, Cechova E, et al: Maternal alloimmunization against fetal platelet antigens: A prospective study. Br J Haematol 1995;90:655–660.

Patterson BJ, Freedman J, Blanchette V, et al: Effect of premedication guidelines and leukoreduction on the rate of febrile nonhaemolytic platelet transfusion reactions. Transfus Med 2000;10:199–206.

Petz LD: Clinical Practice of Transfusion Medicine, 3rd edition. New York: Churchill Livingstone, 1996.

Pink J, Thomson A, Wylie B: Infectious disease markers in autologous and directed donations. Transfus Med 1994;4:135–138.

Rosse WF, Telen MJ, Ware RE: Transfusion Support for Patients with Sickle Cell Disease. Bethesda, MD: AABB Press, 1998.

Schmitz N, Linch DC, Dreger P, et al: Randomised trial of filgrastim-mobilised peripheral blood progenitor cell transplantation versus autologous bone-marrow transplantation in lymphoma patients [see comments] [published erratum appears in Lancet 1996 Mar 30;347:914]. Lancet 1996;347:353–357.

Sloop GD, Friedberg RC: Complications of blood transfusion: How to recognize and respond to noninfectious reactions. Postgrad Med 1995;98:159–162, 166, 169–172.

Spitalnik PF, Spitalnik SL, Telen MJ: Human blood group antigens and antibodies. In Horrman R, Benz EJ Jr, Shattil SJ, et al (eds): Hematology Basic Principles and Practice. Philadelphia: Churchill Livingstone, 2000, pp 2188–2205.

Stehling L, Luban NL, Anderson KC, et al: Guidelines for blood utilization review. Transfusion 1994;34:438–448.

The Trial to Reduce Alloimmunization to Platelets Study Group: Leukocyte reduction and ultraviolet B irradiation of platelets to prevent alloimmunization and refractoriness to platelet transfusions. N Engl J Med 1997;337:1861–1869.

Section III
Evaluation and Treatment of Hematologic and Oncologic Disease

Hematologic Disorders
Hematologic Malignancies
Breast Cancer
Gynecologic Cancer
Gentiourinary Cancer
Gastrointestinal Cancer
Thoracic Cancer
Head and Neck Cancer
Sarcoma
Neuro–Oncology
Cutaneous Malignancies
Endocrine Cancer

Chapter 54
Bone Marrow Failure Syndromes

Elaine Sloand and Jaroslaw Maciejewski

Introduction

In considering treatment options for patients with cytopenias related to bone marrow failure, it is important to differentiate between acquired and congenital forms of the disease, as this distinction will greatly affect therapy. Similarly, it is important to differentiate between acquired aplastic anemia and other bone marrow failure states such as myelodysplasia. The presentation of bone marrow failure syndromes is described in Chapter 39. Aside from iatrogenic pancytopenia, which is easily diagnosed on the basis of clinical history, most acquired aplastic anemia is immune-mediated. The type of therapy and its urgency are dictated by the severity of the disease, the acuity of presentation, clinical symptoms, and comfort of life issues.

Acquired Aplastic Anemia

Acquired aplastic anemia is characterized by pancytopenia and hypocellular bone marrow. In almost all patients, it is immunologically mediated by a T lymphocyte assault on hematopoietic cell precursors. Platelets, erythrocytes, and white cells can be all affected to various degrees. Generally, bone marrow examination shows an acellular or hypocellular marrow, although bone marrow cellularity may fail to correlate with the blood counts and often varies with the location from which the marrow is obtained. The magnetic resonance imaging (MRI) exam may prove useful in estimating marrow cellularity, as generalized hypocellularity and patchy marrow can also be seen in T1-weighted, sagittal images of the thoracic and lumbar spine. Patients either present acutely with severe pancytopenia or experience lengthy periods of mild to moderate cytopenias, which might or might not eventually become severe enough to require treatment.

On the basis of degree of cytopenia, aplastic anemia is classified as severe or moderate. Severe aplastic anemia must fulfill at least two out of three criteria: a platelet count of fewer than 20,000 cells/μL, a reticulocyte count of fewer than 40,000 cells/μL, transfusion dependence, and an absolute neutrophil count of fewer than 500 cells/μL. Patients with aplastic anemia who do not fulfill the criteria for severe disease, that is, those with an absolute neutrophil count below 1200/μL, a reticulocyte count below 60,000/μL, and a platelet count below 80,000/μL, are classified as having moderate aplastic anemia.

Prior to considering the therapy, a thorough clinical evaluation of the patient is required. The presence of karyotypic abnormalities makes the diagnosis of aplastic anemia less likely and is consistent with a diagnosis of myelodysplasia. A test for enhanced chromosomal instability and fragility is recommended in young patients to rule out Fanconi's anemia. These patients do not respond to immunosuppression and require an alternative conditioning regimen, should they receive a bone marrow transplant. Peripheral blood phenotyping may be required to rule out diseases (such as hairy cell leukemia) that can mimic the symptoms of aplastic anemia such as pancytopenia or hypocellular bone marrow. Finally, a patient's suitability as a candidate for the bone marrow transplantation has to be assessed. A proper assessment of these patients includes human leukocyte antigen (HLA) typing of all siblings.

Acute Severe Aplastic Anemia

Untreated, severe aplastic anemia is invariably a lethal disease; however, rare cases of spontaneous remissions in patients receiving only supportive care have been reported. The urgency with which therapy is instituted is dictated by the current neutrophil count and the duration of severe neutropenia. While patients with anemia and thrombocytopenia may be supported by red cell and platelet transfusions, severe neutropenia (absolute neutrophil count less than 500/μL) is associated with a high mortality rate and the risk of life-threatening infection. When patients present with higher neutrophil counts, more time to explore treatment options is available.

Bone Marrow Transplant or Immunosuppression?

The decision about whether to offer a patient a bone marrow transplant or immunosuppression may depend on factors such as the patient's age, the availability of a matched sibling donor, the expense, the patient's insurance coverage, and risk factors such as active infections or heavy transfusion burden (see Chapter 51). Any of these factors might lead the patient and the physician to choose immunosuppression rather than bone marrow transplantation. Most physicians offer bone marrow transplantation to younger patients with a human leukocyte antigen–matched sibling donor, while older patients or patients with significant health problems are generally offered immunosuppression. At least one large study supports this management, finding no differences in survival between bone marrow transplant and immunosuppression (63% versus 61%, respectively) when the overall patient population was analyzed. However, significant differences in survival were noted in favor of bone marrow transplant for patients younger than age 20 years (64% versus 38%, respectively). Patients older than age 20 years with neutrophil counts between 0.2 and 0.5 × 10^9/L appeared to benefit from immunosuppression in comparison to bone marrow transplant (Table 54–1). Another study performed on 1765 aplastic anemia patients receiving either immunosuppression or bone marrow transplant from a human leukocyte antigen–identical sibling confirmed these findings. Again, younger patients fared better with bone marrow transplant, while immunosuppression appeared to be better for older patients. In general, patients with severely depressed neutrophil counts tended to do better with bone marrow transplant, because successful treatment leads to more rapid resolution of neutropenia than occurs after patients receive immunosuppression, wherein improvement of neutropenia may occur as late as six months after initiation of therapy.

Studies comparing treatment survival rates do not

Table 54-1 ■ Difference Between Bone Marrow Transplant and Immunosuppression in Five-Year Failure-Free Survival (%) After Initial Treatment

Neutrophil Count (×10^9/L)	Age (years)				
	10	20	30	40	50
0	24*	20	14	6	–2
0.1	19	14	8	1	–7
0.2	14	9	3	–4	–11
0.3	10	5	–1	–7	–14
0.4	6	1	–4	–10	–16
0.5	3	–2	–7	–12	–17†

Note: Positive values: advantage bone marrow transplant (*24% five-year failure-free survival difference in favor of bone marrow transplant); negative values: advantage immunosuppression (†17% difference in favor of immunosuppression).

From Bacigalupo A, Brand R, Oneto R, et al: Treatment of acquired severe aplastic anemia: Bone marrow transplantation compared with immunosuppressive therapy. Semin Hematol 2000;37:69–80.

always reflect the patient's quality of life or other problems that become apparent with longer follow-up. Patients receiving immunosuppression have a high frequency of relapse that requires retreatment. In addition, some patients receiving immunosuppression develop myelodysplasia or symptomatic hemolysis due to the evolution to paroxysmal nocturnal hemoglobinuria. In contrast, patients undergoing bone marrow transplant have to contend with higher treatment-related mortality and subsequent transplant-related problems such as acute and chronic graft-versus-host disease. Graft-versus-host disease (GVHD) might require continued medical care and is associated with substantial morbidity, which is often not reflected in published studies. In addition, patients who receive radiation as part of their conditioning regimen tend to be infertile and develop cataracts. Solid tumors also can occur within the radiation field.

While therapeutic decisions may be easier for very young and elderly patients, treatment decisions are more difficult for the middle-aged patient. Any decision requires lengthy discussions with patients regarding the risks and benefits of each treatment. For the middle-aged person with a matched sibling donor, the recommendation regarding therapy should be made after considering the general health of the patient, the severity of disease, and the risk tolerance of the patient. Nonneutropenic patients may be supported for long periods of time without substantial morbidity except for problems with iron overload. We generally offer transfusion-dependent middle-aged patients immunosuppression therapy because of its lesser toxicity, requirement for minimal hospitalization, and good response rate.

Immunosuppressive Therapy

Most immunosuppressive regimens employ either rabbit antithymocyte globulin (ATG) or horse anti-lymphocyte globulin (ALG). Combined immunosuppressive regimens are generally superior to single agent therapy. In a German study, the response rate of patients receiving antithymocyte globulin and cyclosporine was superior to that of patients receiving antithymocyte globulin alone (46% versus 70% at six months), although many patients treated with antithymocyte globulin alone responded when cyclosporine treatment was initiated. In a single-center study at the National Institutes of Health (NIH) and in a European study, combining antithymocyte globulin with cyclosporine resulted in response rates close to 80%. The National Institutes of Health regimen consists of horse antithymocyte globulin (40 mg/kg per day for four days) or rabbit antithymocyte globulin (3 to 5 mg/kg/day × five days) and 12 mg/kg/day (in divided doses) of cyclosporine for six months. Corticosteroids are added (1 mg/kg/day of prednisone) during the first two weeks to ameliorate the serum sickness associated with antithymocyte globulin administration. Whether the addition of granulocyte colony-stimulating factor (G-CSF) improves the response rate is unclear. In one Japanese study, there was no difference in the incidence of febrile episodes and documented infections between patients receiving granulocyte colony-stimulating factor and those not receiving it. Response generally occurs within six months in 75% of all responders, but improvement usually occurs after one to two months. Transfusion independence occurs at two to three months, but very late responses are possible. Response rates do not appear to be influenced by the presumed etiology of the disease (posthepatitis, drug or toxin exposure, paroxysmal nocturnal hemoglobinuria/aplastic anemia syndrome, etc). Both antithymocyte globulin and antilymphocyte globulin are immunosuppressive and result in a rapid reduction in the number of circulating lymphocytes to levels less than 10% of the initial value. Significant lymphocytopenia persists for several days following discontinuation of the last infusion. Antilymphocyte globulin administration also is associated with a transient depression in platelet and neutrophil counts. Dramatic but short-lasting decreases in neutrophils have been observed with rabbit antithymocyte globulin. While the number of lymphocytes returns to normal values three months after treatment, the numbers of activated lymphocytes remain decreased. Patients with a severe aplastic anemia (absolute neutrophil count less than 100/μL) generally fare more poorly because of infectious complications. These patients may do better with bone marrow transplant, as bone marrow recovery may be more rapid in patients treated with bone marrow transplant compared to patients treated with immunosuppressive treatment. Responses to immunotherapy frequently do not normally result in completely normal counts, but the response is sufficient to confer transfusion independence and to allow the patient to live normally. Some patients who respond to immunotherapy may continue to be dependent on cyclosporine because cytopenias are exacerbated by discontinuation of the drug. In these patients, the cyclosporine dose should be tapered to the lowest dose possible that will maintain acceptable counts. Although no systematic studies have been conducted, mycophenolate mofetil (500 mg to 1 g bid) can be used in patients who, though dependent on cyclosporine, are experiencing untoward side effects from its use (e.g., azotemia). This drug has been successful in selected cases but may be associated with reversible leukopenia that may limit its use.

Although immunosuppression has relatively few adverse side effects, some patients develop anaphylaxis shortly after receiving antithymocyte globulin. Fever, urticaria, and rigors are common on the first day of treatment and respond to treatment with meperidine and antihistamines. Although commonly used to predict allergic responses, skin testing is not a reliable predictor of an allergic response. Some patients also develop serum sickness, which can be treated by increasing the steroid dose. Cyclosporine toxicity is not uncommon. Hypertension and azotemia are the most common side effects. Both are usually reversible after reduction or withdrawal of the drug. Hirsutism and gingival hypertrophy also are frequent complaints. Also, irreversible renal damage may occur as a result of interstitial fibrosis and tubular atrophy, both of which appear to be related to the duration of therapy and the magnitude of the doses received. Although corticosteroids in modest doses are effective for treatment of serum sickness related to antithymocyte globulin or antilymphocyte globulin, they are not effective when used alone for treatment of aplastic anemia. Very high doses of methylprednisolone have been used in combination with antithymocyte globulin or antilymphocyte globulin in some studies, but it is unclear whether they contribute to the response. Although most studies have examined the effectiveness of horse immunoglobulin, rabbit immunoglobulin has also proved effective. No study currently is available comparing the two preparations.

Efforts to develop tests that predict response to immunotherapy have not met with significant success. Some studies have proposed predictive tests based on hematopoietic colony formation with and without added T cells, in vitro response of progenitor cells to antilymphocyte globulin, interferon-γ mRNA measurements in marrow cells, and measurement of early progenitor cell numbers post-antithymocyte globulin treatment, but no laboratory test to date has been generally accepted that distinguishes prospectively the approximately 30% of patients who fail immunosuppressive therapy. Patients with very severe aplastic anemia (neutrophil counts less than 100 cells/μL) had inferior survivals to those with severe aplastic anemia, and patients who failed to respond to granulocyte colony-stimulating factor also had an inferior response rate. It has been suggested that this subgroup of patients be considered first for bone marrow transplant, should a matched sibling donor be available. Figure 54–1 shows a treatment algorithm for severe aplastic anemia, which should be modified to allow for individual patient requirements.

Relapse among responders to immunosuppressive therapy is common. In one European study, the relapse rate was 35% at 14 years, but about half of these patients responded to a second course of immunotherapy. In the National Institutes of Health study, the risk of relapse was 87% at seven years, with most patients responding to repeated immunosuppressive therapy. In many cases, patients responded after simply increasing the dose of cyclosporine or reinstituting cyclosporine therapy. Because of the high response to a second course of immunosuppression therapy, relapse does not appear to influence survival. However, the response rate after repeated cycles of

intense immunosuppression decreases. In addition, patients who are receiving immunosuppressive therapy are at risk of developing late-onset clonal diseases such as myelodysplastic syndrome or acute myelogenous leukemia. In one large European study, the risk of developing myelodysplasia and leukemia at seven years was 15%. Paroxysmal nocturnal hemoglobinuria, on the other hand, is not a late complication but is frequently present from the time of diagnosis of aplastic anemia when flow cytometry is used to measure expression of glycosylphosphatidylinositol (GPI)-linked proteins (e.g., CD 59). However, the contribution of the paroxysmal hemoglobinuria clone to blood cell production increases over time, and some patients develop frank hemolysis. There have been reports of response to cyclophosphamide in patients with severe aplastic anemia. The National Institutes of Health recently terminated a protocol comparing cyclophosphamide with antithymocyte globulin because of significant infectious complications resulting from prolonged neutropenia in these patients receiving cyclophosphamide.

Moderate Aplastic Anemia

On the basis of the severity of the blood count depression, aplastic anemia has been subcategorized into severe and moderate forms. Although it is not clear whether chronic, moderate aplastic anemia is a separate entity from severe aplastic anemia, it may be clinically indistinguishable early in the disease course. The natural history and prognosis of chronic moderate aplastic anemia have not been defined, making it difficult to make therapeutic recommendations for this group of patients. Several factors have to be considered in choosing the therapy of chronic moderate aplastic anemia. Clearly, patients with moderately depressed counts who do not require transfusion can be observed with no specific therapy given; however, some patients will be uncomfortable with this decision. Their concerns may be justified, as it is not clear whether the extended periods in which cytopenias are observed may be accompanied by an autoimmune process that results in continued destruction of progenitor cells with exhaustion of the stem cell reserve.

Although the conclusion is not supported by rigorous data, it appears that patients with moderate aplastic anemia who develop severe disease may be more refractory to the therapy. Transfusion dependence or a progressive decline in counts appears to be a good indication for the initiation of therapy. As in severe disease, antithymocyte globulin and cyclosporine are the first-line drugs. The doses are equivalent to those used for severe disease (40 mg /kg/day of horse antithymocyte globulin for four days

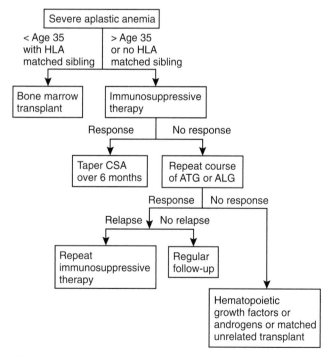

Figure 54-1 ■ Treatment algorithm for severe aplastic anemia.

or 3 to 5 mg/kg/day of rabbit antithymocyte globulin for five days). Androgens also have an established role in the therapy of chronic moderate aplastic anemia. Again, a period of at least six to eight weeks is needed to assess the efficacy of this therapy.

Bone Marrow Transplantation with Matched Related Allogeneic Bone Marrow

The results of bone marrow transplantation have improved greatly over the course of years. Reports of the International Bone Marrow Transplant Registry show that patients with a human leukocyte antigen–matched sibling undergoing transplantation have a five-year survival rate of 77%, and some institutions have recorded five-year year survival rates of greater than 90%. Because a significant portion of morbidity and mortality results from graft-versus-host disease, the availability of cyclosporine has had a significant impact on survival and morbidity. Significant graft-versus-host disease occurs in a minority of patients and decreases with time after transplant. In a recent review of 1759 patients receiving a human leukocyte antigen–matched sibling graft, allogeneic transplant for aplastic anemia, acute graft-versus-host disease greater than grade I was present in only 24%, while grade II or IV was present in 20% of cases. In patients surviving the first 100 days after grafting, chronic graft-versus-host disease was present in only 23%, and graft-versus-host disease of higher grades was present in only 10% of patients. Chronic graft-versus-host disease has been the major factor responsible for the decreased survival rate of adults when compared to children. In one study, 41% of adult patients who survived more than two years had chronic graft-versus-host disease, and their mortality rate was three times higher than that of patients without this complication.

Some transplantation centers use methotrexate in addition to cyclosporine for graft-versus-host disease prophylaxis. In some studies, methotrexate-containing regimens resulted in improvement in survival rates when compared to treatment with cyclosporine alone; however, other studies showed no difference between the two arms. It appears prudent to use methotrexate in patients who are heavily alloimmunized due to transfusion or previous transplantation attempts. However, the most important factor determining success of allogeneic transplantation is the age of the recipient. In a large European study, a significant difference in survival was observed in patients younger than age 20 years compared with those older than 20 years, but there was no difference in survival for patients ages 20 to 30 compared to those ages 31 to 55. In addition, age significantly influenced the risk of graft-versus-host disease. It is possible that the

increase in the rate and severity of graft-versus-host disease with age may be related to the involution of the thymus. Other factors that favorably affect transplantation results include transplantation early in the disease course, effective supportive care, and addition of antithymocyte globulin to the preparative regimen.

Graft rejection constitutes a greater problem in patients with aplastic anemia than in those receiving a transplant for other disorders. The increase in the rate of rejection may be related to the immune pathophysiology of aplastic anemia as well as to the less intensive conditioning regimens that are used in this patient population. Most transplant centers reserve total body irradiation for the unrelated bone marrow transplant, as it has not been shown to confer a survival advantage over cytotoxic therapy alone for the matched related transplant recipient. While intensification of the conditioning regimen results in a lower graft rejection rate, in general, it does not affect the long-term survival.

Bone marrow transplant is associated with several late complications, including occurrence of solid tumors and myelodysplastic syndrome (MDS). While most of these late complications are related to the total body irradiation (e.g., in a French study, solid tumors have developed in the radiation field of five of 147 patients), the risk of solid malignancy remains increased in bone marrow transplant patients who not were not treated with total body irradiation. This risk appears to be equivalent in patients treated with immunosuppressive therapy and those treated with bone marrow transplant without total body irradiation.

Bone Marrow Transplantation with Matched Unrelated Allogeneic Bone Marrow

Only 30% of aplastic anemia patients have a matched sibling donor. Transplantation of patients without an identical sibling donor has been made possible by the establishment of the unrelated bone marrow transplant registry. In a large European study, the survival for phenotypically identical family matches was 45%. For patients with a single mismatch, it is 25%; and for two or three locus mismatches, it is 11%. In a recent study from Seattle, the addition of total body radiation to the conditioning regimen increased the survival rate to 50% in patients receiving a partially matched donor graft. Similarly, improved results have been obtained at Children's Hospital in Milwaukee, where pediatric patients receiving a T-cell-depleted graft were conditioned with a preparative regimen including cytosine arabinoside, cyclophosphamide, and total body irradiation. A survival rate of 54% at three years was achieved. In general, results of unrelated bone marrow transplant for adults have been disappointing owing to higher rates of graft rejection and graft-versus-host disease. In patients receiving matched unrelated donor transplants, factors such as age, degree of match, and type of conditioning regimen have a greater impact on survival than in patients receiving a matched sibling donor graft. In the European registry, the survival of 110 adult recipients of unrelated donor transplants was only 34%. T cell depletion of the donor graft in combination with a rigorous conditioning regimen including total body irradiation increases the survival rate and decreases the prevalence of chronic graft-versus-host disease. However, many adults have difficulty tolerating the conditioning regimen that includes total body irradiation. There is a higher frequency of malignant disease in these patients when compared to those not treated with total body irradiation.

Refractory Severe Aplastic Anemia: Salvage Therapy

Patients not responding to immunosuppression therapy who have a matched sibling donor and no significant medical problems may be offered a bone marrow transplant. Unfortunately, patients with significant transfusion history may have increased transplant morbidity. In addition, prior immunosuppression therapy may affect the results of subsequent bone marrow transplant. However, it is generally believed that an attempt to achieve remission with immunosuppression therapy is warranted in high-risk patients prior to bone marrow transplant.

Generally, refractory patients without a matched related sibling donor and those who do not opt for transplantation should receive another course of antithymocyte globulin. Depending on the availability of horse and rabbit preparations, a different type of antithymocyte globulin should be used in the second attempt to achieve remission, as the risk of recall allergic reaction would be lower if antithymocyte globulin from another species is used. There may also be a chance of more favorable response to alternative forms of antithymocyte globulin. Some investigators have attempted to increase the degree of immunosuppression, but these efforts have led to increased toxicity without significant improvements in responses. Small numbers of patients at Johns Hopkins University have been treated with high-dose cyclophosphamide (50 mg/kg of body weight per day for four consecutive days). Those investigators have reported success in six of seven patients, with no relapses. At the National Institutes of Health, a randomized trial comparing antithymocyte globulin/cyclosporine to cyclophosphamide/cyclosporine was terminated early because of excess toxicity in the cyclophosphamide arm, primarily

as a result of fungal infections. Cyclophosphamide resulted in a more profound and sustained period of neutropenia that necessitated prolonged antibiotic therapy and even granulocyte transfusions. Interestingly, relapse after this therapy has been reported, making this risky and very toxic approach less attractive.

Male anabolic hormones may be used as third-line therapy. Various preparations have given similar results. Nandrolone deconate, oxymetholone, decaduralin, and danazol all have been used in aplastic anemia. Oral doses of oxymetholone (2 to 5 mg/kg/day) may be combined with prednisone (5 to 10 mg) to offset the anabolic effects of anabolic steroids. Increases in hemoglobin are more common than improvements in other cell lines. The toxicity of androgens includes abnormalities of liver function tests. Generally reversible on discontinuation of the drug, androgen toxicity may lead to lasting hepatotoxicity. Other complications of androgens include virilization in females and early epiphyseal plate closure in adolescents. In many patients, these effects are minimal, and androgens tend to be very well tolerated. Patients should receive a three-month trial of androgens prior to being considered nonresponders. There is no justification for treating nonresponding patients with corticosteroids. Patients do not respond and are more prone to complications, including infection, avascular necrosis, and osteoporosis.

Some patients do respond to hematopoietic growth factors, especially when these are chronically administered over prolonged periods of time. Granulocyte colony-stimulating factor and granulocyte macrophage colony-stimulating factor (GM-CSF) may produce responses in patients with moderate disease, although these may be transient in patients with significant aplasia. However, some patients who are refractory to immunosuppressive therapy may achieve durable complete or partial remissions after long cycles of granulocyte colony-stimulating factor and erythropoietin. Clinically, significant responses have also been reported in patients receiving erythropoietin and granulocyte macrophage colony-stimulating factor in a large randomized study in patients with moderate aplastic anemia. One regimen consisted of a 21-day course of granulocyte macrophage colony-stimulating factor (2.5 to 10 µg/kg/day) with a dose escalation if the initial dose was ineffective.

Paroxysmal Nocturnal Hemoglobinuria

Paroxysmal nocturnal hemoglobinuria (PNH) is a disorder resulting from an acquired somatic mutation of a PIG-A gene located on the X chromosome of the affected hematopoietic stem cell. Affected cells lack all glycosylphosphatidylinositol-linked proteins. Deficiency in the expression of CD55 and CD59 on the membrane of erythrocytes results in intravascular hemolysis, the clinical hallmark of the disease. In addition to episodes of hemolysis, patients with paroxysmal nocturnal hemoglobinuria also are at an increased risk for thrombotic events, although patients with underlying aplastic anemia have a very low incidence of thrombosis. In a retrospective European study, thrombosis was found to occur at many locations within the venous side of the circulation, although arterial thrombi have also been reported. Budd-Chiari syndrome occurs with some frequency in the patients with paroxysmal nocturnal hemoglobinuria. A treatment algorithm appears in Figure 54–2.

Treatment of Hemolytic Disease

Many patients with a paroxysmal nocturnal hemoglobinuria clone have chronic low-level hemolysis with periodic exacerbations. In the pure hemolytic paroxysmal nocturnal hemoglobinuria and compensated aplastic anemia/paroxysmal nocturnal hemoglobinuria syndrome, their bone marrow is capable of adequately compensating for the red cell destruction, and they require transfusions only infrequently. These patients do not require treatment for their paroxysmal nocturnal hemoglobinuria, but they, like other patients with hemolytic anemia, should be supplemented with folate (1 mg/day). Iron supplements should be given to patients who are iron deficient. Even patients who have received multiple transfusions may be iron deficient owing to intravascular

hemolysis and urinary loss of iron. Many patients may have spontaneous remissions without treatment. Transfusion of unwashed red cells to patients with paroxysmal nocturnal hemoglobinuria does not present a significant problem and does not exacerbate hemolysis. When hemolysis becomes debilitating, steroids may be used with some success. Chronic use of steroids should be avoided. Steroids are not usually effective and result in significant morbidity. When effective, doses of prednisone in the range of 1 mg/kg/day evoke a rapid response. The dose should be tapered quickly after about two weeks of treatment with reduction to every-other-day dosing.

Therapy of Bone Marrow Failure

Although patients may have purely hemolytic paroxysmal nocturnal hemoglobinuria without evidence of deficient blood cell production, many patients with paroxysmal nocturnal hemoglobinuria present with various degrees of bone marrow failure. In this situation, the bone marrow is unable to compensate for hemolysis, and efforts to treat their cytopenias should be initiated. Responses to antithymocyte globulin/cyclosporine are at least equal to those of patients with aplastic anemia. In fact, the presence of a paroxysmal nocturnal hemoglobinuria clone constitutes a good prognostic factor for the response to antithymocyte globulin therapy. In one study, cyclosporine as a single agent had no beneficial effects. Treatment of aplastic anemia/paroxysmal nocturnal hemoglobinuria syndrome does not appear to affect the size of the paroxysmal nocturnal hemoglobinuria clone, which is rarely eliminated even with high

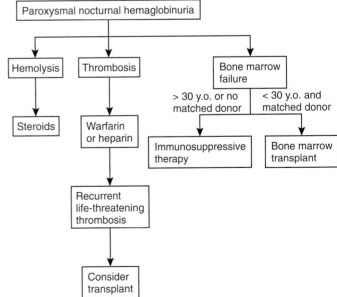

Figure 54-2 ■ Treatment algorithm for paroxysmal nocturnal hemoglobinuria.

doses of cyclophosphamide. In addition, immunosuppressive therapy appears to have little effect on the thrombotic sequela of paroxysmal nocturnal hemoglobinuria. Hematopoietic growth factors and androgens may benefit nonresponders in a similar fashion to that of patients with marrow failure without a paroxysmal nocturnal hemoglobinuria clone. Bone marrow transplantation has been successful in eliminating all sequelae of PNH.

Treatment of Thrombotic Events

Treatment of thrombotic events is very difficult, and patients have been known to continue to exhibit clotting problems despite adequate anticoagulation with heparin or warfarin or use of antifibrinolytic or antiplatelet therapy. No anticoagulation regimen has proved to be superior, although warfarin is the most frequently used agent. Treatment with warfarin may pose a risk to the thrombocytopenic patient and has not proven particularly effective in preventing subsequent thrombosis. Part of the problem is that the mechanism by which thrombosis occurs is not clear. Examination of fibrinolysis, factor V Leiden, and platelet function have failed to provide any insights into the causes of thrombotic events. One might assume that since the paroxysmal nocturnal hemoglobinuria phenotype affects only hematopoietic cells, thrombotic events are mediated by the platelets. However, most platelet disorders preferentially affect the arterial side of the circulation, not the venous side of the circulation as in paroxysmal nocturnal hemoglobinuria. Patients with continued life-threatening thrombotic events should be considered for bone marrow transplant, particularly if they have a matched sibling donor. Complete relief of symptomatology has been reported following a successful transplant.

Fanconi's Anemia

Fanconi's anemia is an autosomal-recessive, inherited condition characterized by sensitivity of chromosomes to agents such as diepoxybutane or mitomycin C. Patients frequently develop aplastic anemia, which is indistinguishable from the acquired form of the disease. They also are at risk for developing acute myelocytic leukemia and myelodysplastic syndrome. The importance of differentiating this diagnosis from acquired aplastic anemia or myelodysplastic syndrome is that immunosuppressive therapy, while effective in patients with acquired aplastic anemia, is not effective in patients with Fanconi's anemia. Allogeneic bone marrow transplant from a sibling donor is the only curative therapy for bone marrow failure related to Fanconi's anemia. The conditioning regimen needs to

be modified, as patients have a heightened sensitivity to cytotoxic agents. Historically, Fanconi's anemia patients undergoing bone marrow transplant had poor survival rates owing to the significant toxicity of standard preparative regimens. French investigators have reported relatively good results (two-year survival rates of 66%) using a preparative regimen including low-dose cyclophosphamide (20 mg/kg) and thoracoabdominal irradiation (5 Gy). Even if patients have a successful bone marrow transplant, the risk of developing secondary tumors, particularly head and neck cancer, is increased, presumably related to the continued general genetic susceptibility to carcinogenesis. Many patients with Fanconi's anemia respond to androgens (2 to 5 mg/kg/day of orally administered oxymetholone or 1 to 2 mg/kg/week of an intramuscular injection of nandrolone decanoate). Approximately 50% of patients respond. Androgens are associated with liver toxicity, and liver function tests should be monitored. Injectable androgens generally are less hepatotoxic.

Pure Red Cell Aplasia

Pure red cell aplasia is characterized by anemia, reticulocytopenia, and a bone marrow that is absent of erythroid precursors. Neutrophil and platelet counts are generally normal. Although most cases are idiopathic, pure red cell aplasia may be associated with autoimmune disorders, thymoma, leukemias, hepatitis, and B19 parvovirus infection. It is particularly important to distinguish patients with parvovirus infection, as the appropriate treatment differs from that of other types of pure red cell aplasia. In many cases of pure red cell aplasia, transfusion independence may be achieved following treatment with some form of immunosuppression. Prednisone alone has been reported to be effective in producing remissions in about 66% of patients, and there is little evidence that treatment with multiple drugs is superior. Cytotoxic drugs including azathiaprine, cyclophosphamide and 6-mercaptopurine have been used for nonresponders. A three- to four-month trial of these should be given to adequately assess responsiveness. As in aplastic anemia, patients have responded to treatment with antithymocyte globulin and cyclosporine. Chronic immunosuppression may be required to maintain transfusion dependence. A small number of patients experience spontaneous remission. Although thymoma is occasionally associated with pure red cell aplasia, its removal is not invariably associated with hematologic improvement. Plasmapheresis has also produced remissions in sporadic cases, but improvements in hematopoiesis have not been durable. Because more than 80% of patients with pure red cell aplasia either respond to treatment or have a sponta-neous remission, efforts should be made to support patients with transfusions in conjunction with immunosuppressive therapy. Patients who have received a substantial number of transfusions (more than 50 units) should be considered for chelation therapy. Desferrioxamine should be administered subcutaneously five days per week.

Parvovirus Infection

Although most patients with normal immunity do not experience detectable changes in hematopoiesis, and the disorder may even be asymptomatic, patients with underlying hemolytic anemias including those with hereditary spherocytosis, thalassemia, sickle-cell anemia, and red blood cell enzymopathies may develop transient aplastic crisis. Patients with HIV-1 infection are susceptible to chronic B19 parvovirus infection, and one study estimated that 14% of transfusion-dependent HIV-1-infected patients had parvovirus infection. Symptomatic patients with parvovirus are often viremic, and the disorder may be diagnosed by DNA studies of the patient's plasma. Therapy of chronic disease consists of infusion of com-mercial immunoglobulin. Most adults have antibody to parvovirus so that parvovirus-specific globulin is not superior to preparations made from pooled plasma. The recommended course is five to ten days of intravenous immune globulin at a dose of 0.4 g/kg. Immunocompromised patients such as those with HIV infection might require repeated treatments.

Diamond-Blackfan Anemia

Congenital pure red cell aplasia, or Diamond-Blackfan anemia, is an inherited disorder associated with an insensitivity to erythropoietin. As in pure red cell aplasia, steroid treatment 1 to 2 mg/day is effective in producing a response in about 70% of patients. There is a substantial relapse rate after steroid withdrawal, and many patients require continued treatment. Unfortunately, some patients do not respond to reini-tiation of treatment, but few of them will respond to androgens. Studies of other immunosuppressive therapy with antithymocyte globulin or cyclosporine are in progress, but preliminary studies do not appear to be promising. Bone marrow transplantation may be considered in patients who are unresponsive to other measures and who have an identical sibling donor available. However, the decision to undergo trans-plantation should be made only when patients clearly understand the complications and weigh these against problems associated with chronic transfusion and chelation therapy.

Pure White Cell Aplasia

Pure white cell aplasia, like pure red cell aplasia, has been associated with thymoma, although, like pure red cell aplasia, it is not always cured by thymectomy. It is sometimes difficult to distinguish between pure white cell aplasia that appears to have an autoimmune etiology and agranulocytosis, which is related to drug exposure. Patients have variably responded to cyclosporine, cyclophosphamide, and intravenous immunoglobulin.

Supportive Treatment in Bone Marrow Failure Syndromes

Transfusions

Red Cells

Patients with aplastic anemia require transfusion support while awaiting institution of definitive therapy. Patients who are being considered for bone marrow transplant should receive as few transfusions as possible, and these components should all be depleted of leukocytes. In addition, blood products from a potential marrow donor or from a family member who shares histocompatibility should be avoided because of the potential of alloimmunization. Despite better conditioning regimens that have decreased the risk of rejection for the heavily trans-fused recipient, this risk still remains significant when compared to the nontransfused recipient. The risk of rejection is 5% for untransfused recipients but is 15% in moderately transfused patients. However, widespread application of effective leukodepletion will more likely further reduce the risk of rejection in the heavily transfused patient.

Patients who are being considered for bone marrow transplantation who test negative for anti-body to cytomegalovirus (CMV) should receive cytomegalovirus-negative blood, although leukode-pleted blood components appear to be equivalent to cytomegalovirus antibody–negative blood and should be used when cytomegalovirus-negative units are unavailable.

Platelets

Although all patients should receive platelets when bleeding is observed and prophylactically when the platelet count drops precipitously or when serious infection is present, there has been considerable dis-agreement regarding the criteria for prophylactic platelet transfusion in the absence of these factors. Data from multiple studies has demonstrated that most patients do not demonstrate significant sponta-neous bleeding when the platelet count is above

10,000/μL, while data from one study showed that 90% of patients bled when the platelet count was below 5,000/μL. These criteria should be applied only to patients with normal platelet function and should not be used for patients with myelodysplastic syndrome or other hematologic malignancies in which platelet function is abnormal.

Despite widespread use of leukodepleted blood products that decrease the risk of alloimmunization, some patients still become alloimmunized. Antibodies most frequently develop against human leukocyte antigens, although antiplatelet antibodies do occur and may be responsible for decreased survival of transfused platelets. The frequency of alloimmunization correlates with the number of transfusions received. However, some patients never become alloimmunized. Besides leukodepletion, the use of single-donor platelets rather than pooled platelet concentrates also decreases the frequency of alloimmunization. Although use of human leukocyte antigen–matched and selectively mismatched donors provide support for the vast majority of patients who fail to respond to unmatched platelets, as many as 20% to 25% of patients fail to respond adequately to human leukocyte antigen–matched platelets. Their failure to respond may be related to other factors that affect platelet survival such as infection, splenomegaly, ABO incompatibility of platelets, platelet-specific antibodies, or antibodies directed against neoantigens that develop as a result of platelet storage. Platelet crossmatching might, in certain instances, be valuable in selecting compatible platelets in certain individuals. Intravenous immunoglobulin has been used in attempts to overcome established alloimmunization with some success, but the effect of intravenous immunoglobulin is transient, and the supply of intravenous immunoglobulin is limited.

Granulocytes

Granulocyte transfusions may be of benefit in selected patients with severe aplastic anemia who have life-threatening infections that are not responsive to antibiotics. Most studies have demonstrated efficacy specifically in neutropenic patients with documented bacterial infections who subsequently experience bone marrow recovery. In contrast, patients with severe persistent neutropenia might not necessarily benefit from granulocyte transfusions and should be selected for this treatment on a case-by-case basis. Similarly, a retrospective study in neutropenic bone marrow transplant recipients with fungal infection failed to demonstrate benefit. Factors that potentially affect the success of granulocyte transfusions are the method for harvesting granulocytes (older filtration methods of harvest are inferior to those obtained by leukopheresis), granulocyte number (a minimum of 2 to 3×10^{10} granulocytes should be transfused), and the length of time the granulocytes are stored prior to infusion (granulocytes should be transfused immediately following harvest). Prophylactic use of granulocytes should be avoided because they are of marginal value and subject the patient to risk.

Most patients receiving granulocyte transfusions from random donors develop antileukocyte antibodies. Antileukocyte antibodies not only mediate transfusion reactions but adversely affect posttransfusion recovery. Severe pulmonary reactions may also occur and are related to the formation of leukoagglutinins in the pulmonary vasculature. Cytomegalovirus infections in patients who are cytomegalovirus antibody negative can be avoided by selecting granulocyte donors who are also cytomegalovirus antibody negative.

Therapy of Iron Overload

Patients with iron overload should be treated aggressively before they exhibit endocrine and hepatic abnormalities. Usually, patients exhibit signs of iron overload when they have received 100 units of blood. For such patients, the iron-chelating agent desferroxamine should be administered subcutaneously over 12 hours with a syringe infusion pump (40 mg/kg/day) for five days each week.

Infections and Antibiotics (See Chapter 115)

Infections are the most important factor determining survival of patients with aplastic anemia and agranulocytosis. The role of prophylactic antibiotics in chronic neutropenic is unclear. No study has demonstrated the benefit of prophylactic antibiotics, and given the potential problems with antibiotic resistance, their use in a noninfected, nonfebrile patient is unclear. However, prompt institution of antibiotic therapy in the febrile neutropenic patient can be life-saving. We treat febrile neutropenic patients with a broad-spectrum antibiotic with good gram-negative and gram-positive coverage. Many different regimens have been studied, and in general, none is clearly superior. Unless an intravenous line infection is suspected, we direct our coverage toward gram-negative coverage. Although anaerobic infections do occur, they are relatively rare in the absence of an intra-abdominal or gingival infection. Therapy should be bacteriocidal if possible. A combination of an aminoglycoside and a beta-lactam antibiotic with *Pseudomonas* coverage is recommended by many.

References

Ayas M, Mustafa MM: Results of allogeneic BMT in 16 patients with Fanconi's anemia. Bone Marrow Transplant 2000; 25:1321–1322.

Bacigalupo A, Brand R, Oneto R, et al: Treatment of acquired severe aplastic anemia: Bone marrow transplantation compared with immunosuppressive therapy—The European Group for Blood and Marrow Transplantation Experience. Semin Hematol 2000;37:69–80.

Bacigalupo A, Oneto R, Bruno B, et al: Current results of bone marrow transplantation in patients with acquired severe aplastic anemia. Acta Haematol 2000;103:19–25.

Ballester OF, Elfenbein GJ: A rational appraisal of bone marrow transplantation and immunosuppressive therapy for severe aplastic anemia. Cancer Causes Control 1994;1:208–212.

Centenara E, Guarnone R, Ippoliti G, Barosi G: Cyclosporin-A in severe refractory anemia or myelofibrosis with myeloid metaplasia: A preliminary report. Il Pensiero Scientifico Editore 1998;83:622–626.

Cockerill GW, Meyer G, Noack L, et al: Characterization of a spontaneously transformed human endothelial cell line. Labor Invest 1994;71:497–509.

Crobak L: Paroxysmal nocturnal hemoglobinuria (membrane defect, pathogenesis, aplastic anemia, diagnosis). Facultas Medica Hradec Kralove University 2000;43:3–8.

Deeg HJ, Leisenring W, Sturb R, et al: Long-term outcome after bone marrow transplantation for severe aplastic anemia. Blood 1998;91:3637–3645.

Dunn DE, Tanawattanacharoen P, Boccuni P, et al: Paroxysmal nocturnal hemoglobinuria cells in patients with bone marrow failure syndromes. Ann Intern Med 1999; 131:401–408.

Elford J, Bolding G, Maguire M, Sherr L: Do gay men discuss HIV risk reduction with their GP? AIDS Care 2000; 12:287–290.

Giri N, Kang E, Tisdale JF, et al: Clinical and laboratory evidence for a trilineage haematopoietic defect in patients with refractory Diamond-Blackfan anaemia. Br J Haematol 2000;108:167–175.

Gustafsson A, Remberger M, Winiarski J, Ringden O: Unrelated bone marrow transplantation in children: Outcome and a comparison with sibling donor grafting. Bone Marrow Transplant 2000;25:1059–1065.

Issaragrisil S, Leaverton PE, Chansung K, et al: Regional patterns in the incidence of aplastic anemia in Thailand. The Aplastic Anemia Study Group: Am J Hematol 1999; 61:164–168.

Issaragrisil S, Kaufman D, Thongput A, et al: Association of seropositivity for hepatitis viruses and aplastic anemia in Thailand. Hepatology 1997;25:1255–1257.

Iwabuchi A, Ohyashiki K, Ohyashiki JH, et al: Trisomy of chromosome 8 in myelodysplastic syndrome. Signifi 70–74.

Kojima S, Hibi S, Kosaka Y, et al: Immunosuppressive therapy using antithymocyte globulin, cyclosporine, and danazol

with or without human granulocyte colony-stimulating factor in children with acquired aplastic anemia. Blood 2000;96:2049–2054.

Leverkus M, Walczak H, McLellan A, et al: Maturation of dendritic cells leads to up-regulation of cellular FLICE-inhibitory protein and concomitant down-regulation of death ligand–mediated apoptosis. Blood 2000;96:2628–2631.

Liu JM, Kim S, Read EJ, et al: Engraftment of hematopoietic progenitor cells transduced with the Fanconi anemia group C gene (FANCC). Hum Gene Ther 1999;10:2337–2246.

Locatelli F, Bruno B, Zecca M, et al: Cyclosporin A and short-term methotrexate versus cyclosporin A as graft versus host disease prophylaxis in patients with severe aplastic anemia given allogeneic bone marrow transplantation from an HLA-identical sibling: results of a GITMO/EBMT randomized trial. Blood 2000;96:1690–1697.

Maciejewski JP, Kim S, Sloand E, et al: Sustained long-term hematologic recovery despite a marked quantitative defect in the stem cell compartment of patients with aplastic anemia after immunosuppressive therapy. Am J Hematol 2000;65:123–131.

Maciejewski JP, Selleri C, Sato T, et al: A severe and consistent deficit in marrow and circulating primitive hematopoietic cells (long-term culture-initiating cells) in acquired aplastic anemia. Blood 1996;88:1983–1991.

Maciejewski JP, Sloand EM, Sato T, et al: Impaired hematopoiesis in paroxysmal nocturnal hemoglobinuria/aplastic anemia is not associated with a selective proliferative defect in the glycosylphosphatidylinositol-anchored protein-deficient clone. Blood 1997;89:1173–1181.

Paquette RL, Tebyani N, Frane M, et al: Long-term outcome of aplastic anemia in adults treated with antithymocyte globulin: Comparison with bone marrow transplantation. Blood 1995;85:283–290.

Pinto LA, Williams MS, Dolan MJ, et al: β-Chemokines inhibit activation-induced death of lymphocytes from HIV-infected individuals. Eur J Immunol 2000;30:2048–2055.

Rosenfeld SJ, Kimball J, Vining D, Young NS: Intensive immunosuppression with antithymocyte globulin and cyclosporine as treatment for severe acquired aplastic anemia. Blood 1995;85:3058–3065.

Sati T, Kim S, Selleri C, et al: Measurement of secondary colony formation after 5 weeks in long-term cultures in patients with myelodysplastic syndrome. Leukemia 1998;12:1187–1194.

Ueda H, Tashiro S, Kojima S, et al: Instability of chromosome 7 in colony forming cells of patients with aplastic anemia. Int J Hematol 1999;70:13–19.

Ward AC, Smith L, de Koning JP, van Aesch Y, Touw IP: Multiple signals mediate proliferation, differentiation, and survival from the granulocyte colony-stimulating factor receptor in myeloid 32D cells. J Biol Chem 1999;274(21): 14956–14962.

Willig TN, Gazda H, Sieff CA: Diamond-Blackfan anemia. Curr Opin Hematol 2000;7:85–90.

Young NS: Acquired aplastic anemia. Ann Intern Med 2002; 136:534–536.

Young NS: Hematopoietic cell destruction by immune mechanisms in acquired aplastic anemia. Semin Hematol 2000;37(1):3–14.

Young NS, Maciejewski J: The pathophysiology of acquired aplastic anemia. N Engl J Med 1997;336(19):1365–1372.

Yu JM, Emmons RVB, Hanazono Y, et al: Expression of interferon-γ by stromal cells inhibits murine long-term repopulating hematopoietic stem cell activity. Exp Hematol 1999;27(5):895–903.

Chapter 55
Red Blood Cell Disorders

Peter W. Marks

Anemia (see also Chapter 37) may reflect a disorder that primarily affects the production of erythrocytes or may be a finding incidental to the pathogenesis of another disease process. This section will focus on the management of selected non-malignant disorders of red blood cells that are encountered in clinical practice (Table 55-1).

Iron Deficiency Anemia

Iron, coordinated by heme in hemoglobin, mediates oxygen transport in blood. It is also required for the function of numerous other proteins, such as the cytochromes. Iron balance is normally regulated, with absorption of about 1 mg of iron daily replenishing the loss that occurs through the loss from the gastrointestinal (GI) tract and other sources. Iron deficiency is relatively prevalent in the United States; it is estimated that 15% of menstruating women are iron deficient and 5% are frankly anemic. (See also Chapters 34 and 37.)

The diagnosis of iron deficiency is facilitated by the finding of a microcytic, hypochromic anemia in conjunction with a low ferritin level. In patients with infection or inflammatory conditions, the ferritin level may be elevated and is therefore of less utility.

All patients who are diagnosed with iron deficiency anemia should be thoroughly evaluated for an underlying cause. Although nutritional deficiency of iron occasionally occurs in vegans and vegetarians, in the vast majority of cases, iron deficiency anemia is due to gastrointestinal or vaginal blood loss. Though empiric treatment with iron replacement may be a reasonable therapy for a menstruating woman without evidence of gastrointestinal blood loss, men and postmenopausal women should undergo evaluation for gastrointestinal bleeding unless another source of blood loss is evident.

Once a decision to initiate therapy with iron is made, an appropriate preparation should be chosen on the basis of the clinical setting. Oral iron preparations generally contain between 50 and 150 mg of elemental iron per tablet; however, only a fraction of that is absorbed. After initiation of therapy in an otherwise healthy iron-deficient patient, the hemoglobin rises at a rate of 0.2 g/dL/week. Repletion of iron stores may take six months or more to accomplish after the anemia has been corrected.

Vitamin B$_{12}$ and Folate Deficiencies

Folate and cobalamin (vitamin B$_{12}$) deficiencies are the major causes of megaloblastic anemia. However, other conditions, such as treatment with the antifolate chemotherapeutic agent methotrexate or other agents that inhibit DNA synthesis, such as hydroxyurea, can also cause a megaloblastic anemia.

Folate is the precursor for tetrahydrofolate that serves as a methyl donor-acceptor in a number of reactions. These reactions include the synthesis of purine nucleic acids as well as the synthesis of methionine. The absorption of folate involves an active transport process that occurs in the jejunum. Without folate intake, body stores of folate can sustain hematopoiesis for up to four months. However, the folate requirement is dramatically increased in severe hemolytic anemias.

Cobalamin is involved in folate metabolism, facilitating the conversion of methyl tetrahydrofolate to tetrahydrofolate and the conversion of homocysteine to methionine. In addition, cobalamin is involved as a hydrogen carrier in fatty acid metabolism. The involvement of cobalamin in fatty acid metabolism, and therefore in the synthesis and maintenance of nerve sheaths, helps to explain the neurologic manifestations of vitamin B$_{12}$ deficiency, called pernicious anemia. In this disorder, but not in folate deficiency, patients develop subacute combined degeneration of the spinal cord, which is largely due to demyelination. The posterior spinal tracts are damaged, causing diminished vibration and position sense in the lower extremities, and lateral tract injury causes impairment of motor function, resulting in spasticity of the leg

Table 55-1 ■ Overview of Selected Disorders of Red Blood Cells

Disorder	Characteristic Laboratory Findings
Iron deficiency	Microcytosis, ↓ ferritin, ↓ iron, ↑ TIBC
B₁₂ and folate deficiency	
folate	Macrocytosis, hypersegmented PMN, ↑ homocysteine
Vitamin B₁₂	Macrocytosis, hypersegmented PMN, ↑ MMA, homocysteine
Anemia of chronic disease	Normocytic-microcytic, ↓ or normal iron & TIBC
Hemoglobinopathies	
Sickle-cell disease	Sickle cells, hemoglobin S > 95%
α-Thalassemias (Hb H disease)	Microcytosis, target cells, Heinz body–like inclusions
β-Thalassemias (intermedia, major)	Microcytosis, target cells, increased hemoglobin A₂
G-6-PD deficiency	Bite cells, spherocytes, Heinz bodies
Membrane abnormalities	
Hereditary spherocytosis	Spherocytes, increased osmotic fragility, ↑ MCHC
Paroxysmal nocturnal hemoglobinuria	Positive acid serum lysis (Ham) test, absent CD59
Autoimmune hemolytic anemias	
Idiopathic/secondary to other causes	Spherocytes, positive direct antiglobulin test
Drug-related	Spherocytes, medication-associated

G-6-PD = glucose-6-phosphate dehydrogenase; MCHC = mean corpuscular hemoglobin concentration; MMA = methylmalonic acid; PMN = polymorphonuclear leukocyte; TIBC = total iron-binding capacity.

TREATMENT

Iron Replacement Therapy

A variety of oral and parenteral iron preparations are available. Oral iron preparations, particularly ferrous sulfate, are often associated with gastrointestinal distress, diarrhea, or constipation. These side effects cause patients to be noncompliant with therapy. However, because they are relatively inexpensive, ferrous sulfate and ferrous gluconate are still most often prescribed. Less gastrointestinal toxicity and constipation may be encountered in using these agents if patients are started on one tablet a day for several days prior to increasing to twice-daily dosing. Oral preparations of iron polysaccharide (Niferex) are often claimed to be better tolerated; however, they are significantly more expensive.

The decision to use parenteral iron replacement should be based on how rapidly improvement in the hematocrit is required. Individuals experiencing debilitating symptoms from iron deficiency anemia may significantly benefit from such therapy, as well as those who do not absorb iron. In these cases, iron dextran (InFed) or ferrous gluconate (Ferrlecit) may be administered. Administration of iron dextran can, on occasion, produce severe allergic reactions. A test dose of 25 mg should be administered prior to the therapeutic dose of iron dextran. Calculation of the appropriate therapeutic dose (usually 1 to 2 grams) is facilitated by a nonogram based on hemoglobin and weight that is available in the manufacturer's prescribing information. By using iron dextran, total body stores can be replenished in one sitting. Ferrous gluconate is an alternative therapy. It is associated with fewer allergic reactions and can be given as 125 mg over 10 minutes by intravenous push. Higher doses are not yet approved, so it is often necessary to have patients return for several treatments.

muscles and a positive Babinski sign. A peripheral neuropathy occurs as well. Vitamin B_{12} absorption requires the binding of the vitamin to intrinsic factor secreted by gastric parietal cells and absorption of the complex in the ileum. Body stores of vitamin B_{12} are generally sufficient to support hematopoiesis for several years. Thus, deficiency usually develops very gradually with time.

Whereas folate deficiency is often due to decreased absorption or nutritional intake, with or without alcoholism, vitamin B_{12} deficiency is generally due to an inability to absorb the vitamin. This may be either due to anti-intrinsic or antiparietal cell antibodies or due to anatomic defects such as intestinal resection or Crohn's disease. Dietary vitamin B_{12} deficiency rarely occurs but can be encountered in vegans.

Folate and vitamin B_{12} deficiency are associated with abnormalities affecting all of the hematopoietic lineages, so pancytopenia may be seen. In addition, ineffective erythropoiesis in the marrow (due to an inability to synthesize sufficient DNA for normal cell division) can lead to a highly elevated lactate dehydrogenase (LDH) and moderately elevated indirect bilirubin. In folate deficiency, the homocysteine level is elevated, whereas in vitamin B_{12} deficiency, both homocysteine and methylmalonic acid levels are increased. The methylmalonic acid level in particular can help to distinguish borderline vitamin B_{12} deficiency from normal. In the past, a Schilling test, with and without administration of intrinsic factor orally, was often performed to determine whether vitamin B_{12} absorption was decreased. It served to document whether the cause of vitamin B_{12} deficiency was decreased dietary intake, intrinsic factor deficiency, decreased absorption, or bacterial overgrowth. However, in part owing to the complexity of this test, the Schilling test is now rarely done.

Folate deficiency is generally treated by administration of 1 mg orally daily. The administration of such high doses of folate (15 to 20 times the normal daily requirement) can also largely correct the megaloblastic anemia caused by vitamin B_{12} deficiency but does not alter the accompanying central nervous system manifestations. The neurologic impairment of vitamin B_{12} deficiency can therefore progress on folate therapy while the clinician is lulled into a false sense of security by the improvement in the blood counts. The clinician has to be wary that the precise cause of the megaloblastic anemia has been properly identified. Administration of vitamin B_{12} does not, however, correct the anemia caused by folate deficiency.

Vitamin B_{12} deficiency can be treated with either oral or parenteral replacement. In either case, care should be taken that patients are folate and iron replete, as repletion of vitamin B_{12} can lead to such vigorous hematopoiesis that borderline stores of these factors may rapidly be depleted. A variety of regimens may be used for initial repletion in vitamin B_{12} deficiency. It is reasonable to give vitamin B_{12} as 1 mg IM for five days, followed by 1 mg IM weekly for three more weeks. This is then followed by monthly injections. Alternatively, high-dose oral vitamin B_{12} (1 to 2 mg crystalline vitamin B_{12} daily) may be administered once the initial repletion with parenteral vitamin is complete. Patients on oral therapy should occasionally have vitamin B_{12} levels monitored to confirm compliance.

There are a few cautionary notes in the management of folate and vitamin B_{12} deficiency. Red blood cell transfusions should be used judiciously, particularly for patients with severe vitamin B_{12} deficiency. These patients have adapted to the gradual onset of the anemia, and they are generally very well compensated and hypervolemic. Correction to a normal hematocrit is generally unnecessary and can even be harmful by precipitating congestive heart failure. Initial therapy with vitamin B_{12} or folate occasionally causes severe hypokalemia, posing a risk of arrhythmia. Hypokalemia is thought to be due to the rapid maturation of the megaloblastic blood cells and abrupt cellular uptake of potassium from the serum.

Anemia of Chronic Disease

The production of red blood cells may be impaired in infection, inflammatory states, or cancer owing to the production of cytokines, such as interleukin-1, tumor necrosis factor, and interferons. These cause anemia by several mechanisms, including direct inhibition of red cell progenitor colony formation, impaired iron mobilization from the reticuloendothelial system, and decreased erythropoietin production. In renal failure, decreased erythropoietin production by the kidney is responsible for the anemia that is observed.

The anemia of chronic disease is usually normochromic and normocytic. Occasionally, it is hypochromic and microcytic, especially in severe inflammatory disease, requiring delineation from iron deficiency anemia. Aside from treatment of the underlying disease, therapy with erythropoietin may be of benefit. The anemia of renal disease in particular readily responds to relatively low doses of erythropoietin. Significant improvement in the hematocrit may be seen in a few weeks. The anemia of chronic disease due to other etiologies may also respond to erythropoietin. In this case, high doses of erythropoietin may be necessary (100 to 150 U/kg SC one to three times weekly), and the response may be less brisk. Unless iron stores are adequate, the response to erythropoietin will be blunted, so in many cases, it is well to administer iron therapy concurrently with erythropoietin.

The Hemoglobinopathies

Hemoglobin Structure and the Hemoglobin Gene Locus

An understanding of the structure of hemoglobin and the globin gene locus is helpful in understanding the pathophysiology and management of the hemoglobinopathies. Hemoglobin is a tetramer composed of two pairs of like polypeptides, α- and β-globin chains, to each of which a heme moiety is bound. In addition to transporting oxygen, hemoglobin transports hydrogen ion and carbon dioxide, and its oxygen affinity, or oxygen dissociation curve, is regulated by both intrinsic factors (the structure of the polypeptide chains) and environmental ones (pH, CO_2, O_2, and 2,3-diphosphoglycerate). The predominant normal hemoglobin is designated hemoglobin A and can be represented as $\alpha_2\beta^A_2$. Other hemoglobins that are normally present in small amounts are hemoglobin A_2, designated as $\alpha_2\delta_2$, and hemoglobin F, designated as $\alpha_2\gamma_2$.

To serve the different requirements of the embryo, fetus, and adult for oxygen delivery, the subunit composition of hemoglobin changes during development. The α genes are located on chromosome 16, and the β genes are located on chromosome 11. As development occurs, synthesis of different members of the α and β gene families results in hemoglobin tetramers having different intrinsic oxygen affinity (Figure 55-1). In the normal adult, hemoglobin A makes up 97% of the total hemoglobin, hemoglobin A_2 makes up approximately 2% to 3%, and hemoglobin F is 1% or less. Though hundreds of abnormal hemoglobin variants have been described, knowledge of only several of these variants is sufficient to manage the most common disorders.

The Thalassemias

Thalassemias are hemoglobinopathies that result from the decreased or absent expression of globin genes. Taken together as a class, the thalassemias represent one of the most common single gene disorders in humans, and over 200 mutations have been identified (over 50 in α-thalassemia and 150 in β-thalassemia). The two major categories to be considered here are the α-thalassemias and the β-thalassemias. Although the α and β chains are homologous, they are not identical; their structural differences lead to unique differences in pathophysiology when one or the other is present in excess. In either case, the resulting impairment or abnormality of globin chain production vari-

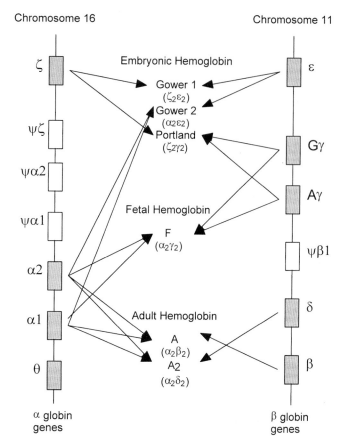

Figure 55-1 ■ Illustration of hemoglobin production during phases of development. The embryonic hemoglobins (primarily Gower 1) are synthesized at detectable levels only for the first 10 weeks of development. After that, fetal hemoglobin (Hb F) becomes the major hemoglobin, dominating the adult hemoglobins that are also synthesized during the fetal period. After birth, Hb F levels decline to their adult levels by age 6 months.

ably reduces hemoglobin in the red blood cell, causing a microcytic, hypochromic anemia.

α-Thalassemia

α-Thalassemia is found in areas throughout the world in which malaria is endemic. Because two α-globin genes are present on chromosome 16, the normal adult has a total of four α genes. Though gene deletion most commonly leads to loss of one or both α-globin genes, point mutations have also been identified. Loss of either one or both α gene copies on a given chromosome can occur. Loss of one copy on a chromosome (α-thalassemia-2 deletion) is generally found in populations with African heritage, and loss of both copies (α-thalassemia-1 deletion) in populations with Southeast Asian heritage.

In the absence of modifying factors, the severity of the clinical presentation in α-thalassemia is rela-

Table 55-2 ■ α-Thalassemia Genotype and Phenotype

Genotype	Disorder	Characteristics
αα/α-	Heterozygous α-thalassemia-2	Clinically silent Near normal MCV Near normal MCH Diagnosis by DNA analysis
α-/α- αα/−	Homozygous α-thalassemia-2 Heterozygous α-thalassemia-1	Asymptomatic Mild anemia with elevated red cell number Microcytosis (MCV ≈ 70 fL) Hypochromia (MCH ≈ 22 pg) Anisocytosis, poikilocytosis Normal Hb A_2 and HbF Diagnosis by globin synthetic studies or by DNA analysis
α-/−	Hb H disease	Jaundice, hepatosplenomegaly, gallstones, leg ulcers Mild to moderate hemolytic anemia Hemoglobin 7 to 10 g/dL Microcytosis, hypochromia Target cells, anisocytosis, poikilocytosis Presence of Hb H (β_4 tetramers) which precipitates in the red cell Hb H inclusion bodies present on supravital staining
−/−	Hydrops fetalis	Death in utero or soon after birth unless transfused or exchange transfused Severe anemia Presence of Hb Bart's (γ_4 tetramers), which is unsuitable for oxygen delivery

MCV = mean corpuscular volume (normal = 80 to 100 fL, age and gender dependent); MCH = mean corpuscular hemoglobin (normal = 26 to 34 pg, age and gender dependent); Hb = hemoglobin.

tively closely linked to the number of missing α gene copies (Table 55-2). Deletion of one or two genes results in only minor abnormalities. Deletion of three α chain genes leads in the adult to production of hemoglobin H (consisting of four β chains) disease associated with a moderately severe hemolytic anemia. Deletion of four α chain genes leads in the fetus to predominant formation of hemoglobin Bart's (consisting of four γ chains) and hydrops fetalis. The absence of α chains in hydrops fetalis produces profound anemia along with congestive heart failure in the fetus, causing third trimester abortion and/or death shortly after birth. In a few cases of hydrops fetalis, measures such as in utero exchange transfusion and chronic transfusion therapy immediately after birth have facilitated survival so that allogeneic bone marrow transplantation could be performed later. Because of the prevalence of loss of both α genes on one chromosome in Southeast Asians, this group is at an especially high risk of having infants with hydrops fetalis. Identification of mothers carrying such affected infants is important, as they may suffer from severe toxemia of pregnancy.

From the perspective of clinical management of affected individuals, the deletion of three α genes that leads to hemoglobin H disease is perhaps most rele-vant. It presents as a hemolytic anemia of mild to moderate severity, with a hemoglobin level between 7 and 11 g/dL. Jaundice and hepatosplenomegaly are frequently seen, and complications may include bilirubin gallstones and leg ulcers. Though there is less ineffective erythropoiesis in Hb H disease than in some of the β-thalassemias because β tetramers are more soluble than α tetramers, the management of Hb H disease is largely the same. Folate supplementation, transfusion therapy, treatment of iron overload, and monitoring for complications such as skin ulcers serve as cornerstones of management.

β-Thalassemia

Similar to the α-thalassemias, β-thalassemias are found in areas where malaria is or once was endemic. Though β-thalassemia is common in the Mediterranean basin and in Africa, mutations responsible for β-thalassemia are sporadically observed in other populations as well. In the endemic areas, gene frequencies of up to 10% can be observed. Though there is only one β-globin gene located on chromosome 11, mutations can lead either to some production of β-globin (β+-thalassemia) or to no production (β0-thalassemia). The result of insufficient β-globin production is α-globin excess. In contrast to α-

TREATMENT

Thalassemia Management Overview

The care of the majority of patients with thalassemia is largely supportive. Management of the body iron burden is one of the most important aspects of this care. Although individuals with homozygous α-thalassemia-2, heterozygous α-thalassemia-1, or β-thalassemia trait should be identified so that they can receive genetic counseling, it is also important to distinguish these individuals from those with iron deficiency anemia, the other major cause of microcytosis. Distinguishing thalassemia trait from iron deficiency anemia can require thoughtful review of the peripheral blood smear and additional laboratory studies. The practice of empirically administering oral iron supplements to individuals with microcytosis on automated blood count can lead to iatrogenic iron overload in those with thalassemia, particularly males and postmenopausal females.

In the forms of thalassemia that are of mild or moderate severity, such as Hb H disease and β-thalassemia-intermedia, a hematocrit in the mid-20s is often well tolerated. Transfusion may be necessary only with intercurrent illness causing marrow suppression. Despite the fact that these individuals do not require regular transfusion, they still need to be monitored for iron overload, as ineffective erythropoiesis causes dysregulation of iron homeostasis. The gastrointestinal tract continues to absorb iron despite adequate iron stores. The need to control the body iron burden is most pressing early on in β-thalassemia major and in more severe cases of β-thalassemia-intermedia that require chronic transfusion therapy either for hematologic support or for prevention of extramedullary hematopoiesis. Iron chelation therapy should be initiated at an appropriate time on a prophylactic basis, long before overt manifestations of iron overload become manifest, at which time it is often too late to intervene.

thalassemia, in which soluble β tetramers generally allow red cell production to proceed to maturity and to be subject to premature destruction in the periphery, in β-thalassemia, the α chains precipitate in developing red cell precursors. These precipitated α chains are toxic and result in intramedullary hemolysis as well as hemolysis in the periphery. Because different β$^+$ mutations result in different β-globin levels and because various combinations of β$^+$ and β^0 alleles are possible, a wide spectrum of disease may be observed in these disorders. With the understanding that there is phenotypic variation that depends on a number factor, including the genotype within each category, a general categorization of the β-thalassemias can be made (Table 55-3).

The two major clinical syndromes requiring active management are β-thalassemia intermedia (Figure 55-2) and β-thalassemia major. Because a large number of potential molecular defects can combine with a variety of modifying factors, the spectrum of disease that is observed in β-thalassemia intermedia can be quite variable. The clinical distinction between β-thalassemia intermedia and β-thalassemia major is therefore generally based on the age of presentation and the transfusion requirement. Individuals with β-thalassemia major generally present within the first year of life with anemia and failure to thrive and subsequently require regular transfusions in order to survive, whereas patients with β-thalassemia intermedia do not.

The pathophysiology observed clinically in β-

thalassemia intermedia and β-thalassemia major is similar (Figure 55-3). A deleterious cycle of increased production in the marrow and destruction in the spleen is set up. However, because the majority of hemolysis occurs in the intramedullary space as red cells are forming, splenectomy is generally of benefit only in select cases of β-thalassemia intermedia. In individuals with β-thalassemia intermedia who are borderline transfusion-dependent, splenectomy can sometimes increase the hemoglobin by 1 to 2 g/dL and thereby abrogate the need for blood transfusion. Although a benefit of chronic transfusion for patients with β-thalassemia major is that such therapy suppresses endogenous ineffective erythropoiesis (and therefore marrow expansion and increasing splenomegaly), it is accompanied by the significant drawback of associated iron overload. Because of such difficulties with lifelong transfusion therapy, children with β-thalassemia major who have suitable donors should be considered potential candidates for bone marrow transplantation. This curative procedure has been found to carry an acceptable risk and to be cost-effective in patients with β-thalassemia major who have normal organ function.

Clinically, all individuals with β-thalassemia intermedia and β-thalassemia major need to be monitored for the complications of ineffective erythropoiesis and marrow expansion, including megaloblastic anemia due to folate deficiency, osteopenia causing skeletal deformities, extramedullary hematopoiesis, and iron overload. The latter of these complications can occur

Table 55-3 ■ β-Thalassemia Genotype and Phenotype

Genotype	Disorder	Characteristics
ββ⁺ $ββ^+$ ββ⁰ $ββ^0$	β-Thalassemia trait	Asymptomatic Mild anemia (hemoglobin 9 to 11 g/dL) Microcytosis (MCV 50 to 70 fL) Hypochromia (MCH 20 to 22 pg) Elevated Hb A_2 level on electrophoresis in patients who are not iron deficient
$β^+β^+$ $β^+β^0$	β-Thalassemia intermedia	Jaundice, hepatosplenomegaly, gallstones, skeletal changes Moderate to severe anemia Microcytosis Hypochromia Target cells, basophilic stipling, nucleated red blood cells Reticulocytosis Elevated Hb F
$β^+β^0$ $β^0β^0$	β-Thalassemia major	As above for β-thalassemia intermedia Failure to thrive Transfusion requirement manifest early in life

even in the absence of transfusion therapy. The normal homeostasis of iron absorption is disturbed in states of ineffective erythropoiesis such as thalassemia. Continued iron uptake from the gastrointestinal tract occurs even in the presence of overloaded total body iron stores. Prevention and treatment of secondary hemochromatosis are therefore crucial in the management of patients with thalassemic disorders to avoid the secondary complications of diabetes mellitus, pituitary dysfunction, cirrhosis, and cardiomy-opathy. In this regard, all patients should be monitored closely for iron overload, especially those who are undergoing chronic transfusion therapy. Serum ferritin levels generally reflect the degree of iron overload, and liver biopsy provides a quantitative measure of the iron burden in the liver.

Despite significant drug discovery effort to date in the development of orally bioavailable iron chelators, none has yet been approved for use in the United

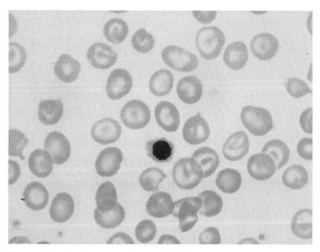

Figure 55-2 ■ Smear of a patient with thalassemia intermedia showing target cells and hypochromia with a nucleated red blood cell (original magnification ×100, oil). (See Color Plate 7, same as Fig. 42-10. Courtesy of Cabello Inchausti B: Chapter 42 of this book.)

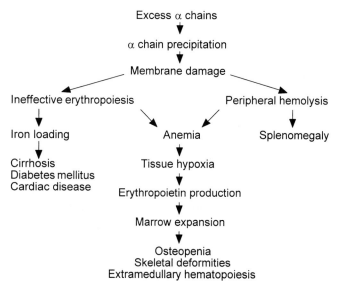

Figure 55-3 ■ Overview of the pathophysiology in β-thalassemia. The α chain excess leads to a deleterious cycle of increased production and increased destruction of erythrocytes.

Deferoxamine Therapy

Unfortunately, given the current state of the art, it is much easier to give iron systemically than it is to take it away. One unit of packed red blood cells contains about 250 mg of elemental iron; in contrast, deferoxamine, the only agent that is currently approved in the United States for chronic iron chelation therapy, can remove only about 50 to 75 mg of iron per gram administered. It also has the disadvantages of the requirement for parenteral administration and a side effect profile that is particularly pronounced when the body iron burden is low.

The decision of when to start chelation therapy with deferoxamine needs to be carefully considered. Determination of hepatic iron concentration through liver biopsy is more reliable than the often used surrogate, serum ferritin. Appropriately administered and monitored, therapy with deferoxamine prevents progression of hepatic fibrosis to cirrhosis. In addition, it can prevent the development of endocrine abnormalities and allow normal sexual maturation in children. However, its administration does not reverse established endocrine abnormalities, such as diabetes mellitus secondary to iron overload.

For adults, after the administration of an initial test dose to identify anaphylactic reactions, 1 to 2 grams of deferoxamine can routinely be administered overnight by subcutaneous continuous infusion on a daily basis. Newer regimens that are under investigation include administration by bolus subcutaneous injection; if proven to be equivalent in efficacy, such regimens may greatly facilitate compliance with therapy.

States. This leaves a sole parenteral agent, deferoxamine, as the only choice available at this time for iron chelation therapy. The conscientious use of deferoxamine in conjunction with judicious transfusion therapy and careful medical monitoring results in significant improvement in the quality of life and survival of patients with the more severe forms of thalassemia.

Sickle-Cell Disease

Sickle-cell disease represents a group of disorders that all have in common the presence of hemoglobin S (Hb S) derived from inheritance of a single point mutation in the normal β^A-globin chain to become a β^S-globin chain. Included are homozygotes for hemoglobin S, who are classically described as having sickle-cell anemia, as well as individuals who have inherited other hemoglobinopathies that, in conjunction with hemoglobin S, lead to syndromes similar to sickle-cell anemia. These include Hb SC disease (Figure 55-4), sickle/β^+-thalassemia, and sickle/β^0-thalassemia (Table 55-4). Sickling syndromes are very common. They are highly prevalent in regions of Africa, India, and the Middle East. About 8% of African-Americans carry the sickle-cell trait, and about one in 600 is affected by sickle-cell disease.

The pathophysiology of sickle-cell anemia results directly from polymerization of deoxygenated hemoglobin S (Figure 55-5). Sickling of cells is facilitated in capillaries after the release of oxygen. In fact, because of the low oxygen tension in the kidney, even heterozygote carriers (Hb AS), who are detectable only on sickle-cell preparation or by hemoglobin electrophoresis, develop isosthenuria (an inability to concentrate urine), and a small percentage may develop hematuria. These individuals are otherwise generally asymptomatic. Pulmonary, or other sites such as splenic, infarction can occasionally occur when the inspired oxygen tension is decreased, for example, at high altitudes. Sickle-cell anemia patients are prone to a number of complications (Table 55-5). Some of these, such as the development of bilirubin gallstones, are similar to those encountered in other chronic hemolytic anemias. Others are specifically related to consequences of vaso-occlusion. Patients with other

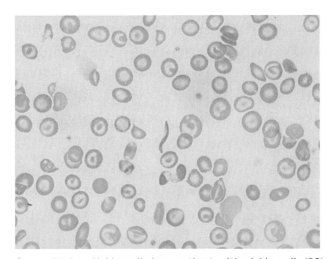

Figure 55-4 ■ Sickle cells in a patient with sickle-cell (SC) disease. Target cells and two red cells showing condensation of hemoglobin toward one side of the cell (original magnification ×60). (See Color Plate 7, same as Fig. 42-11. Courtesy of Cabello Inchausti B: Chapter 42 of this book.)

Table 55-4 ■ Features of Sickling Disorders in Decreasing Order of Relative Overall Severity

Disorder	Characteristics
Hb SS (sickle-cell anemia)	Moderate to severe anemia (hemoglobin 7 to 10 g/dL) Irreversibly sickled cells on blood smear Hb S and Hb F and normal Hb A_2 on electrophoresis
Hb S/β^0 thalassemia	Moderate to severe anemia (hemoglobin 7 to 10 g/dL) Microcytosis with sickle cells and target cells Hb S and Hb F and elevated Hb A_2 on electrophoresis
Hb SC	Mild to moderate anemia (hemoglobin 9 to 13 g/dL) Sickle cells and target cells on blood smear Hb S and Hb C on electrophoresis
Hb S/β^+ thalassemia	Mild to moderate anemia (hemoglobin > 10 g/dL) Microcytosis with sickle cells and target cells Hb S, Hb F, Hb A, and Hb A_2 appear on electrophoresis; the ratio of Hb S/Hb A is more than 1
Hb S/A (sickle-cell trait)	Normal hemoglobin and hematocrit HB S, Hb F, Hb A, and Hb A_2 appear on electrophoresis; the ratio of Hb S/Hb A is less than 1

HbS = sickle hemoglobin; HbF = fetal hemoglobin, Hb = hemoglobin.

sickling syndromes can experience a similar spectrum of complications, although certain of these may be more or less common, and their severity may be different. For instance, although relatively rare in sickle-cell disease (Hb SS), proliferative retinopathy is frequently present in patients with Hb SC disease, requiring close monitoring and occasional ophthalmologic intervention. Patients are at risk for folate deficiency due to increased red blood cell production, and supplementation with folic acid is useful.

Because of the stress associated with surgery, special precautions need to be taken when individuals with sickle-cell disease undergo surgical procedures. These include expanded preoperative evaluation, close perioperative monitoring, and maintaining of adequate oxygenation and hydration. In addition, consideration should be given to transfusion to a hematocrit of approximately 30%. Achieving a hematocrit more than 30% is believed to be counterproductive, as it can increase blood viscosity and paradoxically provoke or worsen crises.

Certain complications deserve special mention. As a consequence of vaso-occlusion, splenic dysfunction, infarction, and eventual atrophy occurs in patients with sickle-cell anemia. Thus, patients are functionally asplenic and are susceptible to infection with encapsulated organisms. Children with sickle-cell anemia should therefore receive appropriate vaccinations against organisms such as *Streptococcus pneumoniae*. In the pediatric population, consideration should also be given to the administration of penicillin prophylaxis. Adults remain at risk and should be counseled regarding the signs and symptoms of acute bacterial infections such as pneumonia and urinary

Figure 55-5 ■ Overview of the pathophysiology in sickle-cell anemia. Polymerization of hemoglobin S leads to membrane damage and irreversible sickling of cells. These cells have altered adherence to other cells such as leukocytes and the endothelium and become trapped in the capillary circulation, causing vaso-occlusive syndromes.

Table 55-5 ■ Complications in Patients with Sickle-Cell Disease

Etiology of Complication	Disorder
Vaso-occlusion	Pain crisis
	Acute chest syndrome
	Stroke (children more frequently symptomatic)
	Avascular necrosis of the hips
	Leg ulcers
	Splenic sequestration (in children)
	Renal insufficiency
	Priapism
	Excess fetal loss
	Proliferative retinopathy (less common in Hb SS than SC)
Chronic hemolytic anemia	Gallstones
	Folate deficiency
	Cardiomegaly
	High-output heart failure
	Liver disease from iron overload (with chronic transfusion)
Infection	Sepsis from encapsulated organisms
	Salmonella and *Staphylococcus aureus* osteomyelitis
	Aplastic crisis (Parvovirus B19 infection)
	Hepatitis B and C (from transfusion)

Hb = hemoglobin.

TREATMENT

Transfusion in Sickle-Cell Anemia

Blood transfusions should be administered very judiciously in sickle-cell disease. Apart from the obvious risk of resulting iron overload, the incompatibility of minor red blood cell antigens can lead eventually to alloimmunization, causing difficulty finding suitably cross-matched units. Patients with uncomplicated sickle-cell anemia generally tolerate hematocrits in the upper teens to low 20s very well. Transfusion simply to normalize the hematocrit is both generally unnecessary and potentially harmful owing to the iron burden that it imposes. Similarly, uncomplicated painful crises and uncomplicated pregnancies do not necessitate transfusion. On the other hand, transfusion for symptomatic anemia, acute chest syndrome, surgical procedures under general anesthesia, and prevention of recurrent stroke in children is certainly indicated.

More controversial is the role of transfusion in the management of prolonged or particularly severe pain crises and complicated obstetric cases. The goal is to raise the hematocrit to about 30%, as this suppresses erythropoiesis without unduly increasing blood viscosity. Whether to perform simple transfusion or to perform exchange transfusion, in which a pheresis machine is used to remove the patients' red cells as transfusion is administered, is still debated. In certain situations, such as stroke in evolution and acute chest syndrome, exchange transfusion with carefully matched, leukocyte-depleted units can produce remarkably rapid clinical improvement. Some hematologists therefore favor its use in such settings.

tract infections. Fever in the setting of bone pain should raise consideration of osteomyelitis. *Salmonella* and *Staphylococcus aureus* are frequent pathogens.

Stroke can be a disastrous complication of sickle-cell disease. Both small-vessel and large-vessel disease can be observed. Though about 10% of children experience this complication, a much higher percentage actually have silent events. A history of stroke is an indication for red cell transfusion to prevent recurrent episodes in children. The technique of transcranial Doppler ultrasonography may help to identify children at risk who might benefit from prophylactic transfusion prior to a first event. Though there are few well-controlled studies in adults, prevention of recurrent stroke in iron overloaded individuals may be a reasonable indication for exchange transfusion.

Acute chest syndrome is a syndrome of progressive hypoxia in the setting of worsening chest infiltrates. It may or may not be triggered by an infection such as pneumonia and can be difficult to diagnose in its early stages. The combination of progressive chest pain with infiltrate on chest X-ray and/or fever in a patient with sickle-cell disease should trigger consideration of this entity, especially in the setting of worsening hypoxia. Early diagnosis and careful management are critical. Broad-spectrum intravenous antibiotics should be administered empirically, along with respiratory support as necessary. Strong suspicion for acute chest syndrome should lead to consideration of transfusion therapy, which can lead to improvement in symptoms.

The most commonly encountered complications of sickle-cell disease, however, are vaso-occlusive crises. These most frequently manifest as pain in the back joints or entire extremities. The severity of such crises is quite variable between individuals. Although some patients with sickle-cell anemia are hospitalized quite frequently for management to receive narcotics intravenously, others never require hospitalization for painful crisis and manage their pain with nonnarcotic analgesics. Though disease-modifying factors undoubtedly exist, as is suggested by the different genotypic backgrounds of patients who have sickle-cell anemia, they remain to be fully defined.

Management of painful crises in the absence of associated symptoms or signs can be challenging because there is no specific marker associated with their severity. In particular, the presence or absence of an increased percentage of sickle cells on peripheral blood smear cannot be used as a marker of disease severity. Patients must be managed on the basis of good clinical judgment in response to their symptoms after a thoughtful evaluation is performed ruling out infection and the potentially life-threatening complications described above. Patients should receive hydration as appropriate for their clinical status. Nonnarcotic and narcotic analgesics should be employed in adequate doses to control pain in the outpatient and inpatient settings. In the absence of clear evidence to the contrary, sickle-cell patients should never be assumed to be narcotic seeking and should receive prompt and adequate management for pain.

A number of prophylactic measures to prevent painful crises have been, and are currently, under investigation. The most deserving of mention is hydroxyurea. Through a mechanism that is not completely understood but that might include elevation of hemoglobin F levels, chronic administration of

---

TREATMENT

Treatment of Painful Sickle-Cell Crises

Painful crises in sickle-cell disease are often treated inadequately. These patients become readily dehydrated when ill owing to inability to concentrate their urine. This contributes to increased viscosity of the blood. Adequate hydration should be established, but the tendency to overhydrate should be avoided, as the dilution of blood beyond euvolemia confers no added benefit. Although mild pain may be adequately managed with nonnarcotic analgesics such as nonsteroidal anti-inflammatory drugs, moderate to severe pain generally requires narcotic analgesics. In the outpatient setting, oxycodone/acetaminophen (Percocet/Roxicet) or immediate-release oral forms of morphine are frequently useful for management of acute crisis pain, whereas in the emergency room or hospital setting, intravenous morphine sulfate or hydromorphone (Dilaudid) is useful. Patients with chronic pain can be managed with longer-acting narcotics such as delayed-release oxycodone (Oxycontin), morphine (MSContin), or methadone. Though effective for moderate pain, use of meperidine (Demerol) should be avoided because its normeperidine metabolites accumulate, especially in patients with renal impairment, and lower the seizure threshold.

After a diagnostic decision has been made that a patient is having a crisis, adequate medication should be administered to bring the pain under control. Regimens may make use of patient-controlled analgesia and incorporate both narcotic and nonnarcotic medications, depending on the severity of the painful episode. In the inpatient setting, a pain regimen should include both routinely scheduled medications for pain and the provision for rescue doses for treatment of breakthrough pain. In the outpatient setting, it is important to track prescriptions for pain medication and to periodically review the pain control regimen. Use of nonsteroidal anti-inflammatory drugs in conjunction with narcotic analgesics can reduce the overall requirement for controlled substances. In addition, review of medication use allows patients requiring pain medication on a very frequent basis to be identified. These individuals often benefit from the use of long-acting agents for baseline pain control.

hydroxurea decreases the number of painful crises in adults. Because the long-term effects of hydroxyurea in patients with sickle-cell anemia are not known, questions remain about its safety. Nonetheless, patients with frequent crises and hospitalizations may benefit. It is not unreasonable to begin hydroxurea at a dose of 15 mg/kg rounded to the nearest 500 mg. Initially, monitoring of blood counts every other week is necessary to titrate the dose to effect. In general, the dose can be raised until a clinical benefit is noted or until a slight suppression in the white blood cell or platelet count is observed. Maximally tolerated doses are generally around 35 mg/kg. Several weeks to months of administration may be necessary, however, to clinically observe a benefit.

Glucose-6-Phosphate Dehydrogenase Deficiency

Though the red blood cell does not have a nucleus, it is metabolically active. Utilization of glucose mainly occurs by glycolysis and the hexose-monophosphate shunt. Proper energy metabolism is critical to maintenance of appropriate levels of ATP, 2,3-DPG, NADH, NADPH, and glutathione. These are involved in the maintenance of red cell shape, in the regulation of oxygen affinity of hemoglobin, and in keeping hemoglobin in the ferrous state. Deficiencies in the more than 20 enzymes involved in glycolysis and the hexose-monophosphate shunt have been described, and a large number of the deficiencies result in hemolytic anemia. Glycolytic enzyme deficiencies are relatively rare; the most common of these is pyruvate kinase deficiency.

The hexose-monophosphate shunt is responsible for the production of concentrations of NADPH and

reduced glutathione that are needed to maintain iron in the ferrous state in the presence of oxidant stress (Figure 55-6). Oxidation of iron on heme from the ferrous (Fe^{2+}) to Ferric (Fe^{3+}) state results in the formation of methemoglobin, which cannot bind oxygen. Although several intermediaries and enzymes are involved in the hexose-monophosphate shunt, the overwhelming majority of genetic abnormalities affect one protein. Several hundred phenotypic variants and over 100 genetically defined mutations have been identified for the enzyme glucose-6-phosphate dehydrogenase (G-6-PD).

The gene that encodes glucose-6-phosphate dehydrogenase is located on the X chromosome. Males who carry a defective copy of the gene are therefore affected. In addition, because of the apparently random nature of X chromosome inactivation (lyonization), females who carry a defective copy of the gene harbor two populations of red cells arising from stem cell mosaicism: those with a normal glucose-6-phosphate dehydrogenase activity and those with an abnormal glucose-6-phosphate dehydrogenase activity. Because the clones of stem cells that harbor the defective activity become predominant over time in some women, the effects of glucose-6-phosphate dehydrogenase deficiency may be observed in females.

The normally functioning glucose-6-phosphate dehydrogenase proteins that have different electrophoretic mobility with 110% and 100% of enzymatic activity are termed A- and B- variants, respectively. Despite the hundreds of abnormal enzymatic activities that have been described, two in particular are responsible for the majority of cases of glucose-6-phosphate dehydrogenase deficiency that are encountered in clinical practice: the A- variant and

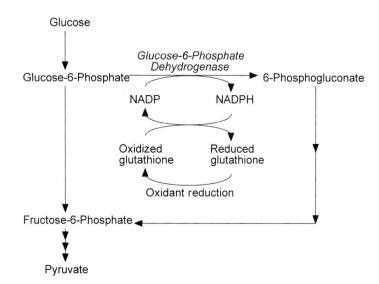

Figure 55-6 ▪ Schematic diagram of the hexose-monophosphate shunt and the role of glucose-6-phosphate dehydrogenase. As the first enzyme in the pathway, glucose-6-phosphate dehydrogenase controls entry into the shunt and therefore its production of NADPH. Superoxide radicals and hydrogen peroxide are two oxidant stressors that are detoxified through a pathway that involves glutathione and NADPH.

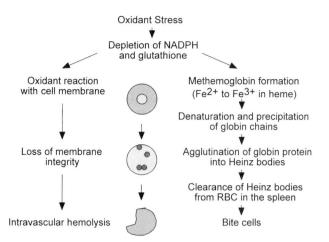

Figure 55-7 ■ Mechanism of oxidant injury in glucose-6-phosphate dehydrogenase deficiency leading to Heinz body hemolytic anemia. Oxidant stress leads to both membrane damage and hemoglobin precipitation. Aggregates of hemoglobin precipitation are visible on supravital staining with methyl or crystal violet as Heinz bodies.

the Mediterranean variant. The pathogenesis of disease is similar in both variants, both leading to a Heinz-body hemolytic anemia (Figure 55-7), but several features of the disease do differ, as described below.

G-6-PD A- Variant

Because it conveys some resistance against the malaria parasite *Plasmodium falciparum*, the prevalence of the A- variant for glucose-6-phosphate dehydrogenase is as high as 25% in some parts of the world, such as sub-Saharan Africa. About 10% of the African-American population carry this allele. The A- variant of the enzyme has an essentially normal activity level when it is first produced, but the activity declines as the cell ages. Thus, reticulocytes and young erythrocytes are relatively resistant to oxidant stress, but older red cells are not. When unchallenged by oxidant stress, red cells live a relatively normal life span, as enzyme activity is not critical. However, a variety of factors, including numerous drugs, cause oxidant stress and can lead to hemolysis (Table 55-6). The ability of an oxidant stress to cause hemolysis in a given individual varies depending on the specific agent, as well as on the specific glucose-6-phosphate dehydrogenase variant of the individual exposed. Fava beans, for instance, infrequently cause hemolytic anemia in persons with the A- variant, whereas they do cause it in individuals with the Mediterranean variant.

Diagnosis of glucose-6-phosphate dehydrogenase deficiency is most commonly made by dye decolorization tests that reflect enzymatic activity. It is crit-

Table 55-6 ■ Common Agents Associated with Oxidant Stress

Antibacterials	Environmental/Foodstuffs
Dapsone	Fava beans
Naladixic acid	Naphthalene (mothballs)
Nitrofurantoin	Toluene blue
Sulfamethoxazole	
Sulfapyridine	**Miscellaneous Agents**
	Doxorubicin
Antimalarials	Methylene blue
	Phenazopyridine (pyridium)
Primaquine	Phenylhydrazine
Pamaquine	Probenecid

ical to emphasize that the diagnosis of glucose-6-phosphate dehydrogenase deficiency in individuals with the A- variant is often not possible during hemolytic episodes. The older erythrocytes containing unstable enzyme are eliminated from the circulation, leaving behind reticulocytes and young cells that have functional enzyme. Thus, though a tentative diagnosis can be made clinically, definitive diagnosis should await recovery from the hemolytic episode.

Therapy for glucose-6-phosphate dehydrogenase deficiency for patients with the A- variant consists of identification of the precipitating cause and, if it is drug-related, the discontinuation of the offending agent whenever possible. Because individuals with a normal hematopoietic reserve will compensate for the hemolysis of older erythrocytes with increased production of younger red cells, the hemolytic anemia that is observed is generally transient. Continuation of an offending agent, though not recommended if at all possible, will lead to a new steady state.

G-6-PD Mediterranean Variant

The Mediterranean variant of glucose-6-phosphate dehydrogenase is present in about 5% of individuals living in this region. It can therefore also be found in individuals of Mediterranean descent who have migrated to other regions. In contrast to the A- variant, in the Mediterranean variant, glucose-6-phosphate dehydrogenase enzymatic activity is lost or minimal in the early developing red blood cell. Therefore, the erythrocytes in patients with the Mediterranean variant are susceptible to hemolysis throughout their life span. The oxidant reserve is low enough that certain bacterial or viral infections, such as hepatitis, can precipitate significant hemolysis. Given a drug that creates an oxidant stress, patients with this variant will continue to hemolyze until the agent is discontinued.

These drugs should be strictly avoided and should be discontinued promptly if this disorder is suspected. Individuals are susceptible to the effects of additional agents as well as those that trigger hemolysis in the A- variant. Chloramphenicol, aspirin, acetophenetidin (Phenacetin), and sulfa-containing antibiotics should not be administered to patients with the Mediterranean variant. Because of the large number of glucose-6-phosphate dehydrogenase variants that are present in different populations, the finding of unexplained hemolysis in a patient receiving any of the medications listed should warrant prompt consideration for this disorder. Prompt diagnosis and discontinuation of offending agents form the mainstay of treatment.

Red Cell Membrane Disorders

Red cell membrane disorders may either be hereditary or acquired. The congenital diseases include hereditary spherocytosis, hereditary elliptocytosis, and hereditary stomatocytosis. Management of these disorders largely consists of supportive care. The acquired disorders include membrane abnormalities associated with immune hemolytic anemias, liver disease, and paroxysmal nocturnal hematuria (PNH). Liver disease may lead to a hemolytic anemia as the red membrane becomes cholesterol loaded and stiff, subject to irreversible deformation and hemolysis.

Hereditary Spherocytosis

Hereditary spherocytosis (HS) is the most common inherited membrane defect; its incidence is one in 2,500 individuals of northern European descent. Alpha and beta spectrin are components of the red cell cytoskeleton and are linked to the membrane at the location of the anion transporter band 3. This linkage is facilitated through ankyrin and band 4.2. A wide variety of different mutations in ankyrin, alpha spectrin, beta spectrin, band 3, and band 4.2 cause disruption of the red cell cytoskeleton and lead to hemolysis. Among these, ankyrin mutations are the most common cause of autosomal-dominant hereditary spherocytosis. However, many different mutations can lead to the hereditary spherocytosis phenotype, and autosomal-recessive cases are observed. Most of these mutations are specific to a given kindred of individuals. The severity of anemia in persons with hereditary spherocytosis can vary widely from asymptomatic to transfusion-dependent. However, cases of severe hereditary spherocytosis with hemoglobin levels less than 6 g/dL are rare.

The diagnosis of hereditary spherocytosis is facilitated by the osmotic fragility test. In this test, the saline content bathing the red cells is lowered from 0.9% (normal) to 0. Most individuals' red blood cells begin to lyse in the range of 0.4% to 0.5% sodium chloride, whereas patients with hereditary spherocytosis do so earlier. Some patients with mild hereditary spherocytosis may have few spherocytes on peripheral smear and an osmotic fragility test performed on fresh blood that is normal or near normal, thus obscuring the diagnosis. The incubated osmotic fragility, in which blood is placed at 37°C for 24 hours prior to the performance of the assay, can be diagnostic in these instances. Note that the osmotic fragility test is abnormal in warm antibody-immune hemolytic anemia because of the development of spherocytes, so this should always be formally excluded.

Mild cases of hereditary spherocytosis require no therapy. Moderate and severe cases may benefit from splenectomy. However, the benefits and risks of splenectomy (i.e., increased risk of overwhelming acute infection if infection by encapsulated bacteria or malarial parasites should occur) should be carefully considered. If a decision to perform splenectomy is reached, then pneumococcal, meningococcal, and *Haemophilus influenzae* B vaccines should be administered in advance. Patients should be cautioned to seek medical attention for high fevers or symptoms that are suggestive of sepsis and to avoid areas where malaria is endemic.

Hereditary Elliptocytosis

In hereditary elliptocytosis, the red blood cells are of elliptical shape owing to abnormalities in the spectrin or other proteins in the red cell membrane. The patterns of inheritance are heterogeneous. The severity of the disease varies within families and within the same patient at different times. It can appear as a silent carrier state, with no clinical illness despite elliptocytes in the peripheral blood, or can exhibit varying intensities of hemolytic anemia. The classic form is not uncommon in patients of African descent. Several morphologic varieties exist, including hereditary pyropoikilocytosis (bizarre red blood cell fragments), hereditary ovalocytosis, and a spherocytic variant that occurs primarily in patients of European extraction.

Paroxysmal Nocturnal Hematuria

An acquired clonal stem cell disorder, paroxysmal nocturnal hemoglobinuria is a chronic hemolytic anemia, with occasional exacerbations of severe complement-mediated intravascular hemolysis. Notwithstanding its name, loss of hemoglobin into the urine at night because of intravascular hemolysis rarely occurs. Leukocytes and platelets are abnormal, and there is a thrombotic predisposition that can lead to severe complications such as hepatic vein thrombosis. The pathophysiology underlying paroxysmal nocturnal hemoglobinuria is an acquired defect in the PIG-A gene (phosphatidylinositol glycan class A gene), an X-linked gene product that plays a key role in the formation of the phosphatidylinositol anchor that links numerous proteins to the cell membrane. The defect predisposes the blood cells to ready activation of complement components on their membrane surfaces, leading to lysis.

Patients with paroxysmal nocturnal hemoglobinuria may present with pancytopenia and suffer from chronic intravascular hemolysis. Over time, they can become iron deficient owing to urinary blood loss. Despite mild to severe thrombocytopenia, thrombotic events (deep venous thrombosis and hepatic vein thrombosis) are among the most common complications observed in individuals with this disorder. The pancytopenia may be accompanied by a hypercellular or hypocellular bone marrow. In the latter case, paroxysmal nocturnal hemoglobinuria should be considered in the differential diagnosis of aplastic anemia. In fact, a small percentage of patients who are treated for aplastic anemia later develop paroxysmal nocturnal hemoglobinuria.

Until recently, the diagnosis was made through use of the sucrose hemolysis test for screening and the acidified serum lysis test (Ham test) for confirmation. In the acidified serum lysis test, the patient's own serum, when acidified, lyses the patient's red blood cells. With the now ready availability of flow cytometry, the diagnosis is facilitated by immunostaining of granulocytes for CD55 and CD59 and of erythrocytes for CD59. The absence of these marker proteins is highly sensitive and specific for the disorder.

Treatment is supportive, except for those individuals who are candidates for curative allogeneic bone marrow transplantation. Supportive care consists of blood transfusions as needed and iron therapy as indicated. Despite the presence of some plasma in packed red blood cell concentrates, there is generally no need to wash the cells free of complement. Drugs that are associated with increased thrombotic risk should be avoided, and thrombotic episodes should be treated aggressively. Though it has been suggested that prophylactic anticoagulation may be of benefit, there are no data to support its use. Both androgens and glucocorticoids have been used for the management of paroxysmal nocturnal hematuria, but they are generally of little clinical benefit, and corticosteroids increase the risk of infectious complications.

Autoimmune Hemolytic Anemia

Immune hemolytic anemia can be divided into disorders caused by autoantibodies and those caused by alloantibodies. In the latter situation, foreign red cell antigen exposure results in the formation of antibodies that are usually directed against a specific antigen and lead to red cell destruction. In contrast, numerous mechanisms can lead to autoimmune hemolytic anemia (AIHA). Although different nomenclatures can be used to describe the types of autoimmune hemolytic anemia, one can categorize these disorders into the subsets of warm antibody autoimmune hemolytic anemia, cold autoimmune hemolytic anemia, paroxysmal cold hemoglobinuria, and drug-induced hemolytic anemia (Table 55-7). Although each of these entities has specific features, they share aspects of clinical presentation.

Destruction of red blood cells in autoimmune hemolytic anemia can occur by extravascular or intravascular hemolysis. Extravascular destruction occurs when red blood cells coated with IgG and/or complement are recognized by macrophages as they pass through the spleen and liver. Interaction of the Fc component of immunoglobulin with the Fc receptors of macrophages leads to removal of a part of the red blood cell membrane and damage to the erythrocyte cytoskeleton. These damaged red blood cells, which take on a spherical appearance (Figure 55-8), are subsequently more sensitive to destruction in the circulation. Intravascular red blood cell destruction occurs when specific types of immunoglobulins that are capable of activating the complement cascade (IgM, IgG_1, and IgG_3) are present at sufficient density on the erythrocyte surface. Attachment of the antibody to the red cell surface leads to deposition of the terminal pore-forming complement components C5 though C9, causing leakage of cellular contents. Because certain immunoglobulins such as IgM can both bind and activate complement, both intravascular and extravascular mechanisms may be involved when they are present.

Presenting manifestations vary. Most commonly noted are symptoms and signs of anemia, accompanied by mild jaundice. In patients who have had a chronic process, the spleen may be enlarged (in one third of cases). Alternatively, at times, the anemia may be essentially asymptomatic and be discovered only through laboratory evaluation. Symptoms and findings may be overshadowed by those of the underlying diseases that are associated with autoimmune hemolytic anemias.

The diagnostic test that is commonly used to diagnose autoimmune hemolytic anemia is the direct antiglobulin test (DAT), formerly known as the direct Coombs' test (Figure 55-9A). In practice, the test involves screening the patient's red cells for the presence of IgG or complement using a reagent of broad specificity. Once a positive test is detected, specific reagents are used to determine whether IgG or C3d is present on the red cell surface. Immunoglobulin, when present, can often be further characterized by

Table 55-7 ■ Classification of Immune Hemolytic Anemia with Selected Examples

Warm Autoimmune Hemolytic Anemia

Primary (idiopathic)
Secondary
    Lymphoproliferative disorders
        Chronic lymphocytic leukemia
        Non-Hodgkin's lymphoma
        Hodgkin's disease
        Multiple myeloma
    Rheumatologic diseases
        Systemic lupus erythematosus
        Rheumatoid arthritis
        Scleroderma

Cold Autoimmune Hemolytic Anemia

Primary (idiopathic)
Secondary
    Lymphoproliferative disorders
    Mycoplasma pneumoniae
    Infectious mononucleosis

Paroxysmal Cold Hemoglobinuria

    Tertiary syphilis
    Postviral

Drug-Induced Immune Hemolysis

    Autoantibody
    Drug adsorption (hapten)
    Immune complex

Alloimmune Hemolysis

    Hemolytic disease of the newborn
    Hemolytic transfusion reactions

washing the antibody off the surface of the red cell and determining the reactivity of this eluate to a defined panel of antigens. The direct antiglobulin test is not absolutely sensitive or specific. Moreover, when the concentration of non-complement-fixing immunoglobulin on the red cell surface is less than a few hundred molecules, the direct antiglobulin test that is used in many screening assays may be negative even in the presence of antibodies that substantially

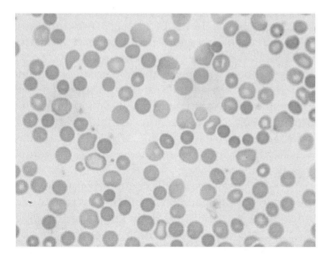

Figure 55-8 ■ Blood smear from a patient with autoimmune hemolytic anemia showing spherocytes. Dense staining shows cells that tend to be microcytic (original magnification ×60). (See Color Plate 8, same as Fig. 42-13. Courtesy of Cabello Inchausti B: Chapter 42 of this book.)

shorten red blood cell survival. This is particularly true for IgA and IgG_4 antibodies.

The indirect antiglobulin test, or indirect Coombs' test, is useful for diagnosing alloantibodies (see Figure 55-9B). Though not directly applicable to the diagnosis of autoimmune hemolytic anemia, it becomes relevant when patients with autoantibodies have been transfused. More than one quarter of patients with autoimmune hemolytic anemia who receive blood transfusions develop alloantibodies to one or more common blood group antigens, which they lack. These can be detected in the indirect antiglobulin test. Since the majority of patients with autoimmune hemolytic anemia have erythrocyte-specific antibodies present free in the serum (as opposed to bound to the red cell surface), special methods can be used to adsorb these so that alloantibodies are not inadvertently missed when there is a requirement for transfusion.

Warm Antibody Autoimmune Hemolytic Anemia

Warm antibody autoimmune hemolytic anemia is the most common autoimmune hemolytic anemia and has an incidence of about 1:50,000 to 1:100,000. It is more common in women than in men and, though it may occur in individuals of any age group, is more prevalent in older individuals. The great majority of warm autoantibodies are polyclonal IgG, though, rarely, IgM and IgA may be involved. Though any red

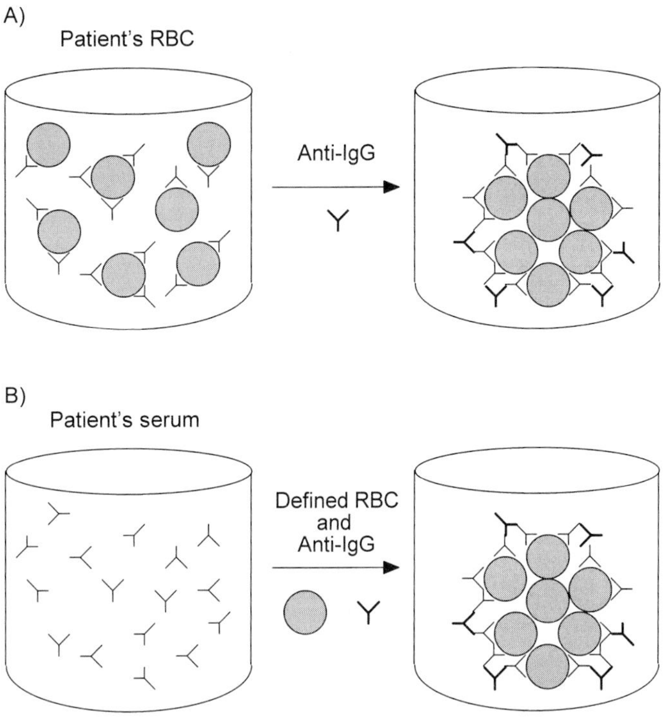

A)

Patient's RBC

Anti-IgG

Figure 55-9 ■ *A*, The direct antiglobulin test. Addition of antihuman globulin or anti-C3d antibody causes agglutination of the patient's red cells that have been coated with antibody at sufficient density. An antibody, if present, can often be eluted from the cell surface and tested on a defined panel of red cells to determine antigenic specificity. *B*, The indirect antiglobulin test. In contrast to the direct antiglobulin test, the indirect antiglobulin test looks for antibodies to the red cell that are present in serum. It uses an analogous strategy to the direct antiglobulin test.

B)

Patient's serum

Defined RBC
and
Anti-IgG

cell surface determinant may be involved, the most common targets are those of the Rh system. Despite the fact that most warm autoantibodies are IgG_1 and IgG_3 subclasses capable of fixing complement, erythrocyte destruction generally occurs via the extravascular mechanism in the spleen and liver.

Although warm antibody autoimmune hemolytic anemia is idiopathic in approximately half of the cases, in the remainder of instances, it is indicative of an underlying disorder or a drug reaction (Table 55-8). In affected patients, the clinician needs to consider potential underlying causes. Of these, the most common are lymphoproliferative disorders such as chronic lymphocytic leukemia (CLL) and B cell lymphomas. An association with other autoimmune diseases, such as systemic lupus erythematosus, is also seen. A wide variety of other conditions may be associated with warm antibody autoimmune hemolytic anemia but are much less common. Identification of underlying disorders is important because treatment for these conditions can be associated with resolution of the anemia.

Treatment of warm antibody autoimmune hemolytic anemia generally involves the judicious use of transfusion, therapy with prednisone, and splenectomy when necessary. For cases in which hemolysis persists after splenectomy, a variety of alternatives exist, none of which are highly effective. These alternatives include immunosuppressive therapy with cytotoxic agents such as cyclophosphamide or azithio-

prine, treatment with the attenuated androgen danazol, and infusion of intravenous gammaglobulin preparations. Many patients continue over time to need chronic low-dose prednisone therapy, which poses its own hazards to the patient. These patients are prone to develop venous thromboembolism, which are a major cause of death. The risk of thrombotic events may be reduced when the rate of hemolysis is slowed by therapy and when oral anticoagulant therapy is continuously administered.

Cold Antibody Autoimmune Hemolytic Anemia

Cold antibody autoimmune hemolytic anemia, or cold agglutinin disease, accounts for perhaps one fifth to one quarter of cases of autoimmune hemolytic anemias. Cold agglutinin disease may be transient (in the postinfectious setting) or chronic. Chronic cases are frequently associated with associated lymphoid malignancies, although some apparently idiopathic cases have been observed. Because of the association with lymphoproliferative disorders, chronic cold agglutinin disease most commonly occurs in individuals who are more than 50 years old.

The pathogenesis of cold antibody autoimmune hemolytic anemia involves antibody binding in the cold and release on warming in conjunction with complement activation. This occurs in the periphery of the circulation (Figure 55-10). In cold antibody

Table 55-8 ▪ Selected Agents Associated with Drug-Induced Hemolysis

Autoantibody Formation

Diclofenac
Ibuprofen
Interferon-α
Methyldopa
Procainamide

Drug Absorption (Hapten)

Acetaminophen
Cefotetan
Cefotaxime
Ceftriaxone
Chlorpromazine
5-Fluorouracil
Hydralazine
Hydrochlorothiazide
Insulin
Isoniazid
Melphalan
Phenacetin
Probenecid
Quinine
Quinidine
Rifampin
Sulindac
Streptomycin
Tetracycline
Tolmetin

Immune Complex

Ampicillin
Carbenicillin
Methicillin
Penicillin
Cefotaxime
Cephaloridine
Cephalothin

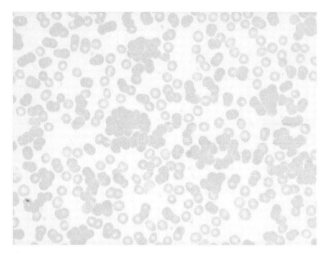

Figure 55-10 ▪ Blood smear. Agglutination of red cells in a patient with cold agglutinins (original magnification ×40). (See Color Plate 6, same as Fig. 42-3. courtesy of Cabello Inchausti B: Chapter 42 of this book.)

autoimmune hemolytic anemia, the antibody is usually an IgM, and rarely an IgG, that optimally binds to the red cell in the cold and falls off the red cell surface at or near physiologic temperature. The transient presence of the antibody on the surface leads to the deposition of complement on the red blood cell, which can lead to complement-mediated lysis.

At the stage of complement activation of C3, an inhibitor can abort the sequence, leaving a deposit of C3d on the red cell surface, protecting the red blood cell from progression of the steps leading to complement-mediated intravascular lysis. The direct antiglobulin test is positive for complement, but no IgM or IgG is detected on the cell surface. The IgM antibody that is responsible is readily washed off the surface of the red blood cell during the performance of the direct antiglobulin test. Cold agglutinin titers are determined by examining for red cell agglutination when the patient's red cells are exposed to serial dilutions of the patient's serum. Cold agglutinins should not be confused with cryoglobulins, which are antibodies that self-associate in the cold, rather than antibodies that directly react to the red blood cell surface.

Very low titer polyclonal cold agglutinins are frequently present in normal individuals and are of no pathologic significance. Significant polyclonal cold agglutinins are transiently observed after infections and in collagen-vascular disorders. Following *Mycoplasma pneumoniae* infection, the target is often the I carbohydrate antigen on the red blood cell surface, whereas in infectious mononucleosis caused by Epstein-Barr virus, the target is frequently the i antigen. The finding of a monoclonal cold agglutinin is frequently, though not invariably, associated with a B-cell lymphoproliferative disorder. Evidence for a B-cell lymphoma should be sought in patients with chronic cold agglutinin disease, because treatment of the underlying disorder with appropriate cytotoxic agents can ameliorate or resolve the anemia.

The management of idiopathic chronic cold agglutinin disease is mainly supportive. Patients should be instructed to avoid cold exposure and keep their extremities warm. This may include wearing gloves when entering the refrigerator or freezer. In cold climates during wintertime, remote starters for automobiles are available to allow warming of the passenger compartment. Blood pack warmers should be used when transfusions are needed. Prednisone and splenectomy are usually ineffective in this disorder. Cytotoxic chemotherapy can be of benefit in some patients.

TREATMENT

Therapy for Warm Antibody Autoimmune Hemolytic Anemia

Instituting appropriate therapy for warm antibody autoimmune hemolytic anemia is predicated on understanding its cause. Potentially offending drugs should be discontinued, and underlying disorders should be diagnosed. Mild anemia is often well tolerated and need not necessarily be treated. However, treatment should be instituted for severe or symptomatic warm antibody autoimmune hemolytic anemia. Initially, red blood cell transfusions may be necessary in cases of severe anemia and when there is comorbid cardiac disease. In such cases, patients should be monitored carefully. Even with careful cross-matching, acute hemolytic transfusion reactions can occur. To identify compatible red blood cell units, careful evaluation and selection requires working in conjunction with the blood bank. First-line therapy for hemolytic anemia is corticosteroids. Therapy may be initiated with 1 mg/kg of prednisone daily. Response may take several weeks. Once an adequate response has been obtained (hematocrit greater than 30%), prednisone can be tapered, and an attempt can be made to discontinue it. The process of very gradually tapering the daily prednisone dose by

10 mg every 1 or 2 weeks, followed by an even slower taper when a daily dose of 10 mg is reached, is believed to lessen the risk of relapse. Relapse is nevertheless common in this disorder, and no data support the value of slow as opposed to more rapid tapering of the dose. For patients who do not respond to prednisone or who relapse after treatment, splenectomy is an option; one half to two thirds of patients will respond to this intervention. For those who fail splenectomy, a number of options of limited utility are available. Immunologic suppression by cytotoxic agents such as cyclophosphamide, azathioprine, or vincristine may be helpful in some patients. The response rate to the administration of high-dose gamma globulin to patients with hemolytic anemia is much lower than when gamma globulin is given to patients with immune thrombocytopenic purpura. Though transiently effective in reducing autoantibodies, plasmapheresis rarely produces a clinically meaningful response, because IgG antibodies are distributed both intravascularly and extravascularly and can readily enter the circulation after intravascular depletion.

References

Iron, Folate and B$_{12}$ Deficiency, and the Anemia of Chronic Disease

Carmel R: Current concepts in cobalamin deficiency. Ann Rev Med 2000;51:357–375.

Goodnough LT, Skikne B, Brugnara C: Erythropoietin, iron, and erythropoiesis. Blood 2000;96(3):823–833.

Hoffbrand AV, Herbert V: Nutritional anemias. Semin Hematol 1999;36(4, Suppl 7):13–23.

Snow CF: Laboratory diagnosis of vitamin B$_{12}$ and folate deficiency: A guide for the primary care physician. Arch Intern Med 1999;159:1289–1298.

Hemoglobinopathies

Brittenham GM, Griffith PM, Nienhuis AW, et al: Efficacy of deferoxamine in preventing complications of iron overload in patients with thalassemia major. N Engl J Med 1994;331:567–573.

Bunn HF: Pathogenesis and treatment of sickle cell disease. N Engl J Med 1997;337:762–769.

Charache S, Terrin ML, Moore RD, et al: Effect of hydroxyurea on the frequency of painful crises in sickle cell anemia. N Engl J Med 1995;332:1317–1322.

Giardini C, Lucarelli G: Bone marrow transplantation for beta-thalassemia. Hematol Oncol Clin N Am 1999;13:1059–1064.

Haberkern CM, Neumayr LD, Orringer EP, et al: Cholecystectomy in sickle cell anemia patients: Perioperative outcome

of 364 cases from the National Preoperative Transfusion Study. Blood 1997;89:1533–1542.

Heller P, Best WR, Nelson RB, Becktel J: Clinical implications of sickle-cell trait and glucose-6-phosphate dehydrogenase deficiency in hospitalized black male patients. N Engl J Med 1979;300:1001–1005.

Koshy M, Burd L, Wallace D, et al: Prophylactic red-cell transfusions in pregnant patients with sickle cell disease: A randomized cooperative study. N Engl J Med 1988; 319:1447–1452.

Ohene-Fremong K, Weiner SJ, Sleeper LA, et al: Cerebrovascular accidents in sickle cell disease: Rates and risk factors. Blood 1998;91:288–294.

Olivieri NF: The β-thalassemias. N Engl J Med 1999;341:99–109.

Steinberg MH: Management of sickle cell disease. N Engl J Med 1999;340:1021–1030.

Steinberg MH, West MS, Gallagher D, et al: Effects of glucose-6-phosphate dehydrogenase deficiency upon sickle cell anemia. Blood 1988;71:748–752.

Vichinsky EP, Haberkern CM, Neumayr L, et al: A comparison of conservative and aggressive transfusion regimens in the perioperative management of sickle cell disease. N Engl J Med 1995;333:206–213.

Vichinsky EP, Neumayr LD, Earles AN, et al: Causes and outcomes of the acute chest syndrome in sickle cell disease. N Engl J Med 2000;342:1855–1865.

Vichinsky EP, Styles LA, Colangelo LH, et al: Acute chest syndrome in sickle cell disease: Clinical presentation and course. Blood 1997;89:1787–1792.

Weatherall DJ: Pathophysiology of thalassaemia. Baillière's Clin Hematol 1998;11:127–146.

G-6-PD Deficiency

Arese P, De Flora A: Pathophysiology of hemolysis in glucose-6-phosphate dehydrogenase deficiency. Semin Hematol 1990;27:1–40.

Beutler E: Glucose-6-phosphate dehydrogenase deficiency. N Engl J Med 1991;324:169–174.

Mason PJ: New insights into G6PD deficiency. Br J Haematol 1996;94:585–591.

Ruwende C, Hill A: Glucose-6-phosphate dehydrogenase deficiency and malaria. J Mol Med 1998;76:581–588.

Membrane Abnormalities

Eber SW, Gonzalez JM, Lux ML, et al: Ankyrin-1 mutations are a major cause of dominant and recessive hereditary spherocytosis. Nature Genet 1993;13:214–218.

Gallagher PG, Tse WT, Forget BG: Clinical and molecular aspects of disorders of the erythrocyte membrane skeleton. Semin Perinatol 1990;14:351–367.

Hillmen P, Lewis SM, Bessler M, et al: Natural history of paroxysmal nocturnal hemoglobinuria. N Engl J Med 1995; 333:1253–1258.

Schubert J, Alvarado M, Uciechowski P, et al: Diagnosis of paroxysmal nocturnal hemoglobinuria using immunophenotyping of peripheral blood cells. Br J Haematol 1991;79:487–492.

Takeda J, Miyata T, Kawagoe K, et al: Deficiency of the GPI anchor caused by a somatic mutation in the PIG-A gene in paroxysmal nocturnal hemoglobinuria. Cell 1993;73:703–711.

Tse WT, Lux SE: Red blood cell membrane disorders. Br J Haematol 1999;104:2–13.

Autoimmune Hemolytic Anemia

Engelfriet CP, Overbeeke MAM, von dem Borne AEG: Autoimmune hemolytic anemia. Semin Hematol 1992;29: 3–12.

Göttsche B, Salama A, Mueller-Eckhardt C: Donath-Landsteiner autoimmune hemolytic anemia in children: A study of 22 cases. Vox Sang 1990;58:281–286.

Jefferies LC: Transfusion therapy in autoimmune hemolytic anemia. Hematol Oncol Clin N Am 1994;8:1087–1104.

Mauro FR, Foa R, Cerretti R, et al: Autoimmune hemolytic anemia in chronic lymphocytic leukemia: Clinical, therapeutic, and prognostic features. Blood 2000;95:2786–2792.

Meyer O, Stahl D, Beckhove P, et al: Pulsed high-dose dexamethasone in chronic autoimmune haemolytic anaemia of warm type. Br J Haematol 1997;98:860–862.

Salama A, Mueller-Eckhardt C: On the mechanisms of sensitization and attachment of antibodies to RBC in drug-induced immune hemolytic anemia. Blood 1987;69: 1006–1010.

Tabbara IA: Hemolytic anemias: Diagnosis and management. Med Clin N Am 1992;76:649–668.

Chapter 56
White Cell Disorders

Laurence Alan Boxer

The differential diagnosis for a patient with recurrent infections is formidable. Similarities in the clinical manifestations of disease can further complicate attempts to establish a diagnosis. Most patients with recurrent infections do not have an identifiable phagocyte defect or immunodeficiency. Given the low probability of identifying a discrete immunologic defect, evaluations should be initiated for those who have within a one-year period at least one of the clinical features: (1) more than two systemic bacterial infections, for example, sepsis, meningitis, or osteomyelitis; (2) serious respiratory infections, for example, pneumonia or sinusitis; (3) bacterial infections, for example, cellulitis, draining otitis media, or lymphadenitis; (4) an infection at an unusual site, for example, hepatic or brain abscess; (5) infections with unusual pathogens, for example, *Aspergillus* pneumonia, disseminated candidiasis, or infection with *Serratia marcescens*, *Nocardia* spp., and *Burkholderia cepacia*; (6) infections of unusual severity; and (7) chronic gingivitis and recurring aphthous ulcers.

Once it has been determined that an evaluation for a white blood cell abnormality is warranted, a thorough clinical history, physical examination, and laboratory testing (Figure 56-1) should provide the diagnosis and help to formulate an appropriate therapeutic plan.

Severe Congenital Neutropenia

Severe chronic neutropenia is a general term for rare conditions with absolute neutrophil counts less than 500/μL documented on three separate occasions during six months of observation. Severe chronic neutropenia and recurrent serious infections are features of heterogeneous group of disorders of myelopoiesis including congenital neutropenia, cyclic neutropenia, and idiopathic neutropenia. The hemoglobin and platelet levels are normal or nearly normal, and the bone marrow shows a selective defect in neutrophil formation with abundant promyelocytes but relatively few myelocytes, metamyelocytes, or neutrophils, leading to what pathologists call "a promyelocytic maturation arrest." Kostmann's syndrome and other congenital disorders associated with severe chronic neutropenia are listed in Table 56-1.

Clinical Manifestations and Diagnosis

These patients have a predictable pattern of infection and inflammation that includes oropharyngeal infection, otitis media, respiratory infections, cellulites, and skin abscesses. These are commonly caused by *Staphylococcus aureus* and *Streptococcus* species. Pneumonias caused by gram-negative or anaerobic bacteria, deep tissue abscesses, and bacteremia occur infrequently but are life-threatening. Because most of these patients have intact monocyte and lymphocyte function and either normal or increased immunoglobulin and complement levels, infections by yeast, fungi, and parasites are unusual. Infections tend to last a long time and are slow to heal, even with optimal antibiotic treatment (Figure 56-2).

The height and weight of affected children are below the fifth percentile for age because repeated infections commence in infancy or early childhood. Physical findings may include scarred tympanic membranes and cervical adenopathy as well as mild hepatosplenomegaly and pallor. Gingivitis is the most common finding. Peripheral blood eosinophilia and monocytosis accompany the profound neutropenia.

Therapy and Disease Course

Before recombinant human granulocyte colony-stimulating factor (G-CSF) was available, half of the children died of infection at a mean age of 2 years. More than 90 percent of patients respond to granulocyte colony-stimulating factor, do not experience life-threatening infections, and survive well beyond childhood. One does have to be wary, however, of the long-term complications of continuous granulocyte colony-stimulating factor therapy, which appear to

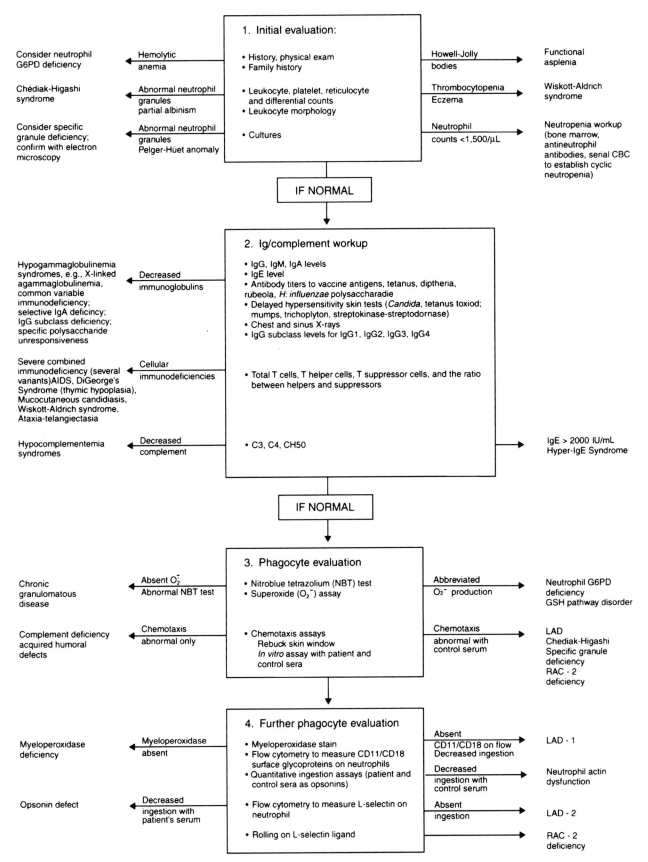

Figure 56-1 ■ Algorithm for the evaluation of patients with recurrent infection. CBC = complete blood count; Ig = immunoglobulin; G6PD = glucose-6-phosphate dehydrogenase; LAD = leukocyte adhesion deficiency; GSH-glutathione. (Modified from Curnutte JT and Boxer LA. Clinically significant phagocytic cell defects. In Current Clinical Topics in Infectious Diseases. JS Remington and MN Swartz, Eds. McGraw-Hill, Inc. New York, p 144, 1985.)

Table 56-1 ■ Classification of Congenital Neutropenia

- Congenital neutropenia (Kostmann's syndrome)
- Glycogen storage disease 1b
- Shwachman-Diamond syndrome
- Hyperimmunoglobulin M (IgM) syndrome

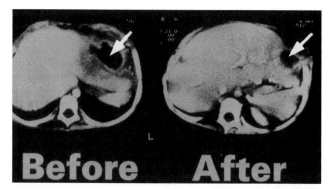

Figure 56-2 ■ Computerized tomography scan of the liver in a patient with severe chronic neutropenia. *Before*, *E. coli* was cultured from the abscess, but the bacteria failed to clear after 10 months of appropriate antibiotic therapy. The arrow delineates the abscess cavity. *After*, Within one month of normalizing the absolute neutrophil count with G-CSF, the abscess began to resolve, and within three months, the CT of the liver was normal. The arrow delineates the resolving abscess cavity.

include a risk of glomerulonephritis, vasculitis, and osteopenic osteoporosis. An added concern is that after a decade of treatment, approximately 10 percent of these patients develop myelodysplasia with increased myeloblasts or acute myeloid leukemia. Approximately one half of the patients who develop myeloid malignancies present with the myelodysplasia, whereas others present with acute myeloid leukemia, usually of the FAB M4 or M5 subtypes, without a preceding myelodysplastic phase. Cytogenetic analysis frequently shows prognostically unfavorable features (see Chapter 60, "Acute Myeloid Leukemia").

The 10 percent of patients who do not respond to granulocyte colony-stimulating factor given even at increased doses (100 μg/kg/day or more) and the subset of patients converting to unfavorable myelodysplasia or acute myeloid leukemia are candidates for stem cell transplantation from an HLA (human leukocyte antigen)-identical sibling.

Cyclic Neutropenia

Cyclic neutropenia is inherited as an autosomal dominant disease in which blood stem cell production from the bone marrow oscillates with 21-day periodicity. Circulating neutrophils vary between almost normal numbers and zero.

Clinical Manifestations and Diagnosis

When their granulocyte count falls, patients with cyclic neutropenia are prone to infections similar to those seen in patients with severe chronic neutropenia. Moreover, until the advent of granulocyte colony-stimulating factor therapy, approximately 10 percent of patients with cyclic neutropenia experienced fatal *Clostridium perfringens* infection, disseminated from gastrointestinal (GI) tract ulcerations, which are common in this disorder. Cyclic neutropenia is often called cyclic hematopoiesis because the platelet and reticulocyte counts also exhibit cycling. Monocyte counts also cycle, but inversely to the neutrophil count, rising as the granulocyte count falls. The diagnosis of cyclic neutropenia is established by obtaining blood counts two to three times per week over a period of two months.

Molecular studies demonstrating mutations in the neutrophil elastase gene on chromosome 19 confirm the diagnosis. It is noteworthy that 90 percent of patients with classic severe chronic neutropenia also have mutations in this gene. Potentially, these abnormalities affect the storage of neutrophil elastase in the primary granules of neutrophils. The defect may contribute to accelerated apoptosis of myeloid precursors found in the bone marrow of both groups of patients.

Therapy and Disease Course

When patients with cyclic neutropenia are treated with granulocyte colony-stimulating factor on a daily basis, their cycle changes from a 21-day interval to a 9- to 11-day interval. On granulocyte colony-stimulating factor, these patients are no longer at risk of fatal infections with *Clostridia* organisms, and the necessity for antibiotic therapy is markedly diminished. Unlike severe chronic neutropenia, none of the patients with cyclic neutropenia are at risk for developing myelodysplasia or acute myeloid leukemia, and complications from granulocyte colony-stimulating factor therapy are much less common than in severe chronic neutropenia.

Disorders of Neutrophil Motility

Chemotaxis directs the migration of neutrophils from the circulation to an inflammatory site. Normal chemotaxis requires that chemotactic factors be generated in sufficient quantities to establish a chemotactic gradient and that the neutrophils express chemotactic agent receptors and have normal mecha-

---

Table 56-2 ■ **Clinical Conditions Associated with Impaired Neutrophil Chemotaxis**

1. Impaired generation of chemotactic agonists. C5a deficiency secondary to congenital deficiency of C3, C5, or dysregulation of complement pathways that can occur in systemic lupus erythematosus and chronic hemodialysis.

2. Acquisition of chemotactic factor inhibitors in cirrhosis, sarcoidosis, and lepromatous leprosy.

3. Inhibition of neutrophil motility that occurs in IgA paraproteinemia, following bone marrow transplantation or thermal injury, and after ethanol ingestions.

4. Intrinsic disorders of neutrophil function as occurs in neutrophil actin dysfunction, leukocyte adhesion deficiency, Chédiak-Higashi syndrome, neutrophil-specific granule deficiency, and glycogen storage disease 1b.

---

nisms for discerning the direction of the gradient. Depressed chemotaxis has been observed in a wide variety of clinical conditions. Table 56-2 outlines some of these disorders classified according to postulated pathophysiologic mechanisms. These include abnormalities in the production or inhibition of chemotactic factors or intrinsic abnormalities of the adhesiveness and locomotion of the phagocyte itself. Hyperimmunoglobulin E syndrome is one of the more frequent abnormalities in which a chemotactic defect plays a major contribution in decreased resistance to bacterial infections.

Hyperimmunoglobulin E Syndrome

Hyperimmunoglobulin E disease has been called Job syndrome because of the nature of the afflictions that these patients experience. Recurrent staphylococcal skin abscesses, pneumonia, chronic dermatitis, chronic otitis media and sinusitis, hyperextensible joints and scoliosis, and markedly elevated IgE levels are characteristic. Both males and females are affected, and the inheritance pattern in familial cases is one of autosomal dominance with variable expression. Patients present initially with an eczematoid rash that usually involves the face and extensor surfaces of the arms and legs. The skin lesions are frequently sharply demarcated and usually lack surrounding erythema. Patients may also develop bacterial arthritis and staphylococcal osteomyelitis at fracture sites, to which these patients are predisposed. Chronic candidiasis at mucosal sites and nailbeds affect the majority of patients with this syndrome.

Clinical Manifestations and Diagnosis

Most patients have characteristic facial features of coarse skin, prominent forehead, deep-set eyes, prognathism, and a thickened lower lip, nose, and ears. Additionally, the majority of patients report delayed shedding of primary teeth, delayed eruption of permanent teeth, or both. Roentgenograms of the oral cavity show two rows of teeth due to retention of primary dentition. Fractures, often due to unrecognized trauma in long bones, ribs, and pelvic bones, occur in 50 percent of patients. In infancy, IgE levels are markedly elevated, frequently exceeding 2500 IU/mL (normal is less than 4 IU/mL). IgD levels are also elevated in greater than 90 percent of the patients, and there is marked eosinophilia in the blood and sputum. Other laboratory abnormalities include positive skin wheal-and-flair response to a variety of food, inhalant, bacterial, and fungal antigens. Anamnestic (IgG) antibody and Tγ lymphocyte mediated responses to neoantigens are impaired.

Therapy and Disease Course

If the syndrome is recognized early in life and the patient is maintained on chronic antistaphylococcal medication, most patients will reach the age of maturity. If the diagnosis is not recognized, chronically infected giant pulmonary pneumatoceles can develop, and lung infections with *Staphylococci* as well as *Candida* and *Aspergillus* may occur. No specific therapy is available. Treatment consists of aggressive antibiotic treatment to minimize infectious complications.

Leukocyte Adhesion Deficiency

Leukocyte adhesion deficiency-1 (LAD-1) is a rare autosomal recessive disorder of leukocyte function wherein expression of β_2 integrins is markedly diminished, owing to a gene mutation on chromosome 21. Leukocyte integrins are responsible for the tight adhesion of neutrophils to the endothelial cell surface, emigration from the circulation, and their adhesion to opsonized, complement-coated microorganisms. Because of decreased adherence characteristics, the neutrophils are unable to attach to endothelium and are therefore unable to undergo chemotaxis to inflammatory sites. The impairment in neutrophil function underlies the propensity for serious and recurrent bacterial function.

Clinical Manifestations and Diagnosis

The disorder is characterized by recurrent bacterial and fungal infections and depressed inflammatory responses despite striking blood neutrophilia. Children who have severe disease present in infancy with recurrent bacterial infections of the skin, mouth, respiratory tract, lower intestinal tract, and genital mucosa. They may have a history of delayed separation of the umbilical cord and often an associated infection of the cord stump. Skin infections may progress to large chronic ulcers. The ulcers heal slowly, requiring months of antibiotic treatment and often skin grafting. Severe gingivitis is common, with early loss of primary and then secondary teeth.

The pathogens affecting these patients are similar to those affecting patients with severe neutropenia, but these patients are also susceptible to fungal infections such as *Candida* and *Aspergillus* spp. Typical signs of inflammation may be lacking. Few neutrophils are identified in biopsy specimens of infected tissue. The circulating neutrophil count during infection typically exceeds 30,000/μL and may on occasion exceed 100,000/μL. The severity of the illness correlates directly with the diminished level of expression of integrin complexes on the neutrophil surface.

The diagnosis is made most readily by flow cytometric measurements of surface integrin expression (CD11b) in stimulated and unstimulated neutrophils.

Therapy and Disease Course

Patients with severe deficiency may die in infancy, and those who survive infancy have a susceptibility to life-threatening systemic infections. Patients with moderate deficiency have infrequent severe infections and a longer (relatively) survival but are at risk for losing their primary and secondary teeth from chronic gingivitis.

Treatment depends on the phenotype. Early allogeneic bone marrow transplantation is the treatment of choice for the severe form of the disease. Other treatment is largely supportive. Patients can be maintained on prophylactic trimethoprim-sulfamethoxazole and should have close surveillance to identify infections at the inception of infection. Determination of the etiologic agent by culture and biopsy is important because prolonged antibiotic treatment is required for infections. Patients with infection are unable to form pus. Pulmonary infiltrates can nevertheless be seen on a chest roentgenogram, because the lung is an organ site where neutrophils are able to migrate independent of expression of surface adhesion molecules.

Chédiak-Higashi Syndrome

Chédiak-Higashi syndrome is a rare autosomal recessive disorder characterized by increased susceptibility to infection due to defective granulation of neutrophils, a mild bleeding tendency, and partial oculocutaneous albinism. The gene for Chédiak-Higashi syndrome encodes for a cytosolic protein named lysosomal-trafficking regulator. Abnormality of this protein results in generalized cellular dysfunction associated with fusion of cytoplasmic granules. Giant cytoplasmic granules, which are fused lysosomal granules, appear in the neutrophils, monocytes, and lymphocytes. The increased susceptibility to infections is explained in part by impaired function of neutrophil chemotaxis, degranulation, and bactericidal activity. Pigmentary dilution involving the hair, skin, and ocular fundi results from pathologic aggregation of melanosomes and is associated with a failure of decussation of the optic and auditory nerves.

Clinical Manifestations and Diagnosis

Affected patients have light skin color and silvery hair. They frequently complain of solar sensitivity and photophobia. Infections of the mucous membranes, skin, and respiratory tract are frequent. Peripheral neuropathy, which can be sensory and/or motor, commonly starts during adolescence and may become the most prominent clinical problem. Ataxia and nystagmus are frequent.

Inclusion bodies are found in all nucleated cells. The diagnosis of Chédiak-Higashi syndrome is established by demonstrating large inclusions in the neutrophils, which are readily seen on Wright-stained blood films (Figure 56-3). The inclusions can be accentuated by performing a peroxidase stain. Giant melanophores are visible in the hair roots of patients. Mild to moderate neutropenia occurs. Platelet aggregation is impaired owing to deficiency of the dense granules in the platelets, leading to prolonged bleeding times despite normal platelet counts.

Therapy and Disease Course

Vitamin C (ascorbic acid) corrects the chemotactic defect in vitro. Although the clinical efficacy of ascorbic acid is debatable, given the safety of the vitamin, most patients are treated with it. High doses of ascorbic acid (200 mg/24 hr for infants and 2000 mg/24 hr for adults) are believed to improve the clinical status of some patients.

The infections are usually mild and respond to antibiotics, and platelet dysfunction rarely causes a clinically significant bleeding problem. In the second decade of life, these patients are at risk of developing

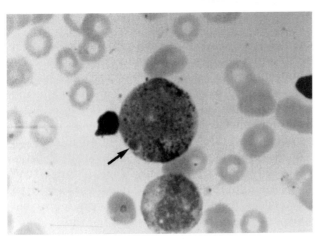

Figure 56-3 ■ Bone marrow film of patient with the Chédiak-Higashi syndrome. The promyelocyte contains large inclusions, one of which is identified by the arrow.

a severe, debilitating peripheral and central neuropathy. The principal concern in these patients, however, is progression to an accelerated phase of disease, characterized by a lymphoma-like syndrome. This eventuates in pancytopenia, recurrent fevers, and lymphohistiocytic infiltration of liver, spleen, and lymph nodes, which mimic the features of the virally mediated hemophagocytic syndrome. Splenic and hepatic enlargement are often massive. The lymphocytic proliferation is polyclonal and appears to be related to the inability of these patients to control Epstein-Barr virus infection. The transition to the accelerated phase predisposes these pancytopenic patients to recurrent bacterial and viral infections, which are ultimately fatal. Cure of the accelerated phase is available only through allogeneic stem cell transplantation from an HLA-compatible donor. Allogeneic transplantation reconstitutes normal hematopoietic and immunologic functions and corrects the natural killer cell deficiency. Unfortunately, allogeneic transplantation does not correct or prevent the progression of peripheral neuropathy, but it may ameliorate central neuropathy to some extent.

Chronic Granulomatous Disease

Patients with chronic granulomatous disease have increased susceptibility to serious infection by bacteria and fungi that are catalase-positive and do not produce hydrogen peroxide. In this disorder, these organisms are not killed after ingestion (phagocytosis) by neutrophils and monocytes. The phagocytes are unable to reduce molecular oxygen and create the reactive oxygen metabolites that are necessary for efficient intracellular microbicidal activity.

Normally, the engulfment of microbes by phagocytic cells stimulates a burst of oxygen consumption accompanied by a unique electron transport chain called the NADPH oxidase. The functional NADPH oxidase is composed of several structural and regulator proteins, including gp91^{phox}, p22^{phox}, p47^{phox}, or p67^{phox}. Two of these (gp91^{phox} and p22^{phox}) are found in the plasma membrane and in the membrane of specific and tertiary granules and make up the cytochrome, b$_{558}$. After ingestion of a pathogen by a phagocytic cell and subsequent fusion of specific granules with a phagocytic vacuole, the cytochrome is translocated to the membrane of a phagocytic vacuole. One or more of the structural or regulator proteins that are defective in chronic granulomatous disease are phosphorylated en bloc and bind to cytochrome b. These assembled elements, called NADPH oxidase, then transfer an electron from NADPH to molecular oxygen, leading to the formation of superoxide. Superoxide is converted into hydrogen peroxide and hypochlorite, both of which aid in microbial killing and digestion.

In chronic granulomatous disease, mutations occur in any of the four major structural components of the NADPH oxidase, thereby impairing efficient microbicidal killing. Seventy percent of patients with chronic granulomatous disease have the X-linked recessive form of the disease characterized by defects in gp91^{phox}, and 22 percent have an autosomal recessive form affecting either p22^{phox}, p47^{phox}, or p67^{phox}. Of the patients with the autosomal recessive form of the disease, 56 percent have a deficiency of p47^{phox}, 12 percent have a deficiency of p67^{phox}, and 8 percent have a deficiency of p22^{phox}. Some patients have defects in the gp91^{phox} that result in the production of a hypofunctional protein retaining small amounts of residual superoxide production. These patients have milder clinical phenotypes.

Apart from their susceptibility to certain infections, patients with chronic granulomatous disease have an increased incidence of chronic inflammatory and/or rheumatic conditions. These include inflammatory bowel disease, discoid and systemic lupus erythematosus, chorioretinitis, Behçet's syndrome, and idiopathic thrombocytopenia purpura. Chronic inflammatory disease can lead to bowel, gastric outlet, or urinary tract obstruction.

Clinical Manifestations and Diagnosis

Although more than three quarters of patients are diagnosed with the disease before the age of 5 years, some patients with milder forms of the disease go unrecognized until the second or third decade of life. The clinical presentation is variable. Chronic granulomatous disease should be considered in any patient with recurrent lymphadenitis and in patients who have bacterial hepatic abscesses, osteomyelitis at multiple sites or in small bones of the hands and feet, a family history of recurrent infections, or unusual catalase-positive microbial infections. The clinical features differ between patients with the X-linked and autosomal recessive forms of disease. For example, compared to the autosomal recessive genetic inheritance, the patients with X-linked inheritance experience infections and are diagnosed at an earlier age; have a higher prevalence of certain infections such as perirectal abscess, suppurative adenitis, and bacteremia/fungemia; have a greater frequency of supervening chronic inflammatory manifestations; and have a higher rate of mortality. The sites of infection and common pathogens are listed in Table 56-3. Abscesses and suppurative adenitis, bacteremia, cellulitis, and meningitis are frequent occurrences in these patients. *B. cepacia* is a common infecting organism. *Chromobacterium violaceum*, a pathogen found in brackish waters, occurs with unusually high frequency in chronic granulomatous disease patients from the southern United States.

The concomitant problems of infection and inflammation in chronic granulomatous disease leads to a variety of clinical problems in patients with established disease; these are listed in Table 56-4.

The test used to confirm the diagnosis involves quantitative determination of the generation of hydrogen peroxide by neutrophils in response to activating stimuli. Flow cytometry monitors the conversion by oxidation of dihydrorhodamine 123 to rhodamine 123. This method not only provides the diagnosis in chronic granulomatous disease, but also suggests whether the inheritance is autosomal recessive (small amounts of hydrogen peroxide are generated) or X-linked recessive (no hydrogen peroxide is generated).

Once the diagnosis of chronic granulomatous disease is made, the genotype can be determined. A mosaic population of NADPH oxidase-positive and oxidase-negative neutrophils in a male patient's mother or sister strongly supports the diagnosis of X-linked chronic granulomatous disease. Molecular methods are used to identify the specific genetic defect.

Prenatal diagnosis of chronic granulomatous disease can be made by analysis of neonatal neutrophil oxidant production from umbilical vein samples obtained by fetoscopy. Alternatively, DNA can be analyzed from amniocytes or chorionic villus samples. Restriction fragment linked polymorphisms have been successful in diagnosing gp91^{phox} and p67^{phox} deficiencies in informative families.

Therapy and Disease Course

Patients with chronic granulomatous disease often do not have typical symptoms or findings of infection. Patients can have mild, nonspecific symptoms or may be asymptomatic in the face of life-threatening infections. Fever and leukocytosis may not be present, and an elevated sedimentation rate may be the only abnormal laboratory test. Therefore it is important to routinely obtain a chest X-ray or computed tomography (CT) scan of the chest when an infection is suspected. The overwhelming majority of infections are caused by only five pathogens: *S. aureus, B. cepacia, Serratia marcescens, Nocardia* spp, and *Aspergillus* spp. Selection of appropriate therapy requires careful microbiologic evaluation. In this regard, fine needle aspiration of pneumonias has proven useful. For liver abscesses, which are commonly caused by *S. aureus,* surgical excision is necessary in the vast majority of cases. Prophylaxis with trimethoprim-sulfamethoxazole is effective in X-linked and autosomal recessive CGD and reduces the rate of infection by at least 50 percent. The drug is generally well tolerated, and its widespread use has not led to an increased frequency of fungal infections or pathogens resistant to trimethoprim-sulfamethoxazole. In patients who are allergic to the drug, prophylaxis with trimethoprim alone or dicloxacillin is useful.

In a European prospective study of itraconazole prophylaxis, the rate of *Aspergillus* infections was reduced in comparison with historical controls, and the drug was well tolerated. Interferon-γ administration also reduces the number of serious infections, adding to the benefit of antibiotic prophylaxis probably by enhancing oxidant-independent antimicrobial activity.

Granulocyte transfusions could provide a small number of normal phagocytes to compensate for the metabolic defect in chronic granulomatous disease. Studies of transfused granulocytes recovered from sites of infection exhibit respiratory burst activity on stimulation and appear to traffic normally. However, the value of granulocyte transfusions in chronic granulomatous disease has not been evaluated in prospective controlled trials. Moreover, granulocyte transfusions have potential side effects such as fever and a transient but hazardous pulmonary capillary leak syndrome that mimics the clinical picture of congestive heart failure.

Allogeneic bone marrow transplantation is a consideration in patients who have recurrent serious infections despite antibiotic and interferon-γ prophylaxis and who have HLA-matched normal siblings.

Corticosteroid therapy is often required to relieve obstruction of the gastrointestinal and genitourinary

Table 56-3 ■ Infections in Chronic Granulomatous Disease: Common Pathogens and Sites of Involvement

Pathogen	Presentation
Bacterial	
Staphylococcus aureus	Soft tissue infection, lymphadenitis, liver abscess, osteomyelitis, pneumonia, sepsis

Burkholderia
  B. cepacia
  B. gladioli
  B. pseudomallei	

Serratia marcescens	Pneumonia, osteomyelitis, sepsis, soft tissue infection

Nocardia species
  N. asteroides
  N. nova
  N. otitidiscaviarum
  N. farcinica
	Pneumonia, osteomyelitis, brain abscess

Chromobacterium violaceum	Soft tissue infection, sepsis
Fungal	

Aspergillus species
  A. fumigatus
  A. nidulans
  A. flavus
  A. terreus
  A. niger
	Pneumonia, osteomyelitis, brain abscess

Paecilomyces species
  P. variotti
  P. lilacinus
	Pneumonia, soft tissue infection, osteomyelitis

Phaeohyphomycete species
  (dark-walled fungi)
  Exophiala sp.
  Bipolaris sp.
  Cladosporium sp.
	Pneumonia, soft tissue infection

Penicillium species	Pneumonia, soft tissue infection
Miscellaneous filamentous Fungi and yeasts *Zygomycete* species *Acremonium* sp. *Trichosporon beigelii* *Trichosporon inkin*	

Candida species
  C. albicans
  Torulopsis (Candida) glabrata
	Sepsis, soft tissue infection, liver abscess

Modified from Segal et al: Genetic, biochemical, and clinical features of granulomatous disease. Medicine 2000;79:155. Used with permission.

tract caused by inflammatory granulomas. The obstruction usually resolves in a few days, but surgery may be required in patients who fail to respond.

The prognosis of patients with chronic granulomatous disease has improved in recent years. More than 25 percent of all living patients with the X-linked form and 42 percent with the autosomal recessive form are age 20 or older. The estimated mortality is approximately 5 percent per year for the patients with the X-linked recessive form of the disorder and 2 percent per year for the patients with the autosomal recessive form of the disease. Both *Aspergillus* and *B. cepacia* account for over half of the deaths. Fatal *Aspergillus* infections are characterized by pneumonia

Table 56-4 ■ Clinical Problems Associated with Chronic Granulomatous Disease Listed in Order of Decreasing Frequency

- Lymphadenopathy
- Hepatomegaly
- Splenomegaly
- Hypergammaglobulinemia
- Anemia of chronic disease
- Underweight
- Chronic diarrhea
- Short stature
- Gingivitis
- Dermatitis
- Pulmonary fibrosis
- Ulcerative stomatitis
- Gastric antral narrowing
- Granulomatosis ileocolitis
- Chorioretinitis
- Urinary outlet obstruction
- Lupus syndromes
- Idiopathic thrombocytopenia purpura
- Behçet's syndrome
- Glomerulonephritis

with direct extension to the ribs, chest wall, and vertebra. Most fatal *B. cepacia* infections result from sepsis and pneumonia.

References

General

Boxer LA, Smolen JE: Neutrophil granule constituents and their release in health and disease. Hematol Oncol Clin North Am 1988;2:101.

Dale DC, Person RE, Bolyard AA, et al: Mutations in the gene encoding neutrophil elastase in congenital and cyclic neutropenia. Blood 2000;96:2317.

Germeshausen M, Ballmaier M, Welte K: Implications of mutations in hematopoietic growth factor receptor genes in congenital cytopenias. Ann N Y Acad Sci 2001;938:305–320.

Lakshman R, Finn A: Neutrophil disorders and their management. J Clin Pathol 2001;54:7–19.

Malech HL, Nauseef WM: Primary inherited defects in neutrophil function: Etiology and treatment. Semin Hematol 1997;34:279–290.

Sieff CA, Nisbet-Brown E, Nathan DG: Congenital bone marrow failure syndromes. Br J Haematol 2000;111:30–42.

Chronic Neutropenia

Ancliff PJ, Gale RE, Liesner R, et al: Mutations in the ELA2 gene encoding neutrophil elastase are present in most patients with sporadic sever congenital neutropenia but only in some patients with the familial form of the disease. Blood 2001;98:2645–2650.

Banerjee A, Shannon KM: Leukemic transformation in patients with severe congenital neutropenia. J Pediatr Hematol Oncol, 2001;23:487–495.

Dale DC, Bonilla MA, Davis MW, et al: A randomized controlled phase III trial of recombinant human G-CSF for treatment of severe chronic neutropenia. Blood 1993;81:2496.

Freedman MH, Bonilla MA, Fier C, et al: Myelodysplasia syndrome and acute myeloid leukemia in patients with congenital neutropenia receiving G-CSF therapy. Blood 2000;96:429–436.

Konishi N, Kobayashi M, Miyagawa S, et al: Defective proliferation of primitive myeloid progenitor cells in patients with severe congenital neutropenia. Blood 1999;94:4077–4083.

Li FQ, Horwitz M: Characterization of mutant neutrophil elastase in severe congenital neutropenia. J Biol Chem 2001;276:14230–14241.

Nakamura K, Kobayashi M, Konishi N, et al: Abnormalities of primitive myeloid progenitor cells expressing granulocyte colony-stimulating factor receptor in patients with severe congenital neutropenia. Blood 2000;96:366–369.

Welte K, Boxer LA: Severe chronic neutropenia: Pathophysiology and therapy. Semin Hematol 1997;34:1.

Zeidler C, Welte K, Barak Y, et al: Stem cell transplantation in patients with severe congenital neutropenia without evidence of leukemia transformation. Blood 2000;95:1195–1198.

Cyclic Neutropenia

Aprikyan AA, Liles WC, Rodger E, et al: Impaired survival of bone marrow hematopoietic progenitor cells in cyclic neutropenia. Blood 2001;97:147–153.

Mutations in the gene encoding neutrophil elastase in congenital and cyclic neutropenia. Blood 2000;96:2317–2322.

Haurie C, Dale DC, Mackey MC: Occurrence of periodic oscillations in the differential blood counts of congenital, idiopathic, and cyclical neutropenia patients before and during treatment with G-CSF. Exp Hematol 1999;27:401–409.

Horwitz M, Benson KF, Person RE, et al: Mutations in ElA2, encoding neutrophil elastase define a 21-day biological clock in cyclic haematopoiesis. Nat Genet 1999;23:433.

Palmer SE, Stephens K, Dale DC. Genetics, phenotype, and natural history of autosomal dominant cyclic hematopoiesis. Am J Med Genet 1996;66:413.

Hyper-IgE Syndrome

Buckley RH: The hyper-IgE syndrome. Clin Rev Allergy Immunol 2001;20:139–154.

Borges WG, Augustine NH, Hill HR: Defective interleukin-12-interferon-γ pathway in patients with hyperimmunoglobulin E syndrome. J Pediatr 2000;136:176.

Grimbacher B, Holland SM, Gallin JI, et al: Hyper-IgE syndrome with recurrent infections: An autosomal dominant multisystem disorder. N Engl J Med 1999;340:692–702.

Stiehm ER: Cytokine dysregulation in the hyperimmunoglobulin E syndrome. J Pediatr 2000;136:141–143.

Leukocyte Adhesion Deficiency

Arnaout MA: Leukocyte adhesion deficiency: Its structural basis, pathophysiology and implications for modulating the inflammatory response. Immunol Rev 1990;114:145.

Arnaout MA, Dana N, Gupta SK, et al: Point mutations impairing cell surface expression of the common β subunit (CD18) in a patient with leukocyte adhesion molecule (Leu-Cam) deficiency. J Clin Invest 1990;85:977.

Bunting M, Harris ES, McIntyre TM, et al: Leucocyte adhesion deficiency syndrome: Adhesion and tethering defects involving beta 2 integrins and selectin ligands. Curr Opin Hematol 2002;9:30–35.

Etzioni A, Doerschuk CM, Harlan JM: Of man and mouse: Leukocyte and endothelial adhesion molecule deficiencies. Blood 1999;94:4281–4288.

Fischer A, Lisowska-Grospierre B, Anderson DC, et al: Leukocyte adhesion deficiency: Molecular basis and functional consequences. Immunodef Rev 1988;1:39.

Shaw JM, Al-Shamkani A, Boxer LA, et al: Characterization of four CD18 mutants in leucocyte adhesion deficient (LAD patients with differential capacities to support expression and function of the CD11/CD18 integrins LFA-11, Mac-1 and p1'50,95. Clin Exp Immunol 2001;126:311–318.

Chédiak-Higashi Syndrome

Creel D, Boxer LA, Fauci AS: Visual and auditing anomalies in Chédiak-Higashi syndrome. Electroencephalogr Clin Neurophysiol 1983;5:252.

Haddad E, LeDeist F, Blanche S, et al: Treatment of Chédiak-Higashi syndrome by allogeneic bone marrow transplantation: Report of 10 cases. Blood 1995;85:3328.

Huizing M, Anikster Y, Gahl WA: Hermansky-Pudlak syndrome and Chédiak-Higashi syndrome: Disorders of vesicle formation and trafficking. Thromb Haemost 2001;86: 233–245.

Kjeldsen L, Calafat J, Borregaard N: Giant granules of neutrophils in Chédiak-Higashi syndrome are derived from azurophilic granules but not from specific and gelatinase granules. J Leukoc Biol 1998;64:72–77.

Merino F, Henle W, Ramerez-Duque P: Chronic active Epstein-Barr virus infection in patients with Chédiak-Higashi syndrome. J Clin Immunol 1986;6:229.

Nagle DL, Karim MA, Woolf EA, et al: Identification and mutation analysis of the complete gene for Chédiak-Higashi syndrome. Nat Genet 1996;14:307.

Chronic Granulomatous Disease

Bielorai B, Toren A, Wolach B, et al: Successful treatment of invasive aspergillosis in chronic granulomatous disease by granulocyte transfusions followed by peripheral blood stem cell transplantation. Bone Marrow Transplant 2000;26: 1025–1028.

Forrest CB, Forehand JR, Axtell RA, et al: Clinical features and current management of chronic granulomatous disease. Hematol Oncol Clin North Am 1988;2:253.

Goldblatt D, Thrasher AJ: Chronic granulomatous disease. Clin Exp Immunol 2000;122:1–9.

Hopkins PJ, Bemiller LS, Curnutte JT: Chronic granulomatous disease: Diagnosis and classification at the molecular level. Clin Lab Med 1992;12:277.

Horwitz ME, Barrett AJ, Brown MR: Treatment of chronic granulomatous disease with non-myeloablative conditioning and a T-cell-depleted hematopoietic allograft. N Engl J Med 2001;344:881–888.

International Chronic Granulomatous Disease Cooperative Study Group: A controlled trial of interferon gamma to prevent infection in chronic granulomatous disease. N Eng J Med 1991;324:509.

Kamani NR, Infante AJ: Chronic granulomatous disease and other disorders of neutrophil function. Clin Rev Allergy Immunol 2000;19:141–156.

Liese J, Kloos S, Jendrossek V, et al: Long-term follow-up and outcome of 39 patients with chronic granulomatous disease. J Pediatr 2000;137:687–693.

Morey R, Veber F, Blanche S, et al. Long-term itraconazole prophylaxis against *Aspergillus* infections in thirty-two patients with chronic granulomatous disease. J Pediatr 1994; 125:998.

Newburger PE, Cohen HJ, Rothchild SB, et al: Prenatal diagnosis of chronic granulomatous disease. N Eng J Med 1979;300:178.

Segal BH, Leto TL, Gallin JI, et al: Genetic, biochemical, and clinical features of chronic granulomatous disease. Medicine 2000;79:170–200.

Winkelstein JA, Marino MD, Johnston RB Jr, et al: Chronic granulomatous disease: Report on a national registry of 368 patients. Medicine 2000;79:155.

Chapter 57
Platelet Disorders: Acquired and Congenital

Christopher L. Carpenter

Platelets are small circulating cells that are specialized for thrombus formation. They originate by release from long cytoplasmic extensions of megakaryocytes. Megakaryocytes are found in many tissues, including the lung, but reside primarily in the bone marrow. Platelets lack organelles such as nuclei and mitochondria but contain dense granules and alpha granules that are unique to platelets. Dense granules contain adenosine diphosphate (ADP), serotonin, and calcium, and alpha granules contain a number of proteins, including fibrinogen and von Willebrand's factor. The average platelet survives eight to ten days in the circulation, and about one third of the total body mass of platelets is in the spleen.

Platelet thrombus formation requires adequate numbers of platelets, platelet activation, and platelet interaction with both the vessel wall and other platelets. In response to tissue injury, platelets adhere to areas of damage through specific receptors, the most important of which is glycoprotein Ib/IX, the von Willebrand's factor receptor. In response to signals generated by these receptors, platelets undergo a change in shape and secrete the contents of their granules. Secretion results in additional platelet stimulation, primarily through the adenosine diphosphate receptor. Stimulation of platelets also leads to activation of the fibrinogen receptor, glycoprotein IIb/IIIa, rendering it able to bind fibrinogen. Fibrinogen bridges glycoprotein IIb/IIIa receptors on different platelets, causing aggregation. Following stimulation, the surface of the platelet also becomes a site for activation of the protein clotting cascade, leading to the formation of fibrin.

Platelet disorders can result in either bleeding or pathologic thrombus formation and are characterized by thrombocytosis, thrombocytopenia, or abnormal platelet function. Thrombocytosis is a risk for thrombus formation in myeloproliferative diseases and is discussed in Chapter 73. Platelet function in myeloproliferative diseases is often abnormal, and patients might experience bleeding as well as thrombosis.

Thrombocytosis occurs after splenectomy and in association with inflammatory disorders, solid tumors, or iron deficiency, but thrombosis or bleeding is uncommon in reactive thrombocytosis.

Thrombocytopenia results from decreased platelet production, reduced platelet survival, or increased splenic sequestration. Splenic sequestration usually causes a mild to moderate reduction in the platelet count (rarely less than 40,000/μL) and does not require therapy that is specific for thrombocytopenia. The primary clinical manifestation of thrombocytopenia or abnormal platelet function is bleeding, but thrombocytopenia is also associated with thrombosis in heparin-induced thrombocytopenia, disseminated intravascular coagulation, or thrombotic thrombocytopenic purpura (TTP). Bleeding resulting from platelet disorders usually involves mucosal membranes: epistaxis, heavy menstrual bleeding, or gum bleeding. Purpura, or bleeding from small capillaries, is characteristic of profound thrombocytopenia.

Thrombocytopenia

Decreased platelet production has many causes, including congenital defects, drugs such as cancer chemotherapy, infections (HIV), and parvovirus or primary bone marrow disorders, such as aplastic anemia, leukemias, or myelodysplasia (see Table 36-1 in Chapter 36). Marrow replacement by fungal or mycobacterial infection, fibrosis, or tumor reduces platelet production, as can deficiencies of iron, folate, or vitamin B_{12}. Amegakaryocytic thrombocytopenia is a rare cause of thrombocytopenia autoimmune disorder that is treated as though it is an immune thrombocytopenia.

Drugs that cause platelet dysfunction, primarily aspirin and nonsteroidal anti-inflammatory agents, should be avoided in thrombocytopenic patients. Platelet transfusion is the primary therapy for most nonimmune causes of thrombocytopenia (see Chapter

DIAGNOSIS

CAUSES OF PLATELET DYSFUNCTION

Congenital Disorders
  Bernard-Soulier disease
  Glanzmann's thrombasthenia
  Storage pool disease
  Gray platelet syndrome
  Release disease
  May-Hegglin anomaly

Acquired Disorders
  Renal insufficiency and renal failure
  Drugs: aspirin, nonsteroidal anti-inflammatory
    agents
  Dysproteinemias
  Immune disorders

---

53). Transfusions are indicated to prevent spontaneous bleeding, to treat bleeding manifestations, or prophylactically, prior to invasive procedures. Prophylactic platelet transfusions should be given to patients who are expected to have prolonged thrombocytopenia from intensive chemotherapy, aplastic anemia, or myelodysplasia. Few patients bleed spontaneously with platelet counts greater than 10,000/µL, and using a threshold value of less than 10,000 platelets/µL as a trigger for prophylactic transfusion is generally safe. Thrombocytopenic patients who are septic or who have other coagulation abnormalities are more likely to bleed and should be transfused when the platelet count falls below 20,000/µL. A pooled pack of platelets from five or six random donors is usually sufficient to raise the platelet count to a safe level. The risks of platelet transfusions include acute febrile reactions, infection, and the development of alloimmunization. The latter risk can be reduced by limiting exposure to foreign leukocytes by using in-line filters, radiation-treated platelet products, or human leukocyte antigen (HLA)–matched platelets. Once alloimmunization develops, increments can be achieved in most patients by transfusing HLA–matched platelets.

Few data are available on the safety of invasive procedures in thrombocytopenic patients. A platelet count of 50,000/µL or greater is safe for most invasive procedures, and platelet counts of greater than 100,000/µL are recommended for neurosurgical or ophthalmologic procedures. Lumbar punctures could be safely done on children with leukemia and platelet counts greater than 10,000/µL.

The plasmin inhibitor ε-aminocaproic acid (EACA) reduces the incidence of bleeding in thrombocytopenic patients and may be useful in patients who either are refractory to platelet transfusions or have minor bleeding for which a transfusion is not

TREATMENT

Posttransfusion Purpura

Posttransfusion purpura is a rare cause of thrombocytopenia but may be catastrophic if not recognized and treated promptly. The characteristics of posttransfusion purpura are as follows:

- Thrombocytopenia, often profound with significant bleeding
- History of a recent transfusion (usually one week prior)
- Transfusion donor expresses an antigen not present on the patient's platelets, usually HPA-1a
- Patient has been previously sensitized to the antigen (usually from pregnancy or a previous transfusion)

The mechanism by which sensitization to an antigen not present on the patient's platelets leads to destruction of the patient's own platelets is obscure. The diagnosis is made on clinical grounds, but typing of the patient's and donor's platelets helps to confirm it. Platelet transfusions are not usually effective and should be reserved for life-threatening bleeding. Both plasma exchange and intravenous immunoglobulin are effective therapies. Because patients are often profoundly thrombocytopenic, intravenous immunoglobulin is safer, since it avoids the placement of a central venous catheter. Intravenous immunoglobulin should be given at a dose of 1 g/kg/day for two days. The platelet count usually increases within two to three days. Relapses may occur, requiring a second course of intravenous immunoglobulin, and some patients remain thrombocytopenic for up to six weeks.

necessary. ε-aminocaproic acid has a short half-life and should optimally be given every two hours; however, patients have responded to doses as low as 1 gram every four hours, decreased to 1 gram every six hours when bleeding stops. A loading dose should be used to treat acute bleeding, and the doses should be titrated on the basis of the patient's response. Side effects include orthostatic hypotension, nausea and vomiting, rhabdomyolysis, and the risk of thrombosis.

Thrombocytopenia resulting primarily from increased platelet destruction may be either immune-based or nonimmune based.

Drug-Induced Thrombocytopenia

Drugs cause thrombocytopenia by either direct marrow toxicity or inducing antibody-mediated platelet destruction. Drug-induced thrombocytopenia may occur soon after a drug is begun or may develop in patients who have been taking a drug for many years. The thrombocytopenia is often profound and accompanied by bleeding. Specific tests to identify drug-mediated antibody binding to platelets are not generally available, so the diagnosis often must be made on clinical grounds. Therapeutic measures, in addition to discontinuing the offending drug, depend on the patient's platelet count and symptoms. In drug-induced, immune-mediated thrombocytopenia, both prednisone and intravenous immunoglobulin speed recovery of the platelet count. Prednisone can be quickly tapered once the platelet count begins to recover. Plasmapheresis can lead to a more rapid resolution of thrombocytopenia, but it poses the risks associated with placement of a central venous catheter.

Heparin-induced thrombocytopenia is a common side effect of heparin administration. Approximately 3% of patients who receive unfractionated heparin for five or more days develop heparin-induced thrombocytopenia, and thrombosis occurs in approximately 50% of these individuals. Fewer than 1% of patients who receive low-molecular-weight heparin develop heparin-induced thrombocytopenia. Venous thrombosis is most common, but arterial thrombosis is also frequent. Some patients with heparin antibodies develop inflamed, sometimes necrotic, skin lesions at sites of heparin injections. Rarely patients with heparin antibodies have an acute systemic reaction to intravenous heparin involving chest pain, shortness of breath, fever, chills, vomiting, and diarrhea, which mandates stopping heparin.

Heparin-induced thrombocytopenia usually occurs between five and ten days after heparin is initiated; however, the onset may be sooner, particularly if the patient received heparin in the recent past.

Thrombocytopenia is usually moderate (50,000 to 100,000/μL) and the platelet count is rarely less than 10,000/μL. A small number of patients with heparin-induced thrombocytopenia have platelet counts that are normal but lower than their preheparin count. Given the potentially severe consequences of heparin-induced thrombocytopenia, it is appropriate to monitor the platelet count for patients who are receiving heparin, and the diagnosis should be suspected if thrombocytopenia develops.

The most common test currently available to detect heparin antibodies is an ELISA-based assay using heparin and platelet factor 4. This test is about 90% sensitive and 90% specific in most patients. Both this test and a test for heparin-dependent platelet activation are much less specific for heparin-induced thrombocytopenia associated with thrombosis if patients have undergone cardiac bypass surgery. In this setting, approximately 20% of patients have a positive activation test, and 50% have a positive platelet factor 4 ELISA test, but only 1% have a thrombosis. One should not be dissuaded from the diagnosis by a negative test if clinical suspicion is high. Tests of platelet activation by heparin in the presence of the patient's serum may correlate better with the clinical syndrome but are not widely available. Tests that rely on heparin-dependent platelet aggregation using platelet-rich plasma are not sufficiently sensitive.

All heparin administration should be stopped if heparin-induced thrombocytopenia is suspected, and platelet transfusions are contraindicated. Low-molecular-weight heparin should not be substituted because it is recognized by the antibody in about 90% of cases. If anticoagulation must be continued, three alternative anticoagulants are available: danaproid, lepirudin, and argatroban (Table 57-1). Lepirudin and argatroban are direct thrombin inhibitors; danaproid binds antithrombin and primarily inhibits Factor Xa. All three drugs are effective in the treatment of heparin-induced thrombocytopenia. Heparin-induced thrombocytopenia antibodies cross-react in vitro with danaproid in 10% to 20% of cases, but this cross-reactivity might not be clinically relevant. Doses of both danaproid and lepirudin must be reduced for patients with renal failure. Currently, danaproid is the drug of choice in pregnant patients with heparin-induced thrombocytopenia. It can be given subcutaneously, has been used successfully in pregnancy, and does not appear to cross the placenta. Lepirudin crosses the placenta, and there is no experience with either lepirudin or argatroban in pregnancy. Since both are administered intravenously, long-term treatment with either drug is complicated. Patients with heparin-induced thrombocytopenia have undergone surgery requiring cardiac bypass using

Table 57-1 ■ Comparison of Danaproid, Lepirudin, and Argatroban for the Treatment of Heparin-Induced Thrombocytopenia*

	Danaproid	Lepirudin	Aragtroban
Mechanism of action	Primarily inhibits Xa in a complex with Antithrombin III	Directly inhibits thrombin	Directly inhibits thrombin
Administration	IV or SC	IV	IV
Half-life	~24 hours	~1.3 hours	~30 minutes
Reversible	No	No	No
Monitoring	Anti-Xa activity, using a danaproid standard	aPTT	aPTT
Use in pregnancy	Several reported cases	No reported experience	No reported experience
Dose adjustment for renal failure	Yes, monitor Xa activity closely in patients with renal insufficiency	Yes, monitor Xa activity closely in patients with renal insufficiency	No
Dose adjustment for hepatic failure	No	No, but monitor aPTT frequently	Yes
Special considerations	Cross-reacts with HIT antibodies in some cases	Antibodies may develop to lepirudin and prolong the half-life	

*All three drugs are effective anticoagulants in patients with heparin-induced thrombocytopenia. The choice of drug depends on personal experience and patient characteristics such as renal or hepatic insufficiency desired route of administration. HIT: heparin-induced antibodies.

either danaproid, lepirudin, or a combination of heparin and the prostaglandin analog iloprost to inhibit platelet aggregation. The method of choice depends on local experience, since all of these methods of antico-agulation during bypass have potential complications, and lepirudin and danaproid are not reversible with protamine.

Warfarin should be initiated gradually for patients with heparin-induced thrombocytopenia who require continuing anticoagulation. High doses of warfarin can precipitously lower proteins C and S before anti-coagulation is achieved, exposing the patient to an increased risk of severe thrombosis. Patients with heparin-induced thrombocytopenia but no thrombo-sis are at increased risk of thrombosis for the next month. Warfarin administration does not reduce this risk.

Autoimmune Thrombocytopenic Purpura

Autoimmune thrombocytopenic purpura (ITP) is characterized by autoantibodies to platelet antigens, leading to platelet destruction by macrophages and the reticuloendothelial system. Immune thrombocytope-nia may be caused by drugs or infections or can occur in association with other autoimmune disorders or malignancies, but many cases are idiopathic. Even in the presence of an underlying disorder, idiopathic thrombocytopenic purpura is a diagnosis of exclusion.

Autoimmune thrombocytopenic purpura may be either acute or chronic. Acute idiopathic thrombocy-topenic purpura resolves within six months, is com-monly associated with viral infection and is most frequent in children and young adults. When the process persists longer than six months, it is termed chronic. This form is present in greater than 90% of adult patients. Until recently, chronic idiopathic thrombocytopenic purpura was thought to be most frequent in women under age 40 years, but it appears to be more common in older patients than previously appreciated and is equally common in older men and women. The primary risk of idiopathic thrombocy-topenic purpura is hemorrhage. The lifetime risk of fatal hemorrhage has been estimated to be approxi-mately 5% for all patients with chronic idiopathic thrombocytopenic purpura (including patients who respond to therapy and those who fail). The risk is increased in patients who have persistently low platelet counts and in elderly patients.

The diagnosis of idiopathic thrombocytopenic purpura should be considered in the evaluation of purpuric or membrane bleeding or if a low platelet count is incidentally discovered on a routine complete blood count. The primary focus of the history is to establish that the type of bleeding is consistent with thrombocytopenia and to identify potential causes of thrombocytopenia. A detailed drug history is important, including illicit drugs, over-the-counter preparations, herbal remedies, and supplements. Risk factors for HIV infection should also be ascertained, since idiopathic thrombocytopenic purpura is a common presentation of HIV infection. Pregnancy raises the possibility of several additional causes of thrombocytopenia. The focus of the physical examination is to be certain that the bleeding is consistent with thrombocytopenia, to determine the severity of any bleeding, and to identify clues to other causes of thrombocytopenia. Except for evidence of bleeding, patients with idiopathic thrombocytopenic purpura have a normal physical examination. The presence of splenomegaly or of lymphadenopathy in patients with idiopathic thrombocytopenic purpura suggests a cause of thrombocytopenia other than idiopathic thrombocytopenic purpura.

The most important laboratory tests in the evaluation of presumed idiopathic thrombocytopenic purpura are the complete blood count and examination of the blood smear. The complete blood count and peripheral smear in idiopathic thrombocytopenic purpura are normal except for the absence or reductions of platelets and increased platelet size. Any additional abnormalities should trigger a search for another cause of thrombocytopenia. Two types of platelet antibody tests have been used: platelet-associated immunoglobulin and antibodies specific for particular platelet antigens. Platelet-associated immunoglobulin is elevated in most cases of idiopathic thrombocytopenic purpura, and the test is about 90% sensitive. However, there are many other causes of increased platelet-associated immunoglobulin, so the test has a specificity of only about 25% and is not clinically useful. In chronic idiopathic thrombocytopenic purpura, antibodies are present to specific platelet antigens, most often glycoproteins IIb, IIIa, or Ib/IX. The presence of one of these antibodies is about 90% specific for idiopathic thrombocytopenic purpura, but the tests are only about 60% to 70% sensitive.

Additional laboratory tests that are useful include evaluation of liver and kidney function and an HIV test, if there are risk factors for infection. Antinuclear antibody tests are not generally helpful in the absence of additional evidence of autoimmune disease. Since solid tumors are associated with idiopathic thrombocytopenic purpura, it is important that routine cancer screening tests be up to date. Preliminary data suggest that *Helicobacter pylori* infection is frequent for patients with idiopathic thrombocytopenic purpura, and treatment of *H. pylori* infection leads to an improvement in platelet counts. If these data are confirmed, screening for and treatment of *H. pylori* infection would be an important aspect of the evaluation and treatment of idiopathic thrombocytopenic purpura. Results of a bone marrow biopsy are not diagnostic for idiopathic thrombocytopenic purpura, although the number of megakaryocytes is often increased. A bone marrow biopsy is not routinely necessary in evaluating patients with idiopathic thrombocytopenic purpura but is indicated if the patient is older than 60 years (because of the frequency of other causes of thrombocytopenia) or if there are unexplained hematologic or physical examination abnormalities. A bone marrow biopsy is often done before splenectomy to be certain that there is no other cause of thrombocytopenia.

Treatment of Idiopathic Thrombocytopenic Purpura

The goal of initial treatment of idiopathic thrombocytopenic purpura is to increase the platelet count to a safe level, allowing time for acute cases of idiopathic thrombocytopenic purpura to resolve. The acute idiopathic thrombocytopenic purpura of childhood usually resolves without therapy. Indications for active treatment in a thrombocytopenic patient include a platelet count below 20,000/μL, active bleeding, or risk factors for bleeding if the platelet count is below 50,000/μL. Patients who have a platelet count greater than 50,000/μL and are asymptomatic do not require active treatment.

Standard initial treatment of idiopathic thrombocytopenic purpura is prednisone 1 mg/kg/day. Responses occur in 70% to 80% of patients within three weeks. To avoid the side effects of prolonged glucocorticoid therapy, once the platelet count has normalized or reached a plateau, prednisone should be tapered over a four- to six-week period. The taper can be delayed if the platelet count begins to drop. When a dose of 10 mg/day is reached, changing to every-other-day prednisone to complete the taper may reduce the effects of prednisone withdrawal and of prednisone side effects. If prednisone is contraindicated or is not effective, intravenous immunoglobulin is given. Anti-D immune globulin can be used for patients who are Rh-positive. These therapies are more expensive than prednisone but no more effective. They should rarely be used for initial treatment. Since neither of these therapies causes immune suppression, they are useful for patients in whom immune suppression is of particular concern. The response to intravenous immunoglobulin or anti-D usually begins within two to four days and lasts three to four weeks. In children, intravenous immunoglobulin is used as initial treatment to prevent prednisone toxicity.

Splenectomy

At most, 20% of adult patients with idiopathic thrombocytopenic purpura have a complete and sustained remission following initial therapy. For patients who fail to respond to treatment and/or who require unacceptable doses of continuing prednisone therapy to maintain a response, splenectomy is the treatment of choice. Although platelet counts might not return to completely normal levels, two thirds of patients require no additional therapy after splenectomy. The likelihood of a good response to splenectomy inversely correlates with the age of the patient. A sustained response is more likely to occur when platelet recovery is rapid. Compared with laparotomy, laparoscopic splenectomy has reduced complications and hospital stay and has a very low operative mortality rate. The primary risk of splenectomy is fulminant sepsis. Prior to splenectomy, the patient should receive pneumococcus, *Haemophilus influenzae* B, and meningococcus vaccines.

Splenectomy Failures

Treatment of patients who do not respond to splenectomy or who subsequently relapse is challenging, and there is no consensus about the best approach. One approach is shown in Figure 57-1. The goal of medical treatment is to maintain the platelet count in an acceptable range with tolerable side effects from the drugs. A discussion with the patient about the goals and side effects of therapies and the risks of thrombocytopenia is important in determining the best therapy. Ideally, a platelet count greater than 30,000/μL could be attained, but this is not always possible. Since significant bleeding is not common with platelet counts greater than 10,000/μL, no therapy, even with platelet counts between 10,000/μL and 20,000/μL, may be the best option for some patients.

A liver/spleen scan should be done to detect an accessory spleen, which may be present and functioning in up to 10% of patients with idiopathic thrombocytopenic purpura following splenectomy. Removal of an accessory spleen may be beneficial and may be associated with a modest long-term effect on platelet counts. Initial medical therapy in refractory cases is prednisone, since some patients maintain a safe platelet count on low dose prednisone (less than 5 to 10 mg/day). Patients who fail to respond to prednisone and have significant bleeding can be treated with chronic intravenous immunoglobulin therapy. Approximately three quarters of patients respond to intravenous immunoglobulin, but one third of patients become refractory. Side effects are usually tolerable, but intravenous immunoglobulin is expensive and in limited supply. Some patients have long-

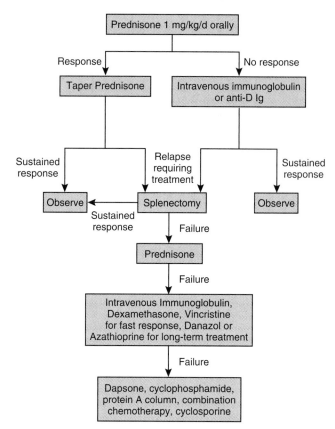

Figure 57-1 ■ Algorithm for the treatment of chronic idiopathic autoimmune thrombocytopenia in adults. Standard initial treatment is prednisone. Patients who do not respond to prednisone or relapse following a taper and require therapy should usually have a splenectomy. Patients who relapse following splenectomy and require therapy should be treated with prednisone. Many therapies have been tried in patients who fail prednisone or require a high maintenance dose, and there are no clear best alternative therapies. A decision should be made balancing toxicity and potential benefit. One approach is presented in the figure, but this might not be optimal for all patients.

term remissions following chronic intravenous immunoglobulin, but for most it is temporizing therapy. Vinca alkaloids can be used for patients who fail to respond to intravenous immunoglobulin or become refractory, but they rarely induce long-term remissions, and vincristine has cumulative neurotoxicity. Anti-D immune globulin does not work well after a splenectomy.

Several options exist for long-term therapy for patients who do not respond to prednisone or require a high maintenance dose of prednisone. Approximately one half of patients with idiopathic thrombocytopenic purpura respond to danazol, and some have long-term remissions. Following a response to danazol, prednisone can be tapered if the patient is also taking prednisone. Danazol should be continued for at least six months because some patients do not respond earlier and relapses are common in responding patients who stop danazol earlier.

A course of high-dose dexamethasone might induce remission, but the success rate has not been high in many studies. Nevertheless, if low-dose prednisone therapy is not adequate, a course of high-dose dexamethasone can be tried and may induce remission or may be substituted as intermittent pulses of therapy instead of chronic prednisone. Approximately half of patients respond to azathioprine, and about 20% have a lasting remission. The response to azathioprine may be delayed, and the drug should be continued for four months before it is deemed a failure. Approximately 60% of patients respond to cyclophosphamide, and 20% to 30% have a sustained remission following completion of therapy. Like azathioprine, cyclophosphamide is not a good choice for women who may become pregnant and cannot be used during pregnancy.

A number of other therapies have been reported to work in idiopathic thrombocytopenic purpura. Thirty percent to 50% response rates to dapsone have been reported, but dapsone appears to work less well for patients who have failed splenectomy. Nearly one third of patients have a sustained response to a course of treatment by means of immunoglobulin removal with protein A columns. Isolated responses to ascorbic acid, colchicine, interferon, and cyclosporins have been reported. Plasma exchange may result in transient increases in the platelet count but not sustained responses.

Life-threatening bleeding should be treated with a combination of high-dose corticosteroids (methylprednisolone 1 g/day for three days), platelet transfusions, and intravenous immunoglobulin (1 gram/kg/day for two days). Although the half-life of transfused platelets is reduced in idiopathic thrombocytopenic purpura, most patients do have a short-term increase in the platelet count following transfusion. Intravenous immunoglobulin and high-dose glucocorticoids may increase the half-life of transfused and endogenous platelets.

Idiopathic Thrombocytopenic Purpura in Pregnancy

Treatment of idiopathic thrombocytopenic purpura during pregnancy is complicated by the risk of fetal and neonatal thrombocytopenia and the side effects of therapy on the fetus. A decision to begin therapy should be based on the same factors as in nonpregnant patients with idiopathic thrombocytopenic purpura. A platelet count lower than 50,000/µL is an indication for treatment in the third trimester. Many anesthesiologists require a platelet count greater than 80,000/µL for epidural anesthesia, and a decision

might need to be made about whether to use alternative forms of analgesia or use intravenous immunoglobulin or prednisone to raise the platelet count to this level. Both glucocorticoids and intravenous immunoglobulin have been used successfully for treatment of idiopathic thrombocytopenic purpura in pregnant women, and there is controversy about which therapy is better. Prednisone is cheaper and easier to administer, but it may cause or worsen gestational diabetes, contribute to hypertension, and lead to premature birth. Intravenous immunoglobulin does not appear to have any affects on the fetus, and side effects for the mother are usually mild. The balance of risks and benefits favors intravenous immunoglobulin as the treatment of choice in pregnant women with idiopathic thrombocytopenic purpura. Splenectomy is avoided during pregnancy, except during the second trimester. In the first trimester, splenectomy is associated with fetal loss and it is technically difficult in the third trimester.

Approximately 10% of babies born to mothers with idiopathic thrombocytopenic purpura have platelet counts less than 50,000/µL, and 5% have a platelet count less than 20,000. About 1.5% of infants born to mothers with idiopathic thrombocytopenic purpura will suffer intracranial hemorrhage or death. The only factor that predicts the baby's platelet count is the platelet count at birth of a sibling. The mother's platelet count does not correlate with the baby's count, and treatment of the mother with prednisone or intravenous immunoglobulin does not appear to affect the fetal platelet count. Since it is not possible to accurately predict which babies will have either thrombocytopenia or bleeding, there is controversy regarding whether the baby's platelet count should be determined before birth and whether a low fetal platelet count is an indication for cesarean delivery.

Fetal platelet counts can be determined either by fetal scalp vein sampling or by percutaneous umbilical blood sampling, but both methods have limitations. Fetal scalp vein sampling can be done only after cervical dilation and gives an interpretable result only about half of the time. In some studies, incorrect results were obtained and acted on. Percutaneous umbilical blood sampling is much more accurate but carries a risk of fetal bleeding and death and should be performed only by very experienced physicians. For most women with idiopathic thrombocytopenic purpura, cesarean section should be done for obstetrical indications. If the mother had a previous infant with a platelet count below 20,000/µL, the risks and benefits of either determining the fetal platelet count or planning a cesarean delivery should be presented to the patient by the consulting hematologist and the obstetrician. The baby may also develop thrombocytopenia following birth, so a platelet count should be checked at birth and repeated for three days if the initial count is normal. If the fetal platelet count is low at birth, it should be followed daily until it begins to increase. Central nervous system ultrasound to rule out intracranial hemorrhage is indicated if the platelet count is less than 50,000/μL.

Idiopathic Thrombocytic Purpura in the HIV-Infected Patient

Autoimmune thrombocytopenic purpura may occur as a presenting illness in HIV infection or early in drug treatment as the immune system reconstitutes. It responds to the same therapies as idiopathic thrombocytopenic purpura. Autoimmune thrombocytopenic purpura also often responds to treatment of underlying HIV infection. Early studies showed a response of platelets to zidovudine, and recent experience indicates that HIV-associated idiopathic thrombocytopenic purpura responds to highly active anti-retroviral therapy (HAART). If thrombocytopenic HIV-positive patients have platelet counts below 20,000/μL or are bleeding, then specific therapy for idiopathic thrombocytopenic purpura should be instituted, as well as highly active antiretroviral therapy. Prednisone is the standard therapy, but if further immune suppression is of particular concern, intravenous immunoglobulin or anti-D immune globulin can be used. Splenectomy is also successful in treating idiopathic thrombocytopenic purpura associated with HIV infection and should be considered if patients relapse after initial therapy and do not respond to antiretroviral therapy.

Thrombotic Thrombocytopenic Purpura

Thrombotic thrombocytopenic purpura (TTP) is characterized by thrombocytopenia, microangiopathic hemolytic anemia, and complications of small-vessel thrombosis. Thrombotic thrombocytic purpura can have a broad spectrum of manifestations, but organ involvement may be limited to renal failure, thrombocytopenia, and anemia (hemolytic uremic syndrome, HUS). The history, physical examination, and laboratory evaluation should focus on identifying a cause of thrombotic thrombocytopenic purpura and the extent of organ involvement. Most cases of thrombotic thrombocytopenic purpura/hemolytic uremic syndrome are idiopathic, but hemolytic uremic syndrome may result from *Escherichia coli* strain O157:H7. The antiplatelet agents ticlopidine and clopidogrel, perhaps the Norplant contraceptive, bone marrow transplantation, cancer chemotherapy, HIV infection, and pregnancy are all associated with thrombotic thrombocytopenic purpura.

Microangiopathic hemolytic anemia is diagnosed by the presence of schistocytes on the peripheral blood smear (Figure 57-2). Other findings include an elevated lactate dehydrogenase level, renal insufficiency, fever, neurologic changes, and abdominal symptoms. Patients with risk factors should be tested for HIV infection. Occasionally, thrombotic thrombocytopenic purpura can be difficult to distinguish from other causes of microangiopathic hemolytic anemia, including malignant hypertension, lupus nephritis, and disseminated intravascular coagulation.

Plasma exchange is the cornerstone of therapy for most cases of thrombotic thrombocytopenic purpura and has made a dramatic difference in patient survival. Daily exchanges of 1 to 1.5 plasma volumes are standard for one week but should be continued if the platelet count has not recovered or if the lactate dehydrogenase level rises. Replacement with cryo-poor supernatant (the supernatant of fresh frozen plasma after cryoprecipitation) may be more effective than replacement with fresh frozen plasma because some patients who failed to respond to fresh frozen plasma did respond to cryo-poor supernatant. Red cell transfusions should be given as needed. Platelet transfusions are contraindicated, except for life-threatening bleeding, since they may worsen the thrombotic complications.

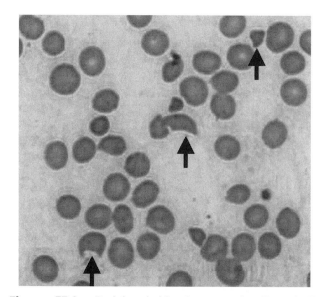

Figure 57-2 ■ Peripheral blood smear in thrombotic thrombocytopenic purpura. The peripheral blood smear in thrombotic thrombocytopenic purpura is characterized by schistocytes and red blood cell fragments (arrows). The number of schistocytes in thrombotic thrombocytopenic purpura can vary greatly and does not correlate well with severity, but they are the sine qua non of thrombotic thrombocytopenic purpura. (See Color Plate 14.)

The roles of corticosteroids and antiplatelet agents in the treatment of thrombotic thrombocytopenic purpura are controversial. Corticosteroids alone have cured some patients with thrombotic thrombocytopenic purpura, and the evidence for an immune basis for thrombotic thrombocytopenic purpura provides theoretical grounds for their use, but there is no evidence to indicate whether they add any benefit to plasma exchange alone. Corticosteroids and aspirin may be used in conjunction with plasma exchange as initial therapy or may be added if patients do not respond to plasma exchange alone.

The most important parameters to follow in assessing response are the patient's clinical status, particularly the neurologic status, and the platelet count. Because schistocytes can persist into remission, the number of schistocytes does not provide a useful index of response. The lactate dehydrogenase level often decreases initially, since it is removed during plasma exchange but also continues to fall in responding patients as tissue damage and hemolysis abate. In many patients, the response to plasma exchange is slow or delayed, and in cases of hemolytic-uremic syndrome, resolution of renal failure may lag hematologic recovery by many days. If the patient does not respond to therapy or worsens, additional measures should be instituted. Corticosteroids and antiplatelet agents should be added if they were not used initially, and if fresh frozen plasma was used during plasma exchange, cryopoor supernatant should be substituted. Patients may also respond to more plasma exchange, either by increasing the frequency to twice daily or by increasing the volume of exchange during a single session.

The three therapies that appear to be most successful for patients who fail plasma exchange are protein A column absorption plasma treatment, vincristine, and splenectomy. Since the response to plasma exchange may be delayed and alternative therapies are not well established, it is reasonable to wait five to seven days to consider alternative therapy unless the patient deteriorates dramatically in spite of plasma exchange. Occasionally, patients with thrombotic thrombocytopenic purpura have frequent relapses, and both splenectomy and combination chemotherapy have been successful in treating chronic relapsing thrombotic thrombocytopenic purpura.

Plasma exchange should continue at least until the platelet count is 100,000/μL, and many continue plasma exchange until the platelet count is normal. Thirty percent of patients with thrombotic thrombocytopenic purpura relapse, and many of these occur early on. Frequent complete blood counts after plasma exchange are warranted to detect recurrence. The interval at which complete blood counts are checked can be progressively lengthened over the first month. Relapses may also occur months and years later. Routine blood counts cannot be expected to detect these recurrences before symptoms develop, but blood counts should be obtained if a patient with a history of thrombotic thrombocytopenic purpura develops any suspicious symptoms.

Not all patients require or benefit from plasma exchange. Children with *E. coli* O157:H7-induced hemolytic uremic syndrome do well with supportive therapy alone, but the survival of older adults with *E. coli* O157:H7-induced hemolytic uremic syndrome is improved by plasma exchange. Most patients with thrombotic thrombocytopenic purpura/hemolytic uremic syndrome secondary to bone marrow transplantation or following cancer chemotherapy do not respond well to plasma exchange. Some patients with thrombotic thrombocytopenic purpura following bone marrow transplantation respond to cyclosporine or intravenous immunoglobulin. Patients with cancer chemotherapy-induced thrombotic thrombocytopenic purpura may respond better to treatment with protein A column adsorption.

Thrombocytopenia in Pregnancy

Any cause of thrombocytopenia may also occur in pregnant women, but some forms of thrombocytopenia are more frequent in or unique to pregnancy. Mild thrombocytopenia occurs in about 7% of pregnant women. This benign thrombocytopenia of pregnancy is a diagnosis of exclusion but is the likely diagnosis when it is associated with the absence of prior thrombocytopenia, onset in the third trimester, and a platelet greater than 80,000/μL. It might not be possible to distinguish benign thrombocytopenia of pregnancy from idiopathic thrombocytopenic purpura, however. In the third trimester of pregnancy, microangiopathic hemolytic anemia due to preeclampsia, HELLP syndrome (hemolysis, elevated liver enzymes, and low platelets), thrombotic thrombocytopenic purpura/hemolytic uremic syndrome, or disseminated intramuscular coagulation may occur. HELLP syndrome or thrombotic thrombocytopenic purpura/hemolytic uremic syndrome may also occur postpartum.

In the obstetrical setting, disseminated intravascular coagulation is easily distinguished from other causes of thrombocytopenia because of the presence of a clear precipitating event such as a retained dead fetus and associated clotting factor consumption, elevated prothrombin time, and partial thromboplastin time, decreased fibrinogen, increased D-dimer, and the appearance of increased fibrin degradation products.

The most important component of therapy is treatment of the precipitating cause. Platelet and fresh frozen plasma transfusion are indicated for bleeding.

HELLP syndrome is a form of preeclampsia, but in 20% of patients with HELLP, hypertension is absent, and in 10%, there is no proteinuria. HELLP syndrome occurs most often between 32 and 34 weeks of pregnancy but may occur earlier. In a significant number of patients, HELLP occurs postpartum. HELLP syndrome is usually detected either when hypertension or right upper quadrant or epigastric pain is evaluated. HELLP syndrome is distinguished from thrombotic thrombocytopenic purpura by the elevation of the liver transaminases and more prominent abdominal symptoms. It is not possible to distinguish thrombotic thrombocytopenic purpura from severe preeclampsia or HELLP syndrome in all cases, and if thrombotic thrombocytopenic purpura cannot be excluded, plasma exchange is indicated.

If HELLP syndrome begins early in the third trimester, the relative merits of temporizing therapies to delay the need for delivery must be weighed against the risks. Recent evidence indicates that high-dose corticosteroids improve the hematologic manifestations of HELLP syndrome, and if blood pressure can be controlled, it may be possible to delay delivery in women with the onset of HELLP syndrome early in the third trimester.

Neonatal Alloimmune Thrombocytopenia

Mismatch of maternal and fetal platelet antigens (most often HPA-1a) can result in destruction of fetal platelets by maternal antibodies. The possibility of neonatal alloimmune thrombocytopenia is usually raised by either a family or personal history of a baby born with thrombocytopenia. Typing of the mother's and father's platelet antigens can confirm the mismatch. The incidence of neonatal alloimmune thrombocytopenia in subsequent pregnancies approaches 90% and appears to be highest with HPA-1a incompatibility. Therapy of neonatal alloimmune thrombocytopenia is complicated and controversial. Effective therapies include fetal platelet transfusions and maternal administration of intravenous immunoglobulin or corticosteroids.

Platelet Function Defects

Normal platelets sense stimuli and activate signaling pathways that lead to secretion, aggregation, and clot formation. Defects in the ability to sense or respond to these signals can cause bleeding disorders. A number of inherited abnormalities of platelet function have been described, and the responsible genetic abnormality has been identified in many cases. Inherited platelet function disorders can be classified by the type of platelet function affected: membrane receptors, granules, or signal transduction pathways. In Glanzmann's thrombasthenia, a defect in GP IIb/IIIa prevents platelet aggregation to all agonists except ristocetin. Defects in the von Willebrand's factor receptor, GP Ib/IX, cause Bernard-Soulier disease and are characterized by lack of aggregation to ristocetin but normal aggregation to other agonists. Disorders of secretion may be due to dense or alpha granule abnormalities or deficiency. Defects in the signal transduction pathways leading to secretion and activation of GP IIb/IIIa may affect both secretion and aggregation. Platelets are also important as a site for activation for generation of fibrin, and this function is deficient in platelets from patients with Scott syndrome.

Patients with inherited defects in platelet function should avoid drugs that affect platelet function. Acute bleeding episodes in many patients with platelet function disorders can be treated with 1-deamino-8-D-arginine vasopressin (DDAVP), in addition to local measures. Defects in granule secretion seem to respond best to DDAVP, and patients with Glanzmann's disease or Scott syndrome do not respond. Before using DDAVP to treat a platelet defect prior to an invasive procedure, the patient's response to DDAVP should be determined in the clinic by measuring the bleeding time before and after DDAVP administration. The usual intravenous DDAVP dose is 0.3 µg/kg. Availability of a preparation of DDAVP that is administered intranasally allows patients to treat bleeding episodes promptly themselves. The mechanism of action of DDAVP in platelet disorders is not known. DDAVP causes the release of von Willebrand's factor from endothelial cells and has a direct effect on platelets that sensitizes them to agonists.

Epsilon-aminocaproic acid is also helpful for minor bleeding episodes. Oral contraceptive pills often significantly reduce menstrual blood loss in women with bleeding disorders. Recent reports suggest that recombinant activated factor VII (rVIIa) is beneficial in the treatment of Glanzmann's, Bernard-Soulier, and pseudo von Willebrand's disease. For treatment of life-threatening bleeding or conditions that do not respond to DDAVP or local measures, platelet transfusions are necessary. The risk of alloimmunization is an important consideration if repeated platelet transfusions will be necessary. Therefore, platelet transfusions should be used only when absolutely necessary, and human leukocyte antigen–matched donors should be used when possible.

Acquired platelet dysfunction is fairly common (aspirin use being the most frequent cause) and usually does not require treatment. Significant bleeding following cardiac bypass surgery may be caused by platelet dysfunction resulting from platelet trauma by the pump. Regardless of the platelet count, platelet transfusions should be given if bleeding occurs. Clinically important bleeding may also result from platelet dysfunction due to uremia. If immediate treatment is not required, dialysis and an increase in the hematocrit reduce the hemorrhagic diathesis. Platelet function can be improved more quickly by administration of DDAVP. Conjugated estrogens can also be used to treat uremic bleeding and work within six hours when given intravenously. Cryoprecipitate has also been used to treat uremic bleeding, but DDAVP is equally effective and does not involve the risks of transfusion. Platelet transfusions are of limited benefit because uremia will also impair their function. Platelet dysfunction may also contribute to bleeding in severe liver disease. DDAVP shortens the bleeding time and may be beneficial prior to invasive procedures but has not been beneficial in treating variceal bleeding.

References

General

Balduini CL, Noris P, Belletti S, et al: In vitro and in vivo effects of desmopressin on platelet function. Haematologica 1999;84:891–896.

Development Task Force of the College of American Pathologists. Practice parameter for the use of fresh-frozen plasma, cryoprecipitate, and platelets: Fresh-Frozen Plasma, Cryoprecipitate, and Platelets Administration Practice Guidelines. JAMA 1994;271:777–781.

Heckman KD, Weiner GJ, Davis CS, et al: Randomized study of prophylactic platelet transfusion threshold during induction therapy for adult acute leukemia: 10,000/microL versus 20,000/microL. J Clin Oncol 1997;15:1143–1149.

Howard SC, Gajjar A, Ribeiro RC, et al: Safety of lumbar puncture for children with acute lymphoblastic leukemia and thrombocytopenia. JAMA 2000;284:2222–2224.

Mannucci PM: Desmopressin (DDAVP) in the treatment of bleeding disorders: The first twenty years. Haemophilia 2000;6(Suppl 1):60–67.

Rath W, Faridi A, Dudenhausen JW: HELLP syndrome. J Perinat Med 2000;28:249–260.

Rebulla P, Finazzi G, Marangoni F, et al: The threshold for prophylactic platelet transfusions in adults with acute myeloid leukemia. Gruppo Italiano Malattie Ematologiche Maligne dell'Adulto. N Engl J Med 1997;337:1870–1875.

The Trial to Reduce Alloimmunization to Platelets Study Group. Leukocyte reduction and ultraviolet B irradiation of platelets to prevent alloimmunization and refractoriness to platelet transfusions. N Engl J Med 1997;337:1861–1869.

Wandt H, Frank M, Ehninger G, et al: Safety and cost effectiveness of a 10 × 10(9)/L trigger for prophylactic platelet transfusions compared with the traditional 20 × 10(9)/L trigger: A prospective comparative trial in 105 patients with acute myeloid leukemia. Blood 1998;91:3601–3606.

HIV Infection

Aboulafia DM, Bundow D, Waide S, et al: Initial observations on the efficacy of highly active antiretroviral therapy in the treatment of HIV-associated autoimmune thrombocytopenia. Am J Med Sci 2000;320:117–123.

Immune Thrombocytopenic Purpura

Bartholomew JR, Salgia R, Bell W: Control of bleeding in patients with immune and nonimmune thrombocytopenia with aminocaproic acid. Arch Intern Med 1989;149:1959–1961.

Bell WR, Braine HG, Ness PM, Kickler TS. Improved survival in thrombotic thrombocytopenic purpura-hemolytic uremic syndrome: Clinical experience in 108 patients. N Engl J Med 1991;325:398–403.

Bussel JB, Pham LC, Aledort L, Nachman R: Maintenance treatment of adults with chronic refractory immune thrombocytopenic purpura using repeated intravenous infusions of gammaglobulin. Blood 1988;72:121–127.

Carr JM, Kruskall MS, Kaye JA, Robinson SH: Efficacy of platelet transfusions in immune thrombocytopenia. Am J Med 1986;80:1051–1054.

Chong BH, Keng TB: Advances in the diagnosis of idiopathic thrombocytopenic purpura. Semin Hematol 2000;37:249–260.

Cohen YC, Djulbegovic B, Shamai-Lubovitz O, Mozes B: The bleeding risk and natural history of idiopathic thrombocytopenic purpura in patients with persistent low platelet counts. Arch Intern Med 2000;160:1630–1638.

Facon T, Caulier MT, Fenaux P, et al: Accessory spleen in recurrent chronic immune thrombocytopenic purpura. Am J Hematol 1992;41:184–189.

Frederiksen H, Schmidt K: The incidence of idiopathic thrombocytopenic purpura in adults increases with age. Blood 1999;94:909–913.

Gasbarrini A, Franceschi F, Tartaglione R, et al: Regression of autoimmune thrombocytopenia after eradication of *Helicobacter pylori*. Lancet 1998;352:878.

George JN, Kojouri K, Perdue JJ, Vesely SK: Management of patients with chronic, refractory idiopathic thrombocytopenic purpura. Semin Hematol 2000;37:290–298.

George JN, Woolf SH, Raskob GE, et al: Idiopathic thrombocytopenic purpura: A practice guideline developed by explicit methods for the American Society of Hematology. Blood 1996;88:3–40.

Gill KK, Kelton JG: Management of idiopathic thrombocytopenic purpura in pregnancy. Semin Hematol 2000;37:275–289.

McMillan R: Therapy for adults with refractory chronic immune thrombocytopenic purpura. Ann Intern Med 1997;126:307–314.

Scaradavou A, Woo B, Woloski BM, et al: Intravenous anti-D treatment of immune thrombocytopenic purpura: Experience in 272 patients. Blood 1997;89:2689–2700.

Thrombotic Thrombocytopenia Purpura

Alessandrino EP, Martinelli G, Canevari A, et al: Prompt response to high-dose intravenous immunoglobulins given as first-line therapy in post-transplant thrombotic thrombocytopenic purpura. Bone Marrow Transplant 2000;25:1217–1218.

Bobbio-Pallavicini E, Gugliotta L, Centurioni R, et al: Antiplatelet agents in thrombotic thrombocytopenic purpura (TTP): Results of a randomized multicenter trial by the Italian Cooperative Group for TTP. Haematologica 1997;82:429–435.

Bobbio-Pallavicini E, Porta C, Centurioni R, et al: Vincristine sulfate for the treatment of thrombotic thrombocytopenic purpura refractory to plasma-exchange. The Italian Cooperative Group for TTP. Eur J Haematol 1994;52:222–226.

Brooker JZ: Clopidogrel and thrombotic thrombocytopenic purpura. N Engl J Med 2000;343:1192,1193–1194.

Dundas S, Murphy J, Soutar RL, et al: Effectiveness of therapeutic plasma exchange in the 1996 Lanarkshire *Escherichia coli* O157:H7 outbreak. Lancet 1999;354:1327–1330.

Egerman RS, Witlin AG, Friedman SA, Sibai BM: Thrombotic thrombocytopenic purpura and hemolytic uremic syndrome in pregnancy: Review of 11 cases. Am J Obstet Gynecol 1996;175:950–956.

Fraser JL, Millenson M, Malynn ER, et al: Possible association between the Norplant contraceptive system and thrombotic thrombocytopenic purpura. Obstet Gynecol 1996;87:860–863.

Furlan M, Robles R, Galbusera M, et al: von Willebrand factor-cleaving protease in thrombotic thrombocytopenic purpura and the hemolytic-uremic syndrome. N Engl J Med 1998; 339:1578–1584.

Gaddis TG, Guthrie TH, Drew MJ, et al: Treatment of plasma refractory thrombotic thrombocytopenic purpura with protein A immunoabsorption. Am J Hematol 1997; 55:55–58.

George JN: How I treat patients with thrombotic thrombocytopenic purpura-hemolytic uremic syndrome. Blood 2000; 96:1223–1229.

Gordon LI, Kwaan HC: Cancer- and drug-associated thrombotic thrombocytopenic purpura and hemolytic uremic syndrome. Semin Hematol 1997;34:140–147.

Page Y, Tardy B, Zeni F, Comtet C, et al: Thrombotic thrombocytopenic purpura related to ticlopidine. Lancet 1991;337:774–776.

Rock GA, Shumak KH, Buskard NA, et al: Comparison of plasma exchange with plasma infusion in the treatment of thrombotic thrombocytopenic purpura: Canadian Apheresis Study Group. N Engl J Med 1991;325:393–397.

Schriber JR, Herzig GP: Transplantation-associated thrombotic thrombocytopenic purpura and hemolytic uremic syndrome. Semin Hematol 1997;34:126–133.

Slichter SJ: Algorithm for managing the platelet refractory patient. J Clin Apheresis 1997;12:4–9.

Snyder HW, Mittelman A, Oral A, et al: Treatment of cancer chemotherapy-associated thrombotic thrombocytopenic purpura/hemolytic uremic syndrome by protein A immunoadsorption of plasma. Cancer 1993;71:1882–1892.

Sutor GC, Schmidt RE, Albrecht H: Thrombotic microangiopathies and HIV infection: Report of two typical cases, features of HUS and TTP, and review of the literature. Infection 1999;27:12–15.

Thompson CE, Damon LE, Ries CA, Linker CA: Thrombotic

microangiopathies in the 1980s: Clinical features, response to treatment, and the impact of the human immunodeficiency virus epidemic. Blood 1992;80:1890–1895.

Tsai HM, Lian EC: Antibodies to von Willebrand factor-cleaving protease in acute thrombotic thrombocytopenic purpura. N Engl J Med 1998;339:1585–1594.

van Ojik H, Biesma DH, Fijnheer R, et al: Cyclosporin for thrombotic thrombocytopenic purpura after autologous bone marrow transplantation. Br J Haematol 1997;96:641–643.

Platelet Dysfunction

Buss DH, Cashell AW, O'Connor ML, et al: Occurrence, etiology, and clinical significance of extreme thrombocytosis: A study of 280 cases. Am J Med 1994;96:247–253.

Thrombocytopenia in Pregnancy

Christiaens GC, Nieuwenhuis HK, Bussel JB: Comparison of platelet counts in first and second newborns of mothers with immune thrombocytopenic purpura. Obstet Gynecol 1997;90:546–552.

Kaplan C, Murphy, Kroll H, Waters AH: Feto-maternal alloimmune thrombocytopenia: Antenatal therapy with intravenous immunoglobulin G and steroids—more questions than answers. European Working Group on FMAIT. Br J Haematol 1998;100:62–65.

Laskin CA, Bombardier C, Hannah ME, et al: Prednisone and aspirin in women with autoantibodies and unexplained recurrent fetal loss. N Engl J Med 1997;337:148–153.

O'Brien JM, Milligan DA, Barton JR: Impact of high-dose corticosteroid therapy for patients with HELLP (hemolysis, elevated liver enzymes, and low platelet count) syndrome. Am J Obstet Gynecol 2000;183:921–924.

Heparin-Induced Thrombocytopenia

Greinacher A, Eichler P, Lubenow N, et al: Heparin-induced thrombocytopenia with thromboembolic complications: Meta-analysis of 2 prospective trials to assess the value of parenteral treatment with lepirudin and its therapeutic aPTT range. Blood 2000;96:846–851.

Magnani HN: Heparin-induced thrombocytopenia (HIT): An overview of 230 patients treated with orgaran (Org 10172). Thromb Haemost 1993;70:554–561.

Popov D, Zarrabi MH, Foda H, Graber G: Pseudopulmonary embolism: Acute respiratory distress in the syndrome of heparin-induced thrombocytopenia. Am J Kidney Dis 1997;29:449–452.

Warkentin TE: Heparin-induced thrombocytopenia: A ten-year retrospective. Annu Rev Med 1999;50:129–147.

Warkentin TE, Elavathil LJ, Hayward CP, et al: The pathogenesis of venous limb gangrene associated with heparin-induced thrombocytopenia. Ann Intern Med 1997; 127:804–812.

Warkentin TE, Hirte HW, Anderson DR, et al: Transient global amnesia associated with acute heparin-induced thrombocytopenia. Am J Med 1994;97:489–491.

Warkentin TE, Sheppard JA, Horsewood P, et al: Impact of the patient population on the risk for heparin-induced thrombocytopenia. Blood 2000;96:1703–1708.

Warkentin TE, Sikov WM, Lillicrap DP: Multicentric warfarin-induced skin necrosis complicating heparin-induced thrombocytopenia. Am J Hematol 1999;62:44–48.

Platelet Dysfunction

Griesshammer M, Bangerter M, Sauer T, et al: Aetiology and clinical significance of thrombocytosis: Analysis of 732 patients with an elevated platelet count. J Intern Med 1999;245:295–300.

Poon MC, d'Oiron R: Recombinant activated factor VII (Novo-Seven) treatment of platelet-related bleeding disorders: International Registry on Recombinant Factor VIIa and Congenital Platelet Disorders Group. Blood Coagul Fibrinolysis 2000;11(Suppl 1):S55-S68.

Rao AK: Congenital disorders of platelet function: Disorders of signal transduction and secretion. Am J Med Sci 1998; 316:69–76.

Chapter 58
Coagulation Disorders: Acquired and Congenital

Craig M. Kessler and Arafat Tfayli

Hemostasis consists of a complex series of mechanisms that maintains the integrity of a closed circulatory system. When hereditary or acquired qualitative or quantitative defects occur in these pathways, bleeding or bruising may present either spontaneously or following trauma. Injury to the vascular endothelium activates blood coagulation, and each biochemical reaction contributes to the immediate reduction of blood loss and the formation of a fibrin clot. Simultaneously, thrombus propagation is modulated by multiple endogenous inhibitors of thrombin formation and by the fibrinolytic system.

Five main components are critical to achieving hemostasis. These include platelets, the blood vessel wall, the plasma blood coagulation proteins, the fibrinolytic system, and the natural circulating anticoagulants. The diagnosis of the etiology of bleeding depends on a methodical search for clinical, historical, and genetic features that are characteristically associated with specific defects in each of these systems. The physical exam and history coupled to the laboratory evaluation allows diagnosis of the specific abnormality in the hemostatic process (see Chapter 41). Abnormal results in global assays that assess the function of each pathway leads to the performance of specific assays, thereby defining the specific nature of the defect and establishing a diagnosis.

In this chapter, we discuss the most common hereditary and acquired coagulation disorders encountered by internists and hematologists. Platelet disorders are discussed in Chapter 57.

Hemophilia A

Hemophilia A is the most common inherited coagulation protein deficiency, occurring in approximately one in 10,000 live births in the United States or 20.6 per 100,000 males. This coagulopathy is due to the hereditary deficiency of factor VIII activity. Because the gene encoding for factor VIII is located on the X chromosome, hemophilia A is transmitted in an X-linked recessive manner. Hemophilia A occurs in the absence of a positive family history in about 30% of cases, presumably secondary to spontaneous mutations in the gene that is located in a particularly fragile portion of the X chromosome. The degree of bleeding correlates with the severity of factor VIII deficiency, leading to the classification of hemophilia A as mild (factor VIII activity level of 5% to 20% of normal), moderate (factor VIII activity level of 1% to 5% of normal), or severe (factor VIII activity level less than 1% of normal levels). Thus, those with severe disease and without documented family histories may present at birth with an intracranial hemorrhage or shortly thereafter at circumcision. Intracranial bleeding is a potentially lethal complication during delivery of newborns with hemophilia and probably adversely influences the child's cognitive development. It is not clear whether cesarian section decreases the incidence of intracranial bleeding compared to vaginal delivery. Prolonged labor, forceps delivery, and the use of suction extraction increase the risk of intracranial bleeding. Although excessive bleeding after circumcision should raise the suspicion of hemophilia A or B, fewer than one half of children with hemophilia experience this complication.

Spontaneous hemarthroses, bleeds into muscles and soft tissues, and bleeding from mucosal surfaces, all unassociated with significant trauma, are the features of severe hemophilia A but are not pathognomonic (Figure 58-1). In contrast, patients with disease of mild or moderate severity and without documented family histories might not be diagnosed until around the toddling age of 2 to 5 years. Common manifestations of their disease include easy bruisability; soft tissue bleeding; and excessive bleeding after trauma, dental procedures, loss of deciduous teeth, or intramuscular injections. The differential diagnosis of hemophilia A includes platelet disorders, von Willebrand disease (vWD), and other coagulation factor deficiencies. The pattern of inheritance and family history should narrow the differential

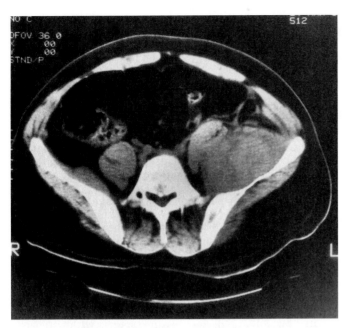

Figure 58-1 ■ Radiographic changes associated with hemophilic arthropathy. (From Flaumenhaft R, Furie B: Biochemistry of factor X and molecular biology of hemophilia A. In Hoffman R et al: Hematology, 3rd ed. Philadelphia, Churchill Livingstone, 2000, p 1888.)

diagnosis to a X-linked coagulopathy consistent with and suggestive of hemophilia A or B. An autosomal-recessive or autosomal-dominant genetic pattern should lead one to consider other coagulopathies or von Willebrand disease.

Hemarthroses and intramuscular hemorrhages, so-called bulky bleeds, are more suggestive of the hemophilias than of qualitative and quantitative platelet disorders or von Willebrand disease, which are most characteristically accompanied by bleeding from mucosal surfaces and cutaneous bruising. It is not possible to distinguish on clinical grounds between hemophilia A and hemophilia B; specific clotting assays are required. Bleeding into the closed joint space produces severe pain, swelling, and decreased joint range of motion. Repeated bleeds lead to synovial scarring and destruction of cartilage with permanent deformation and compromise of joint function.

The laboratory evaluation of individuals who are suspected of having hemophilia reveals a prolonged partial thromboplastin time (PTT) in the face of a normal prothrombin time. The increased partial thromboplastin time corrects with mixing studies in which a mixture of patient plasma and normal pooled plasma is incubated. The detection of an isolated decrease in factor VIII coagulant activity in the presence of normal factor IX, factor XI, and factor XII identifies hemophilia A. A normal bleeding time, normal platelet aggregation studies, and negative evaluation for von Willebrand disease, including a normal von Willebrand factor (vWF) antigen and activity, are consistent with the diagnosis of hemophilia A. An exception to this laboratory algorithm is von Willebrand variant type 2 Normandy (2N), which is characterized by normal von Willebrand factor activity and multimeric composition but low levels of factor VIII coagulant activity. These individuals might appear to be phenotypically identical to patients with hemophilia A, but the defect is due to a point mutation in the von Willebrand factor at the factor VIII binding site. Factor VIII synthesis is normal. The von Willebrand factor therefore lacks the capacity to complex with and chaperone the factor VIII coagulant protein in the plasma circulation, resulting in increased factor VIII degradation in vivo.

The mainstay of hemophilia A management is predicated on replacement of factor VIII to levels that are adequate to support normal hemostasis. This can be achieved by administration of exogenous purified factor VIII derived from plasma or recombinant genetically engineered protein expressed in tissue culture. Alternatively, in moderate and mild hemophilia A, factor VIII activity levels can be increased by the release of endogenously synthesized storage pools in response to the administration of arginine desmopressin (DDAVP), a synthetic vasopressin analog.

The decision to use either plasma-derived or recombinant factor VIII preparations is based on multiple medical, economic, and subjective issues. Some of these include the HIV and hepatitis status of the patient, the presence or absence of alloantibody inhibitors, whether treatment is for surgery, prophylaxis, or treatment of an acute bleeding event, the reimbursement allowed by the patient's health insurance mechanism, and patient preference, based on personal perception of incremental viral safety and product innovation.

Factor VIII is administered in various regimens depending on the primary purpose of treatment. In the vast majority of patients, factor VIII is administered as an intravenous bolus to control and reverse an acute bleeding episode or as prophylaxis to prevent bleeding during surgery and invasive procedures (Figure 58-2). General guidelines for the levels of factor VIII activity that are needed to control or prevent bleeding have been largely derived from clinical experience rather than randomized, controlled studies. Therefore, these should be considered practical recommendations but do not represent minimal levels necessary to achieve adequate hemostasis. Factor VIII activities of 25% to 30% of normal are usually sufficient to treat minor bleeding events, such as spontaneous hemarthroses and dental procedures, whereas 80% to 100% factor VIII activity levels are

The Role of Arginine Desmopressin in the Management of Hemophilia A

Arginine desmopressin is useful only in the treatment of individuals whose hemophilia is mild or moderate in degree. It has no benefit in severe hemophilia A or hemophilia B. Intravenous administration of 0.3 µg arginine desmopressin/kg in 50 mL of normal saline over 20 minutes usually raises the factor VIII activity by twofold to fourfold and may decrease or eliminate the need for factor VIII concentrate. Alternatively, arginine desmopressin can be administered intranasally as a spray (150 µg per nostril for adults). The incremental factor VIII increases are lower with the spray than with intravenous preparation, and nasal absorption may be compromised by concurrent nasal membrane inflammation. In Europe, subcutaneous regimens are utilized. These formulations may be given every 12 hours if necessary. However, patients develop tachyphylaxis with multiple dosing. In unusual circumstances, the antidiuretic effects of arginine desmopressin may mediate onset of hyponatremia and seizures. Therefore, fluid restriction and close monitoring of serum sodium levels are recommended. Arginine desmopressin is also a potent vasoconstrictor and hence should be used cautiously in older patients with preexisting atherosclerotic heart disease. Significant blood pressure elevations may occur as well. All patients will develop a facial flush, which usually is inconsequential. In addition, arginine desmopressin causes the systemic release of tissue plasminogen activator from endothelial cells; antifibrinolytic agents (such as ε aminocaproic acid or tranexamic acid) can be administered simultaneously for treatment of bleeding from mucosal surfaces, such as the gastrointestinal tract, naso-oropharynx, and genitourinary tract, and may be continued for several days thereafter. Because of interindividual variability to arginine desmopressin effects, patients should be electively tested for arginine desmopressin response with one or more formulations before it is to be used for treatment or preoperative prophylaxis.

Recombinant Versus Plasma-Derived Factor VIII: Approach to Product Choice

The primary advantages of administering recombinant factor VIII to individuals with hemophilia versus plasma-derived factor VIII include (1) the virtual elimination of the risk of transmitting human blood-borne pathogens; (2) the significantly higher specific activity of the recombinant products allowing for smaller replacement volumes, more rapid infusions for acute bleeds, and ease of implementation of continuous infusion regimens; (3) the fact that recombinant factor VIII should guarantee an unlimited supply of factor VIII, theoretically at lower cost, and thus circumvent the need and expense for large numbers of plasma donors. The major disadvantage of recombinant factor VIII is its current cost per unit, which is substantially higher than plasma-derived concentrates. In addition, recombinant factor VIII products and the ultra-high-purity, monoclonal antibody purified plasma-derived concentrates (specific activities >150 units of factor VIII activity/mg protein) do not contain sufficient intact von Willebrand factor protein to be useful in the treatment of severe type 3 von Willebrand disease or 2N von Willebrand disease. Current treatment philosophy in North America, Western Europe, and Japan recommends prescription of recombinant factor VIII products to all newly diagnosed individuals or previously untreated patients, who are HIV- and HCV-seronegative. Plasma-derived products may be recommended for HCV- and HIV-seropositive patients to lower their overall cost of care, since many are receiving expensive HAART therapy and alpha-interferon/ribavirin for chronic hepatitis. The decision regarding the type and brand of replacement product also depends on clinical scenarios, patient preference, physician interpretation of the literature as to perceived or real differences in viral safety, and the existence of restrictions on reimbursement for the more expensive products. For example, it may be reasonable to recommend that an HIV/HCV-positive individual be given recombinant products in the surgical setting to facilitate continuous infusion but to continue on-demand therapy with a plasma-derived product. Detailed discussions with the patient are necessary, and patient preference has to be taken into consideration. Recent studies have indicated that the cost of care and the mortality associated with hemophilia are substantially reduced when care is provided within a hemophilia treatment center, where expertise in coagulation, blood banking, and pharmacy are concentrated

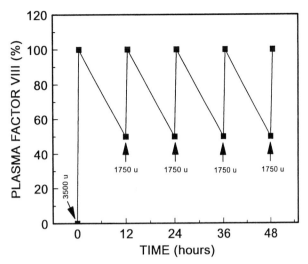

Figure 58-2 ■ Factor VIII administration in hemophilia A. (From Furie B, Limetani SA, Rosenfield CG: A practical guide to the evaluation and treatment of hemophilia. Blood, 1994; 84:6.)

desired for life-threatening or serious bleeding events, for major surgical procedures, or for visceral or intramuscular bleeds. A unit of factor VIII activity is the amount of factor VIII in 1 mL of normal plasma. Dosing of factor VIII for replacement in hemophilia A can be calculated by assuming the rule of thumb that each unit of factor VIII administered per kilogram of body weight will raise the plasma factor VIII activity by 2%. This incremental rise in factor VIII activity should be confirmed in the patient prior to any emergent bleeding episode by administering the calculated dose of factor VIII and then measuring the factor VIII level within 15 to 30 minutes. Redosing 8 to 12 hours later (the half-life of factor VIII) is indicated if acute bleeding does not subside. For surgery, factor VIII is administered before surgery and then continued at lower doses (to achieve 50% factor VIII levels) for 7 to 14 days postoperatively to ensure adequate wound healing. A test dose followed by measured factor VIII activity is appropriate prior to elective surgery to ensure that the approximate factor VIII levels are obtained and that the recovery and half-life of factor VIII are as anticipated.

On-demand administration of factor VIII with each acute bleeding episode is the most common treatment regimen for hemophilia A. Longitudinal trials of primary prophylaxis, in which the factor VIII trough level is constantly maintained between 1% and 5%, have demonstrated fewer spontaneous hemarthroses and preservation of joint mobility. There is enthusiasm for adopting this regimen as the standard of care beginning after the first or second joint bleed. Factor VIII is usually administered thrice weekly. Recent

studies also have demonstrated that continuous infusion of factor VIII in the postoperative scenario avoids the peaks and troughs of factor VIII activity that are observed with intermittent dosing. This reduces the bleeding complications, decreases the factor consumption needed for replacement, and substantially reduces the overall cost of the procedure. Continuous infusion is preceded by a bolus of factor VIII to achieve 100% activity followed by infusion at 2 units/kg/hour, with titration of the rate to maintain the desired factor VIII level.

There is no difference in clinical efficacy among the plasma-derived and recombinant factor VIII concentrates. The recombinant factor VIII preparations are safe from the transmission of human blood-borne viruses by virtue of their production in transfected mammalian cells maintained in tissue culture lines. All currently available plasma-derived factor VIII preparations have various single or multiple viral inactivation steps inserted into their production processes, such as heat inactivation in dry and wet conditions and solvent detergent treatment, and therefore appear safe from the transmission of blood-borne lipid-enveloped viruses, including hepatitis B, hepatitis C, and HIV. This safety is enhanced by extensive viral screening of individual donors and donated plasma pools. Unfortunately, because of the lack of effective universal viral elimination processes, these products have been associated with the transmission of nonenveloped viruses, such as hepatitis A and parvovirus B19. The recent introduction of specific polymerase chain reaction testing and nucleic acid testing for these viruses in the plasma pools that are ultimately used to purify these products should minimize these risks. Although there has never been a documented case of new variant Creutzfeld-Jacob transmission and because these prions are not eliminated by any available means, many clinicians are concerned about the theoretical risks to patients using plasma-derived factor VIII. Cryoprecipitate is not indicated for hemophilia treatment unless factor VIII concentrates are unavailable in emergency situations, because viral safety cannot be guaranteed.

Hemophilia A with Factor VIII Alloantibody Inhibitors

Individuals with severe hemophilia A may develop alloantibody inhibitors that neutralize exogenously administered factor VIII. This probably represents a natural immune response against a foreign antigen, since they have been detected in up to 50% of patients with severe hemophilia at some time during their lifetimes.

The Bethesda assay is a functional assay to quan-

TREATMENT

Management Options for Joint Disease in Hemophilia A

Repetitive bleeding into a specific joint leads to significant deformity and subsequently affects the mobility and quality of life of hemophilia A patients. The source of bleeding is usually the subsynovial venous plexus. Acute management requires the administration of factor VIII to arrest the bleeding process. The pain usually requires short-term narcotic analgesics, but the use of large amounts of codeine or hydrocodone compounds containing acetaminophen should be avoided in those patients with chronic hepatitis C. Aspirin is contraindicated. The use of the nonsteroidal anti-inflammatory drugs, such as ibuprofen and naproxen, may be used judiciously, particularly for treatment of the chronic arthritis, which results from recurrent hemarthroses. Preliminary studies suggest that inhibitors of cyclooxygenase type 2 may be safe in hemophilic arthropathy and pain. If increased bleeding or bruising occurs with any of the nonsteroidal anti-inflammatory drugs, they should be terminated immediately. Increased frequency and severity of joint bleeds have been reported in hemophiliacs on HAART therapy and with chronic hepatitis. Orthotics are indicated to improve the mobility of the patients by stiffening the limb around a weak subluxed joint. They are generally used in an attempt to delay joint replacement.

Several surgical interventions can be performed to decrease morbidity and pain. As the implementation of primary prophylaxis regimens becomes more ubiquitous, joint function may be preserved so that these approaches are unnecessary:

■ Synovectomy is indicated to relieve persistent synovitis and the pain of hemophilic arthropathy in a specific joint. It is not intended to improve articulation around that joint. Mobility may actu-

ally worsen after the procedure. Careful patient selection is necessary. Although synovectomy removes the primary source of blood vessels in the joint, it does not prevent progression of the joint destruction. Recently, successful synovectomies have been accomplished in hemophiliacs without surgery by employing the intra-articular administration of radionuclides.

■ Arthroplasties (joint replacement) have been developed for all joints, although the most experience in hemophilia focuses on knees and hips. The success of these procedures depends on maintaining adequate hemostasis intraoperatively and postoperatively and throughout the aggressive physical therapy rehabilitation period. The goal is to achieve normalcy in the range of motion of the joint. Success in ankle, shoulder, and elbow replacements is limited, since the full range of motion of these prostheses is difficult to achieve. Pain is substantially reduced in most patients following these procedures, and the use of factor VIII may decrease. In hip replacement, the prosthesis is reported to loosen after 10 to 15 years, depending on surgical technique. Newer prosthetic composites and metals may extend the life of the joint in the future. There is controversy as to the utility of arthroplasties in HIV-seropositive hemophiliacs. With effective HAART therapy and undetectable viral loads, there appears to be little risk of joint infections.

■ Arthrodesis (joint fixation) is commonly used for ankle joints to stabilize the foot, reduce pain, and improve mobility. With the introduction of effective ankle prostheses, the frequency of this procedure may decrease in the future.

---

titate factor VIII neutralization by the alloantibody inhibitor. One Bethesda unit is arbitrarily defined as the reciprocal of inhibitor dilution required to sustain a 50% residual factor VIII activity in a mixture of patient plasma and a pooled normal plasma. Thus, if a 1/100 dilution of patient plasma is required to accomplish this, the patient has an inhibitor level of 100 Bethesda units.

The majority of factor VIII inhibitors are so-called low-titer inhibitors (less than 5 Bethesda units) and may be short-lived with spontaneous disappearance. There is no anamnestic antibody response (low responder) on reexposure to factor VIII. Many patients with low-titer inhibitors have a subclinical response to factor VIII replacement therapy. This is in contrast to

high-titer inhibitor patients (>10 Bethesda units) in whom large doses of factor VIII are unable to overcome the neutralizing effects of the alloantibody. High-titer inhibitor patients typically display an anamnestic rise (high responder) on reexposure to any source of factor VIII (Figure 58-3). Prospective studies indicate that most inhibitors develop within a median of nine exposure days to factor VIII concentrate. There is debate as to whether users of high-purity, plasma-derived, and recombinant factor VIII products have a greater incidence of inhibitor formation than do patients receiving intermediate-purity, plasma-derived factor VIII. Alloantibodies are most commonly associated with hemophilia A caused by nonsense gene mutations and the intron 22 inversion.

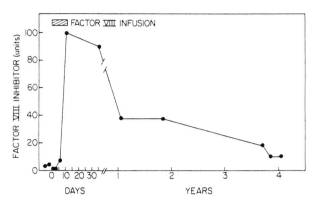

Figure 58-3 ■ Induction of Factor VIII inhibitor on reexposure to factor VIII in a patient with severe hemophilia. (From Furie B: In Williams RH et al: Williams Textbook of Endocrinology, 3rd ed. New York: McGraw-Hill, 1983, p 142.)

Alloantibody formation in moderate hemophiliacs is very uncommon.

Typically, factor VIII alloantibody inhibitors are oligoclonal IgG (subclass 1 or 4), directed predominantly against both the A2 domain of factor VIII and the C2 domain of factor VIII. Patients with alloantibody inhibitors against factor VIII present with a normal prothrombin time but prolonged partial thromboplastin time, which may show correction immediately after mixing the inhibitor plasma with normal plasma. However, if the mixture is allowed to incubate at 37°C for one to two hours, the partial thromboplastin time will be prolonged since the kinetics of factor VIII neutralization by the alloantibody are relatively slow. Specific factor VIII assays confirm the presence of the inhibitor, which can be quantitated with a Bethesda assay. Alloantibody inhibitors follow type I kinetics in which factor VIII activity is totally neutralized. This is in sharp contrast to the lupus anticoagulant, for which the degree of partial thromboplastin time prolongation in the mixing study at time zero does not lengthen after two hours of incubation.

Management of acute bleeding episodes associated with factor VIII alloantibody inhibitors is determined by the titer of inhibitor activity. Recently, immune tolerance induction regimens have been initiated for eradication of alloantibody inhibitors. These are most successful (>50%) for recently diagnosed low titer inhibitors and require daily administration of a desensitization regimen of factor VIII (25 to 50 U/kg daily). For high-titer inhibitors, much larger doses of factor VIII are needed (up to 200 U/kg/day) to suppress the inhibitor. Porcine factor VIII has been used successfully in immune tolerance induction regimens.

TREATMENT

Acute Bleeding Episodes Associated with Factor VIII Alloantibody Inhibitors

Individuals with high-titer inhibitors (>10 Bethesda units) should be treated with agents that initiate coagulation by bypassing the effects of the neutralizing alloantibody. These include the activated formulations of the prothrombin complex concentrates (FEIBA or Autoplex HT), which are administered as 75 to 100 units/kg intravenously every 8 to 12 hours until bleeding subsides. Repetitive infusions may lead to thrombotic complications due to the effects of activated clotting enzymes in these products. Activated prothrombin complex concentrates are monitored by clinical parameters, since laboratory assays are inaccurate. These agents have about an 80% chance of successful reversal of bleeding events. Alternative treatment approaches include the use of recombinant factor VIIa (Novo-7) and porcine factor VIII concentrate (Hyate:C). The former is dosed at 90 μg/kg intravenously every 2.5 to 3 hours, with a single dose after bleeding terminates. Because of its relatively high cost, Novo-7 has been typically reserved as a second-line agent despite its approximately 70% success rate. The choice of product is usually dictated by availability, cost, and the familiarity and personal experiences of the prescribing physician with one or more of the products.

Infusions of porcine factor VIII can be justified only if the coagulation laboratory can confirm that there is little (<15 Bethesda units) or no neutralizing cross-reactivity between the patient's alloantibody inhibitor and the porcine factor VIII coagulant protein. Dosed at 50 to 100 units/kg every 8 to 12 hours until bleeding subsides, porcine factor VIII is the only replacement product for inhibitor treatment that will allow for specific monitoring of factor VIII. Both products should be safe from transmission of human pathogenic viruses.

Low-titer inhibitors (<5 Bethesda units) can usually be overwhelmed successfully by administering large enough quantities of human factor VIII. The factor VIII that is required to neutralize the alloantibody and then provide adequate plasma levels is calculated. Doses might need to be increased to achieve adequate factor VIII levels for hemostasis. For some low-titer inhibitors, adequate factor VIII levels have been achieved after the administration of arginine desmopressin (0.3 μg/kg in 50 mL normal saline infused over 20 minutes).

Anamnestic responses may occur in these high-titer inhibitor patients, and acute bleeds may ensue. Treatment of these events are approached according to standard practice. Once tolerance is achieved, maintenance factor VIII should be administered three times weekly.

Hemophilia B

Hemophilia B is the hereditary deficiency of factor IX. As with hemophilia A, hemophilia B is transmitted in an X-linked inheritance pattern, but it is less common than hemophilia A. In the United States, the prevalence of hemophilia B is estimated at 5.3 per 100,000 male births. The clinical features of hemophilia B are identical to and indistinguishable from those of hemophilia A. It is not possible to differentiate between the two without specific laboratory assays. These patients commonly present with soft tissue (intramuscular) and joint bleeding and posttraumatic or operative bleeding.

The laboratory profile for hemophilia B patients includes normal platelet count and function. The prothrombin time, thrombin time, von Willebrand factor activities, and factor VIII activity are normal. Individuals have a prolonged partial thromboplastin time, which corrects with mixing studies. Factor IX activity levels correlate with the severity of the disease, as with hemophilia A.

Both recombinant and plasma-derived factor IX are available for therapeutic and prophylactic replacement of factor IX. Recombinant factor IX is safe from the transmission of blood-borne pathogens but is more expensive. Plasma-derived factor IX concentrates are available as low purity or high purity. Repeated administration of intermediate-purity factor IX concentrates in large amounts over a short interval has been associated with an increased incidence of thrombotic complications.

Factor IX is distributed equally between the intravascular plasma compartment and the extravascular space. Therefore, administration of 1 unit of factor IX per kilogram raises the plasma activity by 1% as compared to 2% in hemophilia A. The plasma half-life of factor IX is 18 to 24 hours, and repeated dosing should be done at 18- to 24-hour intervals. Cryoprecipitate, while rich in factor VIII, does not contain factor IX and has no role in the management of patients with hemophilia B.

The guidelines for management of acute bleeding episodes and for preoperative prophylaxis are very similar for hemophilia A and hemophilia B. Also, the indications for surgical interventions for arthropathy are the same. The development of alloantibody inhibitors against factor IX is unusual, occurring in

about 1% to 3% of cases. The administration of any factor IX–containing product may trigger acute anaphylaxis with life-threatening laryngospasm and/or nephrotic syndrome in a small percentage of individuals with anti–factor IX alloantibody inhibitors. This is probably due to precipitation of factor IX antigen-antibody complexes in various organs, a phenomenon that does not occur with factor VIII–alloantibody complexes. Because factor IX replacement therapy is contraindicated in such patients, recombinant factor VIIa is the treatment of choice. Factor IX replacement options include intermediate-purity, plasma-derived products (Konyne-80, Bebulin); high-purity, plasma-derived (AlphaNine SD); ultra-high-purity, monoclonal-purified, plasma-derived factor IX (Mononine); and recombinant factor IX (Benefix). Cryoprecipitate does not contain factor IX and should not be used as replacement therapy for hemophilia B. Arginine desmopressin does not increase factor IX levels and should not be used to treat hemophilia B.

Factor XI Deficiency

Factor XI deficiency (hemophilia C) is inherited in an autosomal-recessive manner, being most prevalent in Ashkenazic Jews with a 4.3% gene frequency. The disease can occur in other ethnic groups, has no sex predilection, and should be considered in the differential diagnosis for anyone with a family history of bleeding involving both males and females. Homozygotes and compound heterozygotes may have hemorrhagic manifestations and have factor XI activity levels less than 20% of normal. Spontaneous bleeding events, including hemarthroses and intramuscular bleeds, which are commonly encountered in severe hemophilia A and B, rarely occur in factor XI deficiency. Typically, these patients bleed excessively with trauma, surgery (usually oral, postpartum, and genitourinary), and menses (menorrhagia). Heterozygotes tend to have modest factor XI deficiency (about 40% to 50% normal activity) but do not manifest any clinical bleeding symptoms. They may be detected incidentally when a routine preoperative partial thromboplastin time is prolonged and subsequent evaluation reveals a specific factor XI deficiency. As a rule of thumb, clinical bleeding cannot be predicted following surgery or trauma based on the degree of factor XI deficiency. A prior history of bleeding in the patient or in their family members appears to be the optimal indicator of bleeding potential. This uncertainty produces a clinical conundrum for the clinician, who might be required to prepare a factor XI-deficient patient for major surgery in the absence of prior challenges. Acute bleeding episodes can be treated adequately in most patients with fresh frozen plasma

---

TREATMENT

When Is Replacement Therapy Indicated for Patients with Factor XI Deficiency?

Bleeding potential in factor XI deficiency cannot be predicted accurately by the factor XI plasma activity, even in severely deficient individuals. Although family medical history and personal prior history of bleeding with surgery and trauma may be more predictive, even a negative history provides little solace to the physician who is preparing the patient for major surgery. The risk:benefit ratio favors replacement therapy with fresh frozen plasma to achieve factor XI levels of 40% to 50% before major surgery and 30% for minor surgery. Postoperative factor XI levels of 20% are usually adequate for hemostasis, and this level should be maintained for 7 to 10 days to facilitate wound healing. In selected individuals, arginine desmopressin may raise mildly decreased factor XI levels into an adequately hemostatic range for minor surgery or to reverse extreme menorrhagia. Patients must be pretested to determine their response. Antifibrinolytic agents (ε-aminocaproic acid or tranexamic acid) may be beneficial as single agents or in combination with factor XI replacement therapy, particularly for mucosal-based bleeds. In addition, fibrin sealants can be used to treat localized bleeding during surgery.

---

dosed at 20 mL/kg body weight, repeated if necessary according to the factor XI activity level. Because of the long half-life of factor XI (up to 50 hours), daily dosing with smaller amounts of plasma may be appropriate. Plasma-derived factor XI concentrates are available in Europe. However, their popularity has been tempered somewhat by their propensity to induce hypercoagulable complications. Plasmapheresis and exchange, platelet transfusions (platelets contain factor XI in their alpha granules), and use of antifibrinolytic agents such as ε-aminocaproic acid may be very useful as adjunctive therapies when bleeding is not controlled by fresh frozen plasma alone. Factor XI deficiency can occur concomitantly with other inherited coagulopathies such as von Willebrand disease, factor VIII or factor IX deficiencies, and qualitative platelet disorders. Factor XI deficiency can also be acquired in conjunction with development of autoantibody inhibitors, most commonly associated with systemic lupus erythematosus. Alloantibody inhibitors have been reported in severe factor XI deficiency (<1% activity) treated with fresh frozen plasma. In these situations, recombinant factor VIIa concentrate may be used to treat acute bleeding episodes.

Laboratory findings include normal platelet count and function. The prothrombin time and thrombin time are normal, while the partial thromboplastin time, which corrects in mixing studies, is prolonged. A specific assay for factor XI activity confirms the diagnosis.

Von Willebrand Disease

Von Willebrand disease is the most common hereditary bleeding disorder, occurring in approximately 1% of the population without ethnic predilection. A prolonged bleeding time in an individual with easy bruisability, menorrhagia, or abnormal bleeding from mucosal surfaces should trigger an evaluation for von Willebrand disease. Type 1 (classical) von Willebrand disease, the most common type of von Willebrand disease, typically has a slightly prolonged partial thromboplastin time because of modest concomitant factor VIII deficiency, decreased von Willebrand factor antigen and activity, measured as ristocetin cofactor activity, and abnormal ristocetin-induced platelet aggregation. Individuals with type O red blood cells may have von Willebrand factor and factor VIII coagulant activities significantly reduced below the normal range. Although there is debate whether such individuals actually have mild von Willebrand disease, mild hemophilia A, or an otherwise undefined coagulopathy, such individuals may bruise easily, bleed profusely, and respond to von Willebrand disease and hemophilia treatment modalities. A recently described variant of von Willebrand disease, designated 2 Normandy, is due to a point mutation in the von Willebrand factor gene on chromosome 12 at the site that encodes factor VIII binding for complex formation. Individuals with von Willebrand disease 2N appear phenotypically to have moderate or mild hemophilia A, with low factor VIII levels but normal von Willebrand factor activities. However, the factor VIII gene is normal. This disorder is inherited in an autosomal manner, and women may be affected. The von Willebrand factor multimeric structure is normal on SDS-polyacrylamide gel electrophoresis. The diagnosis of von Willebrand disease 2N hinges on assays to quantitate the ability of the patient's von Willebrand factor to bind factor VIII.

Von Willebrand disease and its variants are classified according to platelet aggregation studies and von Willebrand factor multimeric analysis. Ristocetin-induced platelet aggregation responses are suboptimal in types 1, 2A, and severe type 3 von Willebrand disease. Variant type 2B von Willebrand disease is characterized by hyperaggregation responses at low concentrations of ristocetin (0.6 mg/mL) and normal aggregation patterns with standard ristocetin concentrations (1.2 mg/mL). This variant is associated with variable degrees of thrombocytopenia and rare thrombotic complications due to spontaneous platelet agglutination in vivo. Multimeric analysis of the von Willebrand factor structure, accomplished by SDS-polyacrylamide gel electrophoresis, reveals a pattern of absent high-molecular-weight multimers in von Willebrand disease type 2B. The type 2B von Willebrand factor protein has abnormally increased affinity for the glycoprotein Ib/IX complex on the platelet membrane. Von Willebrand disease variant type 2A is defined by loss of the highest and intermediate-molecular-weight multimers of von Willebrand factor, accompanied by decreased ristocetin-induced platelet aggregation. Type 1 von Willebrand disease is characterized by the uniform decrease of all molecular weight multimers of von Willebrand factor, as observed by electrophoresis. However, each multimer is qualitatively normal. In type 3 von Willebrand disease, the von Willebrand factor protein concentration is so markedly decreased that no multimers can be visualized on electrophoretic gel analysis.

In addition to raising the plasma level of factor VIII, arginine desmopressin causes substantial elevation in von Willebrand factor activity levels and constitutes the mainstay of treatment in patients with type 1 von Willebrand disease and approximately 50% of those with type 2A disease. Von Willebrand disease type 2B might not respond to arginine desmopressin, and the thrombocytopenia might worsen, leading to thrombotic complications. Arginine desmopressin is therefore contraindicated for type 2B disease. The same dosage recommendations and precautions that are used in the management of mild and moderate hemophilia A are applicable here, including the adjunctive use of antifibrinolytic agents.

Von Willebrand disease patients who cannot tolerate or benefit from arginine desmopressin or whose response is not adequate to sustain hemostasis for major bleeds or for surgeries are best managed by administering factor VIII concentrates containing von Willebrand factor. The two most commonly used products are Alphanate SD/HT and Humate-P, both of which are viral-attenuated for lipid-enveloped viruses. These concentrates are dosed according to ristocetin cofactor activity units per kilogram (60 units/kg bolus prior to surgery) or titrated to achieve and maintain ristocetin cofactor activities in the 50% to 100% range. If these products are not available in an emergent situation, cryoprecipitate is a reasonable alternative but is not viral safe. Oral estrogens, which are physiologic inducers of von Willebrand factor synthesis, often ameliorate menorrhagia exacerbated by von Willebrand disease, particularly type 1.

Accidental and Intentional Anticoagulation Induced by Ingestion of Vitamin K Antagonists

Warfarin is the most commonly prescribed oral anticoagulant, administered to millions daily for a variety of medical conditions associated with thrombotic tendencies. The anticoagulation effects of chronic warfarin use may be enhanced significantly by polypharmacy, drug interactions, and comorbid conditions such as malnutrition, cancer, or hepatic insufficiency. The incidence of major bleeding complications when the International Normalized Ratio (INR) is beyond the therapeutic International Normalized Ratio of 2 to 3 is about 2% per year in younger individuals and exceeds 4% per year in those over 80 years old. The frequency and severity of life-threatening bleeding events and easy bruising rise dramatically when the International Normalized Ratio exceeds the therapeutic range. When antiplatelet agents are combined with warfarin to prevent embolization in chronic atrial fibrillation, the hemorrhagic stroke incidence may approach a rate of 8% per year, even with low-intensity warfarin therapy targeting the International Normalized Ratio to 1.2 to 1.5.

Easy bruisability and abnormal bleeding may also occur in otherwise normal individuals who ingest warfarin surreptitiously. These patients frequently are affected by psychiatric disorders, such as schizophrenia, obsessive-compulsive disorder, and personality disorders. Often, their ecchymoses are self-inflicted (factitious purpura), a situation that is suspected when bruises occur only over body areas that are accessible to reach and by their unusual or geometric shapes. These patients have a variant of Münchhausen's syndrome in which they inflict harm on themselves using warfarin. Occasionally, a young child (or elderly individual) may present with these same symptoms as a result of warfarin or superwarfarin (present in rodenticides) administration by a mentally ill parent (or relative), so-called Münchhausen's by proxy.

Acute management of warfarin ingestion is fundamentally different depending on whether a patient who is taking warfarin for therapeutic purposes has an inappropriately high International Normalized Ratio, a patient with psychiatric disease, occult or obvious, has ingested warfarin surreptitiously, or a normal individual is accidentally poisoned with warfarin. In all cases, the appropriate treatment depends on whether the patient is bleeding and the prolongation of the prothrombin time.

All patients who are taking therapeutic warfarin will occasionally have an International Normalized Ratio that is supertherapeutic. In the presence of a markedly prolonged International Normalized Ratio (for example, greater than 6) that is not associated with bleeding, withholding of additional warfarin is usually adequate to prevent bleeding. Warfarin should not be restarted until the International Normalized Ratio is in the therapeutic range. Vitamin K$_1$ supplementation is usually not necessary, and its use will induce warfarin resistance when anticoagulation is resumed. Patients with an exceptional International Normalized Ratio, for example, in the 6 to 10 range, but without bleeding should have warfarin withheld and should receive small doses of vitamin K$_1$ (1 to 2 mg) administered subcutaneously or orally. When there is clinically significant bleeding, a high risk of potential bleeding, or an International Normalized Ratio in excess of 10, two to three units of fresh frozen plasma should be administered for rapid reversal of anticoagulant effects. Vitamin K$_1$ supplementation (5 to 10 mg) should be given, ideally via the intravenous route. When patients cannot tolerate the large volume of fresh frozen plasma or when a rapid reversal of the International Normalized Ratio is necessary to treat acute bleeds, the use of bolus recombinant factor VIIa (20 to 50 µg/kg) might be considered.

Patients who ingest warfarin surreptitiously do not acknowledge the cause of their prolonged prothrombin time, deficiency of the vitamin K–dependent blood clotting proteins, or ecchymoses. The diagnosis of surreptitious or accidental ingestion of warfarin is secured by determination of the serum warfarin level. The prolonged prothrombin time can be reversed by administration of intravenous vitamin K. Typically, 10 to 15 µg intravenously over two to three days will completely correct warfarin-induced prolongation of the prothrombin time. Only if clinically significant bleeding is an issue should fresh frozen plasma be administered, as described previously. There is no role for factor VIIa in the treatment of this problem. The ultimate challenge is, without confrontation, to indicate to the patient the need for psychiatric care.

In the patient with a prolonged prothrombin time, ecchymoses, deficiency of the vitamin K–dependent proteins when other coagulation proteins are normal, and a serum warfarin level that is negative, super-warfarin ingestion—either surreptitious or accidental—should be considered. Although superwarfarins, such as brodifacoum, can be measured in serum in some commercial laboratories, this test is not as readily available as serum warfarin levels. If super-warfarins, the active ingredient in most rodenticides, is suspected of causing the coagulopathy, oral vitamin K at doses of 50 to 100 mg/day might be necessary to reverse the prolonged prothrombin time (Figure 58-4). The prothrombin time should be normalized with intravenous vitamin K, then the patient should be switched to oral vitamin K at the lowest doses adequate to keep the prothrombin time at normal levels. Treatment may be necessary for months or years.

Coagulopathy of Liver Disease

The hepatocyte is the major site of synthesis for most of the blood coagulation factors with the exception of factor VIII, which is produced at low levels in many cells. Acute and chronic hepatic dysfunction can lead to significant decreases in multiple coagulation factor levels, which may or may not give rise to clinical symptoms despite prolongations in the prothrombin time or partial thromboplastin time. Specific coagulation factor measurement define the deficiencies, which include decreased levels of prothrombin, factor V, factor VII, factor IX, factor X, factor XI, and factor XII. Factor VIII, in contrast, is normal or elevated in

Figure 58-4 ■ Response of brodifacoum poisoning to vitamin K. (From Weitzel JN et al: Surreptitious ingestion of a long-acting vitamin K antagonist/rodenticide, brodifacoum: Clinical and metabolic studies of three cases. Blood 1990;76:2555–2559.)

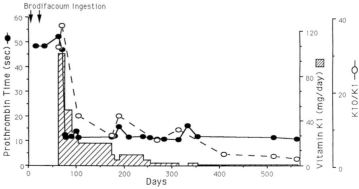

DIAGNOSIS

Detection of Anticoagulation Effects Induced by the Superwarfarins

Occasionally, patients present with signs, symptoms, and laboratory results that are typical of warfarin ingestion but deny having access to the anticoagulant medication. Routine laboratory testing with the prothrombin time, partial thromboplastin time, and mixing studies cannot distinguish between warfarin or superwarfarin ingestion. If there is a strong clinical suspicion, serum warfarin levels can be obtained. However, patients who have been exposed to rodenticides containing superwarfarins will have a negative warfarin assay. Specific testing for superwarfarins through commercial laboratories can be pursued. This is of clinical significance because the superwarfarins have a longer half-life and are more potent than warfarin. Prolonged vitamin K_1 supplementation with higher daily doses than are used for warfarin is required. Adequate psychiatric evaluation and treatment are essential in these patients, many of whom have medical backgrounds and can use sophisticated means to hide their sociopathic behavior.

liver disease. Hypofibrinogenemia and/or dysfibrinogenemia may occur in hepatic failure and end-stage disease and may be associated with a prolonged thrombin time, Reptilase time, and discordance between fibrinogen levels measured as total clottable protein and specific immunologic levels. Dysfibrinogenemia may be the first coagulation defect detected in the course of advanced liver disease, although it may also appear in association with hepatocellular carcinoma. The dysfibrinogen of liver disease is characterized by its high sialic acid content and its asymptomatic nature. Bleeding manifestations are not increased, and no specific treatment is necessary.

The liver is also the main synthetic site of proteins involved in the endogenous fibrinolytic mechanism. Thus, liver disease may be associated with decreased levels of plasminogen, tissue plasminogen activator, and $\alpha2$ antiplasmin. Thus, some of the hyperfibrinolytic features of liver disease can be attributed to excessive plasmin generation by tissue plasminogen activator released from damaged hepatocytes and compromised inhibition of plasmin activity by $\alpha2$ antiplasmin deficiency. In addition, since the dysfunctional liver cannot degrade activated clotting factors efficiently or synthesize adequate levels of proteins C or S, excessive thrombin generation occurs with subsequent low-grade disseminated intravascular coagulation (DIC), characterized by fibrinogen consumption and production of D-dimers. Another laboratory feature of hyperfibrinolysis is an accelerated euglobulin clot lysis time. In disseminated intravascular coagulation, antithrombin III levels and platelet counts are decreased via consumption, and schistocytes may be detected on the peripheral blood smear secondary to microangiopathic hemolysis. Portal hypertension with secondary hypersplenism may exacerbate the thrombocytopenia. Qualitative platelet disorders have also been observed in liver disease and may contribute to the development of mucosal bleeding symptoms.

The management of acute bleeding episodes associated with liver dysfunction should start with replacement of the deficient coagulation proteins with infusions of fresh frozen plasma. Prothrombin complex concentrates or recombinant factor VIIa may be considered in an emergency if bleeding persists. Cryoprecipitate may be necessary to replenish low fibrinogen levels, and platelet transfusions may control mucosal bleeding. Arginine desmopressin has also been a useful adjunctive therapy to reverse qualitative platelet defects caused by liver disease. Aprotonin has been utilized to inhibit hyperfibrinolysis. Bleeding due to an anatomic lesion, such as bleeding varices, requires definitive local measures to be taken concurrently. Vitamin K supplementation has little benefit in severe liver disease but is often administered in large doses (10 mg subcutaneously). Orthotopic or living-donor liver transplantation is associated with its own spectrum of bleeding complications.

Hemostatic Abnormalities of Renal Disease

Patients with chronic renal disease have multiple hematologic disorders that may predispose them to bleeding. Most important is the well-documented qualitative platelet dysfunction whose etiology remains unclear. Platelet dysfunction may respond to arginine desmopressin or high-dose estrogen therapy. The nephrotic syndrome may be associated with bleeding or thromboembolic disease, although the molecular basis is not known.

Disseminated Intravascular Coagulation

Disseminated intravascular coagulation is one of the most common acquired coagulopathies and is associated with a variety of disease states, such as obstetri-

TREATMENT

Preparing a Patient with Chronic Renal Failure for Surgery

In addition to electrolyte abnormalities and fluid status, patients with chronic renal failure may have bleeding complications. Platelet dysfunction is a prominent feature of chronic renal failure and predisposes patients to potential bleeding complications during surgery. The primary approach to prepare this patient for invasive diagnostic or therapeutic procedures includes intensive preoperative hemodialysis or peritoneal dialysis to remove the toxins that are thought to be responsible for the platelet dysfunction. Second, recombinant erythropoietin with supplemental iron should be administered to raise the hematocrit into the normal range. If time does not allow for this or if the patient does not respond adequately, transfusions of packed red cells might be necessary. Arginine desmopressin has been frequently successful in reversing the platelet dysfunction of chronic renal failure. It can be administered intravenously (0.3 µg/kg) in 50 mL of normal saline over 20 minutes. The peak effect should occur in approximately one hour and be sustained over four hours, although individual variability can be expected. The use of high-dose estrogens (Premarin 10 to 50 mg/day PO or a single intravenous bolus of conjugated estrogen 0.6 mg/kg) provides an alternative approach to reversal of platelet dysfunction in chronic renal failure. Improvement of platelet function might not occur for at least three days, but complete normalization is not required for adequate hemostasis. If all else fails, platelet transfusions may provide adequate coverage during and after surgery and can be combined with any of the above approaches.

cal catastrophes, sepsis, trauma, and malignancies. Disseminated intravascular coagulation is a secondary complication induced by the activation of the blood coagulation, with consumption of clotting proteins and subsequent generation of thrombin, activation of platelets, and secondary activation of the fibrinolytic system. Therefore, clinical manifestations consist of either thrombotic complications or abnormal bleeding, typically occurring at any site of trauma, surgery, venipuncture, and arterial stick sites and from mucosal surfaces, such as the bladder, oropharynx, and gastrointestinal tract.

The laboratory evaluation reveals a decrease in platelet count, circulating schistocytes and microangiopathic red cell changes (Figure 58-5), an increased thrombin time, decreased fibrinogen levels, and elevated D-dimers. An isolated prolonged prothrombin time may be present early in the course of disseminated intravascular coagulation, but as the process accelerates, the partial thromboplastin time also becomes prolonged. The fibrinogen level is a strong predictor of bleeding tendency and should be maintained above 100 mg/dL. Depletion of antithrombin, protein C, and plasminogen during DIC is associated with poor prognosis.

Management of DIC depends on the dominant clinical manifestation. Most important, treatment of the underlying disease state that incited the DIC should be initiated rapidly to avoid the progression of DIC into multiorgan failure, which mediates development of end-organ failure and mortality. This could include evacuation of the uterus to reverse obstetrical complications, administration of antibiotics for sepsis, chemotherapeutic intervention for malignancies, and so on. Because the benefits of these measures might not become apparent for hours to days, the thrombotic or hemorrhagic complications may require urgent action. If the major symptom is bleeding, systemic blood pressure should be stabilized. Administration of transfusions of fresh frozen plasma for replenishment of blood-clotting proteins, cryoprecipitate for restoration of fibrinogen levels to over 100 mg/dL, and platelets to achieve and maintain a count greater than 50,000/µL should be initiated. In the exceptional case

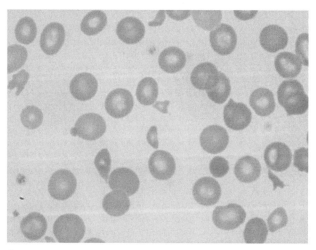

Figure 58-5 ■ Microangiopathic changes in disseminated intravascular coagulation) (See Color Plate 7, same as Fig. 42-7.) (Courtesy of Cabello Inchausti B: Chapter 42 of this book.)

in which the underlying cause of DIC cannot be effectively treated, this replacement strategy may be instituted in conjunction with the inhibition of blood coagulation to avoid fueling the fire. This can be accomplished with a simultaneous infusion of unfractionated heparin, administered at low doses, for example, 40 to 50 units/kg bolus followed by 10 units/kg/hour, titrated upward until the fibrinogen level and platelet counts begin to recover.

If thrombosis is the predominant feature of DIC, anticoagulation with unfractionated heparin should be maintained until the underlying disease process is contained. Adjunctive use of antifibrinolytic agents is controversial and should be used only in conjunction with heparin. Antifibrinolytic therapy may be particularly useful to prevent hemorrhagic complications precipitated by the DIC associated with acute promyelocytic leukemia and accompanying decreased levels of α-2-antiplasmin.

Bleeding in the Surgical Patient

Bleeding complications in the surgical patient can often be avoided with careful preoperative assessment for bleeding potential. A detailed personal and familial bleeding history should be elicited, and a comprehensive medication history is imperative. In the otherwise normal individual with no personal or family history of bleeding, routine laboratory testing beyond the platelet count, prothrombin time, and partial thromboplastin time is not necessary and has been shown in prospective trials to be a poor predictor of perioperative bleeding. However, for patients with a moderate or high risk of bleeding based on their medical history or with positive family histories, laboratory screens are essential to identify patients with coagulopathies, von Willebrand disease, hyperfibrinolysis, and platelet disorders. Prolonged bleeding times do not predict surgical bleeding, even in those patients who have ingested aspirin or nonsteroidal anti-inflammatory drugs (NSAIDs), except inpatients with von Willebrand disease.

If intraoperative bleeding occurs, the first step is to establish whether it is due to an anatomic defect related to the surgery itself or due to an undetected congenital or acquired hemostatic defect. Bleeding at the surgical site only is most often due to vascular damage and should be managed accordingly. On the other hand, more generalized bleeding accompanied by mucocutaneous and venipuncture site oozing is typical of a systemic coagulopathy, including disseminated intravascular coagulation. This warrants further laboratory evaluation, including prothrombin time, partial thromboplastin time, thrombin time or D-dimer assay, fibrinogen, platelet count, review of the peripheral smear for schistocytes, and renal and liver function studies. Subsequently, mixing studies, platelet aggregation studies, and specific assays for individual clotting factors and for von Willebrand factor activities may be needed. It is not uncommon for mild von Willebrand disease or factor XI deficiency to become clinically apparent for the first time during surgery, particularly when bleeding involves the mucous membranes, for example, oropharyngeal or genitourinary. If bleeding occurs hours to days postoperatively, factor XIII deficiency, dysfibrinogenemia, and hyperfibrinolysis should be considered. Ehlers-Danlos syndrome, an inherited defect in collagen structure, may also be associated with perioperative and delayed postoperative bleeding by virtue of poor wound healing. Management is focused ideally on the specific abnormality identified. Clotting factor supplementation with fresh frozen plasma and factor concentrates and platelet transfusions are the mainstays of therapy. If von Willebrand disease or hemophilia A carrier state is suspected, arginine desmopressin administration might be adequate. Typically, however, the results of the laboratory assessment are delayed, and empirical treatment measures must be instituted to stem bleeding. Fresh frozen plasma is usually given immediately, but intravenous arginine desmopressin should also be administered, since it appears to reverse platelet dysfunction produced by a wide variety of causes. Antifibrinolytic agents and fibrin sealants may be useful adjunctive measures. Recombinant factor VIIa has also been used for rapid reversal of an undefined coagulopathy in desperate situations.

References

Adjusted-dose warfarin versus low-intensity, fixed-dose warfarin plus aspirin for high-risk patients with atrial fibrillation: Stroke Prevention in Atrial Fibrillation III randomised clinical trial. Lancet 1996;348:633–638.

Cohen AJ, Kessler CM: Treatment of inherited coagulation disorders. Am J Med 1995;99:675–682.

Furie B, Limentani SA, Rosenfield CG: A practical guide to the evaluation and treatment of hemophilia. Blood 1994;84:3–9.

Mannucci PM, Chédiak J, Hanna W, et al: Treatment of von Willebrand disease with a high-purity factor VIII/von Willebrand factor concentrate: A prospective, multicenter study. Blood 2002;99(2):450–456.

Rapaport SI: Coagulation problems in liver disease [Review]. Blood Coagul Fibrinolysis 2000;11(Suppl 1):S69–S74.

Weitzel JN, Sadowski JA, Furie BC, et al: Surreptitious ingestion of a long-acting vitamin K antagonist/rodenticide, brodifacoum: Clinical and metabolic studies of three cases. Blood 1990;76:2555–2559.

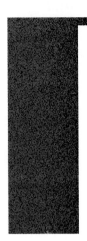

Chapter 59
Venous Thromboembolism

Jeffrey I. Weitz

Venous thromboembolism, which includes deep-vein thrombosis and pulmonary embolism, is a common problem that needs to be treated to reduce mortality from pulmonary embolism and to prevent recurrent deep-vein thrombosis and the postphlebitic syndrome.

Evaluation for Venous Thromboembolic Disease

At least 75% of patients who present with suspected venous thromboembolism do not have this disorder. Objective testing is necessary because clinical diagnosis alone is unreliable, and untreated venous thromboembolism can lead to fatal pulmonary embolism. A pretest probability of venous thromboembolism can be established on the basis of the history and physical examination, but further testing is required to confirm the diagnosis.

Deep-Vein Thrombosis

Patients with suspected deep-vein thrombosis can be classified as having high, intermediate, or low pretest probability of disease based on simple clinical criteria (see Chapter 43). Patients with a high pretest probability of deep-vein thrombosis are those with typical symptoms and signs, including localized pain and swelling in the affected limb, as well as risk factors for deep-vein thrombosis, such as recent immobilization, surgery in the past three months, or cancer that is being treated with chemotherapy or radiation therapy. Those who have an alternative explanation for their symptoms can be assigned a low pretest probability. Common alternative causes of pain and swelling in the leg include superficial phlebitis, cellulitis, muscle or tendon tear, or ruptured Baker's cyst.

Compression ultrasonography is the objective test that is most often used to exclude deep-vein throm-

bosis in the popliteal or more proximal veins. The inability to compress a vein with gentle pressure from the ultrasound transducer indicates the presence of deep-vein thrombosis. Compared with venography, the reference standard for deep-vein thrombosis diagnosis, compression ultrasonography has a sensitivity and specificity for proximal deep-vein thrombosis of 96% and 98%, respectively. Compression ultrasonography is less sensitive for detecting calf vein thrombosis because the calf veins are smaller in caliber and are buried deep in the calf muscles.

If the initial compression ultrasound is positive, the diagnosis of deep-vein thrombosis is established because the test has a positive predictive value over 90%. A negative compression ultrasound does not exclude the possibility of calf deep-vein thrombosis, and one of three approaches can be taken (Figure 59-1). Studies have shown that it is safe to withhold anticoagulant therapy in these individuals and to repeat the test in one week. Approximately 2% of patients with a negative initial ultrasound examination will have a positive result on repeat testing, likely reflecting proximal extension of calf vein thrombi. A second strategy can obviate the need for serial testing. The diagnosis of deep-vein thrombosis can be reliably excluded in patients with a negative initial ultrasound examination who have a low to moderate pretest probability of deep-vein thrombosis if the D-dimer test is negative. A plasmin-derived product of cross-linked fibrin, D-dimer can be measured in whole blood or in plasma. Rapid D-dimer assays are now available to simplify deep-vein thrombosis diagnosis. Because these tests vary in their performance characteristics, however, it is important to use a D-dimer assay that has been validated for deep-vein thrombosis diagnosis. Only assays with negative predictive values over 90% should be used in this setting.

The third strategy is reserved for patients with a high pretest probability of deep-vein thrombosis, particularly those with a positive D-dimer. If the initial ultrasound examination is negative, venography

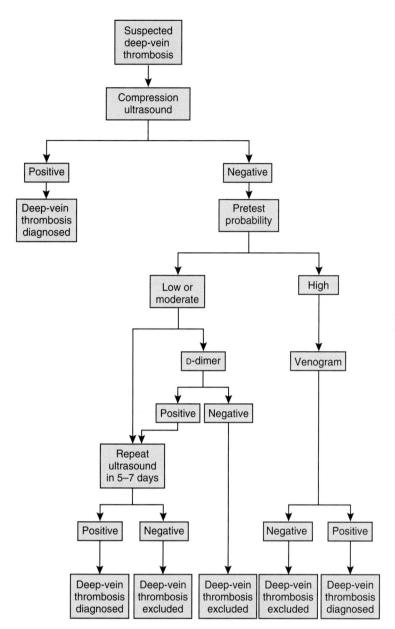

Figure 59-1 ■ Approach to patients with clinically suspected deep-vein thrombosis.

should be considered to document calf vein thrombosis or nonocclusive proximal vein thrombi that can be missed by ultrasonography. Early diagnosis of symptomatic calf vein thrombosis is worthwhile because anticoagulant therapy is the only modality that will afford symptom relief.

Diagnosis of recurrent venous thrombosis is problematic. Symptoms of postphlebitic syndrome often mimic those of recurrent deep-vein thrombosis, and objective test results can be abnormal as a consequence of previous disease. Recurrence is readily diagnosed when ultrasonography or venography shows new abnormalities. The diagnosis by ultrasonography can be complicated because a high proportion of

patients with previous deep-vein thrombosis have persistently noncompressible veins. Likewise, venographic evidence of recurrent thrombosis can be masked by obliteration or recanalization of veins as a result of previous disease. A positive D-dimer test can help to establish the diagnosis of recurrence in this setting.

Pulmonary Embolism

Clinical diagnosis of pulmonary embolism is difficult, but a pretest probability can be derived on the basis of symptoms and signs (see Chapter 43).

The diagnosis of pulmonary embolism must be

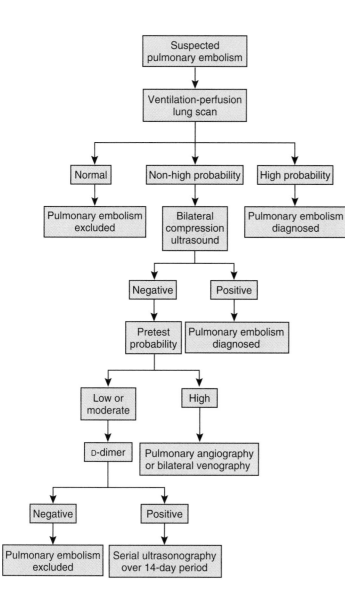

Figure 59-2 ■ Approach to patients with clinically suspected pulmonary embolism.

established by using objective testing (Figure 59-2). The first step is radionuclide lung imaging. If the test is normal, the diagnosis of pulmonary embolism is excluded, whereas a high-probability scan, one that shows a nonventilated perfusion defect that is segmental or larger, establishes the diagnosis. Over 50% of patients have a nondiagnostic scan and require further investigation because at least 25% will have pulmonary embolism. Although fewer than 20% of patients with proven pulmonary embolism have symptoms or signs suggestive of deep-vein thrombosis, about 70% of such patients have evidence of deep-vein thrombosis if venography is performed. Consequently, the next step in the diagnostic evaluation of patients with a nondiagnostic scan is to determine whether there is evidence of deep-vein thrombosis. This can be accomplished by performing bilateral compression ultrasonography. If the test is positive, the diagnosis is established. Normal results, however, do not exclude the possibility of pulmonary embolism. In this instance, the diagnostic strategy is guided by the pretest probability of pulmonary embolism and the result of the D-dimer test. For patients with a low to moderate pretest probability of pulmonary embolism, particularly those with a negative D-dimer test, it is safe to withhold anticoagulant therapy and to perform serial compression ultrasonography. Patients with a high pretest probability of pulmonary embolism require either pulmonary angiography, the reference standard, or bilateral venography. If these tests are negative, anticoagulation therapy can be withheld. Spiral computed tomography (CT) of the chest does not have sufficient sensitivity to exclude pulmonary embolism, although the technology is improving. A positive test, however, can establish the diagnosis.

Table 59-1 ▪ Indications for Various Treatment Modalities in Patients with Venous Thromboembolism

Treatment	Indications
Anticoagulant therapy	Majority of patients with venous thromboembolism
Thrombolytic therapy	Massive pulmonary embolism with hemodynamic compromise; selected patients with extensive iliofemoral thrombosis
Intracaval filter	Bleeding or high risk of bleeding; noncompliant with anticoagulants; pulmonary embolism despite adequate doses of anticoagulants; prophylaxis in patients with massive pulmonary embolism who cannot tolerate more emboli
Venous thrombectomy	None; high rates of recurrent thrombosis limit long-term effectiveness
Acute pulmonary embolectomy	Massive pulmonary embolism in patients with contraindications to thrombolytic therapy or failure of thrombolytic drugs
Pulmonary endarterectomy	Selected patients with chronic large-vessel thromboembolic pulmonary hypertension

Treatment

Therapeutic modalities that are available for the treatment of venous thromboembolism are shown in Table 59-1. Most patients are given anticoagulant therapy. Thrombolytic therapy is reserved for selected patients with extensive iliofemoral thrombosis or pulmonary embolism. An intracaval filter is indicated in patients with contraindications to anticoagulants, including active bleeding or a high risk for bleeding, or in anticoagulated patients who are noncompliant. Pulmonary embolectomy is rarely performed in the acute setting and should be considered only in patients with massive pulmonary embolism who are not candidates for thrombolytic therapy or who fail to respond to this treatment.

Anticoagulant Therapy

Initial Treatment of Venous Thromboembolism

Once the diagnosis of venous thromboembolism has been established, heparin or low-molecular-weight heparin therapy should be started, provided that there are no contraindications to anticoagulant therapy. Adequate doses of anticoagulants must be given to prevent pulmonary embolism and recurrent deep-vein thrombosis. If heparin is used, doses sufficient to produce an activated partial thromboplastin time (PTT) that is twofold to threefold greater than the control value should be given. Although a partial thromboplastin time ratio of 1.5 to 2.5 was recommended in the past, with the more sensitive partial thromboplastin time reagents in current use, a partial thromboplastin time ratio below 2.0 results in a heparin level below the therapeutic target of 0.3 to 0.7 antifactor Xa units/mL or 0.2 to 0.4 units/mL by protamine titration of the thrombin clotting time.

The likelihood of achieving a therapeutic anticoagulant response with heparin is increased with the use of heparin dosing nomograms. A therapeutic partial thromboplastin time is achieved more rapidly, and the risk of recurrent venous thromboembolism is lower, with a weight-adjusted heparin nomogram than with a fixed-dose regimen. The low rates of recurrent venous thromboembolism in contemporary studies that used a variety of therapeutic ranges for the partial thromboplastin time and different reagents and coagulometers for monitoring suggest that heparin therapy is likely to be effective, provided that starting doses are adequate and the partial thromboplastin time is monitored.

Heparin therapy must be monitored because the anticoagulant response to heparin varies among patients. This variability reflects the nonspecific binding of heparin to plasma proteins, endothelium, and macrophages within the reticuloendothelial system. Binding of heparin to plasma proteins and cells reduces the anticoagulant effect of heparin by limiting the amount of heparin that is available to interact with antithrombin. This effect varies among patients because some heparin-binding proteins, such as fibronectin and vitronectin, are acute-phase reactants whose levels increase with illness, whereas others, such as platelet factor 4 and high-molecular-weight multimers of von Willebrand's factor, are released from activated platelets during clotting.

If the plasma levels of heparin-binding proteins are excessive, high doses of heparin may be required to achieve a therapeutic partial thromboplastin time. The antifactor Xa level should be measured in patients who have a subtherapeutic partial thromboplastin time despite daily heparin doses that exceed 35,000 units. If the antifactor Xa level also is subtherapeutic, a situation that is indicative of high levels of heparin-binding proteins, the heparin dose can be increased until a therapeutic partial thromboplastin time or antifactor Xa level is obtained. In contrast, if the antifactor Xa level is therapeutic in the face of a subtherapeutic partial thromboplastin time, a reflection of the presence of high levels of factor VIII that shorten the partial thromboplastin time, then the antifactor Xa level should be used for subsequent heparin monitoring.

Heparin binding to plasma proteins and cells is chain-length-dependent, longer chains having higher affinity than shorter chains. Consequently, low-molecular-weight heparin, which has a mean molecular mass about one third that of unfractionated heparin, exhibits less binding. Reduced binding to endothelium and macrophages endows low-molecular-weight heparin with greater bioavailability and a longer half-life than heparin and dose-independent clearance. Less binding to plasma proteins results in a more predictable anticoagulant response with low-molecular-weight heparin than with heparin. On the basis of these characteristics, low-molecular-weight heparin can be given subcutaneously once or twice daily in weight-adjusted doses without laboratory monitoring (Table 59-2). Because low-molecular-weight heparin is cleared by the kidneys, however, the dose should be adjusted in patients with renal dysfunction. Although data are limited, a therapeutic range of 0.5 to 1.2 antifactor Xa units/mL has been recommended.

Unmonitored subcutaneous low-molecular-weight heparin is at least as safe and effective as intravenous heparin for the treatment of deep-vein thrombosis and pulmonary embolism. Two trials in patients with proximal deep-vein thrombosis compared out-of-hospital twice-daily subcutaneous low-molecular-weight heparin with conventional heparin therapy given in hospital by continuous intravenous infusion. The two treatments resulted in similar rates of recurrent venous thromboembolism and bleeding. On the basis of these findings, unmonitored outpatient treatment with low-molecular-weight heparin appears to be as safe and effective as intravenous heparin in patients with proximal deep-vein thrombosis. Given the health care savings associated with out-of-hospital treatment, low-molecular-weight heparin is more cost-effective than heparin and is rapidly becoming the drug of choice for initial venous thromboembolism treatment.

Unmonitored low-molecular-weight heparin also is as safe and effective as intravenous heparin for treatment of patients with submassive pulmonary embolism. Patients with minimal symptoms of pulmonary embolism can be safely treated as outpatients. Those with comorbid illnesses, extensive iliofemoral deep-vein thrombosis, venous gangrene, symptomatic pulmonary embolism, or high risk of bleeding might need hospitalization, but early discharge may be possible once their condition stabilizes.

Heparin or low-molecular-weight heparin therapy should be given for at least five days on the basis of the results of two randomized trials demonstrating that a four- to five-day course of heparin is as effective as a nine- to ten-day course. With the shorter duration of heparin therapy, oral anticoagulants are started within 24 hours of initiation of heparin treatment. On the basis of the four- to five-day delay necessary to obtain an antithrombotic effect with warfarin, it is recommended that heparin be given for at least five days and be discontinued only when the International Normalized Ratio (INR) has been therapeutic for two consecutive days. Although this streamlined approach can be used for most patients with venous thromboembolism, those with extensive iliofemoral thrombosis or massive pulmonary embolism might benefit from a longer course of heparin treatment.

Long-Term Treatment of Venous Thromboembolism

After an initial course of heparin treatment, long-term anticoagulant therapy with warfarin is needed to prevent recurrent venous thromboembolism. Warfarin is given in doses sufficient to produce an Inter-

---

Table 59-2 ■ Once- or Twice-Daily Dosing Regimens for Low-Molecular-Weight Heparins

Agent	Once-daily (U/kg)	Twice-daily (U/kg)
Dalteparin	100	200
Enoxaparin	100	150
Tinzaparin	175	—

*The doses of enoxaparin are calculated based on a specific antifactor Xa activity of 100 U/mg.

national Normalized Ratio of 2 to 3 on the basis of evidence that this intensity of anticoagulation is not only as effective as higher-intensity treatment that results in International Normalized Ratio of 3 to 4, but also safer. Some investigators have recommended an International Normalized Ratio of 3 to 4 for treatment of patients with antiphospholipid antibody syndrome.

Doses of twice-daily subcutaneous heparin sufficient to produce a therapeutic midinterval partial thromboplastin time are as safe and effective as warfarin for secondary prophylaxis. Likewise, low-molecular-weight heparin is effective for secondary prophylaxis.

The optimal duration of anticoagulant therapy depends on the balance between the risk of bleeding and the risk of recurrent venous thromboembolism (Figure 59-3). Patients with symptomatic calf deep-vein thrombosis complicating surgery or medical illness should be treated for six weeks to three months, while those with proximal deep-vein thrombosis in these settings should be treated for three months. Treatment can be stopped at these points, provided that precipitating factors have resolved and the patient is fully ambulatory. The risk of recurrence after stopping anticoagulant therapy is higher in patients who develop venous thromboembolism in the absence of obvious risk factors, and these patients should be treated for at least six months. At this point, decisions regarding continued anticoagulation therapy can be based on patient preference and careful analysis of the bleeding risk. Long-term anticoagulation is indicated for patients with recurrent venous thromboembolism or ongoing risk factors, such as metastatic cancer or thrombophilia secondary to homozygous factor V

Leiden or presence of antiphospholipid antibodies or a lupus anticoagulant. Patients with a single episode of idiopathic venous thromboembolism who are heterozygous for the factor V Leiden or the prothrombin gene mutation and those with antithrombin, protein C, or protein S deficiency should be treated for at least six months, although some recommend longer-term treatment.

Treatment of Venous Thromboembolism in Pregnancy
Neither heparin nor low-molecular-weight heparin crosses the placenta, and both have been successfully used in pregnancy. In contrast, coumarin derivatives should be avoided because they cross the placenta and can cause fetal malformations if given in the first trimester, central nervous system abnormalities if used in any trimester, and an increase in the risk of fetal bleeding when given in the third trimester. Venous thromboembolism in pregnancy should be treated with continuous intravenous heparin in therapeutic doses for five days followed by twice-daily subcutaneous heparin in doses sufficient to produce a therapeutic mid-interval partial thromboplastin time. Low-molecular-weight heparin appears to be a reasonable alternative and has the advantages of once-daily administration and possibly a lower risk of heparin-induced osteoporosis. After delivery, intravenous heparin or subcutaneous low-molecular-weight heparin can be given along with warfarin. Once the International Normalized Ratio is therapeutic, heparin is discontinued, and warfarin is given for four to six weeks or until patients with venous thromboembolism have had a minimum of three months of anticoagulation treatment. Warfarin does not pass

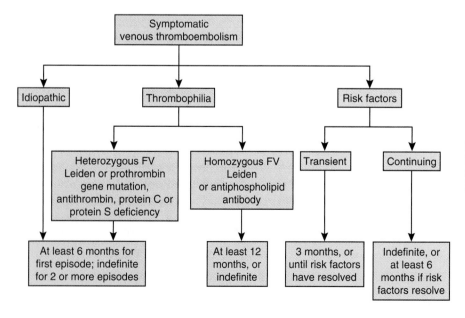

Figure 59-3 ■ Duration of anticoagulation therapy for patients with venous thromboembolism FV = Factor V.

into breast milk and is safe for infants of nursing mothers.

The risk of recurrent venous thromboembolism in pregnancy is low in women with a history of prior venous thromboembolism that occurred in the setting of known risk factors. Consequently, routine antepartum thromboprophylaxis is not warranted. However, these individuals should receive a four- to six-weeks course of warfarin therapy postpartum.

The risk of recurrence is higher if the prior episode of venous thromboembolism was unprovoked or if there is an underlying biochemical abnormality. In patients who are not given antepartum anticoagulation, about 5% develop recurrent venous thromboembolism during pregnancy. Consequently, these patients may benefit from antepartum thromboprophylaxis with prophylactic doses of heparin or low-molecular-weight heparin in addition to a four- to six-weeks course of warfarin therapy postpartum.

Complications of Anticoagulant Therapy

Patients who are treated with anticoagulants are subject to complications. These include recurrent venous thromboembolism, bleeding, heparin-induced thrombocytopenia, osteoporosis, and skin necrosis.

Recurrent Thromboembolism Despite Anticoagulant Therapy

Recurrent venous thromboembolism early in the course of treatment may reflect inadequate dosing of anticoagulants or may complicate heparin-induced thrombocytopenia. The former requires increased doses of anticoagulants, whereas the latter is best managed by discontinuation of heparin and use of an alternative anticoagulant drug. Recurrent venous thromboembolism in patients receiving therapeutic doses of warfarin most often occurs in patients with cancer or antiphospholipid antibodies. These patients can usually be managed with therapeutic doses of heparin or low-molecular-weight heparin.

Bleeding

Approximately 5% of patients who are treated with full-dose heparin have major bleeding. Although excessive prolongation of the partial thromboplastin time may increase the risk of bleeding, comorbid conditions such as recent surgery, hepatic dysfunction, severe thrombocytopenia, or concomitant antiplatelet therapy are better predictors. Meta-analyses comparing rates of major bleeding with therapeutic doses of heparin or low-molecular-weight heparin suggest that the rates are lower with low-molecular-weight heparin.

Although protamine sulfate neutralizes heparin, it incompletely neutralizes the antifactor Xa activity of low-molecular-weight heparin because smaller heparin chains do not bind protamine sulfate. Despite this limitation, protamine sulfate should be given to low-molecular-weight heparin-treated patients with major bleeding because protamine sulfate completely neutralizes the antithrombin activity of low-molecular-weight heparin and neutralizes at least two thirds of its antifactor Xa activity. With either heparin preparation, 1 mg of protamine neutralizes 100 units of heparin.

The risk of bleeding with long-term warfarin therapy increases when the International Normalized Ratio is excessively prolonged. Comorbid conditions associated with an increased risk of warfarin-induced bleeding include age over 65 years, a previous stroke or gastrointestinal bleeding, atrial fibrillation, concomitant antiplatelet therapy, or coexisting hepatic or renal failure. Patients who present with gastrointestinal or genitourinary bleeding when their International Normalized Ratio is 3.0 or less should be investigated for an underlying lesion.

Warfarin-treated patients with International Normalized Ratio values of 4.5 to 10 who are asymptomatic should have their warfarin held. Compared with placebo, administration of 1 mg of vitamin K sublingually more rapidly lowers the International Normalized Ratio into the therapeutic range without compromising further warfarin therapy. Patients who are bleeding should be given vitamin K and plasma to normalize the International Normalized Ratio. For life-threatening or serious bleeding (e.g., intracranial or intraocular), recombinant factor VIIa or prothrombin complex concentrates can be given in place of plasma to effect more rapid hemostasis. Although recombinant factor VIIa is expensive, it is a better choice than prothrombin complex concentrates for this indication because there is no risk of viral transmission.

Heparin-Induced Thrombocytopenia

Approximately 3% of patients who are given heparin develop heparin-induced thrombocytopenia, a disorder that is caused by IgG antibodies directed against complexes of platelet factor 4 and heparin. The incidence of heparin-induced thrombocytopenia is lower with low-molecular-weight heparin than with heparin because low-molecular-weight heparin has lower affinity for platelet factor 4. The diagnosis of heparin-induced thrombocytopenia should be suspected when the platelet count falls to less than $100,000/mm^3$ or to 50% of the baseline value 5 to 15 days after heparin therapy is started, or sooner if the patient has received heparin in the past three months. Extension of existing venous thromboembolism or new arterial thrombosis can complicate heparin-induced thrombocytopenia, so early diagnosis is important. Unfortunately, diagnostic tests for antibodies against complexes of platelet factor 4 and heparin or assays of heparin-induced release of serotonin from platelets are not widely available, and the turnaround times for these tests are long. Consequently, empiric therapy often is needed. Thus, in patients with suspected heparin-induced thrombocytopenia, heparin or low-molecular-weight heparin should be stopped, and treatment with an alternative drug should be initiated. Suitable alternative agents include danaparoid sodium, hirudin, or argatroban. Danaparoid sodium is given as an intravenous bolus of 2500 units followed by an infusion of 400 units/hour, for four hours, 300 units/hour for four hours, and a maintenance infusion of 200 units/hour thereafter. The dose of drug is then titrated to achieve an antifactor Xa level of 0.5 to 0.8 units/mL. Hirudin is given as an intravenous bolus of 0.4 mg/kg followed by a continuous infusion of 0.15 mg/kg/hour, whereas argatroban is given as an infusion of 2 µg/kg/hour. In both cases, the doses are then titrated to achieve a 1.5- to 2.5-fold prolongation of the partial thromboplastin time.

Heparin-Induced Osteoporosis

Therapeutic doses of heparin given for a month or more can cause osteoporosis. Although the risk of fractures is low, a partly reversible reduction in bone density occurs in about 30% of patients who are given long-term heparin. The risk is likely to be lower with low-molecular-weight heparin.

Warfarin-Induced Skin Necrosis

This uncommon side effect most often occurs in patients with protein C or protein S deficiency. Skin necrosis also can occur in patients with heparin-induced thrombocytopenia who are given warfarin without concomitant danaparoid sodium, hirudin, or argatroban because these individuals have acquired protein C deficiency as a consequence of thrombin-induced protein C activation and consumption. Skin necrosis starts two to five days after initiation of warfarin therapy and likely reflects the rapid decrease in protein C or S levels that precedes the reduction in the levels of prothrombin and factor X that mediates the antithrombotic effect of warfarin (Figure 59-4). To avoid this complication in patients with known protein C or protein S deficiency, warfarin should be started in low doses only after therapeutic doses of heparin or low-molecular-weight heparin have been given. Heparin or low-molecular-weight heparin should be continued until the International Normalized Ratio is therapeutic for at least two consecutive days. For patients with heparin-induced thrombocytopenia, initiation of warfarin therapy should be

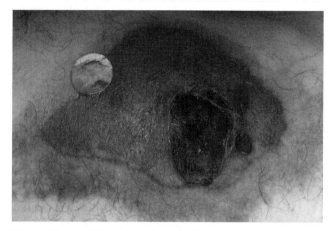

Figure 59-4 ■ Warfarin-induced skin necrosis. Central area of necrosis is surrounded by a well-circumscribed area of erythema. Circular defect at the margin is the biopsy site. (See Color Plate 14.)

delayed until the platelet count is near normal with danaparoid sodium, hirudin, or argatroban therapy.

Thrombolytic Therapy

Thrombolytic therapy has been advocated in patients with massive pulmonary embolism who have syncope, hypotension, severe hypoxemia, or clinical or echocardiographic evidence of right heart failure. It also should be considered in patients with submassive pulmonary embolism who are clinically compromised because of underlying cardiac or pulmonary disease and in selected patients with proximal deep-vein thrombosis.

The goal of thrombolytic therapy in patients with pulmonary embolism is to produce rapid dissolution of pulmonary thrombi so as to improve pulmonary perfusion and reverse right ventricular dysfunction. Compared with anticoagulants, thrombolytic therapy produces greater improvement in hemodynamic abnormalities and defects seen on perfusion lung scans or pulmonary angiograms when follow-up tests are done within 24 hours. By five to seven days, however, perfusion lung scans are similar in patients who are given thrombolytic therapy and those who are given anticoagulants. Although long-term follow-up studies suggest that patients who are given thrombolytic therapy have higher diffusion capacity and lung capillary volume at one year and lower pulmonary pressures at seven years than those who are given heparin, the clinical significance of these findings is uncertain.

A small study comparing thrombolytic therapy with anticoagulant therapy in 46 patients with pulmonary embolism demonstrated improved right ventricular function in 39% and 19%, respectively, and worsened right ventricular function in 2% and 17%, respectively. These findings require confirmation in patients with more massive pulmonary embolism and greater hemodynamic compromise.

Regional catheter-directed thrombolysis has been advocated for selected patients with extensive iliofemoral thrombosis to reduce symptoms more rapidly and to minimize valve destruction, thereby lowering the risk or severity of postphlebitic syndrome. Although successful thrombolysis can improve symptoms, evidence that it enhances long-term outcome is lacking. Thrombolytic therapy is expensive, requires specialized equipment, and produces a twofold to fourfold increase in the risk of bleeding. Consequently, it should be reserved for patients with extensive iliofemoral thrombosis who are not at high risk of bleeding.

Intracaval Filters

An intracaval filter should be considered in patients with proximal deep-vein thrombosis or pulmonary embolism who are actively bleeding or at high risk of bleeding. Patients on anticoagulant therapy who are noncompliant, those with objectively diagnosed pulmonary embolism despite therapeutic doses of anticoagulants, and those with chronic large-vessel thromboembolic hypertension who cannot tolerate further emboli may also benefit from an intracaval filter. Because intracaval filters may increase the risk of recurrent venous thromboembolism, patients without ongoing contraindication to anticoagulation should receive anticoagulant therapy after filter insertion.

Surgical Thrombectomy or Embolectomy

Thrombectomy is often complicated by acute recurrent thrombosis despite anticoagulant therapy because the damaged vein wall is highly thrombogenic. Consequently, this procedure is of no long-term benefit and is rarely performed. Although pulmonary embolectomy can be life-saving, the procedure is associated with a high mortality rate and requires special facilities and highly trained personnel. Pulmonary embolectomy should be reserved for patients with massive pulmonary embolism who are not candidates for thrombolytic therapy or who fail to respond to thrombolytic drugs.

In contrast to acute pulmonary embolectomy, elective pulmonary endarterectomy relieves morbidity by reducing pulmonary hypertension in selected patients with chronic large-vessel thromboembolic pulmonary hypertension. The success of this procedure, however, depends on the experience of the personnel performing the operation.

Summary and Conclusions

Increased availability of compression ultrasonography and introduction of rapid D-dimer testing have simplified the diagnosis of venous thromboembolism. The advent of low-molecular-weight heparin has shifted venous thromboembolism treatment to the outpatient setting, thereby reducing health care costs.

References

General

Becker DM, Philbrick JR, Selby B: Inferior vena cava filters: Indications, safety, effectiveness. Arch Intern Med 1992; 152:1985–1994.

Comerota AJ, Aldridge SC, Cohen G, et al: A strategy of aggressive regional therapy for acute iliofemoral venous thrombosis with contemporary venous thrombectomy or catheter-directed thrombolysis. J Vasc Surg 1994; 20:244–254.

Decousus MN, Leizorovicz A, Parent F, et al: A clinical trial of vena cava filters in the prevention of pulmonary embolism in patients with proximal deep-vein thrombosis. N Engl J Med 1998;338:409–415.

Ginsberg JS: Management of venous thromboembolism. N Engl J Med 1996;335:1816–1828.

Ginsberg JS, Wells PS, Brill-Edwards P, et al: Antiphospholipid antibodies and venous thromboembolism. Blood 1995;86: 3685–3691.

Khamashta MA, Cuadrado MJ, Mujic F, et al: The management of thrombosis in the antiphospholipid-antibody syndrome. N Engl J Med 1995;332:993–997.

Levine JS, Branch DW, Rauch J: The antiphospholipid syndrome. N Eng J Med 2002;346:752–763.

Plate G, Akesson H, Einarsson E, et al: Long-term results of venous thrombectomy combined with temporary arteriovenous fistula. Eur J Cardiovasc Surg 1990;4:483–489.

Deep-Vein Thrombosis

Birdwell B, Raskob GE, Whitsett TL, et al: The clinical validity of normal compression ultrasonography in outpatients suspected of having deep-vein thrombosis. Ann Intern Med 1998;128:1–7.

Brill-Edwards P, Lee A: D-dimer testing in the diagnosis of acute venous thromboembolism. Thromb Haemost 1999;82: 688–694.

Cogo A, Lensing AW, Koopman MM, et al: Compression ultrasonography for diagnostic management of patients with clinically suspected deep-vein thrombosis: prospective cohort study. BMJ 1998;316:17–20.

Couturaud F, Kearon C: Long-term treatment for venous thromboembolism. Curr Opin Hematol 2000;7:302–308.

Lensing AWA, Prandoni P, Prins MH, et al: Deep-vein thrombosis. Lancet 1999;353:479–485.

Prandoni P, Cogo A, Bernardi E, et al: A simple ultrasound approach for detection of recurrent proximal-vein thrombosis. Circulation 1993;88:1730–1735.

Prandoni P, Lensing AWA, Piccioli A, et al: Recurrent venous thromboembolism and bleeding complications during anticoagulant treatment in patients with venous thrombosis. Blood 2002;100:3484–3488.

Wells PS, Hirsh J, Anderson DR, et al: Accuracy of clinical assessment of deep-vein thrombosis. Lancet 1995;345: 1326–1330 [erratum, Lancet 1995;346:516].

Heparin

Alving BM: How I treat heparin-induced thrombocytopenia and thrombosis. Blood 2003;101:31–37.

Anand S, Bates SM, Ginsberg JS, et al: Recurrent venous thrombosis and heparin therapy: An evaluation of the importance of early activated partial thromboplastin times. Arch Intern Med 1999;159:2029–2032.

Bates SM, Weitz JI, Johnston M, et al: Use of a fixed activated partial thromboplastin time ratio to establish a therapeutic range for unfractionated heparin. Arch Intern Med 2001;161:385–391.

Brill-Edwards P, Ginsberg JS, Gent M, et al: Safety of withholding heparin in pregnant women with a history of venous thromboembolism. N Engl J Med 2000;343:1439–1444.

Goldhaber SZ, Haire WD, Feldstein ML, et al: Alteplase versus heparin in acute pulmonary embolism: Randomised trial assessing right-ventricular function and pulmonary perfusion. Lancet 1993;341:507–511.

Gould MK, Dembitzer AD, Doyle RL, et al: Low-molecular-weight heparins compared with unfractionated heparin for treatment of acute deep venous thrombosis: A meta-analysis of randomized, controlled trials. Ann Intern Med 1999;130:800–809.

Hirsh J: Heparin. N Engl J Med 1991;324:1565–1584.

Hull RD, Delmore T, Carter C, et al: Adjusted subcutaneous heparin versus warfarin sodium in the long-term treatment of venous thrombosis. N Engl J Med 1982;306:189.

Hull RD, Raskob GE, Rosenbloom D, et al: Heparin for 5 days as compared with 10 days in the initial treatment of proximal venous thrombosis. N Engl J Med 1990;322:1260–1264.

Koopman MMW, Prandoni P, Piovella F, et al: Treatment of venous thrombosis with intravenous unfractionated heparin administered in the hospital as compared with subcutaneous low-molecular-weight heparin administered at home. N Engl J Med 1996;334:682–687.

Levine MN, Gent M, Hirsh J, et al: A comparison of low-molecular-weight heparin administered primarily at home with unfractionated heparin administered in the hospital for proximal deep-vein thrombosis. N Engl J Med 1996;334:677.

Monreal M, Lafoz E, Olive A, et al: Comparison of subcutaneous unfractionated heparin with a low-molecular-weight heparin (Fragmin) in patients with venous thromboembolism and contraindications to coumarin. Thromb Haemost 1994;71:7–11.

Pini M, Aiello S, Manotti C, et al: Low-molecular-weight heparin in the prevention of recurrences after deep-vein thrombosis. Thromb Haemost 1994;72:191–197.

Raschke RA, Reilly BM, Guidry JR, et al: The weight-based heparin dosing nomogram compared with a "standard care" nomogram: A randomized controlled trial. Ann Intern Med 1993;119:874–881.

Sanson BJ, Lensing AW, Prins MH, et al: Safety of low-molecular-weight heparin in pregnancy: A systematic review. Thromb Haemost 1999;81:668–672.

Weitz JI: Low-molecular-weight heparin. N Engl J Med 1997;337:688–698.

Pulmonary Embolism

Hull RD, Hirsh J, Carter CJ, et al: Pulmonary angiography, ventilation lung scanning, and venography for clinically suspected pulmonary embolism with abnormal perfusion lung scan. Ann Intern Med 1983;98:891–899.

Hull RD, Raskob GE, Ginsberg JS, et al: A noninvasive strategy for the treatment of patients with suspected pulmonary embolism. Arch Intern Med 1994;154:289–297.

Sharma GVRK, Burleson VA, Sasahara AA: Effect of thrombolytic therapy on pulmonary capillary blood volume in patients with pulmonary embolism. N Engl J Med 1980;303:842–845.

Sharma GVRK, Folland ED, McIntyre KM, et al: Long-term hemodynamic benefit of thrombolytic therapy in pulmonary embolic disease. J Am Coll Cardiol 1990;15:65A.

The PIOPED Investigators: Value of the ventilation/perfusion scan in acute pulmonary embolism: Results of the prospective investigation of pulmonary embolism diagnosis (PIOPED). JAMA 1990;263:2753–2759.

Warfarin

Crowther MA, Julian J, McCarty D, et al: Treatment of warfarin-associated coagulopathy with oral vitamin K: A randomised controlled trial. Lancet 2000;356:1551–1553.

Gallus A, Jackaman J, Tillet J, et al: Safety and efficacy of warfarin started early after submassive venous thrombosis or pulmonary embolism. Lancet 1996;2:1293–1296.

Chapter 60
Acute Myeloid Leukemia

Larry D. Cripe and Martin S. Tallman

Introduction

Acute myeloid leukemia (AML) is a heterogeneous group of disorders that arise from the neoplastic transformation of the hematopoietic stem cell. Such malignant cells either do not differentiate or differentiate abnormally (Figure 60-1). These immature cells proliferate and accumulate primarily in the bone marrow and peripheral blood but may also invade visceral tissues such as the liver, lung, and skin. The accumulation of immature cells inhibits normal hematopoiesis, resulting in neutropenia, anemia, and thrombocytopenia, with the corresponding clinical consequences of infection, fatigue, and bleeding. The disease is rapidly fatal if untreated. The etiology of acute myeloid leukemia appearing de novo is unknown in the majority of cases. However, secondary acute myeloid leukemia can evolve from either an antecedent hematologic disorder or prior exposure to certain chemotherapeutic agents. This secondary form is an increasingly important problem because the improved cure rate of patients who have a primary malignancy leaves them vulnerable to late effects of their therapy, which include leukemic transformation. Moreover, secondary forms of acute myeloid leukemia tend to proliferate rapidly and be resistant to chemotherapy. These patients may respond to initial therapy, but the responses are generally short-lived despite additional intensive chemotherapy.

Recent advances in immunophenotyping, karyotype analysis, and DNA analysis have led to important developments in tailored and targeted therapy. Some examples are the use of all-trans retinoic acid (ATRA) and arsenic trioxide for patients with acute promyelocytic leukemia, the anti-CD33-calicheamicin immunoconjugate gemtuzumab ozogamicin for patients whose leukemia cells express the CD 33 antigen, and high-dose cytarabine for patients with core binding factor leukemias. Further insights into the mechanisms of cell cycle control, apoptosis, differentiation, and cellular antigen expression should expand the armamentarium of targeted therapy.

Epidemiology

Acute myeloid leukemia accounts for 15% to 20% of acute leukemias in children and approximately 80% of the acute leukemias in adults. The disease occurs with an incidence of approximately 2.3 per 100,000 population and increases with age such that there are 2.6 cases per 100,000 population overall but the incidence increases to 12.6 cases per 100,000 in individuals who are older than age 65 years. Interestingly, acute promyelocytic leukemia is one subtype of acute myeloid leukemia whose incidence is constant regardless of age. This variety of acute myeloid leukemia also occurs more frequently in individuals of Latino origin, a finding suggesting a possible genetic link. In 2002, an estimated 10,600 new cases of acute myeloid leukemia will occur in the United States with a slight predominance in women (5,900 estimated new cases in women and 4,700 in men). An estimated 7,400 patients with acute myeloid leukemia will die in 2002. The median age of patients with acute myeloid leukemia is 63.

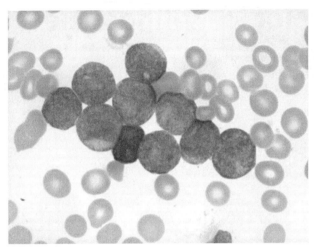

Figure 60-1 ■ Acute myeloid leukemia. These blasts have fine chromatin, prominent nucleolus, and very little cytoplasm (original magnification ×100, oil). (See Color Plate 10, same as Fig. 42-26. Courtesy of Cabello Inchausti B: Chapter 42 of this book.)

Risk Factors

A number of risk factors are reasonably well established in the genesis of acute myeloid leukemia. These include genetic factors, occupational exposure to benzene, prior exposure to chemotherapy, the presence of an antecedent hematologic disorder, such as a myelodysplastic syndrome or a myeloproliferative disorder, and exposure to radiation. Smoking of tobacco is associated with an increased risk, probably from the exposure to benzene in cigarette smoke.

Genetic Factors

The incidence of acute myeloid leukemia is increased in patients with a variety of congenital disorders associated with chromosomal abnormalities, such as Down syndrome and Klinefelter's syndrome and disorders associated with chromosomal instability, such as Fanconi's anemia, Bloom syndrome, and ataxia telangiectasia. Acute megakaryocytic leukemia is an uncommon variant in the general population but occurs more often in patients with Down syndrome.

Although most patients who develop acute myeloid leukemia have no identified predisposing factor, the majority, if not all, affected patients exhibit acquired clonal chromosomal abnormalities. These abnormalities are more common in cases of secondary acute myeloid leukemia.

Prior Chemotherapy Exposure

Detailed information about secondary acute myeloid leukemia comes from patients who have been treated with alkylating agents (mechlorethamine or cyclophosphamide) as part of combination chemotherapy for Hodgkin's disease. Such patients are at a more than 5% risk of developing acute myeloid leukemia within 2 to 12 years after completing chemotherapy (Figure 60-2). Acute myeloid leukemia also develops after exposure to inhibitors of topoisomerase II, such as etoposide. Acute myeloid leukemia that develops after alkylating agent exposure characteristically has a long latency, usually is preceded by a myelodysplastic phase, and is often associated with deletions and/or partial loss of chromosomes 5 and/or 7. In contrast, acute myeloid leukemia developing after exposure to topoisomerase II inhibitors have a relatively short latency period, myelomonocytic or monocytic differentiation, and frequent translocations involving chromosome 11q23.

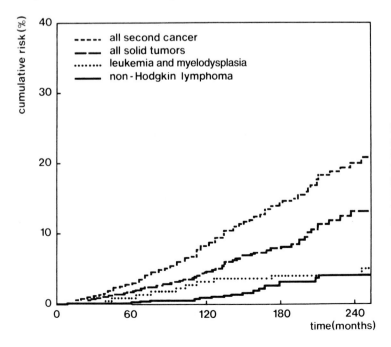

Figure 60-2 ■ Actuarial risk of developing a second malignancy following treatment for Hodgkin's disease (29% of patients received only radiation therapy and 71% both chemotherapy and radiation therapy). (From van Leeuwen FE, Klokman WJ, Hagenbeek A, et al: Second cancer risk following Hodgkin's disease: A 20-year follow-up study. J Clin Oncol 1994;12:312–325.)

Therapy-related myelodysplasia and acute myeloid leukemia also occur after high-dose treatment used in autologous hematopoietic stem cell transplantation. In one analysis, the estimated cumulative probability of developing these disorders was approximately 9% at six years among patients undergoing autologous transplantation for Hodgkin's disease and non-Hodgkin's lymphoma (Figure 60-3). The most important risk factor is the cumulative dose of alkylating agents. Increased patient age and previous radiation therapy, particularly total body irradiation, as part of the conditioning regimen, are additional risk factors.

Radiation Exposure

Survivors of radiation exposure from the atomic bomb blasts in Hiroshima and Nagasaki exhibited an increased incidence of acute myeloid leukemia, as did patients who had been treated with radiation therapy for ankylosing spondylitis or menorrhagia and radiation workers and radiologists prior to the institution of proper safeguards.

Viruses

The only clearly identified etiologic role for virally induced acute leukemia is the lymphoid leukemia that develops in the adult T cell leukemia and lymphoma of the Caribbean region and Japanese patients infected with the human T cell leukemia virus type 1 (HTLV-1) retrovirus.

Classification Systems

French-American-British Classification

The French-American-British (FAB) Classification was initially described in 1976 and was based solely on morphologic and cytochemical features of the leukemia cell. Although cytogenetics and immunophenotyping have emerged as important markers of the diagnosis and prognosis of acute myeloid leukemia, the FAB classification remains in use today. The frequency and characteristics of each variant are outlined in Table 60-1.

World Health Organization Classification

A new classification system was generated by the World Health Organization (WHO) to incorporate morphologic features and cytochemistry of the FAB classification along with the data from immunophenotyping, molecular genetics studies, and clinical features. The category of refractory anemia with excess blasts in transformation (RAEBt), which was associated with 20% to 30% blasts in the bone marrow and considered to be part of the spectrum of myelodysplasia, is now categorized as acute myeloid leukemia because the lower limit of bone marrow blast cells that is sufficient to establish the diagnosis of acute myeloid leukemia was lowered to 20% from 30% (Table 60-2). Acute myeloid leukemias are classified into four categories, which include those (1) with well-characterized cytogenetic or molecular abnormalities, (2) those with multilineage dysplasia, (3) those that are therapy-related, and (4) others, such as the morphologic subtypes of acute basophilic leukemia, acute panmyelosis and fibrosis, and acute biphenotypic leukemia.

Cytogenetics and Molecular Genetics

Clonal chromosomal abnormalities represent the most important independent prognostic factor at diagnosis. Numerical or structural abnormalities of the chromosomes can be identified with high-resolution banding

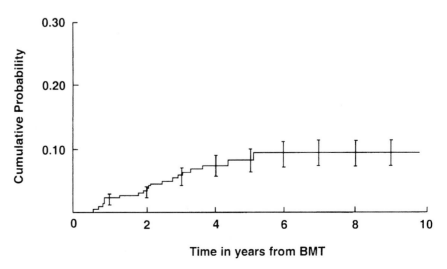

Figure 60-3 ■ Cumulative probability of the occurrence of therapy-related myelodysplastic syndrome or acute myeloid leukemia among 612 patients at the City of Hope Medical Center undergoing high-dose chemotherapy and autologous stem cell transplantation (BMT) for Hodgkin's disease and non-Hodgkin's lymphoma. (From Krishnan A, Bhatia S, Slovak ML, et al: Predictors of therapy-related leukemia and myelodysplasia following autologous transplantation for lymphoma: An assessment of risk factors. Blood 2000;95:1588–1593.)

Table 60-1 ■ French-American-British (FAB) Classification of Acute Myeloid Leukemia

FAB Subtype	Morphologic and Cytochemical Characteristics	Frequency (%)
M0	Large, agranular myeloblasts, sometimes resembling lymphoblasts of FAB subtype L2. Myeloperoxidase stain negative. Express CD13 or CD33 antigens on cell surface.	2–3
M1	Acute myeloblastic leukemia without maturation to at least promyelocyte stage: large, poorly differentiated myeloblasts represent ≥90% of the nonerythroid cells. At least 3% of the myeloblasts stain positive for myeloperoxidase.	20
M2	Acute myeloblastic leukemia with maturation, 30–89% of the nonerythroid cells are myeloblasts having abundant cytoplasm with moderate-to-many granules. Auer rods are often visible. Myeloblasts are myeloperoxidase positive.	25–30
M3	Leukemia cells usually contain heavy azurophilic granulation. Nuclear size varies greatly. Nuclei are often bilobed or kidney-shaped. Some cells contain bundles of Auer rods. Leukemia cells strongly positive for myeloperoxidase. Microgranular variant. Usually HLA-DR negative.	8–15
M4	Myeloblasts, promyelocytes, myelocytes, and other granulocytic precursors comprise over 30% of the nonerythroid cells but do not exceed 80%. Monocytic cells account for up to 20% of the nonerythroid cells. Nonspecific esterase and chloroacetate esterase cytochemical reactions are positive. Auer rods may be present.	20–25
M4Eo	Myelomonoblasts with cytochemically and morphologically abnormal eosinophils.	5
M5	Monoblasts, promonocytes, or monocytes make up ≥80% of the nonerythroid cells. In M5$_a$, ≥80% of all monocytic cells are monoblasts; negative for myeloperoxidase and usually positive for nonspecific esterase. In the well-differentiated subtype M5$_b$, <80% are monoblasts. Nonspecific esterase positivity is lost after exposure to sodium fluoride.	10
M6	>50% of the nucleated marrow cells are erythroid. Erythroblasts usually strongly PAS positive. Myeloblasts represent 30% or more of the nonerythroid cells.	5
M7	Large and small megakaryoblasts with high nuclear/cytoplasm ratio. Cytoplasm is pale and agranular. Standard cytochemical stains not definitive. Platelet peroxidase and platelet-specific antibodies often positive. Factor VIII may be positive.	1–2

Adapted from Bennett JM et al: Br J Haematol 1976;33:451 and Bennett JM et al: Am J Med 1985;103:620.

techniques in the majority of patients with acute myeloid leukemia. A number of specific cytogenetic abnormalities correlate with particular morphologic and clinical features of acute myeloid leukemia, which together define characteristic clinical syndromes of acute myeloid leukemia, including t(15;17) in acute promyelocytic leukemia, called FAB type M3 in the FAB classification, inv(16) or t(15;16) in acute myelomonocytic leukemia (FAB type M4EO) and t(8;21) in acute myelocytic leukemia (FAB type M2).

Many specific chromosomal abnormalities in patients with acute myeloid leukemia involve rearrangements and often fusion of specific genes that have been implicated in the pathogenesis of acute myeloid leukemia (Table 60-3). Some of these genes function as oncogenes; others act as tumor-suppressors. Knowledge of the molecular features of

the different acute myeloid leukemia types provides insight into mechanisms of leukemogenesis and drug resistance.

Fluorescence in Situ Hybridization

Fluorescence in situ hybridization (FISH) has become an important method of detecting clonal chromosomal abnormalities in patients with acute myeloid leukemia because it does not require dividing cells, can be done on either bone marrow or peripheral blood, is highly sensitive and specific, and can be carried out rapidly (4 to 24 hours). A DNA probe is designed to identify a target in the nuclear DNA of interphase or metaphase cells. Probes are now available to identify many of the common chromosome abnormalities in acute myeloid leukemia, including

Table 60-2 ■ Proposed WHO Classification of Acute Myeloid Leukemias

1. AML with recurrent cytogenetic translocations:
   AML with t(8;21)(q22;q22)
   Acute promyelocytic leukemias with t(15;17)(q22;q11) and variants
   AML with abnormal bone marrow eosinophils inv(16)(p13q22) or t(16;16)(p13;q11)
   AML with 11q23 abnormalities

2. AML with multilineage dysplasia
   With prior myelodysplastic syndrome
   Without prior myelodysplastic syndrome

3. AML and myelodysplastic syndromes, therapy-related
   Alkylating agent-related
   Epipodophyllotoxin-related (some may be lymphoid)
   Other types

4. AML not otherwise categorized
   AML minimally differentiated
   AML with maturation
   AML without maturation
   Acute monocytic leukemia
   Acute erythroid leukemia
   Acute panmyelosis with myelofibrosis

5. Acute biphenotypic leukemias

From Harris NL, Jaffee ES, Diebold J, et al: World Health Organization classification of neoplastic diseases of the hematopoietic and lymphoid tissues: Report of the Clinical Advisory Committee Meeting–Airlie House, Virginia, November, 1997. J Clin Oncol 1999;17:3835–3849.

t(8;21), t(16;16), inv(16), t(15;17), 11q23, −5/del5q, −7/del7q, trisomy 8, and t(12;21). This technique has become particularly useful in establishing the diagnosis and monitoring patients with acute promyelocytic leukemia.

Cytogenetic Prognostic Groups

The correlation of specific cytogenetic abnormalities with outcome has defined three groups (Table 60-4), whose outcomes from therapy strikingly differ (Figure 60-4).

Favorable Chromosomal Abnormalities

This group includes patients with acute myeloid leukemia whose leukemia cells exhibit balanced reciprocal translocations, namely, t(8;21); t(15;17) or t(16;16) or inv(16). These have a high likelihood (greater than 80%) of achieving remission (Table 60-5), and disease-free and overall survival is lengthy after conventional chemotherapy. The overall survival rate is 60% to 70% at five years. The majority of patients with these translocations are young and present with de novo acute myeloid leukemia. The

favorable prognostic implication also extends to the uncommon older patient or patient with therapy-related acute myeloid leukemia who presents with one of these favorable abnormalities.

FAB M2 with t(8;21) is one of the most frequent subtypes of acute myeloid leukemia (Table 60-6), occurring in 20% of adults and 40% of pediatric patients. The disease is associated with a younger median age at onset, extramedullary manifestations, and a relatively favorable prognosis in the absence of extramedullary disease.

Molecular Features of Acute Myeloid Leukemia with t(8;21)

AML FAB M2 with t(8;21), FAB M4 with inv(16) or t(16;16), and t(12;21) are all classified as core-binding factor (CBF) leukemias (Table 60-7). The balanced reciprocal translocation between chromosomes 8 and 21 results in the fusion of the AML-1 and ETO genes. The AML-1 gene codes for the DNA-binding component of core-binding factor, which activates transcription of a number of genes important in hematopoiesis. Core-binding factor contributes to transcriptional repression and DNA replication; the AML-1 gene thus plays a major role in the control of normal hematopoiesis. The normal function of the ETO gene remains elusive, but the gene is expressed as a nuclear phosphoprotein in brain tissue and in CD34+ hematopoietic progenitor cells. In healthy cells, ETO functions within the nuclear complex to stabilize the interaction of corepressor proteins. The chimeric fusion protein AML-1/ETO therefore appears to repress transcription of genes that are normally activated by the AML-1 gene.

Molecular Features of Acute Myeloid Leukemia with t(15;17)

The translocation between chromosomes 15 and 17 in acute promyelocytic leukemia (FAB type M3) produces a fusion between the retinoic acid receptor α (RARα) gene normally located on chromosome 17 and the PML (promyelocyte) gene normally located in chromosome 15. The RARα gene is a retinoic acid–dependent transcription factor that is important in normal myeloid differentiation. Similar to the molecular pathogenesis in acute myeloid leukemia with t(8;21), changes in the function of the PML and RARα genes that occur as a result of their fusion result in the recruitment of nuclear corepressors that bind histone deacetylase leading to transcriptional repression. Therefore, the chimeric fusion protein arrests normal differentiation at the promyelocytic stage of myeloid maturation. The administration of pharmacologic doses of the vitamin A derivative all-trans retinoic acid results in terminal differentiation of the

Table 60-3 ■ Recurring Structural Rearrangements in Acute Myeloid Leukemia

Disease	Chromosome Abnormality	Involved Genes
AML-M2	t(8;21)(q22;q22)	ETO-AML1
APL-M3, M3v	t(15;17)(q22;q12)	PML-RARA
Atypical APL	t(11;17)(q23;q12)	PLZF-RARA
AMMoL-M4Eo	inv(16;16)(p13;q22) or t(16;16)(p13;q22)	MYH11-CBFB
AMMoL-M4/AmoL-M5	t(6;11)(q27;q23)	AF6-MLL
	t(9;11)(p22;q23)	AF9-MLL
AMegL-M7	t(1;22)(p13;q13)	
AML	t(3;3)(q21;q26) or inv(3)(q21;q26)	RPN-EVI1
	t(3;5)(q21;q31)	
	t(3;5)(q25;q34)	MLF1-NPM1
	t(6;9)(p23;q34)	DEK-CAN (NUP214)
	t(7;11)(p15;p15)	HOXA9-NUP98
	t(8;16)(p11;p13)	MOZ-CBP
	t(9;12)(q34;p13)	TEL-ABL
	t(12;22)(p13;q13)	TEL-NM1
	t(16;21)(p11;q22)	TLS(FUS)-ERG
	−5 or del(5q)	
	−7 or del(7q)	
	del(20p)	
	del(12p)	TEL,?p27^{KIP1}
Therapy-related AML	−7 or del(7q) and/or −5 or del(5q)	IRF1:
	t(11q23)	MLL
	t(3;21)(q26;q22)	EAP/MDS1/EVI1-AML1

From Rowley JD: The role of chromosome translocations in leukemogenesis, Semin Hematol 1999;36:59–76.

leukemic promyelocytes into mature granulocytes, leading to clinical remission.

Unfavorable Chromosomal Abnormalities

Patients whose leukemic cells have abnormalities of chromosome 5 or 7 such as 5q-, 7q-, or monosomy 5 or 7; complex karyotypes (with more than three clonal abnormalities); and most 11q23 abnormalities have very unfavorable prognoses. These abnormalities are associated with a diminished chance of achieving a complete remission, and remission duration is brief. Five-year survival rates are 5% to 15%.

The translocations involving chromosome 11q23 most commonly are t(6;11), t(9;11), and t(11;19). A significant proportion of patients with acute myeloid leukemia and 11q23 abnormalities will have received therapy with topoisomerase II–reactive drugs. The Cancer and Leukemia Group B found that patients with t(9;11) (p22;q23) have a better outcome than do patients with other translocations involving band 11q23. Translocations involving the breakpoint at 11q23 occur frequently in infants with leukemia (80% in those younger than age one year) and in those developing acute myeloid leukemia following exposure to chemotherapeutic agents that interact with topoisomerase II. A mixed lineage leukemia (MLL)

Table 60-4 ■ Cytogenetic Risk Groups

Favorable	inv(16); t(15;17) with any abnormality t(8;21) lacking del(9q) or complex karyotype
Intermediate	Normal or +8 or +21 or other numerical abnormalities
Unfavorable	−5/del(5q), −7/del(7q), inv(3q) Abnormality of 11q, 20q, 21q, 17p del(9q), t(6;9), t(9;22) Complex karyotypes with ≥3 abnormalities

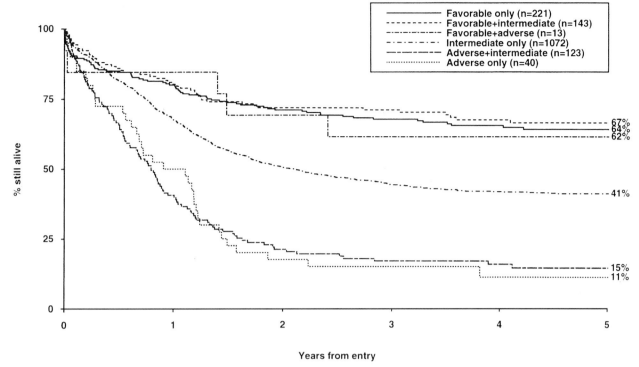

Figure 60-4 ■ Survival data of patients with acute myeloid leukemia based on cytogenetic prognostic groups. (From Grimwade D, Walker H, Oliver F, et al: The importance of diagnostic cytogenetics on outcome in AML: Analysis of 1,612 patients entered into the MRC AML 10 trial. Blood 1998;92:2322–2333.)

Table 60-5 ■ Complete Remission Rates by Cytogenetic Prognostic Groups

Therapy	Cytogenetic Prognostic Groups		
Groups	**Favorable**	**Intermediate**	**Unfavorable**
U.S. Intergroup	84%	76%	55%
MRC	90%	84%	57%
GOELAM	87%	76%	58%
Italy	88%	65%	36%

From Slovak ML et al: Karyotypič analysis predicts outcome of preremission and postremission therapy in adult acute myeloid leukemia: A Southwest Oncology Group/Eastern Cooperative Oncology Group Study. Blood 2000;96:4075–4083; Harousseau JL, et al: Comparison of autologous bone marrow transplantation and intensive chemotherapy as postremission therapy in adult acute myeloid leukemia. The Groupe Ouest Est Leucemies Myeloblastiques (GOELAM). Blood 1997;90:2978–2986; Visani G, et al: The prognostic value of cytogenetics is reinforced by the kind of induction/consolidation therapy in influencing the outcome of acute myeloid leukemia–analysis of 848 patients. Leukemia 2001;15:903–909.

Table 60-6 ■ Clinical, Biologic, and Molecular Characteristics of FAB Subtype M2 with t(8;21)

Clinical Features

Young median age at onset
20% of adult and 40% of pediatric FAB subtype M2
Extramedullary disease is not uncommon
Favorable prognosis

Biologic Features

Most common cytogenetic abnormality associated with extramedullary disease
Presence of extramedullary disease worsens prognosis
Expression of AML1-ETO fusion protein
Leukocytosis may indicate a poor prognosis
Loss of sex chromosome common
Extramedullary disease associated with CD56 expression

Molecular Features

AML1 activates transcription
ETO binds corepressor-HDAC complex
HDAC removes hydrophobic acetyl groups from histones, suppressing transcription of AML1 target promoters
AML1-ETO represses transcription

Table 60-7 ■ Core-Binding Factor Leukemias

Translocation	Genes Involved
t(8;21)	AML1-ETO
t(3;21)	AML1-EAP, MDS1, EVI1
t(12;21)	TEL (ETV6)
inv(16) or t(16;16)	CBFβ-MYH11

gene has been identified in this chromosomal region. Reciprocal translocations or insertions involving 11q23 have been demonstrated to occur with 25 different chromosomal bands on 14 different chromosomes. Approximately 95% of these translocations involve the mixed lineage leukemia gene. These patients can have the phenotypic picture of either acute myeloid leukemia or acute lymphoblastic leukemia or manifestations of both forms simultaneously as occurs typically in the t(4;11) translocation.

The most common abnormalities in therapy-related myelodysplasia or acute myeloid leukemia involve loss of part or all of chromosomes 5 and/or chromosome 7. Other unfavorable cytogenetic findings are associated with specific clinical characteristics. A balanced reciprocal translocation between chromosomes 6 and 9 is associated with basophilia and abnormalities of chromosome 3, including inversion [inv(3)] or translocation [t(3;3)], and tend to present with thrombocytosis.

Chromosomal Findings of Intermediate Prognosis

Patients with leukemic cells having a normal karyotype, trisomy 8, or other numeric changes, including trisomy 21 and trisomy 22, have an intermediate prognosis and an overall survival rate of 30% to 60% at five years.

Other Prognostic Markers

Age

Age remains an important prognostic factor in acute myeloid leukemia. Many older adults have significant comorbidities that reduce tolerance to chemotherapy and its resulting myelosuppression and increase the likelihood of death from induction therapy. The intrinsic biology of the leukemia cells in older adults offers an additional explanation for their unfavorable outcome. The frequency of unfavorable cytogenetics and of expression of multidrug resistance genes is directly correlated with advancing age.

Secondary and Therapy-Related Acute Myeloid Leukemia

Patients with acute myeloid leukemia who have an antecedent hematologic disorder or prior exposure to cytotoxic agents or radiation are considered to have secondary acute myeloid leukemia or therapy-related acute myeloid leukemia, respectively. The outcome for such individuals is generally inferior to that for individuals with de novo acute myeloid leukemia, attributable in part to the acquisition of unfavorable cytogenetic abnormalities and the expression of multidrug resistance.

Multidrug Resistance (MDR1) Protein Expression

The multidrug resistance (MDR1) gene encodes a transmembrane protein that serves as an efflux pump to expel lipophilic substances from the cell such as anthracyclines and vinca alkaloids. The expression of the MDR1 gene correlates with CD34 expression. Approximately 75% of patients with secondary acute myeloid leukemia express the MDR1 gene compared to approximately 25% of patients with de novo acute myeloid leukemia. The frequency of MDR1 gene expression directly correlates with advancing age and with the likelihood of poor prognosis cytogenetics.

Molecular Markers

Internal tandem duplications of the Flt3 gene located on chromosome 13 are an important predictor of outcome in acute myeloid leukemia. The presence of Flt3 gene mutations correlates with higher circulating blast cell counts, normal cytogenetics, a lower percentage of CD34-positive blasts, and less resistant disease. However, the impact on overall survival has been variable. Mutations in the Wilms' tumor gene (WT1) occur in approximately 15% of patients with acute myeloid leukemia and 20% of those with biphenotypic leukemia. Some leukemia cells with apparently normal karyotypes exhibit molecular gene rearrangements that are usually associated with specific karyotype abnormalities. For example, in certain patients with acute promyelocytic leukemia, the PML-RARα fusion transcript is detectable, even though the t(15;17) translocation is absent on routine karyotype analysis. These patients have the same favorable prognosis as patients with an identifiable t(15;17).

Clinical Presentation

The majority of patients with acute myeloid leukemia present with symptoms resulting from the effects of variable cytopenias, anemia, and/or neutropenia and/or thrombocytopenia. Thus, patients may exhibit fatigue or dyspnea, fever from infection, or bleeding manifestations, such as petechiae, ecchymoses, or epistaxis.

Extramedullary Disease

Patients with acute myeloid leukemia may also present with extramedullary disease. Leukemia cutis

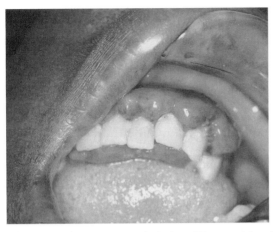

Figure 60-5 ■ Gingival hyperplasia in a 55-year-old patient presenting with monocytic acute myeloid leukemia, FAB type M5. (See Color Plate 14.)

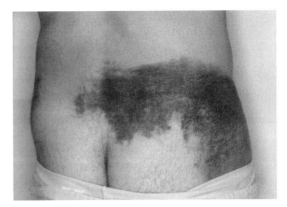

Figure 60-7 ■ Extensive cutaneous ecchymosis and bleeding in a patient presenting with acute promyelocytic leukemia.

and infiltration of the gingiva are particularly common in patients whose leukemia cells demonstrate monocytic differentiation including FAB type M5a and M5b (Figure 60-5). The frequency of leukemic infiltration of the central nervous system is increased in the monocytic subtypes and in FAB type M4EO. Leukemic meningitis is the most common manifestation of central nervous system involvement. Cranial nerve palsy from entrapment and chloroma deposits (focal collections of myeloblasts) also occur. Some patients with FAB type M2 and t(8;21) develop extramedullary disease, particularly orbital chloromas (Figure 60-6). Chloromas are extramedullary collections of leukemia cells, also referred to as granulocytic sarcomas. Chloromas may be associated with expression of CD56, the neural crest adhesion molecule, which is believed to play a role in trafficking of leukemia cells. The expression of this antigen confers an unfavorable prognosis.

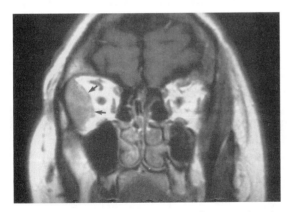

Figure 60-6 ■ Computerized tomography scan showing an orbital chloroma (arrows) in a 25-year-old patient with acute myeloid leukemia, FAB type M2 with t(8;21). (From Tallman MS, Hakimian D, Shaw J, et al: Granulocytic sarcoma is associated with the 8;21 translocation in acute myeloid leukemia. J Clin Oncol 1993;11:690–697.)

Hyperleukocytosis and Leukostasis

Patients may also present with hyperleukocytosis, a poor prognostic finding that is associated with an increased risk of central nervous system involvement and death from leukostasis. Hyperleukocytosis is most commonly associated with the microgranular variant of acute promyelocytic leukemia (FAB type M3v) and monocytic subtypes of acute myeloid leukemia and is also found with the 11q23 abnormality, inv(16) (p13;q22), and chromosome 6 abnormalities. Leukostasis is most likely to develop when the circulating blast cells number greater than 75,000 to 100,000/μL, because of the limited flexibility of myeloblasts navigating the microcirculation. This leads to obstruction of blood flow and hypoxemia with the potential for distal hemorrhagic necrosis. Overt symptoms develop primarily in the lungs and brain.

A single leukapheresis procedure can reduce the blast cell count by 50%. Although this technique is frequently employed as a treatment for markedly increased peripheral blast counts, whether the risk of leukostatic complications is reduced is uncertain. Hydroxyurea is also commonly given, while the initial evaluation of the patient is underway, but hydroxyurea takes 48 hours or more to have an effect. The most rapid (within 24 hours) and profound reduction results from initiation of anthracycline therapy.

Coagulopathy

In addition to thrombocytopenia, patients may also present with disseminated intravascular coagulation. This is particularly common in patients with acute promyelocytic leukemia who have evidence of both disseminated intravascular coagulation as well as fibrinolysis. This poses the risk of life-threatening bleeding (Figure 60-7). Disseminated intravascular coagulation may also be seen in patients whose acute myeloid leukemia cells show monocytic differentiation (FAB types M4 and M5).

Metabolic Abnormalities

Metabolic abnormalities are common at presentation and during treatment. Patients may present with the tumor lysis syndrome manifested by hyperuricemia, hyperkalemia, hyperphosphatemia, renal insufficiency, and hypocalcemia. Lactic acidosis can occur even in the absence of sepsis. Rarely, patients with monocytic variants can present with hypouricemia and hypokalemia because of proximal renal tubular dysfunction, a result of the excessive production of lysozyme (muramidase) by these cells.

Clinical Evaluation

The diagnosis of acute myeloid leukemia is confirmed by bone marrow aspirate and biopsy. Studies of the leukemia cells should include routine morphologic review of stained material (such as Wright-Giemsa stain), immunophenotypic analysis, karyotype analysis, and, in selected cases, molecular genetic analysis. The diagnosis of acute myeloid leukemia is established by the demonstration of at least 20% myeloid blasts in the marrow (World Health Organization criteria) or occasionally by the biopsy of a chloroma (called a myeloid sarcoma by World Health Organization).

Cytologic Findings

Myeloblasts typically exhibit great variability in size, abundant pale blue cytoplasm with azurophilic granules, nuclei with fine open chromatin, and distinct nucleoli with a punched-out appearance on Wright-Giemsa stained aspirate smears. The presence of Auer rods, red azurophilic splinter-shaped cytoplasmic inclusions, indicates that the blast is myeloid in origin. Only one or two Auer rods are usually found in a blast cell, and they appear in some cells in only 20% of the cases of acute myeloid leukemia. In acute promyelocytic leukemia, however, Auer rods are frequently seen and may be numerous such that they appear as bundles of sticks. Cytochemical stains for myeloperoxidase and α-naphthyl butyrate esterase are routinely performed. If more than 3% of the blasts are myeloperoxidase-positive, the diagnosis of acute myeloid leukemia is established, and the esterase stain is used to help determine the FAB subtype. If fewer than 3% of the blasts are myeloperoxidase-positive, then an α-naphthyl butyrate esterase stain is performed. A positive esterase stain is compatible with the diagnosis of acute myeloid leukemia.

Immunophenotype Findings

Although there is considerable heterogeneity in the cell surface marker expression of acute myeloid leukemia cells, the myeloid markers CD13 and CD33 are commonly detected. Leukemia cells in acute myeloid leukemia often also express CD11, CD14, and CD15, but there is no leukemia-specific antigen expression. The identification of cell surface phenotype, usually by flow cytometry, is especially critical in myeloperoxidase-negative, esterase-negative cases. The diagnosis of acute myeloid leukemia FAB type MO (M zero) can be definitively established only by immunophenotyping, which serves to distinguish these cases from acute lymphoblastic leukemia. Criteria necessary to establish the diagnosis of FAB type MO include (1) negative myeloperoxidase stain, (2) reactivity with monoclonal antibodies that recognize the myeloid antigens CD13 or CD33, and (3) no reactivity with monoclonal antibodies that recognize lymphoid restricted antigens, such as CD19 and CD5.

Aberrant Expression of Lymphoid Markers

Aberrant expression of lymphoid markers on the leukemic cells from patients with acute myeloid leukemia is not uncommon. For example, the lymphoid marker terminal deoxynucleotidyl transferase (Tdt) may be expressed in approximately 25% of patients with acute myeloid leukemia, and CD7 may be expressed in 30% of patients. Expression of lymphoid markers may be associated with 11q23 abnormalities and immunoglobulin heavy chain (IgH) or T cell receptor gene rearrangements. These variants are associated with markedly elevated white blood cell counts at presentation and carry a poor prognosis.

Correlation of Surface Antigen Expression with Morphology, Karyotype, and Outcome

A number of cell surface markers have been associated with specific morphologic subtypes and karyotypes. Some examples include B-lineage antigen positivity and t(9;22) or 11q23 abnormalities, absence of CD13 and FAB type M2 and the t(8;21) karyotype, and CD13 and CD34 positivity and inv(16). Immunophenotyping may be useful in detecting minimal residual disease in patients who are in apparent complete remission. One study used multiparametric flow cytometry to estimate the level of minimal resistant disease (MRD). The extent of residual disease was then correlated with the likelihood of relapse. Four risk categories were identified: (1) very low-risk patients with fewer than 10^{-4} cells, of whom none had relapsed; (2) low-risk patients with 10^{-3} cells, for whom the relapse rate was 14%; (3) intermediate-risk

Table 60-8 ■ General Treatment Strategies for Adults with Acute Myeloid Leukemia

Induction Therapy

Chemotherapy including anthracycline plus cytarabine
Differentiation therapy for acute promyelocytic leukemia;
all-trans retinoic acid plus anthracycline-based chemotherapy

Postremission Therapy

Intensive consolidation chemotherapy
Autologous hematopoietic stem cell transplantation
Allogeneic hematopoietic stem cell transplantation (human
leukocyte antigen–matched sibling)
Alternative donor transplantation (matched unrelated;
haploidentical, umbilical cord)
Maintenance chemotherapy
Low-dose chemotherapy in older adults
All-trans retinoic acid + low-dose chemotherapy for acute
promyelocytic leukemia

patients with 10^{-3} to 10^{-2} cells, for whom the relapse rate was 50%; and (4) high-risk patients with more than 10^{-2} cells, for whom the relapse rate was 84% (P = 0.0001). The risk categories also predicted for overall survival.

Treatment

Overview

Once the diagnosis of acute myeloid leukemia has been established, treatment needs to be initiated expeditiously but rarely emergently except in the settings of hyperleukocytosis, with or without leukostasis, and acute promyelocytic leukemia because of the risk of hemorrhage from disseminated intravascular coagulation. The contemporary strategies for the treatment of acute myeloid leukemia are outlined in Table 60-8. With the exception of acute promyelocytic leukemia, which is treated with all-trans retinoic acid, the subtypes of acute myeloid leukemia in adults are treated with remission induction chemotherapy followed by multiple cycles of intensive postremission therapy (in younger adults) to eradicate minimal residual disease.

Intensive antileukemic treatment is divided into the remission induction and postremission phases. The goal of the initial induction chemotherapy is to induce complete remission by reducing the leukemic clone. This allows the normal blood cell precursors to repopulate the marrow. Complete remission is defined as the absence of morphologic evidence of leukemia on examination of the bone marrow (less than 5% blasts identifiable) with peripheral blood count

recovery, and the absence of extramedullary disease. The failure to achieve complete remission can be due to death from complications during the period of chemotherapy-induced hypoplasia, chemotherapy resistance of the leukemia, or rapid proliferative and repopulation rates of the leukemic clone. Postremission therapy is administered to prevent or delay relapse of the leukemia and generally consists of multiple cycles of intensive chemotherapy, including the administration of high-dose cytarabine, whose toxicity is only tolerable in adults under age 60 years.

Despite this strategy, the majority of adults with acute myeloid leukemia die of their disease. Among patients younger than age 55 years, 20% to 30% are disease-free at five years. Of patients older than age 55 years, only 10% to 15% are disease-free at five years.

Supportive Care of Patients with Acute Myeloid Leukemia

During the initial phase of treatment, one needs to be vigilant for metabolic complications related to lysis of leukemic cells. Tumor lysis syndrome is most common in the monocytic acute myeloid leukemia subtypes FAB M5a and M5b (see Chapter 117, Tumor Lysis Syndrome). Infections or hemorrhagic complications of therapy or the underlying disease are the predominant causes of death during induction therapy. The prolonged neutropenia related to the underlying disease and treatment and mucosal injury are major risk factors for infections. Prolonged thrombocytopenia is the major risk factor for hemorrhage, but patients may also have additional coagulation abnormalities such as disseminated intravascular coagulation and fibrinolysis in acute promyelocytic leukemia and in the monocytic variants of acute myeloid leukemia. Finally, patients who receive high-dose cytarabine as part of their therapy are at risk for unique complications including cerebellar dysfunction, keratitis, and rash. Table 60-9 presents a summary of recommendations concerning the supportive care of patients with acute myeloid leukemia. All blood products that are administered to patients with acute myeloid leukemia should be administered through a filter to remove white blood cells and decrease alloimmunization and should be radiated prior to use to prevent transfer of viable lymphocytes to an immunosuppressed patient and the possibility of graft-versus-host disease (GVHD). To prevent sensitization to minor familial human leukocyte antigens (HLA), family members should not be used as blood donors if there is any possibility that the patient will be a candidate at some point for allogeneic hematopoietic stem cell transplantation.

Table 60-9 ■ Supportive Care of Acute Myeloid Leukemia Organized by Problem

Clinical Problem	Treatment Option	Comment
Vascular access	Semipermanent central venous catheter	
Hyperleukocytosis	Therapeutic cytapheresis	Indicated if signs of microvascular compromise or if blast cell count is >100,000/μL
Disseminated intravascular coagulation	Replacement of factors with FFP and fibrinogen with cryoprecipitate Platelet transfusions	If factor replacement is not successful, consider low-dose heparin therapy
Tumor lysis syndrome	Preventive measures	Allopurinol and saline hydration to ensure adequate urinary output. Careful attention to serum electrolytes
Anemia	Packed red blood cells	Erythropoietin of no benefit
Neutropenia	Protective isolation	May reduce prevalence of disseminated aspergillosis
	Hematopoietic colony-stimulating factors: G-CSF or GM-CSF	Use reduces median duration of neutropenia Inconsistent effect on morbidity or hospital stay
	Prophylactic antibiotics	Antifungals reduce risk of candida infections
Fever and neutropenia	Empiric antibiotics	Broad-spectrum antibacterial agents initiated at time of fever. Choice dictated by nosocomial infection data. May require empiric antifungal therapy if prolonged or recurrent fever.
Thrombocytopenia	Transfusions	Single donor or random donor pooled units Prophylactic transfusions indicated for level <10,000/μL
Transfusion-refractory thrombocytopenia	Transfusions	Human leukocyte antigen–compatible units or cross-match-compatible units
	Other	Consider amino-caproic acid if no evidence of disseminated intravascular coagulation and bleeding is significant

Metabolic Complications

All individuals should receive allopurinol 100 to 300 mg a day depending on renal function for the first seven days of induction therapy. To reduce the likelihood of tumor lysis syndrome, an average urinary output of 150 mL per hour should be established with a combination of saline intravenous hydration and diuretics, depending on the patient's cardiopulmonary and renal status.

Neutropenia (See also Chapter 52)

Multiple randomized trials have assessed the benefits of either granulocyte colony-stimulating factor (G-CSF) or granulocyte-macrophage colony-stimulating factor (GM-CSF) in the treatment of acute myeloid leukemia. These studies differed as to when in the course of induction therapy the administration of the colony-stimulating factor was begun. An effect on relevant endpoints, such as the complete remission rate, remission duration, survival, or a reduction in treatment-related morbidity and mortality, length of hospitalization, or resource utilization, was not uniformly demonstrated. The aggregate experience derived from these data indicate that hematopoietic growth factors do shorten the period of neutropenia after induction therapy in acute myeloid leukemia. There is no evidence to support prior concerns that these factors have adverse effects by stimulating the growth of the leukemic clone.

To reduce the incidence of bacterial and fungal infections, many clinicians use prophylactic oral quinolones and antifungal agents, such as fluconazole. Neutropenic fevers are discussed in Chapters 2 and 115. In general, broad-spectrum coverage is initiated after appropriate cultures are obtained. Coverage is modified on the basis of culture results and/or response of the fever. Persistent fever in the face of broad-spectrum antibiotic coverage in the neutropenic patient requires intravenous antifungals, such as amphotericin, on an empiric basis for presumed fungal superinfection. Transfusions of granulocytes are currently being revisited. However, a recent pilot study in neutropenic patients with invasive fungal infections resistant to amphotericin B suggests that this approach has promise.

Thrombocytopenia

The only commercially available thrombopoietic hematopoietic growth factor is recombinant human interleukin-11, which is a pleiotropic cytokine. It is approved by the FDA for use in reducing the likelihood of thrombocytopenia or platelet transfusions in patients receiving chemotherapy for nonmyeloid malignancies. Few studies have evaluated the role of thrombopoietic agents during induction therapy in acute myeloid leukemia. In one randomized trial, patients with newly diagnosed acute myeloid leukemia were randomized to receive either 2.5 or 5.0 µg/kg/day of pegylated recombinant human megakaryocytic growth and development factor (PEG-rHuMGDF) or placebo following the completion of induction chemotherapy. The cytokine was well tolerated, and a biologic effect was noted in that patients receiving rHu-MGDF did achieve a higher maximal platelet count when bone marrow function recovered. There was no difference, however, in the time required to reach self-sustaining platelet counts of greater than 20×10^9/L or in the number of times that platelet transfusions were required. Another randomized study from Europe reported similar results. Therefore, there is no role for the administration of thrombopoietic agents in the treatment of acute myeloid leukemia.

Platelet transfusion therapy reduces the likelihood of bleeding. There are two indications for transfusion: therapeutic or prophylactic. Therapeutic platelet transfusions are given whenever bleeding manifestations occur in a patient with thrombocytopenia. Prophylactic transfusions are administered on the basis of the platelet count and the assessment of the potential for bleeding. Randomized trials demonstrated that the administration of platelet transfusions when a threshold value for the platelet count of 10,000/µL or less is reached is as safe as using a threshold value of 20,000/µL.

High-Dose Cytarabine

High-dose cytarabine is frequently used in the treatment of acute myeloid leukemia. Its use can cause acute cerebellar dysfunction, including ataxia, dysarthria, dysmetria, or dysdiadochokinesis. It usually occurs after completion of a course of cytarabine and clears after three to five days. The incidence of this toxicity is greater in older patients, related to decreased renal function and decreased clearance, and in patients receiving doses of greater than 2 gm/m². Daily observation of the patient for early signs of cerebellar dysfunction is warranted to detect the occasional patient who develops the syndrome during the course of cytarabine administration. In this event, the cytarabine must be discontinued to avoid irreversible cerebellar damage. High-dose cytarabine also causes keratitis, and patients should receive prophylactic corticosteroid eyedrops during therapy and for 24 to 48 hours after the completion of therapy.

Induction Therapy

Clinical trials have established that the combination of an anthracycline and cytarabine is the most effective regimen in inducing complete remission. Overall, about two thirds of patients achieve remission. The likelihood of achieving remission is inversely correlated with age. Patients younger than age 50 years old have a complete remission rate in excess of 70%, whereas in patients older than age 60 years, the complete remission rate is 50%. The most widely used induction chemotherapy regimen consists of daunorubicin 45 to 60 mg/m²/day intravenously for three days and a continuous intravenous infusion of cytarabine at a dose of 100 mg/m²/day for seven days. Addition of other chemotherapeutic agents in induction therapy and/or intensifying the doses of drugs has failed to improve the complete remission rate. Whatever gains occurred in overcoming leukemia resistance or increasing leukemia cell kill were canceled by increasing morbidity and mortality. Conversely, in older patients, anthracycline dosage reduction from the usual levels in an attempt to diminish toxicity led to reduction in the complete remission rate.

Anthracyclines

Anthracyclines include daunorubicin, doxorubicin, aclarubicin, the synthetic agent 4-demethoxy-daunorubicin (idarubicin), and the synthetic anthracenedione, mitoxantrone. Idarubicin offers some potential advantages over daunorubicin, namely, increased cellular uptake, more DNA single-strand breaks, conversion to an active metabolite with a prolonged plasma half-life, and lesser P-glycoprotein mediated efflux. Mitoxantrone is associated with a relatively steep dose-response curve in clonogenic assays of leukemia cells and has a favorable extramedullary toxicity profile. Mitoxantrone and aclarubicin have theoretical advantages because their uptake and outward transport are largely unaffected in multidrug-resistant cell lines.

The Eastern Oncology Group conducted a prospective randomized three-arm trial in older adults comparing cytarabine plus either daunorubicin, idarubicin, or mitoxantrone as induction therapy. The complete remission rates did not differ among the anthracyclines, although a trend toward a decrease in the induction mortality rate was noted with mitoxantrone. The AML-12 trial of the United Kingdom's Medical Research Council randomized patients ages

15 to 59 to receive cytarabine plus either daunorubicin or mitoxantrone for induction therapy. The complete remission rate, percentage of patients dying in remission, frequency of chemotherapy drug resistance, relapse rate, and disease-free and overall survival rates did not differ. A European randomized trial compared cytarabine, etoposide, and intermediate-dose cytarabine plus either daunorubicin, mitoxantrone, or idarubicin and found no differences in complete remission rate or disease-free or overall survival rate. Therefore, there is no definitive evidence that one anthracycline is better than another for induction therapy.

Cytarabine Dosage in Induction Therapy

Cytarabine is one of the most active single agents for the treatment of acute myeloid leukemia. A randomized trial of intermediate-dose cytarabine at 500 mg/m^2/day versus 200 mg/m^2/day, each given with daunorubicin, yielded similar complete remission rates and disease-free survival rates. These trials failed to show an improvement in complete remission rate, but the high-dose regimens exhibited increased hematologic and extramedullary toxicity, including nausea, emesis, and cerebellar and ophthalmologic toxicity. Two of these studies showed a longer disease-free survival rate but no increase in overall survival in the patients receiving high-dose therapy. These studies were not constructed to show whether the same improvement in disease-free survival would have resulted from administering high-dose cytarabine as part of postremission, rather than induction, therapy.

Use of Additional Chemotherapeutic Agents During Induction Therapy

The Australian Leukemia Study Group gave standard-dose cytarabine for seven days plus daunorubicin for three days with or without etoposide 75 mg/m^2/day for seven days, followed by intensive postremission therapy and maintenance therapy. Although the disease-free survival rate was significantly longer in patients receiving etoposide, the overall survival rate did not improve. However, the overall survival rate among patients younger than age 55 years was significantly longer, at 5 and 10 years in the patients who received etoposide than those who did not, approximately 25% versus 15%, respectively. Older patients experienced significantly more toxicity and no benefit. In younger patients with acute myeloid leukemia, intensified induction may improve the duration of complete remission and survival without improving the complete remission rate. However, caution in interpretation is required, because there was no

stratification at randomization on the basis of age. A Medical Research Council's randomized study of the addition of etoposide in induction therapy showed no improvement in either remission duration or survival rate.

Standard-Dose Cytarabine Followed by High-Dose Cytarabine in Induction Therapy

Adding high-dose cytarabine for three days immediately following standard doses of cytarabine plus daunorubicin is another approach to intensifying induction therapy. Phase II studies by the Eastern Cooperative Oncology Group and the Southwest Oncology Group observed no difference in remission rate from the results in historical control patients who received conventional induction therapy. The German AML Cooperative Group randomized newly diagnosed patients to either two courses of standard-dose cytarabine plus daunorubicin and 6-thiogranine or one course of the same chemotherapy followed by high-dose cytarabine and mitoxantrone on day 21 regardless of the marrow findings (Table 60-10). No differences in remission rate, induction mortality rate, or relapse-free survival rate were noted, although review of their data subsets suggested that high-risk patients seemed to do better with intensified therapy.

Taken altogether, there is no clear evidence that any induction regimen is better than the standard regimen of anthracycline plus cytarabine. Nevertheless, clinical trials continue to examine the potential efficacy of variations in dose, timing, or combinations of treatment regimens in induction (Table 60-11).

Postremission Therapy

A number of strategies are employed after patients are in complete remission to prevent or delay the otherwise inevitable regrowth of occult remaining leukemia cells and subsequent relapse. These approaches include intensive consolidation therapy or high-dose chemotherapy or chemoradiotherapy, with either human leukocyte antigen–matched sibling allogeneic or autologous hematopoietic stem cell rescue or low-dose maintenance therapy.

Intensive Consolidation Chemotherapy

Early studies demonstrated that, in comparison to no postremission treatment, low-dose lengthy maintenance therapy prolonged remission and intensive postremission therapy over a short period further improved the outcome compared to maintenance therapy. In contrast to the lack of benefit from intensifying induction therapy, intensifying postremission therapy prolongs remission duration and improves

Table 60-10 ▪ Intensified Therapy in Adults with Newly Diagnosed Acute Myeloid Leukemia and Adverse Prognostic Features

Endpoint	Remission Rate		Median Event-Free Survival (months)		Median Overall Survival (months)	
Assigned treatment	TAD-TAD	TAD-HAM	TAD-TAD	TAD-HAM	TAD-TAD	TAD-HAM
All analyzed patients	65%	71%	9	10	19	18
Poor-prognosis subgroup (represented 39% of trial population)	49%	65%	3	7	8	13

TAD = cytarabine 100 mg/m² by continuous infusion daily days 1–2; every 12 hours days 3–8; Daunorubicin 60 mg/m²/d days 3–5; plus 6-thioguanine 100 mg/m² orally every 12 hours days 3–9.
HAM = cytarabine 3 g/m² every 12 hours days 1–3 plus mitoxantrone 10 mg/m²/day days 3–5.
From Buchner T, et al: Double induction strategy for acute myeloid leukemia: The effect of high-dose cytarabine with mitoxantrone instead of standard-dose cytarabine with daunorubicin and 6-thioguanine: A randomized trial by the German AML Cooperative Group. Blood 1999;93:4115–4124.

overall survival, but only in patients who are younger than age 60 years. Older patients poorly tolerate intensive treatment after remission and experience increased morbidity and mortality. The Cancer and Acute Leukemia Group B randomly assigned patients in complete remission to receive four monthly courses of cytarabine at one of three doses: 100 mg/m²/day by continuous intravenous infusion for five days, 400 mg/m²/day by continuous intravenous infusion for five days, or 3 g/m² as a three-hour intravenous infusion twice daily on days 1, 3, and 5. The high-dose cytarabine produced unacceptable rates of central

Table 60-11 ▪ Common Combination Chemotherapy Regimens for Induction Therapy In Acute Myeloid Leukemia

"7 + 3" (Conventional therapy with 7 days of cytarabine and 3 days of anthracycline)	Cytarabine 100 mg/sq m/d for 7 days as a continuous IV infusion **and** Daunorubicin 45–60 mg/sq m/d for 3 days (days 1–3) brief IV infusion **or** Mitoxantrone 12 mg/sq m/d for 3 days (days 1–3) brief IV infusion **or** Idarubicin 12 or 13 mg sq/m/d for 3 days (days 1–3) brief IV infusion
"ADE" (Medical Research Council of the United Kingdom)	Cytarabine 100 mg/sq m/d for 10 days as an IV infusion every 12 hours **and** Daunorubicin 30–50 mg/sq m/d for 3 days (days 1, 3, 5) brief IV infusion **and** Etoposide 100 mg/sq m/d as a 1-hour IV infusion for 5 days (days 1–5)
"TAD-HAM" (German AML Study Group)	Cytarabine 100 mg/sq m/d on days 1–2 as a continuous IV infusion **then** Cytarabine 100 mg/sq m twice daily on 3–8 days brief IV infusion **and** Daunorubicin 60 mg/sq m/d on days 3–5 brief IV infusion **and** 6-Thioguanine 100 mg/sq m orally every 12 hours days 3–9 **No chemotherapy until day 21, then** Cytarabine 3 mg/sq m twice daily over 3 hours IV infusion days 1–3 **and** Mitoxantrone 10 mg/sq m/d brief IV infusion on days 3–5

Table 60-12 ■ Complete Remission Duration by Cytogenetic Group According to Cytarabine Dose Randomization

Cytogenetic Group	Cytarabine Dose	Number of Patients	Median Duration of Complete Remission (months)	% in Complete Remission at Five Years
Favorable	$3 g/m^2$	18	NR	78
	$400 mg/m^2$	20	NR	57
	$100 mg/m^2$	19	14.3	16
Normal	$3 g/m^2$	45	18.2	40
	$400 mg/m^2$	48	21.4	37
	$100 mg/m^2$	47	12.5	20
Other	$3 g/m^2$	27	13.3	21
	$400 mg/m^2$	31	10.6	13
	$100 mg/m^2$	30	9.6	13

From Bloomfield CD, Lawrence D, Byrd JC, et al: Frequency of prolonged remission duration after high-dose cytarabine intensification in acute myeloid leukemia varies by cytogenetic subtype. Cancer Res 1998;58:4173–4179.

nervous system toxicity in patients older than age 60 years, leading to discontinuation of this part of the randomized study in older patients. The four-year disease-free survival rate was 21% in the 100-mg group, 25% in the 400-mg group, and 39% in the 3-g group. The results were most significant in patients with favorable cytogenetics (Table 60-12). This trial demonstrated a dose-response effect for cytarabine in patients undergoing postremission therapy.

Data from a Medical Research Council study suggest that high-dose cytarabine may not be an essential component of postremission therapy. In their AML-10 trial, patients not undergoing allogeneic hematopoietic stem cell transplantation were treated after complete remission with one course of amsacrine, cytarabine, and etoposide followed by a course of mitoxantrone and cytarabine. Patients were then randomized to either autologous transplantation or no further therapy. The highest dose of cytarabine was $1 g/m^2$ every 12 hours for three days. The long-term disease-free survival rate was 40%, similar to the results reported by the Cancer and Acute Leukemia Group B. In patients not undergoing hematopoietic stem cell transplantation, the critical factor may be the administration of multiple cycles of intensive chemotherapy rather than that cytarabine be given in very high doses (usually defined as $3 g/m^2$ per dose).

The number of courses required for optimal postremission therapy is uncertain and remains an important question. The Finnish Leukemia Group randomized patients younger than age 65 years who were in remission after two courses of high-dose cytarabine-containing chemotherapy to receive an additional four courses of chemotherapy or no further treatment. No benefit accrued to those receiving the lengthier postremission therapy, suggesting that a limited number of courses may suffice. At present, the

standard of care is to administer two to four courses of intensive treatment postremission in patients younger than age 60 years. Such treatment usually contains intermediate-dose or high-dose cytarabine alone or in combination with other agents. Intensifying postremission therapy for patients older than age 60 years is of no value. In general, increasing the degree or duration of postremission therapy in older patients contributes to increasing toxicity without improving outcome.

Some data suggest that patients in the favorable cytogenetic subset (the core-binding factor leukemias) do well when three or four cycles of high-dose cytarabine ($3 g/m^2$ per dose) are administered. For example, in one of these subtypes, acute myeloid leukemia FAB M2 with the t(8;21), a retrospective review found a five-year disease-free and overall survival of greater than 70% in patients receiving more than one course of high-dose cytarabine postremission versus approximately 40% for patients receiving only one course (Figure 60-8).

Hematopoietic Stem Cell Transplantation in Acute Myeloid Leukemia

Autologous and allogeneic hematopoietic stem cell transplantation are useful modalities in the postremission treatment of acute myeloid leukemia (see Chapter 51, Hematopoietic Stem Cell Transplantation). Both forms of transplantation provide intensive antileukemic chemotherapy (or chemoradiotherapy), while allogeneic transplantation additionally exploits a graft-versus-leukemia (GVL) effect. Although allogeneic hematopoietic stem cell transplantation reduces the relapse rate, long-term survival is not substantially improved in comparison to autologous transplantation because of the morbidity and mortality of graft-versus-host disease and of the immuno-

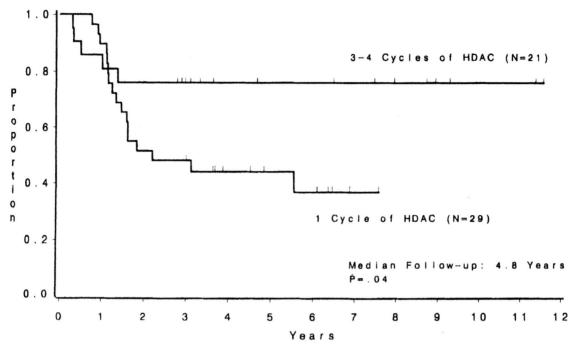

Figure 60-8 ■ Overall survival for patients with acute myeloid leukemia and t(8;21) (q22;q22). The projected five-year overall survival rate was 44% for patients who received one cycle of high-dose cytarabine compared to 76% (95% confidence interval: 48% to 92%) for those who received three or four cycles (*P* = 0.04). HDAC = high-dose cytarabine. (From Byrd JC, Dodge RK, Carroll A, et al: Patients with t(8;21) (q22;q22) and acute myeloid leukemia have superior failure-free and overall survival when repetitive cycles of high-dose cytarabine are administered. J Clin Oncol 1999;17:3767–3775.)

suppressive therapy that is needed to modulate its effects. Autologous hematopoietic stem cell transplantation also decreases the relapse rate, albeit to a lesser extent than allogeneic transplantation does, but was itself associated with an 8% to 15% transplant-related mortality when bone marrow was used as the stem cell source. Previous randomized studies comparing either form of transplantation to intensive postremission therapy have yielded conflicting results about changes in the disease-free survival rate and no significant differences in the overall survival rate. Because of changes in medical management, further study of transplantation in acute myeloid leukemia is warranted. For example, transplant-related mortality from autologous transplantation has declined to less than 3% now that stems cells from peripheral blood instead of bone marrow are used. Moreover, methods to abrogate some of the morbidity of graft-versus-host disease may improve survival from allogeneic transplantation.

Allogeneic Hematopoietic Stem Cell Transplantation

Human Leukocyte Antigen–Matched Sibling Transplantation
Initial studies in allogeneic transplantation of patients with far advanced acute myeloid leukemia who were given high-dose cyclophosphamide and total body irradiation followed by human leukocyte antigen–matched sibling bone marrow–derived stem cells demonstrated that 10% to 15% of these patients who would otherwise have died of their disease were cured. Subsequently, allogeneic transplantation was evaluated in patients earlier in the course of their disease, for example, in initial complete remission. At this time, the leukemia cells would not be chemotherapy resistant, and the less heavily pretreated patients would be better conditioned to tolerate the procedure. The apparent cure rate increased to approximately 50% despite a treatment-related mortality rate of approximately 20% to 30% in studies of large numbers of patients (Table 60-13). An important component of allogeneic transplantation's benefit is attributable to the fact that the graft-versus-host disease also results in a cytocidal attack on the leukemia cells by the donor lymphocytes, producing a graft-versus-leukemia effect.

Nonmyeloablative Transplantation
Current studies investigate whether more modest chemotherapy can facilitate allogeneic transplantation. As one example, administration of the immunosuppressive agent fludarabine can be combined with

Table 60-13 ■ Allogeneic Hematopoietic Stem Cell Transplantation for Acute Myeloid Leukemia in First Complete Remission

Author, Year	Number of Patients	Treatment-Related Mortality Rate	Relapse Rate	Disease-Free Survival Rate	Overall Survival Rate
Forman, 1987	69	30%	16%	51% at 4 years	NA
Clift, 1987	231	25%	25%	46% at 5 years	48% at 5 years
Fagioli, 1994	91	26%	29%	NA	53% at 5 years
Keating, 1996	169	22%	23%	60% at 3 years	NA
Mehta, 1996	85	33%	25%	48% at 10 years	NA
Ferrant, 1997*	346	NA	22%	57% at 3 years	59% at 3 years

*Results for standard-risk patients.
NA = not available.

nonmyeloablative cytotoxic chemotherapy and still permit engraftment of the donor stem cells and promote chimerism and a graft-versus-leukemia effect while reducing treatment-related morbidity and mortality. If successful, this strategy could expand the population of patients who are eligible for allogeneic transplantation to include older adults and those with comorbidities. Although this approach is feasible, because it allows engraftment of donor cells to occur with rapid hematologic recovery, graft-versus-host disease remains a problem.

The identification of alternative donor sources of hematopoietic stem cells also increases the opportunity for patients to undergo allogeneic transplantation.

Matched Unrelated Donors

National transplant registries in the United States and Europe contain a large number of human leukocyte antigen–typed potential stem cell donors for use in allogeneic transplantation as matched but unrelated donors (MUD). However, there are limitations to this strategy. These include donor availability, length of time to identify the donor, and substantial treatment-related mortality due to graft-versus-host disease, which is more frequent and severe than after sibling human leukocyte antigen–matched donors are used. The exact role of matched, unrelated donor transplant in patients with acute myeloid leukemia has not been defined. All transplantation procedures have the best opportunity for cure when they are employed early in the disease, the leukemia cells are sensitive to chemotherapy, and tumor burden is low. However, because of the toxicity of the procedure, matched, unrelated donor transplant is usually reserved for patients with acute myeloid leukemia who have no sibling donor and who have failed to achieve a complete remission initially or after relapse, who have far advanced disease, and who have failed several attempts at chemotherapy. Whether this procedure should be used early on in patients without a matched

sibling donor who have poor prognosis acute myeloid leukemia that is in initial complete remission remains uncertain. The tendency for such patients is to attempt autologous transplantation or intensive chemotherapy instead.

Haploidentical Transplantation

Almost every patient will have a haploidentical family member (parent or child) who could serve as a donor when a fully matched donor is unavailable. A group from the University of Perugia, Italy, explored this approach in a number of patients, using a relatively nontoxic conditioning regimen consisting of the alkylating agent thiotepa, a single dose of 800-cGy total body irradiation, fludarabine, and antithymocyte globulin. To avoid extensive graft-versus-host disease, T-lymphocytes were depleted from the donor cells. To ensure engraftment, which requires the presence of T cells, a large number of donor cells were required (more than 10×10^6 CD34 cells/kg). This group reported a treatment-related mortality rate of approximately 10%. Among 27 high-risk patients with acute myeloid leukemia in first complete remission, the five-year event-free survival rate was 45%. This treatment is associated, not unexpectedly, with delayed immunologic reconstitution, and patients are at substantial risk for opportunistic infections, particularly cytomegalovirus.

Umbilical Cord Transplants

Hematopoietic stem cells procured from umbilical cords from related and unrelated donors can also restore hematopoiesis with acceptable risks of graft-versus-host disease. Such stem cells have advantages compared to stem cells procured from adults, including the capacity to form more colonies in cultures, a higher cell cycle rate, and autocrine production of growth factors. The immaturity and lack of antigenic exposure of the lymphocytes from the fetus theoretically reduce the risks of graft-versus-host disease and allow for more successful human leukocyte antigen–mismatched transplants. The small yield of stem cells from the umbilical cord generally has limited the procedure to children or to adults of low body weight. Ex vivo expansion of stem cells is an area of active research that may expand the application of umbilical cell transplantation.

Autologous Hematopoietic Stem Cell Transplantation

For the great majority of patients with acute myeloid leukemia who lack a suitable, human leukocyte antigen–matched donor and are eligible for allogeneic transplantation, autologous hematopoietic stem cell transplantation is a viable alternative that is associated with low morbidity and mortality rates. Peripheral blood stem cells can be collected when the patient achieves complete remission and cryopreserved until they are needed for transplantation, whether in first or later remission. Although occult remaining leukemia cells may contaminate the reinfused stem cells, there is no evidence that in vitro attempts to purge leukemia cells improves the outcome. Despite the absence of a graft-versus-leukemia effect, this approach results in three- to five-year disease-free survival rates of approximately 50% (Table 60-14). These Phase II study results, like those of allogeneic transplantation, need to be considered in light of the fact that substantial selection bias exists. These series comprise a favorable subset of patients who have achieved complete remission, are healthy enough to undergo transplantation, and have not relapsed prior to the time of the procedure.

Prospective Studies of Intensive Postremission Chemotherapy, Allogeneic Hematopoietic Stem Cell Transplantation, and Autologous Bone Marrow Transplantation

Several studies have compared prospectively the benefits of postremission therapy with high-dose cytarabine, autologous transplantation, and allogeneic transplantation. The randomization occurs in patients after initial complete remission. Patients younger than age 60 years with a human leukocyte antigen–matched sibling donor are assigned to allogeneic transplantation, and the remaining patients are randomized to receive either intensive chemotherapy or autologous transplantation (Table 60-15). In one such study, the EORTC and GIMEMA groups noted that only 74% of patients who were randomized to undergo autologous transplantation actually received the treatment because of early relapse, patient refusal, or persisting toxicity after induction chemotherapy. This has been a problem in all the randomized studies, wherein only 50% to 75% of patients actually undergo their assigned autologous transplantation. This is in contrast to the observation in the same studies that virtually all patients receive their assigned chemotherapy and approximately 80% of patients who are eligible for sibling-matched allogeneic transplantation undergo the procedure. For comparison purposes, to compensate in part for the failure to receive the assigned autologous transplantation, an intent-to-treat analysis is used, including all patients in their assigned group regardless of whether the therapy was actually given. In the Zittoun study, the disease-free survival rate was approximately 50% after either allogeneic and autologous bone marrow transplantation, compared to 30% for patients receiving chemotherapy. However, the overall survival rate of all three treatment groups—allogeneic transplant, autologous transplant, and chemotherapy—did not differ. This was because patients who relapsed after chemotherapy could still be salvaged for cure by undergoing transplantation. The other studies in Table 60-15 were of similar design, and the differences in disease-free and overall survival rates varied. In summary, the overall survival rate of patients with acute myeloid leukemia in first remission does not appear to be different whether hematopoietic stem cell transplantation is used early on or saved for use later

Table 60-14 ■ Autologous Hematopoietic Stem Cell Transplantation for Acute Myeloid Leukemia in First Complete Remission

Author, Year	Number of Patients	Transplant-Related Mortality Rate	Relapse Rate	Disease-Free Survival Rate	Overall Survival Rate
Linker, 1993, 1998	50	4%	27%	76% at 3 years	72% at 5 years
Cahn, 1995[1]	111	28%	50%	34% at 4 years	35% at 4 years
Miggiano, 1996	51	0%	24%	71% at 5 years	77% at 5 years
Stein, 1996	44	8%	33%	61% at 2 years	NA

NA = not available.
[1]Patients ≥ 50 years old.

Table 60-15 ■ Randomized Trials of Postremission Chemotherapy Versus Autologous Bone Marrow Transplantation Versus Assignment to Allogeneic Bone Marrow Transplantation in Acute Myeloid Leukemia in First Complete Remission

	Postremission Therapy					
	Intensive Chemotherapy		Autologous Bone Marrow Transplantation		Allogeneic Bone Marrow Transplantation	
Author	Four-Year Disease-Free Survival Rate	Four-Year Overall Survival Rate	Four-Year Disease-Free Survival Rate	Four-Year Overall Survival Rate	Four-Year Disease-Free Survival Rate	Four-Year Overall Survival Rate
Zittoun, 1995	30%	46%	48%	56%	55%	59%
Cassileth, 1998	34%	52%	34%	43%	43%	46%
Harrouseau, 1997	43%	59%	48%	52%	49%	55%
Burnett, 1998	40%*	57%*	54%	45%	NA	NA

*Survival at seven years.
NA = not available.

in patients who relapse after conventional intensive chemotherapy. It may be that this statement should be modified for specific acute myeloid leukemia subsets. Either autologous or allogeneic transplantation seems to be of most benefit in the favorable prognostic group of patients. In poor prognosis patients, only allogeneic transplantation offers a means to improve the cure rate. Changing technology in transplantation, the development of novel agents, and the use of prognostic factors to apply risk-adapted therapy may alter therapeutic approaches.

Therapy of Older Adults

Characteristics of Acute Myeloid Leukemia in Older Adults

The treatment of older adults (greater than age 55 to 60 years) deserves separate consideration. Compared to younger patients, older patients have a substantially increased frequency of unfavorable prognostic factors, including a history of antecedent hematologic disorders, poor prognosis cytogenetic abnormalities, expression of the multidrug resistance gene, and the lack of tolerance for intensive antileukemic chemotherapy. For example, in a Southwest Oncology Group trial of older patients with acute myeloid leukemia (median age 68 years), unfavorable cytogenetics were present in 32% of patients and 71% of patients expressed a quantitatively determined increase in multidrug resistance gene expression. Those older patients who had de novo acute myeloid leukemia with favorable or intermediate risk cytoge-

netics and multidrug resistance gene expression responded well to therapy. In this group the complete remission rate was 81%.

Treatment Strategies for Older Adults

The outcome for older adults in complete remission with conventional-dose therapy is generally poor. But attenuating the doses of induction therapy reduced the complete remission rate and survival rate of these patients without substantially reducing the toxicity of treatment. Thus, older adults, who are suitable candidates, should be offered either investigational treatments on a clinical trial or conventional-dose induction chemotherapy.

After complete remission is induced, the best postremission approach is uncertain. Multiple studies of intensified dosage chemotherapy or increased numbers of chemotherapeutic agents have not improved the disease-free or overall survival rate in older patients. Low-dose, long-term maintenance chemotherapy may in fact be the most beneficial approach. It has minimal toxicity and improves the disease-free survival rate.

Therapy of Relapsed/Refractory Disease

Induction Therapy in the Adult with Relapsed or Refractory Acute Myeloid Leukemia

Despite many advances, the majority of adults with acute myeloid leukemia who achieve a remission will ultimately relapse. The options for reinduction therapy include (1) intensive chemotherapy with conventional chemotherapeutic agents, (2) investigational therapy on a clinical trial, (3) immediate hematopoietic stem cell transplantation for the individual who has a suitable allogeneic donor, or (4) intensive salvage chemotherapy followed by autologous transplantation with previously cryopreserved autologous stem cells or with autologous stem cells obtained after induction of a complete remission.

The general medical condition of the patient, toxicity from preceding therapy, the length of the preceding remission, and the age of the patient are all factors in selecting subsequent therapeutic approaches. For very elderly patients or those who are refractory to even salvage chemotherapy, supportive care may be the best option. Patients older than age 60 years who are in relapse can be considered for additional induction therapy if their general medical condition permits and their preceding remission has been longer than six months. The likelihood of achieving a second remission and the subsequent survival duration directly correlates with the length of the first remission (Figure 60-9). Remission of short duration makes achievement of another remission with chemotherapy unlikely. In these cases, if the patient is an eligible candidate, allogeneic stem cell transplantation should be done as soon as possible. Approximately 50% of individuals whose preceding remission has been longer than six months can achieve another remission after intensive chemotherapy. Such therapy can be either the previous induction therapy regimen or one of several salvage regimens such as mitox-antrone and etoposide or a high-dose cytarabine-containing combination.

The selection of conventional salvage therapy, the optimal dose of cytarabine, and the benefits of the addition of an anthracycline or other agents are important unanswered questions. Results of three selected trials for patients with relapsed disease are summarized in Table 60-16. The randomized trial conducted by the Southwest Oncology Group failed to demonstrate increased benefit from the addition of mitoxantrone to cytarabine 3 g/m² every 12 hours for six doses. The German AML Cooperative group trial compared cytarabine 3 g/m² versus cytarabine 1 g/m² administered twice daily on days 1, 2, 8, and 9 in patients younger than age 60 years. All patients received mitoxantrone. There was no substantial difference in the remission rate or the overall survival rate. Thus, dose-intense cytarabine should probably be viewed as an essential component of a conventional salvage program, but escalation to 3 g/m² is probably not justified given the increased toxicity. There may be little additional value to escalating doses of cytarabine above 500 mg/m² to 1 g/m².

There appears to be no value to adding standard-dose anthracyclines to high-dose cytarabine. The third trial in Table 60-16 evaluated the concept of time-sequential administration of chemotherapy. It was reasonably well tolerated and produced a complete remission rate and survival rate comparable to those of other regimens. It is critical to minimize the toxicity and likelihood of persistent complications, since many individuals will be offered hematopoietic stem cell transplantation if remission is achieved.

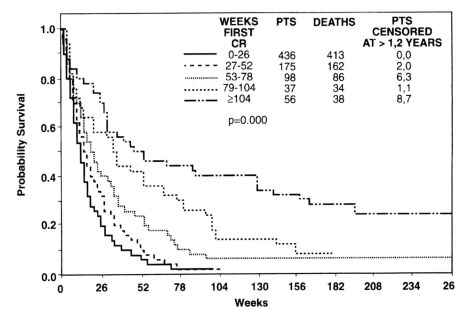

Figure 60-9 ■ Probability of survival for 802 patients by length of initial duration of complete remission in patients with relapsed acute myeloid leukemia treated generally with high-dose cytarabine containing regimens at the MD Anderson Cancer Center. (From Estey E: Treatment of refractory AML. Leukemia 1996;10:932–936.)

WEEKS FIRST CR	PTS	DEATHS	PTS CENSORED AT > 1,2 YEARS
0-26	436	413	0,0
27-52	175	162	2,0
53-78	98	86	6,3
79-104	37	34	1,1
≥104	56	38	8,7

p=0.000

Table 60-16 ▪ Results of Selected Trials of Conventional Salvage Therapy in Adults with Relapsed or Refractory Acute Myeloid Leukemia

Trial Design	SWOG Randomized Phase III		German AML Group Randomized Phase III		EMA-86 Phase II
Therapy	HiDAC	HiDAC + Mito	S-HAM cytarabine 3g	S-HAM cytarabine 1g	EMA
Number of patients	81	81	73	65	133
Complete remission rate	32%	44%	52%	45%	60%
Median disease-free survival rate (months)	9	5	5	3	8
Mortality rate	10%	16%	23%	11%	11%

SWOG = Southwest Oncology Group; HiDAC = High-dose cytarabine; Mito = Mitoxantrone; S-HAM = High-dose cytarabine + mitoxantrone; EMA = Etoposide, mitoxantrone, cytarabine.

New Agents for Relapsed or Refractory Acute Myeloid Leukemia

New approaches to the treatment of acute myeloid leukemia include chemotherapy combined with inhibitors of multidrug resistance P-glycoprotein, such as cyclosporine, the cyclosporine analog PSC833; topotecan, which inhibits topoisomerase I, an enzyme critical for DNA replication; angiogenesis inhibitors; and farnesyl transferase inhibitors. Other targeted therapy depends on antibodies to acute myeloid leukemia surface markers, such as monoclonal antibody-immunoconjugates, exemplified by gemtuzumab ozogamicin. The latter is the first of these agents approved by the U.S. Food and Drug Administration for the treatment of relapsed or refractory acute myeloid leukemia and represents a new therapeutic paradigm.

Unconjugated monoclonal antibodies directed at CD33 produce only a transient decrease in the number of circulating blast cells. Human antimouse antibodies often develop, some of which block the activity of the antibody. These antibodies have substantially reduced immunogenic potential. The antibodies can kill leukemia cells by harnessing a number of immune effector mechanisms. Monoclonal antibodies can also be linked to a cytotoxic agent. This creates another mechanism for leukemia cell destruction, provided that the agent is internalized after binding of the antibody to the leukemia cell surface antigen. Safety considerations require that the toxic conjugate not be released into the circulation causing nonspecific injury to normal tissues.

The antigen that is identified by CD33 is present on mature normal hematopoietic cells, on the majority of leukemia cells from patients with acute myeloid leukemia, but not on normal hematopoietic stem cells. After intravenous administration of radioiodinated anti-CD33 antibodies, rapid saturation of leukemia cells in the peripheral blood and bone marrow occurs, followed by rapid internalization of the antibody.

Gemtuzumab ozogamicin (Mylotarg) is a conjugate of a humanized anti-CD33 antibody covalently linked to a cytotoxic antibiotic, calicheamicin. In the cell, hydrolases cleave calicheamicin from the antibody. Calicheamicin binds to DNA and induces double-stranded DNA breaks and subsequent cell death.

Patients who were entered in Mylotarg trials had a relatively favorable prognosis because entry requirements for study included a first remission duration greater than six months and de novo acute myeloid leukemia. Of 142 patients who were treated in first relapse, remission was achieved in 30% of patients, 16% achieved a complete remission, and 13% had all criteria for complete remission satisfied, including self-sustaining platelets, but incomplete platelet count recovery to less than 100,000/µL. The median time to complete remission was 60 days. The median relapse-free survival for patients achieving a complete remission was 6.8 months. Grade 1 or 2 infusion-related toxicity was noted as follows: chills (11%), fever (7%), and hypotension (4%). Severe (grade 3 or 4) toxicities were as follows: sepsis (16%), fever (15%), chills (13%), nausea and hypertension (9%), hypotension (8%), pneumonia (7%), and asthma (7%). Essentially all patients sustained grade 3 or 4 myelosuppression. Grade 3 or 4 hyperbilirubinemia was observed in 23%. This agent appears to be equally effective in patients in all cytogenetic risk groups. Studies evaluating gemtuzumab ozogamicin in combination with conventional antileukemic chemotherapy, as consolidation and/or maintenance and as a single agent, and in combination with other agents in previously untreated patients are underway.

Treatment of Acute Promyelocytic Leukemia

Initial Therapy for Newly Diagnosed Patients

Acute promyelocytic leukemia merits separate consideration from the other acute myeloid leukemia subtypes because of its unique biologic features, different therapeutic requirements, and higher likelihood of cure (Table 60-17). The leukemic clone in acute promyelocytic leukemia is highly sensitive to anthracyclines. These cells are also readily induced to differentiate when exposed to all-trans retinoic acid and to undergo differentiation and apoptosis upon exposure to arsenic trioxide.

A number of clinical trials have confirmed the effectiveness of all-trans retinoic acid in this disease (Table 60-18). Two prospective randomized trials (European and North American) compared all-trans retinoic acid, with or without chemotherapy, to chemotherapy alone for induction therapy. Following complete remission, patients in both trials received an additional course of conventional induction therapy followed by a course of daunorubicin plus increased-dose cytarabine. In the North American trial, patients were randomized to either one year of daily maintenance all-trans retinoic acid or observation. The complete remission rate was the same with all-trans retinoic acid or chemotherapy induction, but the event-free survival, disease-free survival, and overall survival rates were markedly improved with all-trans retinoic acid, such that approximately 70% of patients remained disease free at four years. This benefit was attributable to a decrease in the relapse rate. The outcome was the same for patients who received all-trans retinoic acid during induction therapy, in maintenance therapy, or in both settings.

The principal, and potentially life-threatening, toxicity of all-trans retinoic acid is the development of the retinoic acid syndrome during induction therapy (Table 60-19). The cardiorespiratory distress syndrome consists of interstitial pulmonary infiltrates, pleural or pericardial effusions, hypoxemia, episodic hypotension, and otherwise unexplained weight gain. The syndrome may be related to the rapid development of

Table 60-17 ■ Unique Biologic Features of Acute Promyelocytic Leukemia

Low expression of multidrug resistance P-glycoprotein
Sensitivity to anthracyclines
Potential for complete remission without interval phase of marrow aplasia
t(15;17) and PML-RARα fusion transcript
Sensitivity to differentiation with all-trans retinoic acid (ATRA)
Sensitivity to apoptosis with arsenic trioxide (As_2O_3)

hyperleukocytosis, which can be observed with all-trans retinoic acid induction. The syndrome usually resolves quickly if high-dose dexamethasone is administered at the earliest sign or symptom.

The European APL93 trial showed that administering all-trans retinoic acid concurrently with chemotherapy reduces the relapse rate compared to giving all-trans retinoic acid as induction therapy, followed by chemotherapy. This was not due to abrogation of the retinoic acid syndrome. The benefit accrued even to patients presenting with very low white blood cell counts who are not prone to the syndrome. Standard induction therapy for acute promyelocytic leukemia therefore includes all-trans retinoic acid plus chemotherapy. Because acute promyelocytic leukemia is exquisitely sensitive to anthracyclines, it might not be necessary to use cytarabine in induction therapy at all. The optimal chemotherapy regimen postremission is not yet established. On the basis of completed clinical trials, postremission therapy should consist of two courses of either anthracycline + cytarabine, anthracycline + cytarabine followed by high-dose cytarabine, or intermediate-dose cytarabine + idarubicin, followed by mitoxantrone + etoposide + cytarabine + 6-thioguanine. The value of maintenance therapy with all-trans retinoic acid is uncertain, but continuing therapy with all-trans retinoic acid plus low-dose chemotherapy (6-mercaptopurine and methotrexate) may be beneficial. Autologous or allogeneic hematopoietic stem cell transplantation in first remission is not warranted because the treatment programs described above have such a favorable outcome and cure rate.

Treatment of Relapsed and Refractory Acute Promyelocytic Leukemia

Patients who have relapsed some time after completing treatment with all-trans retinoic acid can be retreated with this agent with a good expectation of achieving another complete remission. Anthracyclines and/or arsenic trioxide can be used for reinduction

Table 60-18 ▪ Randomized Trials in Acute Promyelocytic Leukemia

Trial	Number of Patients	Induction	Complete Remission Rate	Long-Term Disease-Free Survival
APL91	54	ATRA(+ChemoRx) versus	97%	79%
	47	ChemoRx	81%	50%
APL93	109	ATRA→ChemoRx versus	95%	75%
	99	ATRA+ChemoRx	94%	86%
North American Intergroup	172	ATRA versus	72%	69%
	174	ChemoRx	69%	29%
MRC	119	ATRA(5d)→ChemoRx versus	70%	59%
	120	ATRA+ChemoRx	87%	78%

MRC = Medical Research Council; ATRA = all-trans retinoic acid; ChemoRx = chemotherapy; APL = acute promyelocytic leukemia trial number.

Table 60-19 ▪ Comparison of Incidence and Outcome of Retinoic Acid Syndrome

Study Group	Number of Patients	Induction Therapy	Incidence of RAS	Mortality Rate of Patients with RAS	Mortality Rate of All Treated Patients
North American Intergroup	167	ATRA	26%	5%	1%
APL93	413	ATRA ± ChemoRx	15%	8%	1%
JALSC	196	ATRA ± ChemoRx	6%	9%	0.5%
GIMEMA	480	ATRA + ChemoRx	9%	4%	0.4%
PETHEMA	123	ATRA + ChemoRx	6%	17%	0.8%

ATRA = all-trans retinoic acid; ChemoRX = chemotherapy; RAS = retinoic acid syndrome; APL = acute promyelocyte leukemia; GIMEMA = Gruppo Italiano Mallattie Ematologiche Maligne dell'Adulto; JALSC = Japan Adult Leukemia Study Group.

if all-trans retinoic acid is ineffective. Once another complete remission is obtained, cure is obtainable by means of allogeneic or autologous hematopoietic stem cell transplantation. Autologous transplantation can employ stem cells that were harvested and preserved in first remission or obtained after reinduction of remission.

Arsenic Trioxide

Arsenic trioxide induces antiangiogenesis at relatively high concentrations (1.0 to 2.0 µmol/L), apoptosis at medium concentrations (0.5 to 2 µmol/L), and partial differentiation at low concentrations (0.1 to 0.5 µmol/L). Arsenic trioxide, in low concentrations in acute promyelocytic leukemia, either directly degrades the fusion protein PML-RARα or interferes with

messenger RNA synthesis. Experimental evidence suggests that it is the PML moiety that serves as a target for arsenic trioxide, because the leukemia cells of patients with acute promyelocytic leukemia who exhibit the t(11;17) variant karyotype, which results in a different fusion transcript with RARα, are insensitive to arsenic.

In 1996, investigators in China reported that 73% of 30 patients with previously untreated acute promyelocytic leukemia and 52% of 42 patients with relapsed or refractory disease achieved complete remission. Additional studies in the United States and elsewhere confirmed these results (Table 60-20). In the United States trial, 11 of 12 patients with relapsed disease who received 12 to 39 days (median 33 days) of arsenic trioxide at 10 to 15 mg/day achieved complete remission. Moreover, 8 of these 11 patients in

Table 60-20 ■ Phase II Trials of Arsenic Trioxide in Acute Promyelocytic Leukemia

Treatment Site	Number of Patients	Complete Remission Rate
Previously Treated		
Harbin	42	52%
Shanghai	47	85%
MSKCC	12	92%
US Multicenter	40	85%
Previously Untreated		
Harbin	30	73%
Shanghai	11	73%

MSKCC = Memorial Sloan Kettering Cancer Center.

complete remission also tested negative molecularly by RT-PCR for the PML-RARα transcript. In a subsequent multicenter Phase II trial, 34 (85%) of 40 patients with relapsed or refractory disease who were treated with arsenic trioxide at a dose of 0.15 mg/kg/day achieved complete remission at a median of 53 days (range 28 to 35). An important observation was that 78% of patients exhibited molecular conversion from positive to negative by RT-PCR for the PML-RARα transcript. Patients who had failed multiple chemotherapy regimens and hematopoietic stem cell transplantation responded equally well. The two-year relapse-free survival rate was 50%. Patients who achieved complete remission were able to tolerate subsequent stem cell transplantation.

Adverse reactions included leukocytosis and the acute promyelocytic leukemia-differentiation syndrome (in one quarter of patients), dizziness, hyperglycemia, musculoskeletal pain, and skin rash (in 20% of patients). The differentiation syndrome is similar to the retinoic acid syndrome and responds readily to dexamethasone. Neuropathy occurred with time but was reversible and generally mild. The most important toxicity was prolongation of the QTc interval on the electrocardiogram, presenting a risk of ventricular arrhythmias. The electrocardiogram and electrolytes should be monitored at intervals. Potassium and magnesium levels should be kept well within the normal range, because hypokalemia and hypomagnesemia contribute to QTc prolongation and predispose to ventricular arrhythmias. Other medications that may prolong the QTc interval by inducing hypokalemia, such as amphotericin and diuretics, should be avoided if at all possible. In the clinical trials reported from China, severe hepatic toxicity occurred, and some fatalities were noted. In clinical trials in other countries, hepatic toxicity has not been a significant problem.

Arsenic trioxide is a highly useful agent in acute promyelocytic leukemia, and studies are underway to establish its role in initial therapy and in combination with all-trans retinoic acid and anthracyclines. Because of its pleiotropic antineoplastic effects, arsenic trioxide may be of value in other cancers, such as multiple myeloma.

TREATMENT

Current Recommendations for Primary Treatment of Acute Promyelocytic Leukemia

Initial induction therapy consists of all-trans retinoic acid plus an anthracycline, such as daunorubicin. A dose of at least 50 mg/m² of daunorubicin is given intravenously daily for three to four days. If disseminated intravascular coagulation is severe at presentation and the white blood cell count is low (<10,000/µL), it may be advantageous to first administer all-trans retinoic acid alone for three to five days to ameliorate the coagulopathy. If the white blood cell count is high (≥10,000/µL), chemotherapy is administered first to reduce the count before commencing all-trans retinoic acid therapy, which is continued throughout induction until complete remission is achieved. Early in therapy, at the first symptom or sign of dyspnea, pulmonary infiltrates, or pleural or pericardial effusion, the retinoic acid syndrome should be suspected. Dexamethasone is begun 10 mg intravenously twice daily for at least three days. An additional course of postremission chemotherapy is given. Maintenance therapy with all-trans retinoic acid with or without 6-mercaptopurine and methotrexate is of benefit, especially for patients who are at high risk of relapse, such as older adults and patients whose initial white blood cell count is greater than 10,000/µL. Since children may have more toxicity with all-trans retinoic acid, a reduced dose of 25 mg/m² daily is recommended. The best maintenance schedule is not known. Either all-trans retinoic acid 45 mg/m² daily for 15 days out of every three months with 6-mercaptopurine 50 mg/m² daily plus methotrexate 10 mg/m² weekly for two years or all-trans retinoic acid 45 mg/m² daily for one year is most commonly used at present.

Routine Follow-up of Patients in Complete Remission

Unless patients are being treated on a clinical trial, routine follow-up generally includes a periodic history and physical examination and a complete blood count with differential count. Evaluations should be monthly for one year, every two to three months in the second and third years, and every six months thereafter. The chances of relapse after three years of complete remission is very small. Morphologic evidence of bone marrow relapse precedes blood count abnormalities by only one month on average. Bone marrow examinations therefore are not routinely necessary and are done only when a change in the peripheral blood counts raises the question of a relapse. In patients in remission, the reverse-transcription (RT)-polymerase chain reaction (PCR) can reliably detect minimal residual disease (the presence of the PML-RARα fusion transcript). A positive test predicts for eventual hematologic relapse. Because there is no evidence that therapeutic intervention early on in a preclinical stage of relapse improves results of treatment for relapsed patients, the reverse-transcription–polymerase chain reaction test, which requires otherwise unnecessary bone marrow aspirates, is best reserved for the clinical trials setting.

References

General Information

Krishnan A, Bhatia S, Slovak ML, et al: Predictors of therapy-related leukemia and myelodysplasia following autologous transplantation for lymphoma: An assessment of risk factors. Blood 2000;95:1588–1593.

Lowenberg B, Downing JR, Burnett A: Acute myeloid leukemia. N Engl J Med 1999;341:1051–1062.

Rowe JM: Treatment of acute myelogenous leukemia in older adults. Leukemia 2000;14:480–487.

Steins MB, Padro T, Bieker R, et al: Efficacy and safety of thalidomide in patients with acute myeloid leukemia. Blood 2002;99:834–839.

Acute Promyelocytic Leukemia

Asou N, Adachi K, Tamura J, et al: Analysis of prognostic factors in newly diagnosed acute promyelocytic leukemia treated with all-trans-retinoic acid and chemotherapy: Japan Adult Leukemia Study Group. J Clin Oncol 1998;16:78–85.

Avvisati G, Petti MC, Lo-Coco F, et al: Induction therapy with idarubicin alone significantly influences event-free survival duration in patients with newly diagnosed hypergranular acute promyelocyte leukemia: Final results of the GIMEMA randomized study LAPO389 with 7 years of minimal follow-up. Blood 2002;100:3141–3146.

Burnett AK, Grimwade D, Solomon E, et al: Presenting white blood cell count and kinetics of molecular remission predict prognosis in acute promyelocytic leukemia treated with all-trans retinoic acid: Results of the randomized MRC trial. Blood 1999;93:4131–4143.

De Botton S, Dombret H, Sanz M, et al: Incidence, clinical features, and outcome of all-trans retinoic acid syndrome in 413 cases of newly diagnosed acute promyelocytic leukemia. Blood 1998;92:2712–2718.

Fenaux P, Chastang C, Chevret S, et al: A randomized comparison of all-trans retinoic acid (ATRA) followed by chemotherapy and ATRA plus chemotherapy and the role of maintenance therapy in newly diagnosed acute promyelocytic leukemia. The European APL Group. Blood 1999;94:1192–1200.

Jurcic JG, Nimer SD, Scheinberg DA, et al: Prognostic significance of minimal residual disease detection and PML/RAR-α isoform type: Long-term follow-up in acute promyelocytic leukemia. Blood 2001;98:2651–2656.

Latagliata R, Pettti MC, Fenu S, et al: Therapy-related myelodysplastic syndrome—acute myelogenous leukemia in patients treated for acute promyelocytic leukemia: An emerging problem. Blood 2002;99:822–824.

Mandelli F, Diverio D, Avvisati G, et al: Molecular remission in PML/RARα-positive acute promyelocytic leukemia by combined all-trans retinoic acid and idarubicin (AIDA). Blood 1997;90:1014–1021.

Niu C, Yan H, Yu T, et al: Studies on treatment of acute promyelocytic leukemia with arsenic trioxide: remission induction, follow-up, and molecular monitoring in 11 newly diagnosed and 47 relapsed acute promyelocytic leukemia patients. Blood 1999;94(10):3315–3324.

Sanz MA, Martin G, Rayon C, et al: A modified AIDA protocol with anthracycline-based consolidation results in high antileukemic efficacy and reduced toxicity in newly diagnosed PML/RAR-alpha-positive acute promyelocytic leukemia. PETHEMA group. Blood 1999;94:3015–3021.

Shen Z-X, Chen G-Q, Ni J-H, et al: Use of arsenic trioxide (As₂O₃) in the treatment of acute promyelocytic leukemia (APL). II: Clinical efficacy and pharmacokinetics in relapsed patients. Blood 1997;89:3354–3360.

Soignet SL, Frankel SR, Douer D, et al: United States multicenter study of arsenic trioxide in relapsed acute promyelocytic leukemia. J Clin Oncol 2001;19:3852–3860.

Specchia G, LoCoco F, Vignetti M, et al: Extramedullary involvement at relapse in acute promyelocytic leukemia patients treated or not with all-trans retinoic acid: A report by the Gruppo Italiano Malattie Ematologiche dell'Adulto. J Clin Oncol 2001;19:4023–4028.

Tallman MS, Andersen JW, Schiffer CA, et al: All-trans retinoic acid in acute promyelocytic leukemia. N Engl J Med 1997;337:1021–1028.

Tallman MS, Andersen JW, Schiffer CA, et al: Clinical description of 44 patients with acute promyelocytic leukemia who developed the retinoic acid syndrome. Blood 2000;95:90–95.

Tallman MS, Nabhan C, Feusner JH, Rowe JM: Acute promyelocytic leukemia: Evolving therapeutic strategies. Blood 2002;99:759–767.

Hematopoietic Stem Cell Transplantation

Burnett A, Goldstone AH, Stevens RMF, et al: Randomized comparison of addition of autologous bone-marrow transplantation to intensive chemotherapy for acute myeloid leukemia in first remission: Results of MRC AML10 trial. Lancet 1998;351:700–708.

Cahn JY, Labopin M, Mandelli F, et al: Autologous bone marrow transplantation for first remission acute myeloblastic leukemia in patients older than 50 years: A retrospective analysis of the European Bone Marrow Transplant Group. Blood 1995;85:575–579.

Cassileth P, Harrington D, Appelbaum FR, et al: Chemotherapy compared with autologous or allogeneic bone marrow transplantation in the management of acute myeloid leukemia in first remission. N Engl J Med 1998; 339:1649–1656.

Clift RA, Buckner CD, Thomas ED, et al: The treatment of acute non-lymphoblastic leukemia by allogeneic marrow transplantation. Bone Marrow Transplant 1987;2:243–258.

Fagioli F, Bacigalupo A, Frassoni F, et al: Allogeneic bone marrow transplantation for acute myeloid leukemia in first complete remission: The effect of FAB classification and GVHD prophylaxis. Bone Marrow Transplant 1994; 13:247–252.

Ferrant A, Labopin M, Frassoni F, et al: Karyotype in acute myeloblastic leukemia: prognostic significance for bone marrow transplantation in first remission: A European Group for Blood and Bone Marrow Transplantation study. Blood 1997;90:2931–2938.

Forman SJ, Krance RA, O'Donnell MR, et al: Bone marrow transplantation for acute nonlymphoblastic leukemia during first complete remission: An analysis of prognostic factors. Transplant 1987;43:650–653.

Gondo H, Harada M, Miyamoto T, et al: Autologous peripheral blood stem cell transplantation for acute myelogenous leukemia. Bone Marrow Transplant 1997;20:821–826.

Gorin NC: Autologous stem cell transplantation in acute myelocytic leukemia. Blood 1998;92:1073–1090.

Harousseau J-L, Cahn JY, Pignon B, et al: Comparison of autologous bone marrow transplantation and intensive chemotherapy as postremission therapy in adult acute myeloid leukemia. Blood 1997;90:2978–2986.

Keating S, Suciu S, de Witte T, et al: Prognostic factors of patients with acute myeloid leukemia (AML) allografted in first complete remission: An analysis of the EORTC GIMEMA AML 8A Trial. Bone Marrow Transplant 1996;17:993–1001.

Kollman C, Howe CWS, Anasetti C, et al: Donor characteristics as risk factors in recipients after transplantation of bone marrow from unrelated donors: The effect of donor age. Blood 2001;98:2043–2051.

Linker CA, Ries CA, Damon LE, et al: Autologous bone marrow transplantation for acute myeloid leukemia using busulfan plus etoposide as a preparative regimen. Blood 1993; 81:311–318.

Linker CA, Ries CA, Damon LE, et al: Autologous bone marrow transplantation for acute myeloid leukemia using 5-hydroperoxycyclophosphamide-purged bone marrow and the busulfan/etoposide preparative regimen: A follow-up report. Bone Marrow Transplant 1998;22:865–872.

Mehta J, Powles R, Treleaven J, et al: Long-term follow-up of patients undergoing allogeneic bone marrow transplantation for acute myeloid leukemia in first complete remission after cyclophosphamide-total body irradiation and cyclosporine. Bone Marrow Transplant 1996;18:741–746.

Miggiano MC, Gherlinzoni F, Rosti G, et al: Autologous bone marrow transplantation in late first complete remission improves outcome in acute myelogenous leukemia. Leukemia 1996;10:402–409.

Stein AS, O'Donnell MR, Chai A, et al: In vivo purging with high-dose cytarabine followed by high-dose chemoradio-therapy and reinfusion of unpurged bone marrow for adult acute myelogenous leukemia in first complete remission. J Clin Oncol 1996;14:2206–2216.

Tallman MS, Rowlings PA, Milone G, et al: Effect of post-remission chemotherapy prior to HLA-identical sibling transplantation for acute myelogenous leukemia in first complete remission. Blood 2000;96(4):1254–1258.

Zittoun RA, Mandelli F, Willemze R, et al: Autologous or allogeneic bone marrow transplantation compared intensive chemotherapy in acute myeloid leukemia. N Engl J Med 1995;332:217–223.

Classification of Acute Myeloid Leukemia

Bennett JM, Catovsky D, Daniel MT, et al: Proposals for the classification of the acute leukemias. Br J Haematol 1976;33:451–458.

Bennett JM, Catovsky D, Daniel MT, et al: Proposed revised criteria for the classification of acute myeloid leukemia: A report from the French-American-British Group. Ann Intern Med 1985;103:620–625.

Harris NL, Jaffe ES, Diebold J, et al: World Heath Organization classification of neoplastic diseases of the hematopoietic and lymphoid tissues: Report of the Clinical Advisory Committee meeting—Airlie House, Virginia, November 1997. J Clin Oncol 1999;17:3835–3849.

Induction Therapy

Bishop JF, Lowenthal RM, Joshua D, et al: Etoposide in acute nonlymphocytic leukemia: Australian Leukemia Study Group. Blood 1990;75:27–32.

Bishop JF, Matthews JP, Young GA, et al: A randomized trial of high-dose cytarabine in induction in acute myeloid leukemia. Blood 1996;87:1710–1717.

Bishop JF, Matthews JP, Young GA, et al: Intensified induction chemotherapy with high-dose cytarabine and etoposide for acute myeloid leukemia: A review and updated results from the Australian Leukemia Study Group [Review]. Leukemia Lymphoma 1998;28:315–327.

Buchner T, Hiddemann W, Wormann B, et al: Double induction strategy for acute myeloid leukemia: The effect of high-dose cytarabine with mitoxantrone instead of standard-dose cytarabine with daunorubicin and 6-thioguanine: A randomized trial by the German AML Cooperative Group. Blood 1999;93:4116–4124.

Löwenberg B, Suciu S, Archimbaud E, et al: Mitoxantrone versus daunorubicin in induction-consolidation chemotherapy: The value of low-dose cytarabine for maintenance of remission, and an assessment of prognostic factors in acute myeloid leukemia in the elderly: final report. European Organization for the Research and Treatment of Cancer and the Dutch-Belgian Hemato-Oncology Cooperative Hovon Group. J Clin Oncol 1998;16:872–881.

Rai KR, Holland JF, Glidewell OJ, et al: Treatment of acute mye-locytic leukemia: A study by Cancer and Leukemia Group B. Blood 1981;58:1203–1212.

Rowe JM, Tallman MS: Intensifying induction therapy in acute myeloid leukemia: Has a new standard of care emerged? Blood 1997;90:2121–2126.

Rowe JM, Neuberg D, Friedenberg W, et al: A Phase III study of daunorubicin vs idarubicin vs mitoxantrone for older adult patients (>55 years) with acute myelogenous leukemia (AML): A study of the Eastern Cooperative Oncology Group (E3993) [abstract]. Blood 1998;92:1284a.

Schiller G, Gajewski J, Nimer S, et al: A randomized study of intermediate-dose cytarabine as intensive induction for acute myelogenous leukemia. Br J Haematol 1992;81:170–177.

Weick JK, Kopecky KJ, Appelbaum DR, et al: A randomized investigation of high-dose versus standard-dose cytosine arabinoside with daunorubicin in patients with previously untreated acute myeloid leukemia: A Southwest Oncology Group Study. Blood 1996;88:2841–2851.

Yates J, Glidewell O, Wiernik P, et al: Cytosine arabinoside with daunorubicin or adriamycin for therapy of acute myelocytic leukemia: A CALGB study. Blood 1982;60:454–462.

Zittoun R, Suici S, Dewitte T, et al: Comparison of three intercalating agents in induction and consolidation in acute myelogenous leukemia (AML) followed by autologous or allogeneic transplantation: Preliminary results of the EORTC-GIMEMA AML-10 randomized trial [abstract]. Blood 1999;94:2923a.

Myeloid Growth Factor Therapy in Acute Myeloid Leukemia

Dombret H, Chastang C, Fenaux P, et al: A controlled study of recombinant human granulocyte colony-stimulating factor in elderly patients after treatment for acute myelogenous leukemia. New Engl J Med 1995;332:1678–1683.

Godwin JR, Kopecky KJ, Head DR, et al: A double-blind placebo-controlled trial of granulocyte colony-stimulating factor in elderly patients with previously untreated acute myeloid leukemia: A Southwest Oncology Group Study (903). Blood 1998;91:3607–3615.

Löwenberg B, Suciu S, Archimbaud E, et al: Use of recombinant GM-CSF during and after remission induction chemotherapy in patients aged 61 years and older with acute myeloid leukemia: Final report of AML-11, a phase III randomized study of the Leukemia Cooperative Group of the European Organization for the Research and Treatment of Cancer and the Dutch-Belgium Hemato-Oncology Cooperative Group. Blood 1997;90:2952–2961.

Rowe JM, Andersen J, Mazza JJ, et al: A randomized placebo-controlled study of granulocyte-macrophage colony stimulating factor in adult patients (>55–70 years of age) with acute myelogenous leukemia (AML): A study of the Eastern Cooperative Oncology Group (E1490). Blood 1995;86:457–462.

Stone RM, Berg DT, George SL, et al: For the Cancer and Leukemia Group B: Granulocyte-macrophage colony-stimulating factor after initial chemotherapy for elderly patients with primary acute myelogenous leukemia. New Engl J Med 1995;332:1671–1677.

Zittoun R, Suciu S, Mandelli F, et al: Granulocyte-macrophage colony-stimulating factor associated with induction treatment of acute myelogenous leukemia: A randomized trial by the European Organization for Research and Treatment of Cancer and Leukemia Cooperative Groups. J Clin Oncol 1996;14:2150–2159.

Postremission Chemotherapy

Byrd JC, Dodge RK, Carroll A, et al: Patients with t(8;21) (q22;q22) and acute myeloid leukemia have superior failure-free and overall survival when repetitive cycles of high-dose cytarabine are administered. J Clin Oncol 1999;17:3767–3775.

Elonen E, Almqvist A, Hanninen A, et al: Comparison between four and eight cycles of intensive chemotherapy in adult acute myeloid leukemia: A randomized trial of the Finnish Leukemia Group. Leukemia 1998;12:1041–1048.

Mayer RJ, Davis RB, Schiffer CA, et al: For the Cancer and Leukemia Group B: Intensive postremission chemotherapy in adults with acute myeloid leukemia. N Engl J Med 1994;331:896–903.

Prognostic Factors

Baudard M, Beau Champ-Nicoud A, Delmer A, et al: Has the prognosis of adult patients with acute myeloid leukemia improved over years? A single institution experience of >84 consecutive patients over a 16-year period. Leukemia 1999;13:1481–1490.

Bennett JM, Young ML, Andersen JW, et al: Long-term survival in acute myeloid leukemia: The Eastern Cooperative Oncology Group experience. Cancer 1997;80:2205–2209.

Dastugue N, Payen C, Lafage-Pochitaloff M, et al: Prognostic significance of karyotype in de novo adult acute myeloid leukemia: The BGMT group. Leukemia 1995;9(9):1491–1498.

Frohling S, Skelin S, Liebisch C, et al: Comparison of cytogenetic and molecular cytogenetic detection of chromosome abnormalities in 240 consecutive adult patients with acute myeloid leukemia. J Clin Oncol 2002;20:2480–2485.

Grimwade D, Walker H, Oliver F, et al: The importance of diagnostic cytogenetics on outcome in AML: Analysis of 1,612 patients entered into the MRC AML 10 trial. Blood 1998;92:2322–2333.

Grimwade D, Walker H, Harrison G, et al: The predictive value of hierarchical cytogenetic classification in older adults with acute myeloid leukemia (AML): Analysis of 1065 patients entered into the United Kingdom Medical Research Council AML 11 trial. Blood 2001;98:1312–1320.

Chapter 61
Acute Lymphoblastic Leukemia

Richard A. Larson

Acute lymphoblastic leukemia (ALL) is a malignant neoplasm of lymphocytes characterized by the clonal accumulation of immature blood cells in the bone marrow. These abnormal cells are generally arrested in the lymphoblast stage of the normal maturation pathway. Aberrations in proliferation and differentiation of these cells are common, and normal hematopoiesis is eventually suppressed. Symptoms result from varying degrees of anemia, neutropenia, and thrombocytopenia or from infiltration of acute lymphoblastic leukemia cells into tissues. Although virtually any organ system may become involved by circulating leukemia cells, the lymph nodes, liver, spleen, central nervous system (CNS), and skin are the most common sites that are detected clinically.

The first recognition of leukemia as a distinctive entity is usually accorded independently to Virchow in Berlin and Bennett in Scotland in 1845. In 1847, Virchow coined the term "leukemia" (from the Greek *leuk* = white cells, *emia* = in the blood) to replace "weisshäme," a German term. Leukemic disorders are classified by their presumed cell of origin. Thus, acute lymphoblastic leukemia is a malignant disease of early precursor cells of the B cell and T cell lymphocytic lineages. In contrast, acute myeloid leukemia results from the malignant transformation of a bone marrow (myeloid) progenitor cell or "stem cell" that is the normal precursor for granulocytes, erythrocytes, or megakaryocytes.

Epidemiology

Although leukemia can occur at any age, its incidence is strongly related to increasing age. Across the entire age spectrum, acute lymphoblastic leukemia and acute myeloid leukemia (AML) are nearly equal in overall incidence, but acute lymphoblastic leukemia predominates among children, whereas acute myeloid leukemia is more common in adults. The age-adjusted overall incidence of acute lymphoblastic leukemia in the United States is 1.5 per 100,000 in whites and 0.8 per 100,000 in blacks. Acute lymphoblastic leukemia accounts for approximately 20% of adult acute leukemias and thus is relatively rare, whereas it is by far the most common malignant disease in childhood.

Childhood leukemia is distinctly different from acute lymphoblastic leukemia in adults. The peak incidence of acute lymphoblastic leukemia occurs between ages two to five years. Although the median age for adults with acute lymphoblastic leukemia who are entered into clinical trials is about 35 years, it is very likely that older patients are underrepresented in these reports. Registry data suggest that the incidence of acute lymphoblastic leukemia increases steadily above the age of 50 years. There are marked differences among the various subtypes of leukemia that occur in children, young adults, and older adults (Table 61-1).

Acute leukemia is more common among whites than among blacks at all ages. Jews are more commonly affected than are non-Jews, but it is unclear whether this disparity is the result of genetic or environmental factors. Geographic variations in incidence are likely related to a number of factors including socioeconomic status and ethnicity. These may in part relate to the higher frequency of acute lymphoblastic leukemia reported in industrialized countries and urban areas. Some cytogenetic abnormalities have been reported more frequently from some countries than from others. Acute lymphoblastic leukemia is slightly more common among males than among females.

Etiology

Although the cause of acute leukemia in humans is unknown, a variety of hereditary and environmental factors appear to play an etiologic role. The pathogenesis of acute leukemia involves complex interactions between host susceptibility, chromosomal damage secondary to physical or chemical exposure, and possibly the incorporation of genetic information

549

Table 61-1 ■ Immunophenotypic Subtypes of Acute Lymphoblastic Leukemia in Children and Adults

Type	Frequency		Five-Year Disease-Free Survival Rate	
	Children	Adults	Children	Adults
B lineage acute lymphoblastic leukemia				
Burkitt-type	2%	3–5%	75–85%	50%
Precursor B	80–85%	75–80%	80%	30–40%
T cell acute lymphoblastic leukemia	15%	20–25%	65–75%	60%

transmitted virally into susceptible progenitor cells. Much of the evidence is indirect and has been inferred from epidemiologic studies and animal models of leukemogenesis.

Characteristic leukemic disorders can be generated in animal models by transfecting fusion genes such as *BCR/ABL* into germ cells. The *BCR/ABL* fusion gene results from the translocation of the *ABL* gene from chromosome 9 to lie in juxtaposition with the *BCR* gene on chromosome 22. This fusion gene results in a novel and abnormal protein, which has enhanced tyrosine kinase activity, responsible for the phosphorylation of a number of other proteins involved in intracellular signaling pathways. The translocation also results in an abnormal chromosome 22 that is called the Philadelphia chromosome. This rearrangement is found in the malignant cells of about one third of adults with acute lymphoblastic leukemia as well as nearly all patients with chronic myeloid leukemia (see Chapter 71).

Radiation

The leukemogenic potential of ionizing radiation is well recognized. Leukemias associated with ionizing radiation generally derive from the myeloid lineage but often have trilineage features that are characteristic of multipotential stem cells. Much of the epidemiologic evidence implicating radiation in the etiology emanates from observations on humans who have been exposed to nuclear explosions, therapeutic or diagnostic tests, or occupational radiation sources. The incidence of acute lymphoblastic leukemia was increased among survivors of the atomic bomb explosions in Japan who received total body irradiation greater than 1 Gy. Current diagnostic X-ray imaging studies do not increase the risk of leukemia, except in the circumstance of fetal exposure in utero. Moreover, the mother's diet during pregnancy may expose the fetus to leukemogenic substances. Although alleged in the past, there is no credible evidence that electromagnetic fields cause acute lymphoblastic leukemia.

Chemicals

Acute myeloid leukemia is the usual type of leukemia that results from exposure to chemicals, such as benzene, and cancer chemotherapy. Exposure to alkylating agents, such as melphalan or nitrogen mustard, is associated with the development of therapy-related acute myeloid leukemia after a latency of three to seven years. The risk is greater in patients receiving both chemotherapy and radiotherapy. A specific subset of these "secondary" leukemias occurs after treatment with the epipodophyllotoxins, etoposide or teniposide, or with other agents that also inhibit topoisomerase II activity, such as doxorubicin. The latency is short, often only one to two years, and the leukemia presents acutely with a high leukocyte count, monoblastic morphology, and often a cytogenetic abnormality of the long arm of chromosome 11 at band q23 involving the gene. A number of secondary cases of acute lymphoblastic leukemia also occur. Most of these arise after therapy with topoisomerase II inhibitors. Some of the cases also have chromosomal rearrangements involving band 11q23.

Viruses

Viruses are known to cause acute leukemia in several nonhuman species. At present, although none of the common types of acute lymphoblastic leukemia in humans are of viral origin, some infrequent varieties are associated with viral infections. The Epstein-Barr virus, a DNA virus of the herpes family, has been implicated as a cause of Burkitt's leukemia/lymphoma. An uncommon form of human leukemia, adult T cell leukemia, largely restricted to southern Japan and the Caribbean regions, is closely linked to infection by a leukemogenic virus, HTLV-1 (see Chapter 70). Infection with the virus is endemic in these regions, but only a small percentage of infected individuals ever develop adult T cell leukemia.

Heredity and Genetics

Several observations suggest that hereditary factors play a role in the development of leukemia. There is an increased incidence of acute leukemia among members of certain high-susceptibility families and among individuals with genetic disorders. The risk of early appearance (before age 8 years) of leukemia is high in the identical twin of a child who has leukemia. The disease usually develops within one year of the first twin's diagnosis. Nonidentical siblings of those affected by leukemia have a lesser risk, but it is still greater than that observed among the general population. Whether this is genetically determined and/or related to common source environmental exposures is not clear.

Children with Down syndrome, a disease characterized by chromosome 21 trisomy caused by chromosomal nondisjunction, have an increased risk of both acute myeloid and acute lymphoblastic leukemia. Interestingly, their prognosis is more favorable than that for children of the same age with acute leukemia but without Down syndrome. Bloom syndrome and Fanconi's anemia are hereditary disorders associated with chromosomal fragility and breakage. The risk of leukemia is increased in these children as well. Acute lymphoblastic leukemia occurs in some individuals with Li-Fraumeni syndrome, a hereditary disorder characterized by inactivating mutations of the *P53* tumor suppressor gene. Other genetic conditions that are not usually associated with detectable chromosomal abnormalities, such as ataxia telangiectasia and congenital agammaglobulinemia, also are at increased risk for acute leukemia. In these conditions, the deficiencies in cellular and humoral immunity may increase the susceptibility to leukemogenesis.

Clinical Presentation

The clinical onset of acute lymphoblastic leukemia in adults is usually abrupt. Symptoms are generally present for only a few days or weeks prior to diagnosis. Malaise, lethargy, weight loss, fevers, and night sweats are common but are not typically severe. Bone pain and arthralgias, mimicking a rheumatic disorder, can occur but less frequently in adults than in children. Infection and hemorrhage are present in one third of patients at diagnosis but are less severe than in patients with acute myeloid leukemia. Lymphadenopathy, splenomegaly, and hepatomegaly are substantially more common than in acute myeloid leukemia, affecting half of the adults with acute

lymphoblastic leukemia. Chest radiographs show thymic enlargement in 10% to 15% of adults. Most of these patients have T cell acute lymphoblastic leukemia.

Acute lymphoblastic leukemia can involve the central nervous system in adults, but clinical manifestations are uncommon at diagnosis. Cranial nerve palsies most often involve the sixth and seventh cranial nerves. Headache and papilledema resulting from meningeal infiltration and obstruction of the outflow of cerebrospinal fluid, which causes elevated intracranial pressure, may occur but are rare. Retinal hemorrhages can result from severe thrombocytopenia.

Varying degrees of neutropenia, anemia, and thrombocytopenia are detected on the peripheral blood studies. In adult cases, the granulocyte count is relatively well preserved in comparison to acute myeloid leukemia and is less than 1500/μL in only one of five patients. The total leukocyte count is reduced in one third of patients and is normal or only moderately elevated in one half of patients. Characteristic lymphoblasts can be identified in the peripheral blood in more than 90% of cases. Marked leukocytosis (greater than 100,000/μL) occurs in approximately 15% of patients at diagnosis, but symptomatic leukostasis (plugging up by lymphoblasts) of capillary beds in the lungs and brain is uncommon in acute lymphoblastic leukemia even at these levels. Mild to moderate reductions in hemoglobin level are typical, and almost one third of patients have a hemoglobin level lower than 8 g/dL. Thrombocytopenia is frequent, and more than 50% of patients have a platelet count less than 50,000/μL.

Clinical and Laboratory Evaluation

Precision in diagnosis of acute lymphoblastic leukemia requires a combined evaluation, which includes morphology, cytochemistry, immunophenotyping, and karyotyping of the leukemia cells in the bone marrow and peripheral blood. Bone marrow aspiration and biopsy are standard diagnostic procedures. Aspiration may be difficult and is sometimes impossible (i.e., "a dry tap") in patients with very high marrow cellularity ("a packed marrow"). Most diagnostic testing can be performed adequately on lymphoblasts from fresh blood samples.

The traditional classification of the acute leukemias relied on morphologic description, determining the predominant cell type within the bone marrow population and relating that cell to its normal hematopoietic counterpart. In 1976, a group of hematopathologists formed the French-American-British (FAB) group with the aim of establishing a system to classify the acute leukemias into morphologic subsets and clearly distinguish acute lymphoblastic leukemia from acute myeloid leukemia. This system was initially based solely on light microscopic evaluation of routinely stained blood and marrow smears, supplemented by a limited number of cytochemical stains. The system was revised in 1985 to provide clarification and include new diagnostic techniques. Recently, a committee of the World Health Organization (WHO) described a comprehensive classification scheme that utilizes morphology, immunophenotyping, and cytogenetics. This system helps to clearly define acute lymphoblastic leukemia, acute myeloid leukemia, myelodysplastic syndromes, and chronic myeloproliferative disorders.

Morphology and Cytochemistry

The FAB classification system described three subtypes of acute lymphoblastic leukemia (L1, L2, and L3) based on cytologic features, such as cell size, nuclear chromatin pattern, nuclear shape, nucleoli, and amount of basophilia in the cytoplasm. The subtype L1 accounts for over 80% of the acute lymphoblastic leukemia cases in children and consists largely of small leukemia cells, up to twice the diameter of a small lymphocyte. The majority of adult cases of acute lymphoblastic leukemia are L2. These cells are bigger than those in L1 and are often heterogeneous in size. The distinction between L1 and L2, however, is often arbitrary and provides no guidance for the management of individual patients. Subsetting patients into groups carrying the L1 or L2 variants is therefore no longer used.

The least common type of acute lymphoblastic leukemia, seen in approximately 3% to 4% of both children and adults, is termed L3 or, more commonly, Burkitt-type leukemia. This subtype is morphologically identical to the neoplastic cells in Burkitt's lymphoma. These cells are large and uniform with finely stippled chromatin and regular nuclear shape. Nucleoli are often prominent. The cytoplasm is moderately abundant, deeply basophilic, and frequently vacuolated.

Cytochemical evaluation of blast cells in acute lymphoblastic leukemia reveal characteristic patterns. By definition, stains for lysosomal enzymes such as myeloperoxidase or the Sudan black reaction must be negative to exclude acute myeloid leukemia and support the diagnosis of acute lymphoblastic leukemia. The periodic acid-Schiff (PAS) reaction reveals positively stained clumps due to glycogen deposition in the cytoplasm of acute lymphoblastic leukemia blasts (except in L3, which reacts negatively). It is a poor discriminator of cell lineage,

however, because many cells in acute myeloid leukemia also react positively (although the deposits are usually finer). Chloroacetate esterase and lysozyme stains are negative in acute lymphoblastic leukemia, but α-naphthyl acetate esterase may be positive in T lymphoblasts. Acute lymphoblastic leukemia blast cells contain the enzyme terminal deoxynucleotidyl transferase (TdT). When it is present in the great majority of cells, it is a fairly reliable marker for acute lymphoblastic leukemia, except in the L3 subtype, which usually show no TdT reactivity. L3 leukemia cells often stain positively with oil red O due to neutral lipid within cytoplasmic vacuoles.

Immunophenotyping of Acute Lymphoblastic Leukemia

Morphologic examination of blood or bone marrow smears sometimes fails to provide an unequivocal diagnosis. However, identification of various differentiation antigens on the surface of the abnormal cells by flow cytometry studies or immunohistochemical techniques on slides can rapidly provide this critical information (Table 61-2).

Approximately 80% of acute lymphoblastic leukemia cases arise from the B cell lineage, express B cell differentiation antigens (CD19 or CD20), and have heavy- and/or light-chain immunoglobulin gene rearrangements. The blast cells from many of these cases also express the common acute lymphoblastic leukemia antigen (CALLA), designated CD10. Lymphoblasts from patients with progenitor B cell acute lymphoblastic leukemia, an earlier stage of B cell differentiation, do not express CD10. CD10-bearing cells can be further divided on the basis of the presence in the cytoplasm of the mu heavy chain of IgM (cμ). Most cases of acute lymphoblastic leukemia do not express the cytoplasmic mu heavy chain in their blast cells and are termed progenitor-B acute lymphoblastic leukemia (if CD10 negative) or common acute lymphoblastic leukemia (if CD10 positive). Approximately 20% of CD10-positive cases express the cytoplasmic mu heavy chain and are designated pre-B acute lymphoblastic leukemia. Although the immunoglobulin genes are always clonally rearranged in B lineage acute lymphoblastic leukemia, surface immunoglobulin (SIg) expression occurs in only 2% to 5% of acute lymphoblastic leukemia cases. These are termed mature B cell acute lymphoblastic leukemia or Burkitt-type acute lymphoblastic leukemia and typically display the FAB type L3 morphology.

Approximately 15% of acute lymphoblastic leukemia cases arise from the T cell lineage. These cells express early T cell antigens such as CD2, CD5, and CD7. CD10 may also be present, but CD19 and CD20

Table 61-2 ■ Characteristic Immunophenotypes of Acute Lymphoblastic Leukemia

Subset	Markers Typically Present	Markers Typically Absent
B lineage acute lymphoblastic leukemia	CD19	
Progenitor B	CD19, CD22, CD79a, CD15, CDw65	CD10
Common B-precursor	CD19, CD20, CD10, CD34	
Pre-B	CD19, CD10, cμ	CD34
Burkitt-type (mature B cell)	CD19, CD20, CD22, CD24, SIg	CD34, TdT
T lineage acute lymphoblastic leukemia	CD2, CD7, CD1a, CD5, CD3	

cμ = cytoplasmic mu heavy chain; SIg = surface immunoglobulin; CD10 = common acute lymphoblastic leukemia antigen.

are not. In the majority of cases, one or more of the T cell receptor (TCR) genes is rearranged. Further sub-classification of T cell acute lymphoblastic leukemia into early, intermediate, or mature thymocyte types is based on the expression of various patterns of T cell differentiation antigens. T cell acute lymphoblastic leukemia (T-ALL) is more common in younger adults, and those cases with more mature T cell markers appear to have a better prognosis. Many of these patients have a thymic mass in the anterior mediastinum, whose histology on biopsy is identical to T cell lymphoblastic lymphoma.

The application of both immunophenotyping and molecular probes reveals a number of cases in which leukemia cells display characteristics of both myeloid and lymphoid cells. Certain antigens that are normally present only on myeloid cells can be expressed by malignant lymphoblasts of either B or T cell origin. These cases are called myeloid antigen (My) positive acute lymphoblastic leukemia and probably have no special significance once the correct diagnosis is made. It is important, however, to differentiate these My+ acute lymphoblastic leukemia cases from acute myeloid leukemia without differentiation (FAB type M0). The latter also lacks myeloperoxidase activity and has myeloid antigen expression; but in contrast to the My+ acute lymphoblastic leukemia, it lacks lymphoid antigen expression.

In some instances, a single neoplastic cell may coexpress multiple features of two distinct lineages (biphenotypic), or, alternatively, two distinct subpopulations of leukemia cells may coexist and express either myeloid or lymphoid features separately (bilineal). Various hypotheses (lineage infidelity, lineage promiscuity, and lineage switching) have been advanced to explain the occurrence of these hybrid leukemias. In lineage infidelity, the leukemia cell displays aberrant gene expression by virtue of its neoplastic transformation. Lineage promiscuity proposes that normally differentiating cells sometimes express characteristics of more than one distinct lineage and that the leukemia cell is merely reflecting that particular phase in a cell's development. Lineage switching considers that leukemia is a malignancy of a pluripotent stem cell that is capable of differentiation along either a myeloid or lymphoid lineage. Thus, any individual case may express one or both phenotypes. Regardless of the explanation, the patients who are affected by such lineage infidelity tend to have poor outcomes regardless of whether therapy directed at acute lymphoblastic leukemia or acute myeloid leukemia is employed.

Cytogenetic and Molecular Evaluation

Cytogenetic analysis of the leukemia cells is an essential component in the initial evaluation. Karyotype findings are the strongest determinants of prognosis for the patient and are used to guide therapy. An adequate (greater than 2 mL) sample of bone marrow aspirate from a fresh puncture site should be submitted for cytogenetic analysis in all patients who are suspected of having leukemia. Metaphase cells are stained, and the chromosome number and banding pattern are determined. Specific and well-characterized recurring chromosomal abnormalities facilitate diagnosis, confirm subtype classification, and have major prognostic value for treatment planning (Tables 61-3 and 61-4).

Cytogenetic abnormalities in leukemia are acquired somatic (rather than germline) mutations that have contributed to our understanding of leuke-

Table 61-3 ■ Cytogenetic and Molecular Subtypes of Acute Lymphoblastic Leukemia

Subtype	Karyotype	Frequency		Disease-Free Survival Rate at 3–5 Years	
		Children	Adults	Children	Adults
Burkitt cell	t(8;14)	2%	3–5%	75–85%	50%
Hyperdiploid	>50 chromosomes	25%	2–5%	80–90%	40–50%
TEL/AML1	t(12;21)	20–25%	1–3%	85–90%	?
E2A/PBX1	t(1;19)	5–6%	1–3%	70–80%	10–50%
MLL/AF4	t(4;11)	2–3%	3–6%	10–35%	10–40%
BCR/ABL	t(9;22)	3–4	25–30%	20–40%	<10%
Hypodiploid	< 45 chromosomes	7%	4–5%	25–40%	10%
T cell acute lymphoblastic leukemia	t(14q11), et al	15%	20–25%	65–75%	60%

mogenesis at a molecular level. A number of genes appear to play an integral role in the development of a leukemia clone. Chromosomal localization and analysis of the chromosomal breakpoints associated with leukemia-specific cytogenetic abnormalities have permitted identification of a large number of these oncogenes. Many are involved in intracellular signaling pathways and the control of cellular proliferation and differentiation. Structural chromosomal changes may lead to activation or perturbation of oncogene expression, resulting in disturbance of cellular regulation (proliferation, quiescence, or apoptosis) and eventually malignant transformation. Deletions or loss of DNA may eliminate genes that have tumor suppressor functions. Gains of additional chromosomes may lead to gene dosage effects that provide transformed cells with survival advantages. Translocations of chromosomal DNA yield new (abnormal) protein products from the resultant fusion genes. These proteins, in turn, are responsible for the cellular dysregulation that leads to the malignant clone.

Cytogenetic data allow mapping of chromosomal breakpoints at a molecular level. This allows the use of probes for fluorescence in situ hybridization (FISH) techniques as well as primers for reverse transcriptase polymerase chain reaction (RT-PCR) methods for the detection of tumor cells. Fluorescence in situ hybridization and reverse transcriptase polymerase chain reaction can detect molecular genetic rearrangements that are not apparent in examining chromosomal banding patterns by conventional methods. Both of these methods, however, test only for specific, defined genetic mutations and cannot easily be used for screening purposes or for a comprehensive evaluation. Fluorescence in situ hybridization analysis is more sensitive than conventional karyotypic analysis and can be performed on both metaphase and interphase cells. The morphology of the positive cells can be determined concurrently, and the proportional involvement by leukemia of all of the hematopoietic cells can be evaluated.

Reverse transcriptase polymerase chain reaction is

Table 61-4 ■ Survival on CALGB Clinical Trials of Adult Acute Lymphoblastic Leukemia by Cytogenetic Subset

Karyotype	Number of patients	Complete Remission (%)	Overall Survival		
			Median (years)	At 5 years (%)	P value*
Normal	79	82	2.9	37	
t(9;22)	67	78	1.3	11	<0.001
+8	23	87	1.3	12	0.004
t(4;11)	17	76	0.8	18	<0.001
−7	14	57	1.3	14	0.01
+21	32	84	1.5	26	0.06
del(9p) or t(9p)	28	89	1.3	38	0.58
del(12p) or t(12p)†	11	82	6.8	82	0.10
t(14q11)†	9	100	>7.4	78	0.04

* P value from the logrank test for the difference in survival for each cytogenetic subset compared to patients with a normal karyotype.
† Excluding patients with t(9;22).
CALGB = Cancer and Acute Leukemia Group B

the most sensitive method available for detecting occult leukemia cells. Its sensitivity is approximately 1 in 10^5 cells. Using reverse transcriptase polymerase chain reaction, the method is now quantitative. A positive assay confirms the presence of residual leukemia cells with the specific genetic abnormality but does not necessarily indicate that these cells have neoplastic growth potential. For example, a positive reverse transcriptase polymerase chain reaction assay after treatment appears to predict leukemia relapse reliably in patients with acute promyelocytic leukemia (APL) and a t(15;17) or PML/RARα fusion gene but not in those with AML-M2 and a t(8;21) or AML1/ETO rearrangement. The significance of a positive result after clinically successful treatment is therefore under study.

It is now possible to characterize subsets of acute lymphoblastic leukemia by distinctive genetic features, and these more homogeneous subgroups have important clinical differences in their response to specific treatment regimens. Table 61-3 includes B lineage, Burkitt cell leukemia, and T cell acute lymphoblastic leukemia cases. However, the precursor B cell group has been subdivided according to cytogenetic and molecular features. Two important subgroups have a more favorable outcome. Hyperdiploid cases of acute lymphoblastic leukemia with more than 50 chromosomes account for 25% of childhood acute lymphoblastic leukemia and have an 80% to 90% cure rate. Similarly, another 20% to 25% of childhood acute lymphoblastic leukemia cases have the *TEL/AML1* fusion gene (also called *ETV6/CBFA2*), which results from the cryptic (12;21) translocation, and these children also have an 85% to 90% cure rate. Unfortunately, these genetic subtypes are rarely seen in adult series. Instead, the single largest subgroup among adult acute lymphoblastic leukemia cases are those that are Philadelphia chromosome positive (Ph+). They make up 25% to 30% of adult acute lymphoblastic leukemia and might not be curable with conventional chemotherapy alone.

In contrast, patients with a translocation involving chromosome band 14q11 usually have T cell acute lymphoblastic leukemia and have a relatively good prognosis with conventional multiagent regimens. As will be described later, patients with Burkitt cell acute lymphoblastic leukemia usually have an 8;14 translocation (*MYC/IGH* fusion gene) and also have a good prognosis, but they require chemotherapy that is quite different from the regimens used for the more common types of acute lymphoblastic leukemia.

It is important to note that the considerable differences in long-term outcome between these various cytogenetic subgroups are not as apparent in examining the initial complete remission (CR) rate (Table 61-4). With current intensive induction programs, 80% of patients with poor risk cytogenetics nevertheless achieve a complete remission compared to 90% of those with normal karyotypes or more favorable abnormalities. The long-term outcomes identifies the poor-risk patients. Such patients, after responding to initial treatment, are candidates for early allogeneic hematopoietic stem cell transplant to increase the likelihood of a cure.

Prognostic Factors

Several clinical and biologic factors have a major influence on complete remission rates and on remission duration and survival. In multivariate analyses, patients presenting with white blood cell counts greater than 30,000/µL have significantly shorter remission duration than do patients with lower leukocyte counts. Among patients with T cell acute lymphoblastic leukemia, however, extreme leukocytosis in some studies has not adversely affected the outcome. Other minor adverse factors that have been identified in trials of varying treatment regimens include a high percentage of circulating blast cells and of marrow blasts, the presence of hepatomegaly, splenomegaly, or lymphadenopathy; elevated lactate dehydrogenase (LDH) levels; central nervous system involvement at presentation; and increased time between the start of induction therapy and achieving a complete remission, that is, greater than four to six weeks.

Advancing age is another unfavorable characteristic. It is associated with a progressively decreasing frequency of complete remission, duration of remission, and overall survival. The increased likelihood of unfavorable cytogenetic features in older patients explains, in part, their poor long-term outcome. For example, the incidence of the Philadelphia chromosome among patients with acute lymphoblastic leukemia increases with each decade and may account for more than 40% of cases in older adults. In addition to having more treatment-resistant subtypes of acute lymphoblastic leukemia, comorbid diseases in older patients reduce their ability to tolerate intensive therapies. Fewer than 20% of older patients survive more than three years.

Treatment of Acute Lymphoblastic Leukemia

Overview

The aims of modern acute lymphoblastic leukemia treatment regimens are the rapid restoration of normal bone marrow function, the use of multiple chemotherapeutic drugs at acceptable toxicities to prevent the emergence of resistant subclones; the prophylactic treatment of sanctuary sites such as the central nervous system; and the elimination of minimal (undetectable) residual disease by continuing therapy once complete remission is achieved. The term "complete remission" is reserved for patients who have full recovery of normal peripheral blood counts and bone marrow cellularity with less than 5% residual blast cells (Table 61-5). Induction therapy aims to reduce the total body leukemia population from approximately 10^{12} cells at diagnosis to approximately 10^9 cells, a level that is below clinical and cytologic detection. The leukemia cells in a small fraction of patients exhibit primary drug resistance and ultimately prove to be refractory to one or more courses of remission induction therapy. It is generally assumed, however, that even in those patients who achieve a complete remission, a substantial burden of leukemia cells persist undetected. These residual cells then lead to relapse within a few weeks or months (depending on their growth rate) if no further therapy is administered. Intensive postremission, so-called consolidation therapy, usually includes several additional courses of chemotherapy and is designed to eradicate or reduce residual leukemia, increasing the possibility of cure. Multiple chemotherapy drugs in high doses are typically used to prevent the emergence of resistant subclones and to limit cumulative and overlapping toxicities. Lower doses of continuing, maintenance therapy are usually given over a one- to three-year period to prolong remission duration and increase the cure rate.

Induction Therapy

Treatment schemas from two large clinical trials using intensive induction and postremission therapies for acute lymphoblastic leukemia in adults are shown in Tables 61-6 and 61-7. Four or five drugs are typically used for remission induction followed by similar agents plus antimetabolites for remission consolidation treatment. Most modern induction therapy regimens have in common the use of vincristine, steroids, and an anthracycline (usually daunorubicin) plus either L-asparaginase or cyclophosphamide or both. The outcomes from different induction therapy programs are similar. Approximately 80% to 90% of patients achieve a complete remission, and in at least some studies, one half of the patients are still alive 36 months later (Table 61-8). Because the complete remission rate is already so high in adults with acute lymphoblastic leukemia, it has become increasingly difficult to demonstrate statistically significant improvement in initial response rates with modification of existing therapies. Some data suggest that early use of high doses of cytarabine or cyclophosphamide may add particular benefit for patients with T cell acute lymphoblastic leukemia and for some high-risk subsets and that high-dose methotrexate may have enhanced utility in B lineage acute lymphoblastic leukemia. Some investigators believe that more rapid cytoreduction during the induction phase of therapy by incorporating high-dose chemotherapy may lead to

Table 61-5 ■ Terminology Used in Leukemia Treatment

Remission induction therapy	Initial chemotherapy treatment aimed at achieving a complete remission
Remission consolidation (intensification) therapy	Postremission therapy aimed at destroying clinically occult disease
Maintenance (continuation) therapy	Lower dose of chemotherapy aimed at preventing reemergence of leukemia
Complete remission	Disappearance of leukemia after treatment, with full regeneration of normal hematopoiesis
Cytogenetic (or molecular) complete remission	Inability to detect residual leukemia using genetic methods
Minimal residual disease (MRD)	Persistent leukemia, not detectable by light microscopy
Refractory disease	Leukemia resistant to chemotherapy, preventing complete remission
Relapsed disease	Clinically overt recurrence of leukemia after complete remission
Immunophenotype	Pattern of expression of cell surface or cytoplasmic markers
Cytogenetics	Analysis of chromosomes in metaphase cells for additions, losses, or rearrangements
Multidrug resistance (MDR)	Biologic feature that protects cells from certain classes of chemotherapy drugs through different membrane mechanisms
Stem cell transplantation (SCT)	Transfusion of hematopoietic stem cells from the patient (autologous) or a normal donor (allogeneic) after high-dose chemotherapy ± radiation therapy

Table 61-6 ▪ Chemotherapy Regimen for Acute Lymphoblastic Leukemia in Adults

Course I: Induction (4 weeks)

Cyclophosphamide*	IV	1,200 mg/m^2	Day 1
Daunorubicin*	IV	45 mg/m^2	Days 1, 2, 3
Vincristine	IV	2 mg	Days 1, 8, 15, 22
Prednisone*	PO/IV	60 mg/m^2/d	Days 1–21
L-Asparaginase (*E. coli*)	SC/IM	6,000 IU/m^2	Days 5, 8, 11, 15, 18, 22

*For patients ≥ 60 years old, reduce doses as follows:

Cyclophosphamide	800 mg/m^2	Day 1
Daunorubicin	30 mg/m^2	Days 1, 2, 3
Prednisone	60 mg/m^2/day	Days 1–7

Patients receive G-CSF 5 μg/kg subcutaneously once daily, starting on day 4 and continuing until the absolute neutrophil count is ≥1000/μL on two consecutive determinations >24 hours apart.

Course IIA: Early Intensification (4 weeks; repeat once for Course IIB)

Intrathecal methotrexate	IT	15 mg	Day 1
Cyclophosphamide	IV	1,000 mg/m^2	Day 1
6-Mercaptopurine	PO	60 mg/m^2/day	Days 1–14
Cytarabine	SC	75 mg/m^2/day	Days 1–4, 8–11
Vincristine	IV	2 mg	Days 15, 22
L-Asparaginase (*E. coli*)	SC/IM	6,000 IU/m^2	Days 15, 18, 22, 25

Course III: CNS Prophylaxis and Interim Maintenance (12 weeks)

Cranial irradiation		2,400 cGy	Days 1–12
Intrathecal methotrexate	IT	15 mg	Days 1, 8, 15, 22, 29
6-Mercaptopurine	PO	60 mg/m^2/day	Days 1–70
Methotrexate	PO	20 mg/m^2	Days 36, 43, 50, 57, 64

Course IV: Late Intensification (8 weeks)

Doxorubicin	IV	30 mg/m^2	Days 1, 8, 15
Vincristine	IV	2 mg	Days 1, 8, 15
Dexamethasone	PO	10 mg/m^2/day	Days 1–14
Cyclophosphamide	IV	1000 mg/m^2	Day 29
6-Thioguanine	PO	60 mg/m^2/day	Days 29–42
Cytarabine	SC	75 mg/m^2/day	Days 29–32, 36–39

Course V: Prolonged Maintenance (Monthly until 24 Months from Diagnosis)

Vincristine	IV	2 mg	Day 1 of every 4 weeks
Prednisone	PO	60 mg/m^2/day	Days 1–5 of every 4 weeks
6-Mercaptopurine	PO	60 mg/m^2/day	Days 1–28
Methotrexate	PO	20 mg/m^2	Days 1, 8, 15, 22

See Larson RA et al: A randomized controlled trial of filgrastim during remission induction and consolidation chemotheraphy for adults with acute lymphomia leukemia: CALGB Study 9111. Blood 1999; 92:1556–1564.

prolongation of the subsequent complete remission even though no change is demonstrable in the complete remission rate.

Complications of initial cytotoxic therapy include tumor lysis syndrome with urate nephropathy and electrolyte imbalance (hyperkalemia, hypocalcemia, and hyperphosphatemia), gastrointestinal injury (mucositis and diarrhea), thrombocytopenic bleeding, and neutropenic infections. Prophylactic measures and supportive care are critically important during the

treatment period. Patients must receive adequate intravenous hydration. Allopurinol and alkalinization of the urine reduce the likelihood of uric acid precipitation in the renal tubules. Xanthine oxidase (rasburicase) given intravenously can rapidly lower the serum concentration of uric acid. At the same time, however, overhydration should be assiduously avoided. Measuring the patient's weight daily provides a sensitive indicator of developing volume overload that requires diuresis. Blood products are transfused

Table 61-7 ■ Hyper-CVAD Treatment Program for Acute Lymphoblastic Anemia in Adults

Course A (Hyper CVAD Induction)

Cyclophosphamide	IV	300 mg/m^2 over 3 hours every 12 hours on days 1–3
Adriamycin	IV	50 mg/m^2 over 2 hours on day 4
Vincristine	IV	2 mg on days 4 and 11
Dexamethasone	PO/IV	40 mg daily on days 1–4 and 11–14
Intrathecal methotrexate	IT	12 mg on day 2
Intrathecal cytarabine	IT	100 mg on day 8
G-CSF	SC	10 µg/kg/day starting 24 hours after chemotherapy

Antibiotic prophylaxis with ciprofloxocin/levaquin, fluconazole, acyclovir/valcyclovir

Course B (HD MTX/ARA-C)

Methotrexate	IV	1,000 mg/m^2 over 24 hours on day 1 with leucovorin rescue
Cytarabine	IV	3,000 mg/m^2 over 3 hours every 12 hours on days 2 and 3

Same intrathecal therapy, G-CSF therapy, and antibiotic prophylaxis as Course A.

Course C (CNS Prophylaxis)

High-risk patients	16 IT injections
Unknown risk	8 IT injections
Low-risk patients	4 IT injections

Course D (POMP Maintenance) for two years

6-Mercaptopurine	PO	50 mg TID
Methotrexate	PO	20 mg/m^2 once per week
Vincristine	IV	2 mg once per month
Prednisone	PO	200 mg daily on days 1–5 each month

See Kantarjian et al: Results of the Hyper-CVAD program, a dose-intensive regimen, in adult lymphoblastic leukemia. J Clin Oncol 2000;18:547–563.

to maintain a platelet count greater than 10,000/µL in a nonbleeding patient and a hematocrit greater than 25%. Broad-spectrum antibiotics are begun empirically whenever a fever exceeds 38.5° C in a neutropenic patient (neutrophils less than 500/µL), and antifungal therapy is added for patients who are persistently febrile despite antibiotic administration. Antifungal agents are often used prophylactically, especially for older patients or those with diabetes, or during prolonged courses of corticosteroids.

Remission Consolidation Treatment of Acute Lymphoblastic Leukemia

Postremission consolidation therapy is designed to eradicate the rapidly proliferating neoplastic cells that are thought to be responsible for early relapse. Drugs given for this purpose are usually cell cycle phase–specific antimetabolites. The need for intensive consolidation therapy to achieve a cure, unlike that of remission induction therapy, is controversial, however. In randomized trials, increasing the doses of

chemotherapy during consolidation therapy did not improve the results. The relative benefit of any particular consolidation therapy, however, may well be inversely proportional to the intensity and efficacy of the initial induction therapy. That is, intensive consolidation treatment may add less benefit after an intensive induction regimen than after a less intensive one. In adults, stem cell transplantation has not been proven to be better than intensive chemotherapy for acute lymphoblastic leukemia in first complete remission in general, but it clearly leads to cures that are unobtainable after conventional chemotherapy in patients with chemotherapy-resistant subtypes of acute lymphoblastic leukemia.

Maintenance Therapy

A prolonged period of treatment with low doses of chemotherapy drugs, called remission maintenance therapy, is still standard in acute lymphoblastic leukemia. This approach stands in marked contrast to most other "curable cancers," such as Hodgkin's disease, large-cell lymphoma, or testicular cancer, in

Table 61-8 ■ Treatment Outcome for Adults Receiving Chemotherapy for Acute Lymphoblastic Leukemia

Disease Subset	Complete Remission Rate	Five-Year Disease-Free Survival Rate
Acute lymphoblastic leukemia, overall	80–90%	30–40%
T cell acute lymphoblastic leukemia	90–95%	60%
Precursor B-cell acute lymphoblastic leukemia	75–85%	30–40%
Ph+ acute lymphoblastic anemia	70–75%	0–10%
Burkitt cell leukemia	75%	50%
≥60 years old	75–80%	10–15%

which cure follows the initial intensive cytoreductive therapy and low-dose maintenance chemotherapy provides no additional benefit. The necessity for prolonged maintenance therapy for adults with acute lymphoblastic leukemia may also be a function of the intensity and the success of initial chemotherapy. Traditionally, one to three years of 6-mercaptopurine and methotrexate, often with monthly short courses or "pulses" of vincristine and prednisone, have been given. As yet, the need for maintenance therapy has not been proven in adults, but it is likely to be important at least for some subtypes of acute lymphoblastic leukemia.

Stem Cell Transplantation

Myeloablative therapy followed by transplantation of bone marrow or hematopoietic stem cells (SCT) using a human leukocyte antigen (HLA) identical sibling donor is an established treatment modality in acute leukemia and is indicated for suitable high-risk (poor prognosis) patients in first remission or for any young or middle-aged patient in first relapse or second remission. Allogeneic stem cell transplantation has two therapeutic components (see Chapter 51). Intensive myeloablative therapy is used to eradicate all tumor cells if possible. Second, T cells in the donor marrow can produce a graft-versus-leukemia immune response that can destroy remaining leukemia cells; this effect has been correlated with improved disease-free survival. Unfortunately, this beneficial immune response is closely associated with acute and chronic graft-versus-host disease, a major cause of morbidity and mortality following allogeneic stem cell transplantation. Graft-versus-host disease can be reduced by T cell depletion from the donor stem cells, but only

at the cost of increased rates of both graft failure and relapse of leukemia. Because the risk of treatment-related mortality increases with age, most centers restrict allogeneic stem cell transplantation to patients younger than age 60 years. As yet, few data exist on the use of nonmyeloablative or "mini"-dose allogeneic stem cell transplantation approaches for older patients with acute lymphoblastic leukemia. This technique attempts to reduce toxicity of preparative therapy for allogeneic stem cell transplantation, while stimulating a graft-versus-leukemia effect after relatively mild immunosuppressive therapy. The use of allogeneic stem cell transplantation is also limited in part by donor availability. Patients have only a 30% chance that they will have a sibling who has inherited the identical human leukocyte antigen alleles needed in order to serve as a donor. However, unrelated volunteers who are suitably matched for the human leukocyte antigen alleles can also serve as allogeneic stem cell donors.

Autologous stem cell transplantation allows the use of myeloablative therapy in patients who lack an allogeneic stem cell donor. This treatment modality's role and place in therapy remain unclear. Because treatment-related morbidity and mortality (less than 5%) are relatively low, autologous stem cell transplantation can be used in older patients. Relapse rates are high, however, and overall outcomes are not clearly better than those in patients who receive intensive but nonablative therapy.

Central Nervous System Prophylaxis

Although rarely clinically apparent at diagnosis, the manifestations of central nervous system involvement by leukemia can occur at any time, at the time of systemic relapse or as an isolated site of recurrence (in which case it is frequently the herald of a coming systemic relapse). The meninges may harbor occult leukemia cells at diagnosis, and the blood-brain barrier may shelter them from systemic chemotherapy. Preventive treatment (central nervous system prophylaxis) against the possibility of later central nervous system involvement is routinely administered in both children and adults with acute lymphoblastic leukemia. Randomized clinical trials established its value in childhood acute lymphoblastic leukemia, leading to its application in adults. Although the frequency of unsuspected central nervous system leukemia may be lower in adults than children, it is clear that central nervous system leukemia is much more easily prevented than treated. Once it becomes clinically overt, it is highly likely that central nervous system involvement will recur despite successful treatment.

Central nervous system prophylaxis typically consists of cranial irradiation plus intrathecal methotrexate. Cytarabine and hydrocortisone are sometimes added to the methotrexate for triple intrathecal therapy. In lieu of cranial irradiation, some investigators substitute intravenous high-dose systemic chemotherapy with either methotrexate or cytarabine, because prolonged leukemocidal levels of these drugs in the cerebrospinal fluid can be achieved. Overall, the superiority of any one particular approach to central nervous system prophylaxis therapy has not been established.

The summated data from four consecutive studies by the German multicenter acute lymphoblastic leukemia study group (GMALL), showed that of 1433 patients who achieved a complete remission, 47 (3%) experienced an isolated central nervous system relapse, and 34 (2%) had a combined central nervous system and bone marrow relapse. Risk factors for either an isolated central nervous system relapse or combined central nervous system and systemic relapse included a white blood cell count of >30,000/μL at diagnosis (8% versus 4% for those with a lower white blood cell count, $p = 0.007$), T cell versus B lineage acute lymphoblastic leukemia (8% versus 4%, $p = 0.006$), and lactate dehydrogenase > 500 units/L versus lower values (8% versus 1%, $p = 0.001$). Involvement of the cerebrospinal fluid at diagnosis, patient age, time to achieve complete remission, or the presence of the Philadelphia chromosome or t(4;11) did not correlate with the risk of subsequent central nervous system leukemia. Isolated or combined central nervous system and systemic relapses occurred more rapidly (median, 238 days from complete remission) than did relapses only in the bone marrow (median, 375 days, $p = 0.004$). Survival at eight years

was only 12% for patients with an isolated central nervous system relapse and 9% for those with a combined central nervous system/bone marrow relapse. Although 24 (83%) of the patients with an isolated central nervous system relapse achieved a second complete remission, only four of these, all of whom underwent allogeneic stem cell transplantation, survived.

Kantarjian and coworkers also identified several characteristics associated with an increased risk of central nervous system involvement. Patients with mature B cell acute lymphoblastic leukemia (Burkitt-type), lactate dehydrogenase greater than 600 units/L, or greater than 14% of cells in the S+G2M compartment of the cell cycle were more likely to have central nervous system involvement ($p < 0.01$). These investigators noted a trend (not significant) toward the association of central nervous system involvement and high white blood cell counts at diagnosis. High lactate dehydrogenase levels are often seen at diagnosis with Burkitt-type acute lymphoblastic leukemia, and the white blood cell count is often very high in patients with T cell acute lymphoblastic leukemia. Thus, patients in the highest risk groups are easily recognized by clinical means. Cell cycle analysis is not widely available and probably adds little predictive value.

The Southeastern Cancer Study Group demonstrated benefit from central nervous system prophylaxis in adults in a clinical trial. After achieving initial complete remission, patients were randomized to receive either intrathecal (IT) methotrexate and cranial irradiation (24 Gy in 12 fractions) or no central nervous system prophylaxis. The rate of central nervous system relapse was reduced from 32% to 10% in the patients who received chemoradiotherapy prophylaxis ($p = 0.03$). Craniospinal radiotherapy may be even more effective, but it causes severe and long-lasting myelosuppression as well as considerable growth retardation in children. The spinal cord is rarely irradiated in adults.

In an analysis by the GMALL study group, a statistically significant decrease in central nervous system relapses was noted when the intensity of intrathecal and systemic therapy was increased. Among those who are judged to be at high risk of central nervous system relapse, patients who received nine additional doses of triple intrathecal therapy (methotrexate, cytarabine, and hydrocortisone) plus high-dose systemic therapy had significantly lower rates of central nervous system relapse overall than did those who received only four intrathecal injections of methotrexate plus 24 Gy of cranial radiotherapy (2% versus 7%, $p = 0.001$).

The necessity for including cranial radiation in

central nervous system prophylaxis has been questioned. At the MD Anderson Cancer Center, four different central nervous system prophylaxis strategies were used in sequential adult acute lymphoblastic leukemia trials: (1) no prophylaxis, (2) high-dose systemic chemotherapy with methotrexate and cytarabine alone, (3) high-dose systemic chemotherapy (cytarabine) plus intrathecal cytarabine, and (4) high-dose systemic chemotherapy (methotrexate and cytarabine) plus intrathecal methotrexate and cytarabine. Among patients who were judged to be at high risk for central nervous system relapse, the rates of relapse were found to be 42%, 26%, 20%, and 2%, respectively ($p < 0.001$). The central nervous system relapse rates among patients in the low-risk group were not significantly different. Although not a randomized trial, this evaluation suggests that central nervous system prophylaxis is a necessary component of acute lymphoblastic leukemia therapy. Moreover, hus, high-dose intravenous cytarabine and/or methotrexate, combined with intrathecal chemotherapy, appear to be as effective as cranial radiation plus intrathecal chemotherapy in preventing central nervous system relapses. Although these treatments are generally well tolerated, the long-term neurologic sequelae of either brain radiation or high-dose intravenous methotrexate/cytarabine + intrathecal chemotherapy are not known in adults.

As an increasing fraction of adults survive after treatment of acute lymphoblastic leukemia, the potential for late complications becomes an especially important consideration. In this regard, a randomized trial of different modalities of central nervous system prophylaxis would be informative. Given the low incidence (approximately 5%) of central nervous system relapse after prophylaxis, such a trial would require a very large number of patients to document the presence (or absence) of a significant difference in outcome. In ongoing studies, continued analysis should seek to determine whether combined chemoradiation therapy or chemotherapy alone is optimal for different subsets of disease.

Burkitt Cell Acute Lymphoblastic Leukemia

The first of the high-risk subsets that warrants special attention is Burkitt cell acute lymphoblastic leukemia, also known as FAB type L3 or mature B cell acute lymphoblastic leukemia. This subset makes up 3% to 5% of adult acute lymphoblastic leukemia cases. The ubiquitous biologic features are the presence of monoclonal surface immunoglobulin (SIg) and the 8;14 translocation or one of its two variants [t(2;8) or t(8;22)]. It is relatively easily recognized at

diagnosis from the characteristic clinical findings of hepatosplenomegaly and lymphadenopathy. The lactate dehydrogenase and uric acid levels are usually markedly elevated, and there is often leptomeningeal involvement. The lymphoblasts usually lack TdT reactivity. In the past, few if any of these patients survived following standard acute lymphoblastic leukemia treatment regimens. More recently, the use of short course intensive chemotherapy programs for Burkitt cell leukemia resulted in a high complete remission rate and an apparent plateau in the survival curve at 50%. These regimens, which may require as few as 16 to 18 weeks of treatment, use high doses of methotrexate, cytarabine, and cyclophosphamide or ifosfamide together with other acute lymphoblastic leukemia drugs. One such regimen appears in Table 61–9. Because the opportunity for cure rests upon the initial treatment regimen, it is critically important that Burkitt-type acute lymphoblastic leukemia be recognized at diagnosis and treated appropriately. Regimens that were developed for the more common precursor B cell acute lymphoblastic leukemia should not be used in this circumstance.

Philadelphia Chromosome–Positive Acute Lymphoblastic Leukemia

Philadelphia chromosome–positive acute lymphoblastic leukemia is currently the major challenge to the cure of acute lymphoblastic leukemia, since it makes up 25% to 30% of all adult cases and perhaps half of all B-lineage acute lymphoblastic leukemia. Approximately 75% of these patients have the p190 transcript of *BCR/ABL* most often seen in children, whereas the remaining 25% have a p210 transcript identical to that seen with chronic myeloid leukemia (CML).

Some progress has been made in treating this acute lymphoblastic leukemia variant. Although 70% of these patients achieve a complete remission, the remission durations are markedly shorter (median: seven months) compared to a median of almost three years for those patients with acute lymphoblastic leukemia whose leukemia cells lack the Philadelphia chromosome. Although no conventional chemotherapy regimen alone appears to have the potential to cure the Philadelphia chromosome–positive acute lymphoblastic leukemia, allogeneic stem cell transplantation does cure about one third of patients. However, even after allogeneic stem cell transplantation with its graft-versus-leukemia effect, the relapse rate is high (approximately 30% to 50%), further attesting to the resistant nature of this disease. A novel enzyme inhibitor called imatinib mesylate (Gleevec) demonstrated remarkable activity in inducing apoptosis in Philadelphia chromosome–positive acute lymphoblas-

Table 61-9 ■ Treatment of Burkitt's Leukemia/Lymphoma (FAB Type L3 ALL)

Agent	Route	Dose (mg/m²/day)	Day of Treatment
Cycle 1			
Cyclophosphamide	PO or IV	200	Days 1–5
Prednisone	PO or IV	60	Days 1–7
Cycles 2, 4, and 6			
Ifosfamide	IV over 1 hour	800	Days 1–5
Mesna	IV	200	Days 1–5 at 0, 4, and 8 hours after ifosfamide
Methotrexate	CIVI	1,500	Day 1 over 24 hours
Leucovorin	IV	50	36 hours after initiation of methotrexate, then 15 mg/m² q 6 hr until methotrexate $< 10^{-8}$ M
Vincristine	IV	2 mg	Day 1
Cytarabine	CIVI	150	Days 4 and 5
Etoposide	IV over 1 hour	80	Days 4 and 5
Dexamethasone	PO or IV	10	Days 1–5
Cycles 3, 5, and 7			
Cyclophosphamide	IV	200	Days 1–5
Methotrexate	CIVI	1,500	Day 1 over 24 hours
Leucovorin	IV	50	36 hours after initiation of methotrexate, then 15 mg/m² q 6 hr until methotrexate $< 10^{-8}$ M
Vincristine	IV	2	Day 1
Adriamycin	IV	25	Days 4 and 5
Dexamethasone	PO or IV	10	Days 4 and 5
Intrathecal Therapy (Cycles 2–7)			
Methotrexate	IT	15 mg	Day 1
Cytarabine	IT	40 mg	Day 1
Hydrocortisone	IT	50 mg	Day 1

Cranial Irradiation (only if bone marrow positive)

2,400 cGy given in 12 fractions after completion of all chemotherapy

CIVI = continuous intravenous infusion; See Lee et al, 2001; Hoelzer et al, 1996.
See Hoelzer D et al: Improved outcome in adult B-cell acute lymphoblastic leukemia. Blood 1996;87:495–508.

tic leukemia cells. Unfortunately, clinical responses to this oral drug in Philadelphia chromosome–positive acute lymphoblastic leukemia have been of short duration (two to three months) when the drug was used as a single agent for relapsed disease.

Treatment for patients with Philadelphia chromosome–positive acute lymphoblastic leukemia should include an intensive remission induction chemotherapy program, followed by early allogeneic stem cell transplantation in the first complete remission if the patient is young enough to tolerate the procedure and a source of stem cells, from either a matched sibling, matched unrelated donor, or partially matched umbilical cord blood, is available. If allogeneic stem cell transplantation is not feasible, then investigative regimens should be explored, because of the dismal results in these patients after standard therapy.

Progenitor B Cell Acute Lymphoblastic Leukemia with the t(4;11)

Acute lymphoblastic leukemia patients with a t(4;11)(q21;q23) represent another cytogenetic subset (3% to 6% of adult acute lymphoblastic leukemia) that has a poor outcome after conventional therapy. Allogeneic stem cell transplantation should be employed early on if at all possible. The involved gene on chromosome 11 was named "MLL," for "mixed lineage leukemia," and the gene on chromosome 4 is *AF4*. The immunophenotype is progenitor-B cell (CD19, CD22, and HLA-DR positive and CD10 negative). Among adults, these patients are often older females (more than half are over age 50 years) with high leukocyte counts. Morphologically, the circulating blast forms have a mixed appearance, some resembling lymphoid cells and others resembling monocytic cells.

Follow-up Evaluation and Rescue Treatment After Relapse

The period with the highest risk for relapse begins during the maintenance therapy and extends for about one year after the completion of therapy. During this time, patients are generally seen and evaluated with blood counts once per month. Surveillance bone marrow examinations are unnecessary, because they rarely detect an impending relapse if the complete blood count remains normal. Relapses are less common after patients have remained in continuous complete remission for more than three years, but follow-up visits should continue nevertheless every three months for several more years. The purpose of the continuing follow-up is the early detection not only of a late relapse of acute lymphoblastic leukemia but also of delayed treatment-related complications. These include avascular necrosis of hip or shoulder joints, cardiomyopathy, endocrinopathies such as hypothyroidism or ovarian failure, chronic pulmonary insufficiency or renal dysfunction, and the development of a second neoplasm.

Rescue therapy after relapse of adult acute lymphoblastic leukemia remains unsatisfactory. In patients who achieve a second complete remission after salvage chemotherapy, the probability of long-term event-free survival remains very poor, even after postremission treatment with allogeneic or autologous stem cell transplantation.

Despite major advances in the treatment of adults with acute leukemia in the past decade, many patients still die either from their disease or from complications of its treatment. A number of novel experimental and clinical approaches hold promise for the future. Methods of circumventing multidrug resistance, exploiting immune antileukemia mechanisms, or

TREATMENT

How Should Isolated Extramedullary Relapses Be Managed?

Extramedullary relapses that occur during treatment or after completion of primary therapy pose several challenges. Two common sites of extramedullary relapse in adults are the central nervous system and the testes. If the bone marrow shows systemic relapse at the same time as the extramedullary relapse, patients should be treated with reinduction chemotherapy followed by allogeneic stem cell transplantation, if possible.

Choosing the appropriate treatment for a patient with an isolated extramedullary relapse is problematic. Most of the available data come from clinical studies on children, and the recommendations for treatment (similar to other aspects of care for adults with acute lymphoblastic leukemia) have been extrapolated to adults. Studies in children support the need for systemic as well as local therapy for adults with isolated extramedullary relapse of acute lymphoblastic leukemia, but the optimal regimen and intensity of treatment are not known. There is a strong rationale for the use of drugs such as methotrexate and cytarabine that are known to penetrate the central nervous system and other extramedullary sites when given intravenously in high doses, in addition to local radiation and/or intrathecal therapy. Therapy needs to be individualized on the basis of the adequacy of primary treatment, the site and timing of relapse, and the patient's candidacy for allogeneic stem cell transplantation.

Isolated central nervous system relapse should be treated with intrathecal chemotherapy, using preservative-free methotrexate (15 mg) plus hydrocortisone (50 mg) twice per week until the cerebrospinal fluid is clear of blast cells. The intrathecal therapy continues weekly until six injections have been given and then monthly for one year. An alternative regimen is triple therapy, which also adds cytarabine (50 mg per intrathecal dose). An Ommaya reservoir should be placed in the skull, since this not only makes the treatment easier to administer, but also provides better distribution of the chemotherapy in the cerebrospinal fluid. In general, 1800 to 2400 cGy of radiation should be delivered to the whole cranium and the upper spinal cord to the level of C2. Patients with new cranial neuropathies or a magnetic resonance imaging (MRI) scan showing gross disease around the base of the brain should always receive brain radiation. At the completion of the radiation therapy, high-dose chemotherapy with methotrexate and/or cytarabine should be given to coincide with the continuing intra-Ommaya therapy. Adults with isolated testicular relapse should also receive local radiotherapy (2400 cGy) plus high-dose antimetabolite therapy.

After an isolated extramedullary relapse, an allogeneic stem cell transplantation should be performed in second complete remission if a human leukocyte antigen–matched donor is available. For patients who are not transplant candidates, we generally repeat our intensive induction/consolidation sequence and place the patient back on another year of maintenance chemotherapy.

altering the control of malignant cell growth are under study. Application of modern molecular technologies designed to detect minimal residual leukemia may aid clinicians in monitoring disease during and after chemotherapy.

Because acute lymphoblastic leukemia is an uncommon disease, multicenter clinical trials are necessary to rapidly test new therapies. Acute lymphoblastic leukemia is a heterogeneous disease, so large numbers of patients must be treated to detect an improvement in outcome among the small proportion of patients in individual prognostic subgroups. As has been noted, improvement in the already high complete remission rate will be difficult to demonstrate. Because the median survival is two to three years, lengthy follow-up is required to detect long-term benefit. Taken all together, these facts suggest that short of new therapeutic breakthroughs, further progress in adult acute lymphoblastic leukemia will be slow and perhaps not quickly recognized.

References

General

American Society of Clinical Oncology: Recommendations for the use of hematopoietic colony-stimulating factors: Evidenced-based clinical practice guidelines. J Clin Oncol 1994;12:2471–2508.

Drapner GF, Heaf MM, Kinnear Wilson LM: Occurrence of childhood cancers among sibs and estimation of familial risks. J Med Genet 1977;14:81.

Hoelzer DF: Diagnosis and treatment of adult acute lymphoblastic leukemia. In Wiernik PH, Canellos GP, Kyle RA, Schiffer CA (eds): Neoplastic Diseases of the Blood, 3rd edition. New York: Churchill Livingstone, 1996, pp 295–319.

Hoelzer D, Gokbuget N: Recent approaches in acute lymphoblastic leukemia in adults. Crit Rev Oncol Hematol 2000;36:49–88.

Linet MS: The Leukemias: Epidemiologic Aspects. New York: Oxford University Press, 1985.

Pui CH, Evans WE: Acute lymphoblastic leukemia. N Engl J Med 1998;339:605–615.

Pui CH, Ribeiro RC, Hancock ML, et al: Acute myeloid leukemia in children treated with epipodophyllotoxins for acute lymphoblastic leukemia. N Engl J Med 1991;325:1682.

Roberts WM, Estrov Z, Ouspenskaia MV, et al. Measurement of residual leukemia during remission in childhood acute lymphoblastic leukemia. N Engl J Med 1997;336:317–323.

Sandler DP, Ross JA: Epidemiology of acute leukemia in children and adults. Semin Oncol 1997;24:3–16.

Classification

Bennett JM, Catovsky D, Daniel MT, et al: Proposals for the classification of the acute leukemias. Br J Haematol 1976;33:451.

Bennett JM, Catovsky D, Daniel MT, et al: The morphologic classification of acute lymphoblastic leukemia: Concor-dance among observers and clinical correlations. Br J Haematol 1981;47:553.

Crist W, Grossi CE, Pullen DJ, Cooper MD: Immunologic markers in childhood acute lymphoblastic leukemia. Semin Oncol 1985;12:105.

First MIC Cooperative Study Group: Morphologic, immunologic, and cytogenetic (MIC) working classification of acute lymphoblastic leukemia. Cancer Genet Cytogenet 1986;23:189.

Harris NL, Jaffe ES, Diebold J, et al: The World Health Organization Classification of Tumors. Pathology and Genetics. Tumors of Haematopoietic and Lymphoid Tissues. Lyon, France: IAKC Press, 2001.

Terstappen LWMM: Cell differentiation and maturation in normal bone marrow and acute leukemia. In Macey MG (ed): Flow Cytometry: Clinical Applications. Oxford, Engl: Blackwell Scientific Publications, 1995, p 101.

Chemotherapy

Evans WE, Crom WR, Abromowitch M, et al: Clinical pharmacodynamics of high-dose methotrexate in acute lymphoblastic leukemia. N Engl J Med 1986;314:471.

Finiewicz KJ, Larson RA: Dose-intensive therapy for adult acute lymphoblastic leukemia. Semin Oncol 1999;26:6–20.

Gottlieb AJ, Weinberg V, Ellison RR, et al: Efficacy of daunorubicin in the therapy of adult acute lymphoblastic leukemia: A prospective randomized trial by Cancer and Leukemia Group B. Blood 1984;64:267.

Hoelzer D, Ludwig WD, Thiel E, et al: Improved outcome in adult B-cell acute lymphoblastic leukemia. Blood 1996;87:495–508.

Kantarjian HM, Hoelzer D, Larson RA (eds): Advances in the Treatment of Adult Acute Lymphoblastic Leukemia, Part I. Hematology/Oncology Clinics of North America, Vol 14. Philadelphia: WB Saunders, 2000.

Kantarjian HM, Hoelzer D, Larson RA (eds): Advances in the Treatment of Adult Acute Lymphoblastic Leukemia, Part II. Hematology/Oncology Clinics of North America, Vol 15. Philadelphia: WB Saunders, 2001.

Kantarjian HM, O'Brien S, Smith TL, et al: Results of the HYPER-CVAD program, a dose intensive regimen, in adult acute lymphoblastic leukemia. J Clin Oncol 2000;18:547–561.

Laport GF, Larson RA: Treatment of adult acute lymphoblastic leukemia. Semin Oncol 1997;24:70–82.

Larson RA, Dodge RK, Burns CP, et al: A five-drug remission induction regimen with intensive consolidation for adults with acute lymphoblastic leukemia: Cancer and Leukemia Group B study 8811. Blood 1995;85:2025–2037.

Larson RA, Dodge RK, Linker CA, et al: A randomized controlled trial of filgrastim during remission induction and consolidation chemotherapy for adults with acute lymphoblastic leukemia: CALGB study 9111. Blood 1999;92:1556–1564.

Larson RA, Fretzin MH, Dodge RK, Schiffer CA: Hypersensitivity reactions to L-asparaginase do not impact on the remission duration of adults with acute lymphoblastic leukemia. Leukemia 1998;12:660–665.

Lee EJ, Petroni GR, Schiffer CA, et al: Brief duration high-intensity chemotherapy for patients with small non-cleared cell lymphoma or FAB L3 acute lymphocytic leukemia: Results of Cancer and Leukemia. Group B Study 9251. J Clin Oncol 2001;19:4014–4022.

Linker CA, Levitt LJ, O'Donnell M, et al: Treatment of adult acute lymphoblastic leukemia with intensive cyclical chemotherapy: A follow-up report. Blood 1991;78: 281–822.

Millot F, Suciu S, Philippe N, et al: Value of high-dose cytarabine during interval therapy of a Berlin-Frankfurt-Munster-based protocol in increased-risk children with acute lymphoblastic leukemia and lymphoblastic lymphoma: Results of the European Organization for Research and Treatment of Cancer 58881 randomized Phase III trial. J Clin Oncol 2001;19:1935–1942.

Ottmann OG, Hoelzer D, Gracien E, et al: Concomitant rmetHuG-CSF (Filgrastim) and intensive chemoradiotherapy as induction treatment in adult acute lymphoblastic leukemia: A randomized multicenter phase III trial. Blood 1993;82:1938.

Central Nervous System Leukemia

Borgmann A, Hartmann R, Schmid H, et al: Isolated extramedullary relapse in children with acute lymphoblastic leukemia: A comparison between treatment results of chemotherapy and bone marrow transplantation. BFM Relapse Study Group. Bone Marrow Transplant 1995;15:515–521.

Cortes J, O'Brien SM, Pierce S, et al: The value of high-dose systemic chemotherapy and intrathecal therapy for central nervous system prophylaxis in different risk groups of adult acute lymphoblastic leukemia. Blood 1995;86:2091–2097.

Kantarjian HM, Walters RS, Smith TL, et al: Identification of risk groups for development of central nervous system leukemia in adults with acute lymphoblastic leukemia. Blood 1988;72:1784–1789.

Ribeiro RC, Rivera GK, Hudson M, et al: An intensive re-treatment protocol for children with an isolated CNS relapse of acute lymphoblastic leukemia. J Clin Oncol 1995;13: 333–338.

Ritchey AK, Pollock BH, Lauer SJ, et al: Improved survival of children with isolated CNS relapse of acute lymphoblastic leukemia: A Pediatric Oncology Group study. J Clin Oncol 1999;17:3745–3752.

Cytogenetics

Bloomfield CD, Goldman AI, Alimena G, et al: Chromosomal abnormalities identify high-risk and low-risk patients with acute lymphoblastic leukemia. Blood 1986;67:415.

Le Beau MM, Larson RA: Cytogenetics and neoplasia. In Hoffman R, Benz EJ Jr, Shattil SJ, Furie B, Cohen HJ, Silberstein LE, McGlave P (eds): Hematology: Basic Principles and Practice, 3rd edition. New York: Churchill Livingstone, 2000, pp 848–869.

Thandla S, Aplan PD: Molecular biology of acute lymphoblastic leukemia. Semin Oncol 1997;24:45–56.

Thirman MJ, Gill HJ, Burnett RC, et al: Rearrangement of the MLL gene in acute lymphoblastic and acute myeloid leukemias with 11q23 chromosomal translocations. N Engl J Med 1993;329:909.

Westbrook CA, Hooberman AL, Spino C, et al: Clinical signifi-

cance of the BCR-ABL fusion gene in adult acute lymphoblastic leukemia: A Cancer and Leukemia Group B study (8762). Blood 1992;80:2983–2990.

Wetzler M, Dodge RK, Mrozek K, et al: Prospective karyotype analysis in adult acute lymphoblastic leukemia: The Cancer and Leukemia Group B experience. Blood 1999;93:3983–3993.

Prognostic Features

Buchner T, Hiddemann W, Wormann B, et al (eds): Acute Leukemias VIII: Prognostic Factors and Treatment Strategies. Hematology and Blood Transfusion. Berlin: Springer-Verlag, 2001.

Cave H, van der Werff ten Bosch J, Suciu S, et al: Clinical significance of minimal residual disease in childhood acute lymphoblastic leukemia: European Organization for Research and Treatment of Cancer—Childhood Leukemia Cooperative Group. N Engl J Med 1998;339:591–598.

Crist W, Boyett J, Jackson J, et al: Prognostic importance of the pre-B-cell immunophenotype and other presenting features in B-lineage childhood acute lymphoblastic leukemia: A Pediatric Oncology Group study. Blood 1989;74:1252.

Crist W, Pullen J, Boyett J, et al: Acute lymphoid leukemia in adolescents: Clinical and biologic features predict a poor prognosis—A Pediatric Oncology Group study. J Clin Oncol 1988;6:34.

Czuczman MS, Dodge RK, Stewart CC, et al: Value of immunophenotype in intensively treated adult acute lymphoblastic leukemia: Cancer and Leukemia Group B study 8364. Blood 1999;93:3931–3939.

Hoelzer D, Thiel E, Löffler H, et al: Prognostic factors in multicenter study for treatment of acute lymphoblastic leukemia in adults. Blood 1988;71:123.

Ludwig W-D, Rieder H, Bartram CR, et al: Immunophenotypic and genotypic features, clinical characteristics, and treatment outcome of adult pro-B acute lymphoblastic leukemia: Results of the German multicenter trials GMALL 03/87 and 04/89. Blood 1998;92:1898–1909.

Stem Cell Transplantation

Appelbaum FR: Allogeneic hematopoietic stem cell transplantation for acute leukemia. Semin Oncol 1997;24:114–123.

Ball ED, Rybka WB: Autologous bone marrow transplantation for adult acute leukemia. Hematol Oncol Clinics North Am 1993;7:201–231.

Barrett AJ, Horowitz MM, Ash RC, et al: Bone marrow transplantation for Philadelphia chromosome-positive acute lymphoblastic leukemia. Blood 1992;79:3067–3070.

Dombret H, Gabert J, Boiron JM, et al: Outcome of treatment in adults with Philadelphia chromosome—Positive acute lymphoblastic leukemia: Results of the prospective multicenter LALA-94 trial. Blood 2002;100:2357–2366.

Fiere D, Lepage E, Sebban C, et al: Adult acute lymphoblastic leukemia: A multicentric randomized trial testing bone marrow transplantation as postremission therapy. J Clin Oncol 1993;11:1990–2001.

Horowitz MM, Messerer D, Hoelzer D, et al: Chemotherapy compared with bone marrow transplantation for adults with acute lymphoblastic leukemia in first remission. Ann Intern Med 1991;115:13.

Chapter 62
Myelodysplasia

Jeanne E. Anderson

Myelodysplasia, also referred to as myelodysplastic syndrome (MDS), is a chronic myeloid malignancy that occurs most often in elderly individuals. The defining characteristic of this disease is clonally derived, dysplastic hematopoiesis that is ineffective and results in peripheral cytopenias and a high risk of evolving into acute leukemia. Myelodysplasia is an age-related disorder, with the peak incidence in the eighth decade of life. Although most cases of myelodysplastic syndrome have no known etiology, prior exposure to alkylating chemotherapy is an established cause of myelodysplasia. The diagnosis of myelodysplastic syndrome is based on

1. the presence of dysplasia and peripheral cytopenia(s),
2. the persistence of these abnormalities over time, and
3. the exclusion of other causes of these abnormalities.

Traditionally, the disease is categorized according to the French-American-British (FAB) morphological categories. Currently, however, classification according to the International Prognostic Scoring System (IPSS), which uses blast percentage, number of peripheral cytopenias, and karyotype, is the best way to determine an individual patient's expected survival and risk of progression into acute myeloid leukemia (AML). For the majority of patients, myelodysplasia is an incurable disease with few effective therapies. The mainstay of treatment is supportive care with transfusions and antibiotics as needed. Hematopoietic growth factors are appropriate in carefully selected individuals. Intensive induction chemotherapy, such as is used in patients with acute myeloid leukemia, can result in a temporary remission in some patients, but elderly patients tolerate therapy poorly and experience substantial morbidity and mortality. The occasional young patient with myelodysplastic syndrome can be considered for curative therapy by means of intensive chemotherapy and allogeneic hematopoietic stem cell transplantation.

Pathobiology

The occurrence of clonality in an early hematopoietic stem cell has implications for the diagnosis, clinical manifestations, and management of patients with myelodysplastic syndrome. The pluripotent hematopoietic stem cell has the capacity for self-renewal and production of more differentiated progeny (Figure 62-1). With progressive maturation of the pluripotent stem cell, the first level of restriction is at the level of lymphoid vs. myeloid commitment. The earliest myeloid stem cell differentiates into red blood cells, platelets, granulocytes, monocytes, eosinophils, and basophils.

Neoplastic, or clonal, transformation of hematopoietic cells can occur at various levels of stem cell differentiation. In myelodysplastic syndrome, clonal transformation occurs at either the pluripotent stem cell or the myeloid stem cell. If the transformation occurs at the pluripotent stem cell, then myeloid *and* lymphoid progeny will be clonally derived. If the transformation occurs at the myeloid stem cell, then only myeloid progeny (e.g., red blood cells, platelets, granulocytes, monocytes, etc.) and *not* lymphoid progeny will be clonally derived. Cytogenetic analysis evaluates chromosomal abnormalities by conventional karyotyping or by fluorescence in-situ hybridization. X-inactivation studies are based on the process of random X-inactivation, or Lyonization, that occurs in female fetuses during embryogenesis. Because X-inactivation is accompanied by differential methylation, one can distinguish paternal from maternal and active from inactive X-chromosomes. These studies have consistently demonstrated the clonal origin of all myeloid cells and, in some cases, of lymphoid cells in myelodysplasia. Following the initial transformation into clonal hematopoiesis, it is likely that additional genetic events supervene, including alterations of oncogenes (e.g., the ras family of genes), tumor suppressor genes (e.g., p53, IRF-1), anti-apop-

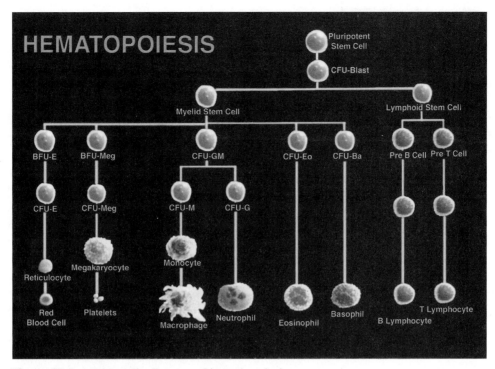

Figure 62-1 ■ Schematic diagram of hematopoiesis.

totic genes (e.g., Bcl-2), and cell cycle regulator genes (e.g., p15). Shortening of telomere (the end caps on the chromosomes) length might contribute to genomic instability that leads to cytogenetic evolution and disease progression.

Impaired maturation of hematopoietic cells in the marrow in myelodysplasia typically results in the paradoxical occurrence of a hypercellular marrow in the presence of peripheral cytopenias. Factors proposed to contribute the marrow failure of myelodysplastic syndrome include

1. decreased production of and sensitivity to hematopoietic colony-stimulating factors, which diminish the growth and maturation of progenitor cells;
2. increased production of inhibitors of hematopoiesis (e.g., tumor necrosis factor alpha, interferon gamma, interleukin 1 beta);
3. increased rate of programmed cell death, or apoptosis, of hematopoietic precursors; and
4. T-cell mediated immune dysregulation.

The mature blood cells that do ultimately arise from the clonal stem cell in myelodysplastic syndrome are often dysfunctional. For example, neutrophils and monocytes can have defective adhesion, phagocytosis, and myeloperoxidase and microbicidal activity, causing an increased risk of infection even if the absolute neutrophil count is normal. Similarly, bleeding can occur from abnormal platelet function, even in the setting of a relatively normal platelet count.

Incidence

Because myelodysplastic syndrome is not a reportable disease in the United States, incidence figures of approximately 4 to 12 per 100,000 population are obtained from European studies. This incidence is clearly greater than that of the acute leukemias and chronic myeloid disorders (i.e., chronic myeloid leukemia, polycythemia vera, and essential thrombocytosis) and approaches that of chronic lymphocytic leukemia. Because of the shorter survival in myelodysplasia compared with chronic lymphocytic leukemia, however, the prevalence of myelodysplastic syndrome is probably considerably lower than that of chronic lymphocytic leukemia. As is true of many other hematologic malignancies, males (representing approximately 60% of patients) are more often affected than females. The effect of race and ethnicity on the incidence of myelodysplastic syndrome has not been studied. The incidence of myelodysplastic syndrome increases with increasing age of the population evaluated (Figure 62-2). Therefore, myelodysplasia is predominantly a disease of the elderly, and the median age at diagnosis is approximately 70 years.

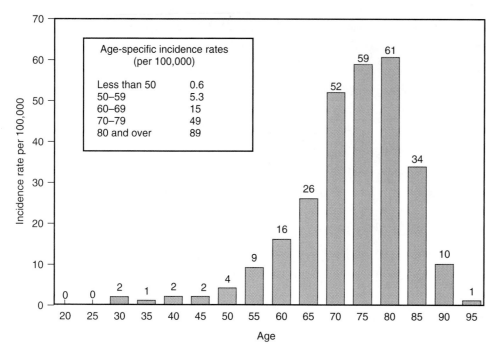

Figure 62-2 ■ Age-specific incidence rates of myelodysplastic syndrome per 100,000 at diagnosis. (From Williamson PJ, Kruger AR, Reynolds PJ, et al: Establishing the incidence of myelodysplastic syndrome. Br J Haemat 1994;87:743–745.)

Etiology

The vast majority of cases of myelodysplastic syndrome (>90%) have no known etiology. In the remaining patients, certain conditions and exposures are accepted as causes (Table 62-1). Consideration of risk factors is important because it influences the screening of "at-risk" populations (for example, patients exposed to prior alkylator chemotherapy). Risk factors also bear on the therapy of myelodysplasia; for example, patients with chromosomal fragility (congenital or secondary to exposure) experience increased toxicity from intensive chemotherapy.

Several rare, congenital diseases are associated with chromosomal fragility, including Fanconi's anemia, ataxia telangiectasia, and Bloom's syndrome. These patients are at increased risk of solid and hematologic malignancies, including myelodysplastic syndrome. Although these disorders usually come to diagnosis in early childhood, occasionally an affected young adult's initial presentation is unexplained pancytopenia. The full-blown phenotype of the congenital disorder might not be apparent. Therefore, in young adults with newly diagnosed myelodysplasia, appropriate genetic screening for such diseases—Fanconi's anemia in particular—should be considered.

Survivors of some prior hematologic disorders (e.g., paroxysmal nocturnal hemoglobinuria or aplastic anemia) are also at increased risk. For example, patients who recover from aplastic anemia have a 15% to 50% actuarial probability of subsequently developing a clonal hematopoietic disorder such as myelodysplasia, paroxysmal nocturnal hemoglobinuria, or acute myeloid leukemia. Whether the risk is entirely due to the preceding marrow injury state or in part due to the intense immunosuppression used in its treatment is unclear.

Exposure to benzene in chemicals, therapeutic chemotherapy, and ionizing radiation are well-established risk factors for what is called "therapy-related" or "secondary" myelodysplasia. Although some clinicians assume that prior cytotoxic exposure (either iatrogenic or environmental) actually causes all cases of myelodysplastic syndrome, it is possible in

---

Table 62-1 ■ Risk Factors for Myelodysplasia

Inherited Chromosomal Fragility State

  Fanconi's anemia
  Ataxia telangiectasia
  Bloom's syndrome

Antecedent Hematologic Disorder

  Aplastic anemia
  Paroxysmal nocturnal hemoglobinuria

Exposure to Hematopoietic Stem Cell Toxins

  Benzene
  Ionizing radiation
  Chemotherapy, especially alkylating agents, and
    epipodophyllotoxins

Table 62-2 ■ Therapy-Related Myelodysplastic Syndrome and Acute Myeloid Leukemia

Agent[1]	Latency Period	Myelodysplastic Syndrome Phase	Karyotype	Prognosis
Alkylating agents and ionizing radiation	Median 4 to 5 years	Yes	Complex, chromosomes 5/7 abnormal	Poor
Topoisomerase II inhibitors	Median 2 to 3 years	Usually no	11q23, 21q22 translocations	May respond to chemotherapy, but poor survival

[1]See text for list of specific agents

some cases that myelodysplasia develops because of the patient's intrinsic susceptibility to malignancy and not because of exogenous exposure.

Therapy-related myelodysplastic syndrome occurs most commonly after alkylating agent therapy, with a peak incidence at 4 to 5 years (range, 2 to 20 years) after exposure (Table 62-2). Mechlorethamine, chlorambucil, and melphalan are more leukemogenic than other alkylators, such as cyclophosphamide. Other alkylators implicated in therapy-related myelodysplastic syndrome include the nitrosoureas (carmustine, lomustine, and semustine), procarbazine, and dacarbazine. The elevation in risk correlates directly with the intensity of exposure and increasing patient age. In Hodgkin's disease survivors, the 10-year cumulative incidence of therapy-related myelodysplastic syndrome or leukemia is in a range of 1.5% to 10%. Intensive therapy, such as occurs in autologous stem cell transplantation for non-Hodgkin's lymphoma and Hodgkin's disease, carries a risk of later therapy-related myelodysplasia as high as 18%.

Patients treated with ionizing radiation alone have a lower risk of developing therapy-related myelodysplastic syndrome than do patients treated with alkylators. However, whether combined modality therapy (radiation therapy and chemotherapy) increases the risk above that occurring after alkylating agents alone is not clear. Therapy-related myelodysplastic syndrome is associated with poor-risk cytogenetic features (usually complex abnormalities and/or abnormalities of chromosomes 5 and/or 7 along with a high risk of early progression to acute myeloid leukemia), poor response to chemotherapy, and short survival. In contrast, intensive exposure to topoisomerase II inhibitors (e.g., etoposide, teniposide, anthracyclines) is associated with a risk of developing therapy-related acute myeloid leukemia, without a phase of preceding myelodysplastic syndrome. The latency period is short (only 2 to 3 years), and the characteristic chromosomal abnormality is an 11q23 or 21q22 translocation. Therapy-related myelodysplasia appears to be increasing in frequency, probably because of escalating inten-

sity of treatment for the original malignancy and improved survival, which provides the opportunity for delayed complications of treatment to develop.

Clinical Presentation

Symptomatology at presentation of myelodysplasia is variable (as outlined in Table 62-3) and related to the number and degree of varying cytopenias. Among patients with myelodysplastic syndrome who present with isolated cytopenias, one finds that anemia is more common than thrombocytopenia, and isolated neutropenia is very rare. Combinations of two or more cytopenias are common. Typically, an elderly patient with anemia observes the gradual onset over months of progressive fatigue, weakness, and decrease in exercise tolerance. Because of the slow progression of marrow failure, patients often compensate well and can present with minimal symptoms despite advanced age and severe anemia (e.g., hemoglobin <7 g/dL). Angina and/or dyspnea on exertion occur for the most

Table 62-3 ■ Presenting Symptoms in Patients with Myelodysplasia

Symptoms of Anemia (Most Common)

Fatigue
Weakness
Exercise intolerance
Angina
Dyspnea

Symptoms of Thrombocytopenia

Bruising
Epistaxis
Gum bleeding
Bleeding from other sites

Symptoms of Neutropenia

Fever with or without obvious infection
Infection

part in patients who have underlying cardiac and/or pulmonary disease. Physical finding abnormalities other than those from the effects of anemia (such as pallor) are unusual. In the form of myelodysplasia known as chronic myelomonocytic leukemia, tissue infiltration by leucocytes can cause hepatosplenomegaly, adenopathy, or chloromas (focal collections of blast cells).

A substantial fraction (perhaps as much as 50%) of patients with myelodysplastic syndrome have no symptoms at diagnosis. Rather, they come to medical attention because blood count abnormalities are noted in routine screening tests.

The signs and symptoms of myelodysplasia are non-specific. They can occur in a wide range of hematologic, oncologic, or benign illnesses. Because so many diseases can be associated with defective production and/or increased destruction of blood cells, ruling out other causes can be difficult, especially when the only laboratory abnormality is anemia. The diagnosis rests on evaluation of the peripheral blood and bone marrow morphology and on marrow cytogenetics. The morphologic changes of marrow dysplasia and peripheral blood abnormalities seen in myelodysplastic syndrome appear in Table 62-4 and Figure 62-3. Taken individually, each of these findings is also consistent with other diseases (Table 62-5). These can be ruled out by appropriate studies. In most cases, the characteristics of routine blood tests and chemistries combined with the findings on physical examination suffice to rule out other causes. One has to be wary of the possibility, however, that the patient with myelodysplastic syndrome has a concomitant clinical problem—such as gastrointestinal bleeding, inflammatory disease, or another malignancy—that complicates the evaluation.

Clinical Evaluation

The diagnosis of myelodysplasia is established by the finding of dysplasia in the bone marrow of one or more cell line precursors in association with peripheral blood cytopenia(s). Dysplasia refers to morphologically abnormal and aberrant maturation of the blood cells in the marrow. In some cases, the finding of cytopenia(s) with a marrow cytogenetic abnormality typical of myelodysplasia (discussed following) is considered to be sufficient for the diagnosis of myelodysplastic syndrome, even in the absence of clear morphologic evidence of marrow dysplasia. Unfortunately, the degree of dysplasia required to make a diagnosis of myelodysplasia is not well defined. Some hematologists require that at least 10% of the cells in a particular lineage show dysplastic features, whereas others require that dysplasia be demonstrable in at least two lineages. In early phases of the disease, dysplastic changes can be subtle. Morphologic analysis of the presence and/or degree of dysplasia is highly subjective, sometimes rendering it difficult to make the diagnosis of myelodysplastic syndrome definitively. Therefore, when the diagnosis of myelodysplasia is uncertain after initial evaluation, it is mandatory to observe the patient over time, correct potentially reversible causes, and make a diagnosis of

---

Table 62-4 ■ Peripheral Blood and Bone Marrow Abnormalities Typical of Myelodysplastic Syndrome

Red Blood Cell Series

Peripheral blood	Oval macrocytes. anisopoikilocytosis, basophilic stippling, nuclear blebs and fragments
Bone marrow	Megaloblastoid appearance (i.e., dysynchronous nuclear/cytoplasmic maturation), ring sideroblasts, binuclearity

White Blood Cell Series

Peripheral blood	Hypogranular neutrophils, hypolobated neutrophils (acquired, pseudo-Pelger-Huet anomaly, monocytosis
Bone marrow	Dysplastic changes (megaloblastoid), increase in precursors (including blasts), Auer rods

Megakaryocytic Series

Peripheral blood	Large platelets (megakaryocyte fragments), hypogranular platelets
Bone marrow	Micro-megakaryocytes, hypogranular megakaryocytes, hypolobulated nuclei in megaryocytes, odd (rather than even) number of megakaryocyte nuclei

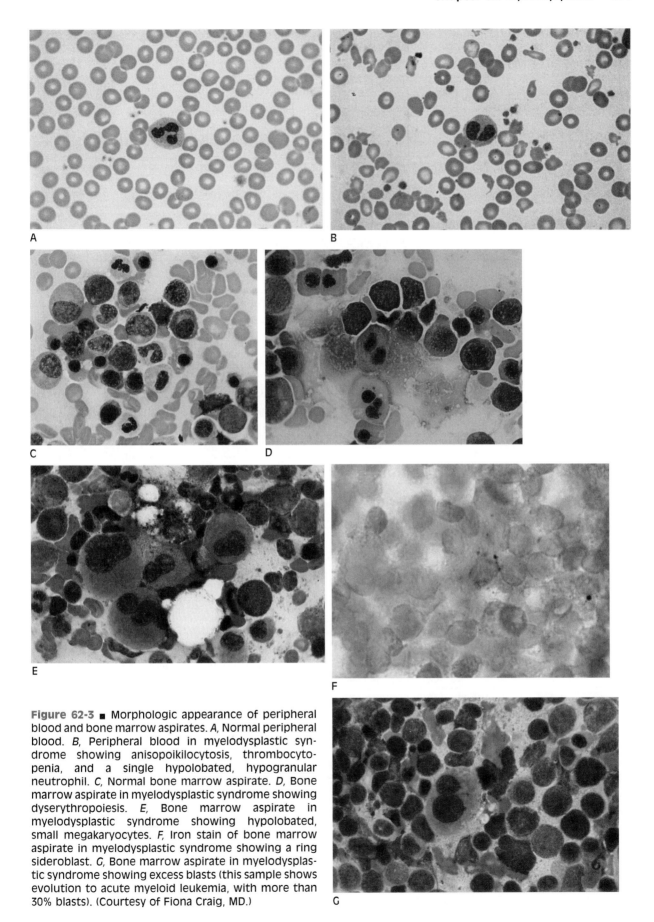

Figure 62-3 ■ Morphologic appearance of peripheral blood and bone marrow aspirates. *A,* Normal peripheral blood. *B,* Peripheral blood in myelodysplastic syndrome showing anisopoikilocytosis, thrombocytopenia, and a single hypolobated, hypogranular neutrophil. *C,* Normal bone marrow aspirate. *D,* Bone marrow aspirate in myelodysplastic syndrome showing dyserythropoiesis. *E,* Bone marrow aspirate in myelodysplastic syndrome showing hypolobated, small megakaryocytes. *F,* Iron stain of bone marrow aspirate in myelodysplastic syndrome showing a ring sideroblast. *G,* Bone marrow aspirate in myelodysplastic syndrome showing excess blasts (this sample shows evolution to acute myeloid leukemia, with more than 30% blasts). (Courtesy of Fiona Craig, MD.)

Table 62-5 ■ Differential Diagnosis of Peripheral Blood and Bone Marrow Abnormalities Found in Myelodysplastic Syndrome

Finding	Other Causes to Be Considered
Minimal reticulocyte response to anemia	Bone marrow failure states, bone marrow infiltration by malignancy, iron, folate, or B_{12} deficiency
Macrocytosis	Folate and B_{12} deficiency; hypothyroidism; liver disease; markedly elevated reticulocyte count
Hypochromia	Iron deficiency; thalassemia; lead poisoning; anemia of chronic disease
Hypogranulated, hypolobated neutrophils	Acute myeloid leukemia, myeloproliferative syndromes
Dysplastic changes in the bone marrow	Nonmalignant disease: Vitamin B_{12} or folate deficiency; HIV infection, severe liver disease, excessive ethanol consumption, recent chemotherapy exposure Malignancies: myeloproliferative disorders; acute myeloid leukemia

myelodysplasia only if cytopenias persist. Observation also provides the opportunity to clinically assess the intrinsic pace of the disease, which is important in devising appropriate management strategies.

The bone marrow is usually hypercellular, although it is hypocellular in perhaps 10% of cases. In the latter event, the diagnosis of aplastic anemia can be excluded by demonstrating the presence of marrow dysplasia in the remaining marrow cells and identifying a specific clonal karyotypic abnormality by cytogenetic analysis.

Classification and Prognosis

Morphologic Classification

Between 1950 and 1982, myelodysplasia was recognized by numerous terms, including subacute or smoldering leukemia, preleukemia, and refractory anemia. In 1982, a French, American, and British (FAB) consensus conference devised a classification system, the term myelodysplastic syndrome was established as the preferred name, and five categories of myelodysplastic syndrome were defined using morphologic criteria

(Table 62-6). The main distinguishing features are the percentage of blasts in marrow and blood, percentage of ring sideroblasts, peripheral monocyte count, and the presence of Auer rods. Increasing numbers of bone marrow blasts showed a direct correlation with increasing of transformation to acute leukemia and progressively shortened survival. Thus, patients with refractory anemia (RA) and refractory anemia with ring sideroblasts (RARS) have the best survival (approximate median survival, 26 to 50 and 34 to 83 months, respectively) and the lowest risk of leukemia progression (approximate risk, 15% to 25%). In contrast, patients with refractory anemia with excess blasts (RAEB) have a median survival of 9 to 18 months and a 50% risk of leukemic progression. The variant called RAEB in transformation (RAEB-T) has a median survival of 6 months and virtually 100% chance of conversion to acute leukemia. Outcomes for patients with chronic myelomonocytic leukemia (CMML) lie between those of patients with refractory anemia and refractory anemia with excess blasts and depend primarily on the percentage of marrow blasts.

The French, American, and British system has a

Table 62-6 ■ French, American, and British Classification of Myelodysplastic Syndrome

Classification	% Marrow Blasts		% Peripheral Blood Blasts		Auer Rods	Ring Sideroblasts (>15%)	Monocytes (>1,000/μL)
RA	<5		<1		–	–	–
RARS	<5		<1		–	+	–
RAEB	5–20		≤5		–	±	–
RAEB-T	21–30	or	>5	or	+	±	±
CMML	≤20		<5		–	±	+

FAB = French, American, and British Classification; + = always present; – = always absent; ± = variable
From Bennett JM, Catovsky D, Daniel MT, et al: Proposals for the classification of the myelodysplastic syndromes. Brit J Haemat 1982;51:189.

number of limitations, however. Features of chronic myelomonocytic leukemia overlap with the criteria for myeloproliferative disorders, including leukocytosis, monocytosis, and marrow features suggestive of chronic myeloid leukemia. The French, American, and British system creates an arbitrary boundary between myelodysplastic syndrome (less than 30% marrow blasts) and acute myeloid leukemia (30% or greater marrow blasts) and does not include information from karyotype analysis. The extent of dysplasia is also at issue. Refractory anemia and refractory anemia with ring sideroblasts are defined as dysplasia in the erythroid lineage with concomitant anemia, not allowing for the inclusion of patients with dysplasia in other lineages and variants with isolated neutropenia or thrombocytopenia. The precise definition used is prognostically important because in refractory anemia or refractory anemia with ring sideroblasts, patients with multilineage dysplasia have a lower survival and a higher rate of leukemic transformation than do those whose dysplasia is confined to the erythroid series. Nor does the French, American, and British classification take into account other morphologic factors, such as marrow fibrosis and marked hypocellularity. In 1999, the World Health Organization (WHO) proposed modifications to the French, American, and British system, but the utility of these changes is also controversial, and they are not discussed here.

Cytogenetic Classification

In cases of minimal dysplasia or an aplastic marrow, the finding of an acquired abnormality (at least two or three metaphases showing the same abnormality) indicates clonal hematopoiesis and supports the diagnosis of myelodysplasia. Approximately 50% of patients with myelodysplastic syndrome, however, have a normal karyotype. Common abnormalities seen in the other half of the patients are listed in Table 62-7. These include complete or partial loss of chromosome 7 (i.e., −7, or del[7q]), trisomy 8 (+8), loss of the long arm of chromosome 5 (i.e., del[5q]), and loss of the long arm of chromosome 20 (i.e., del[20q]). Patients with complex (three or more abnormalities) or chromosome 7 anomalies have a particularly poor prognosis (independent of French, American, and British classification or morphology). Patients with normal cytogenetics, or isolated del(5q), del(20q), or loss of the Y chromosome have a comparatively better prognosis, and patients with other single or double abnormalities have an intermediate prognosis. The del(5q) abnormality, as an isolated finding, is associated with a distinctive clinical presentation of myelodysplasia. The great majority of patients with this form of myelodysplasia are women; the pace of

Table 62-7 ■ Risk Classification and Frequency of Clonal Abnormalities in Myelodysplastic Syndrome

Risk Group/Specific Finding	Frequency
Good	
Normal	60%
del(5q) sole finding	6%
-Y sole finding	2%
del(20q)	2%
Intermediate	
+8	5%
Other single abnormality	9%
Double abnormality	5%
Poor	
Chromosome 7 abnormal	1%
Complex	10%

From Greenberg P, Cox C, LeBeau MM, et al: International scoring system for evaluating prognosis in myelodysplastic syndromes. Blood 1997;89:2079–2088.

the disease is indolent; less than one-quarter of cases evolve to acute leukemia; neutropenia is uncommon and minimal, if present; platelet counts are frequently increased; and bone marrow shows numerous micromegakaryocytes with hypolobulated nuclei. In some patients, cytogenetic abnormalities accumulate progressively as the disease progresses to acute myeloid leukemia.

Prognostic Scoring Systems

Important prognostic variables include age, percentage of marrow blasts, karyotype, lactate dehydrogenase level, number and degree of peripheral cytopenias, and gender. The International Prognostic Scoring System was developed from data on 816 patients from six countries as an approach to incorporate a number of prognostic indicators into a single prognostic score. One should recognize that criteria for inclusion of patients in the analysis required the presence of dysplasia in at least two lineages (in contradistinction to the FAB definition of RA as dyserythropoiesis only), no treatment with aggressive interventions such as induction chemotherapy or transplantation, and no known etiology. Therefore, the scoring system is not validated for therapy-related myelodysplastic syndrome. The score depends on percentage of blasts in the marrow, cytogenetic findings, and number of peripheral cytopenias (Table 62-8). There are four possible scores, and the risk of transformation into acute myeloid leukemia and survival rates are distinct for each group (Figure 62-4). The

Table 62-8 ■ International Prognostic Scoring System (IPSS) for Myelodysplastic Syndrome

Risk Group	Score*	Median Survival (years)		Time to 25% Risk of Acute Myeloid Leukemia Evolution (years)	
		All patients	≤60 years	All patients	≤60 years
Low	0	5.7	11.8	9.4	>9.4
Intermediate-1	0.5–1.0	3.5	5.2	3.3	6.0
Intermediate-2	1.5–2.0	1.2	1.8	1.1	0.7
High	≥2.5	0.4	0.3	0.2	0.2

*Total score is based on sum of individual scores for marrow blast percentage, karyotype, and peripheral cytopenias. For marrow blast percentage, a score of 0 is given for blasts <5%; 1 for ≥5%–10%; 1.5 for 11–20%; and 2.0 for 21–30%. For karyotype, a score of 0 is given for normal; -Y, del(5q), or del(20q); 1.0 for ≥3 abnormalities or chromosome 7 anomalies; and 0.5 for other abnormalities. For peripheral cytopenias, a score of 0 is given for none or a single cytopenia and 0.5 for 2 or 3 cytopenias. Cytopenia is defined as neutrophil count <1,800/μL, hemoglobin <10 gm/dl, and platelet count <100,000/μL.
From Greenberg P, Cox C, LeBeau MM, et al. International scoring system for evaluating prognosis in myelodysplastic syndromes. Blood 1997;89:2079–2088.

International MDS Risk Classification

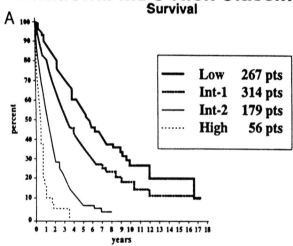

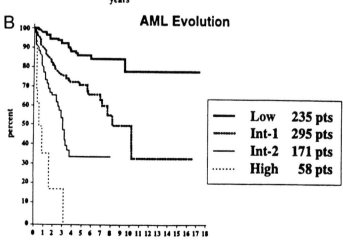

Figure 62-4 ■ Survival (*A*) and freedom from AML evolution (*B*) for myelodysplastic syndrome patients according to their classification by the International Prognostic Scoring System for myelodysplastic syndrome: Low, INT-1, INT-2, and High (Kaplan-Meier curves). (From Greenberg P, Cox C, LeBeau MM, et al: International scoring system for evaluating prognosis in myelodysplastic syndromes. Blood 1997;89:2079–2088.)

outcome is significantly worse for patients over 60 years old than for patients younger than 60 years old in the intermediate-1 and low-risk groups.

Natural History of Myelodysplastic Syndrome

In some patients the disease is indolent for years with easily manageable cytopenias (predominantly anemia); in other patients, it progresses rapidly to acute myeloid leukemia or life-threatening/lethal cytopenias. Many elderly affected patients die of causes unrelated to myelodysplasia. Overall, 40% to 60% of patients die of cytopenic complications, 20% to 50% die of acute myeloid leukemia and its treatment, and 20% die of unrelated causes. Red cell transfusion dependency is common and leads to iron overload, with associated organ failure (e.g., heart, liver, and pancreas). Platelet transfusion dependency is less common but can result in refractoriness to platelet transfusions and life-threatening bleeding. Chronic neutropenia, when it is severe, presents a continuous risk of overwhelming bacterial or fungal infections.

Treatment

There are very few effective therapies for myelodysplasia. Allogeneic bone marrow transplantation is the only curative modality, but this option is available only to the small proportion of patients who are young and have an appropriate (related or unrelated) stem cell donor. Most patients, because of their advanced age, are treated with supportive care, which consists of red blood cell transfusions, antibiotics, and iron chelation therapy for iron overload. Several studies

---

TREATMENT

Considerations in Therapy of Myelodysplastic Syndrome

Allogeneic Stem Cell Transplantation in Myelodysplastic Syndrome

1. Soon after the diagnosis of myelodysplastic syndrome is made, the patient and physician need to determine the goals of therapy. For relatively "young" patients (less than age 60 years) who have a good performance status, it is imperative to refer the patient promptly to an experienced allogeneic stem cell transplant center to discuss this option and its timing.

2. In transplant-eligible patients who wish to maximize their long-term survival, early allogeneic stem cell transplantation, despite its high near-term morbidity and mortality, is worth considering. Nonrelapse mortality is lower and survival greater for patients with shorter disease duration. Front-line therapy with allogeneic stem cell transplantation is appropriate for patients with International Prognostic Scoring System intermediate-1, intermediate-2, or high-risk disease because the relapse rate after transplantation increases as the disease progresses. Transplantation for patients with low-risk disease should be advised only for those with severe, life-threatening cytopenias or for children.

Supportive Care

1. Anemia: The threshold level of anemia below which the patient with myelodysplastic syndrome should be transfused should be individualized, based on symptoms rather than on a specific hematocrit or hemoglobin value. The threshold will be higher in patients with cardiac or pulmonary disease and lower in otherwise healthy individuals. Red cell transfusions should generally be leukoreduced to help prevent alloimmunization. Iron chelation therapy with parenteral desferrioxamine (5 to 7 days per week) should be considered for transfusion-dependent patients without other imminently life-threatening complications, once a threshold of 30 units of blood have been administered (or once ferritin is greater than 1,000 μg/L). Preliminary studies suggest that subcutaneous bolus infections (1 gm twice daily) could be the most practical way of administering desferrioxamine.

2. Bleeding: Patients with myelodysplastic syndrome might have bleeding due to thrombocytopenia and/or dysfunctional platelets. Platelet transfusions in these situations (preferably using leukoreduced product) are appropriate. In patients with serious or life-threatening bleeding (e.g., gastrointestinal bleeding), transfusion to a platelet count of 50,000/μL is desirable. A lower threshold is appropriate for mucocutaneous bleeding. Treatment with anti-fibrinolytic agents can also be considered. Prophylactic therapy of the asymptomatic patient with chronic thrombocytopenia is controversial. Some clinicians transfuse only when bleeding manifestations (purpura or petechiae, for example) appear, whereas others transfuse platelets whenever they are less than 5000 to 10,000 cells/μL.

have shown that cytopenias improve in some patients who receive iron chelation therapy. Treatment options are discussed in the following sections, but it should be noted that no agent is approved by the Federal Drug Administration for use in these patients.

Low-Intensity Therapy

A large number of agents have been tested in treatment, but until recently no drug or combination of drugs has been shown to improve survival compared to supportive care alone. In one study of chronic myelomonocytic leukemia, patients were randomized to receive etoposide or hydroxyurea, demonstrating that the latter had an improved response rate and a survival benefit. A demethylating agent, 5-azacytidine, was randomly compared with observation in patients with myelodysplasia by Cancer and Leukemia Group B (Silverman et al.) and was found to provide a statistically significant subcutaneous 5-azacytidine achieved a delay of leukemic transformation and death. The results with 5-azacytidine alone may be improved by combinations with other agents and/or cytokines.

Three hematopoietic growth factors—granulocyte/macrophage colony-stimulating factor (GM-CSF), granulocyte colony-stimulating factor (G-CSF), and erythropoietin (EPO)—have been used to improve cytopenias in myelodysplastic syndrome. Although in some patients, granulocyte/macrophage colony-stimulating factor and granulocyte colony-stimulating factor each has raised the neutrophil count, this does not occur consistently, granulocyte/macrophage colony-stimulating factor and granulocyte colony-stimulating factor should not be employed routinely in these patients until the absolute granulocyte count falls to low levels (<500/μL) and is associated with clinically significant infections. There is no advantage to prophylactic administration of these agents. The patient should be observed to see whether the absolute granulocyte count improves substantially and the infection risk abates. When, as frequently occurs, the growth factors are shown to be ineffective, they should be discontinued.

Erythropoietin is generally associated with a 15% to 20% increase in responders. The responses to erythropoietin can be improved if iron supplementation is given to patients without iron overload. Response is better among patients with refractory anemia (it is particularly poor for refractory anemia with ring sideroblasts patients), patients with no or infrequent transfusions (e.g., less than two units per month), and patients with low endogenous serum erythropoietin level (e.g., less than 200 U/L). The combination of erythropoietin and G-CSF is synergistic in stimulating erythroid response in some subsets of patients. For example, the erythroid response rate is 74% in patients with serum erythropoietin levels less than 500 U/L and less than two units transfused per month, whereas when only one of these two relatively favorable features is present, the response rate is 23%. Moreover, the response rate falls to 7% among patients when both the serum EPO level is greater than 500 U/L and transfusion of at least two units per month are used.

The National Comprehensive Cancer Network has proposed guidelines for the use of hematopoietic growth factors to support anemic patients, as outlined in Figure 62-5. Currently, there is no thrombopoietic growth factor that is effective in myelodysplasia.

Many other agents show variable response rates, usually at the levels of 20% or less. None of these is considered to be established, recommended therapies for myelodysplasia. These include glucocorticoids, anabolic steroids; low-dose cytarabine; oral low-dose melphalan, antithymocyte globulin, cyclosporine, amifostine, retinoids, sodium phenylbutyrate, and thalidomide.

Intensive Therapy

Intensive acute myeloid leukemia-like combination chemotherapy for patients with myelodysplasia and myelodysplastic syndrome-related acute myeloid leukemia has been the subject of numerous studies. No randomized study compared such treatment with supportive care, and it is quite possible that there is no survival benefit from its use. Compared to patients with de novo acute myeloid leukemia, patients with myelodysplasia and myelodysplastic syndrome-related acute myeloid leukemia have a lower complete remission (CR) rate, a higher toxic death rate, and shorter survival. This adverse outcome is likely to be due to the advanced age of the patients, to increased frequency of intrinsic drug resistance, and to poor-risk karyotypic abnormalities. Most reported studies of induction chemotherapy in myelodysplastic syndrome have excluded patients older than age 65 years because of the unacceptable toxicity and low complete remission rate found in elderly patients. The complete remission rate for patients with myelodysplasia after induction chemotherapy ranges from 15% to 74%. The variability is explained by differences in the population with myelodysplastic syndrome under study. Responses decline with increasing patient age, long disease duration before treatment, and increased percentage of poor-prognosis karyotypes. Even when therapy is successful, the duration of remission is brief, and almost all patients relapse within 12 months.

Induction therapy most commonly uses conventional regimens for acute myeloid leukemia, such as 7

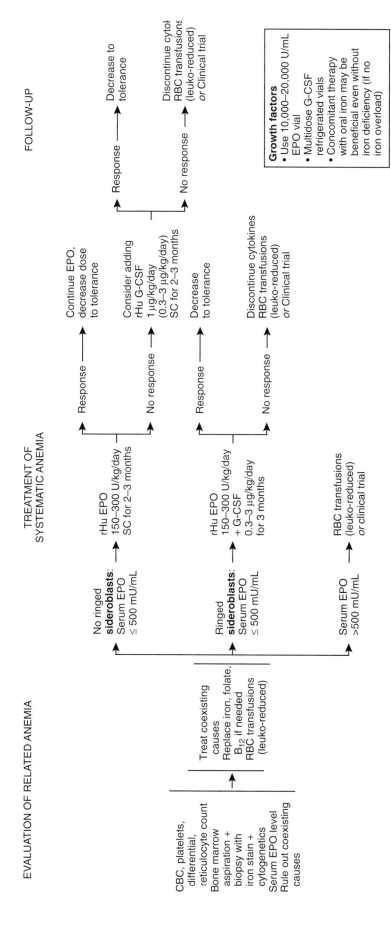

EVALUATION OF RELATED ANEMIA

TREATMENT OF
SYSTEMATIC ANEMIA

FOLLOW-UP

Figure 62-5 ■ The National Comprehensive Cancer Network Practice Guidelines Version 1.0 for Management of Anemia in Myelodysplastic Syndrome. (From NCCN practice guidelines for the myelodysplastic syndromes. Oncology 1998;12(11A):53–80.)

days of cytarabine and 3 days of an anthracycline. Alternative regimens include: topotecan and cytarabine; fludarabine and cytarabine; and high-dose cytarabine as a single agent. Some studies indicate that the period of marrow aplasia after chemotherapy is longer in patients with myelodysplasia than in de novo acute myeloid leukemia.

Given the poor outcome with intensive chemotherapy in myelodysplasia patients, it is difficult to definitively recommend such therapy for most patients with myelodysplasia. Due consideration must be given in an individual patient to the risks and limited benefits of treatment, to the age of the patient, and to any comorbid conditions that could prejudice the outcome. The physician must discuss quality-of-life issues with the patient, including the likelihood of a prolonged, complicated hospital stay if intensive therapy is given.

A subgroup of patients with myelodysplasia does appear, however, to respond to conventional induction therapy and to have long-term outcomes that are equivalent to those of patients with de novo acute myeloid leukemia. This subgroup consists of young patients (less than age 55 years) with newly diagnosed refractory anemia with excess blasts or refractory anemia with excess blasts in transformation, no antecedent lengthy history of abnormal blood counts, and no documented etiologic exposure. This minority of select patients with myelodysplasia should be treated expectantly with acute myeloid leukemia treatment regimens.

Although it is a high-risk procedure, allogeneic hematopoietic stem cell transplantation represents the only known curative therapy for these patients. Its use is restricted to young patients (less than age 60 years) who have a suitable related or unrelated donor. Mortality rates are high among older patients and those with therapy-related myelodysplastic syndrome or long disease duration. Relapse rates are substantially higher in patients with increased blasts than in those with refractory anemia or refractory anemia with ring sideroblasts, without progression. In the latter circumstances, the relapse rate is less than 5%. There is no documented benefit for the use of induction chemotherapy prior to allogeneic transplantation for patients at high risk of relapse. Currently, allogeneic transplantation results in cure for about 40% of patients with myelodysplasia, approximately 25% of those with advanced myelodysplasia, and for more than 50% of the patients with refractory anemia.

Follow-up Evaluation

The frequency of visits and laboratory testing must be individualized and is predominantly dependent on the patient's symptoms. For patients who are transfusion dependent, determination of blood counts is performed at appropriate intervals to permit adequate timely blood product support. Typically, patients who are dependent on red blood cell transfusions have visits every three weeks for blood counts and transfusions. For patients without severe cytopenias, the frequency of visits and blood counts depends on the stability of the disease and generally ranges from one to three months. Frequent bone marrow examinations are unnecessary. For the most part, a repeat bone marrow examination is warranted only when the disease appears to progress clinically and when the results will alter patient care.

References

General Information

Germing U, Gattermann N, Aivado M, et al: Two types of acquired idiopathic sideroblastic anaemia (AISA): A time-tested distinction. Br J Haematol 2000;108:724–728.

Pruneri G, Bertolini F, Soligo D, et al: Angiogenesis in myelodysplastic syndromes. Br J Cancer 1999;81:1398–1401.

Rosenfield C, List A: A hypothesis for the pathogenesis of myelodysplastic syndromes: Implications for new therapies. Leukemia 2000;14:2–8.

Santini V, Ferrini PR: Differentiation therapy of myelodysplastic syndromes: Fact or fiction? Br J Haematol 1998;102:1124–1138.

Bone Marrow Transplantation

Anderson JE: Bone marrow transplantation for myelodysplasia. Blood Rev 2000;14:63–77.

Gassmann W, Schmitz N, Löffler H, et al: Intensive chemotherapy and bone marrow transplantation for myelodysplastic syndromes. Semin Hematol 1996;33:196–205.

Classification

Albitar M, Beran M, O'Brien S, et al: Differences between refractory anemia with excess blasts in transformation and acute myeloid leukemia. Blood 96:372–373.

Bennett JM, Catovsky D, Daniel MT, et al: Proposals for the classification of the myelodysplastic syndromes. Br J Haematol 1982;51:189–199.

Bennett JM, Catovsky D, Daniel MT, et al: The chronic myeloid leukaemias: Guidelines for distinguishing the chronic granulocytic, atypical chronic myeloid and chronic myelomonocytic leukaemias. Br J Haematol 1994;87:746–754.

Boultwood J, Lewis S, Wainscoat JS: The 5q-syndrome. Blood 1994;84:3253–3260.

Gardais J: Dyshaemopoiesis in adults: A practical classification for diagnosis and management. Leuk Res 2000;24:641–651.

Germing U, Gatterman N, Minning H, et al: Problems in the classification of CMML: Dysplastic versus proliferative type. Leuk Res 1998;22:871–878.

Germing U, Gatterman N, Strupp C, et al: Validation of the WHO proposals for a new classification of primary myelodysplastic syndromes: A retrospective analysis of 1600 patients. Leuk Res 2000;24:983–992.

Greenberg P, Anderson J, de Witte T, et al: Problematic WHO reclassification of myelodysplastic syndromes. J Clin Onc 2000;18:3447–3448.

Harris NL, Jaffe ES, Diebold J, et al: World Health Organization classification of neoplastic diseases of the hematopoietic and lymphoid tissues: Report of the Clinical Advisory Committee Meeting—Airlie House, Virginia, November 1997. J Clin Oncol 1999;17:3835–3849.

Kouides PA, Bennett JM: Morphology and classification of the myelodysplastic syndromes and their pathologic variants. Semin Hematol 1996;33:95–110.

Ramos F, Fernández-Ferrero S, Suárez D, et al: Myelodysplastic syndrome: A search for minimal diagnostic criteria. Leuk Res 1999;23:283–290.

Rosati S, Anastasi J, Vardiman J: Recurring diagnostic problems in the pathology of the myelodysplastic syndromes. Semin Hematol 1996;33:111–126.

Rosati S, Mick R, Xu F, et al: Refractory cytopenia with multilineage dysplasia: Further characterization of an "unclassifiable" myelodysplastic syndrome. Leukemia 1996; 10:20–26.

Tuzuner N, Cox C, Rowe JM, et a: Hypocellular myelodysplastic syndromes (MDS): New proposal. Br J Haematol 1995;91:612–617.

Epidemiology and Risk Factors

Aul C, Germing U, Gattermann N, et al: Increasing incidence of myelodysplastic syndromes: real or fictitious? Leuk Res 1998;22:93–100.

Björk J, Albin M, Mauritzson N, et al: Smoking and myelodysplastic syndromes. Epidemiol 2000;11:285–291.

Phillips MJ, Cull GM, Ewings M: Establishing the incidence of myelodysplasia syndrome. Br J Haematol 1994;88: 896–897.

Rådlund A, Thiede T, Hansen S, et al: Incidence of myelodysplastic syndromes in a Swedish population. Eur J Haematol 1995;54:153–156.

Thirman MJ, Larson RA: Therapy-related myeloid leukemia. Hematol/Oncol Clin N Am 1996;10:293–320.

Williamson PJ, Kruger AR, Reynolds PJ, et al: Establishing the incidence of myelodysplastic syndrome. Br J Haematol 1994;87:743–745.

Prognosis

Aul C, Gattermann N, Heyll A, et al: Primary myelodysplastic syndromes: Analysis of prognostic factors in 235 patients and proposals for an improved scoring system. Leukemia 1992;6:52–59.

Balduini CL, Guarnone R, Pecci A, et al: Multilineage dysplasia without increased blasts identifies a poor prognosis subset of myelodysplastic syndromes. Leukemia 1998;12: 1655–1656.

Estey E, Thall P, Beran M, et al: Effect of diagnosis (refractory anemia with excess blasts, refractory anemia with excess blasts in transformation, or acute myeloid leukemia [AML]) on outcome of AML-type chemotherapy. Blood 1997;90:2969–2977.

Hellström-Lindberg E, Robèrt K-H, Gahrton G, et al: A predictive model for the clinical response to low dose ara-C: A study of 102 patients with myelodysplastic syndromes or acute leukaemia. Br J Haematol 1992;81:503–511.

Morel P, Hebbar M, Lai J-L, et al: Cytogenetic analysis has strong independent prognostic value in de novo myelodysplastic syndromes and can be incorporated in a new scoring system: A report on 408 cases. Leukemia 1993;7: 1315–1323.

Solé F, Espinet B, Sanz GF, et al: Incidence, characterization and prognostic significance of chromosomal abnormalities in 640 patients with primary myelodysplastic syndromes. Br J Haemat 2000;108:346–356.

Therapy

Berstein SH, Brunetto VL, Davey FR, et al: Acute myeloid leukemia-type chemotherapy for newly diagnosed patients without antecedent cytopenias having myelodysplastic syndromes as defined by French-American-British criteria. A Cancer and Leukemia Group B study. J Clin Oncol 1996;14:2486–2494.

Cazzola M, Anderson JE, Ganser A, et al: A patient-oriented approach to treatment of myelodysplastic syndromes. Haematologica 1998;83:914–939.

Chabannon C, Molina L, Pégourié-Bandelier B, et al: A review of 76 patients with myelodysplastic syndromes treated with Danazol. Cancer 1994;73:3073–3080.

De Witte T, Suciu S, Peetermans M, et al: Intensive chemotherapy for poor prognosis myelodysplasia (MDS) and secondary acute myeloid leukemia (sAML) following MDS of more than 6 months duration. A pilot study by the Leukemia Cooperative Group of the European Organisation for Research and Treatment in Cancer (EORTC-LCG). Leukemia 1995;9:1805–1811.

Denzlinger C, Bowen D, Benz D, et al: Low-dose melphalan induces favourable responses in elderly patients with high-risk myelodysplastic syndromes or secondary acute myeloid leukaemia. Br J Haemat 2000;108:93–95.

Estey EH: Topotecan for myelodysplastic syndromes. Oncol 1998;12:81–86.

Ferrini PR, Grossi A, Vannucchi AM, et al: A randomized double-blind placebo-controlled study with subcutaneous recombinant human erythropoietin in patients with low-risk myelodysplastic syndromes. Br J Haemat 1998;103:1070–1074.

Greenberg P, Taylor K, Larson R: Phase III randomized multicenter trial of G-CSF vs. observation for myelodysplastic syndromes (MDS). Blood 1995;82(Suppl)1:196a.

Greenberg P, Bishop M, Deeg J, et al: NCCN practice guidelines for the myelodysplastic syndromes. Oncol 1998;12:53–80.

Grossi A, Fabbri A, Santini V, et al: Amifostine in the treatment of low-risk myelodysplastic syndromes. Haematologica 2000;85:367–371.

Heaney ML, Golde DW: Myelodysplasia. N Engl J Med 1999;340:1649–1660.

Hellström-Lindberg E, Negrin R, Stein R, et al: Erythroid response to treatment with G-CSF plus erythropoietin for the anaemia of patients with myelodysplastic syndromes: Proposal for a predictive model. Br J Haemat 1997;99:344–351.

Hellström-Lindberg E: Efficacy of erythropoietin in the myelodysplastic syndromes: A meta-analysis of 205 patients from 17 studies. Br J Haemat 1995;89:67–71.

Hurtado RM, Sosa RC, Majluf AC, et al: Refractory anaemia (RA) type I FAB treated with oxymetholone (OXY): Long-term results. Br J Haemat 1993;85:235–236.

Jensen PD, Heickendorff L, Pedersen B, et al: The effect of iron chelation on haemopoiesis in MDS patients with transfusional iron overload. Br J Haemat 1996;94:288–299.

List AF, Brasfield F, Heaton R, et al: Stimulation of hematopoiesis by amifostine in patients with myelodysplastic syndrome. Blood 1997;90:3364–3369.

Mellibovsky L, Díez A, Pérez-Vila E, et al: Vitamin D treatment in myelodysplastic syndromes. Br J Haemat 1998; 100:516–520.

Miller KB, Kyungmann K, Morrison FS, et al: The evaluation of low-dose cytarabine in the treatment of myelodysplastic syndromes: A phase-III intergroup study. Ann Hematol 1992;65:162–168.

Molldrem JJ, Caples M, Mavroundis D, et al: Antithymocyte globulin for patients with myelodysplastic syndrome. Br J Haemat 1997;99:699–705.

Schuster MW, Larson RA, Thompson JA, et al: Granulocyte-macrophage colony-stimulating factor (GM-CSF) for myelodysplastic syndrome (MDS): Results of a multi-center randomized controlled trial. Blood 1990;76(Suppl 1):318.

Silverman LR, Demakos EP, Peterson B, et al: Randomized controlled trial of azacitidine in patients with the myelodysplastic syndrome: A study of the Cancer and Leukemia Group B. J Clin Oncol 2002;20:2429–2440.

Wattel E, De Botton S, Laï JL, et al: Long-term follow-up of *de novo* myelodysplastic syndromes treated with intensive chemotherapy: Incidence of long-term survivors and outcome of partial responders. Br J Haemat 1997;98:983–991.

Wattel E, Guerci A, Hecquet B: A randomized trial of hydroxyurea versus VP16 in adult chronic myelomonocytic leukemia. Blood 1996;88:2480–2487.

Wijermans P, Lübbert M, Verhoef, et al: Low-dose 5-aza-2-deoxycytidine, a DNA hypomethylating agent, for the treatment of high-risk myelodysplastic syndrome: A multicenter phase II study in elderly patients. J Clin Oncol 2000;18:956–962.

Chapter 63
Multiple Myeloma, Macroglobulinemia, and Amyloidosis

Mohamad A. Hussein and Martin M. Oken

A clonal increase in an immunoglobulin molecule, called a monoclonal gammopathy, can be detected as a result of evaluation of specific symptoms or on routine serum protein electrophoresis. Monoclonal gammopathies can be caused by multiple myeloma or one of its variants—monoclonal gammopathy of undetermined significance, amyloidosis, lymphoma or lymphoplasmacytoid malignancy. The differential diagnosis of monoclonal gammopathies and the biology of immunoglobulin molecules is discussed in Chapter 33, which should be read in conjunction with this chapter.

Multiple Myeloma

Epidemiology

Multiple myeloma is a clonal B-cell malignancy of slowly proliferating plasma cells within the bone marrow. Among hematologic malignancies, it constitutes 10% of the cancers and ranks as the second most frequently occurring hematologic cancer in the United States (14,000 cases annually) after non–Hodgkin's lymphoma. The population-based annual United States mortality is 4 in 100,000. Approximately 40,000 persons are currently living with myeloma in the United States today. The median age at diagnosis is in the range of 65 to 68 years.

The incidence of myeloma is twice as high among African-Americans as it is in whites. Potential dietary contributory factors were analyzed in a population-based case-control study of multiple myeloma in three areas of the United States. It appeared that the greater use of vitamin C supplements by whites and the higher frequency of obesity among African-Americans might explain part of the higher incidence of multiple myeloma among African-Americans. The increasing prevalence of obesity might have contributed to the upward trend in the incidence of multiple myeloma in recent decades.

The etiology of multiple myeloma is unknown, but several agents have been associated with the development of this disease. Ionizing radiation is a clearly established, albeit weak, risk factor. Nickel, dioxin, Agent Orange, petroleum products and other aromatic hydrocarbons, benzene, and silicon have been considered potential (but not proven) risk factors. The BALB/c mouse model is highly susceptible to multiple myeloma based on genetic factors. An inflammatory stimulus readily induces multiple myeloma in these animals. Clear-cut familial myeloma in humans, however, accounts for no more than 1% of cases. Human herpesvirus-8 (HHV-8) has yet to be convincingly established as an etiologic agent for myeloma. Infection with human immunodeficiency virus (HIV), however, is associated with a 4.5-fold increased risk of developing multiple myeloma and could be implicated, directly or indirectly, in its causation in some patients.

Monoclonal gammopathy of undetermined significance (MGUS) occurs in 2% of people over 50 years of age (see Chapter 33). It is generally considered to be a premalignant condition. Patients with this disorder have a 25-fold greater risk of developing multiple myeloma than an age- and gender-matched population without monoclonal gammopathy of unknown significance. The risk of progression to myeloma is about 1% per year.

Disease Pathogenesis

Cytogenetic and Molecular Genetic Alterations

Cytogenetic alterations have major prognostic and therapeutic implications in acute leukemia. Due to the low proliferative activity of the mature B-cell clone in multiple myeloma, standard cytogenetic studies yield abnormal karyotypes in only 30% to 50% of the cases. The "normal" karyotypes that are sometimes reported are usually from the normal hematopoietic cells and not from the malignant clone. Complex karyotypes, often involving more than three chromosomes, occur in 80% of patients when tested with sensitive techniques. Although no consistent genetic abnormality is associated with multiple myeloma, several genetic abnormalities are frequently found, some with important clinical implications. On careful analysis using fluorescence in situ hybridization (FISH) probes, 54% of 325 previously untreated patients were found to have molecular abnormalities in the long arm of chromosome 13 (13q). Patients with chromosome 13 abnormalities have a lower response rate to conventional chemotherapy and a 16-month reduction in median survival compared with patients whose plasma cells lack these genetic alterations. Although cytogenetic and molecular deletion of chromosome 13 is associated with a poor prognosis, a tumor suppressor gene for multiple myeloma has not yet been identified. Intriguingly, deletion of 13q is also found in monoclonal gammopathy of undetermined significance, often years before transition to multiple myeloma.

Cytokines, Adhesion Molecules, and Angiogenesis

Interleukin-6 (IL-6) is an important cytokine in myeloma cell growth and proliferation. Close cell-to-cell contact between myeloma cells and the bone marrow stromal cells triggers a large amount of interleukin-6 production, which supports the growth of these cells and protects them from apoptosis induced by dexamethasone or other chemotherapeutic agents. Interleukin-6, however, is not an absolute requirement for the proliferation of myeloma cells, and anti-interleukin-6 antibody treatment has not been shown to provide meaningful clinical benefit.

Vascular endothelial cell growth factor, in addition to its known stimulation of bone marrow angiogenesis, also has direct effects on myeloma cells. Vascular endothelial cell growth factor stimulates proliferation and migration of myeloma cells through both autocrine and paracrine mechanisms. Within the bone marrow, vascular endothelial cell growth factor is produced by both myeloma cells and bone marrow stromal cells. Interleukin-6 secreted by bone marrow stromal cells enhances the production and secretion of vascular endothelial cell growth factor by myeloma cells; conversely, vascular endothelial cell growth factor secreted by myeloma cells enhances interleukin-6 production by bone marrow stromal cells. Moreover, binding of myeloma cells to bone marrow stromal cells enhances both interleukin-6 and vascular endothelial cell growth factor secretion, suggesting an autocrine vascular endothelial cell growth factor loop. Treatment strategies targeting the different cytokines involved in the growth and development of the myeloma cell are currently being investigated.

Clinical Presentation

The clinical features of multiple myeloma develop from skeletal destruction, complications caused by the monoclonal protein, and from an increased vulnerability to infections due to depression of normal immunoglobulins as well as depletion of bone marrow reserves. These clinical abnormalities provide the first clues to the diagnosis and form the basis for defining the stage and prognosis.

Symptoms

Bone pain, especially back pain, is the most common symptom affecting two out of three patients at the time of diagnosis (see Chapter 26). It results from bony lesions and severe osteoporosis, which is often complicated by pathologic fractures (see Chapter 25). Compression fractures of the thoracic and lumbar vertebral bodies usually result in severe spasms and back pain. Multiple compression fractures often lead to painless dorsal kyphosis and loss of several inches in height. Pleuritic pain from pathologic rib and clavicular fractures is also common and is associated with local tenderness. Destruction of the proximal bones of the extremities is less frequent but important because it can lead to fractures and immobilization. Band-like or bilateral radicular pain should alert the clinician to the risk of spinal cord compression that requires urgent diagnosis and treatment. Hypercalcemia is a complication of the profound skeletal disorder that leeches calcium from bones (see Chapter 31). Hypercalcemia can present with nausea, confusion, polyuria, and constipation. Easy fatigability or dyspnea on exertion is usually secondary to anemia. When immunoglobulins are present at concentrations greater than 5 g/dL, some immunoglobulin G- (IgG) or immunoglobulin A- (IgA) producing myeloma cells can produce features of a hyperviscosity syndrome. Lassitude, confusion, headache, transient disturbances of vision, and an increased bleeding tendency can be related to this syndrome. Recurrent bacterial infection is a major cause of illness and is the most common cause of death in patients with advanced multiple myeloma. Usually, these infections are located in the urinary or respiratory tracts and are caused by common organisms. Systemic amyloidosis with or without multiple myeloma can present with symptoms referable to the gastrointestinal tract (weight loss), neurologic damage (paresthesias), nephrotic syndrome (edema), and cardiac involvement (cardiomyopathy with congestive heart failure and arrhythmias). Aching in the hands, particularly at night, can be caused by the carpal tunnel syndrome. This develops due to amyloid infiltration of the transverse carpal ligament, compressing the median nerves at the wrist.

Findings

Physical findings can be sparse. Pallor from anemia is the most common physical finding. Patients with symptomatic myeloma can have tenderness on pressure over an involved bone, kyphosis, or a pathologic fracture. In a small percentage of patients, firm plasma cell tumors (due to focal collections of malignant plasma cells, called plasmacytomas) may be palpated on the skull, sternum, clavicles, and ribs. Carpal tunnel syndrome can be demonstrable. Fundoscopic examination in patients with a hyperviscosity syndrome shows segmental dilatation ("sausageing") of the retinal veins with retinal hemorrhages. Pleural and/or cardiac involvement can be evident on examination of the chest. Skin plaques and/or joint effusions secondary to amyloid deposit can be presenting findings.

Prognosis

The median survival for multiple myeloma patients who receive no treatment is seven months. Since the introduction of chemotherapy, the median survival rate has improved to 36 to 48 months. For patients who are candidates for high-dose therapy with hematopoietic stem cell transplantation, the median survival is five years, whether or not the transplant is carried out. Cure, however, continues to be elusive in this disease.

The staging system of Durie and Salmon, which is based on hemoglobin, serum calcium, and monoclonal protein concentration as well as on the characteristics of the bone survey, classifies patients into three stages that correlate with the extent of the myeloma cell body burden and survival (Table 63-1). Serum creatinine level does not correlate closely with tumor burden, but its elevations presage shortened survival. It is included in the Durie, Salmon system as a stage modifier for survival prognosis. Although widely used, this staging system does not take into account other independent prognostic indicators. For example, patients with stage III disease by bone criteria alone tend to survive as long as patients with lower-stage multiple myeloma. Other factors of substantial (and unfavorable) prognostic import include chromosome 13 abnormalities, elevated serum beta-2 microglobulin level, bone marrow plasmacytosis greater than 40%, and elevated plasma cell labeling index. Interleukin-6, C-reactive protein, circulating CD19 and CD4 positive cells, interleukin-2, and serum interleukin-6 receptor are other measures that bear on outcome.

Complications

Bone Destruction

Approximately 20% of patients with multiple myeloma have bone demineralization only. Radiographs of the axial skeleton, which must include both

Table 63-1 ■ Durie-Salmon Staging System for Multiple Myeloma

Stage I: Low Myeloma Cell Mass
All of the Following

Hemoglobin more than 10 g/dL
Serum calcium normal
Normal bone structure or solitary plasmacytoma on radiographs
Low level of monoclonal protein: if immunoglobulin G, then less than 5 g/dL and if immunoglobulin A, then less than 3 g/dL
Urinary monoclonal protein less than 4 g/24 hr

Stage II: Intermediate Myeloma Cell Mass

Fits neither stage I nor stage III criteria

Stage III: High Cell Mass
Any One or More of the Following

Hemoglobin less than 8.5 g/dL
Serum calcium more than 12 mg/dL
Advanced lytic bone lesions
Elevated level of monoclonal protein: if immunoglobulin G, then more than 7 g/dL and if immunoglobulin A, more than 5 g/dL
Urinary monoclonal protein more than 12 g/24 hours

Subclassification

A: Serum creatinine less than 2.0 mg/dL
B: Serum creatinine equal to or more than 2.0 mg/dL

femurs, will support the diagnosis of multiple myeloma in approximately 70% of patients. In 10% of patients, the skeletal survey will be normal, presumably because at least 30% of bone calcium must be lost before radiographic changes are evident. Magnetic resonance imaging and bone mineral density studies readily demonstrate disease in nearly all of these patients, however. The bone lesions in the overwhelming majority of patients are osteolytic. In approximately 1% of patients, osteoblastic lesions are present. This finding should lead to consideration of the POEMS syndrome described later in this chapter, a myeloma variant that is associated with osteosclerotic changes and a relatively favorable survival compared with other patients with multiple myeloma.

Bone destruction in multiple myeloma seems to be mediated by a local, not a systemic, mechanism that stimulates osteoclast growth and activation. There are many osteoclast activating factor (OAF) candidates in multiple myeloma, but the leading ones seem to be enhanced RANK ligand production by the bone marrow stromal cells. This appears to act in consort with interleukin-6 and a macrophage inflammatory protein (MIP-1α) produced by the myeloma cells to stimulate osteoclast formation and bone resorption. Myeloma cells produce macrophage inflammatory protein and induce marrow stromal cells to release interleukin-6 and RANK ligand, leading to a self-amplifying process. The central role of RANK ligand is intriguing in that it can be blocked by a decoy receptor, osteoprotegerin, which is currently under evaluation as a treatment for myeloma skeletal disease.

Hypercalcemia

At diagnosis, one-fourth of patients have serum calcium concentrations greater than 11.5 mg/dL after correction for serum albumin. Some hypercalcemic patients might not show bone destruction on radiographs. Hypercalcemia must be diagnosed and treated promptly in patients with multiple myeloma. It is important to recognize the symptom complex of polydypsia, polyuria, nausea, constipation, and loss of appetite that is sometimes associated with drowsiness, somnolence, and confusion. It is common to ascribe mild complaints to an intercurrent illness. The physician should have a high index of suspicion for this serious presenting sign of multiple myeloma and be wary of its later occurrence in patients with an established diagnosis. It is easier to treat multiple myeloma-induced hypercalcemia before renal damage occurs. If the creatinine is elevated, then volume depletion is present due to the hypercalcemic impairment of the renal concentrating mechanism. The hypovolemia further amplifies the serum calcium level. Therefore, normal saline should be given. Only after adequate rehydration should loop diuretics like furosemide be used to promote natruresis and correction of hypercalcemia. Bisphosphonates have become standard in the treatment of hypercalcemia of malignancy and should be used early on, obviating to some extent the need for excessive attempts at rehydration.

Unlike the hypercalcemia of hyperparathyroidism, the hypercalcemia induced by multiple myeloma is readily reversed by administration of high-dose glucocorticoids. Treatment with glucocorticoids should not be delayed because of concerns about side effects. Rapid and sustained improvement of hypercalcemia can be obtained at doses of 60 mg of prednisone daily. Prompt, effective therapy will minimize the severity of hypercalcemia-induced renal failure and reverse or stabilize renal function abnormalities.

Renal Failure

Renal failure occurs in approximately 25% of patients and is common in patients with extensive disease. Most patients with mild azotemia have no symptoms. Fatigability, nausea, vomiting, and confusion appear when the renal damage is severe. The pathogenesis is multifactorial, including renal infection, light chain deposition in the renal tubules, hypercalcemia, hy-peruricemia, nephrotoxic agents, and dehydration. The aggregate of these effects results in what has been called a myeloma kidney.

Patients with renal failure due to multiple myeloma usually have Bence-Jones proteinuria greater than 1 g every 24 hours. If recognized early on, renal failure is often reversible. Failure to institute therapy can lead to chronic renal insufficiency, which limits therapy and causes unnecessary morbidity and early mortality. Patients with Bence-Jones proteinuria are especially susceptible to the development of a myeloma kidney, when nonsteroidal anti-inflammatory agents and certain antibiotics are given. These agents should be avoided in patients with Bence-Jones proteinuria.

Infection

Recurrent bacterial infections are a major cause of illness and are the most frequent cause of death in patients with advanced myeloma. Infections result primarily from the marked hypogammaglobulinemia that develops in most patients with multiple myeloma as the production of normal immunoglobulins declines. *Streptococcus pneumoniae* and *Hemophilus influenzae* are the most common pathogens in previously untreated myeloma patients and in non-neutropenic patients who respond to chemotherapy. However, in neutropenic patients and in those with refractory disease, *Staphylococcus aureus* and gram-negative bacteria are the predominant organisms. Pneumococcal vaccination is worth attempting, as some patients respond. Most patients, however, are unable to muster an antibody response to neoantigens. The incidence of infection within the first two months of chemotherapy is 10-fold higher than later on in the disease course, when a response to treatment has been achieved.

Hyperviscosity Syndrome

Very high concentrations of monoclonal proteins can result in hyperviscosity problems. It is more likely to occur in Waldenström's macroglobulinemia (see later in this chapter) than in multiple myeloma because of the large size of the immunoglobulin M proteins. It is more likely to occur in multiple myeloma that produces monoclonal protein of the immunoglobulin A type than of the immunoglobulin G type. The former (more readily than the latter) forms complexes of individual molecules, resulting in aggregates of large molecular size. Symptoms and signs of this condition are generally not seen unless the relative serum viscosity is greater than 4.0 units (normal range 1.4 to 1.8 units as measured in a simple viscosimeter). The full-blown syndrome is usually not observed unless the viscosity is greater than 5.0 units. The signs and symptoms include lassitude, confusion, blurred vision, dizziness, vertigo, diplopia, and a bleeding tendency, especially oronasal bleeding.

Neurologic Manifestations

Thoracic or lumbosacral radiculopathy is the most frequent neurologic complication. Root pain results from compression of the nerve by the vertebral lesion or by the collapsed bone itself. Characteristically, the pain is movement related and is aggravated by cough, sneeze, and strain. Patients can walk stiffly and have great difficulty getting onto and off the examining table or X-ray table. Vertebral body collapse or cord compression from an extradural plasma cell tumor results in back pain with radicular features, weakness, or paralysis, necessitating rapid diagnosis by magnetic resonance imaging to rule out impending spinal cord compression and to facilitate prompt treatment before irreversible neurologic damage occurs.

Occasionally, patients with multiple myeloma experience peripheral neuropathy that can be quite severe and unexplained by bone involvement or malignant plasma cell collections. Electromyographic studies suggest that this complication occurs more frequently than is generally recognized. Although the pathogenesis is unclear, the neuropathy might be caused by associated amyloid infiltration of the nerves or by toxicity from therapeutic agents, such as vincristine or thalidomide. Severe motor neuropathy is not uncommon in young patients with localized or osteosclerotic multiple myeloma.

Secondary Leukemia and Myelodysplastic Syndrome

Secondary myelodysplastic syndrome, with or without evolution to acute myeloid leukemia, is a devastating complication of the treatment of multiple myeloma. The characteristic cytogenetic pattern associated with alkylating agent-induced myelodysplasia/acute myeloid leukemia is a deletion of the long arm of chromosome 5 or 7 (del 5q or del 7q) or total loss of the chromosome (−5 or −7). Other clonal cytogenetic changes occur as well. Secondary myelodysplasia/ acute myeloid leukemia occurs even when alkylating agents have not been employed in therapy; that is, in patients receiving adriamycin or etoposide. Here, the characteristic cytogenetic lesion is an 11q23 deletion. The duration from initial treatment of multiple myeloma to the diagnosis of secondary myelodysplasia/acute myeloid leukemia is three to seven years; the leukemia is usually preceded by a period of myelodysplasia. With 11q23 deletion-associated leukemia, an intervening phase of myelodysplasia is not recognized and the interval from treatment to the development of acute myeloid leukemia is often less than two years.

An Eastern Cooperative Oncology Group study of 653 patients treated with regimens that included vincristine, BCNU, melphalan, cyclophosphamide, prednisone, and sometimes interferon identified 31 patients with myelodysplasia/acute myeloid leukemia (4.7%). The median time from treatment to onset of myelodysplasia/acute myeloid leukemia was 42 months; the actuarial risk was 6% at 5 years and 19% at 10 years.

The relationship of secondary myelodysplasia/ acute myeloid leukemia to high-dose therapy with hematopoietic stem cell transplantation was reported in 857 patients followed for at least two years after transplantation (Table 63-2). Age more than 50 years and the administration of more than 12 months of conventional therapy before transplantation emerged as risk factors for the development of secondary myelodysplasia/acute myeloid leukemia.

Clinical Evaluation

Basic Studies

Routine laboratory tests, such as the complete blood count and platelet count, serum creatinine, electrolytes, calcium, albumin, uric acid, lactate dehydrogenase (LDH), liver function tests, urinalysis, and chest X-ray provide nonspecific results in establishing the diagnosis, but they are helpful in the overall evaluation of the patient. Anemia is common

Table 63-2 ■ Myelodysplasia After High-Dose Melphalan and Hematopoietic Stem Cell Transplantation

Number of Patients	Preceding Therapy Administered for More Than 12 Months	Age More Than 50 Years	Incidence of Secondary Myelodysplasia
227	−	−	2%
267	−	+	7%
140	+	−	11%
223	+	+	9%

From Govindaragan R et al: Preceding standard therapy is the likely cause of myelodysplasia after auto-transplant in multiple myeloma. Br J Haematol 1996;95:349–353.

Table 63-3 ▪ Differential Diagnosis of Monoclonal Gammopathies

	Monoclonal Gammopathy of Undetermined Significance	Smoldering Multiple Myeloma	Multiple Myeloma	Solitary Plasmacytoma of Bone	Extramedullary Myeloma
Monoclonal protein	Less than 3 g/dL	More than 3 g/dL	More than 3 g/dL	Variable	Variable
Bone marrow plasma cells	Less than 10%	More than 10%	More than 10%	Less than 10%	Less than 10%
Functional impairment*	None	None	Present	Isolated	Isolated

*Functional impairment includes clinical symptoms or abnormalities such as anemia (hemoglobin 2 g/dL below normal or less than 10 g/dL), hypercalcemia (more than 11 mg/dL), lytic bony lesions or osteoporosis with compression fractures, renal insufficiency (creatinine more than 2 mg/dL).

and could be the presenting manifestation of multiple myeloma. High levels of serum immunoglobulin A or immunoglobulin G frequently increase the plasma volume, artificially lowering the hematocrit level, which can be as much as 6% below the value that would be expected if the red blood cell volume were measured. Thrombocytopenia is uncommon at the time of diagnosis but tends to develop over time. Mild granulocytopenia occurs frequently for reasons that are unclear; it usually persists throughout the clinical course. Twenty percent of myeloma patients will have B_{12} deficiency, which appears to be more prevalent in IgA myeloma. Moreover, folic acid deficiency occurs either alone or with B_{12} deficiency with both occurring in 30% of patients. Both of these vitamins might influence presenting counts and tolerance to therapy. Hypercalcemia, hyperuricemia, and an increased serum creatinine are often found at diagnosis. An increased lactate dehydrogenase is noted in 10% to 15% of patients and signifies a poor prognosis. The serum alkaline phosphatase is usually normal. The purely lytic bone lesions that characterize skeletal involvement by myeloma fail to elicit an osteoblastic reaction, so the alkaline phosphatase does not rise despite extensive bony disease; this distinguishes multiple myeloma from other cancers that metastasize to bone. Cardiomegaly may occur due to amyloid deposition.

Differential Diagnosis

When a plasma cell dyscrasia is suspected, the tests about to be described can be used to confirm the diagnosis, detect complications, assist in the staging of the disease, and establish baseline values to gauge the response to treatment. The diagnosis requires the demonstration of

1. plasmacytosis of 10% or more in the bone marrow, plasma cells in sheets in the bone marrow, or biopsy-proven plasmacytoma, and
2. either monoclonal protein in the serum or urine or characteristic osteolytic lesions of bone.

The differential diagnosis includes consideration of other forms of monoclonal gammopathies, which are listed in Table 63-3.

Patients with multiple myeloma must be differentiated from those with monoclonal gammopathy of undetermined significance and smoldering multiple myeloma (SMM) (see Chapter 33). Asymptomatic patients who have a monoclonal protein that is less than 3 g/dL, fewer than 10% bone marrow plasma cells, and no osteolytic lesions, anemia, hypercalcemia, or renal function impairment usually have monoclonal gammopathy of undetermined significance. Asymptomatic patients who have both an M-component higher than 3 g/dL and more than 10% but less than 30% bone marrow plasma cells fulfill the criteria for smoldering multiple myeloma. These patients do not have anemia, renal failure, hypercalcemia, osteolytic bone lesions, or other clinical manifestations related to the monoclonal protein. The patients with smoldering multiple myeloma are clinically and biologically more similar to patients with monoclonal gammopathy of undetermined significance than to patients with overt multiple myeloma. The recognition of smoldering multiple myeloma is extremely important because they should not be treated with chemotherapy until progression occurs or they should be enrolled in well diagnosed trials. No laboratory parameter or clinical factor specifically differentiates patients with monoclonal gammopathy of undetermined significance/smoldering multiple myeloma from overt multiple myeloma. The presence of hypogammaglobulinemia is not useful in this regard, because it occurs in 30% to 40% of patients with monoclonal gammopathy of undetermined significance. Although Bence-Jones proteinuria suggests a diagnosis of multiple myeloma, it is not unusual to find small amounts of urinary monoclonal light chains in monoclonal gammopathy of undetermined significance. In patients newly diagnosed with monoclonal gammopathy of undetermined significance, serum protein electrophoresis should be repeated after three months and then followed serially to detect evidence in favor of multiple myeloma. Patients should be aware that the evolution to multiple myeloma can be abrupt, and prompt reexamination is required if clinical signs suggestive of myeloma develop.

Myeloma Proteins (M-Proteins)

Serum and/or urine protein electrophoresis demonstrates a peak or localized band in 80% of patients, hypogammaglobulinemia in 10%, and no apparent abnormalities in the remainder. In virtually all patients with hypogammaglobulinemia, either urinary light-chain or minute quantities of serum monoclonal proteins can be detected by sensitive methods. Immunofixation is a very sensitive means of detecting monoclonal proteins, identifying the type of protein, with conventional electrophoretic studies quantitating the level in the serum and urine. In 99% of cases of multiple myeloma, a monoclonal protein in the serum or the urine or both is detectable. The remaining 1% of patients with no demonstrable monoclonal protein have nonsecretory multiple myeloma caused by a defect in the synthesis or assembly of the light or heavy chains by the malignant plasma cells. During the course of treatment, serial immunofixation determinations are not routinely necessary, but subsequent testing is useful in documenting the degree of response, especially in the circumstances of patients thought to be in complete remission because a monoclonal protein is no longer present on conventional electrophoretic studies.

Bone Marrow Aspirate and Biopsy

This procedure is crucial for the diagnosis of multiple myeloma and for studies of the plasma cell morphology and biology that contribute important prognostic information. The diagnosis of myeloma requires more than 10% plasma cells in the bone marrow. Bone marrow plasmacytosis is not uniform throughout the bone marrow, but an increase in the number of plasma cells is usually apparent on inspection of the bone marrow aspirate. The bone marrow biopsy allows sampling of several different depths of bone marrow, enhancing the likelihood of establishing the diagnosis.

Reactive plasmacytosis secondary to connective tissue disorders, liver disease, viral and bacterial infec-

tions, or carcinoma is polyclonal and can be differentiated from the monoclonal plasma cell proliferation of multiple myeloma or monoclonal gammopathy of undetermined significance by performing immune staining on the bone marrow. Although increased plasma cells (including binucleate and trinucleate forms) are nonspecific for multiple myeloma, some morphologic changes are indicative of the disease. Bizarre plasmablasts (Figure 63-1) or plasma cells occurring in sheets are not usually found in reactive plasmacytosis.

The bone marrow plasma cell labeling index is performed in some centers to provide a measure of plasma cell turnover and proliferation. A high labeling index confers an adverse prognosis.

Urinary Protein Analysis

Monoclonal protein excretion in the urine is detected in approximately 65% of patients with multiple myeloma. Although renal damage can lead to excretion of the whole monoclonal protein into the urine, the normal kidney only clears the light-chain fraction of the monoclonal protein. The recognition of light chain protein (called the Bence-Jones protein) depends on the demonstration of the monoclonal light chain by immune electrophoresis or immune fixation. Quantitating the 24-hour urinary light-chain excretion is useful in following the response to therapy.

Radiologic Studies

A complete bone survey is an important part of the evaluation of monoclonal gammopathies. The skeletal survey should include the skull, ribs, complete spine, pelvis, and long bones of the arms and legs. The most commonly affected skeletal organ is the spine. Approximately 20% of patients will have bone demineralization alone. Radiographs of the axial skeleton, which

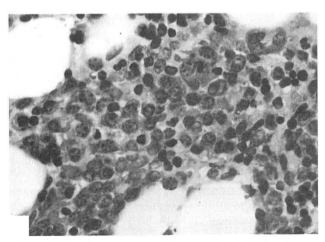

Figure 63-1 ■ Bone marrow biopsy section demonstrates clusters of immature, blast-like plasma cells (plasma blasts). (From Naeim F: Atlas of Bone Marrow and Blood Pathology. Philadelphia: WB Saunders, 2001.) (See Color Plate 14.)

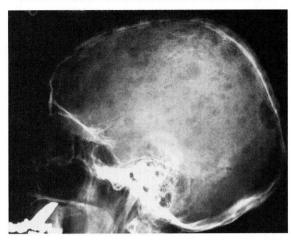

Figure 63-2 ▪ Lateral radiograph of the skull, showing multiple osteolytic bony lesions in a patient with multiple myeloma. (From Mettler FA Jr: Essentials of Radiology. Philadelphia: WB Saunders, 1996.)

must include bone femurs, will support the diagnosis of multiple myeloma in approximately 70% of the patients. Punched-out lesions are best seen on lateral skull radiographs (Figure 63-2). The skeletal survey will appear normal in 10% of the patients at the time of diagnosis. Radionuclide scans of bones show enhanced uptake based on osteoblast activation by metastatic deposits to bone. The absence of an osteoblastic response in multiple myeloma results in negative bone scans, except in the very rare osteosclerotic myeloma or at sites of pathologic fractures, where healing is attempted. Bone scans are not useful in the evaluation of patients with multiple myeloma, but they can be helpful in detecting occult pathologic fractures that are inapparent on routine bone radiographs.

Computed Tomography and Magnetic Resonance Imaging

Computed tomography scan is very sensitive in identifying areas of bone destruction and particularly useful in judging the extent of extramedullary soft tissue lesions adjacent to vertebral compression fractures. Magnetic resonance imaging of the lumbar spine and pelvis provides an intense signal in T2-weighted images of bone marrow involvement by myeloma. Magnetic resonance imaging can assess the extent of disease in asymptomatic indolent multiple myeloma or in patients who have an apparently localized plasmacytoma. It is an excellent way to visualize intramedullary plasma cell tumors. Positron emission tomography (PET scan) can also be useful in the detection of extramedullary disease.

Beta-2 Microglobulin

The beta-2 microglobulin protein is the light chain of the major histocompatible complex in the cell membrane of all nucleated cells. The level of the protein in the serum is particularly increased in states of lymphocyte activation and plasma cell turnover. Serum beta-2 microglobulin levels are elevated in patients with active multiple myeloma. A close relationship exists between the serum beta-2 microglobulin (uncorrected for serum creatinine) and myeloma cell mass. Levels greater than 4 mg/dL are indicative of a large tumor mass and poor prognosis. When combined with the results of the bone marrow plasma cell labeling index, beta-2 microglobulin forms a powerful prognostic system as accurate as clinical staging in predicting survival.

Therapy of Multiple Myeloma

Melphalan and Prednisone

Intermittent courses of melphalan and prednisone have been standard therapy for patients with multiple myeloma for many years. Each month, orally and daily for four days, the patient is given melphalan 8 mg/m² before breakfast and prednisone 60 mg/m² after breakfast. Gastrointestinal absorption of melphalan is unpredictable. Three weeks after each course, it is well to confirm that mild granulocytopenia (1000 to 2000 granulocytes/μL) and/or thrombocytopenia (<100,000 platelets/μL) has occurred in order to ensure that an effective dose (and a not excessive dose) has been administered. If the myeloma is not responding and there is no myelosuppression, the dose should be increased in 20% increments. Response develops slowly and could require six or more cycles before remission or resistance is confirmed.

Intermittent courses of melphalan and prednisone induce a remission in approximately 40% of patients, using the Southwest Oncology Group's (SWOG) criteria of response, consisting of at least a 75% decrease in the production of serum myeloma protein, a 95% decrease in Bence-Jones urinary protein, and less than 5% residual bone marrow plasma cells. Using the criteria of the Eastern Cooperative Oncology Group (ECOG) and other groups—namely, a 50% decrease in the serum monoclonal protein level and 90% decrease in urinary light-chain excretion—the objective response rate to melphalan and prednisone is 50%. The median duration of remission is 18 to 24 months, the median survival is 30 months, and the five-year survival rate is 15% to 19%. Fewer than 5% of patients live more than 10 years, and there is no evidence that even a small subgroup is cured.

Vincristine, Adriamycin (Doxorubicin), and Dexamethasone (VAD)

The combination of vincristine, doxorubicin (Adriamycin), and dexamethasone is given every four

Therapy of Multiple Myeloma

Until cure becomes possible, the goal of primary treatment for myeloma is to prolong life, relieve symptoms, and maintain a good quality of life. In this regard, administration of erythropoietin to correct anemia, focal radiation therapy and adequate analgesia for bone pain, prophylactic antibiotics for inpatients with recurrent infections, and protection against compromising skeletal events by use of bisphosphonates all form part of the supportive care for the patient as well as an active physical therapy program that includes swimming and/or water exercises.

Therapy for multiple myeloma can consist of pulses of high-dose glucocorticoids, monthly oral melphalan and prednisone, dexamethasone and 4-day continuous infusion of doxorubicin and vincristine (VAD), or other combination chemotherapy regimens. Although early and intermediate endpoints are achieved at different rates, there is little to recommend one regimen over the other because survival is the same. Selection of therapy should be based on considerations of the patient's age, severity of the disease, and tolerance of side effects. Therapy should be continued to the point of maximum improvement; after one year without relapse, therapy can be interrupted awaiting subsequent relapse for its reinstitution. Alternatively, interferon can be used for maintenance therapy, but whether the small benefit is worth the side effects warrants careful consideration.

Thalidomide is an active agent in advanced and early multiple myeloma. Thalidomide, along with other therapy such as high-dose dexamethasone, is likely to prove to be part of the standard of care for initial treatment of the disease and/or in maintenance therapy.

For patients under age 70, the possible use of high-dose therapy with autologous stem cell transplantation should be discussed with the patient. In the event that it can be employed, hematopoietic stem cells should be harvested when a substantial response to initial therapy has been achieved. Although frequently used as part of initial therapy in the community, autologous transplantation is as effective if used later in the course of the disease and does not represent a cure of the disease. Tandem autologous transplantation offers greater long-term benefit over a single transplantation procedure and should be considered in patients able to tolerate the toxicity.

---

weeks. Each cycle consists of vincristine, 0.4 mg/day and doxorubicin, 9 mg/m^2/day as a continuous infusion through a central venous catheter for four days, plus high-dose dexamethasone, 20 mg/m^2 orally daily for four days, commencing on days 1, 9, and 17 of each cycle. In practice, the dexamethasone is restricted to administration on days 1 through 4 of the even-numbered cycles, and the three full four-day courses are employed only on odd-numbered cycles. Although the overall response rate is 15% higher and the onset of remission more rapid in the patients treated with this regimen compared with patients receiving melphalan and prednisone, neither remission duration nor survival rate is improved. Notwithstanding this fact, there are several advantages to this regimen:

- Rapid remission induction is an advantage in patients with hypercalcemia or renal failure.
- Absorption of these agents is ensured when compared with oral chemotherapy administration.
- Vincristine, doxorubicin, and dexamethasone are safe in patients with renal failure, as these drugs are not excreted by the kidneys.

The same regimen of dexamethasone used alone also induces a rapid remission, but the response rate is 15% lower than when vincristine and adriamycin are added. Primary or secondary resistance to vincristine, adriamycin, and dexamethasone can develop, and the treatment program carries the risk of corticosteroid toxicity from dexamethasone, of neurotoxicity from vincristine (especially in patients more than age 60 years), and of cardiac toxicity from doxorubicin. Because of the rapid remission induced by either vincristine, adriamycin, and dexamethasone or dexamethasone alone, usually only two courses are necessary to determine whether the myeloma is responding to treatment. In considering complex chemotherapy regimens in multiple myeloma, one needs to be aware of the fact that regardless of the regimen implemented here, long-term survival results are equivalent. Moreover, no conventional regimen has demonstrated the ability to cure the disease in even a small proportion of patients.

For example, a multidrug, alkylating agent-based combination chemotherapy protocol called BCMVP has been developed. The regimen consists of five-week cycles of vincristine 2 mg/m^2 IV on day 1, BCNU 30 mg/m^2 intravenously on day 1, melphalan 8 mg/m^2 PO on days 1 through 4, cyclophosphamide 400 mg/m^2 intravenously on day 1 and prednisone 40 mg/m^2 PO on days 1 through 7. This combination of chemotherapy provides a superior response rate compared with melphalan and prednisone but no survival advantage.

Pegylated Doxorubicin

By encapsulating doxorubicin in a synthetic liposome, the pegylated form of this drug (Doxil) could potentially extend the duration of malignant plasma cell exposure to therapeutic levels of doxorubicin. In a phase II study, pegylated liposomal doxorubicin, 40 mg/m^2 intravenously over two to three hours on day 1, was combined with vincristine, 2.0 mg intravenously on day 1, and a high-dose dexamethasone, 40 mg/day for four days, was given to 33 patients newly diagnosed with advanced multiple myeloma. This regimen was repeated every four weeks. The overall response rate was 88%, median time to progression was 24.1 months, and survival at three years was 67%. No patients discontinued treatment due to adverse events. The most common toxicities were grade 3 palmar-plantar erythrodysesthesia, mucositis, and neutropenia. Only one patient at the age of 80 years received a total dose of Doxil at 520 mg/m^2 and experienced cardiotoxicity. It could be that when compared with the combination of vincristine, doxorubicin, and frequent Decadron dosing, the use of pegylated liposomal doxorubicin and reducing the number of courses of high-dose dexamethasone in each cycle can improve the safety profile and convenience of the treatment regimen without compromising efficacy.

Thalidomide

Thalidomide, marketed in the late 1950s and early 1960s to prevent morning sickness in pregnant women, was arguably the greatest drug disaster of all time and resulted in a major overhaul of the drug testing and approval process. Nevertheless, thalidomide was approved by the Food and Drug Administration (FDA) in 1998 for the treatment of erythema nodosum leprosum, an inflammatory condition associated with leprosy. It is an active drug in multiple myeloma and is also under study as an immunomodulatory agent in a variety of inflammatory conditions (such as chronic graft-versus-host disease and rheumatoid arthritis) and as an antiangiogenic agent in multiple nonhematologic cancers.

The immunomodulatory action of thalidomide is multifaceted and not fully understood. Thalidomide inefficiently, but selectively, inhibits the production of tumor necrosis factor-α (TNF-α) in human monocytes in a dose-dependent fashion, exerting no effect on total protein synthesis or the production of other cytokines. The inhibitory action of thalidomide on tumor necrosis factor-α occurs by enhanced messenger RNA (mRNA) degradation. Thalidomide has complex effects on T-lymphocytes, stimulating proliferation and inducing the secretion of IFN-β. Thalidomide also induces cytokine production by type 2 helper T-lymphocytes and inhibits cytokine production by type 1 helper T-lymphocytes, but its principal effect appears to be on the regulation of the expression of adhesion molecules. The antiangiogenic activity is probably by inhibition of fibroblast growth factor and vascular endothelial growth factor.

In relapsed and refractory multiple myeloma, thalidomide as a single agent induces responses in 25% of patients and in a greater fraction of patients when it is used as part of a combination therapy program. Some of these responses in advanced disease have been durable. Barlogie et al reported an overall two-year survival rate of 60% and a significant dose-response effect, with superior response and survival rates occurring in patients receiving higher doses of the drug.

The side effects of thalidomide are usually mild to moderate. The most common of these include sedation, fatigue, constipation, and skin rash. Peripheral neuropathy also occurs and can become irreversible after chronic administration.

A Mayo Clinic pilot study of the combination of thalidomide, 200 mg/day orally with pulses of high-dose dexamethasone 40 mg/day orally for four days on days 1, 9, and 17 of repeated four-week cycles in previously untreated patients demonstrated a response rate of 64% and good patient tolerance. This combination with thalidomide and others are under evaluation. Whether the addition of thalidomide improves survival remains undetermined. The combination of thalidomide with high-dose dexamethasone is appealing, because it is less toxic and stem cell sparing in comparison to chemotherapeutic combinations, allowing for increased application of stem cell transplantation (see the relevant section later in this chapter).

Interferon

Interferon-α2 has been widely tested in multiple myeloma as part of initial or maintenance therapy. Although some trials showed increased response duration and time to disease progression, no survival benefit was apparent. A meta-analysis evaluating independent patient data from 4012 patients in 24 randomized trials found a statistically significant, but slight, improvement in response rate, progression-free survival, and median survival when interferon was added to other drugs in induction therapy or used after chemotherapy as maintenance. Nevertheless, interferon has not gained popularity in the United States because of its expense and toxicity, which include fever with initial doses, chronic fatigue, anorexia, and weight loss. One has to weigh whether the relatively short increase in disease control makes the toxicity acceptable. The maintenance dose is usually 3 to 5 million units subcutaneously, three days each week.

Immunomodulatory Drugs

A novel group of thalidomide analogues has been developed, which are up to 50,000 times more potent as inhibitors of tumor necrosis factor than is the parent molecule. Immunomodulatory agents can inhibit the proliferation of myeloma cells as well as reverse their resistance to melphalan, doxorubicin, dexamethasone, or vincristine.

PS-341

Proteasomes are large complexes of proteolytic enzymes that are involved in the intracellular degradation of proteins and the turnover of many regulatory proteins via the ubiquitin-proteasome pathway. Ubiquitin marks the proteins scheduled for degradation. Selectively inhibiting proteasome activity "stabilizes" the regulatory proteins, thus disrupting cell proliferation and resulting in apoptosis. PS-341 is a synthetic proteasome inhibitor with good selectivity. It halts susceptible cells in culture in the G2-M phase of the cell cycle, causing cell death. Proteasome inhibition also blocks the activity of the transcription factor, NF-κB. This results in reduced expression of cell-surface adhesion molecules and the NF-κβ–dependent increase in interleukin-6 production in stromal cells, thereby inhibiting the paracrine stimulation of myeloma cell growth. Clinical data suggest that PS341 might have significant clinical activity in advanced myeloma.

Arsenic Trioxide

Arsenic trioxide inhibits the growth of cultured myeloma cell lines at concentrations of 1–2 μm and has shown activity against multiple myeloma in some patients. The *in vitro* effects are relatively selective against myeloma cells, as normal myeloid cells isolated from the bone marrow are much less sensitive. This raises the possibility of combining arsenic trioxide with other myelosuppressive agents in the treatment of multiple myeloma.

Autologous Hematopoietic Stem Cell Transplantation

(See also Chapter 51)

High-dose therapy with autologous hematopoietic stem cell transplantation can be accomplished with a low (less than 2%) mortality rate. The failure to cure patients by conventional means, the relative safety of the procedure, and the potential value of escalating the intensity of treatment has led to increased use of autologous transplantation after securing a response to initial chemotherapy.

The French Myeloma Group treated patients with initial chemotherapy until a response was achieved and then randomized 200 previously untreated patients with multiple myeloma under age 65 to receive either high-dose chemotherapy and autologous bone marrow transplantation or to continue conventional chemotherapy. The data were analyzed on an intent-to-treat basis, because 25% of those patients randomized to autologous transplantation did not actually undergo the procedure. Although only 75% of the intended transplants were performed, the overall response rate (81% versus 57%), complete response rate (22% versus 5%), five-year event-free survival rate (28% versus 10%), and overall survival rate were superior in the transplant group compared with the chemotherapy-treated patients. However, multivariant analysis on different factors affecting survival showed only B_2 macroglobulin to be the factor determining survival and *not* bone marrow transplantation.

The long-term value of autologous stem cell transplantation remains controversial. Autologous transplantation is not curative, because relapses continue to occur without a plateau in the disease-free survival curve after the procedure. In a study of 77 patients with multiple myeloma who fulfilled the criteria for autologous transplant (age less than 66 years, stage II or III disease, good performance status, and disease responsive to initial chemotherapy) and who were treated with conventional chemotherapy, the median survival was five years, which is similar to that seen for autologous stem cell transplantation. It could be that patients who meet the eligibility criteria for transplantation are a selected group with a highly favorable prognosis.

Whether autologous stem cell transplantation should be performed as part of the initial therapy or reserved for relapsed or resistant disease is another unresolved issue in autologous transplantation. In a multicenter, randomized trial, newly diagnosed patients were first treated with three to four courses of vincristine, doxorubicin, and methylprednisolone and then randomized to receive high-dose therapy and autologous stem cell transplantation or to continue with conventional chemotherapy. In both groups stem cells were obtained after the initial chemotherapy. In the latter group autologous stem cell transplantation was only performed later on if resistance to chemotherapy developed or if relapse occurred. Data were analyzed on an intent-to-treat basis. The estimated median survival in both groups was approximately 5 years. This calls into question whether transplantation early in the course of therapy is necessary.

The low morbidity and mortality of autologous transplant has led to investigation of benefit from two sequential transplant procedures, called a tandem transplant. Although nonrandomized studies suggest that two transplants achieve better results than one transplant, the benefit could be a function of the selection of a favorable prognostic subset of patients identified by their ability to undergo the second procedure. A randomized study recently confirmed the value of tandem over single autologous transplantation in a subgroup of patients that receives the second transplant in a timely fashion. Nevertheless, longer follow-up is needed before tandem transplantation can be recommended as a standard of therapy in multiple myeloma.

Allogeneic Bone Marrow Transplantation (See also Chapter 51)

Compared with autologous transplantation, allogeneic stem cell transplantation makes possible the use of stem cells for bone marrow reconstitution that are not contaminated by residual myeloma cells and the added benefit of a graft-versus-myeloma effect. Unfortunately, more than 90% of patients with multiple myeloma are not candidates for allogeneic stem cell transplantation, because they are elderly, lack a human leukocyte antigen (HLA)–matched sibling donor, or have inadequate renal, pulmonary, or cardiac function. A graft-versus-myeloma effect has been demonstrated; it reduces the relapse rate. But the morbidity of the procedure and its accompanying graft-versus-host disease in patients with multiple myeloma is substantial, and the procedure-related mortality rate is more than 30%. The European Blood and Bone Marrow Transplantation registry reported on 266 patients who had a 51% complete response, but treatment-related mortality occurred in approximately 40%. The net result was an actuarial survival of 30% at 4 years and 20% at 10 years. As a result, allogeneic stem cell transplantation is usually reserved for investigative studies or for patients who have failed conventional modalities of treatment.

Treatment of Complications of Multiple Myeloma

Infections

The value of intravenous immunoglobulin as prophylaxis against infection was assessed in a double-blind, placebo-controlled, multicenter trial. Patients with stable multiple myeloma received monthly infusions of intravenous immunoglobulin, 0.4 gm/kg body weight or an equivalent volume of placebo (0.4% albumin) for one year. No episodes of septicemia or pneumonia occurred in patients receiving intravenous immunoglobulin (compared with 25% in patients receiving placebo [P = 0.002]), and the days spent with serious infections were reduced significantly. Those patients who failed to demonstrate even a minimal increase in antibody titer after pneumococcal vaccination (Pneumovax) were the most immunologically

impaired and benefited most from intravenous immunoglobulin. Intravenous immunoglobulin therapy is very expensive and, when the risk of infection is very low, it is unnecessary in most patients once a response to chemotherapy has been obtained.

Antibiotic prophylaxis is as effective as intravenous immunoglobulin in nearly all patients and is much cheaper. Apart from the terminal phases of the disease, patients with multiple myeloma are at highest risk for bacterial infection during the first two months of initial chemotherapy. The rate of infection is twice that experienced during the remainder of the disease course. As many as one-third of these early infections are fatal, and many more prevent adequate administration of chemotherapy. The role of prophylactic antibiotics was studied in a trial, which randomized patients just starting chemotherapy to receive trimethoprim/sulfamethoxazole 160/800 mg orally every 12 hours for the first two months of treatment or to receive a placebo. In comparison with the control group, the patients receiving antibiotic prophylaxis had a statistically significant reduction in bacterial infections and in severe infections. Toxicity (primarily skin rash) was not severe, but it led to discontinuation of the antibiotic in 25% (7/28) of patients. Trimethoprim/sulfamethoxazole or one of the fluoroquinolone derivatives is a highly effective prophylactic antibiotic agent in patients with multiple myeloma who exhibit a propensity for recurrent bacterial infections. As long as the development of allergy or idiosyncratic toxicity remain absent, these drugs can be given for years chronically in a once-daily dose. Moreover, trimethoprim/sulfamethoxazole (but not the quinolones) also represents effective prophylaxis against *Pneumocystis carinii* infection and toxoplasmosis. The risk of these infections is increased in patients with multiple myeloma when they receive, not uncommonly, prolonged therapy with high-dose corticosteroids.

Skeletal Complications

Bisphosphonates

Biphosphonates are inhibitors of osteoclastic activity that are used in the treatment of multiple myeloma in combination with chemotherapy. In 62 patients with newly diagnosed multiple myeloma, pamidronate, a bisphosphonate, was evaluated for its effects on markers of bone resorption, new bone formation, disease activity (β2-microglobulin and monoclonal protein level), and the signs and symptoms of bone disease. Patients were randomly assigned to receive chemotherapy plus or minus pamidronate. Addition of pamidronate to chemotherapy provided a statistically significant improvement in markers of bone resorption (decreased N-telopeptide derived from type I collagen) and bone formation (increased alkaline phosphatase and interleukin-6) and disease activity (reduction in C-reactive protein, β2-microglobulin, and monoclonal protein level). These changes correlated with a reduction in bone pain and skeletal related events in the pamidronate-treated group. These data suggest that pamidronate could act synergistically with chemotherapy to improve disease response.

Zoledronic Acid

Zoledronic acid (4 mg intravenously), another bisphosphonate, was compared with pamidronate3 (90 mg intravenously) in a randomized trial in patients with the hypercalcemia of malignancy. Zoledronic acid was superior to pamidronate in the initial treatment of hypercalcemia. In another randomized trial, zoledronic acid proved to be as efficacious and as safe as pamidronate in preventing skeletal-related events in patients with multiple myeloma at thirteen months follow-up. Treatment is given monthly and, based on long-term studies of pamidronate, can and should be continued indefinitely over years with both agents, however, close monitoring of renal function is critical especially over the long term.

Kyphoplasty

Kyphoplasty is a new technique that involves the introduction of inflatable bone tamps into a vertebral body to stabilize it. Even though bisphosphonates significantly decrease skeletal morbidity, skeletal damage already sustained at the time of diagnosis and the resultant pain limit patient mobility, decreasing the quality of life even if the multiple myeloma is brought under control. Once the bone tamps are inserted and inflated, they restore the vertebral body towards its original height, while creating a cavity that can be filled with highly viscous bone cement. Kyphoplasty has been employed without major complications in patients with vertebral compression fractures. Approximately one-third of lost height was restored, with marked decrease in pain and improved performance status. With the spine being the most afflicted skeletal organ and the longer survival of myeloma patients, this procedure should be considered in all affected myeloma patients to prevent worsening spine mechanics and morbidity/mortality from resulting kyphosis.

Osteoprotegerin

Osteoprotegerin is a potent inhibitor of bone resorption *in vivo*. It acts as a decoy receptor, binding and inactivating its ligand, which is an essential factor for osteoclast differentiation. Transgenic overexpression of osteoprotegerin in mice produces an osteopetrotic phenotype due to the inhibition of growth-related bone resorption. Conversely, in the osteoprotegerin gene-knockout mouse, severe osteoporosis develops.

Osteoprotegerin is important in normal bone physiology and is capable of opposing the bone resorptive effects of parathyroid hormone, vitamin D, interleukin-1, tumor necrosis factor, and estrogen withdrawal after oopherectomy. These factors are the main mediators of metabolic, inflammatory, and cancer-related bone diseases. Osteoprotegerin also prevents and reverses hypercalcemia in a murine model of hypercalcemia of malignancy. This compound is under investigation for its use to prevent or reverse bone disease due to malignancy.

POEMS

POEMS is a syndrome that is characterized by the association of polyneuropathy, organomegaly, endocrinopathy of various forms, monoclonal protein, and skin changes. The complex of abnormalities is secondary to the underlying plasma cell dyscrasia. Apart from the panoply of abnormalities, POEMS' most striking feature is that the bone lesions are extensive and are osteosclerotic rather than osteolyic. Electromyography and nerve biopsy demonstrate changes varying from demyelination to axonal degeneration. Deposition of immunoglobulins on the nerves is rare. Organomegaly can include splenomegaly, hepatomegaly, or enlarged lymph nodes. Endocrinopathic disease can take on any of multiple forms, including mild to insulin-requiring diabetes mellitus, amenorrhea, hyperprolactinemia, hyperestrogenemia, and hypothyroidism. The last is usually present in 40% to 60% of the cases. Nearly all monoclonal proteins show lambda light-chain specificity. The skin lesions (either local or general) also vary widely, ranging from hyperpigmentation to telangiectatic changes. Thrombocytosis occurs in 40% of the patients and polycythemia in 20% of the patients. The bone marrow usually contains less than 5% plasma cells, and the serum monoclonal protein is only modestly elevated. Although patients experience substantial morbidity from neuropathy and other disease manifestations, survival is much longer than in other patients with multiple myeloma.

Plasmacytomas

Focal collections of malignant plasma cells can present as a solitary plasmacytoma of bone or as a solitary soft-tissue plasmacytoma. The former is virtually always the forerunner of disseminated multiple myeloma, whereas the latter can be truly localized and should be viewed as a potentially curable lesion.

Solitary Plasmacytoma of Bone

The relative frequency of multiple myeloma to solitary plasmacytoma of bone is 20:1, and the male:female ratio is 2:1. The median age is approximately 55 years—ten years younger than in multiple myeloma.

Less than 1% of patients with monoclonal gammopathy of undetermined significance develop solitary plasmacytoma of bone.

Diagnostic Criteria

The criteria for the diagnosis vary, but generally include the following:

- a single area of bone destruction due to a clonal collection of plasma cells
- normal bone marrow without evidence of clonal plasma cell disease
- normal skeletal survey and normal magnetic resonance imaging of the spine, pelvis, proximal femurs, and humeri
- no anemia, hypercalcemia, or renal impairment attributable to multiple myeloma
- low concentration of serum or urine monoclonal protein, with uninvolved immunoglobulins usually normal

Clinical Picture

Solitary plasmacytoma of bone can involve any bone but has a predisposition for the red marrow-containing axial skeleton. Spine disease is seen in 50% of patients. The thoracic vertebrae are most commonly involved, followed by lumbar, sacral, and cervical vertebrae. The rib, the sternum, the clavicle, or the scapula are involved in 20% of cases.

The most common symptom is pain due to bone destruction by the infiltrating plasma cell tumor, but patients with vertebral involvement can also have evidence of spinal cord or nerve root compression, and pathological fractures of the long bones can occur. Rarely, patients with solitary plasmacytoma of bone present with peripheral polyneuropathy or with features consistent with POEMS syndrome (see preceding section).

Laboratory Findings and Histopathology

Serum protein electrophoresis reveals a low level of monoclonal protein in the serum or urine in only slightly more than one-half of the patients, reflecting the low tumor burden. The uninvolved immunoglobulin levels are usually normal. The peripheral blood cell counts, renal function, and calcium are normal.

Although the bone marrow biopsy is normal, biopsy of the lesion itself shows infiltration of the bone by monoclonal plasma cells that can be documented by their kappa or lambda light-chain specificity.

Imaging Studies

Solitary plasmacytoma of bone has a lytic appearance on plain radiographs, with clear margins and a narrow zone of transition to normal surrounding bone. Rarely, a cystic, trabeculated lesion resembling a giant-cell tumor or an aneurysmal bone cyst is seen. Sclerotic lesions can be seen in the POEMS syndrome. Computed tomography (CT) depicts the extent of the infiltrating lesion, but magnetic resonance imaging is the preferred imaging study. The magnetic resonance imaging appearance of solitary plasmacytoma of bone resembles that of other primary or secondary malignancies that produce lytic lesions of bone and focal areas of bone marrow replacement. The signal intensity is similar to muscle on T1-weighted images and hyperintense relative to muscle on T2-weighted images. An extraosseous soft-tissue component can be identified extending into the spinal cord or spinal nerve roots.

Treatment

Local radiation therapy is the treatment of choice. Treatment fields should be designed to encompass all disease seen on magnetic resonance imaging and a margin of surrounding apparently normal tissue. For spinal lesions, the margins should include at least one uninvolved vertebra above and below the lesion. Local control is achieved in 88% to 100% of patients, and the local tumor recurrence rate is less than 10%. On plain radiographic evaluation, resolution of the lesion will be accompanied in approximately one-half of the patients by sclerotic changes and bone remineralization. On follow-up magnetic resonance imaging studies, however, abnormalities of the bone and surrounding soft tissue can persist in spite of a good response to treatment. The optimal dose of radiation therapy is not established, but most centers use approximately 4000 cGy for spinal lesions and 4500 cGy for other bone lesions. The local recurrence rate increases from 10% to 36% if doses less than 4000 cGy are used. Although the level of the protein markedly diminishes after radiation therapy in the majority of patients, it disappears in less than one-half of the patients, which indicates that residual malignant plasma cells remain outside of the radiation treatment field.

Rarely, rapid neurologic dysfunction leads to anterior laminectomy in the case of spinal lesions and, on occasion, vertebral instability can require surgical fixation. Chemotherapy does not improve the prognosis or prevent subsequent development of multiple myeloma.

Prognosis

Despite the high rate of local control with radiation therapy, the majority of solitary plasmacytomas of bone progress inexorably to multiple myeloma. The median time to the diagnosis of multiple myeloma is 2 to 5 years, and 65% to 84% of patients have developed the disease at 10 years.

Prognostic features favoring the early development of multiple myeloma include the following:

- lesion size equal to or more than 5 cm
- age greater than 40 years
- elevated levels of monoclonal protein in the serum or urine
- persistence of the monoclonal protein after treatment
- spinal lesions

Soft-Tissue Plasmacytoma

Soft-tissue plasmacytomas (STP) constitute 3% of all plasma-cell neoplasms. Although this type of tumor can occur in any site, 90% develop in the head and neck and principally involve areas of the upper respiratory tract, such as the paranasal sinuses, pharynx, nasal cavity, or oral mucosa. Chronic inflammation from inhaled irritants and/or viruses might play a role in the pathogenesis. The median age at presentation is 50 to 60 years, and men account for three-quarters of the cases.

Diagnosis

The differential diagnosis includes reactive plasmacytosis, poorly differentiated cancer, immunoblastic lymphoma, marginal zone B-cell lymphoma, and plasma cell granuloma. Criteria for the diagnosis of soft tissue plasmacytoma include:

- biopsy of tissue showing monoclonal plasma cells
- bone marrow plasma cells are equal to or less than 5% of all nucleated cells
- absence of osteolytic bone lesions or other tissue involvement
- absence of hypercalcemia, anemia, or renal failure
- serum monoclonal protein present in relatively low concentration

Clinical Picture

Because the usual location of the lesion is in submucosal lesions in the upper aerodigestive tract, nasal discharge, epistaxis, nasal obstruction, sore throat, hoarseness, dysphonia, dysphagia, or hemoptysis are common clinical manifestations. Isolated cases of involvement of the central nervous system, gastrointestinal tract, or other organs as well as of the mediastinum (associated with myasthenia gravis) or thyroid gland (associated with Hashimoto's thyroiditis) have been reported. In 30% to 40% of cases, the first echelon of lymph node is involved at presentation or at relapse.

Laboratory Findings and Histopathology

A monoclonal protein is present in less than one-quarter of cases, and hypogammaglobulinemia is very rare. The peripheral blood cell counts, renal function, and calcium are normal, and the bone marrow biopsy shows less than 5% plasma cells without evidence of clonality. Biopsy of the lesion reveals infiltration by monoclonal plasma cells. Because of the submucosal growth, deep or open biopsies or (depending on the location) even complete excision of the tumor could be required to establish the diagnosis.

Imaging Studies

Radiographic assessment shows local bone destruction in most of the patients with nasal cavity or maxillary sinus involvement. Computed tomography and magnetic resonance imaging and a complete endoscopic examination of the aerodigestive and gastrointestinal tracts are required to determine the exact extent of tumor and its resectability.

Treatment

The goal of therapy in this disease is cure. Radiation therapy alone, given the radiation sensitivity of plasma-cell tumors, is an accepted treatment. Surgery, when a lesion can be completely resected, achieves the same results as radiation therapy. Combined modality therapy using surgery and radiation therapy can also be employed, depending on the location and respectability of the lesion. Combination treatment might even provide the best results. The optimal dose for local control is 5000 cGy (higher than in solitary plasmacytoma of bone) given in 200 cGy fractions. Because of the high rate of regional lymph node involvement, the first lymph node echelon should be included in the radiation field. Local control rates are 80% to 100%. The most common sites of spread outside of the primary are to bone and soft tissues, predominantly lymph nodes. When soft-tissue plasmacytoma progresses to multiple myeloma, bony lesions do not show a predilection for the axial skeleton. As in solitary plasmacytoma of bone, there is no role for chemotherapy unless progression to multiple myeloma ensues.

Prognosis

The 10-year disease-specific survival rate is 50% to 90%. Progression to multiple myeloma is lower than in solitary plasmacytoma of bone. In a review of 721 cases, Alexiou et al noted that 65% of patients were free of recurrence, 22% recurred locally, and 15% evolved into multiple myeloma. Overall prognosis for these patients is much better than for patients with solitary plasmacytoma of bone, even after conversion to multiple myeloma.

Amyloidosis

Amyloidosis can occur on a secondary basis from chronic infections or chronic inflammatory states. In these circumstances, a protein A is produced that is deposited progressively in the form of amyloid. Protein A is not related to immunoglobulins. In primary amyloidosis, the variable portion of the immunoglobulin light chain is the source of the protein in amyloid. It is more often derived from a monoclonal lambda light chain than from kappa light chain in a ratio of 3:1. This form of amyloidosis results from a clonal plasma cell proliferative process. The disease is called light-chain amyloidosis; it is called primary amyloidosis when it is associated with a monoclonal gammopathy without evidence of underlying multiple myeloma. Amyloid has a homogeneous, amorphous appearance under the light microscope and stains pink with hematoxylin and eosin. Congo red stains positively under a polarizing microscope.

Amyloid infiltration can cause hepatomegaly, splenomegaly, and macroglossia. Involvement of different organs produces varying symptoms and findings. For example, amyloid deposition can occur in the heart (cardiomyopathy), kidneys (nephrotic syndrome), vasa vasorum of peripheral nerves (neuropathy), gastrointestinal tract (malabsorption), and skin (cutaneous plaques). Amyloidosis should be considered when any of the clinical events above occur with insidious onset. Weakness, fatigue, and weight loss are the most frequent symptoms. Symptoms of congestive heart failure can predominate, and light-headedness and syncope can appear due to cardiac arrhythmias or orthostatic hypotension that often accompanies the disease.

Aspiration of the abdominal fat and histologic stains (such as Congo red) for amyloid are useful, as this aspirate is positive in more than 80% of patients. A bone marrow aspirate and biopsy specimen should be obtained to determine the degree of plasmacytosis and the likelihood of multiple myeloma or one of its variants. Congo red stain of the bone marrow biopsy is positive in more than 50% of patients with amyloidosis. If the abdominal fat and bone marrow biopsies are negative, a rectal biopsy should be taken that includes the submucosa. This biopsy is positive in approximately 80% of the patients. If all these sites are negative, tissue should be obtained from an involved organ. Approximately 10% of patients with multiple myeloma develop amyloidosis, and 15% to 20% of patients with primary amyloidosis ultimately prove to have multiple myeloma.

The presence of amyloidosis in a patient with multiple myeloma worsens the prognosis. The median survival for amyloidosis is approximately two years. More than one-half of the patients die secondary to cardiac involvement. Treatment with chemotherapy, such as is used in multiple myeloma, can reduce the amount of monoclonal protein secretion in primary or secondary amyloidosis, but it rarely has any substantial clinical impact on the amyloid deposition that has occurred previously. Recent reports from single centers show a decrease in amyloid deposition and its symptoms and an apparent increase in survival in patients with primary amyloidosis who undergo high-dose therapy and autologous stem cell transplantation.

Macroglobulinemia

In the normal response to antigenic stimulation, lymphocytes proliferate and produce polyclonal immunoglobulins M (IgM) and D in the first weeks. In time, a wide range of plasma cells differentiate from the lymphocytes and produce durable levels of polyclonal antibodies of the immunoglobulin G, A, and E types. In neoplastic transformation of these cells, a monoclonal protein is secreted. Given the normal sequence, it is no surprise that monoclonal production of a monoclonal immunoglobulin M protein is a result of a lymphoid or lymphoplasmacytic neoplasm. Monoclonal immunoglobulin M is detectable on serum protein electrophoresis in a number of circumstances (Table 63-4). In surveys of laboratory results of protein electrophoresis and immunofixation, without regard to clinical findings, the incidence of diagnoses associated with an immunoglobulin M monoclonal protein is: monoclonal gammopathy of undetermined significance in approximately 55%; Waldenström's macroglobulinemia in 30%; non–Hodgkin's lymphoma in 10%; chronic lymphocytic leukemia in 4%; and amyloidosis in 1%. As immunoglobulin M is a large multimer, its accumulation in the serum can cause hyperviscosity changes that result in clinical symptomatology, called Waldenström macroglobulinemia. Clinically and biologically, Waldenström macroglobulinemia behaves like a lymphoma rather than like myeloma. Immunoglobulin M-producing multiple myeloma is very rare, requiring the presence of lytic bone lesions and a biopsy showing an exclusively plasma cell infiltrate.

Table 63-4 ■ Causes of Monoclonal Macroglobulinemia

Monoclonal gammopathy of undetermined significance
Chronic lymphocytic leukemia
Non-Hodgkin's lymphoma, usually of the diffuse small lymphocytic type
Cold agglutinin disease
Waldenström macroglobulinemia
Amyloidosis
Immunoglobulin M-secreting multiple myeloma (very rare)

Waldenström Macroglobulinemia

Under the Revised European-American Lymphoma classification of lymphoid neoplasms, Waldenström's macroglobulinemia is included in the low-grade lymphomas, under the classification of lymphoplasmacytoid lymphoma/immunocytoma. Waldenström macroglobulinemia is an infrequent disease that affects approximately 1500 Americans each year. The median age of the affected patients is about 65 years, and the disease is significantly more common among whites than blacks, with a slight male preponderance. The etiology of Waldenström macroglobulinemia is unknown, but a genetic predisposition has been suggested by the identification of family clusters and by the concordance of the disease in monozygotic twins. Occupational exposure may play a role, but clear-cut associations are not established.

Clinical Features

Presenting symptoms usually relate to one or more of the processes, such as the hyperviscosity syndrome, described shortly. Physical examination is consistent with a lymphoma, with hepatosplenomegaly and lymphadenopathy occuring in 30% and 40% of patients, respectively. Hepatomegaly without splenomegaly is relatively uncommon. Unlike multiple myeloma, bone pain and lytic lesions of bone are rarely seen. The complete blood count often shows varying degrees of cytopenias, in part due to marrow infiltration, the anemia of chronic disease, and hypersplenism. Levels of normal immunoglobulins are reduced.

Hyperviscosity Syndrome

Immunoglobulin M is a large pentameric molecule, two-thirds of which is in the intravascular space. An increased concentration of this monoclonal protein can result in an increase of plasma viscosity and an expansion of plasma volume; blood circulation becomes sluggish, and the hyperviscosity syndrome occurs. Symptoms usually appear when the relative serum or plasma viscosity is above 5 centipoise (normal values: 1.4 to 1.8 centipoise), and in such cases, the corresponding serum immunoglobulin M level is virtually always above 3 g/dL. The symptomatic threshold, however, varies from patient to patient, and some patients can tolerate higher levels without developing the hyperviscosity syndrome. At diagnosis, the hyperviscosity syndrome is clinically evident in approximately 20% of patients at presentation with Waldenström macroglobulinemia. Hyperviscosity results in congestive heart failure, bleeding from the mucous membranes of the gums and nose, blurring of vision, sensorineural hearing loss, and unsteadiness. Vascular changes of hyperviscosity can

be appreciated on fundoscopic examination, which reveals "sausageing" of the retinal veins. Paradoxically, although patients are at risk for hemorrhage, the hyperviscosity state also increases the risk of thrombosis, including myocardial infarction and stroke. Prompt correction of most of the abnormalities can be obtained by plasmapheresis to decrease the immunoglobulin M level. Plasmapheresis alleviates the symptoms and reduces the complication rate. This allows time for the institution of specific therapy and the development of a response. Typically, plasmapheresis of one to two blood volumes is performed over two successive days, then once or twice a week until therapy takes effect.

Cryoglobulinemia

Cryoglobulins are serum proteins or protein complexes that undergo reversible precipitation at low temperatures, such as exist in the skin and acral appendages. Type I cryoglobulins consist of monoclonal immunoglobulin M and are detected by laboratory studies in 10% to 20% of patients with Waldenström macroglobulinemia. The clinical syndrome of symptomatic cryoglobulinemia, which causes Raynaud's phenomenon, vasculitic lesions causing palpable purpura, or glomerulonephritis, occurs in less than 5% of patients with Waldenström macroglobulinemia.

Cold Agglutinin Disease

In approximately 10% of patients, the monoclonal immunoglobulin M has the characteristics of an antibody directed at the I antigen on the red blood cell surface. The antibody exhibits thermal amplitude demonstrated by a progressively increasing antibody titer (measured by red blood cell aggregation) as the temperature of the reaction is decreased. Patients may develop acrocyanosis or Raynaud's phenomenon along with an episodic or chronic hemolytic process, usually of moderate severity.

Neurologic Manifestations

Polyneuropathy develops in 10% of patients with Waldenström macroglobulinemia. The etiology of the neuropathies is multifactorial and includes lymphoplasmacytic infiltration of the nerves, development of antibodies directed against neural glycoproteins or glycolipids, cryoglobulinemia, and amyloid deposition. Of the various causes, demyelinating polyneuropathy due to immunoglobulin M antimyelin-associated glycoprotein (MAG) antibodies is the most common form, and the form most likely to be reversible with therapy.

In this circumstance, the monoclonal immunoglobulin M acts as an antibody directed against myelin-associated glycoprotein, a 100-kDa glycoprotein of the central and peripheral-nerve myelin, as well as against other glycoproteins or glycolipids that share antigenic determinants with myelin-associated glycoprotein. Most patients with antimyelin-associated glycoprotein antibodies present with sensory complaints of numbness, paresthesias, imbalance, and gait ataxia caused by lack of proprioception. Some patients experience aching discomfort, dysesthesias, or lancinating pains. Weakness of the distal leg muscles with variable atrophy occurs as the illness advances. Nerve conduction studies are consistent with demyelination characterized by slow conduction velocity and by prolonged distal motor and sensory latencies. Conduction block is uncommon. The amplitude of the muscle action potential can be diminished by a progressive loss of axons as the disease progresses. The needle electromyogram often shows denervation potentials caused by a concomitant axonal degeneration.

Laboratory Findings

The malignant B cells express monoclonal surface and cytoplasmic immunoglobulin M, and a variable proportion of cells can coexpress immunoglobulin D. The level of surface immunoglobulin correlates with the morphology of the neoplastic cells; small lymphocytes express high levels, lymphoplasmacytoid cells express low levels, and plasma cells express no surface immunoglobulin. A number of B-cell antigens (CD19, CD20, CD21, CD22, and CD24) are expressed on the cells; the CD23 antigen is usually absent.

Bone marrow aspirate and biopsy show a variable mixture of malignant lymphocytes, plasma cells, and lymphoplasmocytic cells. Bone marrow cell cytogenetics disclose trisomies or deletions of chromosomes 10, 11, 12, 15, 20, and 21 in 30% of patients, and many of these are complex (multiple) karyotypic abnormalities. Translocations involving the 14q32 band where the immunoglobulin heavy chain gene resides have been found as well, including the t(14;18)(q32;q21) found in follicular lymphomas and the t(8;14)(q24;q32) noted in Burkitt's-type lymphomas.

Therapy

Except for the management of disease-specific manifestations like the hyperviscosity syndrome, therapy conforms to that used in other low-grade lymphomas (see Chapter 66). Chemotherapy with alkylating agents with or without corticosteroids has been the standard primary therapy for patients with symptomatic macroglobulinemia. The agent most commonly used is oral chlorambucil. Daily oral chlorambucil or intermittent pulses of oral chlorambucil are equally effective, resulting in a median survival of 5.4 years. The combination of chlorambucil and prednisone is associated with response and survival rates similar to those obtained by single-agent chlorambucil. Corticosteroids can be helpful if a warm antibody hemolytic anemia is present, but cold agglutinin disease is rarely responsive to this therapy. The anti-CD20 antibody rituximab and the purine analog fludarabine are also effective in Waldenström macroglobulinemia and will probably replace alkylating agent therapy in the future, decreasing the risks of secondary myelodysplasia/acute myeloid leukemia. Fludarabine has to be used with care. Fludarabine decreases the population of T-lymphocytes, adding impaired cellular immunity to the humoral immunity already compromised by the disease process.

References

Multiple Myeloma

General Information

Alexiou C, Kau RJ, Dietzfelbinger H, et al: Extra medullary plasmacytoma: Tumor occurence and therapeutic concepts. Cancer 1999;85:2305–2314.

Anderson KC, Lust JA: Role of cytokines in multiple myeloma. Semin Hematol 1999;36:14.

Bartl R, Frisch B, Fateh-Moghadam A, et al: Histologic classification and staging of multiple myeloma. A retrospective and prospective study of 674 cases. Am J Clin Pathol 1987;87:342.

Brown LM, Gridley G, Pottern LM, et al: Diet and nutrition as risk factors for multiple myeloma among blacks and whites in the United States. Cancer Causes Control 2001; 12:117–125.

Kyle RA, Therneau TM, Rajkumar SV, et al: A long-term study of prognosis in monoclonal gammopathy of undetermined significance. N Engl J Med 2002;346:564–569.

Roodman GD: Biology of osteoclast activation in cancer. J Clin Oncol 2001;19:3562–3571.

Bone Disease and Hypercalcemia

Berenson JR, Lichtenstein A, Porter L, et al: Efficacy of pamidronate in reducing skeletal events in patients with advanced multiple myeloma. The Myeloma Aredia Study Group. N Engl J Med 1996;334:488–493.

Berenson JR, Lichtenstein A, Porter L, et al: Long-term pamidronate treatment of advanced multiple myeloma patients reduces skeletal events. The Myeloma Aredia Study Group. J Clin Oncol 1998;16:593–602.

Dudeney S, Lieberman IH, Reinhardt M-K, et al: Kyphoplasty in the treatment of osteolytic vertebral compression fractures as a result of multiple myeloma. J Clin Oncol 2002;20:2382–2387.

Lacey DL, Timms E, Tan H-L, et al: Osteoprotegerin ligand is a cytokine that regulates osteoclast differentiation and activation. Cell 1998;93:165–176.

Major P, Lortholary A, Hon J, et al: Zoledronic acid is superior to pamidronate in the treatment of hypercalcemia of malignancy: A pooled analysis of two randomized, controlled clinical trials. J Clin Oncol 2001;19:558–567.

Morony S, Capparelli C, Lee R, et al: A chimeric form of osteoprotegerin inhibits hypercalcemia and bone resorption induced by IL-1B, TNFa, PTH, PTHrP, and 1,25-dihydroxyvitamin D3. J Bone Mineral Res 1999; 14:1478–1485.

Shalhoub V, Faust J, Boyle WJ, et al: Osteoprotegerin and osteoprotegerin ligand effects on osteoclast formation from human peripheral blood mononuclear cell precursors. J Cellular Biochem 1999;72:251–261.

Cytogenetics

Avet-Loiseau H, Facon T, Daviet A, et al: 14q32 Translocations and monosomy 13 observed in monoclonal gammopathy of undetermined significance delineate a multi-step process for the oncogenesis of multiple myeloma. Intergroupe Francophone du Myelome. Cancer Res 1999;59:4546.

Fonseca R, Harrington D, Oken MM, et al: Biological and prognostic significance of interphase fluorescence in situ hybridization detection of chromosome 13 abnormalities (Δ13) in multiple myeloma: An Eastern Cooperative Oncology Group Study. Cancer Res 2002;62:715–720.

Shaughnessy J, Barlogie B: Chromosome 13 deletion in myeloma. Curr Top Microbiol Immunol 1999;246:199.

Shaughnessy J, Tian E, Sawyer J, et al: High incidence of chromosome 13 deletion in multiple myeloma detected by multiprobe interphase FISH. Blood 2000;96:1505–1511.

Smadja NV, Bastard C, Brigadeau C, et al: Hypoploidy is a major prognostic factor in multiple myeloma. Blood 2001;98: 2229–2238.

Tricot G, Sawyer J, Jagannath S, et al: Poor prognosis in multiple myeloma is associated only with partial or complete deletion of chromosome 13 or abnormalities involving 11 q and not with other karyotype abnormalities. 1995;Blood 86:4250.

High-Dose Therapy and Allogeneic or Autologous Stem Cell Transplantation

Alyea E, Weller E, Schlossman R, et al: T-cell-depleted allogeneic bone marrow transplantation followed by donor lymphocyte infusion in patients with multiple myeloma: Induction of graft-versus-myeloma effect. Blood 2001; 98:934–939.

Attal M, Herousseau JL, Stoppa AM, et al: A prospective, randomized trial of autologous bone marrow transplantation and chemotherapy in multiple myeloma. Intergroupe Francais du Myelome. N Engl J Med 1996;335:91–97.

Badros A, Barlogie B, Siegel E, et al: Autologous stem cell transplantation in elderly multiple myeloma patients over the age of 70 years. Br J Haematol 2001;114:600–607.

Badros A, Barlogie B, Siegel E, et al: Improved outcome of allogeneic transplantation in high-risk multiple myeloma patients after nonmyeloablative conditioning. J Clin Oncol 2002;20:1295–1303.

Bellucci R, Alyea EP, Weller E, et al: Immunologic effects of prophylactic donor lymphocyte infusion after allogeneic marrow transplantation in multiple myeloma. Blood 2002; 99:4610–4617.

Bkorkstrand B, Svensson H, Goldschmidt H, et al: Alpha-interferon maintenance treatment is associated with improved survival after high-dose treatment and autologous stem cell transplantation in patients with multiple myeloma: a retrospective registry study from the European Group for Blood and Marrow transplantation (EBMT) Bone Marr Transplant 2001;27:511–515.

Blade J, San Miguel JF, Fontanillas M, et al: Survival of multiple myeloma patients who are potential candidates for early high-dose therapy intensification/autotransplantation and who were conventionally treated. J Clin Oncol 1996;14:2167–2173.

Fermand JP, Ravaud P, Chevret S, et al: High-dose therapy and autologous peripheral blood stem cell transplantation in multiple myeloma: Up-front or rescue treatment? Results of a multicenter sequential randomized clinical trial. Blood 1998;92:3131–3136.

LeBlanc R, Montminy-Metivier S, Belanger R, et al: Allogeneic transplantation for multiple myeloma: Further evidence for a GVHD-associated graft-versus-myeloma effect. Bone Marr Transplant 2001;28:841–848.

Moreau P, Facon T, Attal M, et al: Comparison of 200 mg/m² melphalan and 8 Gy total body irradiation plus 140 mg/m² melphalan as conditioning regimens for peripheral blood stem cell transplantation in patients with newly diagnosed multiple myeloma: final analysis of the Intergroupe Francophone du Myelome 9502 randomized trial. Blood 2002;99:731–735.

Stewart AK, Vescio R, Schiller G, et al: Purging of autologous peripheral-blood stem cells using CD 34 selection does not improve overall or progression-free survival after high-dose chemotherapy for multiple myeloma: Results of a multicenter randomized controlled trial. J Clin Oncol 2001;19:3771–3779.

Vesole DH, Simic A, Lazarus HM: Controversy in mutltiple myeloma transplants: tandem autotransplants and mini-allografts. Bone Marr Transplant 2001;28:725–735.

Thalidomide Therapy

Barlogie B, Zinger M, Spencer T, et al: Thalidomide in the management of multiple myeloma. Semin Hematol 2001; 38:250–259.

Davies FE, Raja N, Midshipman T, et al: Thalidomide and immunomodulatory derivatives augment natural killer cell cytotoxicity in multiple myeloma. Blood 2001;98:210–216.

Kyle RA, Rajkumar SV: Therapeutic application of thalidomide in multiple myeloma. Semin Oncol 2001;28:583–587.

Mitsiades N, Mitsiades CS, Poulaki V, et al: Apoptotic signaling induced by immunomodulatory thalidomide analogs (Imids) in human multiple myeloma cells: Therapeutic implications [abstract 3224]. Blood 2001;98:775a.

Moehler TM, Nebenm K, Benner A, et al: Salvage therapy for multiple myeloma with thalidomide and CED chemotherapy. Blood 2001;98:3846–3848.

Rajkumar SV, Witzig TE: A review of angiogenesis and antiangiogenic therapy with thalidomide in multiple myeloma. Cancer Treat Rev 2000;26:351–362.

Singhal S, Mehta J, Desikan R, et al: Antitumor activity of thalidomide in refractory multiple myeloma. N Engl J Med 1999;341:1565–1571.

Zangan M, Anaissie E, Barlogie B, et al: Increased risk of deep-vein thrombosis in patients with multiple myeloma receiving thalidomide and chemotherapy. Blood 2001; 98:1614–1615.

Therapy

Adams J, Palombella VJ, Elliott PJ: Proteasome inhibition: A new strategy in cancer treatment. Invest New Drugs 2000;18:109–121.

Alexanian R, Barlogie B, Dixon D: High-dose glucocorticoid treatment of resistant myeloma. Ann Intern Med 1986; 105:8–11.

Alexanian R, Haut A, Khan AU, et al: Treatment for multiple myeloma: Combination chemotherapy with different melphalan dose regimens. JAMA 1969;208:1680–1685.

Berenson JR, Crowley JJ, Grogan TM, et al: Maintenance therapy with alternate-day prednisone improves survival in multiple myeloma patients. Blood 2002;99:3163–3168.

Govindarajan R, Jagannath S, Flick J, et al: Preceding standard therapy is the likely cause of myelodysplasia after autotransplant for multiple myeloma. Br J Haematol 1996; 95:349.

Hussein MA: Arsenic trioxide: A new immunomodulatory agent in the management of multiple myeloma. Med Oncol 2001;18:239–242.

Hussein MA, Wood L, Hsi E, et al: A phase II trial of pegylated liposomal doxorubicin, vincristine, and reduced-dose dexamethasone combination therapy in newly diagnosed multiple myeloma patients. Cancer 2002;95:2160–2168.

Oken MM, Pomeroy C, Weisdorf D, Bennett JM: Prophylactic antibiotics for the prevention of early infection in multiple myeloma. Am J Med 1996;100:624–628.

Samson D, Gaminara E, Newland A, et al: Infusion of vincristine and doxorubicin with oral dexamethasone as first-line therapy for multiple myeloma. Lancet 1989;2:882–885.

Sirohi B, Kulkami S, Powles R: Some early phase II trials in previously untreated multiple myeloma. The Royal Marsden experience. Semin Hematol 2001;38:209–218.

Amyloidosis

Bellotti V, Mangione P, Merlini G: Review: immunoglobulin light chain amyloidosis: The archetype of structural and pathogenic variability. J Struct Biol 2000;130:280–289.

Cabelleria J, Bruguera N, Sole M, et al: Hepatic familial amyloidosis caused by a new mutation in the apoliprotein A1 gene: clinical and pathological features. Am J Gastroenterol 2001;96:18772–18776.

Comenzo RI, Gertz MA: Autologous stem cell transplantation for primary systemic amyloidosis. Blood 2002;99: 4276–4282.

Cunnane G: Amyloid precursors and amyloidosis in inflammatory arthritis. Curr Opin Rheumatol 2001;13:67–73.

Danesh F, Ho LT: Dialysis-related amyloidosis: history and clinical manifestations. Semin Dial 2001;14:80–85.

Dispenzieri A, Lacy MQ, Kyle RA, et al: Eligibility for hematopoietic stem-cell transplantation for primary systemic amyloidosis is a favorable prognostic factor for survival. J Clin Oncol 2001;19:3350–3356.

Gertz MA, Lacy MQ, Gastineau DA, et al: Blood stem cell transplantation as therapy for primary systemic amyloidosis. Bone Marrow Transplant 2000;26:963–969.

Gertz MA, Rajkumar SV: Primary systemic amyloidosis. Curr Treat Options Oncol 2002;3:261–271.

Hull KM, Kastner DL, Balow JE: Hereditary periodic fever. N Engl J Med 2002;346:1415–1416.

Kyle RA, Therneau TM, Rajkumar SV, et al: A long-term study if prognosis in monoclonal gammopathy if undetermined significance. N Engl J Med 2002;346:564–569.

Nestle FO, Burg G: Bilateral carpal tunnel syndrome as a clue for the diagnosis of systemic amyloidosis. Dermatol 2001; 202:353–355.

Waldenström Macroglobulinemia

Bueso-Ramos CE: Cytogenetic findings in lymphoplasmacytic lymphoma/Waldenström macroglobulinemia. Chromosome abnormalities are associated with the polymorphous subtype and an aggressive clinical course. Am J Clin Pathol 2001;116:543–549.

Desikan KR, Dhodapkar MV, Barlogie B: Waldenström macroglobulinemia. Curr Treat Opt Oncol 2000;1:97–103.

Dhodapkar MV, Jacobson JL, Gertz MA, et al: Prognostic factors and response to fludarabine therapy in patients with Waldenström macroglobulinemia: Results of United States intergroup trial (Southwest Oncology Group S90003). Blood 2001;98:41–48.

Dimopoulos MA, Panayiondis P, Moulopoulos LA, et al: Waldenström macroglobulinemia: Clinical features, complications, and management. J Clin Oncol 2000;18: 214–226.

Dimopoulos MA, Zomas A, Viniou NA, et al: Treatment of Waldenström macroglobulinemia with thalidomide. J Clin Oncol 2001;19:3596–3601.

Dimopoulos MA, Zervas C, Zomas A, et al: Treatment of Waldenström macroglobulinemia with rituximab. J Clin Oncol 2002;2327–2333.

Drew MJ: Plasmapheresis in the dysproteinemias. Therap Apheresis 2002;6:45–52.

Leblond V, Levy V, Maloisel F, et al: Multicenter, randomized comparative trial of fludarabine and the combination of cyclophosphamide-doxorubicin-prednisone in 92 patients with Waldenström macroglobulinemia in first relapse or with primary refractory disease. Blood 2001;98: 2640–2644.

Libow LF, Mawhinney JP, Bessinger GT: Cutaneous Waldenström macroglobulinemia: report of a case and overview of the spectrum of cutaneous disease. J Am Acad Dermatol 2001;45(6 Suppl):S202–206.

Owen RG, Barrans SL, Richards SJ, et al: Waldenström macroglobulinemia. Development of diagnostic criteria and identification of prognostic factors. Am J Clin Pathol 2001;116:420–428.

Syms MJ, Arcila ME, Holtel MR: Waldenström macroglobulinemia and sensorineural hearing loss. Am J Otolaryngol 2001;22:349–353.

Tetrault SA, Saven A: Delayed onset of autoimmune hemolytic anemia complicating cladribine therapy for Waldenström macroglobulinemia. Leuk Lymph 2000;37:125–130.

Treon SP, Anderson KC: The use of rituximab in the treatment of malignant and non-malignant plasma cell disorders. Semin Oncol 2000;27:79–85.

Chapter 64
Diagnosis of Malignant Lymphoma and Hodgkin's Disease

Gerald E. Byrne, Jr. and Clarence C. Whitcomb

Classifications of malignant lymphoma (non-Hodgkin's lymphoma) and of Hodgkin's disease have become more complex as our understanding of their biology has improved. In 1966, the Rappaport classification of non-Hodgkin's lymphoma included only eight distinct entities, each of which was defined solely by histopathologic features observed in sections of fixed tumor tissue. Today, immunophenotypic characteristics of the neoplastic cells are used for diagnosis as well as morphologic features. A current classification, the Revised European-American Lymphoma (REAL) classification developed by the European-American Lymphoma Study Group, includes more than 28 categories. Many of the entities that are recognized in this and other classification systems were unknown 30 years ago. Classification of Hodgkin's disease has remained essentially unchanged since the Rye conference modification of the Lukes-Butler classification in 1966, but recent studies have led to refinements in the nomenclature of this disorder as well.

A new nosology of hematolymphoid neoplasia, the World Health Organization (WHO) Classification of Lymphoid Neoplasms, has been published (Table 64-1). This comprehensive classification incorporates most of the entities defined within the current REAL system, organizing individual diagnostic entities into three major groups: B cell neoplasms, T cell and NK cell neoplasms, and Hodgkin's disease. Within each group, individual entities are distinguished by their immunophenotypic as well as histopathologic features. For some entities, cytogenetic characteristics may also be needed for accurate diagnosis. This discussion will review diagnostic features of Hodgkin's disease and of the more frequently encountered types of non-Hodgkin's lymphoma with specific reference to the concepts and terminology embodied in the new World Health Organization classification.

Accurate and complete diagnosis of lymphoid neoplasms using this new classification will require integration of findings from several different studies. Traditional histopathologic observations alone may suffice for diagnosis of some entities, but in many cases, immunohistochemical staining techniques or flow cytometry analysis of intact tumor cells is needed to characterize the immunophenotype of the abnormal cells. In some cases, molecular analysis of DNA extracted from tumor tissue may be required as well. To ensure that materials appropriate for all necessary diagnostic studies will be available, careful handling of biopsy tissues at the outset is of critical importance. Issues of tissue preparation are discussed in the accompanying management box.

Malignant Lymphoma

Neoplasms of Lymphoid Precursor Cells

This category includes precursor B cell lymphoblastic leukemia/lymphoma (precursor B cell acute lymphoblastic leukemia) and precursor T cell lymphoblastic leukemia/lymphoma (precursor T cell acute lymphoblastic leukemia) (see Chapter 61).

The term *lymphoblastic* denotes an immature lymphoid precursor cell. Both lymphoblastic leukemia and lymphoblastic lymphoma are neoplasms of lymphoid precursor cells. The neoplastic cells may be of either B cell or T cell lineage, and the cellular proliferation may present clinically either as acute lymphoblastic leukemia or as a tissue tumor without conspicuous peripheral blood or bone marrow involvement. In the tumoral form (lymphoblastic lymphoma), the neoplastic cells are almost always of T cell lineage; lymphoblastic lymphomas of precursor B cells is extremely rare. In lymphoblastic leukemia, the neoplastic cells are most often precursor B cells, but precursor T cell acute lymphoblastic leukemia is by no means uncommon.

Histologic and cytologic features are similar in both precursor B and precursor T lymphoblastic leukemia/lymphoma. The lymphoblastic cells have

Table 64-1 ■ Proposed WHO Classification of Lymphoid Neoplasms

B cell neoplasms
Precursor B cell neoplasm
   Precursor B lymphoblastic leukemia/lymphoma (precursor
      B cell acute lymphoblastic leukemia)
Mature (peripheral) B cell neoplasms
   B cell chronic lymphocytic leukemia/small lymphocytic
      lymphoma
   B cell prolymphocytic leukemia
   Lymphoplasmacytic lymphoma
   Splenic marginal zone B cell lymphoma (+/– villous
      lymphocytes)
   Hairy cell leukemia
   Plasma cell myeloma/plasmacytoma
   Extranodal marginal zone B cell lymphoma (+/– monocytoid
      B cells)
   Nodal marginal zone B cell lymphoma (+/– monocytoid
      B cells)
   Follicular lymphoma
   Mantle cell lymphoma
   Diffuse large B cell lymphoma
      Mediastinal large B cell lymphoma
      Primary effusion lymphoma
   Burkitt's lymphoma/Burkitt cell leukemia
T cell and NK cell neoplasms
Precursor T cell neoplasm
   Precursor T lymphoblastic leukemia/lymphoma (precursor
      T cell acute lymphoblastic leukemia)
Mature (peripheral) T cell neoplasms
   T cell prolymphocytic leukemia
   T cell granular lymphocytic leukemia
   Aggressive NK cell leukemia
   Adult T cell lymphoma/leukemia (HTLV1+)
   Extranodal NK/T cell lymphoma, nasal type
   Enteropathy-type T cell lymphoma
   Hepatosplenic gamma-delta T cell lymphoma
   Subcutaneous panniculitislike T cell lymphoma
   Mycosis fungoides/Sézary syndrome
   Anaplastic large cell lymphoma, T/null cell, primary
      cutaneous type
   Peripheral T cell lymphoma, not otherwise characterized
   Angioimmunoblastic T cell lymphoma
   Anaplastic large cell lymphoma, T/null cell, primary systemic
      type
Hodgkin's disease
Nodular lymphocyte predominant Hodgkin's disease
Classical Hodgkin's disease
   Nodular sclerosis Hodgkin's disease (grades 1 and 2)
   Lymphocyte-rich classical Hodgkin's disease
   Mixed cellularity Hodgkin's disease
   Lymphocyte depletion Hodgkin's disease

scant cytoplasm, finely dispersed nuclear chromatin, and inconspicuous nucleoli. The cells may expand the paracortex (the T-zone) of involved lymph nodes or may diffusely obliterate normal nodal architectural features (Figure 64-1A). The nuclei may be ovoid, or they may have prominent nuclear invaginations, which impart a convoluted cytologic appearance (Figure 64-1B). Mitotic figures are typically abundant, and phagocytic histiocytes may be intermingled among the neoplastic cells, imparting a so-called starry-sky appearance.

Immunophenotype

Diagnosis of precursor B (or precursor T) lymphoblastic leukemia or lymphoma requires evidence of cellular immaturity, typically demonstrated by expression of either terminal deoxynucleotidyl transferase (TdT) or CD34 in the abnormal cells. Lineage associated markers are variably expressed. In precursor T lymphoblastic leukemia/lymphoma the cells usually express CD7, CD5, or CD2. If expressed on the cell surface CD3 is usually of low intensity, and in some cases, only cytoplasmic expression of this marker is seen. In many cases, CD4 and CD8 are both absent, but in others, both of these two markers may be coexpressed. Expression of CD1 in conjunction with other T cell markers may also be seen.

In precursor B lymphoblastic leukemia/lymphoma, the abnormal cells exhibit no surface immunoglobulin. Other B cell associated markers (CD19, CD79a, CD22) may be expressed, but CD20, if expressed, is typically of low intensity, as is the pan-leukocyte marker CD45. CD10 is often expressed and is an important prognostic marker in cases of precursor B acute lymphoblastic leukemia. Aberrant expression of CD13 does not exclude the diagnosis. Cells with "blastic" features may be seen in other hematolymphoid tumors. Histopathologic differential diagnosis of specimens with "blastic" features include large cell lymphoma, Burkitt's lymphoma, a "blastic" variant of mantle cell lymphoma, and granulocytic sarcoma (chloroma). Immunophenotypic characterization of the cells is essential for discriminating these entities.

Mature B Cell Neoplasms

B Cell Chronic Lymphocytic Leukemia/Small Lymphocytic Lymphoma

Three different types of B cell lymphoma, each composed predominantly of small lymphocytic cells, are recognized in the World Health Organization classification. Discrimination of these entities—B cell chronic lymphocytic leukemia/small lymphocytic lymphoma, mantle cell lymphoma, and nodal or extranodal marginal zone B cell lymphoma—can

DIAGNOSIS

Establishing a Pathologic Diagnosis for Malignant Lymphoma

Histopathologic examination of tissue sections from excised tumor tissue is still the primary method for establishing a pathologic diagnosis. In many cases, histologic sections with appropriate immunohistochemical stains will adequately demonstrate cell lineage (B cell or T cell) as well as characteristic cellular attributes used in diagnosing these neoplasms. In other cases, however, ancillary studies such as immunophenotyping by flow cytometry and/or analysis of cellular DNA for lymphocyte antigen receptor gene rearrangements may be required. Proper handling of diagnostic biopsy tissue to facilitate all necessary diagnostic techniques is critical to accurate and complete diagnosis.

The following are important in transporting the biopsy tissue:

Tumor tissue must remain unfixed until examined.
The tissue should be transported as rapidly as possible to the site of examination.
The tissue must not be allowed to desiccate; it may be transported in saline to prevent drying.
The tissue must not be frozen; viable cells are required if flow cytometric analysis is necessary.
Transportation on wet ice will retard degradation of DNA by endogenous nucleases.

When the specimen is sufficiently large, imprint preparations for cytologic evaluation should be prepared.

Imprints ("touch preps") are prepared by gently touching a glass slide to the surface of a portion of the fresh tissue. Separate "touches" may be made on each of several slides. Some of these slides may be fixed in alcohol for later Papanicolau staining, but others should be allowed to dry in air for subsequent staining with a polychrome stain (e.g., Wright or Wright-Giemsa).

The unfixed tissue is then apportioned into aliquots sufficient for the different studies:

1. An aliquot for histopathologic examination should be placed into neutral buffered formalin. If sufficient tissue is present, additional portions may be placed into B-5 or a zinc-based fixative, both of which provide superior morphologic detail.
2. An aliquot for flow cytometry analysis should be placed into sterile tissue culture medium and then transported as rapidly as possible to the laboratory where the examination will be performed. The tissue should not be subjected to extremes of temperature, and it must not be frozen.
3. An aliquot for DNA studies should be frozen without delay. The tissue may be directly immersed in liquid nitrogen or it may be immersed in isopentane, which is then rapidly cooled by liquid nitrogen. Once frozen, this aliquot may be safely stored at $-70°$ C to $-20°$ C for several years.

The diagnostic studies are selected as follows:

1. Histomorphologic examination with immunohistochemical staining can suffice in many cases, especially for lymphomas comprised of large lymphoid cells, for follicular lymphomas, and for Hodgkin's disease.
2. Flow cytometry analysis is most useful when the neoplastic cells are of B cell lineage and are small. Monoclonal B cell populations, characterized by immunoglobulin light chain restriction, as well as the expression by abnormal B cells of characteristic immunophenotypic features (e.g., CD5 or CD23) together with a useful quantification of antigen expression, are often more readily demonstrated by flow cytometry than by immunostaining.
3. DNA analysis for lymphoid cell antigen receptor gene rearrangements (e.g., immunoglobulin gene and T cell receptor gene rearrangements) are needed when an unequivocal determination of neoplasia cannot be made from the morphologic features. DNA analyses are particularly useful for tumors comprised of admixed small and large cells, or when a determination of cell lineage (B cell or T cell) cannot be established by other techniques.

be difficult. Differences between the three entities in their tempo of progression and response to chemotherapeutic regimens are significant concerns for clinical management. An association of extranodal marginal zone lymphoma, particularly gastric marginal zone lymphoma of mucosal-associated lymphoid tissue (MALT) type, with *Helicobacter pylori* infection provides a rationale for use of antimicrobial therapy in this particular type of lymphoma as well.

Chronic lymphocytic leukemia and small lymphocytic lymphoma of B cell lineage are considered to be the same disorder, differing only in clinical presentation (see Chapter 72). Lymph nodes in this disorder are diffusely effaced by a monotonous proliferation of small lymphocytes having round nuclei (Figure 64-1C). Larger lymphoid cells—called prolymphocytes or paraimmunoblasts—are typically intermingled and aggregates of these larger cells, termed pseudofollicles or growth centers, may be conspicuous. In some cases, the nuclei of the small lymphocytes may be slightly irregular in con-figuration; in such cases, distinction of B cell chronic lymphocytic leukemia/small

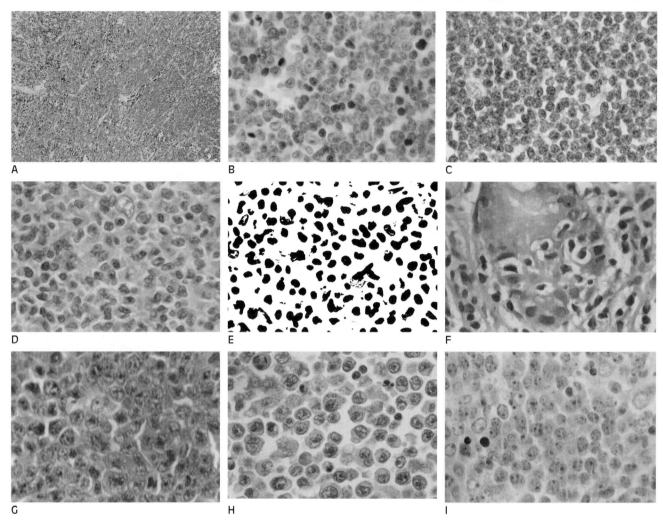

Figure 64-1 ■ *A*, Lymphoblastic lymphoma with diffuse pattern. *B*, Precursor T cell lymphoblastic lymphoma. *C*, B cell small lymphocytic lymphoma. *D*, Mantle cell lymphoma. *E*, Nodal marginal zone lymphoma (monocytoid cells). *F*, Lymphoepithelial lesion in extranodal marginal zone lymphoma of mucosal-associated lymphoid tissue type. *G*, Diffuse large B cell lymphoma. *H*, Diffuse large B cell lymphoma (plasma cell variant). *I*, Burkitt's lymphoma. (See Color Plate 15.)

lymphocytic lymphoma from other neoplasms of small lymphocytes will necessitate immunophenotypic characterization of the cells (Table 64-2).

Immunophenotype
The tumor cells in B cell chronic lymphocytic leukemia/small lymphocytic lymphoma express B cell associated antigens (CD19, CD20, CD79a) and monotypic surface immunoglobulin (SIg), but the intensity of expression of CD20 and SIg is typically rather weak. The cells characteristically express CD5 and usually CD23 as well but do not express CD10 (Table 64-2). The immunophenotype can be determined either by flow cytometry analysis of cell suspensions or by immunohistochemical staining of tissue sections.

Table 64-2 ■ **Flow Cytometric Immunophenotypes in the Small Lymphocytic Lymphoma Category**

	SIg	CD5	CD23	CD10
SLL/CLL	+	+	+	−
Mantle cell	+	+	−	−
Marginal zone	+	−	−/+ *	−
Follicular	+	−	−/+	+

*−/+ = less than 50% of cells are positive; SIg = surface immunoglobulin; SLL = small cell lymphocytic lymphoma; CLL = chronic lymphocytic leukemia.

Mantle Cell Lymphoma

The neoplastic cells may diffusely efface lymph nodes in mantle cell lymphoma, or the abnormal cells may expand the mantle zones surrounding germinal centers, creating a vague "nodular" appearance. The abnormal cells are small to medium in size. The nuclei are irregular and indented (Figure 64-1D). Large lymphoid cells are extremely rare in mantle cell lymphoma, and pseudofollicles/proliferation centers are not seen (see Chapter 67).

Immunophenotype

The neoplastic cells express B cell associated antigens (CD19, CD20, CD79a) and SIg with intermediate to strong intensity. The cells characteristically express CD5, but expression of CD10 and CD23 expression is not observed (Table 64-2). The cellular immunophenotype may be demonstrated either by flow cytometry or by immunohistochemical staining of tissue sections.

Demonstration of the nuclear protein cyclin D1 can be helpful for diagnosis of this entity. This protein is expressed strongly in mantle cell lymphoma but is not expressed strongly in other lymphomas of small lymphocytes (small B lymphocytic lymphoma or nodal marginal zone lymphoma). Cyclin D1 expression can be demonstrated by immunohistochemical staining. This feature of mantle cell lymphoma has been attributed to overexpression of the PRAD1 gene, which can result from a chromosomal translocation t(11;14). Demonstration of this cytogenetic abnormality may also be helpful for the diagnosis of mantle cell lymphoma.

Marginal Zone B Cell Lymphoma

Marginal zone B cell lymphoma may occur either as a nodal or extranodal tumor. Extranodal marginal zone B cell lymphoma frequently involves mucosal-associated lymphoid tissue. Gastrointestinal mucosal tissue is frequently involved, but this neoplasm has also been observed in the orbit, salivary gland, breast, spleen, skin, and lung. The category of marginal zone B cell lymphoma includes tumors that have been called monocytoid B cell lymphoma in the past (see Chapter 66).

The cellular population in marginal zone B cell lymphoma is usually heterogeneous. Small lymphocytes predominate, but plasma cells and occasionally larger lymphoid cells are often admixed. The nuclei of the small lymphocytes usually have an irregular configuration. The term *centrocytelike* has been used to describe these lymphocytes.

In some cases of marginal zone B cell lymphoma, the abnormal lymphocytes may exhibit a zone of clear cytoplasm. These distinctive cells have been called "monocytoid lymphocytes" (Figure 64-1E). Germinal centers may be present and are often infiltrated by the small centrocytelike cells (so-called follicular colonization). In extranodal marginal zone B cell lymphoma the centrocytelike cells may infiltrate surface or glandular epithelium. Collections of such cells within epithelial structures are called lymphoepithelial lesions (Figure 64-1F).

Immunophenotype

The neoplastic cells express B cell associated antigens (CD19, CD20, and CD79a) and surface immunoglobulin. Monotypic cytoplasmic immunoglobulin (CIg) may be demonstrable in approximately 40% of cases. The cells do not express CD5, CD23, or CD10. The plasma cells may be either polyclonal or monoclonal.

Differentiation among Small Lymphoid Tumors

Correct classification of lymphoid tumors in which the predominating cells are small lymphocytes of B cell lineage requires correlation of morphologic and immunophenotypic features. Expression of several different B cell associated markers—CD5, CD23, and CD10 in particular—must be characterized to accurately differentiate these lymphomas (see Table 64-2). For example:

1. A predominant population of small cells with round nuclei admixed with a minor population of larger immunoblasts, which may be apparent as vague aggregates (pseudofollicles), strongly suggests B cell chronic lymphocytic leukemia/small lymphocytic lymphoma. This diagnosis should be confirmed by demonstrating a typical immunophenotypic profile for the neoplastic cells (CD5+, CD23+, CD10−, with monoclonal SIg of low intensity).

2. A small lymphocytic proliferation in which the cells have irregular nuclei and a vaguely nodular pattern or in which germinal centers with an expanded mantle zone are apparent suggests mantle cell lymphoma. Demonstration of the characteristic immunophenotype is extremely important in this situation. The neoplastic cells should express CD5 with high-intensity monoclonal SIg, and demonstration of cyclin D1 expression will be very helpful. No expression of either CD10 or CD23 is expected.

3. A nodal tumor of small lymphocytic cells with irregular nuclei and including monocytoid cells suggests marginal zone B cell lymphoma. Another morphologic clue for a diagnosis of marginal zone B cell lymphoma is the presence of follicular colonization. If neither monocytoid cells nor germinal centers are apparent, however, discrimination

between marginal zone lymphoma and mantle cell lymphoma is not possible from the morphologic features alone. Immunophenotypic characterization of the small lymphocytic cells is essential for proper diagnosis in this situation.

Diffuse Large B Cell Lymphoma

Tumors that are composed of a diffuse proliferation of large lymphoid cells, the "large cell lymphomas," are the most common type of malignant lymphoma in most reported series (see Chapter 67). The term *large* refers to the size of the neoplastic lymphoid cells. Specifically, the diameter of the nuclei in the abnormal cells must be equal to or greater than that of nuclei in macrophages (histiocytes) or endothelial cells within the surrounding tissue. The nuclear chromatin in the large lymphoid cells is well dispersed, imparting a clear or "vesicular" appearance, and nucleoli are easily seen. The amount of cytoplasm is also visible. The large cells may be of either B cell or T cell lineage, and the large cell lymphomas are classified within separate categories depending upon the immunophenotype.

Considerable morphologic variation may be seen within the large cell lymphomas of B cell lineage. The large cells may have cleaved, ovoid (Figure 64-1G), or lobulated nuclei; nucleoli may vary in size; and cytoplasm can be quite variable in amount. Cells with abundant cytoplasm have been called immunoblasts in previous classification systems. In some cases of large B cell lymphoma, the abnormal cells may resemble plasma cells (so-called plasmacytoid immunoblasts) (Figure 64-1H). In other cases, the cytoplasm may be optically clear. Variable numbers of small lymphocytes, which may have either round or irregular nuclei, may be admixed with the large B cells. No strong associations between the morphologic variants of large B cell lymphoma and clinical characteristics of therapeutic significance have been established, however, and in the World Health Organization classification system, all of the large cell lymphomas of B cell phenotype have been grouped into a single category.

Immunophenotype

The tumor cells express B cell associated antigens (CD19, CD20, CD79a), but surface immunoglobulin expression is variable. In some cases, only cytoplasmic immunoglobulin may be demonstrable. Expression of CD10 may be seen in some cases. Expression of CD5 is less common. Immunophenotypic characterization sufficient for diagnosis can be achieved by immunohistochemical staining of tissue sections in most cases. Flow cytometry can also be used but may not be definitive in all cases.

Discrimination of diffuse large B cell lymphoma from nonlymphoid tumors (e.g., poorly differentiated carcinoma, malignant melanoma, etc.) is a common diagnostic problem. Immunohistochemical stains are extremely useful to this end. Immunostains for cytokeratin and other nonlymphoid cellular markers as well as B lymphocyte and T lymphocyte markers will suffice for diagnosis in many cases, but interpretation of an immunostain profile is not always straightforward. For example, plasmacytoid neoplastic cells are usually CD45 and CD20 negative but express epithelial membrane antigen (EMA), a pattern suggesting an epithelial neoplasm. Stains for cytoplasmic immunoglobulin are usually needed to correctly identify such plasmacytoid lymphomas.

Burkitt's Lymphoma

Burkitt's lymphoma (see Chapter 67) was called small noncleaved cell lymphoma in the Lukes-Collins and Working Formulation classifications that were used in the past. This type of lymphoma is usually seen as a diffuse proliferation. The nuclei are ovoid and have multiple, small nucleoli, and a rim of amphophilic cytoplasm is visible (Figure 64-1I). Mitotic figures are usually numerous, and phagocytic histiocytes may be intermingled among the neoplastic cells, imparting a so-called starry sky appearance. Although the cells in Burkitt's lymphoma exhibit some of the cytologic features seen in diffuse large B cell lymphoma, the nuclei are slightly smaller (medium size) and are remarkably homogeneous (monotonous) in appearance. In tissue imprint preparations, the cells exhibit a characteristic cytologic appearance, having deep blue cytoplasm with conspicuous vacuoles.

Immunophenotype

The neoplastic cells express B cell related antigens (CD19, CD20, CD22, and CD79a), and may express CD10. No expression of CD5 is seen. Monoclonal surface immunoglobulin expression is usually evident by flow cytometry but might not be demonstrable by immunohistochemical staining of tissue sections.

Lymphomas in which the morphologic features are suggestive of Burkitt's lymphoma but in which there is more variability in nuclear size and shape (nuclear pleomorphism) or in which nucleoli are more prominent than in typical cases are difficult to classify. In some previous classifications, such cases were designated as non-Burkitt's lymphoma. A category designated Burkitt-like lymphoma was introduced in the REAL classification, but in the World Health Organization classification, such cases are considered to be a variant of Burkitt's lymphoma.

The neoplastic cells in Burkitt's lymphoma and in the Burkitt-like variant have a very high rate of proliferation. Demonstration of a high S-phase fraction by flow cytometry or of a high proliferative fraction by immunostaining of tissue sections for expression of the proliferation-associated antigen Ki67 may be useful for discrimination of these entities from the more common diffuse large B cell lymphoma. In children, both typical Burkitt's lymphoma and the Burkitt-like variant are treated similarly, but in adult patients, this has not been the case. Discrimination between "typical" Burkitt's lymphoma and Burkitt-like lymphoma has never been successfully accomplished by morphologic observation alone, however, and imunophenotypic criteria for separating these two entities have not yet been defined. Because of this diagnostic difficulty, use of an additional diagnostic parameter, specifically demonstration of a translocation involving the c-myc gene, such as t(8:14) (q24:q32) or its variants t(2;8) or t(8;22), has been proposed for definitive diagnosis of Burkitt's lymphoma. Presence of a c-myc oncogene translocation would favor a diagnosis of the Burkitt-like variant rather than a large B cell lymphoma. The variant form may respond equally well to conventional therapy as does B cell large cell lymphoma, sparing the affected patients the rigors of therapy for Burkitt's lymphoma.

Follicular Lymphoma

Follicular lymphoma is extremely common, constituting the second most prevalent type of lymphoma in many series (see Chapter 66). The neoplastic cells in follicular lymphoma are derived from the cells of germinal centers (follicular center cells). Aggregates of neoplastic cells (nodules or follicles) are distributed throughout the lymph node (Figure 64-2A). The neoplastic nodules may vary in size, but they are usually round or ovoid in configuration. The neoplastic nodules are usually sharply demarcated from the surrounding interfollicular tissues, but in some cases, the nodular pattern can be rather indistinct.

Varying proportions of small lymphocytes with cleaved nuclei (small cleaved cells or centrocytes) and larger cells with ovoid nuclei (large noncleaved cells or centroblasts) make up the neoplastic nodules. Three subtypes of follicular lymphoma—designated grade 1, grade 2, and grade 3—are defined on the basis of the cellular composition of the neoplastic nodules. In follicular lymphoma, grade 1 small cleaved cells predominate within the neoplastic nodules (Figure 64-2B). In follicular lymphoma, grade 2 small cleaved cells are again numerous but larger cells are also conspicuous, creating a mixed population. In follicular lymphoma, grade 3 large cells make up an obvious and significant proportion of the cells (Figure 64-2C).

Experience with previous classification systems suggests that discrimination of grade within follicular lymphoma may be problematic. In particular, separation of grade 1 from grade 2 follicular lymphoma may be poorly reproducible. Use of a method devised by Mann and Berard for counting the number of large cells within the neoplastic nodules has been recommended to improve diagnostic reproducibility. With this method, an average of 0 to 5 large cells per high-power field are found in grade 1 follicular lymphoma, while 6 to 15 large cells per high-power field are found in grade 2, and more than 15 large cells per high power field are found in grade 3.

Immunophenotype

The abnormal cells in follicular lymphoma express B cell markers CD19, CD20, CD22, and CD79a and SIg of strong intensity. In the majority of cases, CD10 is expressed, but CD5 is not expressed. The cells within the neoplastic nodules typically express BCL-2 protein in abundance, and demonstration of strong BCL-2 expression by immunohistochemical staining can be helpful in distinguishing follicular lymphoma from follicular lymphoid hyperplasia.

Mature T Cell Neoplasms

Neoplasms of mature T cells, called "peripheral T cell lymphoma," are morphologically heterogeneous. Separate diagnostic categories such as angioimmunoblastic (AILD-like) T cell lymphoma, lymphoepitheliod cell (Lennert's) lymphoma, and angiocentric T cell lymphoma have been included within previous classifications. One particular subtype, angioimmunoblastic T cell lymphoma, is specifically designated within the World Health Organization classification, but several of the others have been collectively grouped into a single category called peripheral T cell lymphoma, not otherwise characterized.

Peripheral T Cell Lymphoma, Not Otherwise Characterized (See Chapter 69)

A relatively common histopathologic feature among cases of peripheral T cell lymphoma is a heterogeneous cellular composition including small T lymphocytes, larger cells (T immunoblasts), and varying numbers of eosinophils, plasma cells, and epithelioid histiocytes. The neoplastic T cells often have irregular nuclei (Figure 64-2D). In some cases, the T immunoblasts may resemble the abnormal cells of Hodgkin's disease (see below). Indeed, histologic discrimination of peripheral T cell lymphoma from Hodgkin's disease may be difficult.

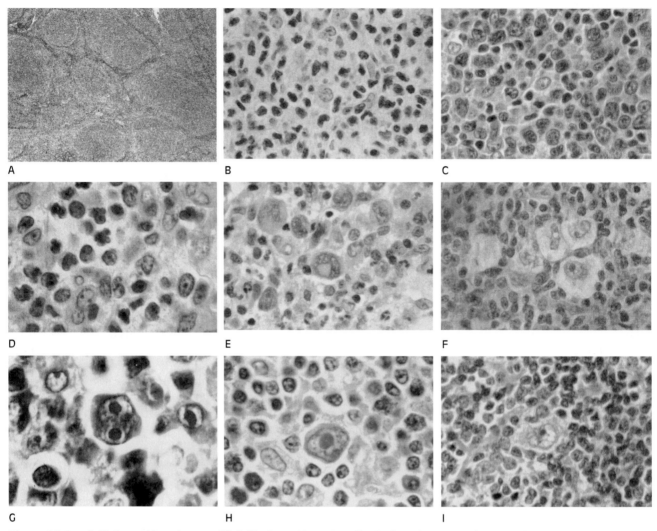

Figure 64-2 ■ *A*, Malignant lymphoma with follicular pattern. *B*, Follicular lymphoma, grade 1. *C*, Follicular lymphoma, grade 3. *D*, Peripheral T cell lymphoma. *E*, Anaplastic large cell lymphoma. *F*, Lacunar cell. *G*, Reed-Sternberg cell. *H*, Mononuclear Hodgkin's cell. *I*, L & H cell. (See Color Plate 16.)

Immunophenotype

Demonstration of a T cell phenotype for the abnormal cells is the minimal requirement for a diagnosis of peripheral T cell lymphoma. This can be achieved by either immunohistochemical staining of tissue sections or by flow cytometric analysis of cell suspensions. Neoplastic T cells express a variety of T cell–associated antigens (e.g., CD2, CD3, CD5, and CD7), but aberrancy of marker expression is often demonstrable. For example, absence of an antigen normally expressed by a T cell, or coexpression of markers (e.g., CD4 and CD8) not usually expressed on the same cell, would constitute an aberrant immunophenotype. Flow cytometry is generally more useful than immunostaining for demonstrating aberrancy of marker expression. For discrimination of peripheral T

cell lymphoma from Hodgkin's disease, however, immunohistochemical staining of tissue sections is most useful.

Analysis of cellular DNA for clonal rearrangements of T cell receptor genes is frequently required for diagnosis of peripheral T cell lymphoma, because neither flow cytometric analysis nor immunostaining can definitively demonstrate the presence of clonal T cell populations. Analysis of DNA restriction fragments by Southern blotting for rearrangement(s) of the T cell receptor beta chain gene can be performed using material extracted from frozen, unfixed biopsy tissue. Alternatively, polymerase chain reaction amplification of the T cell receptor gamma chain gene and subsequent analysis for clonality can be performed using DNA extracted from formalin-fixed, paraffin-embedded tissue, which is routinely used for histopathologic interpretation.

Anaplastic Large Cell Lymphoma, T/Null Cell

Expression of CD30 by large "anaplastic" cells is the characteristic feature of malignant lymphoma, anaplastic large cell type. The terms *Ki-1-positive lymphoma* or *CD30-positive lymphoma* have been used in the past for this type of lymphoma. Anaplastic large cell lymphoma may present as a primary cutaneous lymphoma or as a systemic disorder with lymph node involvement. The systemic form is common in children. Extranodal tumors, including involvement of the skin, may be seen in the systemic form as well.

In typical cases of anaplastic large cell lymphoma, the abnormal cells have abundant cytoplasm, and the nuclei are large and indented. Multilobulated nuclei or multinucleated cells may be present (Figure 64-2E). Aggregates of CD30-positive cells may be located within lymph node sinuses, creating a histologic pattern that mimics that of lymph node involvement by a metastatic neoplasm. Several morphologic variants of anaplastic large cell lymphoma have been described, including a monomorphic variant, a lymphohistiocytic variant, a small cell variant, a sarcomatoid variant, and a Hodgkin's-like variant. The relationship of these variants to the typical form is unclear at this time.

The abnormal CD30-positive cells exhibit a B cell immunophenotype in about one third of cases, exhibit a T cell immunophenotype in another one third of cases, but do not express markers of either lineage in the remaining cases, which are designated as null. Because clinical features in cases of CD30-positive lymphoma of B cell immunophenotype are similar to those found in cases diagnosed as large B cell lymphoma, such lymphomas are included within the category of large B cell lymphoma in the World Health Organization classification. The specific diagnosis of anaplastic large cell lymphoma, therefore, is restricted to cases in which the CD30-positive cells either exhibit a T cell phenotype or are null.

A chromosomal translocation—t(2;5) (p23:q35), in which the nucleophosmin gene (NPM) on chromosome 5 is fused with the anaplastic lymphoma kinase (ALK) gene on chromosome 2, has been found in many cases of anaplastic large cell lymphoma, but this translocation is not completely specific for this type of lymphoma. The translocation results in the production of an abnormal, chimeric NPM-ALK protein. This abnormal anaplastic lymphoma kinase protein, demonstrable by immunostaining using monoclonal antibodies, has been identified in as many as 51% of cases. Cases that do not express anaplastic lymphoma kinase are also common, and this biologic variation limits the diagnostic usefulness of anaplastic lymphoma kinase expression as a primary diagnostic parameter. Prognostic implications of anaplastic lymphoma kinase expression need more study, however.

Hodgkin's Disease (See Chapter 65)

Tumors of Hodgkin's disease differ from those of the non-Hodgkin's lymphomas discussed previously. The cellular proliferation in Hodgkin's disease is comprised predominantly of nonneoplastic, reactive lymphoreticular elements rather than clonal neoplastic cells. Characteristic abnormal cells—Reed-Sternberg cells, Hodgkin cells, and variants—must be present for a diagnosis of Hodgkin's disease, but these are found in varying numbers within the four morphologic subtypes defined in the Rye modification of the Lukes-Butler classification for Hodgkin's disease, which has been in general use since 1966. In this traditional classification, differing admixtures of cells and associated tissue reactions (e.g., fibrosis) are used to define the familiar categories of mixed cellularity, nodular sclerosis, lymphocyte depletion, and lymphocte predominant Hodgkin's disease.

The nature of the abnormal cells in Hodgkin's disease has long been elusive, but within the past decade, evidence has emerged suggesting that in most cases, the cells are abnormal B lymphoid cells. Several different investigators have used microdissection to isolate individual Reed-Sternberg and Hodgkin cells and have studied DNA from these cells for the presence of antigen receptor gene rearrangements. Clonal rearrangements of the immunoglobulin heavy chain gene have been found in the majority of cases. Characterization of this genomic DNA suggests a relationship of the abnormal B cells to lymphoid follicles. In addition, differences in the degree of somatic hypermutation present have been observed in DNA extracted from the cells of nodular lymphocyte predominant Hodgkin's disease as compared with that observed in DNA from other subtypes. These studies provide justification for inclusion of Hodgkin's disease among the other clonal proliferations of lymphoid cells—the non-Hodgkin's lymphomas—as well as a rationale for recognizing nodular lymphocyte predominant form as a distinct entity separate from the other morphologic subtypes. The World Health Organization classification for Hodgkin's disease retains most of the traditional morphologic concepts and categories but refines the Rye system to incorporate contemporary concepts relating to the pathobiology of the disorder.

Table 64-3 ▪ Immunophenotype of Atypical Cells

	Nodular Lymphocyte Predominant Hodgkin's Disease	Classical Hodgkin's Disease
CD15	–	+
CD30	–	+
B cell–associated antigens (CD19, 20, 22, 79a)	+	–/+
Epithelial membrane antigen	+	–
CD45	+	–

Classical Hodgkin's Disease

The categories of nodular sclerosing Hodgkin's disease, mixed cellularity Hodgkin's disease, and lymphocyte depletion Hodgkin's disease are included under the general designation of classical Hodgkin's disease. Another included subset of classical disease is a lymphocyte-rich rariant which occurs in 5% of patients. These subtypes are still defined by morphologic criteria, which include the nature and proportions of the nonneoplastic background cells and associated features such as fibrosis, but all share a common characteristic. In each of these variants, the Reed-Sternberg and Hodgkin cells typically express CD30 and CD15 while exhibiting an absence of expression of the pan-leukocyte antigen CD45 and, in most cases, no expression of common markers of either B cell or T cell lineage. This CD30-positive, CD15-positive, CD45-negative immunophenotype, which is characteristic for classical Hodgkin's disease, is readily characterized by immunohistochemical stains (Table 64-3). Flow cytometry is not useful for detecting or characterizing these abnormal cells.

Nodular Sclerosis Hodgkin's Disease

The nodular sclerosis subtype is the most common form of classical Hodgkin's disease in the United States. It is characterized by broad bands of fibrous connective tissue that extend inward from a thickened capsule and surround nodules of parenchymal tissue. The cellular nodules are composed of lymphocytes, histiocytes, plasma cells, eosinophils, and neutrophils in varying proportions. Typical Reed-Sternberg cells are present but are often quite rare. A characteristic abnormal cell, the lacunar cell, is present in variable numbers. This is a large cell with a multilobulated nucleus and has abundant cytoplasm, which, in for-

malin-fixed tissue, retracts inward to create a space: the "lacuna" around the nucleus (Figure 64-2F). The Reed-Sternberg and lacunar cells exhibit the typical immunophenotype for classical Hodgkin's disease as discussed above.

European workers have subdivided nodular sclerosis Hodgkin's disease into two grades based on the relative abundance of the lacunar and Reed-Sternberg cells. Only a few Reed-Sternberg cells are found within the cellular nodules in nodular sclerosis Hodgkin's disease, grade 1, while such cells are more numerous in nodular sclerosis, grade 2. The variant of nodular sclerosis Hodgkin's disease that has been called syncytial or fibroblastic Hodgkin's disease in the past is included within the grade 2 form. In the World Health Organization classification system, this grading system will not be required.

Mixed Cellularity Hodgkin's Disease

Mixed cellularity Hodgkin's disease is only slightly less common than nodular sclerosis in most series in this country. It is characterized by a diffuse proliferation of small lymphocytes, histiocytes, eosinophils, and plasma cells with classic Reed-Sternberg cells (Figure 64-2G) and mononuclear Hodgkin cells (Figure 64-2H) admixed. The proliferation typically expands involved lymph nodes and obliterates normal nodal structures. Focal involvement, in which small aggregates of cells including diagnostic Reed-Sternberg cells are found within interfollicular areas, may occur, often in association with follicular hyperplasia. The Reed-Sternberg and Hodgkin cells exhibit the typical immunophenotype for classical Hodgkin's disease (Table 64-3).

The polymorphous composition of mixed cellularity Hodgkin's disease often makes discrimination from reactive lymphoid proliferation or from a non-Hodgkin's lymphoma challenging. In particular, mixed cellularity Hodgkin's disease can mimic peripheral T cell lymphoma. Demonstration of the characteristic immunophenotype in the abnormal cells is important in such problem cases. Flow cytometry analysis is not useful to this end, but immunohistochemical staining of tissue sections for the characteristic markers CD30 and CD15, as well as other B cell and T cell markers, is extremely helpful. In particularly difficult cases analyses of DNA for T and B cell antigen receptor gene rearrangements should be performed as well (see below).

Lymphocyte Depletion Hodgkin's Disease

The lymphocyte depletion subtype is an uncommon form of classical Hodgkin's disease, making up fewer than 1% of cases in most series. Two morphologic variants have long been recognized. In the reticular variant, the tumor masses are composed of abundant abnormal cells with relatively few reactive lymphocytes as a background. Typical Reed-Sternberg cells are numerous, and bizarre sarcomatous variants may be present. In contrast, in the diffuse fibrosis form, the dominant histologic feature is a diffuse proliferation of disorganized fibrous tissue within which abnormal cells are embedded.

Accurate diagnosis of lymphocyte depletion Hodgkin's disease can be quite difficult. The histopathologic differential diagnosis includes large B cell lymphoma, peripheral T cell lymphoma, anaplastic large cell lymphoma, and nonlymphoid neoplasms. Careful immunophenotypic characterization of the abnormal large cells is critical. The abnormal cells should exhibit an immunophenotype that is typical for classical Hodgkin's disease. Immunohistochemical staining of tissue sections for the characteristic markers CD30 and CD15 as well as for T and B lymphoid antigens and markers for nonhematolymphoid cells is of paramount importance. Flow cytometry analysis is not useful to this end. Analyses of DNA extracted from frozen biopsy tissue for T and B cell antigen receptor gene rearrangements are often necessary for accurate diagnosis in these cases. Demonstration of a prominent clonal lymphoid cell population by Southern blot analysis is more compatible with a diagnosis of a non-Hodgkin's lymphoma than of lymphocyte depletion Hodgkin's disease. The significance and interpretation of clonal populations demonstrated by polymerase chain reaction amplification of DNA from fixed and embedded tissues are more problematic, however.

Nodular Lymphocyte-Predominant Hodgkin's Disease

Specifically designated in the World Health Organization classification system as a separate entity distinct from classical Hodgkin's disease, nodular lymphocyte predominant Hodgkin's disease is relatively uncommon, making up only 4% to 5% of cases of Hodgkin's disease in most series. The tumors in this type of Hodgkin's disease are composed of a predominant population of small lymphocytes with varying numbers of histiocytes admixed. Small aggregates of epithelioid histiocytes are often present. Characteristic abnormal cells, the L & H cells (so-called popcorn cells), are interspersed among the background lymphocytes, but classic Reed-Sternberg cells are extremely rare. The characteristic L and H cells have large, polylobulated nuclei with small nucleoli (Figure 64-2I).

The immunophenotypic characteristics of nodular lymphocyte-predominant Hodgkin's disease are distinctly different from those found in classical Hodgkin's disease. The small lymphocytes that make up the background cell population in this subtype are predominantly B cells, while the background lymphocytes in the variants of classical Hodgkin's disease are predominantly T cells. In addition, the L & H cells express neither CD30 nor CD15 but do express CD45 and CD20, in contrast to the immunophenotype of Reed-Sternberg cells, Hodgkin cells, or the variants found in classical Hodgkin's disease (see Table 64-3).

The histopathologic differential diagnosis of nodular lymphocyte predominant Hodgkin's disease includes progressive transformation of germinal centers, the non-Hodgkin's lymphomas of small lymphocytic cells, and so-called T cell rich B cell lymphoma, a variant of diffuse large B cell lymphoma. In addition, distinction of nodular lymphocyte predominant Hodgkin's disease from mixed cellularity Hodgkin's disease in which small lymphocytes form a very conspicuous proportion of the background cells— a so-called lymphocyte-rich classical Hodgkin's disease—can be very difficult. Flow cytometry analyses to demonstrate the presence or absence of clonal B cell populations, immunostains to characterize the atypical large cells, and in difficult cases analyses of DNA for B and T cell antigen receptor gene rearrangements are often required for accurate diagnosis.

Summary

Classifications of the non-Hodgkin's lymphomas have changed as new diagnostic techniques have been incorporated into routine practice. Thirty years ago, the Rappaport classification used only morphologic criteria—histologic patterns and cytologic characteristics of cells in tissue sections—to define eight types of malignant lymphoma. Immunologic characteristics of the neoplastic cells—the B cell or T cell immunophenotype—were used in addition to morphologic features in the classification of Lukes-Collins in America and in the Kiel classification, which was popular in Europe. Both systems recognized several specific variants of large cell lymphoma, which had been subsumed within a single category in the Rappaport system. The Working Formulation, introduced in 1981, compared entities defined morphologically within each of several classification systems that were in general use at that time with then current clinical characteristics (e.g., response to therapy) in an attempt to define clinically meaningful groups of low-grade, intermediate-grade, and high-grade non-Hodgkin's lymphoma. This clinicopathologic system is still in widespread use.

During the past two decades, new types of malignant lymphoma that were not specifically identified within the Working Formulation have been characterized through the use of modern morphologic and immunophenotypic techniques. The REAL system has incorporated these more recently characterized entities into a comprehensive but complex nosology of hematolymphoid neoplasms within a framework based on the previous Kiel classification. The latest system, the World Health Organization classification, simplifies the REAL system, retaining clinically useful categories as identified by the Working Formulation and refining the morphologic and immunophenotypic criteria for the defined entities.

The World Health Organization classification retains the original Rappaport concept of nodular lymphoma and its three variants, but this entity is renamed follicular lymphoma, and the variants are identified as grades 1, 2, and 3. The immunologic distinction of B cell from T cell lymphoma, used in the Lukes-Collins and Kiel systems, is also retained, but several of the morphologically distinctive variants of B cell large cell lymphoma, which were previously accorded individual categorical status, are gathered into a single category. Several variants of peripheral T cell lymphoma are similarly subsumed into a single category. In contrast, the more recently recognized neoplasms of small lymphocytic cells—small B cell lymphocytic lymphoma, mantle cell lymphoma, and marginal zone lymphoma—are accorded specific categorical status.

More refinements will undoubtedly be suggested as newer investigative techniques are incorporated into routine diagnostic practice. Studies using this new system will be needed to assess the clinical usefulness of the categories now defined. As with previous systems for classification of the malignant lymphomas and Hodgkin's disease, however, some cases will still present diagnostic problems. Particular problematic issues include the following:

1. Discrimination among the lymphomas of small lymphocytes. Accurate diagnosis of small B cell lymphocytic lymphoma, mantle cell lymphoma, and marginal zone lymphoma will require detailed immunophenotypic characterization of the neoplastic cells. Morphologic observations, even if supplemented by immunohistochemical staining, might not suffice. Flow cytometry analysis will be particularly useful in these cases to provide evidence for monoclonal B cell populations by demonstrating immunoglobulin light chain restriction and to more fully characterize the immunophenotypic profiles of the abnormal cells.

2. Discrimination of nodular lymphocyte predominant Hodgkin's disease from non-Hodgkin's lymphomas of small lymphocytic cells. Clonal populations of lymphoid cells are not observed in Hodgkin's disease by flow cytometry or by Southern blot analysis of DNA restriction fragments but should be easily demonstrable in non-Hodgkin's lymphomas with which this entity may be confused. Flow cytometry or DNA analysis will often be necessary for definitive diagnosis in cases in which small lymphocytes comprise a predominant population.

3. Discrimination of Hodgkin's disease from peripheral T cell lymphoma. Clonal populations of T cells are usually not demonstrable by routine molecular analyses in Hodgkin's disease but are often found in peripheral T cell lymphoma. While flow cytometry may demonstrate an "atypical" T cell immunophenotype in cases of peripheral T cell lymphoma, this finding alone does not definitely establish the presence of a clonal T cell population. Analysis of DNA for T cell receptor gene rearrangements will frequently be needed to definitively discriminate between these entities.

4. Diagnosis of anaplastic large cell lymphoma. Heterogeneity among the "CD30-positive" lymphoid neoplasms complicates this diagnosis. At the present time, demonstration of CD30 expression by cells of T cell or null immunophenotype is required. Immunostaining and flow cytometric analysis might not suffice, however, and analysis of DNA for both T cell and B cell antigen receptor gene rearrangements will be necessary in many cases to definitively establish this diagnosis. Demonstrations of a t(2;5) translocation or of anaplastic lymphoma kinase protein expression may also be useful, but owing to lack of specificity of the chromosomal abnormality and to heterogeneity of anaplastic lymphoma kinase expression, these adjunctive procedures will not resolve diagnostic problems in all cases. In addition, the clinical implications of anaplastic lymphoma kinase expression have not been sufficiently studied at this time.

5. Diagnosis of Burkitt's lymphoma and the Burkitt-like variant. Demonstration of a high proliferative rate by flow cytometric determination of S-phase fraction or by immunohistochemical staining for proliferation-associated antigens will be useful for recognizing these entities. Cytogenetic analyses for abnormalities involving the c-myc oncogene have been recommended as a useful adjunct for diagnosing Burkitt's lymphoma specifically, but morphologic and immunophenotypic criteria to clearly separate Burkitt's and Burkitt-like lymphoma have not yet been established.

A complete diagnostic workup using the new World Health Organization classification will require integration of data from ancillary techniques with traditional morphologic observations. Careful processing of diagnostic tissue to ensure that all necessary studies are expeditiously and accurately completed is critical. Thoughtful application of all diagnostic modalities currently available should permit accurate and complete diagnosis in most cases.

References

Lymphoma Classification

Harris NL, Jaffe ES, Diebold J, et al: World Health Organization Classification of Neoplastic Diseases of the Hematopoietic and Lymphoid Tissues: Report of the Clinical Advisory Committee Meeting—Airlie House, Virginia, November 1997. J Clin Oncol 1999;17:3835.

Harris NL, Jaffe ES, Stein H, et al: A Revised European-American Classification of Lymphoid Neoplasms: A proposal from the International Lymphoma Study Group. Blood 1994;84:1361.

Lennert K: Malignant Lymphomas Other Than Hodgkin's Disease. New York: Springer-Verlag, 1978.

Lukes RJ, Carver LF, Hall TC, et al: Report of the Nomenclature Committee. Cancer Res 1966;26:1311.

Lukes RJ, Collins RD: Immunologic characterization of human malignant lymphomas. Cancer 1974,34:1488.

Mann R, Berard C: Criteria for the cytologic subclassification of follicular lymphoma: A proposed alternative method. Hematol Oncol 1982;1:187.

Non-Hodgkin's Lymphoma Pathologic Classification Project. National Cancer Institute-sponsored study of classifications of non-Hodgkin's lymphomas: Summary and description of a working formulation for clinical usage. Cancer 1982; 49:2112.

Rappaport H: Tumors of the Hematopoietic System. In: Atlas of Tumor Pathology, 1st series, fascicle 8. Washington, DC: Armed Forces Institute of Pathology, 1966.

World Health Organization Classification of Neoplastic Diseases of the Hematopoietic and Lymphoid Tissues. In: Kleinus P, Sobin LH (eds): World Health Organization International Histological Classfication of Tumors. Lyon, France: IARC Press, 2001.

Molecular and Immunophenotypic Studies

Arber DA, Sun LH, Weiss LM: Detection of the t(2;5) (p23; q35) chromosomal translocation in large B cell lymphomas other than anaplastic large cell lymphoma. Hum Pathol 1996;27:590.

Borowitz MJ, Bray R, Gascoyne R, et al: U.S.-Canadian consensus recommendations on the immunophenotypic analysis of hematologic neoplasia by flow cytometry: Data analysis and interpretation. Cytometry 1997;30: 236.

Jennings CD, Foon KA: Recent advances in flow cytometry: applications to the diagnosis of hematologic malignancy. Blood 1997;90:2863.

Karkas DH, Kaul KL, Wiedbrauk DL, et al: Specimen collection and storage for diagnostic molecular pathology investigation. Arch Pathol Lab Med 1996;120:591.

Medeiros LJ, Carr J: Overview of the role of molecular methods in the diagnosis of malignant lymphomas. Arch Pathol Lab Med 1999;123:1189.

Ngan B, Chen-Levy Z, Weiss L, et al: Expression in non-Hodgkin's lymphoma of the bcl-2 protein associated with the t(14;18) chromosomal translocation. N Engl J Med 1988;318:1638.

Weisenberger DD, Gordon BG, Vose JM, et al: Occurrence of the t(2;5) (p23;q35) in non-Hodgkin's lymphoma. Blood 1996;87:3860.

Non-Hodgkin's Lymphomas

Benharroch D, Mequerian-Bedoyan Z, Lamant L, et al: ALK-positive lymphoma: A single disease with a broad spectrum of morphology. Blood 1998;91:2076.

Chan JKC: Peripheral T cell and NK cell neoplasms: An integrated approach to diagnosis. Mod Pathol 1999;12:177.

Gascoyne RD, Aoun P, Wu D, et al: Prognostic significance of anaplastic lymphoma kinase (ALK) protein expression in adults with anaplastic large cell lymphoma. Blood 1999;93:3913.

Hutchison R, Murphy S, Fairclough D, et al: Diffuse small noncleaved cell lymphoma in children, Burkitt's versus non-Burkitt's types. Cancer 1989;64:23.

Isaacson PG: Mucosa-associated lymphoid tissue lymphoma. Semin Hematol 1999;6:139.

Kinney MC, Kadin ME: The pathologic and clinical spectrum of anaplastic large cell lymphoma and correlation with ALK gene dysregulation. Am J Clin Pathol 1999;111:556.

Lopez-Guillermo A, Cid J, Salar A, et al: Peripheral T cell lymphomas: Initial features, natural history, and prognostic factors in a series of 174 patients diagnosed according to the R.E.A.L. Classification. Ann Oncol 1998;9:849.

Nathwani B, Kim H, Rappaport H: Malignant lymphoma, lymphoblastic. Cancer 1976;38:964.

Sheibani K, Burke J, Swartz W, et al: Monocytoid B cell lymphoma: Clinicopathologic study of 21 cases of a unique type of a low-grade lymphoma. Cancer 1988,62:1531.

Swerdlow SH: Small B cell lymphomas of the lymph nodes and spleen: Practical insights to diagnosis and pathogenesis. Mod Pathol 1998;12:125.

Weisenberger DD, Vose JM, Greiner TC, et al: Mantle cell lymphoma: A clinicopathologic study of 68 cases from the Nebraska Lymphoma Study Group. Am J Hematol 2000;64:190.

Wright DH: What is Burkitt's lymphoma and when is it endemic? [Letter]. Blood 1999;93:758.

Hodgkin's Disease

Chan WC: Cellular origin of nodular lymphocyte-predominant Hodgkin's lymphoma: Immunophenotypic and molecular studies. Semin Hematol 1999;36:242.

Fosis HD, Reusch R, Demel G, et al: Frequent expression of the B cell specific activator protein in Reed-Sternberg cells of classic Hodgkin's disease provides further evidence for its B cell origin. Blood 1999;94:3108.

Harris NL: Hodgkin's disease: Classification and differential diagnosis. Mod Pathol 1999;12:159.

Harris NL: Hodgkin's lymphomas: Classification, diagnosis, and grading. Semin Hematol 1999;36:220.

Lukes R, Butler J, Hicks E: Natural history of Hodgkin's disease as related to its pathologic picture. Cancer 1966;19:317.

Seitz V, Hummel M, Marafioti T, et al: Detection of clonal T cell receptor gamma-chain gene rearrangement in Reed-Sternberg cells of classic Hodgkin's disease. Blood 2000; 95:3020.

Stein H, Hummel M: Cellular origin and clonality of classic Hodgkin's lymphoma: Immunophenotypic and molecular studies. Semin Hematol 1999;36:233.

Chapter 65
Hodgkin's Disease

Thomas M. Habermann and Joseph P. Colgan

Introduction

In 1832, Sir Thomas Hodgkin described the disease that later bore his name in a paper entitled "On Some Morbid Appearances of the Absorbent Glands and Spleen." The disease was then universally fatal. The successful treatment of Hodgkin's disease has been one of the most significant accomplishments in cancer therapy over the last century. Curative treatment regimens vary, including radiation therapy, multiagent chemotherapy regimens, and high-dose therapy with autologous transplantation used alone or in combined modality treatment programs. With modern therapy, approximately 75% of patients are cured, although patients over age 65 years continue to fare less well than younger patients.

Further progress and refinements in the evaluation and treatment of Hodgkin's disease occurred in the last decade. The standard staging studies and approaches to therapy have been substantially altered. For example, routine laparotomy to stage the extent of abdominal disease was discarded, and the treatment of patients with stages I and II Hodgkin's disease is in evolution away from the former standard of extended-field radiation therapy. The malignant cell in Hodgkin's disease is the Reed-Sternberg cell. Its cell of origin was long in question but has now been established as a B cell lymphocyte. ABVD [doxorubicin (Adriamycin), bleomycin, vinblastine, and DTIC (dacarbazine)] chemotherapy has replaced MOPP [nitrogen mustard (Mustargen), vincristine (Oncovin), procarbazine, and prednisone] as the standard of care for advanced disease. High-dose therapy followed by stem cell transplantation is increasingly used for recurrent disease, and its role in initial therapy of poor prognosis disease is under study. With the dramatic improvement in cure rates, attention in clinical trials has shifted to focus on approaches to reducing immediate and long-term morbidity of treatment without sacrificing the benefits that have been achieved.

The appropriate evaluation, management, and follow-up of patients with Hodgkin's disease require mastery of a complex body of information about the benefits and toxicities of treatment for initial and relapsed disease. Decision making about therapy involves the synthesis of multiple pieces of data, including the age and general medical status of the patient, tempo of disease progression, epidemiology, histology, staging, prognostic indicators, and the potential for long-term complications in patients who are cured.

Epidemiology

In the United States, approximately 7500 new cases of Hodgkin's disease occur annually, and 1500 patients die. The five-year relative survival diminishes with increasing age, ranging from a 90% survival in patients less than age 45 years to 65% in patients age 55 to 64 years and to 40% in patients over 75 years old. Over the last two decades, the incidence has decreased in Caucasians and African-Americans. There is a greater risk of contracting Hodgkin's disease among Jews than among other groups. A bimodal age incidence is seen in economically advantaged Westernized countries' populations. The first peak of incidence is at age 25, the trough is at age 40, and the second peak occurs at age 65. In young adults, an increased incidence occurs in those of high socioeconomic status and educational level, associated particularly with the nodular sclerosis histologic subtype, whereas in low socioeconomic status populations, mixed cellularity and lymphocyte depletion histologic subtypes predominate. The frequency of mixed cellularity histology increases to 50% in men with Hodgkin's disease who are older than age 70 years.

Familial aggregation occurs in Hodgkin's disease, and the risk of developing the disease is increased in siblings of young adult patients. The increased risk is ninefold in siblings of the same sex, fivefold in siblings of the opposite sex, and 100-fold in monozygotic twins.

Evidence of a recessive susceptibility gene that is tightly linked to the human leukocyte antigen (HLA) complex was reported from a study of family pedigrees. Because Hodgkin's disease is such an uncommon disease, the incidence in the general population is very low, and families should be informed that the risk of the disease among siblings is very small in absolute terms.

The Epstein-Barr virus (EBV), which causes infectious mononucleosis, is the strongest risk factor for Hodgkin's disease. The Epstein-Barr virus genome is expressed as a restricted latent phenotype in one third to one half of the Reed-Sternberg cells in Hodgkin's disease. In a multivariate analysis of factors, Epstein-Barr virus–positive Hodgkin's disease was associated with the mixed cellularity histologic subtype, younger age (15 to 49 years versus older patients), young male adults, patients of Hispanic background, and children from less economically developed areas. Most patients with HIV-associated Hodgkin's disease are Epstein-Barr virus positive. Data also suggest an increased risk of Hodgkin's disease in other circumstances of immunologic dysfunction, such as congenital primary immunodeficiency states and immunosuppression after solid organ transplantation.

There are no established occupational risk factors. Studies on occupational exposures to wood and woodworking, herbicides (such as Agent Orange), and other chemicals have provided inconsistent results regarding their putative contribution to the development of Hodgkin's disease. Hodgkin's disease is not associated with radiation exposure, and there is no compelling evidence to support geographical clustering (common source exposures) of cases.

Clinical Presentation

Hodgkin's disease usually presents as local limited enlargement of peripheral lymph nodes, but virtually any organ or tissue may be involved with the exception of the central nervous system. Many other manifestations of the disease are present at the time of the initial diagnosis or at relapse (Table 65-1). Approximately one half of patients have mediastinal lymphadenopathy, which might not be evident on routine chest X-ray. Computed tomography studies of the chest, abdomen, and pelvis may demonstrate unexpected lymphadenopathy. Splenic involvement occurs in 20% to 25% of patients at diagnosis, but palpable splenomegaly is extremely rare. Hodgkin's disease in the spleen is usually in the form of macroscopic but small deposits that are not usually large enough to produce filling defects or splenic enlargement on computed tomography (CT) scan.

Approximately one half of patients also have "B" symptoms at the time of the initial diagnosis. "B"

Table 65-1 ■ Initial Presentation or Relapse Presentations of Hodgkin's Disease

Painless lymphadenopathy
"B" symptoms (night sweats, fever, >5% weight loss)
Pruritus (without cutaneous lesions)
Extranodal involvement: lungs, bone, liver, etc.
Hematologic findings
  Eosinophilia
  Coombs' positive hemolytic anemia
  Immune thrombocytopenia
  Cytopenias secondary to bone marrow infiltration
  Autoimmune neutropenia
  Thrombotic thrombocytopenic purpura
Neurologic
  Spinal cord compression
  Paraneoplastic cerebellar degeneration
  Peripheral neuropathy
  Cranial neuropathy
  Subacute motor neuropathy
  Subacute myelopathy
  Central pontine myelinolysis
  Stiff-man syndrome
  Limbic encephalitis
  Guillain-Barré syndrome
Renal
  Glomerulonephritis
    Minimal disease change
    Membranous glomerulonephropathy
    Focal sclerosing glomerulonephropathy
    Crescentic glomerulonephropathy
  Amyloidosis
  Renal parenchymal involvement
Dermatologic
  Infectious varicella zoster
  Nonspecific
    Erythematous
    Urticarial
    Vesicular
    Bullous
  Erythema nodosum
  Rare:
    Psoriasiform lesion
    Acrokeratosis paraneoplastica
    Granulomatous slack skin disorder
    Prurigo nodularis
    Follicular necrosis
    Necrobiotic xanthogranuloma
Nails
  Transverse white lines
  Hypertrophic osteoarthropathy
Endocrinologic
  Hypercalcemia
  Hypoglycemia
  Lactic acidosis
Alcohol-induced pain (in areas of bone or lymph node involvement)
Hepatic involvement
Jaundice (secondary to external biliary tract obstruction or to cholestasis on a paraneoplastic basis)

symptoms include unexplained fever (temperature greater than 38°C), night sweats, and unexplained loss of greater than 10% body weight within the preceding six months. Fever may be continuous or intermittent and may be low-grade or greater than 104°F; it is frequently unrecognized by the patient, and the only symptoms may be fatigue and malaise. Symptomatic night sweats should be drenching and characterized by soaking nightclothes or sheets and not limited to perspiration and a damp neck. Pruritus (Chapter 3) is not a "B" symptom. Although, stage for stage, it does not confer an adverse prognosis, pruritus is more often associated with advanced-stage disease than with limited-stage disease. The itching is not due to skin involvement by Hodgkin's disease, but skin changes can occur owing to excoriation. Pruritus resolves with the treatment of Hodgkin's disease; its recurrence can be the initial symptom of relapse.

Extranodal disease is less common. The lung is a frequent site of extranodal disease, usually occurring as a direct extension from enlarged perihilar lymph nodes; however, isolated single or more commonly multicentric nodules, and, uncommonly, cavitary lesions can be seen. Patients with pulmonary parenchymal Hodgkin's disease commonly present with cough. Rare neurologic manifestations include brachial plexopathy, cranial neuropathy, peripheral neuropathy, and cerebral or spinal manifestations of granulomatous angiitis. Involvement of the liver at initial diagnosis occurs in fewer than 10% of patients and is almost always associated with "B" symptoms. Conversely, abnormal liver function tests (elevated alkaline phosphatase with minimal increase in the transaminase values) are often nonspecific manifestations of extrahepatic Hodgkin's disease, occurring not infrequently in patients who have "B" symptoms and no direct liver involvement. An increased bilirubin level is usually due to extrahepatic causes, such as common bile duct compression by enlarged lymph nodes in the porta hepatis, increased red blood cell turnover in autoimmune hemolytic anemia, or, rarely, intrahepatic cholestasis as a distant effect of symptomatic Hodgkin's disease. Other Hodgkin's disease–associated abnormalities include the broad range of manifestations in Table 65-1. The most common of these include eosinophilia, cytopenias, autoimmune hemolytic anemia, immune thrombocytopenia, nephrotic syndrome, and nonspecific dermatologic presentations. Hodgkin's disease thus has the capacity for a variety of distant effects secondary to cytokine release or immunologic dysfunction. In fewer than 10% of patients, alcohol ingestion causes pain in areas of involved lymph nodes or bone. Alcohol-induced pain in disease sites is virtually pathognomonic of Hodgkin's disease.

Biopsy for Diagnosis

Biopsy is a diagnostic, not a therapeutic, procedure. Extensive lymph node dissection and removal are therefore not warranted. Peripheral lymph node biopsy may be accomplished by four different methods: (1) fine-needle aspiration, (2) core biopsy, (3) open incisional biopsy, and (4) open excisional biopsy. Fine-needle aspirate and core biopsy may be inadequate to provide a diagnosis because of the limited sample size and the necessity to identify Reed-Sternberg cells and/or the patterns of involvement that are found in Hodgkin's disease. Excisional biopsy is the procedure of choice for lymph nodes measuring 1 to 3 cm in diameter, whereas incisional biopsy is preferred for lymph nodes greater than 3 cm in diameter. In patients who have a mediastinal mass and no readily available peripheral lymph nodes for biopsy, mediastinoscopy (cervical or anterior), anterior mediastinotomy, median sternotomy, and thoracoscopy have been used to obtain a tissue diagnosis. Since complete surgical extirpation is not indicated therapeutically, median sternotomy (or thoracotomy) for greater exposure is rarely performed. Mediastinoscopy, which can be performed on an outpatient basis, is preferred over thoracoscopy. In the fewer than 10% of patients who present only with abdominal disease, laparoscopic lymph node biopsy has a high yield and minimal morbidity.

The surgeon who is performing the lymph node biopsy should notify pathology in advance. The tissue should be sent to the pathology laboratory in sterile saline. This allows studies, such as flow cytometry or gene rearrangement, to be performed on fresh tissue if indicated. A portion can then be placed by the pathologist in fixative and snap frozen. Monoclonal antibody studies can be subsequently performed on frozen tissue or paraffin-embedded tissue.

Pathology

The World Health Organization (WHO) Classification of Neoplastic Diseases of the Hematopoietic and Lymphoid Tissues: Report of the Clinical Advisory Committee recognizes three major categories of lymphoid neoplasms: B cell neoplasms, T cell/natural killer (NK) cell neoplasms, and Hodgkin's disease. This system is based on the premise that a classification should attempt to define distinct disease entities using all currently available information, including morphology, immunophenotype, genetic features, and clinical features. The details from a histologic perspective are discussed in Chapter 64. Clinical observations that are relevant to the revised classification for Hodgkin's disease (Table 65-2) are discussed in this chapter.

Table 65-2 ▪ Proposed World Health Organization Classification of Hodgkin's Disease Lymphomas

Hodgkin's lymphoma (Hodgkin's disease)
  Nodular lymphocyte-predominant Hodgkin's lymphoma
  Classical Hodgkin's lymphoma
    Nodular sclerosis Hodgkin's lymphoma (grades 1 and 2)
    Lymphocyte-rich classical Hodgkin's lymphoma
    Mixed cellularity Hodgkin's lymphoma
    Lymphocyte depletion Hodgkin's lymphoma

Modified from Harris NL, Jaffe ES, Diebold J, et al: World Health Organization Classification of Neoplastic Diseases of the Hematopoietic and Lymphoid Tissues: Report of the Clinical Advisory Committee Meeting—Airlie House, Virginia, November 1997. J Clin Oncol 1999;17:3835–3849.

Two histologies predominate: nodular sclerosing (40% to 70% of cases) and mixed cellularity (20% to 40% of cases). Lymphocyte depletion Hodgkin's disease represents fewer than 15% of cases. The World Health Organization committee separated lymphocyte-rich classical Hodgkin's disease from nodular lymphocyte-predominant Hodgkin's disease because of their distinguishing clinical, immunologic, and biologic characteristics. This classification correlates with the clinical observation that lymphocyte-predominant Hodgkin's disease may be indolent. Lymphocyte-rich Hodgkin's disease is a new histologic subtype of classical Hodgkin's disease. Patients with lymphocyte-predominant Hodgkin's disease and lymphocyte-rich classical Hodgkin's disease have similar disease characteristics at presentation and no difference in overall survival rates. However, compared to lymphocyte-rich classical Hodgkin's disease, lymphocyte-predominant Hodgkin's disease exhibits a pattern of multiple relapses after remission induction, involves fewer patients older than age 50 years (18% versus 32%), presents less often with stage III disease (14% versus 24%), and has a lower incidence of mediastinal lymph node enlargement (7% versus 15%). At the same time, lymphocyte-rich classical Hodgkin's disease itself has a lower frequency of mediastinal disease compared to the mixed cellularity (40%) and nodular sclerosis (80%) subtypes. Limited-stage disease is more likely to occur in lymphocyte-rich classical Hodgkin's disease (46%) versus 10% in nodular sclerosis and 21% in mixed cellularity.

Immunohistochemical studies facilitate separation of Hodgkin's disease from other possible diagnoses. The present panel of antibodies routinely included in the diagnosis of Hodgkin's disease includes CD45, CD30, CD15, CD20, CD3, and the keratin stain. The differential diagnosis of Hodgkin's disease can include sarcoma, malignant melanoma, carcinoma, peripheral T cell non-Hodgkin's lymphoma, T cell rich non-Hodgkin's lymphoma, B cell diffuse large cell lymphoma of the mediastinum, reactive lymphoid hyperplasia, and necrotizing granulomatous lymphadenitis. A negative keratin stain excludes carcinoma. The Reed-Sternberg cells react with the Hodgkin's disease-associated markers, CD15 (Leu-M1) and CD30, and not with B or T cell markers. Flow cytometry studies may be misleading. The results may be consistent with a reactive lymph node picture because the diagnostic Reed-Sternberg cells are too sparse and/or too large so that they are gated out. On paraffin sections, testing for CD45, a molecule that is present on virtually all hematopoietic lymphoid cells, is very useful because it is expressed in only 7% of Hodgkin's disease cells. The delineation of anaplastic large cell lymphoma, which is also CD 30+, from Hodgkin's disease remains problematic (see the discussion in Chapter 64).

The distinction between a diagnosis of Hodgkin's disease and non-Hodgkin's lymphoma can, at times, be quite a diagnostic challenge. The resolution is critical for the clinician, because therapeutic strategies for the two entities differ significantly.

Composite Lymphoma

Composite lymphoma is defined as the simultaneous occurrence of non-Hodgkin's lymphoma and Hodgkin's disease. Most composite lymphomas reflect the incidence of the types of non-Hodgkin's lymphoma in the general population. Follicular lymphoma and diffuse large B cell lymphoma are therefore the most common, but marginal zone and mantle-cell lymphoma have also been reported. Nodular lymphocyte-predominant Hodgkin's disease may transform into diffuse large B cell lymphoma in 2% to 3% of cases. This conjunction with diffuse large cell lymphoma may occur some years after, concurrently with, or before the diagnosis of nodular lymphocyte-predominant Hodgkin's disease is made. The histologies may be clonally related by phenotypic and genotypic analysis. Epstein-Barr virus expression is concordant in most cases. Some investigators prefer to reserve the term *composite lymphoma* for circumstances in which the two histologies are clonally unrelated. The prognosis depends fundamentally on the histology of the non-Hodgkin's lymphoma component.

Secondary Non-Hodgkin's Lymphoma

The risk of developing a subsequent non-Hodgkin's lymphoma after successful treatment of Hodgkin's disease is approximately 5%. Most commonly, the secondary disease is a diffuse B cell large cell non-

Hodgkin's lymphoma. Secondary low-grade non-Hodgkin's lymphomas occur more frequently after lymphocyte-predominant Hodgkin's disease than after the other histologic subtypes. Conversely, on occasion, Hodgkin's disease develops in a patient with a previously diagnosed non-Hodgkin's lymphoma. Hodgkin's disease has also been reported in association with chronic lymphocytic leukemia.

Staging

Hodgkin's disease in many patients appears to be of unifocal origin and to undergo orderly spread and dissemination. During the era when exploratory laparotomy and splenectomy were performed for surgical staging of the disease, the patterns of spread became apparent. Occult splenic disease was found in up to one third of patients with early-stage disease. Hodgkin's disease in the liver and bone marrow was infrequent, and rarely occurred in the absence of Hodgkin's disease in the spleen. Similarly, the retroperitoneal nodes rarely contained disease unless the spleen was involved. It thus seemed that disease in the neck and/or chest spread via the lymphatics from one lymph node–bearing area to the next adjacent area, whereas abdominal and visceral disease developed from hematogenous dissemination (the splenic architecture playing a role in filtering and initially retaining Hodgkin's disease cells circulating in the blood). To some extent, the stage of the disease correlates with the histologic pattern at presentation. For example, nodular lymphocyte-predominant Hodgkin's disease is associated with disease in the upper neck and lymphocyte depletion is associated with advanced disease, including abdominal and extranodal disease. Liver involvement at presentation is more commonly associated with mixed cellularity and lymphocyte-depletion histologies than with the other types.

The Cotswolds Staging Classification of Hodgkin's disease is the most recent staging system based on the anatomic distribution of disease (Table 65-3). Three important considerations contributed to the revised staging system: (1) there were doubts about the necessity for surgical staging by laparotomy, (2) the prognosis for patients who relapsed after radiation therapy was good, and (3) bulky disease, especially in the mediastinum, carried a significant adverse prognosis. The new staging classification is a clinical one, based on the physical examination and the results of routine radiographs and computed tomography scans. This classification includes the evaluation of the number of involved sites, defines bulky disease, subdivides stage III, establishes precise criteria for the diagnosis of spleen and liver involvement, and adds

Table 65-3 ■ The Cotswolds Staging Classification of Hodgkin's Disease

Classification	Description
Stage I	Involvement of a single lymph node region or lymphoid structure
Stage II	Involvement of two or more lymph node regions on the same side of the diaphragm (the mediastinum is considered a single site, but the right and left hilar lymph nodes are considered separately)
Stage III	Involvement of lymph node regions or structures on both sides of the diaphragm
Stage III-1	With or without involvement of splenic, hilar, celiac, or portal nodes
Stage III-2	With involvement of para-aortic, iliac, and mesenteric nodes
Stage IV	Involvement of one or more extranodal sites in addition to a site for which the designation "E" has been used
	Designations applicable to any stage
A	No symptoms
B	Fever (temperature >38°C), drenching night sweats, unexplained loss of >10% of body weight within the preceding six months
X	Bulky disease: maximum transverse mediastinal tumor mass >1/3 of the intrathoracic diameter of the chest measured at T5–T6 interspace or a nodal mass with a maximal dimension >10 cm)
E	Involvement of a single extranodal site that is contiguous or proximal to the known nodal site
CS	Clinical stage
PS	Pathologic stage (as determined by laparotomy)

Modified from Kaufman D, Longo DL: Hodgkin's disease. In Abeloff MD, Armitage JO, Lichter AS, Niederhuber JE (eds); Clinical Hematology. New York: Churchill Livingstone, 1995, pp 2075–2107.

a response category, namely, unconfirmed/uncertain complete remission (CRu). The Cotswolds committee defined bulky mediastinal disease as a 1/3 or greater ratio between the maximum (mediastinal) transverse tumor mass diameter and the internal thoracic diameter measured at the level of the T5–6 interspace. Criteria for the definition of mediastinal bulky disease by use of computed tomography scan measurements have not yet been established.

Because staging is now clinical rather than surgical, one needs to be aware in treatment planning that the risk of occult splenic or upper abdominal lymph node involvement not detected by computed tomography scan of the abdomen and pelvis, magnetic resonance imaging (MRI), or gallium scanning is 20% to 30% in stages IA and IIA and approximately 35% in stages IB and IIB.

Standard staging studies include history, physical examination, complete blood count with differential, sedimentation rate, chemistry analyses (liver and renal function studies, and electrolytes), lactase dehydrogenase (LDH) levels, chest X-ray, computed tomography scan of the chest, and computed tomography scan of the abdomen. Abdominal computed tomography has replaced bipedal lymphangiography for the assessment of involvement of abdominal lymph nodes. Intravenous contrast media should be administered as a bolus with rapid scanning during the early phase of arterial contrast enhancement. This approach increases the likelihood of detecting splenic involvement by Hodgkin's disease. The current Cotswolds guidelines recommend that the finding of multiple focal splenic defects (after excluding cystic and vascular lesions) should be confirmed by at least one other imaging technique.

Bone marrow involvement occurs in fewer than 10% of patients overall and is not found in patients who have early-stage disease. Bone marrow aspiration and biopsy need only be routinely done therefore in the following circumstances: patients with stage III or IV disease, "B" symptoms, bulky disease, blood count abnormalities (anemia, thrombocytopenia, or leukopenia), and prior to consideration of high-dose therapy. Reed-Sternberg cells are very rarely seen on bone marrow aspirate or biopsy even when the bone marrow is involved. If Hodgkin's disease involves the bone marrow, the biopsy will, however, often disclose surrogate markers for the presence of Reed-Sternberg cells, such as variant mononuclear Reed-Sternberg cells, atypical mononuclear forms, and fibrosis.

Gallium scanning is not of benefit in the majority of patients with newly diagnosed Hodgkin's disease, because its sensitivity is lower than that of computed tomography and magnetic resonance imaging. A pretreatment gallium scan can be useful, however, in the initial staging of Hodgkin's disease in those patients who have a bulky mediastinal mass. Approximately 80% of such patients have a positive scan in the mediastinum pretreatment. Commonly, full regression of these masses does not occur after treatment, leaving a residual mass of uncertain significance on scan or X-ray. If the gallium scan was positive before treatment, then a positive scan after treatment indicates that the residual mass contains Hodgkin's disease rather than fibrosis. Positron emission tomography (PET) may now obviate the use of gallium scans for this purpose. Magnetic resonance imaging scanning of the chest provides minimal additional information after computed tomography scan results, but it can be helpful in following osseous disease. Bone scans are of value in cases of suspected osseous disease with bone pain, joint pain, or elevated bone fraction of the alkaline phosphatase. The technetium liver/spleen scan on occasion may be helpful in confirming nodular visceral deposits of Hodgkin's disease.

Staging laparotomy is no longer routinely utilized in Hodgkin's disease. The EORTC H6 trial randomized clinical stage I and II patients to receive subtotal nodal and splenic radiation therapy without a laparotomy or staging laparotomy followed by radiation therapy or radiation therapy plus chemotherapy depending on the results of the laparotomy. After 10 years, there was a small overall survival advantage for the no-laparotomy arm compared to the laparotomy arm. A staging laparotomy includes the following: splenectomy, core biopsies and surgical wedge biopsies of the liver, removal of abnormal lymph nodes in the retroperitoneum, surgical wedge biopsy of bone/bone marrow from the iliac crest, and sampling of even apparently normal lymph nodes. After splenectomy, patients are not more susceptible to infection than other patients, but when infections with certain encapsulated organisms do occur, they can be rapidly overwhelming and lethal. Prior to splenectomy, therefore, patients should routinely receive polysaccharide-conjugate vaccines against pneumococcus, *Haemophilus influenzae* type B, and meningococcus type C. Current recommendations are that the vaccinations be repeated once at two to six years and then every six years thereafter. Daily oral penicillin, which is given to children after splenectomy, is not recommended in adults who have a lower risk of acquiring these infections and exhibit poor compliance.

Prognostic Factors

Using a large population database, the International Database on Hodgkin's Disease and the International Prognostic Factors Project on Advanced Hodgkin's Disease developed prognostic scoring systems based on the accumulation of adverse prognostic features at presentation. The endpoint was freedom from progression from initial treatment. Overall survival encompasses patients who underwent salvage therapy for potential cure, deaths related to complications of treatment, and deaths unrelated to Hodgkin's disease. The limitation on the data is that these patients received a variety of different treatments. Seven factors were associated independently with an adverse prognosis. These included a serum albumin level of less than 4 g/dL; a hemoglobin level of less than 10.5 g/dL, male gender; age greater than or equal to 45 years; stage IV disease; total white blood cell count greater than or equal to 15,000/μL; and lymphocytopenia (lymphocyte count less than 600/μL and/or lymphocytes less than 8% of the total white blood cell count). The freedom from progression based on the number of negative factors was 84% with 0 factors (7% of the patients), 77% for one factor (22% of the patients), 67% for two factors (29% of the patients), 60% for three factors (23% of the patients), 51% for four factors (12% of the patients), and 42% for five or more factors (7% of the patients). This scoring system is now used in the design of trials in Hodgkin's disease. For example, the Southwest Oncology Group is conducting a randomized study comparing early high-dose chemotherapy and an autologous stem cell transplant versus conventional-dose ABVD chemotherapy for patients with advanced-stage Hodgkin's disease and a poor prognosis, defined as the presence of three or more of the unfavorable prognostic indicators.

The sedimentation rate, although a nonspecific acute phase reactant, does correlate with disease activity and aggressiveness. Elevations of the sedimentation rate to more than 50 or more than 70 mm/hour were used as markers of unfavorable early-stage disease in a number of European studies. Following the sedimentation rate serially with treatment and after treatment can provide a relatively sensitive index of response and relapse, respectively.

Initial Treatment

One needs to be wary of the results of studies whose endpoints are remission duration and/or survival

---

TREATMENT

Suggested Initial Therapy of Hodgkin's Disease Based on Clinical Stage of Disease

Stage	Treatment (Number of Monthly Cycles of Chemotherapy and Dose of Radiation Therapy)
IA	
Limited to high neck (0, 1 risk factors)	Involved or extended field RT 36–40 Gy
Nonbulky disease	ABVD × 3 + involved field RT 20–24 Gy
Bulky mediastinal or >2 risk factors	ABVD × 6–8 + involved field RT 24–30 Gy
IB	
Nonbulky and ≤2 risk factors	ABVD × 6–8
Bulky mediastinal disease or >2 risk factors	ABVD × 6–8 + involved field RT 24–30 Gy
IIA	
Nonbulky and ≤2 risk factors	ABVD × 4–6: +/– involved field RT 20–24 Gy
Bulky mediastinal disease or >2 risk factors	ABVD × 6–8 + involved field RT 24–30 Gy
IIB	
Nonbulky	ABVD × 6–8
Bulky mediastinal or other bulky disease	
plus extranodal disease or >2 risk factors	ABVD × 6–8 + involved field RT 24–30 Gy
IIIA	ABVD × 6–8
IIIB	ABVD × 6–8
IVA	ABVD × 6–8
IVB	ABVD × 6–8

ABVD + doxorubicin (Adriamycin), bleomycin, vinblastine, and DTIC (see Table 65-4).
Adverse Risk Factors: serum albumin <4 g/dL, hemoglobin <10.5 g/dL, male sex, age ≥ 45 years, stage IV, white blood cell count ≥15,000/μL, and lymphocytes <8% of the total white blood cell count and/or <600/μL. (Hasenclever D, Diehl V: A prognostic score for advanced Hodgkin's disease. International Prognostic Factors Project on Advanced Hodgkin's Disease: New Engl J Med 1998;339:1506–1514.)

Authors' Notes: No international consensus on the optimal initial therapy exists. The reader should recognize that treatment recommendations for Hodgkin's disease vary even among experienced clinicians. Before the course of therapy is determined, the suggestions provided here should be considered against recommendations made elsewhere by other investigators.

Because of continuing therapeutic controversies, patients who are eligible for well-designed clinical trials should be invited to participate whenever feasible.

When anthracyclines are contraindicated owing to cardiac disease, BCVPP or MOPP is a reasonable alternative for initial chemotherapy.

curves that only fall as deaths from Hodgkin's disease occur. In various reports, deaths in the first 5 to 10 years are most frequently due to progressive Hodgkin's disease, whereas deaths occurring after 10 years are more likely from causes other than Hodgkin's disease. Many different therapeutic approaches are available in the initial treatment of Hodgkin's disease, and patients who relapse can be salvaged for cure with appropriate therapy. Toxicities from therapy can appear early or late and can cause death in patients who are in remission. The summated value of treatment (including initial and any necessary salvage therapy) is best reflected in the overall survival data (including all deaths from any cause) and a comparison with a demographically matched control population.

Radiation Therapy in Early-Stage Disease

A landmark paper in 1950 by Dr. Peters from the Toronto General Hospital in Canada reported on the treatment of patients with limited-stage disease by means of high doses of radiation therapy (using the low-voltage machines of that era) to involved and adjacent sites. Dramatic improvement in outcome, compared to historical data, occurred, resulting in 5-year and 10-year survival rates of 88% and 79%, respectively. In 1966, Dr. Kaplan reported excellent results and reduced toxicity when treating patients on the Stanford Linear Accelerator with supervoltage range (1 MeV or greater).

Radiation treatment fields are defined as follows. An *involved field* encompasses enlarged lymph nodes and other regional lymph nodes in the same lymph node region. *Extended field* includes the involved field and all adjacent lymph node regions. *Mantle field* involves all supradiaphragmatic lymph nodes, including cervical, supraclavicular, axillary, infraclavicular, mediastinal, and hilar nodes. *Minimantle field* includes the bilateral cervical, supraclavicular, infraclavicular, and axillary nodes but excludes the mediastinum entirely. The *para-aortic field* involves the upper abdominal lymph nodes ± the spleen. *Extended mantle field* involves the mantle and upper abdominal fields. The *inverted-Y field* involves the para-aortic, pelvic, and inguinal-femoral fields ± the spleen. *Total lymphoid* and *total nodal irradiation* involve treatment of all major lymph node regions above and below the diaphragm.

Kaplan determined from a retrospective review of treated patients that the probability of Hodgkin's disease recurring within an irradiated field was less than 5% when a total dose greater than or equal to 35 Gy was used. The German Hodgkin's Study Group trial is the only trial that prospectively randomized patients to evaluate doses of radiation therapy and their impact on areas of subclinical disease. Patients were randomized to receive 40 Gy to an extended field or 30 Gy to an extended field followed by an additional 10 Gy to involved lymph node regions. They reported that a radiation dose of 30 Gy was adequate to eliminate recurrence of Hodgkin's disease from clinically uninvolved lymph node areas. The five-year freedom from treatment failure favored the 30 Gy extended field plus 10 Gy arm (81% versus 70%, $p = .026$).

In the past, patients with early-stage Hodgkin's disease (stage I or II without "B" symptoms or bulky disease) were surgically staged by a staging laparotomy, thereby eliminating from this group a number of patients who had occult disease below the diaphragm. After laparotomy, the early-stage patients were treated with radiation therapy alone to the mantle, para-aortic, and splenic pedicle fields. Long-term freedom from relapse was greater than 80%. In the modern era, in the absence of information that was formerly provided by a staging laparotomy, stages IA–IIA may have unsuspected disease in the abdomen, and this possibility has to be factored into the design of therapy for these clinically staged patients.

Meta-analysis of studies of more-extensive and less-extensive radiation therapy fields have revealed a higher recurrence rate in less-extensive treatment field patients, but the 10-year survival rates (approximately 75%) were not statistically significantly different, a finding suggesting that chemotherapy for relapse after radiation therapy is effective. Patients who relapse are more likely to be cured with chemotherapy if they were initially treated with radiation therapy alone rather than chemotherapy or combined chemotherapy and radiation therapy.

Chemotherapy in Advanced-Stage Disease

For maximal effectiveness, chemotherapy should be delivered at the full, intended doses and on time as established by the treatment protocol. Deviations from the schedule decrease the likelihood of a successful outcome. If myelosuppression and declining blood counts threaten to cause departures from the treatment schedule, then colony-stimulating factors and/or blood product support should be employed so that interruptions in therapy and dosage reduction are minimized. Prophylactic antibiotics, such as a quinolone or trimethoprim/sulfamethoxazole, should be considered for high-risk patients such as the elderly and those with impaired performance status. Fertility issues should be addressed before treatment in young patients, especially when alkylating agents are used. Sperm banking in men and cryopreservation of ova in women are options to be considered. It is unlikely that the time delay in the institution of therapy to allow for storage will prejudice the results of therapy, because the pace of progression of most cases of Hodgkin's disease is not very rapid.

Nitrogen mustard was the first effective chemotherapeutic agent for Hodgkin's disease. Nitrogen mustard's lympholytic effects were identified as a byproduct of secret government research on mustard gases during World War II. Subsequently, a number of additional drugs were shown to cause regression of Hodgkin's disease. These included vincristine, vinblastine, cyclophosphamide, prednisone, chlorambucil, melphalan, procarbazine, bleomycin, dacarbazine (DTIC) and BCNU (carmustine). As these drugs became available, they were used initially in a sequential fashion, each drug (or two in combination) being administered until the therapeutic response waned. As disease progression became apparent, another single agent was then substituted. The overall response to the individual drugs was approximately 60% to 70%, but complete remission (CR) was achieved in only 15% of patients. Dr. DeVita of the National Cancer Institute developed the combination of drugs known as the MOPP regimen. It capitalized on the use of highly effective drugs with differing toxicities so that the drugs could be given in full doses and yet allow for repeated courses of therapy. The intent was that Hodgkin's disease that was resistant to one of the drugs would still have an independent opportunity to respond to one or more of the other drugs in the combination, since their mechanisms of action were different. Of the initial series of patients with stages III and IV disease, 80% (159/198) achieved a complete remission. Complete remission was achieved in 100% of asymptomatic patients and in 78% of patients with "B" symptoms. Of the patients who achieved a complete remission, 55% remained free of relapse 10 years or more after completion of therapy. Toxicities included nausea, vomiting, neutropenia, thrombocytopenia, vincristine-induced peripheral neuropathy, azoospermia in all males, amenorrhea in 41% of women over age 25 years, and acute leukemia in 13 patients (12 of these 13 had also received radiation therapy during the course of the disease). Approximately one third of patients relapsed by the fifth year. Of 98 deaths, 23 (24%) had no evidence of disease. Subsequent, multi-institutional studies showed somewhat lower rates of complete remission and disease-free survival, but the favorable results led to exploration of other combination therapies in Hodgkin's disease and other cancers (the first-generation regimens listed in Table 65-4). The guidelines for the original MOPP chemotherapy was that monthly cycles were to be given until complete remission was achieved, followed by treatment with two additional cycles of therapy. Subsequent randomized studies showed no advantage to adding lengthy programs of maintenance therapy after completion of the prescribed course of MOPP chemotherapy. As with most other cancers except acute lymphoblastic leukemia, the benefit of chemotherapy is derived entirely from the initial administration of a highly effective treatment regimen.

Bonadonna developed an alternative regimen to MOPP called ABVD (Adriamycin, bleomycin, vinblastine, and DTIC), which was given parenterally every two weeks (the second-generation regimens listed in Table 65-4). His early studies showed that approximately 70% of patients who had failed MOPP therapy (initially or at relapse) could achieve complete remission after ABVD treatment, indicating no cross-resistance between MOPP and ABVD. Randomized studies sought to combine the two regimens. Patients with stages III and IV disease were randomized to receive 12 cycles of MOPP or six cycles of MOPP alternating with six cycles of ABVD. The complete remission rate in the alternating therapy (89%) was superior to the MOPP treatment (74%) alone, but no difference in survival was demonstrable. The Cancer and Leukemia Group B (CALGB) randomized patients with stages III and IV disease were to receive MOPP, ABVD, or MOPP/ABVD. The vincristine dose was limited to a total of 2 mg. The ABVD-containing regimens were superior to MOPP in complete remission rates (approximately 80% versus 70%), and the failure-free survival rate was improved as well (60% versus 50%), but overall survival did not differ significantly.

A hybrid regimen was constructed consisting of portions of MOPP and of ABVD (Table 65-4). The MOPP/ABV hybrid regimen is made up of MOPP on day 1 and ABV on day 8 of a 28-day cycle. Dacarbazine was omitted, and the dose of doxorubicin was increased from 25 to 35 mg/m². MOPP/ABV appeared in initial studies to provide results superior to those of ABVD. A randomized intergroup compared MOPP/ABV hybrid to ABVD. Preliminary results from this study showed equivalence of the regimens in complete remission rate and freedom from progression. The study was terminated prematurely, however, because of increased toxicity of the MOPP/ABV therapy compared to ABVD and an increase in the development of secondary cancers. Currently, ABVD is the treatment of choice for advanced Hodgkin's disease. The risk of infertility and the leukemogenic potential is much lower after ABVD than after alkylating agent–containing regimens, which carry a 5% to 10% risk of subsequent acute myeloid leukemia in patients who are cured of their Hodgkin's disease.

The Stanford V regimen (the third-generation regimens listed in Table 65-4) is a shorter, yet more intensive, regimen than ABVD. Therapy is given weekly for

Table 65-4 ■ Hodgkin's Disease Treatment Regimens

	mg/m³/day	Day(s) 1	8	15	22	29	43	57
First Generation								
MOPP						New cycle		
M (mechlorethamine)	6	●	●					
O (vincristine, Oncovin)	1.4	●	●					
P (procarbazine)	100	● (1–14)						
P (prednisone)	40	● (1–14)						
ChIVPP						New cycle		
Chl (chlorambucil)	6	● (1–14)						
V (vinblastine)	6	●	●					
P (procabazine)	100	● (1–14)						
P (prednisone)	40	● (1–14)						
BCVPP						New cycle		
B (BCNU, carmustine)	100	●						
C (cyclophosphamide)	600	●						
V (vincristine)	1.4	●						
P (procarbazine)	100	● 1–10						
P (prednisone)	60	● 1–10						
Second Generation								
ABVD						New cycle		
A (doxorubicin)	25	●		●				
B (bleomycin)	10	●		●				
V (velban)	6	●		●				
D (DTIC)	375	●		●				
MOPP/ABVD								Repeat cycle
M (nitrogen mustard)	6	●	●					
O (vincristine)	1.4	●	●					
P (procarbazine)	100	● 1–14						
P (prednisone)	40	● 1–14						
A (doxorubicin)	25					●	●	
B (bleomycin)	10					●	●	
V (velban)	6					●	●	
D (DTIC)	375					●	●	
MOPP/ABV						New cycle		
M (nitrogen mustard)	6	●						
O (vincristine)	1.4	●						
P (procarbazine)	100	● 1–7						
P (prednisone)	40	●						
A (doxorubicin)	35		●					
B (bleomycin)	10		●					
V (velban)	6		●					
Third Generation								
Stanford V[1,2]						New cycle		
Doxorubicin	25	●						
Vinblastine	6	●						
Mechlomethamine	6	●						
Vincristine	1.4		●					
Bleomycin	5		●					
Etoposide	60			●				
Prednisone	40	● 1–28						
BEACOPP (Escalate dose)					New cycle			
B (bleomycin)	10		●					
E (etoposide)	100 (200)	● 1–3						
A [Adriamycin (doxorubicin)]	25 (35)	●						
C (cyclophosphamide)	650 (1250)	●						
O [Oncovin (vinblastine)]	1.4		●					
P (procarbazine)	100	● 1–7						
P (prednisone)	40	● 1–14						

1. Radiation therapy to bulky residual disease.
2. Treatment repeated every 28 d for a total of 3 cycles. Vinblastine dose decreased to 4 mg/m², and vincristine dose decreased to 1 mg/m² during cycle 3 for patients ≥50 y of age. Tapered by 10 mg qod starting at week 10. Maximum dose, 2.0 mg. Followed by 36 Gy radiation therapy.

12 weeks. All patients receive daily oral trimethoprim/sulfamethoxazole and granulocyte colony-stimulating factor. After initial regression, radiation therapy is administered to sites of initial bulky disease or to areas where radiologic abnormalities persist after chemotherapy. The three-year failure-free survival rate was 100% for stage II patients with bulky mediastinal disease and 82% in patients with stages III and IV disease. An ongoing Eastern Cooperative Oncology Group trial randomizes patients to the Stanford V regimen versus ABVD. The intent is to compare their effectiveness and, of special importance, their toxicities. The concern remains that the nitrogen mustard, albeit in attenuated total dose compared to MOPP, in the Stanford V therapy may be associated with an increased risk of leukemogenesis, second malignancies, and infertility.

The German Hodgkin's Lymphoma Study Group developed BEACOPP (see Table 65-4), which achieved a complete remission rate of 83%. The HD9 clinical trial randomized patients to four cycles of COPP (the same as MOPP but with cyclophosphamide substituted for nitrogen mustard)/ABVD, eight cycles of BEACOPP in standard dose, or eight cycles of BEACOPP in escalated doses. Chemotherapy was followed in each instance by limited-field radiation therapy, consisting of 30 Gy to bulky initial sites and 40 Gy to sites of residual disease. The COPP/ABVD arm was closed to further accrual when interim analysis showed that the combined BEACOPP arms were superior in complete response rate (89% versus 76%) and freedom from treatment failure (85% versus 74%). The risk of long-term complications increases when dose-intensive regimens such as these are used. For example, an interim analysis showed an increased incidence of secondary leukemia in the heavily treated patients.

Combined Modality Treatment

In clinically evaluated (no-laparotomy) patients with early-stage disease who are treated with radiation therapy alone, the risk of relapse in nonirradiated sites (occult areas of disease) is 20% to 30%. Many of these relapsing patients can nevertheless be cured by chemotherapy. It therefore became of interest to determine whether combined modality therapy would improve on the results of either modality used alone. In early- or advanced-stage Hodgkin's disease, in comparison with single-modality therapy, combined modality therapy improves disease control and the complete remission rate, reduces the relapse rate, and improves the failure-free survival rate; however, the overall survival rate does not change.

A meta-analysis of 1,740 patients with advanced Hodgkin's disease who were treated on 14 randomized trials showed no improvement in overall survival with combined modality therapy. Two groups of patients receiving combined modality therapy were evaluated. One group of patients had received the same chemotherapy (most of whom were treated with MOPP-type regimens) ± additional radiation therapy, and another group compared chemotherapy + additional radiation therapy to those who received chemotherapy (most were treated with ABVD or MOPP/ABV) + additional chemotherapy. When doxorubicin chemotherapy was used (in ABVD or MOPP/ABV), the addition of radiation therapy did not improve disease control or the disease-free survival rate. Moreover, the overall survival rate actually decreased by 8% at 10 years compared to chemotherapy alone owing to an increased risk of dying from causes other than Hodgkin's disease. There thus appears to be no established role at present for the addition of radiation therapy to chemotherapy in advanced disease.

The International Hodgkin's Disease Collaborative Group performed a meta-analysis on 1666 patients with early-stage Hodgkin's disease from 13 randomized trials comparing chemotherapy added to radiation therapy versus radiation therapy alone. The addition of chemotherapy reduced the risk of treatment failure from 33% to 16% ($p < .00001$), but the 10-year overall survival rate was not improved (79% versus 77%). These full-dose combined modality approaches do not provide a survival benefit. Nevertheless, current studies of therapy in early-stage Hodgkin's disease continue to use combined modality therapy with the primary aim of reducing the long-term toxicities by decreasing the dose and duration of each modality. A number of such studies are underway, and/or some of these approaches have already been incorporated into clinical practice. For example, the German Hodgkin's Disease Study Group HD10 trial randomizes early-stage patients to receive one of the four following therapies: four cycles of ABVD followed by 30 Gy involved-field radiation therapy, four cycles of ABVD followed by 20 Gy involved-field radiation therapy, two cycles of ABVD followed by 30 Gy involved-field radiation therapy, or two cycles of ABVD followed by 20 Gy involved-field radiation therapy. The use of the initial courses of chemotherapy has the salutary effect of reducing the radiation field volume (by shrinking the mass of disease) while treating subclinical occult disease in the abdomen. This study also addresses what reduction in the dose/duration of each modality can be employed without loss of efficacy.

An alternative approach, taken in the National Cancer Institute of Canada CTG HD6 trial, evaluates whether short-course chemotherapy may be as effective as, and less toxic than, large-field radiation therapy. In this study, clinically staged patients who have limited disease and a good prognosis (nodular sclerosis or lymphocyte-predominant histology, age younger than 40 years, a sedimentation rate less than 50 mm/hour, and three sites or less of involvement) are randomized to receive subtotal nodal and splenic radiation therapy versus four cycles of ABVD.

Combined modality therapy using ABVD chemotherapy and no alkylating agents does not appear to increase delayed cardiac (from doxorubicin) or pulmonary (from bleomycin) toxicity.

Issues in Early-Stage Disease

The standard of care for clinical stages IA and IIA HD with a favorable prognosis (young age, female gender, involvement of fewer than four nodal sites, no systemic symptoms, nonbulky disease, and a normal erythrocyte sedimentation rate) remains controversial. One option is mantle-field radiation therapy. Because of concern about radiation therapy-induced delayed pulmonary and cardiac toxicity and increased risk of breast cancer, the trend has been to treat such patients with combination chemotherapy and radiation therapy, reducing the number of cycles of chemotherapy and radiation dose and fields as previously discussed. The long-term freedom from treatment failure in favorable prognosis, clinically staged IA–IIA Hodgkin's disease is 80% to 90%. It will therefore be difficult to demonstrate improvement in the cure rate of Hodgkin's disease in these patients. What remains are a number of questions, such as what approach best reduces short- and long-term toxicity without reduction in efficacy, what the salvage rates are for patients previously treated with a limited number of cycles of ABVD, and whether those patients who relapse can be salvaged with chemotherapy treatment alone or require high-dose therapy and peripheral blood stem cell transplantation.

Treatment of Patients with a Large Mediastinal Mass

Mediastinal bulky disease is the most common unfavorable prognostic factor in patients who have stage I and II Hodgkin's disease. In patients treated with radiation therapy alone, the relapse rate in the mediastinum was 2% if the mediastinal mass was one third or less of the maximum intrathoracic diameter, whereas the mediastinal relapse rate was 40% if the ratio was greater than one third (bulky disease). Combining full doses of chemotherapy with mantle radiation therapy in patients with bulky mediastinal masses increases the disease-free survival rate to 75% from

50% for radiation therapy or chemotherapy alone. No evidence of improved survival occurs, however, from the use of combined modality therapy, most likely because of the efficacy of chemotherapy in patients who relapse after radiation therapy. The long-term overall survival rate in patients with bulky mediastinal disease remains approximately 50%. Although combined modality therapy is routinely used in these patients, the fact that one half of these patients ultimately die of the disease or its treatment means that new therapeutic approaches are needed in the circumstances of bulky mediastinal disease.

Follow-up Evaluations

Evaluations prior to each cycle during treatment include a history, especially for pain, constitutional symptoms, performance status assessment, and treatment toxicity, and a physical examination focused on cardiopulmonary status and lymph node or organ enlargement. A complete blood count and chemistry analysis are appropriate prior to each chemotherapy cycle. Abnormal pretreatment laboratory results, such as an elevated sedimentation rate (ESR) and/or lactase dehydrogenase level should be monitored with each cycle. Chest X-rays are of value to assess for disease response, occult infection, and toxicities of treatment such as bleomycin lung injury.

After therapy and documentation of response, patients should be evaluated at approximately three-month intervals for the first two years, four-month intervals in the third year, six-month intervals in years four and five, and annually thereafter. Nearly all relapses that will occur become apparent in the first four years after therapy is completed. Patients are encouraged to return at any time if new signs or symptoms occur. Tests at each visit include a complete blood count, sedimentation rate, chemistry panel, and chest X-ray. A clinical assessment of the complications of therapy should be carried out and explored if clinically indicated. Repeat computed tomography scans should be obtained at 6 and 12 months after therapy to establish a posttreatment baseline. The routine continuing use of computed tomography scans and gallium scanning in follow-up has no utility and is not cost-effective. Most relapses are detected on the basis of symptoms reported by patients or abnormalities noted on blood tests. It is exceedingly rare for a routinely scheduled computed tomography scan to detect relapse in the absence of symptoms, abnormal physical examination findings, or abnormal blood studies. In patients who have undergone mantle radiation therapy, a thyroid-stimulating hormone (TSH) assay should be done annually to detect at an early stage the not infrequent occurrence of hypothyroidism secondary to thyroid damage from neck irradiation. In women, annual mammograms should commence 8 to 10 years after radiation therapy in patients who were younger than 25 to 30 years old at the time of treatment.

The Treatment of Initial Relapse After Chemotherapy

Patients whose duration of initial remission lasts more than one year after combination chemotherapy can occasionally be cured by combination chemotherapy after relapse. Highly selected patients with localized relapse following a complete remission from chemotherapy can be cured with radiation therapy. For most patients, however, who relapse after combination chemotherapy (as well as those who fail initial chemotherapy), high-dose therapy with hematopoietic stem cell transplantation, either allogeneic or autologous, is now the standard of care.

After autologous stem cell transplantation, the five-year time to treatment failure rate is 45%, and the five-year survival rate is 55%. Chemotherapeutic responsiveness and the number of prior therapeutic attempts strongly influence the outcome of autologous stem cell transplantation. The degree of sensitivity of the disease to conventional chemotherapy administered immediately prior to autologous stem cell transplantation is the most important determinant of outcome. For example, the five-year time to treatment failure and survival rate is approximately 65%; it is 70% for patients who achieve a complete remission prior to stem cell transplantation versus 40% and 45% for patients with chemotherapy-sensitive disease and 15% and 20% for patients with chemotherapy-resistant Hodgkin's disease, respectively. The greater the number of prior attempts with conventional chemotherapy, the worse the outcome with autologous stem cell transplantation. Because of this, autologous stem cell transplantation has taken the place of chemotherapy in salvage treatment of patients with relapsed Hodgkin's disease.

The most frequently used high-dose regimens in autologous stem cell transplantation are CBV [cyclophosphamide, carmustine (BCNU), and etoposide (VP-16)] and BEAM [carmustine (BCNU), etoposide, cytosine arabinoside, and melphalan]. The doses and schedules vary somewhat from institution to institution. For example, the doses that are employed in CBV vary from 4.8 to 7.2 g/m^2 for cyclophosphamide to 300 to 600 mg/m^2 for carmustine and 750 to 2400 mg/m^2 for etoposide. The higher doses are not more effective, and they are associated with increased toxicity, which is most evident in the risk of pulmonary injury from high-dose carmustine. Total body radia-

tion as a component of the high-dose therapy is rarely used. It is contraindicated in patients who were previously treated for their Hodgkin's disease with conventional radiation therapy fields, because of the increased risk of fatal pulmonary toxicity.

Most transplant centers do try to induce a partial or complete remission by salvage chemotherapy prior to proceeding to autologous stem cell transplantation, because patients with extensive disease at the time of stem cell transplantation do worse than those with minimal disease. Patients with minimal disease at the time of relapse can go directly to autologous stem cell transplantation without preliminary cytoreduction with the expectation of a good result. The results of autologous stem cell transplantation are so poor in patients who have bulky disease that is unresponsive to conventional salvage chemotherapy regimens that many clinicians believe it is inappropriate to take such patients through autologous stem cell transplantation.

The value of posttransplantation radiation therapy is unknown. Nevertheless, most centers do administer radiation therapy (when feasible) to sites of bulky disease after recovery from transplantation, because these are the most frequent sites of subsequent relapse.

Whether high-dose therapy with autologous stem cell transplantation may be of benefit in the initial treatment of patients with poor prognosis disease is under investigation in several randomized clinical trials.

Allogeneic stem cell transplantation is an alternative to autologous stem cell transplantation in patients with relapsed and refractory disease. The treatment-related mortality rate of allogeneic stem cell transplantation is substantially higher than that of autologous stem cell transplantation (approximately 30% versus less than 5%), but the graft-versus-host disease (GVHD) effect results in a decreased incidence of relapse. Allogeneic stem cell transplantation is a consideration, especially when the patient is young and has a human leukocyte antigen–matched histocompatible sibling and the Hodgkin's disease is resistant to conventional chemotherapy.

Optimal therapy for patients who relapse after stem cell transplantation is unclear, but there is no evidence that these patients are potentially curable. Treatment is therefore palliative, consisting of administering single-agent chemotherapy (such as vinblastine or prednisone) and supportive care measures. Alternative measures for such patients may include rituximab (Rituxan). Its activity in Hodgkin's disease is dependent on the histology. Responses have been seen in lymphocyte-predominant Hodgkin's disease at the standard dose of 375 mg/m^2 administered intravenously on a weekly basis, and some activity has been noted in patients in relapse after transplantation.

Infradiaphragmatic Hodgkin's Disease

Approximately 7% of patients with Hodgkin's disease present with disease below the diaphragm, usually consisting of inguinal and/or femoral lymph node enlargement. Occasionally, an abdominal mass is detected. Approximately one half of patients with stage I presentations have lymphocyte-predominant histology. In patients with para-aortic disease, splenic involvement is common. Some years ago, stage IA disease was treated with radiation to an "inverted-Y" field (paraortic, iliac, inguinal, and femoral lymph nodes), and patients had an 80% likelihood of cure. Because so much bone marrow is irradiated in the treatment field, impaired marrow reserve develops, compromising the ability to deliver chemotherapy subsequently to patients who relapse. For this reason and in the absence of specific studies of this small subset of patients, most patients are now treated with systemic chemotherapy with or without local radiation therapy to initial sites of disease.

HIV-Related Hodgkin's Disease

Hodgkin's disease was recently added to the list of AIDS-defining malignancies (see Chapter 113). Hodgkin's disease has a poor prognosis in patients with AIDS. Hodgkin's disease more commonly occurs in patients with AIDS who are drug abusers and homosexual men, whereas the incidence is not increased in HIV-infected women or hemophiliacs. Compared to patients with Hodgkin's disease who do not have AIDS, HIV-infected patients with Hodgkin's disease exhibit an increased incidence of mixed cellularity and lymphocyte depletion histologies, higher frequency of association with Epstein-Barr virus–infected lymphocytes (80% to 100%), advanced stage of disease at presentation, "B" symptoms, noncontiguous patterns of spread, and poor prognosis. At presentation in these patients, liver involvement can occur without splenic involvement. In contrast to HIV-related non-Hodgkin's lymphoma, the CD4+ (helper T lymphocytes) median counts are greater than 200/μL. Opportunistic infections complicate treatment and include *Pneumocystis carinii*, cytomegalovirus, extrapulmonary tuberculosis, candidiasis, cryptococcal meningitis, and cerebral toxoplasmosis.

The optimal treatment for AIDS-related Hodgkin's disease is not known. The complete response rates to standard therapy are worse than those in non–AIDS-related Hodgkin's disease. The already low CD4+ counts drop with chemotherapy, leukopenia occurs, and tolerance to chemotherapy is poor, prejudicing the outcome because of treatment-related complications. The overall median survival is 1.5 years. Reducing the viral load and increasing CD4+ counts with antiretroviral medications may improve the outcome. These patients should be encouraged to participate in innovative clinical trials.

Hodgkin's Disease in Pregnancy

Although Hodgkin's disease occurs in young patients, its presentation during pregnancy is rare. In most cases, Hodgkin's disease is a slowly progressive cancer, and every effort should be made to carry the fetus to term. Moreover, Hodgkin's disease in the mother is not an indication for delivery by cesarian section. These women should be treated as high-risk obstetrics cases. Radiographic staging studies are necessarily limited to avoid or minimize exposure of the developing fetus to radiation. Acceptable studies include a single posteroanterior chest film with adequate abdominal shielding and abdominal magnetic resonance imaging of the abdomen in place of computed tomography scans. Gallium scans and positron emission tomography are contraindicated during pregnancy. Termination of the pregnancy is very rarely necessary.

Fetal risk from radiation or chemotherapy is greatest·in the first trimester. It is therefore reasonable to delay therapy until after the first trimester unless patients are symptomatic or have bulky disease. Although the data are limited on the long-term effects of chemotherapy exposure in utero, there is no evidence that chemotherapy with MOPP or ABVD after the first trimester increases the risk of fetal malformations, congenital anomalies, or of cancer in childhood or adolescence.

It is difficult to find a consensus on specific recommendations for pregnant patients. The management of each patient must be individualized, taking into account the anxiety of the patient and the rest of the family, the stage of disease, the patient's symptoms, the location and extent of involvement, the trimester of pregnancy when the diagnosis is made, and the recommendations that are made for nonpregnant women with Hodgkin's disease. Pregnancy does not worsen the prognosis, and stage for stage, the outcome is the same as in nonpregnant patients. Radiation therapy can be safely administered above the diaphragm to limited-stage disease. However, most clinicians turn to chemotherapy for treatment of these patients. Depending on the circumstances, after the first trimester, one can initiate a full course of chemotherapy during the pregnancy or give only one or two courses of treatment to tide the patient over until after delivery, when comprehensive evaluation and definitive treatment can be given safely.

Long-Term Complications in Patients with Hodgkin's Disease

Although 75% of patients with Hodgkin's disease are cured with present treatment modalities, their survival rate is not the same as that of the age-matched general population. Years after treatment, the mortality rate from complications and naturally occurring disease exceeds the mortality rate from Hodgkin's disease itself. These complications may be due to the toxicity of therapy, impaired immunity, or genetic susceptibility.

Secondary Malignancies

The risk of developing acute leukemia or myelodysplasia is 1% to 4%. These secondary disorders are generally refractory to therapeutic intervention; the median survival is two to five months, and the five-year survival rate is less than 5%. Risk factors for developing this complication include alkylating agent chemotherapy, radiation therapy, splenectomy, age, advanced stage, and female gender. Nitrogen mustard is the most significant association with these complications. The risk of these disorders is decreasing since ABVD has replaced MOPP as the primary choice for chemotherapy. Limited-field radiation therapy alone does not predispose patients to these complications, but the combination of radiation therapy with alkylating agent chemotherapy does increase the risk. The only intervention that can lead to cure of these secondary malignancies is allogeneic stem cell transplantation.

The risk of developing secondary solid tumors is greater than that for other hematologic malignancies. Solid tumors represent 55% to 75% of secondary malignancies in Hodgkin's disease. Skin, breast, and thyroid cancers are the most common second malignancies. The risks of secondary malignancy are increased in women and in older patients. Primary initial radiation therapy to a mantle field increases the likelihood of breast cancer (in women), esophageal cancer, lung cancer, and thyroid cancer that is, in organs within the treatment field.

Non-Hodgkin's lymphoma develops in 1% to 2% of patients with Hodgkin's disease, more often in those who received extensive treatment initially and in patients older than age 40 years. The lymphocyte-predominant histologic subtype has a higher association with the development of non-Hodgkin's lymphoma than do the other histologic subtypes of Hodgkin's disease. Responses and even cures can be obtained in this circumstance, the choice of therapy and the outcome being dependent on the histology of the non-Hodgkin's lymphoma and the extent of disease.

Immunologic Impairment in Hodgkin's Disease

An impaired immune response was first recognized by Dorothy Reed in 1902. The lymphocytic and plasma cell infiltration of the neoplastic nodes have always suggested that an immunologic response to Hodgkin's disease is occurring. At the same time, patients with Hodgkin's disease frequently have impaired delayed hypersensitivity responses to common antigens. Anergy to mumps, *Candida albicans*, and tuberculosis is a common finding and is more likely to be present in advanced and/or symptomatic Hodgkin's disease. Another manifestation is the absence of an effective cytotoxic response against the Epstein-Barr virus in patients with Epstein-Barr virus–positive lymph nodes.

Because the cell-mediated immunologic response is defective in Hodgkin's disease, patients are predisposed to a variety of viral, bacterial, parasitic, and fungal infections. This inherent risk is amplified in patients who develop cytopenias from therapy or from extensive bone marrow involvement. The infectious complications include pneumonia, bacteremia, skin infections, and meningitis. The most common bacterial infections are *Streptococcus pneumonia*, *Staphylococcus aureus*, and *Staphylococcus epidermidis*. Among viral illnesses, herpes zoster and cytomegalovirus infections can occur by reactivation in patients who have had prior, now latent, infection. Fungal infections tend to occur late in the disease course as a complication of myelosuppression and further immunosuppression induced by the disease and aggressive treatment for relapse.

Cardiovascular Complications of Treatment

The most common causes of excess morbidity and mortality in long-term survivors of Hodgkin's disease are cardiovascular diseases, which account for approximately 15% of the deaths. Complications that can be caused by radiation therapy to a mantle field include acute pericarditis, chronic constrictive pericarditis, valvular heart disease, premature coronary artery disease, acute myocardial infarction, arrhythmias secondary to conduction abnormalities, and myocardial fibrosis. The likelihood of coronary artery disease events increases in patients who are smokers and exhibit hypertension, obesity, or hyperlipidemia. Valvular heart disease usually consists of tricuspid and/or mitral regurgitation and is more common in young patients. Mediastinal radiation therapy can potentiate the cardiac toxicity of anthracyclines. Because false-negative and false-positive results occur, the role of routine noninvasive cardiac screening after radiation therapy or anthracycline chemotherapy has not been defined. The risk of cerebral vascular disease is increased in patients who have received radiation therapy to the neck.

Pulmonary Complications of Treatment

Radiation therapy or chemotherapy can cause lung damage. Radiation pneumonitis and fibrosis in the septa are the acute and chronic phases, respectively, of radiation-induced lung injury. Pneumonitis symptoms include a dry hacking cough, dyspnea on exertion, and occasionally fever. Acute pneumonitis can occur in the early months following mantle-field radiation therapy, which encompasses 20% to 30% of the lung volume despite careful lead shielding. On long-term follow-up, some restrictive impairment is characteristic, but clinically significant impairment of pulmonary function is uncommon.

Bleomycin, which is a component of ABVD and other chemotherapy regimens, can cause similar changes. Much less often, cyclophosphamide can itself cause pneumonitis. Dyspnea, nonproductive cough, and fever characteristically present 4 to 10 weeks after treatment with bleomycin, but the reaction can occur earlier or as late as six months after discontinuing therapy. The chest radiograph shows bilateral basilar reticulonodular infiltrates, which may progress to involve the middle and upper lobes, but computed tomography scans are more sensitive in detecting this complication. The DLCO (diffusing capacity for carbon monoxide) and vital capacity are useful tests to establish the degree of injury and monitor for recovery. The risk of bleomycin-induced interstitial fibrosis is approximately 10% at a cumulative dose of bleomycin of 450 to 550 mg and generally does not become apparent until a cumulative dose of 200 mg is reached. However, this complication can occur on some occasions with total doses as low as 20 to 50 mg. Acute, severe bleomycin-induced lung injury is reversible if treated with high-dose corticosteroids with a slow taper.

References

General Information

Aisenberg AC: Problems in Hodgkin's disease management. Blood 199;3:761–779.

Brada M, Eeles R, Ashley S, et al: Salvage radiotherapy in recurrent Hodgkin's disease. Ann Oncol 1992;3:131–135.

Brown RS, Haynes HA, Foley HT, et al: Hodgkin's disease: Immunologic, clinical and histologic features of 50 untreated patients. Ann Intern Med 1967;67:291–302.

Buzaid A, Lippman SM, Miller TP: Salvage therapy of advanced Hodgkin's disease. Critical appraisal of curative potential. Am J Med 1987;83:523–532.

Dolginow D, Colby TV: Recurrent Hodgkin's disease in treated sites. Cancer 1981;48:1124–1126.

Habermann TM, Steensma DP: Lymphadenopathy. Mayo Clin Proc 2000;75:723–732.

Hellman S: Thomas Hodgkin and Hodgkin's disease: Two paradigms appropriate to medicine today. JAMA 1991;265:1007–1010.

Lucas JB, Hoppe RT, Horwitz SM, et al: Rituximab is active in lymphocyte-predominant Hodgkin's disease [Abstract]. Blood 2000;96:831a, 2000.

Molrine D, George S, Tarbell N, et al: Antibody responses to polysaccharide and polysaccharide-conjugate vaccines following treatment for Hodgkin's disease. Ann Intern Med 1995;123:824–828.

Radford JA, Eardley A, Woodman C, et al: Follow-up policy after treatment for Hodgkin's disease: Too many clinic visits and routine tests? A review of hospital records. Br Med J 1997;314:343–346.

Rosenberg SA, Kaplan HS: Evidence for an orderly progression in the spread of Hodgkin's disease. Cancer Res 1966; 26:1225–1231.

Roskrow MA, Suzuki N, Gan Y, et al: Epstein-Barr virus (EBV)-specific cytotoxic T lymphocytes for the treatment of patients with EBV-positive relapsed Hodgkin's disease. Blood 1998;91:2925–2934.

Sextro M: Differences in clinical presentation and course between adult patients with Hodgkin's disease older and younger than 60 years [Abstract]. Blood 1997;88(Suppl 1):227a.

Wilks S: Cases of enlargement of the lymphatic glands and spleen (or Hodgkin's disease) with remarks. Guy's Hosp Red 1865;11:56–67.

Younes A, Romaguera J, Hagemeister F, et al: A pilot study of rituximab in patients with relapsed Hodgkin's disease of classical type [Abstract]. Blood 2000;96:733a.

Chemotherapy

Bonadonna G: Chemotherapy strategies to improve the control of Hodgkin's disease: The Richard and Hinda Rosenthal Award Lecture. Cancer Res 1982;42:4309–4320.

Bonadonna G, Beretta G, Tancini G, et al: Adriamycin (NSC-123127) studies at the Instituto Nazionale Tumori, Milan. Cancer Chemother Rep 1975;6:231–245.

Bonadonna G, Valagussa P, Santoro A: Alternating noncross-resistant combination chemotherapy or MOPP in Stage IV Hodgkin's disease: A report of the 8-year results. Ann Intern Med 1986;104:736–746.

Canellos GP, Anderson JR, Propert KJ, et al: Chemotherapy of advanced Hodgkin's disease with MOPP, ABVD, or MOPP alternating with ABVD. N Engl J Med 1992;327:1478–1484.

Connors JM, Klimo P, Adams G, et al: Treatment of advanced Hodgkin's disease with chemotherapy-comparison of

MOPP/ABV hybrid regimen with alternating courses of MOPP and ABVD: A report from the National Cancer Institute of Canada Clinical Trials Group. J Clin Oncol 1997;15:1638–1645.

DeVita VT, Serpick AA, Carbone PP: Combination chemotherapy in the treatment of advanced Hodgkin's disease. Ann Intern Med 1970;73:891–895.

Diehl V, Sieber M, Ruffler U, et al: BEACOPP: An intensified chemotherapy regimen in advanced Hodgkin's disease. Ann Oncol 1997;8:143–148.

Duggan DB, Petroni GR, Johnson JL, et al: Randomized comparison of ABVD and MOPP/ABV hybrid for the treatment of advanced Hodgkin's disease: Report of an Intergroup Trial. J Clin Oncol 2003;21:607–614.

Glick JH, Barnes JM, Bakemeier RF, et al: Treatment of advanced Hodgkin's disease: 10 years experience in the Eastern Cooperative Oncology Group. Cancer Treat Rep 1982;66:855–870.

Little R, Wittes RE, Longo DL, et al: Vinblastine for recurrent Hodgkin's disease following autologous bone marrow transplant. J Clin Oncol 1998;16:584–588.

Lewis BM, Izbicki R: Routine pulmonary function tests during bleomycin therapy. JAMA 1980;243:347–351.

Longo DL, Duffey PL, Young RC, et al: Conventional-dose salvage combination chemotherapy in patients relapsing with Hodgkin's disease after combination chemotherapy: The low probability for cure. J Clin Oncol 1992; 10:210–218.

Longo DL, Young RC, Wesley M, et al: 20 years of MOPP therapy for Hodgkin's disease. J Clin Oncol 1986;4:1295–1306.

Rodriguez J, Rodriguez MA, Fayad L, et al: ASHAP: A regimen for cytoreduction of refractory or recurrent Hodgkin's disease. Blood 1999;93:3632–3636.

Santoro A, Bonadonna G, Bonfante V, et al: Alternating drug combinations in the treatment of advanced Hodgkin's disease. N Engl J Med 1982;306:770–775.

Silvestri F, Fanin R, Velisig M, et al: The role of granulocyte colony-stimulating factor (filgrastim) in maintaining dose intensity during conventional-dose chemotherapy with ABVD in Hodgkin's disease. Tumori 1994;80:453–458.

Tesch H, Diehl V, Lathan B: Moderate dose escalation for advanced stage Hodgkin's disease using the bleomycin, etoposide, adriamycin, cyclophosphamide, vincristine, procarbazine, and prednisone scheme and adjuvant radiotherapy: A study of the German Hodgkin's Lymphoma Study Group. Blood 1998;92:4560–4567.

Tesch H, Diehl V, Lathan B, et al: Interim analysis of the HD9 study of the German Hodgkin Study Group (GHSG)-BEACOPP is more effective than COPP-ABVD in advanced stage Hodgkin's disease. Leuk Lymphoma 1998;29:2–8.

Combined Modality Therapy

Horning SJ, Williams J, Bartlett NL, et al: Assessment of Stanford V regimen and consolidative radiotherapy for bulky and advanced Hodgkin's disease: Eastern Cooperative Oncology Group Pilot Study E1492. J Clin Oncol 2000;18:972–980.

Hughes-Davies L, Tarbell NJ, Colemen CN, et al: Stage IA-IIB Hodgkin's disease: Management and outcome of extensive thoracic involvement. Int J Radiat Oncol Biol Phys 1997;39:361–369.

Loeffler M, Brosteanu O, Hasenclever D, et al: Meta-analysis of chemotherapy versus combined modality treatment trials in Hodgkin's disease. J Clin Oncol 1998;6:818–829.

Loeffler M, Diehl V, Pfreundschuh M, et al: Dose-response relationship of complementary radiotherapy following four cycles of combination chemotherapy in intermediate-stage Hodgkin's disease. J Clin Oncol 1997;15:2275–2287.

Longo DL, Glatstein E, Duffey PL, et al: Alternating MOPP and ABVD chemotherapy plus mantle-field radiation therapy in patients with massive mediastinal Hodgkin's disease. J Clin Oncol 1997;15:3338–3346.

Mauch P: What is the role for adjuvant radiation therapy in advanced Hodgkin's disease [Editorial]? J Clin Oncol 1998;6:815–817.

Santoro A, Bonadonna G, Valagussa P, et al: Long-term results of combined chemotherapy-radiotherapy approach in Hodgkin's disease: Superiority of ABVD plus radiotherapy versus MOPP plus radiotherapy. J Clin Oncol 1987;5:27–37.

Early-Stage Disease

Biti GP, Cimino G, Cartoni C, et al: Extended-field radiotherapy is superior to MOPP chemotherapy for the treatment of pathologic stage I-IIA Hodgkin's disease: Eight-year update of an Italian prospective randomized study. J Clin Oncol 1992;10:378–382.

Carde P, Hagenbeek A, Hayat M, et al: Clinical staging versus laparotomy and combined modality with MOPP versus ABVD in early-stage Hodgkin's disease: The H6 twin randomized trials from the European Organization for Research and Treatment of Cancer Lymphoma Cooperative Group. J Clin Oncol 1993;11:2258–2272.

Cooper DL: Treatment of early-stage Hodgkin's disease: Lessons from recent studies. PPO Updates Princ Pract Oncol 1999;13:1–10.

Duhmke E, Diehl V, Loeffler M, et al: Randomized trial with early-stage Hodgkin's disease testing 30 Gy vs. 40 Gy extended field radiotherapy alone. Int J Radiat Oncol Biol Phys 1996;36:305–310.

Duhmke E, Franklin J, Pfreundschuh M, et al: Low-dose radiation is sufficient for the noninvolved extended-field treatment in favorable early-stage Hodgkin's disease: Long-term results of a randomized trial of radiotherapy alone. J Clin Oncol 2001;19:2905–2914.

Gospodarowicz M, Sutcliffe S, Clark R, et al: Analysis of supra-diaphragmatic clinical stage I and II Hodgkin's disease treated with radiation alone. Int J Radiat Oncol Biol Phys 1992;22:859–865.

Hoppe RT, Coleman CN, Cox RS, et al: The management of stage I-II Hodgkin's disease with irradiation alone or combined modality therapy: The Stanford experience. Blood 1982;59:455–465.

Hutchison GB, Alison RE, Fuller LM, et al: Radiotherapy of stage I and II Hodgkin's disease. Cancer 1984; 54:1928–1942.

Longo DL, Glatstein E, Duffey PL, et al: Radiation therapy versus combination chemotherapy in the treatment of early-stage Hodgkin's disease: Seven-year results of a prospective randomized trial. J Clin Oncol 1991;9:906–917.

Mauch P, Tarbell N, Weinstein H, et al: Stage IA and IIA supra-diaphragmatic Hodgkin's disease: Prognostic factors in surgically staged patients treated with mantle and para-aortic irradiation. J Clin Oncol 1988;6:1576–1583.

Rueda A, Alba E, Ribelles N, et al: Six cycles of ABVD in the treatment of stage I and II Hodgkin's lymphoma: A pilot study. J Clin Oncol 1997;15:1118–1122.

Specht L, Gray RG, Clarke MJ, et al: Influence of more extensive radiotherapy and adjuvant chemotherapy on long-term outcome of early-stage Hodgkin's disease: A meta-analysis of 23 randomized trials involving 3,888 patients. International Hodgkin's disease Collaborative Group. J Clin Oncol 1998;16:830–843.

Torrey MJ, Poen JC, Hoppe RT: Detection of relapse in early-stage Hodgkin's disease: Role of routine follow-up studies. J Clin Oncol 1997;15:1123–1130.

Tubiana M, Henry-Amar M, Carde P, et al: Toward comprehensive management tailored to prognostic factors of patients with clinical stages I and II Hodgkin's disease: The EORTC Lymphoma Group controlled clinical trials: 1964–1987. Blood 1989;73:47–56.

Wirth A, Choa M, Corry C, et al: Mantle irradiation alone for clinical stage I–II Hodgkin's disease: Long-term follow-up and analysis of prognostic factors in 261 patients. J Clin Oncol 1999;17:230–240.

Epidemiology

Boice JD Jr, Land CE, Preston DL: Ionizing radiation. In Schottenfeld D, Fraumeni JR Jr (eds): Cancer Epidemiology and Prevention, 2nd ed. New York: Oxford University Press, 1996.

Chakravarti A, Halloran SL, Bale SJ, et al: Etiological heterogeneity in Hodgkin's disease: HLA linked and unlinked determinants of susceptibility independent of histological concordance. Genet Epidemiol 1986;3:407–415.

Dolcetti R, Frisan T, Sjoberg J, et al: Identification and characterization of an Epstein-Barr virus–specific T-cell response in the pathologic tissue of a patient with Hodgkin's disease. Cancer Res 1995;55:3675–3681.

Ferraris AM, Racchi O, Rapezzi D, et al: Familial Hodgkin's disease: A disease of young adulthood? Ann Hematol 1997;74:131–134.

Filipovich AH, Mathur A, Kamat D, et al: Primary immunodeficiency: Genetic risk factors for lymphoma [Abstract]. Cancer Res 1992;52:5465a.

Frisan T, Sjoberg J, Dolcetti R, et al: Local suppression of Epstein-Barr (EBV)–specific cytotoxicity in biopsies of EBV-positive Hodgkin's disease. Blood 1995;86:1493–1501.

Glaser SL, Ruby JL, Stewart SL, et al: Epstein-Barr virus–associated Hodgkin's disease: Epidemiologic characteristics in international data. Int J Cancer 1997;70:375–382.

Grufferman S: Clustering and aggregation of exposures in Hodgkin's disease. Cancer 1977;39:1829–1833.

Grufferman S, Cole P, Levitan PR: Evidence against transmission of Hodgkin's disease in high schools. N Engl J Med 1979;300:1006–1011.

Gutensohn N, Cole P: Childhood social environment and Hodgkin's disease. N Engl J Med 1981;304:135–140.

Henderson BE, Dworsky R, Pike MC, et al: Risk factors for nodular sclerosis and other types of Hodgkin's disease. Cancer Res 1979;39:4507–4511.

Kingma DW, Medeiros LJ, Barletta J, et al: Epstein-Barr virus is infrequently identified in non-Hodgkin's lymphoma associated with Hodgkin's disease. Am J Surg Pathol 1994;18:48–61.

Mack TM, Cozen W, Shibata DK, et al: Concordance for Hodgkin's disease in identical twins suggesting genetic susceptibility to the young-adult form of the disease. New Engl J Med 1995;332:413–418.

MacMahon B: Epidemiology of Hodgkin's disease. Cancer Res 1966;26:1189–1201.

Miller RW, Beebe GW: Infectious mononucleosis and the empirical risk of cancer. J Natl Cancer Inst 1973;50:315–321.

Mueller NE, Hodgkin's disease: In Schottenfeld D, Fraumeni JR Jr (eds): Cancer Epidemiology and Prevention, 2nd ed. New York: Oxford University Press, 1996.

Razis DV, Diamond HD, Craver LF: Familial Hodgkin's disease: Its significance and implications. Ann Intern Med 1959;51:933–937.

Ries LAG, Kosary CL, Hankey BF, et al. (eds): SEER cancer statistics review: 1973–1994. NIH Publ. No. 97-2789. Bethesda, MD: National Cancer Institute, 1997.

Smith PG, Pike MC, Kinlen LJ, et al: Contacts between young patients with Hodgkin's disease: A case-controlled study. Lancet 1977;2:59–62.

Vianna NJ, Greenwald P, Davies JNP: Extended epidemic of Hodgkin's disease in high school students. Lancet 1971;1:1209–1211.

Pathology

Aguilera NS, Howard LN, Brissette MD, et al: Hodgkin's disease and an extranodal marginal zone B-cell lymphoma in the small intestine: An unusual composite lymphoma. Mod Pathol 1996;9:1020–1026.

Anagnostopoulos I, Hansmann ML, Franssila K, et al, on behalf of the European Task Force on Lymphoma: European Task Force on Lymphoma Project on lymphocyte-predominant Hodgkin's disease histologic and immunohistologic analysis of submitted cases reveals 2 types of Hodgkin's disease with a nodular growth pattern and abundant lymphocytes. Blood 2000;96:1889–1899.

Colby TV, Warnke RA: The histology of the initial relapse of Hodgkin's disease. Cancer 1980;45:289–292.

Gonzalez CL, Medeiros LJ, Jaffe ES: Composite lymphoma: A clinicopathologic analysis of nine patients with Hodgkin's disease and B-cell non-Hodgkin's lymphoma. Am J Clin Pathol 1996;96:81–89.

Hansmann ML, Zwingers T, Boske A, et al. Clinical features of nodular paragranuloma (Hodgkin's disease, lymphocyte-predominance type, nodular). J Cancer Res Clin Oncol 1984;108:321–330.

Harris NL, Jaffe ES, Diebold J, et al: World Health Organization classification of neoplastic diseases of the hematopoietic and lymphoid tissues: Report of the Clinical Advisory Committee Meeting—Airlie House, Virginia, November 1997. J Clin Oncol 1999;17:3835–3849.

Harris NL, Jaffe ES, Stein H, et al: A revised European-American classification of lymphoid neoplasms: A proposal from the International Lymphoma Study Group. Blood 1994;84:1361–1392.

Hell K, Hansmann ML, Prongle JH, et al: Combination of Hodgkin's disease and diffuse large cell lymphoma: An in-site hybridization study for immunoglobulin light chain messenger RNA. Histopathol 1995;27:491–499.

Marafioti T, Hummel M, Anagnostopoulos I, et al: Origin of nodular lymphocyte-predominant Hodgkin's disease from a clonal expansion of highly mutated germinal–center B cells. N Engl J Med 1997;337:453–458.

Poppema S, Bhan AK, Reinherz EL, et al: In situ immunologic characterization of cellular constituents in lymph nodes and spleens involved by Hodgkin's disease. Blood 1982;59:226–232.

Travis LB, Gonzalez CL, Hankey BF, et al: Hodgkin's disease following non-Hodgkin's lymphoma. Cancer 1992;69:2337–2342.

Williams J, Schned A, Cotelingam JD, Jaffe ES: Chronic lymphocytic leukemia with coexistent Hodgkin's disease: Implications for the origin of the Reed-Sternberg cell. Am J Surg Pathol 1991;15:33–42.

Pregnancy in Hodgkin's Disease

Aviles A, Diaz-Maqueo JC, Talavera A, et al: Growth and development of children of mothers treated with chemotherapy during pregnancy: Current status of 43 children. Am J Hematol 1991;36:243–248.

Doll DC, Ringenberg QS, Yarbro JW: Antineoplastic agents and pregnancy. Semin Oncol 1989;16:337–346.

Jacobs C, Donalson SS, Rosenberg SA, et al: Management of the pregnant patient with Hodgkin's disease. Ann Intern Med 1981;95:669–675.

Yahalom J: Treatment options for Hodgkin's disease during pregnancy. Leuk Lymphoma 1990;2:151–161.

Prognosis

Front D, Bar-Shalom R, Mor M, et al: Prediction of outcome of patients with Hodgkin's disease (HD) by Ga-67 scintigraphy after one cycle of chemotherapy. J Nucl Med 1998;39:101–118.

Gobbi PG, Comelli M, Grignani GE, et al: Estimate of expected survival at diagnosis in Hodgkin's disease: A means of weighting prognostic factors and a tool for treatment choice and clinical research. A report from the International Database on Hodgkin's Disease (IDHD). Haematol 1994;79:241–255.

Guinee VF, Giacco GG, Durand M, et al: The prognosis of Hodgkin's disease in older adults. J Clin Oncol 1991;9:947–953.

Hasenclever D, Diehl V for the International Prognostic Factors Project on Advanced Hodgkin's Disease: A prognostic score for advanced Hodgkin's disease. N Engl J Med 1998;339:1506–1514.

Henry-Amar M, Friedman S, Hayat M, et al: Erythrocyte sedimentation rate predicts early relapse and survival in early-stage Hodgkin's disease. Ann Intern Med 1991;114:361–365.

Lee CKK, Bloomfield CD, Goldman AI, et al: Prognostic significance of mediastinal involvement in Hodgkin's disease treated with curative radiotherapy. Cancer 1980;46:2403–2409.

Leibenhaut M, Hoppe R, Efron B, et al: Prognostic indictors of laparotomy findings in clinical stage I–II supradiaphragmatic Hodgkin's disease. J Clin Oncol 1989;7:81–91.

Leslie NT, Mauch PM, Hellman S: Stage IA to IIB supradiaphragmatic Hodgkin's disease: Long-term survival and relapse frequency. Cancer 1985;55(Suppl 9):2072–2078.

Mauch P, Goodman R, Hellman S: The significance of mediastinal involvement in early stage Hodgkin's disease. Cancer 1978;42:1039–1045.

Mauch P, Larson D, Osteen R, et al: Prognostic factors for positive surgical staging in patients with Hodgkin's disease. J Clin Oncol 1990;8:257–265.

Specht L: Tumour burden as the main indicator of prognosis in Hodgkin's disease. Eur J Cancer 1992;28A:1982–1985.

Tubiana M, Attie E, Flamant R, et al: Prognostic factors in 454 cases of Hodgkin's disease. Cancer Res 1971;31:1801–1810.

Radiation Therapy

Hoppe R, Hanlon A, Hanks G, et al: Progress in the treatment of Hodgkin's disease in the United States, 1973 versus 1983: The Patterns of Care Study. Cancer 1994;74:3198–3203.

Kaplan HS: Evidence for a tumoricidal dose level in the radiotherapy of Hodgkin's disease. Cancer Res 1966;26:1221–1224.

Kaplan HS: Long-term results of palliative and radical radiotherapy of Hodgkin's disease. Cancer Res 1966;26:1250–1252.

Kaplan HS, Rosenberg SA: Extended-field radical radiotherapy in advanced Hodgkin's disease: Short-term results of 2 randomized clinical trials. Cancer Res 1966;26:1268–1276.

Kinzie J, Hanks G, Maclean C, et al: Patterns of care study: Hodgkin's disease relapse rates and adequacy of portals. Cancer 1983;52:2223–2226.

MacMillan CH, Bessell EM: The effectiveness of radiotherapy for localized relapse in patients with Hodgkin's disease (IIB–IVB) who obtained a complete response with chemotherapy alone as initial treatment. Clin Oncol (Royal Coll Radiol) 1994;6:147–150.

Peters MV: A study of survivals in Hodgkin's disease treated radiologically. Am J Roentgenol Radium Ther 1950;63:299–311.

Staging

Blackledge G, Best JJ, Crowther D, et al: Computed tomography (CT) in the staging of patients with Hodgkin's disease: A report on 136 patients. Clin Radiol 1980;31:143–147.

Castellino RA, Hoppe RT, Blank N, et al: Computed tomography, lymphography, and staging laparotomy: Correlations in the initial staging of Hodgkin's disease. Am J Radiol 1984;143:34–41.

Devizzi L, Bonafante V, et al: Comparison of gallium scan, computed tomography, and magnetic resonance in patients with mediastinal Hodgkin's disease. Ann Oncol 1997;18:53–56.

Ertel IJ, Boles ET Jr, Newton WA Jr: Infection after splenectomy [Letter]. N Engl J Med 1997;296:1174.

Hopper KD, Diehl LF, Lesar M, et al: Hodgkin's disease: Clinical utility of CT in initial staging and treatment. Radiology 1988;169:17–22.

Kluin-Nelemans HC, Noordijk EM: Staging of patients with Hodgkin's disease: What should be done? Leukemia 1990;4:132–135.

Larcos G, Farlow DC, Antico VF, et al: The role of high dose Ga-67 scintigraphy in staging untreated patients with lymphomas. Aust NZ J Med 1994;24:5–8.

Lister TA, Crowther D, Sutcliffe SB, et al: Report of a committee convened to discuss the evaluation and staging of patients with Hodgkin's disease: Cotswolds Meeting. J Clin Oncol 1989;7:1630–1636.

Mauch P, Kalish LA, Kadin M, et al: Patterns of presentation of Hodgkin disease. Cancer 1993;71:2062–2071.

Munker R, Hasenclever D, Brosteanu O, et al: Bone marrow involvement in Hodgkin's disease: An analysis of 135 consecutive cases. J Clin Oncol 1995;13:403–409.

Rhodes M, Rudd M, O'Rourke N, et al: Laparoscopic splenectomy and lymph node biopsy for hematologic disorders. Ann Surg 1995;222:43–46.

Stem Cell Transplantation

Armitage JO, Bierman PJ, Vose JM: Autologous bone marrow transplantation for patients with relapsed Hodgkin's disease. Am J Med 1991;91:605–611, 1991.

Bierman PJ, Anderson JR, Freeman MB, et al: High-dose chemotherapy followed by autologous hematopoietic rescue for Hodgkin's disease patients following first relapse after chemotherapy. Ann Oncol 1996;7:151–156.

Carella AM, Cartier P, Congiu A, et al: Autologous bone marrow transplantation as adjuvant treatment for high-risk Hodgkin's disease in first complete remission after MOPP/ABVD protocol. Bone Marrow Trans 1991;8:99–103.

Chopra R, McMillan AK, Linch DC, et al: The place of high-dose BEAM therapy and autologous bone marrow transplantation in poor-risk Hodgkin's disease: A single-center eight-year study of 155 patients. Blood 1993;81:1127–1145.

Colwill R, Crump M, Couture F, et al: Mini-BEAM as salvage therapy for relapsed or refractory Hodgkin's disease before intensive therapy and autologous bone marrow transplantation. J Clin Oncol 1995;13:396–402.

Demirer T, Weaver CA, Buckner CD, et al: High-dose cyclophosphamide, carmustine, and etoposide followed by allogeneic bone marrow transplantation in patients with lymphoid malignancies who had received prior dose-limiting radiation therapy. J Clin Oncol 1995;13:596–602.

Gajewski JL, Phillips GL, Sobocinski KA, et al: Bone marrow transplants from HLA-identical siblings in advanced Hodgkin's disease. J Clin Oncol 1996;14:572–578.

Linch DC, Winfield D, Goldstone AH, et al: Dose intensification with autologous bone marrow transplantation in relapsed and resistant Hodgkin's disease: Results of a BNCI randomized trial. Lancet 1993;341:1051–1054.

Poen JC, Hoppe RT, Horning SJ: High-dose therapy and autologous bone marrow transplantation for relapsed/refractory Hodgkin's disease: The impact of involved field radiotherapy on patterns of failure and survival. Int J Radiat Oncol Biol Phys 1996;36:3–12.

Sureda A, Arranz R, Iriondo E, et al: Autologous stem-cell transplantation for Hodgkin's disease: Results and prognostic factors in 494 patients from the Grupo Espanol de Linfomas/Transplante Autologo de Medula Osea Spanish Cooperative group. J Clin Oncol 2001;19:1395–1404.

Yuen AR, Rosenberg SA, Hoppe RT, et al: Comparison between conventional salvage therapy and high-dose therapy with autografting for recurrent or refractory Hodgkin's disease. Blood 1997;89:814–822.

Toxicity and Late Effects

Bastion Y, Coiffier B: Pulmonary toxicity of bleomycin: Is G-CSF a risk factor? [Letter]. Lancet 1994;344:474.

Glanzmann C, Kaufmann P, Jenni R, et al: Cardiac risk after mediastinal irradiation for Hodgkin's disease. Radiother Oncol 1998;46:51–62.

Hancock SL, Cox RS, McDougall IR: Thyroid diseases after treatment of Hodgkin's disease. N Engl J Med 1991;325:599–605.

Hancock SL, Hoppe RT: Long-term complications of treatment and causes of mortality after Hodgkin's disease. Semin Radiat Oncol 1996;6:225–242.

Hassink E, Souren T, Boersma L, et al: Pulmonary morbidity 10–18 years after irradiation for Hodgkin's disease. Eur J Cancer 1993;29A:343–347.

Henry-Amar M: Second cancers after the treatment for Hodgkin's disease: A report from the International Database on Hodgkin's Disease. Ann Oncol 1992;3(Suppl 4):117–128.

Henry-Amar M, Somers R: Survival outcome after Hodgkin's disease: A report from the International Database on Hodgkin's disease. Semin Oncol 1990;17:758–768.

Hoppe RT: Hodgkin's disease: Complications of therapy and excess mortality. Ann Oncol 1997;8(Suppl 1):115–118.

Jensen B, Carlsen NL, Nissen NI: Influence of age and duration of follow-up on lung function after combined chemotherapy for Hodgkin's disease. Eur Respir J 1990;3:1140–1145.

Jules-Elysee K, White DA: Bleomycin-induced pulmonary toxicity. Clin Chest Med 1990;11:1–20.

Krikorian JG, Burke JS, Rosenberg SA, et al: Occurrence of non-Hodgkin's lymphoma after therapy for Hodgkin's disease. N Engl J Med 1979;300:452–458.

Lund MB, Kongerud J, Boe J, et al: Cardiopulmonary sequelae after treatment for Hodgkin's disease: Increased risk in females? Ann Oncol 1996;7:257–264.

Maher J, Daly PA: Severe bleomycin lung toxicity: Reversal with high-dose corticosteroids. Thorax 1993;48:92–94.

Mauch P, Kalish L, Marcus KC, et al: Second malignancies after treatment for laparotomy staged IA-IIIB Hodgkin's disease: Long-term analysis of risk factors and outcome. Blood 1996;87:3625–3632.

Miettinen M, Franssila KO, Saxen E: Hodgkin's disease, lymphocyte predominance nodular: increased risk for subsequent non-Hodgkin's lymphomas. Cancer 1983;51: 2293–2300.

Rueffer U, Josting A, Franklin J, et al: Non-Hodgkin's lymphoma after primary Hodgkin's disease in the German Hodgkin's Lymphoma Study Group: Incidence, treatment, and prognosis. J Clin Oncol 2001;19:2026–2032.

Swerdlow AJ, Douglas AJ, Hudson GV, et al: Risk of second primary cancers after Hodgkin's disease by type of treatment: Analysis of 2846 patients in the National British Lymphoma Investigation. Br J Med 1992;304:1137–1143.

Tucker MA, Coleman CN, Cox RS, et al: Risk of second cancers after treatment for Hodgkin's disease. N Engl J Med 1988;318:76.

Van Leeuwen FE, Klokman WJ, Veer MB: Long-term risk of second malignancies in survivors of Hodgkin's disease treated during adolescence or young adulthood. J Clin Oncol 2000;18:487–497.

Van Rijswijk R, Verbeek J, Haanen C, et al: Major complications and causes of death in patients treated for Hodgkin's disease. J Clin Oncol 1987;5:1624–1633.

White DA, Stover DE: Severe bleomycin-induced pneumonitis: Clinical steroids and response to corticosteroids. Chest 1992;86:723–728.

Zarate-Osorno A, Medeiros LJ, Longo DL, et al: Non-Hodgkin's lymphoma arising in patients successfully treated for Hodgkin's disease: A clinical, histologic, and immunophenotypic study of 14 cases. Am J Surg Pathol 1992;16:885–895.

Chapter 66
Low-Grade Non-Hodgkin's Lymphoma

R. Gregory Bociek and James O. Armitage

Introduction

Non-Hodgkin's lymphoma is the fifth most common tumor diagnosed annually in the United States. For unknown reasons, the incidence has been rising for the last 25 years. The Survival, Epidemiology, and End Results (SEER) databases demonstrate approximately a twofold rise in incidence between 1973 and 1995. The relative magnitude of increase in the crude mortality rate has been less than the increase in incidence, suggesting that current treatment has improved the survival of patients with this illness. Non-Hodgkin's lymphoma is largely a disease of older adults, the peak incidence being in patients older than 60 years old. Predisposing circumstances that increase the risk of developing non-Hodgkin's lymphomas are listed in Table 66-1. No clear evidence is available to support the concept that specific heritable genetic defects are associated with non-Hodgkin's lymphomas.

Pathology/Classification of Low-Grade Non-Hodgkin's Lymphoma

Low-grade lymphomas were previously classified (in the Working Formulation) in three subsets as small lymphocytic lymphoma (the nodal morphologic equivalent of chronic lymphocytic leukemia), follicular predominantly small cleaved cell, and follicular mixed small cleaved and large cell lymphomas.

In 1994, the Revised European American Lymphoma (REAL) classification was developed and later modified by the World Health Organization (WHO) (see Chapter 64). Change in the system of classification was driven in part by the discovery of new histologic entities not described or included within the Working Formulation (e.g., mantle cell lymphoma, splenic and extranodal marginal zone B cell lymphomas) and the addition to conventional morphologic evaluation of evolving techniques to accurately determine the immunophenotype of the malignant cells and to identify unique cytogenetic abnormalities within the tumor cells.

Table 66-2 provides a summary of the information regarding morphology and immunophenotype of the most common forms of low-grade lymphoma, using the grading system proposed by Mann and Berard. The distinction between subtypes of follicular lymphoma is to some extent arbitrary and not consistently reproducible. Follicular small cleaved and follicular mixed small cleaved and large cell lymphomas (follicular grades 1 and 2) in particular are difficult to distinguish. They exhibit similar biology and are treated in a similar fashion. In contrast, the clinical characteristics of follicular large cell lymphomas (follicular grade 3 in the grading system) differ from those of the low-grade lymphomas. Follicular large cell lymphomas are treated similarly to the diffuse large B cell lymphomas, whose characteristics are similar. As is true in chronic lymphocytic leukemia, transformation to a diffuse large B cell lymphoma (Richter's syndrome) can occur in any of the low-grade lymphomas, often pursuing an aggressive and rapidly fatal course.

Clinical Presentation/Biology of Low-Grade Lymphomas

Small Lymphocytic Lymphoma

Patients with small lymphocytic lymphoma usually present with painless lymph node enlargement and often have bone marrow and peripheral blood involvement. (By convention, patients who have 5000/μL or more of circulating malignant small lymphocytes are considered to have chronic lymphocytic leukemia.) Some patients have a detectable paraprotein (a complete or partial monoclonal immunoglobulin that is secreted by the malignant B cell clone).

Follicular Low-Grade Lymphoma

Low-grade follicular lymphomas constitute as much as 40% of all non-Hodgkin's lymphomas and tend to

Table 66-1 ■ Factors Associated in the Development of Non-Hodgkin's Lymphoma

1. Congenital Immune Deficiency Diseases
   a. Wiskott-Aldrich syndrome
   b. Severe combined immune deficiency disease
2. Acquired Immune Deficiencies
   a. Human immunodeficiency virus (HIV) infection
   b. Postallogeneic solid organ or hematopoietic stem cell transplantation
   c. Autoimmune disorders: rheumatoid arthritis, systemic lupus erythematosus, Sjögren's syndrome, Hashimoto's thyroiditis
3. Physical Agents
   a. Noninfectious: herbicides, ionizing radiation, chemotherapy
   b. Infectious
      Human T-lymphotrophic virus I (HTLV-1)
      Human herpes virus 8 (HHV-8)
      Helicobacter pylori
      Epstein-Barr virus (posttransplant lymphoproliferative disorders)

present with painless waxing and waning lymphadenopathy. Most patients have advanced disease at diagnosis, and bone marrow involvement is frequent. Circulating cells may occasionally be seen on blood smear or detected as a clonal population by flow cytometry. These lymphomas tend to have a relatively slow growth fraction compared to more aggressive lymphomas and are generally exquisitely chemosensitive, at least early on in their course. More than 90% of follicular low-grade lymphomas are associated with

a unique cytogenetic abnormality, the t(14;18) translocation. This brings the immunoglobulin heavy chain locus on chromosome 14 and the *bcl*-2 gene on chromosome 18 into juxtaposition. This results in the constitutive production of *bcl*-2 protein, which blocks apoptosis and likely confers a lengthy survival on the lymphoma cells. Remission in follicular lymphomas can often be achieved with simple low intensity therapy, but maintenance of a durable remission is difficult to achieve. The course of the illness therefore tends to be one of repeated relapses with progressively shorter disease-free intervals over time.

Marginal Zone Lymphoma

Marginal zone lymphomas are divided clinically into nodal and extranodal presentations. These are low-grade B cell neoplasms with a heterogeneous cellular morphology characterized by small lymphocytes with monocytoid B cells intermixed with varying numbers of large cells. Extranodal presentations generally involve mucosal tissues and are therefore referred to as lymphomas of mucosa-associated lymphoid tissue (MALT lymphomas). Common sites of involvement are the thyroid, orbit, and gastrointestinal tract, especially the stomach. It appears as though these lymphomas may be driven by antigenic stimulation, since it is not unusual to find underlying Hashimoto's thyroiditis in thyroid presentations or evidence in 90% of gastric mucosal–associated lymphoid tissue lymphomas of *Helicobacter pylori* infection and gastritis. Similarly, nodal presentations of marginal-zone B cell lymphomas also develop in patients with autoimmune inflammatory disorders (e.g., Sjögren's syndrome) and

Table 66-2 ■ Distinguishing Features of Low-Grade Lymphomas

Lymphoma Subtype	Morphologic Features	Immunophenotype	Cytogenetics
Follicular grade 1	Follicular pattern 0–5 large cells/hpf	Surface Ig + CD 19, 20 + CD 10+/– CD 5–	t(14;18) + in 70–90%
Follicular grade 2	Follicular pattern 6–15 large cells/hpf	Surface Ig + CD 19, 20 + CD 10+/– CD 5–	t(14;18)+ in 70–90%
Small lymphocytic lymphoma	Diffuse pattern Small lymphocytes Clumped chromatin Pseudofollicles	Surface IgM + CD 19, 20, 5, 23 + CD 10 –	Trisomy 12 t(14;18) bcl-1
Splenic marginal-zone lymphoma	Small lymphocytes	Surface Ig CD 20, 22 + CD 5 –, usually	t(11;14)

may represent nodal spread of a mucosa-associated lymphoid tissue lymphoma. Bone marrow involvement and occasionally peripheral blood involvement may be seen with nodal presentations.

Clinical Evaluation

The clinical evaluation of patients with low-grade lymphomas should include a detailed history and physical examination supplemented with laboratory and imaging studies to stage the extent of disease (Table 66-3). The history should detail the patient's functional status (e.g., Karnofsky or ECOG [Eastern Cooperative Oncology Group] performance status) and the presence or absence of systemic "B" symptoms (see Table 66-3). Symptoms and signs related to bone marrow dysfunction (unexplained anemia; frequent, protracted, or unusual infections; and easy bruising/bleeding) should be elicited. Symptomatology may also provide a clue to involvement of the gastrointestinal tract, sinus, or oropharynx. The physical examination should include a careful inspection of Waldeyer's ring and palpation of all superficial node-bearing areas, liver, and spleen. Musculoskeletal examination should include percussion/palpation of the axial skeleton, including the sternum, to detect areas of tenderness, which might need further exploration and/or imaging studies. Involvement of certain sites that is seen more commonly in aggressive lymphomas (e.g., testes, sinuses) is uncommon in low-grade lymphomas, but these areas should nevertheless be screened by history and physical examination.

Laboratory studies include a complete blood count with differential and platelet count, serum elec-

trolytes, calcium and uric acid levels, renal and hepatic function studies, lactic dehydrogenase, and serum protein electrophoresis for monoclonal proteins and the presence of hypogammaglobulinemia. Anemia, if present, requires evaluation of single or multiple causes, such as marrow involvement, anemia of chronic disease, concomitant iron deficiency, and warm or cold antibody hemolytic anemia. Imaging studies include a chest radiograph, contrast-enhanced computed tomography (CT) of the chest if the chest film is abnormal, and contrast-enhanced computed tomography scans of the abdomen and pelvis. Because lymphoma in Waldeyer's ring is frequently associated with gastrointestinal tract involvement, patients with lymphoma in the tonsillar ring require gastrointestinal imaging studies and endoscopy even in the absence of gastrointestinal symptoms. Patients with gastric mucosal–associated lymphoid tissue lymphomas should be evaluated for evidence of *H. pylori* infection. A bone marrow aspirate and biopsy are performed to complete the staging evaluation. Imaging by gallium scan is optional. Because it has only moderate sensitivity and specificity, with as much as 30% false positives and 30% false negatives, it is an imprecise study to stage the disease. Gallium-avid lesions at diagnosis can be reimaged at the completion of therapy to help document a complete remission if this confirmation is essential to subsequent treatment considerations. The use of positron emission tomography (PET) is not part of the routine staging evaluation, but current studies may establish a role for it.

Staging and Prognostic Factors in Low-Grade Lymphomas

The Ann Arbor system (see Table 66-3), which was initially developed for Hodgkin's disease, remains the most commonly used staging system for the non-Hodgkin's lymphomas. The system was based on the partly flawed concept that as Hodgkin's disease develops, it consistently extends to anatomically contiguous adjacent lymph node sites before hematogenous distant dissemination occurs. This concept had limited value in the low-grade non-Hodgkin's lymphomas, which tend to undergo early and widespread hematogenous spread to multiple sites. For treatment planning purposes, it usually suffices to categorize patients as early stage (nonbulky stage I and II disease) versus advanced stage (the presence of bulky disease or stage III or IV disease). It is important to recognize the distinction between patients with early-stage disease involving an extralymphatic site (stage "E" disease) and stage IV disease. For example, a patient with lymphoma involving the hilar region plus an

---

Table 66-3 ▪ Ann Arbor Staging System for Lymphomas

Stage	Anatomic Description
Stage I	Involvement of a single lymph node region (I) or a single extralymphatic organ or site (IE)
Stage II	Involvement of two or more lymph node regions on the same side of the diaphragm (II) or localized involvement of an extralymphatic organ or site (IIE)
Stage III	Involvement of lymph node regions on both sides of the diaphragm without (III) or with (IIIE) localized involvement of an extralymphatic organ or site
Stage IV	Diffuse involvement of one or more extralymphatic organ or site, with or without lymphatic involvement

Use of the letter "A" after the stage description denotes the absence of systemic symptoms (unexplained fevers >38°, drenching night sweats, weight loss of 10% or more of body weight over previous six months). Use of the letter "B" after the stage description denotes the presence of systemic symptoms.

ipsilateral solitary pulmonary nodule (implicitly contiguous localized spread) has stage IIE disease. A patient with hilar involvement plus multiple bilateral pulmonary nodules (implicitly hematogenous spread) has stage IV disease.

The International Prognostic Index (IPI), which was designed to predict outcome in patients with aggressive (e.g., diffuse large B cell) lymphomas, also provides excellent delineation of prognostic subsets of patients with low-grade lymphomas. The Index, both elegant and simple, utilizes baseline clinical factors (favorable versus unfavorable): age (60 years or younger versus older than 60 years), stage (I or II versus III or IV), performance status (0 or 1 versus 2 or greater), lactate dehydrogenase (LDH) level (normal versus high), and number of extranodal sites (one or fewer versus more than one) to predict outcome. The greater the accumulation of unfavorable factors, the worse is the prognosis. Based on the Index, the projected eight-year survival in low-grade lymphomas is 70% in the low-risk group (no or one risk factor), 50% in the intermediate-risk group (two or three risk factors), and 20% in the high-risk group (four or five risk factors). In patients who present with a poor prognosis, one should consider whether trials of aggressive or novel initial therapies are warranted instead of the conventional approaches.

Treatment

Early-Stage Disease

Approximately 10% to 20% of patients present with true early-stage disease (nonbulky clinical stage I and II). For these patients, particularly those with follicular lymphomas, radiation therapy has traditionally been used as the single modality of treatment. A retrospective review of patients with early-stage low-grade follicular lymphomas who received radiation therapy alone showed a relapse-free survival rate of 44% at 10 years and 37% at 20 years and an overall survival rate of 64% at 10 years and 35% at 20 years. Very few patients who were followed for greater than 10 years relapsed. Increasing the extent of the radiation therapy fields did not improve survival but did increase the risk of secondary malignancy. In multivariate analysis, older patients (above age 60 years) and those with stage II disease (compared to stage I disease) had an increased risk of both relapse and death. Because the number of patients who have been followed for prolonged periods of time is very small, it is difficult to know whether the reported apparent plateau on the survival curves is meaningful. Moreover, the presence of competing causes of death (other than lymphoma) in the elderly population of patients

make it uncertain whether in fact any substantial proportion of patients are truly cured by radiation therapy. Nevertheless, patients presenting with apparently localized low-grade lymphomas disease can achieve long disease-free intervals and survival with limited-field radiation therapy alone.

Frequent acute toxicities from radiation therapy include fatigue, erythema, and inflammation at the site of treatment. Desquamation of the skin occasionally occurs, requiring interruption of treatment. Radiation therapy to the head and neck region can lead to salivary gland destruction. Mucositis can occur, and xerostomia (dry mouth) can become a chronic problem with troubling symptoms and increase in dental caries and loss of teeth. Cytopenias can also develop during treatment if the treatment portal includes a large volume of bone marrow. Other major late toxicities include a risk of accelerated atherosclerosis (if the mediastinum is in the treatment field) and hypothyroidism (if the neck is irradiated). Careful follow-up is necessary to monitor for these potential toxicities.

Mucosa-Associated Lymphoid Tissue (MALT) Lymphoma

In the absence of randomized prospective trials, therapy of mucosa-associated lymphoid tissue lymphoma is based on retrospective analysis of varying treatment approaches. Although these data carry the usual bias created by nonrandomized treatment assignment, a consensus view has emerged.

Stage I nongastric mucosa-associated lymphoid tissue lymphomas are most often treated with local radiation therapy. It is not known whether the addition of adjuvant chemotherapy benefits these patients. The five-year probability of freedom from relapse and of overall survival is approximately 70% and 95%, respectively. Stage II to IV nongastric mucosa-associated lymphoid tissue lymphomas are treated in a fashion similar to other low-grade lymphomas.

Patients with nonbulky stage IAE gastric mucosa-associated lymphoid tissue lymphomas who have evidence of *H. pylori* infection represent a unique clinical situation. In these patients, antibiotic therapy is commonly used as initial treatment, because eradication of *H. pylori* can induce regression of the lymphoma. These patients should be restaged with upper endoscopy and gastric biopsy three months after antibiotic therapy to document elimination of the infection and the degree of response by the lymphoma. Patients who are still *H. pylori* positive at three months may be treated with a second-line antibiotic regimen and re-endoscoped in three months. Patients who are *H. pylori* negative at three months may be followed with observation if there is no evidence of lymphoma or may be offered local radiation therapy if residual lymphoma is detected. Treatment of patients with advanced-stage gastric mucosa-associated lymphoid tissue lymphoma follows the same principles that are used to guide therapy of advanced-stage follicular lymphoma. It is important to emphasize that the treatment principles outlined here for mucosa-associated lymphoid tissue lymphomas are for patients with true histologic low-grade lymphomas. Patients with mucosa-associated lymphoid tissue lymphomas that are histologically diffuse large B cell lymphomas should be treated as such.

General Considerations in Advanced-Stage Disease

The optimal treatment strategy for patients with advanced-stage low-grade lymphomas remains highly controversial, and decision-making is often complex. Since advanced-stage, low-grade lymphomas are thought to be incurable by conventional chemotherapy, a number of different therapeutic perspectives need to be considered. One is obliged to determine the goals of treatment in the individual patient and to assess the risks and benefits of alternative approaches. For example, whether to treat at all initially is an issue. When should treatment be initiated and how intensive should it be? Should aggressive therapy by means of allogeneic or autologous hematopoietic stem cell transplantation be a part of the treatment plan in some patients or be reserved for the time of treatment failure? Other factors are involved in the treatment assessment, such as the age of the patient, quality of life with and without therapy, the intrinsic pace of the illness, speed of recurrences, and the specific manifestations of disease progression in a given patient. All of these issues require lengthy exploration with the patient and the patient's family; inevitably the most satisfactory treatment plan is the one that the patient and clinician comfortably settle on together (Figure 66-1).

Observation Without Treatment

The early institution of therapy does not substantially alter the natural history of advanced-stage, low-grade lymphomas. A group of patients at Stanford University were followed from the time of diagnosis without any therapy being administered until symptoms, laboratory abnormalities (cytopenias), or progressive lymph node enlargement developed. After a median follow-up period of less than four years, the median time to institution of therapy was three years, and the median survival for the entire group was 11 years.

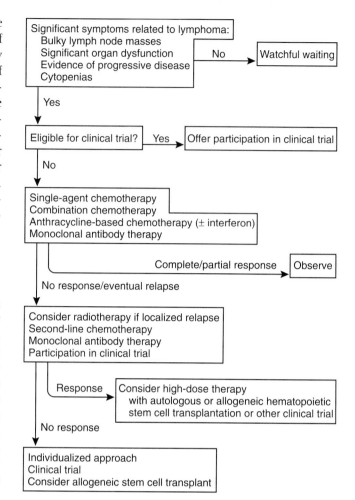

Figure 66-1 ■ Treatment of advanced low-grade non-Hodgkin's lymphoma.

Low-grade lymphomas are known to wax and wane without intervention, and 25% of the patients at Stanford actually experienced spontaneous regression of disease to the point of a clinical complete remission. When the initially untreated patients by histologic type were compared to a group of similar patients at Stanford who were treated at the time of diagnosis, the overall survival and the risk of later transformation to a higher grade of lymphoma were found to be essentially identical. Moreover, although intensive initial therapy with anthracycline-based chemotherapy (CHOP: cyclophosphamide, doxorubicin, vincristine, prednisone) resulted in a complete remission rate of 64%, the median survival was only 6.9 years, and the Kaplan-Meier plot of survival did not convincingly demonstrate evidence of a plateau, that is, cure, at the tail of the curve. These observational studies support the inference that early, as opposed to delayed, institution of therapy does not improve outcome. The lack of data on large numbers of patients in randomized studies, however, makes a definitive conclusion difficult.

One randomized study by the National Cancer Institute evaluated 104 patients with low-grade lymphomas; of these, 89 were considered appropriate for deferral of initial therapy. These patients were then randomly assigned either to initial aggressive combined modality therapy ($N = 45$) or to observation without therapy until warranted by the clinical circumstances ($N = 44$). The median delay before the observation group began systemic chemotherapy was approximately three years. Patients who were randomized to initial therapy received ProMACE-MOPP (procarbazine, methotrexate, doxorubicin, cyclophosphamide, etoposide, mechlorethamine, vincristine, and prednisone) followed by total nodal irradiation. Toxicity, mainly due to cytopenias, was substantial but manageable. Despite a median duration of remission of more than 45 months in these initially intensively treated patients, the five-year survival of the two groups did not differ. It thus appears that conventional chemotherapy of advanced-stage, low-grade lymphomas is palliative, not curative. The current consensus therefore is to observe asymptomatic patients until such time as the development of symptoms, rapidly growing tumor masses, cytopenias, or organ impairment signals the necessity for therapy to control the disease.

Choices of Initial Therapy

The choice of initial therapy is perplexing, because no survival advantage is apparent among treatment regimens as different as the following: the established standard of daily oral alkylating agent (e.g., chlorambucil or cyclophosphamide); combination chemotherapy, such as triple therapy with cyclophosphamide, vincristine, and prednisone (COP) or with added anthracycline, such as Adriamycin (CHOP); combination chemotherapy in escalated doses; maintenance chemotherapy; or radiation therapy used alone or as part of a combined modality approach. More recently, the purine analogues (e.g., fludarabine, cladribine), monoclonal antibodies directed at CD20 on the lymphoma cells (e.g., rituximab, tositumomab), and monoclonal antibodies linked to radionuclides have shown their effectiveness in inducing responses. Although response rates with the newer approaches appear to be high, particularly when studied in selected patients in phase II trials, no clear survival advantage has yet emerged. Therefore, one needs to be wary about selecting alternatives to daily oral alkylating agent therapy, because additional toxicity is introduced without evidence of durable benefit. For example, the purine analogues cause prolonged T cell suppression, exposing patients to the risks of opportunistic infection and the necessity for viral, fungal, and bacterial prophylaxis. Moreover, attempts to combine fludarabine or cladribine with other chemotherapeutic drugs escalate the risks of treatment-induced complications.

Interferon-α has been extensively evaluated in low-grade lymphomas for nearly two decades. Interferons are inducible glycoproteins with antiviral, antitumor, and immunomodulatory properties. The exact mechanism(s) of action remain unclear but likely include direct antiproliferative effects, antiangiogenic effects, induction of maturation/differentiation in tumor cells, induction of apoptosis, and activation of nonspecific cellular cytotoxic immune responses. Phase II trials reported response rates in the range of 30% to 50%, including patients with bulky tumor, and there was a suggestion of prolongation of remission when interferon was continued after response was achieved. Randomized trials of non-anthracycline-based regimens showed borderline benefit from the addition of interferon. Although it did not improve complete response rates or the overall survival rate, prolongation of time to disease progression was observed in some studies. The Groupe d'Etude des Lymphomes Folliculaires (GELF) studied an anthracycline-containing regimen, CHVP (cyclophosphamide, doxorubicin, teniposide, prednisone), for six cycles versus (in a randomized trial) the same therapy plus interferon (5×10^6 units subcutaneously tiw) given for 18 months. Response rate (69% versus 85%), median event-free survival (19 months versus 34 months), and the three-year overall survival rate (69% versus 86%) all favored the interferon-containing treatment arm. Interferon was stopped in 11% of patients, primarily due to abnormal liver function tests and fatigue. After lengthy follow-up (six years), this study continues to show an increased median duration of progression-free survival and overall survival of 1.5 years and 5.6 years, respectively, for the patients receiving chemotherapy alone versus 2.9 years and median not yet reached, respectively, for the patients receiving added interferon. The Southwestern Oncology Group (SWOG) treated patients with stage III or IV low-grade lymphoma with induction chemotherapy using six cycles of ProMACE-MOPP, plus involved-field radiation therapy for patients achieving only a partial response. Patients were then randomly assigned to receive either interferon 2×10^6 units/m^2 tiw for two years or no further therapy. With a median follow-up of 6.2 years, progression-free survival and overall survival rates did not significantly differ. A meta-analysis that excluded the negative results of the SWOG trial reported that a survival advantage accrued when interferon was added to doxorubicin-containing regimens. The variation in clinical trial experience is likely to be due to differences in interferon doses and schedules, chemotherapy regimens used (anthracycline-based or not), statistical power, and differences in risk groups (e.g., the GELF trial enrolled only patients with a large tumor burden, whereas 50% of patients in the SWOG study were low risk by the International Prognostic Index). Because the controversy is not resolved and because interferon administration produces constitutional symptoms, lethargy, and fatigue, interferon often has not been incorporated as part of the treatment of choice. A polyglycosylated form of interferon may improve both tolerance and efficacy by providing more continuous levels, fewer injections, and perhaps a lower frequency of side effects.

Monoclonal antibodies offer a new approach to the treatment of low-grade lymphomas. The CD20 antigen is expressed on approximately 90% of B cell non-Hodgkin's lymphomas and on normal B cells. Monoclonal antibodies that bind to the CD20 antigen have been developed for use as both unconjugated and conjugated (e.g., bound to *Pseudomonas* exotoxin, radioactive iodine, or yttrium) molecules. Unconjugated forms (e.g., rituximab) rely on a relatively intact host immune system to be effective, whereas conjugated antibodies (e.g., tositumomab, ibritumomab) offer a means to target cytotoxic effects to the lymphoma cells. The humanized antibodies that are used reduce the potential for a host immune response to the antibody, either neutralizing its effect or causing adverse reactions. What makes these monoclonal antibodies such valuable additions to the therapeutic armamentarium for low-grade lymphomas is the evidence that these antibodies can induce responses in patients who have failed one or more prior chemotherapy regimens, that second and third responses can occur after their readministration to patients who relapse after a prior response, and that the radiolabeled antibodies can be effective even in patients who fail to respond to unlabeled antibody.

Rituximab is an unconjugated chimeric monoclonal antibody directed against the CD20 antigen. It contains human IgG1 antibody and kappa constant regions complexed to murine variable regions. This combination seems to maximize antitumor activity while minimizing autoimmunogenicity. Its mechanisms of action are several, including antibody-dependent, cell-mediated cytotoxicity, complement-dependent cytotoxicity, and the induction of apoptosis. Toxicity is generally limited to the time of infusion. Fever and chills are common and usually mild reactions, but on occasion, acute bronchospasm and hypotension may occur, as well as full-blown anaphylaxis. Infusional side effects are most pro-

Table 66-4 ▪ Summary Results of Rituximab Trials

Trial Characteristics	N	Response Rates	Median Time to Progression
Multidose	37	46%	10 months
Pivotal trial	166	48%	13 months
Eight weekly infusions	37	57%	>19 months
Bulky disease	31	43%	8 months
Retreatment	58	40%	>17 months
CHOP/rituximab	40	95%	>29 months
Initial therapy	41	54%	82% progression free at 8 months

N = number of patients treated. CHOP = cyclophosphamide, doxorubicin, vincristine, prednisone.

nounced with the initial infusion and decrease with each successive administration. A dose of 375 mg/m^2 intravenously weekly is most often used.

Table 66-4 displays the results of several phase II studies of low-grade lymphomas, demonstrating the substantial response rate achieved when this agent is alone. The table also includes data from a trial of rituximab in combination with CHOP in patients (low-grade/follicular lymphoma) who had not previously received an anthracycline. In these patients, responses occurred in 95% of patients; with a median follow-up duration of nearly two years, 75% of patients remain free from disease recurrence or progression. Toxicity did not appear to be different than that associated with CHOP alone, with the exception of the expected first dose effects seen with rituximab.

Data from a French randomized trial showed that the combination of CHOP and rituximab can prolong survival in elderly patients with aggressive non-Hodgkin's lymphoma. This should prompt further studies of these agents in conjunction with other therapies that are effective in low-grade lymphoma. A number of studies have also demonstrated significant activity for conjugated antibodies such as tositumomab ([131]iodine) and ibritumomab ([90]yttrium). These radiolabeled antibodies can cause myelosuppression, but they are effective even in far advanced disease. How they will be incorporated with other therapy or in the sequence of therapy is as yet uncertain.

Monoclonal antibody therapy is a form of passive immunotherapy, whereas active immunotherapy involves stimulating the host to produce autologous immunoglobulin in response to a specific antigenic challenge. Active immunotherapy has been limited immunologically by the inability of the host to recognize tumor antigens as foreign, since they are self-derived. In the case of lymphomas, a tumor-specific, patient-specific tumor antigen is represented by the idiotype (unique antigenic array) of the monoclonal surface immunoglobulin produced by the malignant B cell clone. The generation of an anti-idiotype antibody (to the surface immunoglobulin) could provide a therapy, which potentially recognizes only that patient's tumor cells. Investigators at Stanford generated such patient-specific anti-idiotype antibodies in patients with non-Hodgkin's lymphoma. After treating them with initial chemotherapy until the point of maximum response, five subcutaneous immunizations of the lymphoma idiotype (which included a nonspecific adjuvant) were given over five months. Patients in first remission who mounted demonstrable anti-idiotype responses to the vaccine (14 of 32 patients) experienced both prolonged median freedom from progression (7.9 years versus 1.3 years) and median overall survival (not yet reached versus 7 years) compared with patients in first remission who failed to develop a specific immune response. Whether these results represent a therapeutic effect of vaccination or simply a surrogate marker demonstrating the presence/benefit of an intact host immune system requires randomized trials.

Patients failing initial therapies become candidates for any of a number of aggressive conventional-dose salvage chemotherapy regimens (Table 66-5). No one regimen appears to be superior to the others, and clinicians appropriately choose the treatment with which they are most familiar. These treatment programs are commonly used in an attempt to reduce the body burden of tumor prior to an attempt at cure by high-dose chemotherapy/stem cell transplantation.

Hematopoietic Stem Cell Transplantation

The concept of dose-intensification in patients with low-grade lymphomas, especially patients with follicular lymphoma, arose as an extension of the observation that patients with relapsed aggressive lymphomas have superior disease-free and overall survival when treated with high-dose therapy/autologous hematopoietic stem cell transplantation compared with conventional salvage therapy only. Studies of transplantation for patients with refractory/relapsed low-grade lymphoma have reported high complete response rates with only limited evidence to suggest better freedom from progression when compared to historical controls. Only a single trial conducted by Schouten was a randomized study. Patients with relapsed follicular non-Hodgkin's lymphoma received three cycles of chemotherapy (usually CHOP). Those who achieved a partial or complete response were randomized to receive one of three additional therapies, consisting of three further cycles of chemotherapy, unpurged autologous stem cell transplantation, or purged autologous stem cell transplantation. Only 89 patients out of an intended 300 were randomized due to poor accrual, which forced early closure of the study. With a short median follow-up of 26 months, 66% of patients randomized to conventional-dose chemotherapy had progressed/relapsed versus 39% of patients randomized to unpurged stem cell transplantation, and 37% of patients randomized to purged stem cell transplantation. A trend toward improved survival with transplantation was also observed in this trial. Because this study was underpowered (small patient sample size) and terminated prematurely, its results should be viewed with some skepticism. This is especially warranted in view of the results of multiple unrandomized studies of autologous transplantation in low-grade lymphomas. The event-free survival curves in virtually all of these studies fail to demonstrate the occurrence of a plateau. Instead they exhibit a continuing decline over time, due to relapse and/or death. As with conventional chemotherapy, whether autologous transplantation can cure a fraction of these patients remains uncertain.

Concern about the role of lymphoma cell contamination of the reinfused stem cells in autologous stem cell transplantation led to a number of approaches to purge the tumor cells ex vivo by stem cell selection or exposure of the stem cell population to chemotherapy or cytotoxic antibody or antibodies directed at lymphoma antigens. That studies of stem cell purging have failed to show decreased relapse rates compared to patients receiving unpurged stem cells, suggests that this potential problem contributes little, if at all, to the relapses that occur after autologous stem cell transplantation. Allogeneic stem cell transplantation, using matched related donors, produces high response rates and appears to have a lower relapse rate than autologous stem cell transplantation. Because the absence of tumor cell contamination does not adequately explain

Table 66-5 ■ Common Salvage Chemotherapy Regimens Used in Non-Hodgkin's Lymphoma

Regimen	Chemotherapeutic Agents
DHAP	Dexamethasone, cytarabine, cisplatin
ESHAP	Etoposide, methylprednisolone, cytarabine, cisplatin
MINE	Mesna, ifosfamide, mitoxantrone, etoposide
ICE	Ifosfamide, carboplatin, etoposide
Mini-BEAM	Carmustine, etoposide, cytarabine, melphalan

this difference, one can infer the possibility of a graft-versus-lymphoma effect in allogeneic stem cell transplantation. Moreover, correlation of tumor responses with the temporal development of graft-versus-host disease (GVHD) offers direct confirmation of graft-mediated immunologic attack on the lymphoma. Event-free survival curves in the range of 40% to 60% have been reported in the allogeneic setting, with some studies suggesting the existence of a survival plateau. It is possible that allogeneic transplantation offers the best possibility of achieving prolonged disease-free survival for this illness and may be the best (or only) therapy with the potential to actually cure a proportion of patients. However, toxicity resulting from allogeneic transplantation (regimen related, infectious, and graft-versus-host disease) results in a higher risk of transplant-related morbidity and mortality, which restricts the application of this therapy to young patients with good functional status.

Nonmyeloablative allogeneic stem cell transplant preparative regimens demonstrate that it is possible to generate stable mixed chimeric (host and donor cells present) engraftment, often leading to eventual complete donor cell engraftment, in patients with lymphoid and other malignancies. Less regimen-related morbidity occurs, but the major toxicities of infections and graft-versus-host disease remain. In such a setting, once stable chimerism has been attained, other therapies (e.g., cytokine therapy, specific targeted cellular therapies, donor leukocyte infusions) can be used in an attempt to improve antitumor effects or to modulate the immunologic effect of the graft, hopefully reducing or eliminating residual disease in the host.

Allogeneic stem cell transplantation, using a non-myeloablative regimen, showed that tumor regression in metastatic renal cell carcinoma could take months to occur. Response coincided with discontinuation of cyclosporine immunosuppression, the development of complete donor engraftment, and the appearance of acute graft-versus-host disease. Generation of adequate numbers of the cytotoxic lymphocytes required to kill host malignant cells may therefore be much delayed after this allogeneic transplantation approach. If this holds true in low-grade lymphoma, then such nonmyeloablative therapy would be best employed as a form of consolidative therapy after a response is achieved by other means, rather than as initial therapy in relapsed patients.

Follow-up Evaluation for Patients on Therapy

Follow-up is directed at both the results of therapy (i.e., is there subjective or objective evidence of disease regression?) as well as an assessment of toxicity. The principal toxicities of the chemotherapeutic agents should be reviewed with the patient prior to each cycle of therapy. Restaging evaluation is usually performed part way through a course of therapy (e.g., after three to four cycles of treatment) to ensure that an objective response is occurring, as well as to decide on how many courses of therapy to administer (generally two courses past the occurrence of a complete remission or best response for patients with advanced disease), then again at the completion of therapy. A positive bone marrow biopsy need not be repeated during therapy if other measurable sites of disease exist, but it is a useful study to obtain to document a complete remission at the end of therapy.

Follow-up Evaluation for Patients in Remission

Follow-up evaluation for patients with low-grade lymphomas should concentrate on the same aspects of history/physical examination that were important in the initial evaluation. Since most patients will present with advanced-stage disease, management should be focused on helping patients understand how to live with their disease, with the expectation that they will likely experience multiple recurrences over time and will not necessarily require urgent therapy at relapse. This helps the patient and clinician come to an understanding of how to best follow the patient for relapse. Patients with no new symptoms of concern, no new abnormalities on physical examination or screening blood tests are unlikely to have significant abnormalities on routinely obtained imaging studies that would mandate urgent therapy. Some patients may prefer episodic computed tomography scanning for some measure of reassurance that their illness remains stable or in remission. Follow-up visits can be planned with the patient; every three months for two years (gradually lengthening the interval afterwards) is a reasonable frequency. Patients who have received irradiation to the head and neck region need to be followed for the occurrence of hypothyroidism. Patients who relapse should be considered for a new tissue biopsy if they were previously in complete remission, if they develop abnormalities at sites that could represent a new or nonneoplastic diagnosis, or if there is clinical suspicion of transformation to a higher-grade lymphoma. A bone marrow biopsy on occasion can be used to prove the existence of recurrent disease, thereby obviating the need for a lymph node biopsy. A bone marrow biopsy will, however, rarely be sufficient to determine whether high-grade transformation has occurred, since subtyping of lymphomas based on bone marrow specimens can be extremely difficult.

Late Sequelae of Treatment

Long-term effects of radiation result from injury to normal tissues in the radiation field, causing alopecia, cataracts, skin changes, hypothyroidism, accelerated coronary artery disease, xerostomia, and second malignancies. The late effects of chemotherapy may include late infections (e.g., herpes zoster), infertility (especially with the use of alkylating agents), cardiac (doxorubicin) and pulmonary (bleomycin) toxicity, and second malignancies (e.g., treatment-related myelodysplastic syndrome/acute leukemia). All patients should be followed by a hematologist or oncologist at least annually for life. Later visits should emphasize the detection of the delayed complications, the signs and symptoms of which may occasionally be subtle (e.g., hypothyroidism, early myelodysplasia).

Summary

Low-grade lymphomas continue to represent a challenge to the clinician, from the standpoint of both diagnosis and therapy. The ever-growing list of agents that are active in the treatment of these lymphomas has increased uncertainty about which particular approach to therapy is in fact the optimal choice for the individual patient. The clinician can draw marginal reassurance from the knowledge that no one therapy at present has consistently demonstrated superiority over others in the setting of a clinical trial. It is likely that future trials will concentrate on sequential combined or multimodal therapies (e.g., chemotherapy, monoclonal antibody therapy, active or maintenance immunotherapy) to improve outcomes. But it will continue to be difficult to be certain of patient benefit in the absence of simple, definitive, highly powered randomized trials.

Suggested Reading

General Information

Anonymous: A predictive model for aggressive non-Hodgkin's lymphoma: The International Non-Hodgkin's Lymphoma Prognostic Factors Project. N Engl J Med 1993;329:987–994.

Carbone PP, Kaplan HS, Musshoff K, et al: Report of the committee on Hodgkin's disease staging. Cancer Res 1971;31:1860–1861.

Greenlee RT, Murray T, Hill-Harmon MB, Murray T, et al: Cancer statistics 2001. CA Cancer J Clin 2001;51:15.

Harris NL, Jaffe ES, Diebold J, et al: World Health Organization classification of neoplastic diseases of the hematopoietic and lymphoid tissues: Report of the clinical advisory committee meeting—Arlie House, Virginia, November 1997. J Clin Oncol 1999;17:3835–3849.

Harris NL, Jaffe ES, Stein H, et al: A revised European-American classification of lymphoid neoplasms: A proposal from the international lymphoma study group. Blood 1994;84:1361–1392.

Johnson PWM, Rohatiner AZS, Whelan JS, et al: Patterns of survival in patients with recurrent follicular lymphoma: A 20-year study from a single center. J Clin Oncol 1995;13:140–147.

Lopez-Guillermo A, Montserrat E, Bosch F, et al: Applicability of the International Index for aggressive lymphomas to patients with low-grade lymphoma. J Clin Oncol 1994;12:1343–1348.

MacManus MP, Hoppe RT: Is radiotherapy curative for stage I and II low-grade follicular lymphoma? Results of a long-term follow-up study of patients treated at Stanford University. J Clin Oncol 1996;14:1282–1290.

Mikhaeel NG, Timothy AR, Hain SF, et al: 18-FDG-PET for the assessment of residual masses on CT following treatment of lymphomas. Ann Oncol 2000;11(Suppl 1):147–150.

SEER cancer statistics review, 1973–1997. 2000.

Spaepen K, Stroobants S, Dupont P, et al: Prognostic value of positron emission tomography (PET) with fluorine-18 fluorodeoxyglucose ([^{18}F]FDG) after first-line chemotherapy in non-Hodgkin's lymphoma: Is ([^{18}F]FDG-PET a valid alternative to conventional diagnostic methods? J Clin Oncol 2001;19:414–420.

Mucosa-Associated Lymphoid Tissue Lymphoma

Roggero E, Zucca E, Pinotti G, et al: Eradication of *Helicobacter pylori* infection in primary low-grade gastric lymphoma of mucosa-associated lymphoid tissue. Ann Intern Med 1995;122:767–769.

Starostik P, Patzner J, Greiner A, et al: Gastric marginal zone B cell lymphoma of the MALT type develop along 2 distinct pathogenetic pathways. Blood 2002;99:3–9.

Thieblemont C, Bastion Y, Berger F, et al: Mucosa-associated lymphoid tissue gastrointestinal and nongastrointestinal lymphoma behaviour: Analysis of 108 patients. J Clin Oncol 1997;15:1624–1630.

Zinzani PL, Magagnoli M, Galieni P, et al: Non-gastrointestinal low-grade mucosa-associated lymphoid tissue lymphoma: analysis of 75 patients. J Clin Oncol 1999;17:1254.

Chemotherapy

Dana BW, Dahlberg S, Nathwani BN, et al: Long-term follow-up of patients with low-grade malignant lymphomas treated with doxorubicin-based chemotherapy or chemo-immunotherapy. J Clin Oncol 1993;11:644–651.

Hochster HS, Oken MM, Winter JN, et al: Phase I study of fludarabine plus cyclophosphamide in patients with previously untreated low-grade lymphoma: Results and long-term follow-up—A report of the Eastern Cooperative Oncology Group. J Clin Oncol 2000;18:987–994.

Horning SJ, Rosenberg SA: The natural history of initially untreated low-grade non-Hodgkin's lymphomas. N Engl J Med 1984;311:1471–1475.

Jacobs P, King HS: A randomized prospective comparison of chemotherapy to total body irradiation as initial treatment for the indolent lymphoproliferative diseases. Blood 1987; 69:1642–1646.

Lepage E, Sebban C, Gisselbrecht C, et al: Treatment of low-grade non-Hodgkin's lymphomas: Assessment of doxorubicin in a controlled trial. Hematol Oncol 1990;8:31–39.

McLaughlin P, Hagemeister FB, Romaguera JE, et al: Fludarabine, mitoxantrone, and dexamethasone: An effective new regimen for indolent lymphoma. J Clin Oncol 1996;14: 1262–1268.

Peterson BA, Petroni GR, Frizzera G, et al: Prolonged single-agent versus combination chemotherapy in indolent follicular lymphomas: A study of the Cancer and Leukemia Group B. J Clin Oncol 2003;21:5–15.

Saven A, Emanuele S, Kosty M, et al: 2-Chlorodeoxyadenosine activity in patients with untreated, indolent non-Hodgkin's lymphoma. Blood 1995;86:1710–1716.

Steward WP, Crowther D, McWilliam LJ, et al: Maintenance chlorambucil after CVP in the management of advanced stage, low-grade histologic type non-Hodgkin's lymphoma: A randomized prospective study with an assessment of prognostic factors. Cancer 1988;61:441–447.

Young RC, Longo DL, Glatstein E, et al: The treatment of indolent lymphomas: Watchful waiting vs. aggressive combined modality treatment. Semin Hematol 1988;25:11–16.

Zinzani PL, Magagnoli M, Moretti L, et al: Randomized trial of fludarabine versus fludarabine and idarubicin as frontline treatment in patients with indolent or mantle cell lymphoma. J Clin Oncol 2000;18:773–779.

Interferon

Arranz R, Garcia-Alfonso P, Sobrino P, et al: Role of interferon alfa-2b in the induction and maintenance treatment of low-grade non-Hodgkin's lymphoma: Results from a prospective, multicenter trial with double randomization. J Clin Oncol 1998;16:1538–1546.

Fisher RI, Dana BW, LeBlanc M, et al: Interferon alfa consolidation after intensive chemotherapy does not prolong the progression-free survival of patients with low-grade non-Hodgkin's lymphoma: Results of the Southwest Oncology Group randomized phase III study 8809. J Clin Oncol 2000;18:2010–2016.

Foon SA, Sherwin SA, Abrams PG, et al: Treatment of advanced non-Hodgkin's lymphoma with recombinant leukocyte A interferon. N Engl J Med 1984;311:1148.

Hagenbeek A, Carde P, Meerwaldt JH, et al: Maintenance of remission with human recombinant interferon alfa-2a in patients with stages III and IV low-grade malignant non-Hodgkin's lymphoma. J Clin Oncol 1998;16:41–47.

McLaughlin P, Cabanillas F, Hagemeister F, et al: CHOP-Bleo plus interferon for stage IV low-grade lymphoma. Ann Oncol 1993;4:205–211

Peterson BA, Petroni G, Oken MM, et al: Cyclophosphamide versus cyclophosphamide plus interferon alpha-2b in follicular low-grade lymphomas: A preliminary report of an intergroup trial (CALGB 8691 and EST7486). Proc ASCO 1993;12:366.

Price CG, Rohatiner AZ, Steward W, et al: Interferon-alpha 2b in the treatment of follicular lymphoma: preliminary results of a trial in progress. Eur J Cancer 1991;27(Suppl 4):534–536.

Rohatiner AZ, Richards MA, Barnett MJ, et al: Chlorambucil and interferon for low-grade non-Hodgkin's lymphoma. Br J Cancer 1987;55:225–226.

Solal-Celigny P, Lepage E, Brousse N, et al: Doxorubicin-containing regimen with or without interferon alfa-2b for advanced follicular lymphomas: Final analysis of survival and toxicity in the Groupe d'Etude des Lymphomes Folliculaires 86 trial. J Clin Oncol 1998;16:2332–2338.

Antibody Therapy

Czuczman MS, Grillo-Lopez AJ, White CA, et al: Treatment of patients with low-grade B cell lymphoma with the combination of chimeric anti-CD20 monoclonal antibody and CHOP chemotherapy. J Clin Oncol 1999;17:268–276.

Davis TA, Grillo-Lopez AJ, White CA, et al: Rituximab anti-CD20 monoclonal antibody therapy in non-Hodgkin's lymphoma: Safety and efficacy of re-treatment. J Clin Oncol 2000;18:3135–3143.

Davis TA, White CA, Grillo-Lopez AJ, et al: Single-agent monoclonal antibody efficacy in bulky non-Hodgkin's lymphoma: Results of a phase II trial of rituximab. J Clin Oncol 1999;17:1851–1857.

Hainsworth JD, Burris HA, Morrissey LH, et al: Rituximab monoclonal antibody as initial systemic therapy for patients with low-grade non-Hodgkin's lymphoma. Blood 2000;95:3052–3056.

Hsu FJ, Caspar CB, Czerwinski D, et al: Tumor-specific idiotype vaccines in the treatment of patients with B cell lymphoma: Long-term results of a clinical trial. Blood 2000; 89:3129–3135.

Kaminski MS, Zelenetz AD, Press OW, et al: Pivotal study of iodine ^{131}I tositumomab for chemotherapy-refractory low-grade or transformed low-grade B cell non-Hodgkin's lymphomas. J Clin Oncol 2001;19:3918–3928.

Maloney DG, Grillo-Lopez AJ, Bodkin DJ, et al: IDEC-C2B8: Results of a phase I multiple-dose trial in patients with relapsed non-Hodgkin's lymphoma. J Clin Oncol 1997;15: 3266–3274.

McLaughlin P, Grillo-Lopez AJ, Link BK, et al: Rituximab chimeric anti-CD20 monoclonal antibody therapy for relapsed indolent lymphoma: Half of patients respond to a four-dose treatment program. J Clin Oncol 1998;16: 2825–2833.

Maloney DG, Grillo-Lopez AJ, White CA, et al: IDEC-C2B8 (rituximab) Anti-CD20 monoclonal antibody therapy in patients with relapsed low-grade non-Hodgkin's lymphoma. Blood 1997;90:2188–2195.

Maloney DG, Liles TM, Czerwinski DK, et al: Phase I clinical trial using escalating singe-dose infusion of chimeric anti CD20 monoclonal antibody (IDEC-C2B8) in patients with recurrent B cell lymphoma. Blood 1994;84:2457–2466.

Piro LD, White CA, Grillo-Lopez AJ, et al: Extended rituximab (anti-CD20 monoclonal antibody) therapy for relapsed or refractory low-grade or follicular non-Hodgkin's lymphoma. Ann Oncol 1999;10:655–661.

Rambaldi A, Lazzari M, Manzoni C, et al: Monitoring of minimal residual disease after CHOP and rituximab in previously untreated patients with follicular lymphoma. Blood 2002; 99:856–862.

Vose JM, Wahl RL, Saleh M, et al: Multicenter phase II study of iodine-131 tositumomab for chemotherapy-relapsed/refractory low-grade and transformed low-grade B cell non-Hodgkin's lymphomas. J Clin Oncol 2000;18:1316–1323.

Autologous Stem Cell Transplantation

Apostolidis J, Gupta RJ, Grenzelias D, et al: High-dose therapy with autologous bone marrow support as consolidation of remission in follicular lymphoma: Long-term clinical and molecular follow-up. J Clin Oncol 2000;18:527–536.

Philip T, Guglielmi C, Hagenbeek A, et al: Autologous bone marrow transplantation as compared with salvage chemotherapy in relapses of chemotherapy-sensitive non-Hodgkin's lymphoma. N Engl J Med 1995;333:1540–1545.

Rohatiner AZS, Freedman A, Nadler L, et al: Myeloablative therapy with autologous bone marrow transplantation as consolidation therapy for follicular lymphoma. Ann Oncol 1994;5(Suppl 2);143–146.

Schouten HC, Colombat P, Verdonck LF, et al: Autologous bone marrow transplantation for low-grade non-Hodgkin's lymphoma: The European Bone Marrow Transplant Group experience. Ann Oncol 1994;5(Suppl 2):147–149.

Schouten HC, Kvaloy S, Sydes M, et al: The CUP trial: A randomized study analyzing the efficacy of high dose therapy and purging in follicular non-Hodgkin's lymphoma (NHL). Ann Oncol 200;11(Suppl 1):91–94.

Allogeneic Stem Cell Transplantation

Childs R, Chernoff A, Contentin N, et al: Regression of metastatic renal cell carcinoma after nonmyeloablative allogeneic peripheral-blood stem cell transplantation. N Engl J Med 2000;343:750–758.

Khouri IF, Keating M, Korbling M, et al: Transplant-lite: Induction of graft-versus-malignancy using fludarabine-based nonablative chemotherapy and allogeneic blood progenitor cell transplantation as treatment for lymphoid malignancies. J Clin Oncol 1998;16:2817–2824.

van Besien KW, de Lima M, Giralt SA, et al: Management of lymphoma recurrence after allogeneic transplantation: The relevance of graft-versus-lymphoma effect. Bone Marrow Transplant 1997;19:977–982.

van Besien K, Sobocinski KA, Rowlings PA, et al: Allogeneic bone marrow transplantation for low-grade lymphoma. Blood 1998;92:1832–1836.

Verdonck LF, Dekker AW, Lokhorst HM, et al: Allogeneic versus autologous bone marrow transplantation for refractory and recurrent low-grade non-Hodgkin's lymphoma. Blood 1997;90:4201–4205.

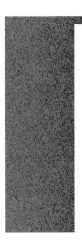

Chapter 67
Intermediate- and High-Grade Lymphoma

Ann Mellott and Leo I. Gordon

Introduction

Topics relevant to the intermediate-grade and high-grade lymphomas are also discussed in other chapters of this textbook. The reader is referred to Chapter 64 (biopsy approaches, handling of tissues for diagnosis, and lymphoma histology), Chapter 66 (mantle cell lymphoma and transformation from low-grade lymphoma), Chapter 68 (extranodal presentations of lymphoma), Chapter 69 (dermal and other manifestations of anaplastic large cell lymphoma), and Chapter 113 (lymphoma in the immunocompromised host and posttransplant lymphoproliferative disease). Although mantle cell lymphoma has been considered to be a low-grade lymphoma in the past, its clinical and biologic characteristics warrant its consideration here as an aggressive variant of non-Hodgkin's lymphoma. It is discussed under intermediate-grade lymphoma. Conversely, immunoblastic lymphoma was once thought to be a high-grade neoplasm but is now considered as an intermediate-grade lymphoma, a variant of large cell lymphoma.

Epidemiology

Non-Hodgkin's lymphomas are a heterogeneous group of malignant lymphoproliferative disorders, which represent 4% of the newly diagnosed cancers in the United States. In the year 2000, 54,900 new cases of non-Hodgkin's lymphoma were diagnosed. The incidence has been slowly increasing since the 1940s, but the cause is unclear. The increment is not completely explained by the advancing average age of the United States population, the progressive growth in the number of HIV-infected individuals who are at high risk for the development of lymphomas, or improved diagnostic techniques. A component of this epidemiologic change is an increase in extranodal presentations, primarily in the central nervous system and the eye. Improved capability to biopsy lesions in unusual locations may account in part for increased detection. Studies have attributed exposure to phenoxyacetic pesticides, metal fumes, organic solvents, and prior chemotherapy as risk factors for non-Hodgkin's lymphoma; however, the role of these factors in the genesis of the disease remains uncertain.

The incidence of non-Hodgkin's lymphoma increases in patients over age 40 years and continues to rise steadily with age. The diagnosis is more common in men than in women. An increased incidence of non-Hodgkin's lymphoma occurs in immunodeficiency states, whether congenital or acquired. Congenital disorders include ataxia-telangiectasia, Wiskott-Aldrich syndrome, common variable immunodeficiency, Bruton-type agammaglobulinemia, and Chédiak-Higashi syndrome. Acquired immunodeficiency states predisposing to non-Hodgkin's lymphoma include the immunosuppression that results from therapy to prevent graft rejection in organ transplantation, autoimmune disorders, and acquired immunodeficiency due to HIV infection. The incidence of non-Hodgkin's lymphoma is 40-fold to 100-fold greater then expected in renal allograft patients, for example. The immmunologic dysfunction associated with rheumatoid arthritis, Sjögren's syndrome, Hashimoto's thyroiditis, systemic lupus erythematosus, and celiac sprue is also associated with an increased incidence of lymphoma. There appears to be an indirect relationship between the CD4 (helper T cell) count and the increased risk of non-Hodgkin's lymphoma in HIV-infected individuals.

Epstein-Barr Virus and Lymphoma

The Epstein-Barr virus is a human herpes virus that has the ability to immortalize normal resting B-lymphocytes in vitro, converting them to permanently growing lymphoblastoid cells. The virus can be detected by in situ hybridization, by polymerase chain reactions, and indirectly by immunohistochemical analysis targeted to specific Epstein-Barr virus–

associated antigens. The precise role of Epstein-Barr virus in oncogenesis remains unclear. In endemic Burkitt's lymphoma in Africa, essentially all of these lymphomas developing in immunocompetent individuals are Epstein-Barr virus positive. In sporadic cases of Burkitt's lymphoma in Western countries, fewer than 20% of the lymphomas are positive for the virus. Epstein-Barr virus may increase the risk of neoplastic mutation by establishing a population of long-lived, dividing cells as they go through the cell cycle. Epstein-Barr virus also plays a role in the development of lymphoproliferative disorders in immunoincompetent individuals, as, for example, in patients receiving immunosuppressive therapy after solid organ transplantation. The epidemiology of lymphomas in this circumstance is discussed in Chapter 113.

Diagnosis

With an easily palpable peripheral lymph node, an excisional biopsy should be done. In some cases (very large nodes), an incisional biopsy may suffice. Fine needle aspiration is often inadequate and, especially in the large cell lymphomas, can be difficult to distinguish from a poorly differentiated carcinoma. There are instances when a fine-needle biopsy may be the least morbid procedure for an extremely ill patient or when lymphadenopathy is limited to abdominal or thoracic sites. In these cases, it is important to obtain a core-needle biopsy for histologic examination.

Although the extent of the patient's disease is an important consideration, the prognosis and choice of therapy in non-Hodgkin's lymphomas are determined largely by the histology. Precise diagnosis requires an adequate biopsy specimen and proper processing of the tissue for a number of sophisticated studies as well as microscopic evaluation. Because of the intricacies of differentiating among lymphomas, the services of a pathologist who is experienced in evaluating hematologic disorders are of great benefit. The details of histologic pathology observed in non-Hodgkin's lymphomas are discussed in Chapter 64.

This chapter focuses on the intermediate-grade and high-grade non-Hodgkin's lymphomas. The intermediate-grade lymphomas include

1. Follicular large cell
2. Diffuse small cleaved cell (most of these are currently classified as mantle cell lymphoma)
3. Small cleaved and large cell (diffuse mixed)
4. Diffuse large cell or its immunoblastic morphologic variant (immunoblastic variant) and the diffuse large cell (cleaved).

The high-grade lymphomas include

1. Diffuse small noncleaved cell lymphoma (Burkitt's or Burkitt's-like)
2. Lymphoblastic lymphoma.

Clinically and therapeutically, the management of the different subsets of the intermediate-grade non-Hodgkin's lymphomas (primarily B cell neoplasms) does not differ substantially. These are discussed as a group, with the exception of the special circumstances that distinguish mantle cell lymphoma. Because the management of Burkitt's lymphoma differs from that employed for the other B cell, intermediate-grade lymphomas, it is discussed separately. In almost all cases, lymphoblastic lymphoma is derived from T cells and is histologically identical to T cell acute lymphoblastic leukemia. Therapy for lymphoblastic lymphoma is the same as that used for T cell acute lymphoblastic leukemia, which is described in Chapter 61.

Clinical Presentation and Evaluation

Intermediate-grade lymphomas typically arise in the nodal tissues, bone marrow, and spleen. Masses in the neck, axillae, and abdomen are common. Cough or chest pain can result from mediastinal lymphadenopathy. Constitutional ("B") symptoms of fevers, chills, night sweats, and weight loss may be pronounced at the time of diagnosis, even in the absence of overtly palpable disease. "B" symptoms are noted at presentation in 20% to 25% of patients. As a result, it is important to keep lymphoma in mind when evaluating a patient with these systemic complaints. Other, less frequent, sites of primary presentation include the skin, small intestine, stomach, oral cavity, breast, and testes.

The physical exam should focus on evaluation of lymph node sites, that is, cervical, axillary, epitrochlear, and inguinal areas and the tonsillar tissues in Waldeyer's ring. Local areas of invasion or pressure can produce specific symptomatic problems. For example, obstruction of the superior vena cava, which is present in 3% to 8% of patients with large cell lymphoma, causes distended neck veins, facial swelling, and suffusion of the eyelids that is increased in the early morning. A thrombus can form owing to the compression of the superior vena cava, but this event occurs more often in carcinomas of the lung than in lymphomas. Superior vena cava syndrome is a potentially lethal complication (see Chapter 17). It can compromise respiration owing to pressure on the trachea. Neurologic symptoms at presentation, such as unilateral muscle weakness or cranial nerve palsies, suggest spinal cord compression or leptomeningeal disease, respectively.

Table 67-1 ▪ Staging Procedures in the Evaluation of Non-Hodgkin's Lymphomas

1. Complete physical examination with special attention to nodal sites, liver, spleen, and Waldeyer's ring
2. Query the presence of constitutional symptoms: fever, night sweats, weight loss of >10% of premorbid weight.
3. ECOG Performance Status (PS) assessment: PS 0 (no symptoms), PS 1 (mild symptoms), PS 2 (moderate symptoms), PS 3 (confined to bed <50% of the day), PS4 (confined to bed >50% of the day)
4. Laboratory studies: complete blood count, platelet count, BUN, creatinine, lactate dehydrogenase, bilirubin, AST, ALT, alkaline phosphatase, uric acid, calcium, beta-2 microglobulin, pregnancy test (in fertile women), HIV test (if risk factors are present)
5. CT scans of chest, abdomen, and pelvis. CT scan of neck if indicated
6. Positron emission tomography (PET) scan or gallium scan
7. Chest X-ray: PA and lateral
8. Bone marrow aspirate and biopsy
9. Consider lumbar puncture, CT or magnetic resonance imaging (MRI) scans of the brain
10. Endoscopy if risk of gastrointestinal tract involvement is high

The extent of disease is an important determinant of the patient's prognosis and is used as a guide to therapy. Tests involved in staging the disease are shown in Table 67-1. Waldeyer's ring involvement occurs in 5% to 10% of patients with intermediate-grade non-Hodgkin's lymphoma and is associated with lymphomatous involvement of the gastrointestinal (GI) tract. Patients with tonsillar disease should therefore undergo radiographic and endoscopic studies of the gastrointestinal tract. Bone marrow involvement is noted in 15% to 25% of cases. Elevations of the lactate dehydrogenase (LDH) level and/or the beta-2 microglobulin level reflect unfavorably on prognosis and are directly related to the total lymphoma body burden and the rate of proliferation or cell turnover of the malignant cells. Patients whose history places them in the high-risk category for HIV infection because of prior blood transfusions, homosexuality, or intravenous drug abuse need to be tested for HIV. In locations where HIV infection is endemic, HIV testing should be performed in any patient with non-Hodgkin's lymphoma even in the absence of a suggestive history. In some circumstances, it may be reasonable to also evaluate the cardiac ejection fraction and/or pulmonary function tests if chemotherapy will include intensive treatment with chemotherapy that is potentially toxic to the heart and lungs.

In patients who are HIV positive, have Burkitt's lymphoma or neurologic findings or symptoms, or whose lymphoma involves the testes or orbit, a lumbar puncture is indicated because of the increased likelihood of central nervous system (CNS) involvement.

Intermediate-Grade Non-Hodgkin's Lymphomas

Staging the Disease

The extent of the patient's disease is usually staged according to the Ann Arbor staging system (Table 67-2). The International Prognostic Index assembles salient clinical characteristics to create an informative risk profile at the time of diagnosis. The index utilizes five prognostic features: age, lactate dehydrogenase, performance status, the number of extranodal sites of disease, and the stage of the disease (Table 67-3). The International Non-Hodgkin's Lymphomas Prognostic Factors Project found that five-year survival rates were 73% with zero to one adverse prognostic features, 51% with two adverse features, 43% with three adverse features, and 26% with four or five adverse features. Other molecular and cellular markers that have been reported to be associated with reduced overall survival and increased recurrence rates include elevated levels of Ki-67; a nuclear proliferation antigen; T cell phenotype; lack of HLA-DR expression; decreased number of $CD8^+$ tumor lymphocytes; increased β-2 microglobulin; and overexpression of bcl-2. Moreover, patients whose lymphomas exhibited greater than 60% overexpression of Ki-67 antigen had a median survival of 8 months compared with 39

Table 67-2 ▪ Ann Arbor Staging System

Stage	Involvement of
I	one lymph node site, or one single extranodal organ or site (Stage IE)
II	two or more lymph node sites on the same side of the diaphragm or multiple extranodal sites on the same side of the diaphragm (Stage IIE)
III	lymph node sites on both sides of the diaphragm; can include an extranodal site or the spleen
IV	the bone marrow or disseminated disease in nodal sites and infiltration of nonlymphoid organs, such as skin, liver, lung, or bone

Add "B" as suffix to the stage designation if constitutional symptoms are present.

Table 67-3 ■ International Prognostic Index (IPI)

One Point Is Given for Each of the Following Adverse Prognostic Factors

1. Age >60 years (versus younger patients)
2. Stage III or IV disease (versus stage I or II)
3. Involvement of >1 extranodal sites (versus none or one extranodal site)
4. Performance status 2, 3, or 4 (versus performance status 0 or 1)
5. Lactate dehydrogenase higher than normal limit (versus normal lactate dehydrogenase level)

Table 67-4 ■ Combination Chemotherapy Regimens Used in Intermediate-Grade Non-Hodgkin's Lymphoma

Eponym	Agents
CHOP	cyclophosphamide, doxorubicin, vincristine, prednisone
COPP	cyclophosphamide, procarbazine, vincristine, prednisone
COMLA	cyclophosphamide, cytarabine, vincristine, methotrexate, leukovorin
m-BACOD	cyclophosphamide, doxorubicin, vincristine, bleomycin, dexamethasone, methotrexate, leukovorin
MACOP-B	cyclophosphamide, doxorubicin, vincristine, prednisone, bleomycin, methotrexate, leukovorin
ProMACE-CytaBOM	cyclophosphamide, doxorubicin, vincristine, prednisone, bleomycin, cytarabine, etoposide, methotrexate, leukovorin

months for those with lower levels of Ki-67 antigen expression.

Treatment

Chemotherapy, with or without radiation therapy, is the mainstay of therapy. The treatment plan depends on the stage, pace of the disease, age of the patient, and concomitant medical problems. When chemotherapy is initially used in a patient with extensive or rapidly proliferating disease, destruction of the lymphoma cells may be so rapid and substantial that the patient manifests the tumor lysis syndrome. The breakdown products of these cells are released into the circulation, resulting in hyperuricemia, hypocalcemia, hyperkalemia, hyperphosphatemia, and metabolic acidosis. Renal insufficiency and renal failure result. Prevention is the best treatment and includes aggressive hydration to maintain renal blood flow and renal clearance, allopurinol to lower the uric acid, and alkalinization of the urine to increase the solubility of uric acid and prevent urinary sludging.

The recurrence rate in stage I or IE patients treated with radiation therapy alone is 30% to 50%. These recurrences usually occur outside the radiation field. The local control rate with a dose of 4400 cGy of radiation therapy is 80% to 90%. Radiation therapy used alone is unsatisfactory in patients who have more than stage I disease.

The Eastern Cooperative Oncology Group randomized patients with stages I/IE and nonbulky II/IIE disease to receive eight cycles of CHOP (cyclophosphamide, hydroxydaunorubicin [Adriamycin], vincristine [Oncovin], and prednisone) with or without radiation therapy to initial sites of disease. The combined modality therapy achieved an increased complete remission rate and increased progression-free survival compared to patients who received chemotherapy alone. The Southwest Oncology Group randomized a similar subset of patients to receive either eight cycles of CHOP or three cycles of CHOP followed by local radiation therapy to the sites of initial disease. The five-year progression-free survival rate was 64% for CHOP alone and 77% for CHOP and radiation therapy, and the five-year overall survival rate was 72% and 82%, respectively. Thus a survival advantage and diminished toxicity were seen in patients receiving combined-modality therapy. The long-term benefit of the combined modality regiment compared to lengthier chemotherapy has been questioned. Nevertheless, because of its lower toxicity, standard therapy for stage I nonbulky intermediate-grade lymphoma is three cycles of CHOP followed by radiation therapy.

For more advanced disease—bulky stage II or stages III or IV disease—chemotherapy with CHOP alone is effective, resulting in long-term survival in approximately 40% of patients. All of the combination chemotherapy regimens shown in Table 67-4 are active in intermediate-grade lymphomas. The regimens vary in the number of active agents used, the intensity of the doses, and the frequency of administration of chemotherapy. In the 1980s, it appeared from reports of nonrandomized trials of different therapeutic regimens (see Table 67-4) that escalating the intensity of therapy improved five-year survival compared to results of CHOP treatment. Randomized studies failed to document benefit, however. Thus a randomized trial of CHOP versus m-BACOD in patients with advanced non-Hodgkin's lymphoma showed no difference in outcome, and treatment with m-BACOD resulted in significantly worse toxicity, especially grade 3 or 4 pulmonary toxicity. The actual intensity of the delivered doses of CHOP was greater than of the drugs in the more intensive schedule used in m-BACOD therapy, because dose reductions for nonhematologic toxicity were more often required with the latter treatment. These results were confirmed in a subsequent trial randomizing patients to CHOP, m-BACOD, MACOP-B, or Pro-MACE-CytaBOM. Three-year survival rates were 44% overall. No significant differences in response rate, time to treatment failure, or overall survival were noted among the regimens, and CHOP exhibited a significantly lower rate of toxicity. These trials established that for diffuse large cell non-Hodgkin's lymphoma (the most frequent type of intermediate-grade non-Hodgkin's lymphomas), CHOP remains the treatment of choice among chemotherapy regimens. It has been difficult to demonstrate that increasing the intensity of chemotherapy by various means, such as by the use of hematopoietic growth factors, provides greater benefit than conventional doses of CHOP given monthly for six to eight cycles to patients with advanced disease.

The French lymphoma trials group compared standard chemotherapy with standard chemotherapy followed by autologous bone marrow transplantation. Overall, there was no significant difference in disease-free or overall survival. Subset analysis of 236 poor-risk patients showed that the three-year disease-free survival rate improved from 39% in patients receiving conventional chemotherapy alone compared to 59% in patients undergoing chemotherapy plus autologous bone marrow transplantation. The five-year overall survival rate showed a similar improvement, increasing from 52% to 65%. A subsequent study that combined autologous stem cell transplantation with chemotherapy in high-risk young patients demonstrated a lower overall and event-free survival than that reported from the subset analysis. Further discussion of the role of stem cell transplantation appears in Chapter 51.

In patients at high risk of central nervous system involvement, prophylactic intrathecal therapy is recommended as part of initial therapy. No studies have clearly documented what constitutes optimal central nervous system prophylaxis, or central nervous system therapy for that matter. A regimen that is in common use for central nervous system prophylaxis in patients with lymphoma is intrathecal instillation of methotrexate, cytarabine, or both, given on four occasions. If lymphomatous meningitis is present, then intrathecal cytarabine or methotrexate can be administered every other day until the cerebrospinal fluid cytology is negative, then weekly for four weeks, followed by monthly evaluation of the spinal fluid and intrathecal administration of chemotherapy for one year. For lymphomatous deposits causing cranial nerve palsies, cranial radiation therapy is also given.

Follow-up Evaluation

After the completion of successful treatment, each visit to the office by the patient is highly stressful because of the fear that the physician will detect recurrence that is not apparent to the patient. Patients should be seen frequently enough to detect recurrence to initiate salvage therapy, to treat late-occurring toxicities, and to allow surveillance for second malignancies but not so often as to burden the patient. One such balanced approach would include follow-up visits every three months for the first two years, every six months for an additional two years, and then yearly thereafter. The risk of recurrent disease declines progressively with time, and the great majority of recurrences occur within the first two years after therapy. Recurrences usually occur within the first 18 to 24 months and become less frequent thereafter. Although clinicians tend to do repeated computed tomography (CT) scans and other imaging studies on each visit, these are unnecessary. Most recurrences are detected because the patient notes a new finding or symptom or because routine laboratory studies become abnormal. The overwhelming majority of recurrences become apparent between routinely scheduled imaging studies rather than at the time of the visit.

Relapse should be documented by a repeat biopsy, if feasible, to confirm the recurrence. Thorough repeat staging studies with computed tomography scans and bone marrow biopsy are warranted when relapse occurs. Recurrence is treated by reducing the tumor burden with chemotherapy followed by autologous stem cell transplantation in eligible patients with the appropriate performance status and end-organ function. The long-term survival rate after the procedure varies from 20% to 50%.

New Therapies

Monoclonal antibodies of several different types have been utilized in the treatment of non-Hodgkin's lymphomas. Rituximab (Rituxan) is a chimeric monoclonal antibody that targets CD20 antigen on normal and malignant B cells. At this writing, it is the only FDA-approved monoclonal antibody therapy for recurrent low-grade lymphoma; it is not approved for use in intermediate-grade non-Hodgkin's lymphoma. This antigen is an attractive target because it is not shed or internalized following exposure to the ligand (rituximab). Anti-CD20 has multiple mechanisms of activity against CD20-positive lymphomas. These include complement-dependent cytotoxicity, antibody-dependent cytotoxicity, and activation of death signals leading to apoptosis. Immediate depletion of normal B cells in the peripheral blood occurs following infusion. Antibody can be detected for up to six months in patients after treatment. B cells begin to return to normal levels in approximately nine months.

Radiolabeling the antibodies, such as in ^{90}yttrium ibritumomab (Zevalin) and tositumomab/^{131}iodine (Bexxar), adds another mechanism of lymphoma cell killing. Local radiation emission also can destroy adjacent lymphoma cells even if the antibody is not directly bound to those cells. Ibritumomab tiuxetan, a murine anti-CD20 monoclonal antibody, is covalently bound to the chelator tiuxetan and can chelate yttrium-90, thereby delivering radiation directly to the CD20 cells. Tositumomab uses iodine-131 as the radioisotope. The range of response rates and remission rates are variable owing to the extensive pretreatment that many of these patients have had. Side effects of these agents include myelosuppression, immunosuppression, and infection. In all cases, it is necessary to administer cold antibody prior to radioimmunotherapy to maximize tumor uptake. It is clear that the radioactive antibodies can induce good responses, even complete responses, in patients who are resistant to unlabeled antibody. How the radiolabeled or unlabeled antibody should best be employed in the treatment of the intermediate-grade lymphomas, which subsets will be responsive, and whether these agents are best employed in combination with chemotherapy or as part of stem cell transplantation are unclear.

Lymphoma in the Elderly

The treatment of lymphoma in the elderly is a difficult clinical problem. Approximately one third of new cases in the Western hemisphere are diagnosed in people over age 70 years. Advanced age not only is an adverse prognostic factor (International Prognostic Index), but also is associated with a manyfold increase in morbidity from and intolerance of chemotherapy. Performance status is an important prognostic factor that is influenced by comorbid conditions that are commonly found in the elderly, such as cardiovascular or pulmonary disease. Extranodal disease, another adverse prognostic factor, occurs with increasing frequency in the elderly.

The toxicity of therapy poses challenges in elderly patients. Enhanced drug toxicity is believed to be a result of altered drug metabolism and the natural reduction in reserve capacity in organs such as the heart, lungs, and kidneys that occurs with increasing age. In a study of CHOP chemotherapy, the Southwest Oncology Group specified automatic dose reductions in cyclophosphamide and doxorubicin to minimize toxicity in patients over age 65 years. Only a 37% complete remission rate was achieved. Whether the low remission rate was related to dose reduction or other factors such as disease resistance and comorbid conditions is uncertain. The French randomized trial of rituximab plus CHOP versus CHOP alone in patients 60 years old or older who had intermediate-grade lymphoma showed statistically significant improvement in complete response rate, progression-free survival, and overall survival for the combined modality therapy group.

Mantle Cell Lymphoma

Mantle cell lymphoma represents fewer than 10% of all non-Hodgkin's lymphomas. Although previously included in the category of small cell lymphoma of intermediate differentiation, it is now clearly defined as a distinctive entity. In mantle cell lymphoma, a homogenous population of small lymphoid cells with irregular nuclear borders arises from and expands the mantle zone surrounding the germinal centers in the lymph nodes, overrunning the centers and spreading diffusely throughout the node. The lymphocytes usually express surface immunoglobulin IgM or IgD, but in greater density than is noted in chronic lymphocytic leukemia. Like chronic lymphocytic leukemia, mantle cell lymphoma is derived from B cells, yet both express the T cell marker CD5. Nevertheless, although occasional cases of mantle cell lymphoma behave as a low-grade lymphoma or chronic lymphocytic leukemia clinically, the great majority of cases exhibit aggressive clinical characteristics and inexorable disease progression through multiple chemotherapy regimens. The immunophenotypic pattern that is specific for mantle cell lymphoma is CD5+, CD23−, and FMC7+. Translocation of the long arms of chromosome 11 and 14 (t(11;14)(q13;q23)) is found in most cases of mantle cell lymphoma. This abnormality juxtaposes the bcl-1 gene to the immunoglobulin heavy chain gene, leading to overexpression of bcl-1. This gene codes for the cell cycle regulatory protein, cyclin D1, which is believed to play a role in lymphomagenesis. Cyclin D1 overexpression is not found in normal lymphocytes and rarely occurs in other B cell malignancies.

Compared to low-grade lymphomas, patients with mantle cell lymphoma are older (median age 64 years), are predominantly male (75% of patients), and have more widespread disease (liver, spleen, and bone marrow involvement are common at diagnosis), extranodal manifestations are more often present (50%), and the number of affected regional node sites is increased. Patients therefore typically present with diffuse lymphadenopathy and splenomegaly, but constitutional symptoms are initially present in fewer than one half of the patients. Circulating lymphoma cells appear in the peripheral blood in approximately one third of cases. The wall of the gastrointestinal tract can be infiltrated, resulting in a pattern of involvement called multiple lymphomatous polyposis. If gastrointestinal symptoms are present, then colonoscopy and/or esophogastroduodenoscopy are warranted to assess disease extent.

Elevation of lactate dehydrogenase, β-2 microglobulin, decreased albumin, advanced age, and poor performance status are unfavorable prognostic indicators. Overall response rates to traditional chemotherapy, such as CHOP (see Table 67-3) or COP (cyclophosphamide, vincristine, and prednisone), are 50% to 60%, but complete remissions are infrequent. Median response duration (8 months) is short, requiring repeated treatment for progression and the development of chemoresistance. Median overall survival is approximately three years. Conventional chemotherapy yields no apparent cures, and the long-term survival rate is less than 10%. Autologous stem cell transplantation is of limited value in this disease. Fludarabine is substantially less effective in mantle cell lymphoma than in the low-grade lymphomas. Responses to antibodies have been of marginal value, but radioisotopically labeled antibodies and combined chemotherapy and antibody therapy regimens may improve on current results. Mantle cell lymphoma remains a therapeutically challenging illness. There is no clear consensus about the optimal approach to therapy.

Gastrointestinal Lymphomas

Lymphomas of the gastrointestinal tract are uncommon and account for 1% to 10% of gastrointestinal malignancies. In the Western world, the most common sites of gastrointestinal involvement in descending order of frequency are the stomach, small intestine (ileum>jejunum>duodenum), large intestine, and esophagus. In the Middle East, small bowel lymphomas are more common then gastric lymphomas, owing to the high incidence of immunoproliferative small intestinal disease that is part of the malabsorptive defect that develops in tropical sprue.

Gastric lymphoma often presents with symptoms similar to a peptic ulcer or gastritis, including abdominal pain or gastrointestinal bleeding. Fevers and night sweats are uncommon; when they are present, the underlying lymphoma often has a T cell phenotype. Nonhealing gastric ulcers or gastritis may prove on follow-up to be lymphoma. The diagnosis can be dif-

ficult to make by endoscopic biopsy because the malignant cells are often submucosal. The diagnosis is therefore frequently made at the time of exploratory surgery when the surgeon performs a partial or total gastrectomy. An aggressive lymphoma histology is common, most frequently of large cell or mixed cell type. Lymphomas of mucosa-associated lymphoid tissue (MALT) are also seen. These are predominantly low-grade lymphomas and are treated according to the guidelines outlined in Chapters 66 and 68. Antibiotic therapy to eliminate *Helicobacter pylori* infection, which is involved in the pathogenesis of mucosa-associated lymphoid tissue lymphomas, achieves remission in a majority of patients with low-grade mucosa-associated lymphoid tissue lymphomas. Responses to antibiotic therapy are less consistent in high-grade mucosa-associated lymphoid tissue lymphomas, perhaps reflective of transformation to a lymphoma that proliferates autonomously independent of the *H. pylori* stimulus. Thus histological large cell mucosa-associated lymphoid tissue lymphomas, even those associated with *H. pylori* infection, require the same therapy as other large cell lymphomas.

The Ann Arbor system of staging is not as useful for gastrointestinal lymphomas as it is for other non-Hodgkin's lymphomas. The alternative staging system described by Blackledge and colleagues is often used (Table 67-5). The optimal therapy for gastrointestinal lymphoma is not defined. Some investigators recommend gastrectomy as the primary treatment for intermediate-grade gastric lymphoma, but recent data indicate that patients are effectively treated with chemotherapy (CHOP) for up to six cycles, followed by local radiation therapy to the stomach. This approach conserves gastric function. Chemotherapy does, however, carry a less than 5% risk of causing gastrointestinal perforation due to resulting weakness of the wall of the stomach, when chemotherapy lyses

---

Table 67-5 ■ Blackledge Staging System for Gastrointestinal Non-Hodgkin's Lymphomas

Stage	Description
I	Tumor confined to GI tract without serosal penetration; single or multiple sites
II	Tumor extending into the abdomen from primary site
	1 Local node involvement, such as gastric or mesenteric
	2 Distant node involvement, such as para-aortic or paracaval
III	Penetration into adjacent structures, such as pancreas or intestines
IV	Disseminated disease or supradiaphragmatic involvement

extensive transmural deposits of lymphoma. Compared to surgery, however, it affords an opportunity to treat occult lymphoma elsewhere in the body.

Primary Central Nervous System Lymphoma

Primary central nervous system lymphoma refers to lymphoma confined to the craniospinal axis. This category does not include systemic non-Hodgkin's lymphoma that incidentally involves the central nervous system. Primary central nervous system lymphoma develops in both immunocompetent and immunoincompetent patients and is associated with a poorer prognosis in the latter group. Primary central nervous system lymphoma represents fewer than 1% of all brain tumors, but in the past 20 years, the incidence has tripled. In part, this is due to an increase in immunocompromised states such as HIV infection, but this does not explain the increased incidence in immunocompetent patients. Chapter 113 provides a detailed discussion of primary central nervous system lymphoma in immunocompromised patients.

The incidence is greater in men and typically is more common in men in their fifties and sixties. Computed tomography scans of the brain can reveal single or multiple isodense or hypodense lesions; contrast enhancement is frequently observed. The SPECT scan has a high degree of sensitivity and specificity for the diagnosis of central nervous system lymphoma. Stereotactic biopsy is the best means of diagnosis. Corticosteroids are useful in therapy but should be avoided, if feasible, until after biopsy confirmation of the diagnosis has been obtained. The administration of corticosteroids prior to a biopsy can obscure the diagnosis, because up to two thirds of patients exhibit a striking response to the lympholytic effects. These lymphomas in immunocompetent patients are usually of the large B cell type. Other histologic types, such as Burkitt's, immunoblastic, or Burkitt's-like lymphomas, are more common in HIV-positive patients. Primary central nervous system lymphoma is distinguished from other large cell lymphomas because it arises outside of the conventional lymphoid system and its prognosis is much worse than that in systemic large cell lymphomas.

Treatment can be by radiation therapy alone, chemotherapy alone, or combined modality therapy. Radiation therapy alone is associated with a median survival of approximately one year. Whole-brain radiation therapy is usually administered to a total dose of 40 Gy. Local recurrence in the brain is a common event, and neurologic damage from therapy not uncommonly occurs in the small percentage of long-term survivors.

A number of studies have demonstrated that high-dose methotrexate-based chemotherapy improves median progression-free survival to approximately 1.5 years and median survival to 40 months, resulting in a five-year survival rate of 25%. Systemically administered high-dose cytarabine, like high-dose methotrexate, establishes lymphomacidal concentrations of the drug in the central nervous system and is an alternative chemotherapeutic approach, but high-dose methotrexate is most commonly used in treatment regimes. Although some treatment programs include intraventricular therapy via an Ommaya reservoir, neurotoxicity is increased. In some reports, combined radiation therapy and chemotherapy has improved the outcome, but this combination therapy is not well tolerated by elderly patients, and the frequency of long-term cognitive defects is substantial. Moreover, the value of aggressive therapy for patients over age 65 years is debatable, since the prognosis for survival is so poor. It may be that the combination of high-dose methotrexate combined with focal gamma knife radiation therapy will improve results without increasing neurotoxicity.

Ki-1+ Anaplastic Lymphoma

Primary Ki-1 (CD30+) anaplastic large cell lymphoma is now recognized as a distinct clinical pathologic entity. Prior to this demarcation, the Ki-1+ lymphomas were characterized as lymphocyte-depleted Hodgkin's disease, reactive lymphadenopathy, or malignant histiocytosis. The relatively undifferentiated large cells can appear similar to melanoma or carcinoma on light microscopy. Leukocyte common antigen (CD45+) and epithelial membrane antigen are expressed in 65% of patients. If epithelial membrane antigen is present, it separates anaplastic lymphoma from the other non-Hodgkin's lymphomas, which are usually negative. Conversely, CD15 is rarely expressed in anaplastic lymphomas, whereas it is positive in 70% of cases of Hodgkin's disease. Anaplastic large cell lymphoma cells express CD30, CD25, and HLA-DR, which are lymphocyte activation markers. The presence or absence of the t(2;5)(p23;q25) translocation distinguishes two phenotypic subsets of anaplastic lymphoma that are morphologically similar ("horseshoe" or "wreath-shaped" appearance, prominent nucleoli and basophilic cytoplasm) but have different clinical and immunophenotypic features. This translocation results in the expression of the CD30+ phenotype and encodes for an 80-kD tyrosine kinase. This protein results from the fusion of the nucleophosmin (NPM) gene on chromosome 5 and the anaplastic lymphoma kinase (ALK) gene on chromosome 2. The fusion protein is present in three quarters of patients, is more often identified in children (80%) than in adults (60%), and is rare in other forms of non-Hodgkin's lymphoma. Because Hodgkin's disease is also CD30 positive, the presence of the fusion protein or demonstration of the gene translocation helps to diagnose anaplastic large cell lymphoma. The absence of t(2;5) and anaplastic lymphoma kinase negativity are associated with a worse prognosis.

Systemic anaplastic lymphoma is more frequent in children and adolescents than in adults. In adults, the median age is 44 years (range, 16 to 86). It is a T cell malignancy in approximately one half of patients, B cell in one third, and non-B-, non-T cell in the remainder. Lymph nodes are characteristically tender and soft. Extranodal sites of involvement are common, occurring in two thirds of patients, most often in the skin. Cutaneous involvement is present in one third of patients at diagnosis. Fevers, night sweats, and weight loss are noted in 40% of patients. Although stages II and IV disease occur in two thirds of patients, bone marrow and central nervous system involvements are unusual.

More often in adults than children, anaplastic large cell lymphoma can present initially with involvement only of the skin. Raised, nodular deposits, seldom larger than 2 cm, are seen. These can progress to necrosis and ulceration. Nevertheless, the lesions tend to wax and wane and can even spontaneously resolve without therapy. This form of the disease is difficult to distinguish from benign lymphomatoid papulosis. Progression to systemic disease occurs in only 25% of patients. The course in many patients is indolent, and individual lesions may not require treatment. When they persist or advance, local superficial radiation therapy causes regression. Chemotherapy is reserved for symptomatic treatment when systemic disease supervenes.

Patients with systemic disease are treated with chemotherapy with curative intent. Chemotherapy with CHOP as for large cell lymphomas or with ABVD (Adriamycin, bleomycin, vinblastine, and DTIC) as for Hodgkin's disease are both effective. Results of treatment are similar to those for large cell lymphomas of equivalent stage and prognosis. The overall complete response rate is approximately 45%. In contrast to other non-Hodgkin's lymphomas, relapses after successful chemotherapy tend to occur in anaplastic large cell lymphoma at new, rather than previous, sites of disease. Autologous stem cell transplantation may improve on the results of chemotherapy alone, and anti-CD30 antibody may prove to be a viable therapeutic option in the future.

High-Grade Non-Hodgkin's Lymphoma

The high-grade non-Hodgkin's lymphomas include small noncleaved cell lymphomas (Burkitt's and Burkitt's-like) and lymphoblastic lymphoma.

Lymphoblastic Lymphoma

This lymphoma is a T cell neoplasm that is identical morphologically and phenotypically to the T cell variant of acute lymphoblastic leukemia (Chapter 61). Lymphoblastic lymphoma is rare in adults. It is characterized histologically by immature lymphoid cells with fine chromatin and indistinct nuclei that are indistinguishable from the cells of T cell acute lymphoblastic leukemia. This disorder is also clinically indistinguishable from T cell acute lymphoblastic leukemia. Lymphoblastic lymphoma is primarily a disease of adolescents and children and is an infrequent variety of lymphoma in adults.

The treatment of this disorder consists primarily of high-dose chemotherapy but includes central nervous system prophylaxis and long-term maintenance and so is more similar to treatment of acute lymphoblastic leukemia than it is to treatment of other lymphomas. When the disease presents occasionally in a limited form, treatment as for intermediate-grade non-Hodgkin's lymphomas is a satisfactory approach. In general, however, these patients present with extensive stage III or IV disease with bulky involvement, especially in the mediastinum. Therapeutic studies of this low-incidence form of lymphoma have been limited. Because of the propensity for lymphoblastic lymphoma to involve the bone marrow and central nervous system, these patients are best treated with regimens designed for acute lymphoblastic leukemia, which are especially effective in the T cell variant.

Burkitt's and Burkitt's-like Lymphoma

The small noncleaved cell lymphomas account for fewer than 1% of adult lymphomas and are the most rapidly proliferating of the non-Hodgkin's lymphomas. Morphologically, the cells are indistinguishable from the B cell FAB L3 variant of acute lymphoblastic leukemia. Although classification schemes have attempted to separate the form called Burkitt's lymphoma from the form called Burkitt's-like, they are histologically similar, both bearing mature B cell markers. Concordance among pathologists in separating the two entities is very low. This fact confounds analysis of series purporting to show clinical and therapeutic differences between the two forms. Biologic differences do exist in that among these lymphomas is a subset that can be defined by the lack of c-myc overexpression usually found in Burkitt's lymphoma. Whether this absence can be used to identify a Burkitt's-like variant remains uncertain.

In all Burkitt's lymphomas, whether positive or negative for Epstein-Barr virus, the c-myc oncogene on chromosome 8 undergoes reciprocal translocation with one of the genetic sites of the immunoglobulin genes. The great majority of cases (more than three quarters) exhibit the t(8;14)(q24;q32), linking c-myc to the site of the immunoglobulin heavy chain gene on chromosome 14. A t(8;22)(q24;q11) is found in some cases, involving the lambda light chain immunoglobulin gene on chromosome 22, and, rarely, in the (2;8)(p13;q24), the kappa light chain on chromosome 2 is involved. How the translocation triggers c-myc overexpression is unclear, but c-myc is known to play a role in cell cycle progression and cellular transformation. Translocation of c-myc occasionally occurs in other non-Hodgkin's lymphomas and in B cell acute lymphoblastic leukemia.

Clinically and epidemiologically, there are two forms of Burkitt's lymphoma. The epidemic form occurs in Africa and is almost always associated with a latent EBV infection. The disease is most common in young children, presenting with bulky peripheral lymph nodes, especially in the head and neck region, and a proclivity for involvement of the maxilla and mandible. The American form occurs in sporadic fashion. It more commonly occurs in young adults than in children, and Epstein-Barr viral DNA is found in the neoplastic clone in only approximately 20%. In the American Burkitt's lymphoma, the disease tends to present less often with peripheral node enlargement and more often with bulky intra-abdominal disease and involvement of extranodal sites, especially the gastrointestinal tract. In both African and American Burkitt's lymphoma, males are more often affected than females.

Young adults usually present with stage IV disease and a high lactate dehydrogenase. Patients often exhibit bulky tumor deposits, marked elevations of the lactate dehydrogenase, and involvement of the bone marrow or central nervous system, each of which is an unfavorable prognostic finding. Patients must be evaluated and treated as quickly as possible owing to rapid growth rate of this lymphoma. Particular attention should be paid to the likelihood of tumor lysis syndrome following initial treatment of patients with small noncleaved lymphomas, as the high cell turnover and high response rate make patients especially susceptible to tumor lysis syndrome with resultant fluid and electrolyte imbalances and renal dysfunction. Careful hydration and lowering of the uric acid level by administration of allopurinol are important prophylactic measures against this complication. Despite these efforts, tumor lysis may be so profound that renal failure nevertheless occurs, requiring dialysis while recovery is awaited.

Adults are treated with aggressive chemotherapy regimens. These are usually based on regimens developed for use in children. They include high-dose systemic combination chemotherapy, which includes methotrexate or cytarabine in doses that produce lymphomacidal levels of the drugs in the cerebrospinal fluid, as well as intrathecal therapy with cortisone, cytarabine, and methotrexate. Because of the likelihood of central nervous system disease, central nervous system prophylaxis needs to be aggressive and given early on in therapy to prevent overt lymphomatous meningitis. Chemotherapy causes complete remission in 70% to 80% of adults, but most relapse later, except for the small subgroup without adverse prognostic factors. The overall five-year survival rate for adults is approximately 40%. Owing to these results and because allogeneic or autologous stem cell transplantation can achieve cures in patients with relapsed disease, many clinicians advocate the application of transplantation shortly after the initial response to therapy.

Suggested Reading

General Information

Rodriguez J, McLaughlin P, Hagemeister FB, et al: Follicular large cell lymphoma: An aggressive lymphoma that often presents with favorable prognostic features. Blood 1999;93:2202–2207.

Weeks JC, Yeap BY, Canellos GP, Shipp MA: Value of follow-up procedures in patients with large cell lymphoma who achieve a complete remission. J Clin Oncol 1991;9:1196–1203.

Anaplastic Large Cell Lymphoma

Deconick E, et al: Autologous stem cell transplantation for anaplastic large cell lymphomas: The results of a prospective trial. Br J Haematol 2000;109:736–742.

Falini B, Pileri S, Zinzani PL, et al: ALK+ lymphoma: Clinicopathologic findings and outcome. Blood 1999;93:2697–2706.

Fanin R, Silvestri F, Geromin A, et al: Primary systemic CD30 (Ki-1)-positive anaplastic large cell lymphoma of the adult: Sequential intensive treatment with F-MACHOP regimen (± radiotherapy) and autologous bone marrow transplantation. Blood 1996;87:1243–1248.

Filippa DA, Ladanyi M, Wollner N, et al: CD30 (Ki-1)-positive malignant lymphomas: Clinical, immunophenotypic, histologic, and genetic characteristics and differences with Hodgkin's disease. Blood 1996;87:2905–2917.

Shiota M, Nakamura S, Ichinohasama R, et al: Anaplastic large cell lymphomas expressing the novel chimeric protein p80$^{NPM/ALK}$: A distinct clinicopathologic entity. Blood 1995;86:1954–1960.

Stein H, Foss H-D, Durkop H, et al: CD30+ anaplastic large cell lymphoma: A review of its histopathologic, genetic, and clinical features. Blood 2000;96:3681–3695.

Zinzani PL, Bendandi M, Martelli M, et al: Anaplastic large cell lymphoma: Clinical and prognostic evaluation of 90 adult patients. J Clin Oncol 1996;14:955–962.

Zinzani PL, Martelli M, Magagnoli M, et al: Anaplastic large cell lymphoma Hodgkin's-like: A randomized trial of ABVD versus MACOP-B with and without radiation therapy. Blood 1998;92:790–794.

Lymphoma in the Elderly

Carbone A, Volpe R, Gloghini A, et al: Non-Hodgkin's lymphoma in the elderly. I: Pathologic features at presentation. Cancer 1990;66:1991–1994.

Gomez H, Hidalgo M, Casanova L, et al: Risk factors for treatment-related death in elderly patients with aggressive non-Hodgkin's lymphoma: Results of a multivariate analysis. J Clin Oncol 1998;16:2065–2069.

Lichtman SM. Aggressive lymphoma in the elderly. Crit Rev Oncol Hematol 2000;33:119–128.

Vose JM, Armitage JO, Weisenberger DD, et al: The importance of age in survival of patients treated with chemotherapy for aggressive non-Hodgkin's lymphoma. J Clin Oncol 1988;6:1838–1844.

Gastric Lymphoma

Chen L-T, Lin J-T, Shyu R-Y, et al: Prospective study of *Helicobacter pylori* eradication therapy in stage IE high-grade mucosa-associated lymphoid tissue lymphoma of the stomach. J Clin Oncol 2001;19:4245–4251.

D'Amore F, Brincker H, Grouback K, et al: Non-Hodgkin's lymphoma of the gastrointestinal tract: A population-based analysis of incidence, geographic distribution, clinico-pathological presentation features and prognosis. J Clin Oncol 1994;12:1673–1684.

Hammell P, Haioun C, Chaumette MT, et al: Efficacy of single-agent chemotherapy in low-grade B cell mucosa-associated lymphoid tissue lymphomas with prominent gastric expression. J Clin Oncol 1995;13:2524–2529.

Morgner A, Miehlke S, Fischbach W, et al: Complete remission of primary high-grade B cell gastric lymphoma after cure of *Helicobacter pylori* infection. J Clin Oncol 2001;19:2041–2048.

Schecter NR, Portlock CS, Yaholm J. Treatment of mucosa-associated lymphoid tissue lymphoma of the stomach with radiation alone. J Clin Oncol 1998;16:1916–1921.

Zucca E, Bertoni F, Roggero E, et al: The gastric marginal zone B cell lymphoma of MALT type. Blood 2000;96:410–419.

High-Grade Lymphoma

Haddy TB, Addie MA, McCalla J, et al: Late effects in long-term survivors of high-grade non-Hodgkin's lymphoma. J Clin Oncol 1998;16:2070–2079.

Lee EJ, Petroni R, Schiffer CA, et al: Brief-duration high-intensity chemotherapy for patients with small noncleaved lymphoma or FAB L3 acute lymphocytic leukemia: Results of Cancer and Acute Leukemia Group B Study 9251. J Clin Oncol 2001;19:4014–4022.

MacPherson N, Lesack D, Klasa R, et al: Small noncleaved, non-Burkitt's (Burkitt-like) lymphoma: Cytogenetics predict outcome and reflect clinical presentation. J Clin Oncol 1999;17:1558–1567.

Magrath I, Adde M, Shad A, et al: Adults and children with small non-cleaved lymphoma have a similar excellent outcome when treated with the same chemotherapy regimen. J Clin Oncol 1996;14:925–934.

Magrath IT, Haddy TB: Treatment of patients with high-grade non-Hodgkin's lymphoma and CNS involvement: Is radiation an essential component of therapy? Leuk Lymphoma 1996;21:99–105.

Thomas DA, Cortes J, O'Brien S, et al: Hyper-CVAD program in Burkitt's-type adult acute lymphoblastic leukemia. J Clin Oncol 1999;17:2461–2470.

Intermediate Grade Non-Hodgkin's Lymphoma

Ashraf A, Abou-Elella A, Weisenberger D, et al: Primary mediastinal large B cell lymphoma: A clinicopathologic study of 43 patients from the Nebraska Lymphoma Study Group. J Clin Oncol 1999;17:784–790.

Coiffier B, Lepage E, Briere J, et al: CHOP chemotherapy plus rituximab compared with CHOP alone in elderly patients with diffuse large B cell lymphoma. N Engl J Med 2002;346:235–242.

Cosset JM: Chemoradiotherapy for localized non-Hodgkin's lymphoma. N Engl J Med 998;339:44–45.

Dana BW, Dahlberg D, Miller TP, et al: m-BACOD treatment for intermediate- and high-grade malignant lymphomas: A Southwest Oncology Group Phase II trial. J Clin Oncol 1990;8:1155–1162.

Fisher RI, Gaynor ER, Dahlberg S, et al: Comparison of a standard regimen (CHOP) with three intensive chemotherapy regimens for advanced non-Hodgkin's lymphoma. N Engl J Med 1993;328:1002–1008.

Gaynor ER, Fisher RI: Chemotherapy of intermediate-grade non-Hodgkin's lymphoma: Is "more" or "less" better? Oncol 1995;9:1273–1286.

Gordon LI, Harrington D, Andersen J, et al: Comparison of a second-generation combination chemotherapeutic regimen (m-BACOD) with a standard regimen (CHOP) for advanced diffuse histiocytic lymphoma. N Engl J Med 1992;327:1342–1349.

Guglielmi C, Gomez F, Philip T, et al: Time to relapse has prognostic value in patients with aggressive lymphoma enrolled onto the PARMA trial. J Clin Oncol 1998;16:3264–3269.

Gutierrez M, Chabner BA, Pearson D, et al: Role of a doxorubicin-containing regimen in relapsed and resistant lymphomas: An 8-year follow-up study of EPOCH. J Clin Oncol 2000;18:3633–3642.

Haioun C, Lepage E, Gisselbrecht C, et al: Survival benefit of high-dose therapy in poor-risk aggressive non-Hodgkin's lymphoma: final analysis of the prospective LNH87–2 protocol: A Groupe d'Etude des Lymphomas de l'Adulte study. J Clin Oncol 2000;18:3025–3030.

Kaminski MS, Estes J, Zasadny KR, et al: Radioimmunotherapy with iodine ^{131}I tositumomab for relapsed and refractory B cell non-Hodgkin's lymphoma: Updated results and long-term follow-up of the University of Michigan experience. Blood 2000;96:1259–1266.

Lazzarino M, Orlandi E, Paulli M, et al: Treatment outcome and prognostic factors for primary mediastinal (thymic) B cell lymphomas: A multicenter study of 106 patients. J Clin Oncol 1997;15:1646–1653.

Lee AYY, Connors JM, Klimo P, et al: Late relapse in patients with diffuse large cell lymphoma treated with MACOP-B. J Clin Oncol 1997;15:1745–1751.

Longo DL, DeVita VT Jr, Duffey PL, et al: Superiority of ProMACE-CytaBOM over ProMACE-MOPP in the treatment of advanced diffuse aggressive lymphoma: Results of a prospective randomized trial. J Clin Oncol 1991;9:25–38.

Meyer RM, Quirt IC, Skillings JR, et al: Escalated as compared with standard doses of doxorubicin in BACOP therapy for patients with non-Hodgkin's lymphoma. N Engl J Med 1993;329:1770–1776.

Miller TP, Dahlberg S, Cassady JR, et al: Chemotherapy alone compared with chemotherapy plus radiotherapy for localized intermediate- and high-grade non-Hodgkin's lymphoma. N Engl J Med 1998;339:21–26.

Rodriguez MA, Cabanillas FC, Velasquez W, et al: Results of a salvage treatment program for relapsing lymphoma: MINE consolidated with ESHAP. J Clin Oncol 1995;13:1734–1741.

Shipp MA, for The International Non-Hodgkin's Lymphoma Prognostic Factors Project: A predictive model for aggressive non-Hodgkin's lymphoma. N Engl J Med 1993;329:987–994.

Sparano J, Wiernik PH, Leaf A, Dutcher JP: Infusional cyclophosphamide, doxorubicin, and etoposide in relapsed and resistant non-Hodgkin's lymphoma: Evidence for a schedule-dependent effect favoring infusional administration of chemotherapy. J Clin Oncol 1993;11:1071–1079.

Tirelli U, Errante D, Van Glabbeke M, et al: CHOP is the standard regimen in patients ≥70 years of age with intermediate-grade and high-grade non-Hodgkin's lymphoma: Results of a randomized study of the European Organization for Research and Treatment of Cancer Lymphoma Cooperative Study Group. J Clin Oncol 1998;16:27–34.

Tondini C, Zanini M, Lombardi C, et al: Combined modality treatment with primary CHOP chemotherapy followed by locoregional irradiation in stage I and II histologically aggressive non-Hodgkin's lymphoma. J Clin Oncol 1993;11:720–725.

Velasquez WS, McLaughlin P, Hagemeister FB, et al: ESHAP—an effective chemotherapy regimen in refractory and relapsing lymphoma: A 4-year follow-up study. J Clin Oncol 1994;12:1169–1176.

Vitolo U, Lortellazzo S, Liberati AM, et al: Intensified and high-dose chemotherapy in poor risk patients with granulocyte colony-stimulating factor and autologous stem cell transplantation support as first-line therapy in high-risk diffuse large cell lymphoma. J Clin Oncol 1997;15:491–498.

Vose JM, Link BK, Grossbard ML, et al: Phase II study of rituximab in combination with CHOP chemotherapy in patients with previously untreated, aggressive non-Hodgkin's lymphoma. J Clin Oncol 2001;19:389–397.

Wendum D, Sebban C, Gaulard P, et al: Follicular large cell lymphoma treated with intensive chemotherapy: An analysis of 89 cases included in the LNH87 trial and comparison with the outcome of diffuse large B cell lymphoma. J Clin Oncol 1997;15:1654–1663.

Mantle Cell Lymphoma

Coiffier B: Which treatment for mantle cell lymphoma patients in 1998? J Clin Oncol 1998;16:3–5.

Decaudin D, Bosq J, Tertian G, et al: Phase II trial of fludarabine monophosphate in patients with mantle cell lymphomas. J Clin Oncol 1998;16:579–583.

Fisher RI, Dahlberg S, Nathwani BN, et al: A clinical analysis of two indolent lymphoma entities: Mantle cell lymphoma and marginal zone lymphoma (including the mucosa-associated lymphoid tissue and monocytoid B cell subcategories): A Southwest Oncology Group Study. Blood 1995;85:1075–1082.

Freidman AS, Neuberg D, Gribben JG, et al: High-dose chemoradiotherapy and anti-B cell monoclonal antibody-purged autologous bone marrow transplantation in mantle cell lymphoma: No evidence for long-term remission. J Clin Oncol 1998;16:13–18.

Hiddemann W, Unterhalt M, Herrmann R, et al: Mantle cell lymphomas have more widespread disease and a slower response to chemotherapy compared with follicle-center lymphomas: Results of a prospective comparative analysis of the German Low-Grade Lymphoma Study Group. J Clin Oncol 1998;16:1922–1930.

Howard OM, Gribben JG, Neuberg DS, et al: Rituximab and CHOP induction therapy for newly diagnosed mantle-cell lymphoma: Molecular complete responses are not predictive of progression-free survival. J Clin Oncol 2002;20:1288–1294.

Leonard JP, Schaltner EJ: Biology and management of mantle cell lymphoma. Curr Opin Oncol 2001;13:342–347.

Majlis A, Pugh WC, Rodriguez MA, et al: Mantle cell lymphoma: correlation of clinical outcome and biologic features with three histologic variants. J Clin Oncol 1997;15:1664–1671.

Weisenberger DD, Armitage JO: Mantle cell lymphoma: An entity comes of age. Blood 1996;87:4483–4494.

Chapter 68
Extranodal Non-Hodgkin's Lymphoma

David P. Schenkein

The word lymphoma implies that it is a malignancy arising from lymph nodes. A substantial number of patients with lymphoma, however, present with a malignant proliferation of lymphocytes that appears to originate in nonnodal tissue. These lymphomas are termed primary extranodal non-Hodgkin's lymphoma. They should be distinguished from lymphomas that arise in a lymph node and then directly extend out of the node to invade adjacent nonnodal tissue. Primary extranodal lymphoma is here distinguished from lymphomas that arise concomitantly in both nodal and extranodal sites in an individual patient and from lymphomas where the extranodal site is presumed not to be the site of origin.

Primary extranodal lymphomas represent approximately 15% of all lymphomas. They can present in many different tissues, with a frequency of distribution shown in Figure 68-1. The cause of the increasing incidence of all non-Hodgkin's lymphomas (NHL) is unknown, but the rising number of affected patients includes those who do not have underlying immunodeficiency as well as those who do. Primary extranodal presentations are much more common, however, in those non-Hodgkin's lymphomas that arise against a background of immunodeficiency, such as occurs in patients who are HIV-infected, receiving immunosuppressive medication after organ transplantation (post-transplant lymphoproliferative disorder, or PTLD), or who have associated autoimmune disorders. Infections can also play a role in primary extranodal non-Hodgkin's lymphomas. For example, *Helicobacter pylori* is associated with mucosa-associated lymphoid tumors (MALT) of the stomach, and the Epstein-Barr virus has been implicated in primary central nervous system (CNS) lymphoma and in post-transplant lymphoproliferative disorders. The herpes virus, which is associated with Kaposi's sarcoma, could also play a role in the primary effusion lymphomas seen in HIV-infected patients. The primary extranodal non-Hodgkin's lymphomas are not characterized by a specific histology or unique genetic marker, but the usual mutations (such

as gene translocations) that characterize the different histologic subtypes of nodal lymphomas are also present in the setting of extranodal disease.

Clinical Presentation

Because the primary extranodal non–Hodgkin's lymphomas are such a heterogeneous group, clinical presentations vary. Affected patients are no more likely to have constitutional symptoms than patients with primary nodal lymphomas. The specific symptoms and/or signs are directly related to the site of origin. For example, symptoms of visual disturbance occur in ocular non-Hodgkin's lymphoma, mental status changes in central nervous system non-Hodgkin's lymphoma, and abdominal pain in gastrointestinal non-Hodgkin's lymphoma. For this reason, the diagnosis is often initially suspected by the subspecialist (dentist, ophthalmologist, neurologist, and gastroenterologist) rather than by the generalist. The clinical pace of the disease is, as is true of other non-Hodgkin's lymphomas, determined primarily by the histology rather than by the site of involvement. Follicular lymphomas typically progress slowly over a period of months to years, whereas the more aggressive histologies show rapid development. In considering the clinical presentation, it is important to bear in mind that there is a high incidence of the following:

- involvement of the contralateral structure when the presentation is in the breast or testes
- central nervous system spread in patients presenting with aggressive histologies involving the testes, breast, and, perhaps, the sinuses
- central nervous system lymphoma as the presenting feature in AIDS lymphoma and post-transplant lymphoproliferative disorder
- gastrointestinal lymphoma in patients with primary disease in Waldeyer's ring or thyroid gland

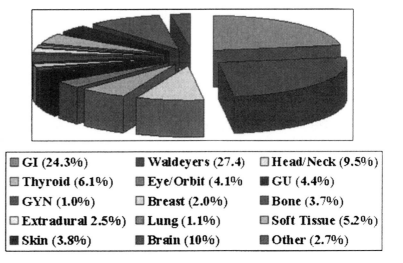

Figure 68-1 ■ Sites of primary extranodal lymphoma. (Adapted from Sutcliffe SB, Gospodarowicz MK: Localized extranodal lymphomas. In Keating A, Armitage J, Burnett A, et al [eds]: Haematological Oncology. Cambridge, Mass., Cambridge University Press, 1992, pp 189–222. Reprinted with the permission of Cambridge University Press.) (See Color Plate 16.)

- GI (24.3%)
- Thyroid (6.1%)
- GYN (1.0%)
- Extradural 2.5%)
- Skin (3.8%)
- Waldeyers (27.4)
- Eye/Orbit (4.1%
- Breast (2.0%)
- Lung (1.1%)
- Brain (10%)
- Head/Neck (9.5%)
- GU (4.4%)
- Bone (3.7%)
- Soft Tissue (5.2%)
- Other (2.7%)

Clinical Evaluation

The evaluation and staging of patients with a primary extranodal lymphoma is the same as for nodal lymphomas. Thus, staging includes a thorough physical examination, complete history, computed tomography (CT) scans, laboratory studies (complete blood count, blood chemistries, and lactate dehydrogenase [LDH]), and a bone marrow aspirate and biopsy. As histology is a critically important prognostic factor, good-quality tissue samples are required for analysis, even if a rebiopsy is necessary. Because of the associations previously noted, some additional staging procedures are warranted in the evaluation of certain presentations:

- Spinal fluid examination is advisable for lymphoma in patients with testicular, bilateral breast, and sinus lymphoma and in patients with HIV-associated lymphomas. Intrathecal chemotherapy should be instilled at the time of the procedure to avoid an additional lumbar puncture for treatment should central nervous system involvement be documented.
- Computed tomography or magnetic resonance imaging of the brain is recommended for patients with HIV-associated lymphoma or post-transplant lymphoproliferative disease, to rule out a mass.
- Upper endoscopy of the gastrointestinal tract and mucosal biopsies are recommended for patients with lymphoma of Waldeyer's ring or thyroid gland.

Staging and Prognosis

The Ann Arbor staging system developed for Hodgkin's disease remains the standard for both nodal and extra-nodal presentations of non-Hodgkin's lymphoma. All cases of primary extranodal lymphoma are typically staged using the "E" (for extranodal) designation. Thus, even though Waldeyer's ring, thymus, spleen, and small intestine are all lymphoid tissues, lymphomas that arise in these locations are designated as extranodal (E). The prognosis for patients with extranodal lymphoma is dictated by the same factors that affect prognosis for nodal lymphomas. The most important factors remain the histology and the integration of findings into the International Prognostic Index formulation (see Table 67-3 in Chapter 67). The prognosis of extranodal vs. nodal lymphomas with comparable risk factors is similar. In the primary extranodal non-Hodgkin's lymphomas, as for the nodal presentation lymphomas, an increasing number of extranodal sites of involvement confer a worse prognosis.

Treatment

The treatment strategy for the extranodal lymphomas is based on the same principles that govern the management of the nodal lymphomas. Options for treatment depend on a careful review of the histology, staging evaluation, prognostic factors, sites of involvement, and any immunologic impairment (e.g., HIV infection). Because occult systemic disease is likely to be present even in patients presenting with apparently localized extranodal disease, combined modality therapy is usually employed; e.g., short course chemotherapy (three to four months) followed by involved-field radiation. This approach appears to be highly effective in patients who have limited-stage nodal lymphomas, but few randomized clinical trials of therapy have been conducted. The heterogeneity of presentation creates numerous subsets of small numbers of patients, making adequate accrual for statistical analysis problematic. Despite the limitations imposed by the lack of confirmed data to guide therapy, some specific considerations apply to individual sites of extranodal presentation.

Primary Central Nervous System Lymphoma (Including Optic Nerve, Retina, and Vitreous)

Central nervous system lymphomas are usually aggressive, high-grade tumors with poor prognoses. Therapy, therefore, includes high-dose cytosine arabinoside and methotrexate (to cross the blood-brain barrier) and whole-brain radiation. The latter is frequently omitted for elderly patients because of its toxicity in this group.

Gastrointestinal Lymphoma

Mucosa-associated lymphoid tumor of the stomach is associated with *H. pylori* infection and the appearance of the t(11;18) or t(1;14) translocation. The lymphoma can be of several different histologies, but usually it is of a marginal zone B cell lymphoma. In early phases of disease development, the translocations are rarely found, and antibiotic therapy directed at *Helicobacter* offers an opportunity to induce remissions, which can be durable. In later phases, the translocations appear, and eradication of *Helicobacter* is less likely. Chemotherapy and radiation therapy are indicated for antibiotic failures or for patients with aggressive histologies. Alternatives include adjuvant chemotherapy after surgical resection of high-grade tumors. Radiation alone is effective in the low-grade counterparts.

Waldeyer's Ring Lymphoma (Tonsil, Base of Tongue, and Nasopharynx)

Waldeyer's ring lymphoma patients typically present with diffuse large cell (B cell) lymphoma with a substantial frequency of associated and unsuspected gastrointestinal tract involvement. These patients are usually treated with anthracycline-containing combination chemotherapy until radiographic complete remission is achieved, followed by involved-field radiation. Central nervous system prophylaxis is not needed, and prognosis for non-bulky tumors is excellent (greater than 60% overall survival at five years).

Sinus Lymphoma

Sinus lymphomas typically present as intermediate or high-grade (B cell) tumors (T cell type in Asian populations) that are approached with combined modality therapy using anthracycline-based chemotherapy and involved-field radiation. Intrathecal prophylaxis is administered by some physicians because of the concern about the potential for central nervous system involvement.

Testicular Lymphoma

Testicular lymphoma generally occurs in older men (median age, approximately 70 years), displays an aggressive histology (diffuse large B cell), and carries a significant risk for contralateral involvement. Even in localized presentations, systemic therapy is required. The best reported results occurred in patients treated with anthracycline-based chemotherapy and radiation to the scrotum. The need for central nervous system prophylaxis with intrathecal chemotherapy remains controversial, despite the fact that the central nervous system is a principal site of recurrent disease, which, in general, occurs frequently at extranodal sites.

Orbital Lymphoma

Involvement of the conjunctiva, eyelid, lacrimal gland, and retrobulbar tissues are common in orbital lymphoma. Histologically, these are commonly low-grade tumors (most often, marginal zone B cell lymphomas) and have a better prognosis than the ocular lymphomas. Early-stage disease with low-grade histology is best managed by low-dose radiation therapy

---

TREATMENT

CENTRAL NERVOUS SYSTEM LYMPHOMA TREATMENT CONSIDERATIONS

Ocular lymphoma (excluding lid, conjunctiva, and orbit) should be treated as a primary central nervous system lymphoma.

Extranodal lymphoma of the sinus can directly extend and involve the base of the brain and spinal fluid. In patients with intact sinus walls, however, it is not proven that central nervous system prophylaxis is required despite the proximity of the sinus to the central nervous system.

to preserve vision. Chemotherapy is indicated in conjunction with radiation for the high-grade lesions. Prophylactic central nervous system treatment is not indicated.

Breast Lymphoma

Breast lymphoma tends to present in older women and is often bilateral. Although low-grade lymphomas occasionally occur in this location, they are most often of diffuse, large B cell histology. Combined modality therapy is warranted in patients with aggressive lymphomas, whereas the considerations for treatment of low-grade, isolated lesions follows the recommendations for systemic presentations of these histologies (see Chapter 66). Diffuse bilateral involvement with high-grade disease is associated with central nervous system spread, and prophylaxis is indicated. Mastectomy is seldom necessary.

Cutaneous Lymphoma

See Chapter 69.

Thyroid Lymphoma

Patients affected with thyroid lymphoma are frequently elderly, and the histology is often, of the diffuse large cell (B cell) type. A history of prior thyroiditis is a predisposing risk factor. Combined modality therapy is used because occult systemic disease is common.

Follow-up Evaluation

After therapy, patients with extranodal lymphoma are evaluated in a fashion similar to those with nodal disease, but with special attention to the primary site of disease. It is important to remember to evaluate untreated paired organs (breast, testes, kidney, eye, and lung), as contralateral involvement is common. In patients with gastric mucosa-associated lymphoid tumors, evaluation with endoscopy is necessary to assess remission status and to monitor for recurrence.

References

Abrey LE, Yahalom J, DeAngelis LM: Treatment for primary CNS lymphoma: the next step. J Clin Oncol 2000; 18:3144–3150.

Brogi E, Harris NL: Lymphomas of the breast: pathology and clinical behavior. Semin Oncol 1999;26:357–364.

Fonseca R, Habermann TM, Colgan JP, et al: Testicular lymphoma is associated with a high incidence of extranodal recurrence. Cancer 2000;88:154–161.

Shahab N, Doll DC: Testicular lymphoma. Semin Oncol 1999;26:259–269.

Siegel RS, Pandolfino T, Guitart J, et al: Primary cutaneous T cell lymphoma: review and current concepts. *J Clin Oncol* 2000;18:2908–2925.

Sutcliffe SB, Gospodarowicz MK: Primary extranodal lymphomas. In Canellos G, Lister TA, Sklar JL (eds): The Lymphomas. Philadelphia: WB Saunders, 1998, pp 449–479.

Sutcliffe SB, Gospodarowicz MK: Localized extranodal lymphomas. In Keating A, Armitage J, Burnett A, et al (eds): Haematological oncology. Cambridge Mass, Cambridge University Press, 1992, pp 189–222.

Yuen A, Jacobs C: Lymphomas of the head and neck. Semin Oncol 1999;26:338–345.

Zucca E, Bertoni F, Roggero E, Cavalli F: The gastric marginal zone B cell lymphoma of MALT type. Blood 2000; 96:410–419.

Chapter 69
Peripheral T Cell Lymphomas

Stephen M. Ansell

Introduction

Peripheral T cell lymphoma refers to a morphologically, immunologically, and clinically heterogeneous group of T cell lymphomas with a postthymic, mature immunophenotype. The term *peripheral T cell lymphoma* is used to distinguish these diseases from central, immature, or thymic lymphomas, such as lymphoblastic lymphomas. In this chapter, the term peripheral T cell lymphomas refers to non-Hodgkin's lymphomas with a T cell immunophenotype but does not include adult T cell leukemia/lymphoma, which because of its distinctive features is discussed separately in Chapter 70.

The Revised European American Lymphoid (REAL) classification as well as the proposed World Health Organization (WHO) classification (Table 69-1) defines a number of distinct immunologic and clinical entities within the spectrum of peripheral T cell lymphomas.

Mycosis Fungoides and Sézary Syndrome

Mycosis fungoides and Sézary syndrome (MF/SS) are uncommon, indolent T cell lymphomas that predominantly involve the skin. In its early stages, mycosis fungoides causes cutaneous patches that later progress to plaques. Subsequently, patients can develop cutaneous tumors (nodules) with involvement of lymph nodes as well as visceral sites. Sézary syndrome is an erythrodermic variant of mycosis fungoides in which the malignant T cells are seen circulating in the peripheral blood. Although mycosis fungoides and Sézary syndrome are often referred to as cutaneous T cell lymphomas, they should be distinguished from other non-Hodgkin's lymphomas that can involve the skin, such as other peripheral T cell lymphomas and adult T cell leukemia/lymphoma.

Epidemiology

Mycosis fungoides and Sézary syndrome typically affects middle-aged adults with a median age of 55 years. The annual incidence is estimated to be 1 per 100,000 population. The incidence of the disease is increasing for unknown reasons, and young patients make up an increasing fraction of those affected. The disease is more common in men than in women and more common among African-Americans than among other groups.

The etiology of mycosis fungoides and Sézary syndrome is uncertain. Genetic, environmental, and infectious agents have been implicated as possible factors triggering lymphocyte activation or transformation. Familial cases of this disease are rare. Chronic stimulation by antigens—specifically, chemicals, infection, smoking, and sun exposure—have been considered, but multiple studies show no clear association of these putative risk factors with the disease. A mouse model suggests that interleukin-7 (IL-7) might play a role. Over time, mice overexpressing interleukin-7 develop a cutaneous T cell infiltration that mimics mycosis fungoides.

Pathophysiology

The diagnosis of mycosis fungoides and Sézary syndrome rests on the clinical presentation in association with histopathologic findings of an epidermotropic lymphoma. The characteristic atypical lymphocytes in mycosis fungoides and Sézary syndrome are dysplastic cerebriform T cells with enlarged hyperchromatic nuclei and complex nuclear folding. The essential criteria for diagnosis are a bandlike lymphocytic infiltrate in the superficial papillary dermis and atypical T cells in the dermal and epidermal infiltrates. Pautrier microabscesses (small clusters of cells surrounded by a clear zone) are characteristic of mycosis fungoides and Sézary syndrome but are often absent in patch-stage lesions and erythroderma. Definitive diagnosis

Table 69-1 ■ Proposed World Health Organization Classification of Peripheral T Cell Lymphomas

Mycosis fungoides and the Sézary syndrome
Adult T cell leukemia/lymphoma (HTLV-1+)
Extranodal NK/T cell lymphoma, nasal type*
Angioimmunoblastic T cell lymphoma
Systemic anaplastic large cell lymphoma (T and null cell types)
Primary cutaneous anaplastic large cell lymphoma
Subcutaneous panniculitis-like T cell lymphoma
Enteropathy-type intestinal T cell lymphoma
Hepatosplenic γ/δ T cell lymphoma
Peripheral T cell lymphoma (unspecified)

*Called "angiocentric lymphoma" in the R.E.A.L. classification.

can be difficult in early phases of the disease, despite multiple biopsies of separate skin lesions, immunophenotyping, and T cell receptor gene rearrangement studies.

The malignant cells usually have a mature CD4+ T-helper cell phenotype, but some cases have been described with clonal populations expressing predominantly a suppressor cytotoxic CD8+ phenotype. The lymphocytes can express the cutaneous lymphocyte-associated antigen and lymphocyte function-associated protein that bind to the intercellular adhesion molecule (ICAM-1 or CD54). The binding to ICAM on epidermal keratinocytes may explain the homing of mycosis fungoides and Sézary syndrome cells to the skin.

Clinical Presentation

The expanding, ulcerating, mushroom-like tumors noted in the original case described by Alibert in 1806 led to the use of the term *mycosis fungoides*. The patch phase is the earliest manifestation of the disease and is characterized by the presence of erythematous, flat patches with slight scaling. As the patches become more infiltrated, they evolve into palpable plaques that are red, raised, and have well-marginated borders (Figure 69-1). These lesions, in turn, subsequently evolve into tumors. Rarely, the tumor phase of mycosis fungoides and Sézary syndrome presents without the preceding patch and plaque phases (d'emblee variant). Although some patients who have minimal skin involvement by cutaneous patches never show progression, most patients inexorably proceed to the advanced stages of the disease. Progression of the skin lesions is highly variable; it is common for a patient to exhibit simultaneously the patch, plaque, and tumor stages of disease on different areas of the skin.

Intense pruritus and cutaneous pain are common in patients with Sézary syndrome, materially compromising their quality of life. Intense reddening (Figure 69-2) of the skin (erythroderma) and/or or pruritic exfoliation are accompanied by circulating Sézary cells. Erythroderma might be the only manifestation, but other plaque-like lesions or tumors might be present. Although the Sézary cells are readily seen in the peripheral blood smear (Figure 69-3), bone marrow involvement is rare.

Spread to other sites occurs in the late stages of disease, as the cutaneous lesions progress. The major sites of extracutaneous involvement are the regional lymph nodes, followed by the spleen, liver, and other viscera. Infection due to excoriation of the skin is a common and potentially life-threatening complication of mycosis fungoides and Sézary syndrome.

Staging and Prognosis

A subset of patients with minimal skin involvement (less than 10% of the surface) by plaques or patches

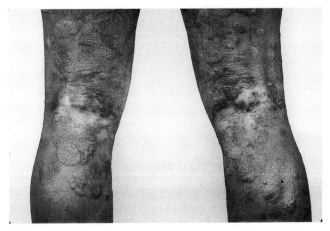
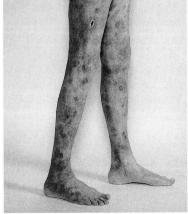

Figure 69-1 ■ Plaque stage of mycosis fungoides.

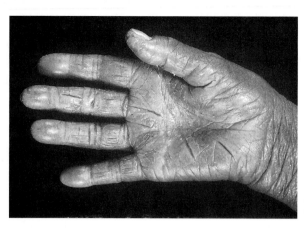
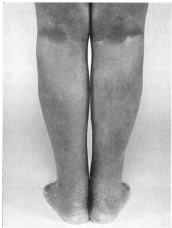

Figure 69-2 ▪ Erythroderma associated with Sézary syndrome.

has a survival similar to a matched control population. Good-risk patients are those who have cutaneous patches only, without lymph node, blood, or visceral involvement; their median survival is greater than 12 years. For intermediate-risk patients (those with tumors, erythroderma, or plaque disease with lymph node or blood involvement but no visceral involvement), the median survival is approximately 5 years. Poor-risk patients have visceral involvement or lymph node effacement and a poor prognosis with a 2.5-year median survival.

Treatment

Treatment of the disease is palliative rather than curative and is therefore geared toward providing symptom control and cosmesis with the least toxicity. Randomized studies demonstrate that administration of intensive therapy early in the disease course, rather than later when the disease progresses, does not improve survival.

Patients with Predominant Skin Involvement

Patients with disease limited to the skin are generally managed with topical therapy. Chemotherapy, such as nitrogen mustard, applied to all affected skin surfaces in early stage disease causes disease regression in 65% to 90% of patients. Adverse reactions to this therapy, which might limit its use, include contact irritant dermatitis, dry skin, hyperpigmentation, and telangiectasia.

Psoralen plus ultraviolet light (PUVA) is a useful therapy. This involves the ingestion of 8-methoxypsoralen, a photoactivated (by ultraviolet light) compound that inhibits both DNA and RNA synthesis. Response rates with this therapy range from 55% to 85%. Side effects, such as nausea, dry skin, and erythema, are less frequent and severe with PUVA than with topical chemotherapy.

Mycosis fungoides is highly radiosensitive. External electron beam radiation therapy provides good palliation in 55% to 95% of patients with early disease. Because it only superficially penetrates the skin, it can be administered over the whole body surface without damage to the underlying tissues and organs. It thus can be safely given to patients with erythroderma in the Sézary syndrome and to those with thick plaques and tumors in the advanced stages of mycosis fungoides.

Sézary Syndrome

Extracorporeal photophoresis with or without the addition of interferon-alpha is frequently used in patients with Sézary syndrome. Extracorporeal photophoresis involves the ingestion of psoralens and the

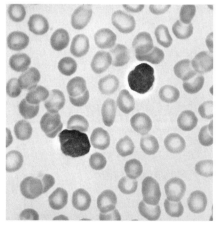

Figure 69-3 ▪ Sézary cells in the peripheral blood. (See Color Plate 17.)

extracorporeal exposure of the blood cells to ultraviolet light, which kills the irradiated malignant cells. Moreover, the reinfused cells apparently stimulate an autologous immune response against the Sézary cells, because the extent of cancer reduction is greater than can be accounted for by the number of cells irradiated by the ultraviolet light. Photophoresis has a response rate of approximately 70%, and this response rate might possibly be increased by the addition of alpha interferon. Interferon-alpha is itself active in the treatment of mycosis fungoides and Sézary syndrome. Response rates in heavily pretreated patients range from 45% to 65%.

Extensive Disease and Visceral Involvement

A wide range of chemotherapeutic agents elicits short-lived responses in approximately 30% of patients. Prednisone alone can induce a partial response in approximately 50% of patients. Combination chemotherapy with cyclophosphamide, Adriamycin, vincristine, and prednisone produces modest responses in a substantial percentage of patients for short periods of time. Intensive therapy is usually reserved for patients with advanced disease, at a time when they are debilitated by disease and prone to infection, especially due to the breakdown of the skin. Because of these problems, patients tolerate chemotherapy poorly.

Agents effective in low-grade lymphomas and chronic lymphocytic leukemia are increasingly being used in the treatment of mycosis fungoides and Sézary syndrome with good effect. These agents include the purine analogs fludarabine, pentostatin, cladribine, and CAMPATH-1H.

Other Peripheral T Cell Lymphomas

Peripheral T cell lymphomas are less common than B cell lymphomas, comprising approximately 10% to 15% of the non-Hodgkin lymphomas in the United States and Western Europe. Although their presentation is similar to B cell lymphomas, they are morphologically, immunologically, and clinically heterogeneous. Accurate diagnosis of these disorders usually requires immunophenotypic studies, because T cell lymphomas can have morphologic features similar to those seen in B cell lymphomas and Hodgkin's disease. Due to their relative rarity, diversity, and variable geographic distribution, few clinical studies of the peripheral T cell lymphomas have been conducted. The result is that for some of the subsets of peripheral T cell lymphoma, the clinical course, natural history, and appropriate therapy are not well defined.

Epstein-Barr virus has a clear association with certain peripheral T cell lymphomas, particularly the angioimmunoblastic type and some peripheral T cell lymphomas associated with the hemophagocytic syndrome. The Epstein-Barr virus is also related to the development of extranodal T cell lymphomas originating in the nose or nasal sinuses (nasal type).

Clinical Presentation

Recognition of various constellations of the presenting symptoms and findings is helpful in considering whether a peripheral T cell lymphoma is the cause of the patient's illness (Table 69-2). As is true for B cell lymphomas, the commonest of these presentations of peripheral T cell lymphoma is that of a nodal or extranodal tumor. The other presentations listed in Table 69-2, however, are much more common in the peripheral T cell lymphomas than in the B cell variants. The hemophagocytic syndrome presents with fever, hepatosplenomegaly, liver function abnormalities, cytopenia(s) or pancytopenia, and erythrophagocytosis. The latter is readily demonstrable morphologically on bone marrow biopsy or biopsy of other organs. Although some viral illnesses can initiate this syndrome, the association with peripheral T cell lymphoma is sufficiently strong to recommend an evaluation that excludes this lymphoma as the cause.

Other unusual presentations are the appearance of pulmonary infiltrates and/or central nervous system involvement, usually associated with systemic symptoms, or the combination of peripheral neuropathies, granulomatous liver disease, angioedema, and diffuse pulmonary infiltrates. Patients can also present with destructive, necrotic facial or sinus tumors and an angiocentric proliferation of T cells on histologic examination or with systemic symptoms, liver dysfunction, and unusual organ infiltration by mature T cells.

Immunologic dysfunction not infrequently forms the background for the development of peripheral T cell lymphomas, which occur in patients with a variety of autoimmune diseases (especially immune-mediated arthritis) and other immunologic abnormalities. Peripheral T cell lymphomas also occur in patients with HIV infection or who are immunosuppressed after solid-organ transplantation. Peripheral T cell

---

Table 69-2 ■ Presenting Manifestations of Peripheral T Cell Lymphomas

Nodal or extranodal involvement similar to B cell lymphomas
Hemophagocytic syndrome
Facial/nasal/sinus disease
Systemic illness with atypical organ infiltration

Table 69-3 ■ Common Clinical Characteristics of Peripheral T Cell Lymphomas

Male predominance
Preceding immunologic abnormality or disorder
Elevated lactate dehydrogenase (LDH) at diagnosis
B-symptoms (fever, weight loss, night sweats)
Stage IV (advanced) disease

lymphomas also are noted in some patients with congenital immune deficiency syndromes or after the administration of rituximab (a monoclonal anti-CD20 antibody) as therapy for B cell lymphomas.

Patients with adult celiac disease appear to have an increased risk for developing intestinal peripheral T cell lymphoma. Other clinical circumstances that carry an increased risk include systemic vasculitis and profound eosinophilia, myelodysplasia, or hairy cell leukemia. The common specific clinical characteristics at presentation are listed in Table 69-3.

Angioimmunoblastic T Cell Lymphoma

Affected patients are most often adults who typically are noted to have generalized lymphadenopathy, polyclonal hypergammaglobulinemia, constitutional B-symptoms, a skin rash, and various autoimmune phenomena, including warm-antibody-induced hemolytic anemia. Most angioimmunoblastic T cell lymphomas have a CD4+ (T-helper cell) phenotype, and many cases have aberrant T cell antigen expression. They usually demonstrate T cell receptor gene rearrangements, and the Epstein-Barr virus genome has been detected in both B and T cells in this disease. Although it masquerades as a systemic immunologic disorder, this is usually an aggressive lymphoma that often follows a rapidly fatal course.

Anaplastic Large T Cell Lymphoma

Anaplastic large T cell lymphoma (ALCL) is characterized by an infiltrate of CD30+ (formerly called Ki-1+) lymphocytes. A characteristic chromosomal abnormality, t(2;5)(p23;q35), is frequently associated with this subtype of lymphoma. This translocation is due to the fusion of the nucleophosmin (NPM) gene on chromosome 5q35 to the anaplastic lymphoma kinase (ALK) gene on chromosome 2p23. The t(2;5) can be detected in approximately one-half to three-quarters of patients with anaplastic large T cell lymphoma. The incidence is bimodal, with the largest peak in adolescence and a smaller peak in older patients. Primary anaplastic large T cell lymphoma can be subdivided into systemic and cutaneous forms. A secondary form of anaplastic large T cell lymphoma results from the transformation of another lymphoma, such as mycosis fungoides.

Systemic anaplastic large T cell lymphoma is a moderately aggressive tumor that presents with peripheral lymphadenopathy and extranodal disease that often includes the skin. Other extranodal sites of involvement include bone, gastrointestinal tract, lung, and muscle. Most anaplastic large T cell lymphomas have a T cell phenotype, but some express B cell antigens or lack both T cell and B cell antigens (null cell type). The malignant lymphocytes of most systemic anaplastic large T cell lymphomas demonstrate cytotoxic granule proteins and express epithelial membrane antigen (EMA). The ALK+ variant occurs more often in young patients than in the elderly. Despite the frequent presentation in these ALK+ young patients of advanced disease at diagnosis, systemic symptoms, and extranodal sites of involvement, the overall survival is better than in patients who have ALK– disease. Moreover, overall this type of anaplastic large T cell lymphoma responds more frequently to combination chemotherapy than do other large cell lymphomas, when corrected for age, stage, and symptom status. A small subset of patients has fulminant, advanced lymphoma, refractory to therapy; their lymphomas usually exhibit multiple cytogenetic abnormalities.

Primary cutaneous anaplastic large T cell lymphoma typically occurs in adults who have localized disease at the time of diagnosis and generally has an indolent clinical course. Primary cutaneous anaplastic large T cell lymphoma is usually epithelial membrane antigen (EMA) negative and lacks the t(2;5) chromosomal abnormality, suggesting that it has a pathogenesis different from that of systemic anaplastic large T cell lymphoma. The skin lesions tend to wax and wane, even regressing spontaneously without treatment, only to reappear later. Combination chemotherapy causes responses, but their duration is brief. Treatment consists of observation for regression and/or local, low-dose superficial radiation therapy to the skin lesions until the disease becomes generalized.

Hepatosplenic Gamma/Delta T Cell Lymphoma

This lymphoma preferentially infiltrates the cords and sinuses of the splenic red pulp, hepatic sinusoids, and marrow interstitium. A leukemic phase can develop as the disease progresses, and hemophagocytosis by benign histiocytes can be observed. NK cell-associated antigens, such as CD16 and CD56, and cytotoxic granule-associated proteins are often expressed. T cell receptor gamma and delta chain gene rearrangements are observed, sometimes with beta-chain gene rearrangements as well. Karyotypic studies often show isochromosome 7q, which may be accompanied by trisomy 8 and loss of the Y chromosome. Most cases involve young adult males with no lymphadenopathy, but rather with significant constitutional symptoms, massive hepatosplenomegaly, anemia, and marked thrombocytopenia. The disease is aggressive, and most patients die within two years of the original diagnosis, even if they respond favorably to initial therapy.

Subcutaneous Panniculitis-like T Cell Lymphoma

Subcutaneous panniculitis-like T cell lymphoma principally involves the subcutaneous adipose tissue. Most cases have alpha/beta T cell receptors, and there is heterogeneous expression of CD4 and CD8. These lymphomas contain cytotoxic granule-associated proteins, and some also express NK cell-associated antigens, usually CD56. This lymphoma usually presents as multiple erythematous subcutaneous nodules on the extremities and/or trunk, which vary in size. This lymphoma tends to be moderately aggressive but remains localized to the subcutis. A severe (and often fatal) hemophagocytic syndrome can complicate the clinical course. Patients with single or limited numbers of lesions may, however, have a far more benign clinical course.

Enteropathy-Type Intestinal T Cell Lymphoma

Primary intestinal T cell lymphomas are rare, tending to occur in patients with a history of celiac disease or other malabsorptive problems. A common presentation includes abdominal pain, weight loss, and diarrhea. These lymphomas are regarded as "enteropathy-associated" if there is villous atrophy of the mucosa or clinical evidence of malabsorption. The small intestine is usually involved, and most patients have multifocal disease in the jejunum. The neoplastic cells involve the mucosa, often causing ulceration and villous destruction and, at times, resulting in acute small bowel obstruction or spontaneous perforation of the bowel wall. These T cell lymphomas are aggressive, and most patients die of their disease within two years of diagnosis.

Extranodal NK/T Cell Lymphoma, Nasal Type

Called angiocentric lymphomas in the Revised European American Lymphoid classification, these lymphomas are a heterogeneous group that shares similar morphologic features. They are angiocentric and angioinvasive and have angiodestructive lesions composed of a lymphoid infiltrate that often occludes vessels, resulting in areas of ischemic necrosis. These lymphomas are rare in the United States and Europe and are most often seen in East Asia. Any age group can be affected. These patients can respond to effective combination chemotherapy regimens with or without radiation therapy. Most cases express natural killer (NK) cell-associated antigens, particularly CD56, and some contain cytotoxic granules. Most of these lymphomas are EBV-associated. A number of T cell or NK cell lymphomas involving the nasopharynx lack demonstrable angiocentricity, but the term "extranodal T/NK cell lymphoma, nasal type" is applied to all of these tumors.

Cutaneous, pulmonary, and other non-nasal angiocentric lymphomas can also be called nasal-type T/NK cell lymphomas because they share many of the features of T/NK cell lymphomas in the nasal region. Some cutaneous/subcutaneous angiocentric lymphomas could represent secondary spread from nasal T/NK cell lymphomas. Cutaneous cases are generally true NK cell lymphomas or peripheral T cell lymphomas. A high degree of association exists with EBV, particularly those lymphomas of apparent true NK cell origin.

Peripheral T Cell Lymphoma—Unspecified

Despite the advances in defining subtypes of peripheral T cell lymphomas immunophenotypically and clinically, many subsets remain unclassified. This group constitutes approximately 60% to 70% of all peripheral T cell lymphomas and presents with disseminated disease as nodal or extranodal tumors. The unspecified peripheral T cell lymphomas are distinguishable from B cell lymphomas only on the basis of immunophenotypic studies.

These lymphomas generally exhibit a diffuse pattern of growth histologically, but rare cases can appear follicular (nodular). Diverse and often aberrant T cell phenotypes are expressed, usually involving alpha/beta T cell receptors and T cell receptor gene rearrangements. The Revised European American Lymphoid classification (but not the proposed World Health Organization classification) stratifies these unspecified peripheral T cell lymphomas into three categories based on the number of large cells present: medium-sized cell; mixed medium- and large cell; and large cell types. No clinical significance has been attached thus far to this poorly reproducible cytological grading approach.

Clinical Evaluation

The diagnosis of a peripheral T cell lymphoma depends on identifying that the tumor cells have a mature T cell immunophenotype. Some diffuse, large cell B cell lymphomas are highly infiltrated by reactive T-lymphocytes. To avoid confusion between these lymphomas and peripheral T cell lymphomas, it might be necessary on occasion to prove T cell clonality by documenting a monoclonal T cell receptor gene rearrangement.

The specific immunophenotype of peripheral T cell lymphomas shows considerable variability. Most cases have a helper/inducer phenotype, whereas approximately 10% to 30% have a cytotoxic/suppressor immunophenotype. The remaining cases demonstrate T cell antigens, such as CD3 and/or CD4 and/or CD8.

Many patients with peripheral T cell lymphoma have been found to have cytogenetic abnormalities. Besides the specific chromosomal translocation t(2;5) (p23;q35) associated with Ki-1-positive anaplastic large cell lymphomas, a number of other specific chromosomal abnormalities have been identified in patients with T cell malignancies. Trisomies 3 and 5 have been correlated with angioimmunoblastic T cell lymphoma, and isochromosome 7q with trisomy 8 have been associated with hepatosplenic lymphomas. Other abnormalities include +5, +21, −13, −6q, −1q, −7q, inv(14), t(8;14), and t(11;14).

Prognostic Features and Outcome

Clinical characteristics in patients with peripheral T cell lymphomas, like those in B cell lymphomas, predict patient outcome. The International Index of Prognostic Factors (see Chapter 67) is thus of value in assessing the future course of peripheral T cell lymphomas. Patients in the low-risk group as defined by the International Index had a 76% survival rate at 5 years, compared with 32%, 28%, and 9% for those patients in the low-intermediate, high-intermediate, and high-risk groups, respectively. Some investigators also believe that high tumor growth fraction and bone marrow involvement are independent predictors of a poor outcome.

The prognostic significance of a T cell phenotype rather than a B cell phenotype remains somewhat controversial. Some studies suggest that the outcome is similar when comparable clinical features are present, but the majority of analyses indicate that compared with B cell lymphomas, patients with peripheral T cell lymphomas have a somewhat poorer progression-free survival and an inferior overall survival rate.

Therapeutic Concepts

The lack of controlled trials to evaluate therapy in these patients leaves the optimal management of peripheral T cell lymphomas poorly defined. In the absence of definitive studies to guide treatment planning, the current consensus is to apply the same principles that are used in therapy of B cell lymphomas. That is, peripheral T cell lymphomas need to be diagnosed as early as possible, and therapy should be based on the stage of disease as well as the specific immunopathologic disease entity.

The staging evaluation procedures for patients with peripheral T cell lymphomas are the same as for patients with other non-Hodgkin's lymphomas. Evaluation should include a careful history and physical examination, complete blood count, chemistry profile (including a serum lactate dehydrogenase), chest radiograph, computed tomograms of the abdomen and pelvis, and bone marrow biopsy. Careful attention should be directed to any historical or physical finding that suggests unusual sites of extranodal involvement, and these sites should be biopsied if necessary.

Combination chemotherapy can cure some patients with peripheral T cell lymphoma, but the complete response rate in these patients might be lower than in similarly treated patients with B cell lymphomas. Due to the paucity of comparative trials, no one regimen has been shown to be superior to others. It is therefore reasonable to use an anthracycline-containing regimen similar to those used in B cell lymphomas as front-line therapy in this disease.

Certain disease entities deserve special consideration. Patients with nasal T/NK cell lymphomas commonly present with localized disease, and treatment usually consists of combination chemotherapy followed by involved-field radiation therapy. Other disease entities, such as hepatosplenic T cell lymphomas and intestinal T cell lymphomas, often have a very poor prognosis, and affected patients should be considered for autologous stem cell transplantation early on, if they respond well to initial therapy. Surgical intervention might be required in the case of intestinal T cell lymphoma, when it presents as a gastrointestinal emergency such as obstruction, perforation, or hemorrhage. In the past, the angioimmunoblastic type was regarded as minimally aggressive and its immune, inflammatory symptoms were treated with prednisone alone. Yet survival was short, and retrospective analyses comparing conservative therapy (prednisone as a single agent) with combination chemotherapy found a significantly superior complete response rate for the latter. Although combination chemotherapy is now the recommended treatment of choice, whether it improves survival remains uncertain.

Salvage Therapy

Patients with peripheral T cell lymphoma who are not cured by initial combination-chemotherapy treatment have a dismal outlook. The possibility remains, however, that some relapsed patients, as is true in B cell lymphomas, can be salvaged for cure by autologous stem cell transplantation. Some comparative studies show that the peripheral T cell lymphomas have the same response to and overall survival rate after the procedure as do B cell lymphomas.

References

General Information

Ansell SM, Habermann TM, Kurtin PJ, et al: Predictive capacity of the International Prognostic Factor Index in patients with peripheral T cell lymphoma. J Clin Oncol 1997;15: 2296–2301.

Ascani S, Zinzani PL, Gherlinzoni F, et al: Peripheral T cell lymphomas. Clinico-pathologic study of 168 cases diagnosed according to the R.E.A.L. Classification. Ann Oncol 1997;8:583–592.

Harris NL, Jaffe ES, Diebold J, et al: World Health Organization classification of neoplastic diseases of the hematopoietic and lymphoid tissues: report of the clinical advisory committee meeting—Airlie House, Virginia, November 1997. J Clin Oncol 1999;17:3535–3849.

Lepretre S, Buchonnet G, Stamatoullas A, et al: Chromosome abnormalities in peripheral T cell lymphoma. Cancer Genet Cytogenet 2000;117:71–79.

Pileri SA, Ascani S, Sabattini E, et al: Peripheral T cell lymphoma: a developing concept. Ann Oncol 1998;9:797–801.

Winberg CD: Peripheral T cell lymphoma. Morphologic and immunologic observations. Am J Clin Pathol 1993;99: 426–435.

Mycosis Fungoides and Sézary Syndrome

Bunn PA Jr, Lamberg SI: Report of the Committee on Staging and Classification of Cutaneous T cell Lymphomas. Cancer Treat Rep 1979;63:725–728.

Chuang TY, Su WP, Muller SA: Incidence of cutaneous T cell lymphoma and other rare skin cancers in a defined population. J Am Acad Dermatol 1990;23:254–256.

de Coninck EC, Kim YH, Varghese A, et al: Clinical characteristics and outcome of patients with extracutaneous mycosis fungoides. J Clin Oncol 2001;19:779–784.

Diamandidou E, Cohen PR, Kurzrock R: Mycosis fungoides and Sézary syndrome. Blood 1996;88:2385–2409.

Evans AV, Wood BP, Scarisbuck JJ, et al: Extracorporeal photopheresis in Sézary syndrome: Hematologic parameters as predictors of response. Blood 2001;98:1298–1301.

Kim YH, Hoppe RT: Mycosis fungoides and the Sézary syndrome. Semin Oncol 1999;26:276–289.

Minna JD, Roenigk HH Jr, Glatstein E: Report of the Committee on Therapy for Mycosis Fungoides and Sézary Syndrome. Cancer Treat Rep 1979;63:729–733.

Olsen E, Duric M, Fankel A, et al: Pivotal phase III trial of two dose levels of denileukin diftitox for the treatment of cutaneous T cell lymphoma. J Clin Oncol 2001;19:376–388.

Sausville EA, Eddy JL, Makuch RW, et al: Histopathologic staging at initial diagnosis of mycosis fungoides and the Sézary syndrome. Definition of three distinctive prognostic groups. Ann Intern Med 1988;109:372–382.

Siegel RS, Pandolfino T, Guitart J, et al: Primary cutaneous T cell lymphoma: review and current concepts. J Clin Oncol 2000;18:2908–2925.

Willemze R, Kerl H, Sterry W, et al: EORTC classification for primary cutaneous lymphomas: a proposal from the Cutaneous Lymphoma Study Group of the European Organization for Research and Treatment of Cancer. Blood. 1997;90:354–371.

Willemze R, Meijer CJ: EORTC classification for primary cutaneous lymphomas: a comparison with the R.E.A.L. Classification and the proposed WHO Classification. Ann Oncol 2000;11(Suppl. 1):11–15.

Peripheral T Cell Lymphomas

DeCoteau JF, Kadin ME: New insights into peripheral T cell lymphomas. Curr Opin Oncol 1995;7:408–414.

Falini B, Pileri S, Zinzani PL, et al: ALK+ lymphoma; clinico-pathological findings and outcome. Blood 1999;93: 2697–2706.

Gale J, Simmonds PD, Mead GM, et al: Enteropathy-type intestinal T cell lymphoma: clinical features and treatment of 31 patients in a single center. J Clin Oncol 2000;18:795–803.

Gordon BG, Weisenburger DD, Sanger WG, et al: Peripheral T cell lymphoma in children and adolescents: role of bone marrow transplantation. Leuk Lymph 1994;14:1–10.

Jaffe ES, Chan JK, Su IJ, et al: Report of the Workshop on Nasal and Related Extranodal Angiocentric T/Natural Killer Cell Lymphomas. Definitions, differential diagnosis, and epidemiology. Am J Surg Pathol 1996;20:103–111.

Jaffe ES, Krenacs L, Kumar S, et al: Extranodal peripheral T cell and NK cell neoplasms. Am J Clin Pathol 1999;111(Suppl. 1):S46–55.

Kwong YL, Chan AC, Liang R, et al: CD56+ NK lymphomas: clinicopathological features and prognosis. Br J Haematol 1997;97:821–829.

Nakamura S, Suchi T, Koshikawa T, et al: Clinicopathologic study of 212 cases of peripheral T cell lymphoma among the Japanese. Cancer 1993;72:1762–1772.

Rodriguez J, Munsell M, Yazji S, et al: Impact of high-dose chemotherapy on peripheral T cell lymphomas. J Clin Oncol 2001;19:3766–3770.

Stein H, Foss H-D, Durkop H, et al: CD30+ anaplastic large cell lymphoma: a review of its histopathologic, genetic, and clinical features. Blood 2000;96:3681–3695.

Wang CC, Tien HF, Lin MT, et al: Consistent presence of isochromosome 7q in hepatosplenic T gamma/delta lymphoma: a new cytogenetic-clinicopathologic entity. Genes Chrom Cancer 1995;12:161–164.

Weidmann E: Hepatosplenic T cell lymphoma: A review on 45 cases since the first report describing the disease as a distinct lymphoma entity in 1990. Leukemia 2000; 14:991–997.

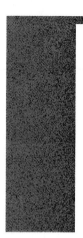

Chapter 70
Adult T Cell Leukemia/Lymphoma

R. Judith Ratzan

Epidemiology

In 1977, Uchiyama reported an unusual constellation of symptoms and findings that established the diagnosis of an entity now called adult T cell leukemia/lymphoma (ATL/L). The initial reports indicated that all affected patients lived in the islands that constitute southern Japan. In 1980, viral particles were found in the cells from a patient who was thought to have cutaneous T cell lymphoma but who actually had adult T cell leukemia/lymphoma. The virus, subsequently termed human T cell lymphotropic virus 1 (HTLV-1), is identified in more than 90% of patients with adult T cell leukemia/lymphoma and was the first retrovirus directly associated with human malignancy. In a small number of cases, HTLV-1 is not found in patients who have all of the features consistent with adult T cell leukemia/lymphoma.

HTLV-1 infection, confirmed by antibody testing or measurement of viral load, is endemic in southern Japan. The prevalence in southern Japan is approximately 15% for men and 18% for women; the lifetime risk for infected patients to develop adult T cell leukemia/lymphoma is approximately 5%. Seroprevalence increases with advancing age, as does the incidence of conversion to a symptomatic disease state. HTLV-1 infects the CD4+ T lymphocyte, and transmission involves cellular transfer. Unlike human immunodeficiency virus-1 (HIV-1), HTLV-1 is not free in the plasma but is localized intracellularly in CD4+ helper lymphocytes. Viral load is measured by the number of proviral copies per 100 peripheral-blood mononuclear cells.

Infection is transmitted primarily through sexual intercourse, more effectively from male to female than vice versa. Maternal transfer of viral infection to the child occurs during prolonged breast feeding and from cross-contamination of individuals by administration of infected blood transfusions and through the use of shared needles, as occurs among drug addicts.

The virus is also endemic in the Caribbean basin, the southeastern United States, central and south Africa, and areas of South America, particularly Brazil.

Retroviral Oncogenesis

HTLV-1 is an RNA virus. The virus binds to the surface of CD4+ cells, and after transport into the cell, the viral RNA is directly transcribed to double-stranded DNA by viral reverse transcriptase. Retroviral integrase then irreversibly integrates the DNA into the host cell chromosome, where it exists as a provirus. Viral infection immortalizes the T cell, making continued replication in vitro possible, provided that interleukin-2 is available.

Immortalizing the cell is not identical to malignant transformation, which requires a number of additional steps. The virus consists of three structural genes—gag, pol, and env—and the regulatory proteins tax and rex, which control viral replication and expression of viral proteins. The tax protein activates the long terminal repeats at the end of the structural genes, thereby stimulating transcription of the provirus. It also transactivates production of interleukin-2 and the interleukin-2 receptor as well as granulocyte-macrophage colony-stimulating factor (GM-CSF). Tax also inactivates several cell cycle-related proteins and suppresses activity of p53 and thus p53-induced apoptosis. The tax protein is critical to, but not sufficient for, the process of malignant transformation. The rex regulatory protein is also required. Perpetuation of replication is achieved in part by secretion of interleukin-2, allowing for paracrine stimulation of T cell proliferation.

A number of nonspecific clonal cytogenetic abnormalities occur. The most frequent of these involve translocations of chromosome 14 at sites q32 and q11. The q11 site is also the locus for the alpha and beta T cell receptors. Not all of the events necessary for viral infection to cause malignancy are known, but the HTLV-1 provirus titer does strongly correlate with the risk of progression to adult T cell leukemia/lymphoma. In adult T cell leukemia/lymphoma, the virus resides in a clonal population of malignant T-lymphocytes. Since most HTLV-1-infected individuals in endemic areas do not suffer adverse consequences of the infection, other factors must be involved in malignant transformation. Nevertheless, there is a relationship between length of time of infection and risk of conversion to malignancy; the average latency period for adult T cell leukemia/lymphoma after viral infection is 20 years.

Disease Manifestations Associated with HTLV-1 Infection

Two major illnesses can develop after HTLV-1 infection, either adult T cell leukemia/lymphoma or an immune-mediated spinal cord injury, called tropical spastic paresis (TSP) in the Caribbean area and HTLV-1-associated myelopathy (HAM) in Japan. HTLV-1 has also been associated with an infectious dermatitis in children and uveitis.

Tropical Spastic Paresis/HTLV-1–Associated Myelopathy

Patients with tropical spastic paresis/HTLV-1-associated myelopathy have a high viral load, a level of provirus in their lymphocytes that is 16 times greater than that found in asymptomatic carriers of HTLV-1. Symptoms of tropical spastic paresis/HTLV-1-associated myelopathy are caused by the insidious and slowly progressive development of a spastic paraplegia or paraparesis. This primarily involves upper motor neurons, but there may be an associated mild sensory deficit and sphincter abnormalities. Although the predominant clinical features of this syndrome are due to spinal cord involvement, especially of the thoracic region, magnetic resonance imaging (MRI) abnormalities similar to the white matter damage seen in multiple sclerosis also occur in the brains of affected patients. The process is in fact an encephalomyelitis. Virus can be demonstrated in lymphocytes in the cerebrospinal fluid. Histologic examination at autopsy reveals chronic inflammation of the spinal cord with perivascular cuffing and parenchymal lymphocytic infiltration by CD4+ and CD8+ cells. The role of the CD8+ cell is of interest. Although the virus preferentially invades CD4+ cells, CD8 cells from patients with tropical spastic paresis/HTLV-1-associated myelopathy have been found to contain provirus as well, and these cells are increased in number. The disease is thought to be autoimmune in etiology on the basis of the formation of antibody to neuron-specific antigens that are similar to those of the HTLV-1 tax protein.

In contrast to adult T cell leukemia/lymphoma, the increased viral load is not as high in tropical spastic paresis/HTLV-1-associated myelopathy, the latency is shorter, as brief as two years after an infected blood transfusion, and the disorder is not a malignancy, since the viral integration in lymphocytes does not result in clonal abnormalities.

Adult T Cell Leukemia/Lymphoma

Because of the long latency period after infection, adult T cell leukemia/lymphoma patients have a median age of approximately 40 years in Caribbean patients and 55 years in the Japanese population.

Common presenting features and their approximate frequency among patients are as follows: lymphadenopathy in three fourths, skin lesions in half, hepatomegaly in half, and splenomegaly in one fourth. Hypercalcemia occurs in more than 90% of cases that occur outside of Japan. Lymph node enlargement is usually not massive. The retroperitoneal lymph nodes and the hilar nodes are commonly involved, but mediastinal masses are rarely seen. The malignant T cells in adult T cell leukemia/lymphoma carry the following immunophenotype: CD3+, CD4+, CD8−, and CD25+. The latter marker is the alpha chain for the interleukin-2 receptor. Table 70-1 contains the diagnostic criteria and subtypes of adult T cell leukemia/lymphoma proposed by Shimoyama.

Acute Form

This variant accounts for approximately 60% of patients and is a highly aggressive disease with a medial survival time of six months and a five-year sur-

---

Table 70-1 ■ Subtypes of Adult T-Cell Leukemia/Lymphoma and Criteria for Diagnosis

Subsets

Acute
Smoldering
Chronic
Lymphoma

Diagnostic Criteria

Histologic and/or cytologic demonstration of a T-cell lymphoid malignancy
Demonstration of abnormal T lymphocytes in all of the subtypes except the lymphoma variant
Seropositivity for HTLV-1 by ELISA, Western blot
Demonstration of clonality of proviral DNA and clonal integration by Southern blot or polymerase chain reaction

vival rate of 5%. Such patients frequently present with skin lesions, lymph node enlargement, and evidence of diffuse organ infiltration, especially of the liver, spleen, and lung. They may have symptoms of abdominal pain, diarrhea, and cough. Laboratory studies usually show an elevated white blood cell count and atypical pleomorphic cells that have lobulated nuclei, known as "flower" or "cloverleaf" cells. The serum calcium level is often elevated, as are the lactate dehydrogenase (LDH) and alkaline phosphatase levels.

Hypercalcemia is multifactorial in origin. The malignant cells of some patients produce a parathormonelike molecule. Osteoclast-activating factor, tumor necrosis factors (TNF-α and TNF-β), and interleukin 1 (IL-1α and IL-1β) are secreted by cell lines from patients. These can enhance bone resorption and cause hypercalcemia. Osteoclast-activating factor can cause multiple lytic lesions of bone that are not due to local tumor cell collections. Bone marrow involvement is common, occurring in 50% of patients. Despite extensive disease and circulating malignant cells, cytopenias are rare, and the bone marrow infiltration is patchy, not diffuse as it is in other lymphoid malignancies. Skin biopsies often show Pautrier's microabscesses that are difficult to distinguish from those present in mycosis fungoides or Sézary syndrome.

Smoldering and Chronic Forms

These variants account for approximately 25% of patients and are characterized by a more indolent course than the acute form. Smoldering adult T cell leukemia/lymphoma may have disease limited to the skin for a substantial period of time, whereas the chronic form tends to exhibit multiple organ involvement. The number of circulating T cells is lower in patients with smoldering adult T cell leukemia/lymphoma than in chronic adult T cell leukemia/lymphoma and carries a better prognosis. Unfortunately, both forms ultimately terminate in the acute form of the disease.

Lymphoma Form

This group of patients does not have circulating abnormal T-lymphocytes but does have predominant lymph node enlargement due to malignant infiltration. The clinical presentation is consistent with a non-Hodgkin's lymphoma, but the clinical and laboratory findings, including frequent hypercalcemia, are similar to those in the acute form. This subtype accounts for approximately 20% of patients with adult T cell leukemia/lymphoma, and the median survival is 10 months.

Prognosis

Age greater than 40 years, poor performance status, elevated lactate dehydrogenase, hypercalcemia, and the presence of four or more involved areas indicate a poor prognosis for all types of this disease. In the chronic subtype, normal values of lactate dehydrogenase, serum albumin, and blood urea nitrogen indicate a relatively favorable prognosis.

Treatment

Treatment of adult T cell leukemia/lymphoma has so far been of limited value. Treatment goals can vary, depending on the intent, which can be to cure aggressive disease, prevent disease progression from a smoldering or chronic course to the acute form, or palliate symptomatic manifestations of disease. The first of these goals, cure of disease, is not attainable.

Standard cytotoxic regimens, such as cyclophosphamide, vincristine, prednisone, and doxorubicin, that are used in large B cell lymphomas are generally ineffective in adult T cell leukemia/lymphoma. Although complete remissions can occur in as many as 45% of patients, relapses are virtually inevitable and occur rapidly. Intensifying treatment by the addition of other agents does not improve the median survival. Treatment by continuous infusion of chemotherapeutic agents rather than by bolus administration may be somewhat more effective. Adenosine deaminase inhibitors, such as deoxycoformycin, are effective, but the incidence of infectious complications increases owing to immunosuppression, and responses are of short duration. A small number of patients have received high-dose therapy followed by autologous or allogeneic stem cell transplantation. Both approaches achieve transient responses, but infectious complications are a major problem, and long-term survival is poor.

Arsenic trioxide induces apoptosis in HTLV-1-infected cells in vitro and may prove to be an effective agent when used alone or in combination. The importance of retroviral infection in disease pathogenesis has led to some intriguing studies of antiviral agents, such as the combination of α-interferon and zidovudine. Responses have been demonstrated, and some of these have been durable on continuation of therapy. Approaches that combine antiviral therapy with conventional chemotherapy may improve on these results. Although the responses to antiviral therapy may be due to viral suppression, it is also possible that some antivirals (zidovudine, for example, was initially developed as an anticancer drug) are directly toxic to the malignant cells or that they act to enhance the patient's autologous cytotoxic T cell response against the malignant lymphocytes.

Because adult T cell leukemia/lymphoma cells express the interleukin-2 receptor on their surface, antibodies to the receptor represent a potential means of therapy. A monoclonal antibody to the interleukin-2 receptor, called anti-Tac, is a monoclonal mouse IgG2a that prevents the growth of certain cell lines in vitro. In clinical trials, anti-Tac achieved a 30% overall response rate with response durations of 1 to 30 months. Radiolabeling the antibody slightly improved the response, but the relapse rate and survival remained poor.

References

General Information

Bangham, CRM: HTLV-I infections. J Clin Pathol 2000;53:581–586.

Daenke S, Kermode AG, Hall SE, et al: High activated and memory cytotoxic T cell responses to HTLV-1 in healthy carriers and patients with tropical spastic paresis. Virology 1996;2217:139–146.

Lymphoma Study Group: Major prognostic factors of patients with adult T cell leukemia-lymphoma: A cooperative study. Leukemia Res 1991;15:81–90.

Lyons SF, Liebowitz DN: The roles of human viruses in the pathogenesis of lymphoma. Semin Oncol 1998;25:461–475.

Manns A, Hisada M, La Grenade L: Human T-lymphotropic virus type I infection. Lancet 1999;353:1951–1958.

Nagai M, Usuku K, Matsumoto W, et al: Analysis of HTLV-1 proviral lead in 202 HAM/TSP patients and 243 asymptomatic HTLV-1 carriers: High proviral load strongly predisposes to HAM/TSP. J Neurovirol 1998;4:586–593.

Nagai M, Jacobson S: Immunopathogenesis of human T cell lymphotropic virus type I-associated myelopathy. Curr Opin Neurol 2001;14:381–386.

Nakamura T: Immunopathogenesis of HTLV-1-associated myelopathy/tropical spastic paraparesis. Ann Med 2000;32:600–607.

Ohshima K, Ohgami A, Matsuoka M, et al: Random integration of HTLV-1 provirus: Increasing chromosomal instability. Cancer Lett 1998;132:203–212.

Poiesz BJ, Ruscetti FW, Gazdar AF, et al: Detection and isolation of type C retrovirus particles from fresh and cultured lymphocytes of a patient with cutaneous T cell lymphoma. Proc Natl Acad Sci USA 1980;77:7415–7419.

Richard V, Lairmore MD, Green P, et al: Humoral hypercalcemia of malignancy. Am J Pathol 2001;158:2219–2228.

Shimoyama M: Diagnostic criteria and classification of clinical subtypes of adult T cell leukemia-lymphoma: A report from the lymphoma study group 1984–1987. Br J Haematol;1991;79:428–437.

Tsukasaki K, Kreb J, Nagai K, et al: Comparative genomic hybridization analysis in adult T cell leukemia/lymphoma. Blood 2001;97:3875–3881.

Uchiyama T, Yodoi J, Sagawa K, et al: Adult T cell leukemia: Clinical and hematologic features of 16 cases. Blood 1977;50:481–492.

Zucker-Franklin D: The role of human T cell lymphotropic virus type I in the development of cutaneous T cell lymphoma. Ann NY Acad Sci 2001;941:86–96.

Therapy

Bazarbachi A, El-Sabban ME, Nasr R, et al: Arsenic trioxide and interferon-α synergize to induce cell cycle arrest and apoptosis in human T cell lymphotropic virus type I-transformed cells. Blood 1999;93:278–283.

Bazarbachi A, Nasr R, El-Sabban ME, et al: Evidence against a direct cytotoxic effect of alpha interferon and zidovudine in HTLV-1 associated adult T cell leukemia/lymphoma. Leukemia 2000;14:716–721.

Bazarbachi A, Hermine O: Treatment of adult T cell leukaemia/lymphoma: current strategy and future perspectives. Virus Res 2001;78:79–92.

El-Sabban ME, Nasr R, Dbaibo G, et al: Arsenic–interferon-α-triggered apoptosis in HTLV-1 transformed cells is associated with TAX down-regulation and reversal of NF-κB activation. Blood 2000;96:2849–2855.

Gill PS, Harrington W, Kaplan MK, et al: Treatment of adult T cell leukemia-lymphoma with a combination of interferon alpha and zidovudine. N Engl J Med 1995;332:1744–1748.

Machua A, Rodes B, Soriano V: The effect of antiretroviral therapy on HTLV infection. Virus Res; 2001;78:93–100.

Matutes E, Taylor GP, Cavenagh J, et al: Interferon α and zidovudine therapy in adult T cell leukaemia lymphoma: Response and outcome in 15 patients. Br J Haematol 2001;113:779–784.

Taguchi H, Kinoshita KI, Takatsuki K, et al: An intensive chemotherapy of adult T cell leukemia/lymphoma: CHOP followed by etoposide. Vindesine, ranimustine, and mitoxantrone with granulocyte colony-stimulating factor support. J Acquir Immun Defic Syndr Hum Retrovirol 1996;12:182–186.

Tan C, Waldmann TA: Proteasome inhibitor PS-341, a potential therapeutic agent for adult T cell leukemia. Cancer Res 2002;62:1083–1086.

Yamada Y, Tomonaga M, Fukuda H, et al: A new G-CSF-supported combination chemotherapy, LSG15, for adult T cell leukaemia-lymphoma: Japan clinical oncology group study 9303. Br J Haematol 2001;113:375–382.

Chapter 71
Chronic Myeloid Leukemia

Richard T. Silver

Introduction

The *myeloproliferative disorders* are clonal disorders that include chronic myeloid leukemia (CML), polycythemia vera, essential thrombocythemia, and agnogenic myeloid metaplasia. These disorders are grouped together because they have similar clinical characteristics, namely splenomegaly and an increase in one or more of the formed elements of the blood—either red blood cells, white blood cells, or platelets. In these diseases, the bone marrow is usually hypercellular at presentation and contains varying amounts of fibrous tissue (collagen, reticulin). All of these diseases can terminate in an aggressive phase that clinically resembles an acute leukemia. This occurs commonly in chronic myeloid leukemia and is observed in order of decreasing frequency in agnogenic myeloid metaplasia, polycythemia vera, and essential thrombocythemia. The clone that characterizes chronic myeloid leukemia contains a specific cytogenetic abnormality known as the Philadelphia (Ph) chromosome, which is directly involved in its pathogenesis. It is this specific abnormality that now permits a targeted therapeutic approach to the pathophysiology of this disease—an approach that could represent a new paradigm for the treatment of other, more common, cancers.

Epidemiology and Incidence

The annual incidence of chronic myeloid leukemia is 1 case per 100,000 population. It accounts for approximately 15% of all adult patients with leukemia.

Etiology

The trigger mechanism for the generation of the Philadelphia chromosome is unknown, but excess exposure to radiation is clearly an etiologic factor in some cases. For example, individuals exposed to radiation from the atomic bombing of Hiroshima and Nagasaki subsequently demonstrated an increase not only in acute leukemia but also in chronic myeloid leukemia. Similarly, years ago, radiologists who performed radiographic studies without appropriate lead shielding had an increased incidence of both acute and chronic myeloid leukemia.

Presenting Clinical and Hematologic Characteristics

The peak incidence of the disease occurs between the ages of 50 to 60 years, but no age group is exempt. There is no sex preference. The first phase of the disease, the *chronic phase*, is relatively indolent with few, if any, symptoms. Because automated blood count studies are usually performed routinely during physician encounters, as many as half of the patients with chronic myeloid leukemia are diagnosed while asymptomatic, based on unsuspected blood count abnormalities. In most cases, symptoms develop insidiously and are related to the increase in spleen size or to anemia. The spleen is palpable in approximately one-half of the patients; otherwise, no other abnormalities are generally found on physical examination. In some patients, the enlarged spleen causes discomfort in the left side of the abdomen and/or early satiety due to pressure effects on the stomach. Weight loss can occur because of the cachexia seen in cancer patients and/or because of a compromised stomach size due to compression by the enlarged spleen.

Peripheral Blood Findings

About one-half of the patients are anemic at presentation. Thrombocytosis and large platelets are not uncommon, but thrombotic complications are rare. Thrombocytopenia occurs in a minority of patients when first diagnosed. When present, this is an unfavorable prognostic sign. The white blood cell count ranges from 20,000 to 400,000/µL with a median of 200,000/µL at diagnosis; higher white blood cell counts are sometimes seen. The granulocytic leukocytosis in the peripheral blood shows all levels of differentiation, from the myeloblast to the segmented neutrophil, with myelocytes predominating. Basophils and eosinophils can also be increased in number. Red cell morphology is usually normal, and red blood cell precursors are rarely seen in the blood. An acquired Pelger-Hüet anomaly can appear, consisting of hyposegmented neutrophilic leukocytes demonstrating only two nuclear lobes, rather than the usual three or four lobes.

Bone Marrow Findings

The bone marrow is hypercellular and devoid of fat. During the chronic phase, the myelocyte predominates; myeloblasts and promyelocytes account for less than 10% of the marrow cells. Early in the disease, megakaryocytes may be increased in number. Cells morphologically indistinguishable from true Gaucher cells can be seen in about 10% of cases. These pseudo-Gaucher cells occur due to accumulation of glucocerebrosides (derived from rapid white blood cell turnover) in bone marrow histiocytes. As in other myeloproliferative disorders, biopsy sections can show an increase in reticulin fibers. The fibroblasts responsible for deposition of the fibers are not part of the malignant clone. Evidence suggests that the marrow fibrosis is a secondary phenomenon, relating to interaction between the proliferative clone of chronic myeloid leukemia megakaryocytes and the elements that regulate marrow fibrosis, collagen, and collagen deposition. These elements include, at least, platelet-derived growth factor, transforming growth factor-beta, basic fibroblastic growth factor, and other cytokines not yet completely defined.

Differential Diagnosis of Chronic Phase Chronic Myeloid Leukemia

The evaluation of a patient with chronic myeloid leukemia includes a complete blood count, assessment of renal and hepatic function, and consideration of the consequences of hyperuricemia (due to increased white blood cell turnover), including acute gouty arthritis and gouty renal colic. A bone marrow aspiration and biopsy may be performed to evaluate morphology, obtain cytogenetic studies, and determine the degree of fibrosis. The clinical picture and peripheral blood examination usually strongly indicate the diagnosis. The most important distinction in the differential diagnosis is between chronic myeloid leukemia and a myeloid (granulocytic) leukemoid reaction, i.e., an elevated blood cell count and the appearance of white blood cell precursors in the peripheral blood in response to inflammation or infection. In leukemoid reactions, the white blood cell count is rarely greater than 50,000/μL, whereas higher levels are commonly found in chronic myeloid leukemia. In most cases, the underlying stimulus for the leukocytosis is clinically apparent when a leukemoid reaction is present. When the cause is treated and subsides, the white blood cell count rapidly returns to normal levels. In the absence

DIAGNOSIS

Blast Cells in Chronic Myeloid Leukemia

The white blood cell count in chronic myeloid leukemia can rise to 300,000 to 400,000/μL or even higher without the patient being at risk for leucostasis (plugging up of small vessels in the brain and/or lung, causing hemorrhagic infarction). In contrast, blast cell counts of 75,000 to 100,000/μL create this hazard. The difference lies in the fact that the blast cell forms circulating in chronic phase chronic myeloid leukemia are usually only 2% to 3% of the total (representing an absolute blast cell count of only 8000 to 12,000/μL if the white blood cell count is 400,000/μL). The blast forms, not the later white blood cell precursors, are poorly deformable in their passage through the blood vessels, obstructing the flow.

When the white blood cell count in chronic myeloid leukemia is greater than 400,000 to 500,000/μL, a hyperviscosity syndrome can develop, with tinnitus, decreased hearing, and symptoms of congestive heart failure. Lowering the white blood cell count by leukapheresis or treatment with hydroxyurea corrects the problem. Patients presenting with this problem are usually very anemic. Until the white blood cell count is lowered, these patients should not be transfused with packed red blood cells for fear of exacerbating the hyperviscosity.

In patients with chronic phase chronic myeloid leukemia, the development of a focus of severe unexplained pain (usually in a bone) is often a herald of transformation to the blast phase of chronic myeloid leukemia, even though the peripheral blood and bone marrow findings might be unchanged and X-rays and scans are negative. The pain is usually due to a focal collection of rapidly expanding blast cells.

of overt signs of inflammation or infection and with only modest elevations of the white blood cell count of 10,000 to 15,000/μL, an occult malignancy should be considered. In general, marked increases in myelocytes and lesser increases in promyelocytes are more commonly seen in chronic myeloid leukemia than in leukemoid reactions. The presence of splenomegaly favors the diagnosis of chronic myeloid leukemia.

At times, other myeloproliferative syndromes present with clinical characteristics (e.g., enlarged spleen, leukocytosis with immature white blood cells, and thrombocytosis) that are similar to those observed in chronic myeloid leukemia. In all cases, demonstration of the Philadelphia chromosome or its molecular equivalent, the BCR-ABL chimeric gene, from cells in the peripheral blood and/or bone marrow is readily accomplished and establishes the diagnosis.

Natural History of Chronic Myeloid Leukemia

The chronic phase lasts for a variable period but ultimately terminates in all patients in an aggressive acute illness, called the *blast phase* of the disease. Usually the change is abrupt, and the illness assumes the characteristics of a de novo acute leukemia with greater than 30% myeloblasts and promyelocytes in the marrow. Survival from the time of the blast phase is usually about three to six months. An intervening phase, called the *accelerated phase*, can develop for a variable period (three to six months) between the chronic and blast phases of chronic myeloid leukemia. The accelerated phase is defined by less precise criteria, but it is associated with a gradual increase in myeloblasts and promyelocytes in the peripheral blood and bone marrow, increasing splenomegaly, fever of undetermined origin, basophilia, progressive anemia, thrombocytopenia, and decreased responsiveness of the elevated white blood cell count and/or platelet count to agents that were previously effective in the treatment of the chronic phase. Published reports concerning the terminal phase of chronic myeloid leukemia use differing definitions of the clinical and laboratory findings requisite for recognizing the transition from the chronic phase.

The blast phase can be either myeloid, lymphoid, or biphenotypic (mixed lymphoblastic-myeloblastic). A lymphoid blast crisis occurs in approximately one-third of patients. The blast cells resemble those seen in acute lymphocytic leukemia and often contain terminal deoxynucleotidyl transferase, CD10 (common lymphocytic leukemia antigen), CD20, and other markers of the lymphoid phenotype. Although most lymphoblastic crises in chronic myeloid leukemia are of B cell origin, a few cases of T cell blast crises have

been described. Myeloid blast crisis can mimic acute myeloid leukemia. Rarely, patients present in myeloid blast crisis without a recognized antecedent chronic phase; the demonstration of the Philadelphia chromosome, molecular abnormalities, and splenomegaly of significant degree help to distinguish this condition from de novo acute myeloid leukemia (AML). Acute megakaryoblastic and erythroblastic transformations, and blast crisis marked by extreme basophilia (greater than 20%) have also been reported. The mechanism underlying the change from the chronic into the blast phase is not understood. Cytogenetic abnormalities in addition to the Philadelphia chromosome appear, but it is not clear that they specifically initiate the dramatic change from the relatively clinically indolent chronic phase.

The Molecular Biology of Chronic Myeloid Leukemia

The cytogenetic hallmark of chronic myeloid leukemia is the Philadelphia chromosome, so-called because it was first detected in a patient living in Philadelphia. The Philadelphia chromosome involves a shortening of chromosome 22 due to a reciprocal translocation [t(9;22)(q34;q11)] of genetic material between the long arms of chromosomes 9 and 22 (Figure 71-1). This transposes the 3′ segment of the ABL gene from chromosome 9 to the 5′ segment of the BCR gene on chromosome 22, resulting in a fusion or chimeric BCR gene. The ABL designation stands for the Abelson variant of a virus that can cause cellular transformation in murine systems. The viral oncogene is homologous with the protooncogene located in all normal human cells on chromosome 9. The protein product of this gene is 140 kd; it exhibits modest protein kinase activity in most normal cells, but its precise function is unknown. The BCR (breakpoint cluster region) gene refers to the limited segment of DNA on chromosome 22 where the breaks occur in patients with the Philadelphia chromosome. The BCR gene is also widely distributed in human cells, and its normal function is obscure. The BCR-ABL gene produces a cytoplasmic protein, known as a p210 kilodalton protein (expressed as p210$^{bcr-abl}$) that has markedly increased and unregulated tyrosine kinase activity. This in turn affects intracellular signaling pathways, causing cellular proliferation and differentiation to occur independently of normal regulatory mechanisms. One principal effect of the protein is to decrease apoptosis (normal programmed cell death). That the BCR-ABL rearrangement is a major factor in the pathophysiology of chronic myeloid leukemia has been demonstrated experimentally. Transfection of cells in vitro or of mouse embryos in vivo with the

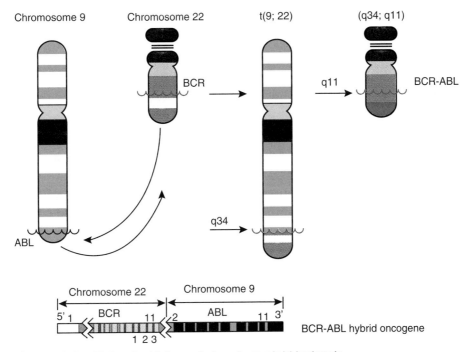

Figure 71-1 ■ Molecular biology of chronic myeloid leukemia.

BCR-ABL gene results in alterations that are morphologically, cytogenetically and clinically similar to the changes noted in chronic myeloid leukemia in humans.

Virtually all patients with chronic myeloid leukemia express only the p210$^{bcr-abl}$ protein. Philadelphia chromosome–positive patients with de novo acute lymphocytic leukemia, however, express either the p210$^{bcr-abl}$ protein or a variant p190$^{bcr-abl}$ protein. The latter is more common, being present in 50% of adults and 80% of children with acute lymphocytic leukemia who are Philadelphia chromosome-positive.

The Philadelphia chromosome is detected by karyotyping studies in approximately 95% of patients with chronic myeloid leukemia, in children (5%) and adults (30%) who have acute lymphocytic leukemia; and in a small number of patients (1% to 2%) with newly diagnosed acute myeloid leukemia. In the remaining 5% of patients with the clinical picture of chronic myeloid leukemia, the Philadelphia chromosome is not demonstrable by metaphase analysis, but molecular studies show the BCR-ABL chimeric gene rearrangement. Some patients with the Philadelphia chromosome have variant complex translocations of other chromosomes with chromosomes 9 and 22. There is no difference in survival between patients who present with the standard Philadelphia chromosome compared with variant or complex translocations.

Karyotyping involves the examination of 20 metaphases and is a reliable technique as long as the frequency of the Philadelphia clone among the cells studied is more than 5% to 10%. A number of molecular studies have been developed that are more sensitive in detecting the BCR-ABL rearrangement. For example, reverse transcriptase polymerase chain reaction (RT-PCR) technology detects BCR-ABL at the messenger RNA level. RT-PCR can detect the presence of 1/10,000 to 1/1,000,000 cells that carry the BCR-ABL rearrangement, but it is not used for diagnosis on a routine basis. Monoclonal antibodies can detect BCR and ABL by Western blot or immunoprecipitation but are used for research purposes only.

Fluorescence In Situ Hybridization Test

A number of other tests based on molecular technology have been used in clinical practice to substitute for cytogenetic testing, which nevertheless remains the gold standard in most trials. Various modifications of the fluorescence in situ hybridization (FISH) technique have been developed, and experience with them has been increasing rapidly.

The fluorescence in situ hybridization test has expanded the sensitivity of the standard karyotype analysis and permits the detection of submicroscopic abnormalities that might occur at low frequency. With this new method, targeted DNA sequences are visualized, permitting analysis and quantification of disease at the molecular level. This test is more sensitive than standard cytogenetics because many more cells are surveyed. Satisfactory results can be obtained from the analysis of peripheral blood samples or of bone marrow. This technique is thus especially useful in situations in which the marrow is packed with cells, making aspiration difficult, or when the marrow is hypoplastic following chemotherapy—a time when it is also often impossible to obtain adequate marrow specimens for cytogenetic studies.

Fluorescence in situ hybridization techniques use colored dyes that are directly labeled to the BCR and ABL sequences. The interphase fluorescence in situ hybridization test is done on peripheral blood, thereby avoiding the necessity for a bone marrow aspiration, and it can be done rapidly, using dual-color BCR-ABL probes. Fluorescence in situ hybridization tests are excellent for diagnostic purposes. One needs to be aware, however that the frequency of false positives can be as high as 10%, which makes this test not reliable in patients with a low burden (less than 10%) of Philadelphia chromosome cells. The hypermetaphase fluorescence in situ hybridization test, because it permits the examination of more than 500 cells for the BCR-ABL rearrangement, is more sensitive, but the procedure is time consuming and is done only on bone marrow samples after stem cell transplantation using painted probes for chromosome 9 and 22. Using BCR-ABL extrasensitive probes, however, the technique detects and quantifies the BCR-ABL gene at diagnosis and at all times during treatment from either blood or marrow. Indeed, this probe easily detects residual disease when the frequency of positive cells is as low as 1%.

Detection of BCR-ABL employing a triple-color code is of value because it detects patients with deletion of chromosome 9 at the site of the Philadelphia chromosome breakpoint; this deletion has been associated with a poor prognosis.

The clinical progression of chronic myeloid leukemia from the chronic to the accelerated or acute phase is accompanied by additional cytogenetic abnormalities in approximately 80% of patients. These changes occur much more commonly in the myeloid than in the lymphoid transformation. In the latter type, new specific, nonrandom clonal markers are generally absent, and hypodiploidy is common. In myeloid crisis, the most common changes—gain of chromosomes 8, 19, or the second Philadelphia chromosome, and i(17q)—frequently occur in combination to produce modal chromosome numbers of 47 to 50. When patients have only a single new chromosome change, this most commonly involves gain of (in descending order of frequency) a second Philadelphia chromosome, an i(17q), +8, or a +19. Isochromosome 17q occurs almost exclusively in myeloid blast crisis. Other rearrangements, occurring less frequently, include monosomies of chromosomes 7, 17, and Y, trisomies of chromosomes 17 and 21, and t(3;21)(q26;q22).

Although molecular abnormalities correspond to cytogenetic changes in blast crisis of chronic myeloid leukemia, the genetic events responsible for transformation are poorly understood. They include mutations of P53 (on 17p13), N-ras (1p36), and RB1 (13q14), although they are rare. Up to 50% of patients with lymphoid transformation have homozygous deletions of p^{16INK} (9p21).

Treatment

Chemotherapy with Hydroxyurea and Busulfan

The standard of treatment for many years was the daily oral administration of chemotherapy, either of busulfan or hydroxyurea. Moreover, as the interferon rIFN-α alone or in combination with chemotherapy is not tolerated by 30% to 40% of patients, these two drugs remain as valuable therapeutic agents. Despite long use, only recently has the superiority of hydroxyurea over busufan been established in a randomized clinical comparative trial. The median survival was significantly less with busulfan compared with hydroxyurea (45 versus 58 months, respectively), as was the five-year survival (32% versus 44%).

Hydroxyurea

Hydroxyurea is S-phase and cell-cycle specific and functions as an antimetabolite. It has a short duration of action, with 90% of the drug excreted in 24 hours. Hydroxyurea can be started at a dose of 15 to 50 mg/kg/day orally depending on the white blood cell count and increasing, if necessary, or decreasing the dose as the white blood cell and/or platelet count falls. The drug should be discontinued when the white blood cell count falls to less than 15,000/μL. A rapid decrease in the platelet count in relation to the white blood cells requires prompt dose modification. On the other hand, additional treatment is sometimes required after the white cell count is normalized, if the platelet count remains substantially elevated. A handy guide is to halve the dose of hydroxyurea as the white blood cell count is halved. Maintenance doses usually range from 500 to 2,500 mg daily, with appropriate dose adjustment based on blood counts. Hydroxyurea side effects are rare and include a maculopapular rash, stomatitis, nausea and vomiting, nephrotic syndrome, and pretibial and ankle skin ulcers.

Busulfan

A standard initial daily dose of the alkylating agent busulfan is 4.0 to 6.0 mg/m^2 body surface (0.06 to 0.1 mg/kg) orally, with a maximum daily dose of 8 mg. Similar to the guide for hydroxyurea, the daily dose of drug should be halved as the white blood cell count falls serially by half. Myelosuppressive effects of busulfan can be durable, and it is well to avoid dropping blood counts below normal levels.

Bone marrow hypoplasia in patients receiving busulfan is usually dose-related but can be idiosyncratic. Thus, this agent should not be used in patients for whom marrow transplantation is being considered. Exfoliative cytologic studies of the cervix, sputum, and (less often) urine may reveal dysplastic changes, suggesting the presence of a secondary malignancy. In this circumstance, it might be necessary to discontinue the drug and/or undertake other studies to evaluate the significance of the cytologic changes. Other toxic effects of busulfan include amenorrhea, increased skin pigmentation, a wasting syndrome with features of Addison's disease, cataracts, "busulfan lung" (a form of interstitial fibrosis), and endocardial fibrosis.

Either hydroxyurea or busulfan causes excellent clinical and hematologic remissions in 80% to 90% of patients with chronic myeloid leukemia, but the fundamental abnormality, the Philadelphia chromosome, persists nevertheless. Thus, remission after conventional chemotherapy in chronic myeloid leukemia reflects quantitative, not qualitative, changes. Refractoriness to either drug is uncommon in the chronic phase of chronic myeloid leukemia, and its occurrence usually signifies impending terminal- or blast-phase disease.

Extramedullary myeloblastomas, which can occur during hydroxyurea or busulfan treatment, usually portend an ensuing frank blast crisis. They occur in the bones, skin, lymph nodes, and elsewhere and respond readily to locally directed external beam radiation therapy.

Important advances in the treatment of chronic myeloid leukemia in the past two decades include the use of the recombinant interferons and bone marrow transplantation, and, most recently, the signal transduction inhibitor, STI-571 or Gleevec.

Treatment with Interferon and Other Drugs

Because interferons have a wide range of biologic activities—including antiviral, antiproliferative, immunomodulatory, antiangiogenic, and oncogene regulatory properties—they were evaluated in chronic myeloid leukemia. This decision was fortunate because until then, the therapeutic notion existed that the natural course of chronic myeloid leukemia could not be altered except by the use of bone marrow transplantation. There is now general agreement that recombinant interferon-α (rIFN-α) combined with chemotherapy with either hydroxyurea or cytarabine (cytosine arabinoside, ara-C), and probably with other chemotherapeutic agents as well, can prolong life in chronic myeloid leukemia by causing durable suppression of the Philadelphia chromosome-positive clone.

Most of the evidence for the effectiveness of interferon relates to the use of rIFN-α therapy and consists of at least 30 uncontrolled observational studies. In some cases, complete and durable cytogenetic remission after rIFN-α based therapy required months of treatment and resulted in a small number of patients with sustained cytogenetic remission lasting many years, suggesting that they might have been cured. The largest number of patients has been followed at the M. D. Anderson Cancer Center in observational studies in which complete and partial hematologic remission rates with interferon therapy were reported to be 70% to 80% and 6% to 10%, respectively. Remission rates reported by others have been lower.

More important than hematologic response after rIFN-α, however, is the production of *cytogenetic response*, which, unfortunately, occurs significantly less often. Assessment of cytogenetic response is based on the analysis of the most favorable karyotype, employing the M. D. Anderson criteria. Complete cytogenetic response is defined as 0% Philadelphia chromosome-positive metaphases, partial cytogenetic response as 5% to 34% Philadelphia chromosome-positive metaphases, and minor response as 35% to 95%. At the M. D. Anderson Cancer Center, approximately 15% to 20% of the patients have had a complete cytogenetic response, and another 15% to 20% have had a partial response. Cytogenetic responses reported by others approximate half of these values, related to differences in case mix, age, stage of disease, elapsed time from diagnosis to treatment, and prognostic factors that differ among the various centers. In most cases, cytogenetic response occurs more frequently in patients who have low/normal platelet counts, a low percentage of blasts, and a nonpalpable spleen. These patients are defined as "good," "favorable," or "low risk;" their risk status can be quantified using a Sokal or Hasford score.

The achievement of a cytogenetic remission is important because it is accompanied by superior survival compared with those patients who have an intermediate response or none at all. In most studies showing a survival advantage for interferon alone, the maximum tolerated doses of rIFN-α have been used, driving leukocyte counts down to 2000 to 4000/μL. All other studies of interferon therapy have included hydroxyurea and/or cytarabine during induction and during some phase of the maintenance program.

Responses to interferon therapy occur slowly. The time to maximum hematologic response is approximately 6 months. The time to cytogenetic response is usually 9 to 12 months, but it can take up to 18 months. A major cytogenetic response might require two years of therapy. No studies have determined the optimal duration of administration of interferon. The current consensus is to continue treatment indefinitely in responding patients who have less than a complete cytogenetic response.

The side effects of rIFN-α include fever, chills, malaise, headache, anorexia, joint pain, vomiting, low backache, myalgia, various types of neuropathy, changes in mood and concentration and depression, abnormalities of liver enzymes, retinal vein thrombosis, leukopenia, and thrombocytopenia. Long-term therapy can be associated with autoimmune effects, including immune-mediated thrombocytopenia, hypothyroidism, and hemolytic anemia. Varying degrees of impotence can occur in about one-quarter of men. At least 30% of patients cannot tolerate interferon over the long term.

For many years, an unresolved issue was whether rIFN-α actually prolonged life or only identified those patients whose survival was predetermined to be good. In this case, the cytogenetic response was considered an epiphenomenon. The Italian Study Group on Chronic Myeloid Leukemia finally resolved this question. Patients were randomized to receive rIFN-α or hydroxyurea only and were stratified according to risk factors. Patients in the interferon arm were also allowed to receive hydroxyurea if the response was considered "sluggish." This occurred in one-third of the patients. After a median follow-up of 68 months, the frequency of clinical and hematologic remission was the same in both arms. In the interferon arm, however, a complete cytogenetic response was seen in 8% of the complete responders and a major response (67% to 99% Ph negative) in 11%. This compared with 0% and 1%, respectively, for the hydroxyurea-treated group. The time to progression from the chronic phase of leukemia to accelerated or blastic phase was 72 months in the interferon group, as compared with 45 months in the conventionally treated group. Overall median survival was 72 months in the rIFN-α + hydroxyurea arm compared with 52 months in the hydroxyurea-treated group. Cytogenetic response (complete, major, or minor) correlated with survival. At a median of 112 months, in the interferon arm 30% of the patients were still alive, and 8% maintained a complete or major cytogenetic remission. In the chemotherapy arm, 18% of the patients were alive, with a minor cytogenetic response in one case.

In order to improve the results of interferon therapy, cytarabine (cytosine arabinoside, ara-C) was added in a variety of doses and schedules. Two prospective studies have demonstrated the superiority of the combination of cytarabine and interferon over hydroxyurea and rIFN-α. The best results occurred in a French trial employing a combination of rIFN-α, five

million U/m² daily and cytarabine, 20 mg/m² for 10 days each month. In a randomized trial, a complete cytogenetic response was seen in 15%, and a partial cytogenetic response was seen in 26% of patients treated with rIFN-α and cytarabine. In comparison, complete cytogenetic responses occurred in 9% and partial cytogenetic responses in 15% of patients treated with rIFN-α and hydroxyurea. A recent Italian randomized trial of 837 newly diagnosed chronic myeloid leukemia patients, however, did not confirm the superiority of the rIFN-α and cytarabine in combination. The causes of these differences could be related to differences in the doses of drugs administered in these studies.

Even in patients with a complete cytogenetic response, molecular studies using reverse transcriptase polymerase chain reaction technology indicates that BCR-ABL chimerism persists, albeit in low frequency, in most patients. Thus, interferon therapy with or without low-dose cytarabine is not curative, but the concept of *biologic remission* has now been established—a term that applies to long-lived patients with persisting, low-titer BCR-ABL positivity. This is especially true if the patient was initially categorized as low-risk. Moreover, some patients who have had therapy discontinued in complete cytogenetic remission have had prolonged clinical remissions even though they remain BCR-ABL positive as determined by reverse transcriptase polymerase chain reaction.

Summary of the Efficacy of Interferon-Based Treatment

Interferon improves survival compared with busulfan and hydroxyurea, but only when it is combined with other agents such as hydroxyurea and probably cytarabine. The 5-year survival for all patients treated with rIFN-α is 57%, compared with 43% for patients treated with hydroxyurea. In patients with advanced disease or a poor prognosis (patients with a high Sokal or Hasford score), survival is not improved with rIFN-α compared with hydroxyurea. Overall, interferon increases survival by about 20 months, although achievement of a major cytogenetic response is an important correlate of prolonged survival. Even in patients with a complete cytogenetic response, however, molecular studies as determined by reverse transcriptase polymerase chain reaction for BCR-ABL chimerism continue to demonstrate residual leukemic cells in most of these patients, in contrast to the majority of successfully transplanted patients who become BCR-ABL negative by reverse transcriptase polymerase chain reaction testing.

Treatment of Blast Crisis

No substantial progress has been made in the treatment of blast phase disease except for the use of

Gleevec. In the past 20 years, a large number of drugs and drug regimens, particularly those useful in the treatment of the acute leukemias, have been tested; yet the treatment of blast phase chronic myeloid leukemia remains unsatisfactory. Using a combination of hydroxyurea, 6-mercaptopurine, and prednisone, a hematologic response rate (complete and partial remission) of approximately 30% has been achieved. This modest improvement in response is characterized by a median remission duration of seven months as compared with a survival time of two to three months for patients with no response.

Although a vincristine/prednisone combination is especially useful in other lymphatic malignancies and can induce remission in chronic myeloid leukemia, survival in lymphoid blast crisis was not significantly improved over that of myeloid blast crisis. In one study, patients with either lymphoid or myeloid blast crises were given courses of vincristine, prednisone, and cytarabine. Median survival for patients with responses was 201 days, compared with 65 days for patients without response. Most of the patients with clinical responses had a remission after a single course of therapy. These results suggest that therapeutic responsiveness in the blast crisis might depend on the intrinsic sensitivity of the blast cells regardless of type, rather than on the inherent effectiveness of the therapeutic regimen.

Allogeneic Bone Marrow (Stem Cell) Transplantation

Allogeneic stem cell transplantation (see Chapter 51) after intensive chemotherapy with cyclophosphamide and busulfan or total body irradiation (TBI) is a successful therapy for chronic myeloid leukemia in the chronic phase, because it results in cures of suitably selected patients with histocompatible siblings. There is a finite risk of near-term mortality (within the first 100 days of transplant) from treatment-related complications, a risk which increases in frequency with advancing patient age from approximately 10% for patients under age 20 years to greater than 35% to 40% in patients age 50 years or older, depending upon the transplant center and the overall physical status of the patient. Moreover, graft versus host disease also increases in frequency and severity in older patients, resulting in substantial morbidity and an impaired quality of life in 10% to 15% of potentially cured patients. The results of allogeneic stem cell transplantation are less favorable in patients who are beyond one to two years from the time of diagnosis. It is generally agreed that stem cell transplantation in accelerated and/or blast phase disease is relatively unsatisfactory. Nevertheless, 5% to 10% of patients can survive more than five years.

The true efficacy of allogeneic stem cell transplantation in the treatment of chronic phase chronic myeloid leukemia has not been evaluated in a strict fashion. Projected annual three- to five-year survival rates range from 38% to 80%, with the higher values reported from more experienced centers. In general, most studies report values around 50% to 60% and slightly lower probability for disease-free survival. Projected survival curves appear to plateau or taper more slowly after three to seven years, suggesting that allogeneic bone marrow transplantation (BMT) offers eligible patients—especially young adults with a histocompatible sibling—a prospect for cure. One must be aware, however, that most reported allogeneic stem cell trials are retrospective and nonrandomized, lack complete documentation of the clinical characteristics of the patient population (such as the status of the Philadelphia chromosome at the time of transplantation), and provide few details of the methods of patient selection. In many of these studies, the treated population had mean ages of 30 to 35 years, and few elderly patients were included. Yet, frequently, the treatment algorithms recommended for allogeneic transplantation extend to age 50 years. Large studies of registry data include patients treated variably in the chronic phase and on differing transplant protocol regimens (preparative regimens, stem cell sources, and graft-versus-host disease prophylaxis).

Strategies for when to offer allogeneic stem cell transplantation vary depending on the age of the patient, the availability of a tissue-typed matched donor, risks of the procedure, and the projected prognosis in the individual patient. Factors unfavorable for survival include early features of accelerated and blast phase disease, prior treatment with busulfan, and long duration in chronic phase.

In general, allogeneic stem cell transplantation is reserved for patients under age 55 years, although some transplant centers also treat carefully selected patients beyond this age. There is probably little reduction in benefit or increase in risk to the patient if allogeneic stem cell transplantation is deferred for one to two years. Young patients (under age 30 years), regardless of risk status, are referred early for allogeneic stem cell transplantation because of the relative effectiveness and safety of the procedure for them.

It is difficult to determine the precise benefit of allogeneic stem cell transplantation in early chronic phase chronic myeloid leukemia, because the data accrued are derived from a group of patients who have favorable characteristics. On the other hand, it is clear that for patients between 30 and 55 years old with unfavorable prognosis factors, early allogeneic stem cell transplantation provides a better prospect of survival than interferon-based therapy.

The patient's response to interferon therapy after

diagnosis provides additional helpful prognostic data. Those patients who experience a complete or major response without early relapse after interferon therapy have a lengthier survival than those who do not. Many physicians, therefore, defer a decision about allogeneic stem cell transplantation until they have had time to assess the maximum response to interferon therapy in patients who are at low risk, a process that can take up to 18 months. Because recent data suggest that interferon administration immediately prior to transplant prejudices the outcome, interferon is usually discontinued 90 days before the transplant procedure.

The efficacy of allogeneic stem cell transplantation is due in major part to the development of a graft versus leukemia (GVL) effect. The impact of an immune cellular response is apparent from several observations. Attempts to reduce the frequency of graft-versus-host disease (by depleting T-lymphocytes from the stem cell product used in transplantation) increases the relapse rate. Relapses after stem cell transplantation are less frequent in patients who have graft-versus-host disease than in those without it. Intravenous infusion of lymphocytes from the stem cell donor (without additional chemotherapy) can salvage and even cure patients who relapse after transplant. After donor lymphocyte infusion, complete cytogenetic and hematologic remission are achieved in up to three-quarters of patients, and the three-year survival is 40% to 60%.

After stem cell transplantation, complete cytogenetic responses are frequently seen. Molecular studies (e.g., reverse transcriptase polymerase chain reaction) often show persistence of the BCR-ABL gene, but this tends to disappear over the first 12 months after transplant. Subsequent reappearance of the gene after serial quantitative molecular studies usually suggests impending relapse. This is important because it is an indication for the use of donor lymphocyte infusions at a time when they are most effective, i.e., before overt hematologic relapse occurs.

The fact that only 30% of patients will have a histocompatible sibling is another limitation to allogeneic stem cell transplantation. For a fraction of patients, however, bone marrow transplant registries can identify a matched unrelated stem cell donor, although the mortality and morbidity of the procedure is increased by the use of such unrelated donors. Patients in the chronic phase of chronic myeloid leukemia can be considered for this treatment, depending upon the desires and risk tolerance of the patient and the skills of the transplant center, among other factors. These transplants, compared to those from matched sibling donors, have a higher incidence of graft failure, severe acute graft-versus-host disease, and extensive chronic graft-versus-host disease. A good-risk patient for a matched unrelated donor transplant would be a patient younger than age 30 years, early in the chronic phase, cytomegalovirus negative, and matched at the HLA-DRB1 locus. Improved molecular matching of donor-recipient matching will reduce the toxicities of a matched unrelated donor transplant but also will reduce the number of potential donors. Because of the increased risks of these transplants, most physicians reserve them for patients who present with adverse prognostic findings or for patients in the later stages of chronic myeloid leukemia.

Autologous Stem Cell Transplantation

The marrow of patients with chronic myeloid leukemia at diagnosis is a mosaic of both Philadelphia chromosome-positive and Philadelphia chromosome-negative cells. Investigators have tried multiple approaches to take advantage of this observation by attempting to separate the Philadelphia chromosome-positive cells from the Philadelphia chromosome-negative cells. The "purged" stem cells can then be used for reinfusion after high-dose chemo/radiation therapy. Techniques to obtain the proliferating normal stem cell population have included long-term stem cell cultures of hematopoietic cells (stromal cells replace growth factors, stimulating normal cell proliferation, while the Philadelphia chromosome-positive cells disappear with time in vitro) and antisense oligonucleotides directed against the BCR-ABL genomic DNA or messenger RNA. Although these in vitro studies are informative about chronic myeloid leukemia biology, they have not yielded useful clinical responses.

Imatinib Mesylate (STI-571 Gleevec)

Abnormalities of cell-signaling pathways occur in a number of human cancers. One example is the deregulated activity of enzymes known as protein tyrosine kinases, which play a key role in signal transduction. Thus, specific inhibitors of tyrosine kinases have potential therapeutic application.

BCR-ABL, the chimeric gene, is the product of the Philadelphia chromosome and the causative molecular abnormality of chronic myeloid leukemia. BCR-ABL produces a novel, constitutively activated intracellular enzyme, a specific tyrosine kinase that is necessary for its abnormal functions. An inhibitor of BCR-ABL kinase activity could thus be an ideal and specific therapy for chronic myeloid leukemia. Gleevec, a phenylaminopyrimidine, is a "small molecule" that preferentially inhibits the unphosphorylated form of the kinase domain of *ABL*. It functions through competitive inhibition at the ATP binding site of the enzyme, leading to inhibition of tyrosine phosphorylation of proteins involved in BCR-ABL signal transduction. This results in antiproliferative and apoptotic effects.

Imatinib mesylate has proven to be the most effective and least toxic of the agents used in the treatment of chronic myeloid leukemia. In chronic phase disease a randomized trial compared imatinib mesylate against the combination of cytarabine and interferon (Larson, 2002). The results with imatinib were statistically significantly better than with the combination. The drug produced a complete hematologic response in 94% of patients, a major cytogenetic response in 82%, and a complete cytogenetic response in 68%, compared to 55%, 20%, and 7%, respectively, with the combination. Progression-free survival at two years was also significantly better with imatinib. A number of patients who failed cytarabine and interferon were then given imatinib as part of the study. Responses were obtainable in the majority of patients but at a lower rate than that achieved when imatinib was the initial therapy. Other studies of patients in chronic phase who had failed interferon showed a 90% to 95% overall response rate and major cytogenetic responses in 30% to 60%.

In the accelerated phase of disease, responses were achieved by 82% of patients, with major cytogenetic responses in 24% and complete cytogenetic responses in 17%. Although the conventional dose of imatinib is 400 mg/day orally, this last study suggested that better responses could be achieved with higher doses (600 to 800 mg) without any substantial increase in toxicity. Toxicities include nausea, myalgias, edema, diarrhea, and decreased platelet and granulocyte counts.

In the blastic phase of chronic myeloid leukemia, the overall response rate was 50%; complete hematologic remission was achieved in 10% to 20% and complete cytogenetic responses in 8%.

Imatinib is also of value in treating patients who relapse after allogeneic hematopoietic stem cell transplantation. In this circumstance the complete hematologic response rate was 74% and complete cytogenetic response rate was 35%. As expected, patients who had been transplanted in chronic phase responded better to imatinib than did patients in accelerated or blast phase. However, graft-versus-host disease exacerbated in approximately one-third of patients, and severe neutropenia and thrombocytopenia eventuated in 40% of patients.

In advanced stage disease, resistance to imatinib develops after a variable period of time—and few of these responses are durable—whereas in chronic phase, durable remissions occur. Although it is too early to precisely assess the length of long-term survival from imatinib administration in chronic phase disease, the time to disease progression and early survival are better than after other forms of medical treatment. Long-term survival may prove to be much prolonged because of the substantial rate of major and complete cytogenetic responses, but there is no data available at this time. Imatinib's therapeutic efficacy, ease of oral administration, potential favorable impact on survival, and decreased morbidity and mortality associated with its use make clinical decision-making about the role and timing of allogeneic stem cell transplantation in this disease more involved. In this situation, shared decision-making and the wishes of the patient, as always, remain most important.

Treating the Patient and the Disease

Every option for the treatment of chronic phase chronic myeloid leukemia involves discussion between physician and patient of the balance between the relative benefits of different approaches and their associated risks. The choice that is selected depends on

TREATMENT

Treating the Patient and the Disease

In the context of treating the patient and the disease, how should one advise a young patient with chronic myeloid leukemia about therapy? For a relatively young individual, for whom cure is the chief objective, hematopoietic stem cell transplantation must remain a serious option until it becomes clear that Gleevec (or the combination of Gleevec with other agents) can cure a high proportion of patients or at least prolong life more than rIFN-α. If short-term survival is higher priority for the patient than is cure, then initial treatment with Gleevec seems logical, because the estimated transplant-related mortality exceeds 15% to 20%. Allogeneic stem cell transplantation should be considered as an option soon after the diagnosis of chronic myeloid leukemia is made and should not be delayed in these patients who are appropriate candidates for the procedure. If, however, Gleevec is shown to reduce progression to blast crisis and to obliterate all molecular evidence of residual leukemia, the role of transplantation in chronic myeloid leukemia will have to be reevaluated.

objective clinical variables including patient age, stage of disease, comorbid conditions, and the subjective variables related to personal preferences. The issue of trading short-term risks (including mortality), for long-term benefits is never easy. An expert panel on chronic myeloid leukemia agreed that no treatment option should be pressed on any patient without thoroughly discussing the risk and benefits involved. Shared decision-making between patient and physician is playing a more important role each day, not only in chronic myeloid leukemia, but in other diseases as well.

References

General Information

Brunstein CG, McGlave PB: The biology and treatment of chronic myelogenous leukemia. Oncol 2001;15:23–32.

Chomel J-C, Brizard F, Veinstein A, et al: Persistence of BCR-ABL genomic rearrangement in chronic myeloid leukemia patients in complete and sustained remission after interferon-α therapy or allogeneic stem cell transplantation. Blood 2000;95:404–409.

Derderian PM, Kantrjian HM, Talpaz M, et al: Chronic myelogenous leukemia in the lymphoid blastic phase: Characteristics, treatment responses and prognosis. Am J Med 1993;94:69–74.

Faderl S, Talpaz M, Estrov Z, et al: Chronic myelogenous leukemia: Biology and therapy. Ann Intern Med 1999;131:207–219.

Faderl S, Talpaz M, Estrov Z, et al: The biology of chronic myeloid leukemia. N Engl J Med 1999;341:164–172.

Faderl S, Talpaz M, Kantarjian HM, et al: Should polymerase chain reaction analysis to detect minimal residual disease in patients with chronic myelogenous leukemia be used in clinical decision making? Blood 1999;93:2755–2759.

Hehlmann R: Trial of IFN or ST1571 before proceeding to allografting for CML? Leuk 2000;14:1560–1562.

Kantarjian HM, O'Brien S, Anderlini P, et al: Treatment of chronic myelogenous leukemia: Current status and investigational options. Blood 1996;87:3069–3081.

Kurxrock R, Bueso-Ramos CE, Kantarjian H, et al: BCR rearrangement: Negative chronic myelogenous leukemia revisited. J Clin Oncol 2001;19:2915–2926.

Kvasnicka HM, Thiele J, Schmitt-Graeff A, et al: Bone marrow features improve prognostic efficiency in multivariate risk classification of chroni-phase Ph¹⁺ chronic myelogenous leukemia: A multicenter trial. J Clin Oncol 2001;19:2994–3009.

Silver RT, Woolf SH, Hehlmann R, et al: An evidence-based analysis of the effect of busulfan, hydroxyurea, interferon, and allogeneic bone marrow transplantation in treating the chronic phase of chronic myeloid leukemia. Blood 1999;94:1517–1536.

Sokal JE, Baccarani M, Russo D, et al: Staging and prognosis in chronic myelogenous leukemia. Semin Hematol 1988;25:49–61.

Tanabe T, Kuwabara T, Warashina M, et al: Oncogene inactivation in a mouse model. Nature 2000;406:473–474.

The Italian Cooperative Study Group on Chronic Myeloid Leukemia: Monitoring treatment and survival in chronic myeloid leukemia. J Clin Oncol 1999;17:1858–1868.

Bone Marrow Transplantation

Carella AM, Chimirri F, Podesta M, et al. High dose chemoradiotherapy followed by autologous Philadelphia chromosome-negative blood progenitor cell transplantation in patients with chronic myelogenous leukemia. Bone Marrow Transplant 1996;17:201–205.

Clift RA, Radich J, Appelbaum FR, et al: Long-term follow-up of a randomized study comparing cyclophosphamide and total body irradiation with busulfan and cyclophosphamide for patients receiving allogeneic marrow transplants during chronic phase of chronic myeloid leukemia. Blood 1999;94:3960–3962.

Falkenburg JHF, Smit WM, Willemze R: Cytotoxic T-lymphocyte (CTL) responses against acute or chronic myeloid leukemia. Immunol Rev 1997;157:223–230.

Giralt S, Hester J, Hugh Y, et al: CD8-depleted donor lymphocyte infusion as treatment for relapsed chronic myelogenous leukemia after allogeneic bone marrow transplantation. Blood 1995;86:4337–4343.

Mackinnon S, Papadopoulos EB, Carabasi MH, et al: Adoptive immunotherapy evaluating escalating doses of donor leukocytes for relapse of chronic myeloid leukemia after bone marrow transplantation: Separation of graft-versus-leukemia responses from graft-versus-host disease. Blood 1995;86:1261–1268.

McGlave PB, Shu XO, Wen W, et al: Unrelated donor marrow transplantation for chronic myelogenous leukemia: 9 years' experience of the National Marrow Donor Program. Blood 2000;95:2219–2225.

McGlave PB, De Fabritiis P, Deisseroth A, et al: Autologous transplants for chronic myelogenous leukemia: Results from eight transplant groups. Lancet 1994;343:1486–1488.

Molldrem JJ, Lee PP, Wang C, et al: Evidence that specific T lymphocytes may participate in the elimination of chronic myelogenous leukemia. Nature (Med) 2000;6:1018–1023.

Olavarria E, Kanfer E, Szydlo R, et al: Early detection of BCR-ABL transcripts by quantitative reverse transcriptase-polymerase chain reaction predicts outcome after allogeneic stem cell transplantation for chronic myeloid leukemia. Blood 2001;97:1560–1565.

Savage DG, Szydio RM, Chase A, et al: Bone marrow transplantation for chronic myeloid leukemia: The effects of differing criteria for defining chronic phase on probabilities of survival and relapse. Br J Haematol 1997;99:30–35.

Chemotherapy

Bolin RW, Robinson WA, Sutherland J, et al: Busulfan versus hydroxyurea in long-term therapy of chronic myelogenous leukemia. Cancer 1982;50:1683.

Coleman M, Silver RT, Pajak RF, et al. Combination chemotherapy for terminal-phase chronic granulocytic leukemia: Cancer and Leukemia Group B studies. Blood 1980;55:22.

Chronic myeloid leukemia trialists collaborative group: Hydroxyurea versus busulphan for chronic myeloid leukaemia: An individual patient data meta-analysis of three randomized trials. Br J Haematol 2000;110:573–576.

Hehlmann R, Heimpel H, Hasford J, et al: Randomized comparison of busulfan and hydroxyurea in chronic myelogenous leukemia: Prolongation of survival by hydroxyurea. Blood 1993;82:398.

Imatinib Mesylate

Beham-Schmid C, Apfelbeck U, Sill H, et al: Treatment of chronic myelogenous leukemia with the tyrosine kinase inhibitor STI571 results in marked regression of bone marrow fibrosis. Blood 2002;99:381–383.

Coutre P, Mologni L, Cleris L, et al: In vivo eradication of human BCR/ABL-positive leukemia cells with an ABL kinase inhibitor. J Natl Cancer Inst 1999;91:163–168.

Druker BJ, Talpaz M, Resta DJ, et al: Efficacy and safety of a specific inhibitor of the BCR-ABL tyrosine kinase in chronic myeloid leukemia. N Engl J Med 2001; 344:1031–1037.

Kantarjian HM, Cortes J, O'Brien S, et al: Imatinib mesylate (STI571) therapy for Philadelphia chromosome-positive chronic myelogenous leukemia in blast phase. Blood 2002;99:3547–3553.

Kantarjian HM, O'Brien S, Cortes JE, et al: Imatinib mesylate therapy for relapse after allogeneic stem cell transplantation for chronic myelogenous leukemia. Blood 2002; 100:1590–1595.

Kantarjian HM, Sawyers C, Hochhaus A, et al: Hematologic and cytogenetic responses to imatinib mesylate in chronic myelogenous leukemia. N Engl J Med 2002;346:645–652.

Larson RA: Imatinib (STI571, Gleevec) as initial therapy for patients with newly diagnosed Ph+ chronic myeloid leukemia (CML): results of a randomized phase III study vs. interferon-alpha + cytarabine (IFN + AraC). Blood 2002; 100:4a (Abstract).

Marley SB, Deininger MW, Davidson RJ, et al: The tyrosine kinase inhibitor ST1571, like interferon-alpha, preferentially reduces the capacity for amplification of granulocyte-macrophage progenitors from patients with chronic myeloid leukemia. Exp Hematol 2000;28:551–557.

Sawyers CL, Hochhaus A, Feldman E, et al: Imatinib induces hematologic and cytogenetic responses in patients with chronic myelogenous leukemia in myeloid blast crisis: results of a phase II study. Blood 2002;99:3530–3539.

Talpaz M, Silver RT, Druker BJ, et al: Imatinib induces durable hematologic and cytogenetic responses in patients with accelerated phase chronic myeloid leukemia: results of a phase 2 study. Blood 2002;99:1928–1937.

Interferon Therapy

Guihot F, Chastang C, Michallet M, et al: Interferon alfa-2b combined with cytarabine versus interferon alone in chronic myelogenous leukemia: French Chronic Myeloid Leukemia Study Group. N Engl J Med 1997;337:223–229.

Hehlmann R, Hochhaus A, Kolb HJ, et al: Interferon-α before allogeneic bone marrow transplantation in chronic myelogenous leukemia does not affect outcome adversely, provided it is discontinued at least 90 days before the procedure. Blood 1999;94:3668–3677.

The Italian Cooperative Study Group on Chronic Myeloid Leukemia: Long-term follow-up of the Italian trial of interferon-α versus conventional chemotherapy in chronic myeloid leukemia. Blood 1998;92:1541–1548.

Kurzrock R, Estrov Z, Kantarjian H, et al: Conversion of interferon-induced, long-term cytogenetic remissions in chronic myelogenous leukemia to polymerase chain reaction negativity. J Clin Oncol 1998;16:1526–1531.

MacKinnon S: Who may benefit from donor leucocyte infusions after allogeneic stem cell transplantation? Br J Haematol 2000;110:12–17.

Mahnon FX, Faberes C, Pueyo S, et al: Response at three months is a good predictive factor for newly diagnosed chronic myeloid leukemia patients treated by recombinant interferon-alpha. Blood 1998;92:4059–4065.

Ozer H, George SL, Schiffer CA, et al. Prolonged subcutaneous administration of recombinant alpha2b interferon in patients with previously untreated Philadelphia chromosome-positive chronic-phase chronic myelogenous leukemia: Effect on remission duration and survival. Cancer and Leukemia Group B Study 8583. Blood 1993;82:2975.

Talpaz M, Kantarjian HM, McCredie KB, et al: Hematologic remission and cytogenetic improvement induced by recombinant human interferon alpha in chronic myelogenous leukemia. N Engl J Med 1986;314:1065–1069.

Talpaz M, O'Brien S, Cortes J, et al: Phase I study of pegylated-interferon α-2A (PEGASYS) in patients with chronic myelogenous leukemia (CML). Blood 1999;94(Suppl 1):530a.

The Italian Cooperative Study Group on Chronic Myeloid Leukemia: Long-term follow-up of the Italian trial of interferon-alpha versus conventional chemotherapy in chronic myeloid leukemia. Blood 1998;92:1541–1548.

Philadelphia Chromosome

Barbany G, Hagberg A, Olsson-Stromberg U, et al: Manifold-assisted reverse transcription-PCR with real-time detection for measurement of the BCR-ABL fusion transcript in chronic myeloid leukemia patients. Clin Chem 2000;46: 913–920.

Dewald GW, Wyatt WA, Juneau AL, et al: Highly sensitive fluorescence in situ hybridization method to detect double BCR/ABL fusion and monitor response to therapy in chronic myeloid leukemia. Blood 1998;91:3357–3365.

Guo JQ, Wang JYG, Arlinghaus RB: Detection of BCR-ABL proteins in blood cells of benign phase chronic myelogenous leukemia patients. Cancer Res 1991;51:3048–3051.

Heisterkamp N, Jenster G, ten Hoeve J, et al: Acute leukemia in BCR/ABL transgenic mice. Nature 1990;344:251–253.

Muhlmann J, Thaler J, Hilbe W, et al: Fluorescent in situ hybridization (FISH) on peripheral blood smears for monitoring Philadelphia chromosome-positive chronic myeloid leukemia (CML) during interferon treatment: a new strategy for remission assessment. Genes Chrom Cancer 1998;21:90–100.

Nowell P, Hungerford D: A minute chromosome in human granulocytic leukemia. Science 1960;132:1497.

Verma RS, Chandra P: Clinical significance of reverse BCR/ABL gene rearrangement in Ph-negative chronic myelogenous leukemia. Leuk Res 2000;24:631–635.

Chapter 72
Chronic Lymphocytic Leukemia and Hairy Cell Leukemia

Bruce D. Cheson

Chronic Lymphocytic Leukemia

Epidemiology

Chronic lymphocytic leukemia (CLL) is the most common adult leukemia in Western countries; approximately 7500 to 12,500 new cases are diagnosed in the United States each year. It appears more often in Jewish people of Russian or Eastern European ancestry and is not often seen in Asians. Chronic lymphocytic leukemia is more common in men than in women and increases in incidence with age. The median age at diagnosis is 65 years, and fewer than 20% of patients are under age 55 years. Young patients tend to die from chronic lymphocytic leukemia–related events, whereas older patients more frequently succumb to secondary malignancies and causes unrelated to chronic lymphocytic leukemia. Although the incidence is increased in family members of patients with chronic lymphocytic leukemia, the etiology of the disease is unknown. No risk factors have been identified.

Cytogenetics

Conventional banding techniques detect cytogenetic abnormalities in approximately one-half of the cases, but fluorescent in situ hybridization (FISH) now identifies abnormalities in more than 80% of cases. The most common cytogenetic abnormality involves deletions of 13q, which is present in more than half of cases either alone or in combination with other abnormalities. Patients with 13q14 abnormalities tend to have a benign course and experience a normal life span. Deletions of 11q23 are found in 18% of cases and are associated with massive lymphadenopathy that is often out of proportion to the peripheral blood lymphocytosis. Trisomy 12 occurs in 16% of cases. The leukemia cells in these cases have an atypical morphology, and patient outcome is poor.

Cytogenetic studies provide useful prognostic information, but they are expensive, not readily available, and cannot as yet be used to guide the choice of therapy. Therefore, cytogenetic analysis is not part of the routine evaluation of patients with chronic lymphocytic leukemia.

Molecular Biology

The malignant lymphocytes in chronic lymphocytic leukemia are not in a state of abnormally rapid proliferation; rather, the disease results from the progressive accumulation of immunologically incompetent cells because of a defect in apoptosis (normal programmed cell death). BCL-2 gene expression blocks apoptosis, and the gene is overexpressed in more than 70% of cases, even in the absence of the chromosomal rearrangements. No single oncogene has been implicated in the pathogenesis of chronic lymphocytic leukemia. The translocations associated with BCL-2 [t(14;18)(q32;q21)] and BCL-3 [t(14;19)(q32;q13.1)] are detected in only 5% to 10% of cases. Abnormalities of the tumor suppressor oncogene, p53, occur in at least 15% of patients. These patients have a high percentage of circulating prolymphocyte forms, advanced clinical stage at presentation, chemotherapy resistance, and a poor prognosis.

Clinical Presentation

Most patients with chronic lymphocytic leukemia are diagnosed based on blood counts obtained during routine evaluation or during an examination for another medical disorder. More than half of patients are asymptomatic at diagnosis, and the physical examination is initially normal in 20% to 30%. Approximately one quarter of patients seek medical attention because of an enlarged lymph node (see Chapter 35), which is often mistaken for an infectious process and treated initially with antibiotics. Only when the enlargement persists and the blood counts are examined is the diagnosis of chronic lymphocytic leukemia made. As the disease progresses, generalized lymphadenopathy and splenomegaly become common. Although the lymphocytes of chronic lymphocytic leukemia pass freely through the circulation, they rarely damage other organs.

Clinical Features

Infections

Hypogammaglobulinemia is a common occurrence in chronic lymphocytic leukemia, increasing in frequency with the passage of time and the development of advanced disease. Increased susceptibility to infection results from a diminished antibody response to bacterial antigens, coupled with abnormal activation of the complement system. Common pathogens are those that require opsonization for bacterial killing, such as *S. pneumoniae, S. aureus,* and *H. influenzae.* Treatment with one of the nucleoside analogs (fludarabine, cladribine [2-chlorodeoxyadenosine] and pentostatin [deoxycoformycin]) heightens the risk of opportunistic infections with *Candida, Listeria,* pneumocystis, cytomegalovirus, *Aspergillus,* herpes viruses, and others that were rarely encountered before these chemotherapeutic agents were in common use. A febrile patient with chronic lymphocytic leukemia receiving one of these drugs could require aggressive diagnostic measures. Moreover, despite the expense, many physicians employ prophylactic antibiotics in all patients receiving fludarabine, including sulfamethoxazole/trimethoprim (two days each week to prevent pneumocystis), fluconazole (antifungal), and in some cases, acyclovir (to prevent herpes virus infection). Prophylactic antibiotics are especially indicated in the treatment of elderly or frail patients, prior treatment failures, patients who have had previous serious infections, or those who are on corticosteroids.

In patients who are hypogammaglobulinemic and who experience recurrent severe infections such as pneumonia and sinusitis, intravenous administration of immunoglobulins every three weeks reduces the incidence of bacterial infections. This measure is rarely necessary because in most such patients, daily oral antibiotics are safe and protective, even when administered over long periods of time.

Aggressive Transformation

In most patients with chronic lymphocytic leukemia, symptoms are initially absent or minimal, and the disease pursues an indolent pace. One-half of the patients continue to have relatively slow-growing or stable manifestations of disease over many years and require no treatment. In the other patients, the disease progresses more rapidly and is associated with increasing lymphocytosis, enlarging lymph nodes, increasing splenomegaly, anemia, and thrombocytopenia. Chemotherapy is needed for this group. Constitutional symptoms of fever, night sweats, and weight loss can supervene. Once these symptoms appear, median disease-free survival is only 12 to 18 months. Usually, the evolution to increasingly aggressive disease is not accompanied by changes in lymphocyte morphology.

In some patients, however, the morphology itself is altered. The most common transformation is to the appearance of a large cell lymphoma known as Richter's syndrome. Patients characteristically present with increasing lymphadenopathy, hepatosplenomegaly, fever, abdominal pain, weight loss, progressive anemia, and thrombocytopenia, associated with a rapid rise in the peripheral blood lymphocyte count, which can contain circulating lymphoma cells. A lymph node biopsy is often required to confirm the transition. Richter's syndrome responds poorly to the usual systemic therapy (cyclophosphamide, Adriamycin, vincristine, and prednisone) administered for large cell lymphomas, and the median survival is four to five months. Nucleoside analog-based regimens might provide longer survival.

Chronic lymphocytic leukemia can also evolve into prolymphocytic leukemia, which is associated with at least 55% prolymphocytes (large lymphocytes with increased cytoplasm and prominent nucleoli) in the peripheral blood, progressive lymphadenopathy, hepatosplenomegaly, worsening anemia, thrombocytopenia, a wasting syndrome, and increasing resistance to therapy.

Autoimmunity

The immunologic dyscrasia that is part of the picture of chronic lymphocytic leukemia not only causes reduced production of immunoglobulins but also is associated with autoimmune phenomena. For example, a direct antiglobulin (Coombs' test) is positive at diagnosis in 20% to 30% of patients with chronic lymphocytic leukemia. Despite the high frequency of positive laboratory tests, clinically significant hemolysis occurs in only 10% to 25% of these patients. Autoimmune thrombocytopenia occurs in approximately 2% of patients.

Immune hemolytic anemia and thrombocytopenia respond readily to the same therapies employed in the management of patients without chronic lymphocytic leukemia who have these disorders. Responses to corticosteroids such as prednisone (60 to 100 mg/day orally) are frequent, usually allowing subsequent tapering to low maintenance-dose levels. Patients who are unresponsive to corticosteroids might respond to high-dose intravenous immunoglobulins using an initial loading dose of 2 g/kg over two days, followed by repeated courses at lower doses every two to three weeks as needed. Impressive results have been noted following therapy with rituximab given at 375 mg/m² weekly for four consecutive weeks. As the principal site of clearance of antibody (IgG)-coated red blood cells and platelets is the spleen, splenectomy can be helpful when systemic approaches fail. Splenic irradiation induces only transient responses and causes myelosuppression.

Pure red cell aplasia is an uncommon disorder characterized by severe anemia, without neutropenia or thrombocytopenia. The bone marrow is nearly devoid of red blood cell precursors, and the reticulocyte count is almost zero, reflecting the total absence of red blood cell production. Although this clinical picture can result transiently from parvovirus infection, it also occurs due to the development of antibodies that bind to determinants on red blood cell precursors in the bone marrow and destroy them. Corticosteroids alone or with cyclosporine are often effective in restoring erythropoiesis.

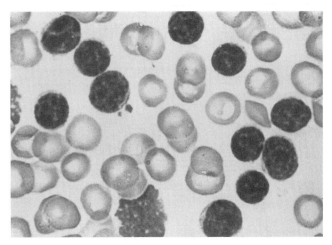

Figure 72-1 ■ Peripheral blood smear from a patient with chronic lymphocytic leukemia demonstrating small, mature-appearing lymphocytes with smudge cells.

Second Malignancies

Secondary malignancies occur with increased frequency in patients with chronic lymphocytic leukemia, a feature related to the immune defects of this disease as well as to the consequences of therapy. The most frequently diagnosed conditions are lung cancers and melanomas, but other solid tumors and hematologic malignancies also occur. The astute clinician needs to be alert to the possibility of this development in order to avoid the error of attributing any alterations to the chronic lymphocytic leukemia itself.

Clinical Evaluation

The possibility of chronic lymphocytic leukemia should be suspected when the complete blood count and differential detects at least 5000/μL small, mature-appearing lymphocytes (Figure 72-1). The nuclear chromatin is condensed, and nucleoli are not visible. These cells are fragile, easily rupturing from the shearing stress of making the peripheral blood film, resulting in cellular debris called smudge cells (see Figure 72-1). These findings are diagnostic of chronic lymphocytic leukemia, even in the absence of a bone marrow examination or immunophenotypic characterization. A small percentage of patients present with atypical lymphocyte forms in the blood and/or atypical clinical findings, raising the possibility of other diagnoses. The differential diagnosis includes prolymphocytic leukemia, hairy cell leukemia, or the leukemic phase of non-Hodgkin's lymphomas. Immunophenotyping (Figure 72-2) is of substantial value in distinguishing among these disorders and also permits the identification of the small number of patients (5%) who present with T cell rather than B cell chronic lymphocytic leukemia. Chronic lymphocytic leukemia cells are characterized by the expression of the B cell markers CD19, CD20, CD23, and, paradoxically in this B cell disorder, by CD5, which is a T cell marker. Surface immunoglobulins are expressed with low intensity.

The bone marrow in chronic lymphocytic leukemia is infiltrated by greater than 30% lymphocytes. A bone marrow aspirate and biopsy are generally not required for the diagnosis of chronic lymphocytic leukemia, however, because the peripheral blood smear examination is usually definitive. Nevertheless, bone marrow examination, by revealing the extent and pattern of infiltration, does provide prognostic information and can be used as a point of comparison to measure response to therapy.

Clinical evaluation (Table 72-1) includes a careful physical examination with particular attention to the location and size of enlarged lymph nodes. Helpful laboratory tests are a complete blood count, white blood cell count and differential, platelet count, and blood chemistries to assess hepatic and renal function. Other tests include a direct antiglobulin test to assess the possibility that an overt hemolytic anemia could supervene. A reticulocyte count is useful even when the hemoglobin is normal to rule out ongoing compensated hemolysis, and a quantitative immunoglobulin determination provides a measure of immunologic impairment. A chest X-ray serves as a baseline for comparison with subsequent films, especially when questions of infection later arise; however, computed tomography (CT) and other scans are not

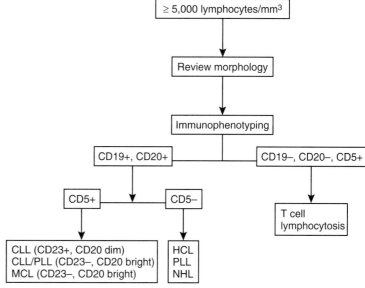

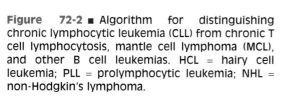

Figure 72-2 ■ Algorithm for distinguishing chronic lymphocytic leukemia (CLL) from chronic T cell lymphocytosis, mantle cell lymphoma (MCL), and other B cell leukemias. HCL = hairy cell leukemia; PLL = prolymphocytic leukemia; NHL = non-Hodgkin's lymphoma.

Table 72-1 ■ Recommendations for Evaluation and Monitoring of Chronic Lymphocytic Leukemia Patients

Pretreatment Evaluation

History and physical examination	Yes
Complete blood and platelet counts; reticulocyte count; blood smear examination; blood chemistries; direct antiglobulin test; quantitative immunoglobulins	Yes
Immunophenotyping	Yes
Bone marrow aspiration/biopsy	No
Cytogenetic/molecular studies	No
Computed tomography scans, magnetic resonance imaging, gallium scan	No

needed for routine initial evaluation. They should be obtained only for specific clinical indications. A lymph node biopsy is not appropriate and adds nothing to the evaluation.

Prognosis

Chronic lymphocytic leukemia can exhibit a highly variable clinical course. Some patients might not require therapy for many years and eventually die of unrelated causes, whereas others die from disease-related complications within a few months of diagnosis despite appropriate therapy. The first widely accepted prognostic grouping of patients was the Rai classification (Table 72-2). The median survival for each individual stage is 12.5 years for stage 0, seven years for stages I and II, two years for stage III, and 1.5 years for stage IV. This system was recently simplified to three categories: "low-risk" (stage 0); "intermediate-risk" (stages I to II); and "high-risk" (stages

DIAGNOSIS

Clinical Observations: Chronic Lymphocytic Leukemia

Because the percentage of neutrophils in the peripheral smear is low in chronic lymphocytic leukemia, patients are frequently thought to be neutropenic. If the patient has a white blood cell count of 50,000/μL and the differential shows 3% neutrophils, however, then the absolute neutrophil count is 1500/μL, and the patient is in fact not neutropenic.

One has to be wary in chronic lymphocytic leukemia not to conclude inappropriately that advancing disease, rather than an occult infection, is causing fever.

Similarly, when anemia progresses in chronic lymphocytic leukemia, one must always consider whether iron deficiency is present in order not to miss an occult concurrent gastrointestinal cancer.

Table 72-2 ▪ The Rai System for Clinical Staging of Chronic Lymphocytic Leukemia

Stage	Clinical Features	Three-Stage System	Median Survival (Years)
0	Lymphocytosis in blood and bone marrow	Low-Risk Category	12.5
I	+ Lymphadenopathy	Intermediate-Risk Category	7
II	+ Splenomegaly ± Hepatomegaly		
III	+ Anemia	High-Risk Category	1.5 to 4
IV	+ Thrombocytopenia		

III to IV). The Binet system (Table 72-3) designates stage A as involvement of less than three node-bearing areas (median survival greater than 12 years); stage B, three or more node-bearing areas (median survival seven years); stage C, anemia and/or thrombocytopenia (median survival two to four years). The Rai classification is most commonly used in the United States, while the Binet system is in common use in Europe. A major difference between the two classification systems is that the Binet system fails to identify Rai stage 0 patients. The two systems have similar prognostic value.

Because the outcome for individual patients is variable within each clinical stage, other prognostic indicators are sought to separate patients into clinically meaningful risk groups, with a view to tailor treatment recommendations to each patient's outlook. An algorithm for the initial evaluation and treatment of chronic lymphocytic leukemia appears in Figure 72-3. Poor prognostic factors include male gender, African American race, impaired performance status, diffuse bone marrow infiltration, and rapid lymphocyte doubling time. Laboratory findings that predict for a poor outcome include cytogenetic abnormalities, elevated serum β_2-microglobulin or soluble CD23, unmutated variable region of the heavy chain genes, and expression of CD38. Not all of these tests are routinely available.

Therapy

Initial Treatment

Chronic lymphocytic leukemia is usually responsive to initial therapy but is not curable. Many patients with this disease do not require therapy for months or years after diagnosis. Moreover, randomized trials have failed to show a survival advantage for early intervention in patients with limited-stage, asymptomatic disease. Therefore, identifying the optimal time to treat is an important decision. Initiation of therapy is warranted in the setting of disease-related symptoms (e.g., fevers, chills, weight loss, pronounced fatigue), increasing bone marrow failure with anemia and/or thrombocytopenia, autoimmune anemia or thrombocytopenia, massive or progressive hepatosplenomegaly or lymphadenopathy, or recurrent infections. A lymphocyte count that doubles in less than 6 months is an unfavorable sign of the disease's aggressive behavior and supports the decision to treat. One should be wary of tumor lysis syndrome with initial therapy even though it is extremely rare in chronic lymphocytic leukemia (see Chapter 117). It can be fatal and is not consistently prevented by the use of prophylactic allopurinol and/or hydration.

Alkylating Agents

The oral alkylating agent chlorambucil has been the treatment of choice for decades. When administered

Table 72-3 ▪ The Binet System for Clinical Staging of Chronic Lymphocytic Leukemia

Group	Clinical Features
A	<3 involved node areas; no anemia or thrombocytopenia
B	≥3 involved node areas; no anemia or thrombocytopenia
C	Hemoglobin <10 g/dL and/or platelets <100,000/μL

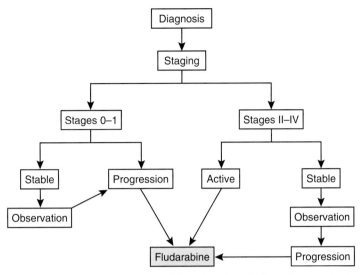

Figure 72-3 ■ Treatment algorithm for chronic lymphocytic leukemia.

at a dose of 4 to 8 mg/m^2 daily for four to eight weeks, or as pulsed doses of 15 to 30 mg/m^2 every two to four weeks, responses occur in approximately 30% to 70% of patients; complete responses are rarely seen. Cyclophosphamide appears to have similar activity but is more often used in combination chemotherapy regimens.

Corticosteroids

Although they are lympholytic, corticosteroids are less active than alkylating agents and should be reserved to treat autoimmune complications because of the risks of infections, diabetes, and osteoporosis that accompany their prolonged administration.

Fludarabine

Fludarabine is the treatment of choice because it is the most active agent for the treatment of chronic lymphocytic leukemia with an overall response rate of 70%, including 30% complete remissions. Fludarabine is administered as an intravenous bolus of 25 mg/m^2 daily for five consecutive days once a month for approximately six months. Patients failing to show any response to two to three courses should be

---

TREATMENT

Initial Therapy of Chronic Lymphocytic Leukemia

Treatment of chronic lymphocytic leukemia is not curative. Moreover, treatment in early-stage asymptomatic chronic lymphocytic leukemia does not prolong survival, and many patients live normally for years without any treatment. Therefore, therapy is generally deferred until the presence of one or more of the following indications:

- Disease-related symptoms
- Massive and/or progressive lymphadenopathy
- Recurrent infections
- Bone marrow compromise with cytopenias
- Autoimmune hemolytic anemia or thrombocytopenia

An increase in the lymphocyte count by itself is not justification for treatment. In chronic lymphocytic leukemia, unlike chronic myeloid leukemia, the increasing white blood cell count does not impose a metabolic burden. Even elevation of the white blood cell count to 300,000/μL or higher, when unaccompanied by other alterations in disease status, does not produce any symptoms. The small size of the chronic lymphocytic leukemia lymphocytes and their deformability poses no risk of microvascular obstruction (such as can occur in the acute leukemias), and hyperviscosity syndrome does not occur in chronic lymphocytic leukemia until the white blood cell count is greater than 1,000,000/μL.

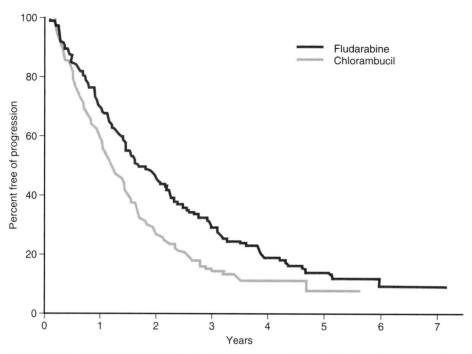

Figure 72-4 ■ Progression-free survival in randomized trial of fludarabine versus chlorambucil. (From Rai KR, Peterson BL, Appelbaum FR, et al: Fludarabine compared with chlorambucil as primary therapy for chronic lymphocytic leukemia. N Engl J Med 2000;343:1750–1757.)

offered alternate treatment. Patients who achieve a complete remission probably do not warrant additional treatment. For those patients achieving a partial remission, therapy is generally continued to the time of maximal response plus two additional courses, not to exceed six to nine months because of concern about cumulative myelotoxicity. Other schedules have not been as active. The oral bioavailability of fludarabine is about 50%, and an oral formulation is in clinical trials.

In several randomized trials, fludarabine induces higher response rates than alkylating agents, with a longer disease-free survival and time to progression (Figure 72-4). No survival advantage has been observed, however (Figure 72-5). This observation is related, in part, to the ability to salvage alkylating agent failures by the later administration of fludarabine. Elderly patients with a reduced performance status may be treated with chlorambucil or reduced doses of fludarabine (30 mg/m^2/day for three days). Although this treatment is not as effective as the standard schedule, toxicity is substantially reduced.

The major toxicities associated with fludarabine are moderate myelosuppression and severe immunosuppression, with occasional neurotoxicity, particularly at higher than recommended doses. Lymphocyte counts, particularly the CD4 cells, decrease within weeks and do not return to normal for a year or longer after treatment is discontinued. Fludarabine is not significantly more myelotoxic than alkylating agents, but it is associated with an increased risk of opportunistic infections because of its immunosuppression, leading to consideration of antifungal and pneumocystis prophylaxis. In some patients with chronic lymphocytic leukemia, fludarabine seems to evoke autoimmune hemolytic anemia and/or immune thrombocytopenia. It might be advisable to consider alternative therapy in patients who have a positive direct antiglobulin test or are actively hemolyzing. The increased frequency of secondary malignancies in patients with chronic lymphocytic leukemia is not further augmented by therapy with fludarabine.

The other nucleoside analogs, cladribine and pentostatin, are less active than fludarabine in chronic lymphocytic leukemia and, therefore, are less often used.

Combination Chemotherapy

Compared with chlorambucil therapy as a single agent, most randomized trials have failed to demonstrate a benefit for combination regimens such as cyclophosphamide and prednisone (CP), cyclophosphamide, vincristine, and prednisone (CVP), or cyclophosphamide, Adriamycin (hydroxydaunorubicin), vincristine, and prednisone (CHOP). Similarly, combinations of fludarabine with chlorambucil, anthracyclines or related compounds, cytarabine, and

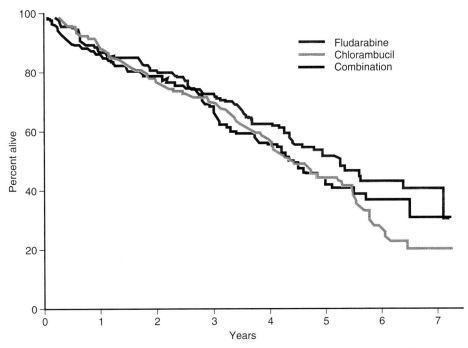

Figure 72-5 ■ Survival in randomized trial of fludarabine versus chlorambucil. (From Rai KR, Peterson BL, Appelbaum FR, et al: Fludarabine compared with chlorambucil as primary therapy for chronic lymphocytic leukemia. N Engl J Med 2000;343:1750–1757.)

alpha-interferon are not clearly superior to fludarabine alone. The addition of prednisone to fludarabine does not increase the response rate but is associated with increased toxicity, consisting of more frequent opportunistic and other infections. Clinical trials of the combination of fludarabine and cyclophosphamide suggest an improved response rate. Toxicity is increased as well, however; fevers of unknown origin, pulmonary toxicity, and pneumonia occur in a substantial percentage of patients. The value of this combination is being tested in ongoing randomized trials.

Second-Line Therapy

Second-line treatment for chronic lymphocytic leukemia patients poses its own challenges because of diminished bone marrow reserves from the disease and prior therapy. In patients with chronic lymphocytic leukemia who relapse after or are refractory to initial treatment, referral for inclusion in a clinical research study should be considered. For patients who are not eligible for or are unwilling to participate in clinical trials, salvage therapy is determined by the choice of and response to initial treatment.

Patients who responded to an alkylating agent might respond again to the same drug. Significant responses are uncommon, however, and response duration will be shorter than after the initial treatment. Fludarabine is now the standard secondary agent for patients initially treated with an alkylating agent-based regimen. Complete clinical and hematologic remissions are achieved in 3% to 13% of such patients, with an overall response rate of 40% to 50% that varies with patient age, performance status, and other factors.

Most patients who are initially treated with fludarabine and whose disease response persists for more than one year experience a second response to fludarabine readministration. For these patients, the median time to progression is 18 months; median survival is 29 months for relapsed patients and less than half as long in treatment-refractory patients. Indeed, few effective therapeutic options are available for patients whose disease is refractory to fludarabine. The use of an alternative nucleoside generally does not result in a meaningful response but can result in significant toxicity.

Other Treatment Approaches

New cytotoxic drugs are being studied in patients with chronic lymphocytic leukemia, as are new biologic therapies such as CAMPATH-1H and rituximab.

CAMPATH-1H

CAMPATH-1H is a chimeric humanized monoclonal antibody that recognizes the CD52 antigen, which is present on 95% of B cells and T cells. Responses occur in one-third of patients who have failed other treatments, including fludarabine. CAMPATH-1H causes profound and durable T cell depletion, increasing the risk of opportunistic infections. In relapsed patients, CAMPATH-1H is more active in clearing peripheral blood and bone marrow involvement than disease in the lymph nodes. Changing the dose and duration of administration has given preliminary evidence of decreasing lymph node size.

Rituximab

Rituximab is an anti-CD20 antibody that induces responses in 50% of patients with follicular/low-grade non-Hodgkin's lymphomas. At the dose and schedule used in lymphomas, it has not demonstrated much activity in patients with chronic lymphocytic leukemia, where response rates are in the range of 10% to 15% and few complete remissions are seen. Higher response rates are seen when the antibody is used as initial therapy. Rituximab might sensitize tumor cells to chemo-therapy agents, and combinations of the antibody with fludarabine appear to be additive or synergistic. Patients with chronic lymphocytic leukemia who are treated with this antibody are at risk for potentially life-threatening toxicities characterized by abrupt release of multiple cytokines on intravenous administration, as this agent binds to the large numbers of cells that are present. These effects decrease with time, and long treatment courses improve rituximab's effectiveness.

Allogeneic Stem Cell Transplantation

Allogeneic bone marrow transplantation is not often performed in chronic lymphocytic leukemia because many affected patients are elderly and unacceptable candidates. Of those younger patients who undergo this therapy, approximately one-half experience prolonged leukemia-free survival. The occurrence of late relapses, however, raises questions about the curative potential of this approach. Moreover, the treatment-related death rate is 25% to 50%. Patients should be carefully selected for allogeneic bone marrow transplantation because of the risks. In general, it is reserved for younger patients who have failed fludarabine and who have an HLA-identical sibling.

Splenectomy

Splenectomy might provide effective palliation in patients with chronic lymphocytic leukemia who have failed systemic treatment and have persistent splenomegaly and/or persistent cytopenias that preclude further therapy. Of the cytopenias, thrombocy-topenia is the most likely to respond to splenectomy. When performed by an experienced surgeon, the mortality of the procedure is less than 10%.

Erythropoietin Therapy

This option can ameliorate anemia in chronic lymphocytic leukemia. In many patients with advanced chronic lymphocytic leukemia, the etiology of the anemia is multifactorial, including splenic sequestration, hemolysis, and bone marrow replacement by chronic lymphocytic leukemia cells. Nevertheless, erythropoietin may reduce transfusion requirements in selected patients who are first documented to have low circulating endogenous levels of erythropoietin.

Assessment of Response to Therapy in Chronic Lymphocytic Leukemia

In order to standardize the conduct of clinical trials, the National Cancer Institute–sponsored Working Group has defined the criteria for treatment of chronic lymphocytic leukemia, response to therapy, and assessment of toxicity. Moreover, the Group established guidelines for dose modifications for drug-related myelosuppression and a grading system for infectious complications. Although this consensus was developed for the purpose of clinical trials, the outline in Table 72-4 also provides a useful framework for the clinician.

Follow-up Evaluation

The frequency with which patients with chronic lymphocytic leukemia are followed is determined by the extent and level of activity of the disease. Following initial evaluation, patients who appear to be clinically stable should be seen again in two to three months to assess the pace of their disease. Patients whose blood counts remain stable and who are asymptomatic can then be seen every four to six months. For patients with advancing disease, the frequency of visits is determined by clinical indications.

Prolymphocytic Leukemia

B Cell Type

Patients with B cell prolymphocytic leukemia (PLL) tend to be older (median age in the 70s) than those with chronic lymphocytic leukemia and are usually symptomatic. Virtually all present with advanced-stage disease at diagnosis, with a much larger spleen and a higher white blood cell count, but with less pronounced lymphadenopathy than in chronic lymphocytic leukemia. Examination of the peripheral blood reveals large cells with a round nucleus and a prominent nucleolus. In de novo prolymphocytic leukemia,

Table 72-4 ■ Revised NCI-Working Group Guidelines for Chronic Lymphocytic Leukemia

Diagnosis

Absolute lymphocyte count: Greater than 5000/μL
Immunophenotype: One or more B cell markers (CD19, CD20, CD23) + CD5
"Atypical" cells (e.g., prolymphocytes): <55%
Duration of lymphocytosis: None required
Bone marrow lymphocytes: Equal to or greater than 30%

Staging

Modified (three stage) Rai

Response Criteria*

Complete Response	
Physical examination	Normal
Symptoms	None
Lymphocyte count	Equal to or greater than 4000/μL
Neutrophil count	Equal to or greater than 1500/μL
Platelet count	Greater than 100,000/μL
Hemoglobin (untransfused)	Greater than 11 g/dL
Bone marrow lymphocytes	Less than 30%; no nodules

Partial Response	
Physical examination	At least a 50% decrease in nodes, liver, and spleen. Plus one or more of the following:
Neutrophils	Equal to or greater than 1500/μL
Platelets	Greater than 100,000/μL
Hemoglobin	Greater than 11 g/dL or 50% improvement from baseline

*To qualify, response must persist for more than two months.

most of the peripheral blood mononuclear cells tend to be prolymphocytes. In the less common setting of transformation from chronic lymphocytic leukemia, a dimorphic population is noted. The presence of the t(11;14) clonal chromosomal abnormality in a number of cases of de novo prolymphocytic leukemia suggests a relationship of this disease to mantle cell lymphoma, which frequently carries the same translocation.

Patients with prolymphocytic leukemia respond poorly to single-agent or combination chemotherapy, with overall response rates of less than 25% and rare complete responses. The median survival for de novo prolymphocytic leukemia is three years. Survival is much shorter for patients whose disease arises as a secondary transformation from chronic lymphocytic leukemia. Small series suggest impressive activity for nucleoside analogs, and anecdotal responses have been reported with CAMPATH-1H.

T cell Type

Patients with T cell prolymphocytic leukemia present with massive splenomegaly, lymphadenopathy (in 40% of patients), and skin infiltration (in 20% of patients). The initial white blood cell count is usually greater than 100,000/μL. The prognosis is poor, and median survival is seven months. Pentostatin results in complete responses in 5% to 10% of patients and partial responses in 33%. CAMPATH-1H also appears to be a promising agent in this disease. Of 15 patients, most of whom had failed pentostatin, major responses occurred in 11 (70%) and complete responses in 9 (60%).

Hairy Cell Leukemia

Hairy cell leukemia is a rare illness. Approximately 500 new patients are diagnosed each year in the United States—generally older persons, with a strong male predominance. Patients most often present with symptoms referable to cytopenias, including infections in 29% and weakness or fatigue in 27%. Less common presentations include left upper quadrant pain related to splenomegaly (5%) or bleeding related to thrombocytopenia (4%). The most common findings include palpable splenomegaly (80%), hepatomegaly (15%), "hairy" cells in the peripheral blood, thrombocytopenia (50%), anemia (75%), and neutropenia (absolute neutrophil count less than 500/μL in 35%). These patients experience an increased incidence of second malignancies.

The cells in the peripheral blood have an eccentric, spongiform, kidney-shaped nucleus, with charac-

DIAGNOSIS

Monocytopenia in Hairy Cell Leukemia

Most infections, inflammatory disorders, and neoplasms (including hematologic malignancies) are associated with an increase in circulating monocytes. Hairy cell leukemia is one of the few disorders associated with monocytopenia, and its presence is a helpful clue to the diagnosis.

teristic filamentous cytoplasmic projections. The bone marrow exhibits dense reticulin fibrosis, making bone marrow inaspirable. Bone marrow biopsy is therefore required to make the diagnosis. Bone marrow biopsy discloses heavy infiltration with small lymphocytes of relatively benign appearance (no nucleoli and compacted chromatin) with large clear zones around each nucleus. For a skilled hematopathologist, these findings are pathognomonic of the disease. The malignant cells are of B cell origin, expressing CD19, CD20, and the monocytic antigen CD11c. The cells also stain for tartrate-resistant acid phosphatase (TRAP). Perhaps the most specific marker is CD103 (Bly-7).

A hairy cell leukemia variant has been identified. The variant form is associated with a high circulating white blood cell count, cells with bilobed nuclei and prominent nucleoli, a bone marrow showing interstitial infiltration of clumped cells, and resistance to treatment with alpha-interferon, cladribine, and pentostatin, to which classical hairy cell leukemia readily responds.

Therapy

Hairy cell leukemia is a very slowly developing neoplasm in most patients. It can run an indolent course, and 10% of patients might never require therapy. Treatment is instituted because of massive or progressive splenomegaly, severe or worsening cytopenias, recurrent infections, more than 20,000/μL hairy cells in the peripheral blood, or bulky lymphadenopathy. Splenectomy was formerly the standard treatment because it relieved symptoms related to splenomegaly and improved peripheral blood counts, but it did not affect the extensive infiltration of the bone marrow and lymph nodes. Splenectomy is now reserved for the rare patient who is refractory to other therapies.

Interferon-alpha was the first active systemic therapy in hairy cell leukemia. At doses of $2 \times 10^6 \, U/m^2$/daily or $3 \times 10^6 \, U/m^2$ three times each week administered subcutaneously, interferon-alpha induces responses in 80% of patients, but only 10% of these are complete responses. The disease inevitably recurs after interferon-alpha is discontinued. Maintenance therapy is, however, associated with excessive toxicity and expense without apparent survival benefit. Many patients who recur will respond when retreated.

The purine analogs have revolutionized the treatment of these patients. Pentostatin at doses of $4 \, mg/m^2$ intravenously every other week for four to six months results in complete remissions in 60% to 89% of patients (including those who have failed interferon-alpha) and overall response rates of 80% to 90%. Moreover, only 30% of patients relapse even after prolonged (greater than 10 years) of follow-up. In a randomized trial of 350 previously untreated patients with hairy cell leukemia, the complete remission rate was 11% in the patients receiving interferon-alpha versus 76% for those receiving pentostatin, with a significant benefit for the latter in the duration of the response.

Patients treated with cladribine, given as a seven-day continuous intravenous infusion or as a two-hour infusion for five to seven days, achieve a response in 80% to 90% of patients, including 65% to 80% complete remissions. Strikingly, in the great majority of patients, a single course of therapy suffices to bring about complete remission. Responses tend to be durable, with only 20% to 30% of patients relapsing. As is true after pentostatin treatment, relapse is often characterized only by an increase in bone marrow hairy cells, with no indication for treatment. Most patients who require retreatment achieve a second durable response to the same or alternate nucleoside analog. Although the toxicity may be somewhat greater than pentostatin, cladribine's shorter duration of treatment and the fact that it can also be given subcutaneously make it the preferred choice for initial therapy for many physicians. Nevertheless, the response rates of pentostatin and cladribine are comparable.

References

Chronic Lymphocytic Leukemia

General Information

Cheson BD, Bennett JM, Grever M, et al: National Cancer Institute–Sponsored Working Group guidelines for chronic lymphocytic leukemia: Revised guidelines for diagnosis and treatment. Blood 1996;87:4990–4997.

Kitada S, Andersen J, Akar S, et al: Expression of apoptosis-regulating proteins in chronic lymphocytic leukemia: Correlations with in vitro and in vivo chemoresponses. Blood 1998;91:3379–3389.

Mauro FR, Foa R, Gianarelli D, et al: Clinical characteristics and outcome of young chronic lymphocytic leukemia patients: A single institution study of 204 cases. Blood 1999;94:448–454.

Mauro FR, Foa R, Cerretti R, et al: Autoimmune hemolytic anemia in chronic lymphocytic leukemia: Clinical, therapeutic, and prognostic features. Blood 2000;95:2786–2792.

Robertson LE, Pugh W, O'Brien S, et al: Richter's syndrome: A report on 39 patients. J Clin Oncol 1993;11:1985–1989.

Yuille MR, Matutes E, Marossy A, et al: Familial chronic lymphocytic leukaemia: A survey and review of published studies. Br J Haematol 2000;109:794–799.

Prognosis

Binet JL, Auquier A, Dighiero G, et al: A new prognostic classification of chronic lymphocytic leukemia derived from a multivariate survival analysis. Cancer 1981;48:198–206.

Juliusson G, Oscier DG, Fitchett M, et al: Prognostic subgroups in B cell chronic lymphocytic leukemia defined by specific chromosomal abnormalities. New Engl J Med 1990;323:720.

Rai KR, Sawitsky A, Cronkite EP, et al: Clinical staging of chronic lymphocytic leukemia. Blood 1975;46:219–234.

Zwiebel J, Cheson BD: Prognostic factors in chronic lymphocytic leukemia. Sem Oncol 1998;25:42–59.

Therapy

Anaissie EJ, Kontoyiannis DP, O'Brien S, et al: Infections in patients with chronic lymphocytic leukemia treated with fludarabine. Ann Intern Med 1998;129:559–566.

Batille M, Ribera JM, Oriol A, et al: Successful response to rituximab in a patient with pure red cell aplasia complicating chronic lymphocytic leukaemia. Br J Haematol 2002;118:1192–1193.

Bosch F, Ferrer A, Lopez-Guillermo A, et al: Fludarabine, cyclophosphamide and mitoxantrone in the treatment of resistant or relapsed chronic lymphocytic leukaemia. Br J Haematol 2002;119:976–984.

Bowen AL, Zomas A, Emmett E, et al: Subcutaneous CAMPATH-1H fludarabine-resistant/relapsed chronic lymphocytic and B-prolymphocytic leukemia. Br J Haematol 1997;96:617–619.

Byrd JC, Waselenko JK, Maneatis T, et al: Rituximab therapy in hematologic malignancy patients with circulating tumor cells: Association with increased infusion-related side effects and rapid blood tumor clearance. J Clin Oncol 1999;17:791–795.

Cheson BD: Immunologic and immunosuppressive complications of purine analogue therapy. J Clin Oncol 1995;13:2431–2448.

Cheson BD, Frame JN, Vena D, et al: Tumor lysis syndrome: an uncommon complication of fludarabine therapy of chronic lymphocytic leukemia. J Clin Oncol 1998;16:2313–2320.

Cheson BD, Vena D, Barrett J, et al: Second malignancies as a consequence of nucleoside analog therapy of chronic lymphoid leukemias. J Clin Oncol 1999;17:2454–2460.

CLL Trialists' Collaborative Group: Chemotherapeutic options in chronic lymphocytic leukemia: A meta-analysis of the randomized trials. J Natl Cancer Inst 1999;91:861–868.

Dighiero G, Maloum K, Desablens B, et al: Chlorambucil in indolent chronic lymphocytic leukemia. French Cooperative Group on Chronic Lymphocytic Leukemia. New Engl J Med 1998;338:1506–1514.

Dihiero G, Binet J-L: When and how to treat chronic lymphocytic leukemia. N Engl J Med 2000;343:1799–1801.

Dillman RO, Mick R, McIntyre OR: Pentostatin in chronic lymphocytic leukemia: A phase II trial of Cancer and Leukemia Group B. J Clin Oncol 1989;7:433–438.

Doney KC, Chauncey T, Appelbaum FR: Allogeneic related donor hematopoietic stem cell transplantation for treatment of chronic lymphocytic leukemia. Bone Marrow Transplant 2002;29:817–823.

Flinn IW, Byrd JC, Morrison C, et al: Fludarabine and cyclophosphamide with filgrastim support in patients with previously untreated indolent lymphoid malignancies. Blood 2000;96:71–75.

French Cooperative Group on CLL, Johnson S, Smith AG, et al: Multicentre prospective randomized trial of fludarabine versus cyclophosphamide, doxorubicin, and prednisone (CAP) for treatment of advanced-stage chronic lymphocytic leukemia. Lancet 1996;347:1432–1438.

Hallek M, Schmitt B, Wilhelm M, et al: Fludarabine plus cyclophosphamide is an efficient treatment for advanced chronic lymphocytic leukaemia (CLL): results of a phase II study of the German CLL Study Group. Br J Haematol 2001;114:342–348.

Hegde UP, Wilson WH, White T, Cheson BD: Rituximab treatment of refractory fludarabine-associated immune thrombocytopenia in chronic lymphocytic leukemia. Blood 2002;100:2260–2262.

Keating MJ, Cazin M, Coutré S, et al: Campath-1H treatment of T cell prolymphocytic leukemia in patients for whom at least one prior chemotherapy regimen has failed. Blood 2001;20:205–215.

Keating MJ, O'Brien S, Lerner S, et al: Long-term follow-up of patients with chronic lymphocytic leukemia (CLL) receiving fludarabine regimens as initial therapy. Blood 1998;92:1165–1171.

Kennedy B, Rawstron A, Carter C, et al: Campath-1H and fludarabine in combination are highly active in refractory chronic lymphocytic leukemia. Blood 2002;99:2245–2247.

Khouri IF, Keating M, Körbling M, et al: Transplant-lite: Induction of graft-versus-malignancy using fludarabine-based nonablative chemotherapy and allogeneic blood progenitor cell transplantation as treatment for lymphoid malignancies. J Clin Oncol 1998;16:2817–2824.

Leporrier M, Chevret S, Cazin B, et al: Randomized comparison of fludarabine, CAP, and ChOP in 938 previously untreated stage B and C chronic lymphocytic leukemia patients. Blood 2001;98:2319–2325.

McLaughlin P, Grillo-López AJ, Link BK, et al: Rituximab chimeric anti-CD20 monoclonal antibody therapy of relapsed indolent lymphoma: Half of patients respond to a four-dose treatment program. J Clin Oncol 1998;16:2825–2833.

Michallet M, Archimbaud E, Bandini G, et al: HLA-identical sibling bone marrow transplantation in younger patients with chronic lymphocytic leukemia. Ann Intern Med 1996;124:311–315.

O'Brien S, Kantarjian H, Beran M, et al: Results of fludarabine and prednisone therapy in 264 patients with chronic lymphocytic leukemia with multivariate analysis-derived prognostic model for response to treatment. Blood 1993;82:1695–1700.

O'Brien S, Kantarjian H, Estey E, et al: Lack of effect of 2-chlorodeoxyadenosine therapy in patients with chronic lymphocytic leukemia refractory to fludarabine therapy. New Engl J Med 1994;330:319–322.

O'Brien SM, Kantarjian HM, Cortes J, et al: Results of the fludarabine and cyclophosphamide combination regimen in chronic lymphocytic leukemia. J Clin Oncol 2001;19:1414–1420.

Osterborg A, Dyer MJ, Bunjes D, et al: Phase II multicenter study of human CD52 antibody in previously treated chronic lymphocytic leukemia. European Study Group of CAMPATH-1H Treatment in Chronic Lymphocytic Leukemia. J Clin Oncol 1997;15:1567–1574.

Pawson R, Dyer MJS, Barge R, et al: Treatment of T cell prolymphocytic leukemia with human CD52 antibody. J Clin Oncol 1997;15:2667–2672.

Provan D, Bartlett-Pandite L, Zwicky C, et al: Eradication of polymerase chain reaction-detectable chronic lymphocytic leukemia cells is associated with improved outcome after bone marrow transplantation. Blood 1996;88:2228–2236.

Rai KR, Freter CE, Mercier RJ, et al: Alemtuzumab in previously treated chronic lymphocytic leukemia patients who also had received fludarabine. J Clin Oncol 2002;20:3891–3897.

Rai KR, Peterson BL, Appelbaum FR, et al: Fludarabine compared with chlorambucil as primary therapy for chronic lymphocytic leukemia. N Engl J Med 2000;343:1750–1757.

Saven A, Lemon RH, Kosty M, et al: 2-Chlorodeoxyadenosine activity in patients with untreated chronic lymphocytic leukemia. J Clin Oncol 1995;13:570–574.

Seymour JF, Cusack JD, Lerner SA, et al: Case/control study of the role of splenectomy in chronic lymphocytic leukemia. J Clin Oncol 1997;15:52–60.

Silverman JA, Franssen E, Buckstein R, Imrie KR: The development of marked elevation in white blood cell count does not predict inferior outcome in chronic lymphocytic leukemia. Leuk Lymph 2002;43:1245–1251.

Ward JH: Autoimmunity in chronic lymphocytic leukemia. Curr Treat Opt Oncol 2001;2:253–257.

Wierda WG, Cantwell MJ, Woods SJ, et al: CD-40 ligand (CD154) gene therapy for chronic lymphocytic leukemia. Blood 2000;96:2917–2925.

Hairy Cell Leukemia

Flinn IW, Kopecky KJ, Foucar MK, et al: Long-term follow-up of remission duration, mortality, and second malignancies in hairy cell leukemia patients treated with pentostatin. Blood 2000;96:2981–2986.

Grever M, Kopecky K, Head D, et al: Randomized comparison of deoxycoformycin (DCF) versus alpha-2a interferon (IFN) in previously untreated patients (pts) with hairy cell leukemia (HCL): An updated report on the NCI-sponsored intergroup study (SWOG, ECOG, CALGB, NCIC CTG). Blood 1993;82:199 (Abstract 782).

Grever M, Kopecky K, Foucar MK, et al: A randomized comparison of pentostatin versus alpha-interferon in previously untreated patients with hairy cell leukemia: An intergroup study. J Clin Oncol 1995;13:974–982.

Juliusson G, Heldol D, Hippe E, et al: Subcutaneous injections of 2-chlorodeoxyadenosine for symptomatic hairy cell leukemia. J Clin Oncol 1995;13:989–995.

Kreitman RJ, Cheson BD: Treatment of hairy cell leukemia at the close of the 20th century. Hematology 1999;4:283–303.

Kreitman RJ, Wilson WH, Robbins D, et al: Responses in refractory hairy cell leukemia to a recombinant immunotoxin. Blood 1999;94:3340–3348.

Maloisel F, Benboubker L, Gardenbas M, et al: Long-term outcome with pentostatin treatment in hairy cell leukemia patients: A French retrospective study of 238 patients. Leukemia 2003;17:45–51.

Saven A, Piro LD: Newer purine analogues for the treatment of hairy cell leukemia. N Engl J Med 1994;330:691–697.

Seymour JF, Kurzrock R, Freireich EJ, et al: 2-chlorodeoxyadenosine induces durable remissions and prolonged suppression of CD4+ lymphocyte counts in patients with hairy cell leukemia. Blood 1994;83:2906–2911.

Tallman MS, Hakimian D, Variakojis D, et al: A single cycle of 2-chlorodeoxyadenosine results in complete remission in the majority of patients with hairy cell leukemia. Blood 1992;80:2203–2209.

Tallman MS, Hakimian D, Rademaker AW, et al: Relapse of hairy cell leukemia after 2-chlorodeoxyadenosine: Long-term follow-up of the Northwestern University experience. Blood 1996;88:1954–1959.

Thomas DA, O'Brien S, Cortes J, et al: Pilot study of rituximab in refractory or relapsed hairy cell leukemia. Blood 1999;94:705a (Abstract 3116).

Chapter 73
Polycythemia Vera, Idiopathic Myelofibrosis, and Essential Thrombocythemia

Jerry L. Spivak

Polycythemia vera, idiopathic myelofibrosis, essential thrombocythemia, and chronic myeloid leukemia have been classified together as the chronic myeloproliferative disorders because they share in common an origin in a multipotent hematopoietic stem cell and dominance by the affected clone as manifested by overproduction of one or more of the formed elements of the blood. Initially, some investigators postulated that these disorders involved different expressions of a basic abnormality of an early precursor stem cell, and that transitions among these illnesses could occur. Each disorder is now believed, however, to be a distinct entity. The apparent transitions in their natural history are actually the result of the phenotypic mimicry that characterizes this group of diseases. For example, isolated thrombocytosis or leukocytosis can be the presenting manifestation of polycythemia vera or chronic myeloid leukemia, and myelofibrosis can also be present in both of these disorders either at the time of diagnosis or later in the disease course. Even so, no seeming transitions occur between polycythemia vera and chronic myeloid leukemia, and myelofibrosis does not evolve into any of the other disorders.

Of the four myeloproliferative states, only chronic myeloid leukemia has a consistent clonal marker, namely the 9–22 translocation and a resulting defined molecular abnormality (see Chapter 71). If chronic myeloid leukemia is not treated successfully by bone marrow transplantation, it usually terminates in acute leukemia. By contrast, acute leukemia is an uncommon terminal event in polycythemia vera, idiopathic myelofibrosis, and essential thrombocythemia in the absence of exposure to mutagens such as ^{32}P, irradiation, hydroxyurea, or alkylating agents. This undoubtedly reflects the differences in pathogenesis between chronic myeloid leukemia and the other three chronic myeloproliferative disorders. Indeed, their generally indolent course suggests that more subtle molecular lesions are involved and, as a corollary, that their treatment should be guided by their natural history.

Polycythemia Vera

Polycythemia vera is a clonal hematopoietic disorder that causes accumulation of morphologically normal red blood cells, white blood cells, platelets, and their progenitors. The overproduction occurs in the absence of a definable stimulus and to the exclusion of normal polyclonal hematopoiesis. Polycythemia vera is the most common of the chronic myeloproliferative disorders. Its incidence is estimated to be approximately 20 per 1 million population, but the frequency varies depending on the age and ethnic status of the populations studied. Polycythemia vera is rare in children but spares no age group among adults; the median age of onset is 55 years. A male predominance is notable, because this is not seen in secondary forms of erythrocytosis. The disorder is less common among Asians and African-Americans than among Caucasians and is occasionally noted in families, but evidence for familial transmission is not well established. No risk factors for the development of the disease are known. Nonrandom cytogenetic abnormalities are present in less than 30% of patients at the time of diagnosis. Chromosomes 1, 5, 8, 9, 12, 13, and 20 are commonly involved, but none of these findings is specific for polycythemia vera. The 13q deletion, which occurs in idiopathic myelofibrosis and is also associated with increased bone marrow angiogenesis in multiple myeloma, is found when myelofibrosis complicates preexisting polycythemia vera.

Clinical Presentation

The manifestations of polycythemia vera are protean and largely nonspecific. The usual complaints result from increased blood viscosity due to the expanded red blood cell mass. The cerebral circulation is highly susceptible to the effects of circulatory stasis. Headache, malaise, weakness, and vertigo are the most common presenting symptoms, followed by visual disturbances, paresthesias of the extremities,

DIAGNOSIS

Clinical Notes on the Myeloproliferative Disorders

In polycythemia vera, stainable iron in the bone marrow is depleted and disappears as iron is used for the increased production of red blood cells. If iron is visible on iron stains of the marrow, then the diagnosis of polycythemia vera is unlikely.

Phlebotomy is the principal form of therapy for polycythemia vera. Each unit of blood removed leads to depletion of approximately 200 mg of iron. With time, the MCV and the MCH decrease, visible as hypochromic, microcytic red blood cells on peripheral smear. Iron therapy is, however, not indicated; it would lead to a need for increased frequency of phlebotomy to maintain the intended hematocrit levels.

Myeloid metaplasia in the myeloproliferative disorders does not result from simple reactivation of sites of embryonic hematopoiesis in the liver and spleen in response to progressive failure of bone marrow pro-duction. Rather, it results from an intrinsic defect that causes circulating stem cells to reside in these organs (and/or extramedullary sites) and generate white and red blood cell precursors and megakaryocytes. The burgeoning cell mass causes organ enlargement.

Marrow fibrosis in the myeloproliferative disorders develops as an epiphenomenon due to the generation of factors (such as transforming growth factor B_1) that stimulate fibroblast proliferation and the deposition of reticulin and collagen.

Pruritus in polycythemia vera can be so severe as to be disabling in some patients. It can be resistant to all standard measures and is not relieved by phlebotomy. The occasional case of severe, unrelieved pruritus, especially in the elderly patient, could warrant therapy with interferon-α, PUVA light therapy, or hydroxyurea to control this distressing symptom.

abdominal pain, aquagenic pruritus (see Chapter 3), and easy bruising or mucous membrane bleeding. The headache and visual complaints might be indistinguishable from those associated with migraine and, occasionally, a single symptom such as pruritus, joint pain due to gout, or extremity pain (erythromelalgia) could predominate, obscuring the underlying hematologic disorder. Indeed, although erythemia and warmth of the affected limb are the typical manifestations of erythromelalgia, it can also present as a burning sensation, isolated pain without a significant rash, or digital ulceration with good pulses.

The circulatory stasis due to increased blood viscosity can lead to venous or arterial thrombosis as the first manifestation of the disease. Any blood vessel can be affected, but obstruction of either the cerebral, cardiac, or mesenteric vessels is most common in newly diagnosed patients. Arterial thrombosis is more frequent than venous thrombosis. Because greater than 10% of patients have a history of prior thrombosis before diagnosis, polycythemia vera is an important consideration in the differential diagnosis of a hypercoagulable state. Myocardial infarction, ischemic stroke, and transient ischemic attacks are the most common arterial thrombotic events, while peripheral venous thrombosis—often complicated by pulmonary embolization—is the most common venous thrombotic event. Polycythemia vera is the commonest cause of hepatic vein thrombosis (Budd-Chiari syndrome). This catastrophic event can be the initial manifestation of the disease, particularly in women under age 40 years. Peculiarly, in these young patients, both the frequency of splenomegaly and the extent of splenic enlargement is greater than in older patients. For uncertain reasons, the incidence of peptic ulcer disease is increased in patients with polycythemia vera, who might present with the combination of iron-deficiency anemia (from bleeding) and splenomegaly. If thrombocytosis is extreme, spontaneous bruising and mucous membrane hemorrhage could be the first manifestation of the illness. Rarely, the disease presents with acute gout or a renal stone secondary to hyperuricemia from increased blood cell turnover. Given its insidious onset and slow progression, the disease is often identified as an incidental finding when blood counts are routinely obtained in the course of a medical evaluation.

Clinical Evaluation

Erythrocytosis is the hallmark of polycythemia vera, but unless the red blood cell mass is markedly elevated, excessive redness of the skin might not be obvious. Splenomegaly is detectable on physical examination in approximately 65% of patients at the time of diagnosis. Some clinicians have advocated ultrasound studies or scanning of the spleen in order to improve diagnostic accuracy in patients suspected of having polycythemia vera whose spleens are impalpable. But, because both false positives and false negatives occur, diagnostic precision is not improved. Hepatomegaly (in approximately 25% to 30% of patients) is half as commonly detectable as is splenomegaly and rarely occurs in the absence of

Table 73-1 ■ **The Diagnosis of Polycythemia Vera**

Three Findings Required

Elevated red blood cell mass ($\geq$ 36 mL/kg in men; $\geq$ 32 mL/kg in women)
Normal arterial oxygen saturation
Splenomegaly

Plus Any Two of the Following If the Spleen Is Not Palpable

Leukocytosis > 12,000/µL
Thrombocytosis > 400,000/µL
Elevated leukocyte alkaline phosphatase (in the absence of infection)
Elevated vitamin B_{12} > 900 pg/mL or
Unbound B_{12} binding capacity > 2200 pg/mL

splenomegaly. Substantial hepatomegaly should suggest the presence of portal hypertension, hepatic vein thrombosis, or another hepatic disease. Hypertension, most often modest and usually systolic in nature, is present in approximately 40% of untreated patients.

The laboratory evaluation is the most important aspect of the workup for polycythemia vera. Sir William Osler first suggested a set of diagnostic criteria for polycythemia vera. Because there is no clinically applicable clonal marker for polycythemia vera, in 1967 the Polycythemia Vera Study Group extended Osler's criteria to improve diagnostic accuracy (Table 73-1). The problem is that many patients do not manifest all the classical features of the disease. Early in its course, for example, palpable splenomegaly is absent in greater than 30% of patients, and approximately 20% of patients have normal white blood cell and platelet counts.

Diagnostic evaluation begins with separating true erythrocytosis from pseudoerythrocytosis due to plasma volume contraction. This can be accomplished by direct measurement of the red blood cell mass and plasma volume. It is generally not possible to estimate the red blood cell mass accurately from the venous hematocrit. The distribution of red blood cells and plasma in the circulatory system is not uniform. With disease, changes can occur independently in the plasma volume and the red blood cell mass or their distribution, particularly if there is splenomegaly. The sine qua non to establish the presence of an absolute erythrocytosis is to determine the red blood cell mass using the patient's own ^{51}chromium-labeled cells. Greater precision is obtainable by also measuring the plasma volume using isotopically labeled albumin. The red cell mass can be elevated even in the face of a hemoglobin and

hematocrit in the normal range. In polycythemia vera, as the red blood cell mass expands, the plasma volume also usually expands, thereby masking the otherwise rising hematocrit. Splenomegaly also contributes to blunting the rise in the hematocrit. If erythrocytosis is suspected, then confirmation of its presence requires a red blood cell mass determination. In the case of polycythemia as the cause of erythrocytosis, the red blood cell mass level also provides information about the number of phlebotomies necessary to adequately reduce the volume of red blood cells. At the same time, patients presenting with very high hematocrits (greater than 60% in men and greater than 56% in women) do in fact have true erythrocytosis, because reduction in plasma volume sufficient to elevate the hematocrit to these levels does not occur in otherwise well, ambulatory patients.

After the diagnosis of an absolute erythrocytosis is made, evaluation proceeds to distinguish secondary forms of erythrocytosis from the autonomous red blood cell proliferation of polycythemia vera (Table 73-2). When the diagnosis of polycythemia vera is uncertain, assessment of pulmonary function by arterial oxygen saturation, serum erythropoietin levels, and scanning of the kidneys and liver for tumors or vascular anomalies should suffice to uncover a secondary form of erythrocytosis (see Chapter 40). A normal or low erythropoietin level does not necessarily exclude hypoxia as a cause for erythrocytosis. Rare cases of congenital hemoglobin disorders have been reported that cause erythrocytosis because of tight binding of oxygen to hemoglobin and impaired oxygen release to the tissues. Bone marrow aspirate and biopsy are unnecessary for diagnostic purposes, and the abnormalities noted are not always distin-

Table 73-2 ■ **Causes of Erythrocytosis**

Relative Erythrocytosis

Hemoconcentration due to decreased plasma volume (e.g., dehydration, excessive diuresis, androgen administration, or tobacco abuse)

Absolute Erythrocytosis

Decreased arterial oxygen saturation (e.g., high altitude, pulmonary disease, right-to-left shunts, sleep apnea)
High oxygen affinity of hemoglobin (e.g., carbon monoxide intoxication, congenital hemoglobinopathies)
Renal disease (e.g., cysts, renal artery stenosis, hydronephrosis, focal sclerosing glomerulitis, renal transplantation)
Tumors (e.g., hypernephroma, hepatoma, cerebellar hemangioblastoma, uterine fibromyomas, adrenal tumors)
Polycythemia vera
Androgen use

Table 73-3 ■ Complications of Polycythemia Vera

Complication	Cause
Thrombosis, hemorrhage, hypertension	Elevated red blood cell mass
Organomegaly	Myeloid metaplasia
Pruritus, acid-peptic disease	Release of inflammatory mediators
Erythromelalgia	Thrombocytosis
Hyperuricemia, gout, renal stones	Increased cell turnover
Myelofibrosis	Reaction to neoplastic clone
Acute leukemia	Therapy-relayed or clonal evolution

guishable from those found in the other myeloproliferative disorders. Cytogenetic studies are not specifically diagnostic for polycythemia vera, but clonality can be established in a small percentage of patients. Endogenous erythroid colony formation in vitro in the absence of added erythropoietin is a feature of polycythemia vera, but this test is done only in research laboratories.

Staging, Prognostic Features, and Outcome

The manifestations of polycythemia vera vary at the time that the diagnosis is made. Thus, some patients might be diagnosed when a complete blood count is obtained for another reason, whereas others might present with substantial splenomegaly or marrow fibrosis. Clinical findings such as leukocytosis, splenomegaly, or thrombocytosis have no adverse prognostic significance with respect to longevity or bone marrow function. Longevity, however, can be compromised by certain complications of the disease, such as arterial or venous thromboses.

Although much has been written about the adverse effects of marrow fibrosis that is said to occur in the "spent" phase of polycythemia vera, myelofibrosis is not an inevitable complication of polycythemia vera, nor are there any data proving that marrow fibrosis *per se* is deleterious.

Treatment

The guiding principle in the management of the chronic myeloproliferative disorders is to do no harm. These are indolent illnesses and need to be approached therapeutically with that in mind. Table 73-3 lists the complications of polycythemia vera, and Table 73-4 provides information about the management of these complications. The most pressing issue is to reduce the red blood cell mass by phlebotomy to achieve a hematocrit of 45% (hemoglobin 14.0 g/dL) or less in men and 42% (hemoglobin 12.0 g/dL) in women. Pregnancy, with its plasma volume expansion, can mask red blood cell mass elevation and accordingly, a hematocrit of 35% or less (hemoglobin 11.0 g/dL) should be the goal in pregnant women. In newly diagnosed patients, phlebotomy can be performed on a daily basis to reach the desired hematocrit. In frail or elderly patients, small amounts of blood should be removed less frequently and replaced in the initial phlebotomies with crystalloid solution. Once the appropriate hematocrit is reached, the role of phlebotomy is to maintain this level. The frequency of phlebotomy is dependent entirely on the patient's body iron stores and is not a measure of disease activity. Once an iron-deficient state is reached, it takes approximately 3 months for sufficient iron to be absorbed to require another phlebotomy. If a site of

Table 73-4 ■ Management of Polycythemia Vera

Problem	Therapy
Erythrocytosis	Phlebotomy
Pruritus	Antihistamines, PUVA, interferon, hydroxyurea
Splenomegaly	Interferon, hydroxyurea, splenectomy, splenic irradiation
Thrombocytosis	Anagrelide, interferon, hydroxyurea
Hemorrhage	Reduce platelet count, Epsilon-aminocaproic acid
Erythromelalgia or migraine	Aspirin, anagrelide, interferon, hydroxyurea
Hyperuricemia	Allopurinol

venous access is available, one should not rely on chemotherapy or alpha interferon to control erythropoiesis, as neither approach effects an immediate reduction in red blood cell mass or iron stores.

The previously reported poor results with phlebotomy therapy early in the treatment of polycythemia vera was due solely to the failure to lower the red blood cell mass sufficiently. The initial Polycythemia Vera Study Group guidelines stipulated a hematocrit of 50% as a treatment goal. This relatively limited reduction in hematocrit meant that essentially all women with polycythemia vera and approximately 20% of men were being inadequately treated by contemporary standards of care. This may well have accounted for the adverse results of the early experience with phlebotomy therapy. There is no occult hypercoagulable state in polycythemia vera beyond the presence of hyperviscosity and circulatory stasis. Iron deficiency in the absence of anemia is not deleterious in polycythemia vera other than to induce pica in some patients. Furthermore, thrombocytosis in polycythemia vera is not exacerbated by phlebotomy. Repeated phlebotomy also will not accelerate the disease, as bone marrow function is by definition autonomous in this disorder, and phlebotomy reduces the risk of bleeding in those patients whose platelets do not function normally.

Aquagenic pruritus and myeloid metaplasia are the two most difficult complications of polycythemia vera to manage. Pruritus occasionally responds to phlebotomy, but the usual symptomatic measures are unavailing (see Chapter 3). Chemotherapy (hydroxyurea) or alpha interferon therapy can alleviate pruritus, but each of these carries its own risks and side effects. PUVA light therapy is also effective.

Although acute leukemia has been considered to occur as part of the natural history of the late stages of polycythemia vera, it is, in fact, a rare occurrence in the absence of exposure to mutagens such as ^{32}P, alkylating agents, or hydroxyurea. Without such treatment, the development of acute leukemia is rare, generally occurring in men age 60 years or older and within the first six years of the disease. Therefore, one should avoid the use of leukemogenic agents in the management of this disease if it is feasible.

Splenomegaly occurs due to extramedullary hematopoiesis in the spleen. It can be distressing when it compromises stomach size or is associated with painful splenic infarcts, abdominal distention, and portal hypertension. Alpha-interferon is the treatment of choice, but it is not always effective. Its onset of action is slow, and any benefit is lost rapidly when the drug is discontinued. Splenic irradiation is sometimes a transiently effective palliative measure, but it can

result in protracted pancytopenia. Splenectomy is a major undertaking, to be performed only by a skilled surgeon due to the mechanical difficulties associated with adhesions and the size of the splenic artery and vein. A large splenic vein remnant is usually not preventable and is a potential initiating site for postoperative mesenteric vein thrombosis. Postsplenectomy leukocytosis and thrombocytosis can be extreme and difficult to control, and occasionally, rapid hepatic enlargement ensues, requiring chemotherapeutic intervention.

Leukocytosis is an inevitable feature of polycythemia vera, but it rarely reaches levels greater than 30,000/μL. It is not harmful per se, nor does it usually require therapy. White blood cell turnover can cause hyperuricemia and gout. This is controllable with allopurinol. Thrombocytosis can be an initial or later manifestation of polycythemia vera. In polycythemia vera, although thrombocytosis is associated with the risk of microvascular arteriolar thrombosis, the level of thrombocytosis has never been shown to correlate with the likelihood of thrombosis. Moreover, very high platelet counts (greater than 1,000,000/μL) paradoxically predispose to hemorrhage. No specific platelet-related abnormality has been correlated with the risk of either a hemorrhagic diathesis or thrombosis.

Lowering the platelet count is effective in reducing the risk of bleeding, but the count need not be lowered to the normal range. Although erythromelalgia is usually responsive to a single aspirin tablet, daily aspirin might be necessary for a short period. Anagrelide is useful for this purpose but not always effective; it has some cardiovascular side effects and can cause severe headache. Dosing, therefore, should be incremental, using the smallest dose possible to achieve the desired effect. Alpha-interferon, followed by hydroxyurea, are the next agents of choice.

Although large-vessel thrombosis in polycythemia vera is inevitably due to inadequate control of the red blood cell mass and not to the platelet count, it is important to remember that many of these patients are elderly and, hence, prone to other causes of thrombosis. One must recognize, however, that in the absence of red blood cell mass control, anticoagulant therapy will not be effective.

The role of bone marrow transplantation in polycythemia vera is not yet defined, but in a patient younger than age 40 years who has a histocompatible donor, this appears to be an option to consider.

By being judicious with therapy—including adequate hematocrit reduction by phlebotomy and avoidance of mutagens—it should be possible to assist patients with polycythemia vera to achieve a prolonged and productive life span.

Follow-up Evaluation

Once the red blood cell mass has been reduced to normal, follow up evaluations, primarily directed at maintaining the hematocrit at the correct level, need not be scheduled more frequently than once a month. When a state of iron deficiency has been achieved, the hematocrit can be monitored every two to three months. In the absence of symptoms or the need to institute specific therapy, clinical evaluation at six-month intervals should be adequate. The most difficult problems to confront the physician are the management of symptomatic thrombocytosis and splenomegaly.

Idiopathic Myelofibrosis

Idiopathic myelofibrosis (also called myelofibrosis with myeloid metaplasia, agnogenic myeloid metaplasia, and primary myelofibrosis) is characterized by abnormalities in red blood cell, white cell, and platelet production in association with extramedullary hematopoiesis in the spleen and liver and marrow fibrosis. Idiopathic myelofibrosis is the least common of the myeloproliferative disorders, with an estimated incidence of approximately 1 to 3 per million population. In contrast to the male predominance noted in polycythemia vera and the female predominance in essential thrombocytosis, males and females are equally likely to develop idiopathic myelofibrosis. With the exception of previous exposure to radiation, there are no known predisposing factors. The median age of patients with idiopathic myelofibrosis is 62 years, but young adults can be affected also (age range, 17 to 89 years), and the incidence increases with advancing age.

The clonal origin of idiopathic myelofibrosis in a multipotent hematopoietic stem was established by analysis of G-6PD isoenzyme expression and X-linked gene inactivation patterns in informative women patients. In one patient in whom an N-Ras mutation was detected, T lymphocytes as well as myeloid cells were affected, suggesting that in this instance, the disease involved a totipotent hematopoietic stem cell. Nonrandom cytogenetic abnormalities are present in approximately 40% of patients at the time of diagnosis, but these abnormalities—most commonly deletions of 13q or 20q and partial trisomy 1q—are not specific for the disorder. In some patients, the retinoblastoma gene (Rb) is deleted, and mutations of other genes, such as N-Ras, are observed occasionally. Fibroblasts have not been demonstrated to be part of the affected clone.

Clinical Presentation

Symptoms of idiopathic myelofibrosis are nonspecific, and approximately 30% of patients are asymptomatic at the time of diagnosis. Fatigue is the commonest complaint, followed by dyspnea, weight loss, anorexia, early satiety, abdominal fullness or discomfort, gout and renal stones, and easy bruising.

Clinical Evaluation

Varying degrees of splenomegaly are found in most patients on physical examination. The rate of splenic enlargement over time is also quite variable. Therefore, contrary to earlier clinical impressions, spleen size cannot be used as an indicator of disease duration. If splenomegaly is not present, another cause should be sought for the myelofibrosis (Table 73-5). Hepatomegaly is found in more than 50% of patients but is usually of a lesser degree than the splenomegaly; lymphadenopathy is uncommon. Weight loss can be a prominent feature if splenic enlargement is substantial.

All hematopoietic cell lines are affected in idiopathic myelofibrosis. Anemia is the commonest abnormality; the hemoglobin is less than 10 g/dL at presentation in approximately 40% of patients. The causes for anemia in idiopathic myelofibrosis are frequently multifactorial, but it is not simply a matter of a crowding out of precursor cells in the bone marrow by fibrosis. Anemia can be in part due to folic acid deficiency, iron deficiency, hemodilution, gastrointestinal bleeding secondary to portal hypertension, hemolysis,

---

Table 73-5 ■ Causes of Myelofibrosis

Malignant Disorders Associated with Marrow Fibrosis

Acute myeloid leukemia, FAB M7 (megakaryocytic) type
Acute lymphocytic leukemia
Hairy cell leukemia
Hodgkin's disease
Non–Hodgkin's lymphoma
Idiopathic myelofibrosis
Chronic myeloid leukemia
Polycythemia vera
Systemic mastocytosis
Metastatic carcinoma

Non-Malignant Disorders Associated with Marrow Fibrosis

HIV infection
Hyperparathyroidism, renal osteodystrophy
Granulomatous infections involving the bone marrow
Thorium dioxide exposure
Gray platelet syndrome

ineffective erythropoiesis, and decreased production of erythropoietin. Extramedullary hematopoiesis occurs in the liver and spleen. Red blood cell, white blood cell, and platelet production at these sites is ineffective and does not make a substantial contribution to the blood cells in the circulation. Leukoerythroblastic changes in the peripheral blood smear are frequent and striking, usually suggesting the diagnosis. Myelocytes and metamyelocytes are present. Red cell morphology is highly varied with abnormal forms, such as tear-drop forms, red cell fragments, and schistocytes; nucleated red blood cells are usually found as well (Figure 73-1). Giant platelets are also seen. These alterations occur from distortion of the marrow architecture by fibrotic bands and by the release of cells from extramedullary sites. The changes are so common in idiopathic myelofibrosis that if they are not identified, one should strongly consider another diagnosis. The leukocyte and platelet counts can be low, normal, or elevated. The leukocyte alkaline phosphatase score is variable and not useful diagnostically.

Abnormalities of liver function tests, such as a reduction in serum albumin and an elevation of the serum alkaline phosphatase, are common. After splenectomy, there is a substantial increase in the alkaline phosphatase level. The lactate dehydrogenase (LDH) level is usually elevated, and hyperuricemia is not uncommon. Laboratory markers of autoreactivity, without clinical evidence of an autoimmune disorder, can appear. These markers include red blood cell autoantibodies, elevated titers of rheumatoid factor, antinuclear antibodies, and circulating immune complexes.

In a small number of patients with long-standing myelofibrosis, osteosclerosis is seen on conventional skeletal X-rays. An evaluation for portal hypertension is mandatory in patients with substantial splenomegaly. Reticulin fibrosis with inability to aspirate bone marrow is a hallmark of idiopathic myelofibrosis. Although demonstration of myelofibrosis on bone marrow biopsy is essential to the diagnosis, fibrotic changes in the bone marrow can occur in

other disorders also. Given the nonspecific nature of marrow fibrosis (see Table 73-5), the presence of myelofibrosis per se does not establish a diagnosis of idiopathic myelofibrosis. Marrow cellularity can vary from hypercellular to hypocellular. The latter is usually associated with a marked increase in collagen fibrosis and disruption of marrow architecture. Dilated sinuses, intravascular hematopoiesis, and increased bone marrow vascularity are other distinctive abnormalities in idiopathic myelofibrosis. Erythropoiesis is generally diminished relative to myelopoiesis, and megakaryocytes are increased in number, usually occurring in clusters. Many of the megakaryocytes have atypical morphologic features, such as coarse chromatin, increased frequency of single nuclei and/or hyperlobulation, and the presence of odd numbers of nuclei, rather than the even number that normally results from nuclear division and replication.

The degree of myelofibrosis does not correlate with the extent of extramedullary hematopoiesis. The latter is an intrinsic component of the disease process and is not secondary to an attempt to compensate for reduced blood cell production by the bone marrow. Myeloid metaplasia is usually confined to the spleen and liver, but any organ or tissue can be involved. Thus, involvement of the skin, lymph nodes, pleura, peritoneum, lungs, spinal cord, brain, retroperitoneum, and kidney have been reported. Extensive extramedullary hematopoiesis or its presence outside of the spleen and liver is a sign of advanced, accelerating disease.

Because of the nonspecific nature of the clinical and histologic features of idiopathic myelofibrosis and the absence of a clonal marker, various diagnostic criteria have been proposed (Table 73-6). There is no clear consensus, however, about the criteria required to make a definitive diagnosis. The clinical and laboratory findings previously described make it feasible, in most cases, to arrive at the diagnosis with substantial certainty. It should, at least, be possible to rule out other potential causes in the differential diagnosis. One must be wary of missing the diagnosis in the occasional patient with polycythemia vera who exhibits splenomegaly and myelofibrosis without apparent elevation of the hemoglobin and hematocrit. A red cell mass is usually definitive. If it is not, then before repeating it, iron therapy should be administered to rule out a complicating iron deficiency that is blunting the expected erythrocytosis.

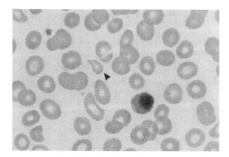

Figure 73-1 ■ Teardrops (dacryocytes) in myelofibrosis. (See Color Plate 17.)

Staging, Prognostic Features, and Outcomes

Once thought to be a disorder with a survival not superior to chronic myeloid leukemia, it has since

Table 73-6 ∎ Diagnostic Criteria for Idiopathic Myelofibrosis

Necessary Criteria

Diffuse bone marrow fibrosis
Absence of Philadelphia chromosome or BCR-ABL
   rearrangement in peripheral blood

Plus Any Two of the Following with Splenomegaly, or any Four of the Following If Splenomegaly Is Absent

Anisopoikilocytosis with teardrop erythrocytes
Circulating immature white blood cells
Circulating nucleated red blood cells
Atypical and/or clustered megakaryocytes on bone marrow
   biopsy
Myeloid metaplasia

Table 73-7 ∎ Two Prognostic Scoring Systems in Idiopathic Myelofibrosis

Scoring Method Based on the Following Prognostic Factors:

Hemoglobin < 10 g/dL
White Blood Cell Count < 4000/μL or > 30,000/μL

Number of Factors	Risk Group	Median Survival (mos.)
0	Low	93
1–2	High	17

Scoring Method Based on the Following Prognostic Factors:

Hemoglobin < 10 g/dL
Constitutional Symptoms
Circulating Blast Cells > 1%

Number of Factors	Risk Group	Median Survival (mos.)
0–1	Low	99
2–3	High	21

Cervantes F, Barosi G, Demory JL, et al: Myelofibrosis with myeloid metaplasia in young individuals: Disease characteristics, prognostic factors, and identification of risk groups. Br J Haematol 1998;102:684–690; Dupriez B, Morea P, Demory JL, et al: Prognostic factors in agnogenic myeloid metaplasia: A report on 195 cases with a new scoring system. Blood 1996;88:1013–1018.

been recognized that in idiopathic myelofibrosis, substantial variability in survival from diagnosis can occur, depending on its clinical manifestations. Retrospective analysis of a large number of patients identified a number of prognostic features, including patient age, hemoglobin level, the leukocyte and platelet counts, the percentage of circulating blast cells, cytogenetic abnormalities, and fever in the absence of infection. Other circumstances, such as hepatomegaly, splenomegaly, circulating immature leukocytes, male gender, and extent of bone marrow abnormalities, do not adversely influence the outcome for patients. Scoring systems predictive of prognosis have been devised. Two of these, applicable to both young and old patients, are illustrated in Table 73-7. Cytogenetic abnormalities are not used in either scoring system, because karyotypes have been obtained in only a limited number of patients. Nevertheless, cytogenetic abnormalities and a white blood cell count greater than 30,000/μL do appear to identify those patients at the greatest risk of leukemic transformation.

Treatment

There is no specific treatment for idiopathic myelofibrosis, and no therapy has been shown to improve survival. These facts increase the importance of diagnosing the disorder accurately and excluding other, more readily treatable, entities. Allogeneic bone marrow transplantation provides the only potentially curative therapy for idiopathic myelofibrosis. Transplantation of an unmanipulated, human leukocyte antigen (HLA)–matched allograft offers a 54% probability of five-year survival and a transplant-related mortality of 22%. Anemia, a transfusion requirement, and osteomyelosclerosis are adverse risk factors for survival after marrow transplantation, whereas increased age at transplant and abnormal cytogenetics increase the risk of treatment failure. For these reasons, allogeneic bone marrow transplantation is best reserved for high-risk patients who are less than age 50 years and have a histocompatible, related donor.

Progressive anemia and splenic enlargement are the two most troublesome complications of idiopathic myelofibrosis and are difficult to treat satisfactorily. With respect to anemia, exclusion of correctable causes such as iron, folic acid, or pyridoxine deficiency, hemorrhage, or the presence of red blood cell antibodies is the first consideration. Massive splenomegaly amplifies the problem because of red blood cell sequestration and an expanded plasma volume. These changes also limit the elevation of the hemoglobin and hematocrit in response to packed red blood cell transfusions. Androgens are occasionally employed, but the infrequent and modest responses probably reflect the resulting decrease in plasma volume and not increased red blood cell production. Erythropoietin therapy has been used successfully in some patients but can cause an unacceptable, but reversible, increase in splenomegaly or hepatomegaly as well as splenic infarction.

Chemotherapy, with either an alkylating agent or hydroxyurea, can reduce symptomatic splenomegaly and marrow fibrosis but has undesirable mutagenic effects. Alpha-interferon can decrease splenomegaly in approximately 50% of patients and occasionally reduce the extent of marrow fibrosis, but it can worsen anemia and thrombocytopenia. The role of splenic radiation or splenectomy to alleviate the burden and symptoms of massive splenomegaly and eliminate its contribution to anemia and thrombocytopenia is controversial. Radiation is an effective but temporary form of palliation. It should be reserved for patients who are unable to tolerate alpha-interferon or are unfit for surgery. Surgery can be a helpful approach to palliation. Parenteral alimentation to correct cachexia should be employed preoperatively to decrease postoperative morbidity. Splenectomy for anemia or other cytopenias is predicated on the likely contribution of splenic sequestration to their manifestation. Recent analyses indicate that splenectomy does not precipitate blastic (leukemic) transformation as was once thought. A role for thalidomide is currently under investigation.

Follow-Up Evaluation

Idiopathic myelofibrosis is generally an indolent process. Only periodic monitoring is required in the absence of a change in clinical status, such as progressive splenomegaly or the development of constitutional symptoms. Periodic serial evaluation of the marrow by repeated bone marrow biopsies is not warranted. Because acute leukemia more frequently develops in idiopathic myelofibrosis than in the other myeloproliferative disorders, bone marrow examination and cytogenetic analysis should be obtained whenever a substantial unexplained change in clinical status or blood counts occurs.

Essential Thrombocythemia

Essential thrombocythemia is a clonal hematopoietic progenitor cell disorder, which results in the overproduction of platelets in the absence of a physiologic stimulus. Its epidemiology is not well defined. Data on the natural history of the disease are limited because until recently, platelet counts were not obtained routinely as part of the complete blood count. The exact incidence of the disease is also obscured by ascertainment bias.

Central to the epidemiology of essential thrombocythemia are the platelet count threshold chosen, the degree of myelofibrosis allowed as consistent with the diagnosis, and the frequency of use of red blood cell mass and plasma volume determinations to rule out polycythemia vera. Including patients with platelet counts less than 600,000/μL risks the loss of diagnostic specificity. Including patients regardless of the degree of marrow fibrosis and not considering the possibility of occult erythrocytosis introduces diagnostic inaccuracy, vis à vis myelofibrosis and polycythemia vera, respectively.

Nevertheless, the incidence of essential thrombocythemia does appear to increase with age. The diagnosis is now more frequently made, probably because of the incorporation of the platelet count into routine blood studies. A biphasic variation in incidence is noted in women, with peaks at 30 to 40 years and at 70 years. When a platelet count of greater than 600,000/μL is used as a threshold, the annual incidence of essential thrombocythemia is between 1 to 3 per million population, with a female:male predominance of 1.5:1 and a median age of onset of 62 years (range 17 to 90 years). Familial thrombocythemia is well documented but uncommon, and it is generally asymptomatic and uncomplicated. Some of these families could represent instances of dysregulation of thrombopoietin production.

Because definitive tests are unavailable, the diagnosis of essential thrombocytosis is often made by excluding other potential causes. It can be difficult to distinguish essential thrombocythemia from the many nonclonal causes of thrombocytosis (Table 73-8). In an attempt to improve diagnostic accuracy, a number of diagnostic criteria have been proposed. The two most widely accepted versions are described in Table 73-9.

Nonrandom chromosomal abnormalities at the time of diagnosis are uncommon—occurring in approximately 5% to 10% of patients—and nonspecific, usually involving chromosomes 8 or 9 (trisomies)

Table 73-8 ■ Causes of Thrombocytosis

Inflammatory disease (e.g., collagen vascular disease, inflammatory bowel disease)
Malignancy (e.g., Hodgkin's disease and various solid tumors)
Iron-deficiency anemia
Myeloproliferative disorders:
    Polycythemia vera
    Idiopathic myelofibrosis
    Essential thrombocytosis
Chronic myeloid leukemia
Myelodysplasia—the 5q-variant
Acute hemorrhage
Infection
Post-splenectomy or hyposplenism
Rebound phenomenon (e.g., transiently, after initiation of therapy for folate or B_{12} deficiency or after alcohol withdrawal in severe alcoholics)

Table 73-9 ■ Diagnostic Criteria for Essential Thrombosis

Polycythemia Vera Study Group Criteria:

Platelet count > 600,000/μL

Hemoglobin < 13 g/dL or normal red blood cell mass for gender

Stainable iron in bone marrow or failure of hemoglobin to increase > 1 g/dL after a 1-month trial of iron therapy

Megakaryocytic hyperplasia

Absence of substantial marrow fibrosis

Absence of the Philadelphia chromosome

Absence of a cause for reactive thrombocytosis

No more than two of the following:

 Mild myelofibrosis (less than one-third of marrow biopsy area)

 Splenomegaly

 Leukoerythroblastic reaction

Rotterdam Thrombocythemia Study Group Criteria

Diagnostic

Platelet count > 400,000/μL

No other known cause of thrombocytosis

Increase and clustering of enlarged mature megakaryocytes with hyperploid nuclei on bone marrow biopsy

Confirmatory

Normal or elevated leukocyte alkaline phosphatase score, normal sedimentation rate, and no fever or infection

Normal or increased cellularity of the bone marrow

Splenomegaly on palpation or on ultrasound or scan

Spontaneous erythroid and/or megakaryocyte colony formation

Michiels JJ: Proposal for revised diagnostic criteria of essential thrombocythemia and polycythemia vera by the thrombocythemia vera study group. Semin Thromb Hemost 1997;23:339–347.

or 20 and 21 (deletions of 20q and 21p). Cytogenetic abnormalities, particularly 17p, are common following exposure to agents such as hydroxyurea. No single clinical or laboratory finding distinguishes clonal from nonclonal thrombocytosis. In vitro cell culture studies in essential thrombocytosis demonstrate endogenous erythroid and megakaryocyte colony formation, but this phenomenon is variably demonstrable. Thrombocytosis can be the presenting manifestation of the other myeloproliferative diseases. It is important that the care of these patients be planned with due regard for the potential uncertainties in diagnosis and lack of fundamental knowledge about the molecular basis of this clinical syndrome.

Clinical Presentation

Essential thrombocythemia is asymptomatic in greater than 50% of patients at diagnosis. In the remainder of patients, spontaneous (and usually superficial) hemorrhage, arterial or venous thrombosis, or erythromel-

algia leads to laboratory studies. Cerebral, myocardial, and peripheral arteries are the most frequently affected. Venous events most often involve the cerebral sinuses, intraabdominal veins, and the deep venous system of the extremities. Erythromelalgia (see the description in the previous section on polycythemia vera) is the most common complication, followed by arterial thrombosis, superficial hemorrhage, and venous thrombosis. Neurologic symptoms from microvascular occlusion include headache (often of the migraine type), visual disturbances, dizziness, and transient ischemic attacks. These symptoms are not specific for essential thrombocytosis, because they also occur in hyperviscosity syndromes, such as in polycythemia vera and macroglobulinemia.

Clinical Evaluation

On physical examination, splenomegaly is usually the only abnormality; it is found in 30% of patients and generally extends approximately 2 cm below the left costal margin. The presence of hepatomegaly, marked splenomegaly, or lymphadenopathy should suggest another diagnosis. The hemoglobin level is usually normal. If it is elevated, polycythemia vera becomes a diagnostic consideration. A hemoglobin level lower than normal suggests either another disorder or the presence of occult iron deficiency. Low-grade gastrointestinal bleeding can occur in these patients as a hemorrhagic manifestation. Conversely, uncomplicated iron deficiency itself can be associated with a substantial reactive thrombocytosis, which resolves on repletion with iron. Leukocytosis is common, usually mild in degree, and virtually never greater than 30,000/μL. The lactate dehydrogenase and serum alkaline phosphatase may be elevated. Bone marrow aspiration and biopsy reveal increased cellularity with abundant megakaryocytes, occurring in clusters and lacking the nuclear atypia of idiopathic myelofibrosis or myelodysplasia. Although some diagnostic classifications permit a small increase in marrow reticulin, an increase in reticulin out of proportion to cellularity or to an extent that prevents aspiration is more compatible with the presence of another disorder, such as idiopathic myelofibrosis or chronic myeloid leukemia.

The increased frequency of hemorrhagic and thrombotic events in essential thrombocythemia is related to abnormalities in platelet function. Impaired platelet aggregation in vitro in response to one or more stimuli is present in the majority of patients. Similar laboratory abnormalities can be seen in the thrombocytosis of polycythemia vera but are not often found in chronic myeloid leukemia or secondary forms of thrombocytosis. The bleeding is usually normal, and there is no correlation between either the presence of abnormal platelet aggregation studies or the elevation of the platelet count and the risk of thrombosis or hemorrhage. Every patient with essential thrombocytosis should be evaluated for BCR-ABL expression using the fluorescence in situ hybridization technique to identify the 5% of patients with chronic myeloid leukemia who present with isolated thrombocytosis. Although platelet counts of greater than 1,000,000/μL usually indicate the presence of a myeloproliferative disorder, reactive thrombocytosis can reach these levels as well.

Staging, Prognostic Features, and Outcomes

Otherwise astute clinicians who usually follow evidence-based guidelines tend to act reflexively in deciding to treat a patient who is found to have a markedly elevated platelet count. The overwhelming concern is to prevent thrombosis by promptly lowering the platelet count. This reaction results from an understandable intuition that an elevated platelet count places the patient at high risk for a thrombotic event. No controlled study has ever validated this belief, however, and several studies have discredited it.

The published literature is flawed in a number of ways. In patients with essential thrombocythemia who have thrombotic events, the reported patients have not been evaluated for concomitant causes of vascular disease, such as diabetes, cardiac and peripheral vascular disorders, hyperviscosity, or a non–thrombocytosis-related hypercoagulable state. The previously noted ascertainment bias of these largely retrospective studies intrinsically selects certain patients for publication, and the appropriateness of generalizing to the larger world of patients in the community is questionable. A contributing factor to the controversy is the predilection of women to develop essential thrombocythemia. A substantial proportion of female patients in most series are reported to have hemoglobins that are too high, raising the question of whether a number of them actually have polycythemia vera (with thrombocytosis) and have been misdiagnosed. Moreover, in many reports no distinction is made between major-vessel thrombotic events and the microvascular syndrome known as erythromelalgia; this lack of distinction leads to a bias with respect to disease morbidity, as microvascular events are neither life-threatening nor irreversible. Given these issues, it is not surprising that there is little consensus in essential thrombocytosis about prognostic factors, survival, and therapeutic recommendations. It is nevertheless quite clear that evolution to acute leukemia is rare in essential thrombocytosis in the absence of exposure to mutagens such as ^{32}P, alkylating agents, and hydroxyurea.

A reasonable conclusion from the published literature on essential thrombocytosis is that the most important risk factor for a thrombotic complication is a prior history of such an event. Of course, this same increased risk would be true of any patient without thrombocytosis who had a similar history. What needs to be emphasized is that the risk does not correlate with the elevation of the platelet count. In fact, in a seeming paradox, patients with a platelet count greater than 1,500,000/μL are at a greater risk of hemorrhage than those with a lower platelet count. Neither the platelet count, patient age, nor splenomegaly is prognostic for survival, and platelet function studies do not predict the risk of hemorrhage or thrombosis. Venous thrombosis is uncommon (occurring in approximately 6% of patients), whereas arterial and microvascular thrombosis occur in 18% and 26% of patients, respectively. Superficial hemorrhage occurs in approximately 14%, Although there are conflicting reports, lifespan appears to be normal in essential thrombocythemia, and there are no data indicating that a reduction in the platelet count improves survival. Adverse cardiovascular risk factors such as tobacco use and hypercholesterolemia are also important risk factors for thrombosis in essential thrombocytosis, just as they are in the absence of this finding. Unfortunately, the role of oral contraceptives and other causes of hypercoagulability have not been investigated thoroughly. It has also been suggested that an elevation in reticulated platelets—presumably representing an increase in platelet turnover—is a prethrombotic marker, but this supposition requires confirmation. Finally, clonality does not predict morbidity, and a spontaneous reduction of the platelet count can occur over time and during pregnancy.

Treatment

Thrombocytosis per se is never an indication for therapy and should not be assumed to be the cause of thrombosis without the appropriate evaluation of all possible causes. The strongest indication for therapy is a prior thrombotic event, and there is no indication that age should dictate the institution of therapy or even the type of therapy. The neurologic manifestations of erythromelalgia need to be distinguished from arterial thrombosis, as their treatment is different and the possibility that the patient has polycythemia vera must always be considered. Based on the published literature, there is no "safe" platelet count. With respect to thrombosis, it is not the platelet count that needs correction. In this situation, venous or arterial thrombosis requires the same type of anticoagulation as would be given if the platelet count were normal.

Aspirin or another COX-1 inhibitor is the treatment of choice for the microvascular syndrome. These should only be employed as needed, as there is a risk of bleeding, particularly when high doses are administered. Reduction in the platelet count can be accomplished safely with anagrelide or alpha-interferon. These drugs, however, are not always effective, and responses, when obtained, might not be durable. Anagrelide has a number of undesirable side effects such as tachycardia, headache, fluid retention, gastric distress, diarrhea, anemia, and thrombocytopenia. Gradual titration of the dose should be used. Alpha-interferon also has many side effects, such as flulike symptoms, fatigue, myalgias, suppression of thyroid function, cardiac arrhythmias, and neurotoxicity. Either of these drugs, if tolerable, is preferable to hydroxyurea, which is a mutagen and should never be considered as a first-line agent.

Essential thrombocythemia is not infrequent in women in the reproductive age, but there is as yet no consensus concerning the impact of the disorder and its treatment in the pregnant patient. Anecdotal reports suggest that first-trimester abortion, intrauterine death, or fetal growth retardation due to placental infarction are the major consequences of essential thrombocytosis during pregnancy, with abortion occurring in approximately 35% of patients. At the same time, a regression of the disease has also been associated with pregnancy followed by its reemergence postpartum. Furthermore, in several series, essential thrombocytosis had no effect on pregnancy outcome and in others, only maternal hemorrhage was observed. The roles of salicylates during pregnancy and of anticoagulants postpartum are unresolved. Alpha-interferon is both safe and effective when given during pregnancy. The possibility of other causes for spontaneous abortion or placental insufficiency, such as the antiphospholipid syndrome or polycythemia vera, has never been adequately evaluated, and prior medical history has not been predictive of complications. With the present level of knowledge, a conservative approach is best.

Follow-up Evaluation

Most patients with essential thrombocytosis are asymptomatic or require only intermittent treatment for erythromelalgia. Therefore, follow-up evaluation need be no more frequent than at six-month intervals to ensure that the thrombocytosis is not the marker of another chronic myeloproliferative disorder. There is no need for serial marrow evaluation in the absence of a change in blood counts or clinical findings. Cardiac risk factors need to be addressed prophylactically, but in the absence of symptoms,

manipulation of the platelet count is neither necessary nor desirable.

References

Polycythemia Vera

Adamson JW, Fialkow PJ, Murphy S, et al: Polycythemia vera: Stem cell and probable clonal origin of the disease. N Engl J Med 1976;295:913–916.

Kessler CM, Klein HG, Havlik RJ: Uncontrolled thrombocytosis in chronic myeloproliferative disorders. Br J Haematol 1982;50:157–167.

Kurzrock R, Cohen PR. Erythromelalgia and myeloproliferative disorders. Arch Intern Med 1989;149:105–109.

Morison WL, Nesbitt JA. Oral psoralen photochemotherapy (PUVA) for pruritus associated with polycythemia vera and myelofibrosis. Am J Hematol 1993;42:409–410.

Nand S, Messmore H, Fisher SG, et al: Leukemic transformation in polycythemia vera: analysis of risk factors. Am J Hematol 1990;34:32–36.

Pearson TC, Weatherly-Mein G: Vascular occlusive episodes and venous haematocrit in primary proliferative polycythaemia. Lancet 1978;2:1219–1221.

Rector WG, Fortuin NJ, Conley CL: Non-hematologic effects of chronic iron deficiency: A study of patients with polycythemia vera treated solely with venesections. Medicine 1982;61:382–389.

Roberts BE, Miles DW, Woods CG: Polycythaemia vera and myelosclerosis: a bone marrow study. Br J Haematol 1969;16:75–85.

Rozman C, Giralt M, Feliu E, et al: Life expectancy of patients with chronic nonleukemic myeloproliferative disorders. Cancer 1991;67:2658–2663.

Silver RT: Interferon alfa: effects of long-term treatment for polycythemia vera. Semin Hematol 1997;34:40–50.

Spivak JL: Polycythemia vera: Myths, mechanisms, and management. Blood 2002;100:4272–4290.

Spivak JL: The optimal management of polycythemia vera. Br J Haematol 2002;116:243–254.

Swolin B, Weinfeld A, Westin J: A prospective long-term cytogenetic study in polycythemia vera in relation to treatment and clinical course. Blood 1988;72:386–395.

Myelofibrosis

Barosi G, Ambrosetti A, Finelli C, et al: The Italian consensus conference on diagnostic criteria for myelofibrosis with myeloid metaplasia. Br J Haematol 1999;104:730–737.

Barosi G: Myelofibrosis with myeloid metaplasia: Diagnostic definition and prognostic classification for clinical studies and treatment guidelines. J Clin Oncol 1999; 17:2954–2970.

Cervantes F, Barosi G, Demory JL, et al: Myelofibrosis with myeloid metaplasia in young individuals: Disease characteristics, prognostic factors and identification of risk groups. Br J Haematol 1998;102:684–690.

Dupriez B, Morea P, Demory JL, et al: Prognostic factors in agnogenic myeloid metaplasia: A report on 195 cases with a new scoring system. Blood 1996;88:1013–1018.

Elliott MA, Chen MG, Silverstein MN, et al: Splenic irradiation for symptomatic splenomegaly associated with myelofibrosis with myeloid metaplasia. Br J Haematol 1998; 103:505–511.

Guardiola P, Anderson JE, Bandini G, et al: Allogeneic stem cell transplantation for agnogenic myeloid metaplasia: A European Group for Blood and Marrow Transplantation, Societe Francaise de Greffe de Moelle, Gruppo Italiano per il Trapianto del Midollo Osseo, and Fred Hutchinson Cancer Research Center Collaborative Study. Blood 1999;93:2831–2838.

Mesa RA, Li C-Y, Schroeder G, et al: Clinical correlates of splenic histopathology and splenic karyotype in myelofibrosis and myeloid metaplasia. Blood 2001;97:3665–3667.

Murphy S, Davis JL, Walsh PN, et al: Template bleeding time and clinical hemorrhage in myeloproliferative disease. Arch Intern Med 1978;138:1251–1253.

Reilly JT, Snowden JA, Spearing RL, et al: Cytogenetic abnormalities and their prognostic significance in idiopathic myelofibrosis: a study of 106 cases. Br J Haematol 1997;98:96–102.

Tefferi A, Mesa RA, Nagorney DM, et al: Splenectomy in myelofibrosis with myeloid metaplasia: a single-institution experience with 223 patients. Blood 2000;95:2226–2233.

Ward HP, Block MH: The natural history of agnogenic myeloid metaplasia (AMM) and a critical evaluation of its relationship with the myeloproliferative syndrome. Medicine 1971;50:357–420.

Wolf BC, Neiman RS: Myelofibrosis with myeloid metaplasia: pathophysiologic implications of the correlation between bone marrow changes and progression of splenomegaly. Blood 1985;65:803–809.

Thrombocythemia

Anonymous: Anagrelide, a therapy for thrombocythemic states: experience in 577 patients. Anagrelide Study Group. Am J Med 1992;92:69–76.

Beressi AH, Tefferi A, Silverstein MN, et al: Outcome analysis of 34 pregnancies in women with essential thrombocythemia. Arch Intern Med 1995;155:1217–1222.

Griesshammer M, Bangerter M, Sauer T, et al: Aetiology and clinical significance of thrombocytosis: Analysis of 732 patients with an elevated platelet count. J Intern Med 1999;245:295–300.

Harrison CN, Gale RE, MacHin SJ, et al: A large proportion of patients with a diagnosis of essential thrombocythemia do not have a clonal disorder and may be at lower risk of thrombotic complications. Blood 1999;93:417–424.

Jensen MK, de Nully BP, Nielsen OJ, et al: Incidence, clinical features and outcome of essential thrombocythaemia in a well defined geographical area. Eur J Haematol 2000; 65:132–139.

Kaushansky K: Thrombopoietin. N Engl J Med 1998; 339:746–754.

Michiels JJ: Proposal for revised diagnostic criteria of essential thrombocythemia and polycythemia vera by the thrombocythemia vera study group. Semin Thromb Hemost 1997;23:339–347.

Michiels JJ, Koudstaal PJ, Mulder AH, et al: Transient neurologic and ocular manifestations in primary thrombocythemia. Neurology 1993;43:1107–1110.

Ruggeri M, Finazzi G, Tosetto A, et al: No treatment for low-risk thrombocythaemia: results from a prospective study. Br J Haematol 1998;103:772–777.

Sacchi S, Gugliotta L, Papineschi F, et al: Alfa-interferon in the treatment of essential thrombocythemia: Clinical results and evaluation of its biological effects on the hematopoietic neoplastic clone. Italian Cooperative Group on ET. Leukemia 1998;12:289–294.

Soren EC, Tefferi A: Long-term use of anagrelide in young patients with essential thrombocythemia. Blood 2001; 97:863–866.

Sterkers Y, Preudhomme C, Lai JL, et al: Acute myeloid leukemia and myelodysplastic syndromes following essential thrombocythemia treated with hydroxyurea: High proportion of cases with 17p deletion. Blood 1998;91:616–622.

Stoll DB, Peterson P, Exten R, et al: Clinical presentation and natural history of patients with essential thrombocythemia and the Philadelphia chromosome. Am J Hematol 1988;27:77–83.

Tefferi A, Fonseca R, Pereira DL, et al: A long-term retrospective study of young women with essential thrombocythemia. Mayo Clin Proc 2001;76:22–28.

van Genderen PJ, Budde U, Michiels JJ, et al: The reduction of large von Willebrand factor multimers in plasma in essential thrombocythaemia is related to the platelet count. Br J Haematol 1996;93:962–965.

Chapter 74
Breast Cancer: Staging and Prognosis

Craig A. Bunnell, Eric P. Winer, and Judy E. Garber

Staging

An effective staging system should accurately reflect prognosis and thereby inform therapeutic decisions. More than 25 years ago, the American Joint Committee on Cancer published its first staging manual to codify the extent of disease at a number of cancer sites and to group patients into similar prognostic categories. This system has been modified over the last three decades, most recently in 2002, to reflect accumulating outcome data and advances in diagnostic techniques. The most recent version differs from the prior edition primarily by (1) reclassifying axillary nodal status according to the number of involved lymph nodes; (2) discriminating between macrometastases, micrometastases, and isolated tumor cells identified in lymph nodes; (3) indicating which techniques were used for identifying lymph node metastases; and (4) no longer classifying as distant metastases spread to certain nonaxillary lymph nodes.

The changes in the American Joint Committee on Cancer staging system help to more accurately estimate prognosis. The improved prognostic relevance of the modified staging system contributes to clinical decision making about therapy, which requires careful consideration of the balance between the potential benefit from systemic therapy to reduce the risk of disease recurrence and the attendant concomitant morbidities. Some apparently predictive factors have only limited application because of lack of standardized methodologies, nonuniform reporting of results, and dearth of prospective studies confirming their value. Several of these are likely to have a future role in the evaluation of patients with early-stage breast cancer and are therefore discussed here.

Staging systems group patients according to the extent of disease. Their ultimate utility lies in the ability to (1) estimate an individual's prognosis, (2) determine appropriate treatment options, (3) enhance uniform data collection, and (4) facilitate the conduct of clinical trials.

Breast cancer staging has traditionally employed TNM nomenclature, which is based largely on tumor size (T); presence, location, and number of involved lymph nodes (N); and the presence or absence of distant metastatic disease (M). The need for changes in the staging system arose because of the development of new methods of breast cancer diagnosis and management and the recognition that previous staging criteria did not adequately differentiate among different prognostic subsets of patients. The sixth edition of the American Joint Committee on Cancer breast cancer staging system was implemented in January 2003. The revised TNM staging system is shown in Table 74-1. The final stage groupings and their relationship to long-term survival appear in Table 74-2.

Primary Tumor (T)

Tumor size is clinically assessed by whatever method is most accurate for a particular case (e.g., physical examination or imaging). Pathologic tumor size refers to measurement of only the *invasive* component of the tumor mass. Therefore, a tumor with 5 cm of intraductal carcinoma, containing only 0.4 cm of invasive disease, is classified as T1a. With increasing tumor size, the "T" designation increases from T1 to T2 to T3 and so forth. The designation "Tx" is used when the extent of tumor cannot be assessed, which may occur if a

Table 74-1 ■ TNM Staging System for Breast Cancer

Primary Tumor (T)

TX	Primary tumor cannot be assessed
T0	No evidence of primary tumor
Tis	Carcinoma in situ
Tis (DCIS)	Ductal carcinoma in situ
Tis (LCIS)	Lobular carcinoma in situ
Tis (Paget)	Paget's disease of the nipple with no tumor
	Note: Paget's disease associated with a tumor is classified according to the size of the tumor.
T1	Tumor ≤2 cm in greatest dimension
T1mic	Microinvasion ≤0.1 cm in greatest dimension
T1a	Tumor >0.1 cm but not >0.5 cm in greatest dimension
T1b	Tumor >0.5 cm but not >1 cm in greatest dimension
T1c	Tumor >1 cm but not >2 cm in greatest dimension
T2	Tumor >2 cm but not >5 cm in greatest dimension
T3	Tumor >5 cm in greatest dimension
T4	Tumor of any size with direct extension to
	(a) chest wall or
	(b) skin, only as described below
T4a	Extension to chest wall, not including pectoralis muscle
T4b	Edema (including peau d'orange) or ulceration of the skin of the breast, or satellite skin nodules confined to the same breast
T4c	Both T4a and T4b
T4d	Inflammatory carcinoma

Regional Lymph Nodes (N)

NX	Regional lymph nodes cannot be assessed (e.g., previously removed)
N0	No regional lymph node metastasis
N1	Metastasis in movable ipsilateral axillary lymph node(s)
N2	Metastases in ipsilateral axillary lymph nodes fixed or matted, or in clinically apparent* ipsilateral internal mammary nodes in the absence of clinically evident axillary lymph node metastasis
N2a	Metastasis in ipsilateral axillary lymph nodes fixed to one another (matted) or to other structures
N2b	Metastasis only in clinically apparent* ipsilateral internal mammary nodes and in the absence of clinically evident axillary lymph node metastasis
N3	Metastasis in ipsilateral infraclavicular lymph node(s), or in clinically apparent* ipsilateral internal mammary lymph node(s) and in the presence of clinically evident axillary lymph node metastasis; or metastasis in ipsilateral supraclavicular lymph node(s) with or without axillary or internal mammary lymph node involvement
N3a	Metastasis in ipsilateral infraclavicular lymph node(s) and axillary lymph node(s)
N3b	Metastasis in ipsilateral internal mammary lymph node(s) and axillary lymph node(s)
N3c	Metastasis in ipsilateral supraclavicular lymph node(s)

Regional Lymph Nodes: Pathologic Classification

PNX	Regional lymph nodes cannot be assessed (e.g., previously removed or not removed for pathologic study)
pN0	No regional lymph node metastasis histologically, no additional examination for isolated tumor cells
pN0(i–)	No regional lymph node metastasis histologically, negative IHC
pN0(i+)	No regional lymph node metastasis histologically, positive IHC, no IHC cluster >0.2 mm
pN0(mol–)	No regional lymph node metastasis histologically, negative molecular findings (RT-PCR)
pN0(mol+)	No regional lymph node metastasis histologically, positive molecular findings (RT-PCR)
pN1mi	Micrometastasis (>0.2 mm, none >2.0 mm)
pN1	Metastasis in one to three axillary lymph nodes and/or in internal mammary nodes with microscopic disease detected by sentinel lymph node dissection but not clinically apparent*
pN1a	Metastasis in one to three axillary lymph nodes
pN1b	Metastasis in internal mammary nodes with microscopic disease detected by sentinel lymph node dissection but not clinically apparent*
pN1c	Metastasis in one to three axillary lymph nodes and in internal mammary lymph nodes with microscopic disease detected by sentinel lymph node dissection but not clinically apparent*,
pN2	Metastasis in four to nine axillary lymph nodes or in clinically apparent* internal mammary lymph nodes in the absence of axillary lymph node metastasis
pN2a	Metastasis in four to nine axillary lymph nodes (at least one tumor deposit >2.0 mm)
pN2b	Metastasis in clinically apparent* internal mammary lymph nodes in the absence of axillary lymph node metastasis

Distant Metastases (M)

Mx	Distant metastases cannot be assessed
M0	No distant metastases
M1	Distant metastases

*Clinically apparent is defined as detected by imaging studies (excluding lymphoscintigraphy) or by clinical examination.
From Singletary SE, Allred C, Ashley P, et al: Revisions of the American Joint Committee on Cancer staging system for breast cancer. J Clin Oncol 2002;20:3628–3636.

Table 74-2 ■ TNM Stage Grouping for Breast Cancer

Stage Grouping	Tumor Size	Nodal Status	Distant Metastases	10-Year Risk of Death
0	Tis	N0	M0	<2%
I	T1*	N0	M0	<10%
IIA	T0	N1	M0	10% to 30%
	T1*	N1	M0	
	T2	N0	M0	
IIB	T2	N1	M0	30% to 50%
	T3	N0	M0	
IIIA	T0, T1*,	N2	M0	50% to 75%
	T2	N2	M0	
	T3	N1, N2	M0	
IIIB	T4	N0, N1, N2	M0	75% to 90%
IIIC	Any T	N3	M0	75% to 90%
IV	Any T	Any N	M1	>90%

*T1 includes T1mic tumors, which have a similar prognosis to stage IIA tumors if they are histologic grade 3.
This table is modified from the AJCC Prognostic Factors Consensus Conference, published in Cancer 1999;86:2436–2446.

---

microscopic tumor is found at the margin of resection. If multiple, synchronous, ipsilateral, primary carcinomas are present, the largest primary carcinoma is used for determining T, but the multicentric nature should be documented in the record, and each tumor should be analyzed separately. Inflammatory carcinoma (T4A) is an entity characterized pathologically by dermal lymphatic invasion or clinically by an inflammatory or infectious appearance, with erythema and induration of the skin, often without an underlying mass.

Regional Lymph Nodes (N)

Changes to the staging system focus on establishing new categories based on the extent of regional lymph node involvement by breast cancer. Because the number of involved lymph nodes is inversely correlated with survival duration, the staging system no longer designates the nodes simply as positive or negative for cancer. Rather, an increase in the number of involved lymph nodes increases the stage as well. Micrometastatic disease in lymph nodes is distinguished from both macrometastatic disease on one end of the spectrum and isolated tumor cells on the other. In addition, the techniques by which these metastatic foci are detected (e.g., sentinel lymph node dissection versus standard dissection or hematoxylin and eosin versus immunohistochemistry versus reverse transcriptase-polymerase chain reaction are also noted. In addition, consistent with current outcomes data and clinical practice, patients with certain nonaxillary lymph node involvement, such as in-

volvement of the supraclavicular, infraclavicular, or internal mammary lymph nodes, have had their disease reclassified from metastatic to nonmetastatic status. In this way, the manner in which lymph node involvement affects stage reflects the manner in which it affects clinical outcome in practice.

Micrometastases and Isolated Tumor Cells

The number of immunohistochemical and molecular techniques for detecting microscopic metastatic tumor deposits is increasing. Micrometastatic lymph node involvement, at the level of isolated tumor cells, can thus now be routinely detected. Unfortunately, the databases of the past perforce did not contain this information, and the relationship of micrometastatic disease to recurrence and survival is unknown. Nevertheless, some clinicians treat patients with immunohistochemical or reverse transcriptase-polymerase chain reaction (rt-PCR)–detected tumor cell deposits as if they had macrometastatic disease, thereby confounding attempts to collect data about their prognostic significance in untreated patients. Future studies will have to determine whether a lower size limit exists for micrometastases, below which clinical prognostic relevance disappears, and distinguish between the identification of micrometastases and isolated tumor cells according to uniform quantitative criteria.

With time, the new staging system should provide these data, because it does identify the type of metastatic deposits and the method used in their detection. Micrometastasis is defined as a deposit that is larger than 0.2 mm and no larger than 2.0 mm. Such lesions are recognized as clinically meaningful and classified as pN1, in the absence of larger lymph node metastases. Any lesions smaller than 0.2 mm are classified as isolated tumor cell deposits and classified as pN0 (i.e., lymph node–negative). In addition, a descriptor is added in cases in which the tumor cell deposits or micrometastases are identified by methods other than standard hematoxylin and eosin-stained histologic specimens.

If the lesions are identified by immunohistochemistry, the descriptor "(i+)" is added. For lesions identified by molecular methods (e.g., rt-PCR), the descriptor "(mol+)" is added. For example, a lesion that is histologically negative by hematoxylin and eosin staining but greater than 0.2 mm by immunohistochemistry would be designated pN1(i+). If the deposit is not greater than 0.2 mm, it is designated "pN0(i+)." Similarly, a lesion negative by hematoxylin and eosin staining, which reveals positive cells by rt-PCR, is designated "pN0(mol+)." By subcategorizing the method of detection of node positivity, the staging system acknowledges the potential importance and possible confounding influences of the methodology used in making the diagnosis of lymph node involvement.

Sentinel Lymph Node Dissection

Sentinel lymph node dissection has rapidly become a diagnostic standard of care for women with no palpable axillary lymph nodes on physical examination. Not uncommonly, the sentinel node is the only positive lymph node. In many cases, the sentinel node is positive only by immunohistochemical staining and not by hematoxylin and eosin staining, raising the question of whether a complete axillary dissection is indicated. The significance of the findings in the sentinel node and its implications for adjuvant chemotherapy are under study. Cases in which the lymph node classification is based solely on the results of sentinel lymph node dissection are given the additional descriptor of "(sn)" for "sentinel node." For example, involvement of a sentinel lymph node by metastatic disease in the absence of a subsequent axillary dissection is designated "pN1(sn)." This specification will allow data collection on the outcome in the circumstances when axillary lymph node dissection is omitted.

Number of Axillary Lymph Nodes Involved

The number of axillary lymph nodes involved by metastatic disease remains one of the most important prognostic factors in breast cancer. Treatment approaches in the clinic and in clinical trials are based on the number of involved axillary lymph nodes; the new staging criteria now mirror this stratification.

Patients with one to three axillary lymph nodes involved by metastatic disease, in which at least one tumor deposit is > 2.0 mm, are classified as "pN1a." Patients with four to nine positive axillary lymph nodes are classified as "pN2a," and those with 10 or more positive lymph nodes are classified as "pN3a." The "upstaging" of patients who have increasing numbers of involved lymph nodes reflects the worsening prognosis.

Metastases to Nonaxillary Lymph Nodes

Lymphatics from the breast generally drain to the axillary lymph nodes but may also drain to the internal mammary, infraclavicular, and supraclavicular lymph nodes. The internal mammary lymph nodes lie in the intercostal spaces along the edge of the sternum in the endothoracic fascia. The infraclavicular lymph nodes are medial to the medial aspect of the pectoralis minor muscle. The supraclavicular lymph nodes are located in the supraclavicular fossa, bounded by the omohyoid muscle and tendon, the internal jugular vein, and the clavicle and subclavian vein.

The prognostic implications of internal mammary lymph node involvement are in part dependent on the status of the axillary lymph nodes. In a small series of patients (Valagussa, 1978) undergoing extended radical mastectomy who had metastases to the internal mammary lymph nodes, the 10-year survival rate of patients whose axillary lymph nodes were negative was 45% (similar to the results for patients who have spread only to the axillary lymph nodes), whereas it was 20% for patients with internal mammary lymph node–positive/axillary lymph node–positive findings. Prognosis is also inversely correlated with increasing size of internal mammary lymph nodes. To reflect these complex but important distinctions, both the number of involved axillary lymph nodes and the size of the internal mammary lymph nodes are considered in staging. Internal mammary lymph nodes that are found to be positive by sentinel node dissection but not by imaging studies are classified as "pN1b" in the absence of axillary lymph node involvement. If one to three axillary lymph nodes are involved, however, the staging becomes "pN1c," and if four or more lymph nodes are positive, it becomes "pN3b." If the internal mammary lymph nodes are detected clinically, by examination or imaging studies, they are classified as "N2b/pN2b" if axillary nodes are negative or as "N3b/pN3b" if axillary nodes are positive.

Though previously considered part of the axillary lymph node group, infraclavicular lymph node involvement is now recognized as being associated with a particularly poor prognosis and is classified as N3 disease, reflecting the adverse outcome in these patients.

The prognosis of metastases to the supraclavicular lymph nodes is so poor that earlier staging systems classified such patients as M1, that is, the same as distant metastases and hence incurable disease. Recent data, however, suggest that with aggressive therapy, the outlook is similar to that of patients with stage IIIB disease. As a result, supraclavicular lymph node involvement has been reclassified as N3 disease. A new stage, IIIC, has been added for patients with any T designation, N3, M0 disease to indicate that this high-risk subset is still potentially curable.

Prognostic Factors

Once the diagnosis of breast cancer has been established, the patient and her clinician confront a number of therapeutic choices. The selection of treatment or indeed of no further therapy depends largely on the risk of recurrent disease in a particular patient. Prognostic factors are the measurements or characteristics available at the time of diagnosis or surgery that are associated with disease-free or overall survival. These factors strongly influence whether and how much therapy should be given. In contrast, predictive factors are those characteristics or measurements that help to determine how efficacious a specific therapy is likely to be. An example is the increased likelihood of a response to hormonal therapy when the estrogen receptor is expressed in breast cancer cells.

Prognostic factors fall into three categories: patient characteristics independent of the disease (e.g., age), disease characteristics (e.g., tumor size, histologic grade), and biomarkers (measurable parameters in tissues, cells, or fluids) such as hormone receptors and measures of cell proliferation or invasiveness.

In November 2000, the National Institutes of Health held a consensus conference on the adjuvant therapy of breast cancer. Age, tumor size, lymph node involvement, histologic tumor type, histologic grade, and hormone receptor status were approved as accepted prognostic factors. Overexpression of HER-2/neu, the presence or absence of lymphovascular invasion or bone marrow micrometastases, and other measures of proliferation or invasiveness were believed to be worthy of further evaluation but not to have an established role in patient management. The lack of well-designed clinical studies based on standardized protocols with adequate power has limited the validation of most of these factors. Novel technologies, such as tissue and expression microarrays and proteonomics, were recognized for their future potential application but were deemed not ready for use in clinical practice (Table 74-3).

Axillary Lymph Node Involvement

Because of the paramount importance of accurately determining axillary lymph node involvement, axil-

lary dissection should contain six to 10 lymph nodes to provide adequate sampling. Prognostically, patients are generally categorized into those without any axillary lymph node involvement or in three groups of patients depending on whether there are one to three, four to nine, or 10 or more involved nodes (Table 74-4). In fact, one can demonstrate a direct correlation between the exact number of nodes and the risk of relapse and death; that is, patients with three positive nodes do worse than those with one positive node, and those with seven positive nodes do worse than those with four positive nodes. A dramatic decrease in survival occurs when 10 or more nodes are involved. As indicated in Table 74-4, deaths from breast cancer continue well beyond five years.

The significance of micrometastatic axillary lymph node involvement or the presence of isolated tumor cells in axillary nodes remains controversial. Retrospective studies and uncontrolled, unblinded prospective studies have yielded conflicting data, rendering treatment decisions difficult. Ongoing, prospective, randomized trials should resolve these issues.

Tumor Size and Histopathologic Subtype

Tumor size correlates with the likelihood of lymph node involvement but is also an independent prognostic factor. It becomes of particular importance when deciding whether to use adjuvant chemotherapy in patients with negative lymph nodes. Among patients with tumor size <1 cm, the likelihood of recurrence at 10 years is ≤10%. This risk rises precipitously with increasing tumor size. Survival at 10 years falls dramatically as one looks at tumor sizes more than 2 cm or 5 cm (Figure 74-1).

Certain histopathologic subtypes of breast cancer are associated with relatively favorable prognoses, including tubular, mucinous, and typical medullary carcinomas. Guidelines for systemic therapy relate to joint consideration of tumor size and histopathologic subtype. In general, systemic therapy is not recommended for tumors that are less than 1 cm and have a favorable histology. In contrast, systemic therapy should be considered in the case of unfavorable histology if the tumor size exceeds 5 mm, particularly if other unfavorable outcome characteristics are present.

Tumor Grade

Tumor grade is another prognostic factor. The unfavorable long-term effects of advancing tumor grade appear in the outcome data of Figure 74-2, from a study of patients with axillary lymph node metastases. The applicability of tumor grading in treatment decisions has been questioned because of variable reproducibility of results. In an attempt to minimize interobserver variability and make grading criteria more quantitative,

Table 74-3 ▪ Overview of Prognostic Factors in Breast Cancer

Finding	Prognosis Favorable	Unfavorable
Axillary lymph nodes*	Negative	Positive
Tumor size*	Small	Large
Histologic grade*	Grade 1 (well-differentiated)	Grade 3 (poorly differentiated)
Hormone receptors*	Positive	Negative
Lymphovascular invasion†	Present	Absent
HER-2/neu overexpression†	Negative	Positive
Epidermal growth factor Receptor overexpression	Negative	Positive
Mitotic index†	Low	High
DNA ploidy	Diploid	Aneuploid
S-phase fraction†	Low	High
Thymidine-labeling Index	Low	High
Ki-67	Low	High
Urokinase-type Plasminogen activator	Low	High
Age*	<35 years	≥35 years
Ethnicity*	Caucasian, Hispanic	African-American

*Established as an independent prognostic factor.
†Accepted as a prognostic factor, but use is limited by technical issues, such as lack of standardized methodologies and/or confirmed reproducibility among investigators.

a new system, called the Nottingham Combined Histologic Grade, was devised. It is based on the evaluation of three morphologic features: the percentage of tubule formation, degree of nuclear pleomorphism, and mitotic index in a defined field area. Each component is scored on a scale of 1 to 3. The numerical score for each feature is used to calculate an overall grade. Validation studies have confirmed the system's robust prognostic ability and reproducibility. Though the current American Joint Committee on Cancer staging system does not yet include grade in determining stage, it is likely that it will do so in the future.

Lymphatic/Vascular Invasion

Lymphatic and vascular invasion indicates an unfavorable prognosis. In single-institution studies, the presence of lymphatic or blood vessel invasion in the breast confers a prognosis similar to that of patients with one to three positive axillary lymph nodes. Its use as a determinant is hampered, as is tumor grading, by poor concordance among pathologists, primarily because of the difficulty of confirming that tumor cells are in a vessel rather than a duct. Moreover, most series have not quantitated the degree of lymphatic or

Table 74-4 ▪ Percent Overall Survival by Axillary Lymph Node Status

Number of Involved Nodes	Approximate Percent of Patients Surviving at:			
	2 Years	5 Years	8 Years	10 Years
None	>95	85	80	75
1 to 3	>95	80	65	60
4 to 9	90	65	50	40
10 or more	80	45	25	15

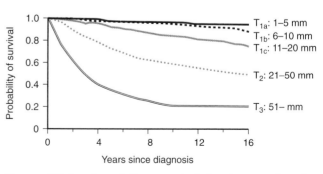

Figure 74-1 ▪ Cumulative survival by tumor size for women ages 40 to 74 years. (From Tabar L, Duffy S, Vitak B, et al: The natural history of breast carcinoma: What have we learned from screening? Cancer 1999;86:449–462.)

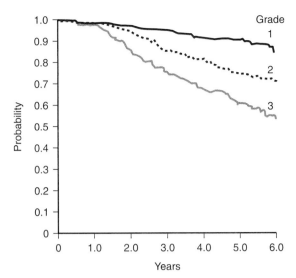

Figure 74-2 ■ Overall survival of 786 pre/perimenopausal women by tumor grade (*P* = <0.0001). (From Davis BW, Gelber RD, Goldhirsch A, et al: Prognostic significance of tumor grade in clinical trials of adjuvant therapy for breast cancer with axillary lymph node metastasis. Cancer 1986;58:2662.)

blood vessel invasion to determine whether there is a correlation between the degree of vessel involvement and prognosis.

Hormone Receptor Status

Estrogen and progesterone receptor status is a potent predictive factor for response to endocrine therapy. The presence of hormonal receptors is also a favorable, albeit weaker, prognostic factor for overall survival. Some studies report, however, that disease-free survival curves for patients with or without hormone receptors, while significantly different at five years, begin to merge with longer follow-up. In addition, hormone receptor levels are inversely correlated with DNA ploidy, S-phase fraction, and other measures of proliferation. These data suggest that receptor positivity may be more a measure of proliferative capacity than of metastatic potential.

Interestingly, when hormone receptor–positive disease recurs, it is usually in the bone or soft tissues and less often in the central nervous system or visceral organs. In addition, if analyzed according to site of recurrence, hormone receptor–positive patients tend to have improved survival over patients with hormone receptor–negative tumors recurring at the same site. Both of these observations attest to the biologic differences between hormone receptor–positive and hormone receptor–negative tumors. The noted survival differences are confounded by the potential effects of hormonal therapy used in the treatment of patients with hormone receptor–positive disease. That the pres-

ence of hormonal receptors is associated with a more indolent disease course than is their absence is likely to be due to the tumor biology, which is associated with a lower level of proliferative activity (prognostic implication) and responsiveness to endocrine maneuvers (predictive implication). This illustrates the interactions between predictive and prognostic factors.

Growth Factors and Receptors

Epidermal growth factor receptor (EGFR) and HER-2/neu are transmembrane glycoproteins present on normal breast epithelial cells that are overexpressed in a subset of breast cancers. Their overexpression tends to be associated with breast cancer that is high-grade, demonstrates increased indices of proliferation, and is hormone receptor–negative. Most studies show that overexpression of the epidermal growth factor receptor or HER-2/neu is associated with poorer disease-free and overall survival in univariate analyses, particularly among lymph node–positive patients. Unfortunately, it is among lymph node–negative patients that the need for prognostic factors is most acute. The results of multivariate analyses have been less consistent. The lack of standardization of assay methods has hindered the validation and wider application of the epidermal growth factor receptor and HER-2/neu as prognostic factors.

Despite the limitations to their use as prognostic factors for the natural history of breast cancer, both the epidermal growth factor receptor and HER-2/neu are useful predictive factors for response to hormone therapy and to chemotherapy. The overexpression of the epidermal growth factor receptor is associated with increased antiestrogen resistance, although the mechanisms that govern this relationship are not yet known. Similarly, overexpression of HER-2/neu may also confer increased resistance to tamoxifen, but these data are much more limited; are largely from nonrandomized, retrospective analyses; and at present should not be used to obviate the use of tamoxifen in patients with tumors that overexpress HER-2/neu.

Evidence continues to accumulate for the role of HER-2/neu as a predictor for relative resistance to non-anthrocycline chemotherapy. Several large, retrospective analyses show decreased benefit from non-anthracycline-containing adjuvant chemotherapy regimens in patients with tumors overexpressing HER-2/neu compared with nonoverexpressors. In contrast, similar analyses of large, multicenter trials demonstrate improved outcomes among patients whose breast cancers overexpress HER-2/neu when they are treated with anthracycline-containing chemotherapy. As further proof of principle, patients with high levels of HER-2/neu expression, but not those with low levels of expression, showed a dose-response relationship in terms of disease-free and overall survival to a regimen consisting of cyclophosphamide, doxorubicin, and 5-fluorouracil (Figure 74-3). These data suggest an important predictive role for HER-2/neu in the selection of adjuvant chemotherapy, though its routine application awaits consensus about the most appropriate and standardized method for determining HER-2/neu status.

Proliferative Indices

A plethora of measures of tumor cell proliferative rate are widely available. Each of the measures demonstrates prognostic significance in univariate analyses. But for a variable to have independent prognostic value, its statistical significance must persist in multivariate analyses, which exclude the impact of other potent prognostic factors that may be highly correlated with the variable in question. Even though a number of prognostic factors fail multivariate tests of significance or lack reproducible precision between laboratories, they may still be useful in improving the understanding of tumor biology or in making therapeutic decisions. A number of techniques that are used to measure breast cancer cellular proliferation are in this category.

Mitotic Index

The mitotic index is the most widely accepted, quickest, and least expensive of the methods used to assess tumor cell proliferative rates. The mitotic index, as was previously noted, is used in establishing the histologic grade of a tumor. In this method, paraffin-embedded tumor specimens are stained with hematoxylin and eosin, and the mitotic figures are counted, using light microscopy. The number of cells in active mitosis is variably reported relative to the number of tumor cells, high-power fields, tumor volume, or unit area. Each of these methods has demonstrated prognostic significance by univariate analysis and in some multivariate analyses. If the number of cells appearing in each high-power field is known, then the mitotic index includes a measure of both proliferation and cellularity, which enhance its prognostic utility. The mitotic index is therefore usually reported as the number of mitotic figures per high-power field.

Flow Cytometry for DNA Ploidy and S-Phase Fraction

Flow cytometry can be used to assess DNA ploidy and S-phase fraction. DNA ploidy measures the DNA content of cells. Cells with apparently normal DNA content are diploid, because they contain two copies of DNA. Cells that have an abnormal content of DNA are aneuploid, reflecting a more poorly differentiated state. Aneuploid DNA content correlates with shortened disease-free and overall survival compared to patients whose breast cancers are diploid.

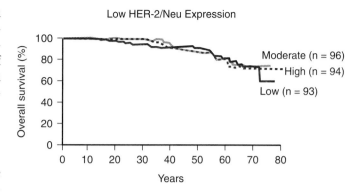

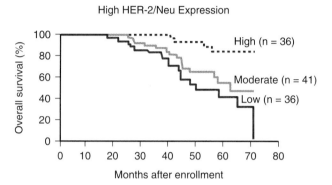

Figure 74-3 ▪ Overall survival according to treatment group receiving high-dose, moderate-dose, or low-dose chemotherapy (cyclophosphamide, doxorubicin, and 5-fluorouracil) and levels of HER-2/neu expression. (From Muss HB, Thor AD, Berry DA, et al: c-erbB-2 expression and response to adjuvant therapy in women with node-positive early breast cancer. N Engl J Med 1994;330:1260–1266.)

The S-phase fraction estimates the proportion of tumor cells undergoing active DNA synthesis in preparation for mitosis. The S-phase fraction is highly directly correlated with other prognostic factors, including histologic grade, degree of lymph node involvement, tumor size, and DNA aneuploidy. The S-phase fraction is a continuous variable, and levels demarcating high from low levels are lacking, causing inconsistency in separating patients into different risk groups. Moreover, tumors generally consist of a mixture of benign and malignant cell subpopulations, each of which exhibits varying cell cycle kinetics. The changing proportion of these cell subpopulations causes large variations in the reported S-phase fraction.

Ki-67

Ki-67 is a monoclonal antibody directed against a nuclear antigen expressed in proliferating cells, that is, cells that are not in the resting G_0 phase of the cell cycle. Ki-67 expression directly correlates with other prognostic factors including tumor size, lymph node status, histologic grade, and lymphovascular invasion.

Thymidine-Labeling Index

The thymidine-labeling index (TLI) measures the proliferative rate of a tumor by counting the number of radiolabeled nuclei on a microsection of tumor after incubation with tritiated thymidine. As with Ki-67 and S-phase fraction, the thymidine-labeling index is a continuous variable; establishing standardized methodologies and cutoff values and ensuring reproducibility remains problematic.

Plasminogen Activators and Inhibitors

The interaction between urokinase-type plasminogen activator and its inhibitor is one of the systemic axes that is potentially involved in cancer invasion and metastasis. Urokinase-type plasminogen activator is a proteolytic enzyme that catalyzes the conversion of plasminogen to plasmin. Plasmin activates type IV collagenase, which degrades collagen and proteins of the basement membrane, thereby fostering tumor cell invasion through vessel walls. Several studies demonstrate that the balance between urokinase-type plasminogen activator and plasminogen activator inhibitors (e.g., PAI-1) correlate with an unfavorable prognosis. Unfortunately, at present, the routine clinical assay of these factors remains impractical, requiring fresh frozen tissue and specialized laboratory techniques.

Gene Expression Profiling

Gene expression profiling using DNA microarrays allows measurement of thousands of genes simultaneously. Using this approach, one can identify distinct patterns of gene expression that correlate with clinical outcome measures. The successful use of such "molecular fingerprinting" was reported by van de Vijver et al. (2002). Using microarray analysis, a 70-gene prognostic profile was determined in a test population of 78 young women with lymph node–negative breast cancer. Using this profile, 295 women were subsequently classified as having either a poor or a good prognosis. All patients had stage I or II disease, and approximately half of patients had no axillary lymph node involvement. The prognostic signatures obtained by microarray of gene expression were capable of identifying patients at low or high risk of recurrent disease, with finer delineation of risk groups than is available from current histologic and clinical criteria. The study results were potentially compromised by inclusion of patients in the validation study sample who were used to construct the original profile and the confounding effect of treatment on disease outcome. Nevertheless, microarray technology holds significant promise for our ability to select patients who could benefit from adjuvant systemic treatment. It could provide a means to reduce both the undertreatment and overtreatment of

TREATMENT

Clinical Use of Prognostic Factors in Breast Cancer

A staging system's raison d'etre is, at least in part, to help estimate an individual's prognosis. This estimate largely informs the decision of whether or not to use systemic therapy. Patients whose tumor sizes are very small (≤0.5 cm) and who do not have lymph node metastases rarely receive systemic adjuvant therapy. If the tumor is larger than 0.5 cm, histologic type and grade become relevant factors in determining whether the prognosis has changed sufficiently to warrant treatment. Once size exceeds 1 cm, in the absence of very favorable histologic grade or type, systemic treatment is recommended. Involvement of lymph nodes, regardless of tumor size, usually leads to systemic therapy. The presence or absence of hormone receptors influences choice of therapy (chemotherapy, endocrine therapy, or both). In practice, the threshold for hormonal therapy, because of its lesser toxicity, is lower than that for chemotherapy. Therefore, patients with low-risk, hormone receptor–positive disease are more likely to receive systemic therapy (in the form of hormonal therapy) than are patients with low-risk, hormone receptor–negative disease (for whom chemotherapy would be the only systemic option), even if they share a similar favorable prognosis.

Despite its shortcomings as a prognostic factor, HER-2/neu overexpression is widely accepted as an unfavorable finding. Its ability to predict response to treatment is its principal value in practice. Although the NIH Consensus Conference on adjuvant therapy for breast cancer did not find the data sufficient to base treatment on the HER-2/neu status of tumors, many clinicians use it to determine the type of therapy. Patients whose tumors overexpress HER-2/neu and have a prognosis that warrants the use of systemic chemotherapy are treated preferentially with anthracycline-containing regimens. At present, however, the HER-2/neu status is not used to decide whether or what hormonal therapy should be employed.

patients with breast cancer, thereby enhancing the opportunity to deliver patient-specific therapy.

Patient Characteristics

Age

Young age in patients with breast cancer is an important adverse prognostic factor, especially for women younger than 35 years old. Other poor prognostic factors occur frequently in such young patients, including large tumor size, high-grade histology, extensive axillary lymph node involvement, hormone receptor negativity, lymphatic vessel invasion, and higher S-phase fraction. Nevertheless, multivariate analyses that control for these and other factors consistently find that the prognosis is worse for younger than older patients. This suggests that breast cancer may be biologically more aggressive in young women than in women older than age 35.

Ethnicity

African-American women tend to have overall poorer prognoses than white women, probably occasioned by both socioeconomic factors and differences in tumor cell biology. Cultural barriers and decreased access to breast cancer screening and medical care among non-white women play a role in the increased frequency of their presentation with locally advanced disease. Compared to African-American women, white women at presentation more often are older and have less axillary lymph node involvement, higher incidence of estrogen-receptor positivity and lower S-phase fraction. These data suggest that biologic differences exist as well. When analyses have accounted for these factors, however, systemic treatment appears to confer similar benefits, regardless of ethnicity.

References

Albain KS, Allred DC, Clark GM: Breast cancer outcome and predictors of outcome: Are there age differentials? J Natl Cancer Inst Monogr 1994;16:35–42.

Carter CL, Allen C, Henson DE: Relation of tumor size, lymph node status, and survival in 24,740 breast cancer cases. Cancer 1989;63:181–187.

Clark GM: Should selection of adjuvant chemotherapy for patients with breast cancer be based on erbB-2 status? J Natl Cancer Inst 1998;90:1320–1321.

Clark GM: Prognostic and predictive factors. In Harris J, Lippman M, Morrow M, et al (eds): Diseases of the Breast, 2nd ed. Philadelphia: Lippincott Williams & Wilkins, 2000.

Clark GM, Dressler LG, Owens MA, et al: Prediction of relapse or survival in patients with node-negative breast cancer by DNA flow cytometry. N Engl J Med 1989;320:627–633.

Clayton F: Pathologic correlates of survival in 378 lymph node-negative infiltrating ductal breast carcinomas. Cancer 1991;68:1309–1317.

Contesso G, Mouriesse H, Friedman S, et al: The importance of histologic grade in long-term prognosis of breast cancer: A study of 1,010 patients, uniformly treated at the Institut Gustave-Roussy. J Clin Oncol 1987;5:1378–1386.

Cote RJ, Peterson HF, Chiawun B, et al: Role of immunohistochemical detection of lymph-node metastases in management of breast cancer. International Breast Cancer Study Group. Lancet 1999;354:896–900.

Dalton LW, Page DL, Dupont WD: Histologic grading of breast carcinoma: A reproducibility study. Cancer 1994;73:2765–2770.

Davis BW, Gelber RD, Goldhirsch A, et al: Prognostic significance of tumor grade in clinical trials of adjuvant therapy for breast cancer with axillary lymph node metastasis. Cancer 1986;58:2662–2666.

Diab SG, Clark G, Osborne CK, et al: Tumor characteristics and clinical outcome of tubular and mucinous breast carcinomas. J Clin Oncol 1999;17:1442–1448.

Donegan WL: Tumor-related prognostic factors in breast cancer. CA Cancer J Clin 1997;47:28–517.

Dressler LG, Eudey L, Gray R, et al: Prognostic potential of DNA flow cytometry measurements in node-negative breast cancer patients: Preliminary analysis of an intergroup study (INT 0076). J Natl Cancer Inst Monogr 1992;11:167–172.

Early Breast Cancer Trialists' Collaborative Group: Polychemotherapy for early breast cancer: an overview of the randomised trials. Lancet 1998;352:930–942.

Eifel P, Axelson JA, Costa J, et al: National Institutes of Health Consensus Development Conference Statement: Adjuvant therapy for breast cancer, November 1–3, 2000. J Natl Cancer Inst 2001;93:979–989.

Eley JW, Hill HA, Chen VW, et al: Racial differences in survival from breast cancer. JAMA 1994;272:947–954.

Elledge RM, Clark GM, Chamness GC, Osborne CK: Tumor biologic factors and breast cancer prognosis among white, Hispanic, and black women in the United States. J Natl Cancer Inst 1994;86:705–712.

Elledge RM, Green S, Ciocca D, et al: HER-2 expression and response to tamoxifen in estrogen receptor-positive breast cancer: A Southwest Oncology Group Study. Clin Cancer Res 1998;4:7–12.

Elston CW, Ellis IO, Pinder SE: Pathological prognostic factors in breast cancer. Crit Rev Oncol Hematol 1999;31:209–223.

Fisher B, Bauer M, Wickerham DL, et al: Relation of number of positive axillary nodes to the prognosis of patients with primary breast cancer: An NSABP update. Cancer 1983;52:1551–1557.

Fisher B, Slack NH, Bross ID: Cancer of the breast: Size of neoplasm and prognosis. Cancer 1969;24:1071–1080.

Fisher E, Anderson S, Redmond C, et al: Pathologic findings from the National Surgical Adjuvant Breast Project Protocol B-06. Cancer 1993;71:2507–2514.

Fitzgibbons PL, Page DL, Weaver D, et al: Prognostic factors in breast cancer: College of American Pathologists Consensus Statement 1999. Arch Pathol Lab Med 2000;124:966–978.

Foekens JA, Schmitt M, van Putten WL, et al: Prognostic value of urokinase-type plasminogen activator in 671 primary breast cancer patients. Cancer Res 1992;52:6101–6105.

Fox S, Smith K, Hollyer J, et al: The epidermal growth factor receptor as a prognostic marker: Results of 370 patients and review of 3009 patients. Breast Cancer Res Treat 1994;29:41–47.

Goldhirsch A, Glick JH, Gelber R, et al: Meeting highlights: International consensus panel on the treatment of primary breast cancer. J Clin Oncol 2001;19:3817–3827.

Greene FL, Page DL, Fleming ID, et al: AJCC Cancer Staging Manual, 6th ed. New York: Springer-Verlag, 2002.

Hayes DF, Trock B, Harris AL: Assessing the clinical impact of prognostic factors: When is "statistically significant" clinically useful? Breast Cancer Res Treat 1999;52:305–319.

Hedley D: DNA flow cytometry and breast cancer. Breast Cancer Res Treat 1993;28:51–58.

Hedley DW, Clark GM, Cornelisse CJ, et al: Consensus review of the clinical utility of DNA cytometry in carcinoma of the breast: Report of the DNA Cytometry Consensus Conference. Cytometry 1993;14:482–485.

Isaacs C, Stearns V, Hayes DF: New prognostic factors for breast cancer recurrence. Semin Oncol 2001;28:53–67.

Joslyn SA, West MM: Racial differences in breast carcinoma survival. Cancer 2000;88:114–123.

Lauria R, Perrone F, Carlomagno C, et al: The prognostic value of lymphatic and blood vessel invasion in operable breast cancer. Cancer 1995;76:1772–1778.

Lee A, DeLellis R, Silverman M, et al: Prognostic significance of peritumoral lymphatic and blood vessel invasion in node-negative carcinoma of the breast. J Clin Oncol 1990; 8:1457–1465.

Lee A, Loda M, Mackarem G, et al: Lymph node negative invasive breast carcinoma 1 centimeter or less in size (T1a,bN0M0). Cancer 1997;79:761–771.

Leitner SP, Swern AS, Weinberger D, et al: Predictors of recurrence for patients with small (one centimeter or less) localized breast cancer (T1a,bN0M0). Cancer 1995;76:2266–2274.

Leitzel K, Teramoto Y, Konrad K, et al: Elevated serum c-erbB-2 antigen levels and decreased response to hormone therapy of breast cancer. J Clin Oncol 1995;13:1129–1135.

McGuire WL, Clark GM: Prognostic factors and treatment decisions in axillary-node-negative breast cancer. N Engl J Med 1992;326:1756–1761.

Moon TE, Jones SE, Bonadonna G, et al: Development and use of a natural history data base in breast cancer studies. Am J Clin Oncol (CCT) 1987;10:396–403.

Muss HB, Thor AD, Berry DA, et al: c-erbB-2 expression and response to adjuvant therapy in women with node-positive early breast cancer. N Engl J Med 1994;330:1260–1266.

Nixon A, Neuber D, Hayes D, et al: Relationship of patient age to pathologic features of the tumor and prognosis for patients with stage I or II breast cancer. J Clin Oncol 1994;12:888–894.

O'Reilly SM, Camplejohn RS, Barnes DM, et al: Node-negative breast cancer: Prognostic subgroups defined by tumor size and flow cytometry. J Clin Oncol 1990;8:2040–2046.

Paik S, Bryant J, Park C, et al: erbB-2 and response to doxorubicin in patients with axillary lymph node-positive, hormone receptor-negative breast cancer. J Natl Cancer Inst 1998;90:1361–1367.

Rosen PP, Groshen S, Kinne DW, et al: Factors influencing prognosis in node-negative breast carcinoma: Analysis of 767 T1N0M0/T2N0M0) patients with long-term follow-up. J Clin Oncol 1993;11:2090–2100.

Rosen PP, Groshen S, Saigo PE, et al: Pathological prognostic factors in stage I (T1N0M0) and stage II (T1N1M0) breast carcinoma: A study of 644 patients with median follow-up of 18 years. J Clin Oncol 1989;7:1239–1251.

Sigurdsson H, Baldetorp B, Borg A, et al: Indicators of prognosis in node-negative breast cancer. N Engl J Med 1990; 322:1045–1053.

Silvestrini R, Daidone MG, Luisi A, et al: Biologic and clinico-pathologic factors as indicators of specific relapse types in node-negative breast cancer. J Clin Oncol 1995; 13:697–704.

Singletary SE, Allred C, Ashley P, et al: Revision of the American Joint Committee on Cancer staging system for breast cancer. J Clin Oncol 2002;20:3628–3636.

Spyratos F, Martin PM, Hacene K, et al: Multiparametric prognostic evaluation of biological factors in primary breast cancer. J Natl Cancer Inst 1992;84:1266–1272.

Stal O, Dufmats M, Hatschek T, et al. S-phase fraction is a prognostic factor in stage I breast carcinoma. J Clin Oncol 1993;11:1717–1722.

Tabar L, Duffy S, Vitak B, et al: The natural history of breast carcinoma: What have we learned from screening? Cancer 1999;86:449–462.

Valagussa P, Bonadonna G, Veronesi U: Patterns of relapse and survival following radical mastectomy. Cancer 1978; 41:1170–1178.

van de Vijver MJ, He YD, van't Veer LJ, et al: A gene-expression signature as a predictor of survival in breast cancer. N Engl J Med 2002;347:1999–2009.

Van't Veer LJ, Dai J, van de Vijver MJ, et al: Gene expression profiling predicts clinical outcome of breast cancer. Nature 2002;415:530–536.

Weigand R, Isenberg WM, Russo J, et al: Blood vessel invasion and axillary lymph node involvement as prognostic indicators for human breast cancer. Cancer 1982;50:962–969.

Wenger CR, Beardslee S, Owens MA: DNA ploidy, S-phase, and steroid receptors in more than 127,000 breast cancer patients. Breast Cancer Res Treat 1993;28:9–20

Yarboro JW, Page DL, Fielding LP, et al: American Joint Committee on Cancer prognostic factors consensus conference. Cancer 1999;86:2436–2446.

Chapter 75
Noninvasive Breast Cancer

Virginia Borges and Steven E. Come

The hallmark of noninvasive breast cancer is the aberrant proliferation of malignant epithelial cells within the walls and lumens of ducts and/or lobules in the absence of evidence of invasion through the underlying basement membrane. Two main subcategories comprise noninvasive breast cancer: ductal carcinoma in situ (DCIS) and lobular carcinoma in situ (LCIS). The advent of routine screening mammography has had a dramatic effect on the incidence and presentation of both of these disorders, which once were thought to be uncommon findings. According to the National Cancer Institute's Surveillance Epidemiology and End Results (SEER) database, in 1973 the annual incidence of ductal carcinoma in situ was approximately 2 in 100,000, increasing to approximately 15 in 100,000 by 1992. The rate of change correlated with the advent of screening mammography in approximately 1982. During the period 1983 to 1992 compared with the period 1973 to 1982, the rate of detection of ductal carcinoma in situ increased 138% and 235% for women less than age 50 years and older than age 50 years, respectively, while the rate of detection of invasive breast cancer increased by only 50%. The rates of lobular carcinoma in situ also increased during this time (although not as dramatically), with the rate of new diagnosis four times higher for ductal carcinoma in situ than for lobular carcinoma in situ. Rather than a mammographic finding, lobular carcinoma in situ is usually an incidental finding on biopsies done for other indications.

Ductal carcinoma in situ and lobular carcinoma in situ are clinically quite distinct in their presentations, pathologic appearances, and implications for future invasive breast cancer. Thus, current treatment recommendations for ductal carcinoma in situ and lobular carcinoma in situ differ as well. This chapter focuses on the clinical presentations, significant histological patterns, and current management concepts for the two disorders.

Ductal Carcinoma in Situ
Presentation

Ductal carcinoma in situ has been a recognized pathologic entity since the 1930s, when its presentation was commonly that of a clinically detectable mass. Nipple discharge, with or without an underlying detectable mass, was the other common presentation of the early twentieth century. Occasionally, ductal carcinoma in situ was an incidental finding on a biopsy done for a benign cause. Although these presentations are still seen today, the implementation of screening mammography has altered the typical presentation of ductal carcinoma in situ to a much earlier diagnosis. Now, new or increased microcalcifications on mammography are the most common findings, although a nonpalpable mass might be seen as well.

Issues of multicentric disease and concomitant microinvasion are confounding aspects of ductal carcinoma in situ presentation that have significant impact on treatment and prognosis. Early series done in the premammographic era showed an incidence of multicentric disease as high as 53%; however, this was found to relate directly to the size of the ductal carcinoma in situ lesion. Small lesions (less than 2.5 cm) exhibited multicentric disease only 14% of the time. Earlier studies are difficult to interpret due to the variable definition of multicentricity and sampling issues. A contemporary study that examined mastectomy specimens from mammographically detected lesions defined multicentricity as foci of disease separated by 4 cm or more and found only one instance in the 82 cases surveyed. Similarly, the risk of occult microinvasive disease has also been dependent upon tumor size and method of detection (clinical presentation versus mammographic finding). In one series, ductal carcinoma in situ lesions greater than 2.5 cm showed microinvasion 29% of the time, whereas microinvasion was detected in only 2% of smaller lesions. Thus, two common and important features in ductal carcinoma in situ presentation—namely, multicentricity and microinvasion—are now rarely seen in cases that are detected mammographically.

The risk factors for presentation of ductal carcinoma in situ in women undergoing screening mammography appear to mimic those for invasive carcinoma. Family history, nulliparity or age of first childbirth over 30 years, and early menarche were associated with an increased risk of both ductal carcinoma in situ and invasive cancer for women over age 50. Women in this series who were diagnosed with ductal carcinoma in situ were significantly younger (54 versus 59 years old) and less likely to have had a palpable mass than women diagnosed with an invasive cancer. The similar pattern of risk and earlier age at presentation support the view that ductal carcinoma in situ is a preinvasive lesion with clearly malignant potential.

Pathologic and Mammographic Features

The traditional classification of ductal carcinoma in situ is based upon architectural appearance and can be divided into five major groupings: papillary, micropap-illary, cribriform, solid, and comedo. Papillary ductal carcinoma in situ (Figure 75-1D) is characterized by projections of small- to intermediate-sized cells arranged along a fibrovascular core, forming the hallmark papillae. In the micropapillary form, the fibrovascular core is not present, and the projections are also smaller in size (Figure 75-1C). Cribriform ductal carcinoma in situ is characterized by the ductal lumen being nearly full with a monotonous small- to intermediate-sized cell population and only small, well-rounded areas of open lumen remaining. Mitotic figures are rare, and necrosis is not present to any significant extent (Figure 75-1B). In the solid classification, the entire lumen is filled with tumor cells (Figure 75-1E). The cells can be of any size and can have variable morphologic appearances. Again, little or no necrosis is seen. Lastly, comedo-type ductal carcinoma in situ (Figure 75-1A) is characterized by large, heterogeneous-appearing cells and a prominent feature of necrosis in the center of the solid area of cellular proliferation. The necrotic center is the hallmark of this type and can often be extruded from the lesion as a soft, cheesy material after surgical removal. In contrast to the other forms, in the comedo type many mitotic figures are often present. Ductal carcinoma in

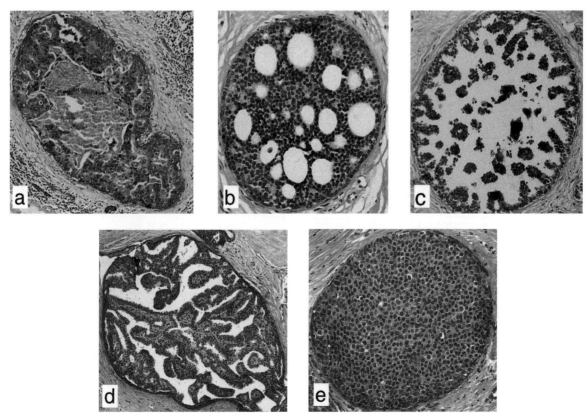

Figure 75-1 ■ Architectural classifications of ductal carcinoma in situ. *A*, Comedo pattern. *B*, Cribriform pattern. *C*, Micropapillary pattern. *D*, Papillary pattern. *E*, Solid pattern. (See Color Plate 17.) (From Schnitt S: Pathology of breast cancer. In Hayes DF (ed): Atlas of Breast Cancer, 2nd ed. St. Louis: Mosby, 2000.)

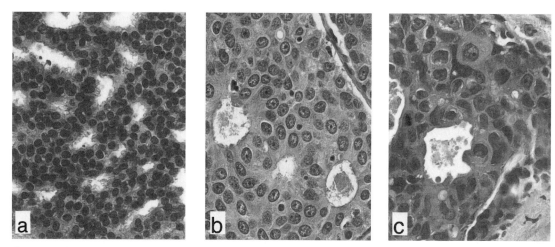

Figure 75-2 ■ Nuclear grading of ductal carcinoma in situ. *A*, Low nuclear grade. *B*, Intermediate grade. *C*, High nuclear grade. (See Color Plate 17.) (From Schnitt S: Pathology of breast cancer. In Hayes DF (ed): Atlas of Breast Cancer, 2nd ed. St. Louis: Mosby, 2000.)

situ is often separated by nuclear grading into low-, intermediate-, and high-grade classifications based on the degree of nuclear pleomorphism (Figure 75–2). Comedo ductal carcinoma in situ, with a prevalence of mitotic figures, is frequently of a high nuclear grade, while the other classifications are usually of an intermediate or low nuclear grade.

Calcification is most often associated with the comedo form of ductal carcinoma in situ because calcium deposition correlates with rapid growth and necrosis. A pattern of linear branching calcifications following along the ductal tree as it fills with necrotic debris is the predominant mammographic appearance for this type of ductal carcinoma in situ. However, coarse granular calcifications can also be seen in comedo ductal carcinoma in situ. In the low-grade forms of ductal carcinoma in situ, calcifications can also occur but are predominantly granular areas often clustered in groups (Figure 75-3). These are called *psammoma* calcifications and are less suggestive of ductal carcinoma in situ than the linear type, which can be found in many benign breast conditions as well. The difference in calcifications seen with high-grade vs. low-grade ductal carcinoma in situ also alters the ability to assess extent of disease by mammogram, with the branching pattern of comedo-form ductal carcinoma in situ more reliably correlating with disease size by standard two-view imaging. The low-grade forms are more often underestimated with this approach, but the use of additional magnification views can overcome this discrepancy.

Prognostic Correlation

The classification system of ductal carcinoma in situ is limited by a number of factors and is, therefore, not of ideal clinical utility. The classification is not uni-formly defined. A lack of reproducibility in the interpretation exists between pathologists. Further, overlap or mixed lesions are common; the biology of the disease is not so neat as to fit into one of the five distinct categories. In an attempt to provide a more practical and meaningful system, ductal carcinoma in situ has been dichotomized into comedo and noncomedo subtypes by some authors. This is based on the higher incidence of malignant features with comedo or high-grade lesions when compared with the other forms or with low-grade lesions. Table 75-1, adapted from Connolly and Nixon, outlines

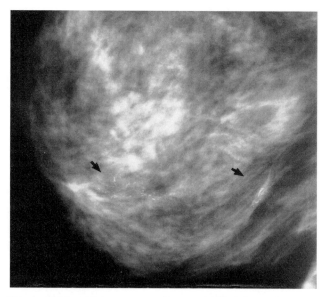

Figure 75-3 ■ Mammogram demonstrating two areas (see arrows) of granular clusters suggestive of ductal carcinoma in situ.

Table 75-1 ■ Biologic Differences Among Cases of Ductal Carcinoma in Situ Based on Grade/Comedo Status

Characteristic	High-Grade (Comedo Type)	Low-Grade (Non-Comedo Type)
Estrogen Receptor Positive	Infrequent	Frequent
Necrosis	Frequent	Infrequent
Nuclear Cytology	High-grade	Low-grade
Aneuploidy	Frequent	Infrequent
Proliferative Rate	High	Low
HER-2/neu+	Frequent	Infrequent
p53+	More common	Less common
Microvessel Density	High	Low
Microinvasion	More common	Less common
Calcifications	Coarse granular	Fine granular

Reprinted and adapted with permission from Connolly JL, Nixon AJ: Ductal carcinoma in situ of the breast: Histologic subtyping and clinical significance. Updates Prin Pract Oncol 1996;10:3.

the differences seen, providing a biologic rationale for this stratification.

Other groups have proposed classification systems that seek to provide more prognostic information and therefore better serve to guide treatment decisions. These classification systems focus primarily on predictors of recurrence after breast-conserving therapy, such as nuclear grade, margin status, and presence of comedo-type features or necrosis. These classification systems use similar factors, with the common theme being a split of ductal carcinoma in situ into low-, intermediate-, and high-risk categories. A consensus conference was held in 1997 to address ductal carcinoma in situ classification, but no single existing method was adopted. An agreement, however, was reached on the features of ductal carcinoma in situ that should be reported by pathologists and used by clinicians in interpretation of disease risk. These features include nuclear grade (low, intermediate, or high), cell polarization, architectural pattern, and the presence of necrosis.

Unfortunately, even with some consensus on the important features of ductal carcinoma in situ, a true prognostic mechanism to determine those lesions that will ultimately progress to invasive cancer within a woman's lifetime does not currently exist. Small retrospective series from the 1970s to 1980s demonstrate that the risk of subsequent invasive cancer for untreated ductal carcinoma in situ averages 31%. Although the current methods of classification do impart some understanding of the prognosis for a given ductal carcinoma in situ lesion, improved iden-

tification of important molecular markers will be an important step in refining this process.

Differential Diagnosis

As ductal carcinoma in situ represents one point in a spectrum of malignant change, diagnostic challenges often lie at the edges of the disease category. Distinguishing certain cases of low-grade ductal carcinoma in situ from atypical ductal hyperplasia can be challenging, and expert review of the specimen could be necessary for any degree of certainty. Likewise, some cases of ductal carcinoma in situ can be difficult to distinguish from invasive carcinoma, particularly if the lesion is large or the specimen demonstrates any distortion of the tissue from either inflammation in the lesion or fixation artifact. Determining ductal carcinoma in situ with microinvasion from more extensive invasive cancer can be another area of difficulty. The American Joint Committee on Cancer (AJCC) Cancer Staging Manual now defines microinvasion as the extension of cancer cells beyond the basement membrane by no more than 0.1 cm in greatest dimension ($T1_{mic}$). Furthermore, when multiple foci of microscopic invasion are present, only the largest area is used to determine size, rather than the sum of multiple areas. Finally, if ductal carcinoma in situ extends up into the terminal lobules (a phenomenon known as "cancerization of the lobules"), the diagnosis can be confused with lobular carcinoma in situ, and there are also lesions with true overlap between these two entities.

Management of Ductal Carcinoma in Situ

Therapeutic Options

From the earliest descriptions of ductal carcinoma in situ, it was recognized that the disease was highly curable by mastectomy, and so this procedure remained the standard of care for many decades. The combined data for 14 published studies comprising over 1061 women who underwent mastectomy for ductal carcinoma in situ demonstrates a cancer-related mortality of 1.7%. Follow-up time in these studies ranged from two to more than 15 years, and the pattern of disease recurrence was typical for metastatic breast cancer presentations in general: local recurrence on the chest wall and axilla or distant metastasis. Although the theoretical rate of cure for mastectomy in a noninvasive lesion should be 100%, these studies demonstrate that occult invasion can exist and become (albeit rarely) clinically significant.

As it became increasingly apparent and accepted that women with invasive breast cancer could be treated adequately by breast-conserving surgery, this technique was applied to ductal carcinoma in situ. One problem with this approach for ductal carcinoma

TREATMENT

Overview of Ductal Carcinoma in Situ Therapy

The treatment of ductal carcinoma in situ is best approached in a multidisciplinary setting, where the radiologist, pathologist, surgeon, and radiation oncologist have the opportunity for careful review of all mammograms and pathologic specimens available at the time of presentation. First, ensuring that adequate mammographic views have been obtained—including magnification films aimed at delineating all suspicious areas—is extremely important at the outset of therapy. For lesions with extensive calcifications, the use of two wires bracketing the area can help ensure an adequate excision. Postexcision specimen mammograms are important to ensure that all calcifications have been addressed adequately. Follow-up mammogram of the breast is indicated if the specimen mammogram is not conclusive or if the area of disease was extensive. Once the diagnosis of ductal carcinoma in situ is certain, assessment of the pathologic subtype, extent of disease, assurance of ability to receive radiation therapy, and preference of the patient must be considered before a treatment plan is recommended and decided upon. With all members of the breast care team present (including the patient), rapid clarification of any outstanding issues or test needs is possible, allowing for expeditious planning of the woman's remaining therapy. The decision regarding systemic therapy with tamoxifen can be delayed until after definitive local treatment has occurred, thereby allowing the woman to face one decision at a time.

Although many women will be candidates for lumpectomy and radiation therapy, certain situations render this an inappropriate form of therapy. One such case is where the extent of calcifications on mammography encompasses the majority of the breast or is located in disparate regions of the breast, such that lumpectomy would not allow for complete removal of all areas with tumor-free margins and/or provide for adequate cosmesis. If clear margins cannot be obtained or residual calcifications remain after reexcision(s), mastectomy should be strongly encouraged. Finally, any women for whom radiation therapy would be contraindicated (i.e., history of prior radiation therapy or significant connective tissue disease) should undergo mastectomy unless the lesion merits inclusion in an investigative protocol that uses wide excision alone.

In the majority of cases, sampling of the lymph nodes is not a necessary step. Any large lesion (4–5 cm or greater), however, raises a concern about the risk of microinvasion, particularly if the lesion is of high-grade histology. In such situations, sampling of the lymph nodes is important to ensure that the planned therapeutic intervention is appropriate.

Women who have had a diagnosis of ductal carcinoma in situ are at increased risk for future breast cancer. A careful program of follow-up is essential, particularly if a conservative treatment approach was used. Quarterly examination of the breast with mammograms performed at 6-month follow-up and then annually is one approach. Women who have had mastectomy need only resume their annual contralateral screening program but should still be physically examined quarterly to semiannually as well.

in situ centers on the risk for increased cancer-related mortality as a trade-off for breast conservation. Although the risk of death from pure ductal carcinoma in situ is very low, recurrence as an invasive cancer in a preserved breast carries the associated risk of metastasis and subsequent increased breast-cancer mortality.

Unfortunately, no prospectively designed study comparing the use of mastectomy to breast-conserving surgery for ductal carcinoma in situ has ever been done. In the National Surgical Adjuvant Breast Project (NSABP) B-06 protocol, a randomized study of invasive breast cancer treated with mastectomy, lumpectomy and radiation, or lumpectomy alone, review of the pathologic specimens revealed 78 patients with pure ductal carcinoma in situ who were initially thought to have had invasive disease. It is noteworthy that the ductal carcinoma in situ lesions were mostly clinically apparent rather than detected by mammog-

raphy alone. The rate of local recurrence for the 29 patients that had received lumpectomy and radiation was 7%, or two cases, of which one was invasive. The 21 patients who had received lumpectomy alone had a 23% risk at the initial point of 39 months of mean observation. Subsequently, 76 of these patients were then followed for a mean of 83 months. The rate of local recurrence for the lumpectomy plus radiation group remained 7%, however, the lumpectomy alone group had an increase to 43%, with 3 of 9 cases being invasive. Nonetheless, the overall outcome across the three groups were similar, with one patient in the mastectomy arm and one patient in the lumpectomy arm having died of disease at the time of the 1991 presentation.

Two approaches to breast-conserving therapy for ductal carcinoma in situ have been investigated. One attempt has been to identify patients for whom wide excision alone would be appropriate. The other has been to treat unselected cases of ductal carcinoma in situ with lumpectomy followed by radiation therapy, analogous to the management of invasive breast cancer. Two large randomized trials directly comparing the role of lumpectomy with or without radiation therapy have been reported and are discussed in the following sections.

A number of studies examined wide excision alone as an appropriate therapy for selected cases of ductal carcinoma in situ. Table 75-2 summarizes the results of some of these studies, all of which were retrospective series. Typically, these studies required small lesions (less than 2.5 cm) and consisted of mostly mammographically detected lesions. The study by Lagios et al has the longest length of median follow-up time, with 124 months for the initial 20 enrolled patients and 48 months for the remaining 59 patients. Their local recurrence rate of 20% for the initial group is somewhat higher than in the other studies with shorter follow-up duration.

Nonetheless, the local recurrence rate of the initial group can be contrasted to the 43% rate seen in the B-06 study, where patients had not been preselected for small lesions. In the largest of the nonrandomized studies (Table 75-2), 256 patients were treated with excision alone and followed for a mean of 72 months. Special attention was given to the processing of samples at the time of excision, with total sequential evaluation of the tissue specimen and detailed determination of lesion size and margin extent. The recurrence rate of 15%, half of which was invasive disease, is consistent with the other series.

A large, nonrandomized study retrospectively evaluated postlumpectomy radiation therapy in 270 cases of ductal carcinoma in situ from 10 European and U.S. institutions. Outcomes were reported at 15 years of actuarial follow-up. The majority of cases were 2 cm or less in size, but documentation of tumor-negative margins were known for only 35% of cases. All cases had undergone lumpectomy, with 15%

receiving reexcision and 32% undergoing axillary lymph node dissection. All sampled cases were node-negative. Radiation was given according to local institutional protocol, and 65% of cases received a boost to the tumor site. The interpretation of the results is hindered by the lack of consistent treatment across the institutions. The 15-year actuarial local failure rate was 19%. This is more than twice the value reported at the 5-year mark (7%), which is usually reported in other, smaller studies with shorter follow-up time. Nonetheless, the actuarial cause-specific survival rate was 96%. This study emphasizes the need for long-term follow-up for such therapies, as recurrences were documented up to 15 years or longer after treatment (Figure 75-4).

The National Surgical Adjuvant Breast Project B-17 protocol randomized 818 women to lumpectomy versus lumpectomy plus a fixed program of radiation therapy at 50 Gy. The results were initially presented in 1993 and subsequently updated in 1998 with 90 months of median follow-up. The European Organization for Research and Therapy of Cancer (EORTC) Trial 10853 prospectively randomized 1010 women to lumpectomy vs. lumpectomy with radiation therapy fixed at 50 Gy. The results of this study have been presented with four years of follow-up (Table 75-3). Overall, the use of radiation significantly decreases the risk of local recurrence to about one-half that for lumpectomy alone. Similar to other nonrandomized studies of both lumpectomy alone and lumpectomy followed by radiation therapy, approximately one-half of all recurrences in the EORTC study were invasive.

Table 75-2 ■ Non-Randomized Retrospective Studies of Wide-Excision Alone as Therapy for Selected Cases of Ductal Carcinoma in Situ

Author	# of Patients	% Local Recurrences	% Invasive Recurrences
Lagios et al	79	20	50
Schwartz et al	70	15.3	27
Arnesson et al	38	13	40
Silverstein et al	256	14.8	42

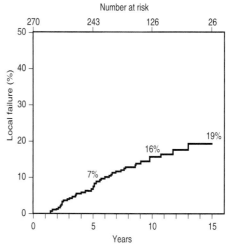

Figure 75-4 ■ Actuarial local failure for all 270 treated breasts. (From Solin LJ, Kurtz J, Fourquet A, et al: Fifteen-year results of breast-conserving surgery and definitive breast irradiation for the treatment of ductal carcinoma in situ of the breast. J Clin Oncol 1996;14:754.)

Table 75-3 ■ Results of the Randomized NSABP and EORTC Trials of Lumpectomy +/− Radiation Therapy for Ductal Carcinoma in Situ

			% Local Recurrences	
Study	Number of Patients	Median Follow-up (Months)	Radiation Therapy	No Radiation Therapy
NSABP B-17	818	96	11.4	25.8
EORTC 10853	1010	51	10.5	16.6

In contrast, in the National Surgical Adjuvant Breast Project trial, only one-third of recurrences were invasive in the group that received radiation therapy, compared to one-half of the recurrences in the group treated by lumpectomy alone. These results suggest an increased benefit for radiation in the reduction of subsequent invasive disease. Despite this observation, no survival difference was noted in either study to date.

Salvage Therapy

The risk of local recurrence is twice as high among patients treated by lumpectomy alone as for those treated by lumpectomy with radiation, and it is considerably higher for both groups when compared with treatment by mastectomy (where there is little chance of recurrence in the minimal residual breast tissue). The ability to treat recurrent disease adequately, therefore, becomes extremely important. In a retrospective study by Solin et al, 42 cases of disease recurrence after lumpectomy and radiation therapy in 274 cases of ductal carcinoma in situ were examined in detail. Forty cases were local disease alone, of which 55% were invasive cancer. All but two of these patients were treated with mastectomy. Four of 22 cases of invasive local recurrence progressed to and died from

metastatic disease. All of these cases had presented initially with clinically detectable disease, whereas none of the mammographically detected lesions have recurred. In another series of 74 cases of recurrent disease from a pool of 707 cases, the cases included both lumpectomy with radiation and excision alone as initial treatment. Of the 35 patients who had a local invasive recurrence, the rate of subsequent metastatic disease was 20% at 69 months of follow-up. No case of noninvasive recurrence developed distant spread. The breakdown by stage at time of disease recurrence is shown in Figure 75-5. In both of these studies, the relatively low rates of recurrence coupled with a relatively high likelihood of successful salvage with mastectomy led to a cause-specific mortality after breast-conserving therapy for ductal carcinoma in situ treatment of 1.8% and 2.1%, respectively.

Systemic Therapy

The focus of systemic therapy in ductal carcinoma in situ is not to eradicate micrometastatic disease (which is the case in the adjuvant treatment of patients with invasive disease) but rather, to reduce the risk of local recurrence in patients treated with breast conserving approaches and to decrease the risk of contralateral

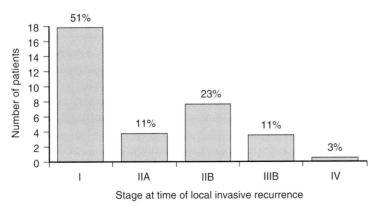

Figure 75-5 ■ The number of patients with a prior diagnosis of ductal carcinoma in situ by stage of disease at the time of invasive breast cancer recurrence. (From Silverstein M, Lagios M, Martino S, et al: Outcome after invasive local recurrence in patients with ductal carcinoma in situ of the breast. J Clin Oncol 1998;16:1367.)

breast cancer. Tamoxifen, a selective estrogen receptor modulator, is established potent breast cancer therapy and also has an evolving role in breast cancer prevention. Women with a history of invasive breast cancer had a 47% reduction in the development of contralateral disease when treated with tamoxifen for five years for reduction of the risk of recurrence of their primary cancer. Tamoxifen also reduced the risks of noninvasive and invasive breast cancer for women determined to be at high risk of developing the disease. The National Surgical Adjuvant Breast Project conducted the B-24 trial (Figure 75-6), which randomized 1804 patients with ductal carcinoma in situ to receive either tamoxifen 20 mg daily or placebo for 5 years, showed significant benefit for tamoxifen. The risk of invasive ipsilateral recurrence declined in the study from 3.4% to 2.1%, for a relative risk of 0.53, and the relative risk for recurrent ipsilateral ductal carcinoma in situ was reduced to 0.85. The overall risk of any recurrence of disease (ipsilateral and contralateral) declined from 13% to 9%. In the setting of a patient with ductal carcinoma in situ who was treated by mastectomy instead of lumpectomy, tamoxifen would mainly be expected to have a preventive benefit on the contralateral breast, as risk of local or distant disease recurrence is extremely low. For women treated with wide excision alone, the role of tamoxifen is the subject of investigation.

Tamoxifen does have potential risks and side effects that need to be considered. The common side effects from tamoxifen are not life threatening and seldom lead to discontinuation of the drug. These include hot flashes, mild nausea, weight gain, fluid retention, vaginal discharge, and irregular menses or induction of menopause in pre- or perimenopausal women. The more serious side effects of thrombotic events and uterine cancer are relatively uncommon and appear to be directly age-related in frequency. In the primary prevention study, the relative risk of thrombotic events, including deep-vein thrombosis and pulmonary embolism, were 1.7% and 3.0%, respectively. The increased risk was confined to patients 50 years of age or more. The risk of endometrial cancer over 5 years of therapy is increased by 2.5%. This translated into a change in incidence of endometrial cancer from 5.4 of 1000 cases seen in postmenopausal women on placebo to 13.0 out of 1000 cases on tamoxifen therapy. Again, the increased risk predominated in the population of women over 50, where the relative risk represented a fourfold increase.

Treatment Selection

The appropriate recommendations for a woman with ductal carcinoma in situ depend upon several factors, all of which must be taken into careful consideration and discussed fully with the patient. Total mastectomy offers the lowest risk of disease recurrence, but the overall survival benefit compared with breast-conserving approaches is very small. Clearly, most women can be treated safely with lumpectomy and radiation. It is important, however, that the patient understand the ongoing, long-term risk for local disease recurrence, including invasive disease, to ensure compliance with follow-up screening. Whether women with the best prognostic features of ductal carcinoma in situ can be treated safely without radiation therapy by lumpectomy alone or by lumpectomy with tamoxifen merits further investigation. The studies completed to date with breast-conserving surgery and no radiation demonstrate a higher risk of local disease recurrence, approximately one-half of which is seen to be invasive disease. Whether longer-term follow-up in this patient population will continue to demonstrate little or no survival difference will be important information to help guide treatment selection.

Lobular Carcinoma in Situ

Presentation

Lobular carcinoma in situ, the other major type of noninvasive breast cancer, is characterized by the abnormal proliferation of cells arising in the lobules and terminal ducts of the breast without invasion through the basement membrane. Unlike its counterpart, ductal carcinoma in situ, lobular carcinoma in situ does not have a distinguishing appearance on clinical presentation or radiologic imaging. Due to its occult presentation, the true incidence of lobular carcinoma in situ is very difficult to determine. A review of 6,000 mammographically triggered biopsy specimens showed lobular carcinoma in situ present in 2% of all cases, representing 10% of those lesions classified as malignant. Lobular carcinoma in situ is seen

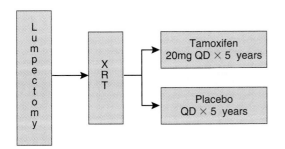

Figure 75-6 ■ Schema of the National Surgical Adjuvant Breast Project B-24 trial comparing tamoxifen to placebo after lumpectomy and radiation therapy for ductal carcinoma in situ.

most frequently in premenopausal women with a mean age of 45 years. Among American women, lobular carcinoma in situ is diagnosed 12 times more frequently in Caucasian women than in African-American women. Lobular carcinoma in situ itself, however, is considered a risk factor for future invasive breast cancer.

Pathology

The pathologic features of lobular carcinoma in situ were first reported by Foote and Stewart in 1941, and theirs continues to be the definitive description. Microscopically, the involved lobules contain abnormally large cells with proportionally increased nuclear size. The nuclei tend to be bland, uniform, and somewhat pale in appearance, without the presence of mitotic figures or hyperchromatism. The cytoplasm is often dense and acidophilic appearing, with some vacuolation occasionally seen. Early in the development of lobular carcinoma in situ, "pagetoid" cells can be recognized, whereby abnormal cells line the area between the basement membrane and the epidermal cells, mimicking the appearance of Paget's disease. As the process progresses, the involved lobules contain a spectrum of disordered, noncohesive cell layers. Cellular polarity is lost throughout these layers, and ultimately, they progress to obliterate the lumen and even distend the lobule (Figure 75-7).

The multifocal nature of lobular carcinoma in situ has long been recognized. Moreover, lobular carcinoma in situ may be bilateral in up to 45% of cases, which influences treatment recommendations. More contemporary studies of lobular carcinoma in situ have sought to characterize the entity on a molecular basis. They have recognized its almost uniform expression of the estrogen receptor and complete absence of overexpression of the HER-2/neu oncogene.

Prognosis

Lobular carcinoma in situ was once thought to be a precursor lesion to future invasive cancer at the site of disease detection. Hence, the original recommendation for treatment was unilateral mastectomy. Several studies have subsequently evaluated the prognosis after biopsy alone for women with lobular carcinoma in situ. The largest series, compiled by Haagensen et al, followed 287 cases for a mean of more than 16 years. The researchers noted that 21% of the subjects developed subsequent invasive cancer, with the numbers equally split between the ipsilateral and contralateral breasts. In another study, invasive cancer was documented in 35% of 84 cases, and the recurrences were equally likely in the ipsilateral and contralateral breasts. Both studies demonstrated a 7- to 10-fold increased risk for the development of invasive breast cancer after lobular carcinoma in situ when compared with the general population. Although most of these subsequent invasive lesions were of ductal pathology, there was also an overall increased percentage of invasive lobular tumors. Taken together, these studies demonstrate the nature of lobular carcinoma in situ as a significant risk factor for future breast cancer that is both bilateral and of either ductal or lobular histologic subtype. The length of time that

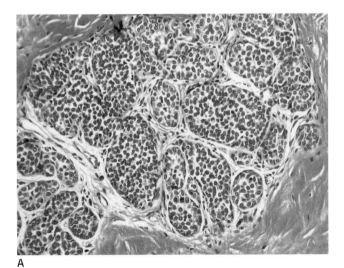
A

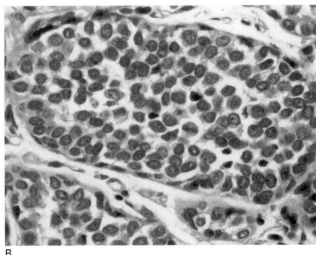
B

Figure 75-7 ■ Lobular carcinoma in situ. *A,* Low-power view showing replacement of the lobule. *B,* High-power view demonstrating the relative uniform nuclei and lack of mitotic figures.

patients with lobular carcinoma in situ are at risk for the subsequent development of invasive disease persists at least up to 15 years.

Treatment

The treatment of lobular carcinoma in situ must take into consideration the elevated risk of future invasive breast cancer of any histologic subtype and the bilateral nature of that risk. The earlier concept of lobular carcinoma in situ as a precursor lesion for invasive cancer, as ductal carcinoma in situ is known to be, has not held true. Thus, treatment strategies aimed at unilateral breast management are not logical. Margin status is not an issue, and lymph node sampling is not indicated because axillary involvement is not seen. As the majority of women with lobular carcinoma in situ will not go on to develop invasive disease, a conservative approach is appropriate, provided that the woman can participate in a program of close follow-up. For women whose fear of breast cancer precludes peace of mind under such a plan or in whom the requirements of a close follow-up program cannot be met, then bilateral simple mastectomy is the other option. Ultimately, only the woman facing such a choice can determine which is the better plan for her. Further understanding of the molecular basis of lobular carcinoma in situ that could identify those lesions destined to become invasive would be helpful in advising patients about treatment.

If observation is chosen, follow-up examination of the breasts should be performed quarterly to biannually, and annual mammography is needed. This strategy must be adhered to for the remainder of the woman's life, as the increased risk appears to persist indefinitely.

Women with a history of lobular carcinoma in situ were included in the National Surgical Adjuvant Breast Project's study of tamoxifen for breast cancer prevention in patients at risk. Among these women, 26 invasive breast cancers developed in the lobular carcinoma in situ subgroup; 18 had received placebo and 8 received tamoxifen, resulting in a risk ratio of 0.44 favoring tamoxifen therapy. As is true in ductal carcinoma in situ, the decision to use tamoxifen as a preventative measure for women with lobular carcinoma in situ must take into account a careful assessment of the risks of therapy versus the intended benefit. The ongoing study of tamoxifen and raloxifene (STAR) trial randomizes postmenopausal women at high risk for breast cancer to receive 5 years of either tamoxifen or raloxifene, a selective estrogen reception modulator compound. This study will help clarify the role of systemic hormonal therapy in the reduction of invasive cancer risk after lobular carcinoma in situ.

References

General

Bradley SJ, Weaver DW, Bouwman DL: Alternatives in the surgical management of in situ breast cancer: A meta-analysis of outcome. Am Surg 1990;56:428.

Bur ME, Zimarowski MJ, Schnitt SJ, et al: Estrogen receptor immunohistochemistry in carcinoma in situ of the breast. Cancer 1992;69:1174.

Fisher B, Costantino J, Wickerham D, et al: Tamoxifen for the prevention of breast cancer: Report of the National Surgical Adjuvant Breast and Bowel Project P-1 study. J Nat Canc Inst 1998;90:1371.

Fleming I, Cooper J, Henson D, et al (eds): AJCC cancer staging handbook. Philadelphia: Lippincott-Raven, 1998.

Kessler LG, Fuer EJ, Brown MJ: Projections of the breast cancer burden to US women 1990–2000. Prev Med 1991;20:170.

Rosner D, Bedwani RN, Vane J, et al: Noninvasive breast cancer: Results of a national survey by the American College of Surgeons. Ann Surg 1980;192:139.

——: Tamoxifen for early breast cancer: an overview of the randomized trials. Early Breast Cancer Collaborative Group. Lancet 1998;15:1451.

Ductal Carcinoma in Situ

Arnessen LG, Smeds S, Fagerberg G, et al: Follow-up of two treatment modalities for ductal cancer in situ of the breast. Br J Surg 1989;76:672.

Betsill WL, Rosen PP, Lieberman PH, et al: Intraductal carcinoma: long-term follow-up after treatment by biopsy alone. JAMA 1978;239:1863.

Connolly JL, Nixon AJ: Ductal carcinoma in situ of the breast: Histologic subtyping and clinical significance. Updates Prin Pract Oncol 1996;10.

Ernester L, Barclay J, Kerlikowske K, et al: Incidence of and treatment for ductal carcinoma in situ of the breast. JAMA 1996;275(12):913.

Fisher B, Dignam J, Wolmark N, et al: Lumpectomy and radiation treatment for the treatment of intraductal breast cancer: Findings from National Surgical Adjuvant Breast and Bowel Project B-17. J Clin Oncol 1998;16:441.

Fisher B, Dignam J, Wolmark N, et al: Tamoxifen in the treatment of intraductal breast cancer: National Surgical Adjuvant Breast and Bowel Project B-24 randomized controlled trial. Lancet 1998;353:1993.

Fisher E, Leeming R, Anderson S, et al: Conservative management of intraductal carcinoma of the breast. J Surg Oncol 1991;47:139.

Fisher ER, Sass R, Fisher B, et al: Pathologic findings from the National Surgical Adjuvant Breast Project (protocol B06): intraductal carcinoma (DCIS). Cancer 1986;57:197.

Frykberg ER, Bland KI: Overview of the biology and management of ductal carcinoma in situ of the breast. Cancer 1994;74(1 suppl):350.

Holland R, Hendricks J, Verbeek A, et al: Extent, distribution, and mammographic/histologic correlations of breast ductal carcinoma in situ. Lancet 1990;335:519.

Julien JP, Bijker N, Fentiman IS, et al: Radiotherapy in breast conserving treatment for ductal carcinoma in situ: First results of EORTC randomized phase III trial 10853. Lancet 2000;355:528.

Kerlikowske K, Barclay J, Grady D, et al: Comparison of risk factors for ductal carcinoma in situ and invasive breast cancer. J Nat Can Inst 1997;89:76.

Lagios MD, Margolin FR, Westdahl PR, et al: Mammographically detected ductal carcinoma in situ: frequency of local recurrence following tylectomy and prognostic effect of nuclear grade on local recurrence. Cancer 1989;63:618.

Lagios MD, Westdahl PR, Margolin FR, et al: Ductal carcinoma in situ: Relationship of extent of noninvasive disease to the frequency of occult invasion, multicentricity, lymph node metastasis, and short term treatment failures. Cancer 1982;50:1309.

Morrow M, Schnitt S: Ductal carninoma in situ. In: Harris JR, Lippman ME, Morrow M, et al (eds): Diseases of the breast, p 355. Philadelphia: Lippincott-Raven, 1996.

Page DL, Dupont WD, Rogers LW, et al: Intraductal carcinoma of the breast: Follow-up after biopsy only. Cancer 1982;49:751.

Schwartz GF, Finkel GC, Garcia JC, et al: Subclinical ductal carcinoma in situ of the breast: Treatment by local excision and surveillance alone. Cancer 1992;70:2468.

Silverstein MJ, Lagios MD, Martino S, et al: Outcome after invasive local recurrence in patients with ductal carcinoma in situ of the breast. J Clin Oncol 1998;16:1367.

Silverstein MJ, Lagios MD, Craig PH, et al: Prognostic index for ductal carcinoma in situ of the breast. Cancer 1996;77:2267.

Siverstein MJ, Lagios MD, Groshen S, et al: The influence of margin width on local control of ductal carcinoma in situ of the breast. N Engl J Med 1999;340:1455.

Solin L, Fourquet A, McCormick B, et al: Salvage treatment for local recurrence following breast-conserving surgery and definitive irradiation for ductal carcinoma in situ (intraductal carcinoma) of the breast. Int J Rad Oncol Biol Phys 1994;30:3.

Solin LJ, Kurtz J, Fourquet A, et al: Fifteen-year results of breast-conserving therapy and definitive breast irradiation for the treatment of ductal carcinoma in situ of the breast. J Clin Oncol 1996;14:754.

Stomper PC, Connolly JL: Ductal carcinoma in situ of the breast: Correlation between mammographic calcification and subtype. Am J Roentgenol 1992;159:483.

The Consensus Conference Committee: Consensus conference of the classification of ductal carcinoma in situ. Cancer 1997;80:1798.

Lobular Carcinoma in Situ

Andersen JA: Lobular carcinoma in situ of the breast: an approach to rational treatment. Cancer 1977;39:2597.

Foote FW, Stewart FW: Lobular carcinoma in situ: a rare form of mammary cancer. Am J Pathol 1941;17:491.

Haagensen CD, Bodian C, Haagensen DE: Lobular neoplasia (lobular carcinoma in situ) breast carcinoma: Risk and detection, p 238. Philadelphia, WB Saunders, 1981.

Page DL, Kidd TE, Dupont WD, et al: Lobular neoplasia of the breast: higher risk for subsequent invasive cancer predicted by more extensive disease. Hum Pathol 1991;22:1232.

Porter PL, Garcia R, Moe R, et al: C-erb-B2 oncogene protein in situ and invasive lobular breast neoplasia. Cancer 1991;68:331.

Rosen PP, Leiberman PH, Braun DW Jr, et al: Lobular carcinoma in situ of the breast: A detailed analysis of 99 patients with average follow-up of 24 years. Am J Surg Pathol 1978;2:225.

Chapter 76
Locally Invasive Breast Cancer

Julie J. Olin and Hyman B. Muss

Introduction

As many as 800,000 women worldwide will develop invasive breast cancer this year; 210,000 new diagnoses will occur in the United States alone. For the first time in decades, the mortality rate for breast cancer is declining in the United States. This decline is attributable to multiple factors, including earlier diagnosis and better treatment of the primary lesion, radiation therapy, and adjuvant systemic therapy. Breast cancer diagnosis, staging, prognostic factors (see Chapter 74), and management of noninvasive disease (see Chapter 75) are discussed elsewhere in this text. This chapter focuses on issues related to the management of invasive breast cancer, that is, patients with stage I through III breast cancer.

Numerous randomized clinical trials performed over the past three decades have been instrumental in establishing current adjuvant therapy guidelines. Options for adjuvant therapy include chemotherapy, hormonal therapy, combined chemohormonal therapy, and breast and chest wall irradiation.

Initial Evaluation

Initial evaluation of all patients starts with a complete history and physical examination. The patient should be carefully queried for symptoms of metastases, including bone pain, abdominal pain, dyspnea, and weight loss. Comorbid illness that is likely to have an adverse effect on survival, such as cardiovascular disease, should be kept in mind. For patients who are in generally good health, the routine preoperative workup should include a complete blood count, chemistry profile, and chest X-ray. Patients with a large primary breast mass 5 cm or greater or with palpable axillary nodes are at higher risk for distant metastases and, even in the absence of symptoms, should undergo additional studies for metastatic disease, such as radionuclide bone scan and hepatic imaging via ultrasound or computed tomography

(CT). If these tests are not performed preoperatively, they should be done after surgery in patients who are found to have large primary lesions and/or four or more positive axillary lymph nodes. Extensive imaging in patients with T1 or T2 lesions or 0 to 3 positive nodes is unnecessary unless such imaging is used to evaluate symptoms, signs, or abnormalities in screening laboratory tests that suggest metastases. Except when required for clinical trials, tumor marker assessment (CEA, CA 15-3, CA 27-29, and others) is not recommended. The basis for treatment selection in patients with invasive breast cancer is the pathologic stage, estrogen and progesterone receptor status, and tumor grade as described in the pathology report (Table 76-1).

Breast-Conserving Therapy for the Primary Lesion: Lumpectomy and Radiation Therapy

For patients who choose breast preservation, the invasive lesion and any in situ component should be surgically excised with clear margins. Close surgical margins (1 mm or greater) for invasive lesions do not increase the risk of ipsilateral breast tumor recurrence. When possible, the in situ component associated with invasive lesions should have margins of 1 cm or more. All patients with invasive breast cancer who are treated with lumpectomy benefit from postoperative breast radiation. In addition to lowering the risk of ipsilateral breast tumor recurrence, data suggest that postoperative breast radiation is associated with improved survival. After breast radiation, the incidence of ipsilateral breast tumor recurrence in these patients is less than 5%.

The timing of the radiation therapy was thought to be an issue in the care of these patients. Concern existed that delaying breast radiation following lumpectomy for periods longer than three months would be associated with an increased risk of ipsilateral breast tumor recurrence. A randomized trial

Table 76-1 ▪ Elements of a Pathology Report on Breast Cancer

1. Tumor size is based on the greatest dimension of the invasive component only. When there is more than one distinct invasive lesion, the greatest dimension of only the largest lesion is used for staging.
2. At least six and preferably 10 or more nodes are needed in an axillary dissection for an accurate sample size.
3. Estrogen and progesterone receptors should be obtained on all patients. The proportion of cells staining for each receptor should be part of the report.
4. Tumor grade should be estimated.
5. Tumor margins should be clear.
6. c-erbB-2 (HER-2) overexpression should be evaluated on every primary breast cancer either at the time of initial diagnosis or on subsequent recurrence.

showed that the sequence of chemotherapy followed by breast radiation was associated with a significantly lower risk of distant metastases than the sequence of radiation therapy followed by chemotherapy. At five years, the crude rate for first recurrence at regional or distant sites was 20% in patients treated with chemotherapy first compared with 32% in patients receiving radiation therapy first. Thus, where adjuvant chemotherapy is appropriate, women undergoing lumpectomy should receive chemotherapy prior to breast irradiation.

Postmastectomy Radiation Therapy

Radiation therapy to the chest wall is increasingly being employed in the treatment of patients even after mastectomy. In addition to decreasing locoregional recurrence by about two thirds, there is now good evidence that radiation therapy after mastectomy confers a significant survival benefit. Two recent trials in premenopausal women whose axillary lymph nodes were involved by cancer received CMF (cyclophosphamide, methotrexate, and 5-fluorouracil) adjuvant chemotherapy and were randomized to receive after mastectomy either radiation therapy or no further treatment. The addition of radiation therapy was associated with an 8% to 10% improvement in the overall survival rate. The American Society of Clinical Oncology's (ASCO) clinical practice guidelines suggest that postmastectomy radiation therapy should be given to women with T3 lesions and to women with four or more positive axillary nodes. The ASCO panel believed that the current evidence is insufficient to recommend the routine use of postmastectomy radiation therapy in patients with one to three positive

nodes. Patients who are not eligible for a clinical trial but who do have high-risk features (T2 primary, two to three positive nodes, or aggressive histologies) should be considered for postmastectomy radiation therapy as well.

Adjuvant Chemotherapy

Landmark clinical trials that christened the age of adjuvant chemotherapy began in the early 1970s in patients with axillary node–positive breast cancer. Early randomized studies of single-agent melphalan versus CMF revealed a significant disease-free survival advantage for adjuvant chemotherapy and a trend toward improved survival. Subset analysis found that the disease-free survival was limited to patients under 50 years of age, the majority of whom were premenopausal.

To determine the effectiveness of numerous diverse adjuvant therapy trials, four major meta-analyses have been performed by the Early Breast Cancer Trialists' Collaborative Group. The first overview, in 1988, led to three major conclusions that have been reinforced by three subsequent overviews. First, adjuvant chemotherapy provides a statistically significant reduction in the risk of relapse and death at five years of follow-up. Second, combination chemotherapy (polychemotherapy) displays greater efficacy than does single-agent therapy. Third, adjuvant chemotherapy given for four to six months is as effective as lengthier treatment lasting eight to 24 months.

The last published overview in 1998 broadened the role of chemotherapy in early breast cancer. In this analysis, the comparison of polychemotherapy versus no chemotherapy incorporated 47 trials in 17,723 women. Considering patients of all ages, polychemotherapy of several months' duration produced a 23.8% proportional risk reduction in annual recurrence and a 15.2% proportional risk reduction in annual mortality. Thus, roughly one of every four recurrences and one of every seven deaths is avoided each year because of adjuvant polychemotherapy.

Subset analysis of the 1998 overview provided information on the quantitative differences in the benefits derived from chemotherapy. The greatest benefit of polychemotherapy occurred in the youngest patients; more then one third of recurrences and one fourth of deaths each year prevented were in patients under 50 years of age. While less benefit was seen in patients between 50 and 69 years of age, the reduction in annual odds of both recurrence and death was still significant between the chemotherapy-treated and untreated groups. Thus, only one of every

10 deaths is avoided per year with chemotherapy in the older, clearly postmenopausal, category. Too few elderly women age 70 years and older participated in clinical trials to draw conclusive results regarding benefits of polychemotherapy in this age group. The proportional reductions in recurrence and mortality with chemotherapy were similar in both node-positive and node-negative disease. For women under age 50 at the time of randomization, polychemotherapy improved the 10-year survival rate from 71% to 78% in node-negative patients and from 42% to 53% in node-positive patients, an absolute survival benefit of 7% and 11% in node-negative and node-positive patients, respectively. For women age 50 to 69 years, polychemotherapy improved the 10-year survival rate from 67% to 69% in node-negative patients and from 46% to 49% in node-positive patients. Estrogen receptor status had only a small impact on the overall benefit of chemotherapy in women younger than 50 years old. However, in women age 50 to 69 years, polychemotherapy significantly reduced both recurrence and mortality in both estrogen receptor–positive and estrogen receptor–negative tumors, but the reduction in recurrence in patients whose breast cancer lacked estrogen receptors was almost double that of estrogen receptor–positive disease.

Two additional analyses included in the 1998 overview help to guide the choice of chemotherapeutic regimens. Comparison of longer versus shorter duration of polychemotherapy was based on 11 trials of 6104 women. While a nonsignificant 7% further reduction in recurrence was noted with treatment durations longer than six months, no survival advantage was associated with the use of polychemotherapy for more than three to six months. Anthracycline-based regimens (polychemotherapy containing doxorubicin or epirubicin) were compared to CMF in 11 trials involving 5942 women. The results showed a 12% reduction in recurrence and an 11% reduction in mortality for the anthracycline-based regimens. This translated into an approximate absolute risk reduction of 3% for both recurrence and mortality. Of note, approximately 70% of the women composing the overview trials were premenopausal, thus making it difficult to fully access the impact of the anthracyclines on the older population.

Three recent trials that were not included in the 1998 meta-analysis bear review regarding anthracycline-based therapy. The Intergroup INT 0102 trial evaluated cyclophosphamide, doxorubicin, and 5-fluorouracil (CAF) versus CMF in approximately 4000 high-risk node-negative patients. The five-year relapse-free survival rate was 85% in the CAF-treated group compared with 82% in the CMF-treated group. In contrast, the National Surgical Adjuvant Breast and Bowel Project study number B-23 showed no survival difference in approximately 2000 women with high-risk node-negative cancer treated with doxorubicin and cyclophosphamide (AC) versus CMF. In the National Cancer Institute of Canada (NCIC) trial, approximately 700 premenopausal node-positive patients were randomly assigned to either CMF or moderately dose-intensified cyclophosphamide, epirubicin, and 5-fluorouracil (CEF). The five-year relapse-free survival rate was 53% in CMF-treated patients and 63% in CEF-treated patients. Debate continues regarding the impact of 5-fluorouracil in the anthracycline-containing regimens and the overall duration of adjuvant therapy, which was six months for the three-drug combinations, such as CEF, versus three months for the two-drug Adriamycin + cyclophosphamide combination.

The role of taxane therapy in the adjuvant setting remains controversial. Cancer and Leukemia Group B Protocol 9344 randomly assigned 3170 premenopausal and postmenopausal patients with node-positive breast cancer to one of three dose levels of doxorubicin combined with standard-dose cyclophosphamide for four cycles followed by a second randomization comparing four cycles of paclitaxel at 175 mg/m^2 and no further treatment. Patients with estrogen receptor–positive disease also received adjuvant tamoxifen for five years following completion of chemotherapy. At a median follow-up of 21 months, paclitaxel-treated patients showed a statistically significant improvement in disease-free survival rates (90% versus 86%) and overall survival rates (97% versus 95%). However, a retrospective subset analysis failed to show a significant reduction in risk of disease recurrence in the estrogen receptor–positive paclitaxel-treated group. Thus, current U.S. Food and Drug Administration guidelines recognize the use of paclitaxel only in the node-positive, hormone recetor–negative setting. An update on this trial after five years of follow-up suggests a persistent improvement in disease-free survival in paclitaxel-treated patients with hormone-receptor negativity.

In a second major trial (National Surgical Adjuvant Breast and Bowel Project B-28), 3060 women with node-positive breast cancer were randomly assigned to receive doxirubicin and cyclophosphamide every three weeks for four cycles or doxirubicin and cyclophosphamide for four cycles followed by paclitaxel for four cycles at 225 mg/m^2. With three years of follow-up, this study failed to show a benefit from the addition of paclitaxel to standard doxirubicin + cyclophosphamide. While the value of adjuvant paclitaxel continues to be explored, the optimal regimen and disease characteristics most likely to respond to the taxanes requires further study.

Dose Intensification and Dose Density

Dose intensification, achieved either by increasing the dose of chemotherapy (dose escalation/intensity) or by increasing the frequency of administering a standard dose (dose density), has been and continues to be evaluated. The rationale for dose intensification is based on alkylating agents' steep dose-response curve and their effectiveness in overcoming drug resistance in the adjuvant setting when a minimal tumor burden is present. Two pivotal National Surgical Adjuvant Breast and Bowel Project trials have carefully evaluated dose intensification of cyclophosphamide in the setting of node-positive breast cancer. Conversely, Cancer and Acute Leukemia Group B Protocol 9344 held the dose of cyclophosphamide constant and randomized patients to receive varyingly increased doses of doxorubicin. None of these studies revealed improved disease-free or overall survival in response to increasing doses of either agent.

Further dose intensification with high-dose myeloablative chemotherapy requiring autologous stem cell support was studied in very high-risk patients with 10 or more positive axillary nodes. While initial enthusiasm was generated by impressive results from a dose-intensified regimen from South Africa, the trial results were subsequently discredited because of scientific misconduct. Several cooperative group randomized trials have failed to confirm the value of this approach to high-dose therapy.

The dose-density approach administers single agents in sequential fashion with shortened intervals between treatments. Theoretic advantages of a dose-density approach include avoidance of overlapping toxicities and minimization of periods of tumor regrowth between treatments. The Cancer and Leukemia Group B protocol 9741 compared concurrent doxirubicin/cyclophosphamide and paclitaxel with sequential doxirubicin-paclitaxel-cyclophosphamide in an every-two-week dose-dense administration schedule or in an every-three-week conventional schedule in women with node-positive operable breast cancer. Four-year disease-free survival was 82% for the dose-dense regimens and 75% for the conventionally-administered treatments. Overall survival was 92% with dose-dense therapy versus 90% with conventionally-scheduled therapy. Patients treated with the dose-dense approach received prophylactic filgrastim (Neupogen) and experienced less grade IV neutropenia. Further long-term follow-up of this pivotal trial may strongly influence dosing schedules of standard adjuvant chemotherapy.

Neoadjuvant Chemotherapy

Neoadjuvant therapy involves the administration of chemotherapy prior to definitive breast surgery. The National Surgical Adjuvant Breast and Bowel Project Protocol B-18 randomly assigned 1523 women with palpable breast cancers to receive either neoadjuvant Adriamycin and cyclophosphamide for four cycles followed by breast surgery or breast surgery followed by adjuvant Adriamycin and cyclophosphamide for four cycles. Because of shrinkage of the primary breast cancer, the patients who received chemotherapy before surgery were more likely (68% versus 60%) to undergo breast-conserving surgery. The patients who received neoadjuvant chemotherapy achieved an 80% combined partial or complete clinical response; no residual palpable disease was found in 36%. Nine percent of the patients (all with complete clinical responses) had no evidence of invasive carcinoma on histologic examination of the breast tissue. Rates of ipsilateral breast tumor recurrence following lumpectomy were similar in both groups, although local recurrence among women less than 50 years old was higher in those receiving chemotherapy preoperatively (13%) than in those receiving chemotherapy postoperatively (8%). Only 3% of patients who were more than 49 years old had an ipsilateral breast tumor recurrence, probably reflecting the protective effects of adjuvant tamoxifen given to postmenopausal patients whose cancers were estrogen receptor–positive.

Although neoadjuvant therapy provided downstaging of the breast cancer and a higher rate of breast conservation, it failed to improve disease-free survival or overall survival. Nevertheless, this trial and others of neoadjuvant therapy have confirmed that the response to chemotherapy is a powerful predictor of the patient's subsequent clinical course. Patients with little or no residual disease following neoadjuvant therapy have a favorable outlook, while those with large residual primary lesions or extensive nodal involvement following neoadjuvant therapy are at very high risk for metastases.

Endocrine Therapy

Tamoxifen

Tamoxifen is a selective estrogen receptor modulator (SERM) that displays both estrogen agonist and antagonist properties. The 1995 Early Breast Cancer Trialists' Collaborative Group overview reviewed 37,000 patients with early-stage breast cancer entered in 55 randomized trials comparing tamoxifen to no adjuvant. The data from a large number of randomized trials clearly show that adjuvant tamoxifen therapy should be considered in all cases of hormone receptor–positive breast cancer regardless of age, menopausal status, tumor size, or nodal involvement. In these patients treated with tamoxifen for five years, the annual odds of recurrence are reduced by approximately 50%, and the annual odds of death decline by 26%. In contrast, no reduction in the annual odds of recurrence or death was noted in the approximately 8000 women with estrogen receptor–negative tumors who received adjuvant tamoxifen therapy.

Randomized studies of the optimal duration of tamoxifen therapy demonstrate that survival improves if tamoxifen is administered for five years instead of one to two years. Prolonged tamoxifen usage of 10 years or more was addressed in the randomized, placebo-controlled National Surgical Adjuvant Breast and Bowel Project Protocol B-14 and the Scottish Tamoxifen Trial. In both trials, no survival advantage accrued to the premenopausal and postmenopausal women who had axillary node–negative, estrogen receptor–positive breast cancer when tamoxifen therapy was continued beyond five years. The Scottish trial also contained postmenopausal women whose axillary nodes were positive. In this subset of patients as well, after a median follow-up of 15 years, no additional benefit was observed in those who continued tamoxifen beyond five years.

A secondary but important benefit of five years of adjuvant tamoxifen therapy is that the annual incidence rate of a subsequent contralateral breast cancer is halved. This protective effect was confirmed in the tamoxifen prevention trial in individuals who were at high risk for the development of a primary breast cancer.

Aromatase Inhibitors

Aromatase inhibitors inhibit the synthesis of estrogen from androgens in postmenopausal women. Anastrozole (Arimidex) is one such compound that is an orally administered, highly potent suppressor of estrogen production. It is at least as effective as, if not slightly more effective than, tamoxifen in the treatment of estrogen receptor–positive metastatic breast cancer. Thus aromatase inhibitor therapy has moved into the adjuvant treatment setting of receptor-positive early-stage breast cancer in postmenopausal women.

In the multinational Arimidex, Tamoxifen Alone or in Combination (ATAC) trial, over 9000 postmenopausal women were randomized to receive tamoxifen alone, anastrozole alone, or a combination of both drugs for five years. With a median follow-up of 33 months, disease-free survival at three years was 89.4% in the anastrozole-treated group and 87.4% in the tamoxifen-treated group. Results with the combination were not significantly different from those with the tamoxifen alone. Tamoxifen usage was more likely associated with hot flashes, vaginal bleeding and discharge, endometrial cancer, and thromboembolic events, whereas anastrozole usage led to more musculoskeletal complaints and higher vertebral fracture rates.

A 2002 American Society of Clinical Oncology technology assessment considered results of the ATAC trial to be promising but insufficient to change the gold-standard usage of tamoxifen in the adjuvant care of estrogen receptor-positive breast cancer. The panel found no data to support substituting an aromatase inhibitor for tamoxifen in those women already taking tamoxifen, although one might consider anastrozole in patients with intolerable side effects or serious complications felt to be secondary to tamoxifen. The Food and Drug Administration has approved anastrozole for use in the adjuvant setting in postmenopausal hormone receptor-positive patients.

Ovarian Ablation

Adjuvant ovarian ablation was initially accomplished by either oophorectomy or ovarian irradiation and was shown to be effective in premenopausal women. A 1995 meta-analysis incorporated data from 12 randomized trials of ovarian ablation in 2102 patients under age 50. Seven trials compared ovarian ablation with no adjuvant therapy, and five trials compared ovarian ablation and chemotherapy with the same chemotherapy alone. The 15-year survival rate was significantly improved in patients who underwent ovarian ablation compared with those who did not (52% versus 46%). Both node-positive and node-negative premenopausal patients benefited from ovarian ablation. In the trials of ovarian ablation plus chemotherapy versus chemotherapy alone, the benefit from ovarian ablation was much smaller and not statistically significant. This portion of the meta-analysis contained slightly more than 900 premenopausal women; the sample size was too small to allow for definitive statements about the combination of ovarian ablation and chemotherapy.

The development of luteinizing hormone releasing hormone (LHRH) analogs, such as goserelin, to chemically induce ovarian failure renewed interest in the combination of ovarian ablation and chemotherapy. In one study of this approach, the Eastern Cooperative Oncology Group Protocol 5188 randomly assigned 1504 premenopausal patients with node-positive, estrogen receptor–positive breast cancer to three treatment groups: adjuvant chemotherapy with CAF alone, with added goserelin, or with added goserelin and tamoxifen. With a median follow-up of six years, the chemotherapy and goserelin/tamoxifen-treated group experienced improved disease-free survival. Overall survival rates, however, were identical. Although some trials did not use estrogen receptor positivity as a prerequisite for participation, the data suggest that ovarian ablation is likely to be effective only in premenopausal women with estrogen receptor–positive cancers. In premenopausal women whose breast cancers are estrogen receptor–positive and maintain their menses despite receiving adjuvant chemotherapy and tamoxifen, it remains uncertain whether ovarian ablation would improve the outcome.

Chemohormonal Therapy

A combined chemohormonal approach in women with estrogen receptor–positive breast cancer represents the current adjuvant therapy of choice for many women. Except in the setting of extensive comorbidity, advanced age, or low-risk breast primaries measuring 1 cm or less, patient age, menopausal status, and nodal status should not preclude the use of combined chemohormonal therapy in estrogen receptor–positive patients.

Several studies justify the use of combined chemotherapy and tamoxifen. National Surgical Adjuvant Breast and Bowel Project Protocol B-20 randomly assigned 2363 premenopausal and postmenopausal patients with node-negative, estrogen receptor–positive breast cancer to tamoxifen alone or in combination with either methotrexate and 5-fluorouracil (MFT) or cyclophosphamide, methotrexate, and 5-fluorouracil (CMFT). Chemotherapy plus tamoxifen resulted in significantly better disease-free survival and overall survival than tamoxifen alone. The greatest benefit for both chemotherapy regimens was observed in the premenopausal subset of women. Nevertheless, a 20% reduction in the risk of death following MFT and a 43% reduction with CMFT were found in the postmenopausal patients.

Another randomized trial of chemotherapy with and without tamoxifen focused on high-risk, axillary node–negative breast cancer in both premenopausal and postmenopausal women. Both estrogen receptor–positive and –negative breast cancers were included. The addition of tamoxifen to chemotherapy demonstrated significant benefit in both disease-free survival and overall survival in receptor-positive patients of all ages. It was noteworthy that premenopausal patients treated with tamoxifen who had estrogen receptor–negative breast cancer actually fared significantly worse in both disease-free survival and overall survival. Tamoxifen should not be routinely given to estrogen receptor–negative patients.

Toxicity

Both acute and long-term toxicities associated with adjuvant therapy must be carefully considered in maintaining a proper perspective on the risk-benefit ratio that is involved in the treatment of early-stage breast cancer. Numerous toxicities may be caused by breast surgery, radiation therapy, chemotherapy, and tamoxifen (Table 76-2).

Although chemotherapy is perceived by many to be highly toxic, chemotherapy-related death in patients with breast cancer is rare, occurring in 0.2% to 0.9% of patients treated with standard-dose adjuvant therapy. Although anthracycline therapy raised concerns about cardiac damage, clinically significant cardiomyopathy occurs in only 0.5% to 1% of patients treated with standard cumulative doxorubicin of 300 mg/m² or less. In a 14-year follow-up study of 1000 patients with early-stage breast cancer treated with either CMF or a doxorubicin-containing regimen, only six cases of congestive heart failure and three cases of myocardial infarction were reported for an overall cardiac mortality rate of 0.4%. Premature ovarian failure is often considered an unavoidable consequence of chemotherapy, yet its incidence varies extensively according to patient age, cytotoxic agents used, and cumulative cyclophosphamide dosage. With CMF for six months, the risk of permanent amenorrhea is 35% in women under age 40 and 90% in women over 40. In contrast, the anthracycline-containing regimens may produce little if any amenorrhea in women under age 30 years. Recovery of menstrual function after temporary amenorrhea occurs in approximately half of women under age 40 years; reinitiation of menses can occur as long as two years after completion of chemotherapy.

Similar concern regarding extensive toxicity associated with tamoxifen has also been expressed, especially in the lay press. Although tamoxifen-induced vasomotor instability can be very bothersome in some patients; one large randomized trial showed 64% of tamoxifen-treated patients experienced hot flashes compared with 48% of placebo-treated patients. Although tamoxifen may be associated with varying degrees of loss of bone mineral density in premenopausal patients, tamoxifen preserves and perhaps even increases bone density in postmenopausal women. Several studies show that tamoxifen does not cause significant weight gain, sexual dysfunction, or depression.

Treatment Selection

Recommendations for systemic adjuvant therapy are based on the Early Breast Cancer Trialists' Collaborative Group overview of numerous published clinical trials. Our recommendations for therapy of stages I to III breast cancer parallel National Comprehensive Cancer Network (NCCN) practice guidelines version 2000 (Figures 76-1, 76-2, and 76-3). Treatment deci-

Table 76-2 ■ Toxicities of Therapy Used in Locally Invasive Breast Cancer

Treatment	Toxicity	Incidence*	Comment
Surgery	Local pain, numbness	Common	
	Lymphedema	Common	Greater risk with extensive surgery, radiation therapy, obesity, weight gain
Radiation therapy	Localized erythema, moist desquamation	Common	Occurs acutely and resolves quickly
	Pneumonitis, pulmonary fibrosis	Uncommon	Greater risk with larger fields or concurrent chemotherapy
	Contralateral breast cancer	Uncommon	Increased incidence in women ≤45 years old
	Brachial plexopathy	Rare	Usually associated with axillary doses >50 Gy or large radiation therapy fields
	Secondary cancers	Rare	Sarcoma, lung, esophageal, leukemia
Chemotherapy			
Acute	Nausea, vomiting	Common	More evident with anthracyclines
	Stomatitis	Common	Usually mild to moderate
	Alopecia	Common	Partial loss is common, but is total after anthracyclines
	Myelosuppression	Common	Very low incidence of neutropenic fever and serious bleeding
	Fatigue	Common	Usually resolves within months
	Psychological distress	Common	Frequently associated with alternative therapies
	Weight gain	Common	Usually mild (2–3 kg)
Chronic	Ovarian failure	Common	Higher incidence in women > 40 years old, may contribute to early osteoporosis
	Cognitive dysfunction†	Common	Acute or chronic; usually subtle and difficult to quantify; may be dose-related; may be associated with psychological distress
	Cardiomyopathy	Rare	Acute or delayed; risk increases after total doxorubicin dose >550 mg/m², preexisting heart disease, left breast radiation, age >70
	Acute myeloid leukemia/myelodysplasia	Rare	Higher incidence with dose-intensified cyclophosphamide
Tamoxifen	Hot flashes, vaginal discharge, menstrual irregularity	Common	
	Osteopenia	Uncommon	Premenopausal subset
	Hypercoagulability	Uncommon	Deep-vein thrombosis, pulmonary embolism, cerebrovascular accident
	Uterine cancer	Rare	Usually low-grade endometrial carcinoma; uterine sarcomas very rare occurrences

*Common = >10%, uncommon = 1–10%, rare = <1%.
†Only limited data currently available.
Adapted with permission from Burstein H, Winer E: Primary care for survivors of breast cancer. N Engl J Med 2000;343:1086–1094. Copyright 2000. Massachusetts Medical Society. All rights reserved.

sions need to be individually tailored for each patient on the basis of the characteristics of the primary tumor, comorbid illness, and the willingness of the patient to undergo toxicity for variable levels of potential benefit.

Patients should be given precise data concerning their risk for recurrence without systemic therapy and with selected adjuvant treatments. As was described in earlier sections of this chapter, the benefits of adjuvant therapies are routinely given in terms of annual proportional reductions in the risks of either recur-rence or death due to breast cancer. While such terminology may be readily conceptualized by the clinician, it often is poorly understood by the patient. Recently, two readily understandable and accessible computer programs have been developed by Ravdin (*Adjuvant!*, available at http://www.adjuvantonline.com), and Loprinzi and Thome (*Numeracy*, available at http://mhs.mayo.edu/adjuvant) that allow for accurate estimation of 10-year survival with and without adjuvant therapy. Two simplified tables have been thoughtfully constructed by Loprinzi and Thome

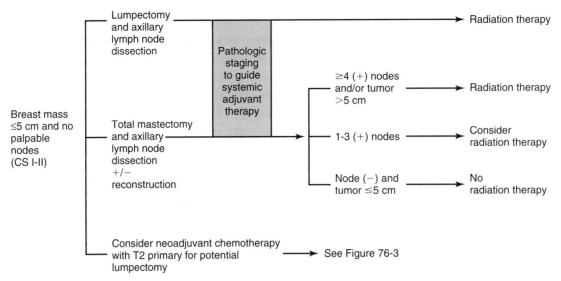

Figure 76-1 ■ Algorithm for locoregional therapy for stage I to IIB breast cancer. CS = clinical stage. (Adapted with permission from Authors: NCCN Practice Guidelines for Breast Cancer (Version 2000). Oncology 2000;14:33–49. Copyright © National Comprehensive Cancer Network, Inc. To view the most recent and complete version of the Guideline, go online to www.nccn.org. These Guidelines are a work in progress that will be refined as often as significant data becomes available.)

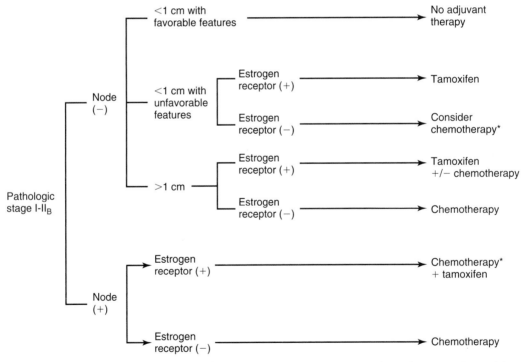

Figure 76-2 ■ Systemic adjuvant therapy guidelines for stage I to IIB breast cancer. Favorable features may include low histologic/nuclear grade, low S-phase, and no angiolymphatic invasion; unfavorable features may include high histologic/nuclear grade, high S-phase, or angiolymphatic invasion. *Consider ovarian ablation in premenopausal women with hormone receptor positivity. (Adapted with permission from Authors: NCCN Practice Guidelines for Breast Cancer (Version 2000). Oncology 2000;14:33–49. Copyright © National Comprehensive Cancer Network, Inc. To view the most recent and complete version of the Guideline, go online to www.nccn.org. These Guidelines are a work in progress that will be refined as often as significant data becomes available.)

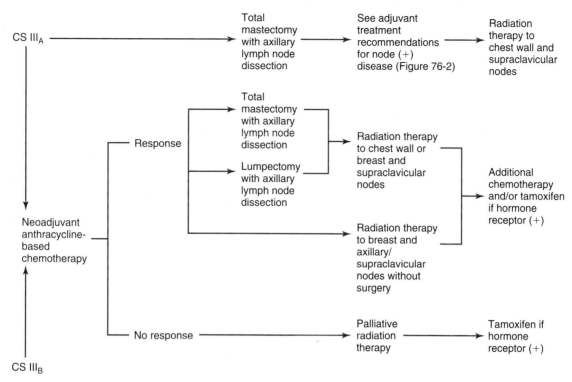

Figure 76-3 ■ Treatment guidelines for clinical stage III breast cancer. CS = clinical stage. (Adapted with permission from Authors: NCCN Practice Guidelines for Breast Cancer (Version 2000). Oncology 2000;14:33–49. Copyright © National Comprehensive Cancer Network, Inc. To view the most recent and complete version of the Guideline, go online to www.nccn.org. These Guidelines are a work in progress that will be refined as often as significant data becomes available.)

based on prognostic factors including patient age, nodal status, tumor size, and estrogen-receptor status (Tables 76-3 and 76-4). In addition to discussing the 10-year survival percentages both with and without adjuvant therapy, the patient must also be presented with detailed information regarding expected toxicities from such therapy. Clinicians are strongly encouraged to invest the time and effort to provide every woman with newly diagnosed breast cancer with detailed information to make her aware of the risk-benefit ratio of various adjuvant therapies. A recent study indicated that patients prefer precise data concerning treatment benefit.

Currently, there is intense interest in predictive factors, markers that predict response to treatment. The estrogen receptor remains the most helpful marker in this regard. Only patients who are estrogen or progesterone receptor–positive will benefit from adjuvant endocrine therapy. Data also suggest that patients with more rapidly proliferating tumors as defined by higher-grade (poorly differentiated), high S-phase, high MIB-1 expression, or high thymidine-labeling index are more likely to benefit from chemotherapy than are patients with more slowly proliferating cancers. Such data may be helpful in con-

sidering overall prognosis but should not be used as criteria to select specific chemotherapy regimens.

The c-erbB-2 gene (HER-2 or HER-2/*neu*) has become a widely used marker in determining prognosis and predicting response to treatment. C-erbB-2 gene amplification is observed in 20% to 40% of breast cancers and confers an overall poorer prognosis. According to the American Society of Clinical Oncology clinical practice guidelines 2000 update on tumor marker usage, c-erbB-2 overexpression should be evaluated on every primary breast cancer either at the time of initial diagnosis or on subsequent recurrence. C-erbB-2 appears to be a weak to moderately negative predictive factor for response to endocrine therapy. The guidelines suggest, however, that the evidence is insufficient to routinely use c-erbB-2 to select hormone receptor–positive patients who should not receive tamoxifen. Thus, we recommend the use of adjuvant tamoxifen in hormone receptor–positive patients regardless of their HER-2 status. The c-erbB-2-positive patients appear to be more likely to benefit from anthracycline-containing regimens than from non-anthracycline-based therapy. We recommend that patients with HER-2-positive lesions be treated with anthracycline-based therapy unless this is

Table 76-3 ■ Estimated 10-Year Disease-Free Survival Percentages for Estrogen Receptor–Positive Women

No. of Positive Nodes	<1 cm ∅	T	AC/T	1–2 cm ∅	T	AC/T	2–3 cm ∅	T	AC/T	3–4 cm ∅	T	AC/T	4–5 cm ∅	T	AC/T	>5 cm ∅	T	AC/T
Women ≤50 years																		
0	90	92	94	81	85	89	75	81	86	69	76	82	63	71	78	56	65	73
1–3	60	68	76	56	65	73	50	60	69	47	57	67	42	53	63	37	48	59
4–6	46	56	66	42	53	63	38	49	59	35	46	57	31	42	53	27	38	50
6–9	36	47	58	32	43	54	29	40	52	26	37	49	21	32	44	18	28	40
≥10	22	33	45	19	30	42	17	27	39	16	26	38	14	24	36	13	23	34
Women >50 years																		
0	90	92	93	81	85	87	75	81	83	69	76	79	63	71	74	56	65	69
1–3	60	68	72	56	65	69	50	60	64	47	57	62	42	53	57	37	48	53
4–6	46	56	61	42	53	57	38	49	54	35	46	51	31	42	47	27	38	44
6–9	36	47	52	32	43	48	29	40	46	26	37	42	21	32	37	18	28	34
≥10	22	33	38	19	30	35	17	27	33	16	26	32	14	24	29	13	23	28

Abbreviations: ∅ = no systemic adjuvant therapy; AC = standard primary adjuvant chemotherapy such as doxorubicin/cyclophosphamide; T = tamoxifen; AC/T = standard primary adjuvant chemotherapy and tamoxifen.
Adapted with permission from Loprinzi C, Thomé S: Understanding the utility of adjuvant systemic therapy for primary breast cancer. J Clin Oncol 2001;19:972–979.

Table 76-4 ■ Estimated 10-Year Disease-Free Survival Percentages for Estrogen Receptor-Negative Women

No. of Positive Nodes	<1 cm ∅	AC	AC and P*	1–2 cm ∅	AC	AC and P*	2–3 cm ∅	AC	AC and P*	3–4 cm ∅	AC	AC and P*	4–5 cm ∅	AC	AC and P*	>5 cm ∅	AC	AC and P*
Women ≤ 50 years																		
0	90	93	95	81	87	90	75	83	87	69	79	84	63	74	80	56	69	76
1–3	60	72	78	56	69	76	50	64	72	47	62	70	42	57	66	37	53	62
4–6	46	61	69	42	57	66	38	54	63	35	51	61	31	47	57	27	44	54
6–9	36	52	61	32	48	58	29	46	56	26	43	53	21	37	48	18	34	45
≥10	22	38	49	19	35	46	17	33	44	16	32	43	14	29	40	13	28	39
Women >50 years																		
0	90	92	94	81	85	88	75	79	84	69	74	80	63	69	76	56	63	71
1–3	60	67	74	56	63	71	50	58	66	47	55	64	42	50	60	37	46	56
4–6	46	54	63	42	50	60	38	46	57	35	44	54	31	40	50	27	36	47
6–9	36	45	55	32	41	51	29	38	48	26	35	46	21	29	40	18	26	37
≥10	22	30	41	19	27	38	17	25	36	16	24	35	14	21	32	13	20	31

Abbreviations: ∅ = no systemic adjuvant therapy; AC = standard primary adjuvant chemotherapy such as doxorubicin/cyclophosphamide, P = Paclitaxel.
*Based on limited information from a single study.
Adapted with permission from Loprinzi C, Thomé S: Understanding the utility of adjuvant systemic therapy for primary breast cancer. J Clin Oncol 2001;19:972–979.

Table 76-5 ■ American Society of Clinical Oncology Recommendations for Follow-Up After Early Breast Cancer Therapy

Procedure	Frequency
History and Physical Exam	Every 3–6 months for 3 years, every 6–12 months for 2 years, then yearly
Mammography (includes patients who had breast radiation)	Yearly
Pelvic Examination	Yearly

Data are not sufficient to recommend hematologic blood counts, tumor markers, chest radiographs, bone scans, liver sonograms or computed tomography be routinely performed.

contraindicated by underlying cardiac disease. The use of c-erbB-2 as a predictive marker for taxane therapy is not recommended by ASCO guidelines.

Follow-Up After Primary Breast Cancer

The underlying assumption for follow-up of asymptomatic patients after a diagnosis of early-stage breast cancer is that early detection of metastases improves survival; currently, this is not the case. Imaging studies may occasionally precede the development of signs and symptoms of metastases by several months, but this does not translate into improved survival. Two randomized trials have directly compared an intensive follow-up testing program that routinely included extensive imaging and laboratory tests with every scheduled visit against more limited studies. In both trials, asymptomatic recurrence was noted in about 30% of intensively followed patients and 21% of controls. Of note, 30% to 40% of recurrences were detected between routinely scheduled visits after patients developed new signs and symptoms of metastases that were not found on prior routine clinic visits. The survival rate was identical in both trials, and quality of life was not affected by follow-up method.

About 75% of recurrences are detected by the physician or the patient from signs and symptoms even when frequent imaging and laboratory work are done. In one review, locoregional recurrence accounted for 19% to 39%, bone for 16% to 63%, lung for 16% to 25%, and liver for 5% to 22% of documented recurrences. Of note, almost one third of initial recurrences occur in soft tissue and nodal areas for which physical examination remains the mainstay of detection. Elevation of tumor-associated antigens including CEA and mucin-associated antigens (CA 15-3, CA 27-29, and others) may occur an average of three to six months before the development of clinically detectable metastatic disease, but there is no evidence that routine use of marker studies for follow-up improves outcome. The American Society of Clinical Oncology guidelines (Table 76-5) for patients who are followed outside of a clinical trial setting demonstrate how few studies are warranted by the existing data. Patients may feel comfortable with this perspective. They need to be educated to understand that the use of extensive imaging and laboratory studies does not improve survival.

If so little investigation is required with each visit, then why do follow-up at all? Follow-up provides a forum for patients to discuss their fears and concerns, for physicians to provide reassurance, and to make certain that annual mammography is being done. Also, early detection of bone or soft tissue metastases is likely to result in better disease control and presumably a better quality of life.

References

General

Anonymous: Impact of follow-up testing on survival and health-related quality of life in breast cancer patients: A multicenter randomized controlled trial. The GIVIO Investigators. JAMA 1994;271:1587–1592.

Bast R, Ravdin P, Hayes D, et al: 2000 update of recommendations for the use of tumor markers in breast and colorectal cancer: Clinical practice guidelines of the American Society of Clinical Oncology. J Clin Oncol 2001;19:1865–1878.

Burstein H, Winer E: Primary care for survivors of breast cancer. N Engl J Med 2000;343:1086–1094.

Curtis R, Boice J, Stovall M, et al: Risk of leukemia after chemotherapy and radiation treatment for breast cancer. N Engl J Med 1992;326:1745–1751.

Day R, Ganz P, Costantino J, et al: Health-related quality of life and tamoxifen in breast cancer prevention: A report from the National Surgical Adjuvant Breast and Bowel Project P-1 Study. J Clin Oncol 1999;17:2659–2669.

Gage I, Schnitt S, Nixon A, et al: Pathologic margin involvement and the risk of recurrence in patients treated with breast-conserving therapy. Cancer 1996;78:1921–1928.

National Institutes of Health Consensus Development Conference Statement: Adjuvant therapy for breast cancer, November 1–3, 2000. J Natl Cancer Inst 2001;30:1–15.

NCCN Practice Guidelines for Breast Cancer (version 2000). Oncology 2000;14:33–49. To view the most recent and complete version of the Guideline, go online to www.nccn.org.

Ravdin P, Siminoff L, Davis G, et al: Computer program to assist in making decisions about adjuvant therapy for women with early breast cancer. J Clin Oncol 2000;19:980–991.

Roselli Del Turco M, Palli D, Cariddi A, et al: The efficacy of intensive follow-up testing in breast cancer cases. Ann Oncol 1995;6(Suppl 2):37–39.

Smith T, Davidson N, Schapira D, et al: American Society of Clinical Oncology 1998 update of recommended breast cancer surveillance guidelines. J Clin Oncol 1999;17:1080–1082.

Yamauchi H, Stearns V, Hayes D: When is a tumor marker ready for prime time? A case study of c-erbB-2 as a predictive factor in breast cancer. J Clin Oncol 2001;19:2334–2356.

Adjuvant Chemotherapy

Citron M, Berry D, Cirrincione C, et al: Randomized trial of dose-dense versus conventionally-scheduled and sequential versus concurrent combination chemotherapy as postoperative adjuvant treatment of node-positive primary breast cancer: First report of Intergroup trial C9741/Cancer and Leukemia Group B trial 9741. J Clin Oncol 2003;21.

Demark-Wahnefried W, Peterson B, Winer E, et al: Changes in weight, body composition, and factors influencing energy balance among premenopausal breast cancer patients receiving adjuvant chemotherapy. J Clin Oncol 2001;19:2381–2389.

Early Breast Cancer Trialists' Collaborative Group: Polychemotherapy for early breast cancer: An overview of the randomized trials. Lancet 1998;352:930–942.

Fisher B, Anderson D, DeCillis A, et al: Further evaluation of intensified and increased total dose of cyclophosphamide for the treatment of primary breast cancer: Findings from the National Surgical Adjuvant Breast and Bowel Project B-25. J Clin Oncol 1999;17:3374–3388.

Henderson IC, Berry D, Demetri G, et al: Improved disease-free and overall survival from the addition of sequential paclitaxel but not from the escalation of doxorubicin dose level in the adjuvant chemotherapy of patients with node-positive primary breast cancer. Proc Am Soc Clin Oncol 1998;17:101a (abstract 390a).

Henderson IC, Berry D, Demetri G, et al: Improved outcomes from adding sequential paclitaxel but not from escalating doxirubicin dose in an adjuvant chemotherapy regimen for patients with node-positive primary breast cancer. J Clin Oncol 2003;21:976–983.

Hudis C, Seidman A, Baselga J, et al: Sequential dose-dense doxorubicin, paclitaxel, and cyclophosphamide for resectable high-risk breast cancer: Feasibility and efficacy. J Clin Oncol 1999;17:93–100.

Loprinzi C, Thome S: Understanding the utility of adjuvant systemic therapy for primary breast cancer. J Clin Oncol 2001;19:972–979.

McCarthy N, Swain S. Update on adjuvant chemotherapy for early breast cancer. Oncology 2000;14:1267–1280.

Peters W, Rosner G, Vredenburgh J, et al: A prospective, randomized comparison of two doses of combination alkylating agents as consolidation after CAF in high-risk primary breast cancer involving ten or more axillary lymph nodes (LN): Preliminary results of CALGB 9082/SWOG 9114/NCIC MA-13. Proc Am Soc Clin Oncol 1999;18:1a (abstract 2).

Shapiro C, Hardenbergh P, Gelman R, et al: Cardiac effects of adjuvant doxorubicin and radiation therapy in breast cancer patients. J Clin Oncol 1998;16:3493–3501.

van Dam F, Schagen S, Muller M, et al: Impairment of cognitive function in women receiving adjuvant treatment for high-risk breast cancer: High-dose versus standard-dose chemotherapy. J Natl Cancer Inst 1998;90:210–218.

Zambetti M, Moliterni A, Materazzo C: Long-term cardiac sequelae in operable breast cancer patients given adjuvant chemotherapy with or without doxorubicin and breast irradiation. J Clin Oncol 2001;19:37–43.

Adjuvant Hormonal Therapy

ATAC (Arimidex, Tamoxifen Alone or in Combination) Trialists Group: Anastrazole alone or in combination with tamoxifen versus tamoxifen alone for adjuvant treatment of postmenopausal women with breast cancer: First results of the ATAC randomized trial. Lancet 2002;359:2131–2139.

Bines J, Oleske D, Cobleigh M: Ovarian function in premenopausal women treated with adjuvant chemotherapy for breast cancer. J Clin Oncol 1996;14:1718–1729.

Early Breast Cancer Trialists' Collaborative Group: Ovarian ablation in early breast cancer: Overview of the randomized trials. Lancet 1996;348:1189–1196.

Early Breast Cancer Trialists' Collaborative Group: Tamoxifen for early breast cancer: An overview of the randomized trials. Lancet 1998;351:1451–1467.

Fisher B, Dignam J, Bryant J, et al: Five versus more than five years of tamoxifen therapy for breast cancer patients with negative lymph nodes and estrogen receptor-positive tumors. J Natl Cancer Inst 1996;88:1529–1541.

Jakesz R, Hausmaninger H, Sámonigg H, et al: Comparison of adjuvant therapy with tamoxifen and goserelin vs. CMF in premenopausal stage I and II hormone-responsive breast cancer patients: Four-year results of Austrian Breast Cancer Study Group (ABCSG). Proc Am Soc Clin Onc 1999;18:67a (abstract 250).

Lam R, Chlebowski R: Tamoxifen for treatment of premenopausal women with breast cancer. Cancer Invest 2000;18:681–684.

Pritchard K: Endocrine therapy for breast cancer. Oncology 2000;14:483–492.

Ragaz J, Coldman A: Survival impact of adjuvant tamoxifen on competing causes of mortality in breast cancer survivors, with analysis of mortality from contralateral breast cancer, cardiovascular events, endometrial cancer, and thromboembolic episodes. J Clin Oncol 1998;16:2018–2024.

Stewart H, Prescott R, Forrest A: Scottish adjuvant tamoxifen trial: A randomized study updated to 15 years. J Natl Cancer Inst 2001;93:456–462.

Winer E, Hudis C, Burstein H, et al: American Society of Clinical Oncology technical assessment on the use of aromatase inhibitors as adjuvant therapy for women with hormone receptor–positive breast cancer: Status report 2002. J Clin Oncol 2002;20:3317–3327.

Adjuvant Radiation Therapy

Overgaard M, Hansen P, Overgaard J, et al: Postoperative radiotherapy in high-risk premenopausal women with breast cancer who receive adjuvant chemotherapy: Danish Breast

Cancer Cooperative Group 82b Trial. N Engl J Med 1997;337:949–955.

Ragaz J, Jackson S, Le N, et al: Adjuvant radiotherapy and chemotherapy in node-positive premenopausal women with breast cancer. N Engl J Med 1997;337:956–962.

Recht A, Come S, Henderson I, et al: The sequencing of chemotherapy and radiation therapy after conservative surgery for early-stage breast cancer. N Engl J Med 1996;334:1356–1361.

Recht A, Edge S, Solin L, et al: Postmastectomy radiotherapy: Clinical practice guidelines of the American Society of Clinical Oncology. J Clin Oncol 2001;19:1539–1569.

Whelan T, Julian J, Wright J, et al: Does locoregional radiation therapy improve survival in breast cancer? A meta-analysis. J Clin Oncol 2000;18:1220–1229.

Combined Chemohormonal Therapy

Davidson N, O'Neill A, Vukov A, et al: Effect of chemohormonal therapy in premenopausal, node-positive, receptor-positive breast cancer: An Eastern Cooperative Oncology Group Phase III intergroup trial (E 5188, INT-0101). Proc Am Soc Clin Onc 1999;18:67a (abstract 249).

Fisher B, Dignam J, Wolmark N, et al: Tamoxifen and chemotherapy for lymph node-negative, estrogen receptor-positive breast cancer. J Natl Cancer Inst 1997;89:1673–1682.

Fisher B, Redmond C, Legault-Poisson S, et al: Postoperative chemotherapy and tamoxifen compared with tamoxifen alone in the treatment of positive-node breast cancer patients aged 50 years and older with tumors responsive to tamoxifen: Results from the National Surgical Adjuvant Breast and Bowel Project B-16. J Clin Oncol 1990;8:1005–1018.

Neoadjuvant Therapy

Fisher B, Bryant J, Wolmark N, et al: Effect of preoperative chemotherapy on the outcome of women with operable breast cancer. J Clin Oncol 1998;16:2672–2685.

Chapter 77
Metastatic Breast Cancer

Charles L. Shapiro

Approximately 180,000 women are diagnosed with breast cancer annually in the United States, and about 13,000 of them have metastatic disease at the time of initial diagnosis. In addition, many women presenting with localized breast cancer will have metastatic disease that is not evident initially but will manifest itself months to years later. When detected, these are called *recurrences;* it is important to emphasize that these so-called recurrences are actually micrometastases that were already present, albeit occult, at the time of the initial diagnosis of breast cancer.

The natural history of breast cancer is lengthy. Estimates of the time from the first breast cancer cell to grow to the size of the earliest nonpalpable mammographically detectable or palpable cancer range from 5 to 10 years or even longer. During this lengthy preclinical growth period, some breast cancers acquire the biologic properties that enable them to invade and disseminate via the lymphatic or circulatory systems to other organs. Metastases establish themselves through complex biologic interactions with the organ microenvironment. For example, the transforming growth factor-alpha and other growth factors are important regulators of osteoclasts and osteoblasts during normal bone remodeling. These same growth factors stimulate breast cancer growth. This may explain the propensity for breast cancer to metastasize to bone, because the microenvironment is rich in the relevant growth factors.

The management of metastatic disease is complex. These interrelated aspects include clinical and biologic factors that help to determine which treatment option is optimal, psychosocial factors affecting both women with metastatic breast cancer and their families, and evaluating the benefits versus the side effects (Figure 77-1). Potential adverse effects of therapy are of particular importance, because the treatment for metastatic breast cancer is palliative, not curative. However, the natural history of metastatic breast cancer is highly variable, such that some patients live for years and receive successive treatments. For this subgroup, metastatic breast cancer is akin to having a chronic disease; the symptoms wax and wane with long periods of relative stability punctuated by periods in which the disease is no longer controlled.

Presentation of Metastatic Breast Cancer

Metastatic breast cancer usually presents with signs and symptoms that are referable to an organ site (Table 77-1). However, it is important to emphasize that many times metastases do not cause symptoms, or the initial symptoms are subtle, intermittent, and only recognized in retrospect. The skeleton is the most frequent site of first metastasis, followed by lung and liver. Autopsies in women dying of metastatic breast cancer reveal spread to virtually every organ.

Prognostic and Predictive Factors in Metastatic Breast Cancer

Prognostic factors are associated with shorter or longer survival duration in metastatic breast cancer (Table 77-2). Sites of first metastasis (e.g., liver, brain versus skeleton), shorter time interval between the initial diagnosis of breast cancer and first metastasis (also called *disease-free interval*), estrogen receptor (negative versus positive), and history of having received prior adjuvant chemotherapy are all independently associated with shorter survival. By using a combination of these factors, women with metastatic breast cancer can be separated into groups whose median survival varies from as much as four years to as little as 10 months.

Factors that are associated with a likelihood of response to treatment are called predictive factors (see Table 77-2). Women who are apt to benefit from hormonal therapy have estrogen receptors in the primary breast cancer or metastatic site, have had a prior response to hormonal therapy, have skeletal rather

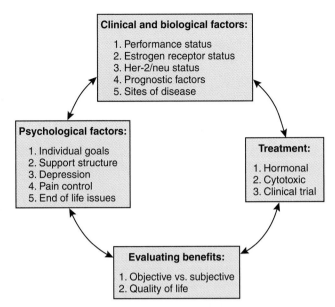

Figure 77-1 ■ Factors in the management of metastatic breast cancer.

than visceral disease, and have had a longer disease-free interval. Factors that predict benefit from chemotherapy are also described in Table 77-2. The most important one is functional status at time of treatment, or performance status (Table 77-3). There is a direct correlation between the response to chemotherapy and better performance status. This correlation reflects the extent of tumor burden, sites of metastases, and host factors that all contribute to the extent of interference with normal activities of daily living. Women with metastatic breast cancer who have performance status of 3 or 4 have a low likelihood of clinical benefit and are less able to tolerate the side effects.

About 20% to 30% of breast cancers will have more than two copies of the HER-2/neu (or Erb-b2) gene, and this gene amplification leads to overexpression of the HER-2/neu protein on the breast cancer cell. This protein is part of family of proteins that function as receptors and are involved in the regulation of cell growth. Trastuzumab (Herceptin) is a monoclonal antibody that alone or in combination with chemotherapy is effective treatment for metastatic breast cancer. HER-2/neu overexpression predicts benefit for trastuzumab and also may be useful in predicting benefit from doxorubicin-containing adjuvant regimens; lack of benefit from adjuvant cyclophosphamide, methotrexate, and fluorouracil (CMF); and possibly resistance to hormonal therapy.

Hormonal Treatment of Metastatic Breast Cancer

In the late nineteenth century, the first successful hormonal treatment was removing the ovaries from

Table 77-1 ■ **Signs and Symptoms of Metastatic Breast Cancer**

Organ	Symptoms	Signs	Treatment
Skeleton	Pain, fracture, hypercalcemia		Systemic treatments including bisphosphonates. Local: radiation, orthopedic stabilization of pathologic fractures.
Spinal cord compression	Pain, weakness, constipation, urinary retention	Weakness, numbness	Systemic: steroids. Local: radiation, surgery for unstable vertebrae or for progression after radiation.
Lung	Cough, dyspnea		Systemic treatments. Local: surgery for a solitary nodule.
Pleura	Cough, dyspnea, chest pain	Pleural effusion	Systemic treatments. Local: chest tube drainage and pleurodesis.
Liver	Abdominal pain, nausea	Hepatomegaly, jaundice	Systemic treatment. Local: consider surgery for solitary metastasis.
Brain	Headaches, altered mental status, focal weakness; seizure, impaired gait	Hemiparesis, cognitive dysfunction, focal weakness, impaired gait, papilledema	Systemic: steroids. Local: whole brain radiation for multiple metastases with surgery or radiosurgery (gamma knife) for solitary metastasis.
Carcinomatous meningitis	Headaches, altered mental status, focal weakness, impaired gait, seizure	Cranial nerve dysfunction, focal weakness, impaired gait	Intrathecal chemotherapy. Local: whole-brain radiation.

Table 77-2 ■ Prognostic and Predictive Factors for Metastatic Breast Cancer

	Metastatic Disease	Hormonal Therapy	Chemotherapy
Favorable Prognostic Factors for Survival			
Good performance status	+++		
First metastasis (nonvisceral versus visceral)	++		
Disease-free interval from primary therapy (longer versus shorter)	++		
Estrogen receptor status (positive versus negative)	++		
Prior adjuvant chemotherapy (no versus yes)	+		
Predictive Factors for Response to Therapy			
Performance status		+++	+++
Estrogen receptor positivity		+++	
HER-2/*neu* (overexpression)			+++
Prior response to hormonal therapy		+++	
Prior response to chemotherapy			+
Disease-free interval from primary therapy (longer versus shorter)		++	
Nonvisceral disease (skeleton, lymph node)		+	

Number of + marks indicates relative strength of prognostic or predictive factor.

young women with advanced breast cancer. Nearly 70 years later, the biologic basis for the hormonal responsiveness of breast cancer was clarified with the discovery of estrogen and progesterone receptor proteins. These receptor proteins are critical to the growth and function of normal breast tissue and also form the basis of breast cancer hormonal treatment.

There are two approaches to hormonal therapy: Use partial agonists or antagonists of estrogen to block the estrogen receptor, or reduce circulating endogenous estrogen levels. The source of estrogen varies with menstrual status. The ovaries are the primary source of estrogen in premenopausal women, whereas in postmenopausal women, estrogens are produced primarily in peripheral adipose and muscle tissue by the action of the aromatase enzyme. This enzyme converts androstenedione derived from the adrenal gland into estrogens. Aromatase is also found within breast tissue and is the source of estrogens produced within breast cancers.

Hormonal treatments are listed in Table 77-4. Aromatase inhibitors are ineffective in premenopausal women because the primary source of estrogen is the ovaries. Likewise, an oophorectomy or reducing the production of ovarian estrogen using a gonadotropin-releasing hormone (GnRH) agonist is ineffective in postmenopausal women because the primary source of estrogen is the adrenal gland and not the ovary. Tamoxifen is effective irrespective of menstrual status because it blocks the estrogen receptor.

Tamoxifen and Other Selective Estrogen Receptor Modulators

Tamoxifen is both an estrogen antagonist and agonist depending on the specific tissue. The antagonist activ-

Table 77-3 ■ Performance Status

Functional ability	ECOG	Karnofsky (%)
Fully active, able to carry on normal activity; no special care is needed.	0	100
Restricted in physically strenuous work but ambulatory and to carry light work.	1	85
Ambulatory and capable of all self-care but unable to carry out any work-related activities; up and about more than 50% of the waking hours.	2	65
Capable of only limited self-care and confined to bed or chair more than 50% of waking hours.	3	40
Completely disabled; cannot carry on any self-care; totally confined to bed or chair	4	15

Table 77-4 ▪ Hormonal Therapy for Metastatic Breast Cancer

	Clinical Benefit (%)	TTP (months)	Side Effects
Estrogen Antagonist			
Tamoxifen	58	6–8	Hot flashes, vaginal discharge, irregular menses, small increased risks of endometrial cancer and thromboembolic events
Fulvestrant (Falsodex)	43	5–6	Hot flashes, nausea/vomiting
Ovarian Ablation			
Oophorectomy	29	5–6	Hot flashes, tumor flare, nausea/vomiting, fatigue
Goserelin (Zoladex)	29	7	
Aromatase Inhibitors			
Anastrozole (Arimidex): first line	56	8–11	Nausea/vomiting, hot flashes, edema, thromboembolic events
Anastrozole: second line (after tamoxifen)	35	5	
Letrozole (Femara): first line	49	10	Hot flashes, nausea/vomiting, thromboembolic events
Letrozole: second line	36	6	
Exemestane: second line	37	5	Hot flashes, nausea, fatigue
Progestin			
Megestrol acetate (Megace): first line	55	8–11	Weight gain, fluid retention, vaginal bleeding, thromboembolic events
Megestrol acetate: first line	37	4–6	

Abbreviations: TTP, median time to progression; Clinical Benefit % = sum of complete response + partial response + stable disease.

ity is the basis of its therapeutic efficacy in all stages of breast cancer and the prevention of breast cancer in high-risk women. Unlike estrogen, when tamoxifen binds to the estrogen receptor, the receptor complex binds to deoxyribonucleic acid but transcription is not activated. Tamoxifen acts as an estrogen agonist in bone, liver, the coagulation system, and the endometrium. Like estrogen, it preserves bone mineral density in postmenopausal women, lowers total and low-density lipoprotein cholesterol, is thrombogenic, and is associated with a small increase in endometrial cancer, respectively.

Two randomized trials demonstrate that tamoxifen and oophorectomy provide similar benefits in premenopausal women with metastatic breast cancer. It is reasonable to consider oophorectomy or medical ovarian ablation in women who have had a prior response to tamoxifen. Several randomized trials in postmenopausal women with metastatic breast cancer compared tamoxifen to megestrol acetate. Tamoxifen was associated with fewer side effects.

The tamoxifen withdrawal response occurs in a small number of postmenopausal women with metastatic breast cancer. It is more likely to occur in women who have had a long duration of response to tamoxifen and then begin to have progressive disease,

especially if they are minimally symptomatic. One potential mechanism for the withdrawal response is that initially tamoxifen-sensitive breast cancers become resistant to and then reliant on tamoxifen for their growth. Perhaps the most difficult aspect of the withdrawal response for clinicians is explaining the concept to the patient. It is a counterintuitive that withdrawing a treatment (and not replacing it with another treatment) might be of some benefit.

A clinical flare syndrome can occur within days to a few weeks after starting tamoxifen. It can result in an increase in skeletal pain, enlargement and erythema of skin metastases (5% to 10%), or hypercalcemia (3% to 5%). Although the mechanism of flare is not well understood, it is thought to represent transient stimulation of tumor growth. The symptoms usually resolve spontaneously over several days or weeks despite continuation of tamoxifen. Clinical flare can be distressing and severe, but it responds to appropriate therapy. Affected patients should be reassured that a clinical flare often predicts a subsequent favorable therapeutic response to tamoxifen.

Radionuclide bone scan obtained within two to three months of starting tamoxifen or other hormonal therapy may show apparent worsening of bone metastases, with increased intensity of uptake or new areas of apparent disease. The dilemma for the clinician is whether this represents disease progression or is scintigraphic flare, which is associated with response to hormonal therapy. Distinguishing scintigraphic flare from progression is important so as not to prematurely abandon a useful treatment. Several clinical findings are useful in making this determination. Assessment of response in extraskeletal sites of metastases may be helpful. Obtaining correlative plain films of the regions of uptake on bone scan may be useful as well. If the plain films demonstrate an enlarging lytic lesion, then this is evidence of progression. Often, the best way to distinguish scintigraphic flare from disease progression is to repeat another bone scan in two or three months. In most cases, the clinical course and response to treatment is the same whether disease progression is recognized and another treatment is instituted or delayed for two to three months, when there is more definitive evidence of progression.

The side effects of tamoxifen in postmenopausal women with metastatic breast cancer include increases in vasomotor symptoms (10% to 20%), vaginal discharge (10%), and rarely thrombotic events (deep vein thrombosis, pulmonary embolism (1% to 2%) and endometrial cancer (1% to 2%)). Many of the side effects of tamoxifen that postmenopausal women experience are reduced in frequency in premenopausal women, but irregular menstrual bleeding or cessation of menses occurs commonly. Contrary to popular belief, observations from placebo-controlled trials in high-risk women and those diagnosed with noninvasive breast cancer suggest that tamoxifen itself does not cause weight gain or depression.

Pure Estrogen Antagonist

Fulvestrant (Faslodex) is a new hormonal treatment approved for postmenopausal women with breast cancer that is administered once a month by intramuscular injection. Unlike tamoxifen, which has both agonist and antagonist activity, when fulvestrant binds the estrogen receptor it is pure receptor antagonist. In randomized trials comparing it to anastrozole as second-line after tamoxifen, fulvestrant had similar activity and side effects. With aromatase inhibitors now replacing tamoxifen as the initial treatment for postmenopausal women with estrogen receptor–positive metastases, additional trials will establish the optimal sequence of hormone treatments. There is insufficient data as yet to use fulvestrant in premenopausal women.

Aromatase Inhibitors

There are two types of aromatase inhibitors: Type I or steroidal inactivators (also called suicide inhibitors) and Type II or nonsteroidal inhibitors. Exemestane (Aromasin) is a Type I inhibitor. It is chemically related to the substrate androstenedione and irreversibly binds to the aromatase enzyme. Anastrozole (Arimidex) and letrozole (Femara) are Type II reversible enzyme inhibitors (see Table 77-4). Both inhibitors suppress circulating levels of estrogen in postmenopausal women. Whether the biologic differences

Table 77-5 ■ Selected Randomized Trials of Hormonal Therapy

	N	Benefit (%)	TTP (months)	Side Effects	Significant Difference
First-line treatment					
Letrozole versus tamoxifen	907	49 versus 38	9 versus 4	=	yes[†]
Anastrozole versus tamoxifen	353	59 versus 46	11 versus 6	↑ Tam	yes[†]
Anastrozole versus tamoxifen	668	56 versus 56	8 versus 8	↑ Tam	no
Second-line treatment					
Exemestane versus megestrol acetate	769	37 versus 35	5 versus 4	↑ MA	yes[‡]
Letrozole versus megestrol acetate	363	35 versus 32	6 versus 6	↑ MA	yes[‡]
Fulvestrant versus anastrozole	451	45 versus 45	6 versus 5	=**	no
Fulvestrant versus anastrozole	400	42 versus 36	5 versus 3	=**	no
Anastrozole versus megesterol acetate	516	42 versus 40	–	↑ MA	yes[¶]

Abbreviations: Median time to progression (TTP); Benefit % = complete response % + partial response % + stable disease %; N = number of patients; ↑Tam = higher rates of thromboembolic events and vaginal bleeding; ↑ MA = higher incidence of side effects with megestrol.
[†]Significant difference in benefit % and TTP.
[‡]Significant difference in TTP.
[¶]Significant difference overall survival.
**Arthralgias more frequent in anastrozole-treated patients.

between the two types of inhibitors will translate into clinically meaningful therapeutic differences is under study.

The role of aromatase inhibitors in the treatment of postmenopausal women with metastatic breast cancer is evolving. As second-line treatment after tamoxifen, they have replaced megestrol acetate based on the more favorable side effect profile with similar therapeutic benefits (Table 77-5). However, results of recent randomized trials in women with metastatic disease demonstrate that the aromatase inhibitors are as good as, or superior to, tamoxifen when used as first-line treatment. Letrozole and anastrozole have recently received approval for this indication and are initial treatment for postmenopausal women with estrogen receptor–positive metastases. Aromatase inhibitors have side effects similar to those of tamoxifen but are less thrombogenic and do not cause endometrial cancer.

Progestin

The mechanism of action of megestrol acetate is not well understood; however, it does not work via the progesterone receptor. Adverse effects of therapy include weight gain (18%), fluid retention (5%), vaginal bleeding (5%), and exacerbation of diabetes. While the benefits are similar to those of tamoxifen (as first-line) or aromatase inhibitors (as second-line), the side-effect profile has relegated megestrol acetate to third-line treatment.

Combined Hormonal Therapy

Combinations of hormonal treatments as opposed to single drugs do not provide significant improvement in clinical benefit but do increase the side effects. There is some evidence that the combination of a GnRH agonist plus tamoxifen might be slightly superior to a GnRH agonist alone in premenopausal women. However, information on quality of life is lacking in these trials, and this becomes increasingly important, as the magnitude of difference favoring the combination is small. Hormonal treatments should be used in sequence rather than combination unless the combination is part of a clinical trial.

Hormonal Versus Chemotherapy as Initial Treatment

In several randomized trials, the combination of chemotherapy and hormonal therapy versus chemotherapy or hormonal therapy alone was evaluated in women with metastatic breast cancer. Often, the combination is associated with a higher response, but the duration of response and overall survival are not improved. The Australian and New Zealand Breast Cancer trial deserves special mention. Two hundred twenty-six women with metastatic breast cancer were randomized to receive either cyclophosphamide and doxorubicin, tamoxifen, or the combination of chemotherapy plus tamoxifen as the initial treatment for metastatic breast cancer. The initial response rates were 51%, 45%, and 22%, respectively. However, those who were treated with chemotherapy alone or tamoxifen alone were crossed to the other therapy on disease progression. After the crossover, the response rates were similar, and there were no differences in overall survival. In a multivariate analysis, initial treatment allocation was not associated with survival. These results support the recommendation of treating with hormonal therapy as initial treatment if factors for hormonal responsiveness (estrogen receptor positivity, long disease-free interval, and nonvisceral disease) are present.

Suggested Approach to Hormonal Therapy

Figure 77-2 describes an approach to hormone therapy. A few points deserve special emphasis.

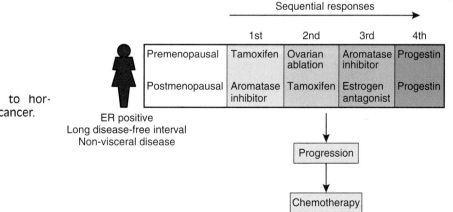

Figure 77-2 ■ Suggested approach to hormonal therapy for metastatic breast cancer.

Table 77-6 ▪ Chemotherapeutic Drugs in Metastatic Breast Cancer

	Response (%)		
	Untreated	Prior treatment	Side Effects
Docetaxel (Taxotere) q3 weeks	50–60	30–50	Myelosuppression, hair loss, arthralgia/myalgia, stomatitis, peripheral neuropathy, fluid retention, nail changes, lacrimation, hypersensitivity reactions
Paclitaxel (Taxol) q3 weeks	35	28	Myelosuppression, hair loss, arthalgia/myalgia, peripheral neuropathy, hypersensitivity reactions
Doxorubicin (Adriamycin)	40–50	33	Myelosuppression, hair loss, nausea/vomiting, cardiomyopathy
Cyclophosphamide (Cytoxan)	36	22	Myelosuppression, hair loss, nausea/vomiting
Capecitabine (Xeloda)	—	25	Diarrhea, hand–foot syndrome, stomatitis, myleosuppression
Vinorelbine (Navelbine)	30–40	20–30	Myelosuppression, peripheral neuropathy, nausea/vomiting, hair loss
Gemcitabine (Gemzar)	18–40	25	Myelosuppression, nausea/vomiting
Trastuzumab (Herceptin)	23	15	Fever, chills, back pain, flulike syndrome, nausea, diarrhea, cough, peripheral edema, cardiomyopathy

Whenever the clinical situation suggests that hormonal therapy is a viable option, take it. Hormonal therapy is directed against a specific target, the estrogen receptor, and relative to chemotherapy, hormone treatment can be as effective with fewer side effects. There are no data to support the notion that chemotherapy, if used as initial treatment, is associated with better survival than hormone therapy, except in the rare instances of those who present with life-threatening liver or lung metastases (so-called visceral crises). Their life span is measured in weeks to months but occasionally can be prolonged by chemotherapy.

Chemotherapy of Metastatic Breast Cancer

Relative to other epithelial cancers, there are many chemotherapy drugs that are active in metastatic breast cancer (Table 77-6). The single most important predictor of benefit from chemotherapy is performance status. The response rate and expectation of clinical benefit decrease with successive chemotherapy treatments such that the National Comprehensive Cancer Center Network treatment guidelines recommend that after failing two standard chemotherapy regimens for metastatic breast cancer, it is appropriate to discontinue any further chemotherapy and emphasize supportive care.

Doxorubicin and Taxanes

The two most active drugs in metastatic breast cancer are doxorubicin and taxanes (see Table 77-6). The use of doxorubicin for metastatic breast is evolving. Doxorubicin-containing chemotherapy regimens were used frequently as initial treatment for metastatic breast cancer, the majority of women having received CMF regimens in the adjuvant setting. During the past 15 years, the use of adjuvant regimens containing doxorubicin has dramatically increased such that the majority of women with metastatic disease will have had between 240 and 360 milligrams per square meter of body surface area (mg/m^2) of prior adjuvant doxorubicin. This limits the amount of doxorubicin they can receive for treatment of metastatic disease because of the cumulative dose-dependent risk of cardiomyopathy. At total cumulative doxorubicin doses typically used in the adjuvant regimens, the risk of cardiomyopathy is less than 1%; however, the risk begins to rise steeply at doses that exceed $450\ mg/m^2$.

A number of strategies to lessen cardiac toxicity have been developed. It is well established that altering the schedule of doxorubicin, either by giving continuous infusion or by using weekly low-dose treatment instead of higher doses every three weeks, increases total cumulative doxorubicin dose before cardiomyopathy ensues. In particular, lower doses of doxorubicin (20 to 25 mg/m^2 weekly) have similar antitumor activity but fewer side effects than higher doses given every three weeks. This is an alternative for women responding to doxorubicin for whom continued treatment would be of benefit.

Another strategy that reduces the risk of cardiomyopathy is the use of derazoxane, a cardioprotectant. Derazoxane is approved for women with

Table 77-7 ■ Selected Randomized Trials of Chemotherapy in Metastatic Breast Cancer

	N	Prior Treatment*	Response (%)	TTP (months)
Docetaxel (D) versus doxorubicin (A)	326	No	47 versus 33	7 versus 5
DA versus CA	429	No	60 versus 47	9 versus 8
Paclitaxel (T) versus A	331	No	25 versus 41	4 versus 8
Paclitaxel (T) 175 versus 135 mg/m^2	471	No	29 versus 22	4 versus 3
T (175 versus 210 versus 250 mg/m^2)	475	Yes	21 versus 28 versus 24	4 versus 4 versus 5
T versus A versus AT	703	No	33 versus 34 versus 46	6 versus 6 versus 8
T versus CMF	209	No	35 versus 35	6 versus 6
Trastuzumab/T versus T	188	No	38 versus 16	7 versus 3

Abbreviations: TTP = median time to progression; response includes complete and partial responses; C = cyclophosphamide.
*Prior treatment for metastatic disease.

metastatic breast cancer who have received a cumulative dose of 300 mg/m^2 and are responding to treatment. Derazoxane in combination with doxorubicin allows for higher cumulative doxorubicin doses before the risk of cardiomyopathy increases. Likewise, liposomal-encapsulated doxorubicins and epirubicin appear to have similar antitumor activity but less risk of cardiomyopathy than doxorubicin per total cumulative dose.

The taxanes, paclitaxel and docetaxel, are increasingly used as front-line treatment for women who recur after adjuvant doxorubicin-containing regimens. The primary side effects of paclitaxel are hair loss, myelosuppression, myalgias and arthralgias, and peripheral neuropathy. It is less emetogenic then either cyclophosphamide or doxorubicin. The hypersensitivity reactions associated with paclitaxel are due to the agent that is used to solubilize the drug. These can be prevented in the great majority of women by giving glucocorticoids and drugs that block histamine 1 and 2 receptors before therapy. These are recommended as part of standard premedication for paclitaxel.

Most women receiving paclitaxel experience mild numbness in the hands and feet that does not interfere with walking, buttoning clothes, writing, or any other activities that require fine sensory or motor nerve function. It is common to have the neuropathy associated with paclitaxel worsen as the cumulative dose increases over successive treatments. Women receiving paclitaxel should be questioned frequently about the degree of numbness and the extent to which the symptoms interfere with function. Dose delays until the symptoms improve or reducing the dose is appropriate. If the paclitaxel is continued despite worsening neurologic symptoms, the consequences may be irreversible and result in permanent loss of function.

Several trials have addressed the optimal dose and schedule of paclitaxel (Table 77-7). Doses of 175 mg/m^2 over a three-hour intravenous infusion repeated every three weeks resulted in slightly better results than 135 mg/m^2, whereas doses of 210 and 250 mg/m^2 did not increase response rates or overall survival but had more side effects, particularly peripheral neuropathy. Phase II trials of paclitaxel administered weekly at doses of 80 to 100 mg/m^2 suggest similar or higher responses than those observed at 175 mg/m^2 every three weeks but less peripheral neuropathy and hematologic toxicity.

Many combinations of doxorubicin and paclitaxel have been reported. Through these efforts, it was discovered that cardiotoxicity of the combination is sequence dependent. Administering paclitaxel before doxorubicin alters the pharmacokinetics of doxorubicin such that it leads to decreased clearance of doxorubicin and a higher incidence of cardiac toxicity. When doxorubicin is given first followed by paclitaxel, such increases in cardiac toxicity do not occur.

An informative trial led by the Eastern Cooperative Oncology Group (ECOG) randomized women with metastatic breast cancer to doxorubicin, paclitaxel, or the combination (see Table 77-7). Although there was a slightly higher response rate favoring the combination over either drug alone, the time to disease progression and overall survival rates were not different among the three groups. As expected, there were more side effects with the combination. The results of the ECOG study are generally consistent with most randomized trials of combinations versus single drugs in metastatic disease; combination chemotherapy usually results in higher response rates, increased side effects, but little or no impact on time to progression or survival with the combination.

Docetaxel (Taxotere) causes myelosuppression, hair loss, fatigue, peripheral neuropathy, mouth sores, nail changes, myalgias and arthralgias. The fluid accumulation and hypersensitivity reactions associated with docetaxel can be reduced by three days of dexamethasone 16 mg orally beginning 24 hours before treatment, the day of treatment, and 24 hours after. The liver metabolizes docetaxel, and the drug clearance is decreased in the presence of elevated transaminases and alkaline phosphatase. Docetaxel doses should be reduced in the presence of elevated liver function tests according to standard guidelines.

In women with metastatic breast cancer, docetaxel provided superior response rates compared to doxorubicin but similar time to disease progression and overall survival in women who were previously untreated with doxorubicin (see Table 77-7). Likewise, the combination of doxorubicin and docetaxel proved superior to doxorubicin and cyclophosphamide (see Table 77-7).

Capecitabine (Xeloda)

Capecitabine is an oral chemotherapy drug that is converted to 5-fluorouracil at the tumor site. It is indicated for women with metastatic breast cancer in whom treatment with an anthracycline and taxane has failed (see Table 77-6). The most common side effects are myelosuppression; diarrhea; mouth sores; and redness, irritation, and pain of the palms of the hands and soles of the feet, called the hand–foot syndrome. These side effects are dose-related and improve with holding the dose until the symptoms resolve and then continuing treatment at a lower dose depending on the severity of side effects. Although the recommended starting dose is 2500 mg/m^2 per day for 14 days, there is some evidence that reducing the dose to 2000 mg/m^2 provides similar benefits but reduces the side effects.

Trastuzumab

Response to trastuzumab depends on breast cancer overexpression of HER-2/*neu* protein. The standard method of evaluating HER-2/*neu* overexpression is the Hercept™ Test using immunohistochemical methods. The results are semiquantitative; 0 and 1+ are negative, 2+ is weakly positive, and 3+ is strongly positive. In clinical trials, it is 3+ breast cancers that respond to treatment with trastuzumab. A more sensitive test is to directly measure gene amplification by fluoresence in situ hybridization (FISH). Up to 70% of the 2+, or weakly positive, breast cancers do not have HER-2/*neu* gene amplification when tested by fluoresence in situ hybridization. These false positive cases do not respond to trastuzumab. It is much less of a problem in 3+ (strongly positive) and 0, 1+ (negative) breast cancers, in which more than 80% do and do not have

gene amplification, respectively. Clinicians who are considering trastuzumab for women with 2+ overexpression should have the tumor evaluated by fluoresence in situ hybridization to confirm HER-2/*neu*.

As a single agent or in combination with chemotherapy, trastuzumab is active in HER-2/*neu*-overexpressing metastatic breast cancers (see Tables 77-6 and 77-7). The combination of trastuzumab and chemotherapy provided superior response rates, increased the time to disease progression, and improved overall survival and was associated with improvements in quality-of-life assessments relative to chemotherapy. However, there was an unacceptably high rate of cardiac problems (about 18%) when trastuzumab was combined with cyclophosphamide and doxorubicin, compared to 3% when it was combined with paclitaxel. Other less cardiotoxic anthracyclines, such as liposomal-encapsulated doxorubicin and epirubicin, are being evaluated in combination with trastuzumab. However, anthracyclines and trastuzumab should not be combined unless it is in the context of a clinical trial with careful cardiac monitoring.

Chemotherapy of the Older Woman with Metastatic Breast Cancer

It is often assumed the older women tolerate chemotherapy less well than younger women, "older" usually being defined as age more than 65 or 70 years. The ability to tolerate and derive benefit from chemotherapy is often confounded by differences in performance status, comorbidity, and end organ function between younger and older women. When these factors are comparable, the side effects and expectation of benefit from chemotherapy are similar irrespective of age. Thus, treatment decisions should be based on physiologic rather than chronologic age.

High-Dose Chemotherapy

Is there a clinically meaningful dose response in metastatic breast cancer? Less than standard doses of chemotherapy proved inferior to standard doses. However, escalating the dose higher than standard doses has not resulted in significant improvements in time to disease progression or overall survival. The results of recent randomized trials show no improvement in overall survival for high-dose chemotherapy with autologous marrow support relative to standard chemotherapy. These observations are most consistent with a threshold effect beyond which there is no benefit to increasing the chemotherapy but there are increased side effects.

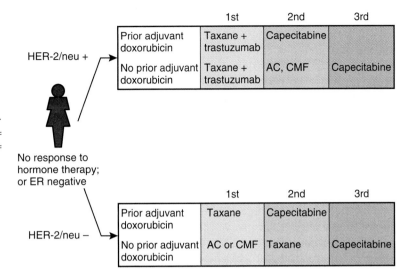

Figure 77-3 ■ Suggested approach to chemotherapy for metastatic breast cancer. A = Adriamycin, C = cyclophosphamide, M = methotrexate, F = 5-fluorouracil.

Suggested Approach to Chemotherapy

There is a multitude of active chemotherapy drugs in breast cancer. The most active are the taxanes and doxorubicin. A general approach to treating metastatic breast cancer is outlined in Figure 77-3. The most important factors are performance status and HER-2/*neu* status.

There are several relevant questions about treating metastatic breast cancer with chemotherapy. Are combinations superior to sequentially administered single drugs? What is the meaning of a response, and is it the best endpoint for evaluating new drugs for metastatic breast cancer? Is a shorter or a longer duration of chemotherapy better? Finally, does treatment with a new experimental drug before using an established drug(s) alter the outcome?

Historically, several randomized trials conducted in the 1970s and early 1980s demonstrated small survival advantages for combination chemotherapy versus single drugs. However, these trials included less-active single drugs compared to the drugs in the combination. More recent randomized trials show superior or similar results for docetaxel or paclitaxel compared with combination chemotherapy (see Table 77-7). Often the individual doses of each drug in a combination are reduced owing to overlapping side effects. On the basis of a model of breast cancer growth kinetics, it might be more effective to treat with single drugs at their maximal tolerated doses as opposed lower doses in the combination. This hypothesis continues to be evaluated in clinical trials.

Newer combinations continue to be tested, and some of them show promising preliminary results. A recent randomized trial of docetaxel and capecitabine versus docetaxel alone showed a superior survival benefit for the combination. However, in most cases, the therapeutic ratio is maximized when single drugs are used sequentially, and this is a viable option for treatment of metastatic breast cancer outside of a clinical trial setting.

Within breast tumors, the individual cancer cells are heterogeneous. There are mixtures of hormone-sensitive and hormone-resistant cells; likewise, there are mixtures of chemotherapy-sensitive and chemotherapy-resistant cells. A complete response (defined as no detectable evidence of metastasis) or a partial response (defined as more than 50% reduction in the size of the metastasis) is dependent on the ratio of sensitive to resistant cancer cells. A cancer that is made up of mostly sensitive cells will manifest a response, whereas the opposite is true of a cancer that is composed primarily of resistant cells. No chemotherapy combination is expected to eliminate 100% of cancer cells, even in cases in which there is a complete response. For this reason, endpoints such as time to disease progression are potentially more important than response rates and may be a better indicator of clinical benefit. This is especially so in evaluating newer biologic agents such as angiogenesis inhibitors that may, by the nature of how they work, not be associated with objective responses.

Several randomized trials show that continuing the chemotherapy until disease progression instead of stopping after three to six cycles of chemotherapy and restarting again when disease progresses, might be a more effective way to provide clinically meaningful benefits. Although overall survival is not improved, the time to disease progression and quality-of-life assessments suggest a benefit for continuing treatment until disease progression. In particular, newer combinations of weekly paclitaxel or vinorelbine in combination with trastuzumab lend themselves to a longer-duration therapy because of their antitumor activity and favorable side-effect profile.

It is axiomatic that the antitumor activity of most drugs in breast cancer will be greater or less depending on the setting in which the drug is evaluated. In addition to the multiple mechanisms of drug resistance already present, breast cancers may acquire new ones when exposed to chemotherapy. This, in combination with the poorer performance status and larger tumor burden of women who have received multiple prior treatments, complicates the evaluation of new drugs. The traditional setting for phase I and II chemotherapy trials is, however, in women who have received multiple prior chemotherapy regimens. In an effort to address this problem, the CALGB reported the results of a trial in which women with metastatic breast cancer were randomized to either a Phase II or "experimental drug" or a standard combination chemotherapy with CAF. After two to four cycles of the experimental drug, the women were crossed over to CAF. The results in this trial demonstrated that the overall survival was not different between the treatment groups. This important trial provides the justification for moving experimental drugs from the traditional position of last-resort treatment to earlier in the treatment course, when they are more likely to show activity.

Management of Skeletal Metastases

Bone is the most frequent initial site of metastases, occurring in 30% to 50% of women with breast cancer, and pain is the predominant symptom. The pain is often chronic, occurs at rest and with movement, and only rarely affects the joints. The majority of breast cancers that metastasize to bone cause increased osteoclast activation, or excess bone resorption. Within most skeletal metastases, there is also osteoblast activation, and this is the basis of the focal uptake imaged on technetium-99 radionuclide bone scans. This tracer is taken up by osteoblasts, and the scan reflects their activity. Rarely, the radionuclide bone scan will be normal in the case of purely lytic lesions.

Bone scans and plain skeletal radiographs are complementary tests in the evaluation of suspected skeletal metastases. A bone scan is a very sensitive test, though it lacks specificity. Nonpathologic fracture, bone infection, and degenerative disease can all cause focal uptake imaged on bone scan. For example, the skeletal radiograph can reveal degenerative changes that correspond to the region of focal uptake. If the skeletal radiograph is normal or does not provide an explanation for the bone scan findings, then the like-lihood of metastasis is increased. Computed tomography (CT) scans or magnetic resonance imaging (MRI) scans are more specific than skeletal radiographs and can be helpful in confirming skeletal metastasis.

Excess bone resorption is responsible for the clinical manifestations associated with skeletal metastases, such as pain, hypercalcemia, and pathologic fracture, which occur in 75%, 17%, and 16% of patients, respectively. It is better to diagnose an impending pathologic fracture and institute treatment than to have to treat a pathologic fracture. There are several characteristics of an impending pathologic fracture: large bone metastasis (≥2.5 cm) located in a weight-bearing bone that is painful or a metastasis that involves one third or more of cortex. Treatment options include orthopedic stabilization of the bone followed by radiation or radiation alone. Orthopedic surgery followed by radiation is usually reserved for those who have a good performance status and reasonable expectation of response to systemic treatment for metastatic breast cancer.

Spinal cord compression and hypercalcemia are relatively rare complications of bone metastases, but it is important to diagnosis them early and initiate treatment promptly. Spinal cord compression can lead to irreversible paralysis, and hypercalcemia can cause death if untreated. The single most important factor in determining neurologic function after treatment for spinal cord compression is neurologic function before treatment, again emphasizing the importance of early diagnosis. The signs and symptoms of spinal cord compression include focal back pain, motor or sensory dysfunction, constipation, and urinary retention or incontinence. However, these are advanced symptoms of spinal cord compression, and many patients will present earlier with more subtle symptoms. Any suspicion of spinal cord compression should prompt an imaging study.

Bisphosphonates are specific inhibitors of osteoclast activity and are indicated for the treatment of hypercalcemia. They are targeted to sites of increased bone resorption, where they inhibit osteoclast-mediated bone resorption. Several randomized double-blind placebo-controlled trials in women with lytic breast cancer metastases show that the intravenous bisphosphonates pamidronate (Aredia) and zoledronic acid (Zometa) in combination with systemic therapy significantly reduce pain and the number of episodes of hypercalcemia, pathologic fractures, and the need for radiation therapy. Thus far, no survival benefit is associated with these bisphosphonates in breast cancer.

Several important questions remain to be answered. The optimal dose and duration of bisphosphonate for the treatment of skeletal metastases in

TREATMENT

Approach to Solitary Sites of Metastases

Not infrequently, metastatic disease occurs initially as a solitary focus in the lung, liver, or brain. Two questions arise: Is it a breast cancer metastasis versus a new primary cancer, and should it be surgically resected? The first problem is manifest in a solitary pulmonary nodule appearing on a chest radiograph in a woman who has received prior treatment for breast cancer. Approximately 50% of resected solitary pulmonary nodules are actually new primary lung cancers, not breast cancer metastases.

There are several series that show prolonged survival in breast cancer and other solid tumors when solitary metastases are surgically resected. It is difficult to sort out whether the survival benefit stems from the resection of a single metastatic site versus the various selection factors (e.g., good performance status) that influence the decision for resection. Nonetheless, it is reasonable to consider resection of solitary lung, liver, and brain metastases in breast cancer both for diagnostic and potential therapeutic value.

breast cancer remain undefined. Zoledronic acid has activity comparable to that of pamidronate but a shorter infusion time, 15 minutes as opposed to 90 to 120 minutes. More important, as yet there are no precise guidelines that define which women with skeletal metastases benefit most from bisphosphonate treatment. A general guideline is that painful skeletal lytic metastases will benefit from continuing bisphosphonate treatment in combination with successive hormonal and chemotherapy treatments.

Psychosocial Aspects and Symptom Management

"Women" rather than "patients" with metastatic breast cancer are referred to throughout this chapter. This is purposeful and designed to emphasize the very important, though often neglected, aspect of providing psychosocial care and symptom management in metastatic breast cancer. (See also Chapters 78, 120, and 122.) There is evidence that oncologists do not treat pain effectively, are uncomfortable with discussing end-of-life issues, and make inappropriate referrals to hospice when death is imminent. Treatment of metastatic breast cancer goes well beyond selection of treatment. Issues of depression, sexuality, anxiety, pain control, end-of-life issues, and hospice are of importance to women with metastatic breast cancer, and clinicians should be willing to discuss them and refer to other health care professionals who have the appropriate expertise in these areas. An integrated approach that involves the use of antidepressants, counseling, and support groups can be helpful to women who are emotionally overwhelmed by living with metastatic breast cancer. It is also important to remember that breast cancer is a disease that affects the entire family. Children may benefit from

specially designed support programs that address their fears and anxieties; husbands too may benefit by seeking counseling and support groups.

The Importance of Clinical Trials

Clinicians and women with metastatic breast cancer are united in a common goal: to improve treatments and quality of life for this disease. During the past 40 years, incremental progress toward this goal has been achieved through properly conducted clinical trials. It is important to remember that the standard treatments outlined in Tables 77-4 and 77-6 and Figures 77-2 and 77-3 were once considered experimental and it was only through evaluating them in clinical trials that they were proven beneficial and then incorporated into standard practice.

It is also important to remember that the results of clinical trials may identify ineffective treatments. Many clinicians and women with metastatic breast cancer assumed that high-dose chemotherapy with autologous marrow support was better than standard-dose chemotherapy on the basis of small preliminary trials. This led to the widespread use of this treatment. However, the results of randomized trials of high-dose versus standard-dose chemotherapy demonstrated that the overall benefit was comparable. Many thousands of women received a treatment outside of the clinical trial setting that had severe side effects, was expensive, and ultimately was no more effective than standard treatment.

The Clinical Trials Support Unit (CTSU) of the National Cancer Institute (NCI) is a mechanism to increase the availability of clinical trials to clinicians. Once registered, a clinician can gain access to cooperative group trials and other trials and offer the option of participating in a clinical trial. More information about the CTSU can be obtained at the National Cancer Institute website at <www.nci.nih.gov> or the CTSU website at <www.CTSU.org>.

References

Anonymous: A randomized trial in postmenopausal patients with advanced breast cancer comparing endocrine and cytotoxic therapy given sequentially or in combination: The Australian and New Zealand Breast Cancer Trials Group, Clinical Oncological Society of Australia. J Clin Oncol 1986;4:186–193.

Bishop JF, Dewar J, Toner GC, et al: Initial paclitaxel improves outcome compared with CMFP combination chemotherapy as front-line therapy in untreated metastatic breast cancer. J Clin Oncol 1999;17:2355–2364.

Buzdar AU: Role of aromatase inhibitors in advanced breast cancer. Endocrine-Related Cancer 1999;6:219–225.

Chan S, Friedrichs K, Noel D, et al: Prospective randomized trial of docetaxel versus doxorubicin in patients with metastatic breast cancer: The 303 Study Group. J Clin Oncol 1999;17:2341–2354.

Cobleigh MA, Vogel CL, Tripathy D, et al: Multinational study of the efficacy and safety of humanized anti-HER2 monoclonal antibody in women who have HER2-overexpressing metastatic breast cancer that has progressed after chemotherapy for metastatic disease. J Clin Oncol 1999;17:2639–2648.

Costanza ME, Weiss RB, Henderson IC, et al: Safety and efficacy of using a single agent or a phase II agent before instituting standard combination chemotherapy in previously untreated metastatic breast cancer patients: Report of a randomized study—Cancer and Leukemia Group B 8642. J Clin Oncol 1999;17:1397–1406.

Ellis MJ, Hayes DF, Lippman ME: Treatment of metastatic breast cancer. In Harris JR, Lippman ME, Morrow M, Osborne CK (eds): Diseases of the Breast. Philadelphia: Lippincott Williams and Wilkins, 2000.

Hayes DF, Henderson IC, Shapiro CL: Treatment of metastatic breast cancer: Present and future prospects. Semin Oncol 1995;22:5–19; discussion 19–21.

Hillner BE, Ingle JN, Berenson JR, et al: American Society of Clinical Oncology guideline on the role of bisphosphonates in breast cancer: American Society of Clinical Oncology Bisphosphonates Expert Panel. J Clin Oncol 2000;18:1378–1391.

Hortobagyi GN: High-dose chemotherapy for primary breast cancer: Facts versus anecdotes. J Clin Oncol 1999;17:25–29.

Hortobagyi GN, Theriault RL, Lipton A, et al: Long-term prevention of skeletal complications of metastatic breast cancer with pamidronate: Protocol 19 Aredia Breast Cancer Study Group. J Clin Oncol 1998;16:2038–2044.

Kaufmann M, Bajetta E, Dirix LY, et al: Exemestane is superior to megestrol acetate after tamoxifen failure in postmenopausal women with advanced breast cancer: Results of a phase III randomized double-blind trial. The Exemestane Study Group. J Clin Oncol 2000;18:1399–1411.

Muss HB: Chemotherapy of breast cancer in the older patient. Semin Oncol 1995;22:14–16.

Muss HB, Case LD, Richards FD, et al: Interrupted versus continuous chemotherapy in patients with metastatic breast cancer: The Piedmont Oncology Association. N Engl J Med 1991;325:1342–1348.

Nabholtz JM, Buzdar A, Pollak M, et al: Anastrozole is superior to tamoxifen as first-line therapy for advanced breast cancer in postmenopausal women: Results of a North American multicenter randomized trial. J Clin Oncol 2000;18:3758–3767.

Nabholtz JM, Gelmon K, Bontenbal M, et al: Multicenter, randomized comparative study of two doses of paclitaxel in patients with metastatic breast cancer. J Clin Oncol 1996;14:1858–1867.

Nabholtz JM, Senn HJ, Bezwoda WR, et al: Prospective randomized trial of docetaxel versus mitomycin plus vinblastine in patients with metastatic breast cancer progressing despite previous anthracycline-containing chemotherapy: 304 Study Group. J Clin Oncol 1999;17:1413–1424.

Sledge GW Jr., Miller KD: Metastatic breast cancer: The role of chemotherapy. Semin Oncol 1999;26:6–10.

Stadtmauer EA, O'Neill A, Goldstein LJ, et al: Conventional-dose chemotherapy compared with high-dose chemotherapy plus autologous hematopoietic stem cell transplantation for metastatic breast cancer: Philadelphia Bone Marrow Transplant Group. N Engl J Med 2000;342:1069–1076.

Vogel CL, Schoenfelder J, Shemano I, et al: Worsening bone scan in the evaluation of antitumor response during hormonal therapy of breast cancer. J Clin Oncol 1995;13:1123–1128.

Chapter 78
Breast Cancer: Supportive Measures and Follow-up Care

Harold J. Burstein

For women of any age, breast cancer diagnosis and treatment are life-altering events, often accompanied by profound physical and psychological consequences. Breast cancer patients need extended medical follow-up and must adjust to the changes in their bodies brought about by medical treatments. Following initial therapies for breast cancer, women must evaluate their other health concerns in light of their cancer history and must manage the uncertainty introduced into their lives and the lives of their family members by the diagnosis of cancer. Thus, breast cancer patients can require extensive supportive measures, often provided or coordinated by their oncology team. The National Cancer Institute estimates that nearly two million women in the United States are breast cancer survivors, a fact that underscores the large magnitude as well as the broad range of supportive measures that breast cancer patients might require.

Local–Regional Management Following Breast Surgery and Radiation

Long-term sequelae of breast surgery and radiation can be common problems for breast cancer patients. These include mild to moderate restrictions in range of motion, numbness, pain, or paresthesias in the chest wall, breast, or axilla, hyperpigmentation in radiation fields, and cosmetic defects from surgery. The more extensive the treatment with either surgery or radiation—in particular, the extent of axillary treatment—the greater the likelihood of these types of musculoskeletal or neurological sequelae. Most patients have symptoms that are not terribly bothersome and that tend to improve over time. Postoperative physical therapy can help patients with range-of-motion limitations following surgery or radiation.

The most dreaded local-regional problem following breast cancer treatment (aside from tumor recurrence) is lymphedema. Lymphedema arises following disruption of axillary lymphatic drainage, and the risk is proportional to the extent of axillary surgery or radiation and tumor involvement of axillary lymph nodes. Lymphedema presents with asymmetric swelling of the ipsilateral arm or hand. Surgical procedures that limit axillary dissection to lymph node sampling or sentinel lymph node mapping, instead of clearing the axilla of lymph nodes, rarely lead to lymphedema. Venous thrombosis (e.g., with an indwelling central venous catheter), infection, and tumor recurrence should be excluded in patients who develop lymphedema.

Prevention of lymphedema remains the best approach to treatment; however, aside from judicious use of surgery and radiation, there are no proven preventative strategies. Widely accepted practices—avoiding trauma, burns, excessive weight bearing, infection, abrasion, and venipuncture—are all reasonable, though the actual value of such practices is not known. For patients who do develop lymphedema, a graduated approach to treatment is warranted. Patients with mild arm swelling could respond well to compressive sleeves and/or gauntlets, compression wraps, and arm elevation. Patients who fail such conservative measures or who have more dramatic symptoms might benefit from referral for individually tailored physical therapy programs.

Most women undergoing mastectomy are potential candidates for reconstructive surgery. There are no data to suggest that breast reconstruction adversely affects the early detection or natural history of tumor recurrence. A variety of techniques, including autologous tissue grafts or prosthetic implants, are available. The optimal procedure for most patients depends on the individual's anatomy and personal preferences. Patients can undergo either immediate or delayed reconstruction, although immediate reconstruction is more common. Surgical reconstruction might require contralateral breast surgery to achieve symmetry. Postmastectomy radiation therapy can influence the choice and timing of breast reconstruction, especially if immediate reconstruction is contemplated.

Radiation therapy often affects the cosmetic results following reconstructive surgery, particularly when prosthetic implants are used in the reconstruction.

Medical Surveillance

Breast cancer patients require medical surveillance for timely detection of systemic or regional recurrences or second cancers in the ipsilateral or contralateral breast. Most recurrences are heralded by symptoms such as cough, shortness of breath, musculoskeletal pain, adenopathy, unexplained alterations in weight, or changes in the breast or chest wall. These symptoms are nonspecific and frequently do not reflect cancer recurrence, even in women with personal histories of breast cancer. Clinicians should inquire about symptoms and evaluate any such complaints appropriately. Intensive surveillance with chest radiographs or computed tomography scans, bone scans, routine laboratory blood tests, or serum tumor markers has not improved survival for women with early-stage breast cancer when compared with less intensive surveillance that does not include screening radiologic or laboratory studies. Nor has intensive surveillance changed the observation that most recurrences are brought to medical attention by patient report. For these reasons, a more focused surveillance strategy that emphasizes elicitation of patient symptoms, physical examination, screening mammography, and screening gynecologic exam with Pap smear, has been advocated by the American Society of Clinical Oncology. Patients often welcome the reassurance of negative test results. However, unnecessary testing can lead to false-positive findings and more elaborate evaluations (including diagnostic procedures). Most patients are satisfied by the more focused surveillance plan when it is properly explained.

Breast cancer patients are at risk for second malignancies, including contralateral breast cancer and gynecological cancers. Patients should undergo annual screening mammography following breast cancer treatment. Tamoxifen therapy has been associated with a small increase in risk of developing uterine cancer. Transvaginal ultrasound, however, is not recommended for asymptomatic patients on tamoxifen, as the absolute incidence of endometrial cancer is low and the sensitivity and specificity of the technique are inadequate for screening. By contrast, postmenopausal patients with vaginal bleeding or premenopausal patients with irregular bleeding should be evaluated with ultrasound and endometrial sampling biopsy. Breast cancer patients merit screening for other malignancies (such as colorectal cancer) in accordance with guidelines for the general population.

DIAGNOSIS

Surveillance After Primary Breast Cancer

Proper surveillance after primary breast cancer provides timely evaluation of symptoms or recurrence and offers reassurance to patients. The following surveillance measures are recommended:

- history and physical exam every three to six months for the first three years
- history and physical exam every six to 12 months for the next two years
- history and physical exam annually thereafter
- mammography (annual)
- pelvic exam (annual)

The history taking should focus on new symptoms (pain, cardiopulmonary complaints, anatomic changes, bleeding including gynecological bleeding), while the physical exam must include evaluation of the breast/chest wall and of lymph node chains in addition to routine assessment. In addition, physicians should inquire about menopausal symptoms and psychosocial function. Annual mammography is valuable in screening for ipsilateral tumor recurrence or second breast cancers. Annual pelvic examination is warranted for detecting gynecological abnormalities, including cancers.

The following evaluations are not recommended for asymptomatic patients:

- routine X-rays, computerized tomography scans, bone scans
- liver function tests, screening chemistry or hematologic blood tests
- serum tumor markers
- transvaginal ultrasound (including patients on tamoxifen)

These tests all have a very low yield in asymptomatic patients and have not been shown to improve survival.

Breast cancer patients merit long-term follow-up by a breast cancer physician in addition to follow-up by primary care provider(s) capable of routine gynecologic examination.

Genetic Testing

The majority of breast cancer cases are sporadic and do not reflect inherited predisposition to cancer. Between 10% and 20% of all breast cancer cases might arise from genetic predisposition, however, and roughly one-half of these cases are attributable to inherited mutations in the autosomal-dominant BRCA1 and BRCA2 genes. Treatment of breast cancer is not currently affected by knowing whether the patient has a genetic susceptibility to cancer. Guidelines for genetic testing suggest that testing might be indicated when the prior probability of a positive result is on the order of 10% or more, or when the clinical information could be valuable to patients or family members. Following these guidelines, circumstances in which cancer susceptibility testing for the BRCA1 and BRCA2 genes might be useful for women with previously diagnosed breast cancer include

- young age at tumor diagnosis (age less than 35 years)
- personal history of breast and/or ovarian cancer
- family history of breast and/or ovarian cancer
- male breast cancer, or multiple family members with breast cancer
- women of Ashkenazi ancestry (particularly if cancer is diagnosed before age 40 and/or a family history of breast cancer is present)

By contrast, BRCA mutations are uncommon in patients with isolated cases of breast cancer, in elderly cancer patients, and in women of African-American ancestry.

Women with known BRCA-associated breast cancer might contemplate different prevention and surveillance strategies for long-term care, including screening for ovarian cancer, which in some instances justifies genetic testing. Modeling studies have suggested, for instance, that young women bearing BRCA1 or BRCA2 mutations who have favorable prognosis for primary breast cancer might benefit from consideration of prophylactic mastectomy or oophorectomy. At present, the complex medical, legal, financial, and social issues surrounding genetic testing warrant patient referral to designated cancer genetics centers.

Management of Menopausal Symptoms and Health

Menopausal symptoms are common among breast cancer patients. In part, this reflects the epidemiology of breast cancer as a disease of middle-aged or older women; however, it also reflects the side effects of breast cancer treatments. In premenopausal women, chemotherapy frequently causes amenorrhea that can be either temporary or permanent. The antiestrogen agent tamoxifen, which is used widely as adjuvant therapy, contributes directly to menopausal symptoms. Finally, because breast cancers might be hormonally sensitive tumors, breast cancer patients have historically been advised not to use hormone replacement therapy.

Clinicians should inquire about menopausal symptoms in all postmenopausal breast cancer patients or women taking tamoxifen. These symptoms include hot flashes, night sweats, vaginal dryness or irritation, dyspareunia, and loss of libido. Many patients have mild symptoms that tend to ameliorate over time. Patients with more pronounced symptoms or with symptoms that interfere with daily function merit consideration of treatments tailored to relieve their discomfort. Patients with urogenital symptoms might benefit from vaginal moisturizers or lubricants that alleviate dryness and dyspareunia. For women with severe vaginal complaints, local estrogen therapy with either estrogen-impregnated rings or estrogen creams might be useful and is associated with less systemic absorption of estrogen than is oral supplementation. The long-term safety of such preparations, however, has not been evaluated in breast cancer patients.

Hot flashes and night sweats are disruptive and uncomfortable for menopausal women. Fortunately, many patients experience gradual improvement in their symptoms. It is useful to have patients keep a diary, noting both the frequency and intensity of such vasomotor symptoms. The use of randomized, placebo-controlled trials has allowed for adequate assessment of many nonhormonal treatments for hot flashes. In almost all instances, a placebo effect can be documented. Several agents have demonstrated significant activity beyond that of a placebo in reducing the severity of hot flashes, and these are worth considering for patients with pronounced symptoms. The optimal duration of therapy has not been established.

Hormone replacement therapy for breast cancer patients remains highly controversial. In contemplating hormone replacement therapy, clinicians and patients must carefully weigh the severity of the indicating symptoms or findings, the realistic clinical benefit, the available nonhormonal alternatives, the natural history of the patient's breast tumor, and the possibility that exogenous hormones might affect cancer outcomes.

Lifestyle and Dietary Changes

For many patients, a breast cancer diagnosis stimulates greater health awareness. Patients can be encouraged

Treating Hot Flashes After Breast Cancer

Randomized, placebo-controlled trials are essential for evaluating claims that interventions improve hot flashes. In most such trials, a well-documented placebo effect can be demonstrated, which might be clinically useful. For patients with mild to moderate symptoms, vitamin E (400 IU orally, twice daily) has been shown to yield modest improvement compared to placebo. Because of the easy availability and few side effects of this intervention, it might be a useful initial therapy.

For patients with more pronounced or persistent hot flashes, the most promising nonhormonal options are the serotonin selective reuptake inhibitors (SSRIs) frequently used to treat affective disorders. In clinical trials, these agents generally reduce the number of hot flashes by about half. Results should be noted within three to four weeks. Treatment options studied in breast cancer patients include:

- venlafaxine 75 mg orally
- fluoxetine 20 mg orally
- paroxetine 20 mg orally

Another treatment option is the antihypertensive agent clonidine, which can reduce hot flashes; however, it causes side effects (including postural hypotension) that make its use more difficult. Progestins can also reduce hot flashes in breast cancer patients, but the long-term safety is not known.

Despite popular interest and anecdotal claims, well-controlled studies have not suggested that either soy supplements or evening primrose oil alleviate hot flashes. The selective estrogen-receptor modulator raloxifene does not affect hot flashes.

---

to practice good general health habits, including reducing alcohol intake, smoking cessation, and moderate exercise programs. For a variety of reasons, breast cancer patients often use alternative or complementary health practices and nutritional supplements. Clinicians should directly ask patients about use of such therapies. To date, there are no compelling data that alternative or complementary therapies have an impact on breast cancer outcome.

There are epidemiologic associations between obesity, alcohol consumption, and lack of physical activity as risk factors for developing breast cancer. It is not known whether behavior modification after breast cancer diagnosis alters a patient's prognosis. The available data do not suggest that dietary consumption of red meat, fiber, or fat changes breast cancer outcomes after initial therapy. Weight gain might accompany adjuvant breast cancer treatment, especially in

Hormone Replacement Therapy After Breast Cancer

Breast cancer has been considered a relative contraindication to hormone replacement therapy (HRT) because of concern that HRT might aggravate the natural history of the disease. Limited experience with HRT in breast cancer survivors has not shown an increased risk of tumor recurrence. These trials, however, involved carefully selected and well-informed women, many of whom had hormone-insensitive breast cancer and/or long disease-free intervals, and none of the studies had adequate power to exclude small adverse effects on tumor outcome. Clinicians should focus on the motivation or indication for HRT in breast cancer patients, as well as the natural history of breast cancer in the particular patient. For patients with disabling menopausal symptoms or refractory osteoporosis, HRT may be a medical necessity. Low-dose treatments for short periods of time (less than six months) probably pose less jeopardy than extended treatment. For other patients, however, many nonhormonal treatment options exist and should be explored before administration of HRT.

Pros	Cons
Alleviate severe menopausal symptoms	Safety not proven in breast cancer patients
	Theoretical concern over effect on tumor
Treat refractory osteoporosis	Possible interference with other hormonal therapy (e.g., tamoxifen)
Could have other health-promoting effects, but not demonstrated to date in prospective trials	Other options often available
	Thorough informed consent required

women with treatment-related menopause. Studies of weight-loss programs in breast cancer patients suggest that multidisciplinary programs combining individualized nutritional counseling with dietary modification and exercise achieve the most favorable results.

Because of the shared epidemiological factor of estrogen exposure, breast cancer patients might be at less risk for osteoporosis and heart disease than the general population. Breast cancer treatments, however, might alter the natural history of these disorders. Chemotherapy-related amenorrhea is associated with loss of bone mineral density. Tamoxifen causes increased bone mineral density in postmenopausal women but could contribute to loss of bone density in premenopausal women. Breast cancer patients who might be at greater risk for osteoporosis include premenopausal women on tamoxifen, postmenopausal women not on tamoxifen, postmenopausal patients taking aromatase inhibitors, women with a family history of osteoporosis, and women with treatment-related premature menopause. These patients might merit assessment of bone mineral density and supplementation with vitamin D and calcium, or consideration of other treatments for osteoporosis if bone mineral density is more than one or two standard deviations less than age-matched controls according to standard guidelines. Bisphosphonates are effective in minimizing the bone mineral density loss that accompanies chemotherapy-related menopause. Radiation therapy (particularly with older techniques) and anthracycline-based chemotherapy might slightly increase the risk of heart disease. There are no recommendations for screening of cardiac function in asymptomatic patients.

Psychosocial Function

Psychosocial distress and dysfunction can affect breast cancer patients (see also Chapter 120 on psychosocial issues). Symptoms are typically most pronounced during the first year after diagnosis. A variety of concerns has been reported by breast cancer patients (Table 78-1). Problems are more frequently reported by younger patients, patients with preexisting psychosocial stressors or lack of supportive environments, or by patients with treatment-related sequelae such as amenorrhea, lymphedema, or perceived disfigurement. Clinicians should assess patients for symptoms of anxiety, mood disturbance, or pain. Fatigue and sexual dysfunction can contribute to impaired quality of life, and symptoms related to these conditions should be elicited by clinicians.

Following chemotherapy, patients often note cognitive disturbances, such as lack of concentration

Table 78-1 ■ Psychosocial Concerns Among Breast Cancer Patients

Impaired body image
Sexual dysfunction
Family and/or marital stress
Sleep disturbance
Somatic symptoms (bodily aches/pains)
Fatigue
Cognitive/memory disturbance
Anxiety/fear of recurrence or death
Depression

or difficulty with memory. The relationship of these complaints to chemotherapy treatment is the subject of active investigation. Interpreting the significance of concentration or memory difficulties is frequently confounded by concurrent pain, anxiety or mood disorders, or by concomitant medications (such as sleeping aids or antiemetics) that can contribute to the symptoms.

Those patients with more acute or profound psychological reactions or sustained psychosocial dysfunction merit referral to mental health care providers when appropriate. Fortunately, most patients find that the impact of breast cancer diagnosis and treatment on well being and social function lessens over time, though anniversaries of treatment dates or follow-up visits can be sources of anxiety. In long-term follow-up studies, breast cancer patients report functioning at social and psychological levels comparable to those of age-matched populations.

References

Lymphedema

Petrek JA, Lerner R: Lymphedema. In Harris JR, Lippman ME, Morrow M, Osborne K (eds). Diseases of the Breast, 2nd ed, pp 1022–1040. Philadelphia, Lippincott Williams & Wilkins, 2000.

Pezner RD, Patterson MP, Hill LR, et al: Arm lymphedema in patients treated conservatively for breast cancer. Relationship to patients' age and axillary node dissection technique. Int J Radiation Oncol Biol Phys 1986;12:2079–2083.

Rockson SG: Precipitating factors in lymphedema: myths and realities. Cancer 1998;83:2814–2816.

Warmuth MA, Bowen G, Prosnitz L, et al: Complications of axillary lymph node dissection for carcinoma of the breast: A patient survey based report. Cancer 1998;83:1362–1368.

Breast Reconstruction

Johnson CH, van Heerden JA, Donohue JH, et al: Oncological aspects of immediate breast reconstruction following mastectomy for malignancy. Arch Surg 1989;124:819–823.

Schuster RH, Kuske RR, Young VL, Fineberg B: Breast reconstruction in women treated with radiation therapy for breast cancer: Cosmesis, complications, and tumor control. Plast Reconstr Surg 1992;90:445–452.

Surveillance

American Society of Clinical Oncology: Recommended breast cancer surveillance guidelines. J Clin Oncol 1997;15:2149–2156.

Burstein HJ, Winer EP: Primary care for survivors of breast cancer. N Engl J Med 2000;343:1086–1094.

Del Turco MR, Palli D, Cariddi A, et al: Intensive diagnostic follow-up after treatment of primary breast cancer. JAMA 1994;271:1593–1597.

Gerber B, Krause A, Muller H, et al: Effects of adjuvant tamoxifen on the endometrium in postmenopausal women with breast cancer: A prospective long-term study using transvaginal ultrasound. J Clin Oncol 2000;18:3464–3470.

GIVIO Investigators: Impact of follow-up testing on survival and health-related quality of life in breast cancer patients. JAMA 1994;271:1587–1592.

Loprinzi CL, Hayes D, Smith T: Doc, shouldn't we be getting some tests? J Clin Oncol 2000;18:2345–2348.

Pandya KJ, McFadden ET, Kalish LA, et al: A retrospective study of earliest indicators of recurrence in patients on Eastern Cooperative Oncology Group adjuvant chemotherapy trials for breast cancer. Cancer 1985;55:202–205.

Suh-Burgmann EJ, Goodman A: Surveillance for endometrial cancer in women receiving tamoxifen. Ann Intern Med 1999;131:127–135.

Genetics of Breast Cancer

Armstrong K, Eisen A, Weber B: Assessing the risk of breast cancer. N Engl J Med 2000;342:564–571.

Burke W, Daly M, Garber J, et al: Recommendations for follow-up care of individuals with an inherited predisposition to cancer. II. BRCA1 and BRCA2. JAMA 1997;277:997–1003.

Schrag D, Kuntz KM, Garber JE, Weeks JC: Life expectancy gains from cancer prevention strategies for women with breast cancer and BRCA1 or BRCA2 mutations. JAMA 2000;283:617–624.

Statement of the American Society of Clinical Oncology: Genetic testing for cancer susceptibility. J Clin Oncol 1996;14:1730–1736.

Menopausal System

Bines J, Oleske DM, Cobleigh MA: Ovarian function in premenopausal women treated with adjuvant chemotherapy for breast cancer. J Clin Oncol 1996;14:1718–1729.

Castiel M: Management of menopausal symptoms in the cancer patient. Oncology (Huntington) 1999;13:1363–1370.

Cobleigh MA: Managing menopausal symptoms. In Harris JH, Lippman ME, Morrow M, Osborne K (eds): Diseases of the Breast, 2nd ed, pp 1041–1050. Philadelphia, Lippincott Williams & Wilkins, 2000.

Couzi RJ, Helzlsouer KJ, Fetting JH: Prevalence of menopausal symptoms among women with a history of breast cancer and attitudes towards estrogen replacement therapy. J Clin Oncol 1995;13:2737–2744.

Eastell R: Treatment of postmenopausal osteoporosis. N Engl J Med 1998;338:736–746.

Goodwin PJ, Ennis M, Pritchard KI, et al: Adjuvant treatment and onset of menopause predict weight gain after breast cancer diagnosis. J Clin Oncol 1999;17:120–129.

Loprinzi CL, Abu-Ghazaleh S, Sloan JA, et al: Phase III randomized double-blind study to evaluate the efficacy of a polycarbophil-based vaginal moisturizer in women with breast cancer. J Clin Oncol 1997;15:969–973.

Loprinzi CL, Kugler JW, Sloan JA, et al: Venlafaxine in management of hot flashes in survivors of breast cancer: A randomised controlled trial. Lancet 2000;356:2059–2063.

Osborne CK: Tamoxifen in the treatment of breast cancer. N Engl J Med 1998;339:1609–1618.

Powles TJ, McCloskey E, Paterson AHG, et al: Oral clodronate and reduction in loss of bone mineral density in women with operable primary breast cancer. J Natl Cancer Inst 1998;90:704–708.

Psychosocial Factors

Aapro M, Cull A: Depression in breast cancer patients: the need for treatment. Ann Oncol 1999;10:627–636.

Bower JE, Ganz PA, Desmond KA, et al: Fatigue in breast cancer survivors: occurrence, correlates, and impact on quality of life. J Clin Oncol 2000;18:743–753.

Brezden CB, Phillips KA, Abdolell M, et al: Cognitive function in breast cancer patients receiving adjuvant chemotherapy. J Clin Oncol 2000;18:2695–2701.

Burstein HJ, Gelber S, Guadagnoli E, Weeks JC: Use of alternative medicine by women with early stage breast cancer. N Engl J Med 1999;340:1733–1739.

Ganz PA, Coscarelli A, Fred C, et al: Breast cancer survivors: psychosocial concerns and quality of life. Breast Cancer Res Treatment 1996;38:183–199.

Ganz PA, Desmond KA, Belin TR, et al: Predictors of sexual health in women after breast cancer diagnosis. J Clin Oncol 1999;17:2371–2380.

Ganz PA, Rowland JH, Desmond K, et al: Life after breast cancer: understanding women's health-related quality of life and sexual function. J Clin Oncol 1998;16(2):501–514.

Holmes MD, Stampfer MJ, Colditz GA, et al: Dietary factors and the survival of women with breast carcinoma. Cancer 1999;86:826–835.

Schag CAC, Ganz PA, Polinsky ML, et al: Characteristics of women at risk for psychosocial distress in the year after breast cancer. J Clin Oncol 1993;11:783–793.

Chapter 79
Carcinoma of the Cervix, Vulva, and Vagina

Michael V. Seiden and AnneKathryn Goodman

Introduction

The lower genital tract is composed predominantly of squamous epithelium as well as of some specialized glandular and neuroendocrine cells. The majority of carcinomas in this region are squamous cell carcinomas, followed in incidence by a smaller subset of adenocarcinomas, and a collection of rarer tumors comprise the remainder. The region is also occasionally a site for metastatic disease. Visual and cytologic screening of the lower genital tract, by detecting preinvasive or early invasive disease, has been effective in reducing morbidity and mortality. Recent epidemiologic, immunologic, and infectious disease research has identified human papilloma virus, other sexually transmitted diseases, and cigarette smoking as predisposing causes, which are potentially treatable and/or modifiable factors.

Cervical Dysplasia

Intraepithelial lesions may be classified as low-grade or high-grade. A low-grade squamous intraepithelial lesion (LSIL) may also be referred to as CIN (cervical intraepithelial neoplasia) I or mild dysplasia. Of Pap smears initially read as showing mild dysplasia, regression to normal occurred in 44% within 2 years, 74% in 5 years, and 88% in 10 years (Holowaty). The diagnosis of LSIL must be based on biopsy rather than cytology on Pap smear, because LSIL may be a manifestation of a more serious lesion. Thus, of women with LSIL on Pap smear, subsequent biopsy showed CIN II in 15% and CIN III (invasive cancer of the cervix) in another 15%.

The diagnosis of LSIL requires prompt referral for colposcopy. Testing for human papilloma virus DNA is not useful since more than 80 percent of these women test positive for high-risk HPV types. If CIN is not found after satisfactory or unsatisfactory colposcopy and biopsies, then a repeat pap smear should be performed in 6 and 12 months. Women with histologically confirmed CIN I may be treated with ablation or excision or followed with serial cytologic smears at 6-month intervals if the entire lesion and limits of the transformation zone are completely visualized.

A high-grade squamous intraepithelial lesion (HSIL) may also be referred to as CIN II or III, severe dysplasia, or carcinoma in situ (CIS). Of women with HSIL on cytology, 1% to 2% will have invasive cancer at the time of further evaluation, and approximately 20 percent of women with biopsy-proven carcinoma in situ develop an invasive cancer if left untreated. HSIL is treated by an excisional procedure, such as cervical cone biopsy or large loop excision of the transformation zone (LLETZ) or ablated by carbon dioxide laser or cryotherapy if the whole lesion can be seen. Despite adequate treatment, 12% of patients exhibit recurrence and the risk in immunocompromised women is in excess of 50%.

Cervical Cancer

There are approximately 15,000 newly diagnosed cases of cervical cancer each year in the United States, and 4800 deaths occur annually from this disease. Advances in viral oncology, molecular biology, and epidemiology have increased the understanding of the etiology and pathogenesis of this disease.

769

Epidemiology and Pathogenesis

The incidence of cervical carcinoma is directly related to the degree of sexual promiscuity and increases in smokers and in immunosuppressed women. The large majority of cases of cervical cancers are associated with infection by the human papilloma virus (HPV), a double-stranded DNA virus. There are at least sixty types of human papilloma virus, which share only limited DNA homology. Epidemiologic data demonstrate that although many types of human papilloma virus can cause genital disease (including benign genital warts), only certain subtypes are strongly associated with the development of invasive cervical carcinoma. Molecular biologic studies show that high-risk human papilloma viruses encode two early genes (E6 and E7) that bind and inactivate p53 and the retinoblastoma (RB) gene, respectively. The inactivation of both p53 and RB serve to remove the normal cell checkpoints within the cell cycle of cervical epithelium. The result is cervical epithelial dysplasia. Infection with high-risk human papilloma virus is frequently necessary, but not sufficient, for the progression from cervical epithelial dysplasia to invasive cancer. Other factors are involved, including coinfection with other viruses or microorganisms and potentially poorly defined immunologic and dietary factors. Curiously, the transition from dysplasia to invasive carcinoma can take several decades in some women or can occur rapidly.

Presentation and Cytology

Localized squamous and nonsquamous cervical carcinomas are often asymptomatic, although a subset of patients might notice postcoital or intermenstrual bleeding or vaginal discharge. Extension of the tumor from the cervix to the parametrial tissue is associated with pelvic pain and/or hydronephrosis, both of which suggest pelvic sidewall disease. Bulky cervical tumors can also lead occasionally to chronic blood loss and anemia at presentation. Postcoital spotting always requires thorough evaluation. Blood and inflammation can obscure cytologic changes, increasing the false negative Pap smear rate. Thus, postcoital spotting should be evaluated by colposcopy (Figure 79-1), regardless of the Pap smear results.

A Pap smear reading of atypical squamous cells of undetermined significance (ASCUS) indicates a significant cervical abnormality in up to 20% of cases. In HIV-positive women, atypical squamous cells of undetermined significance reading represents significant pathology in more than 50% of cases. The standard workup in a low-risk woman is to repeat the smear in three months. If the Pap smear is persistently abnormal, a colposcopy with directed cervical biopsies is recommended. All high-risk women (such as those with

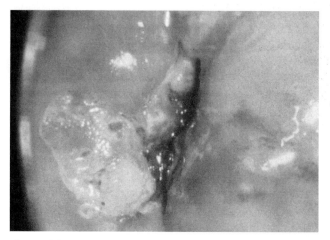

Figure 79-1 ■ Colposcopic view of cervical carcinoma in situ.

HIV infection) should undergo immediate colposcopy. A reading of atypical cells of undetermined significance is more ominous. In up to 45% of women with a cytology report of atypical cells of undetermined significance, a premalignant or malignant lesion is present. The lesion can be either a glandular or a squamous lesion involving endocervical gland crypts.

Pathology

Squamous Cell Carcinoma

The majority of invasive cervical carcinomas are squamous cell in histology. Typically these are subclassified according to both cell type and degree of differentiation.

Important pathologic features include grade, depth of stromal invasion, margin status, and some additional molecular markers discussed in the Prognostic Factors section later in this chapter. The presence or absence of keratin probably carries little prognostic significance and is less important.

Verrucous Carcinoma

These are well-differentiated squamous cell carcinomas, which have a tendency to recur locally but seldom metastasize.

Adenocarcinomas

These tumors arise in the endocervical canal and may not be visible by standard inspection of the cervix. Adenocarcinomas have a propensity to infiltrate deeply into the cervix and have a higher frequency of uterine corpus invasion as well as a higher frequency of nodal metastases than do squamous cell cancers. Several different variants are known; the most common subtype is mucinous followed by endometrioid carcinomas. Mixed subtypes, including adenosquamous carcinomas, are seen also.

Neuroendocrine Carcinomas

Neuroendocrine carcinoma of the cervix includes a number of tumors, such as carcinoids, atypical

Table 79-1 ■ Staging of Cervical Cancer

TNM Classifications		Characteristics
AJCC **T = Primary Tumor**	**FIGO** **Stages**	
TX		Primary tumor not assessed
T0		No evidence of primary tumor
Tis	0	Carcinoma in situ (preinvasive carcinoma)
T1	I	Confined to uterine cervix
T1a	IA	Minimal microscopic stromal invasion
T1a1	IA1	Microscopic invasion (<3 mm deep and <7 mm horizontally)
T1a2	IA2	Tumor invasion < or = to 3 mm in depth and < or = 7 mm horizontally
T1b	IB	Clinically visible, confined to uterine cervix (larger than T1A2)
T1b1	IB1	Largest dimension ≤4.0 cm
T1b2	IB2	Largest dimension >4.0 cm
T2	II	Invades parametrium or upper vagina
T2a	IIA	Upper vaginal involvement without parametrial invasion
T2b	IIB	Limited parametrial invasion (not to pelvic sidewall)
T3	III	Extends to pelvic sidewall or/and lower third of the vagina
T3a	IIIA	Involves lower one-third of the vaginal w/o pelvic sidewall extension
T3b	IIIB	Pelvic sidewall extension or hydronephrosis
T4	IVA	Invades mucosa of bladder or rectum and/or extends beyond true pelvis
Staging by AJCC	**TNM**	
IA	$T_{1a}\ N_0\ M_0$	
IB	$T_{1b}\ N_0\ M_0$	
IIA	$T_{2a}\ N_0\ M_0$	
IIB	$T_{2b}\ N_0\ M_0$	
IIIA	$T_{3a}\ N_0\ M_0$	
IIIB	$T_{1-3b}\ N_1\ M_0 / T_{3b}\ N_0\ M_0$	
IVA	$T_4\ N_{0-1}\ M_0$	
IVB	$T_{0-4}\ N_{0-1}\ M_1$	

N_0 = Regional lymph nodes not involved; N_1 = Regional lymph nodes involved.
M_0 = No distant metastases; M_1 = Distant metastases (also FIGO IVB).

carcinoids, large cell neuroendocrine carcinomas, and small cell carcinomas. These display a wide range of biologic behavior. Small cell variants are highly cellular small, spindled, or oval-shaped tumor cells that demonstrate prominent mitotic activity, often with surrounding areas of necrosis. These are aggressive cancers, and nodal or distant metastases are usually evident at the time of primary diagnosis or soon thereafter.

Rare Histologies

Women exposed in utero to diethylstilbestrol because their mothers were taking the drug during pregnancy are at increased risk for clear cell carcinomas of the cervix. With the current restrictions against nearly all but the most essential medications for pregnant women, these cases are diminishing. Lymphomas occasionally appear to arise in the cervix. Although seemingly confined, most cases prove to be systemic, often requiring multimodality therapy.

Staging

Careful staging of cervical carcinoma is vital to the design of appropriate therapeutic plans. Tumors localized to the cervix or to the cervix and upper vagina can be treated with curative intent by either surgery or radiation therapy. Loco-regional tumors are typically treated primarily by radiation delivered with concurrent chemotherapy, as described in following sections. Computed tomography scans do not accurately determine extracervical extension of these tumors. Therefore, staging is based on clinical assessment, often by gynecologic oncologists in concert with radiation therapists. Comprehensive staging requires examination under anesthesia and can include cystoscopy and sigmoidoscopy. Pelvic magnetic resonance imaging (MRI) and positron emission tomography (PET) scanning are quickly becoming important tools for evaluating pelvic extension and nodal involvement, respectively. Table 79-1 shows the current American Joint Committee on Cancer (AJCC) and

Federation Internationale de Gynecologie et d'Obstetrique (FIGO) staging systems.

Treatment

The majority of cervical cancers are squamous cell carcinomas. Clinical trials have variably been confined to women with squamous cell carcinomas or allowed the inclusion of women with other types of cervical carcinomas. The relative infrequency of these non-squamous subtypes makes it difficult to determine whether treatment recommendations for these less common histologies should differ from those for squamous cell carcinomas. After correction for comparable stage of disease, adenocarcinomas carry the same prognosis as squamous cell carcinomas.

Treatment of cervical carcinoma is stage-based. Either surgery (radical hysterectomy) or radiation therapy (to the pelvis) offers a high probability of cure for stage I and II disease. Short-term and long-term morbidity differ, however, between the two treatment modalities. Radical hysterectomy preserves ovarian function and might be preferred in younger patients. Radiation therapy avoids surgical morbidity but carries the risk of long-term rectal or bladder dysfunction. Both procedures can negatively affect sexual function.

Stage IA1 Cervical Cancer

Microscopic cervical carcinomas can typically be treated with conizations or loop electrosurgical excision procedure as long as the patient is reliable and will return for frequent follow-up. Patients who are beyond child-bearing age or who might not be available for follow-up should be considered for total hysterectomy. Cure rates in this group approach 100%.

Stage IA2 Cervical Cancer

Because conization of the cervix is not universally effective at removing all invasive carcinoma, stage IA2 disease is most often treated with radical hysterectomy. Some centers have begun to gain experience with the use of radical trachelectomy with reanastomosis of the vagina to the uterus. Whether this procedure—which is more limited than radical hysterectomy—provides an adequate cure rate of the cancer and whether subsequent pregnancies have a good record of success and safety are uncertain.

Locally Advanced and Local/Regional Cervical Cancer

Over time, cervical cancer extends progressively from the cervical epithelium into the underlying cervical stroma (Figure 79-2) with subsequent extension to parametrial tissue, the upper vagina, the lower uterine segment, and draining pelvic and periaortic lymph nodes. The management of bulky tumors that are confined to the cervix (stage IB) and extend into the sur-rounding tissues or draining lymph nodes includes concurrent chemotherapy, radiation therapy, and surgery. As shown in Table 79-2, this multimodality approach improves survival when compared with radiation and surgery alone.

Bulky Stage IB, IIA Cervical Cancer

Both radical hysterectomy and radical radiotherapy are acceptable options for patients with stage IB or IIA disease. Patients undergoing radical hysterectomy for stage I disease might be found to have tumor involvement of pelvic or low paraaortic lymph nodes. In these cases, the combination of cisplatin and 5-fluorouracil chemotherapy with concurrent radiation leads to superior overall and disease-free survival compared with patients receiving radiation therapy alone after hysterectomy. Similarly, patients with bulky stage IB tumors who underwent preoperative radiation prior to extrafascial hysterectomy had a superior survival when platinum-based chemotherapy was combined with radiation therapy, compared with patients who underwent radiation therapy without concurrent chemotherapy. Although concurrent therapy increased the incidence of gastrointestinal and hematologic toxicities, these were generally manageable with good supportive care; long-term radiation-associated complications, such as fistula formation or intestinal obstruction, have not occurred.

Stage IIB, IIIB, and IVA Cervical Cancer

Regionally advanced cervical cancer is not managed surgically. The previous standard of care was radical radiation therapy, which can cure patients who have regionally advanced disease. Prospective randomized trials have demonstrated superior disease-free and overall survival when radiation therapy is delivered concurrently with platinum-based chemotherapy or with regimens containing epirubicin and mitomycin

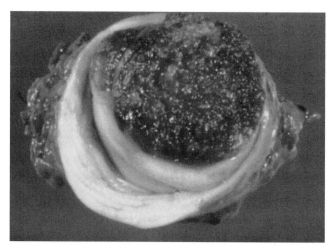

Figure 79-2 ■ Invasive cervical cancer.

Table 79-2 ■ Concurrent Chemotherapy and Radiation Therapy Trials in Locally Advanced Cervix Cancer

Patients	N	Trial	Overall Survival (%)
Bulky stage IB; hysterectomy after treatment	374	Radiation therapy alone	74%
		vs.	P = 0.008
		Radiation therapy plus weekly cisplatin	83%
Stage IIB, III, IVA	526	Radiation therapy plus	
		Hydrea	48%
		vs.	P = 0.004
		Cisplatin	68%
		vs.	
		Hydrea and cisplatin and 5-fluorouracil	68%
Stage IIB, III, IVA	388	Radiation therapy plus	
		Hydrea	43%
		vs.	P = 0.018
		Cisplatin	55%
Bulky IB, IIA, or IIB, III, IVA	403	Radiation therapy alone	58%
		vs.	P = 0.004
		Radiation therapy plus cisplatin and 5-fluorouracil	73%
Postresection or IA2, IB, IIA carcinoma with positive nodes or margins	268	Radiation therapy alone	71%
		vs.	P = 0.03
		Radiation therapy plus cisplatin and 5-fluorouracil	81%
Bulky I, II, III	220	Radiation therapy alone	68%
		vs.	P = 0.04
		Radiation therapy and adjuvant epirubicin	80%

N = number of patients.

C. Most of these studies show improved local control, and some also found a decrease in the incidence of subsequent metastatic disease.

The most appropriate chemotherapy to be combined with concurrent radiation is uncertain. Both weekly and three-week platinum schedules have been evaluated. Some of these regimens contain platinum with 5-fluorouracil; anthracycline, taxanes, and mitomycin C might also play roles as concurrent radiation sensitizers. Standard therapy consists of radiation

TREATMENT

Bulky Cervical Cancer

A barrel cervix, representing a deep endophytic cervical lesion, has a higher incidence of central recurrence, periaortic lymph node metastasis, and distant dissemination than squamous cell carcinomas. Optimal outcome requires multimodality therapy. Radiation alone or in combination with chemotherapy might not encompass all of the tumor adequately. Although extrafascial hysterectomy (Figure 79-3) is advocated to improve therapeutic results, the majority of stage IB2 lesions are treated completely with radiation and concurrent chemotherapy. However, not all cervical cancers are radiosensitive. The maximum response to radiation is seen by six weeks. If tumor persists at that point, an extrafascial hysterectomy should be performed.

Although ovarian ablation is not part of the therapeutic intervention for cervical cancer, radiation therapy destroys ovarian function. In young women, an ovariopexy to move the ovaries outside the radiation field can be offered. Estrogen replacement therapy is a safe alternative. For women who undergo radiation alone, it is important to add a progestin to prevent unopposed estrogen stimulation of the radiated uterus.

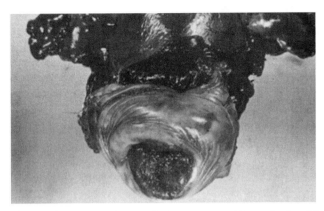

Figure 79-3 ▪ Invasive cervical cancer—en bloc extrafascial hysterectomy specimen.

therapy plus concurrent platinum, delivered either weekly or on a 21-day schedule.

Prognostic Factors

Stage of disease is clearly the most important factor in predicting survival of patients with cervical carcinoma. In patients treated by clinicians with extensive expertise in the management of cervical carcinoma, patients with stage I tumors can expect a five-year survival rate of 90%, while women with stage II tumors can expect survival rates of approximately 75%. Patients with locally advanced disease have a higher risk of death and higher local recurrence rates. For example, patients with stage III tumors have a survival rate of 60% at 5 years. Most recurrences are seen within three years after therapy, although late recurrences do occur.

Increasing tumor size correlates with decreased survival. Other poor prognostic factors include stromal invasion, parametrial extension, and endometrial extension. The presence of lymphatic and vascular involvement has been correlated with an increased risk of lymph node metastases and a worsened clinical outcome.

Clinical staging does not address the issue of occult pelvic lymph node involvement. The detection of positive pelvic or periaortic nodes at surgery adversely affects survival. Prognosis seems to depend directly on the number of lymph nodes involved. Age, when corrected for stage, is not an independent prognostic factor.

Follow-Up Evaluation

After treatment, patients with cervical cancer should be followed for both recurrent tumor and complications of therapy by a gynecologic oncologist. Management of hormonal and sexual issues after therapy require supportive help and counseling. Premenopausal women who have had radiation therapy should receive hormone replacement treatment. Evaluation of pelvic symptoms is difficult both in the surgical and postradiation setting, secondary to fibrosis and obliteration of normal tissue planes. Magnetic resonance imaging and positron emission tomography scans can be useful in identifying residual or recurrent tumor.

Chemotherapy for Recurrent or Advanced Disease

Cervical cancer typically progresses from local to regional to systemic disease. Patients who have received aggressive local/regional therapy for cervical cancer can develop distant metastases (especially to lung and bone) as well as local recurrences within the radiation therapy field. The latter are less responsive to systemic chemotherapy than is disease appearing outside of the radiation therapy portal.

Metastatic disease can be palliated with radiation therapy for focally symptomatic disease. Patients with more extensive disease should be considered for chemotherapy. Squamous cell carcinoma of the cervix is relatively chemotherapy resistant, and most chemotherapeutic agents have only modest activity in

---

TREATMENT

Advanced Cervical Cancer in the Elderly Woman

Twenty-five percent of women diagnosed with cervical cancer are more than age 65 years. Forty percent of all cervical cancer deaths occur in this age group. Older women present with more advanced disease because they do not undergo pelvic examination as frequently as younger women. A recent study of the National Cancer Institute's Surveillance, Epidemiology, and End Results (SEER) program reviewed the data on 10,281 women diagnosed with cervical cancer between 1992 and 1997. Despite the fact that cervical cancer is a highly treatable disease, 22% of women older than 65

who had stage III and IV cancers did not receive treatment. Patient and physician education on the importance of continued pelvic examination is an important public health priority. Without intervention or prevention, these women usually suffer from debilitating pain, necrotic tumor causing socially unacceptable odor, vesicovaginal and rectovaginal fistulas, and chronic bleeding. Causes of death include hemorrhage from the cancer's erosion into arteries, renal failure, and bowel obstruction.

Table 79-3 ■ Single-Agent Chemotherapy in Advanced Cervical Cancer

Single Agent	Number of Responders/Total Number	Percent Responding
Carboplatin	13/55	23
Cisplatin	190/815	22
Irinotecan*	21/110	19
Vincristine	10/55	18
Methotrexate	17/96	18
Navelbine	7/41	17
Doxorubicin*	45/266	15
Cyclophosphamide	38/251	13
Topotecan	5/40	13
Ifosfamide*	10/73	13
Gemcitabine*	2/41	5

*Combination of multiple studies.

the range of 10% to 20% (Table 79-3). In the neoadjuvant setting in untreated patients presenting with advanced disease, combination chemotherapy regimens (Table 79-4) produce higher response rates than does single-agent cisplatin. There is no strong evidence, however, that survival is improved with combination regimens compared with the use of sequential single agents.

Vulvar Cancer

Although vulvar cancer is an uncommon tumor, accounting for only 5% of all gynecologic malignancies, the incidence of preinvasive disease is rising. The annual incidence of invasive vulvar cancers is 1.5 cases per 100,000 women. Ninety percent of vulvar tumors are squamous cell carcinomas. The second most common cancer of the vulva is melanoma, followed by Bartholin gland carcinomas, extramammary Paget's disease of the vulva, and basal cell carcinoma.

Risk factors for vulvar cancer include tobacco use, previous human papilloma virus infection, vulvar intraepithelial neoplasia, and immunosuppression. Although some studies suggest that the disease is more common in women who are obese, hypertensive, diabetic, and nulliparous, a recent case-control study did

Table 79-4 ■ Combination Chemotherapy in Patients with Cervical Carcinoma

Combination Agents	Overall Response		Complete Response	
	N/T	Percent	N	Percent
Irinotecan-Cisplatin*‡	29/42	70%	3	7%
Taxol-Ifosfamide-Cisplatin*	32/38	84%	11	29%
Taxol-Ifosfamide-Cisplatin†‡	42/67	63%	NA	NA
Irinotecan-Cisplatin†	15/29	52%	2	7%
Taxol-Cisplatin†‡	67/125	54%	21	17%
5 FU-Cisplatin‡	12/55	22%	NA	NA
Mitomycin C-Cisplatin‡	22/73	30%	NA	NA
Bleomycin-Vincristine-Mitomycin-Cisplatin	34/103	33%	NA	NA

*Neoadjuvant trials
†Mixed neoadjuvant and postradiation relapse
‡Summary of 2 or more trials
NA = not available, N = number of patients responding, T = number of patients treated; 5 FU = 5-fluorouracil

Diagnostic Evaluation of Vulvar Disease

Vaginal itching and burning are common symptoms. Vulvar disease is diagnosed by a careful visual inspection, palpation of the appendages, and vulvar biopsy. The pain evoked by a biopsy can be avoided by thoughtful planning and discussion. EMLA cream (lidocaine 2.5% plus prilocaine 2.5%) is applied to the biopsy site, and the area is left covered for 45 minutes. Following this, local intradermal application of 1% lidocaine (without epinephrine) makes the biopsy using a small Keyes punch completely painless. Biopsy can reveal benign or malignant disease, as can be seen in the cases that follow.

The punch biopsy shows that lichen sclerosis (Figure 79-4) is a benign chronic skin condition. The etiology is uncertain but possibly has an autoimmune basis. If diagnosed early, many of the disfiguring irreversible changes to the labia and clitoris can be prevented.

A high-potency corticosteroid is applied to the skin once daily, usually at night, until there is improvement. The frequency can then be reduced. It is important to follow a patient with careful examinations every six months. New ulcers or lesions need to be biopsied, as vulvar neoplastic changes can occur over time.

The punch biopsy shows squamous carcinoma in situ (Figure 79-5) involving gland crypts. A Pap smear showed atypical squamous cells of undetermined significance. Cervical and vaginal colposcopy with endocervical curettage are normal. Human immunodeficiency (HIV) testing is negative. *Chlamydia* and gonorrhea cervical testing are negative. A vulvar wide local excision is performed under local anesthesia in the office. A follow-up examination every three months with Pap smear tests is planned.

Lower genital tract neoplasias are associated with human papilloma virus (HPV) infection. When one lesion is discovered, it is important to evaluate the whole lower genital tract for other lesions. In this age group, an atypical squamous cells of undetermined significance Pap smear reading is usually secondary to cytopathic effects of the papilloma virus. New lower genital tract preinvasive lesions can develop over time. Most women develop an immune response and clear the papilloma virus infection within two years. Because papilloma virus is sexually transmitted, the patient must be screened for other sexually transmitted diseases.

---

not confirm these as risk factors. The average age at diagnosis is 65 years; however, there is a bimodal age incidence that is thought to reflect distinct epidemiologies. Younger women (average age of 45 years) present with papilloma virus-associated disease. They have multifocal lesions against a background of preinvasive disease and a history of lesions in the vagina and cervix. In contrast, older women (average age of 75 years), present with a solitary vulvar cancer that can be associated with preexisting or concurrent vulvar dystrophies.

Clinical Presentation

Although 30% of women with preinvasive disease are asymptomatic, more than 99% of women with invasive cancer have symptoms. The most common initial complaint is a vulvar mass or lump. Other common symptoms include pruritus, pain, burning, bleeding, dysuria, and discharge. Appropriate management of vulvar cancer and its predisposing premalignant lesions (vulvar intraepithelial neoplasia) are challenged both by frequent misdiagnosis and delay in diagnosis. Indeed, the onset of symptoms to diagnosis approaches one year with delay related to patient embarrassment, denial, and reluctance to be examined. Additional delay in diagnosis occurs secondary to a tendency among health care practitioners to at first prescribe extended courses of topical medications

to a patient with vulvar complaints without performing careful vulvar inspection and appropriate biopsy of these lesions.

Clinical Evaluation

Careful visual inspection of the vulvar and perianal skin, vulvar appendages, vaginal tube, and cervix are

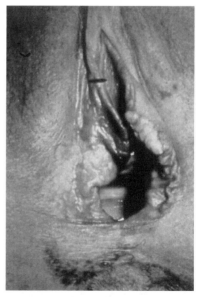

Figure 79-4 ▪ Lichen sclerosis of the vulva.

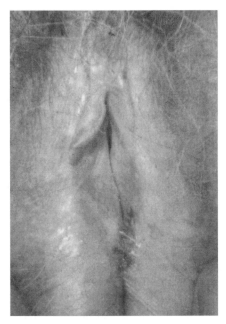

Figure 79-5 ■ Carcinoma in situ of the vulva.

mandatory. Most vulvar cancers are seen easily; however, biopsy is crucial prior to treatment planning. The differential diagnosis of vulvar lesions include condyloma acuminata, manifestations of infectious disease (condyloma lata, chancroid, granuloma inguinale), metastatic malignant lesions (e.g., lymphoma), and manifestations of systemic illness (e.g., inflammatory bowel disease). Palpation of inguinal nodes should be performed but is highly inaccurate in predicting nodal involvement with tumor. A chest X-ray and computerized tomography scan of the abdomen and pelvis are important to rule out metastatic spread. Among patients with extramammary Paget's disease, 12% are associated with an underlying adenocarcinoma of the vulvar appendages, colon, or breast. Patients presenting with Paget's disease should have a mammogram and colonoscopy performed prior to surgery.

Staging and Prognosis

Vulvar cancer is a surgically staged disease (Table 79-5). Five-year survival is dependent on the extent of lymphatic spread. Risk factors for nodal spread include tumor size, depth of invasion of primary lesion, and grade of the tumor. The incidence of nodal involvement is 5% for lesions less than 1 cm, 16% for lesions

Table 79-5 ■ Staging of Vulvar Cancer

AJC TNM Classification	FIGO Staging	Description
Tumor Assessment		
Tx		Primary tumor not assessable
T0		No evidence of primary tumor
Tis		Carcinoma in situ
T1	I	Confined to vulvar/perineum and <2 cm
T2	II	Confined to vulvar/perineum and >2 cm
T3	III	Invades urethra, vagina or anus
T4	IVA	Invades bladder, mucosa, upper urethral mucosa or rectal mucosa or is fixed to bone
Nodal Status		
N0		No lymph node metastases
N1	IVA	Unilateral regional lymph node metastasis
N2	IVA	Bilateral regional lymph node metastases*
Distant Metastases		
M0		No distant metastases
M1	IVB	Distant metastases

Stage	TNM findings
I	T1N0M0
II	T2N0M0
III	T1–3N1M0/T3N0M0
IVA	T1–4N2M0/T4N0–2M0
IVB	T1–4N0–2M1

*Note: Pelvic or peri-aortic lymph node metastases are scored as M1 disease.

between 1 cm and 2 cm, 33% for those between 3 cm and 4 cm, and 53% for those lesions larger than 4 cm. Prognosis is related to the extent of nodal invasion; with less than three involved unilateral inguinal nodes, the chance of cure is still excellent. Survival data from the Gynecologic Oncology Group (GOG) shows a five-year survival of 98% for stage I, 85% for stage II, 74% for stage III, and 31% for stage IV disease.

Treatment

Vulvar intraepithelial neoplasia is typically treated by surgical local excision. Alternative treatments of these lesions depend on their locations. Carbon dioxide laser treatment and 5-fluorouracil cream applications are efficacious. A smoking cessation plan should be included for those patients for whom smoking is a factor.

Vulvar cancer is treated primarily by radical surgery. Prompt diagnosis allows for curative surgical therapy. The standard therapy for tumors localized to the vulva includes radical surgical resection of the primary lesion and of the draining inguinal nodal basin. This procedure, related to the extent of disease, should be individualized and can incorporate wide local excision, hemivulvectomy, or vulvectomy. Inadequate local excision results in high local failure rates and can reduce the possibility of cure significantly. Experience in gynecologic oncology is important in providing appropriate surgical management. Earlier diagnosis of vulvar cancers leads to smaller, localized, less deforming surgery with unilateral lymph node dissection. Complete regional lymph node resection carries substantial morbidity. The value of sentinel lymph node identification and biopsy in obviating the need for extensive lymphadenectomy is under evaluation.

For large vulvar cancers that have spread locally to involve the rectum, vagina, or bladder, a combination of concurrent chemotherapy with radiation therapy followed by surgery should be considered. Because of the relative infrequency of this type of tumor, large randomized trials have not been conducted. Regimens containing cisplatin, 5-fluorouracil, or paclitaxel have been used alone or in combination. Reconstructive surgery with skin grafts, flaps, and pelvic floor repair is frequently necessary.

Unlike squamous cell carcinoma of the cervix, melanoma of the cervix is treated in a manner similar to that employed for melanomas appearing elsewhere on the body. A wide local excision is performed often with lymphatic mapping to assess locoregional nodal involvement. A complete lymphadenectomy is not therapeutic for melanoma in the way that it is for squamous cell carcinomas.

Paget's disease and basal cell carcinomas are treated by local surgical resection. Regional draining lymph nodes are not routinely resected.

The consequences of curative surgery can be psychologically devastating. Sexual dysfunction is common. Anatomic alterations change the urinary stream, alter pelvic vault suspension, and cause sensory loss along the inner thigh, lower abdomen, and vulva. Extensive lymph node dissection can cause lower extremity lymphedema resulting in difficulty in walking, leg pain, recurrent lower extremity cellulitis, and disfigurement. Radiation therapy causes chronic vulvar skin changes and can lead to vaginal stenosis, radiation cystitis and proctitis, and fistula formation. Ovarian failure is to be expected in premenopausal women treated with radiotherapy.

Follow-up Evaluation

Follow up pelvic examinations should be performed every three months for the first two years after treatment and then every six months for the next three years thereafter. As these women are at risk for secondary cancers of the lower genital tract, careful inspection of the vagina and cervix with Pap smear evaluation should be included. Counseling to address issues of body image change and sexual dysfunction is often helpful. After radiation therapy, women are given a vaginal dilator with instructions for daily use to prevent vaginal stenosis. Women made amenorrheic by radiation therapy should be offered hormone replacement therapy. Secondary uterine malignancies are a long-term risk of pelvic radiation. If examination of the cervix and uterus is suboptimal because of the development of vaginal or cervical stenosis after treatment, a transvaginal ultrasound can be used to assist in the evaluation.

Recurrent Disease

Localized recurrences or new primary vulvar cancers can be treated again by surgical excision. Radiation can be used secondarily if there are positive resection margins or involved lymph nodes. Pelvic exenterative surgery is an option for locoregional recurrence after radiation.

Chemotherapeutic agents can be offered for women with distant metastases, but response rates are low, and long-term survival is uncommon in this setting.

Vaginal Cancer

Primary vaginal cancer not involving the vulvar or cervix is one of the least common gynecologic malignancies, representing only about 1% of the total. In some cases, this carcinoma can arise from a precursor intraepithelial lesion, which, like its counterpart in the vulva, can be graded as mild, moderate, or severe. The relative rarity of this malignancy makes it difficult to obtain firm epidemiologic data. Low socioeconomic status, history of genital warts, and prior irradiation have been proposed as risk factors. Diethylstilbestrol (DES) is a risk factor for the subsequent development of clear cell carcinoma. The role of the human papilloma virus as a precursor to vaginal carcinoma is not clear, although patients with vaginal dysplasia can have cytopathic effects consistent with papilloma virus infection. Vaginal Pap smear and/or colposcopic evaluation provide a means to evaluate squamous cell lesions. The close proximity of the vagina to the urethra, rectum, and bladder, as well as its rich and complex lymphatic and vascular supply, make the vagina a site for both metastatic disease and extension from vulvar, cervical, and (less commonly) rectal or urethral malignancies.

Squamous Cell Carcinoma

The most common primary tumor of the vagina is squamous cell carcinoma. These tumors are most common among women between the ages of 50 and 70 years and are usually located in the posterior and upper portions of the vagina. Patients frequently have histories of other squamous cell lesions in the lower genital tract (including carcinoma of the cervix and/or vulva), and it can be difficult to determine whether vaginal squamous cell carcinomas represent new primary carcinomas or tumor recurrences from patients with histories of prior vulvar or cervical malignancies. To reduce ambiguity between primary vaginal cancer and vaginal recurrences from other sites, a 5- to 10-year disease-free interval is defined as necessary to rule out recurrent disease.

Clear Cell Carcinomas

Clear cell carcinomas present in the anterior upper one-third of the vagina. They are seen frequently in very young adults and occasionally in the teenage or preteen population. In utero exposure to diethylstilbestrol, particularly between weeks 16 and 17 of gestation, increases the risk of malignant and premalignant lesions in the vagina. Registry data of diethylstilbestrol-exposed infants suggest that approximately 1 in 1000 girls or young women who had fetal in utero diethylstilbestrol exposure will develop this type of malignancy. These malignancies are more likely to be submucosal and might be missed with Pap smear screening; they require more careful follow up, including regular colposcopy.

Other Tumors

Other tumors of the vagina include malignant melanoma and sarcomas. The vagina can also be the site of botryoid rhabdomyosarcoma in infants and young children as well as of small cell carcinomas arising from neuroendocrine rests within the vagina. Metastatic disease most commonly arises from other gynecologic primary sites.

Clinical Presentation and Staging

The majority of women with vaginal cancers present with postcoital or dysfunctional bleeding. Patients with more locally advanced disease can present with pelvic pain, dysuria, or signs or symptoms of nodal metastases.

Cytology can detect early squamous cell lesions of the vagina but is much less sensitive for clear cell carcinomas, which often are submucosal. Staging requires careful evaluation of the vulva and cervix to distinguish between primary vaginal carcinoma and carcinoma arising in a different portion of the lower genital tract and subsequently extending directly or metastasizing to the vagina. Staging can be done through either the American Joint Committee on Cancer staging system or the Federation Internationale de Gynecologie et d'Obstetrique staging system (Table 79-6).

The clinical staging of newly diagnosed vaginal cancer is performed under general anesthesia (Figure 79-6). Determining the degree of extravaginal extension is important for appropriate radiation therapy planning and/or for determining which patients are appropriate candidates for surgical excision. Upper vaginal lesions metastasize to deep pelvic lymph nodes, while lower vaginal lesions metastasize to pelvic lymph nodes, inguinal lymph nodes, or occasionally to femoral lymph nodes.

Treatment

Patients with stage I or small stage II tumors located in the upper vagina are candidates for radiation therapy or radical hysterectomy. Older patients or patients with bulky stage II or advanced stage disease or patients with middle or lower vaginal tumors are treated with radiation therapy. Dosimetry is planned to include intracavitary and, occasionally, interstitial implants to provide appropriate dosage to the vaginal vault and parametrial tissues. Despite the absence of data, it is probably reasonable to extrapolate from the recent cervical cancer trials and consider the delivery of concurrent cisplatin with radiation therapy, especially for patients with squamous cell malignancies. There is no proven role for neoadjuvant or adjuvant chemotherapy after primary surgical or radiation therapy.

Prognosis and patterns of treatment failure vary, based on stage of the disease at presentation. Women with stage I or II tumors have a 10% to 15% rate of pelvic recurrences and a 7% to 20% chance of distant

Table 79-6 ■ Staging of Vaginal Cancers

AJC TNM Classification	FIGO	
Tumor Assessment		
Tx		Primary tumor cannot be evaluated
Tis	0	Carcinoma in situ
T1	I	Carcinoma confined to mucosa
T2	II	Submucosal infiltration
	IIA	No parametrial extension
	IIB	Parametrial extension but not to sidewall
T3	III	Extension to pelvic sidewall
T4		Extension to bladder or rectum
	IV	Extension to bladder or rectum or distant metastases
Nodal Status		
N0		No nodal involvement
N1		Unilateral groin or pelvic nodes
N2		Bilateral groin or pelvic nodes
Distant Metastases		
M0		No distant metastases
M1		Para-aortic nodal involvement or distant metastases
AJC TNM Staging		
Stage 0	$Tis\ N_0\ M_0$	
Stage I	$T_1\ N_0\ M_0$	
Stage II	$T_2\ N_0\ M_0$	
Stage III	$T_{1-3}\ N_1\ M_0\ T_3\ N_0\ M_0/T_3\ N_0\ M_0$	
Stage IVA	$T_{1-4}\ N_2\ M_0\ T_4\ N_{0-1}\ M_0$	
Stage IVB	$T_{1-4}\ N_{0-2}\ M_1$	

metastases. Long-term survival ranges from 75% for patients with stage I disease to approximately 50% for stage II disease. In comparison, patients with advanced stage III/IV disease have higher rates of both local and distant recurrence. The largest published series of locally advanced vaginal cancers demonstrated a 38%

survival in stage III disease and a similar 10-year survival for stage IV disease. It is noteworthy that some authors have suggested that cancers located in the upper vagina carry a better prognosis than lesions presenting elsewhere.

Metastatic Disease

Recurrences within the vaginal vault can be treated effectively with surgery in patients who were treated previously with radiation therapy, or with radiation therapy in patients who were previously treated with surgery. Surgical salvage often requires partial or total exenterative procedures. The limited data derived from reports of chemotherapy trials support the use of combination chemotherapy incorporating either anthracyclines or platinum.

References

Cervical Cancer

Albores Saaverdra J, Gersell D, Gilks CB, et al: Terminology of endocrine tumors of the uterine cervix: Results of a workshop sponsored by the college of American pathologists in

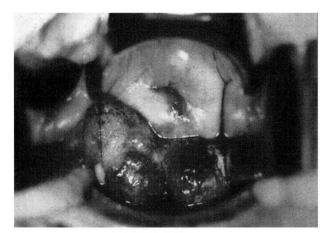

Figure 79-6 ■ Vaginal carcinoma.

the National Cancer Institute. Arch Pathol Lab Med 1997;121:34.

Duska L, Toth T, Goodman A: Fertility options for patients with stages IA2 and IB cervical cancer: Presentation of two cases in discussion of technical and ethical issues. Obstet Gynecol 1998;92:656.

Grogin M, Thomas GM, Melamed I, et al: The importance of hemoglobin levels during radiotherapy for carcinoma of the cervix. Cancer 1999;86:1528.

Holowaty P, Miller AB, Rohan R, To T: Natural history of dysplasia of the uterine cervix. J Natl Cancer Inst 1999;91:252.

Kristensen GB, Abeler VM, Risberg B, et al: Tumor size, depth of invasion and grading of the invasive tumor front are the main prognostic factors in early squamous cell cervical carcinoma. Gynecol Oncol 1999;74:245.

Martin X, Sacchetoni A, et al : Laparoscopic vaginal radical trachelectomy: A treatment to preserve the fertility of cervical carcinoma patients. Cancer 2000;88:1877.

Montz FJ, Monk BJ, Fowler JM, Nguyen L: Natural history of the minimally abnormal Papanicolaou smear. Obstet Gynecol 1992;80:385.

Morris M, Eifel PJ, Jiandong L, et al: Pelvic radiation with concurrent chemotherapy compared with pelvic and para-aortic radiation for high-risk cervical cancer. N Engl J Med 1999;340:1137.

Peppercorn P, Jeyarajah A, Woolas R, et al: Role of MR imaging in the selection of patients with early cervical carcinoma for fertility preserving surgery: initial experience. Radiology 2000;212:395.

Peters III WA, Liu PY, Barrett II RJ, et al: Concurrent chemotherapy and pelvic radiation therapy compared with pelvic radiation therapy alone as adjuvant therapy after radical surgery in high-risk early-stage cancer of the cervix. J Clin Oncol 2000;18:1606.

Rose PG, Blessing JA, Gershenson DM, McGehe R: Paclitaxel and cisplatin as first-line therapy in recurrent or advanced squamous cell carcinoma of the cervix: A gynecologic oncology group study. J Clin Oncol 1999;17:2676.

Rose PG, Bundy BN, Watkins EB, et al: Concurrent cisplatin-based radiotherapy and chemotherapy for locally advanced cervical cancer. N Engl J Med 1999;340:1144.

Sugawara Y, Eisbruch A, Kosuda S, et al: Evaluation of FDG PET in patients with cervical cancer. J Nucl Med 1991;40:1125.

Whitney CW, Sause W, Bundy BN, et al: Randomized comparison of fluorouracil plus cisplatin versus hydroxyurea as an adjunct to radiation therapy in stage IIB–IVA carcinoma of the cervix with negative para-aortic lymph nodes. A Gynecologic Oncology Group and Southwest Oncology Group study. J Clin Oncol 1999;17:1339.

Wright TC Jr, Cox JT, Massad LS, et al: 2001 consensus guidelines for the management of women with cervical cytological abnormalities. JAMA 2002;287:2120.

Zanetta G, Fei F, Parma G, et al: Paclitaxel, ifosfamide and cisplatin (TIP) chemotherapy for recurrent or persistent squamous cell cervical cancer. Ann Oncol 1999;10:1171.

Vulvar Carcinoma

Andersen BL, Hacker NF: Psychological adjustment after vulvar surgery. Obstet Gynecol 1983;62:457.

Brinton LA, Nasca PC, Mallin K, et al: Case control study of cancer of the vulva. Obstet Gynecol 1990;75:859.

Fanning J, Lambert L, Hale TM, et al: Paget's disease of the vulva: prevalence of associated vulvar adenocarcinoma, invasive Paget's disease, and recurrence after surgical excision. Am J Obstet Gynecol 1999;180:24.

Hoffman JS, Kumar NB, Morley GW: Prognostic significance of groin lymph nodes metastases in squamous carcinoma of the vulva. Obstet Gynecol 1985;66:402.

Homesley HD, Bundy BN, Sedlis A, et al: Assessment of current International Federation of Gynecology and Obstetrics staging of vulvar carcinoma relative to prognostic factors for survival. A Gynecologic Oncology Group study. Am J Obstet Gynecol 1991;164:997.

Hording U, Junge J, Daugaard S, et al: Vulvar squamous cell carcinoma and papilloma viruses: indications for two different etiologies. Gynecol Oncol 1994;52:241.

Irvin WP Jr, Legallo RL, Stoler MH, et al: Vulvar melanoma: a retrospective analysis and literature review. Gynecol Oncol 2001;83:457.

Iversen T, Tretli S: Intraepithelial and invasive squamous cell neoplasia of the vulva: trends in incidence, recurrence and survival rate in Norway. Obstet Gynecol 1998;91:969.

Jones R, Joura E: Analyzing prior clinical events at presentation in 10% of women with vulvar carcinoma. Evidence of diagnostic delays. J Reprod Med 1999;44:766.

Joura EA: Epidemiology, diagnosis and treatment of vulvar intraepithelial neoplasia. Curr Opin Obstet Gynecol 2002;14:39.

Podratz KC, Symmonds RE, Taylor WF: Carcinoma of the vulva: analysis of treatment failures. Am J Obstet Gynecol 1982;143:340.

Raspagliesi F, Ditto A, Paladini D, et al: Prognostic indicators in melanoma of the vulva. Ann Surg Oncol 2000;7:738.

Ramirez PT, Levenback C: Sentinel nodes in gynecologic malignancies. Curr Opin Oncol 2001;13:403.

Vaginal Cancer

Cardosi RJ, Bomalaski JJ, Hoffman MS: Diagnosis and management of vulvar and vaginal intraepithelial neoplasia. Obstet Gynecol Clin N Am 2001;28:685.

Chyle V, Zagars GK, Wheeler JA, et al: Definitive radiotherapy for carcinoma of the vagina: outcome and prognostic factors. Intl J Radiat Oncol Biol Phys 1996;35:891.

Doronow RC, Hickman BT, Reagan MT, et al: Combined therapy as an alternative to exenteration for locally advanced vulvo-vaginal cancer. II. Results, complications endo symmetric and surgical consideration. Am J Clin Oncol 1987;10:171.

Hatch VE, Palmer JR, Titus-Ernstoff L, et al: Cancer risk in women exposed to diethylstilbestrol in utero. JAMA 1998;280:630.

Herbst A: Diethylstilbestrol and adenocarcinoma of the vagina. Am J Obstet Gynecol 1999;181:1576.

Tarrazza MH, Munce H, Decain M, et al: Patterns of recurrence of primary carcinoma of the vagina. Eur J Gynaecol Oncol 1991;12:89.

Waggoner SE, Anderson SM, Luce MC, et al: p53 protein expression in gene analysis and clear cell adenocarcinoma of the vagina and cervix. Gynecol Oncol 1996;60:339.

Chapter 80
Endometrial Cancer

Michael G. Muto

Introduction

There are approximately 36,100 new cases of endometrial carcinoma diagnosed in the United States annually. This is a disease largely of perimenopausal and postmenopausal women (median age 61 years) and rarely occurs in women below the age of 40. Incidence rates are 1.5-fold higher among Caucasians than among African Americans, but the death rate is twofold higher among African Americans. The observed racial difference in death rate may be related to a preponderance of aggressive histologic subtypes in African Americans. Caucasians, on the other hand, are more likely to develop a more indolent form of the disease.

The recent introduction of a surgical staging system for endometrial cancer has created considerable confusion regarding the proper management of these cancers. There is little consensus as to the utility of adjuvant radiation therapy following primary surgical management and even less agreement on the use of cytotoxic chemotherapy or hormonal treatment in the setting of recurrent disease. Other controversial issues including the management of cancer precursors and the appropriate surveillance for patients on tamoxifen.

The most common form of endometrial carcinoma, the so-called Type I adenocarcinomas, are principally well-differentiated tumors of endometrioid type. Uncommon and more virulent forms of endometrial adenocarcinomas include the Type II cancers and uterine sarcomas.

Risk Factors

Independent risk factors for Type I endometrial carcinoma include obesity, nulliparity, late menopause, and insulin-dependent diabetes mellitus. Hypertension does not represent an independent risk factor but is linked closely to the risks of diabetes and obesity. Most Type I endometrial carcinomas arise from a field of atypical endometrial hyperplasia. An environment of relative estrogen excess, due to exogenously administered estrogen or exaggerated endogenous production, is the primary event in the development of this disease. Androstenedione, an adrenal androgen, is converted to estrone, a weak estrogen, in adipose tissue. Obese patients have significantly elevated levels of estrone, thereby increasing their risk of developing both atypical hyperplasia and invasive carcinoma of the endometrium.

Unopposed estrogen replacement therapy is known to produce endometrial hyperplasia and is a risk factor for the development of endometrial carcinoma. Tumors arising from exogenous or endogenous estrogen sources and forming in a field of atypical endometrial hyperplasia are often minimally invasive and readily treated. In fact, the life expectancy of patients with endometrial cancers resulting from exogenous estrogen use is the same as that of unaffected women. These data, coupled with the adverse impact androgenic progestins have on high-density lipoprotein profiles, have prompted some primary care physicians to use low-dose continuous estrogen therapy in perimenopausal and postmenopausal patients. The safety of this approach is unproven and is in conflict with the standard of medical care that mandates both estrogen and progesterone administration to women on estrogen replacement therapy who have an intact uterus. If a woman has undergone a hysterectomy, unopposed estrogen replacement is acceptable.

Tamoxifen has estrogenic effects on both endometrial glands and stroma. Its estrogenic potency is roughly equivalent to that of the standard dose of conjugated equine estrogens (Premarin) used in hormone replacement therapy regimens. Therefore, tamoxifen is associated with an increased risk of both endometrial hyperplasia and Type I endometrial cancer. This drug may also contribute to the development of endometrial polyp formation by stimulating the endometrial stroma. There is controversy as to whether or not tamoxifen may also contribute to an increased risk of more aggressive (Type II) endometrial carcinoma and uterine sarcoma. When a woman who is on tamoxifen for the treatment or chemoprophylaxis of breast cancer presents with abnormal bleeding, endometrial pathology should be ruled out with an endometrial biopsy.

Endometrial cancer is the second most common malignancy in women with hereditary nonpolyposis colorectal carcinoma syndrome. In women who meet the modified Amsterdam criteria for the diagnosis of hereditary nonpolyposis colorectal carcinoma syndrome or who have had confirmatory genetic testing, routine endometrial biopsy and ultrasound screening may be indicated.

Oral contraceptives have a strong protective effect against the development of Type I endometrial carcinoma because most formulations are progesterone-dominant. Potent progestins (levonogestrel or norethindrone acetate) drive the endometrium toward atrophy and counteract the effect of endogenous estrogen. Therefore, oral contraceptive users are less likely to develop Type I endometrial cancer. Contraceptives can be particularly helpful in managing anovulatory states in young women that are either due to intrinsic disease, such as polycystic ovarian syndrome, or induced by cytotoxic chemotherapy.

Cigarette smokers also have a significantly reduced risk of developing Type I endometrial cancer because smokers are relatively hypoestrogenic. This hypoestrogenic state results from both an inhibition of the conversion of androstenedione to estrone and increased catabolism of estrone. Smokers also have a lower body fat content, an earlier menopause, and higher levels of sex hormone-binding globulin, which reduces the bioavailability of circulating estrogen. Any beneficial effect in the reduction of endometrial cancer, however, is far outweighed by an increased risk of lung cancer.

Clinical Presentation

The most common presenting symptom of endometrial carcinoma is intermenstrual or postmenopausal bleeding. This symptom is present in 90% of patients with endometrial carcinoma and usually occurs at an early stage. Only 50% of patients with endometrial cancer will have an abnormal Papanicolaou (Pap) smear, making this an unacceptable test for screening. However, among postmenopausal women with normal endometrial cells present on a routine Pap smear, 6% will have endometrial cancer, and 13% will have endometrial hyperplasia. If these cells are atypical endometrial cells, up to 25% of these women will have endometrial cancer. Therefore, the detection of

endometrial cells on a Pap smear in a postmenopausal woman is an indication for endometrial biopsy.

Precursor Lesions

The topic of precursor lesions of endometrial carcinoma has been made needlessly complicated by multiple classification systems. Terms such as *cystic and adenomatous hyperplasia, adenocarcinoma in situ,* and *cystic hyperplasia* should be discarded. In describing hyperplastic lesions, one is concerned with both the architectural and cytologic characteristics of the endometrium. Architectural atypia refers to abnormalities in the number, size, and complexity of the endometrial glands, whereas cytological atypia refers to nuclear pleomorphism in individual cells lining those glands. The degree to which endometrial hyperplasia demonstrates cellular atypia determines malignant potential. In women with nonatypical hyperplasia, the progression rate to invasive carcinoma is only 1% to 5%. Among women with atypical hyperplasia, there is a 30% progression rate to invasive carcinoma. An atypical hyperplasia identified in a perimenopausal or postmenopausal woman carries with it a 15% risk of a coexisting endometrial carcinoma.

Endometrial hyperplasia may also cause heavy vaginal bleeding; therefore, therapy is warranted in all cases. Nonatypical hyperplasia is best managed medically with continuous or cyclic progestin therapy. Atypical hyperplasia in perimenopausal or postmenopausal women is best treated surgically when possible. When fertility is an issue, atypical hyperplasia can also be managed medically with high-dose continual progestin therapy, followed by ovulation induction with cyclic oral contraceptives.

Diagnostic Methods

Ninety percent of endometrial carcinomas are accurately diagnosed with the use of an office endometrial biopsy. Instruments, including the Pipelle, Vabra, or Novac, combine both suction and sharp curettage to achieve an overall accuracy equivalent to that of a formal dilatation and curettage performed under anesthesia. Preceding the endometrial biopsy, endocervical curettage may help in ruling out endocervical involvement and in differentiating an endocervical adenocarcinoma from an endometrial adenocarcinoma. However, endocervical biopsy results are no longer used in endometrial cancer staging because the false-positive rate for endocervical curettage is 40% and therefore will lead to a significant overestimate of clinical stage II endometrial carcinoma. In patients with multiple episodes of perimenopausal or post-menopausal bleeding, a negative endometrial office biopsy might not be reassuring, and a sharp curettage under anesthesia should be considered. There is some evidence to suggest that in these cases, the addition of hysteroscopy will improve the detection rate of polypoid lesions, hyperplasias, and carcinoma, and it is therefore recommended. There is no evidence to suggest that hysteroscopy is of any benefit in determining true endocervical involvement. With the advent of surgical staging, this issue is now of no consequence.

There is a growing body of data that supports the use of high-resolution transvaginal sonography in the evaluation of patients with postmenopausal bleeding. An accurate measure of the thickness of the endometrial stripe can be readily accomplished and is highly predictive of endometrial neoplasia and hyperplasia. Using a cutoff of up to 5 mm, endometrial carcinoma was detected in only 0.3% of women with postmenopausal bleeding, whereas if the endometrial stripe was over 5 mm, the risk of neoplasia or hyperplasia on a subsequent endometrial biopsy approaches 20%. If a woman has a single episode of postmenopausal bleeding, a normal Pap smear, and an endometrial stripe measurement of 5 mm or less on a transvaginal sonography performed by an experienced sonographer, it may be possible to avoid endometrial biopsy. Any woman with an abnormal Pap smear or recurrent bleeding must undergo a biopsy promptly. Unfortunately, women who are on tamoxifen will routinely have thickened endometria due to benign endometrial proliferation or polyp formation, limiting the utility of transvaginal sonography in this population. In addition, Type II endometrial cancer and uterine sarcomas may develop without significantly thickening the endometrium.

There is no role for the routine screening of asymptomatic postmenopausal women for endometrial cancer. Routine endometrial biopsies or transvaginal sonography, even in women who are obese or diabetic, results in an excessive cost per year of life saved. Routine screening should be reserved for patients who are on tamoxifen for chemoprophylaxis of breast cancer, for patients with chronic anovulatory states who are not undergoing regular progesterone-induced menses, and for women with hereditary nonpolyposis colorectal carcinoma syndrome. Since women with hereditary nonpolyposis colorectal carcinoma syndrome are also at risk for developing ovarian cancer, one rational annual screening strategy is to perform an endometrial biopsy followed six months later by a transvaginal sonography both to measure the endometrial stripe and to evaluate the ovaries for the development of suspicious masses.

Serum CA-125 levels may be elevated in women with advanced endometrial cancer. These elevations are usually associated with extensive intrauterine disease and extrauterine spread. An elevated CA-125 level in the presence of biopsy-proven endometrial carcinoma may be an indicator of extensive disease. Patients with elevated CA-125 are candidates for further radiographic evaluation.

Preoperative Imaging

The role of abdominopelvic computed tomography (CT) and magnetic resonance imaging (MRI) in the preoperative evaluation of patients with endometrial cancer is unclear. In asymptomatic patients with well-differentiated lesions, the likelihood of extrauterine spread is so low that radiographic evaluation beyond a routine preoperative chest X-ray is not warranted. When a patient has significant constitutional symptoms, abdominal or lower extremity pain or swelling, or an aggressive histology on endometrial biopsy, a preoperative computed tomography scan of the abdomen and pelvis may be helpful in planning surgery (Figure 80-1).

Recently, pelvic magnetic resonance imaging has been employed to assess the depth of myometrial invasion and to determine whether there has been extension of a uterine fundal lesion into the endocervix (Figure 80-2). Although properly performed magnetic resonance imaging may accurately predict the degree of myoinvasion in up to 90% of cases, it should not be considered a routine examination. The quality of the magnetic resonance imaging estimate is highly dependent on the imaging protocol that is used and the experience of the radiologist. In addition, in older women with thin myometria, the image is very difficult to interpret. The test should be considered only if surgical staging is not planned.

Surgical Staging

Endometrial cancer is now a surgically staged disease. The International Federation of Gynecology and Obstetrics (FIGO) staging system is outlined in Table 80-1. The advantage of surgical staging is that it overcomes the inherent inaccuracies of clinical staging. For example, extension of disease from the fundus to the cervix is a poor prognostic feature in endometrial cancer. Under a clinical staging system, cervical involvement was determined by endocervical curettage. Endocervical curettage is not a reliable indicator of cervical involvement and is associated with a 40% false-positive rate. Therefore, the clinical staging system led to substantial overstaging in this common

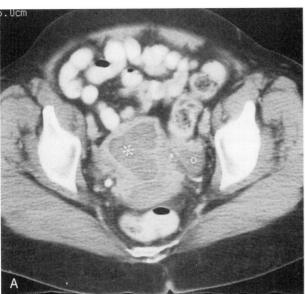
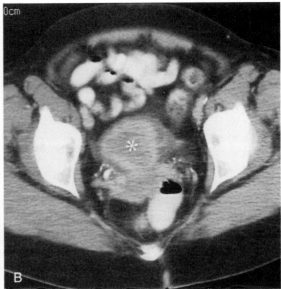

Figure 80-1 ■ Endometrial carcinoma. Contrast-enhanced computed tomography images show an enhancing endometrial mass. (From Boles SM, Hricak H, Rubin P: Carcinoma of the cervix and endometrium. In Bragg DG, Rubin P, Hricak H [eds]: Oncologic Imaging, 2nd ed. Philadelphia: WB Saunders, 2002, p 541.)

circumstance. Surgical staging allows precise evaluation of prognostic factors, including histologic type, grade, and depth of myoinvasion, and is the only reliable method of determining cervical invasion and extrauterine spread.

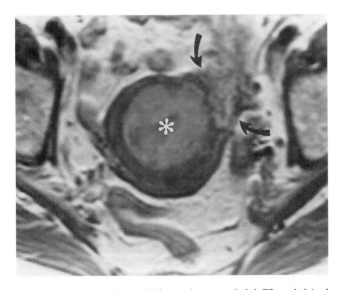

Figure 80-2 ■ Endometrial carcinoma. Axial T2-weighted fast spin echo magnetic resonance image demonstrating extension of the endometrial mass into the myometrium. (From Boles SM, Hricak H, Rubin P: Carcinoma of the cervix and endometrium. In Bragg DG, Rubin P, Hricak H [eds]: Oncologic Imaging, 2nd ed. Philadelphia: WB Saunders, 2002, p 543.)

Endometrial cancer surgery should include a thorough exploratory laparotomy, pelvic washings, omental biopsy, and palpation of pelvic and para-aortic nodes, followed by total abdominal hysterectomy with bilateral salpingo-oophorectomy, resection of grossly enlarged pelvic or para-aortic nodes, and pelvic and para-aortic node biopsy in selected patients. Not all patients with endometrial carcinoma must undergo nodal sampling. Comprehensive descriptive data collected by the Gynecologic Oncology Group

Table 80-1 ■ **FIGO Staging of Cancer of the Uterine Corpus**

Stage	Finding
IA	Tumor limited to endometrium
IB	Invasion to <½ myometrium
IC	Invasion to ≥½ myometrium
IIA	Endocervical glandular involvement only
IIB	Cervical stromal invasion
IIIA	Tumor invades serosa and/or adnexa and/or positive peritoneal cytology
IIIB	Vaginal metastases
IIIC	Metastases to pelvic and/or para-aortic lymph nodes
IVA	Tumor invasion of bladder and/or bowel mucosa
IVB	Distant metastases including intra-abdominal and/or inguinal nodes

Table 80-2 ■ Tumor Grade versus Risk Factors in Stage I Endometrial Cancer

Grade	Lymph Node Metastases (%)	Deep Myoinvasion (%)	Recurrence (%)
1	2	4	4
2	11	15	15
3	27	39	42

(GOG) allow accurate estimates of the likelihood of para-aortic lymph node metastasis and therefore help to determine the need for extended surgical staging. For example, in patients with minimally invasive grade I lesions, there are no reported cases of para-aortic lymph node spread, whereas in the presence of deep myometrial invasion and poor differentiation, para-aortic lymph nodes may be involved in up to 16% of cases (Tables 80-2 and 80-3).

Following removal of the uterus, the specimen should be opened, and the depth of myometrial invasion should be determined. It is difficult to accurately determine the degree of myoinvasion by gross inspection, particularly in poorly differentiated lesions, in which the depth of invasion can be underestimated in up to 50% of cases. Intraoperative frozen section by a pathologist who is experienced in gynecologic pathology is therefore recommended. In the presence of deep myometrial invasion or poor differentiation, pelvic and para-aortic node biopsies are indicated.

Occasionally, patients with well-differentiated carcinomas diagnosed by endometrial biopsy are upgraded to moderately or poorly differentiated lesions at the time of final pathology. An increase of more than one grade is unusual. Conversely, the uterus often contains no evidence of a well-differentiated lesion present on endometrial biopsy. This likely represents a removal of the entire superficial lesion at the time of diagnostic procedure (Table 80-4).

To summarize general guidelines, one should be prepared to perform pelvic and/or para-aortic lymph node biopsies in patients with moderate or poorly differentiated carcinoma with any measurable myometrial invasion and in women with deeply invasive, well-differentiated lesions. Subspecialty consultations should be obtained in the management of patients with the following:

1. Grade 2 or grade 3 lesions on endometrial biopsy
2. Papillary serous, adenosquamous, or clear cell histology
3. Any sarcoma
4. Patients with elevated CA-125 levels
5. Patients with adnexal masses, adenopathy, or an enlarged uterus
6. Patients with severe intercurrent medical problems

Vaginal hysterectomy is an appropriate alternative to laparotomy in patients with well-differentiated adenocarcinomas arising in endometrial hyperplasia. These lesions are likely to be confined to the endometrial cavity, and the advantages of vaginal surgery in obese, hypertensive women are clear. When compared to abdominal hysterectomy, vaginal hysterectomy is associated with a shorter hospital stay, less febrile morbidity, and disability. The disadvantage of the vaginal approach is that it does not allow for extended surgical staging. Recently, however, with the advent of laparoscopically assisted vaginal hysterectomy, pelvic washings and biopsy of pelvic and para-aortic lymph node groups can be accomplished in conjunction with vaginal hysterectomy in the management of patients with higher-grade lesions.

Alternatives to Surgery

There are alternatives to the surgical management of endometrial carcinoma in highly selected patients. Young women with chronic anovulatory states, such as polycystic ovarian syndrome, who develop endometrial cancer may be treated with high-dose progestin therapy. To be a candidate for conservative medical rather than surgical therapy, the patient must wish to retain her fertility and have a well-differentiated cancer of endometrioid type. She must be asymptomatic, have reassuring imaging, preferably magnetic resonance imaging indicating no myometrial invasion, and be willing to undergo serial endometrial biopsies. Continuous high-dose progestin therapy for a period of three to six months is required. Such therapy may be associated with marked weight gain, mild depression, and hair thinning. Persistent endometrial carcinoma despite six months of continuous high-dose progestin administration is an indication for hysterectomy. With

Table 80-3 ■ Pelvic and Para-aortic Node Metastases Relative to Grade in Stage I Endometrial Cancer (GOG Results)

Grade	Pelvic Nodes	Para-aortic Nodes
1 (n = 180)	5 (3%)	3 (2%)
2 (n = 288)	25 (9%)	14 (5%)
3 (n = 153)	28 (18%)	17 (11%)

Table 80-4 ■ Stage I Endometrial Cancer, Tumor Grade and Five-Year Survival

Depth of Invasion	Five-Year Actual Survival		
	Grade 1 (%)	Grade 2 (%)	Grade 3 (%)
No residual (after biopsy)	98	98	80
Endometrium	97	98	80
Myometrium <50%	93	87	61
Myometrium >50%	91	71	26

resolution of the carcinoma, patients may be cycled with oral contraceptives, withdrawn with progestin monthly, or undergo ovulation induction to become pregnant.

In elderly patients or patients with significant intercurrent medical problems that make abdominal or vaginal surgery unacceptably risky, high-dose continuous progestin therapy or primary radiation using intrauterine brachytherapy devices may be employed.

Radiation Therapy in Primary and Recurrent Endometrial Cancer

Radiation therapy is frequently employed to prevent or treat locally recurrent endometrial cancer. The single most important factor in determining whether a patient is a candidate for adjuvant radiation therapy following surgery for endometrial cancer is the likelihood of local or regional recurrence of disease. On the basis of the histologic type, surgical stage, and grade of the cancer, it is possible to define three groups who are at low, intermediate, and high risk for recurrence. Women with well-differentiated, stage I endometrioid tumors are at very low risk for recurrence and are rarely offered additional therapy, whereas patients with poorly differentiated lesions or those who have advanced surgical stage are often treated. Despite the use of adjuvant radiotherapy, prognosis is not altered. Pelvic radiation therapy is very effective at reducing the likelihood of recurrence at the vaginal cuff or in the pelvis but does not seem to impart a survival advantage. Nevertheless, women with a pelvic recurrence of endometrial cancer often suffer severe symptoms, including vaginal hemorrhage, pelvic pain, bowel or ureteral obstruction, and infection. These symptoms dramatically affect the quality of remaining life and are often difficult to palliate. Therefore, adjuvant pelvic radiation plays an important role in maintaining quality of life by effectively reducing the risk of pelvic recurrence.

Patients may be treated with adjuvant radiation therapy following hysterectomy for endometrial cancer in one of four ways: vaginal brachytherapy, whole pelvic radiation, extended field radiation, or whole abdominal radiation. In general, no adjuvant radiation therapy is recommended for minimally invasive, well-differentiated lesions. Patients who have lesions of intermediate differentiation with some measur-able myoinvasion are frequently offered vaginal brachytherapy to reduce the risk of vaginal cuff recurrences. Poorly differentiated or deeply invasive lesions receive whole pelvic radiation therapy with extended field to the para-aortic nodes if those nodes are known to be histologically positive. Extended radiation therapy to incorporate the para-aortic lymph nodes is potentially morbid and therefore is offered only to patients in whom positive para-aortic nodes have been documented. In small retrospective studies, up to 40% of patients with microscopically positive para-aortic nodes who receive para-aortic nodal irradiation survive longer than five years. Whole abdominal radiation therapy is reserved for patients with microscopic upper abdominal disease or with papillary serous histology.

Radiation therapy is effective in the treatment of locally recurrent endometrial cancer, particularly if the recurrence is confined to the vaginal cuff. Over 50% of local cuff recurrences in previously nonirradiated patients can be cured with pelvic or vaginal radiotherapy. Local radiation therapy to recurrences in the pelvic or para-aortic nodes may serve to palliate but rarely cures.

Chemotherapy for Advanced or Recurrent Disease

High-dose progestin therapy is the preferred systemic treatment for women with disseminated endometrial cancer, particularly if the tumor has detectable estrogen and progesterone receptors. Although the response rates are lower for less well-differentiated

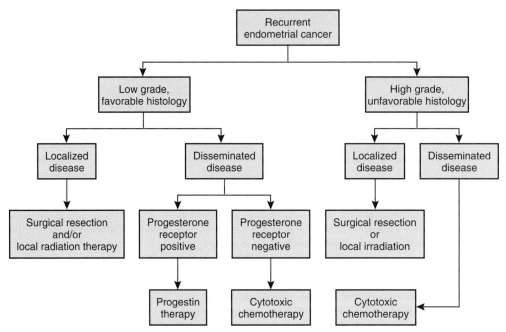

Figure 80-3 ■ Algorithm for treating recurrent endometrial cancer.

lesions, the toxicity profile for progestins make these drugs a logical first choice. Megesterol acetate (Megace) in a daily dose of 80 to 160 mg is both well tolerated and convenient. Higher doses do not seem to increase response rates and are associated with weight gain and depression.

Although frequently used in the treatment of advanced or recurrent disease, cytotoxic chemotherapy has limited activity in endometrial cancer (Figure 80-3). In patients who have failed progestin therapy, chemotherapy may play a palliative role. The most active multiagent therapy regimens all contain cisplatin or derivatives. Doxorubicin and paclitaxel also have activity. In combination with cisplatin, these drugs may induce a partial remission in up to 35% of previously untreated patients. Unfortunately, there is no improvement in overall survival.

in association with papillary serous carcinoma. Papillary serous carcinoma of the endometrium is characterized by intraperitoneal dissemination similar to that of papillary serous carcinoma of the ovary. Despite its similarity to ovarian cancer, response to combination chemotherapy regimens utilized for ovarian cancer is poor. Finally, adenosquamous carcinoma should not be confused with adenocanthoma. Benign squamous metaplasia is commonly found in well-differentiated adenocarcinoma of the endometrium and is of no prognostic significance. When the squamous component is malignant, however, the tumor has a poor prognosis. In general, 90% of adenosquamous carcinomas have a very poorly differentiated squamous component, which may result in deep myometrial invasion, rapid lymphatic and hematogenous dis-

High-Risk Histologic Types

There are three aggressive histologic types of endometrial adenocarcinoma that account for a disproportionate number of recurrences and deaths (Table 80-5). These are clear cell, papillary serous, and adenosquamous carcinoma. Clear cell carcinoma represents 5% of all endometrial carcinomas and has a predilection for vascular space involvement and early hematogenous dissemination. Clear cell cancers are often found as a component of other poorly differentiated histologic types but are most frequently found

Table 80-5 ■ Stage I Endometrial Cancer by Histology and Five-Year Survival

Type by Histology	Alive (%)
Adenoacanthoma	88
Adenocarcinoma	80
Papillary serous	70
Adenosquamous	53
Clear cell	44

semination, and a high risk for recurrent disease. In dealing with these virulent forms of endometrial cancer, deep myometrial invasion, lymphatic involvement, and upper abdominal involvement must be anticipated.

Special Circumstances

Occasionally, a total abdominal hysterectomy will be performed, and an unsuspected endometrial carcinoma will be subsequently identified. Reexploration with bilateral salpingo-oophorectomy and thorough staging are indicated for poorly differentiated lesions. The likelihood of adnexal metastases in patients with stage IA grade 1 lesions is so low that reexploration is not warranted.

Estrogen replacement therapy may safely be offered to patients with noninvasive, well-differentiated lesions. Though there are no data to substantiate it, it may be prudent to add a progestin to this hormone replacement regimen. Hormone replacement therapy is contraindicated in deeply invasive or poorly differentiated carcinomas.

Occasionally, patients have synchronous ovarian neoplasms. The most frequent combination is an endometroid adenocarcinoma of the ovary with an endometroid carcinoma of the endometrium. The excellent prognosis of most of these lesions suggests synchronous primaries as opposed to metastasis from one organ to the other.

Follow-Up Care

Following treatment, the patient should be examined every three to four months for two years, followed by visits at six-month intervals for three additional years. A pelvic examination and Pap smear are crucial at each of these visits, since local recurrences, particularly at the vaginal cuff, can be cured with surgery and/or radiotherapy. Although some practitioners advocate the routine use of imaging (chest X-ray and abdominopelvic computed tomography scans) in asymptomatic women, the lack of effective systemic therapy for disseminated recurrence makes the practice of questionable value.

Uterine Sarcomas

In general, sarcomas commonly demonstrate hematogenous and lymphatic dissemination and have considerable resistance to radiotherapy and combination chemotherapy. As such, they are highly malignant tumors with only a 50% five-year survival rate in early-stage disease and a dismal 20% survival rate in advanced-stage disease. The leiomyosarcoma

and stromal sarcoma bear special mention here (Table 80-6).

The diagnosis of leiomyosarcoma is uncommon, whereas leiomyomas are the most common benign tumors in women and the most common indication for gynecologic surgery in the United States. It is estimated that substantially fewer than 0.1% of all leiomyomas undergo malignant degeneration. The classic teaching that a rapidly enlarging fibroid is a sign of malignancy has proven not to be true. Although leiomyosarcomas are frequently softer and more hemorrhagic than their benign counterparts, there are few gross findings to guide the surgeon. Therefore, these tumors may often be removed at the time of myomectomy or hysterectomy without raising clinical suspicion. To further complicate matters, if there is a clinical suspicion of malignancy, frozen section examination is often inaccurate because the microscopic diagnosis of low- or high-grade leiomyosarcoma is based on the number of mitoses per 10 high-power fields and the presence or absence of cellular atypia. Therefore, it is not uncommon for the diagnosis to be unsuspected and the surgical staging incomplete. A decision regarding reexploration for complete surgical staging must be made on the basis of the degree of differentiation found on final pathologic evaluation.

Stromal sarcomas are also divided into low- and high-grade lesions on the basis of mitotic count. Low-grade stromal sarcomas, formerly called endolymphatic stromal myosis, are indolent tumors, which invade venous channels. They are sensitive to progestin therapy and are readily treated with a combination of surgery and high-dose hormonal treatment. Bilateral salpingo-oophorectomy is a required component of surgical management, and estrogen replacement therapy is prohibited. High-grade stromal sarcomas, like high-grade leiomyosarcomas, carcinosarcomas, and mixed mesodermal sarcomas, are highly malignant tumors that are resistant to all forms of adjuvant therapy.

Table 80-6 ■ Classification of Uterine Sarcomas

Histologic Type	Homologous	Heterologous
Pure	Leiomyosarcoma	Rhabdomyosarcoma
	Stromal sarcoma	Chondrosarcoma
	Low-grade	Osteosarcoma
	High-grade	Liposarcoma
Mixed	Carcinosarcoma	Mixed mesodermal sarcoma

References

Boronow RC: Should whole pelvic radiation therapy become past history? A case for the routine use of extended field therapy and multimodal therapy. Gynecol Oncol 1991; 43:71–76.

Boronow RC, Morrow CP, Creasman WT, et al: Surgical staging in endometrial cancer: Clinical pathological findings of a prospective study. Obstet Gynecol 1984;63:825–832.

Chambers JT, Chambers SK: Endometrial sampling: When? Where? Why? With what? Clin Obstet Gynecol 1992; 35:28–39.

Childers JM, Hatch KD, Tran An, Surwit EA: Laparoscopic para-aortic lymphadenectomy in gynecologic malignancies. Obstet Gynecol 1993;82:741–747.

Childers JM, Spirtos NM, Brainard P, Surwit EA: Laparoscopic staging of the patient with incompletely staged early adenocarcinoma of the endometrium. Obstet Gynecol 1994;83:597–600.

Chu J, Schweid AL, Weiss NS: Survival among women with endometrial cancer: A comparison of estrogen users and nonusers. Am J Obstet Gynecol 1982;143:569–573.

Goff BA, Rice LW: Assessing depth of invasion in endometrial carcinoma: Gross examination of surgical specimens is highly inaccurate. Gynecol Oncol 1990;38:46–48.

Goldchmit R, Katz Z, Blichstein I, et al: The accuracy of endometrial pipelle sampling with and without sono-graphic measurement of endometrial thickness. Obstet Gynecol 1993;82:727–730.

Granberg S, Wikland M, Karlson B, et al: Endometrial thickness as measured by endovaginal ultrasonography for identify-ing endometrial abnormality. Am J Obstet Gynecol 1991;164(1, Pt 1):47–52.

Iossa A, Cianteroni L, Ciatto S, et al : Hysteroscopy and endome-trial cancer diagnosis: A review of 2007 consecutive exam-inations in self referred patients. Tumori 1991;77:479–483.

Kahanpaa KV, Wahlston T, Grohn P, et al: Sarcoma of the uterus: A clinicopathologic study of 119 patients. Obstet Gynecol 1986;67:417–424.

Kurman RJ, Kaminski PF, Norris HJ: The behavior of endome-trial hyperplasia: A long-term study of "untreated" hyper-plasia in 170 patients. Cancer 1985;56:403–412.

Mallipeddi P, Kapps DS, Teng NNH: Long-term survival with adjuvant whole abdominopelvic irradiation for uterine papillary serous carcinoma. Cancer 1993;71:3076–3081.

Morris HJ, Taylor HB: Postradiation sarcomas of the uterus. Obstet Gynecol 1965;26:689.

Morrow CP, Bundy BN, Homesly HD, et al: Doxorubicin as an adjuvant following surgery and radiation therapy in patients with high-grade endometrial carcinoma, Stage I and occult Stage II: A GOG study. Gynecol Oncol 1990;36:166–171.

Morrow CP, Schlaerth JB: Surgical management of endometrial carcinoma. Clin Obstet Gynecol 1982;25:81–92.

Omura GA, Blessing JA, Major E, Silverberg S: A randomized trial of Adriamycin versus no adjuvant therapy in Stage I and II uterine sarcomas. J Clin Oncol 1985;3:1240–1245.

Peters WA III, Andersen WA, Thornton N Jr, Morley GW: The selective use of vaginal hysterectomy in the management of adenocarcinoma of the endometrium. Am J Obstet Gynecol 1983;146:285–289.

Potish RA, Twiggs LB, Adcock LL, Prem KA: The role of whole abdominal radiation therapy in the management of endometrial cancer: Prognostic importance of factors indi-cating peritoneal metastases. Gynecol Oncol 1985; 21:80–86.

Potish RA, Twiggs LB, Adcock LL, et al: Paraaortic lymph node radiotherapy in cancer of the uterine corpus. Obstet Gynecol 1985;65:251–256.

Randall TC, Kurman RJ: Progestin treatment of atypical hyper-plasia and well-differentiated carcinoma of the endo-metrium in women under age forty. Obstet Gynecol 1997; 90:434–440.

Rose PG: Medical progress: Endometrial carcinoma. N Engl J Med 1996;335:630–649.

Suh-Burgmann EJ, Goodman AK: Surveillance for endometrial cancer in women receiving tamoxifen. Ann Intern Med 1999;131:127–135.

Thigpen JT, Blessing JA, DiSaia P, Ehrlich C: Treatment of advanced or recurrent endometrial cancer with medroxy progesterone acetate. Gynecol Oncol 1985;20:250.

Zucker PK, Kasdon EJ, Feldstein ML: The validity of Pap smear parameters as predictors of endometrial pathology in menopausal women. Cancer 1985;56:2256–2263.

Chapter 81
Ovarian Cancer

Stephen A. Cannistra

Introduction

Cancer of the ovary encompasses a broad range of ovarian neoplasms that may originate from either the ovarian epithelial surface, the stromal elements (granulosa and theca cells), or the germ cells. As a general rule, epithelial ovarian cancer usually occurs in women over the age of 50 years and is the most common type of malignant ovarian neoplasm in this age group. As is discussed in the following section, younger women may also develop this disease, especially in the setting of a genetic predisposition. In contrast, stromal cell tumors (such as granulosa or theca cell cancers) may occur in women of reproductive age as well as in the postmenopausal population. Malignant germ cell tumors such as dysgerminomas (the female equivalent of male seminoma) typically occur in the second and third decades. Unless otherwise stated, the term *ovarian cancer* will be used to discuss the more common variety of epithelial malignancy that often affects adult women.

Epidemiology

Epithelial ovarian cancer affects approximately 25,000 U.S. women yearly and is responsible for 15,000 deaths. The sporadic variety occurs with a median age of 60 years and a lifetime risk of 1 in 70. An increased risk for developing this disease is associated with nulliparity, suggesting that incessant ovulation with resultant intermittent proliferation of the ovarian surface epithelium predisposes to malignant transformation. Conversely, a lower risk is associated with pregnancy, birth control pill use, and lactation. The most important risk factor for the development of this tumor, however, is a strong family history of either ovarian and/or breast cancer, suggesting the presence of an inherited germline mutation in either BRCA-1 or BRCA-2. Although such familial ovarian cancer accounts for only 5% of all cases, the clinical presentation of patients with this entity may differ from that

of the sporadic variety in two respects. First, ovarian cancer occurring in the setting of a BRCA-1 or BRCA-2 mutation may present at an earlier age (e.g., 35 to 40 years) compared to the sporadic variety (median age of 60). Second, familial ovarian cancer may behave in a less aggressive fashion in comparison to the sporadic variety, possibly owing to enhanced responsiveness to postoperative chemotherapy, although the data are conflicting in this regard.

Familial Ovarian Cancer

Patients with a strong family history of early-onset breast and/or ovarian cancer are candidates for genetic counseling as a prelude to offering genetic testing. Such counseling should discuss the potential benefits of discovering a germline mutation (including more compulsive mammographic surveillance and screening with a combination of CA-125 plus transvaginal sonography) as well as possible treatment options (including prophylactic mastectomy, prophylactic oophorectomy after childbearing is complete, birth control pill use, and tamoxifen use for possible breast cancer risk reduction). Prophylactic oophorectomy in genetically predisposed individuals does not completely eliminate cancer risk, since malignant transformation of the peritoneal surface may give rise to an intra-abdominal tumor that is histologically indistinguishable from ovarian cancer. Such tumors are referred to as primary peritoneal serous cancers (PPSC) and have a natural history and treatment approach similar to those of epithelial ovarian cancer. Since it is unclear whether any of these approaches confers a survival benefit, and since they are associated with potential medical and psychological morbidity, the patient must be part of the decision-making process. There are also potential negative aspects of knowing the results of genetic testing, including insurance discrimination, survivor guilt (if the test is negative), and anxiety (if the test is positive). Because of the complexity of these issues, individuals with a family history that is suggestive of a genetic predisposition should ideally be referred to a genetics counseling clinic for further evaluation. Other individuals who may be at high risk for familial ovarian cancer include those with a strong family history of right-sided nonpolyposis colon cancer and endometrial cancer (Lynch syndrome II).

Clinical Presentation and Examination

Patients with ovarian cancer often present at an advanced stage, after the tumor has escaped the confines of the ovary and has traveled by peritoneal spread to the upper abdomen (Figure 81-1). Peritoneal nodules often involve the omentum, causing epigastric discomfort, bloating, and early satiety (Figure 81-2). These symptoms are exacerbated by the frequent presence of malignant ascites. For such patients, findings on the general medical examination may include ascites, abdominal masses, an umbilical tumor nodule (Sister Mary Joseph's nodule), and a pleural effusion (the most common site of extra-abdominal spread). When ovarian cancer is suspected in this setting, a pelvic exam may reveal an adnexal mass, although at times, this may be difficult to appreciate in the setting of extensive ascites. Rarely, epithelial ovarian cancer can present as a paraneoplastic syndrome prior to discovery of the primary ovarian neoplasm. Such syndromes include the sign of Leser-Trelat (sudden onset of seborrheic keratoses), Trousseau's syndrome (migratory superficial thrombophlebitis involving

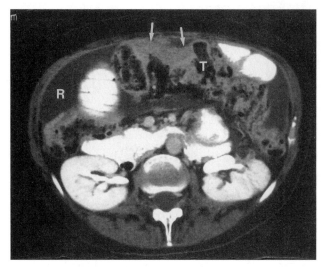

Figure 81-2 ■ Ascites and omental "cake" due to intraperitoneal metastasis from ovarian carcinoma. Computed tomography through the lower abdomen shows ascites in the left and right paracolic gutters and the inframesocolic space. (Right paracolic gutter ascites identified by R.) Omental cake is manifested as an inhomogeneous mass (arrows) abutting the anterior surface of the transverse colon (T). (Courtesy of Stephen E. Rubesin, MD, Hospital of the University of Pennsylvania.)

veins and arteries), and cerebellar degeneration due to the presence of anti-Purkinje cell antibodies. Occasionally, the clear cell and small cell forms of epithelial ovarian cancer may also present with signs and symptoms of hypercalcemia due to secretion of parathyroid hormone–related protein.

In approximately 30% of cases, the disease may be localized to the ovary or to the ovary plus other pelvic structures without upper abdominal involvement. Such patients are often asymptomatic and are detected fortuitously by a mass on routine pelvic exam. Occasionally, early-stage disease causes pelvic pain due to ovarian torsion, which then prompts an unscheduled pelvic exam. Epithelial ovarian cancer of the endometrioid variety may develop in association with a separate uterine cancer, which brings the patient to medical attention owing to postmenopausal vaginal bleeding. In such cases, the ovarian mass is discovered incidentally at the time of pelvic exam or at the time of surgery performed for uterine cancer. Patients with the less common granulosa cell tumor of the ovary may come to medical attention owing to the effects of tumor-derived estrogen secretion. Thus, a postmenopausal woman with a granulosa cell tumor may experience breast tenderness or vaginal bleeding (due to the presence of either endometrial hyperplasia or even endometrial cancer

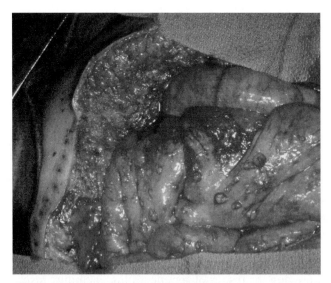

Figure 81-1 ■ Intraoperative appearance of stage III epithelial ovarian cancer. Multiple implants are scattered throughout the peritoneal mesothelial surface of the upper abdomen. (See Color Plate 18.)

as a result of unopposed estrogen secretion by the tumor). Because granulosa cell tumors are highly vascular, they may sometimes rupture and cause hemoperitoneum, resulting in an acute abdomen that can mimic a ruptured ectopic pregnancy.

Finally, it is important to note that the ovaries may be secondarily involved by metastatic tumor from another primary site, in which case the ovarian mass is referred to as a Krukenberg tumor. The most common primary sites that metastasize to the ovaries are the stomach, colorectum, and breast (often the lobular carcinoma variant), in that order of frequency. A history of epigastric discomfort, weight loss, melanotic stools, and iron deficiency anemia should prompt an upper gastrointestinal (GI) tract evaluation to rule out gastric cancer in a patient with ovarian masses.

Clinical Evaluation

Once ovarian cancer is suspected on the basis of the clinical presentation described in the preceding section, a transvaginal ultrasound is often the next most reasonable diagnostic test. Sonography is more sensitive than computed tomography (CT) scanning in the detection of ovarian masses, and it also provides qualitative information about the nature of the mass that may heighten the suspicion for malignancy. For instance, the presence of a complex mass on sonogram, defined as containing both solid and cystic areas, often with internal septations, is highly suspicious for malignancy (Figure 81-3). In contrast, a simple cyst contains only fluid (no mass component), has no septations or internal echogenic material, and is almost never malignant (Figure 81-4). Complex

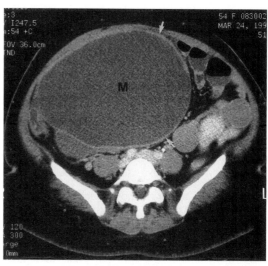

Figure 81-4 ■ Serous cystadenoma. Computed tomography through the pelvis demonstrates a 15-cm low attenuation mass (M) surrounded by a thin rim of contrast-enhancing tissue (arrows). No septations or papillary excrescences are seen. (Courtesy of Stephen E. Rubesin, MD, Hospital of the University of Pennsylvania.)

masses should generally not be biopsied via the percutaneous route, since the cyst could rupture with resultant spillage of tumor contents into the abdominal and pelvic cavities. Because of the need for definitive histologic diagnosis, as well as for tumor debulking (see the next paragraph), the vast majority of patients with a complex mass will require surgical exploration for further evaluation. If the patient is not a good surgical candidate owing to the presence of comorbid disease, a paracentesis or thoracentesis may sometimes reveal an adenocarcinoma of presumed ovarian origin, although it is often difficult to be certain of the primary site under these circumstances. However, for the typical patient who is a good surgical candidate, additional preoperative diagnostic studies such as paracentesis and computed tomography scanning are not generally useful once a complex mass has been discovered by ultrasonography.

Exploratory laparotomy in the hands of an experienced gynecologic cancer surgeon is valuable for several reasons. First, it allows for a definitive tissue diagnosis, thereby establishing the presence of ovarian cancer and excluding Krukenberg metastases from a gastric primary, for instance. Second, it allows for proper staging (Table 81-1), which generally includes a vertical midline incision, inspection of peritoneal and subdiaphragmatic surfaces, omental biopsy, peritoneal washings, and performance of a total abdominal hysterectomy and bilateral salpingo-oophorectomy. Biopsy of para-aortic lymph nodes is

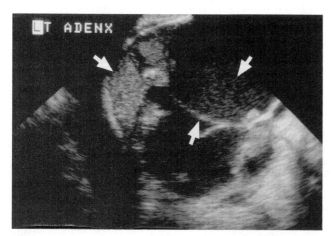

Figure 81-3 ■ Ultrasonography of a complex ovarian cyst. A complex cyst is defined as having both solid (left arrow) and cystic components, often with septations (middle arrow) and internal echoes representing cellular debris (right arrow).

Table 81-1 ∎ **FIGO Surgical Staging and Survival of Ovarian Cancer***

Stage I	Tumor confined to the ovaries
Stage IA (>95%)†	Limited to one ovary, without capsular spread, tumor rupture, positive peritoneal washings, or malignant ascites
Stage IB (>95%)†	Bilateral ovarian involvement, without capsular spread, tumor rupture, positive washings, or malignant ascites
Stage IC (80%)	Capsular spread, tumor rupture, positive washings, or malignant ascites
Stage II	Tumor extends into the pelvis
Stage IIA (80%)	Involvement of the uterus or fallopian tubes
Stage IIB (80%)	Involvement of other pelvic organs (bladder, cul-de-sac implants, vagina, rectum)
Stage IIC (80%)	Pelvic extension, plus findings as indicated for stage IC.
Stage III	Tumor extends to the upper abdomen or involves retroperitoneal lymph nodes
Stage IIIA (50%)	Microscopic seeding outside of the true pelvis (e.g., serosa of the small bowel, undersides of diaphragm, or omental involvement)
Stage IIIB (30%)‡	Gross implants ≤2 cm, prior to debulking
Stage IIIC (20%)§	Gross implants >2 cm, prior to debulking, or the presence of retroperitoneal lymph node involvement (usually para-aortic)
Stage IV (<10%)	Distant organ involvement, including pleural space (most common) or hepatic/splenic parenchyma (unusual)

*The staging system for ovarian cancer is established by the International Federation of Gynecology and Obstetrics (FIGO) and is based on the results obtained at the time of surgery.

†Figures in parentheses reflect estimated five-year survival rates with appropriate postoperative treatment as described in text. Note that 95% survival for stages IA and IB assumes accurate staging and grade I or II histology. For grade III histology (including clear cell), the survival rate for stages IA and IB decreases to 80%.

‡Indicated survival for stage IIIB disease assumes optimal cytoreduction (<1 cm). The survival rate for stage IIIB, suboptimally debulked patients decreases to ≈20%.

§Indicated survival for stage IIIC disease assumes optimal cytoreduction (<1 cm). The survival rate for stage IIIC, suboptimally debulked patients decreases to ≈10–15%.

also performed in patients whose disease appears to be localized to the ovary. (Microscopic nodal disease will be present in 10% to 15% of such cases and may change management as noted below.) Finally, surgery is necessary for tumor debulking, since a strong inverse relationship exists between the amount of residual tumor remaining after surgery and survival. Patients with residual tumor implants measuring less than 1 cm in diameter (optimally debulked) experience a higher response rate and more prolonged survival compared to those with greater than 1 cm residual (suboptimally debulked). It is not known whether debulking has intrinsic therapeutic value or whether the ability to optimally debulk selects for a group of patients with less aggressive tumor characteristics.

Staging, Prognostic Features, and Outcome

Staging

The staging system for ovarian cancer is outlined in Table 81-1 and is defined by the International Federation of Gynecology and Obstetrics (FIGO). It is useful to view ovarian cancer as presenting with either early-stage disease (stages I and II) or advanced-stage disease (stages III and IV), since prognosis and postoperative management considerations differ. Stage I disease is localized to the ovary or ovaries (and assumes that full surgical staging has been performed, including para-aortic nodal biopsy). Stage II disease involves the ovary plus other pelvic structures but without disease extension to the upper abdomen. Within the early-stage group, important substages are identified that have relevance for assigning risk and making treatment decisions. For example, patients with stage IA (unilateral, completely encapsulated) or IB (bilateral, completely encapsulated) tumors, grade I or II, have a greater than 95% cure rate with surgery alone. Higher-risk features within the stage I category include the presence of rupture (especially if it occurs preoperatively), involvement of the ovarian surface by tumor, positive washings, or malignant ascites. Any of these characteristics warrant a stage IC designation and predict five-year disease-free survival rates in the 80% range after adjuvant chemotherapy as described below (see Table 81-1). Any stage II patient is considered to be at relatively high risk for relapse as well. Higher-risk categories within the early-stage group also include patients with grade III histology, including those with the more aggressive clear cell variant

Table 81-2 ■ Common Histologic Types of Epithelial Ovarian Cancer

Histology	Clinical Features
Papillary serous cystadenocarcinoma	The most common type of epithelial ovarian cancer. May also be observed in primary peritoneal serous cancers. Associated with psammoma bodies (see Figure 81-5).
Endometrioid	Resembles endometrial cancer and is sometimes associated with endometriosis. Tends to occur in slightly younger women and at an earlier stage than papillary serous carcinoma. May be associated with a separate endometrial (uterine) cancer in 15% of patients.
Clear cell	Distinguished by cleared-out cytoplasm (due to glycogen) and hobnail nuclei. Also may be associated with endometriosis in 30% to 40% of cases. Humorally mediated hypercalcemia may rarely occur. The most chemoresistant of all epithelial ovarian cancer histologies.
Mucinous	Often with normal or only slightly elevated CA-125 level. The presence of pseudomyxoma peritoneii and bilaterality should suggest an appendiceal primary with metastases to the ovaries.

of epithelial ovarian cancer (discussed later in this chapter and in Table 81-2).

Stages III and IV make up approximately 70% of all ovarian cancer and are characterized by extrapelvic extension (see Figure 81-1). Stage III disease usually involves tumor extension into the upper abdomen but also may be defined as lymph node involvement (usually in the para-aortic region, which is the first drainage site of the ovaries). As is shown in Table 81-1, the prognosis within this group is heterogeneous, depending on the extent of upper abdominal involvement; patients who have microscopic-only disease (stage IIIA) have the best outcome. Stage IV ovarian cancer usually has extended beyond the abdominal cavity to involve the pleural space (not usually the lung parenchyma), other sites of extra-abdominal disease being much less common at presentation. The presence of pulmonary parenchymal disease or other unusual sites such as bone or central nervous system (CNS) metastases at the time of diagnosis should prompt a search for another primary disease such as breast cancer. However, it should be kept in mind that during the course of ovarian cancer, occasional patients with indolent disease may eventually develop metastatic disease in uncharacteristic locations, including the central nervous system (including mass lesions and carcinomatous meningitis). Hepatic or splenic parenchymal tumor (as opposed to local capsular involvement) at the time of diagnosis also qualifies as stage IV disease.

Histology

There are four major histologic subtypes of epithelial ovarian cancer (see Table 81-2). The papillary serous histology is the most common and is sometimes associated with psammoma bodies, which are concentric rings of calcification (Figure 81-5). Psammoma bodies are also observed in other malignancies, such as pap-

illary thyroid cancer and occasionally lung and breast cancer. However, the presence of psammoma bodies in an intra-abdominal malignancy strongly suggests a müllerian-origin source. The papillary serous histologic variant is also observed in patients who develop primary peritoneal serous cancer, as was noted previously. Endometrioid histology is the second most common type of ovarian cancer subtype and is notable for the synchronous occurrence of uterine cancer in 15% of cases, as well as an association with endometriosis. Compared to the papillary serous histology, endometrioid ovarian cancer may occur at an earlier stage and a younger age, even in the absence of a genetic predisposition. Clear cell carcinoma is a relatively chemoresistant histology that confers a worse prognosis, stage for stage, compared to papillary serous ovarian cancer. It is notable for containing

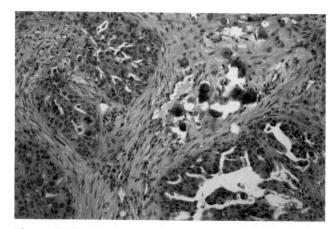

Figure 81-5 ■ Papillary serous ovarian cancer with psammoma bodies. Psammoma bodies are structures composed of concentric rings of calcification, often observed in papillary serous ovarian or primary peritoneal serous cancers. There are several psammoma bodies just to the right of center in this (original magnification ×40) photomicrograph (hematoxylin and eosin stain). (See Color Plate 18.)

characteristic "hobnail" cells and for occasionally producing parathyroid hormone–related protein, resulting in paraneoplastic hypercalcemia. Paradoxically, this tumor is more likely to present with earlier-stage disease than papillary serous cancer, and it may sometimes recur in lymph nodes in the absence of extensive intraperitoneal disease. Like endometrioid ovarian cancer, clear cell cancer may be associated with coexistent endometriosis in up to 30% to 40% of patients. Finally, primary mucinous ovarian cancer is often early stage, although it sometimes can be associated with advanced intra-abdominal spread and rarely with pseudomyxoma peritonei. Such cases are relatively chemoresistant and must be distinguished from primary mucinous adenocarcinoma of gastrointestinal origin, which usually originates in the appendix and is more likely to cause pseudomyxoma peritoneii. The possibility that a mucinous ovarian tumor might represent a metastatic deposit from an occult appendiceal primary should prompt careful evaluation and/removal of the appendix, especially if the ovarian tumor is bilateral.

Prognostic Factors and Outcome

The two most important prognostic factors for patients with epithelial ovarian cancer are stage and residual disease status (Tables 81-1 and 81-3). Adequately treated patients with early-stage disease have five-year survival rates in the range of 80% to 95%, depending on the substage, as is noted in Table 81-1. In contrast, the five-year survival rate of stage III patients with optimally debulked disease (less than 1 cm residual) drops to 25% to 30% after appropriate surgery and postoperative chemotherapy (see the following sections), and the survival rate of patients with

---

Table 81-3 ■ Selected Adverse Prognostic Factors in Epithelial Ovarian Cancer

Advanced disease (stages III/IV)
Suboptimal cytoreduction (>1 cm residual disease after surgery)
High grade
Clear cell histology
Older age (>65 years)
Persistant CA-125 elevation after three cycles of chemotherapy
Failure to achieve a CA-125 level of <15 IU/mL on completion of chemotherapy
Rapid recurrence (within six months of completing first-line therapy)
p53 mutation
Underexpression of the BAX protein (a death-promoting member of the BCL-2 family)
Amplification of the HER-2/*neu* gene (a member of the EGF tyrosine kinase receptor family)

---

suboptimally debulked stage III disease (greater than 1 cm residual) or those with stage IV disease is in the range of 10% to 15% after treatment. Adverse prognostic factors also include a slow rate of CA-125 decline during chemotherapy (i.e., persistent elevation of CA-125 after three cycles), failure to achieve a postchemotherapy CA-125 nadir of less than 15 IU/mL, and high-grade tumors (including clear cell histology) (see Table 81-3).

Primary Postsurgical Treatment

Patient Selection

Almost all patients with epithelial ovarian cancer require postoperative chemotherapy in an attempt to eradicate residual tumor. However, a small subset of patients are diagnosed with low-risk, early-stage ovarian cancer and have an excellent five-year survival rate (greater than 95%) after surgery alone. Such low-risk patients are those with stage IA or IB disease, grade I or II after complete staging, including performance of lymph node biopsy and washings. In contrast, patients with high-risk, early-stage disease are defined as those with stage IC, stage I grade III, and stage II tumors. Without postoperative treatment, this group collectively has a disease-free survival rate of approximately 60%, which increases to the 80% range after treatment with platinum-based chemotherapy. Although there is some debate regarding whether postoperative adjuvant chemotherapy in patients with high-risk early-stage disease actually improves survival (in addition to improving disease-free survival), the current practice in the United States is to offer such therapy to appropriate patients. Essentially all patients with stages III and IV tumors will have residual disease that requires postoperative treatment, with long-term survival for these groups as outlined previously.

Choice of Postoperative Treatment

The standard postoperative treatment for high-risk patients with epithelial ovarian cancer is systemic chemotherapy with paclitaxel and carboplatin for a total of six cycles. The use of intraperitoneal chemotherapy is not a standard approach at present, although this is currently under investigation. There is some debate regarding the minimum amount of chemotherapy required for patients with high-risk early-stage disease (i.e., stage IC, stage I grade III, and stage II tumors). A trial comparing three versus six cycles of paclitaxel and carboplatin in the early-stage setting has been completed, although the results are not yet available. Until the results of this trial are known, it is reasonable to administer six cycles of

Epithelial Ovarian Cancer: First-Line Therapy

Exam	Diagnostic Studies	Surgical Options	Stage	First-Line Chemotherapy
Pelvic mass	Ultrasound, ± CXR, ± CA-125 (CT scanning usually not necessary)	For complex mass on ultrasound that is suspicious for malignancy: Exploratory laparotomy with TAH/BSO and staging (includes washings, omental biopsy, ± para-aortic node biopsies[1] and debulking[2]	Stage I A or B, grade I or II	Observation[3,4]
			Stage I C[5], Stage I, grade III[6], Any stage II	Paclitaxel and carboplatin for six cycles[4,7,8]
			Stages III or IV	Paclitaxel and carboplatin for six cycles[4,8,9]

[1] Information from para-aortic nodes might change management for patients who are otherwise stage IA or IB, grades I or II (i.e., such a patient might be upstaged to stage IIIC disease).

[2] Occasional patients who are very poor surgical candidates may be treated with upfront chemotherapy (without surgery) if deemed to have a müllerian-origin tumor on the basis of a mass on ultrasound and distinctive cytology (pleural or peritoneal).

[3] Assumes adequate staging.

[4] Observation after completion of primary therapy includes exam and CA-125 every three months for the first year, every four months during the second year, every six months for one to two years, then every six to 12 months as clinically indicated thereafter. CT scanning only if clinically indicated.

[5] Stage IC solely on the basis of intraoperative rupture may not represent a high-risk feature under all circumstances. In contrast, preoperative rupture is more strongly associated with risk of relapse.

[6] Clear cell carcinoma is assumed to be grade III.

[7] The comparative effectiveness of three versus six cycles of adjuvant chemotherapy for high-risk, early-stage disease is not yet known. Although platinum-based chemotherapy decreases the risk of relapse in this setting, its impact on overall survival is less clear.

[8] Reasonable dose ranges are paclitaxel 175 mg/m^2 IV over three hours, with standard decadron, benadryl, ranitidine (or equivalent) premedication, followed by carboplatin dosed to achieve an area under the curve (AUC) of 5 to 6. The first-line use of cisplatin is no longer recommended owing to increased toxicity and lack of therapeutic superiority over carboplatin. A switch to cisplatin may be considered if carboplatin is poorly tolerated due to myelosuppression.

[9] Interval cytoreduction may be considered for patients who were suboptimally debulked at initial surgery and who are having a response to the first three cycles of chemotherapy.

CXR = chest X-ray

chemotherapy as tolerated to any patient who qualifies for postoperative adjuvant treatment (early or advanced disease).

Paclitaxel (Taxol) is a taxane that exerts its cytotoxic effects through a novel mechanism of action involving stabilization of the microtubulin polymer, preventing dissociation of the mitotic spindle during M phase, with subsequent mitotic arrest and apoptosis. Paclitaxel was originally isolated from the bark of the Pacific yew tree, *Taxus brevifolia*, although it is now semisynthesized from a precursor called diacetylbaccatin III, obtained from the needles of a related yew tree, *Taxus baccata*. In contrast to taxanes, platinum compounds such as cisplatin and carboplatin exert their cytotoxicity through a mechanism of action that involves formation of intrastrand adducts with DNA at guanine nucleotides. Thus, the nonoverlapping mechanisms of action between platinum and taxanes offer the potential for clinical non-cross-resistance, and the two agents in combination have been shown to be superior to older combinations using platinum and cyclophosphamide. Although initial ovarian cancer trials were performed by using a combination of paclitaxel and cisplatin, this regimen has been largely replaced by the paclitaxel and carboplatin combination, which is equally efficacious, more convenient to administer, and less toxic.

For first-line therapy, paclitaxel is typically administered at a starting dose of 175 mg/m^2 intravenously over three hours, followed by carboplatin at an area under the curve (AUC) of five to six intravenously over 60 minutes, repeated every three weeks as tolerated for a total of six cycles. There is no convincing advantage to the use of paclitaxel doses of greater than 175 mg/m^2 or carboplatin doses greater than a range of AUC 4 to 6 in the treatment of patients with epithelial ovarian cancer. Because paclitaxel may cause a hypersensitivity reaction (perhaps partly due to the Cremaphor vehicle), pretreatment with dexamethasone (e.g., 20 mg orally approximately 12 and six hours prior), diphenhydramine (50 mg intravenously 30 minutes prior), and an H$_2$-blocker such as ranitidine (50 mg intravenously 30 minutes prior) is required. Although paclitaxel is minimally emetogenic, a 5-hydroxytryptamine receptor blocker such as granisetron (Kytril) 30 minutes prior to carboplatin is also advised. Prophylactic use of an agent such as prochlorperazine (Compazine) for two days posthemotherapy is generally effective at preventing delayed platinum-induced nausea. Approximately 20% of patients will experience paclitaxel-induced myalgias and arthralgias, which typically begin 36 to 48 hours after drug administration. Such myalgias are usually mild and may be effectively treated with nonsteroidal anti-inflammatory agents, although occasionally treatment with narcotic analgesics and/or a steroid taper is necessary for more severe cases.

Side Effects and Management

As was noted previously, acute toxicities of this regimen are largely related to paclitaxel and include hypersensitivity, myalgias/arthralgias, and nausea. Hypersensitivity is usually manifested by an anaphylactoid reaction in 5% to 10% of patients, almost always during the first or second cycle of treatment. This reaction does not represent true anaphylaxis and is characterized by diffuse skin erythema, shortness of breath (usually without wheezes), back pain, chest discomfort, and anxiety. In these cases, the blood pressure is almost always elevated and distinguishes this from a true anaphylactic reaction. Management includes temporarily discontinuing paclitaxel, administration of intravenous diphenhydramine and dexamethasone, and patient/nursing staff reassurance. The signs and symptoms of such an anaphylactoid reaction usually subside quickly (within 30 minutes), and it is often possible to restart the paclitaxel infusion at 10% of the original rate, gradually increasing the infusion rate to a more standard level over the next one to two hours, with careful monitoring of vital signs. Rarely, true anaphylaxis may occur in fewer than 1% of patients, characterized by bronchospasm, urticaria, and hypotension. Such reactions are potentially life-threatening and require a management approach that is appropriate for anaphylaxis from any cause. Although a repeat trial of paclitaxel (at a slow infusion rate and with careful monitoring) in a patient who has experienced a severe hypersensitivity reaction (such as true anaphylaxis) may be successful, such an attempt should be preceded by aggressive pretreatment with dexamethasone (e.g., beginning 24 hours prior to rechallenge) and with the knowledge that a life-threatening reaction may still occur. Pretreatment regimens for rechallenging patients with paclitaxel have been published, and suggested reading is provided.

The paclitaxel and carboplatin combination results in predictable subacute toxicity, which is generally self-limited and well tolerated. Absolute neutropenia in the range of 500 neutrophils/μL is not uncommon with this regimen, occurring typically at day 14 of each cycle and lasting only two to four days. Thrombocytopenia rarely occurs below the 75,000 to 100,000/μL range. The short-lived nature of paclitaxel-related myelosuppression is usually well tolerated, although febrile neutropenia requiring hospitalization for parenteral antibiotic therapy may occur in approximately 10% of patients. Rarely, bowel perforation has been associated with paclitaxel use, thought to be due to gastrointestinal mucosal ulceration (although mucositis is unusual with this regimen). The development of abdominal pain in an ovarian cancer patient receiving paclitaxel should prompt consideration of bowel perforation in addition to other possibilities such as tumor-related bowel obstruction. Hair loss is significant with this regimen, usually beginning at day 10 and becoming very noticeable by day 21 of the first cycle. Such hair loss is often characterized by total alopecia, which may involve hair at other sites, including the eyebrows, eyelashes, and pubic regions.

The most common chronic toxicity of the paclitaxel/carboplatin regimen is peripheral neuropathy, which is often mild and reversible, although rarely it may be more severe and irreversible. The neuropathy may affect up to 30% of patients and usually manifests itself as mild numbness and tingling of the fingertips and toes, usually without objective sensory findings on neurologic examination. This side effect generally occurs after three to four cycles of therapy, although it occasionally happens after the first dose. At times, mild tingling is reported several days after treatment, lasts one week, and then spontaneously resolves. At other times, the mild tingling persists but does not interfere with daily activities such as walking, climbing stairs, or buttoning clothing. It is useful to ask the patient direct questions regarding these activities to assess the degree to which neuropathy is interfering with daily functioning. If the neuropathy is mild and nonprogressive and does not interfere with daily activities, then dose reduction of either paclitaxel or carboplatin is usually unnecessary. Some patients believe that the use of pyridoxine (50 mg PO daily) provides benefit in these circumstances, although the value of this agent for reducing neuropathy is not well established. If the neuropathy is progressive or interferes with daily activities, a dose reduction in paclitaxel (or both paclitaxel and carboplatin for more worrisome symptoms) is reasonable. If neuropathy does not respond to these measures, it is sometimes necessary to discontinue paclitaxel and to complete therapy with dose-reduced carboplatin (e.g., AUC of 4) as a single agent (or rarely to discontinue treatment altogether). More severe neuropathy may be associated with painful dysesthesias that are exacerbated by mild pressure, such as when the feet touch bed linens at night. In this instance, the use of a mild narcotic analgesic for pain as well as an agent such as low-dose gabapentin (Neurontin) may be effective. In addition to peripheral manifestations, neuropathy may occasionally result in autonomic dysfunction (e.g., orthostatic hypotension) or hearing loss (the latter toxicity usually being attributed to carboplatin). In elderly patients with a degree of baseline hearing loss, it is good practice to obtain baseline audiograms to avoid potential confusion later in the course of therapy. With the approach outlined above, it is important to realize that mild peripheral neuropathy is generally reversible with time, although it might require up to one year before full recovery is achieved. Recent reports suggest that the combination of docetaxel (Taxotere) and carboplatin is equally efficacious, but associated with less neuropathy (and more myelosuppression), when compared to the paclitaxel and carboplatin regimen.

Interval Cytoreduction

Patients with suboptimally cytoreduced disease (greater than 1 cm in greatest diameter) are at high risk for relapse and death despite treatment with postoperative chemotherapy. In an attempt to improve survival of this high-risk group, a large randomized study has been performed by the European Organization for the Research and Treatment of Cancer (EORTC) in which suboptimally debulked patients were assigned to receive either chemotherapy alone (six cycles) or a repeat attempt at debulking midway through chemotherapy (an "interval" cytoreductive procedure). Patients who were randomized to undergo interval cytoreduction experienced a six-month median survival benefit compared to those who received chemotherapy alone. Since the chemotherapy regimen used in this study was cyclophosphamide and cisplatin, it is not known whether the current widespread use of paclitaxel and platinum might negate the potential benefit of interval cytoreduction demonstrated in this trial. A confirmatory trial of interval cytoreduction in patients treated with paclitaxel and platinum is currently being conducted by the Gynecologic Oncology Group to answer this question. At the present time, it is reasonable to consider the use of interval cytoreduction in any ovarian cancer patient with suboptimally debulked disease (greater than 1 cm) who is a good surgical candidate and who is demonstrating a clinical response to the first three cycles of chemotherapy.

Interval cytoreduction may also be considered for the patient who cannot undergo surgical exploration at the time of initial presentation. Such patients are those who are poor surgical candidates owing to comorbid disease or to deconditioning as a result of poor nutrition. A clinical diagnosis of ovarian or primary peritoneal serous cancer may be suspected on the basis of pleural or peritoneal fluid cytology showing clusters of cells compatible with a Müllerian-origin tumor, an elevated CA-125 level, and a normal CEA level (making a gastrointestinal primary less likely). The absence of breast masses, occult blood in stool, and microcytic/hypochromic anemia also argues in favor of a Müllerian-origin tumor in this setting. It is reasonable to consider treating such patients with paclitaxel and carboplatin, without an initial surgical exploration, with a plan to perform an interval cytoreductive procedure if the patient responds to chemotherapy and her performance status improves.

Follow-up Evaluation and Management of Recurrent Disease

Follow-Up and Detection of Relapse

A CA-125 level greater than 35 IU/mL will be present in at least 80% of patients with advanced-stage disease and 50% of patients with early-stage disease. If initially elevated, the CA-125 level is the most sensitive marker of response to chemotherapy as well as disease recurrence. It is reasonable to serially follow this marker during the duration of chemotherapy (e.g., at the beginning of each cycle) to ensure that the patient is experiencing a response to first-line therapy as well as to obtain prognostic information. Normalization of the CA-125 level to less than 35 IU/mL within three cycles of first-line therapy predicts improved survival, as does achievement of a CA-125 level of less than 15 IU/mL after the completion of therapy.

Most patients who complete first-line therapy with six cycles of paclitaxel and carboplatin will have a normal CA-125 level and a normal physical examination (including pelvic examination). For these patients, it is not usually necessary to obtain a posttreatment computed tomography scan unless the patient has persistent, unexplained symptoms or the patient is participating in a clinical trial that requires this test. The computed tomography scan is relatively insensitive for the detection of small-volume residual disease in this setting, and the chance of finding bulky residual disease in the face of a normal CA-125 level and absence of symptoms is low. After completion of first-line therapy, patients who are asymptomatic and have a normal examination and CA-125 level can be followed by physical examination

TREATMENT

Epithelial Ovarian Cancer: Persistent or Recurrent Disease

Clinical Setting	Surgical Options	Second-Line Therapy
Serologic (marker-only) relapse: Rising CA-125 in the absence of symptoms, exam findings, or CT scan evidence of recurrence	None	Consideration of tamoxifen[1] or arimidex
Clinical relapse (as defined by disease-related symptoms, and/or exam findings, and/or CT scan evidence of recurrence) with a chemotherapy-free interval (CFI) of 6 to 12 months	None, unless indicated for relief of bowel obstruction	Consideration of single-agent carboplatin or paclitaxel (or combination of both for aggressive recurrence)[2]
Clinical relapse with a CFI of >12 months	Consideration of secondary cytoreduction[3]	Consideration of single-agent carboplatin or paclitaxel (or combination of both for aggressive recurrence)[2]
Clinical relapse with a CFI of <6 months	None, unless indicated for relief of bowel obstruction	Consideration of potentially non-cross-resistant agents[4]

[1] Relapsed ovarian cancer is generally incurable. There is no evidence that immediate institution of cytotoxic chemotherapy for treatment of marker-only relapse confers a survival advantage in the asymptomatic patient. Tamoxifen is associated with a response rate of 15% to 20%, although median time to response is two to three months.

[2] Response rate approximately 30%. No evidence that combination therapy (paclitaxel plus carboplatin) is superior to single-agent therapy in the relapsed setting. Combination therapy is reasonable to consider in patients with significant symptoms due to bulky disease.

[3] Patients with a relatively long chemotherapy-free interval who are optimally cytoreduced at the time of relapse may experience longer median survivals than to those who cannot be cytoreduced. However, it is not clear whether this represents a selection phenomenon or an intrinsic therapeutic benefit of the procedure.

[4] Response rate approximately 15% to 20%. Reasonable considerations include liposomal doxorubicin or single-agent topotecan. Other possibilities include gemcitabine, PO etoposide, or navelbine.

and CA-125 levels every three months for the first year, every four months for the second year, and every four to six months thereafter. These are offered as guidelines only, since the frequency of follow-up visits and even the value of serial CA-125 determinations during follow-up have not been extensively investigated. It is reasonable to consider obtaining a follow-up computed tomography scan during the surveillance period for the development of unexplained symptoms (e.g., abdominal bloating or cramps), suspicious exam findings, or a new elevation in the CA-125 level. It is also reasonable to obtain a computed tomography scan during first-line therapy if the CA-125 level does not fall after several cycles of treatment. Although most patients will respond to first-line therapy with paclitaxel and carboplatin, approximately 30% of patients with suboptimally debulked advanced disease will demonstrate primary resistance to this regimen.

Patients with advanced disease who have no clinical or serologic evidence of tumor after completion of first-line chemotherapy have a greater than 50% chance of harboring small-volume residual disease within the abdominal cavity. Consequently, performance of a repeat laparotomy after completion of chemotherapy (i.e., a "second-look" procedure) has been used in the past to identify patients with persistent disease, in hopes of improving outcome through the use of additional chemotherapy. At the present time, the evidence suggests that there is no survival advantage to performing second-look laparotomy, since residual disease almost always means that the patient is incurable with the currently available second-line options described below. Therefore, performance of second-look laparotomy should be restricted to the clinical trial setting and should not generally be used in routine clinical practice.

Relapse Management

Marker-Only Relapse

The CA-125 level generally provides a sensitive and specific marker for relapsed disease in patients with a known diagnosis of ovarian cancer. If the CA-125 is discovered to be newly elevated at the time of a follow-up visit, it should be repeated to confirm the result, and a history, physical exam, and computed tomography scan are reasonable to perform. It is not unusual to detect an elevation in the CA-125 several months prior to the development of signs, symptoms, or radiographic findings of recurrence (i.e., marker-only relapse). The median lead time between CA-125 elevation and development of symptoms or radiographic findings is in the range of three to four months, although some patients may be asymptomatic and have normal computed tomography scans for up to one year before clinically evident disease develops. It should be noted that the CA-125 level may be elevated in nonmalignant conditions, including gastroenteritis, hepatitis, pneumonia, and recent abdominal surgery. In addition, other malignancies may be associated with a CA-125 level elevation, including breast and lung cancers. These issues should be kept in mind when the CA-125 level is found to be newly elevated during follow-up, although the most common reason for a CA-125 elevation in this situation is still relapsed ovarian cancer. Obviously, the CA-125 level might not be a reliable marker of recurrence for patients who never exhibited an elevation at the time of original diagnosis, and rarely it might not be elevated despite overt clinical recurrence (even if it was elevated at the time of original diagnosis). In these cases, the development of signs (pelvic mass, ascites) and/or symptoms (bloating, cramps, change in bowel habits) should prompt performance of computed tomography scanning for further evaluation, regardless of a normal CA-125 level.

Relapsed epithelial cancer of the ovary is almost always incurable. Although a CA-125 elevation is often the earliest sign of relapse, there is no evidence that institution of cytotoxic chemotherapy for marker-only relapse confers a survival advantage. In addition, the use of cytotoxic chemotherapy has the potential for compromising quality of life at a time when the patient is asymptomatic. Thus, marker-only relapse is often managed by avoiding the use of cytotoxic chemotherapy and considering an agent such as tamoxifen, which is capable of inducing responses in approximately 15% to 20% of patients with relapsed disease and is generally well tolerated. It is important to discuss the potential for thrombosis, hot flashes, and nausea with the use of tamoxifen, and it should be avoided in patients with a known clotting diathesis. The median time to response to tamoxifen in the relapsed disease setting is two to three months. If a patient fails a trial of tamoxifen, consideration of cytotoxic chemotherapy is a reasonable next step, as outlined in the following section.

Indications and Options for Cytotoxic Chemotherapy

Patients with relapsed ovarian cancer are reasonable candidates for cytotoxic chemotherapy if they have symptoms that are attributable to recurrent disease (e.g., bloating, cramps, change in bowel habits), and/or exam findings (e.g., pelvic mass, ascites), and/or significant evidence of bulky disease on computed tomography scan. Patients who fail a two- to three-month trial of tamoxifen for marker-only relapse are usually candidates for cytotoxic chemotherapy as well, since they typically develop one or more of the indications listed previously. Prior to instituting chemotherapy for relapsed disease, it is reasonable to consider whether performance of a so-called secondary debulking laparotomy is indicated. Patients who can be successfully cytoreduced to a minimal disease state (e.g., less than 1 cm residual) at the time of relapse tend to have more prolonged survival rates than those who cannot be optimally cytoreduced. However, the value of this procedure in the relapsed setting has not been investigated in a prospective randomized fashion, and it is almost never curative. Patient characteristics that predict for ability to perform a successful secondary cytoreduction include (1) interval of greater than 12 months between end of chemotherapy and time of relapse, (2) localized pelvic relapse without extensive upper abdominal or extra-abdominal disease, and (3) absence of ascites. Since the intrinsic therapeutic value of this procedure has not been formally demonstrated, its use should be limited to those patients who could potentially benefit on the basis of criteria such as those listed previously.

Once a decision has been made to institute cytotoxic chemotherapy for relapsed disease, the choice of agent should be based partly on the chemotherapy-free interval (CFI), defined as the interval of time between the end of first-line chemotherapy and the onset of relapse. Patients who relapse with a chemotherapy-free interval greater than six months are potentially responsive again to first-line treatment with platinum or paclitaxel. Assuming that the patients are otherwise good candidates for these agents, it is reasonable to begin therapy with single-agent carboplatin, reserving single-agent paclitaxel (or other options such as liposomal doxorubicin, gemcitabine, or topotecan) for the development of platinum-resistance. Carboplatin as a single agent (e.g., AUC of 5) is often well tolerated, does not usually cause significant hair loss, and is more active than any other drug, including paclitaxel. In addition, there is no evidence at the present time to suggest a survival advantage to the use of combination chemotherapy in the palliative treatment of patients with recurrent ovarian cancer. If carboplatin fails to induce a response or if resistance to this agent develops, a switch to another agent such as single-agent paclitaxel is then reasonable. Administration of paclitaxel at a dose of 175 mg/m^2 over three hours every three weeks as tolerated (with standard premedication as discussed) is reasonable, although the use of a lower-dose weekly paclitaxel schedule is also an option. Lower-dose weekly paclitaxel (e.g., 80 mg/m^2 on days 1, 8, and 15, with a one-week rest period) is generally well tolerated and less myelosuppressive than the every-three-week dosing schedule, although premedication is still required and neuropathy may be dose limiting. Finally, although many patients with platinum-sensitive relapse (i.e., chemotherapy-free interval greater than six months) are best served by starting with single-agent carboplatin, the use of the paclitaxel/carboplatin combination may occasionally be a better option for those who relapse in an aggressive fashion, with explosive ascites and significant evidence of bulky disease on computed tomography scan.

Patients who have evidence of persistent disease after completion of first-line therapy, recur with a chemotherapy-free interval less than six months, or develop resistance to second-line use of platinum are often treated with a potentially non-cross-resistant agent such as liposomal doxorubicin (Doxil), gemcitabine (Bemzar), or topotecan (Hycamtin). Liposomal doxorubicin and topotecan are equally efficacious in the treatment of platinum-resistant ovarian cancer, with response rates of 15% to 20%, although liposomal doxorubicin is more convenient to administer and often better tolerated. Liposomal doxorubicin is a topoisomerase II inhibitor and is administered at a dose of 40 mg/m^2 once every four weeks, at an infusion rate of less than 1 mg/minute to minimize the risk of an acute hypersensitivity reaction. Occasionally, the cycle length must be prolonged and the dose must be decreased owing to the development of the hand–foot syndrome (palmar–plantar erythrodysesthesia, PPE). Hair loss and myelosuppression are generally not significant problems with this agent, although mucositis can occur, especially in association with palmar-plantar erythrodysesthesia. As with doxorubicin, there is the potential for anthracycline-induced cardiomyopathy, although the risk for developing this problem is less with Doxil. For patients who fail to respond to liposomal doxorubicin or who cannot tolerate the drug owing to severe hand–foot syndrome, topotecan is a reasonable next step. Topotecan is a topoisomerase I inhibitor and is generally administered at a dose of 1.25 mg/m^2/day, days 1 through 5, every three weeks. The drug has potential for myelosuppression, and the dose should be reduced in the presence of significant renal insufficiency.

For platinum-resistant patients who fail to respond to liposomal doxorubicin or topotecan, other options include gemcitabine, oral etoposide, or navelbine. The chance of obtaining a meaningful palliative response to such third- or fourth-line chemotherapy is small and must be balanced against toxicity and quality-of-life considerations. A heavily pretreated patient who has a waning performance status due to progressive intra-abdominal disease may be better served by supportive care measures designed to control pain than by administration of another chemotherapy agent with little hope of benefit.

References

Alberts DS, Liu PY, Hannigan EV, et al: Intraperitoneal cisplatin plus intravenous cyclophosphamide versus intravenous cisplatin plus intravenous cyclophosphamide for stage III ovarian cancer. N Engl J Med 1996;335:1950–1955.

Bast RC, Klug TL, John ES, et al: A radioimmunoassay using a monoclonal antibody to monitor the course of epithelial ovarian cancer. N Engl J Med 1983;309:883–887.

Bolis G, Colombo N, Pecorelli S, et al: Adjuvant treatment for early epithelial ovarian cancer: Results of two randomized clinical trials comparing cisplatin to no further treatment or chromic phosphate. Ann Oncol 1995;6:887–893.

Bookman MA, Malmstrom H, Bolis G, et al: Topotecan for the treatment of advanced epithelial ovarian cancer: An open-label phase II study in patients treated after prior chemotherapy that contained cisplatin or carboplatin and paclitaxel. J Clin Oncol 16:3345–3352.

Bookman MA, McGuire WP, Kilpatrick D, et al: Carboplatin and paclitaxel in ovarian carcinoma: A phase I study of the Gynecologic Oncology Group. J Clin Oncol 1996;14:1895–1902.

Burke W, Daly M, Garber J, et al: Recommendations for follow-up care of individuals with an inherited predisposition to cancer: II. BRCA1 and BRCA2. Cancer Genetics Studies Consortium. JAMA 1997;277:997–1003.

Cannistra SA: Cancer of the ovary. N Engl J Med 1993;329:1550–1559.

McGuire WP, Hoskins WJ, Brady MF, et al: Cyclophosphamide and cisplatin compared with paclitaxel and cisplatin in patients with stage III and stage IV ovarian cancer. N Engl J Med 1996;334:1–6.

Muggia FM, Hainsworth JD, Jeffers S, et al: Phase II study of liposomal doxorubicin in refractory ovarian cancer: Antitumor activity and toxicity modification by liposomal encapsulation. J Clin Oncol 1997;15:987–993.

Ozols RF: Treatment of recurrent ovarian cancer: Increasing options—"recurrent" results. J Clin Oncol 1997;15:2177–2180.

Ozols RF: Paclitaxel plus carboplatin in the treatment of ovarian cancer. Semin Oncol 1999;26:84–89.

Peereboom DM, Donehower RC, Eisenhauer EA, et al: Successful re-treatment with taxol after major hypersensitivity reactions. J Clin Oncol 1993;11:885–890.

Piccart MJP, Bertelsen K, James K, et al: Randomized intergroup trial of cisplatin-paclitaxel versus cisplatin-cyclophosphamide in women with advanced epithelial ovarian cancer: Three-year results. J Natl Cancer Inst 2000;92:699–708.

Rowinsky EK, Donehower RC: Paclitaxel (Taxol). N Engl J Med 1995;332:1004–1014.

Rubin SC, Benjamin I, Behbakht K, et al: Clinical and pathological features of ovarian cancer in women with germ-line mutations of BRCA1. N Engl J Med 1996;335:1413–1416.

Segna RA, Dottino PR, Mandeli JP, et al: Secondary cytoreduction for ovarian cancer following cisplatin therapy. J Clin Oncol 1993;11:434–439.

Struewing JP, Hartge P, Wacholder S, et al: The risk of cancer associated with specific mutations of BRCA1 and BRCA2 among Ashkenazi Jews. N Engl J Med 1997;336:1401–1408.

Van der Burg MEL, Van Lent M, Buyse M, et al: The effect of debulking surgery after induction chemotherapy on the prognosis in advanced epithelial ovarian cancer. N Engl J Med 1995;332:629–634.

Young RC, Walton LA, Ellenberg SS, et al: Adjuvant therapy in stage I and stage II epithelial ovarian cancer. N Engl J Med 1990;322:1021–1027.

Chapter 82
Trophoblastic Tumors

Donald P. Goldstein and Ross S. Berkowitz

Introduction

Any physician who cares for women in the reproductive age is likely to encounter patients with gestational trophoblastic tumors (GTT). Gestational trophoblastic tumors encompass a spectrum of interrelated disease processes originating in the placenta. Other terms that describe this group of diseases include *gestational trophoblastic disease* and *gestational trophoblastic neoplasms*. The histologically distinct disease entities encompassed by this term include complete and partial hydatidiform mole, placental site trophoblastic tumor (PSTT), and choriocarcinoma (CCA). Before the advent of sensitive assays for human chorionic gonadotropin (hCG) and effective chemotherapy, gestational trophoblastic tumors often resulted in substantial morbidity and mortality. However, with the currently available quantitative assays for the beta subunit of hCG (β-hCG) for early diagnosis, monitoring treatment and follow-up, as well as improved diagnostic techniques and advances in chemotherapy, most women with gestational trophoblastic tumors can now be cured, and their reproductive function can be preserved.

Epidemiology

The incidence of molar pregnancy varies dramatically in different regions of the world and appears to be highest in Asia. Japan has a reported incidence of 2 of 1,000 pregnancies, which is twofold to threefold higher than the incidence in Europe and North America. In Ireland, the incidence of complete and partial moles (see following section on distinction between molar types) has been determined to be 1 of 1,945 and 1 of 695 pregnancies, respectively. In the United States, hydatidiform moles are observed in approximately 1 of 600 therapeutic abortions and 1 of 1,000 to 1,200 pregnancies. Some of the variations in worldwide incidence may result from discrepancies between population and hospital-based data. However, the high incidence of molar pregnancies in some populations has been attributed to nutritional and socioeconomic factors. For example, in Korea, the incidence of molar pregnancy has shown a consistent and continuing decrease over the past four decades, presumably due in part to changing social conditions, including completion of childbearing at an earlier age. Low levels of carotene intake may explain some of the global differences in the incidence of complete mole. Regions with a high incidence of complete molar pregnancy correspond to geographic areas with high frequency of vitamin A deficiency. Maternal age has consistently been demonstrated to be a risk factor for complete mole. The risk of complete mole is two times higher for women over the age of 35 and 7.5 times higher for women over age 40 years. The risk for a complete or partial mole is increased two and three times, respectively, after a spontaneous abortion. After two consecutive abortions, the risk of a complete mole increases by a factor of 32. The risk of partial mole appears to be associated with a woman's reproductive history rather than maternal age or dietary factors; these include irregular menstrual cycles and the long-term use of oral contraceptives.

Approximately 20% of patients with complete hydatidiform mole will develop persistent gestational trophoblastic tumors. In contrast, the risk of persistent disease in patients with partial mole is 1% to 5%. Metastatic disease will develop in about 5% of patients with complete hydatidiform mole and rarely after partial moles. Choriocarcinoma occurs in approximately 1 in 20,000 to 40,000 pregnancies; about half of gestational choriocarcinomas develop after term pregnancies, with 25% following molar pregnancies and 25% following other gestations (i.e., miscarriages and ectopics).

Molar Pregnancy
Clinical Presentation

Recent studies have defined two different forms of hydatidiform mole: partial and complete. They are dis-

Table 82-1 ■ Features of Partial and Complete Hydatidiform Moles

Feature	Partial Mole	Complete Mole
Karyotype	Most commonly 69, XXX or 69, XXY	46, XX or 46, XY
Pathology		
Fetus	Often present	Absent
Amnion, fetal red blood cells	Often present	Absent
Villous edema	Variable, focal	Diffuse
Trophoblastic proliferation	Variable, focal, slight to moderate	Variable, slight to severe
Clinical presentation		
Diagnosis	Missed abortion	Molar gestation
Uterine size	Small for dates	50% are large for dates
Theca lutein cysts	Rare	Occur in 25% to 30%
Medical complications	Rare	Frequent
Postmolar gestational trophoblastic tumor	Less than 5% to 10%	20%

tinct cytogenetic disease processes with characteristic clinical and histopathologic findings and do not represent a transition from a normal to a molar gestation. The distinctive features of these two entities are outlined in Table 82-1. However, despite the clinical and pathologic differences, the management of patients with partial and complete moles should be similar.

Partial hydatidiform moles usually have 69 chromosomes derived from two paternal and one maternal haploid sets of chromosomes. Most have 69, XXX or 69, XXY genotype derived from a haploid ovum with dispermic fertilization. Complete hydatidiform moles usually have a chromosomal complement totally derived from the paternal genome while the maternal chromosomes are either inactivated or absent. The 46, XX genotype is most common, representing in most cases reduplication of the haploid genome of one sperm. A smaller proportion of complete moles have a 46, XY karyotype consistent with dispermic fertilization.

The clinical presentation of complete mole has changed considerable over the past few decades and now is similar to partial mole. Prior to the advent of modern sonography and widely available quantitative β-hCG assays, the symptoms of complete molar pregnancy included vaginal bleeding, uterine enlargement greater than expected for gestational dates, absent fetal heart tones, anemia, hyperemesis, preeclampsia, cystic enlargement of ovaries (theca lutein cysts) and abnormally high levels of β-hCG. Complete molar pregnancy is now diagnosed in the first trimester and infrequently presents with these traditional signs and symptoms. Though vaginal bleeding remains the most

common presenting symptom occurring in 85% of patients, it is usually not associated with significant anemia.

Diagnosis

The diagnosis of either a partial or a complete mole can frequently be suggested by transvaginal sonography in conjunction with the β-hCG level. Despite earlier diagnosis and the smaller size of chronic villi, the majority of first-trimester complete moles continue to have an ultrasound appearance similar to those diagnosed later in pregnancy, and the β-hCG level is often markedly elevated. Most first-trimester complete moles continue to appear as complex, echogenic intrauterine masses with many small cystic spaces. Partial moles, on the other hand, will usually reveal focal cystic spaces and a nonviable conceptus. In each instance, however, diagnosis is confirmed pathologically by dilatation and curettage. Most complete molar pregnancies are now evacuated in the first trimester with a mean gestational age of 8.5 to 12 weeks, whereas in the past, the mean gestational age at evacuation was 16 to 17 weeks.

The pathologic findings of complete molar pregnancy have changed significantly owing to earlier uterine evacuation. Whereas cavitation and circumferential trophoblastic hyperplasia were present in three quarters of complete moles in the past, these findings are now present in less than half of cases. Complete moles are now often characterized by subtle morphologic alterations that may result in their misclassification as partial moles of nonmolar hydropic abortions. DNA ploidy studies or karyotyping are useful adjuncts in these circumstances.

Treatment

Suction curettage is the primary treatment for molar pregnancy. Prostaglandins, oxytocin infusion, and hysterectomy are not recommended because they may increase blood loss and the risk of infection. Furthermore, patients frequently require suction curettage after the use of prostaglandins or oxytocin because of retained molar tissue. Occasionally, the diagnosis of hydatidiform mole will be made by the pathologist on the basis of a curettage for an apparent incomplete abortion. In this instance, all patients should have a baseline β-hCG level drawn and chest X-ray performed. In patients in whom molar pregnancy is suspected, the following laboratory studies should be ordered prior to evacuation: complete blood count, blood type and antibody screen, and determination of β-hCG level. A baseline chest X-ray should also be obtained. Patients with uteri that are excessively enlarged (greater than 20 weeks size) and with high hCG levels (greater than 100,000 mIU/mL) are more prone to medical complications such as preeclampsia, hyperthyroidism, and anemia. In patients with hyperthyroidism, beta-blockers should be given prior to anesthesia induction to prevent thyroid storm.

Uterine evacuation is accomplished with the largest cannula that can be introduced into the cervix (usually 12 mm). If brisk bleeding occurs at the time of dilation, proceeding expeditiously with suction evacuation will result in rapid shrinkage of the uterus, thus reducing blood loss. Oxytocin should be used concurrently at the time of evacuation and continued postoperatively for several hours. After completion of suction evacuation, gentle sharp curettage should be performed to remove any residual molar tissue. Patients who are Rh-negative need Rh immune globulin after evacuation because trophoblastic cells express the RhD factor.

Pulmonary complications are occasionally observed around the time of evacuation in patients with marked uterine enlargement. Although the syndrome of trophoblastic embolization has been emphasized as an underlying cause for respiratory distress, there are many other potential causes for respiratory insufficiency in these patients, including high-output congestive heart failure caused by anemia, hyperthyroidism, preeclampsia, or iatrogenic fluid overload. This complication should be treated aggressively with therapy directed by pulmonary artery catheter monitoring and assisted ventilator support as required.

Complete resolution usually occurs in 72 hours. Hyperthyroidism and pregnancy-induced hypertension usually abate promptly after evacuation and might not require specific therapy. Theca lutein ovarian cysts might require months to resolve completely.

Hysterectomy, with or without removal of the ovaries, may be the preferred treatment for a complete mole when the patient no longer wishes to preserve fertility. When this is undertaken, the patient should be counseled that removal of the uterus does not eliminate metastatic disease or obviate the need for follow-up.

After evacuation or hysterectomy, it is important to monitor patients carefully in order to promptly diagnose and treat persistent disease. In all cases of molar pregnancy, careful follow-up with quantitative β-hCG tests should be carried out to detect the presence of persistent disease. It is recommended that β-hCG levels be obtained weekly until normal for three consecutive weeks and then monthly for three consecutive months after partial mole and six consecutive months after complete mole. The average time from evacuation to the first undetectable β-hCG level after the complete mole is 10 weeks and after partial mole is 8 weeks. During the period of β-hCG monitoring effective contraception is required. When the three- to six-month gonadotropin follow-up is completed, the patient may discontinue birth control and try for pregnancy. Oral contraceptives do not increase the incidence of postmolar gestational trophoblastic tumors or affect the pattern of hCG regression. Patients should be counseled that with prior partial or complete molar gestation, there is a 10-fold increased risk (1% to 2% incidence) of a second mole in a subsequent pregnancy. Therefore, all future pregnancies should be evaluated by ultrasound at 10 weeks of gestation.

Although prophylactic chemotherapy has been shown to decrease the incidence of postmolar gestational trophoblastic tumors in patients after evacuation of complete molar pregnancy, it is not routinely recommended. In compliant patients, the low mortality and morbidity achieved by monitoring patients with serial β-hCG determinations and instituting chemotherapy only when indicated outweigh the potential risk and small benefit of routine prophylaxis. As long as the β-hCG values are declining, there does not appear to be any role for chemotherapy. However, if β-hCG values plateau for three or more consecutive weeks or rise, immediate workup and treatment are indicated. Repeat curettage is usually reserved for patients with bleeding due to residual molar tissue.

Persistent Gestational Trophoblastic Tumors

Clinical Presentation

Persistent gestational trophoblastic tumors can occur after any antecedent pregnancy. The clinical presentation is more important in determining prognosis than the precise histologic diagnosis. Infrequently, the diagnosis is made solely on the basis of a rising or plateaued hCG level in the absence of a documented pregnancy or any clinical, radiologic, or pathologic evidence of trophoblastic tissue.

There are three distinct morphologic entities that characterize persistent gestational trophoblastic tumors: invasive mole, choriocarcinoma, and placental site trophoblastic tumor. Invasive mole is characterized by edematous chorionic villi with trophoblastic proliferation invading the myometrium. Since metastases are rare, treatment with either chemotherapy or hysterectomy is usually successful. Choriocarcinoma is made up of both neoplastic syncytioblasts and cytotrophoblasts without chorionic villi that usually metastasizes by the hematogenous route and may require multimodal therapy including chemotherapy, radiation, and surgery. Placental site trophoblastic tumor is a rare trophoblastic neoplasm characterized by absence of chorionic villi and proliferation of intermediate cytotrophoblast cells. Unlike choriocarcinoma, it secretes small amounts of hCG in relation to tumor volume and is relatively insensitive to chemotherapy. Fortunately, placental site trophoblastic tumor infrequently metastasizes beyond the uterus; hysterectomy is the treatment of choice for non-metastatic disease.

Postmolar gestational trophoblastic tumors is diagnosed on the basis of rising (increase of 10%) or plateauing (decline of less than 10% for last three values over 14 days) β-hCG values. Abnormal vaginal bleeding and subinvolution of the uterus and cystic ovaries may be present. Women with gestational trophoblastic tumors following nonmolar pregnancies may present with subtle signs and symptoms making diagnosis difficult. Abnormal bleeding following any pregnancy should be evaluated promptly with HCG testing. Since metastases from choriocarcinoma have been reported in virtually every body site, this diagnosis should be considered in any women in the reproductive age group who present with metastatic disease from an unknown primary site.

Diagnosis and Staging

Once the diagnosis of persistent gestational trophoblastic tumors is suspected or established, immediate evaluation for metastases is mandatory. Along with history and physical examination, the following laboratory studies should be performed: complete blood and platelet count, clotting studies, renal and liver function tests, blood type and antibody screen, and determination of baseline (pretreatment) β-hCG levels. Radiologic studies that may be extremely important in determining prognosis include chest X-ray or computed tomography (CT) scan, pelvic ultrasound, brain computed tomography or magnetic resonance imaging (MRI) scan, and abdominal-pelvic computed tomography scan or magnetic resonance imaging of the liver. In patients with metastases, lung and vaginal involvement is diagnosed in 70% and 30% respectively. Metastases to the brain and liver rarely occur in the absence of pulmonary and/or vaginal involvement. If the chest radiograph is negative, a chest computed tomography scan should be

DIAGNOSIS

Molar Pregnancy and Persistent Gestational Trophoblastic Tumors

The advent of transvaginal ultrasound and sensitive hCG assays has made it possible for clinicians to diagnose molar pregnancy at an early gestational age. This has led to a significant decrease in the incidence of associated medical complications. However, despite earlier diagnosis the incidence of persistent gestational trophoblastic tumors after complete molar pregnancy has not changed. Therefore careful hCG monitoring after molar evacuation is essential for the early detection and successful management of persistent gestational trophoblastic tumors.

Patients with either molar pregnancy or gestational trophoblastic tumors can be reassured that their reproductive function can be preserved despite the use of potent chemotherapeutic agents. Although the risk of subsequent molar gestation is increased, other abnormalities of pregnancy do not seem to be a problem. Following a later pregnancy, hCG testing after delivery or miscarriage is advised to detect the rare case of choriocarcinoma.

Table 82-2 ■ NIH Clinical Classification of Gestational Trophoblastic Tumor

I. Nonmetastatic
II. Metastatic
   A. Good prognosis
      1. β-hCG < 100,000 mIU/24 hours (urine) or <40,000 mIU/mL (serum)
      2. Symptoms present for <4 months
      3. No brain or liver metastases
      4. No prior chemotherapy
      5. Antecedent pregnancy not term
   B. Poor prognosis
      1. β-hCG >100,000 mIU/24 hours (urine) or >40,000 mIU/mL (serum)
      2. Symptoms present for >4 months
      3. Brain or liver metastases
      4. Prior chemotherapeutic failure
      5. Antecedent term pregnancy

obtained because 40% of these patients will have metastatic lesions. If the chest computed tomography scan is positive, the brain and abdomen should be evaluated.

Staging

Three staging systems have been proposed for evaluating patients with persistent gestational trophoblastic tumors to estimate prognosis and help select optimal therapy. The NIH clinical classification system (Table 82-2) separates patients with nonmetastatic disease from those with metastases, because virtually all patients with nonmetastatic disease can be cured with either single-agent chemotherapy or hysterectomy. Patients with metastatic disease are further subdivided into low-risk and high-risk disease based on five risk factors shown to influence prognosis. Patients with poor prognosis disease should be treated initially with multiagent chemotherapy.

The staging system adopted by the International Federation of Gynecologic Oncology (FIGO) (Table 82-3) is an anatomic classification designed to group patients to allow data from difference centers to be compared. It is less useful clinically because it does not take into account risk factors that may influence outcome.

The prognostic scoring system adopted by the World Health Organization (Table 82-4) assigns a

Table 82-3 ■ FIGO Staging System for Gestational Trophoblastic Tumor

Stage

I. Disease confined to the uterus
II. Disease extending outside the uterus but limited to the genital structures (adnexa, vagina, broad ligament)
III. Disease extending to the lungs, with or without known genital tract involvement
IV. Disease at other metastatic sites

Substage

A. No risk factor
B. One risk factor
C. Two risk factors

Risk Factors

■ β-hCG >100,000 mIU/mL
■ Duration from termination of the antecedent pregnancy to diagnosis >6 months

Table 82-4 ■ WHO Prognostic Scoring System for Gestational Trophoblastic Tumor

Parameter	Score			
	0	1	2	4
Age (years)	≤39	>39		
Antecedent pregnancy	Mole	Abortion	Term	
Interval*	<4	4–6	7–12	>12
Pretreatment hCG	$<10^3$	$10^3–10^4$	$10^4–10^5$	$>10^5$
Largest tumor (cm²)		3–4	≥4	
Site of metastases		Spleen, kidney	GI	Brain, liver
Number of metastases		1–4	4–8	>8
Prior chemotherapy failed			Single drug	Two or more drugs

Total score for a patient is obtained by adding the individual scores for each prognostic factor.
Total score ≤6 = low risk; total score >6 = high risk.
*"Interval" is the number of months between the end of the antecedent pregnancy and the start of chemotherapy.

weighted value to individual clinical variables. The total prognostic score has been shown to correlate with prognosis and response to therapy.

In an attempt to overcome the limitations of all three systems and guide clinicians regarding optimal therapy, the International Society for the Study of Trophoblastic Disease (ISSTD) and FIGO have agreed to combine both the FIGO staging and WHO prognostic scoring system. Patients in each stage with a prognostic score of 6 or less are considered low risk and can usually be treated with single-agent chemotherapy with a high degree of success and low morbidity. Patients whose prognostic score is over 6 are considered high risk and treated initially with multiagent chemotherapy.

Treatment

Nonmetastatic Disease

Most patients with nonmetastatic gestational trophoblastic tumors can be cured with single-agent chemotherapy (Figure 82-1). Many chemotherapeutic regimens have been evaluated for the treatment of women with nonmetastatic disease (Table 82-5). Of the available regimens, weekly intramuscular injection of methotrexate is widely used because it is effective, easy to administer, minimally toxic, and cost-effective. Chemotherapy is continued until β-hCG levels become undetectable, and then an additional two weekly doses of methotrexate are administered.

At the New England Trophoblastic Disease Center (NETDC), the majority of patients with nonmetastatic disease achieve remission with one or more courses of methotrexate. The methotrexate infusion regimen is preferred because of its efficacy and reduced total dose

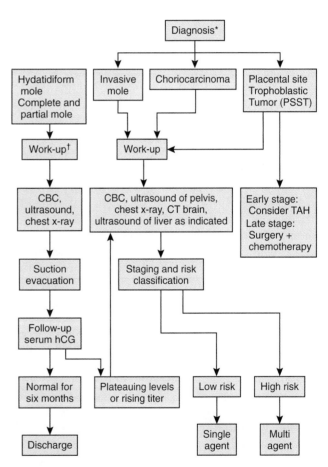

* After miscarriage, ectopic, or term pregnancy: hCG levels persistently elevated and/or pathology shows choriocarcinoma or placental site trophoblastic tumor.

† Additional studies as indicated: thyroid function tests, liver function tests

Figure 82-1 ■ Algorithm for the management of gestational trophoblastic tumor. TAH = total abdominal hysterectomy.

Table 82-5 ■ Chemotherapy Regimens for Nonmetastatic Gestational Trophoblastic Tumors

First-line therapy: methotrexate

    Weekly, 30 mg/m^{2}IM[†], or

    Every two weeks, a five-day regimen of 0.4 mg/kg IM (maximum 25 mg/d), or

    Methotrexate, 1 mg/kg IM, on days 1, 3, 5, and 7 with folinic acid, 0.1 mg/kg IM, on days 2, 4, 6, and 8, or

    Methotrexate, 100 mg/m^2 IV bolus and 200 mg/m^2 IV infusion over 12 hours, followed by folinic acid, 15 mg PO every 6 hours for

        four doses (begun at the end of infusion)

Alternative therapy: dactinomycin[*][†] or etoposide

    Dactinomycin

        For 5 days, 9–13 µg/kg IV (maximum 500 µg/kg), every 2 weeks or

        Bolus, 1.25 mg/m^2 IV, every 2 weeks

    Etoposide

        For 5 days, 200 mg/m^2 PO every 12–14 days[§]

Abbreviations: IM = intramuscularly, IV = intravenously, PO = orally.

[†]A weekly methotrexate regimen is described in Homesley HD, Blessing JA, Rettenmaier M, Capizzi RL, Major FJ, Twiggs LB: Weekly intramuscular methotrexate for nonmetastatic gestational trophoblastic disease. Obstet Gynecol 1988;72:413–418.

[‡]Caution: May produce extravasation injury.

[§]Universal alopecia results.

required. Rather than treating at a set time interval, we determine the number of courses of chemotherapy by the pattern of hCG regression. The β-hCG level is measured weekly after each course of chemotherapy, and the hCG regression curve serves as the primary basis for determining the need for additional treatment. After the first treatment, further chemotherapy is withheld as long as the β-hCG level is falling progressively. A second or additional course(s) of chemotherapy is administered if the β-hCG level plateaus for more than two consecutive weeks, begins to rise again, or if the β-hCG level does not decline by one log within 18 days after completion of the first course of therapy.

When first-line therapy does not produce complete remission, alternative therapy with dactinomycin may be used when methotrexate fails or when liver or renal function abnormalities preclude its use. The small percentage of patients who are resistant to single-agent chemotherapy are generally cured with combination therapy.

In this group of patients, early hysterectomy will shorten the duration and amount of chemotherapy needed to produce remission. Therefore, the patient's desire for further fertility should be evaluated at the onset of therapy. When hysterectomy is elected, a course of adjunctive single-agent chemotherapy should be administered to reduce the likelihood that additional therapy will be required because of occult metastases. Hysterectomy should also be considered when patients with nonmetastatic disease become resistant to single-agent therapy.

Metastatic Disease

Low Risk

Patients with metastatic disease and a prognostic score of 6 or less can be successfully treated with single-agent regimens. Traditionally this has consisted of five-day regimens of sequential methotrexate and dactinomycin but now includes alternative regimens of these drugs (see Table 82-5). In spite of the fact that approximately 35% of patients will require alternative therapy to achieve remission, essentially all patients with low-risk metastatic disease can be cured with conventional chemotherapy. Hysterectomy as primary treatment in conjunction with chemotherapy has been shown to decrease the amount of chemotherapy required to achieve remission when the uterus is involved.

High Risk

Patients with metastatic disease who have a prognostic score of 7 or greater may require some combination of chemotherapy, radiation, and surgery. Optimal survival in trophoblastic disease centers in this group is 60% to 85%. In contrast to patients with non-metastatic and low-risk metastatic disease, primary treatment with hysterectomy does not appear to improve outcome.

Initial multiagent chemotherapy is of primary importance. Triple therapy with methotrexate, dactinomycin, and either chlorambucil or cyclophosphamide has been the standard regimen for many years in the United States. With the identification of etoposide as an active agent in the treatment of gestational trophoblastic tumors, a chemotherapy regimen incorporating etoposide, methotrexate, and dactinomycin alternating with cyclophosphamide and vincristine (EMA/CO) has been used with high success rate in this group of patients.

The management of cerebral and hepatic metastases is still controversial. Radiation therapy (3000 cGy) to the brain has been used with chemotherapy in an attempt to limit acute hemorrhagic complications. Although the use of brain irradiation with systemic chemotherapy is successful in controlling metastases, high remission rates have also been reported when the EMA/CO regimen is used together with intrathecal methotrexate without brain irradiation. Even with extensive chemotherapy, surgery may be necessary to control bleeding, remove isolated metastases, or treat complications from metastatic disease.

When treating patients with high-risk metastatic disease, chemotherapy should be administered intensively at two- to three-week intervals, toxicity permitting, and should be continued until three consecutive normal β-hCG values have been obtained. Most treatment centers recommend two to four additional courses of chemotherapy to eradicate all viable tumors and reduce recurrence rates to a minimum.

Placental Site Trophoblastic Tumors

These are uncommon variants of gestational trophoblastic tumors, which may arise after any type of antecedent pregnancy and are thought to develop from intermediate trophoblasts in the placental bed. Surgery plays a major role in its management owing to its relative chemotherapy insensitivity. Since the majority of cases at diagnosis are nonmetastatic, primary treatment consists of hysterectomy without adjunctive chemotherapy. Spread via the lymphatics occurs; therefore, lymph node sampling is recommended if the disease deeply invades the uterine wall. Patients with extrauterine disease should be treated aggressively with combination chemotherapy consisting of weekly doses of etoposide, methotrexate, and dactinomycin alternating with etoposide and cisplatin.

Surveillance Following Chemotherapy

After hCG remission has been achieved (three consecutive weekly undetectable β-hCG levels), patients should be monitored with determinations of β-hCG values at monthly intervals for one year. Contraception, preferably with oral or injectable contraceptives, may be started during treatment and should be used during the first year of remission. Intrauterine devices should be inserted only after remission is documented.

In patients with nonmetastatic and low-risk metastatic disease, follow-up may be discontinued at this point and pregnancy may be undertaken, since the risk of recurrence after one year of normal β-hCG values is less than 1%. In patients with high-risk metastatic disease, pregnancy should be postponed and monthly follow-up should be continued for two years because of the increased risk of late relapse.

Subsequent Pregnancy Experience

Women who have had a complete or partial molar pregnancy can be reassured that their chances for a normal pregnancy in the future are excellent. However the risk of a later molar gestation is increased to 1% to 2%. For that reason, women with a previous molar gestation should undergo ultrasound in later pregnancies at 9 to 10 weeks of gestation, since most abnormal fetal and placental development is detectable by that time. Women treated for persistent gestational trophoblastic tumors are also likely to have a subsequent normal pregnancy. If a spontaneous miscarriage occurs, the products of conception should be examined to rule out another mole or choriocarcinoma. There does not appear to be any benefit to examine the placenta histologically. It is also recommended that the β-hCG level be tested at the six-week checkup for all women with a history of any type of gestational trophoblastic tumors to rule out postterm or abortal choriocarcinoma.

Long-Term Follow-up

Patients who are treated with combination chemotherapy that includes etoposide are at increased risk of developing secondary tumors, including leukemia, colon cancer, melanoma, and breast cancer. Physicians caring for these patients need to be aware that these secondary tumors might not become apparent for 5 to 25 years after initial treatment for gestational trophoblastic tumors. Therefore, long-term follow-up of these patients is mandatory.

Problems with hCG Measurement

Several case reports have recently highlighted the syndrome of phantom hCG (or phantom choriocarcinoma), in which β-hCG levels are detected despite the lack of radiologic, clinical, or pathologic evidence of gestational trophoblastic tumors. This syndrome is due to the presence of human heterophilic antibodies that interfere with the interpretation of commercial assays. Most of these rare cases present initially as a presumed ectopic pregnancy or missed abortion. Symptoms may be absent and the antecedent pregnancy remote.

While the diagnosis of persistent gestational trophoblastic tumors should always be considered first in patients with an elevated β-hCG level, the phantom hCG syndrome should be considered prior to initiating therapy when the diagnosis is questionable.

References

Berkowitz RS, Bernstein MR, Harlow BL, Rice LW, Lage JM, Goldstein DP: Case control study of risk factors for partial molar pregnancy. Am J Obstet Gynecol 1995;173:788–794.

Berkowitz RS, Cramer DW, Bernstein MR, Cassells S, Driscoll SG, Goldstein DP: Risk factors for complete molar pregnancy from a case-control study. Am J Obstet Gynecol 1985;52:1016–1020.

Berkowitz RS, Goldstein DP: Chorionic tumors. N Engl J Med 1996;335:1740–1748.

Berkowitz RS, Goldstein DP: Presentation and management of molar pregnancy. In Hancock BW, Newlands ES, Berkowitz RS (eds): Gestational Trophoblastic Disease. London: Chapman and Hall, 1997, pp 127–142.

Berkowitz RS, Goldstein DP: The management of molar pregnancy and gestational trophoblastic tumors. In Knapp RC, Berkowitz RS (eds): Gynecologic Oncology, 2nd ed. New York: McGraw-Hill, 1993, pp 328–338.

Berkowitz RS, Goldstein DP, Bernstein MR: Ten years experience with methotrexate and folinic acid rescue as primary therapy for gestational trophoblastic disease. Gynecol Oncol 1986;23:111–118.

Berkowitz RS, Goldstein DP, Marean AR, Bernstein MR: Oral contraceptives and postmolar trophoblastic disease. Obstet Gynecol 1981;58:474–477.

Berkowitz RS, Im SS, Bernstein MR, Goldstein DP: Gestational trophoblastic disease: Subsequent pregnancy outcome, including repeat molar pregnancy. J Reprod Med 1998;43:81–86.

Berkowitz RS, Tuncer ZS, Bernstein MR, Goldstein DP: Management of gestational trophoblastic diseases: subsequent pregnancy experience. Semin. Oncol 2000;27:678–685.

Bower M, Newlands ES, Holder L, Short D, Brock C, Rustin GJ: EMA-CO for high-risk gestational trophoblastic tumors; results from a cohort of 272 patients. J Clin Oncol 1997; 15:2636–2643.

Fine C, Bundy AL, Berkowitz RS, Boswell SB, Berezin AF, Doubilet PM: Sonographic diagnosis of partially hydatidiform mole. Obstet Gynecol 1989;73:414–418.

Finkler NJ, Berkowitz RS, Driscoll SG, Goldstein DP, Bernstein MR: Clinical experience with placental site trophoblastic tumors at New England Trophoblastic Disease Center. Obstet Gynecol 1988;71:805–809.

Goldstein DP, Berkowitz RS: Current management of complete and partial molar pregnancy. J Reprod Med 1994;39:139–146.

Homesley HD: Single agent therapy for nonmetastatic and low-risk gestational trophoblastic disease. J Reprod Med 1998;43:69–74.

Lawlor SDF, Fisher RA, Dent J: A prospective genetic study of complete and partial hydatidiform moles. Am J Obstet Gynecol 1991;164:1270–1277.

Newlands ES, Bower M, Fisher RA, Pardinas FJ: Management of placental site trophoblastic tumors. J Reprod Med 1998; 43:53–59.

Palmer JR: Advances in the epidemiology of gestational trophoblastic disease. J Reprod Med 1994;39:155–162.

Rotmensch S, Cole LA: False diagnosis and needless therapy of presumed malignant disease in women with false-positive human chorionic gonadotropin concentrations. Lancet 2000;355:712–715.

Rustin GJS, Newlands ES, Lutz JM: Combination but not single agent methotrexate chemotherapy for gestational trophoblastic tumors increases the incidence of second tumors. J Clin Oncol 1996;14:2769–2773.

Soto-Wright V, Bernstein MR, Goldstein DP, Berkowitz RS: The changing clinical presentation of complete molar pregnancy. Obstet Gynecol 1995;86:775–779.

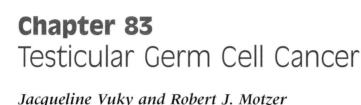

Genitourinary Cancer

Chapter 83
Testicular Germ Cell Cancer

Jacqueline Vuky and Robert J. Motzer

Introduction

Germ cell tumors (GCTs) of the testis account for 95% of all testicular neoplasms. Germ cell tumors infrequently arise from an extragonadal site, such as the retroperitoneum and mediastinum. Ninety-five percent of all newly diagnosed patients are cured, and proper management is required at all stages. Although testicular germ cell cancer accounts for only 1% of cancers in males in the United States, it is the most common malignancy among white men between the ages of 20 and 34. Also, the incidence of testicular cancer has doubled in the past two decades. In 1999, approximately 7400 new cases of testicular germ cell tumors were diagnosed in the United States. Genetic analysis of germ cell tumors has revealed that almost all have abnormalities on chromosome 12, including tandem duplications of 12p, one or more copies of isochrome 12p, and deletions of 12q.

Clinical Presentation

Symptoms of testicular germ cell tumors range from a painless testicular mass to diffuse pain, swelling, and hardness. The differential diagnosis includes testicular torsion, hydrocele, varicocele, spermatocele, epididymitis, and lymphoma. A course of antibiotics may be given if epididymitis is suspected; however, if the testicular discomfort does not abate or findings do not revert to normal within two to four weeks, a testicular ultrasound is indicated. A delay in diagnosis results in more advanced stage at diagnosis and affects survival. The diagnosis should be suspected in patients with an undescended testicle. The failure of descent

does not breed cancer but rather is a marker for the underlying genetic abnormality that increases the predisposition to testicular cancer.

Patients who present with back pain may have enlargement of retroperitoneal lymph nodes. Patients with elevated human chorionic gonadotropin (hCG) may present with nipple tenderness. Chest pain, cough, and shortness of breath or dyspnea on exertion may indicate the presence of an extragonadal germ cell tumor, such as germ cell tumors arising from a primary mediastinal site.

Clinical Evaluation

A radical inguinal orchiectomy is required for all suspected testicular tumors. Simple orchiectomy or testicular biopsy must not be done to avoid disruption of normal routes of spread (important to therapy) and local contamination. Serum tumor marker levels are assessed before, during, and following surgery and throughout follow-up. Elevated levels of α-fetoprotein (AFP) and/or β-hCG without radiographic or clinical findings imply active disease and are sufficient reason to initiate systemic treatment if false-positive cases are excluded. After surgery and/or chemotherapy, serum markers should decrease according to known half-lives (36 hours for hCG, six days for α-fetoprotein). A plateau or slow half-life clearance suggests residual disease. In nonseminomatous germ cell tumors increased serum α-fetoprotein concentration is present in 10% to 20% of patients with clinical stage I disease, 20% to 40% of low-burden clinical stage II disease, and 40% to 60% of high-burden disease. Moreover the B-hCG is elevated in these patients in

Initial Management for Suspected Testicular Cancer

- A two-week trial of antibiotics is reasonable if epididymitis or orchitis is suspected.
- Testicular ultrasound is indicated if the abnormality (swelling, tenderness, palpable mass) does not resolve. If this shows an intratesticular mass, α-fetoprotein and hCG levels should be obtained, followed by a radical inguinal orchiectomy.
- A chest X-ray and computed tomography scan of the abdomen and pelvis are indicated if a germ cell tumor is found.
- If the pathological diagnosis is a nonseminomatous germ cell tumor or computed tomography

scan of the abdomen shows bulky retroperitoneal lymph nodes (>5 cm) in patients with seminoma, a computed tomography scan of the chest is indicated.
- After orchiectomy, previously elevated levels of AFP, hCG, and lactate dehydrogenase (LDH) levels should be obtained followed by serial tests to demonstrate resolution.
- Sperm banking should be performed prior to retroperitoneal lymph node dissection, radiation therapy, and chemotherapy.

approximately 10% to 20% with clinical stage I disease, 20% to 30% with low-volume clinical stage II disease, and 40% of patients with advanced disease. Approximately 15% to 25% of patients with advanced pure seminoma have increased serum concentrations of hCG related to syncytial trophoblastic elements within the tumor.

The serum level of lactate dehydrogenase (LDH) has independent prognostic significance in patients with an advanced germ cell tumor. Increased serum lactate dehydrogenase concentrations are observed in approximately 60% of nonseminomatous germ cell tumor patients with advanced disease and in 80% of patients with advanced seminoma.

Pattern of Metastatic Nodal Spread

The initial route of metastasis for germ cell tumors arising in the testis is to retroperitoneal lymph nodes. Particular attention should be focused on the "landing zones," or lymph node drainage sites. These predict lymph node metastases for left- and right-sided testicular tumors (Figure 83-1). Right-sided testicular tumors typically metastasize to the interaortocaval lymph nodes below the level of the renal vessels, with ipsilateral distribution in the paracaval, preaortic, and right common iliac nodes. Left-sided tumors metastasize to the para-aortic lymph nodes just below the left renal vessels, with ipsilateral distribution to the preaortic and left common iliac nodes.

Imaging

Plain chest radiograph and computed tomography (CT) are the radiological investigations used to determine extent of disease and treatment. Computed tomography is the most effective radiographic technique for identifying metastatic involvement both above and below the diaphragm. The abdominal computed

tomography scan will be normal in 70% of patients with newly diagnosed seminoma and approximately 40% of patients with newly diagnosed nonseminomatous germ cell tumor. Lymph nodes in the primary "landing zones" measuring 10 to 20 mm are involved by germ cell tumors about 70% of the time, and those measuring 4 to 10 mm are involved 50% of the time.

Positron emission tomography (PET) has not been able to detect masses less than 0.5 cm. In addition, positron emission tomography has been unable to distinguish between residual viable germ cell tumors and teratoma and therefore is not currently recommended as part of the initial evaluation or postchemotherapy evaluation.

Pathology

Seminoma accounts for 50% of all testicular germ cell tumors. The definition of pure seminoma excludes the presence of any nonseminomatous histology (Table 83-1). Seminoma may secrete hCG if syncy-

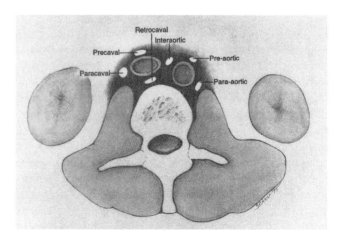

Figure 83-1 ▪ Pattern of metastatic nodal spread.

Table 83-1 ■ Histology of Germ Cell Tumors

Seminoma
    Classic seminoma
    Anaplastic seminoma
    Spermatocytic seminoma

Nonseminoma
    Embryonal carcinoma
    Teratoma (mature and immature)
    Choriocarcinoma
    Yolk-sac tumor
    Teratoma with malignant transformation

tiotrophoblasts are present. However, elevation of α-fetoprotein indicates the presence of a nonseminoma component.

Patients with nonseminoma often present with mixed histology, and seminoma may be a component. Elevated levels of α-fetoprotein and hCG (or both) may be found in embryonal carcinoma. Choriocarcinoma is associated with elevated serum concentrations of hCG. Yolk-sac tumors nearly always produce α-fetoprotein and constitute the most common histology in patients with nonseminoma arising from a primary mediastinal site.

Teratoma is derived from two or more germ cell layers (ectoderm, endoderm, and mesoderm). Mature teratoma refers to adult-type differentiation, while immature teratoma resembles features seen in the fetus. On rare occasions, teratoma may resemble somatic tumors such as enteric adenocarcinoma or rhabdomyosarcomas. This entity is referred to as *teratoma with malignant transformation* and responds poorly to systemic chemotherapy.

TNM Staging Classification

Stage I is defined as disease limited to the testis, stage II is disease limited to the retroperitoneal (regional) lymph nodes, and stage III is disease outside the retroperitoneum, including retrocrural and supradiaphragmatic lymph nodes, and viscera. The revised TNM system of the American Joint Committee on Cancer (AJCC) and the Union Internationale Centre le Cancre (UICC) was adopted in 1997. Serum concentrations of α-fetoprotein, hCG, and lactate dehydrogenase were incorporated because of their independent prognostic significance. Pathological evaluation of retroperitoneal lymph nodes at retroperitoneal lymph node dissection (RPLND) is also included (Table 83-2).

Management

Low-Stage Germ Cell Tumors

Seminoma

Standard therapy consists of abdominal radiotherapy. Ninety-eight percent of patients with stage I and 90% of patients with stage IIA/B seminoma are cured with this approach. The dose of radiation that is recommended for stage I patients (2500 to 3000 cGy) is usually well tolerated. For patients with stage I (T1 to T3) seminoma, a randomized trial showed that a simple para-aortic port, excluding the ipsilateral iliac and pelvic nodes, is as effective as the "dogleg" portal (includes para-aortic and ipsilateral iliac and pelvic lymph nodes), and although more pelvic relapses occur, toxicity is lower.

Radiation therapy using a dogleg portal is the treatment of choice in patients with stage IIA/B seminoma. Fractionation is the same as that in patients with clinical stage I disease, except that a boost of approximately 500 to 750 cGy is administered to involved lymph nodes. Follow-up after radiation therapy for patients with low-stage seminoma is outlined in Table 83-3.

Nonseminoma

For patients with nonseminoma, treatment is based on retroperitoneal lymph node size, location of adenopathy, and presence of elevated serum tumor marker concentrations. The standard approach postorchiectomy has been RPLND for patients with stage I and low-volume stage II (less than 3 cm) disease. In the past, most patients undergoing bilateral RPLND experienced retrograde ejaculation and subsequent infertility. An improved understanding of ejaculatory neuroanatomy, surgical mapping, and the pattern of retroperitoneal metastasis for right- and left-sided tumors have led to nerve-sparing approaches and modification of surgical boundaries within the renal hilum.

Modified, nerve-avoiding RPLND templates were designed to avoid the hypogastric plexus and contralateral sympathetic fibers that are responsible for ejaculation in clinical stage I or IIA disease. This method avoids transection of contralateral nerves and results in preservation of antegrade ejaculation in approximately 50% to 80% of patients. Preservation of ejaculation appears to be more successful when nerves are prospectively identified and spared. With nerve dissection, about 95% of patients retain normal ejaculatory status postoperatively. Regardless of technique, preoperative sperm banking is recommended.

Clinical stage I nonseminoma patients with T1 tumor and serum tumor markers that are normal or normalizing are offered both surgical and observation options. Approximately 25% of patients with T1 N0 M0 disease and normal serum tumor markers relapse

Table 83-2 ▪ TNM Staging of Testis Tumors: American Joint Committee on Cancer

DEFINITION OF TNM

Primary Tumor (T)

pT_X Primary tumor cannot be assessed (if no radical orchiectomy has been performed, T_X is used).

pT_0 No evidence of primary tumor (e.g., histologic scar in testis).

pT_{is} Intratubular germ cell neoplasia (carcinoma in situ).

pT_1 Tumor limited to the testis and epididymis and no vascular/lymphatic invasion. Tumor may invade into the tunica albuginea but not the tunica vaginalis.

pT_2 Tumor limited to the testis and epididymis with vascular/lymphatic invasion or tumor extending through the tunica albuginea with involvement of tunica vaginalis.

pT_3 Tumor invades the spermatic cord with or without vascular/lymphatic invasion.

pT_4 Tumor invades the scrotum with or without vascular/lymphatic invasion.

Regional Lymph Nodes (N)

Clinical

N_X Regional lymph nodes cannot be assessed.

N_0 No regional lymph node metastasis.

N_1 Lymph node mass 2 cm or less in greatest dimension; or multiple lymph nodes, none more than 2 cm in greatest dimension.

N_2 Lymph node mass more than 2 cm but not more than 5 cm in greatest dimension; or multiple lymph nodes, any one mass >2 cm but not more than 5 cm in greatest dimension.

N_3 Lymph node mass more than 5 cm in greatest dimension.

Pathological

pN_0 No evidence of tumor in lymph nodes.

pN_1 Lymph node mass 2 cm or less in greatest dimension and ≤5 nodes positive, none >2 cm in greatest dimension.

pN_2 Lymph node mass more than 2 cm but not more than 5 cm in greatest dimension; more than 5 nodes positive, none >5 cm; evidence of extranodal extension of tumor.

pN_3 Lymph node mass more than 5 cm in greatest dimension.

Distant Metastases (M)

M0   No evidence of distant metastases.

M1   Nonregional nodal or pulmonary metastases.

M2   Nonpulmonary visceral metastases.

Serum Tumor Markers (S)

	LDH	hCG (mIu/mL)	AFP (ng/mL)
S1	$<1.5 \times N$	<5,000	<1,000
S2	$1.5–10 \times N$	5,000–50,000	1,000–10,000
S3	$>10 \times N$	>50,000	>10,000

N indicates the upper limit of normal for the LDH assay.

Stage GROUPING

	T	N	M	S
Stage I				
IA	T_1	N_0	M_0	S_0
IB	T_2	N_0	M_0	S_0
	T_3	N_0	M_0	S_0
	T_4	N_0	M_0	S_0
IS	T_{ANY}	N_0	M_0	S_{ANY}
Stage II				
IIA	T_{ANY}	N_1	M_0	S_0
	T_{ANY}	N_1	M_0	S_1
IIB	T_{ANY}	N_2	M_0	S_0
	T_{ANY}	N_2	M_0	S_1
IIC	T_{ANY}	N_3	M_0	S_0
	T_{ANY}	N_3	M_0	S_1
Stage III				
IIIA	T_{ANY}	N_{ANY}	M_1	S_0
IIIB	T_{ANY}	N_{ANY}	M_0	S_2
IIIC	T_{ANY}	N_{ANY}	M_1	S_3

Note: p refers to pathologic findings.

Table 83-3 ▪ Recommended Follow-up for Seminoma Stage I and II A/B After Radiation Therapy

Follow-up	Physical Examination, Chest X-ray, Serum Tumor Markers: AFP, hCG, LDH	CT Scan of the Abdomen
First year	Every 2–3 months	4–6 weeks postradiation therapy
Second year	Every 3–4 months	*
Third year	Every 5–6 months	*
Fourth year	Every 7–8 months	*
Fifth year and beyond	Every 12 months	*

Not necessary for routine follow-up; to be performed if clinically indicated.

during surveillance. A higher likelihood of retroperitoneal and/or systemic relapse is associated with T2 to T4 tumors. If surveillance is selected, patient compliance is essential, as follow-up is rigorous and includes physical examination; chest X-ray; determinations of α-fetoprotein, lactate dehydrogenase, and hCG levels; and regular computed tomography scans (Table 83-4). When RPLND is chosen, the procedure is a nerve-sparing type.

Patients with clinical stage I and persistently elevated or rising serum tumor markers following orchiectomy are treated with chemotherapy, since the disease is often not limited to the retroperitoneum. Low-tumor-burden clinical stage II nonseminoma includes disease ipsilateral to the primary tumor, at or below the renal hilum, not associated with tumor-related back pain, and limited to the primary landing zone. Unresectable and metastatic disease is often found with lymph nodes greater than 3 cm on computed tomography scan, bilateral retroperitoneal nodal metastases, back pain, suprahilar or retrocrural lymph nodes, or elevated serum tumor markers post-orchiectomy. These patients are treated with primary cisplatin-based chemotherapy.

Adjuvant chemotherapy post-RPLND depends on the pathological findings at RPLND including the number, size, and presence of extranodal extension.

The incidence of relapse is approximately 30% if fewer than six lymph nodes are involved with tumor, the largest lymph node is less than 2 cm, and no extranodal extension is evident. Two cycles of adjuvant cisplatin-based chemotherapy cure approximately 99% of patients. For noncompliant patients or those who do not meet the aforementioned criteria, adjuvant chemotherapy is recommended.

Advanced Metastatic Disease

Cisplatin-combination chemotherapy results in a 70% to 80% complete response (CR) proportion in patients with advanced germ cell tumors. The high cure rate with significant toxicity resulted in an effort to identify patients who are more likely ("good risk") and less likely ("poor risk") to be cured with standard chemotherapy. The International Germ Cell Cancer Collaborative Group (IGCCCG) developed a common classification system based on data from approximately 6000 patients treated with initial chemotherapy. Independent prognostic factors for progression-free survival with advanced nonseminoma were pretreatment levels of lactate dehydrogenase, hCG, α-fetoprotein; site of primary tumor; and the presence of nonpulmonary visceral metastases (bone, brain, or liver). Nonpulmonary visceral

Table 83-4 ▪ Follow-up for Patients on Observation T_1 NSGCT

Follow-up	Physical Examination, Chest X-ray, Serum Tumor Markers: AFP, hCG, LDH	CT Scan of the Abdomen
First year	Every month	Every 3 months
Second year	Every 2 months	Every 4 months
Third year	Every 3 months	Every 6 months
Fourth year	Every 4 months	Every 6 months
Fifth year	Every 6 months	Every year
Sixth year and beyond	Every year	Every year

metastasis was the only significant prognostic factor in patients with seminoma undergoing initial chemotherapy. Investigators agreed on three strata of good, intermediate, and poor prognosis. The IGCCCG grouping is used in clinical trials and treatment decisions.

Patients with good-risk disease achieve response proportions of 90% or greater. The culmination of randomized trials led to two regimens that are considered standard. One is four cycles of etoposide plus cisplatin (EP); the second is three cycles of bleomycin, etoposide, and cisplatin (BEP). Either regimen is effective and, in conjunction with adjunctive surgery, cures approximately 90% of good-risk patients. Therefore, standard therapy for patients with good-risk disease is either four cycles of EP or three cycles of BEP. Follow-up recommendations are listed in Table 83-5.

Approximately 26% and 14% of patients are intermediate and poor risk, respectively. Four cycles of BEP remains the standard regimen for poor-risk disease. Likewise, in intermediate-risk patients by IGCCCG criteria, four cycles of BEP are considered standard therapy. Durable complete responses occur in 75% and 40% of intermediate- and poor-risk patients, respectively.

Reports that high-dose therapy with stem cell rescue cured some patients with refractory germ cell tumors led to the study of dose-intensive regimens as part of first-line therapy. Two studies incorporated high-dose carboplatin plus etoposide into first-line therapy for poor-risk patients. There was less treatment-related toxicity associated with the high-dose therapy in this setting compared to its use in heavily pretreated patients, and survival improved with this approach compared to conventional-dose, cisplatin-combination therapy. An ongoing, national, randomized trial is comparing four cycles of BEP to two cycles of BEP followed by two cycles of carboplatin, etoposide, and cyclophosphamide high-dose therapy in poor- and intermediate-risk patients.

Postchemotherapy Surgery

There is general agreement on the need to resect all measurable residual disease postchemotherapy. Postchemotherapy RPLND is generally considered unnecessary when the postchemotherapy computed tomography scan of the retroperitoneum is interpreted as "normal." In patients with residual radiographic abnormalities, necrosis/fibrotic debris comprises 45% to 50% of pathologic findings, teratoma another 35%, and viable germ cell tumor the remaining 15% to 20%. Residual necrosis cannot be predicted accurately by any single criterion to eliminate the risk of residual teratoma or viable germ cell tumor and obviate the need for postchemotherapy RPLND. The pathologic presence of necrotic debris or mature teratoma at surgery requires no further chemotherapy; between 5% and 10% of patients will relapse. If viable residual germ cell tumor is completely resected, two additional cycles of chemotherapy are given.

TREATMENT

Recommendations for Adjuvant Chemotherapy After Complete Resection of Nonseminoma at RPLND

- Adjuvant chemotherapy is indicated for any of the following findings on pathological node examination since this group has a more than 50% chance of relapse:
  1. More than six lymph nodes are macroscopically or microscopically involved.
  2. Any lymph node with a germ cell tumor more than 2 cm in maximum diameter.
  3. Evidence of extranodal involvement.
- Adjuvant chemotherapy is also recommended for patients with any pathological germ cell tumor on RPLND if the patient cannot meet the frequent periodic follow-up necessary or for those whose psychiatric status might be seriously affected by the development of relapse.
- Regimens recommended for adjuvant chemotherapy:
  Etoposide   100 mg/m^2 IV daily × 5 days
  Cisplatin   20 mg/m^2 IV daily × 5 days

Two cycles administered at 21-day intervals for two cycles
- Adjuvant chemotherapy consists of two cycles of etoposide and cisplatin provided that markers return to normal. If markers are elevated after RPLND, chemotherapy should be initiated with therapy appropriate for good-risk patients.
- Recommended follow-up post-RPLND in patients not receiving adjuvant chemotherapy includes physical examination, tumor markers, chest X-ray every one to two months in the first year, every two to three months in the second year, and less frequently thereafter, with annual visits after five years. A computed tomography scan of the abdomen should be obtained four to six weeks post-RPLND; no further computed tomography scans are recommended unless clinically indicated.

TREATMENT

Management of Patients with Good-Risk Disease

Stage IIB/C and III nonseminomatous, Stage IIC and III seminoma, and patients who relapse from observation of NSGCT Stage I of II or postradiation therapy for seminoma.

	Seminoma germ cell tumors	Nonseminoma germ cell tumors
Good risk	Any hCG	AFP < 1000 ng/mL
	Any LDH	hCG < 5000 mIU/mL
	Nonpulmonary visceral metastases absent	LDH <1.5 × upper limit of normal
	Any primary site	Nonpulmonary visceral metastases absent
		Gonadal or retroperitoneal primary tumor

Etoposide and cisplatin (EP) or bleomycin, etoposide, and cisplatin (BEP), as described following, are standard regimens for good-risk disease.

Etoposide and cisplatin (EP): four cycles administered at 21-day intervals

Etoposide	100 mg/m² IV daily × 5 days
Cisplatin	20 mg/m² IV daily × 5 days

Bleomycin, etoposide, and cisplatin (BEP): three cycles administered at 21-day intervals

Etoposide	100 mg/m² IV daily × 5 days
Cisplatin	20 mg/m² IV daily × 5 days
Bleomycin	30 units IV weekly on days 1, 8, 15

At the start of each cycle of chemotherapy, a CBC, screening profile, AFP, hCG, LDH, serum creatinine, and creatinine clearance should be obtained. An outpatient visit to evaluate potential toxicities (including myelotoxicity) should be obtained between each cycle. For patients with an elevated AFP or hCG level before the start of therapy, the outpatient visit between the first and second cycles of therapy should also include an AFP and hCG level to determine whether markers are falling at the appropriate rate.

Resection of residual mass is more controversial in seminoma, since most resected specimens contain necrosis, and RPLND is technically more difficult. The general recommendation for patients with residual masses 3 cm or less is to observe, since the majority of these patients will not relapse, while residual masses greater than 3 cm are biopsied or resected, since approximately 30% of these patients will relapse or have residual seminoma. Careful observation is an alternative, but salvage chemotherapy has a low cure rate in patients who relapse.

Table 83-5 ■ Recommended Follow-up Post Chemotherapy for Advanced Disease

Follow-up	Physical Examination, Chest X-ray, Serum Tumor Markers: AFP, hCG, LDH	Computed Tomography of Chest/Abdomen/Pelvis
First year	Every one to two months	■ 4–6 weeks after surgical resection of residual disease. ■ For patients who do not undergo post-chemotherapy surgical resection, a CT scan should be performed post-chemotherapy.
Second year	Every 2 months	*
Third year	Every 3 months	*
Fourth year	Every 4 months	*
Fifth year	Every 6 months	*
Sixth year and beyond	Every year	*

*No further computed tomography scans are recommended unless symptoms indicate the necessity for reevaluation.
Note: Day 1 of chemotherapy defines the start of the first year surveillance.

TREATMENT

Intermediate-Risk and Poor-Risk Disease

	Seminoma	Nonseminoma
Intermediate risk	Nonpulmonary visceral metastases present	LDH 1.5 to 10× normal AFP 1000 to 10,000 ng/mL hCG 5000 to 50,000 mIU/mL Absent: nonpulmonary visceral metastases Primary testicular or retroperitoneal site
Poor risk	——	LDH > 10× normal AFP > 10,000 ng/mL hCG > 50,000 mIu/mL Present nonpulmonary visceral metastases Primary mediastinal site

Standard therapy with four cycles of BEP: four cycles administered at 21-day intervals

Etoposide	100 mg/m² IV daily × 5 days
Cisplatin	20 mg/m² IV daily × 5 days
Bleomycin	30 units IV weekly on days 1, 8, 15

■ Pulmonary function tests should be obtained as clinically indicated prior to starting bleomycin. If there is a 25% reduction in DLCO (diffusion capacity), bleomycin should be discontinued.

■ At the start of each cycle of therapy, a CBC, screening profile, AFP, hCG, serum creatinine, and creatinine clearance should be obtained.

■ A weekly outpatient visit to evaluate for potential toxicities and administer bleomycin should be performed during each cycle.

■ At the conclusion of therapy, computed tomography scans of the chest, abdomen, and pelvis are indicated, along with serum tumor markers. If the serum tumor markers are normal, then all sites of residual disease should be resected.

■ For patients with unresectable disease or persistent elevated tumor markers, high-dose chemotherapy with autologous stem cell rescue should be considered.

■ Follow-up as per Table 83-5.

Salvage Chemotherapy

Second-line chemotherapy with ifosfamide plus cisplatin with either etoposide or vinblastine results in a complete response rate of 50% with durable complete response rates in approximately 25% of patients. High-dose chemotherapy with autologous stem cell rescue as second-line salvage therapy results in 15% durable complete response and represents standard therapy in metastatic testicular germ cell tumors following an incomplete response to first-line therapy or relapse/incomplete response to ifosfamide-containing salvage therapy. High-dose chemotherapy consists of etoposide, carboplatin, and cyclophosphamide.

Patients who progress following initial cisplatin induction chemotherapy are grouped according to prognostic factors that predict response for standard-dose versus high-dose chemotherapy with autologous stem cell rescue. Patients with a testicular primary who relapse after complete response and are treated with second-line ifosfamide plus cisplatin-containing salvage chemotherapy have an overall 40% durable complete remission rate. Patients with testicular germ cell tumors who fail to achieve an initial complete response with primary mediastinal nonseminomatous germ cell tumor have a cure rate of less than 10%

with ifosfamide-based therapy and are treated with high-dose etoposide plus carboplatin-based regimens.

These prognostic factors have been used to stratify patients prospectively on two trials incorporating paclitaxel. Paclitaxel has been combined with ifosfamide and cisplatin (TIP) in a first-line salvage program for patients with a testis primary site and a prior history of complete response to cisplatin-based chemotherapy. Eighty percent of evaluable patients achieved complete response or partial response with normal serum tumor markers, and 73% remain progression free with a median follow-up of 33 months. To improve on conventional-dose ifosfamide-based chemotherapy in patients with unfavorable prognostic features, a clinical trial of repetitive cycles of dose-intense therapy consisting of paclitaxel and ifosfamide followed by high-dose carboplatin and etoposide with autologous stem cell rescue was well tolerated and achieved a 41% durable complete response rate with median follow-up of 30 months.

Surgery in the Salvage Setting

Histologic findings of resected masses following second-line chemotherapy in patients with normalized serum tumor markers show viable tumor in

TREATMENT

Management of Patients Who Relapse

Prognostic Factors Favorable for Standard-Dose Ifosfamide Chemotherapy

Testis primary AND previous complete response (CR) to prior cisplatin-based chemotherapy

Prognostic Factors Favorable for High-Dose Chemotherapy with Autologous Stem Cell Rescue

Incomplete response (IR) to cisplatin-based chemotherapy OR extragonadal primary

Standard Ifosfamide-Based Chemotherapy

VeIP

Regimen

Vinblastine* 0.11 mg/kg, days 1 and 2,
Ifosfamide 1.2 gm/m^2 IV day 1 to 5, and Mesna 400 mg/m^2 IV, four hours prior to ifosfamide and q4 hours thereafter × 3 doses/day × 5 days
Cisplatin 20 mg/m^2 IV on days 1 to 5

TIP

Paclitaxel 250 mg/m^2 over 24 hours, day 1
Ifosfamide 1.5 mg/^{2} days 2 to 5 with Mesna 500 mg/m^2, 4 hours prior to ifosfamide and every 4 hours thereafter × 3 doses/day × 4 days
Cisplatin 25 mg/m^2 days 2 to 5

*For the rare patient who might have received vinblastine as part of initial therapy, etoposide 75 mg/m^2 IV days 1 through 5 should be substituted for vinblastine.
A CBC, chest X-ray, creatinine and creatinine clearance, AFP, and hCG levels are needed prior to each cycle of therapy. Cycles are repeated every 21 days for four cycles.
Because of the high frequency of neutropenic fever with both TIP and VeIP, GCSF 5 µg/kg/day SC is self-administered from days 7 through 18 or until the WBC is greater than 10,000/mm^3. While GCSF is being administered, CBC should be obtained twice weekly.

High-Dose Chemotherapy Regimen

Days −5 to −3	Carboplatin 500–600 mg/m^2
	Etoposide 400–600 mg/m^2 IV
	Cyclophosphamide 50 mg/kg IV
Days −2 to −1	No treatment
Day 0	Stem cell infusion

At the completion of therapy, computed tomography scans of the chest, abdomen, and pelvis should be performed. In patients who relapse from complete remission and in whom marker levels have returned to normal, complete excision of all sites of residual disease should be considered. If any site contains viable residual cancer but all sites are resected, then no further treatment is indicated. Routine follow-up as detailed in Table 83-5.

approximately 50% of specimens, teratoma in 40%, and necrosis in only 10%. Additional standard-dose chemotherapy adds no benefit to patients with viable nonseminomatous germ cell tumor in the resected specimen after salvage chemotherapy. This is in contrast to benefit with two additional cycles following complete resection of nonseminomatous germ cell tumor after first-line chemotherapy. In general, surgery should be avoided for patients with elevated serum tumor markers. While this general rule holds true, surgery nonetheless has curative potential in a select group of patients with increased marker levels, even after salvage chemotherapy. Patients with a solitary retroperitoneal mass and increased α-fetoprotein seem to be the best candidates. Technically difficult, this surgery should be performed at a tertiary center. Patients with nonseminomatous germ cell tumors arising from a primary mediastinal primary site have a poor prognosis, with a less than 40% five-year survival rate. In this setting, surgical resection despite postchemotherapy elevated markers may produce durable remissions.

Treatment Sequelae

Acute

Cisplatin is emetogenic, and acute nausea and vomiting frequently occur but are controllable with 5-HT$_3$ antagonist plus dexamethasone. Cisplatin can be

TREATMENT

Special Circumstances

Brain metastases Approximately 5% of germ cell tumor patients will present with or develop brain metastases. For those presenting with a solitary brain metastasis, surgical excision should be considered before the initiation of chemotherapy. Simultaneous radiation therapy and initial chemotherapy for poor-risk disease should then be administered. Heightened myelosuppression might be encountered. If brain metastases are encountered as part of progressive disease, then excision of a solitary site of metastasis should again be considered. If two or more sites of brain metastasis are encountered in this setting, then whole-brain radiation therapy may be administered alone or concurrently with standard salvage chemotherapy or other standard palliative treatment approaches.

Cord compression Approximately 2% of patients with germ cell tumors develop cord compression. Whether this happens as part of the initial presentation (extremely rare) or as part of progression in a relapsed setting (somewhat more common), standard chemotherapy for that stage of disease (initial chemotherapy or first-line salvage chemotherapy) should be administered unless prior chemotherapy has not induced a measurable response. Palliative radiation therapy is indicated if the patient is a candidate only for high-dose therapy with stem cell rescue or has progressed while on other therapy.

Extragonadal Germ Cell Tumors

■ Extragonadal germ cell tumors of the mediastinum and retroperitoneum constitute perhaps 10% of all germ cell tumor presentations (pineal gland germ cell tumors are extremely rare). Retroperitoneal or mediastinal extragonadal tumors generally present with a mediastinal or retroperitoneal mass with an appropriate biopsy showing a germ cell tumor. Rarely, routine histology or immunohistochemistry does not establish the diagnosis. In those cases, repeat biopsy with conventional and/or molecular cytogenetics seeking an i(12p) or increased 12p copy number will be indicated. If either an i(12p) or increased 12p copy number is present, then the mass is a germ cell tumor.

■ All extragonadal pure seminoma should be treated with the chemotherapy approach for good-risk patients. Radiographic, marker, and clinical evaluations should be as outlined for that therapy, and routine follow-up should be initiated when the patient is rendered free of disease (Table 83-5).

Patients with mediastinal NSGCT are treated with chemotherapy as for poor-risk gonadal presentation. More than other germ cell tumors, mediastinal NSGCT is often complicated by the progression of malignant nongerminal components (e.g., embryonal rhabdomyosarcoma or other malignant transformed elements). Therefore, aggressive surgical resection of the mediastinum and retroperitoneum disease must be undertaken in all cases in which the markers normalize. Rarely, acute leukemia complicates the course of patients with mediastinal NSGCT and has a poor prognosis.

---

associated with delayed emesis, and administration of oral metoclopramide and a benzodiazepine plus dexamethasone for two to four days after therapy is sometimes necessary.

Renal toxicity includes decrease in glomerular filtration and hypomagnesemia due to the effect of cisplatin on proximal tubules, particularly after ifosfamide-combination or high-dose salvage chemotherapy.

Neutropenic fever occurs in 10% to 15% of patients receiving etoposide and cisplatin, more frequently with the addition of bleomycin, and in more than 50% of patients receiving salvage chemotherapy. Hematopoietic growth factor support should be used prophylactically from the beginning of ifosfamide salvage therapy. Vinblastine and cisplatin cause symptomatic neuropathy in a minority of patients. Auditory toxicity from cisplatin is associated with reduced high-tone hearing and, less frequently, tinnitus, although patients rarely require hearing aids.

Pulmonary toxicity from bleomycin is rare but can be fatal. In good-risk patients, a reduction in the number of bleomycin doses from 12 to 9 resulted in no bleomycin-related deaths. Vascular toxicity, most prominently manifested as Raynaud's phenomenon, occurs in fewer than 10% of patients receiving bleomycin by weekly bolus.

Long-Term

Diastolic hypertension, cardiac events, increased mean cholesterol levels, and increased low-density and decreased high-density lipoprotein levels have been reported with increased frequency years after chemotherapy for germ cell tumors. Infertility is an important consideration, since patients are young males and the cure rate is high. A standard, modified, bilateral RPLND results in retrograde ejaculation in nearly all patients. Nerve-dissecting and nerve-avoiding RPLND reduce but do not eliminate that risk.

Chemotherapy may affect the germinal epithelium directly, and Leydig cell insufficiency is frequent. After chemotherapy, persistent oligospermia and abnormal forms and motility have been reported, but conception may occur despite oligospermia.

Etoposide causes secondary leukemia characterized by translocations involving chromosome 11q in less than 0.5% of patients receiving a total dose less than 2000 mg/m^2 and as many as 6% of patients receiving total etoposide doses of greater than 3000 mg/m^2. Recent reports showed acute leukemia in 0.8% to 1.3% of patients receiving median cumulative etoposide doses greater than 2400 mg/m^2.

The incidence of gastrointestinal malignancies increases after radiation therapy or the combination of radiation plus chemotherapy. The relative risk increases with time and is greatest after 10 years. An excess of soft tissue sarcoma has also been observed, with radiation therapy implicated as the major cause. This low risk of second malignancies does not outweigh the benefits of primary or salvage therapy and therefore should not influence treatment selection.

Acknowledgments

Supported in part by a grant from the Brian Piccolo Cancer Research Fund and CA-09207-23. The authors thank Carol Pearce for her review of the manuscript.

References

AJCC: AJCC Cancer Staging Handbook. Philadelphia: Lippincott-Raven, 1998.

Bajorin DF, Motzer RJ, Rodriguez E, et al: Acute nonlymphocytic leukemia in germ cell tumor patients treated with etoposide-containing chemotherapy. J Natl Cancer Inst 1993;85:60–62.

Bajorin DF, Sarosdy MF, Pfister DG, et al: Randomized trial of etoposide and cisplatin versus etoposide and carboplatin in patients with good-risk germ cell tumors: A multi-institutional study. J Clin Oncol 1993;11:598–606.

Batata M, Chu F, Hilaris B, Whitmore W, Golbey R: Testicular cancer in cryptorchids. Cancer 1982;49:1023–1030.

Bosl GJ: Germ cell tumor clinical trials in North America. Semin Surg Oncol 1999;17:257–262.

Bosl GJ, Bajorin DF, Sheinfeld J, Motzer RJ: Cancer of the testis. In Devita VT, Hellman S, Rosenberg SA (eds): Cancer Principles and Practice of Oncology. Philadelphia: Lippincott-Raven, 1997, pp 1397–1426.

Bosl GJ, Ilson DH, Rodriguez E, et al: Clinical relevance of the i(12p) marker chromosome in germ cell tumors. J Natl Cancer Inst 1994;86:349–355.

Bosl GJ, Vogelzang NJ, Goldman A, et al: Impact of delay in diagnosis on clinical stage of testicular cancer. Lancet 1981;2:970–973.

Broun ER, Nichols CR, Kneebone P, et al: Long-term outcome of patients with relapsed and refractory germ cell tumors treated with high-dose chemotherapy and autologous bone marrow rescue. Ann Intern Med 1992;117:124–128.

Catalona WJ, Vaitukaitis JL, Fair WR: Falsely positive specific human chorionic gonadotropin assays in patients with testicular tumors: Conversion to negative with testosterone administration. J Urol 1979;122:126–128.

Chaganti RSK, Murty VVVS, Bosl GJ: Molecular genetics of male germ cell tumors. In Vogelzang NJ, Shipley WU, Scardino PT, Coffey DS (eds): Comprehensive Textbook of Genitourinary Oncology. Baltimore: Williams & Wilkins, 1996, pp 932–940.

Davis B, Herr H, Fair W, Bosl GJ: The management of patients with nonseminomatous germ cell tumors of the testis with serologic disease only after orchiectomy. J Urol 1994;152:111–114.

Donohue JP, Foster RS: Retroperitoneal lymphadenectomy in staging and treatment: The development of nerve-sparing techniques. Urol Clin North Am 1998;25:461–468.

Einhorn LH, Williams SD, Troner M, et al: The role of maintenance therapy in disseminated testicular cancer. N Engl J Med 1981;305:727–731.

Ellison MF, Mostofi FK, Flanigan RC: Treatment of the residual retroperitoneal mass after chemotherapy for advanced seminoma. J Urol 1988;140:618–620.

Fossa SD, Horwich A, Russell JM, et al: Optimal planning target volume for stage I testicular seminoma: A Medical Research Council randomized trial. J Clin Oncol 1999;17:1146–1154.

Gels M, Hoekstra H, Sleijfer D, et al: Detection of recurrence in patients with clinical stage I nonseminomatous testicular germ cell tumors and consequences for further follow-up: A single-center 10-year experience. J Clin Oncol 1995;13:1188–1194.

Gels ME, Hoekstra HJ, Sleijfer DT, et al: Thoracotomy for postchemotherapy resection of pulmonary residual tumor mass in patients with nonseminomatous testicular germ cell tumors: Aggressive surgical resection is justified. Chest 1997;112:967–973.

Giwercman A, Muller J, Skakkebaek NE: Prevalence of carcinoma in situ and other histopathological abnormalities in testes from 399 men who suffered sudden unexpected death. J Urol 1991;145:77–80.

Hansen SW, Helweg-Larsen S, Trojaborg W: Long-term neurotoxicity in patients treated with cisplatin, vinblastine, and bleomycin for metastatic germ cell cancer. J Clin Oncol 1989;7:1457–1461.

Harding MJ, Brown IL, MacPherson SG, et al: Excision of residual masses after platinum based chemotherapy for non-seminomatous germ cell tumours. Eur J Cancer Clin Oncol 1989;25:1689–1694.

Hartmann JT, Nichols CR, Droz JP, et al: Hematologic disorders associated with primary mediastinal nonseminomatous germ cell tumors. J Natl Cancer Inst 2000;92:54–61.

Horwich A, Sleijfer D, Fossa S, et al: Randomized trial of bleomycin, etoposide, and cisplatin compared with bleomycin, etoposide, and carboplatin in good-prognosis metastatic nonseminomatous germ cell cancer: A multi-institutional medical research council/European Organization for Research and Treatment of Cancer trial. J Clin Oncol 1997;15:1844–1852.

IGCCCG: International germ cell consensus classification: A prognostic factor-based staging system for metastatic germ cell cancers. J Clin Oncol 1997;15:594–603.

Leibovitch I, Foster R, Kopecky K, Donohue J: Improved accuracy of computerized tomography based clinical staging in low stage nonseminomatous germ cell cancer using size criteria of retroperitoneal lymph nodes. J Urol 1995;154:1759–1763.

Loehrer PJ, Johnson DH, Elson P, et al: Importance of bleomycin in favorable-prognosis disseminated germ cell tumors: An Eastern Cooperative Oncology Group Trial. J Clin Oncol 1995;13:470–476.

Motzer RJ, Amsterdam A, Prieto V, et al: Teratoma with malignant transformation: Diverse malignant histologies arising in men with germ cell tumors. J Urol 1998;159:133–138.

Motzer RJ, Bosl GJ: Testicular germ cell cancer. N Engl J Med 1997;337:242–253.

Motzer RJ, Cooper K, Geller NL, et al: The role of ifosfamide plus cisplatin-based chemotherapy as salvage therapy for patients with refractory germ cell tumors. Cancer 1990;66:2476–2481.

Motzer RJ, Mazumdar M, Gulati SC, et al: Phase II trial of high-dose carboplatin and etoposide with autologous bone marrow transplantation in first-line therapy for patients with poor-risk germ cell tumors. J Natl Cancer Inst 1993;85:1828–1835.

Motzer RJ, Sheinfeld J, Mazumdar M, et al: Etoposide and cisplatin adjuvant therapy for patients with pathologic stage II germ cell tumors. J Clin Oncol 1995;13:2700–2704.

Nichols CR: Treatment of recurrent germ cell tumors. Semin Surg Oncol 1999;17:268.

Nichols CR, Breeden ES, Loehrer PJ: Secondary leukemia associated with a conventional dose of etoposide: Review of serial germ cell tumor protocols. J Natl Cancer Inst 1993;85:36–40.

Nichols CR, Catalano P, Crawford ED, et al: Randomized comparison of cisplatin and etoposide and either bleomycin or ifosfamide in treatment of advanced disseminated germ cell tumors: An Eastern Cooperative Oncology Group, Southwest Oncology Group, and Cancer and Leukemia Group B study. J Clin Oncol 1998;16:1287–1293.

Nicolai N, Pizzocaro G: A surveillance study of clinical stage I nonseminomatous germ cell tumors of the testis: 10-year follow-up. J Urol 1995;154:1045–1049.

Pedersen-Bjergaard J, Hansen ST, Larsen SO, et al: Increased risk of myelodysplasia and leukemia after etoposide, cisplatin, and bleomycin for germ cell tumors. Lancet 1991;338:359–363.

Pont J, Holt W, Kosak D, et al: Risk-adapted treatment choice in stage I nonseminomatous testicular germ cell cancer by regarding vascular invasion in the primary tumor: A prospective trial. J Clin Oncol 1990;8:16–20.

Sharir S, Jewett MAS, Sturgeon JFG, et al: Progression detection of stage I nonseminomatous testis cancer on surveillance: Implications for the followup protocol. J Urol 1999;161:472–476.

Sheinfeld J, Bajorin D: Management of the post chemotherapy residual mass. Urol Clin North Am 1993;20:133–143.

Skakkebaek NE, Berthelsen JG, Giwercman A, Muller J: Carcinoma in situ of the testis: Possible origin from gonocytes and precursors of all types of germ cell tumors except spermatocytoma. Int J Androl 1987;10:19–28.

Stephens AW, Gonin R, Hutchins GD, Einhorn L: Positron emission tomography evaluation of residual radiographic abnormalities in postchemotherapy germ cell tumor patients. J Clin Oncol 1996;14:1637–1641.

Toner GC, Panicek D, Heelan R, et al: Adjunctive surgery after chemotherapy for nonseminomatous germ cell tumors: recommendations for patient selection. J Clin Oncol 1990;8:1683–1694.

van Leeuwen F, Stiggelbout A, van den Belt-Dusebout A, et al: Second cancer risk following testicular cancer: A follow-up study of 1,909 patients. J Clin Oncol 1993;11:415–424.

Vogelzang NJ, Fraley EE, Lange PH, et al: Stage II nonseminomatous testicular cancer: A 10-year experience. J Clin Oncol 1983;1:171–178.

Wanderas EH, Fossa SD, Tretli S: Risk of subsequent non-germ cell cancer after treatment of germ cell cancer in 2006 Norwegian male patients. Eur J Cancer 1997;33:253–262.

Warde P, Gospodarowicz MK, Panzarella T, et al: Stage I testicular seminoma: Results of adjuvant irradiation and surveillance. J Clin Oncol 1995;13:2255–2262.

Weissbach L, Hartlapp JH: Adjuvant chemotherapy of metastatic stage II nonseminomatous testis tumor. J Urol 1991;146:1295–1298.

Williams SD, Birch R, Einhorn LH, et al: Treatment of disseminated germ cell tumors with cisplatin, bleomycin, and either vinblastine or etoposide. N Engl J Med 1987;316:1435–1440.

Williams SD, Stablein DM, Einhorn LH, et al: Immediate adjuvant chemotherapy versus observation with treatment at relapse in pathological stage II testicular cancer. N Engl J Med 1987;317:1433–1438.

Wood DP, Herr HW, Motzer RJ, et al: Surgical resection of solitary metastases after chemotherapy in patients with non-seminomatous germ cell tumors and elevated serum tumor markers. Cancer 1992;70:2354–2357.

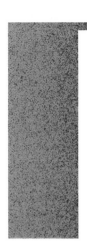

Chapter 84
Renal Cancer

Jared A. Gollob

Epidemiology

Malignant tumors of the kidney, including renal pelvis and ureter, make up 2% of both new cancer diagnoses and deaths each year in the United States. Approximately 30,000 cases and 11,900 deaths were anticipated in 2000. Renal cell cancer accounts for 70% of the total, and occurs more often in men than in women. The mean age at diagnosis is approximately 60 years. The incidence rates for renal cell cancer have been rising each year in the United States since the 1970s, with recent increases more rapid among blacks than whites. The worldwide incidence is highest in Scandinavia and other parts of northern Europe and in North America. The lowest rates are reported in India, China, Japan, and areas of Central and South America.

Risk Factors

Most of the information on risk factors for renal cell cancer has come from case-control studies, the largest comprising 1732 cases and 2309 controls. Cigarette smoking is an established causal risk factor for renal cell cancer, the relative risks among smokers from case-control and cohort studies ranging from 1.2 to 2.3. Approximately 20% to 30% of renal cell cancers among men and 10% to 20% among women can be accounted for by cigarette smoking. Obesity, particularly among women, has been associated with renal cell cancer, as has hypertension. Some studies have suggested that the use of certain drugs, such as thiazide diuretics, and occupational exposure to toxins such as polycyclic aromatic hydrocarbons (among coke oven workers), trichloroethylene, and perchloroethylene (among dry cleaning employees) may be associated with an increased risk of developing renal cell cancer. However, there are as yet no firm data establishing a link between these drugs and toxins and renal cell cancer. Acquired cystic disease of the kidney, occurring in 80% to 95% of patients undergoing hemodialysis and 30% to 45% of those undergoing peritoneal dialysis, predisposes to renal cell cancer. There is a 5% to 30% likelihood that these patients will develop renal cell cancer, and approximately 15% of those who do develop renal cell cancer will present with metastatic disease.

Histologic Subtypes

In 1997, a new classification of renal epithelial tumors was adopted that established distinct subtypes based on morphology, genetic features, and cell of origin (Table 84-1). Conventional (clear cell) renal cell cancer makes up 65% to 70% of renal epithelial tumors and is derived from cells of the proximal convoluted tubule. Most cases are sporadic, unilateral, and unifocal and present in the sixth or seventh decade of life. These tumors tend to show a mixture of cytoplasmic features, with clear or granular-eosinophilic cytoplasm (Figure 84-1A). Approximately 50% of cases exhibit either a solid or acinar growth pattern exclusively; the remaining cases contain a mixture of growth patterns, including cystic, papillary/pseudopapillary, tubular, and sarcomatoid. Papillary renal cell cancer makes up 10% to 15% of renal cell cancers and has a more favorable prognosis than conventional clear cell cancer. The classic papillary pattern is characterized by discrete papillary fronds lined by neoplastic cells and containing a central fibrovascular core (Figure 84-1B). While a papillary growth pattern predominates in the majority of cases, about 25% of tumors exhibit less than 50% papillary growth. Papillary tumors are more likely to have bilateral as well as multifocal disease and derive from cells of the distal convoluted tubule. Chromophobe renal cell cancer makes up 5% to 10% of renal epithelial tumors, is derived from intercalated cells, and tends to be an indolent tumor that grows quite large but usually remains confined to the kidney. The majority of chromophobe tumors demonstrate variable granu-

Table 84-1 ▪ Characteristics of the Major Subtypes of Renal Cell Tumors

Histologic Subtype	Percentage of Total Renal Cell Tumors	Cell of Origin	Genetic Change(s)	Comments
Clear cell (conventional)	65–70%	Proximal convoluted tubule	Deletions and mutations of VHL locus on 3p25	Sarcomatoid and granular variants with worse prognosis.
Papillary	10–15%	Distal convoluted tubule	Trisomy 7 and MET mutation on 7q31–34	Favorable prognosis compared to clear cell; often multifocal.
Chromophobe	5–10%	Intercalated cells	Y-, 1-	Rarely metastasize, even when large.
Collecting duct	<1%	Collecting ducts of renal medulla	1-, 6-, 14-, 15-, 22-	Aggressive, seen in younger patients; early lymph node metastases.
Oncocytoma	5–10%	Intercalated cells	Y-, 1-	Benign tumor.

lar and diffuse blue cytoplasmic staining with Hale's colloidal iron (Figure 84-1*C*).

Collecting duct carcinoma, also known as Bellini duct carcinoma, accounts for fewer than 1% of renal epithelial tumors. The cell of origin is from the collecting ducts of the renal medulla. Collecting duct cancers contain tumor cells with high-grade cytology that are arranged in nests and tubules and associated with stromal desmoplasia. Tumor cells may exhibit a hobnail morphology (Figure 84-1*D*), contain mucin, and demonstrate positive staining for the lectin *Ulex europaeus* agglutinin. These rare cancers tend to present in younger patients and are aggressive, more than 50% of patients presenting with metastatic disease. Medullary carcinoma, like collecting duct carcinoma, is a rare, aggressive tumor derived from the distal portions of the collecting ducts that occurs predominantly in African-American patients with sickle cell trait.

Oncocytomas make up 5% to 10% of all primary renal neoplasms. They are derived from intercalated cells, and are benign tumors. The dominant cell type in this tumor has abundant, densely eosinophilic cytoplasm and a round nucleus with prominent nucleolus and is arranged in nests and tubules. A sarcomalike variant of renal cell carcinoma is also rarely seen (Figure 84-1*E*).

Genetics

The clear cell and papillary subtypes of renal cell cancer are further distinguished by the unique genetic abnormalities that are associated with these histologies. These genetic abnormalities were first identified through studies of familial cancer syndromes.

Von Hippel-Lindau disease (VHL) is an autosomal-dominant multiorgan familial cancer syndrome characterized by the development of cerebellar/spinal hemangioblastomas, retinal angiomas, pheochromocytomas, and renal cysts/tumors. Renal cell cancer develops in 40% to 60% of patients with von Hippel-Lindau disease and is exclusively of the clear cell histologic type. These tumors tend to be multicentric and bilateral and occur at an earlier age. The human VHL gene maps to chromosome subband 3p25. Germline mutations of the VHL gene occur in 100% of the patients presenting with the von Hippel-Lindau disease clinical phenotype, and genetic analysis of von Hippel-Lindau disease–associated clear cell renal cell cancer shows loss of heterozygosity (LOH) at the VHL locus due to deletion of the wild-type allele.

In sporadic clear cell renal cell cancer, loss of heterozygosity at the VHL locus is present in 75% to 80% of cases, along with either simultaneous mutational inactivation of the remaining allele or silencing of the remaining allele by methylation (see Table 84-1). This finding implicates mutations of the VHL gene in the pathogenesis of both hereditary and sporadic clear cell cancers. The VHL gene encodes a tumor suppressor protein with two isoforms that associates with proteins termed elongin B and elongin C that are involved in the control of transcriptional elongation. The von Hippel-Lindau disease protein appears to be involved in the regulation of the expression of hypoxia-inducible proteins. In its absence, these proteins, including vascular endothelial growth factor (VEGF), transforming growth factor-beta 1 (TGF-β1), and platelet-derived growth factor-beta (PDGF-β), are inappropriately overexpressed under normoxic conditions and may contribute to the malignant phenotype of clear cell tumors.

Hereditary papillary renal cell cancer is a rare inherited syndrome. Affected family members tend to develop multifocal, bilateral papillary cancers at a much younger age than those with sporadic renal cell cancer. Trisomy 7 is common in familial papillary car-

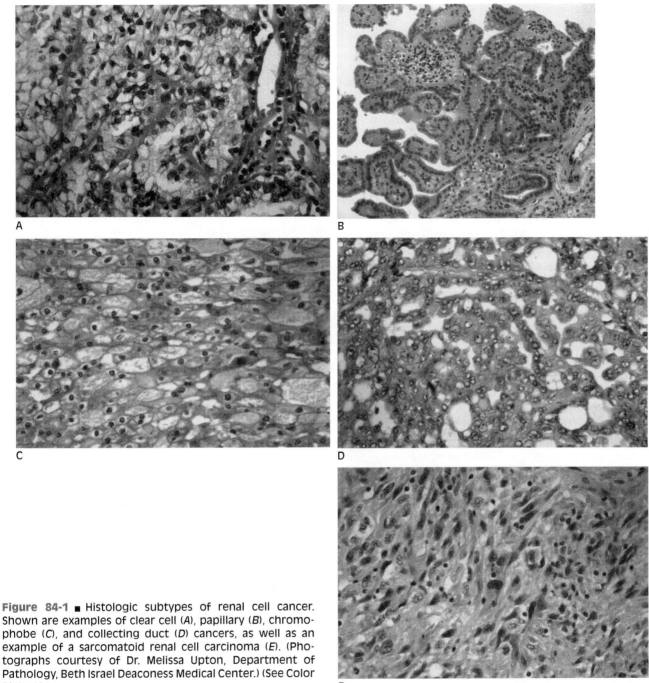

Figure 84-1 ■ Histologic subtypes of renal cell cancer. Shown are examples of clear cell (*A*), papillary (*B*), chromophobe (*C*), and collecting duct (*D*) cancers, as well as an example of a sarcomatoid renal cell carcinoma (*E*). (Photographs courtesy of Dr. Melissa Upton, Department of Pathology, Beth Israel Deaconess Medical Center.) (See Color Plate 19.)

cinomas, and germline mutations of the MET proto-oncogene on 7q31–q34 are found in 80% of cases. Sporadic papillary renal cell cancers are characterized by trisomy involving chromosomes 7, 16, and 17 and loss of the Y chromosome in males (see Table 84-1). The c-met receptor belongs to the tyrosine kinase receptor superfamily, and hepatocyte growth factor/scatter factor (HGF/SF) is the ligand for c-met. Overexpression of c-met through gene amplification or the constitutive activation of c-met caused by muta-

tions may underlie the malignant phenotype of both sporadic and hereditary papillary tumors. Notably, mutations/deletions in the VHL locus are not found in papillary renal cell cancer. Likewise, amplification and/or mutation of the gene encoding c-met is not found in clear cell renal cell cancer.

While collecting duct cancers have a variety of chromosomal abnormalities, none have been classified yet as defining for these histologic subtypes. Both chromophobe tumors and oncocytomas are commonly found to have loss of the Y chromosome and loss of chromosome 1 (see Table 84-1). However, mutations in VHL or c-met have not been seen in these tumors.

Clinical Presentation

Renal cell cancer often remains clinically occult until the primary tumor has grown quite large or until metastases cause constitutional symptoms or pain. As ultrasound and computed tomography (CT) have been used more frequently to evaluate nonspecific abdominal complaints, the incidental diagnosis of renal cell cancer has become more common. At present, approximately 60% to 70% of patients present with localized disease, while 15% to 20% are diagnosed with regional spread, and 15% to 20% are diagnosed with distant metastases. Pain, gross hematuria, and palpable mass are the most common presenting signs and symptoms and are often an indication of locally advanced disease. However, only 5% of patients present with all three (Virchow's triad). Patients with locally advanced disease may also present with bilateral lower extremity edema arising from the growth of a tumor thrombus into the inferior vena cava, as well as full-blown Budd-Chiari syndrome resulting from tumor thrombus extension into the hepatic vein. The lungs, lymph nodes, liver, bone, and adrenal glands are the most common sites of metastases, and patients may initially present with cervical/supraclavicular lymphadenopathy, bone pain, or respiratory symptoms due to hilar/mediastinal adenopathy, pleural effusion, and/or parenchymal lung metastases. Less commonly, patients present with subcutaneous metastases or metastases to unusual sites such as the thyroid gland, orbit, sinuses or other mucosal surfaces. Although 5% to 10% of patients with advanced disease develop central nervous system metastases, brain metastases are rare at presentation.

A variety of paraneoplastic syndromes are associated with renal cell cancer (Table 84-2), and may be observed in patients with either localized or advanced disease. Anemia (often an anemia of chronic disease) and constitutional symptoms such as fever, malaise, anorexia, and weight loss are among the most common findings, present in 20% to 40% of patients at the time of diagnosis. Hepatic dysfunction in the absence of liver metastases (Stauffer's syndrome), characterized by an elevation of the serum alkaline phosphatase and/or hepatic transaminases, is present in 5% to 10% of patients. Polycythemia and hypertension, due to the production by tumor cells of erythropoietin and renin, respectively, can be observed in patients with both localized and advanced disease. Hypercalcemia, seen more commonly in patients

Table 84-2 ▪ Paraneoplastic Syndromes Associated with Renal Cell Cancer

Microcytic anemia
Fever/night sweats
Weight loss/anorexia
Fatigue
Stauffer's syndrome (elevation of hepatic transaminases and/or alkaline phosphatase in the absence of liver metastases)
Hypercalcemia
Polycythemia
Hypertension
Amyloidosis
Neuromyopathy
Dysfibrinogenemia
Trousseau's syndrome

with advanced metastatic disease, is often due to the production of parathyroid hormone–related protein by tumor cells. Other, less common paraneoplastic syndromes include amyloidosis, neuromyopathy, and acquired dysfibrinogenemia. Patients with advanced disease may also develop deep vein thromboses and pulmonary emboli due to hypercoagulability (Trousseau's syndrome) that is associated with metastatic carcinoma.

Clinical Evaluation

Computed tomography scan is the imaging modality of choice for the detection of renal neoplasms. Computed tomography has a sensitivity of 94% for the detection of lesions 3 cm or more in diameter and should be performed both before and after the administration of intravenous (IV) contrast. Enhancement of a mass lesion in the kidney after the administration of intravenous contrast is an indication of a hypervascular tumor and is characteristic, though not diagnostic, of renal cell cancer. There is no pathognomonic feature on computed tomography of renal cell cancer. These neoplasms may arise from either the poles or central region of the kidney (Figures 84-2A and 84-2B) and may encroach on the collecting system like transitional cell cancers of the renal pelvis. The various histologic subtypes of renal cell cancer, as well as transitional cell cancers, may have areas of necrosis or hemorrhage visible on computed tomography. Although the presence of a central stellate scar on computed tomography may be suggestive of oncocytoma, this finding is not pathognomonic. For cystic lesions, the presence on computed tomography of irregular wall thickening or nodularity or of a ragged or blurred margin between the lesion and the

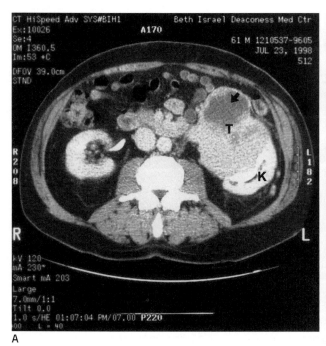

A

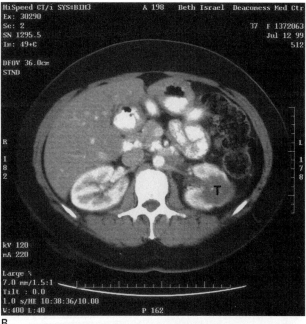

B

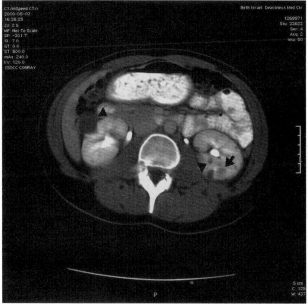

C

Figure 84-2 ■ Computed tomography scan appearance of renal cell cancer. *A,* Clear cell cancer. Large fungating tumor mass (*T*) extends from the upper pole of the left kidney (*K*). The arrow points to a large area of low attenuation indicative of tumor necrosis. *B,* Collecting duct cancer. A centrally located tumor (T) involves the medullary and cortical regions of the kidney and appears to extend into the collecting system. *C,* Clear cell cancer in a young patient with von Hippel Lindau disease. Multiple cysts (arrow heads) are seen, along with a <2 cm tumor in the left kidney (arrow).

renal parenchyma is suggestive of renal cell cancer (Figure 84-2*C*).

For patients who initially present with hematuria and/or flank pain, intravenous urography may be the first test that is performed to rule out nephrolithiasis. If a ureteral stone is not identified, a computed tomography scan should be performed to rule out a renal neoplasm even if the kidney appears normal by intravenous urography, as this test has a low sensitivity for the detection of renal tumors 3 cm or smaller in size. In a study using intravenous urography with linear

tomography, this procedure detected only 52% of renal masses between 2 and 3 cm that were detected by computed tomography.

Ultrasound scanning can be helpful in determining whether a lucent lesion that is seen on intravenous urography is a benign cyst or a solid mass. All solid masses detected by ultrasound should be evaluated with computed tomography scanning. Ultrasound is also a useful screening tool for those who are at high risk for development of renal cell cancer, including patients with VHL gene mutations and their first-

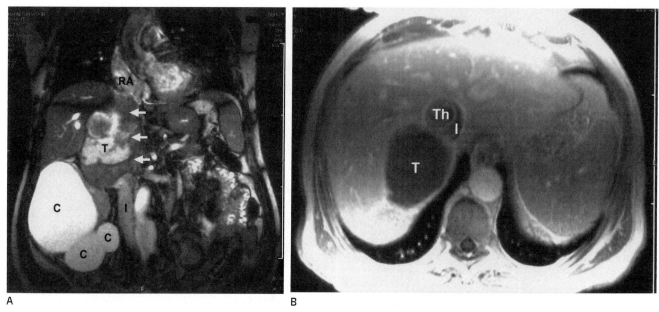

Figure 84-3 ■ Detection by magnetic resonance imaging scan of renal cell cancer extension into the inferior vena cava. *A*, Coronal image shows a large tumor (T) growing out of the upper pole of the right kidney, which also has multiple large cysts (C). The tumor extends into the inferior vena cava (I) and has grown upward (white arrows) above the diaphragm to the level of the right atrium (RA). The pathology of this T3c tumor was clear cell with sarcomatoid features. *B*, Horizontal section through the same patient shows the tumor (T) in the upper pole of the right kidney abutting the liver along with a tumor thrombus (Th) lying within the inferior vena cava (I).

degree relatives, first-degree relatives of patients with hereditary papillary renal cell cancer, and patients with acquired cystic kidney disease.

Contrast-enhanced computed tomography scans can help to determine whether a renal tumor has invaded the renal vein and inferior vena cava. Approximately 23% of renal cell cancers will exhibit extension into the renal vein, and in 7%, there will be extension of tumor thrombus into the inferior vena cava. If the computed tomography scan is equivocal, either Doppler ultrasonography or magnetic resonance imaging (MRI) performed with gadolinium can more fully assess the vasculature for the presence of tumor thrombus (Figures 84-3*A* and 84-3*B*). The magnetic resonance imaging in particular can help to determine the cephalic extent of tumor thrombus within the inferior vena cava, which is important in determining the operability of such a tumor. Magnetic resonance imaging can also help to determine whether a tumor invades or merely abuts an adjacent organ.

Following the identification on computed tomography scan of a suspicious mass lesion in the kidney, patients should undergo a full-torso computed tomography scan to determine whether there are regional nodal and/or distant metastases. As a bone scan is unlikely to be positive in the absence of symptoms, it should be performed only as part of the initial staging workup if the patient has bone pain. Likewise, a head computed tomography scan is not necessary unless there is a clinical suspicion of brain metastases. Routine blood work should include a complete blood count, liver function tests, BUN and creatinine levels to assess renal function, and serum calcium level.

The majority of renal masses (75% to 85%) are renal cell cancers, the remaining being either transitional cell cancers of the collecting system (10% to 15%) or metastatic tumors (fewer than 5%). In the absence of evidence for metastatic disease on computed tomography scan, a computed tomography–guided needle biopsy of the mass should not be performed unless there is a prior diagnosis of another malignancy and a strong suspicion that the renal lesion could represent a metastasis. Instead, the diagnosis should be established through nephrectomy. If there are accessible bulky regional nodal metastases or distant metastases, percutaneous needle biopsy of a metastasis should be performed to establish the diagnosis of renal cell cancer. Alternatively, for patients with advanced disease who are candidates for nephrectomy, the diagnosis can be made from the resected tumor. However, if there is a strong clinical suspicion of a transitional cell cancer (for example, if the tumor appears to be arising from the collecting system or if there is a positive urine cytology), the diagnosis should be established through biopsy, as debulking nephrectomy is not indicated in patients with advanced transitional cell cancer.

Staging, Prognostic Features and Outcomes

The TNM staging system for renal cell cancer (Tables 84-3 and 84-4), which was modified in 1998 by the American Joint Committee on Cancer (AJCC), has largely supplanted the prior staging system. The new staging system takes into account the finding that even large tumors can have a favorable prognosis if confined to the kidney and delineates the incremental worsening of prognosis associated inferior vena cava and lymph node involvement as well as invasion beyond Gerota's fascia into contiguous organs. For stage I patients with tumors 7 cm or smaller that are confined to the kidney, the five-year survival rate is 90% to 95%, while for stage II patients with tumors larger than 7 cm, the five-year survival rate is 70% to 85%. Stage III patients with tumors that extend beyond the renal capsule or into either the renal

Table 84-3 ■ Definition of TNM for Renal Cell Cancer

Primary Tumor (T)

TX   Primary tumor cannot be assessed
T0   No evidence of primary tumor
T1   Tumor ≤7 cm in greatest dimension limited to the kidney
T2   Tumor >7 cm in greatest dimension limited to the kidney
T3   Tumor extends into major veins or invades the adrenal gland or perinephric tissue but not beyond Gerota's fascia
  T3a   Tumor invades the adrenal gland or perinephric fat but not beyond Gerota's fascia
  T3b   Tumor grossly extends into the renal vein or vena cava below the diaphragm
  T3c   Tumor grossly extends into the vena cava above the diaphragm
T4   Tumor invades beyond Gerota's fascia

Regional Lymph Nodes (N)

NX   Regional lymph nodes cannot be assessed
N0   No regional lymph node metastases
N1   Metastasis in a single regional lymph node
N2   Metastases in more than one regional lymph node

Distant Metastasis (M)

MX   Distant metastasis cannot be assessed
M0   No distant metastasis
M1   Distant metastasis

Table 84-4 ■ Correlation of Stage Grouping with Survival in Patients with Renal Cell Cancer

Stage Grouping				Five-Year Survival Rate
Stage I	T1	N0	M0	90–95%
Stage II	T2	N0	M0	70–85%
Stage III	T3a	N0	M0	50–65%
	T3b	N0	M0	50–65%
	T3c	N0	M0	45–50%
	T1	N1	M0	25–30%
	T2	N1	M0	25–30%
	T3	N1	M0	15–20%
Stage IV	T4	N0–1	M0	10%
	T any	N2	M0	10%
	T any	N any	M1	<5%

vein or inferior vena cava (T3a-cN0) have a 45% to 65% five-year survival rate, whereas a metastasis to a single regional lymph node (N1) drops the five-year survival rate down to 25% to 30% for T1–2N1 patients and to 15% to 20% for T3N1 patients. The prognosis is poor for stage IV patients with tumor invasion into contiguous organs or metastases to multiple regional nodes (T4 or N2: 10% five-year survival rate), and fewer than 5% of patients with distant metastases are alive at five years. The median survival for stage IV patients is 9 to 10 months. An exception to the dismal prognosis associated with distant metastases is seen in patients younger than age 60 years who undergo surgical resection of an isolated metastasis to the lung or soft tissue that appears after a disease-free interval of one year or more. These patients, who make up only 2% to 4% of all patients with metastatic disease, have a reported five-year survival rate of 25% to 30%.

Other factors in addition to stage have a bearing on prognosis. For example, chromophobe tumors and oncocytomas rarely metastasize, even when they are large, and therefore have a favorable prognosis. While papillary tumors have a better prognosis than clear cell tumors, collecting duct cancer is an aggressive disease that tends to occur in younger patients (in one series, the mean age was 34) and metastasizes early. Clear cell cancers with sarcomatoid histology or with cytoplasm that is more granular and eosinophilic behave more aggressively, as do clear cell cancers with a high Fuhrman nuclear grade.

Clinical features at the time of presentation that are independent of stage and associated with diminished survival include an Eastern Cooperative Oncology Group (ECOG) performance status of 2 or greater, weight loss of greater than 10% within the past six

Table 84-5 ■ Clinical Features Associated with Diminished Survival

Eastern Cooperative Oncology Group performance status ≥ 2
Weight loss > 10%
Erythrocyte sedimentation rate (ESR) > 50 mm/hour
Hemoglobin < 10 g/dL
Elevated serum lactate dehydrogenase (LDH)
Elevated serum calcium

months, an erythrocyte sedimentation rate (ESR) greater than 50 mm/hour, and hemoglobin less than 10 g/dL (Table 84-5). For patients with metastatic disease, elevation of the serum lactate dehydrogenase (LDH) and serum calcium are also associated with a worse prognosis. Patients with advanced disease who have multiple poor prognostic factors have a median survival of only four months.

Treatment

Surgery

Localized Disease

Radical nephrectomy, involving the en bloc removal of the kidney and perinephric fat outside Gerota's capsule, is the treatment of choice for localized renal cell cancer. Although a radical nephrectomy used to include a complete retroperitoneal lymph node dissection, this is no longer recommended, as it is estimated to be curative in only 2% to 4% of patients. Most surgeons advocate performing only a regional node dissection (ipsilateral great vessel and hilar nodes), largely for prognostic purposes, in patients who are at greater risk for nodal metastases, including those with large tumors (>T1) and renal vein involvement. While radical nephrectomy frequently includes adrenalectomy, the therapeutic advantage of adrenalectomy remains questionable in patients with stage I and stage II disease. In a report of 695 nephrectomies, the incidence of adrenal metastases was 4.3%, and these were more likely to occur in patients whose tumors occupied the whole kidney or the upper pole. Adrenalectomy is therefore recommended only for patients with large tumors, upper pole tumors, or an adrenal abnormality seen on computed tomography scan.

Partial nephrectomy is appropriate in patients with bilateral renal cell cancer, tumors that involve a solitary functioning kidney, patients with chronic renal failure, or unilateral renal cell cancer in patients with a functioning opposite kidney that is at risk for future impairment from an intercurrent disorder such as hypertension, diabetes mellitus, nephropathy, or calculus disease. In a series of 327 patients with sporadic renal cell cancer undergoing nephron-sparing surgery, the five-year recurrence rate was 12%, with only 4% developing recurrences in the remnant kidney. Partial nephrectomy can also be performed in select patients with a normal contralateral kidney. Several studies have shown that for tumors less than 4 cm, the five-year cancer-specific survival rate following nephron-sparing surgery is 95% to 100%, a result comparable with that of radical nephrectomy. The location of the tumor does not appear to be a factor in the success rate of nephron-sparing surgery for patients with small tumors, as five-year cancer-specific survival rates are similar following resection of both peripheral and central tumors. While it is not known whether patients with papillary renal cell cancer have a greater risk of local recurrence following partial nephrectomy, the fact that these tumors are more often multifocal compared to other renal cell cancer histologies argues against its use if papillary cancer has been diagnosed preoperatively through biopsy. Neither lymph node dissection nor adrenalectomy is recommended for patients undergoing partial nephrectomy in the absence of any abnormality on computed tomography scan.

Patients with VHL gene mutations who develop renal cell cancer often have disease that is multifocal and bilateral. For this reason, partial nephrectomy is often advocated to preserve renal function. For these patients, partial nephrectomy is used when the tumors are less than 3 cm in diameter. This is based on a National Cancer Institute study that found no metastases among 54 of these patients who underwent partial nephrectomy for tumors less than 3 cm. The 10-year disease-specific survival rate of these patients with renal cancer is 81%, although the 10-year survival rate free of local recurrence is only 15%. These patients frequently require repeated operations, and most eventually require dialysis. Therefore, it has been suggested that for patients presenting with bilateral renal cancer, bilateral nephrectomies and dialysis may be a better option than repeated partial resections.

Advanced Disease

Radical nephrectomy should be performed in patients with tumor extension into the perinephric fat or adrenal gland (T3a) or invasion of the renal vein or subdiaphragmatic inferior vena cava (T3b), since surgery can be curative in 50% to 65% of these patients. For patients with T3a to T3b tumors and lymph node metastases, the outcome is considerably worse, as many patients will eventually die from distant metastases. However, in a series of 43 patients with regional nodes enlarged to 1 to 2.2 cm on computed tomography scan, only 42% had nodal metastases, whereas 58% had reactive inflammation. Therefore, potentially curative nephrectomy should be offered to patients with T3a to T3b tumors even in the setting of enlarged regional nodes on computed tomography scan.

For patients with tumor extension into the supra-diaphragmatic inferior vena cava (which can include extension into the right atrium), resection requires a thoracoabdominal incision and cardiopulmonary bypass (with or without hypothermic circulatory arrest), with a perioperative mortality rate that can be as high as 10%. While the five-year survival rate has been reported in some series to be as low as 15% to 30% for patients with T3c tumors, other studies have suggested that the outcome might be substantially better (45% to 50% five-year survival rate) if the tumor thrombus is free-floating in the inferior vena cava rather than invasive and if there are no nodal or distant metastases. Therefore, radical nephrectomy and resection of vena cava tumor extension should be considered in patients with a good performance status and no significant cardiopulmonary disease who do not have distant metastases.

The role of debulking nephrectomy in patients with stage IV disease has been controversial. Advocates of this approach have pointed to historic data that suggest a higher rate of response to immune-based therapies such as interleukin-2 (IL-2) and interferon-alpha (IFN-α) in patients who first undergo debulking nephrectomy. Others have argued that debulking nephrectomy can help to prevent pain, blood loss, and worsening constitutional symptoms from an enlarging tumor that is unlikely to respond to medical therapy. There is now evidence from two randomized prospective trials showing that nephrectomy can improve survival in patients with metastatic renal cell cancer. In a Southwest Oncology Group trial, patients with metastatic disease were randomized to immediate IFN-α2b therapy or radical nephrectomy followed by IFN-α2b. Although the response to IFN-α2b was not affected by surgery, the median survival was improved by four months in patients who underwent nephrectomy ($P = 0.033$). On the basis of these findings, patients with a good performance status and metastatic disease that is asymptomatic, small relative to the primary tumor, and slowly progressive should be considered for debulking nephrectomy prior to systemic therapy.

TREATMENT

Selection of Patients with Metastatic Disease for Debulking Nephrectomy

Patients who present with a renal mass and distant metastases should be considered for debulking nephrectomy, which has been shown to improve survival and may also enhance the response to subsequent IL-2-based therapy. However, in selecting patients for nephrectomy, it is important to identify those patients who are likely to remain eligible for immunotherapy following the period of recovery from surgery. In a series of 195 patients with metastatic renal cell cancer, 38% could not receive IL-2 after nephrectomy owing either to substantial disease progression or to postoperative complications.

A needle biopsy of a metastatic site should be performed. If the biopsy reveals renal cell cancer, nephrectomy should be performed in patients who meet the following criteria:

1. More than 75% surgical debulking of total tumor burden is technically feasible
2. No central nervous system, bone, or liver metastases
3. Adequate pulmonary and cardiac function
4. ECOG performance status of 0 or 1
5. No active infection or comorbid condition

Using these criteria for the selection of patients for nephrectomy, one study showed that 93% of patients were able to subsequently receive IL-2-based therapy after recovering from surgery.

For patients with metastatic disease, it is not yet clear whether the histology of the tumor should influence the decision to perform a nephrectomy. As most responses to IL-2 and even to cell-based therapies such as allogeneic nonmyeloablative stem cell transplant occur in patients with predominantly clear cell tumors, an argument can be made against doing a nephrectomy in patients with non–clear cell tumors, who are unlikely to derive a benefit from subsequent immunotherapy. However, as the overall survival benefit observed in patients undergoing nephrectomy has not yet been analyzed according to histologic subtype, histology alone should not be used to select patients for nephrectomy. Nonetheless, for patients who do not meet all of the above criteria and/or have evidence of rapid disease progression, it is prudent to avoid nephrectomy if the biopsy shows an aggressive sarcomatoid or collecting duct histology.

Table 84-6 ■ Response of Renal Cell Cancer to Chemotherapy

Agents(s)	N	Response Rate*
Vinblastine	135	4–16%
5-Fluorouracil (5-FU)	123	5–11%
Floxuridine (FUDR)	165	7–14%
Gemcitabine	48	6–10%
Gemcitabine + 5-FU	39	17%
Doxorubicin	38	5%
Cyclophosphamide	66	0–4%
Navelbine	38	0–4%
Paclitaxel	33	0%
Docetaxel	18	0%
Cisplatin	33	0%
Carboplatin	37	0%

N = population size.
*Ranges represent lowest and highest overall response rates from multiple trials of the indicated agent.

Chemotherapy/Hormonal Therapy

Chemotherapy has had little impact on the course of metastatic renal cell cancer. A wide variety of drugs have been tested in Phase II trials (Table 84-6), with most response rates under 10%. While vinblastine, 5-fluorouracil, and floxuridine have had the most consistent activity in prior trials, the few responses that have been observed have been predominantly partial responses and have had no significant effect on overall survival. A number of mechanisms appear to be involved in the resistance of renal cell cancer to chemotherapy, including the overexpression of the multidrug resistance (MDR) gene product P-glycoprotein, the increased expression of glutathione-S transferase, and the downregulation of topoisomerase-2. Attempts have been made to block the function of P-glycoprotein, using calcium channel blockers and calmodulin inhibitors, to render cells more sensitive to chemotherapy. However, while this approach has been effective in vitro, clinical trials using vinblastine in combination with these P-glycoprotein inhibitors have not demonstrated improved response rates.

Recently, a combination of continuous infusion 5-fluorouracil plus gemcitabine achieved a response rate of 17%, in contrast to response rates of 5% to 10% with either gemcitabine or 5-fluorouracil alone. All responses were partial and occurred primarily in patients with lung and lymph node metastases. This regimen was well tolerated, with only modest hematologic and gastrointestinal toxicity. While the impact of 5-fluorouracil plus gemcitabine on survival remains unclear, it is nonetheless a viable option for patients with predominantly lung and/or lymph node metastases who have either failed or are incapable of receiving immunotherapy.

Because the majority of patients who are enrolled in Phase II chemotherapy trials have had clear cell cancers, the role of chemotherapy in the treatment of other histologic subtypes, such as papillary and collecting duct cancers, is currently unknown.

There is no known effective hormonal therapy for the treatment of metastatic renal cell cancer. While Megace (medroxyprogesterone acetate) was initially reported to have activity, subsequent trials demonstrated a response rate of less than 5%. Although Megace is unlikely to cause tumor regression, it can help to ameliorate the anorexia and cachexia that occur in patients with this disease.

Immunotherapy

Cytokine Monotherapy

Of a number of cytokines, which have antitumor activity in animal models of renal cell cancer, IFN-α and IL-2 have most consistently been shown to induce tumor regression in patients with metastatic renal cell cancer. Although the mechanism of action of these cytokines is incompletely understood, the induction of antitumor responses in mice by IFN-α and IL-2 has been linked both to the direct killing of tumor cells by activated T and natural killer (NK) cells as well as to antiangiogenic effects of these agents.

IFN-α

Phase II trials of IFN-α2a and IFN-α2b in patients with metastatic renal cell cancer have demonstrated response rates of 10% to 20%, the majority of responses being partial and of limited duration. Responses to IFN-α tend to be delayed and are most commonly seen in patients with small-volume metastatic disease in the lungs and lymph nodes. Although there is no clear dose-response relationship, the most commonly used dosing schedules consist of 5 to 18×10^6 U administered by subcutaneous (SC) or intramuscular (IM) injection three times weekly. Treatment for at least three months is recommended, with a maximum duration of one year in responders. The toxicity of IFN-α includes flu-like symptoms such as fever, chills, myalgias, and fatigue, as well as weight loss, altered taste, mental depression, anemia and leukopenia, and elevated liver function tests. Most side effects, especially the flu-like symptoms, tend to diminish with time during chronic therapy, and both Tylenol and nonsteroidal anti-inflammatory drugs (NSAIDs) can help to control flu-like symptoms during the early phase of therapy. While IFN-α clearly does have some activity in renal cell cancer, its overall

Table 84-7 ■ Randomized Trials of IL-2 and IFN-α in the Treatment of Metastatic Renal Cell Cancer

				Patients Responding			
Investigators	N	Dose of IL-2	Dose of IFN-α	Complete Response	Partial Response	Major Response Rate* (%)	Comments
Yang et al (1997)	56	720 (IU/kg × 10³ IVB q8h × 28 doses)	—	4	5	16	Interim analysis in 1997; accrual ongoing.
	55	72 (IU/kg × 10³ IVB q8h × 28 doses)	—	0	2	4	
	53	125 (IU/kg × 10³ SC qd days 1–5 × 6 wks)	—	3	3	11	
Negrier et al (1998)	138	18 (IU/kg × 10⁶ IVCI days 1–5, 12–16)	—	2	7	6.5	No difference in survival rate between groups.
	140	18 (IU/kg × 10⁶ IVCI days 1–5, 12–16)	6 × 10⁶ U SC TIW	1	25	18.6	
	147	—	18 × 10⁶ U SC TIW	0	11	7.5	
Atkins et al (1993)	71	600 (IU/kg × 10³ IVB q8h × 28 doses)	—	4	8	17	Durable complete responses in IL-2 alone group.
	28	360 (IU/kg × 10³ IVB q8h × 28 doses)	3 × 10⁶ U/m² SC q8h	0	3	11	
Dutcher (Cytokine Working Group) (2001)	A	600 (IU/kg × 10³ IVB q8h × 28 doses)	—	8	17	25	Data on survival and durability of responses are forthcoming.
	B	5 × 10⁶ IU/m² SC qd days 1–5 × 4 wks	5 × 10⁶ IU/m² SC TIW × 4 wks	2	10	12	

N = population size.
*Response rate = complete response + partial response.

efficacy as a single agent is quite limited. In a recently published French Immunotherapy Group Phase III trial comparing IFN-α to both IL-2 and IL-2 plus IFN-α, the response to IFN-α was only 7.5% with a one-year event-free survival rate of only 12% (Table 84-7). However, IFN-α may have a modest impact on survival. In a Phase III trial comparing IFN-α2a plus vinblastine to vinblastine alone in patients with metastatic disease, median survival was 67.6 weeks with IFN-α2a plus vinblastine versus 37.8 weeks for vinblastine alone ($P = 0.0049$). In another trial that randomized patients with advanced disease to either Megace or IFN-α, there was a 28% reduction in the risk of death in the IFN-α group (hazard ratio 0.72, $P = 0.017$) and an improvement in median survival of 2.5 months.

IL-2

IL-2 has a central role in the treatment of metastatic renal cell cancer. In particular, high-dose bolus IL-2 is the only therapy that has been shown to consistently induce durable remissions in patients with metastatic disease, and it is this unique feature that led to its approval by the FDA in 1992. This approval was based on data from 255 patients entered into seven Phase II clinical trials involving 21 institutions (Table 84-8). In these studies, 600,000 to 720,000 IU/kg of IL-2 was administered by 15-minute infusion every eight hours × 14 doses, which constituted a cycle of therapy. Patients received a course of therapy consisting of two cycles separated by five to nine days, and courses were repeated every six to 12 weeks in stable or responding patients. With a median follow-up of over five years, the response rate was 15%, including 7% complete remission and 8% partial remission. For patients achieving complete remission (Figures 84-4A and 84-4B), relapses were rare after 20 months, and the median response duration was 80+ months with a 10-year disease-free survival rate of 60% to 70% (Figure 84-5). The median response duration for patients who achieved a partial response was 20 months, and for all major responders, the response duration was 54 months. High-dose IL-2 has also been administered as a 24-hour continuous infusion instead of as an intravenous bolus, but response rates have been generally inferior to those with bolus IL-2, and responses are rarely durable. Lymphokine-activated killer cells (LAK cells), which are autologous lymphocytes activated

Table 84-8 ■ High-Dose Bolus IL-2 in the Treatment of Metastatic Renal Cell Cancer

Investigators	N	Dose of IL-2 IU/kg × 10³ (Schedule)*	Patients Responding		Major Response Rate (%)†	Comments
			Complete Response	Partial Response		
Fisher et al (2000)	255	720 or 600 (q8 hours)	17	20	15	one relapse among complete responses after 20 months.
Rosenberg et al‡ (1998)	277	720 (q8 hours)	21	22	19	80% of complete responses disease-free after 3 years.

N = population size.
* Cycle = IL-2 q8 hrs × 14 doses, Course = 2 cycles separated by 5 to 9 days.
† Response rate = partial response + completed response.
‡ Some of these patients were included in the report by Fisher et al.

ex vivo with IL-2, have also been administered with either bolus or continuous infusion IL-2. However, the response rate of IL-2 plus lymphokine-activated killer cells has not been superior to that of bolus IL-2 alone, whereas the toxicity of IL-2 is augmented with the addition of lymphokine-activated killer cells.

Patients who are most likely to respond to high-dose bolus IL-2 include those with an ECOG performance status of 0 and lung or lymph node metastases (Table 84-9). There also appears to be an association between the development of autoimmune hypothyroidism following high-dose IL-2 therapy and antitumor response. Patients with clear cell cancers, including sarcomatoid variants, are capable of responding to IL-2, whereas responses are rarely observed in patients with papillary, chromophobe, or collecting duct tumors. While the role of prior nephrectomy in the response to IL-2 remains controversial, the majority of responses to IL-2 have been observed in patients who have undergone nephrectomy, and patients who receive IL-2 for metastatic disease more than six months after nephrectomy appear to have a survival advantage compared to those who are treated with IL-2 without having undergone nephrectomy. These findings, along with the survival advantage that nephrectomy confers on patients treated with IFN-α, suggest that patients with clear cell tumors who are likely to recover from surgery with their performance status intact should undergo nephrectomy prior to receiving IL-2-based therapy.

The widespread use of high-dose bolus IL-2 is limited by the considerable toxicity associated with its administration. Two of the most serious toxicities are hypotension, requiring fluid and pressor support in 50% to 75% of patients, and capillary leak syndrome, which results in respiratory dysfunction from pulmonary edema and/or pleural effusions in up to 10% to 20% of patients. Reversible injury to the kidneys, liver, and heart also occur with high-dose IL-2, as does transient central nervous system toxicity. Because patients treated with high-dose IL-2 require intensive-care-unit-level care, its use is limited to treatment centers that have the appropriate clinical expertise and to patients with adequate organ function.

While low-dose IL-2 has less toxicity than high-dose bolus IL-2 and can be administered on either an inpatient or an outpatient basis, its effectiveness relative to high-dose IL-2 is still in question. Although responses have been observed in 10% to 15% of patients treated with low-dose IL-2, the durability of complete responses is undefined. A randomized comparison study of high-dose versus low-dose IL-2 is ongoing at the National Cancer Institute Surgery Branch. Until the results of this study become available, patients treated with IL-2 monotherapy should receive high-dose bolus IL-2 where possible. For elderly patients and patients with renal, cardiac, or pulmonary dysfunction, low-dose IL-2 is a reasonable option.

Combination Cytokine Therapy

The addition of either cis-retinoic acid or vinblastine to IFN-α has not resulted in a significant improvement in either response rate or survival compared to the use of IFN-α alone. The use of IFN-α in conjunction with IL-2 has had mixed results (see Table 84-7). In patients receiving high-dose bolus IL-2, the increased toxicity associated with the addition of IFN-α limited the amount of IL-2 that could be administered and may have contributed to the decrease in the overall response rate observed with IL-2 plus IFN-α compared

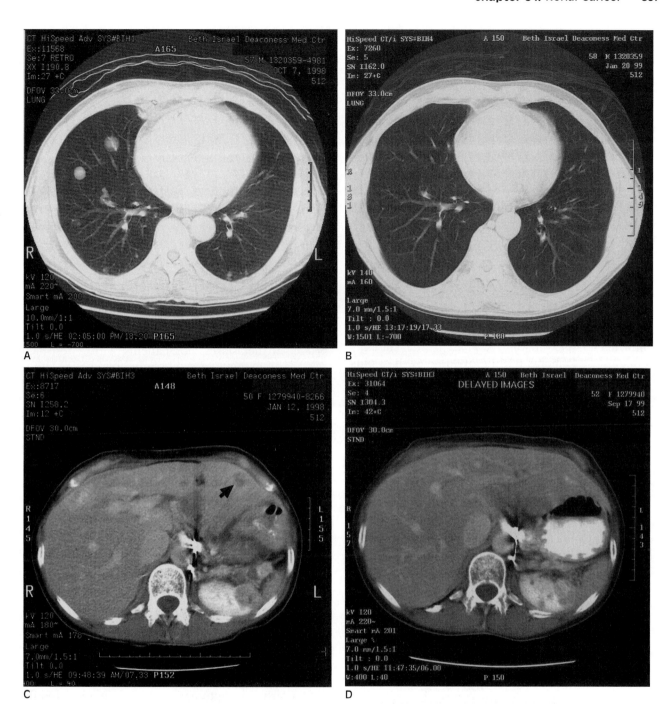

Figure 84-4 ■ Responses of metastatic renal cell cancer to IL-2-based regimens. *A,* A patient with renal cell cancer metastatic to the lungs before therapy. *B,* The same patient after having achieved a complete response to two courses of high-dose IL-2. *C,* A patient with von Hippel-Lindau disease and renal cell cancer metastatic to the liver (arrow) before therapy. *D,* The same patient after having achieved a complete response to six cycles of low-dose IL-2 plus interferon-alpha.

to IL-2 alone. In the French Immunotherapy Group trial, the addition of IFN-α augmented the response rate to intermediate-dose continuous infusion IL-2, but this did not translate into improved survival. The combination of low-dose SC IL-2 plus IFN-α has a response rate of approximately 20%, one quarter of

these being complete responses (Figure 84-4*C* and 84-4*D*). However, the median duration of these responses has been variable, and the durability of responses therefore remains uncertain. The addition of 5-fluorouracil to the regimen of low-dose IL-2 plus IFN-α augmented the toxicity without improving the

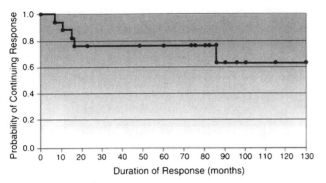

Figure 84-5 ■ Durability of complete responses to high-dose IL-2. Shown is the Kaplan-Meier estimate of response duration for patients with metastatic renal cell cancer achieving a complete response to high-dose IL-2 therapy.

response rate. The Cytokine Working Group recently completed a large, randomized Phase III trial comparing high-dose IV bolus IL-2 to low-dose SC IL-2 plus IFN-α. The preliminary results of this trial show a higher response rate for high-dose IL-2 compared to low-dose IL-2 plus IFN-α (25% versus 12%). The forthcoming data on durability of responses and overall survival should be pivotal in determining which of these two regimens should be used as first-line therapy in the treatment of metastatic renal cell cancer.

Promising new approaches to the treatment of metastatic renal cell cancer include novel cytokine combinations, autologous tumor cell vaccines, allogenic stem cell transplantation, cell-based therapies, antiangiogenic drugs, and signal transduction inhibitors. As these are still experimental, they should be used primarily as salvage therapy in patients who have failed IL-2-based treatments.

Table 84-9 ■ **Factors Associated with Response to High-Dose IL-2 in Patients with Metastatic Renal Cell Cancer**

Eastern Cooperative Oncology Group performance status of 0
Lung or lymph node metastases and absence of bone metastases
One organ with metastases (versus two or more organs)
Prior nephrectomy
Clear cell histology
Autoimmune thyroid dysfunction after IL-2 therapy
Total amount of IL-2 received in first course of therapy
Erythropoietin production by tumor cells

Radiation Therapy

The primary role of external beam radiation therapy is for the palliative treatment of bone or central nervous system (CNS) metastases. There is no evidence to support the use of radiation therapy to prevent recurrences in the renal bed following nephrectomy in patients with locally advanced disease. Radiation therapy given for symptomatic bone metastases often helps to diminish pain but rarely results in any radiographic signs of tumor regression. For patients with large lytic bone lesions in the femoral neck/shaft or in the humerus, surgical stabilization may be necessary to prevent pathologic fracture prior to giving radiation therapy. Spinal metastases resulting in spinal cord compression or symptomatic nerve root compression should be treated with radiation. In addition, radiation may be effective therapy for patients with airway compression or hemoptysis resulting from pulmonary or endo-bronchial metastases. For patients with a resectable solitary brain metastasis, whole-brain radiation should be given following surgery. Solitary central nervous system metastases that are not amenable to resection can be treated with stereotactic radiation therapy. Patients with multiple brain metastases can be treated with whole-brain radiation and/or stereotactic radiation therapy.

Follow-up Evaluation

Patients with pathologic stage I renal cell cancer have a less than 10% risk of relapse, while those with T2 (stage II) or T3aN0 tumors have a 15% to 30% risk of relapse. For patients with T1 tumors, follow-up after nephrectomy should include a semiannual history and physical exam and annual chest X-ray for three years, followed by annual visits thereafter. For T2N0 and T3aN0 tumors, the chest X-ray interval should be increased to every six months for three years and then yearly. Asymptomatic bone, brain, or abdominal metastases are uncommon in these patients, and therefore routine computed tomography imaging and bone scan are not recommended. Patients who are at high risk for relapse, including those with T3b–c or T4 disease, nodal metastases, or isolated metastases resected to no evidence of disease, require more intensive surveillance for both abdominal and lung recurrence using computed tomography scans. Because the majority of recurrences occur within three years of nephrectomy, computed tomography scans of the torso should be performed every three to four months for the first two years, every six months during the third year, and then annually in years 4

TREATMENT

Management of Residual Disease Following IL-2-Based Therapy

Approximately 60% to 70% of complete remissions resulting from high-dose IL-2 therapy are durable in patients with metastatic renal cell cancer. While patients with progressive disease following IL-2-based therapy are candidates for experimental second-line therapies, those with stable disease who are asymptomatic may be observed without additional therapy. In these patients, computed tomography scans of the torso should be performed every three to four months, along with yearly head computed tomography. Some patients with stable disease may go for years without disease progression, and observation is appropriate until there is clinical and/or radiographic evidence of tumor growth or new sites of metastatic disease. A similar approach may be taken with patients who have had either a partial or minor response to IL-2.

For patients who have achieved a partial response to IL-2-based therapy and who have only one or two remaining sites of measurable disease, surgical resection of residual disease should be performed if feasible. Many patients who are rendered disease-free by surgery after a partial response to IL-2 have durable remissions that are qualitatively similar to those occurring in patients achieving a complete response to high-dose IL-2. While metastases to the lung, lymph nodes, and soft tissue are most amenable to this approach, surgery should also be considered for patients with bone, liver, and other visceral metastases. Nephrectomy to remove what remains of the primary tumor may also be performed in patients who were not considered candidates for surgery prior to IL-2 therapy.

Likewise, a solitary metastasis occurring after a complete response to IL-2-based therapy should also be resected, as this can result in a durable remission, especially if more than one year has elapsed since completion of the IL-2.

and 5. Follow-up thereafter should include an annual physical exam, blood work, and chest X-ray.

Patients with metastatic disease who achieve a complete remission to immune-based therapy should be followed in the same manner as high-risk patients. Although the vast majority of relapses occur by 20 months in patients treated with high-dose IL-2, there have been rare relapses as far out as seven to eight years following a complete remission to IL-2. Patients who obtain a partial remission to IL-2 and have no progression of residual disease in the lung, soft tissue, or other isolated site after six to 12 months of follow-up should be considered for surgical resection, as many of these responders to IL-2 that are rendered no evidence of disease by surgery may actually be cured.

References

Chemotherapy

Amato RJ: Chemotherapy for renal cell carcinoma. Semin Oncol 2000;27:177–186.

Childs R, Chernoff A, Contentin N, et al: Regression of metastatic renal cell carcinoma after nonmyeloablative peripheral blood stem cell transplantation. N Engl J Med 2000; 343:750–758.

Eisen T, Boshoff C, Mak I, et al: Continuous low dose thalidomide: A phase II study in advanced melanoma, renal cell, ovarian and breast cancer. Br J Cancer 2000;82:812–817.

Rini BI, Vogelzang NJ, Dumas MC, et al: Phase II trial of weekly intravenous gemcitabine with continuous infusion fluorouracil in patients with metastatic renal cell cancer. J Clin Oncol 2000;18:2419–2426.

Russo P: Renal cell carcinoma: Presentation, staging, and surgical treatment. Semin Oncol 2000;27:160–176.

Interleukin-2 Therapy

Atkins MB, Dutcher J, Weins G, et al: Kidney cancer: The Cytokine Working Group experience (1986–2001). Part I: IL-2-based clinical trials. Med Oncol 2001;18:197–207.

Atkins MB, Mier JW, Parkinson DR, et al: Hypothyroidism after treatment with interleukin-2 and lymphokine-activated killer cells. N Engl J Med 1988;318:1557–1563.

Atkins MB, Sparano J, Fisher RI, et al: Randomized phase II trial of high-dose interleukin-2 either alone or in combination with interferon alfa-2b in advanced renal cell carcinoma. J Clin Oncol 1993;11:661–670.

Bukowski RM, Dutcher JP: Low-dose interleukin-2. In Vogelzang NJ, Scardino PT, Shipley WU, Coffey DS (eds): Comprehensive Textbook of Genitourinary Oncology, 2nd ed. Philadelphia: Lippincott Williams and Wilkins, 2000, pp 218–234.

Dutcher J, Atkins MB, Margolin K, et al: Kidney cancer: The Cytokine Working Group experience (1986–2001). Part II: Management of IL-2 toxicity and studies with other cytokines. Med Oncol 2001;18:209–219.

Dutcher JP, Logan T, Gordon M, et al: Phase II trial of interleukin 2, interferon alpha, and 5-fluorouracil in metastatic renal cell cancer: A cytokine working group study. Clin Cancer Res 2000;6:3442–3450.

Figlin R, Gitlitz B, Franklin J, et al: Interleukin-2-based immunotherapy for the treatment of metastatic renal cell carcinoma: An analysis of 203 consecutively treated patients. Cancer J Sci Am 1997;3:S92–S97.

Fisher RI, Rosenberg SA, Fyfe G: Long-term survival update for high-dose recombinant interleukin-2 in patients with renal cell carcinoma. Cancer J Sci Am 2000;6(Suppl 1):S55–S57.

Fyfe G, Fisher RI, Rosenberg SA, et al: Results of treatment of 255 patients with metastatic renal cell carcinoma who received high-dose recombinant interleukin-2 therapy. J Clin Oncol 1995;13:688–696.

Gollob JA, Atkins MB: Clinical trials of interleukin 12 in oncology. Curr Opin Oncol Endocr Metabol Invest Drugs 1999;1:260–271.

McDermott D, Flaherty L, Clark J, et al: A randomized phase III trial of high-dose interleukin-2 (HD IL-2) versus subcutaneous (SC) IL-2/interferon (IFN) in patients with metastatic renal cell carcinoma (RCC). Proc Amer Soc Clin Oncol 2001;20:172a.

Negrier S, Escudier B, Lasset C, et al: Recombinant human interleukin-2, recombinant human interferon alfa-2a, or both in metastatic renal cell carcinoma. N Engl J Med 1998;338:1272–1278.

Negrier S, Maral J, Drevon M, et al: Long-term follow-up of patients with metastatic renal cell carcinoma treated with intravenous recombinant interleukin-2 in Europe. Cancer J Sci Am 2000;6(Suppl 1):S93–S98.

Rosenberg SA, Lotze MT, Yang JC, et al: Prospective randomized trial of high-dose interleukin-2 alone or in conjunction with lymphokine-activated killer cells for the treatment of patients with advanced cancer. J Natl Cancer Inst 1993;85:622–632.

Rosenberg SA, Yang JC, White DE, Steinberg SM: Durability of complete responses in patients with metastatic cancer treated with high-dose interleukin-2: Identification of the antigens mediating response. Ann Surg 1998;228:307–319.

Weiss GR, Margolin KA, Aronson FR, et al: A randomized phase II trial of continuous infusion interleukin-2 or bolus injection interleukin-2 plus lymphokine-activated killer cells for advanced renal cell carcinoma. J Clin Oncol 1992;10:275–281.

Wiggington JM, Komschlies KL, Back TC, et al: Administration of interleukin 12 with pulse interleukin 2 and the rapid and complete eradication of murine renal carcinoma. J Natl Cancer Inst 1996;88:38–43.

Yang JC, Rosenberg SA: An ongoing prospective randomized comparison of interleukin-2 regimens for the treatment of metastatic renal cell cancer. Cancer J Sci Am 1997;3:S79–S84.

Radiation Therapy

DiBiase SJ, Valicenti RK, Schultz D, et al: Palliative irradiation for focally symptomatic metastatic renal cell carcinoma: Support for dose escalation based on a biological model. J Urol 1997;158 (3, pt 1):746–749.

Surgery

Fallick ML, McDermott DF, LaRock D, et al: Nephrectomy before interleukin-2 therapy for patients with metastatic renal cell carcinoma. J Urol 1997;158:1691–1695.

Flanigan RC, Blumenstein BA, Salmon S, Crawford E: Cytoreduction nephrectomy in metastatic renal cancer: the results of southwest oncology group trial 8949. Proc Am Soc Clin Oncol 2000;19:2a.

Hafez KS, Novick AC, Campbell SC: Patterns of tumor recurrence and guidelines for follow-up after nephron-sparing surgery for sporadic renal cell carcinoma. J Urol 1997;157:2067–2070.

Hatcher BA, Anderson EE, Paulson DF, et al: Surgical management and prognosis of renal cell carcinoma invading the vena cava. J Urol 1991;145:20–24.

Kavolius JP, Mastorakos DP, Pavlovich C, et al: Resection of metastatic renal cell carcinoma. J Clin Oncol 1998; 16:2261–2266.

Landis SH, Murray T, Bolden S, Wingo PA: Cancer statistics, 1999. CA Cancer J Clin 1999;49:8–31.

Levy DA, Slaton JW, Swanson DA, Dinney CP: Stage specific guidelines for surveillance after radical nephrectomy for local renal cell carcinoma. J Urol 1998;159:1163–1167.

Licht MR, Novick AC, Goormastic M: Nephron-sparing surgery in incidental versus suspected renal cell carcinoma. J Urol 1994;152:39–42.

Payne BR, Prasad D, Szeifert G, et al: Gamma surgery for intracranial metastases from renal cell carcinoma. J Neurosurg 2000;92:760–765.

Srougi M: Lymph node dissection in the treatment of renal cell carcinoma. In Vogelzang NJ, Scardino PT, Shipley WU, Coffey DS (eds): Comprehensive Textbook of Genitourinary Oncology, 2nd ed. Philadelphia: Lippincott Williams and Wilkins, 2000, pp 201–206.

Walther MM, Yang JC, Pass HI, et al: Cytoreductive surgery before high dose interleukin-2 based therapy in patients with metastatic renal cell carcinoma. J Urol 1997; 158:1675–1678.

Interferon Therapy

Fossa SD: Interferon in metastatic renal cell carcinoma. Semin Oncol 2000;27:187–193.

Gollob JA, Mier JW, Veenstra K, et al: Phase I trial of twice-weekly intravenous interleukin 12 in patients with metastatic renal cell cancer or malignant melanoma: Ability to maintain IFN-γ induction is associated with clinical response. Clin Cancer Res 2000;6:1678–1692.

Medical Research Council Renal Cancer Collaborators: Interferon-alpha and survival in metastatic renal carcinoma: Early results of a randomized controlled trial. 1999; 353:14–17.

Pizzocaro G, Piva L, Colavita M, et al: Interferon adjuvant to radical nephrectomy in Robson stages II and III renal cell carcinoma: A multicentric randomized study. J Clin Oncol 2001;19:425–431.

Pyrhonen S, Salminen E, Ruutu M, et al: Prospective randomized trial of interferon alfa-2a plus vinblastine versus vinblastine alone in patients with advanced renal cell cancer. J Clin Oncol 1999;17:2859–2867.

Trump DL, Elson P, Propert K, et al: Randomized controlled trial of adjuvant therapy with lymphoblastoid interferon. Proc Am Soc Clin Oncol 1996;15:253.

Epidemiology

Gnarra JR, Tory K, Weng Y, et al: Mutations of the VHL tumour suppressor gene in renal carcinoma. Nat Genet 1994;7:85–90.

Humphrey JS, Klausner RD, Linehan WM: Von Hippel-Lindau syndrome: hereditary cancer arising from inherited mutations of the VHL tumor suppressor gene. Cancer Treat Res 1996;88:13–39.

Iliopoulos O, Eng C: Genetic and clinical aspects of familial renal neoplasms. Semin Oncol 2000;27:138–149.

Lindblad P, Wolk A, Bergstrom R, et al: The role of obesity and weight fluctuations in the etiology of renal cell cancer: A population-based case-control study. Cancer Epidemiol Biomarkers Prev 1994;3:631–639.

McLaughlin JK, Hrubec Z, Heineman EF, et al: Renal cancer and cigarette smoking in a 26-year follow up of U.S. veterans. Public Health Rep 1990;105:535–537.

Muscat JE, Hoffmann D, Wynder EL: The epidemiology of renal cell carcinoma: A second look. Cancer 1995;75:2552–2557.

Perera AD, Kleymenova EV, Walker CL: Requirement for the von Hippel-Lindau tumor suppressor gene for functional epidermal growth factor receptor blockade by monoclonal antibody C225 in renal cell carcinoma. Clin Cancer Res 2000;6:1518–1523.

Schmidt L, Junker K, Weirich G, et al: Two North American families with hereditary papillary renal carcinoma and identical novel mutations in the MET proto-oncogene. Cancer Res 1998;58:1719–1722.

Walther MM, Choyke PL, Glenn G, et al: Hereditary renal cancer: prospective evaluation of tumor size as threshold for renal parenchymal sparing surgery. J Urol 1998; 159(Suppl):149.

Zbar B, Kaelin W, Maher E, Richard S: Third international meeting on von Hippel-Lindau disease. Cancer Res 1999;59:2251–2253.

General Information

Gold PJ, Fefer A, Thompson JA: Paraneoplastic manifestations of renal cell carcinoma. Semin Urol Oncol 1996; 14:216–222.

Kovacs G, Akhtar M, Beckwith BJ, et al: The Heidelberg classification of renal cell tumors. J Pathol 1997;183:131–133.

Kugler A, Stuhler G, Walden P, et al: Regression of human metastatic renal cell carcinoma after vaccination with tumor cell-dendritic cell hybrids. Nat Med 2000;6:332–336.

Matz LR, Latham BI, Fabian VA, Vivian JB: Collecting duct carcinoma of the kidney: A report of three cases and review of the literature. Pathology 1997;29:354–359.

McClennan BL, Deyoe LA: The imaging evaluation of renal cell carcinoma: diagnosis and staging. Radiol Clin North Am 1994;32:55–69.

Moch H, Gasser T, Amin MB, et al: Prognostic utility of the recently recommended histologic classification and revised TNM staging system of renal cell carcinoma: A Swiss experience with 588 tumors. Cancer 2000;89:604–614.

Motzer RJ, Mazumdar M, Bacik J, et al: Survival and prognostic stratification of 670 patients with advanced renal cell carcinoma. J Clin Oncol 1999;17:2530–2540.

Reuter VE, Presti JC Jr: Contemporary approach to the classification of renal epithelial tumors. Semin Oncol 2000;27:124–137.

Tsui KH, Shvarts O, Smith RB, et al: Prognostic indicators for renal cell carcinoma: A multivariate analysis of 643 patients using the revised 1997 TNM staging criteria. J Urol 2000;163:1090–1095.

Warshauer DM, McCarthy SM, Street L, et al: Detection of renal masses: sensitivities and specificities of excretory urography/linear tomography, US, and CT. Radiology 1988;169:363–365.

Wronski M, Maor MH, Davis BJ, et al: External radiation of brain metastases from renal carcinoma: A retrospective study of 119 patients from the M.D. Anderson Cancer Center. Int J Radiat Oncol Biol Phys 1997;37:753–759.

Chapter 85
Superficial Bladder Cancer

Michael A. O'Donnell

Introduction

Bladder cancer is a malignant neoplasm originating from the surface lining (uroepithelium) of the bladder, the most common form of which is transitional cell carcinoma (TCC). Transitional cell carcinoma accounts for approximately 90% of all bladder cancers, the remainder of which are squamous cell carcinomas (7% to 8%), adenocarcinomas (1% to 2%), and rare neuroendocrine, small cell and signet cell carcinomas (less than 1%). When the cancer is confined to the mucosa or submucosa of the bladder, it is referred to as "superficial" because it is defined primarily by its accessibility to local surgical cystoscopic removal rather than by its intrinsic invasive potential. Three quarters of all bladder cancers initially present clinically as superficial disease.

With approximately 54,000 new cases in the United States annually, bladder cancer represents the fourth most common cancer in men and the eighth most common in women, for a net 3:1 male predominance. Furthermore, because of its high recurrence rate, the actual prevalence of active bladder cancer in the United States is estimated to be close to one-half million cases. The highest incidence occurs in men over age 60 and women over 70 years. Even teenage men have a small but finite chance of bladder cancer, but it is very rare to see bladder cancer in a woman under the age of 40. There is also a strong ethnic disparity. The disease is much more common in Caucasians than among those of African, Latino, or Asian decent.

Cigarette smoking is estimated to account for two-thirds of bladder cancers in males and one-third in females. There is strong correlation between the number of pack-years and the risk of developing bladder cancer. Quitting decreases the risk, but it never returns to that of a nonsmoker—a situation not unexpected, given the average 20-year latency between exposure to a carcinogen and the development of bladder cancer. Certain organic chemicals, particularly aromatic amines such as naphthalenes, benzidine, aniline dyes, and 4-aminobiphenyl are known bladder cancer carcinogens. High-risk occupations include petroleum chemical or rubber workers, hair stylists, painters, textile workers, truck drivers, and aluminum electroplaters. Bladder cancer could also result from pelvic radiation therapy, phenacetin use, and cyclophosphamide exposure, particularly when given in a chronic, low-dose format. Cyclophosphamide therapy results in a 16-fold relative increase in the risk of developing bladder cancer.

Familial clustering of bladder cancer is the exception. No bladder cancer susceptibility genes have been identified to date, although it is known that smokers with the slow-acetylator phenotype are at higher risk than those with fast-acetylator phenotypes. There is one rare hereditary form of transitional cell carcinoma in association with Muir-Torre syndrome, a familial multicancer syndrome characterized by sebaceous tumors, various visceral malignancies, and a defect in DNA mismatch repair.

Clinical Presentation and Evaluation

The vast majority of patients with bladder cancer present with gross, painless hematuria that is usually transient in nature. It is too commonly ignored by the patient and often misattributed by physicians to urinary tract infections, gynecological disease, benign prostatic hyperplasia, strenuous exertion/exercise, or anticoagulant use. About 10% of patients report persistent irritative bladder symptoms such as frequency, urgency, and dysuria without any hematuria, whether gross or microscopic. Such cases are particularly problematic because they usually represent a highly aggressive variant of superficial transitional cell carcinoma, known as carcinoma-in-situ (CIS), yet they often are initially misdiagnosed as cystitis or prostatitis.

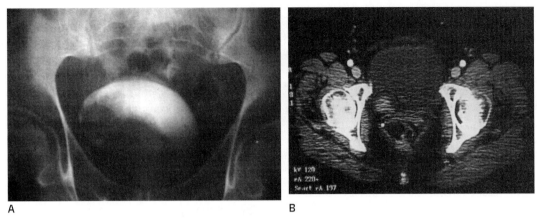

A   B

Figure 85-1 ■ Radiographic appearance of superficial bladder cancer by (*A*) intravenous pyelogram and (*B*) computed tomography scan.

The physical exam is seldom informative for superficial disease. The urinalysis might or might not be positive for blood, given the episodic nature of bladder tumor bleeding. Radiologic studies— ultrasound, intravenous pyelogram (IVP), and computed tomography (CT) scanning—can detect larger lesions (Figure 85-1), but smaller tumors can easily be missed, especially in the corrugated mucosal surface of the nondistended bladder. It cannot be emphasized strongly enough that all patients with a history of gross, painless hematuria require a urological evaluation by cystoscopy to rule out bladder cancer. Urinary cytology is a useful adjunct, especially in diagnosing patients with carcinoma-in-situ that could even be difficult to visualize cystoscopically. Despite the very high specificity of urinary cytology (greater than 95%), however, the poor overall sensitivity (less than 40%) and subjective interpretation mean that a negative cytology is never sufficient to rule out bladder cancer. New FDA-approved urinary marker tests that detect shed nuclear matrix proteins (NMP-22) or bladder tumor-associated antigen (BTA) have become available. Although both tests demonstrate improved sensitivities (in the 60% to 70% range), specificity remains less than 80%, limiting their use primarily to following patients with a history of bladder cancer rather than in screening high-risk patients for the disease.

Staging, Prognostic Features, and Outcomes

Accurate pathological staging and grading of cystoscopically obtained bladder tumor tissue is essential in determining clinical prognosis. In the TMN classification system, superficial bladder cancer can be one of three types: stage Ta (confined to the mucosa), stage T1 (invasive into the submucosa or lamina propria), and CIS (a surface spreading disease) (Figure 85-2). As

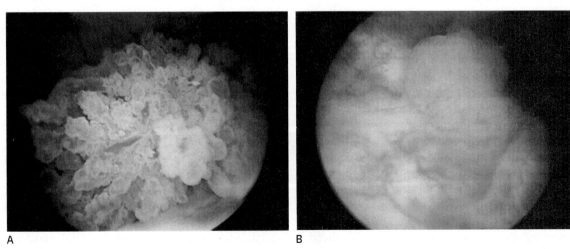

A   B

Figure 85-2 ■ Cystoscopic appearance of common superficial bladder cancers. *A*, Stage Ta grade 1–2. *B*, Stage T1 grade 3. (See Color Plate 20.)

Table 85-1 ■ Rate of Progression and Survival by Tumor Stage and Grade

Stage	Grade	Risk of Progression	Five-Year Survival	10-Year Survival
Ta	1	0–2%	100%	95%
	2	10–20%	95%	89%
	3	40–50%	95%	84%
T1	2	10–20%	90%	78%
	3	40–50%	70%	50%
CIS	N/A	30–50%	70%	55%

CIS = carcinoma-in-situ

it is very rare to have lymph node or distant metastasis with superficial bladder cancer, stage is related to tumor depth. The intrinsic aggressive potential of this malignancy, on the other hand, is strongly associated with tumor grade. Traditionally, a three-tier grading system encompassing low, medium, or high grade (also known as grades 1, 2, or 3, respectively) has been used by most pathologists. Carcinoma-in-situ is a high-grade dysplasia by definition. Some prefer to further identify a highly anaplastic variant, termed grade 4. Yet, inter- and intra-observer variability between grades is about 40%, leading many pathologists to provide a range of grades, such as grade 1–2 out of 3 (commonly notated as 1–2/3). The American Joint Cancer Committee hoped that reclassification of transitional cell carcinoma into three distinct categories would prove clinically useful:

1. tumors of low malignant potential (previously known as papillomas or stage Ta grade 1 tumors)
2. low-grade transitional cell carcinoma
3. high-grade transitional cell carcinoma

Most pathologists and urologists, however, continue to use the traditional nomenclature.

The risk of future disease progression to bladder muscle invasion and death from bladder cancer is strongly linked to tumor stage and grade (Table 85-1). The risk of disease recurrence, however, is significantly affected by several other parameters, including multifocality, size, frequency of prior recurrence, response to therapy, and associated dysplasia, among others (Table 85-2). Although recurrence is not a good surrogate for progression, multiple recurrent superficial tumors do foreshadow a 23% chance of dying from bladder cancer within 20 years. The time to first recurrence by itself is one of the most predictive features for eventual tumor recurrence. Only 30% of first-time (primary) solitary stage Ta grade 1 tumors recur within five years, whereas secondary tumors that have occurred within three months of the primary herald only a 17% chance of remaining disease-free during the same interval. Similarly, failure to have a recurrence within 24 months reduces the chance of ultimate recurrence to under 10%, but persistent recurrence beyond four years practically guarantees continued recurrences over the patient's lifetime. Various molecular markers are now being studied to help provide more objective measures of risk for recurrence and progression (see Table 85-2).

Treatment

For visible tumor lesions of the bladder, the first line of treatment is endoscopic removal through the cystoscope in a procedure commonly referred to as TURB or TURBT (Trans-Urethral Resection of Bladder Tumor). The goals of this procedure are to obtain adequate tissue for pathologic examination and to completely obliterate all visible tumor either by resection or fulguration. Carcinoma-in-situ is not amenable to surgery, due to its diffuse surface-spreading property. Unfortunately, even for visible tumors, the aggregate chance of disease recurrence after surgery alone approximates 60% within five years and 80% within 10 years. Several factors responsible for the high recurrence rate include failure to completely remove the primary tumor, tumor cell reimplantation during resection, microscopic extant disease, and emergence of second primaries due to a generalized carcinogenic "field defect" in the urothelium. For these reasons, adjuvant medical treatment in the form of intravesical drug therapy is commonly used for those tumors assessed to be at high risk for recurrence and/or progression.

Two types of intravesical therapy are commonly employed for the treatment of superficial bladder cancer: chemotherapy and immunotherapy. Both are usually administered two to three weeks after cystoscopic removal of visible tumor using an induction cycle of one treatment per week for six weeks, a two-hour retention time, and variable "maintenance" cycles thereafter. After more than 30 years of empiric testing, only three chemotherapeutic drugs given as single agents have demonstrated acceptable efficacy and toxicity via the intravesical route: thiotepa (and a related alkylating agent used in Europe, ethoglucid), Adriamycin (and its derivatives epirubicin and valrubicin), and mitomycin. In randomized trials, the addition of these chemotherapeutic agents to cytoscopic removal reduced the recurrence rate to 45% from 60% when only cytoscopic removal was performed. No agent was clearly superior in effect. In spite of this statistically significant reduction in recurrence,

Table 85-2 ■ Factors Increasing Risk of Tumor Recurrence and/or Progression

Low Recurrence, Low Progression	Moderate to High Recurrence, Increased Progression	High Recurrence, High Progression
Low-grade	Medium-grade	High-grade
		Grade progression during recurrence
Stage Ta (mucosal only)	Stage progression Ta to T1	Stage T1 (submucosal invasion)
No dysplasia	Moderate dysplasia	CIS
Negative cytology	Abnormal cytology	Highly suspicious or positive cytology
Solitary	Multifocal	
Primary (first time tumor)	Recurrent, especially within three to six months or multi-recurrent	
Papillary configuration		Sessile-nodular configuration
Size <5 cm	Size >5 cm	
Short disease duration	Long (> four years) duration	
Certainty of complete resection	Uncertainty of complete resection	
No prior intravesical therapy	Failed prior intravesical therapy	
Proliferation marker low (e.g., Ki-67)	Proliferation marker high	
Normal DNA ploidy	Abnormal ploidy	Frank DNA aneuploidy
E-cadherin positive		E-cadherin negative
p53 negative		p53 positive
RB positive		RB negative
p21 positive		p21 negative

however, chemotherapy does not reduce the likelihood of ultimate disease progression nor does it improve survival. Used alone, these agents also induce complete responses in 30% to 50% of small-volume tumors (less than 2 cm) and carcinoma-in-situ. The median duration of complete response varies from six months for Adriamycin to nearly two years for mitomycin. All the chemotherapeutic agents cause some degree of irritative cystitis that is generally well tolerated but occasionally necessitates drug withdrawal.

DIAGNOSIS

Practical Guidelines for Interpreting and Utilizing Pathology Reports for Superficial Bladder Cancer

■ The finding of a stage Ta grade 3 or a stage T1 grade 1 tumor is very rare and often the result of misclassification. Similarly, it is unusual to see low-grade tumors mixed with high-grade tumors or low-grade histology with a positive urinary cytology showing highly dysplastic cells. Whenever discordant results are obtained, consultation with a reference pathologist is helpful.

■ Carcinoma-in-situ (CIS) is instead termed by some pathologists as high-grade or severe dysplasia; the variable nomenclature causes confusion in interpretation. At the same time, a report of low, moderate, or reactive dysplasia has no practical clinical significance and should not be used to guide therapeutic decisions. A positive cytology often accompanies carcinoma-in-situ.

■ Stage T1 grade 3 tumors are either incompletely resected or understaged (i.e., actually stage T2+)

30% to 40% of the time, particularly if the tumors are large or multifocal. This is especially problematic when deep muscle biopsies are not included in the resection specimen or the tissue is severely cauterized. Cytoscopic reresection is thus advisable in such cases to achieve accurate staging.

■ From the standpoint of life-threatening disease, one can classify patients into three useful progression risk categories. The aggressive or high-risk category (30% to 50% chance of progression) would include any carcinoma-in-situ, grade 3, or stage T1 disease. The very low-risk category (less than 2% risk of progression) includes only stage Ta, grade 1 disease. The remaining cases fall into the intermediate-risk category (5% to 15% risk of progression).

Unique toxicities include myelosuppression (thiotepa) due to systemic absorption, hypersensitivity (Adriamycin), and a palmar and genital skin rash (mitomycin). Recently, it has been appreciated that a single dose of any of the chemotherapeutic agents given immediately after the completion of transurethral resection of bladder tumor might be just as effective as a traditional six-week course given later after surgery, with attendant decrease in toxicity. The fact that this benefit is reduced even if chemotherapy is delayed more than 24 hours suggests that it works primarily to reduce tumor cell reimplantation.

Immunotherapy with instillation of the live vaccine strain of *Mycobacterium bovis* (bacillus Calmette-Guérin, BCG) into the bladder remains the most successful treatment for superficial bladder cancer. Tumor recurrence using BCG following transurethral resection of bladder tumor (prophylactic use) is diminished by about 30%, which represents roughly twice the success rate of intravesical chemotherapy. Ablation is achieved 55% to 60% of the time for small papillary tumors and up to 75% of the time for carcinoma-in-situ. The median duration of complete response is two to four years in most series. BCG appears to be particularly effective for aggressive superficial lesions; most comparative trials show that it is superior to chemotherapy. Furthermore, prior chemotherapy failures respond well to BCG. At least five studies have demonstrated a clinically meaningful delay in disease worsening, with a reduction in relative risk of progression or need for cystectomy.

Recent refinements in the maintenance phase—consisting of a miniseries of three weekly treatments every three to six months for three years—results in a further 20% improvement in reduction of recurrence compared to absence of maintenance therapy. Unfortunately, the long-term (10-year follow-up) results are not as encouraging, because most patients eventually relapse. No clinical or molecular parameters predict successful response to BCG. Toxicity in the form of symptomatic cystitis occurs in up to 90% of patients. Five percent of patients experience other significant toxicities, including high fevers or systemic BCG infection of the liver or lungs (1%) and frank BCG sepsis in 0.4%. Deaths have occurred in the setting of inadvertent intravascular BCG administration; this risk is increased if BCG is instilled too early after surgery (two to three weeks delay is recommended) or after traumatic catheterization.

Interferon-alpha as an intravesical agent has been used for many years. It has not achieved widespread use, however, due to its high cost and lesser efficacy when compared with both chemotherapy and BCG.

Interferon does not appear to work well against stage T1 tumors and is not effective as a single perioperative dose. Complete responses in carcinoma-in-situ approximates 40% even for patients failing prior chemotherapy or BCG, but high doses in the range of 50 to 100 million units are required. Of all the intravesical agents, interferon has the most favorable local toxicity profile, causing little or no cystitis and only an occasional temporary flu-like illness. It might also be useful in combination with reduced-dose BCG for salvage therapy.

The ability of chemotherapy or alternative immunotherapy to salvage BCG failures is limited. In one small study of 21 patients, only four (19%) were disease-free at three years after mitomycin therapy. In the pivotal trial leading to FDA approval for valrubicin, of 90 high-risk patients treated once weekly for six weeks, only 16 (18%) remained disease-free at six months. With successive follow-up, fewer than one-half the subjects have remained disease-free at two years. Interferon-alpha monotherapy has also been used for BCG failures with limited success. In small series, the one-year disease-free rate is 18% for carcinoma-in-situ and papillary Ta disease. Anecdotal reports on keyhole limpet hemocyanin (KLH) immunotherapy have been encouraging, but the agent is generally available only in a research setting.

External beam radiation therapy, with or without systemic chemotherapy, is rarely appropriate for the treatment of superficial bladder cancer because it can cause significant morbidity while displaying limited efficacy. Carcinoma-in-situ is particularly resistant, and low-grade disease responds more poorly than higher-grade disease. Some benefit might be derived for patients with stage T1 grade 3 tumors, and five-year disease-free survivals are at 30%.

Follow-Up Evaluation

Surveillance after initial diagnosis of superficial bladder cancer involves quarterly cystoscopy for the first two years, followed by semiannual cystoscopy for the next two years, followed by annual cystoscopy thereafter. Any recurrence "resets" the clock. Precystoscopy urinalysis for occult bleeding and urinary cytology should be included in the same schedule for any past history of carcinoma-in-situ, grade 3, or stage T1 disease. Random and/or directed bladder biopsies should be done at the three-month time point for all patients having these aggressive disease characteristics because of the high incidence of associated (and sometimes invisible) carcinoma-in-situ. Thereafter, any suspicious or positive cytology requires rebiopsy. A suspicious or positive cytology with negative bladder

TREATMENT

Recognizing and Treating BCG Toxicity

The toxic effects of BCG can be local, systemic, or both. The vast majority of patients experience a self-limited cystitis, the severity of which escalates with later treatments. Symptoms usually begin two to four hours after instillation, peak between six to ten hours after instillation, and resolve rapidly over the next 24 to 48 hours. Microscopic hematuria and pyuria are common, while occasional gross hematuria and passage of "tissue" (actually white cell aggregates) also occur. Systemic manifestations of the inflammatory response follow a similar time course and include fevers, chills, a flu-like malaise, and occasional arthralgias. During re-induction or maintenance cycles, all of these symptoms tend to be more intense and to occur sooner after the instillation. Most symptoms can be controlled with the appropriate use of acetaminophen, nonsteroidal anti-inflammatory drugs (NSAIDs), urinary analgesics, and antispasmodics. The routine administration of antibiotics with catheterization is unnecessary. If antibiotics are clinically indicated for non-BCG infection, penicillins, cephalosporins, trimethoprim/sulfa, and nitrofurantoin are preferred; fluoroquinolones, azithromycin, and doxycycline are to be avoided, as they are cidal to BCG and could affect the efficacy of the therapy. Conversely, short courses of anti-BCG-specific antibiotics such as isoniazid (INH) and rifampin have not been shown to diminish either the associated symptomatology or the incidence of serious BCG infection.

Clinical signs of a more serious process, such as BCG intravasation into the bloodstream (BCGosis), include exaggerated manifestations of the usual systemic effects associated with instillation. This is likely, especially if the symptoms occur early during the initial course of induction therapy, within two hours after BCG instillation, or in the setting of traumatic catheterization. Although a fever over 102.5°F associated with rigors is cause for concern, this in itself is not a definite sign of BCGosis, especially if it occurs at the expected peak time and resolves within 24 hours. In fact, better therapeutic responses have been reported in patients experiencing significant fevers. Such patients can be retreated with nonsteroidal anti-inflammatory prophylaxis and at a reduced dose of BCG. Conversely, fevers that begin after 24 hours, persist more than 48 hours, or relapse in a diurnal pattern (usually in the early evening) suggest established BCG infection. Organ-specific manifestations—including epididymal-orchitis, pneumonitis, and hepatitis—can occur. These patients usually require hospitalization and the administration of triple drug therapy such as INH, rifampin, and ethambutol. A fluoroquinolone may be added, as it covers most gram-negative rods and has moderate activity against BCG. BCG is resistant to both pyrazinamide and cycloserine. Failure to improve on such therapy or significant clinical deterioration should prompt institution of systemic steroids, which has been shown to be life-saving in such cases. Antituberculosis drugs should be continued for three to six months depending on the severity of the presenting illness.

Prolonged symptomatic BCG cystitis and/or prostatitis (often associated with granulomas) can become a troubling problem during and after therapy. This situation is best avoided by withholding BCG treatment until all significant symptoms from the prior instillation have subsided. A one- to two-week delay does not reduce BCG efficacy in such a setting. Reinstitution of BCG at a lower dose or premature termination of further treatment for that cycle could also be appropriate. If localized severe cystitis does occur and conservative measures fail, this condition can be treated with oral fluoroquinolones (three to 12 weeks) or oral INH. A short two- to three-week oral steroid taper sandwiched between antibiotic coverage has also been shown to be helpful in refractory cases. Rarely, a noninfectious hypersensitivity Reiter's-type syndrome (urethritis, arthritis, conjunctivitis) might occur during BCG treatment. This should prompt the immediate cessation of further treatment.

---

biopsies should prompt bilateral ureteral washings, an upper-tract study (intravenous or retrograde pyelograms), and biopsy of the prostatic urethra because up to 20% of patients with prior aggressive disease eventually relapse outside the bladder—often silently. Upper-tract radiographic studies should otherwise be performed every two years as long as the bladder disease remains active.

There is little question that this intensive monitoring schedule can be modified safely for less aggressive disease. If the first three-month cystoscopy is negative for recurrence, and the disease is low- to intermediate-grade and characterized as stage Ta, then semiannual cystoscopy for the first two years followed by annual cystoscopy thereafter is likely to be sufficient. The chance of developing upper-tract disease is less than 3% in such circumstances, making periodic assessments unnecessary without other indications. The quarterly use of recently available urinary monitoring tools such as the NMP-22 or BTA tests can

TREATMENT

Selecting and Optimizing Proper Intravesical Therapy

- Immediate instillation of one dose of a chemotherapeutic drug retained for one hour should be considered in all but the most benign-appearing primary solitary lesions following TURBT, except for rare cases of significant post-operative bleeding or suspected bladder perforation. Intravenous and oral fluids should be restricted during the period of bladder retention to minimize drug dilution.
- Low- to intermediate-risk groups, especially if their cancers had previously recurred, might benefit from more extended intravesical chemotherapy, especially mitomycin.
- BCG should be considered the primary treatment of choice for all superficial transitional cell carcinomas bearing the aggressive features of CIS, grade 3, or stage T1 disease. It is also an appropriate therapy for intermediate risk patients who have previously failed chemotherapy. BCG is contraindicated in immunocompromised patients or in those taking immunosuppressive drugs.
- Improved tolerance to BCG, especially during the maintenance phases, can be achieved by reducing the BCG dose and/or increasing the interval between treatments from one to two weeks as required.
- Rapid recurrence of high-grade disease or progression despite BCG maintenance usually heralds clinically aggressive disease that should be considered for alternative therapy, including cystectomy.

be especially helpful in such patients to bolster this less rigorous surveillance schedule.

Preventive measures to reduce the long-term risk of bladder cancer recurrence remain provocative but nonetheless worthy of discussion. Smoking cessation should be strongly encouraged. High-dose antioxidant vitamins, especially vitamins A, E, B6, and C, have been found to reduce recurrence of low-intermediate risk papillary lesions substantially following successful BCG therapy.

Because superficial bladder cancer can be a lifelong disease, it is important to discuss the disease with the patient early in the course of therapy in order to set realistic goals and expectations. It is especially helpful to devise a plan appropriate to the level of risk. The very low-grade minimal lesions are considered to be a medical nuisance, whereas the high-risk, aggressive lesions require heightened levels of concern, patient compliance, and preparedness for more aggressive treatment alternatives such as cystectomy.

References

Alexandroff AB, Jackson AM, O'Donnell MA, James K: BCG immunotherapy of bladder cancer: 20 years on. Lancet 1999;353:1689–1694.

Belldegrun AS, Franklin JR, O'Donnell MA, et al: Superficial bladder cancer: The role of interferon-alpha. J Urol 1998;159:1793–1801.

Crawford ED: Diagnosis and treatment of superficial bladder cancer: An update. Semin Urol Oncol 1996;14:1–9.

Esrig D, Freeman JA, Stein JP, Skinner DG: Early cystectomy for clinical stage T1 transitional cell carcinoma of the bladder. Semin Urol Oncol 1997;15:154–160.

Heney NM: Natural history of superficial bladder cancer: Prognostic features and long-term disease course. Urol Clin North Am 1992;19:429–433.

Herr HW, Schwalb DM, Zhang ZF, et al: Intravesical bacillus Calmette-Guérin therapy prevents tumor progression and death from superficial bladder cancer: Ten-year follow-up of a prospective randomized trial. J Clin Oncol 1995; 13:1404–1408.

Klan R, Loy V, Huland H: Residual tumor discovered in routine second transurethral resection in patients with stage T1 transitional cell carcinoma of the bladder. J Urol 1991;146:316–318.

Kurth KH, Denis L, Bouffioux C, et al: Factors affecting recurrence and progression in superficial bladder cancer. Eur J Cancer 1995;31A:1840–1846.

Lamm DL, van der Meijden APM, Akaaza H, et al. Intravesical chemotherapy and immunotherapy: How do we assess their effectiveness and what are their limitations and uses? Int J Urol 1995;2(S2):23–35.

Lamm DL, Riggs DR, Shriver JS, et al: Megadose vitamins in bladder cancer: A double-blind clinical trial. J Urol 1994;151:21–26.

Lamm DL, Blumenstein BA, Crawford ED, et al: A randomized trial of intravesical doxorubicin and immunotherapy with bacille Calmette-Guérin for transitional cell carcinoma of the bladder. N Engl J Med 1991;325:1205–1209.

Lamm DL, Blumenstein BA, Crissman JD, et al: Maintenance BCG immunotherapy for recurrent Ta, T1 and carcinoma in situ transitional cell carcinoma of the bladder: A randomized Southwest Oncology Group study. J Urol 2000;163:1124–1129.

Nseyo UO, Shumaker B, Klein EA, Sutherland K: Photodynamic therapy using porfimer sodium as an alternative to cystectomy in patients with refractory transitional cell carcinoma in situ of the bladder. Bladder Photofrin Study Group. J Urol 1998;160:39–44.

O'Donnell MA: Use of intravesical BCG in treatment of superficial bladder cancer. In Droller M (ed): Bladder cancer: Current Diagnosis and Treatment. Totowa NJ: Humana Press, 2000, pp 225–266.

O'Donnell MA: Intravesical therapy for superficial bladder cancer: a practical guide. In Kursh E, Ulchaker J (eds): Office Urology. Totowa NJ: Humana Press, 2000, pp 185–201.

O'Donnell MA, Downs TM, DeWolf WC: Co-administration of interferon-alpha 2B with BCG is effective in patients with superficial bladder cancer previously failing BCG alone. J Immunother 1999;22:463.

Quilty PM, Duncan W: Treatment of superficial (T1) tumours of the bladder by radical radiotherapy. Br J Urol 1986;58:147–152.

Schwalb MD, Herr HW, Sogani PC, et al: Positive urinary cytology following a complete response to intravesical bacillus Calmette-Guérin therapy: pattern of recurrence. J Urol 1994;152:382–387.

Scher HI, Shipley WU, Herr HW: Cancer of the bladder. In DeVita VT, Hellman S, Rosenberg SA (eds): Cancer: Principles and Practice of Oncology. Philadelphia: Lippincott-Raven, 1997, pp 1300–1321.

Solsona E, Iborra I, Ricos JV, et al: Effectiveness of a single immediate mitomycin C instillation in patients with low risk superficial bladder cancer: short and long-term followup. J Urol 1999;161:1120–1123.

van der Meijden AP: Practical approaches to the prevention and treatment of adverse reactions to BCG. Eur Urol 1995;27(S1):23–28.

Witjes JA, Oosterhof GO, DeBruyne FM: Management of superficial bladder cancer Ta/T1/TIS: intravesical chemotherapy. In Vogelzang NJ, Scardino PT, Shipley WU, et al (eds): Comprehensive Textbook of Genitourinary Oncology. Baltimore: Williams & Wilkins, 1996, pp 416–427.

Wittes R, Klotz L, Kosecka U: Severe bacillus Calmette-Guérin cystitis responds to systemic steroids when antituberculous drugs and local steroids fail. J Urol 1999;161:1568–1569.

Chapter 86
Muscle-Invasive Bladder Cancer

Bruce J. Roth

Muscle-invasive bladder cancer is somewhat of an enigma among solid tumors. Multiple treatment modalities (e.g., surgery, radiation therapy, and chemotherapy) are of benefit to the patient. The standard of care is difficult to ascertain because few definitive phase III randomized trials in this relatively rare form of cancer have been conducted. Of the approximately 50,000 cases of bladder cancer diagnosed in the United States each year, only 10,000 are invasive into the muscle layer of the bladder wall. Reports from specialists in each of the three possible treatment modalities suggest using their approach as the primary modality of therapy and employing the other modalities as adjunctive therapy. These varying points of view, coupled with overstated efficacy claims by some pharmaceutical companies, serve only to confuse practitioners and patients alike.

The more common variety of bladder cancer, the "non–muscle-invasive" tumors, have a much more indolent natural history (see Chapter 85). They characteristically recur frequently with additional non–muscle-invasive lesions, with only a 10% risk of progression to muscle-invasive disease. Local therapies—transurethral resection, fulguration, or intravesical administration of either immunotherapy or chemotherapy—dominate the treatment of this disease, with the intent of decreasing the likelihood of non-invasive recurrences and of progression to muscle-invasive disease. One needs to be aware that the diagnosis of "non–muscle-invasive" disease can be made only if muscle is present in the biopsy specimen. This is particularly critical in high-grade lesions, as depth of penetration and grade are highly correlated. Patients with high-grade "non–muscle-invasive lesions" should, at the very least, undergo a pathology review to confirm that muscle was present in the specimen. Some would advocate rebiopsy of the site if muscle is not present to assess whether invasion has occurred, because the natural history of invasive disease is so significantly different from non–muscle-invasive disease.

Epidemiology

Bladder cancer tends to be a disease of elderly, non-Hispanic white men from the middle socioeconomic level. In the National Cancer Database Report on Bladder Cancer published in 1996, 82% of patients were older than 60 years, 74% were male, 92% were non-Hispanic white, and 78% from a middle-income level. In the United States, transitional cell carcinoma remains the predominant cell type, constituting 94% of cases, with the remaining 6% comprising squamous cell carcinoma, adenocarcinoma (including the signet-ring cell type), and small cell carcinoma.

Worldwide, the most common cell type remains squamous cell carcinoma, because of the high frequency of bladder infection by *Schistosoma heamatobium* in other countries. In Egypt, for example, where approximately 45% of the population is infected with *Schistosoma haematobium*, bladder tumors account for as many as 35% to 40% of malignancies. The risk of transitional cell carcinoma is also increased. Other populations at risk for chronic urinary tract stasis/infection—such as patients who have spinal cord injuries—are at an increased risk for both squamous and transitional histologies. Chronic exposure to chemotherapeutic agents such as cyclophosphamide, whose active metabolite is excreted into the bladder, are predisposed to a particularly aggressive form of urothelial carcinoma.

Among the other known risk factors for bladder carcinoma, the most important is cigarette (but not pipe or cigar) smoking. The relative risk is two- to fourfold among men who smoke cigarettes compared with nonsmokers. It is estimated that approximately 50% of cases in the U.S. are caused by smoking. Occupational exposure accounts for approximately 25% of cases, principally from the dye and rubber industries, because of exposure to 2-napthylamine. Correlations between the risk of bladder cancer and work in other industries, such as leather, textile, clothing, and metal-working, are not well established.

Familial clustering of cases of transitional cell carcinoma has been reported. The early age of onset confirms the likelihood of a genetic component, which appears to be expressed as an autosomal-dominant gene. The relative risk in first-degree relatives of patients with bladder cancer is twofold.

Clinical Presentation and Initial Evaluation

Invasive bladder cancers most commonly present with gross or incidentally discovered microscopic hematuria or bladder irritative symptoms (see Chapter 28). Although hematuria is frequently attributed to a urinary tract infection, all cases of hematuria in men and otherwise not explained hematuria in women require workup, including cystoscopy. In any patient who smokes, the finding of hematuria should raise the question of a primary bladder carcinoma.

Workup should include not only cystoscopy but also radiologic studies of the upper urinary tracts, either by intravenous pyelogram or contrast-enhanced abdominal/pelvic computed tomography (CT) scan. This latter study should be performed prior to cystoscopy, so that any suspicious upper-tract lesion that might occur concomitantly with a bladder lesion can also be evaluated at the time of cystoscopy, either by ureteroscopy, retrograde pyelograms, or ureteral washings.

Endoscopic full-thickness biopsy or complete transurethral resection is undertaken. If muscle-invasive disease is found, subsequent workup includes an abdominal/pelvic computed tomography scan (if not already obtained) and chest X-ray, reserving chest computed tomography scans for suspicious findings on chest films.

Staging and Prognostic Factors

The natural history of invasive bladder cancer is aggressive; it includes early lymphatic and hematogenous metastases and a five-year survival rate of only 50%. The depth of invasion, as outlined in the T-stage defined in the American Joint Committee on Cancer (AJCC) and prognostic factors staging system (Table 86-1) has important prognostic significance. For patients with either superficial (T2a) or deep (T2b) muscle invasion, the five-year survival rate is 65% to 70%, while in patients with either microscopic (T3a) or macroscopic (T3b) extension into the perivesical fat, five-year survival rates decrease to 50% and 25%, respectively. Further local extension into the prostate, uterus, or vagina (T4a) or pelvic/abdominal wall (T4b) results in a further decrease in five-year survival to

15%, a rate comparable to that of patients with node-positive disease.

For staging purposes, regional lymph nodes are considered the nodes of the true pelvis, which are essentially the pelvic nodes below the bifurcation of the common iliac arteries. The number and size of regional nodal metastases is of more prognostic significance than whether disease involves contralateral or bilateral nodal regions. Involvement of common iliac nodes is considered distant metastasis and is classified as M1 disease. Five-year survival for patients with distant metastases is less than 5%. The few long-term survivors of disease considered to be of M1 are those patients who have only lymph node involvement and who have responded to systemic chemotherapy. Visceral spread of disease predicts a diminished potential for response to therapy and short survival. The varying proportion of patients with visceral disease accounts for the sometimes substantial differences among therapeutic trials in response to treatment and survival. This variability should be kept in mind when evaluating the results of published studies. The only certain way to establish the benefit of one treatment program over another is to conduct randomized phase III trials that stratify patients for both performance status and site of metastatic disease.

Other clinical factors—the depth of muscle invasion, World Health Organization grade of the tumor, and the presence of hydronephrosis at presentation—have been used to predict the likelihood of extravesical spread of disease and diminished survival. Recent work has focused on prognostic molecular markers, including expression of proliferation antigens (Ki-67 and PCNA), oncogenes (HER-2/neu), epidermal growth factor receptors, peptide growth factors (EGF, FGF, and TGF-β), cellular adhesion molecules (E-cadherin, integrins), and cell cycle regulatory proteins (Rb gene product, p53, p21). The data on p53 are the most convincing. Increased expression of and/or mutation of p53 appear to predict for diminished survival and might become part of the standard evaluation of patients with bladder tumors within the next several years.

Therapy

Radical cystectomy remains the standard of care for patients with muscle-invasive disease. Surgery provides excellent local control, particularly in patients with low T-stage. Although pelvic failures are more common in patients with more deeply invasive primary tumors, they are usually accompanied by distant recurrence. The lack of pelvic-only recurrences suggests that it is likely that only systemic therapy has a chance to change the natural history of this disease,

Table 86-1 ■ American Joint Committee on Cancer Staging of Bladder Cancer

Primary Tumor (T)

	TX	Primary tumor cannot be assessed
	T0	No evidence of primary tumor
	Ta	Noninvasive papillary carcinoma
	Tis	Carcinoma in situ: "flat tumor"
	T1	Tumor invades subepithelial connective tissue
	T2	Tumor invades muscle
	T2a	Tumor invades superficial muscle (inner half)
	T2b	Tumor invades deep muscle (outer half)
	T3	Tumor invades perivesical tissue
	T3a	Microscopically
	T3b	Macroscopically (extravesical mass)
	T4	Tumor invades any of the following: prostate, uterus, vagina, pelvic wall, abdominal wall
	T4a	Tumor invades prostate, uterus, vagina
	T4b	Tumor invades pelvic wall, abdominal wall

Regional Lymph Nodes (N)

	NX	Regional lymph nodes cannot be assessed
	N0	No regional lymph node metastasis
	N1	Metastasis in a single lymph node, 2 cm or less in greatest dimension
	N2	Metastasis in a single lymph node, more than 2 cm but not more than 5 cm in greatest dimension
	N3	Metastasis in a lymph node more than 5 cm in greatest dimension

Distant Metastasis (M)

	MX	Distant metastasis cannot be assessed
	M0	No distant metastasis
	M1	Distant metastasis

Regional lymph nodes are those within the true pelvis; all others are distant lymph nodes

DIAGNOSIS

Prognostic Factors in Advanced Bladder Cancer

Analysis and comparison of the results of clinical trials in patients with advanced bladder cancer requires delineation of the composition of different subsets of patients based on recognized prognostic factors. Investigators at Memorial Sloan-Kettering Cancer Center reviewed a large database of patients with bladder cancer who had received M-VAC (methotrexate, vinblastine, Adriamycin, and cyclophosphamide) chemotherapy. In a multivariate analysis, only performance status and the presence or absence of visceral metastases emerged as independent prognostic factors. Three groups were identified based on the presence or absence of these two risk factors; those with 0 risk factors (good performance status and no visceral metastases), one risk factor (either poor performance status or visceral metastases), or two risk factors (poor performance status and visceral metastases).

Number of Risk Factors	Fraction of Patients in Each Group	Complete Response Rate	Median Survival in Months	Five-Year Survival
0	32%	35%	33	33%
1	45%	11%	13	11%
2	23%	0	9	0

Although phase II clinical trials control for performance status in the eligibility criteria for entry on study, most do not control for the variable fraction of entering patients who have visceral disease. The differences in the fraction of patients who have visceral disease entered on clinical trials have a major impact on the results; the effect might be greater than any potential differences among the various chemotherapeutic regimens.

and that such change is unlikely to come from additional local measures such as radiation therapy. Because of the relative chemosensitivity of metastatic bladder cancer, chemotherapy has been used in various ways. Potential settings for the application of chemotherapy in patients with muscle-invasive bladder cancer include

1. metastatic disease
2. preoperative (neoadjuvant) chemotherapy in clinically organ-confined disease
3. postoperative (adjuvant) chemotherapy in high-risk muscle-invasive disease
4. primary chemotherapy followed by surgery in locally advanced disease
5. combined chemoradiotherapy in place of cystectomy as an organ-sparing approach

Metastatic Disease

Cisplatin and methotrexate are active agents in bladder cancer. A number of combination chemotherapy regimens have been developed—for example, cisplatin, methotrexate, and vinblastine, or these same agents combined with doxorubicin (M-VAC). M-VAC therapy, given every four weeks, consists of methotrexate (30 mg/m^2 IV on days 1, 15, and 22), vinblastine (3 mg/m^2 IV on days 2, 15, and 22), and doxorubicin (30 mg/m^2 IV) and cisplatin (70 mg/m^2 IV) on day 2. Although the midcycle doses of relatively nonmyelosuppressive agents (methotrexate and vinblastine) were intended to increase the dose-intensity of the regimen, the actual doses delivered were significantly lower. Because of neutropenia and mucositis, only 40% of the day 15 and day 22 doses could be administered. Although the large phase II trial experience at Memorial Sloan-Kettering achieved a 72% response rate, a 36% complete response rate, and a median survival of 13 months, toxicity was substantial. Of patients receiving M-VAC, ≥grade 3 thrombocytopenia was experienced in 21% and neutropenic fever in 25%, leading to septic deaths in 3% and of ≥grade 3 mucositis in 13%. Nevertheless, M-VAC has

been the standard of chemotherapy for more than a decade.

Subsequent phase III trials showed less encouraging results with M-VAC, despite the use of prophylactic granulocyte colony-stimulating factor (G-CSF) to reduce the incidence of neutropenic fever and severe mucositis. For example, in a randomized trial, M-VAC proved to be superior to single-agent cisplatin in every outcome parameter, but the M-VAC-treated group experienced only a 39% response rate and an 11% complete response rate. A similar phase III trial demonstrated superiority of M-VAC over the combination of cisplatin, cyclophosphamide, and doxorubicin. The initial reports of a 20% disease-free survival at more than three years after M-VAC therapy could not be confirmed; in one phase II trial, only 4% of patients were disease-free at more than six years. Attempts to escalate the doses of M-VAC produced significantly more toxicity and no improvement in efficacy.

Given these limitations on the value of M-VAC, new chemotherapeutic agents and new combination regimens have been evaluated. A group of new agents that achieves responses in previously untreated patients and in patients who previously received cisplatin-containing chemotherapy includes paclitaxel, docetaxel, gemcitabine, trimetrexate, piritrexim, and gallium nitrate. Of this group, the two most effective agents appear to be paclitaxel and gemcitabine.

Paclitaxel

In the initial study conducted by the Eastern Cooperative Oncology Group, paclitaxel produced a 42% response rate and a 27% complete response rate, suggesting that this agent might be the most active single agent yet identified. Paclitaxel combined with cisplatin was effective in metastatic bladder cancer, resulting in response rates ranging from 65% to 80%. This regimen, however, appeared to produce more toxicity than was previously seen in patients with nonbladder cancers, causing significant neuropathy, myelosuppression, and treatment-related deaths.

TREATMENT

Treatment of Stage IV Bladder Cancer

A number of chemotherapy regimens—for example, a combination of M-VAC, gemcitabine, and cisplatin, or paclitaxel and a platinum derivative—appear to be equally efficacious. The newer regimens appear to be less toxic than M-VAC. In patients with poor-risk features, in whom palliation is the only real benefit of therapy, consideration of the patient's quality of life in general and the toxicity of therapy in particular, should be given the highest priority when deciding upon treatment.

In part, the toxicity is related to subclinical renal insufficiency. Factors predisposing to impaired renal function in patients with advanced transitional cell carcinoma include high-grade ureterovesical junction obstruction by a large bladder tumor and prior bladder surgery or nephroureterectomy for a primary upper-tract transitional cell carcinoma. These problems are not present in age-matched controls with ovarian cancer or non–small cell lung cancer who receive the identical regimen. Approximately 25% to 30% of patients with transitional cell carcinoma with advanced disease will have a serum creatinine >1.5 mg/dL, and in one study from the University of Pennsylvania, the median creatinine clearance of unselected patients entering a chemotherapy trial was 52 mL/min. Cisplatin is associated with renal toxicity, and both cisplatin and methotrexate are cleared by the kidneys, whereas renal clearance of or renal toxicity from paclitaxel is minimal.

These observations prompted a series of trials substituting carboplatin for cisplatin in combination with paclitaxel. Carboplatin lacks nephrotoxicity, and the doses for individual patients are adjusted to provide a specific clearance (area-under-the-curve, or AUC) based on the patient's estimated glomerular filtration rate. Using carboplatin at doses to provide an area-under-the-curve of 5–6 and paclitaxel doses of 175 to 225 mg/m^2, overall responses were achieved in 60% of patients and complete responses were achieved in 20%.

Gemcitabine

Initial studies of gemcitabine showed a 25% response rate in previously untreated patients. It was extremely well tolerated, with a very low rate of nonhematologic toxicity.

The monthly administration of the combination of cisplatin 70 mg/m^2 IV on day 2, and gemcitabine 1000 mg/m^2 IV on days 1, 8, and 15 achieved a 57% response rate, but myelosuppression was substantial; grade 3 or 4 granulocytopenia occurred in 39% and grade 3 or 4 thrombocytopenia in 55% of patients. Although these results were promising, a randomized phase III trial that compared M-VAC to gemcitabine and cisplatin in patients with advanced disease showed similar response rates, time to progression, quality of life, and survival. The pattern of myelosuppression differed; when compared with M-VAC, gemcitabine and cisplatin cause a significantly higher incidence of anemia and thrombocytopenia but a lower incidence of neutropenia and fewer episodes of neutropenic fever. Despite the fact that the regimens appear to be equivalent, many oncologists have adopted the gemcitabine-plus-cisplatin regimen as

the standard of care, eschewing further use of M-VAC.

Neoadjuvant Chemotherapy

The failure of surgical advances to alter the outcome of radical cystectomy led to attempts to incorporate systemic therapy in the treatment of early stages of disease. The neoadjuvant approach involves administration of chemotherapy prior to definitive therapy by means of cystectomy or radiation therapy. This process provides a potential advantage in downsizing or downstaging a primary tumor and permits determination of whether the patient's primary bladder cancer responds to chemotherapy. This approach, however, is completely dependent on the accuracy of clinical staging, including T-stage as determined by biopsy. Comparison of clinical to pathologic staging in untreated patients shows an error rate of more than 50%, and patients are almost equally likely to be overstaged or understaged based on clinical evaluation. Moreover, 10% to 12% of patients will have no residual tumor following the original diagnostic transurethral resection alone.

The magnitude of the variation makes it difficult to come to definitive conclusions about the efficacy of preoperative chemotherapy. The reported complete response rates as determined by clinical criteria are approximately 20% to 30% higher than those utilizing pathologic criteria. A complete pathologic response (pT0) after chemotherapy alone rarely occurs with lesions that are large or deeply invasive (≥pT3b) at presentation. Nevertheless, this sequence of therapies is well tolerated. Preoperative chemotherapy does not increase the perioperative mortality of radical cystectomy, although perioperative morbidity may be slightly increased.

A number of phase III trials using a variety of combination chemotherapy regimens as neoadjuvant therapy failed to document improvement in survival or other outcome parameters compared with patients who proceeded directly to definitive surgery or radiation therapy. In the largest trial to date involving 1000 patients, the Medical Research Council of the UK and the European Organization for the Research and Treatment of Cancer (EORTC) randomized patients to receive or not receive three courses of cisplatin, methotrexate, and vinblastine prior to definitive therapy and found no significant difference in survival. Particularly disturbing was the observation that although chemotherapy increased the fraction of patients who had a pathologic complete response (T0) at the time of cystectomy, this did not translate into a survival advantage. Achieving a pathologic complete response is thus a poor surrogate measure of long-

TREATMENT

The Patient with Locally Advanced Bladder Cancer

The optimal therapy for patients with newly diagnosed transitional cell carcinoma of the bladder with documented extravesical extension is uncertain. Extravesical extension can be diagnosed during preoperative staging, by visualization of an extravesical mass or regional adenopathy on computed tomography scans, or at the time of laparotomy for planned cystectomy, when a grossly enlarged, frozen section positive adenopathy or direct extension to regional structures in the pelvis is detected.

Neoadjuvant Chemotherapy. In a patient in whom the preoperative computed tomography scan suggests extravesical extension (most commonly enlarged obturator and iliac nodes), a fine-needle aspirate confirmation is mandatory if nonsurgical primary therapy is contemplated. Because the five-year survival is so poor (less than 10%) with cystectomy in patients with N2 or N3 disease, and because adjuvant therapy remains unproven, it is reasonable in this group of patients to give primary chemotherapy and then consider cystectomy in those patients who have a good clinical response to chemotherapy.

Adjuvant Chemotherapy. More problematic is the patient who is found to have extravesical extension only at the time of laparotomy. Many urologists favor proceeding with cystectomy and pelvic lymph node dissection with the intent of sending the patient for postoperative adjuvant chemotherapy. Because the value of such extensive surgery remains unproven, however, and because the value of adjuvant chemotherapy remains questionable, it is difficult to determine whether to proceed first with surgery or chemotherapy as primary therapy. In the latter circumstance, the residual intravesical lesion can be used to gauge whether the cancer is responsive to chemotherapy.

---

term outcome. This finding has profound implications for bladder-sparing strategies, which rely heavily on the achievement of a clinical complete response to determine further therapy.

Adjuvant Chemotherapy

The use of postoperative chemotherapy has the advantage of targeting for therapy high-risk individuals based on pathologic (as opposed to clinical) staging. In this circumstance, however, the patient receives chemotherapy without residual evaluable disease to determine chemosensitivity, exposing some patients who will not derive benefit to the toxicity of a full course of chemotherapy. This approach tends to be more appealing to urologists and patients than neoadjuvant chemotherapy, because "definitive" therapy (i.e., surgery) is not delayed. As noted previously, it is uncertain whether there is benefit to postoperative chemotherapy. The smaller the benefit one would like to demonstrate in a clinical trial, the larger must the patient population be to demonstrate statistical significance. For example, if one expected a probably unrealistic 20% improvement in survival (e.g., from 50% to 70%) from postoperative chemotherapy, 200 patients would be needed in a clinical trial. A 10% improvement in survival is a more realistic expectation, but the trial would have to contain 1000 patients to adequately power the study. Unfortunately, no randomized trial of adjuvant chemotherapy includes even 200 patients. A number of randomized trials with small patient numbers have failed to demonstrate a significant survival benefit from adjuvant chemotherapy given after radiation therapy or chemotherapy.

Despite these negative data, most patients in the United States with demonstrated lymph node involvement routinely receive adjuvant chemotherapy. The unproven belief in the efficacy of adjuvant chemotherapy renders it difficult to conduct randomized clinical trials in the United States that contain a no-treatment control arm. Nevertheless, the trial of the European Organization for the Research and Treatment of Cancer uses a control arm of no therapy for these patients and an investigational arm of chemotherapy with the specific regimen (either gemcitabine and cisplatin, M-VAC, or escalated-intensity M-VAC) left to the discretion of the investigator. It will be some time before this latter trial is completed; until then, the efficacy of adjuvant chemotherapy remains unclear.

Chemoradiotherapy and Bladder Preservation

Chemotherapy in the setting of muscle-invasive disease can also be used not specifically as an attempt to improve survival but rather to assist in organ sparing. These approaches usually involve maximal transurethral resection followed by systemic chemotherapy, followed by combined chemoradiotherapy. After clinical restaging, either cystectomy for incomplete responses or consolidative chemoradiotherapy for clinical complete responses is given. These approaches are based on a series of assumptions. One such assumption is that the quality of life with a native, irradiated bladder is necessarily superior to radical cystectomy. Although this might have been true at a time when the only option for urinary diversion was an ileal conduit, widespread use of continent urinary diversions and orthotopic neobladders call this assumption into question. One study, in fact, found that quality-of-life measures in patients after cystectomy and orthotopic bladder substitution was similar to a matched control population. The proponents of the bladder-sparing approach also assume that recurrences within the preserved bladder will usually be non–muscle-invasive, easily treated with local measures (e.g., fulguration, resection, or intravesical therapy), and will not compromise patient survival. Finally, there is the assumption that clinical staging after induction chemoradiotherapy accurately represents residual disease. Given that initial clinical staging is incorrect 50% of the time, it is unlikely that the precision of the evaluation improves after chemoradiotherapy. In a number of clinical trials, this approach has not improved survival, progression-free survival, or local or distant failure rates. Moreover, bladder resection was ultimately required in more than 50% of the patients. Despite favorable patient selection in some of these studies, this approach failed to preserve the native bladder in the majority of patients. These results should be part of the discussion with patients when they are offered this approach as an alternative treatment option to cystectomy.

The Role of Chemotherapy in Muscle-Invasive Bladder Cancer

Despite the frustration that arises from a 50% survival rate in patients with muscle-invasive disease and the intuitive appeal of the addition of systemic treatment to local therapy, the published data do not establish the value of chemotherapy in a number of presentations of muscle-invasive bladder cancer nor indicate when, if at all, in the course of therapy of early-stage disease chemotherapy should be given. Because chemotherapy carries the burden of toxicity, it is difficult to recommend such therapy outside the confines of a clinical trial. In fact, such trials should be strongly supported, so that the same questions about the role of chemotherapy are not still being asked a decade from now.

References

General Information

Gabrilove JL, Jakubowski A, Scher H, et al: Effect of granulocyte colony-stimulating factor on neutropenia and associated morbidity due to chemotherapy for transitional cell carcinoma of the urothelium. N Engl J Med 1988;318: 1414–1422.

Henningsohn L, Steven K, Kallestrup EB, Steineck G: Distressful symptoms and well-being after radical cystectomy and orthotopic bladder substitution compared with a matched control population. J Urol 2002;68:168–174.

Sternberg CN: Current perspectives in muscle invasive bladder cancer. Eur J Cancer 2002;38:460–467.

Adjuvant Chemotherapy

Freiha F, Reese J, Torti F: A randomized trial of radical cystectomy versus radical cystectomy plus cisplatin, vinblastine and methotrexate chemotherapy for muscle-invasive bladder cancer. J Urol 1996;155:495–500.

Richards B, Bastable JRG, Freedman L, et al: Adjuvant chemotherapy with doxorubicin (Adriamycin) and 5-fluorouracil in T3, NX, M0 bladder cancer treated with radiotherapy. Br J Urol 1983;55:386–391.

Skinner DG, Daniels JR, Russell CA, et al: The role of adjuvant chemotherapy following cystectomy for invasive bladder cancer: A prospective comparative trial. J Urol 1991;145: 459–467.

Stockle M, Meyenburg W, Wellek S, et al: Advanced bladder cancer (stages pT3b, pT4a, pN1 and pN2): improved survival after radical cystectomy and 3 adjuvant cycles of chemotherapy. Results of a controlled prospective study. J Urol 1992;148:302–307.

Stockle M, Meyenburg W, Wellek S, et al: Adjuvant polychemotherapy of non-organ-confined bladder cancer after radical cystectomy revisited: Long-term results of a controlled prospective study and further clinical experience. J Urol 1995;153:47–52.

Studer UE, Bacchi M, Biedermann C, et al: Adjuvant cisplatin chemotherapy following cystectomy for bladder cancer: Results of a prospective randomized trial. J Urol 1994;152:81–84.

Advanced Disease

Bellmunt J, Guillem V, Paz-Ares L, et al: Phase I-II study of paclitaxel, cisplatin, and gemcitabine in advanced transitional cell carcinoma of the urothelium. J Clin Oncol 2000;18:3247–3255.

Burch PA, Richardson RL, Cha SS, et al: Phase II study of paclitaxel and cisplatin for advanced urothelial cancer. J Urol 2000;164:1538–1542.

Culine S: The present and future of combination chemotherapy in bladder cancer. Sem Oncol 2002;29:32–39.

Dreicer R, Manola J, Roth B, et al: Cisplatin and paclitaxel in advanced carcinoma of the urothelium: A phase II trial of the Eastern Cooperative Oncology Group. J Clin Oncol 2000;18:1058–1061.

Harker WG, Meyers FJ, Freiha FS, et al: Cisplatin, methotrexate, and vinblastine (CMV): An effective chemotherapy regimen for metastatic transitional cell carcinoma of the urinary tract. A Northern California Oncology Group study. J Clin Oncol 1985;3:463–1470.

Kaufman D, Raghavan D, Carducci M, et al: Phase II trial of gemcitabine plus cisplatin in patients with metastatic urothelial cancer. J Clin Oncol 2000;18:1921–1927.

Loehrer PJ, Einhorn LH, Elson PJ, et al: A randomized comparison of cisplatin alone or in combination with methotrexate, vinblastine, and doxorubicin in patients with metastatic urothelial carcinoma: A cooperative group study. J Clin Oncol 1992;10:1066–1073.

Loehrer PJ, Elson P, Dreicer R, et al: Escalated dosages of methotrexate, vinblastine, doxorubicin, and cisplatin plus recombinant human granulocyte colony-stimulating factor in advanced urothelial carcinoma. An Eastern Cooperative Oncology Group trial. J Clin Oncol 1994;12:483–488.

Logothetis CJ, Dexeus FH, Finn L, et al: A prospective randomized trial comparing M-VAC and CISCA chemotherapy for patients with metastatic urothelial tumors. J Clin Oncol 1990;8:1050–1055.

Logothetis C, Finn L, Amato R, et al: Escalated M-VAC +/– rhGM-CSF in metastatic transitional cell carcinoma. Proc Am Soc Clin Oncol 1992;10:202 (abstract).

Moore MJ, Tannock IF, Ernst DS, et al: Gemcitabine: A promising new agent in the treatment of advanced urothelial cancer. J Clin Oncol 1997;15:3441–3445.

Moore MJ, Winquist EW, Murray N, et al: Gemcitabine plus cisplatin, an active regimen in advanced urothelial cancer: A phase II trial of the National Cancer Institute of Canada Clinical Trials Group. J Clin Oncol 1999;17:2876–2881.

Murphy BA, Johnson DH, Smith JA, et al: Phase II trial of paclitaxel and cisplatin for metastatic or locally unresectable urothelial cancer. Proc Am Soc Clin Oncol 1996;14:245 (abstract).

Pollera CF, Ceribelli A, Crecco M, Calabresi F: Weekly gemcitabine in advanced bladder cancer: A preliminary report from a phase I study. Ann Oncol 1994;5:182–184.

Redman BG, Smith DC, Flaherty L, et al: Phase II trial of paclitaxel and carboplatin in the treatment of advanced urothelial carcinoma. J Clin Oncol 1998;16:1844–1848.

Roth BJ, Dreicer R, Einhorn LH, et al: Significant activity of paclitaxel in advanced transitional cell carcinoma of the urothelium: A phase II trial of the Eastern Cooperative Oncology Group (E1892). J Clin Oncol 1994;12:2264–2270.

Roth BJ, Bajorin DF: Advanced bladder cancer: the need to identify new agents in the post-M-VAC (methotrexate, vinblastine, doxorubicin, and cisplatin) world. J Urol 1995;153:894–900.

Saxman SB, Propert KJ, Einhorn LH, et al: Long-term follow-up of a phase III Intergroup study of cisplatin alone or in combination with methotrexate, vinblastine, and doxorubicin in patients with metastatic urothelial carcinoma. A cooperative group study. J Clin Oncol 1997;15:2564–2569.

Small EJ, Lew D, Redman BG, et al: Southwest Oncology Group study of paclitaxel and carboplatin for advanced transitional cell carcinoma: The importance of survival as a clinical trial end point. J Clin Oncol 2000;18:2537–2544.

Stadler WM, Kuzel T, Roth B, et al: Phase II study of single-agent gemcitabine in previously untreated patients with metastatic urothelial cancer. J Clin Oncol 1997;15:3394–3398.

Sternberg CN, Yagoda A, Scher HI, et al: M-VAC (methotrexate, vinblastine, doxorubicin, and cisplatin) for advanced transitional cell carcinoma of the urothelium. J Urol 1988;139:461–469.

Sternberg CN, deMulder PH, Schornagel JH, et al: Randomized phase III trial of high-dose-intensity methotrexate, vinblastine, doxorubicin, and cisplatin (M-VAC) chemotherapy and recombinant human granulocyte colony-stimulating factor versus classic M-VAC in advanced urothelial tract tumors. European Organization for Research and Treatment of Cancer Protocol no. 30924. J Clin Oncol 2001;19:2638–2646.

Vaughn DJ, Malkowicz SB, Zoltick B, et al: Paclitaxel plus carboplatin in advanced carcinoma of the urothelium: An active and tolerable outpatient regimen. J Clin Oncol 1998;16:255–260.

von der Maase H, Hansen SW, Roberts JT, et al: Gemcitabine and cisplatin versus methotrexate, vinblastine, doxorubicin, and cisplatin in advanced or metastatic bladder cancer: Results of a large, randomized, multinational, multicenter, phase III study. J Clin Oncol 2000;18:3068–3077.

Bladder Preservation

Kachnic LA, Kaufman DS, Heney NM: Bladder preservation by combined modality therapy for invasive bladder cancer. J Clin Oncol 1997;15:1022–1029.

Kaufman DS, Shipley WU, Griffin PP, et al: Selective bladder preservation by combination treatment of invasive bladder cancer. N Engl J Med 1993;329:1377–1382.

Neoadjuvant Therapy

Cortesi E: Neoadjuvant treatment for locally advanced bladder cancer: A randomized prospective clinical trial. Proc Am Soc Clin Oncol 1995;13:237(abstract).

Herr HW, Scher HI: Neoadjuvant chemotherapy and partial cystectomy for invasive bladder cancer. J Clin Oncol 1994;12:975–980.

Medical Research Council Advanced Bladder Cancer Working Party: Neoadjuvant cisplatin, methotrexate, and vinblastine chemotherapy for muscle-invasive bladder cancer: A randomized controlled trial. Lancet 1999;354:533–540.

Scher HI, Yagoda A, Herr HW, et al: Neoadjuvant M-VAC (methotrexate, vinblastine, doxorubicin, and cisplatin) effect on the primary bladder lesion. J Urol 1988;139:470–474.

Scher H, Herr H, Sternberg C, et al.: Neo-adjuvant chemotherapy for invasive bladder cancer. Experience with the M-VAC regimen. Br J Urol 1989;64:250–256.

Schultz PK, Herr HW, Zhang Z-F, et al: Neoadjuvant chemotherapy for invasive bladder cancer: Prognostic factors for survival of patients treated with M-VAC with 5-year follow-up. J Clin Oncol 1994;12:1394–1401.

Shipley WU, Winter KA, Kaufman DS: Phase III trial of neoadjuvant chemotherapy in patients with invasive bladder cancer treated with selective bladder preservation. J Clin Oncol 1998;16:3576–3583.

Sternberg CN: Neoadjuvant and adjuvant chemotherapy in locally advanced bladder cancer. Sem Oncol 1996;23:621–632.

Tester W, Caplan R, Heaney J: Neoadjuvant combined modality program with selective organ preservation for invasive bladder cancer: Results of Radiation Therapy Oncology Group phase II trial 8802. J Clin Oncol 1996;14:119–126.

Prognosis

Bajorin D, Dodd PM, Mazumdar M, et al: Long-term survival in metastatic transitional cell carcinoma and prognostic factors predicting outcome of therapy. J Clin Oncol 1999;17:3173–3181.

Sarkis AS, Dalbagni G, Cordon-Cardo C, et al: Association of p53 nuclear overexpression and tumor progression in carcinoma in situ of the bladder. J Urol 1994;152:388–392.

Surgery

Hall MC, Swanson DA, Dinney CP: Complications of radical cystectomy: impact of the timing of perioperative chemotherapy. Urol 1996;47:826–830.

Herr HW: Transurethral resection in regionally advanced bladder cancer. Urol Clin North Am 1992;19:695–700.

Chapter 87
Prostate Cancer

Yoo-Joung Ko and Glenn J. Bubley

Introduction

Increased public awareness and widespread prevalence have pushed prostate cancer to the forefront in terms of research funding and clinical trials. Yet this disease, perhaps more than any other solid tumor, lacks definitive and unbiased recommendations for screening, prevention, and therapy. Prevention is an important goal because of the prevalence of this cancer. Although the National Cancer Institute has launched a second major prevention trial, results from this and a previous study will not be forthcoming for years, and men still lack proven guidelines for prevention. Screening for prostate cancer using serum prostate-specific antigen (PSA) values has been ongoing for more than a decade, yet it is not known whether this strategy alters mortality from prostate cancer. The decision regarding what form of primary therapy to choose for the typical newly diagnosed patient can be daunting. Patients can be confronted with several options for therapy that range from radical surgery, various forms of radiation therapy, or even watchful waiting. To make matters even more complex, adjuvant and neoadjuvant hormonal therapy in combination with radiation therapy or surgery might also be proposed as treatment options for these men. Although chemotherapy is believed to be of little value in patients with hormone refractory or androgen-independent prostate cancer, newer chemotherapeutic regimens and a variety of newer nonchemotherapeutic agents hold great promise.

Incidence and Epidemiology

Prostate cancer is the most common malignant tumor in men (excluding non–melanoma skin cancer) and is the second leading cause of cancer death. It is currently estimated that almost one in six men in the United States will be diagnosed with prostate cancer over their lifetimes. In the 1970s and early 1980s, the incidences of prostate cancer and lung cancer in men were similar. From the mid-1980s to 1993, however, there was a dramatic increase in newly diagnosed cases of prostate cancer, with a 108% increase compared with the previous decade. This increase is thought to be due mainly to the introduction of prostate-specific antigen testing and the aging of the population, but other unknown factors may have contributed as well. Interestingly, the incidence of prostate cancer dropped dramatically between 1992 and 1995 and since then has remained stable. The dramatic increase and stabilization is most likely the result of prostate-specific antigen testing identifying men with their first screening and culling them from the population.

Between 1994 and 1997, prostate cancer mortality rates have declined by 4.4% per year. There is controversy as to whether this decline is a real benefit attributable to screening, or merely the result of detecting more cases with indolent disease that might not have required treatment. The latter view is supported by the detection of prostate cancer at autopsy in a great percentage of older men who have died of unrelated causes, indicating the existence of a substantial number of men with an indolent form of the disease.

Worldwide rates of prostate cancer differ dramatically. For instance, the incidence in China and Japan is approximately 50-fold or less than that observed for Western Europe and the United States. The basis for these differences is not known, but it is not wholly due to familial factors. When Asian men immigrate to the United States, they have substantially higher rates of prostate cancer that are thought not to be simply the result of more aggressive screening in this country. The observation that prostate cancer is lower in men living in Asia has sparked interest in the Asian diet as a possible factor in prostate cancer prevention.

The incidence of prostate cancer among African-American men in the United States is twofold that of Caucasian men. African-American men also tend to present with more advanced disease and have a substantially higher death rate. Although it is possible that African-American men have a higher mortality from prostate cancer because of less frequent screening and reduced access to the United States health care system, these are unlikely to be the only causes for this discrepancy. Many experts feel that the disease is biologically more aggressive in African-American men because of a mixture of environmental and familial factors.

Risk Factors and Genetics

Prostate cancer has a distinct familial predisposition. For instance, in a study of the Utah Mormon population, brothers of men with prostate cancer had a relative risk of 2.38 for developing the disease. Men also have an increased risk for prostate cancer risk if their fathers are affected. The highest relative risk is for men who have brothers and fathers diagnosed with prostate cancer at younger than 65 years of age. Family history, often reflecting predominantly genetic factors, is therefore an important component of risk. Although no specific gene has been linked to prostate cancer, an abnormality in chromosome 1 has been detected in some families with an especially strong history of the disease.

The role of androgens, particularly testosterone and dihydrotestosterone (DHT), as risk factors for prostate cancer has been investigated. Despite some controversy, a meta-analysis confirmed that after normalizing for levels of sex hormone-binding globulin and other endocrine hormones, high levels of testosterone are a risk factor for prostate cancer. Androgen levels are likely to be controlled by a number of environmental and inherited factors.

Multiple case-control studies have demonstrated that increased serum levels of insulin-like growth factor 1 (IGF-1) are also associated with an increased risk of prostate cancer. This was first established by a hospital-based case-control study and later confirmed by prospective and population-based case-control studies. Increased serum levels of IGF-1 have also been shown to be a risk factor for lung cancer, childhood leukemia, and in situ ductal carcinoma of the breast. Serum IGF-1 levels are at least partially under the control of growth hormone levels. Like androgen levels, however, IGF-1 levels in men are likely to be the result of multiple environmental and inherited factors.

Increased rates of prostate cancer relative to control populations have been detected in men working in cadmium, rubber, and sheet metal production. However, these increases in risk have been relatively small, and occupational factors are not thought to be a major factor in the etiology of prostate

cancer. There is also no evidence that sexually transmitted diseases play a role. An implication that vasectomy increases prostate cancer risk has not been confirmed.

Several descriptive and case-control studies have demonstrated a positive correlation between intake of animal fat and the risk of prostate cancer. In one review, 10 of 13 studies reported a positive correlation between fat intake and prostate cancer risk. In addition to case-control studies, population-based analyses have shown that dietary intake might influence prostate cancer risk. For instance, Japan has a low death rate from prostate cancer, and the Japanese consume only 18% of their calories from fat, compared with the typical 40% intake in the traditional Western diet. It is difficult to attribute a cause-and-effect relationship to these associations, however, as there are many confounding factors. For example, the intake of soy is also very high in Japan, which could also contribute to the lowered risk of prostate cancer. Soy contains phytoestrogens that have hormonal and perhaps antioxidant properties. Levels of genistein, a key phytoestrogen, have been found to be low in men from Finland, a country with a very high rate of prostate cancer.

Prostate Cancer Prevention

As mentioned in previous sections, an enigma in prostate cancer biology is that a high proportion (greater than 70%) of men over age 80 will have histological evidence of prostate cancer on autopsy examination, although far fewer will ever manifest clinical disease. It is not understood why this specific cancer—unlike colorectal, lung, or other cancers—seems to be so prevalent in an indolent form in the aging male. The prevailing view is that worldwide, the incidence of occult or indolent disease is similar despite dramatic differences in clinically evident prostate cancer. For instance, the incidence of occult prostate cancer detected at autopsy is the same in Japan and the United States, despite the much higher rate of clinical disease in this country. This observation has led to the hypothesis that environmental factors are important in the promotion (as opposed to the initiation) of prostate cancer. If these environmental factors could be recognized and modified, it might be possible to maintain prostate cancer in an indolent state. Many of the prevention strategies discussed in this chapter are based on this hypothesis.

Androgens and Prostate Cancer Prevention

Although androgen exposure is a probable risk factor for prostate cancer, there are no feasible methods of

Table 87-1 ■ TNM Staging of Prostate Cancer

Primary Tumor (T)

Tx	Primary tumor cannot be assessed
T0	No evidence of primary tumor
T1	Clinically inapparent tumor not palpable or visible by imaging
T1a	Incidental surgical finding involving ≤5% of resected tissue
T1b	Incidental surgical finding involving >5% of resected tissue
T1c	Positive blind needle biopsy because of increased PSA
T2	Tumor confined to prostate
T2a	Involves one lobe of prostate gland
T2b	Involves both lobes of prostate gland
T3	Extension through prostate capsule
T3a	Extracapsular extension (unilateral or bilateral)
T3b	Invades seminal vesicle(s)
T4a	Fixed or invades adjacent structures other than seminal vesicles

Regional Nodes (N)

N0	Cannot be assessed
N1	No regional node involvement
N2	Lymph node metastasis(es)

Distant Metastasis (M)

MX	Distant metastasis cannot be assessed
M0	No distant metastasis
M1	Distant metastasis
M1a	Non-regional lymph node(s)
M1b	Bone(s)
M1c	Other site(s)

TNM Stage Grouping:

Stage I	T1a (low grade)	N0	M0
Stage II	T1a (high-grade)–T2	N0	M0
Stage III	T3	N0	M0
Stage IV	T4	N0	M0
	Any T	N1	M0
	Any T	Any N	M1

long-term testosterone depletion without undesirable side effects. Instead, a strategy involving finasteride, an inhibitor of 5-alpha reductase (an intracellular enzyme responsible for converting testosterone to the more potent dihydrotestosterone), is currently being studied in a randomized trial versus placebo.

Vitamin E and Selenium in Prostate Cancer Prevention

A randomized trial of 29,000 smokers tested the effects of alpha-tocopherol (a form of vitamin E) and beta carotene in cancer prevention. Men receiving vitamin E had a 32% decrease in prostate cancer overall. Se-

lenium at 200 µg/day is associated with a significant reduction in mortality from prostate cancer, lung cancer, and colon cancer. In a case control study, decreased selenium intake as measured in toenail clippings was associated with a higher risk of advanced prostate cancer. A randomized study is testing whether supplementation with vitamin E and selenium (alone or together) prevents prostate cancer.

Prostate Cancer Staging

The American Joint Committee on Cancer (AJCC) staging system incorporates the most commonly diagnosed prostate cancer stage, T1C, denoting cancers that are detected by prostate-specific antigen testing only in patients with normal digital rectal exams (Table 87-1).

Adenocarcinoma constitutes the most common histologic subtype of prostate cancer and tends to be multifocal in nature. The histologic grading system most commonly used is the Gleason scoring system, which incorporates the heterogeneous nature of prostate cancer by assigning two grades—one each to the two most predominant patterns that are present on the specimen. The scoring system assigns a grade of 1 (most differentiated) to 5 (poorly differentiated). Prostate cancers of the small cell type often demonstrate neuroendocrine markers such as synaptophysin and chromogranin but account for fewer than 1% of all prostate cancers. These often do not produce prostate-specific antigen and respond poorly to androgen ablation.

Primary treatment recommendations are often based on the use of known prognostic factors, including biopsy Gleason score, prostate-specific antigen, and the TNM clinical stage. Partin et al have constructed nomograms using these three factors to predict the pathologic stage of localized prostate cancer. Specifically, these nomograms can be used to predict organ-confined, established extracapsular extension, seminal vesical invasion, and lymph node disease. Some patients who have pathologically organ-confined disease, however, eventually will develop recurrent disease. Prostate-specific antigen failure-free survival is a surrogate endpoint that is clinically more meaningful than final pathologic stage. D'Amico et al have compiled a pretreatment nomogram to predict two-year prostate-specific antigen failure rates as a function of the pretreatment prostate-specific antigen, biopsy Gleason score, and the AJCC clinical stage for patients undergoing radical prostatectomy or external beam radiation therapy (Table 87-2). Patients with a high prostate-specific antigen (greater than 20 ng/mL) or Gleason score (greater than 8) have a high probability of developing early biochemical recurrence

Table 87-2 ■ Percentage of Prostate-Specific Antigen Failure at Two Years (95% Confidence Intervals), Stratified by Pretreatment Prostate-Specific Antigen, AJCC Clinical Stage, and Biopsy Gleason Score

Pretreatment Prostate-Specific Antigen (ng/mL)	Biopsy Gleason Score	T (Tumor) Category			
		T1C	T2a	T2b	T2c
Surgically Managed Patients at PENN* (n = 892)					
0–4.0					
	6	10 (6–15)	11 (8–14)	19 (11–27)	24 (17–31)
	7	14 (8–20)	15 (11–19)	25 (15–35)	24 (17–31)
	8–10	24 (13–37)	26 (16–36)	42 (24–59)	50 (34–40)
4.1–10.0					
	6	13 (8–18)	14 (11–17)	24 (15–32)	29 (22–37)
	7	17 (11–24)	19 (14–23)	31 (20–42)	37 (28–46)
	8–10	29 (17–44)	32 (20–44)	50 (31–67)	58 (43–72)
10.1–20.0					
	6	18 (11–26)	20 (15–25)	33 (22–43)	39 (31–48)
	7	24 (15–34)	26 (20–33)	42 (29–54)	49 (40–59)
	8–10	39 (24–58)	43 (29–58)	63 (44–80)	72 (56–84)
20.1–50.0					
	6	40 (24–63)	43 (30–63)	63 (47–83)	72 (60–88)
	7	50 (32–74)	53 (39–75)	75 (58–91)	82 (71–95)
	8–10	72 (48–94)	76 (57–94)	92 (77–99)	96 (88–100)
Radiation-Managed Patients at JCRT† (n = 762)					
0–4.0					
	6	10 (6–14)	12 (8–17)	16 (10–23)	17 (11–24)
	7	14 (9–20)	18 (11–25)	23 (15–34)	25 (17–35)
	8–10	29 (17–46)	36 (21–55)	45 (27–68)	48 (29–69)
4.1–10.0					
	6	11 (7–15)	14 (9–19)	18 (12–26)	20 (13–27)
	7	16 (11–23)	20 (13–28)	26 (17–37)	28 (19–39)
	8–10	33 (20–50)	40 (24–59)	50 (31–72)	52 (33–74)
10.1–20.0					
	6	14 (9–19)	17 (11–24)	22 (15–31)	24 (17–33)
	7	20 (13–27)	25 (16–34)	32 (22–44)	34 (24–46)
	8–10	39 (25–57)	47 (30–67)	58 (38–79)	61 (40–81)
20.1–50.0					
	6	23 (15–32)	28 (20–39)	36 (25–49)	38 (27–51)
	7	32 (23–42)	39 (28–51)	49 (36–64)	51 (38–66)
	8–10	58 (41–76)	67 (49–85)	78 (58–93)	80 (62–94)

*University of Pennsylvania
†Joint Center for Radiation Therapy
Adapted from D'Amico AV, Whittington R, Malkowitz SB, et al: Pretreatment nomogram for prostate-specific antigen recurrence after radical prostatectomy or external-beam radiation therapy for clinically localized prostate cancer. J Clin Oncol 1999;17:168–172.

(greater than 50%). Patients who develop early biochemical recurrences are those who have micrometastatic disease at time of local therapy and who eventually relapse at distant sites. Therefore, this nomogram could be useful in identifying patients for adjuvant clinical studies.

Clinical Presentations of Prostate Cancer

Currently, the majority of cases of prostate cancer are detected by prostate-specific antigen screening only. Such patients are entirely asymptomatic, and only

30% have abnormal prostate findings on digital rectal examination. Therefore, as many as 70% of currently diagnosed cases are in men with limited T1 disease. Prior to the use of prostate-specific antigen tests, the majority of prostate cancer patients were detected as a result of abnormal digital rectal examination. Other patients presented with symptoms of metastatic disease or were diagnosed based on histologic examination of specimen from a transuretheral resection of the prostate (TURP) for prostatic hypertrophy. Over the past 15 years, there has also been a commensurate dramatic change in the stage at which men are diagnosed with prostate cancer. Currently, approximately 80% to 90% of patients are diagnosed with early Stage A or B cancer. Less than 5% of men will have symptoms referable to local disease at presentation. It is important to note that these symptoms—urinary frequency, difficulty initiating the urinary stream, and nocturia—are much more likely to be presenting features of benign prostatic hypertrophy than prostate cancer. The remaining 10% of patients present with signs or symptoms of metastatic disease, typically resulting from bone metastasis. Signs and symptoms include bone pain, cord compression from vertebral body involvement, and rarely, pathologic fracture.

Clinical Evaluation of the Newly Diagnosed Patient

In the clinical assessment of a prostate cancer patient, it is important to determine whether the disease is overtly metastatic or is confined to the prostate. If, as in the case of most newly diagnosed patients, the cancer seems to be limited to the prostate gland, it is important to assess the patient's risk for aggressive disease. This risk assessment will help guide treatment decisions.

Evaluation of Metastatic Disease

Patients with metastatic disease at presentation usually are not considered candidates for primary therapy; nonetheless, it is not necessary to perform complete staging studies in every newly diagnosed patient. Bone scans and computed tomography (CT) scans are infrequently positive in patients with prostate-specific antigen values of 10 or less, Gleason

---

TREATMENT

Workup and Management of the Newly Diagnosed Prostate Cancer Patient

One of the most difficult and contentious issues for prostate cancer patients and their providers is deciding on the primary therapy. In the absence of randomized clinical trials, it is difficult to compare the survival data for radical prostatectomy compared with different forms of radiation therapy. Furthermore, a subset of patients might be appropriate for a watchful waiting strategy.

A useful approach to the problem of selecting a specific primary therapy is to assess the risk for aggressive local disease in newly diagnosed patients. In general, patients with the least risk are candidates for brachytherapy or watchful waiting. Patients with intermediate risk are candidates for surgery or radiation. Patients with high risk are candidates for primary therapy combined with hormonal therapy. Other experimental approaches include the use of additive local therapy (such as hyperthermia), combinations of external beam therapy and brachytherapy, or chemotherapy combined with hormonal therapy as an adjunct to surgery or radiation therapy.

The assessment of risk factors in the newly diagnosed patient starts with the digital rectal examination. Patients with easily palpable nodules (T2 disease) are currently not considered to be good candidates for brachytherapy. Furthermore, if a nodule is present, it is important to try to determine whether the nodule seems to protrude beyond the capsule (T3 disease). Patients with T3 disease are at high risk for relapse after either surgery or external beam radiation therapy, and combined therapeutic approaches should be considered. Endorectal magnetic resonance imaging has been used to assess extracapsular invasion but might fail to detect it.

In addition to the evaluation of prostate nodularity, other factors used in the Partin and D'Amico nomograms (see Table 87-2) are important in assessing risk. These include the Gleason sum or score (the combined scores of the differentiation patterns) obtained on the core biopsy. Patients who have Gleason sums of 8 or above or prostate-specific antigen values over 20 are at similar risk for extracapsular disease as patients with clinical T3 involvement.

The optimal patients to consider for watchful waiting are those with stage T1 disease and Gleason combined grades of 6 or less. Furthermore, patients with a life expectancy of less than a decade and low Gleason-grade disease of any stage should be considered for watchful waiting or brachytherapy.

scores of 8 or less, and a clinical stage of less than T3. In fact, in one series of newly diagnosed patients with prostate-specific antigen values of 20 or less, only one patient out of 306 exhibited a bone scan positive for malignancy. Therefore, many physicians perform these radiologic tests only in patients with an increased risk for distant disease.

Assessment of Local Disease

Deciding on the appropriate form of primary therapy can be a consuming and critical issue for newly diagnosed patients and their providers. The estimated risk of local (extracapsular) or regional lymph node spread is an important guide in this decision-making process. Patients at risk for more extensive local disease are generally considered better candidates for external beam radiation therapy (with or without adjuvant hormonal therapy) than for radical prostatectomy. Unfortunately, current modalities are inexact when it comes to staging the extent of local disease.

Only a minority of patients will have prostate abnormalities noted on digital rectal examinations. In these patients, the examiner might be able to assess whether the disease protrudes beyond the prostate capsule (stage C). In some cases, it could be possible during the digital rectal examination to determine whether there is seminal vesicle invasion, although this is often difficult even for the most experienced physician to assess.

Most newly diagnosed patients have had a transrectal ultrasound (TRUS) examination performed as part of a biopsy procedure. Transrectal ultrasound aids in positioning the biopsy needle to peripheral regions of the prostate, but it is neither sensitive nor specific for the detection of prostate cancer. Only one-third of hypoechoic lesions are positive for cancer on core biopsy, and two-thirds of the biopsies positive for cancer are obtained from areas that appeared normal on ultrasound. Furthermore, ultrasound is not very sensitive to the presence of extracapsular disease or seminal vesicle invasion. Endorectal magnetic resonance imaging (MRI) is superior to body magnetic resonance imaging and computed tomography for detecting disease outside the prostate capsule, especially when T2-weighted images are evaluated. However, even in institutions with extensive experience, endorectal magnetic resonance imaging accurately detects extracapsular disease only 70% of the time.

The inaccuracy of current methods to assess capsular invasion or seminal vesicle and lymph node involvement has led to the creation of alternative systems for predicting prostate cancer stage. The nomogram developed by Partin and his colleagues has been shown to predict capsular invasion with 60% accuracy, seminal vesicle involvement with 80% accuracy, and pelvic lymph node involvement with 83% accuracy. The nomogram developed by D'Amico can also be useful for predicting prostate-specific antigen recurrence for both surgically managed and radiation-managed patients. The predictive accuracy of these nomograms often exceeds the accuracy of current radiologic techniques.

Prostate Cancer Screening

Prior to the prostate-specific antigen testing era, prostate cancer was often detected by a digital rectal examination. Unfortunately, many of these cancers were locally advanced and were unlikely to be cured by surgery or radiation therapy. Digital rectal exam by itself is highly inaccurate and poorly reproducible. Therefore, it is recommended by some groups that an annual rectal examination should be combined with a serum prostate-specific antigen. A transrectal ultrasound-guided biopsy is performed if either is found to be abnormal.

Prostate-specific antigen is a prostate-specific (but not a prostate cancer-specific) marker. Although malignant tissue tends to produce more prostate-specific antigen than benign tissue, the lack of cancer specificity imposes a limitation on its use as a screening test. The use of age-specific values has increased the sensitivity of the test for younger men, but only at the expense of lower specificity. Refinements have been made to the ability of prostate-specific antigen to predict prostate cancer by adjusting for the size of the prostate gland (prostate-specific antigen density), adjusting for changes in prostate-specific antigen level over time (prostate-specific antigen velocity), and determining the fraction of free vs. bound protein (free prostate-specific antigen). The added predictive value of these additional tests has not been validated in large prospective randomized studies. The use of these refinements add a significant cost to prostate cancer screening; hence the importance of establishing their utility prior to using them routinely.

Despite the availability of reasonably sensitive and accurate screening tests, the value of prostate cancer screening continues to be debated in both medical and public forums. The lack of consensus for prostate-specific antigen screening is demonstrated by the disparate recommendations of different medical and cancer societies in North America (Table 87-3). Both the American Urological Association (AUA) and the American Cancer Society recommend screening with an annual digital rectal exam and serum prostate-specific antigen in men older than age 50 years who have a life expectancy of greater than 10 years. The

Table 87-3 ■ Recommendations for Prostate Cancer Screening

Organization	Year	Recommendation
American Cancer Society	1992	Annual prostate-specific antigen and digital rectal exam for >50 years of age and for those with life expectancy >10 years; for those at higher risk (family history or African-Americans) >45 years.
American Urological Association	1995	Annual prostate-specific antigen and digital rectal exam for those >50 years or >40 years (high risk).
American College of Radiology	1997	Digital rectal exam and prostate-specific antigen should be used as an initial screen. Transrectal ultrasound recommended for those with an abnormal digital rectal examination or prostate-specific antigen.
American College of Physicians	1997	Physicians should describe potential benefits and known harms of screening, diagnosis, and treatment and individualize decision to screen. Patients should be encouraged to enroll in studies.
National Cancer Institute	1997	Insufficient evidence to establish whether there is decreased mortality from prostate cancer screening by prostate-specific antigen and/or digital rectal exam.
American Association of Family Practitioners	1996	Men ages 50–65 should be counseled about the known risks and uncertain benefits of screening for prostate cancer.
U.S. Preventative Services Task Force	1996	Routine screening not recommended.
Canadian Task Force on the Periodic Health Examination	1994	No routine use of prostate-specific antigen or digital rectal exam as part of a periodic health examination is recommended.

recommended age for initiating screening in African-American men or men with a significant family history is 40. In contrast, the United States Preventative Services Task Force and the Canadian Task Force on Periodic Health Examination do not recommend prostate cancer screening.

Although prostate cancer is an important public health problem in Western nations and prostate-specific antigen testing is relatively cheap and convenient, the controversy over screening is based on the debate over whether early detection and treatment results in improved overall survival. Randomized clinical trials to determine the possible benefits of treatment of early disease have not yet been completed. Furthermore, analyses of potential benefits of screening are complicated by both the lead-time bias (which occurs from earlier detection) and the length-time bias (which produces an apparent improvement in survival). The analysis of the value of prostate cancer screening is also complicated by the potentially mitigating side effects of primary therapy—radical prostatectomy, external beam radiation therapy, and brachytherapy—all of which can affect a patient's quality of life. These attendant morbidities are often seen as minor if treatment leads to prolongation of survival, but they can become unacceptable if screening detects insignificant cancers that would never have caused mortality or even morbidity.

Arguments against screening for prostate cancer have emphasized that screening leads to detection of insignificant prostate cancers and that aggressive treatment of prostate cancer has significant associated morbidity. In addition, older men are subject to competing risks for death, such as cardiovascular disease. On the other hand, only a minority of the prostate cancer that is currently detected with prostate-specific antigen and digital rectal examination and treated with surgery is felt to be clinically insignificant based on histologic grade (Gleason score). Whether a Gleason score of 6 or greater should impel intervention in T1C patients is unclear. Until the results of randomized studies are available, decisions about screening for prostate cancer will have to integrate individual patient preferences with the biases of the treating clinician within the context of conflicting guidelines from the large medical associations. Even though definitive new data is lacking, it is anticipated that an increasingly well-informed public will help shape screening policies at both a local and national level.

Primary Therapy for Newly Diagnosed Prostate Cancer Patients

For both patients and their physicians, one of the more difficult issues in the contemporary management of prostate cancer is the decision regarding primary therapy. Patients are faced with choices ranging from watchful waiting to radical prostatectomy to various forms of radiation therapy. To complicate matters further, primary therapy might be given in conjunction with a course of androgen-ablative therapy. The important criteria for evaluating these alternatives are the rates of cancer-specific survival, side effects, and the natural history of the untreated disease. Unfortunately, randomized studies comparing these different therapeutic options are lacking. Furthermore, during the past few years both surgical and radiation therapy techniques have improved, making historical comparisons of these modalities even more difficult. In this section, options for primary therapy of prostate cancer are discussed, with emphasis on the risks and benefits of each strategy.

Radical Prostatectomy

Radical prostatectomy is often referred to as the "gold standard" for primary therapy, as it serves as the standard by which other therapies are often compared. Currently, more than 50,000 radical prostatectomies are performed yearly in the United States alone.

It is difficult to define precisely who is a candidate for a radical prostatectomy. Many clinicians recommend this procedure for patients who are likely to have organ-confined disease, who are healthy enough to withstand major surgery, and who will live long enough to benefit from this intervention. Many health care providers suggest external beam radiation therapy with or without androgen deprivation therapy (see the section that follows) if there is a high likelihood that the disease has spread beyond the prostate capsule; however, it is possible that patients with extracapsular disease would derive equivalent benefit from prostatectomy. In fact, recent data suggests that even patients with lymph node involvement detected at surgery might benefit from removal of the prostate, especially with the addition of immediate postoperative androgen deprivation therapy. A crucial factor in assessing the value of radical prostatectomy is whether this form of primary therapy increases long-term disease-free survival. Physicians must, for the moment, rely on comparisons between series of patients who often have vastly different selection criteria to determine the relative merits of prostatectomy. In contemporary series, outcome is typically reported as freedom from prostate-specific antigen relapse (Table 87-4). This is a valid surrogate for clinical recurrence, although it needs to be emphasized that prostate-specific antigen relapse can precede clinical relapse by several years.

Radical prostatectomy typically requires at least a three- or four-day hospital stay. The perioperative mortality rate is typically less than 1%. The most frequent long-term complication of radical prostatectomy is impotence from nerve damage sustained during removal of the prostate. Until the advent of the nerve-sparing procedure, impotence occurred in nearly 100% of patients; however, the bilateral nerve-sparing procedure developed by Walsh and colleagues is reported to result in a 74% potency rate. Nerve sparing is an appropriate option for only a subset of men with less aggressive disease characteristics. Even patients who undergo nerve-sparing surgery are impotent in the immediate postoperative period, and it may take them as long as one year to regain sexual function. Return of potency is more frequent for younger men and those with less extensive disease. The effectiveness of nerve-sparing surgery for maintaining potency has been questioned. When patients and their partners were interviewed by a third party, Talcott and his colleagues reported a relatively low potency rate after a nerve-sparing prostatectomy. In contrast, the advent of selective vasodilators like sildenafil (Viagra) can improve reported potency in men after a nerve-sparing operation.

Urinary incontinence is another complication of radical prostatectomy. It is important to stress that almost everyone is incontinent in the immediate postoperative period. By six weeks to six months after surgery, however, most patients have regained significant urinary sphincter function. The frequency of incontinence depends to some degree on how it is defined. For instance, incontinence often is reported as a complication only for those men whose urinary dribbling is severe enough to require wearing pads. The incidence of incontinence ranges from less than 1% to as high as 20%.

Less frequent complications of radical prostatectomy include bladder neck contracture (occurring in less than 5% of patients and amenable to urethral dilatation) and injury to the rectum (which occurs in less than 1% of patients and can typically be repaired successfully during the procedure itself).

Table 87-4 ■ Freedom from Prostate-Specific Antigen Relapse after Radical Prostatectomy

Trial Site	Patient Number	% Undetectable PSA (Five Years)
Washington University	925	78
Duke University	1319	68
Baylor University	500	77
UCLA	601	69
Mayo Clinic	3170	70
Cleveland Clinic	423	59
Johns Hopkins	1623	80
UCSF	543	73

One obvious advantage to surgical removal of the prostate is the amount of staging information obtained. Careful pathological examination of the specimen after surgery can accurately assess margin status, seminal vesicle invasion, and lymph node involvement, all of which can provide important prognostic information. Often this evaluation reveals more extensive disease than had been anticipated preoperatively.

Identification of capsular penetration or seminal vesicle or lymph node involvement raises the question of the need for additional therapy. For patients with positive surgical margins, some advocate radiation to the surgical bed after the patient regains continence. Although patients with positive margins are at increased risk for disease recurrence, it is not known whether adjuvant radiation therapy will decrease the chance of relapse. This question is the focus of an ongoing national study. Although adjuvant radiation therapy is well tolerated, it increases the risk of impotency in men who previously have undergone a nerve-sparing procedure. In addition, positive margins could indicate an increased potential for systemic micrometastatic disease, in which case prostatic bed irradiation would at best only improve local disease control. Adjuvant androgen-ablative therapy might be useful for patients with positive margins or lymph node involvement, but it has not been rigorously evaluated in this setting. Because of the large number of prostatectomies in early-stage disease, positive lymph nodes are detected in less than 10% of radical prostatectomy patients. With minimal apparent disease, many surgeons no longer routinely remove lymph nodes as part of the operation.

External Beam Radiation Therapy

Primary radiation therapy options for localized prostate cancer include both external beam radiation therapy and brachytherapy. Both modalities have been given with and without neoadjuvant hormonal therapy. Although external beam radiation therapy has not been compared directly with radical prostatectomy in a large randomized study, radiation therapy has been accepted widely as an alternative to surgery in both low- and high-risk patients.

Significant improvement in computer technology has allowed better imaging and radiation treatment planning and has minimized the toxicity to normal surrounding tissues, while maximizing dose delivery to cancerous areas. The technique of external beam radiation therapy has evolved to the current standard 3D-conformal approach. Computer-aided planning allows anatomical definition of the prostate and delivery of a prescribed dose of radiation to the target

Table 87-5 ■ Freedom from PSA Relapse after External Beam Radiation Therapy

Group	Five-Year PSA Relapse Free
PSA <9.2	81%
PSA >9.2 and <19.7	69%
PSA >19.7 and Gleason 2–6	47%
PSA >19.7 and Gleason 7–10	29%

tissue in a three-dimensional configuration. Intensity-modulated radiation therapy is a further enhancement that might allow even more focused radiation effect on the tumor.

Radiation therapy is generally given in daily fractions of 1.8 to 2.0 Gy, five days a week, with a variable duration of therapy depending on the cumulative dose. Typically, the total dose delivered ranges from 65 to 70 Gy given over eight weeks. Treatment is confined to the prostate for those with small tumors and low Gleason scores; however, the seminal vesicles and the pelvic lymph nodes are treated with a "boost" for those at a higher risk of progression. Dose escalation could be important for patients with higher Gleason scores, as some retrospective studies suggest.

Reports of long-term outcome for prostate cancer treated with external beam radiation therapy have been limited largely to single-institution studies. The American Society of Therapeutic Radiology, however, conducted a retrospective multi-institutional analysis of 1765 patients with T1b–T2 prostate cancers who were treated between 1988 and 1995. The five-year overall survival rate was 85%, but freedom from prostate-specific antigen failure was 65%. Four risk groups were identified according to prostate-specific antigen at presentation and Gleason score (Table 87-5).

The addition of hormonal therapy to external beam radiation therapy has been studied in several randomized controlled trials. Androgen ablation leads to reduction in the size of the prostate in those patients with large glands (greater than 50 g), thus minimizing the radiation field and its associated toxicity. Furthermore, radiation therapy has been shown to be synergistic with androgen ablation in preclinical models and could lead to elimination of malignant cells that spread beyond the prostate gland. Androgen ablation is usually accomplished with the use of luteinizing hormone-releasing hormone (LHRH) agonists, with or without an antiandrogen. Androgen ablation is often given prior to, during, and after radiation therapy.

One study randomly assigned 415 patients, the majority of whom had stage T3 or higher tumors, to external beam radiation plus or minus androgen ablation for three years. The Kaplan-Meyer estimate of the five-year overall survival was significantly higher for the combined modality (79% versus 62% respectively). The disease-free survival rate was also significantly higher for the combined arm (85% versus 48% respectively). A second study conducted by the Radiation Oncology Therapy Group (RTOG) showed improved disease-free survival for the combination therapy, but no difference in overall survival at five years.

The ability to better define the anatomic borders around the prostate and the shielding of normal tissue reduced radiation toxicity. The acute effects are generally limited to effects on nearby bladder and rectal tissues. As many as 37% of patients experience irritative urinary symptoms such as urinary frequency and dysuria. Symptoms of rectal urgency can occur in 15% of patients during radiation therapy. Chronic effects include proctitis and hematochezia. Severe gastrointestinal toxicity requiring temporary colostomy is rare. The development of impotence is gradual and progressive. As many as 30% to 60% of patients are impotent five years following radiation therapy.

Brachytherapy

Brachytherapy—the implantation of radiation seeds into the prostate gland—was initially performed in the early 1980s. The efficacy of this approach was limited by the poor imaging modalities and relatively poor dosimetry. Advances in computed tomography and magnetic resonance imaging over the last decade have led to evaluation of brachytherapy as a primary therapy for patients with localized prostate cancer.

Seeds can be either Iodine-125 or Pallidium-103. They are now implanted using a transperineal rather than a retropubic approach. The procedure is often performed in an outpatient setting under either spinal or general anesthesia. Retrospective analysis has suggested that the optimal candidates for brachytherapy are patients with stage T1, Gleason score 6 or less, and prostate-specific antigen less than 10 ng/mL. Relative contraindications to brachytherapy include a prostate gland larger than 60 g, a high American Urological Association (AUA) symptom score (measuring the degree of urinary outlet obstruction), and prior pelvic radiotherapy.

Modern-day series of brachytherapy have relatively short follow-up; hence, prostate-specific antigen failure rather than overall or disease-free survival has usually been reported. Most of the published series quote five-year prostate-specific antigen-free recurrence rates of 63% to 84%, because 10-year data are not yet available. Although these rates appear similar to those of surgery and radiation therapy, no randomized studies compare brachytherapy to either radical prostatectomy or external beam radiation therapy.

Complications of brachytherapy are similar to those seen with surgery and external beam radiation therapy. Bladder toxicity includes irritative symptoms, and as many as 40% of patients experience frequency and nocturia requiring medication. Fewer than 5% of patients develop chronic urinary strictures that necessitate dilatation. A "urethral" sparing approach, which preferentially avoids radiation delivery to the central urethral area, might decrease urinary side effects. The incidence of rectal toxicity is lower than that of external beam radiation therapy, with reported rates of proctitis of only 10%. Potency rates have not been studied prospectively but appear to be about 80% in retrospective series.

Brachytherapy can be combined with external beam radiation therapy and hormonal therapy. The addition of brachytherapy to external beam therapy allows the dose of external beam radiation to be reduced significantly, which generally results in better overall treatment tolerance. Neoadjuvant hormonal therapy can reduce the size of the prostate gland, thus improving implant dosimetry, but its value remains uncertain.

Watchful Waiting

For some newly diagnosed patients with prostate cancer, the "watchful-waiting" or "expectant management" approach could be appropriate. This strategy is based on the supposition that for selected patients, primary intervention will adversely affect quality of life and is unlikely to prolong their life spans. Elderly patients, or those with comorbid illnesses who have slowly progressive disease, might benefit from a "watchful-waiting" approach, the assumption being that the chance of problems related to the prostate cancer is likely to be lower than that from other causes. The efficacy of the watchful-waiting strategy is difficult to assess, because studies have not had uniform inclusion criteria and have not been randomized. In practice, patients managed with watchful waiting will often receive some form of therapy (e.g., hormonal therapy), causing some investigators to label this strategy as "deferred" treatment.

To date, several series have been published describing men who chose the watchful-waiting approach. Although these series are often descriptive reports rather than prospective randomized studies, information can be gleaned from this literature that could aid patients facing treatment decisions. Johannson et al followed 223 patients with T0 to T2 disease who did not have any form of primary therapy. With a mean follow-up of approximately ten years, the disease-specific survival was 86.8%. This survival rate is similar to that observed with surgery or radiation therapy. It is important that this study included only patients with well-differentiated prostate cancer. It has also been criticized because it only randomized patients to watchful waiting vs. radiation therapy if they were less than 75 years old, but men over 75 were included in the analysis, even though they were managed routinely by watchful waiting. An analysis of 536 patients from Sweden by Aus et al found younger age to be the strongest predictor of dying from disease in a population of men with well-differentiated or low-stage tumors treated with a non-curative approach. Overall, the investigators determined that prostate cancer contributed to the death of 62% of the men in this study; however, 25% of men over age 85 at diagnosis died from prostate cancer, whereas 100% of men diagnosed at less than 55 year died from prostate cancer. Albertsen et al also assessed the effect of the patient's age at diagnosis in a competing risk analysis of men in the Connecticut Tumor Registry, ages 55 to 74 years, who were managed conservatively. This analysis compared deaths from prostate cancer to deaths from other causes and stratified the results according to age and Gleason score. Patients with tumor Gleason scores of 7 or greater had a higher mortality rate from prostate cancer even when diagnosed between 70 and 74 years old. Conversely, men who had lower Gleason scores had a greater chance of dying from other causes. Surprisingly, even men with moderately differentiated disease (Gleason grade 6) had a 30% risk of dying from prostate cancer when diagnosed between age 70 and 74 years.

Along with Gleason grade, tumor stage is also an important factor in predicting the natural history for patients considering watchful waiting. Aus et al determined that only 10% of men with T1a disease succumbed to prostate cancer, although 47% of men with T1b and 52% of those with T2 died from prostate cancer. Taken together, these studies suggest that as the age at diagnosis increases, the chance of dying from causes other than prostate cancer also increases, especially for patients with lower-grade or -stage disease. For many elderly patients, the decision to choose watchful waiting might be very obvious. Patients with low-grade disease who are physiologically over 75 years are unlikely to benefit from primary therapy. In contrast, for men with higher-grade or -stage disease, primary therapy could be appropriate, even for those older than 75 years at diagnosis.

Hormonal Therapy

Despite primary therapy, many patients will relapse with prostate cancer, first with rising prostate-specific antigen levels alone and ultimately with clinically apparent metastatic disease. Patients who are symptomatic from metastasis and who have not received some form of hormonal therapy are candidates for this intervention. This section discusses the methods and mechanisms of androgen depletion.

Androgen-Ablative and Anti-Androgen Therapies

Both normal and malignant prostate epithelial cells are affected by androgens such as dihydro-testosterone and testosterone. In 1877, Hunter described the effect of orchiectomy on prostate growth in prepubertal rats. In 1941, Huggins and Hodges demonstrated that symptomatic prostate cancer could be ameliorated by treatment with orchiectomy or diethylstilbestrol. Schalley and others investigating the hypothalamic-pituitary gonadal axis discovered luteinizing hormone-releasing hormone. These efforts led to the development of the luteinizing hormone-releasing hormone agonists now commonly used in treating prostate cancer. Orchiectomy, diethylstilbestrol (DES), and luteinizing hormone-releasing hormone agonists all mediate antiprostate effects by the same mechanism of dramatically decreasing serum testosterone levels.

A majority of patients with metastatic prostate cancer respond to androgen-deprivation therapy. Most studies of androgen deprivation demonstrate objective response rates of 50% to 70% and even higher subjective response rates. Because bone is often the only site of metastasis, it is difficult to objectively quantify tumor response, as changes in bone scan are extremely slow to occur. Although about 15% of patients have sites of measurable soft-tissue disease, these sites are often involved either late in the course or in patients with an uncommon and more aggressive form of disease, so it is difficult to extrapolate the response rate of hormonal therapy from this subset of patients. Patients who have bulky adenopathy or visceral disease in the absence of bone metastasis frequently have a neuroendocrine histology. These patients often demonstrate increases in carcino-embryonic antigen levels rather than prostate-specific antigen levels with progression, and they are less responsive to hormonal therapy.

The problem of objectively quantifying therapeutic response has been mitigated by utilizing sequential prostate-specific antigen measurements as a surrogate marker for response. In most (but not all) cases, reductions in prostate-specific antigen have been shown to correspond to objective responses. Improvement in symptoms typically also correlates with prostate-specific antigen decline. However, it is conceivable that prostate-specific antigen measurements might reflect a measure of the androgen status of the cell, rather than strictly a measure of tumor burden. This is because prostate-specific antigen expression is triggered by binding of the activated (androgen-bound) androgen receptor to upstream regulatory DNA sequences.

Unlike breast cancer, in which estrogen and receptor levels are routinely measured from tumor tissue, it is not standard practice to measure androgen receptor levels in prostate cancer tissue. This is because androgen-ablative therapy has a high overall response rate and because tumor specimens uniformly demonstrate substantial levels of androgen receptor expression.

Independent of the method of achieving androgen ablation, therapy usually results in an approximately 12- to 18-month duration of response for patients with stage D2 (distant metastasis) disease. Because all androgen-ablative therapies induce prostatic cancer regression by the same mechanism, they result in equivalent response rates and duration of response.

Methods of Androgen Deprivation

Diethylstilbestrol therapy inhibits the release of luteinizing hormone-releasing hormone from the hypothalamus, which in turn inhibits the release of luteinizing hormone (LH). At a dose of 1 mg orally daily, it was shown to be as effective clinically as other approaches to androgen ablation. Diethylstilbestrol is no longer used because of its significant side effects. It causes fluid retention and painful gynecomastia if not preceded by a short course of prophylactic irradiation to the chest wall. Moreover, the risk of thromboembolic disease is increased. Bilateral orchiectomy is perhaps the most efficient method of decreasing testosterone, resulting in the almost immediate reduction of 90% of circulating androgens. Its disadvantage is that it is irreversible and requires a surgical procedure.

Luteinizing hormone-releasing hormone analogs, such as goserlin acetate and leuprolide, have minor amino acid substitutions compared with native luteinizing hormone-releasing hormone. These substitutions result in decreased enzymatic degradation, increased receptor-binding affinity, and slower plasma clearance. Under normal conditions, the pituitary is stimulated to release luteinizing hormone only by pulsatile exposure to native luteinizing hormone-releasing hormone. The longer serum half-life of luteinizing hormone-releasing hormone and its analogs down-modulates the receptor in the pituitary, resulting in decreased release of luteinizing hormone. Because luteinizing hormone-releasing hormone analogs so closely resemble the native peptide, immediately after the initial injection there is stimulation of

luteinizing hormone secretion, resulting in a short period of higher-than-normal levels of testosterone. The increase in testosterone can be detected in most patients receiving their first luteinizing hormone-releasing hormone analog injection, but it lasts only for the first week of therapy. Although testosterone levels can increase by as much as 50% over baseline, tumor flares during this period are very uncommon unless patients have symptomatic disease at the initiation of therapy. The flare reaction can manifest as increased bone pain, increased propensity to deep-vein thrombosis, or even cord compression in patients with significant spinal column disease. Flares induced by analogs of luteinizing hormone-releasing hormone can be ameliorated by the use of an oral antiandrogen.

The main advantages of luteinizing hormone-releasing hormone agonists over surgery are the psychological benefit of not having to undergo orchiectomy and the potential reversibility of their effects. After discontinuing the analogs, however, recovery of the hypothalamic-pituitary-gonadal axis and secretion of testosterone can take months. In some men treated with luteinizing hormone-releasing hormone analogs for years, appreciable serum testosterone levels might never be achieved even after discontinuation of the analog, although for the treatment of metastatic disease, reversibility is not usually an issue. Furthermore, discontinuing luteinizing hormone-releasing hormone analog therapy may be ill-advised even in patients with documented androgen-independent disease, as renewed testosterone production can accelerate disease progression. The cost of luteinizing hormone-releasing hormone analogs is also an issue, especially considering the long duration of treatment. Fortunately, treatment has become more convenient. Injections can now be given every three or four months as depot preparations.

The final means of interrupting the stimulatory effects of testosterone on prostate cancer cells is to block the androgen receptor on these cells directly with oral nonsteroidal antiandrogens (flutamide, bicalutamide, nilutamide). Antiandrogens can be used as monotherapy, but at conventional doses they have been shown to be inferior to androgen ablation. Antiandrogens have also been used as part of maximum androgen blockade, in which they are combined with either orchiectomy or a luteinizing hormone-releasing hormone analog. Although the combination achieves maximal androgen blockade, no significant survival benefit occurs in comparison with the use of luteinizing hormone-releasing hormone analogs.

Recently, there has been a greater appreciation of the long-term effects of androgen-ablative therapy. In addition to loss of libido and hot flashes, fatigue is also commonly reported. Bone loss and decreased muscle mass can also be significant. An association between androgen-ablative therapy and subtle decreases in cognition has also been reported.

The Timing of Hormonal Therapy

Androgen-ablative therapy is recommended for patients with symptomatic metastatic disease and results in significant palliation in this population. It is uncertain, however, whether any benefit is derived by beginning androgen-ablative therapy in patients with only biochemical (prostate-specific antigen) recurrence or even in patients with asymptomatic metastatic disease. In a study of surgically treated patients followed for a median of 5.3 years, the median time from first detectable prostate-specific antigen elevation to development of clinical metastasis (without early hormonal therapy) was eight years. This study also demonstrated that a prostate-specific antigen doubling time of greater than 10 months or the detection of first measurable prostate-specific antigen levels more than two years after surgery were predictive of a better outcome. Therefore, older patients with relatively long prostate-specific antigen doubling times are less likely to benefit from early hormonal therapy.

What therapy should be instituted for younger men with prostate-specific antigen values that exhibit rapid doubling? If hormonal intervention can improve survival or dramatically delay the onset of clinical disease, its benefits might outweigh its side effects. A randomized trial performed by the British Medical Research Council demonstrated decreases in both morbidity and mortality for patients treated with early hormonal therapy prior to the onset of clinical metastasis. This trial was performed prior to prostate-specific antigen testing, making it difficult to extrapolate its finding for the typical D0 patient. The effects of immediate hormonal therapy vs. observation have also been studied in men with lymph node disease detected at the time of prostatectomy. Patients treated with immediate hormonal therapy demonstrated an improved survival. These studies have methodological limitations, but they suggest that treatment of minimal disease with androgen-ablative therapy could result in improved survival. The decision to treat individual patients with long-term androgen-ablative therapy in this setting must take into account the potential short- and long-term side effects of such therapy and its impact on the quality of life.

Adjuvant and Neoadjuvant Therapy

A contemporary trend in the management of prostate cancer has been to institute neoadjuvant hormonal therapy prior to either radiation therapy or prostatectomy for patients at risk for capsular invasion. Although this strategy decreases the rate of positive tumor margins in patients undergoing prostatectomy, survival does not improve. In contrast, androgen ablation combined with external beam radiation therapy appears to improve local and prostate-specific antigen control and could result in a relapse-free and overall survival advantage. A randomized trial that included mostly T3 patients demonstrated that three years of hormonal therapy combined with radiation led to an improvement in overall survival compared with radiation therapy alone. Overall, however, the optimal neoadjuvant regimen and duration of therapy have not been established. This approach, particularly when combined with surgery, should be reserved for clinical trials.

Intermittent Androgen Suppression

An emerging approach to androgen-ablative therapy is the use of intermittent androgen suppression. It has been postulated that constant low levels of androgen might contribute to the selection of androgen-independent tumor clones. Therefore, intermittent androgen exposure might delay the establishment of androgen-independent disease. Another advantage for intermittent androgen suppression is a reduction in some of the long-term effects of androgen ablation, such as bone loss. Intermittent therapy is accomplished by treating patients with a luteinizing hormone-releasing hormone agonist until the prostate-specific antigen level reaches its nadir, and then discontinuing the agent until prostate-specific antigen rises to an arbitrary level (typically between 10 to 20 ng/mL).

Androgen-Independent Prostate Cancer

Clinical Aspects

Androgen-independent prostate cancer (AIPC) is generally defined as either clinical or biochemical (increase in serum prostate-specific antigen) progression in the setting of serum testosterone levels within the castrate range. In patients receiving luteinizing hormone-releasing hormone analogs, serum testosterone levels will usually not be above eunuchoid levels unless there is a history of noncompliance. Many investigators also refer to this stage of prostate cancer as hormone-refractory disease, despite the fact that secondary hormonal maneuvers can sometimes be useful. Until this issue is answered with a prospective study, continuing androgen suppression for patients on luteinizing hormone-releasing hormone agonists is generally recommended.

The Biology of Androgen-Independent Prostate Cancer

Development of novel treatments and more effective combinations of established agents depends on an improved understanding of prostate tumor biology. The mechanisms responsible for the development of androgen-independent prostate cancer are unknown, but are likely complex and heterogenous.

The androgen receptor has a central role in hormone homeostasis in the prostate. The majority of tumor specimens derived from androgen-independent patients continue to express the androgen receptor, so that down-regulation is not a primary mechanism of escape from androgen ablation. In contrast, it appears that the androgen receptor gene is amplified in as many of 30% of androgen-independent specimens. Importantly, androgen-receptor amplification is not observed in untreated primary tumors, and androgen receptor-regulated genes (e.g., prostate-specific antigen) continued to be expressed in androgen-independent prostate cancer.

Another possible mechanism of androgen-independent prostate cancer is structural alteration in the androgen receptor gene. Point mutations in the androgen receptor gene, although uncommon in early-stage hormone-sensitive cancers, have been detected in androgen-independent prostate cancer. Some of these mutations alter the receptor's functional properties to the extent that normally non-physiologic ligands (e.g., estrogen, progesterone, and the antiandrogen flutamide) become stimulators of mutant androgen receptors. Despite these findings, finding means to inactivate the androgen receptor pathway might not be effective in androgen-independent prostate cancer. Other genetic changes are associated with advanced disease. For instance, the tumor suppressor gene, PTEN, appears to be lost in 70% of patients with advanced prostate cancer. This gene regulates important signal transduction pathways in the cell, and its loss could contribute to alterations in proliferation and cell death. The HER2/neu gene also has been demonstrated to be overexpressed in many patients with androgen-independent prostate cancer. Expression of this gene in vitro has been shown to result in the androgen-independent phenotype.

Secondary Hormonal Manipulations

The provision of additional hormonal therapy appears at first to be paradoxical if the disease has become androgen independent. In fact, a minority of patients on long-term antiandrogens in combination with luteinizing hormone-releasing hormone agonists have been shown to experience a decline in prostate-specific antigen—sometimes accompanied by improvement in clinical symptoms—when the antiandrogen was discontinued. Studies including both steroidal and nonsteroidal antiandrogens have demonstrated that 20% to 25% of these patients experienced a tumor response to an "antiandrogen withdrawal." Molecular analysis of the androgen receptors from patient samples reveal that some of these patients have point mutations in the androgen receptor that resulted in stimulation (rather than inhibition) from flutamide and other antiandrogens.

Megestrol acetate, ketoconazole, and the herbal compound PC-SPES can produce declines in prostate-specific antigen in some patients with androgen-independent prostate cancer. PC-SPES consists of eight different herbs and has estrogen-like effects, including suppression of testosterone production. It has significant activity in patients with androgen-independent disease. Similar to diethylstilbestrol, PC-SPES increases the thromboembolic risk and could warrant concomitant anticoagulant prophylaxis.

Chemotherapy

Prostate cancer has been considered unresponsive to chemotherapeutic agents, because single-agent chemotherapeutic trials revealed response rates of less than 10%. Responses can be difficult to assess in the majority of patients because most prostate cancer metastases are immeasurable bone lesions. Retrospective analyses of chemotherapeutic trials indicated a survival benefit for patients who experience declines of prostate-specific antigen greater than 50%. Consequently, an NIH-sponsored working group recently recommended that a prostate-specific antigen decline of greater than 50% be used as an endpoint in evaluating clinical benefit in chemotherapeutic trials.

The combination of mitoxantrone and prednisone was approved by the U.S. FDA based on a randomized phase III study conducted by Tannock et al (Table 87-6). The primary endpoint of the study was quality of life rather than prostate-specific antigen decline or objective response. Improved quality of life (including palliation of pain) was seen in 29% of patients receiving combined therapy compared with 12% in patients receiving prednisone alone. The combined regimen was extremely well tolerated with minimal cardiac and bone marrow toxicity.

Estramustine, another FDA-approved drug for the treatment of prostate cancer, is a conjugate of nitrogen mustard and estradiol. The drug acts by binding to the nuclear matrix and to microtubular-binding proteins. Preclinical experiments have suggested synergistic interaction with other microtubular inhibitors. Given the potent activity of both docetaxel and paclitaxel on microtubule stabilization, both have

Table 87-6 ■ Contemporary Chemotherapeutic Regimens for Metastatic Prostate Cancer

Study	Year	Regimen	Number of Patients	>50% Decline in PSA	Response in Measurable Disease
Tannock	1996	Mitoxantrone + prednisone	161	33%	NR
Kantoff	1999	Mitoxantrone + hydrocortisone	242	38%	7%
Petrylak	1999	Taxotere + estramustine	34	64%	18%
Picus	1999	Taxotere	35	71%	28%
Hudes	1997	Taxol + estramustine	23	65%	57%
Smith	1999	Taxol + estramustine + etoposide	37	70%	45%
Kelly	1998	Taxol + estramustine + carboplatin	56	63%	45%
Hudes	1999	Vinblastine + oral etoposide	201	25%	20%

NR = not reported
Taxotere = docetaxel; Taxol = paclitaxel

been explored recently in combination with estramustine (see Table 87-6).

Thromboembolic events are being reported with the estramustine-based regimens and could be as high as 10% without anticoagulant prophylaxis. Although taxanes are not known to be thrombogenic, the incidence of thromboembolic events appears to be somewhat higher with the combination of taxanes and estramustine. To decrease the incidence of both arterial and venous thrombosis, low-dose warfarin and acetylsalicilic acid is often recommended. The efficacy and safety of this prophylactic strategy remains to be demonstrated.

Radiation Therapy for Metastatic Disease

Painful bony metastases are often the major source of symptoms for patients with metastatic prostate cancer. Unlike many other cancers, prostate cancer produces predominantly osteoblastic metastases that do not significantly weaken bones, so pathologic fractures are not common. External radiation therapy to areas of painful metastasis is an effective means of palliation. Unfortunately, retreatment of previously irradiated sites is frequently not possible. Moreover, the multiplicity of metastatic sites limits the role of external beam radiation therapy.

An alternative approach uses radionucleotides, chelated radioactive elemental complexes which, when given intraveneously, home in on areas of intense osteoblastic activity. Strontium-89 was approved by the FDA in 1994 based on studies that demonstrated palliation of pain in up to 75% of patients. Pain relief is often described within three to four weeks after treatment, but early flare can be seen in a minority of patients. Complications include myelosuppression—especially thrombocy-

topenia, which is usually reversible. If clinical benefit is observed but the symptoms recur, repeat treatment can be administered 12 to 14 weeks after the initial injection, provided that the myelosuppression has resolved. Samarium-153, an agent that has a lower energy particle emission than strontium, is also approved for use in palliation of painful bone metastases.

References

Delayed Therapy

Adolfsson J, Steineck G, Hedlund PO: Deferred treatment of clinically localized low-grade prostate cancer: Actual 10-year and projected 15-year follow-up of the Karolinska series. Urology 1997;50:722–726.

Albertsen PC: Early-stage prostate cancer. When is observation appropriate? Hematol-Oncol Clin N Am 1996;10:611–625.

Anonymous: Immediate versus deferred treatment for advanced prostatic cancer: Initial results of the medical research council trial. The Medical Research Council Prostate Cancer Working Party Investigators Group. Br J Urol 1997;79:235–246.

Brasso K, Friis S, Juel K, et al: Mortality of patients with clinically localized prostate cancer treated with observation for 10 years or longer: A population based registry study. J Urol 1999;161:524–528.

General Information

Albertsen P, Hanley J, Harlan L, et al: The positive yield of imaging studies in the evaluation of men with newly diagnosed prostate cancer: A population-based analysis. J Urol 2000;63:1138–1145.

Kupelian P, Kupelian V, Witte J, et al: Family history of prostate cancer in patients with localized prostate cancer: An independent predictor of treatment outcome. J Clin Oncol 1997;15:1478–1480.

Hormonally-Dependent Prostate Cancer

Bolla M, Gonzalez D, Warde P, et al: Improved survival in patients with locally advanced prostate cancer treated with radiotherapy and goserlin. N Engl J Med 1997;337: 295.

Caubet JF, Tosteson, T, Dong E, et al: Maximum androgen block-ade in advanced prostate cancer: A meta-analysis of pub-lished randomized controlled trials using nonsteroidal antiandrogens. Urol 1997;49:71–78.

Crawford E, Eisenberger M, McLeod D: Controlled trial of leuprolide with and without flutamide in prostatic carci-noma. N Engl J Med 1989;321:419.

Kelly WK, Sher HI: Prostate specific antigen decline after antian-drogen withdrawal: The flutamide withdrawal syndrome. J Urol 1993;149:607–609.

Hormonally-Independent Prostate Cancer

Bubley G, Carducci M, Dahut W, et al: Eligibility and response guidelines for phase II clinical trials in androgen-independent prostate cancer: Recommendations from the Prostate-Specific Antigen Working Group. J Clin Oncol 1999;17:3461–3467.

Bubley G, Balk S: Treatment of androgen-independent prostate cancer. Oncologist 1996;1:1–6.

Fenton M, Fertig A, Kolvenbag G, et al: Functional characteri-zation of mutant androgen receptors from androgen-independent prostate cancer. Clin Cancer Res 1977;3: 1383–1388.

Hudes G, Einhorn L, Ross E, et al: Vinblastine versus vinblas-tine plus oral estramustine phosphate for patients with hormone-refractory prostate cancer: A Hoosier Oncology Group and Fox Chase Network phase III trial. J Clin Oncol 1999;17:3160–3166.

Kantoff P, Halabi S, Conaway M, et al: Hydrocortisone with or without mitoxantrone in men with hormone-refractory prostate cancer: Results of the cancer and leukemia group B 9182 study. J Clin Oncol 1999;17:2506–2513.

Petrylak DP, Macarthur RB, O'Connor J, et al: Phase 1 trial of docetaxel with estramustine in androgen-independent prostate cancer. J Clin Oncol 1999;17:958–967.

Picus J, Schultz M: Docetaxel (Taxotere) as monotherapy in the treatment of hormone-refractory prostate cancer: Prelimi-nary results. Semin Oncol 1999;26(5 Suppl 17):14–18.

Small E, Frohlich M, Bok R, et al: Prospective trial of the herbal supplement PC-SPES in patients with progressive prostate cancer. J Clin Oncol 2000;18:3595–3603.

Smith DC, Esper P, Strawderman M, et al: Phase II trial of oral estramustine, oral etoposide, and intravenous paclitaxel in hormone-refractory prostate cancer. J Clin Oncol 1999;17: 1664–1671.

Tannock IF, Osoba D, Stockler MR, et al: Chemotherapy with mitoxantrone plus prednisone or prednisone alone for symptomatic hormone-resistant prostate cancer: Canadian randomized trial with palliative end points. J Clin Oncol 1996;14:1756–1764.

Taplin ME, Bubley G, Shuster T, et al: Mutation of the androgen-receptor gene in metastatic androgen-independent prostate cancer. N Engl J Med 1995;332: 1393–1398.

Prognosis

D'Amico AV, Whittington R, Malkowicz SB, et al: Biochemical outcome after radical prostatectomy, external beam radiation therapy, or interstitial radiation therapy for clinically localized prostate cancer. JAMA 1998;280:969–974.

D'Amico AV, Whittington R, Malkowicz SB, et al: Pretreatment nomogram for prostate-specific antigen recurrence after radical prostatectomy or external-beam radiation therapy for clinically localized prostate cancer. J Clin Oncol 1999;17:168–172.

Epstein J, Pizov G, Walsh P: Correlation of pathologic findings with progression after radical retropubic prostatectomy. Cancer 1993;71:3582–3593.

Kattan MW, Eastham JA, Stapleton AME, et al: A preoperative nomogram for disease recurrence following radical prosta-tectomy for prostate cancer. J Natl Cancer Inst 1998;90:766.

Partin AW, Kattan MW, Subong ENP, et al: Combination of prostate-specific antigen, clinical stage, and Gleason score to predict pathological stage of localized prostate cancer: A Multi-institutional update. JAMA 1997;277:1445.

Pound C, Partin A, Eisenberger M, et al: Natural history of progression after PSA elevation following radical pros-tatectomy. JAMA 1999;281:1591–1597.

Screening and Prevention

Candas B, Cusan L, Gomez JL, et al: Evaluation of prostatic spe-cific antigen and digital rectal examination as screening tests for prostate cancer. Prostate 2000;45:19–35.

Catalona W, Smith D, Ratliff T, et al: Measurement of prostate-specific antigen in serum as a screening test for prostate cancer. N Engl J Med 1991;324:1156–1161.

Heinonen OP, Albanes D, Virtamo J, et al: Prostate cancer and supplementation with alpha-tocopherol and beta-carotene: Incidence and mortality in a controlled trial. J Natl Cancer Inst 1998;90:440–446.

Gastrointestinal Cancer

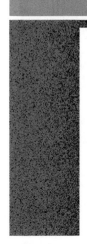

Chapter 88
Esophageal Cancer

David Ilson

Esophageal cancer, an uncommon but highly virulent malignancy in the United States, will be responsible for more than 14,000 deaths in the year 2003. Esophageal cancer represents the seventh leading cause of cancer death in American men, and more than 90% of patients diagnosed with esophageal cancer ultimately will die of their disease.

Epidemiology and Tumorigenesis

The epidemiology of esophageal cancer has changed significantly in the United States and Western Europe over the past 30 years. Adenocarcinoma of the distal esophagus, previously a rare histologic subtype of this cancer, has increased in incidence to a near-epidemic proportion in Western countries. In the mid-1990s, adenocarcinoma overtook squamous cell carcinoma as the predominant histology in the United States. Epidemiologic studies have led to speculation about the potential causes of the rise in incidence of esophageal adenocarcinoma. Barrett's esophagus, the replacement of the squamous epithelium of the esophagus with an intestinal columnar epithelium, is a premalignant precursor of esophageal adenocarcinoma. Given the association of gastroesophageal reflux with the development of Barrett's esophagus, a recent Scandinavian study evaluated chronic esophageal reflux as a potential risk factor for esophageal adenocarcinoma. Depending on the frequency, severity, and years of duration of reflux symptoms in patients on this study, esophageal reflux independently increased the risk of esophageal adenocarcinoma by a factor of 5- to 20-fold. Esophageal reflux appeared to be independent of other lifestyle factors that might predispose

to reflux, including obesity and use of tobacco. Other epidemiologic studies, however, have implicated obesity and tobacco abuse as potential risk factors for the development of esophageal adenocarcinoma. A decline in prevalence of infection by the bacterium *Helicobacter pylori* in Western populations has also been implicated in the increased incidence of esophageal adenocarcinoma. Because infection of the stomach with *Helicobacter pylori* can lead to atrophic gastritis and reduced gastric acidity, some authors have speculated that a decline in *Helicobacter* infection might, paradoxically, increase the development of gastroesophageal reflux disease, and thereby the risk of esophageal adenocarcinoma.

An association between the abuse of tobacco and alcohol and the development of squamous cell carcinoma of the esophagus is generally accepted. Although relatively uncommon in the United States, esophageal squamous cell cancer is a leading worldwide cause of cancer with a particularly high incidence observed in northern China, the Caspian Littoral, and the Transkei province of South Africa. The epidemiologic factors responsible for the geographic variability in incidence of esophageal squamous cancer—including potential dietary factors and environmental carcinogens—remain unclear. In Linxian Province in China, esophageal squamous cancer and gastric cardia cancer are the leading causes of cancer death. In a large nutritional intervention trial conducted in this population, dietary supplementation with selenium, beta carotene, and vitamin E led to a significant 13% reduction in mortality from esophageal and gastric cardia cancer. The study indicated that nutritional deficiencies might play a role in the development of this disease in a poor, rural population and that correcting these deficiencies might have a protective benefit against cancer. A subsequent report from this trial evaluated further the role of selenium deficiency as a potential causative factor for esophageal and gastric cancers in this high-risk population. Patients with the lowest serum selenium levels were found to be at highest risk for developing esophageal squamous and gastric cardia cancer.

Laboratory studies have identified a number of molecular genetic and cytogenetic abnormalities that could lead to the progressive malignant transformation of the esophageal squamous epithelium. These include mutations and loss of heterozygosity of the tumor suppressor gene p53, amplification of the cell cycle regulatory factor cyclin D, and increased expression of the cell surface receptor for epidermal growth factor. In Barrett's esophagus, a sequence of genetic events appears to unfold, leading ultimately to the development of invasive cancer; this sequence includes the acquisition of p53 mutations, the development of aneuploidy, overexpression of cyclin D, and overexpression of the enzyme cyclooxygenase-2 (COX-2). Overexpression of the epidermal growth factor receptor has also been observed in esophageal adenocarcinoma. Pharmacologic agents that target and inhibit these cellular pathways are well into clinical development and evaluation in clinical trials.

Diagnosis and Staging

The typical clinical presentation of esophageal cancer is dysphagia to solid foods, weight loss, and often odynophagia with pain radiating to the epigastrium or back. Because of the lack of screening for this cancer due to its rarity in Western countries, most patients present with an esophageal mass causing mechanical obstruction to swallowing. In consequence, most patients present with locally advanced disease, typically with circumferential or transmural tumor involvement in the majority of patients, and lymph node involvement in more than 50% of patients. Whereas half of patients present with locally advanced disease confined to the chest, the rich vascular and lymphatic supply of the esophagus leads to early systemic dissemination of disease, so that the other half of patients present with extrathoracic metastatic disease at the time of diagnosis. The clinical presentation of patients might also include anemia from blood loss and abnormalities in liver function studies, serum lactate dehydrogenase, or alkaline phosphatase; these findings can be early indicators of visceral or bone metastases in the absence of symptoms of distant metastatic disease.

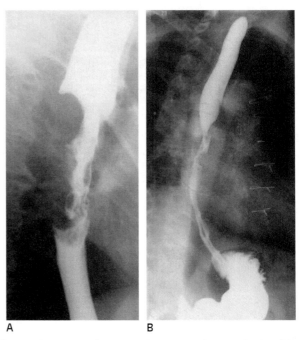

A   B

Figure 88-1 ▪ Barium esophagram of a patient with a midthoracic esophageal squamous cancer. *A,* Esophagram of the patient prior to any therapy. *B,* Esophagram showing a partial response to induction chemotherapy prior to the administration of concurrent chemoradiotherapy.

In addition to upper endoscopy and biopsy, staging of a locally advanced esophageal cancer has included computed tomography (CT) imaging of the chest and abdomen to identify local tumor extent and to assess for metastatic disease. A barium swallow is performed to evaluate local tumor extent within the esophagus. A representative barium esophagram and computed tomography scan image of a patient with a locally advanced squamous esophageal cancer of the midthoracic esophagus are shown in Figures 88-1*A* and 88-2*A*. Given the proximity of the esophagus to the airway, for lesions of the cervical, proximal, or midthoracic esophagus, a bronchoscopy is performed to evaluate for airway invasion by tumor. Endoscopy with ultrasound (EUS) has emerged as a useful local staging technique and appears to be superior to computed tomography for the purpose of determining T stage (depth of tumor penetration into the esophageal wall) and N stage (nodal involvement). A representative endoscopic ultrasound image of a patient with a transmural (T3) and node-positive (N1) gastroesophageal junction cancer is shown in Figure 88-3.

Minimally invasive surgical staging in esophageal cancer—which includes mediastinoscopy and laparoscopy—has also been proposed as preoperative staging. Mediastinoscopy allows sampling and pathologic staging of mediastinal lymph node contents.

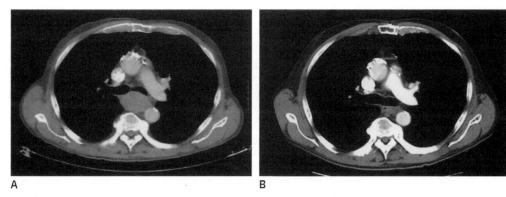

Figure 88-2 ■ Computed tomography scan image of the patient illustrated in Figure 88-1 with a midthoracic esophageal squamous cancer. *A,* Computed tomography scan prior to any therapy showing a midline mass adjacent to the aorta. *B,* Scan after the completion of induction chemotherapy and concurrent chemoradiotherapy. The patient achieved an endoscopic and radiographic complete response to therapy without surgery.

Laparoscopy permits assessment of the peritoneal lining, liver, and celiac lymph nodes for metastatic involvement, which if found would mitigate against therapy with surgery or radiotherapy and would instead direct treatment to palliative chemotherapy. The value of surgical staging over noninvasive radiologic imaging and endoscopic ultrasonography has not yet been determined. Positron emission tomography (PET), which distinguishes tumor tissue from normal tissue by the relatively elevated degree of metabolic activity in tumors, might also be a useful staging technique. Positron emission tomography scanning could have a greater sensitivity for the detection of metastatic disease when conventional imaging studies fail to indicate distant spread of disease, and it also could assist in delineating lymph node disease within the mediastinum and abdomen.

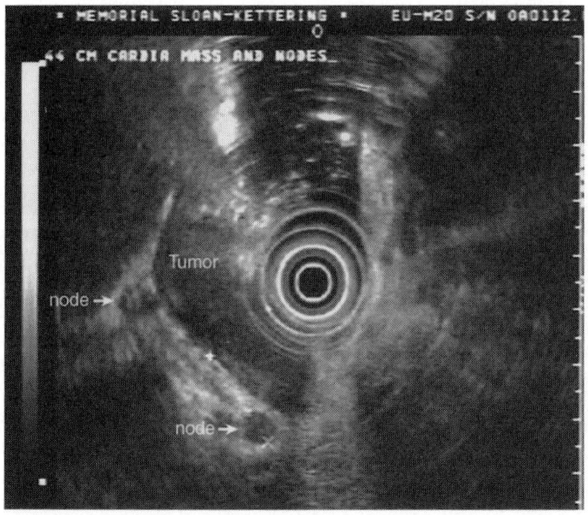

Treatment

Surgery or Radiation Alone

The prognosis for esophageal cancer patients treated with the standard approaches of surgery or radiation therapy is poor. Older retrospective series of patients treated with either surgery alone or radiation therapy alone reported equally poor five-year survivals of 4% to 6%. The operative mortality for surgically treated patients in these older series was as high as 29%. The operative mortality fueled an ongoing debate regarding the relative efficacy of surgery vs. radiation therapy alone for local disease control. More recent surgical series from both single institutions and multicenter cooperative groups, however, have reported surgical mortalities of less than 5% to 10%, and a recent review of the surgical literature reported that 10% of patients achieved a five-year survival. The optimal surgical approach is also debated. Transhiatal esophagectomy avoids thoracotomy by mobilizing the esophagus and stomach and dissecting the mediastinal lymph nodes via abdominal and neck incisions. A combined thoracoabdominal approach with an open thoracotomy is advocated by some surgeons to achieve direct exposure of mediastinal lymph nodes. Other surgeons perform a more radical or *en bloc* resection of mediastinal contents, or an even more extensive resection of lymph nodes beyond the mediastinum to include abdominal and cervical lymph nodes. Regardless of the surgical approach employed to control local disease, ultimately the majority of patients treated with either surgery or

Figure 88-3 ■ Endoscopic ultrasound image of a patient with a transmural (T3) and node-positive (N1) adenocarcinoma of the gastroesophageal junction.

radiation therapy alone are destined to die of their disease.

Surgery or radiation therapy in patients with disease clinically limited to the local-regional area prior to treatment, fails to cure because of locoregional failure and early systemic dissemination of disease. Autopsy series bear out the frequent systemic nature of esophageal squamous cell carcinoma, even at the time of or shortly after initial presentation. Despite the brief duration of illness in patients, the majority were found at autopsy to have evidence of distant metastatic disease whether or not residual local disease was present. Adenocarcinoma of the distal esophagus or gastroesophageal junction appears to have a natural history of disease similar to squamous cell esophageal carcinoma, with equally poor survival after surgical therapy due to a combination of local and systemic disease recurrence. The need to address the problem of early spread of esophageal carcinoma with systemic treatment led to the development of combined modality therapy, which incorporates chemotherapy into surgery- and radiotherapy-based treatment programs. Because one-half of patients diagnosed with esophageal cancer present with overt metastatic disease, chemotherapy is the mainstay of palliation in this setting.

Chemotherapy

The antitumor activity for selected single-agent and combination chemotherapy in esophageal carcinoma is summarized in Table 88-1. Older single agents effective in this disease include cisplatin, 5-fluorouracil, and mitomycin. Paclitaxel has shown favorable results as a single agent in both disease histologies. One-hour weekly paclitaxel, a schedule with little toxicity, could also have activity as a single agent. Irinotecan also appears to be an effective new agent in adenocarcinoma. Modest antitumor activity for a broad range of chemotherapy drugs is seen in esophageal carcinoma, but the duration of response to single-agent chemotherapy is generally brief (four to six months).

Cisplatin has been the cornerstone of combination chemotherapy in esophageal cancer. As a single agent, cisplatin has a response rate of 20% to 30%. Carboplatin, by contrast, has been disappointing, showing a less than 10% response rate in both squamous cell carcinoma and adenocarcinoma. Oxaliplatin is a promising new platinum analog with activity in colorectal cancer, but its efficacy in esophageal cancer has not yet been determined.

Virtually all combination chemotherapy regimens share cisplatin as a common agent. Cisplatin-based combination chemotherapy demonstrates antitumor activity in metastatic squamous cell carcinoma of the

Table 88-1 ■ Single-Agent and Combination Chemotherapy in Esophageal Cancer

	Histology	Patients	Response
Single Agents			
Bleomycin	S	80	15%
Mitomycin	S	58	26%
Fluorouracil	S	26	15%
Cisplatin	S	152	28%
Cisplatin	A	12	8%
Vindesine	S	86	22%
Vinorelbine	S	30	20%
Paclitaxel	S	18	28%
Paclitaxel	A	32	34%
Combination Chemotherapy			
Cisplatin, bleomycin	S	27	17%
Cisplatin, vindesine, bleomycin	S	47	32%
Cisplatin, vinblastine, bleomycin	S	51	29%
Cisplatin, 5-fluorouracil	S	69	35%
Cisplatin, etoposide	S + A	92	48%
Cisplatin, 5-fluorouracil, paclitaxel	S + A	50	45%
Cisplatin, paclitaxel	S + A	32	44%
Cisplatin, irinotecan	S + A	35	57%

S = squamous cell carcinoma, A = adenocarcinoma

esophagus in some 25% to 35% of cases. The response proportion observed in locoregional disease has been consistently higher, on the order of 45% to 75%. Unfortunately, the higher response rates achieved with cisplatin-combinations have not translated into significantly improved response durations or improved survival. In this primarily palliative setting, the potentially greater response rate of combination chemotherapy must be balanced against a frequently higher toxicity and an increasingly complex and time-consuming schedule. Toxicity observed for the combination of cisplatin and 5-fluorouracil, mainly mucositis and myelosuppression, has been substantial but tolerable. Recent trials, employing a more protracted infusion of low-dose 5-fluorouracil in combination with epirubicin and cisplatin, indicated a potential response and survival advantage when compared with a bolus 5-fluorouracil, doxorubicin, and methotrexate regimen. In most other trials, however, the addition of agents such as leucovorin, doxorubicin, and etoposide to 5-fluorouracil and cisplatin has not shown a clear improvement over 5-fluorouracil and cisplatin alone. Combinations of the newer agents— paclitaxel and irinotecan—with cisplatin and with or without 5-fluorouracil, also have resulted in encouraging response rates in phase II trials, but a comparison with the conventional standard chemotherapy of cisplatin and 5-fluorouracil in a phase III trial has not been done. Generally, it appears that adenocarcinoma and squamous cell carcinoma have overlapping response rates to combination chemotherapy, similar to the experience with non–small cell lung cancer.

Palliation

Most chemotherapy trials in metastatic esophageal cancer report on the response rate of single-agent or combination therapy. Secondary endpoints in these trials include median patient survival and toxicity of therapy. Few studies, until recently, have reported on either the symptom palliation or the quality of life achieved in these trials. Recent studies, however, have included symptomatic relief in response assessment, and increasingly, quality-of-life measures are being included in patient assessment on palliative chemotherapy programs. Recent chemotherapy trials have reported significant palliation of patient dysphagia with chemotherapy alone in up to 80% to 90% of patients treated. Dysphagia relief reported in these trials correlated with antitumor response rates ranging from 40% to 50%, and dysphagia relief was often immediate within the course of an initial treatment cycle of chemotherapy. A representative barium swallow of a patient with locally advanced esophageal cancer treated with chemotherapy is shown in Figure 88-1A. After treatment with an induction chemotherapy regimen, the patient had a partial response to therapy (Figure 88-1B) and complete resolution of dysphagia. Given the often substantial toxicity of combination chemotherapy used to palliate metastatic disease, symptom relief and quality-of-life assessment of patients will play an increasing role in the future assessment of the clinical benefit of systemic chemotherapy programs.

In addition to the use of chemotherapy, a number of alternatives exist for the palliation of dysphagia in advanced esophageal cancer. These include endoscopic dilatation of the primary tumor, endoscopic laser ablation of the tumor, or the endoscopic application of photodynamic therapy in conjunction with a systemically administered photosensitizer. The esophagus also can be intubated with a prosthesis. Recent studies favor the use of expansile metal esophageal stents over older plastic prostheses. Endoscopic placement of gastric or jejunal feeding tubes is also a consideration in patients who are unable to maintain oral alimentation or hydration.

Palliative external beam radiation therapy, or endoluminal brachytherapy, has also been used to palliate dysphagia, but these measures generally do not achieve the immediate relief of dysphagia that endoscopic palliation provides. Combined concurrent chemoradiotherapy, usually used in locally advanced disease as a definitive local therapy or as presurgical therapy, might also palliate patient dysphagia significantly. In the setting of metastatic disease, however, concurrent chemoradiotherapy purely for palliation of dysphagia is not often used, given the generally short patient life span and the added complexity, cost, and morbidity of therapy.

Neoadjuvant Therapy

Clinical trials of chemotherapy or radiotherapy given preoperatively in esophageal cancer—termed neoadjuvant therapy—have been undertaken largely because of the disappointing results achieved with conventional surgery or radiation therapy alone. Combined modality trials have taken one of three different approaches:

1. Chemotherapy followed by a planned surgical procedure;
2. Chemotherapy given concurrently with radiation therapy, followed by surgery; and
3. Chemotherapy and radiation therapy as primary treatment without subsequent surgical intervention.

In esophageal cancer, preoperative chemotherapy offers many potential clinical benefits, including enhanced resectability through downstaging of the primary tumor. The ability to assess directly in the primary tumor the response to preoperative chemotherapy makes the endpoint of adjuvant therapy more precise by identifying patients who are responsive to chemotherapy and who might benefit from additional chemotherapy postoperatively. Administering chemotherapy early in the course of the disease also potentially treats subclinical but established micrometastatic disease when chemotherapy is likely to have its greatest impact. A disadvantage of preoperative chemotherapy is the delay in achieving local control of disease—an important issue in patients with dysphagia and restricted nutritional intake. Concurrent chemoradiotherapy given preoperatively potentially enhances local tumor control with the addition of radiotherapy, while simultaneously treating systemic disease with the addition of chemotherapy.

Although neoadjuvant therapy should be reserved for those patients at highest risk for death from disease, most patients in the United States present with high-risk transmural (T3) or lymph-node posi-

TREATMENT

Palliation of Dysphagia in Advanced Esophageal Cancer

Dysphagia is the most common presenting complaint in esophageal cancer, and the inability to swallow leads to considerable morbidity. A number of treatment approaches to the patient with dysphagia are available and include

- systemic chemotherapy
- endoscopic dilatation, laser ablation, or photodynamic therapy
- esophageal intubation with a prosthesis
- endoscopic or surgical placement of a gastrostomy or jejunostomy tube
- radiotherapy
- palliative esophagectomy or bypass

How to best treat dysphagia depends on the severity of the condition, antecedent weight loss, and the overall medical condition of the patient. For example, in patients with less than 10% to 15% weight loss and who are able to tolerate some solid foods, semisolids, or liquid nutritional supplements, systemic chemotherapy could be the optimal initial treatment. This is particularly appropriate in patients with distant metastatic disease, in which chemotherapy could potentially palliate dysphagia as well as systemic disease. In patients with severe weight loss, dysphagia to liquids, or complete esophageal obstruction with intolerance even of oral secretions, endoscopic placement of a feeding tube might be necessary for alimentation and hydration. Endoscopic placement of stent without feeding tube placement may also be considered depending on the degree of nutritional compromise. If the primary tumor is bleeding actively or causing complete obstruction, surgical palliation with esophagectomy or esophageal bypass is also a consideration. Given the morbidity and potential mortality associated with surgery, surgery is rarely resorted to in the setting of metastatic disease. If the patient has a performance status that would permit active therapy, systemic chemotherapy can be used subsequently to palliate both local disease and systemic metastatic disease. Patients with locally unresectable but nonmetastatic disease could be candidates for combined chemotherapy and concurrent radiotherapy, if all disease can be encompassed in a radiotherapy field.

If there is progression of dysphagia symptoms despite the use of systemic chemotherapy, patients might be candidates for endoscopic dilatation and placement of an esophageal stent, or the use of endoscopic laser or photodynamic therapy. A trial of second-line chemotherapy can be considered. External-beam radiation therapy alone can also be considered as a local palliative measure.

---

tive (N1) disease and are therefore candidates for neoadjuvant clinical trials. Results of selected randomized trials of preoperative chemotherapy, preoperative chemoradiotherapy, or definitive chemoradiotherapy without surgery are outlined in Table 88-2.

Preoperative Chemotherapy

The use of preoperative chemotherapy in locally advanced esophageal carcinoma has been the subject of numerous trials. Most of these trials have been single-arm phase II studies evaluating preoperative chemotherapy given from one to up to six cycles, followed by a definitive surgical procedure. More recent trials, however, have given chemotherapy both pre- and postoperatively. Virtually all preoperative chemotherapy trials in esophageal cancer have employed cisplatin-based combination chemotherapy. Whereas earlier trials included predominantly squamous cell carcinoma, with the increased incidence of adenocarcinoma both histologies have been treated on the same preoperative protocols. Phase II trials have demonstrated the safety and feasibility of preoperative chemotherapy. Pathologic complete responses to preoperative chemotherapy, with no residual cancer found in the surgical specimen, are generally rare and occur in less than 5% of patients treated on these trials.

The role of preoperative chemotherapy in the treatment of locoregional esophageal carcinoma can be defined clearly only in the context of random-assignment trials with a surgery-only control arm. The large American Intergroup trial 113 reported by Kelsen is the most definitive trial to date of preoperative chemotherapy in esophageal cancer (see Table 88-2). In this trial, patients were randomized to undergo immediate surgery or to receive three cycles of cisplatin and 5-fluorouracil followed by surgery, followed in turn by two postoperative cycles of cisplatin and 5-fluorouracil. The trial failed to show any benefit for neoadjuvant chemotherapy compared with surgery alone (Figure 88-4). Curative resections with negative surgical margins and surgical mortality were equivalent in both groups. In contrast, the Medical Research Council (MRC) in the United Kingdom reported preliminary results of a larger trial, which compared immediate esophagectomy to two cycles of

Table 88-2 ■ Neoadjuvant Therapy in Locally Advanced Esophageal Cancer: Selected Randomized Phase III Trials

Author	Regimen	Patients	Histology	% Pathologic Complete Response	Overall Survival
Preoperative Chemotherapy					
Kelsen	5-FU/Cisplatin	213	S + A	2.5%	35% 2-year*
	Surgery	227		–	37% 2-year
Clark	5-FU/Cisplatin	802	S + A	not stated	45% 2-year†
	Surgery			–	35% 2-year
Preoperative Chemotherapy + Radiotherapy					
Bosset	Cisplatin + 37 Gy	143	S	26%	48% 2-year*
	Surgery	139		–	43% 2-year
Walsh	5FU/Cisplatin + 40 Gy	58	A	25%	32% 3-year†
	Surgery	55		–	6% 3-year
Urba	5-FU/Cisplatin Vinblastine + 45 Gy	50	S + A	28%	30% 3-year*
	Surgery	50		–	16% 3-year
Definitive Chemotherapy + Radiotherapy					
Herskovic	5-FU/Cisplatin + 50 Gy	61	S + A	–	38% 2-year†
	65 Gy alone	60		–	10% 2-year

S = squamous cancer; A = adenocarcinoma; 5-FU = 5-fluorouracil
*not statistically significant
†statistically significant

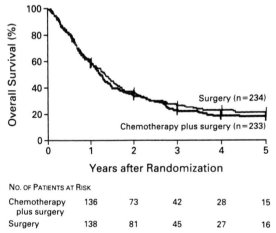

Figure 88-4 ■ Survival in patients with esophageal carcinoma treated with surgery alone or with chemotherapy and surgery combined, on Intergroup Trial 113. The distribution curves represent the results of an intention-to-treat survival analysis involving all registered patients. Patients who received chemotherapy before surgery had a median survival of 14.9 months; in comparison, patients who had only surgery had a median survival of 16.1 months ($P = 0.53$ by the log-rank test). Of the 233 patients receiving preoperative chemotherapy, 180 died; of the 234 not receiving it, 173 died. (From Kelsen DP, Ginsberg R, Pajak T, et al: Chemotherapy followed by surgery compared with surgery alone for localized esophageal cancer. N Engl J Med 1998;339:1979–1984.)

preoperative 5-fluorouracil and cisplatin followed by surgery. Resection rates on this trial were higher after preoperative chemotherapy, and the median and two-year survival were significantly improved with the use of preoperative chemotherapy. A three-month improvement in median survival was achieved, and two-year survival improved to 45% from 35% with the use of preoperative chemotherapy. The larger sample size on this trial might have made possible the detection of a more modest survival improvement achieved with chemotherapy. The trial indicates that currently available chemotherapy might indeed have a favorable impact on surgically treated esophageal cancer. At present, for surgically treated patients, surgery alone remains the standard of care. The use of preoperative chemotherapy with 5-fluorouracil and cisplatin could be a consideration, given the results of the MRC trial; however, further reports of more mature results of this trial are required before this therapy can be recommended as a standard of care.

Preoperative Chemoradiotherapy

The intensification of radiation therapy with concurrent chemotherapy used as a radiation sensitizer, either in the preoperative setting or as definitive local therapy without surgery, has been evaluated in numerous clinical trials. Preoperative radiation therapy alone, without radiosensitizing chemotherapy, has been the subject of a number of randomized trials comparing this approach with surgery alone. None of the trials has demonstrated a survival benefit for preoperative radiotherapy compared with surgery alone, and the use of preoperative radiotherapy by itself cannot be recommended in the surgical management of esophageal cancer.

In the trials combining chemotherapy with concurrent radiation therapy given preoperatively, the chemotherapy most commonly used is a combination of cisplatin or mitomycin with 5-fluorouracil given by continuous infusion. In these trials, consistently 25% or more of patients have achieved a pathologic complete response seen at esophagectomy. Median survival in these series has been disappointing, however, ranging from 11 to 29 months. The contribution of esophagectomy in these trials remains unclear, with some trials indicating long-term survival only in patients achieving a pathologic complete response to chemoradiotherapy. Other trials, however, indicate that surgery for partial responders, with disease remaining in the esophagus after chemoradiotherapy, might also lead to a significant long-term survival in these patients as well. The achievement of a pathologic complete response to preoperative chemoradiotherapy identifies patients with an improved chance of five-year survival in nearly all trials published.

Toxicity for combined chemotherapy and radiation therapy is greater than for preoperative chemotherapy alone. Toxicity has been greatest in the trials in which a higher radiation therapy dose or twice-daily fractionated radiation therapy was given, or in which the radiation therapy overlapped all cycles of chemotherapy given preoperatively. The substantial gastrointestinal toxicity observed using infusional 5-fluorouracil, cisplatin, and radiotherapy (including nausea, mucositis, and esophagitis) led some investigators to mandate the placement of enteral feeding tubes in all patients to provide hydration and nutritional support during therapy. It is unclear whether the addition of agents such as etoposide, leucovorin, or vinblastine to 5-fluorouracil and cisplatin increases rates of resectability, pathologic complete response, or patient survival.

In trials combining preoperative chemoradiotherapy and surgery, local recurrence of disease appears to be uncommon, and distant metastatic disease is the predominant initial site of disease recurrence. To attempt to reduce recurrence of distant metastatic disease, more recent trials have added additional induction chemotherapy cycles prior to radiation

therapy, or additional cycles of postsurgical adjuvant chemotherapy. The use of induction cycles of chemotherapy has the potential advantage of relieving patient dysphagia prior to the start of radiation therapy. This could facilitate administration of scheduled systemic therapy in comparison with the postsurgical chemotherapy, which is difficult to deliver due to patient intolerance. The approach of preoperative concurrent chemotherapy and radiation therapy needs to be validated in the context of a randomized trial comparing preoperative chemoradiotherapy with surgery alone. Recent results from such trials have drawn conflicting conclusions, with some small, randomized trials failing to show a clear benefit for preoperative combined modality therapy (see Table 88-2). Bosset compared surgery alone with preoperative chemoradiotherapy employing single-agent cisplatin. Although no overall survival benefit was observed in this trial, a significant increase in postoperative mortality on the combined modality arm undercut any potential survival benefit that might have accrued to preoperative therapy. A trial reported by Walsh in esophageal adenocarcinoma compared surgery alone with preoperative 5-fluorouracil, cisplatin, and radiotherapy. The trial showed a significant survival benefit for combined modality therapy. A pathologic complete response rate of 25% was observed after preoperative chemoradiotherapy, comparable to reports of other studies. The poor three-year survival of the surgery control arm (less than 10%), raises a question of the validity of the trial, because controlled trials employing a surgery-alone control arm report much higher three-year survival results (15%–25%). The positive results for postoperative combined chemotherapy and radiation therapy in gastric cancer have given great impetus to the further study of preoperative chemoradiotherapy in esophageal cancer.

Although the rates of surgical resection and pathologic complete response to preoperative chemoradiotherapy in esophageal cancer are encouraging, controlled trials have yet to show a clear benefit for the delivery of chemoradiotherapy to patients undergoing surgery. The use of such therapy remains investigational, and the decision to proceed with surgery alone or to use preoperative chemoradiotherapy must be individualized. Whether surgery is obligate after achieving a clinical complete response to chemoradiotherapy is also unclear. Some investigators have argued that surgery should be reserved only as a salvage therapy for patients with residual disease after completion of chemoradiotherapy, or for patients who have local recurrence of disease after achieving a clinical complete response to chemoradiotherapy. Of concern, however, is that endoscopy after completion of chemoradiotherapy showing no obvious residual cancer might not be a guarantee that residual cancer is not present either deep in the wall of the esophagus or in lymph nodes that are inaccessible to evaluation. Because pathologic complete responses and long-term survival can be achieved with chemoradiotherapy alone without surgery, clinical trials also have evaluated the use of definitive chemoradiotherapy without surgery.

Concurrent Chemoradiation without Surgery

A nonoperative approach to the treatment of esophageal cancer has been advocated by some investigators, in light of the significant operative mortality observed in some surgical trials after the delivery of combined modality therapy, and because some trials question whether esophagectomy after combined modality therapy improves long-term survival. Early trials have evaluated chemotherapy with 5-fluorouracil and cisplatin or mitomycin given with concurrent radiation therapy in doses ranging from 4000 to 6000 cGy. Median survival ranged from 18 to 22 months, with some trials reporting five-year survivals approaching that achieved with surgery. A representative computed tomography scan image of a patient with locally advanced esophageal squamous cancer achieving a complete response to combined chemotherapy and radiation therapy without surgery is shown in Figure 88-2B.

Given the curative potential of chemoradiation therapy for locoregional disease, a nonsurgical, random-assignment trial in locoregional esophageal carcinoma comparing radiation therapy alone with radiation given with concurrent 5-fluorouracil and cisplatin was conducted by the Radiation Therapy Oncology Group (Herskovic). A modest but significantly improved median survival was observed for chemoradiation vs. radiation therapy alone (12.5 vs. 8.9 months), but more important, one- and two-year survival were significantly greater for the combined-modality arm (Figure 88-5). The results indicated that the combination of chemotherapy and radiation was superior to radiation therapy alone. The survival benefit for combined chemoradiotherapy was maintained over the long term with a 22% eight-year survival. The biologic effect of chemotherapy added to radiotherapy on this trial was evident. There was a significant reduction in the risk of distant metastatic disease, indicating a systemic biologic effect of chemotherapy on distant disease. There was also a significant reduction in local disease recurrence, suggesting that chemotherapy potentiated the local effects of radiation therapy. A combination of concurrent chemotherapy and radiation therapy

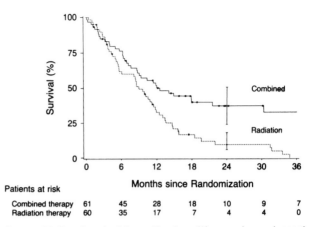

Figure 88-5 ■ Survival in patients with esophageal carcinoma treated with radiation alone or with radiation and chemotherapy combined, on RTOG trial 85-01. Bars indicate 95% confidence intervals at 24 months. (From Herskovic A, Martz LK, Al-Sarraf M, et al: Combined chemotherapy and radiotherapy compared with radiotherapy alone in patients with cancer of the esophagus. N Engl J Med 1992;326:1593–1598.)

without surgery has therefore become the standard of care in patients treated with radiation-based treatment alone.

Management of Esophageal Cancer

Staging of the patient should include endoscopy and computed tomography imaging, with endoscopic ultrasound recommended for more accurate staging of the depth of penetration of the tumor into the esophageal wall and to better assess local lymph node involvement. Positron emission tomography might identify a small number of patients with metastatic disease not evident clinically or imaged via computed tomography, and positron emission tomography might also assist in better defining nodal staging in conjunction with endoscopic ultrasound. Because survival with surgery alone could be fairly good for very early stage (T1) tumors or superficially muscle-invasive (T2) cancers without nodal disease, these patients might be best served with surgery alone if they are medically fit. Chemoradiotherapy could also be a consideration for patients who are not surgical candidates. For patients with transmural (T3) tumors or lymph node positive tumors (who represent the vast majority of patients seen), surgery alone or the use of definitive chemoradiotherapy alone are standard treatment options. If the patient achieves less than a clinical complete response to chemoradiotherapy, surgery should strongly be considered to remove clinically obvious residual disease. Whether a planned surgery

TREATMENT

Management of Locally Advanced Esophageal Cancer

The two treatment approaches for a patient with locally advanced, nonmetastatic esophageal squamous or adenocarcinoma include

- surgery alone or
- definitive concurrent radiation therapy and chemotherapy without surgery.

Procedures for staging of esophageal cancer should include

- endoscopy and biopsy
- computed tomography scan of the chest and abdomen
- barium swallow
- bronchoscopy for cervical tumors or thoracic tumors of the proximal or midthoracic esophagus
- endoscopic ultrasound
- bone scan and brain scan as clinically indicated
- positron emission tomography

Patients with distant metastatic disease should be treated with palliative chemotherapy alone. Patients with locally advanced and either anatomically inoperable or medically inoperable disease should be treated with definitive chemoradiotherapy. Patients with early stage T1 or superficial T2 and node-negative tumors can be considered for surgery alone or for definitive chemoradiotherapy. For patients with transmural T3 or node-positive tumors, either surgery alone or combined chemoradiotherapy alone is a treatment option. Patients with adenocarcinoma of the gastroesophageal junction or gastric cardia can be considered for adjuvant postoperative chemoradiotherapy after surgery, given recent studies that indicate a benefit for adjuvant therapy in gastric cancer.

If less than a complete response has been achieved with definitive chemoradiotherapy, surgical salvage should be considered. Surgical salvage should also be considered for patients who have locally recurrent disease after prior definitive chemoradiotherapy. If initial surgery results in less than a negative margin resection—that is, if surgical margins are positive or gross residual disease is left behind—patients can be considered for treatment with postoperative combined chemoradiotherapy.

after chemoradiotherapy benefits all patients, or whether chemoradiotherapy should be given preoperatively to all higher-risk patients remains unclear. Patients with locally advanced disease are clearly candidates for investigational protocols that evaluate the use of preoperative therapy.

Intensification of Chemoradiotherapy

Recent phase II and III trials have attempted to intensify the delivery of chemoradiotherapy. Trial approaches have included the addition of induction cycles of 5-fluorouracil and cisplatin-based chemotherapy prior to the start of chemoradiation, the escalation of the radiotherapy dose to 6400 cGy, and the addition of a brachytherapy boost given together with concurrent chemotherapy after the completion of conventional chemoradiotherapy. None of these approaches, in particular the escalation of the radiation therapy dose from the standard 5040 cGy to a dose of 6400 cGy, have improved local control of tumor or treatment outcome.

Comparison of Nonsurgical and Surgical Therapy

The selection bias to choose either surgery or radiation therapy-based treatment for a patient with locally advanced esophageal cancer is likely to favor surgery as leading to a better treatment outcome. Patients chosen to undergo surgery are generally medically more fit and have at least clinically resectable disease. Patients chosen to receive nonoperative chemoradiotherapy might be medically unfit for surgery or might have more locally advanced (and in some cases, inoperable) disease. It is difficult, therefore, to make a direct comparison between the results of nonsurgical and surgical approaches in the absence of a randomized trial. Despite the adverse selection factors that could lead to treatment with chemoradiotherapy over surgery, a comparison of the results of these respective treatment approaches from national Intergroup trials reveals that the nonsurgical, radiation therapy-based approach might offer a survival rate that is the same as, if not better than, surgery. Although the results are comparable, it is clear that both the nonsurgical and surgical approaches have limited success, with relatively poor long-term survival rates using either chemoradiotherapy alone or surgery alone. Because pilot trials of preoperative chemoradiotherapy followed by surgery suggest a relatively low incidence of locoregional disease recurrence after chemoradiotherapy and surgery, this treatment strategy is likely to continue to be the primary focus of future research in combined modality therapy in esophageal cancer.

Small Cell Carcinoma

Small cell carcinoma of the esophagus is an uncommon histologic subtype of esophageal carcinoma. The incidence of small cell carcinoma is less than 1% to 3% of cases of esophageal cancer. Staging of small cell cancer of the esophagus is similar to that for small cell cancer of the lung, with limited-stage disease defined as locoregional disease with or without locoregional lymph node involvement (which can potentially be contained in a radiotherapy treatment field). Extensive-stage disease is defined as distant metastatic disease beyond the locoregional area. As with small cell lung cancer, there is a clear association of development of the disease with tobacco use, and distant metastatic disease is frequently present at diagnosis. Like small cell lung cancer, the disease appears to be highly responsive to radiation therapy and to a broad spectrum of chemotherapeutic agents. The almost universal development of metastatic disease in small cell carcinoma of the esophagus indicates that chemotherapy as part of combined modality therapy should be used in the treatment of limited-stage disease. Despite the treatment of limited-stage disease patients with a combination of chemotherapy and surgery and/or radiotherapy, long-term survivors with small cell carcinoma of the esophagus are rare.

References

Ajani J, Ilson D, Daugherty K, et al: Activity of taxol in patients with squamous cell carcinoma and adenocarcinoma of the esophagus. J Natl Cancer Inst 1994;86:1086–1091.

Bani-Hani K, Martin IG, Hardie LJ, et al: Prospective study of cyclin D1 overexpression in Barrett's esophagus: Association with increased risk of adenocarcinoma. J Natl Cancer Inst 2000;92:1316–1321.

Bleiberg H, Conroy T, Paillot B, et al: Randomized phase II study of cisplatin and 5-FU versus cisplatin alone in advanced squamous cell oesophageal cancer. Eur J Cancer 1997; 33:1216–1220.

Blot WJ, Li JY, Taylor PR, et al: Nutrition intervention trials in Linxian, China: Supplementation with specific vitamin/mineral combinations, cancer incidence, and disease-specific mortality in the general population. J Natl Cancer Inst 1993;85:1483–1492.

Bosset JF, Gignoux M, Triboulet JP, et al: Chemoradiotherapy followed by surgery compared with surgery alone in squamous cell cancer of the esophagus. New England radiotherapy for esophageal carcinoma. J Thor Cardiovasc Surg 1992;5:887–895.

Clark PI: Medical Research Council randomized trial of surgery with or without pre-operative chemotherapy in resectable cancer of the oesophagus. Ann Oncol 2000;11(Supplement 4).

Cooper JS, Guo MD, Herskovic A, et al: Chemoradiotherapy of locally advanced esophageal cancer: Long-term follow-up of a prospective randomized trial (RTOG 85-01). JAMA 1999;281:1623–1627.

Devesa SS, Blot WJ, Fraumeni JF Jr: Changing patterns in the incidence of esophageal and gastric carcinoma in the United States. Cancer 1998;83:2049–2053.

Enzinger PC, Ilson DH, Kelsen DP: Chemotherapy in esophageal cancer. Semin Oncol 1999;26(5 Suppl 15):12–20.

Flamen P, Lerut A, Van Cutsem E, et al: Utility of positron emission tomography for the staging of patients with potentially operable esophageal carcinoma. J Clin Oncol 2000;18: 3202–3210.

Gaspar LE, Winter K, Kocha WI, et al: A phase I/II study of external beam radiation, brachytherapy, and concurrent chemotherapy for patients with localized carcinoma of the esophagus (radiation therapy oncology group study 9207): Final report. Cancer 2000;88:988–995.

Herskovic A, Martz LK, Al-Sarraf M, et al: Combined chemotherapy and radiotherapy compared with radiotherapy alone in patients with cancer of the esophagus. N Engl J Med 1992;326:1593–1598.

Ilson DH, Ajani J, Bhalla K, et al: Phase II trial of paclitaxel, fluorouracil, and cisplatin in patients with advanced carcinoma of the esophagus. J Clin Oncol 1998;16:1826–1834.

Ilson DH, Saltz L, Enzinger P, et al: Phase II trial of weekly irinotecan plus cisplatin in advanced esophageal cancer. J Clin Oncol 1999;17:3270–3275.

Kelsen DP, Ginsberg R, Pajak T, et al: Chemotherapy followed by surgery compared with surgery alone for localized esophageal cancer. N Engl J Med 1998;339:1979–1984.

Knyrim K, Wagner HJ, Bethge N, et al: A controlled trial of an expansile metal stent for palliation of esophageal obstruction due to inoperable cancer. N Engl J Med 1993;329:1302–1307.

Lagergren J, Bergstrom R, Lindgren A, et al: Symptomatic gastroesophageal reflux as a risk factor for esophageal adenocarcinoma. N Engl J Med 1999;340:825–831.

Luketich JD, Meehan M, Nguyen NT, et al: Minimally invasive surgical staging for esophageal cancer. Surg Endoscopy 2000;14:700–702.

Macdonald JS, Smalley S, Benedetti J, et al: Postoperative combined radiation and chemotherapy improves disease-free survival (DFS) and overall survival (OS) in resected adenocarcinoma of the stomach and G.E. junction. Results of Intergroup study int-0116(SWOG 9008). Proc ASCO 2000;19:1a.

Mark SD, Qiao YL, Dawsey SM, et al: Prospective study of serum selenium levels and incident esophageal and gastric cancers. J Natl Cancer Inst 2000;92:1753–1763.

Minsky BD, Pajak TF, Ginsberg RJ, et al: INT 0123 (Radiation Therapy Oncology Group 94–05) Phase III trial of combined-modality therapy for esophageal cancer: High-dose versus standard radiation therapy. J Clin Oncol 2002;20:1151–1153.

Muller JM, Erasmi H, Stelzner M, et al: Surgical therapy of oesophageal carcinoma. Br J Surg 1990;77:845–857.

Safran H, Gaissert H, Akerman P, et al: Paclitaxel, cisplatin, and concurrent radiation for esophageal cancer. Cancer Invest 2001;19:1–7.

Spiridonidis CH, Laufman LR, Jones JJ, et al: A phase II evaluation of high dose cisplatin and etoposide in patients with advanced esophageal adenocarcinoma. Cancer 1996;77:2070–2077.

Urba SG, Orringer MB, Turrisi A, et al: Randomized trial of pre-operative chemoradiation versus surgery alone in patients with locoregional esophageal carcinoma. J Clin Oncol 2001;19:305–313.

Walsh TN, Noonan N, Hollywood D, et al: A comparison of multimodal therapy and surgery for esophageal adenocarcinoma. N Engl J Med 1996;335:462–467.

Chapter 89
Gastric Cancer

Jeffrey A. Meyerhardt and Charles S. Fuchs

Introduction

Despite a dramatic decline in the incidence of gastric carcinoma in the United States during the last century, mortality related to the disease remains considerable. In 2003, an estimated 22,400 new cases of gastric cancers will be diagnosed in the United States, and 12,100 people will die of the disease. Worldwide, 755,000 new cases are diagnosed annually. Surgery remains the primary modality of management for patients with gastric cancer. Unfortunately, in the United States and Western Europe, more than 50% of patients with adenocarcinomas of the stomach present with advanced stage III or IV disease. Moreover, among patients undergoing "curative" resection, up to 80% of patients eventually develop either locoregional or distant recurrence.

Epidemiology

In 1930, gastric carcinoma represented the leading cause of cancer-related deaths among American men and the third most common cause among women. Over the subsequent 50 years, the incidence of gastric carcinoma in the United States has dropped from 33 to 10 per 100,000 among men and from 30 to 5 per 100,000 among women. Absolute mortality due to gastric cancer has also decreased, principally as a result of the declining incidence rather than due to marked improvements in therapy. At present, the disease is rare before the age of 40 years, but its incidence increases steadily thereafter, peaking in the seventh decade. In the United States, African-Americans, Hispanic Americans, and Native Americans are 1.5 to 2.5 times more likely to develop the disease than are Caucasians. Furthermore, gastric carcinoma remains approximately twice as common in males as in females.

The declining incidence of gastric carcinoma has also been experienced worldwide, although patterns vary widely. The incidence is highest in Japan, China, South America, and Eastern Europe. In Japan, despite a similar relative decline in incidence, gastric cancer remains the leading cause of cancer death.

Interestingly, gastric cancer incidence by location within the stomach has varied over time. In 1930, gastric carcinoma in the United States originated predominantly in the distal stomach (gastric body and antrum), and the reduction in gastric cancer experienced through 1976 largely reflects a decline in the appearance of distal lesions. Since 1976, however, data from the Surveillance, Epidemiology, and End Results (SEER) program indicate a steady rise in the incidence of adenocarcinoma of the proximal stomach (cardia) and the gastroesophageal junction. In fact, the incidence of adenocarcinoma of the gastroesophageal junction and the gastric cardia has increased at a rate exceeding that for any other cancer (including melanoma and lung cancer). Similar trends in proximal gastric cancers have been observed in Europe.

Pathology

More than 90% of malignant tumors arising in the stomach are adenocarcinomas, with the remaining being lymphomas, leiomyosarcomas, carcinoids, or metastatic disease. Differentiation between gastric adenocarcinoma and other cancers originating in the stomach is critical, as prognosis and treatment differ considerably according to type. This chapter focuses on gastric adenocarcinomas.

On gross inspection and endoscopic examination, gastric cancers can have a wide range of appearances. Early gastric cancers, defined as lesions confined to the mucosa and submucosa, are typically detected incidentally or during screening examinations. Early cancers can appear as superficial plaques, mucosal discoloration, polypoid protrusions, or ulcerations. In contrast, advanced cancers most commonly appear as fungating or ulcerating masses. Another advanced presentation is the diffusely infiltrating *linitis plastica* (thickened "leather bottle"), which is associated with a particularly poor prognosis.

Histologically, gastric adenocarcinomas can be subdivided into two categories: an intestinal type characterized by cohesive neoplastic cells forming glandlike structures, and a diffuse type in which cell cohesion is absent, so that individual cells infiltrate and thicken the stomach wall without forming a discrete mass. Intestinal-type lesions are frequently ulcerative, occur in the distal stomach more often than the diffuse type, and are often preceded by a prolonged precancerous phase. Diffuse carcinomas occur more often in younger patients, develop throughout the stomach but especially in the cardia, and are associated with a poor prognosis.

The decline in gastric cancer incidence observed during this century appears largely attributable to a decrease in the number of intestinal-type lesions. Although assignment of all adenocarcinomas to either diffuse or intestinal histologies is not always possible, this categorization defines two classes of gastric cancer that appear to represent entities reflecting uniquely different epidemiologic and etiologic factors.

Pathogenesis

Precursor Conditions

Reviews of surgical and autopsy specimens have suggested that gastric cancers often develop in the context of other pathological conditions (Table 89-1). Chronic atrophic gastritis and its associated abnormality, intestinal metaplasia, are the precursor lesions most closely linked to an increased risk of gastric cancer, specifically of the intestinal type. Atrophic gastritis usually begins as a multifocal process in the distal stomach. As foci coalesce, gastric acid production declines, which could lead to the sequential progression to metaplasia, dysplasia, and, ultimately, carcinoma. Histologic studies indicate that intestinal metaplasia precedes intestinal-type gastric cancers but not diffuse-type cancers. Nonetheless, only 10% of patients with atrophic gastritis and intestinal metaplasia develop gastric cancer, indicating that atrophic gastritis or achlorhydria as isolated factors are not sufficient causes of gastric carcinoma.

Pernicious anemia and *Helicobacter pylori* (*H. pylori*) infection are two major causes of atrophic gastritis and intestinal metaplasia. Most observational studies of patients with pernicious anemia have demonstrated a two- to threefold excess risk of stomach cancer. In contrast, no study has detected an increased risk for gastric carcinoma in patients with long-term drug-induced achlorhydria (use of parietal cell histamine antagonists or gastric proton pump inhibitors).

Epidemiologic studies have consistently demonstrated an association between *H. pylori* and the risk of

Table 89-1 ■ Risk Factors for Gastric Adenocarcinoma

Predisposing Conditions

Chronic atrophic gastritis with intestinal metaplasia
Pernicious anemia
Helicobacter pylori
Barrett's esophagus (gastroesophageal junction tumors)
History of partial gastrectomy for benign disease
Ménétrier's disease
Gastric adenomatous polyps

Environmental Factors

High-nitrite content foods (meats and fish)
High salt consumption
Low consumption of fruits and vegetables
Low antioxidant intake (vitamins A and C, olive oil, garlic)
Cigarette smoking
Low socioeconomic status
Obesity (particularly proximal cancers)
Low fiber diet

Genetic Factors

Li-Fraumeni syndrome
Familial adenomatous polyposis syndrome
Hereditary nonpolyposis colorectal cancer (Lynch syndrome II)
Hereditary diffuse gastric cancer (including E-cadherin germline mutations)
Family history without known genetic syndrome
Blood type A

gastric cancer. Prospective serological studies have reported that *H. pylori*-infected individuals experience a three- to sixfold increased risk of gastric cancer. A recent study from Japan found a significant risk of gastric cancer in patients with *H. pylori* and either nonulcer dyspepsia, gastric polyps, or active gastric ulcers. In contrast, patients with *H. pylori* and duodenal ulcers do not have an increased risk of gastric cancer. Furthermore, studies suggest a potential protective effect of duodenal ulcers. A link between gastric ulcers and gastric cancer has been shown but most likely relates to common etiological factors (particularly atrophic gastritis and *H. pylori*).

Most patients with *H. pylori* infection will not develop gastric cancer. Recent prospective observational studies do suggest, however, that treatment of *H. pylori* reduces the risk of gastric cancer. A nonrandomized trial of patients with submucosal-only gastric cancer treated by endoscopy showed no recurrence of gastric cancer in patients treated with *H. pylori* eradication therapy compared to 9% recurrence in patients who did not receive treatment.

Distal gastrectomy for benign disorders—particularly peptic ulcer disease—is associated with an increased risk of gastric cancer. The risk remains low until 15 to 20 years after resection of the distal stomach but increases steadily thereafter to a relative risk of 1.5 to 3. This delay in the appearance of gastric cancer is believed to be related to prolonged achlorhydria and enterogastric reflux after antrectomy, leading to a gradual progression from normal mucosa to intestinal metaplasia to dysplasia and malignancy.

Barrett's esophagus is definitively a strong risk factor for distal esophagus and gastroesophageal junction tumors. The incidence of cancer in patients having Barrett's esophagus has been estimated to be 0.5% to 2% per year. Studies linking obesity to gastric cancer likely reflect in part the positive association between Barrett's esophagus and obesity. Furthermore, the increasing incidence of Barrett's in the United States over the past 20 years could partly explain the rise in proximal cancers.

Several case reports link gastric cancer to hypertrophic gastropathy (i.e., Ménétrier's disease) and immunoglobulin deficiency, although the strength of these associations is unclear. Similarly, evidence indicates an increased risk of gastric cancer among individuals with adenomatous polyps of the stomach. The malignant potential for adenomas appears to be directly related to the size of the polyp and degree of dysplasia.

Environmental Factors

A large number of observational studies have suggested certain environmental factors affect the risk of gastric adenocarcinoma (see Table 89-1). Studies of people emigrating from areas of high risk to areas of low risk also point to a substantial environmental influence. Among Japanese immigrants in Hawaii, the risk of gastric cancer remains high, despite adoption of a Western diet. For their second- and third-generation offspring, however, the rates of the disease progressively decline, approaching the rates of the native population. Similar observations have been noted among Eastern European immigrants living in the United States.

Foods that are relatively rich in nitrates, nitrites, and secondary amines can combine to form N-nitroso compounds, which have been shown to induce gastric tumors in laboratory animals. Nitrites are found in many meats and cheeses, while nitrates are derived mainly from vegetables. Fish and meat proteins are a major source of secondary and tertiary amines. Epidemiological studies have examined dietary intakes of meats, cheeses, and vegetables and estimated nitrate and nitrite contents as risk factors for gastric cancer.

Increased intake of foods with high nitrite content is generally positively associated with risk of gastric cancer. In contrast, studies on nitrate content have shown mixed results. The inconsistency in regard to nitrates is thought to be related to the concurrent negative risk factors associated with vegetable intake—in particular, antioxidants (vitamins A and C), high fiber, and micronutrients (selenium, zinc, iron) appear to reduce risk of gastric adenocarcinoma.

Diets rich in salted, smoked, or poorly preserved foods are associated with an increased risk of gastric cancer. Excessive dietary salts have been linked to atrophic changes in the stomach mucosa. Studies in Japan suggest that the decline in gastric cancer mortality parallels a decline in per capita consumption of salted and dried foods. Furthermore, the increased use of refrigeration over the past century, and the subsequent decrease in the use of salt preservation, are most likely related to the lower overall incidence of the disease.

Multiple cohort and case-control studies have shown a 1.5- to 3.0-fold increased risk of gastric cancer among smokers, although most studies have failed to demonstrate a clear dose-response relationship. Similarly, several studies have demonstrated an increased risk of gastric dysplasia and other potentially premalignant lesions among smokers. Studies of the relationship between alcohol consumption and gastric cancer risk have been largely inconclusive.

Throughout the world, the risk of distal gastric cancer is inversely associated with socioeconomic class. Although the link between gastric cancer risk and lower socioeconomic status appears to be independent of occupational exposures, it is difficult to ascertain the relative contribution of other potential confounding factors, such as poor sanitation, inadequate food preservation, and nutrition. In striking contrast, the increasing incidence of adenocarcinoma of the distal esophagus and gastric cardia has been reported to be greater among higher socioeconomic classes, a finding partially explained by diet, obesity, and Barrett's esophagus.

Genetic Predisposition

Familial predisposition to gastric cancer has long been recognized. Most notably, Napoleon Bonaparte, his father, and his grandfather all died of the disease, as did several of Napoleon's siblings. Gastric cancers have been associated with Li-Fraumeni syndrome (p53 germline mutation), familial adenomatous polyposis syndrome (adenomatous polyposis coli [APC], germline mutation), and hereditary non–polyposis colorectal cancer syndrome (mismatch repair gene mutations). Recently, a familial syndrome of gastric cancer with germline mutations of the E-cadherin gene was described. Beyond these well-defined, rare syndromes, case-control studies indicate that first-degree relatives of patients with gastric cancer have a two- to threefold increased risk of developing the disease. Further supporting a genetic influence, several studies have observed a modest increased risk of gastric cancer among individuals with blood type A.

A cascade of pathologic states has been described for gastric cancer. Mucosal changes—including superficial gastritis, atrophic gastritis, metaplasia, and dysplasia—appear to evolve sequentially prior to the development of carcinoma. Unlike a similar pathway seen in colon cancer, the molecular changes at each step are not clear. Overexpression of certain growth factors and oncogenes are described in gastric carcinomas, but their roles in the pathway remain to be defined.

Clinical Presentation

Early-stage gastric carcinoma is typically asymptomatic. Patients might experience vague gastrointestinal symptoms or progressive weight loss; they either do not seek medical attention or are not initially aggressively worked up. Consequently, at the time of presentation, the disease is often locally advanced or metastatic. As the tumor becomes more extensive, patients might complain of an insidious upper-abdominal discomfort varying in intensity from a vague, postprandial fullness to a severe, steady pain. Anorexia, often with slight nausea, is quite common but is usually not the presenting complaint. Weight loss is frequently present and is usually the result of insufficient caloric intake. The American College of Surgeons reviewed 18,365 patients and reported weight loss and abdominal pain as the most frequent symptoms present at diagnosis (Table 89-2). Dysphagia is typical with gastroesophageal junction and cardia lesions, whereas vomiting occurs more often when the tumor invades the pylorus. Occult gastrointestinal bleeding is common, with associated anemia, but frank hematemesis or melena occurs in less than 20% of patients. Overt bleeding is more often associated with other gastric neoplasms, including leiomyomas, leiomyosarcomas, or metastatic melanoma. Direct extension of gastric cancers into the colon may be associated with foul-smelling emesis or the passage of recently ingested material in the stool.

Though no physical examination findings are diagnostic, the clinician can detect abnormalities resulting from lymphatic spread or from the development of "drop" metastasis common in gastric cancer. The disease can spread by lymphatics to involve intra-

Table 89-2 ■ Symptoms at the Time of Initial Diagnosis among 18,365 Patients with Gastric Cancer

Symptom	Frequency
Weight loss	62%
Abdominal pain	52%
Nausea	34%
Anorexia	32%
Dysphagia	26%
Melena	20%
Early satiety	18%
Ulcer-type pain	17%
Lower-extremity edema	6%

abdominal lymph nodes, supraclavicular nodes (Virchow node), and axillary node (Irish node). Spread along peritoneal surfaces can result in a periumbilical nodule (Sister Mary Joseph node), an enlarged ovary (Krukenberg tumor), a mass in the cul-de-sac (Blumer shelf), or frank peritoneal carcinomatosis and malignant ascites. Rarely, patients with gastric carcinoma present with a variety of paraneoplastic conditions such as microangiopathic hemolytic anemia, membranous nephropathy, the sudden appearance of seborrheic keratoses (sign of Leser-Trelat), filiform and papular pigmentation lesions in skin folds and mucous membranes (acanthosis nigricans), chronic intravascular coagulation leading to arterial and venous thrombi (Trousseau's syndrome), and, rarely, dermatomyositis. The liver is the most common site of hematogenous dissemination, although pulmonary metastases are also seen.

Laboratory findings might demonstrate anemia (42% of patients at presentation), hypoproteinemia (26%), and abnormal liver function tests (26%). No test is diagnostic of malignancy, but abnormalities should be pursued by further workup. Measuring tumor markers (carcinoembryonic antigen and CA 19-9) as a means of diagnosis of gastric cancer is not recommended.

Diagnostic Studies

When patients present with vague gastrointestinal symptoms, the clinician often orders an upper gastrointestinal series as the first diagnostic test. When gastric cancer is suspected, however, a double-contrast barium meal will increase sensitivity to detect abnormalities. Double-contrast techniques allow improved visualization of mucosal detail and might indicate diminished distensibility of the stomach, which is often the only indication of a diffuse infiltrative carcinoma. For lesions between 5 and 10 mm, however, false negative rates as high as 25% have been reported. Differentiating between a benign ulcer, a malignant ulcer, and a lymphoma could be impossible, and the anatomic location of the ulcer is not adequately predictive for the presence or absence of malignancy.

The limitations of barium studies provide support for endoscopy as the initial test to evaluate patients. The clinician, however, must weigh the increased cost and potential side effects and risks when choosing a first test. Endoscopy and biopsy should always be performed if an upper gastrointestinal series is suspicious for the presence of malignancy, or if there is not complete healing of an ulcer greater than six weeks after detection. When endoscopy is performed, all ulcers should be biopsied because up to 5% have a malignant component. The combination of fiberoptic endoscopy and biopsy has been reported to provide a diagnostic accuracy of up to 98% when multiple biopsies are performed and evaluated. Because gastric carcinomas can be difficult to distinguish from gastric lymphomas, adequate biopsy depth is important due to the submucosal location of lymphoid neoplasms. The diagnosis of diffuse-type lesions—in particular, *linitis plastica*—can be difficult because such lesions can have a normal endoscopic appearance. Barium testing can demonstrate a stiff-appearing stomach, and deep biopsies should subsequently be performed by endoscopy.

The 1998 guidelines by the American Gastroenterological Association outline an approach to patients with dyspepsia. Patients under age 45 years with new-onset dyspepsia should initially be tested for *H. pylori* by noninvasive serology or urea breath test and treated with empiric medical therapy and *H. pylori*-eradication drugs (if noninvasive tests are positive). Patients who fail this trial of treatment or who initially present with other worrisome symptoms or signs should have an upper endoscopy. In contrast, all patients over age 45 with new-onset dyspepsia should have immediate evaluation with endoscopy.

Once a gastric cancer is detected, staging of the disease is needed to decide upon appropriate treatment. Computed tomography (CT) scan of the abdomen can delineate the extent of the primary tumor as well as the presence of nodal or distant metastases. Comparisons with findings at laparotomy, however, indicate that preoperative computed tomography scans often underestimate the extent of disease, principally as a result of radiographically undetectable metastases to the lymph nodes, liver, and omentum. Endoscopic ultrasound can determine the depth of tumor penetration and presence of nodal metastases with an accuracy of approximately 77% and 69%, respectively. It can also be used to biopsy suspicious nodes detected by computed tomography scan. In practice, endoscopic ultrasound is used in some centers for gastroesophageal junction and proximal cardia tumors in which tumor depth and nodal status can affect decisions regarding neoadjuvant therapy.

Whole body [^{18}F] fluorodeoxyglucose positron emission tomography (PET) scanning is increasingly useful in the evaluation of malignancies. Tumors studied by positron emission tomography scan before and after chemotherapy have demonstrated changes consistent with computed tomography scan findings. Routine preoperative positron emission tomography scanning is not standard. When a suspicious lesion on computed tomography or endoscopic ultrasound raises concern for metastatic disease, however, positron emission tomography scanning can be particularly helpful.

Carcinoembryonic antigen (CEA) levels are less frequently elevated in gastric carcinoma than in colorectal carcinoma. Although an elevated carcinoembryonic antigen (greater than 5 ng/dL) has been observed in 40% to 50% of patients with metastatic gastric carcinomas, similar elevations are noted in only 10% to 20% of patients with surgically resectable disease. Carcinoembryonic antigen might offer some value in the follow-up of patients postoperatively. Alpha-fetoprotein (a marker more commonly used for germ cell and hepatocellular tumors) and CA 19-9 (a marker often associated with pancreatic and biliary cancers) are both elevated in 30% of patients with gastric carcinoma, though usually in late-stage disease.

Screening

Although it is difficult to justify population-based surveillance in the United States, screening for gastric cancer has been advocated in geographic regions where the prevalence of gastric cancer remains high. In Japan, annual screening by radiography or endoscopy has been recommended for persons age 50 years or older. Among Japanese programs using screening endoscopy, 40% to 60% of newly diagnosed patients have early-stage lesions, and such screening is alleged to account for the recent decline in gastric cancer mortality in Japan. To date, population screening for gastric cancer has not been studied in a prospective, controlled manner. Screening for certain high-risk patients, such as those with Barrett's esophagus and pernicious anemia, is warranted, though further trials are necessary to determine optimal timing.

Staging and Prognosis

Pathological stage remains the most important determinant of prognosis. Analyses from multiple clinical trials confirm that the depth of penetration through the wall of the stomach and metastases to regional lymph nodes best predict disease-free and overall survival. The American Joint Committee on Cancer revised the TNM staging of gastric cancer in 1997 to reflect the importance of the number of lymph nodes in prognosis (Table 89-3). It is noteworthy that in contrast to other cancers, stage IV disease for gastric carcinoma includes patients with and without distant metastasis (without distant metastasis is often referred to as stage IV_0).

Survival rates after gastrectomy drop dramatically with increasing depth of disease or number of nodes involved (Table 89-4). As previously discussed, survival is also affected by location of disease, with significantly worse survival rates associated with proximal cancers compared with same-stage distal cancers (Table 89-5). In the United States, proximal cancers account for 31% of all patients, distal cancers 30%, lesser curvature of stomach 16%, and greater curvature 6%. Approximately 12% of cancers involve the entire stomach, usually of diffuse-type pathology.

Beyond surgical stage and location of tumor, intestinal-type cancers are associated with a better five-year survival rate than diffuse forms. Similarly, poorly differentiated tumors and tumors with abnormal DNA content (i.e., aneuploidy) have been associated with diminished survival. Of recent interest has been the correlation of the molecular features of gastric cancers with prognosis. Studies have demonstrated that tumors with overexpression of transforming growth factor –β1 (TGF-β1), epidermal growth factor receptor (EGFR), c-erb B-2, c-met, vascular endothelial growth factor (VEGF), carbohydrate antigens sialyl Le^a (sLe^a), and loss of expression of cyclin-dependent kinase inhibitor $p27^{Kip1}$ have poorer prognosis. Similarly, tumors with higher microvessel count and tumor angiogenic activity have higher recurrence rates and more frequent liver metastases. The applicability of these findings to the prognosis and therapy of individual patients is uncertain. These biologic insights at the molecular level could improve the ability to make rational therapeutic decisions and to develop targeted therapy in the future.

Reports have often cited better prognosis for patients in Japan compared with patients in the United States and Western Europe. In Japan, five-year survival for patients with stage IA and IB gastric cancer

Table 89-3 ■ 1997 American Joint Committee on Cancer Staging of Gastric Cancer

T (Primary Tumor)

Tx	Cannot be assessed
T0	No evidence of tumor
Tis	Carcinoma in situ
T1	Tumor invades lamina propria or submucosa
T2	Tumor invades muscular propria*
T3	Tumor invades adventitia
T4	Tumor invades adjacent structures

N (Regional Nodes†—Recommend at Least 15 Nodes Be Evaluated)

Nx	Cannot be assessed
N0	No regional lymph node metastasis
N1	1–6 regional lymph node metastases
N2	7–15 regional lymph node metastases
N3	>15 regional lymph node metastases

M (Distant Metastasis)

Mx	Cannot be assessed
M0	No distant metastasis
M1	Distant metastasis

Stage Grouping

Stage 0	Tis N0 M0
Stage IA	T1 N0 M0
Stage IB	T1 N1 M0
	T2 N0 M0
Stage II	T1 N2 M0
	T2 N1 M0
	T3 N0 M0
Stage IIIA	T2 N2 M0
	T3 N1 M0
	T4 N0 M0
Stage IIIB	T3 N2 M0
Stage IV	T4 N1–2 M0
	T1–4 N3 M0
	Any T any N M1

*Tumor can penetrate the muscularis propria with extension into the gastrocolic or gastrohepatic ligaments or into the greater or lesser omentum without perforation of the visceral peritoneum covering these structures (these are T2 lesions). If visceral peritoneum covering the gastric ligaments or omentum perforates, the tumor is T3.
†Regional lymph nodes include perigastric nodes along lesser or greater curvature and nodes along the left gastric, common hepatic, splenic, and celiac arteries. Involvement of other nodes (including hepatoduodenal, retropancreatic, mesenteric, and para-aortic nodes) represent distant metastasis.

has been reported as high as 95% and 86%, respectively, compared with 78% and 58% in the United States and Western Europe. Hypotheses about "different disease" between the two regions have been entertained. Thorough analyses suggest that these favorable outcomes for patients in Japan relate to greater fre-

Table 89-4 ▪ Survival Rates for Patients Treated with Gastrectomy from 1985–1996 by Stage at Diagnosis

Stage	Five-Year Survival	10-year Survival
IA	78%	65%
IB	58%	42%
II	34%	26%
IIIA	20%	14%
IIIB	8%	3%
IV	7%	5%

Table 89-5 ▪ Five-Year Stage-by-Stage Survival Rates Based on Location of Disease Following Gastrectomy

Stage	Proximal (Cardia/Fundus)	Distal (Antrum/Pylorus)	Other
IA	64%	81%	84%
IB	42%	65%	65%
II	24%	38%	41%
IIIA	13%	23%	24%
IIIB	6%	6%	10%
IV	6%	9%	8%

quency of earlier-stage disease (perhaps due partly to screening programs), more accurate staging due to extended lymph node dissections, and differences in tumor location (with more proximal cancers in American and European patients). As discussed in the following section, some clinicians have suggested that the more extensive lymph node resections practiced widely in Japan might improve survival, although no prospective study has substantiated that claim.

Therapy

Surgery with Curative Intent

Complete surgical eradication of the primary tumor with resection of adjacent lymph nodes represents the only chance for cure. Because resection of the primary lesion can also offer the most effective means of symptomatic palliation, abdominal exploration with curative intent should be considered unless there is clear evidence of disseminated disease or other contraindications to surgery. The choice of operation depends on stage, location, intestinal- versus diffuse-type lesions, adjacent organ involvement, and clinical practice in regard to extent of node resection.

Endoscopic mucosal resection is used primarily in Japan for disease that has not invaded the submucosa. It is generally reserved for small, superficial lesions with favorable features. Patients with residual or recurrent disease have been salvaged successfully by surgery, thereby justifying attempts for a less morbid procedure in the appropriate patient.

For all other lesions, either a subtotal (partial) or total gastrectomy should be performed. The goal of resection is wide gross margins and complete resection of microscopic disease. Tumors of the cardia and middle third of the stomach generally require a total gastrectomy to achieve negative margins. Studies of proximal tumors have demonstrated that gross negative margins of only 2 cm have up to a 30% chance of microscopically positive margins. At least 6 cm of grossly negative margins are needed to ensure microscopically negative margins for proximal tumors. Among patients with proximal cancers, the Norwegian Stomach Cancer Trial found higher rates of postoperative morbidity (including dumping syndrome, anorexia, and heartburn) and postoperative mortality for proximal gastrectomy versus total gastrectomy.

For distal-only lesions, subtotal gastrectomy with adjacent lymph node removal is appropriate. Several large, prospective randomized trials for distal tumors have demonstrated no difference in survival between total and distal gastrectomies, but distal gastrectomies might have better functional results. Other lesions, including large midgastric tumors, multiple sites, and *linitus plastica*, require total gastrectomy for curative intent resections. The recent International Union Against Cancer TNM classification describes R_0-R_2 resections to denote resection margins (Table 89-6). To avoid confusion, the reader should note that the *R* classifications were used previously to denote extent of node and adjacent organ resection, which are now described by *D* classes.

Controversies in gastric cancer surgery include extent of lymphadenectomy and the roles of splenectomy and pancreatectomy. The better survival rates in Japan compared with those in the United States and Western Europe, especially in early stage disease, have raised questions about the differences in surgical techniques. In particular, surgeons in Japan routinely perform more extensive lymph node dissections (D_2-D_4, see Table 89-6) based on retrospective comparisons showing superior survival rates, when compared with patients who underwent either D_1 or D_2 dissections. In four prospective randomized trials, however, more extensive surgery compared with D_1 resection did not provide a survival advantage. Moreover, length of

Table 89-6 ■ **Surgical Resections for Gastric Cancer**

Procedure	Description
R0	Removal of all detectable tumor with negative microscopic margins
R1	Incomplete removal of tumor, with microscopic positive margins
R2	Incomplete removal of tumor, with macroscopic tumor at site
D1	Removal of all or part of the stomach, with local perigastric nodes
D2	Removal of all or part of the stomach, with local and regional lymph nodes along branches of celiac axis. Spleen and tail of pancreas may be resected for adequate removal of nodes.
D3	Removal of D2 along with hepatoduodenal ligament, retropancreatic, and root of mesentery nodes.
D4	Removal of D3 along with transverse mesocolon and para-aortic nodes

stay, postoperative morbidity, and postoperative mortality were increased with D_2 or D_3 resections.

Similarly, studies have shown no benefit for routine splenectomy or distal pancreatectomy when those organs are not directly invaded by tumor. Surgery with organ removal should be attempted with curative intent in patients who have T4 lesions invading only one organ, without distant or peritoneal metastasis, and few lymph nodes, as there is a limited but definite survival improvement after surgery in these patients. However, resection of a noninvolved spleen or pancreas increases morbidity and mortality rates.

Following resection of gastric cancer, perioperative complications can include anastomotic failure, ileus, pulmonary complications, pancreatitis, thrombophlebitis, bleeding, and infections. Mortality rates of 1% to 10% have been reported, depending on surgical expertise and patient characteristics. Patients can also face potential long-term problems—dumping syndrome and blind-loop syndrome leading to malabsorption and diarrhea, early satiety, iron and vitamin B_{12} deficiency leading to anemia and neurological complications, vitamin D deficiency accelerating osteoporosis, reflux esophagitis, and immune deficiencies.

Data regarding the follow-up of patients after curative resection of gastric cancer are limited. No study has demonstrated that early detection of recurrent disease is beneficial to overall survival. Nonetheless, regular physical exam every three months and routine laboratory tests every six months for the first two years (and then more periodically) are often recommended. Tumor markers in gastric cancer are imprecise (e.g., less than one-half of patients with advanced disease have elevated CEA levels) and thus might not be useful to measure routinely. Imaging with computed tomography scans should be based on symptoms and can be difficult to interpret in patients who receive adjuvant radiotherapy.

Palliative Surgery and Endoscopic Procedures

In the absence of ascites or extensive metastatic disease, patients who are believed to be surgically incurable should be considered for palliative gastric resection, which can be performed with acceptable morbidity and mortality. Although the median survival after palliative resection remains only approximately 8 to 12 months, resection can provide effective relief from obstruction, bleeding, or pain. When resection is not possible, bypass of obstructing lesions can be performed, although symptomatic relief is often modest and transient.

A variety of endoscopic methods are available for palliation of symptoms related to obstruction. Laser ablation of tumor tissue can be effective, although relief from obstruction appears to be brief and requires repeated treatments. The use of plastic and expansile metal stents has been associated with a greater than 85% success rate in selected patients with gastroesophageal and cardia tumors.

Radiation Therapy

Gastric cancer has generally been considered relatively resistant to radiotherapy. As opposed to esophageal cancer, the effectiveness of radiation therapy to the primary tumor with either curative intent or the intent to prolong survival has not been demonstrated. External-beam radiation can be used for relief of obstructive symptoms or for control of excess bleeding in patients unfit for a palliative surgery.

Due to the high incidence of recurrent local and regional disease, the administration of radiotherapy shortly after complete resection of the primary tumor has been assessed as a means of treating clinically undetectable micrometastases. Few trials have examined radiation only as adjuvant treatment. Though local relapse is reduced, no survival benefit is seen with only postoperative radiotherapy. Similarly, studies of intraoperative radiotherapy (IORT) have shown reduced locoregional relapse rates but no difference in survival.

Chemotherapy

With over one-half of patients presenting with advanced disease and three-quarters of patients relapsing following attempts at curative resection, many studies of chemotherapy for gastric cancer have been reported. The use of chemotherapy in patients with gastric cancer has been disappointing. For metastatic disease, complete responses to chemotherapy are rare, and partial responses with single-agent chemotherapies have been limited, with results ranging from 0% to 30% (Table 89-7). The most widely used agent remains 5-fluorouracil, with single-agent response rates ranging from 21% to 30%. Cisplatin also has been associated with moderate response rates of 18% to 22% and frequently is incorporated into combination regimens. Recently, both the taxanes and camptothecins have shown activity as single agents, with response rates of 11% to 30%.

Though objective responses are limited and typically brief in duration, single-agent therapy might be a reasonable approach in patients who would not tolerate combination therapy. In a trial conducted more than a decade ago, single-agent 5-fluorouracil was associated with similar survival when compared with combination therapies of that era.

The history of combination chemotherapy for advanced gastric cancer provides an important lesson

in exercising caution in interpreting initial phase II trial results in patients with advanced solid tumors. Over the years, multiple phase II trials have touted new chemotherapy regimens for gastric cancer, with objective tumor response rates in excess of 50%. When additional phase II or multicenter phase III trials are performed on a larger population of patients, however, both response rates and median survivals frequently decline to much lower levels. Moreover, such confirmatory trials often find far greater toxicity than was reported in initial studies. Examples of regimens initially thought to be of benefit but later abandoned include FAM (5-fluorouracil, mitomycin, and Adriamycin), FAMTX (FAM plus methotrexate), EAP (etoposide, Adriamycin, and cisplatin), and ELF (etoposide, leukovorin, and 5-fluorouracil).

The introduction of epirubicin as an alternative anthracycline to doxorubicin and recognition of its activity in gastric cancer, with potential lower toxicity, led to its incorporation in combination regimens for advanced gastric cancer. Given the activity of cisplatin and 5-fluorouracil in gastric cancer, a group at the Royal Marsden Hospital first described a regimen of epirubicin, cisplatin, and continuous-infusion 5-fluorouracil (ECF), which was well tolerated and had a favorable response rate and median survival. The benefit was confirmed in a randomized trial comparing it with FAMTX. Based on these results, ECF is considered by many oncologists to represent the current standard of care.

Newer regimens incorporating the taxanes and irinotecan (CPT-11) for the treatment of patients with advanced gastric cancers have been reported in phase I/II trials (Table 89-8). In vitro studies suggest that repair of cisplatin-induced DNA damage can be inhibited by exposure to SN-38, the active metabolite of irinotecan. Based on this purported in vitro synergy, several investigators have reported objective response rates of 41% to 51% with irinotecan and cisplatin in patients with gastric cancer. Limited phase II studies of taxanes with cisplatin have shown similar high response rates. Randomized multicenter trials are needed to confirm these results.

Treatment versus Best Supportive Care in Advanced Disease

In light of the limited efficacy of systemic chemotherapy in advanced gastric cancer, there has been considerable debate over whether chemotherapy has any additional benefit beyond best supportive care. Four randomized, prospective studies have been conducted in which patients were assigned to either combination chemotherapy or best supportive care (Table 89-9). Although each trial enrolled a relatively small number

Table 89-7 ■ Single-Agent Chemotherapies for Advanced Gastric Cancer

Drug	Response Rate (%)
5-FU	21–30
Mitomycin	30
Cisplatin	18–22
Methotrexate	11
Triazinate	15
Adriamycin	13–21
BCNU	18
Etoposide	8
Epirubicin	22
Taxol	17–23
Taxotere	17–24
Gemcitabine	4
Irinotecan	18–25
UFT (uracil-tegafur)	20–27

Table 89-8 ■ Predominant and Newer Combination Therapies for Advanced Gastric Cancer

Combination	Response Rate (%)	Median Survival (mo)
5-FU, Adriamycin, mitomycin*	9–39	5.6–8.0
5-FU, Adriamycin, methotrexate*	12–41	5.7–10.5
Etoposide, Adriamycin, cisplatin*	20	6.1
Etoposide, leucovorin, 5-FU*	9	7.2
Epirubicin, cisplatin, 5-FU*	45	8.9
Irinotecan, cisplatin	48	8.9
Irinotecan, 5-FU, leucovorin	22	7.8
Irinotecan, oxaliplatin	20	NR
Gemcitabine, cisplatin	25	>6
Taxotere, cisplatin	56	9
Taxol, 5-FU	66	12
Taxol, 5-FU, cisplatin	51	6
Taxol, 5-FU, leucovorin, cisplatin	51	14

NR = not reported; 5-FU = 5-fluorouracil.

*Results only of randomized trials incorporating regimen.

of patients, they all showed a statistically significant survival advantage for patients randomized to chemotherapy. In two of the studies, a prospective quality-of-life study was conducted; each demonstrated an improvement in either quality of life or pain control among patients assigned to chemotherapy. These data indicate that systemic chemotherapy can offer a modest but significant benefit for patients with advanced gastric cancer and provide a basis for ongoing and future trials to find more optimal regimens.

Adjuvant Therapy

Several meta-analyses have been published to determine whether adjuvant chemotherapy leads to a reduced rate of recurrence and increased survival. Most recently, Earle and Maroun reported a small but statistically significant survival benefit for patients randomized to postoperative chemotherapy compared with surgery alone, with an odds ratio for death in the treated group of 0.80 (95% confidence interval of 0.66 to 0.97). Based on these data, the authors estimated that for a group of patients similar to those included in the analyzed trials, 65% of patients treated with surgery alone would recur and die of gastric cancer compared to 61% of patients treated with surgery followed by adjuvant chemotherapy. Given the marginal nature of this benefit, adjuvant systemic chemotherapy could not be recommended routinely outside of a clinical trial.

Many investigators have explored the combination of chemotherapy and radiation therapy after gastrectomy. Ultimately, a large North American Intergroup trial addressed the benefit of combined modality adjuvant treatment (Figure 89-1). Patients treated with postoperative chemoradiation experienced a significant improvement in both three-year disease-free survival and overall survival (Table 89-10). These results translate into a 44% improvement in relapse-free survival and a 28% improvement in overall survival at three years for patients receiving postoperative therapy. Consequently, postoperative chemoradiation has emerged as a new standard for patients with resected stage IB to $IV_{(mo)}$ gastric cancer. Much of the benefit associated with chemoradiation in this trial appears to relate to improved local control rather than to prevention of distant recurrence. Long-

Table 89-9 ■ Randomized Trials of Chemotherapy Versus Best Supportive Care in Advanced Gastric Cancer

Regimen	# of Pts	Median Survival (mo)	p Value	Comments on Quality of Life
ELF	31	8	<0.02	39% improvement/prolonged high quality of life
BSC*	30	5		20% improvement/prolonged high quality of life
FAMTX	30	10	<0.001	NR†
BSC	10	3		
FEMTX + BSC‡	21	12.3	<0.001	Pain relieved or unchanged
BSC	20	3.1		Majority of patients had worse pain within two months
ELF	18	>7.5	0.05	NR†
BSC	19	4		

E: etoposide; L: leucovorin; F: 5-fluorouracil; A: Adriamycin; MTX: methotrexate; M: mitomycin; BSC: best supportive care.

*In the ELF or 5FU/LCV vs. BSC trial, 12 patients in the BSC arm crossed over to chemotherapy for palliation.

† NR = not reported

‡ In FEMTX vs. BSC trial, both groups received vitamins A and E.

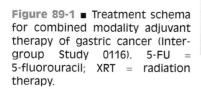

Figure 89-1 ■ Treatment schema for combined modality adjuvant therapy of gastric cancer (Intergroup Study 0116). 5-FU = 5-fluorouracil; XRT = radiation therapy.

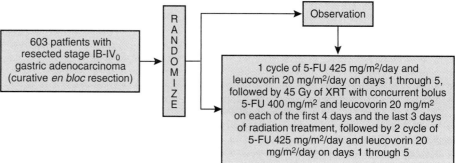

term survival (at 5 years or 10 years) might thus not be improved.

Two notes of caution in regard to aggressive adjuvant combined modality therapy are warranted. First, approximately 35% of patients assigned to the chemoradiation arms required significant modification of their designated radiation fields after central review. Careful attention to the design of radiation fields following gastrectomy is critical. Second, in the experience of these authors, patients have a variable (and often long) recovery time following gastric surgery. Adjuvant therapy can be difficult to administer to these patients. In the Intergroup trial, 36% of patients did not complete the prescribed therapy, in many cases due to toxic side effects.

Neoadjuvant and Intraperitoneal Therapy

Neoadjuvant therapy has been an attractive concept in patients with gastric cancer. Preoperative treatment provides the potential for downstaging patients with advanced disease, identifying patients with rapidly growing disease that will recur early after surgery, and increasing compliance with systemic therapy in patients who often have prolonged postoperative morbidity after en bloc resection. A single randomized trial in China of preoperative radiation therapy followed by surgery versus surgery alone in patients with stage II to IV adenocarcinoma of the gastric cardia demonstrated a statistically significant improvement in five-year survival with neoadjuvant radiation (30% vs. 20%, respectively).

Phase I/II studies have demonstrated the feasibility of preoperative chemotherapy, with downstaging of disease in up to 50% of patients and complete pathology responses in up to 10% of patients. Moreover, operative morbidity and mortality were not increased by the use of preoperative chemotherapy.

The high frequency of peritoneal recurrence after surgical resection has generated considerable interest in postoperative intraperitoneal therapy. Unfortunately, clinical trials fail to demonstrate any

Table 89-10 ■ **Intergroup 0116 Study Results**

Parameter	Surgery Only (*n* = 275 Patients)	Surgery + Adjuvant Chemoradiotherapy (*n* = 281 Patients)	*p* Value
Completed adjuvant therapy	—	65%	
Median overall survival	26 months	35 months	0.01
Three-year overall survival	40%	50%	0.01
Median relapse-free survival	19 months	30 months	<0.0001
Three-year relapse-free survival	30%	48%	<0.0001
Hematological toxicity*	—	54%[†]	
Gastrointestinal toxicity*	—	33%[†]	
Toxicity-related death*	—	1%[†]	
Local recurrence	29% (of 176 patients)	19% (of 112 patients)	
Regional recurrence	72% (of 176 patients)	68% (of 112 patients)	
Distant recurrence	18% (of 176 patients)	35% (of 112 patients)	

*Grade III or greater
[†]Of 273 evaluable patients

significant survival advantage in favor of intraperitoneal therapy.

References

Alexander HR, Kelsen DG, Tepper JG: Cancer of the stomach. In DeVita VT, Hellman S, Rosenberg SA (eds): Cancer: Principles and Practice of Oncology. Philadelphia, Lippincott, 1997, pp 1021–1054.

Bonenkamp JJ, Hermans J, Sasako M: Extended lymph-node dissection for gastric cancer. New Engl J Med 1999;340:908–914.

Bozzetti F, Marubini E, Bonfanti G: Subtotal versus total gastrectomy for gastric cancer: Five-year survival rates in multicenter randomized Italian trial. Ann Surg 1999;230:170–178.

Brennan MF, Karpeh MS: Surgery for gastric cancer: The American view. Semin Oncol 1996;23:352–359.

Craanen M, Dekker W, Blok P: Time trends in gastric carcinoma: Changing patterns of type and location. Am J Gastroenterol 1992;87:572–579.

Cullinan SA, Moertel CG, Fleming TR: A comparison of three chemotherapeutic regimens in the treatment of advanced pancreatitic and gastric carcinoma. Fluorouracil vs. fluorouracil and doxorubicin vs. fluorouracil, doxorubicin, and mitomycin. JAMA 1985;253:2061–2067.

Cuschieri A, Weeden S, Fielding J: Patient survival after D_1 and D_2 resection for gastric cancer: Long-term results of the MRC randomized surgical trial. Br J Cancer 1999;79:1522–1530.

Devesa SS, Blot WJ, Fraumeni JF: Changing patterns in the incidence of esophageal and gastric carcinoma in the United States. Cancer 1998;83:2049–2053.

Earle CC, Maroun JA: Adjuvant chemotherapy after curative resection for gastric cancer in non-Asian patients: Revisiting a meta-analysis of randomized trials. Eur J Cancer 1999;35:1059–1064.

Fuchs CS, Mayer RJ: Gastric cancer. N Engl J Med 1995;333:32–41.

Glimelius B, Ekstrom K, Hoffman K: Randomized comparison between chemotherapy plus best supportive care with best supportive care in advanced gastric cancer. Ann Oncol 1997;8:163–168.

Graham DY: Helicobacter pylori infection in the pathogenesis of duodenal ulcer and gastric cancer: A model. Gastroenterology 1997;113:1983–1991.

Gunderson LL, Sosin H: Adenocarcinoma of the stomach: Areas of failure in a re-operation series (second or symptomatic look) clinicopathologic correlation and implications for adjuvant therapy. Int J Radiat Oncol Biol Phys 1982;8:1–11.

Hundahl SA, Phillips JL, Menck HR: The National Cancer Database Report on poor survival of U.S. gastric carcinoma patients treated with gastrectomy: 5th edition American Joint Committee on Cancer staging, proximal disease, and the "different disease" hypothesis. Cancer 2000; 88:921–932.

Kelsen D, Atiq OT, Saltz L: FAMTX versus etoposide, doxorubicin, and cisplatin: A random assignment trial in gastric cancer. J Clin Oncol 1992;10:541–548.

Lowy AM, Leach SD: Adjuvant/neoadjuvant chemoradiation for gastric and pancreatitic cancer. Oncology 1999; 13(Supp):121–130.

Macdonald JS, Smalley S, Benedetti J: Chemoradiotherapy after surgery compared with surgery alone for adenocarcinoma of the stomach or gastroesophageal junction. New Engl J Med 2001;345:725–730.

Noguchi Y, Yoshikawa T, Tsuburaya A: Is gastric carcinoma different between Japan and the United States: A comparison of patient survival among three institutions. Cancer 2000;89:2237–2246.

Palli D: Epidemiology of gastric cancer: An evaluation of available evidence. J Gastroenterol 2000;35(Suppl XII):84–89.

Preusser P, Achterrath W, Wilke H: Chemotherapy of gastric cancer. Cancer Treat Rev 1988;15:257–277.

Pyrhonen S, Kuitunen T, Nyandoto P: Randomized comparison of fluorouracil, epidoxorubicin, and methotrexate (FEMTX) plus supportive care with supportive care alone in patients with non-resectable gastric cancer. Br J Cancer 1995;71:587–591.

Stein HJ, Sendler A, Fink U: Multidisciplinary approach to esophageal and gastric cancer. Surg Clin North Am 2000;80:659–682.

Uemura N, Okamoto S, Yamamoto S: Heliocobacter pylori infection and the development of gastric cancer. New Engl J Med 2001;345:784–789.

Vanhoefer U, Rougier P, Wilke H: Final results of a randomized phase III trial of sequential high dose methotrexate, fluorouracil, and doxorubicin versus etoposide, leucovorin, and fluorouracil versus infusional fluorouracil and cisplatin in advanced gastric cancer: A trial of the European Organization for Research and Treatment of Cancer Gastrointestinal Tract Cooperative Group. J Clin Oncol 2000;18:2648–2657.

Wanebo HJ, Kennedy BJ, Chmiel J: Cancer of the stomach: A patient care study by the American College of Surgeons. Ann Surg 1993;218:583–592.

Webb A, Cunningham D, Scarffe JH: Randomized trial comparing epirubicin, cisplatin, and fluorouracil versus fluorouracil, doxorubicin, and methotrexate in advanced esophagogastric cancer. J Clin Oncol 1997;15:261–267.

Wils JA, Klein HO, Wagener DJ: Sequential high-dose methotrexate and fluorouracil combined with doxorubicin—A step ahead in the treatment of advanced gastric cancer: A trial of the European Organization for Research and Treatment of Cancer Gastrointestinal Tract Cooperative Group. J Clin Oncol 1991;9:827–831.

Zhang ZX, Gu XZ, Yin WB: Randomized control trial on the combination of preoperative irradiation and surgery in the treatment of adenocarcinoma of gastric cardia (AGC)—Report on 370 patients. Int J Radiat Oncol Biol Phys 1998;42:929–934.

Chapter 90
Hepatobiliary Cancers

Alan P. Venook

Primary cancers of the liver, bile ducts, and gallbladder are often considered together as hepatobiliary cancers, given the fact that they are an anatomically related set of diseases. However, because of the divergent etiologies, presentations, and therapy, they will be considered separately in this chapter.

Primary Liver Cancer

A variety of histologic cancers can arise from the liver, but by far the most common is hepatocellular carcinoma (HCC). The fibrolamellar variant of hepatocellular carcinoma, which tends to occur in young women, is a rare and slow-growing cancer that is often distinguished from hepatocellular carcinoma but may appear to be indolent because of the absence of underlying liver disease. Other cancers, such as angiosarcoma and hepatic lymphoma, are so rare that they will not be discussed further in this chapter.

The vast majority of patients with hepatocellular carcinoma have preexisting underlying liver disease, either cirrhosis or hepatitis. On the basis of observations that hepatocellular carcinoma seemed prevalent in parts of the world with endemic hepatitis, epidemiologists demonstrated in the 1980s that underlying active hepatitis B (HBV) was a cause of hepatocellular carcinoma. Further epidemiologic studies confirmed this finding, and the molecular mechanisms by which chronic hepatitis B infection leads to primary liver cancer are slowly being clarified.

Chronic hepatitis C (HCV) infection is also a risk factor for hepatocellular carcinoma. Hepatitis C virus exposure leads to chronic infection in about 80% of exposed individuals, despite the presence of antibodies to the virus. Although hepatocellular carcinoma is still rare in the United States, it is increasing in incidence, mirroring the development of cirrhosis in patients exposed to hepatitis C virus through transfusions administered before the virus was screened from the blood supply. With an estimated four million people in the United States infected with hepatitis C

virus, the number of cases of hepatocellular carcinoma is certain to rise.

The focus on hepatitis B and C viruses does not mean that other factors do not predispose patients to hepatocellular carcinoma, although these are minor contributors. Alcoholic liver disease, long blamed for hepatocellular carcinoma in some parts of the world, apparently contributes mostly as a cofactor, since evidence of hepatitis C virus infection can be found in many patients who are thought to have alcoholic cirrhosis. Other causes of cirrhosis, such as inborn errors of metabolism (alpha-1 antitrypsin deficiency, for example) or chronic inflammatory diseases such as ulcerative colitis or autoimmune hepatitis, may also lead to hepatocellular carcinoma, although with less regularity.

Clinical Presentation

Patients with hepatocellular carcinoma generally come to medical attention in one of two ways. Patients who have underlying liver disease are often followed closely, perhaps for antihepatitis therapy as well as for surveillance for the development of hepatocellular carcinoma. In these patients, there are often no distinguishing symptoms of hepatocellular carcinoma, which may be detected either through a rise in the serum alpha-fetoprotein (AFP) level or on screening radiologic studies. In these patients, hepatocellular carcinoma may also become apparent through an asymptomatic perturbation of liver function tests.

The presentation of hepatocellular carcinoma in people who are not known to have underlying liver disease may be quite different. Although it is unusual, sudden and intense abdominal pain may be an acute presentation due to tumor rupture. More commonly, right upper quadrant pain of a less dramatic nature occurs, related to internal necrosis of an enlarging tumor or hepatic capsular distension from tumor hemorrhage. These patients may also complain of shoulder pain, referred from diaphragmatic irritation.

Patients may develop evidence of liver dysfunction such as jaundice, edema and/or ascites, or easy bruisability or may present with clinical sequelae of portal hypertension such as variceal bleeding or encephalopathy.

Hepatocellular carcinoma may also present with paraneoplastic phenomena as the first sign of disease. These syndromes are far-ranging, and the diagnosis of hepatocellular carcinoma might not be an initial consideration, particularly if the liver function tests are normal. The most frequent paraneoplastic events include fever, erythrocytosis, hypercalcemia, and pruritus (in the absence of hyperbilirubinemia). Indeed, when questioned, many patients with hepatocellular carcinoma will recall intermittent fevers and night sweats or mild itching. Although very unusual, hepatocellular carcinoma may also first present as an "unknown primary" with distant metastases to the bone and lung, for example.

Clinical Evaluation

Physical findings are variable. Palpable abdominal masses are unusual, whereas subtle evidence of chronic liver disease, such as spider angiomata or palmar erythema, is relatively common. More overt signs of advanced liver disease, such as scleral icterus, jaundice, ascites, caput medusa, or splenomegaly, may also be noted. The classic description of a bruit heard in auscultation over the liver is distinctly unusual in Western countries.

The presentation or physical findings lead to abdominal imaging. The symptomatic patient may be assessed with abdominal ultrasound, computed tomography (CT), or magnetic resonance (MRI) scanning, each of which may disclose a hepatic mass and other associated findings such as ascites or portal vein thrombosis. In patients with cirrhosis, ultrasound is neither sensitive nor specific for hepatocellular carcinoma, and other imaging modalities need to be employed.

The complete and definitive radiologic assessment of patients with hepatocellular carcinoma, however, often requires further tests. Because surgery is the best approach to treatment, precise identification of tumor borders and vascular involvement and the enumeration and site of multiple lesions is required. In general, computed tomography or magnetic resonance imaging is far superior to ultrasound for this level of evaluation. Spiral computed tomography and magnetic resonance imaging appear to be equivalent although sometimes complementary, particularly in characterizing flow through the portal vein. Of course, imaging of the chest and pelvis to exclude metastases is imperative prior to undertaking surgical resection. Because bone metastases are rare in hepatocellular carcinoma, bone scanning is not indicated in the absence of symptoms.

Much of the laboratory evaluation will already have been conducted by the time the diagnosis is made, particularly in the symptomatic patient. Most patients will have had a complete blood count and liver function tests. The commonest finding among these would be thrombocytopenia as well as elevated transaminase or hyperbilirubinemia. Low serum albumin and prolongation of the prothrombin time may also occur. The presence of a hepatic mass in the absence of another known primary cancer, particularly in the setting of cirrhosis, should lead to an alpha-fetoprotein determination. If the alpha-fetoprotein is particularly elevated—above 400 ng/mL in patients without hepatitis B virus and 4000 ng/mL in the presence of hepatitis B virus—biopsy of the mass is not necessary to make the diagnosis of hepatocellular carcinoma.

The other critical laboratory assessment is a search for the underlying etiology of hepatocellular carcinoma. Serological tests for hepatitis B and C viruses are the first step, since these carry treatment as well as public health ramifications. Depending on those findings and on the clinical setting, a search for the more exotic causes of liver disease and hepatocellular carcinoma, such as Wilson disease or alpha-1 antitrypsin deficiency, may be appropriate.

With this information in hand, the definitive diagnosis might not require a biopsy (if the alpha-fetoprotein level is elevated), although one is usually done. While the risk of serious bleeding following core biopsy of hepatocellular carcinoma is often cited as a reason not to get tissue, the risk of a fine-needle aspirate is relatively small. Unfortunately, hepatocellular carcinoma tumors are often necrotic in the center, reflecting internal hemorrhage, and fine-needle aspiration may be surprisingly nondiagnostic despite the computed tomography–guided biopsy. If the diagnosis is in doubt, a laparoscopy or other unusual steps may be required, such as fine-needle aspiration of portal vein thrombus, to confirm the tissue diagnosis.

Staging, Prognostic Features, and Outcomes

The AJCC staging system appears in Table 90-1. This TNM paradigm is based on size, distribution, and number of intrahepatic tumors along with nodal and distant metastases, either of which portends an incurable disease. One unusual aspect of this staging system for hepatocellular carcinoma is the separation of stage IV into an A classification for portal vein involvement and a B subtype to denote distant metastatic disease.

While this staging convention looks good on paper, it is of little independent value in determining

Table 90-1 ▪ AJCC Staging of Liver Cancer: Definition of TNM

Primary Tumor (T)

TX	Primary tumor cannot be assessed
T0	No evidence of primary tumor
T1	Solitary tumor 2 cm or less in greatest dimension without vascular invasion
T2	Solitary tumor 2 cm or less in greatest dimension with vascular invasion, or multiple tumors limited to one lobe, none more than 2 cm in greatest dimension without vascular invasion, or a solitary tumor more than 2 cm in greatest dimension without vascular invasion
T3	Solitary tumor more than 2 cm in greatest dimension with vascular invasion, or multiple tumors limited to one lobe, none more than 2 cm in greatest dimension, with vascular invasion, or multiple tumors limited to one lobe, any more than 2 cm in greatest dimension, with or without vascular invasion
T4	Multiple tumors in more than one lobe or tumor(s) involve(s) a major branch of the portal or hepatic vein(s) or invasion of adjacent organs other than the gallbladder or perforation of the visceral peritoneum

Regional Lymph Nodes (N)

NX	Regional lymph nodes cannot be assessed
N0	No regional lymph node metastasis
N1	Regional lymph node metastasis

Distant Metastasis (M)

MX	Distant metastasis cannot be assessed
M0	No distant metastasis
M1	Distant metastasis

STAGE GROUPING

Stage I	T1	N0	M0
Stage II	T2	N0	M0
Stage IIIA	T3	N0	M0
Stage IIIB	T1	N1	M0
	T2	N1	M0
	T3	N1	M0
Stage IVA	T4	Any N	M0
Stage IVB	Any T	Any N	M1

From American Joint Committee on Cancer, American Cancer Society and American College of Surgeons: AJCC Cancer Staging Manual, 5th ed. Philadelphia: Lippincott Williams & Wilkins, 1997.

prognoses or treatment options for patients even with limited hepatocellular carcinoma, since it does not incorporate any measures of reserve liver function, which is a critical factor that often determines the survival of patients with hepatocellular carcinoma. The Okuda system (Table 90-2) incorporates rough measures of hepatic involvement with objective findings such as ascites, encephalopathy, and bilirubin level and can clinically categorize patients into these prognostic groups. Unfortunately, there is no international consensus on combining the UIJCC and Okuda systems. Ultimately, prognosis is most related to the health of the underlying liver, since the majority of patients with hepatocellular carcinoma succumb to liver failure, which might not be directly related to tumor progression.

A number of independent prognostic factors are related to tumor biology of hepatocellular carcinoma. Since the entire damaged liver may be at risk for developing hepatocellular carcinoma, the presence of a single, isolated tumor confers a superior prognosis to multifocal disease. The development of new tumors in residual liver tissue may be as important as, or more

Table 90-2 ▪ Okuda Staging System

Feature

Tumor size: encompasses > 50% of the liver
Ascites: present or absent
Albumin: >3 g/dL
Bilirubin: >3 mg/dL

Stages (based on number of features present)
Stage I: None of above
Stage II: 1 or 2 of above
Stage III: 3 or 4 of above

important than, the risk of intrahepatic metastases from the original primary. As in most cancers, well-differentiated histology is somewhat favorable. Most experts also believe that the underlying etiology is of biologic importance as well, hepatocellular carcinoma in the setting of hepatitis B virus infection having a poorer prognosis than others. While there is a substantial literature on molecular and other features of both tumor and neighboring nontumorous liver, these have not proven to be of clinical utility.

Survival of patients with hepatocellular carcinoma is a function of the aforementioned variables. Only about 25% of patients are candidates for surgical resection, and just 25% to 30% of those are long-term survivors. The anticipated survival of patients with unresectable disease is highly variable, based on the status of the underlying liver and/or hepatitis, although few patients survive more than three years.

Treatment

Surgical extirpation of hepatocellular carcinoma is the preferred treatment. However, because of the complicating factors that are often associated with hepatocellular carcinoma, the operation may be either technically impossible or unsafe because of inadequate hepatic reserve. If resection is contemplated, the outcomes are superior at centers that perform a large number of such operations.

If a limited-stage hepatocellular carcinoma is not resectable because of underlying cirrhosis, location within the liver, or proximity to critical structures, local ablative measures may be applicable. Cryotherapy (freezing) and radiofrequency hyperthermia (heating) are two methods of tumor destruction that are performed either via the laparoscope or at laparotomy. Ethanol or other necrotizing agents may also be applied percutaneously with ultrasound guidance. Each of these methods can successfully control the targeted tumor, although they are limited by their dependence on visualization and by the same risks of tumor recurrence or tumor dissemination. Some investigators maintain that ablative techniques are as effective as surgical resection, although a direct comparative study has never been conducted.

The optimal treatment for hepatocellular carcinoma (and the underlying liver disease) is orthotopic liver transplant. The outcome of orthotopic liver transplantation in selected patients—those with three or fewer hepatocellular carcinoma tumors, none of which exceeds 5 cm—is as good as that in patients without hepatocellular carcinoma. Furthermore, the liver disease is resolved. However, the unavailability of donor organs and the long waiting list for transplant make this impractical for most patients. Orthotopic

liver transplantation removes the primary, but many patients recur in the abdomen later owing to previously occult micrometastatic disease.

When the hepatocellular carcinoma is multifocal, very large or unresectable, or metastatic or the patient is otherwise not a candidate for transplant, the treatment of hepatocellular carcinoma is palliative. The absence of any one efficacious strategy has led to a proliferation of approaches, none of which is clearly the best and none of which clearly achieves improved outcomes. These treatments include systemic chemotherapy, regional chemotherapy with or without embolization, and a variety of novel methods to deliver treatment selectively to tumors in the liver.

Tamoxifen, a weak estrogen that is used in the treatment of breast cancer, has been tested extensively in hepatocellular carcinoma but appears to be inactive. Somatostatin analog, which is effective in treating hormone-secreting tumors, does not appear to have antitumor effect yet may prolong survival of patients with hepatocellular carcinoma. Systemic chemotherapy is generally considered ineffective. Standard treatment is single-agent doxorubicin, which has not been shown to prolong survival and which has a low objective response rate. Combination chemotherapy protocols have generally been associated with substantial toxicity and little benefit, although recent data suggest that the regimen of cisplatin, doxorubicin, α-interferon, and 5-fluorouracil can induce response in about 25% of patients and can convert some patients' tumors to resectability. Because of the comorbidities that are often seen in patients with hepatocellular carcinoma, particularly baseline liver dysfunction and cytopenias, these systemic chemotherapies are associated with severe toxicities, including mucositis, diarrhea, and sepsis.

Regional chemotherapy via the hepatic artery (HAI) has been studied extensively. Because hepatic tumors get the majority of the blood supply from the hepatic artery, pharmacologic principles make this a logical route of administration. The major response rate for hepatic artery infusion chemotherapy may be as high as 50%, but this approach is applicable to a minority of patients with hepatocellular carcinoma owing to the likelihood of coexistent liver dysfunction. Most often, hepatic artery infusion chemotherapy is coadministered with embolizing particles, which either completely occlude the arterial supply of the tumor or markedly decrease arterial perfusion. Lipidol, a contrast agent that is lipophilic and is employed as a drug carrier, is often included in chemotherapy mixtures. These approaches, called chemoembolization, are associated with tumor necrosis and palliation of symptoms in some patients, but numerous randomized studies have failed to demonstrate a survival advantage from their application.

Because of the multifocal nature of hepatocellular carcinoma and the high risk of recurrence or new primaries in patients treated with resection or tumor ablation, preventive and/or adjuvant treatments have been emphasized. Prevention, the most appealing strategy, can work, as illustrated by the effort in Taiwan to eliminate hepatitis B from a generation of Taiwanese born to mothers with the hepatitis B carrier state. Immediate hepatitis B vaccination has virtually eliminated childhood hepatocellular carcinoma in this very high-risk population. Two adjuvant strategies have demonstrated potential efficacy, although neither is readily available. A Japanese group showed benefit from polyprenoic acid, a semisynthetic retinoid, used for one year following definitive surgery for hepatocellular carcinoma, and investigators in Hong Kong showed improved survival in patients treated with radio-labeled lipiodol into the hepatic artery following hepatocellular carcinoma resection. Both approaches suggest this is an encouraging course to pursue, although neither can be recommended outside of a clinical trial.

Follow-Up Evaluation

Algorithms for follow-up are predicated on the belief that early detection of recurrence may result in improved therapeutic options. A minority of patients—perhaps 10% to 20%—who undergo definitive resection or ablation of hepatocellular carcinoma may still have options for curative therapy at the time of recurrence, particularly if they are otherwise candidates for orthotopic liver transplantation. For that reason, such patients are often followed with serial alpha-fetoprotein levels and liver imaging at three- to six-month intervals. In general, however, the second-chance options are limited, and most patients will fall into the palliative setting even if the new primary hepatocellular carcinoma or recurrence is detected early. These patients are also usually followed closely for evidence of hepatic decompensation, which may occur even in the absence of tumor recurrence.

Biliary Cancers

Cancers of the biliary tree are divided into those of the intrahepatic, perihilar, or distal biliary tree as well as peripheral bile ducts. Chronic biliary inflammatory processes, such as those induced by liver fluke infestation or in the setting of ulcerative colitis, predispose patients to this cancer, although most patients have no apparent predisposing condition.

Clinical Presentation

The majority of bile duct cancers present as painless jaundice. This may be preceded or accompanied by a variety of systemic manifestations, including fever, anorexia, weight loss, or pruritus. Most patients first note changes in the color of their urine, the orange hue reflecting an increasing bilirubin load being excreted through the kidneys. Stools may develop a classic "clay" color due to the absence of bilirubin metabolites. Bile duct cancers almost never present with cholangitic findings, such as chills and bacteremia, because the biliary tract is sterile, at least until it is manipulated for the first time by endoscopy.

In contrast, peripheral cholangiocarcinomas may present as abdominal masses, painful or not, with symptoms such as early satiety or shoulder pain related to diaphragmatic irritation. Because of the efficiency of bile clearance in the uninvolved liver, these peripheral hepatic tumors often present without hyperbilirubinemia.

Clinical Evaluation

There might be no physical findings other than jaundice in patients with obstructing biliary tumors, since the relative acuity of the presentation does not allow development of the stigmata of chronic liver disease. Palpable abdominal masses are extremely unusual except when the tumor is in the periphery and when the patient does not present with jaundice.

The first diagnostic test for a patient with painless jaundice is either an ultrasound of the right upper quadrant or an abdominal computed tomography scan. If dilated biliary ducts are found, the source of the obstruction is then determined. If there is no biliary duct dilatation, the cause of the jaundice is not likely to be obstruction. A computed tomography scan may show a mass lesion in the liver, head of the pancreas, or porta hepatis, each of which raises the probability of cancer. However, only about 20% of patients with biliary tumors have masses that are visualized on scanning, since these tumors are usually quite small and within the ducts.

The next diagnostic step is to visualize the biliary tree, either by percutaneous transhepatic cholangiography (PTC) or through an endoscopic retrograde cholangiopancreatogram (ERCP). The latter procedure offers both diagnostic and therapeutic opportunities, ranging from the identification of the site of obstruction, a biopsy of a mass, or brushings of the suspicious region for cytology and the placement of a temporary stent through the obstruction to drain the biliary system. Biliary obstruction high in the substance of the liver is often first assessed with percutaneous transhepatic cholangiography, while more distal blockage is often approached via endoscopic retrograde cholangiopancreatogram.

Because surgery needs to be considered as the initial option, precise identification of the extent of bile duct involvement, vascular encasement, and the presence of metastases is important. Therefore, the initial diagnostic study will often be just the first of many radiologic procedures targeting the liver.

Much of the laboratory evaluation will already have been conducted by the time the diagnosis is confirmed, since most patients present with jaundice and the initial assessment will have included a variety of blood tests. The finding of laboratory abnormalities other than hyperbilirubinemia and mild elevation of the transaminases and alkaline phosphatase should raise the suspicion of a diagnosis other than biliary cancer, since one would not expect cytopenias or major defects in protein synthesis in these patients.

Patients with peripheral cholangiocarcinoma usually present with an isolated hepatic mass that is large and almost always unresectable. These patients typically undergo an evaluation for adenocarcinoma of unknown primary before the diagnosis is made by exclusion. These rare tumors are then assessed for resectability, just as one would evaluate any isolated hepatic tumor.

Staging, Prognostic Features, and Outcomes

Before addressing staging, the treating physician will often need to proceed with treatment planning in the absence of a tissue diagnosis. Frequently, there is no mass to biopsy, cytologic brushings are nondiagnostic or merely "suspicious," and definitive proof of malignancy is lacking. In such patients, if there is no evidence of metastatic cancer, an operation should be done, either to potentially resect the cancer or to alleviate the cause of the biliary stricture.

Just as in the staging of hepatocellular carcinoma, there is a conventional TNM classification for biliary cancers. This has great relevance for prognosis, since N or M positive patients have incurable tumors and should not be considered for definitive therapy. In the absence of clear-cut nodal or metastatic disease, however, surgical exploration needs to be considered.

Prognosis and the surgical procedure are largely a function of the anatomic location of the biliary tract cancer. Tumors that occur right at the bifurcation of the right and left hepatic bile ducts, called Klatskin's tumor, have a favorable prognosis, probably because they are found very early in the natural history of their progression. Similarly, tumors may arise in the intrapancreatic portion of the bile duct and cause obstructive jaundice early in their course, making them relatively favorable lesions. On the other hand,

bile duct tumors in the remaining portions of the biliary tree are often more extensive and more likely to have involved contiguous structures or have spread to lymph nodes. These tumors are rarely resectable for cure.

Only about 15% to 20% of patients with biliary cancers are deemed respectable, and the long-term disease-free survival rate of such patients is no more than 30%. Patients with unresectable disease have a life expectancy less than two years.

Treatment

Surgery is the only curative therapy for biliary tract cancers and, as was stated previously, is an option for only selected patients. The specific surgery that is required depends on the location of the tumor. Klatskin's tumors may be removed with reconstruction of the bile duct with a Roux-en-Y loop of jejunum. Tumors of the right or left bile duct may be resected en bloc with the lobe of the involved liver. Tumors of the distal bile duct may require a Whipple procedure, which entails the removal of the head of the pancreas, bile duct, gallbladder, and duodenum. The rare peripheral cholangiocarcinoma may be resected with a hepatic lobectomy. Each of these operations carries substantial morbidity and should be performed by experienced surgeons at centers with a long track record of treated patients. Although the majority of these patients will have undergone placement of a stent during their evaluation, there is no consensus on whether patients undergoing these surgeries should have bile duct stenting before the operation takes place.

Once curative surgery is completed, there may be a role for adjuvant chemotherapy and radiation. Tumors in the distal bile duct are often lumped with tumors of the head of the pancreas or ampulla of Vater, and there are some data to support a role for chemoradiation. There are, however, no prospective data arguing for adjuvant therapy following resection of more proximal biliary tumors. Furthermore, the morbidity associated with radiation delivered to the hepatic bed may well be substantial.

The treatment of unresectable biliary tumors is not well studied. Locally advanced tumors are first managed with biliary stenting. Indeed, the ability to normalize bile flow may be the most important predictor for survival in such patients. There are anecdotal reports of long-term survival in a patient after stenting and external beam radiation, but this is not an established therapy, and the morbidity can be substantial. Internal catheters bearing radiation, so-called brachytherapy, is an interesting technique but has never been compared to conventional external beam radiation. Similarly, conformal radiation involving three-dimensional treatment planning can be admin-

TREATMENT

Biliary Drainage

In patients who have bile duct cancers, the quality of life and survival are most often determined by the ability to maintain bile flow. Therefore, while surgery, chemotherapy, and/or radiation therapy have roles, the first order of business is to maximize drainage of the biliary tree.

Biliary drainage (stenting) can be accomplished in many ways and with various appliances:

Endoscopic: Usually done via an endoscopic retrograde cholangiopancreatogram, this is often the preferred choice, since the entire procedure can be done without any external appliance or manipulation. Success is a function of the skill and experience of the endoscopist but also of the anatomic location of the blockage. Lesions that are high up in the biliary tree may be difficult to bypass endoscopically, whereas obstruction at the level of the hilum of the liver or ampulla of Vater may be more readily relieved.

Percutaneous: Transhepatic drainage can be done in almost any patient, although the need for an external appliance makes this unpopular. However, if an endoscopic retrograde cholangiopancreatogram fails and the bile ducts are dilated, the percutaneous approach must be considered. In general, temporary percutaneous catheters can be changed to fully internalized stents in a multistep procedure.

Surgical: Choledochojejunostomy done either at laparotomy or via the laparoscope may be an excellent and better palliative maneuver than biliary stenting, but the morbidity of surgery often outweighs the advantages.

In general, initial efforts at stenting are made with plastic devices. These can be removed or exchanged, a particularly important feature given the risk of biliary tract infections once stenting is done. There are no randomized data showing any clear value to prophylactic stent changes in the biliary tract. Metallic stents may be preferable for the longer term, because the inherent resilience of metallic devices may resist tumor ingrowth. However, metallic stents cannot be removed once they are placed.

This author's approach: If the initial plastic stent is functioning, leave it alone. Exchange for a metallic stent if there is clinical evidence of tumor in-growth or if the plastic stent requires exchanging due to sluggish flow or infection.

istered to biliary tumors but remains an investigational approach.

The role for chemotherapy in biliary tumors is not clear. Anecdotal reports of activity are found for most chemotherapeutic agents, but none has clearly been demonstrated to confer a survival advantage, partly because prospective studies of biliary tumors are not often reported. Gemcitabine, the first-line treatment for pancreatic cancer, has been disappointing in biliary tumors. By default, the treatment that is most often used is a 5-fluorouracil-based chemotherapy.

Follow-up Evaluation

As with other cancers, the intensity of follow-up after definitive therapy should reflect the options that will exist if a tumor recurrence can be found at its earliest stage. For biliary cancers, it is difficult to imagine a scenario in which a curative option could exist at the time of recurrence. For that reason, aggressive surveillance is not recommended.

For patients with indwelling stents, either following definitive surgery or in the palliative setting, the optimal management is controversial. Metallic stents are often employed for malignant strictures and these cannot be removed. Plastic stents may be exchanged regularly by the endoscopists in an effort to avoid cholangitis, although prophylactic stent exchange has not been validated by randomized studies.

Gallbladder Cancer

Carcinoma of the gallbladder is an uncommon tumor with a very poor prognosis. The majority of these are adenocarcinomas, and although other histologies occur, they are all treated in the same way. Gallbladder cancer tends to be a disease of elderly women and may be related to frequent and recurrent cholelithiasis. The clearest risk factor is the so-called porcelain gallbladder, which is calcified following chronic inflammation, prompting some to advocate prophylactic cholecystectomy in such patients. Typhoid carriers also have an increased risk of gallbladder cancer.

Clinical Presentation

Gallbladder cancer may present with findings indistinguishable from those of bile duct cancers, since involvement of the cystic duct may extend to the main hepatic bile duct. It may also present as an abdominal mass, painful or not, with symptoms such as early satiety or shoulder pain related to diaphragmatic irritation. Advanced cases may mimic hepatocellular carcinoma, with ascites, anorexia, and jaundice. Gallbladder cancer may also be an incidental finding when cholecystectomy is performed for what is presumed to be chronic or acute cholelithiasis or cholecystitis.

Clinical Evaluation

The evaluation of these patients is a function of the presenting symptoms. Because this disease may be indistinguishable from hepatocellular carcinoma or biliary tract cancer until the full diagnostic evaluation is completed, the workup follows the previous discussion. The patient who presents with an abdominal mass, anorexia, ascites, or other overt manifestations of advanced gallbladder cancer is first evaluated with abdominal imaging. Identification of a mass or ascites then leads to a biopsy, either via a fine-needle or cytologic assessment of fluid, to make the diagnosis. An endoscopic retrograde cholangiopancreatogram offers both diagnostic and therapeutic opportunities, including the identification of the site of obstruction, a biopsy of a mass, or brushings of the suspicious region for cytology and the placement of a temporary stent through the obstruction to drain the biliary system.

Although it is highly unlikely that surgery will be indicated in an advanced patient such as this, it needs to be considered as the initial option. The precise identification of the extent of bile duct involvement, vascular encasement, and the presence of metastases usually exclude a surgical approach. If that evaluation suggests that surgical resection is still possible, imaging of the chest and pelvis to exclude metastases is done. Because bone metastases are quite unusual in bile duct cancer, bone scanning is not usually indicated.

Staging, Prognostic Features, and Outcome

As with hepatocellular carcinoma and biliary tumors, there is a conventional TNM staging system for cancer of the gallbladder. However, more than half of all patients with gallbladder cancer present with local extension, node-positive disease, or metastatic disease, which is incurable. The TNM staging is more relevant for patients with "incidental" gallbladder cancer, since such patients will be cured on occasion. Unfortunately, conventional techniques for cholecystectomy, particularly via the laparoscope, do not yield important staging information such as peritoneal spread, intrahepatic metastases, or the assessment of regional lymph nodes. Most often, the surgeon is surprised when notified by the pathologist that the gallbladder contained cancer. In that situation, a computed tomography scan of the abdomen is belatedly done to exclude evident metastatic disease and to obtain clinical staging.

Other than this rare event of unexpected diagnosis by surgery, the long-term survival rate of patients with gallbladder cancer is less than 5%. There is no evidence that histology, tumor grade, or other features can identify a different prognostic subset of patients.

Treatment

In most circumstances, the management of patients with gallbladder cancer is palliative. This includes effecting biliary drainage if possible as well as managing the symptoms associated with abdominal involvement of cancer. There is no clear evidence that chemotherapy and/or radiation therapy is beneficial, although there are occasional case reports of patients having long-term survival after such treatment. The most common chemotherapy is 5-fluorouracil-based.

The exceptional patient with an incidental finding of gallbladder cancer is treated aggressively, however. Once the diagnosis is made and radiologic studies do not find evidence of metastatic or advanced cancer, a second operation is warranted. Although it has never been tested in a randomized controlled study, the surgery would appear to improve curability of the disease. At the operation, evaluation for metastatic disease within the peritoneal cavity is done. Once this is grossly excluded, a regional lymph node dissection is carried out. Finally, the gallbladder bed is resected with a rim of liver from that region. This approach appears to account for the occasional patient who survives gallbladder cancer.

References

Hepatocellular Carcinoma

Alter MJ, Kruszon-Moran D, Nainan OV, et al: The prevalence of hepatitis C virus infection in the United States, 1988 through 1994. N Engl J Med 1999;341:556–562.

Beasley RP, Lin C-C, Hwang L-Y, Chien C-S: Hepatocellular carcinoma and hepatitis B virus. Lancet 1981;2:1129–1133.

Begg CB, Cramer LD, Hoskins WJ, Brennan MF: Impact of hospital volume on operative mortality for major cancer surgery. JAMA 1998;280:1747–1751.

Bergsland EK, Venook AP: Hepatocellular carcinoma. Curr Opin Oncol 2000;12:357–361.

Berman MM, Libbey NP, Foster JH: Hepatocellular carcinoma: Polygonal cell type with fibrous stroma—an atypical variant with a favorable prognosis. Cancer 1980;46:1448–1455.

Chang M-H, Chen C-J, Lai M-S, et al: Universal Hepatitis B vaccination in Taiwan and the incidence of hepatocellular carcinoma in children. N Engl J Med 1997;336:1855–1859.

Colombo M, De Franchis R, Del Ninno E, et al: Hepatocellular carcinoma in Italian patients with cirrhosis. N Engl J Med 1991;325:675–680.

Cottone M, Turri M, Caltagirone M, et al: Screening for hepatocellular carcinoma in patients with Child's A cirrhosis: An 8-year prospective study by ultrasound and alphafetoprotein. J Hepatol 1994;21:1029–1034.

Curley SA, Izzo F, Ellis LM et al: Radiofrequency ablation of hepatocellular cancer in 110 patients with cirrhosis. Ann Surg 2000;232:381–391.

Dodd GD, III, Miller WJ, Baron RL, et al: Detection of malignant tumors in end-stage cirrhotic livers: Efficacy of sonography as a screening technique. AJR Am J Roentgenol 1992;159:727–733.

El-Serag HB, Mason AC: Rising incidence of hepatocellular carcinoma in the United States. N Engl J Med 1999; 340:745–799.

Glasgow RE, Showstack JA, Katz PP, et al: The relationship between hospital volume and outcomes of hepatic resection for hepatocellular carcinoma. Arch Surg 1999;134:30–35.

Groupe d'Etude et de Traitement du Carcinome Hepatocellulaire: A comparison of Lipiodol chemoembolization and conservative treatment for unresectable hepatocellular carcinoma. N Engl J Med 1995;332:1256–1261.

Johnson PJ, Williams R, Thomas H, et al: Induction of remission in hepatocellular carcinoma with doxorubicin. Lancet 1978;1:1006–1009.

Kouroumalis E, Skordilis P, Thermos K, et al: Treatment of hepatocellular carcinoma with octreotide: A randomised controlled study. Gut 1998;42:442–447.

Lau W, Leung W, Ho S, et al: Adjuvant intra-arterial iodine-131-labelled lipiodol for resectable hepatocellular carcinoma: A prospective randomised trial. Lancet 1999;353:797–801.

Leung TWT, Patt YZ, Lau W-y, et al: Complete pathological remission is possible with systemic combination chemotherapy for inoperable hepatocellular carcinoma. Clin Canc Res 1999;5:1676–1681.

Livraghi T, Bolondi L, Lazzaroni S, et al: Percutaneous ethanol injection in the treatment of hepatocellular carcinoma in cirrhosis. Cancer 1992;69:925–929.

Llovet JM, Bustamante J, Castells A, et al: Natural history of untreated nonsurgical hepatocellular carcinoma: Rationale for the design and evaluation of therapeutic trials. Hepatology 1999;29:62–67.

Llovet JM, Bruix J, Gores GJ: Surgical resection versus transplantation for early hepatocellular carcinoma: Clues for the best strategy. Hepatology 2000;31:1019–1021.

Marsh JW, Dvorchik I, Bonham CA, Iwatsuki S: Is the pathologic TNM staging system for patients with hepatoma predictive of outcome? Cancer 2000;88:538–543.

Mazzaferro V, Regalia E, Doci R, et al: Liver transplantation for the treatment of small hepatocellular carcinomas in patients with cirrhosis. N Engl J Med 1996;334:693–699.

Muto Y, Moriwaki H, Ninomiya M, et al: Prevention of second primary tumors by an acyclic retinoid, polyprenoic acid, in patients with hepatocellular carcinoma. N Engl J Med 1996;334:1561–1567.

Nishiguchi S, Kuroki T, Nakatani S, et al: Randomised trial of effects of interferon-a on incidence of hepatocellular carcinoma in chronic active hepatitis C with cirrhosis. Lancet 1995;346:1051–1055.

Okuda K, Ohtsuki T, Obata H, et al: Natural history of hepatocellular carcinoma and prognosis in relation to treatment. Cancer 1985;56:918–928.

Tanaka H, Tsukuma H, Kasahara A, et al: Effect of interferon therapy on the incidence of hepatocellular carcinoma and mortality of patients with chronic hepatitis C: A retrospective cohort study of 738 patients. Int J Cancer 2000;87:741–749.

Venook AP: Treatment of hepatocellular carcinoma: Too many options? J Clin Oncol 1994;12:1323–1334.

Bile Duct Cancer

Bismuth H, Malt RA: Carcinoma of the biliary tract. N Engl J Med 1979;301:704–706.

Heslin MJ, Brooks AD, Hochwald SN, et al: A preoperative biliary stent is associated with increased complications after pancreatoduodenectomy. Arch Surg 1998;133:149–154.

Kalser MH, Ellenberg SS: Pancreatic cancer: Adjuvant combined radiation and chemotherapy following curative resection. Arch Surg 1985;120:899–903.

Saini S: Imaging of the hepatobiliary tract. N Engl J Med 1997;336:1889–1894.

Shapiro MJ: Management of malignant biliary obstruction: Nonoperative and palliative techniques. Oncology 1995;9: 493–503.

Gallbladder Cancer

Abi-Rached B, Neugut AI: Diagnostic and management issues in gallbladder carcinoma. Oncology 1995;9:19–24.

Chapter 91
Pancreatic Cancer

Jeffrey W. Clark

Introduction

Pancreatic adenocarcinoma ranks as the fifth leading cause of death from malignancy in the United States. By the time of diagnosis, it is rarely curable. A measure of its dismal prognosis is that annually in the United States, approximately 29,200 new cases of pancreatic adenocarcinoma are diagnosed, and 28,900 patients die from the disease. The only potential for cure lies in surgical excision if this is feasible. Unfortunately, most patients have extensive disease and are not candidates for surgery. Even among the 25% of patients who undergo surgical resection with curative intent, only 20% to 25% are long-term survivors. Thus, overall only approximately 5% of patients are alive and disease-free at five years. Palliative therapy such as biliary tract diversion, chemotherapy, and/or radiation therapy can relieve symptoms in patients with unresectable disease, but therapy does not significantly affect five-year survival rates.

Current trials are evaluating whether optimal integration of surgery, radiation therapy, chemotherapy, and immunotherapy (e.g., vaccines) can improve the survival of patients who can be surgically resected but are at high risk for recurrent or metastatic disease.

Incidence and Epidemiology

As with most solid tumors, the incidence of pancreatic adenocarcinoma rises with increasing age. It is uncommon before the age of 50 but increases in the ensuing decades. Although the incidence of disease in some countries has varied over time, the incidence of pancreatic cancer in the United States and Western Europe has remained unchanged during the past 25 years. Disease prevalence is equal among men and women. In the United States, for uncertain reasons, the incidence among African-Americans is higher than in the Caucasian population.

A number of potential risk factors for the development of pancreatic adenocarcinoma have been identified (Table 91-1). Of these, the best established is cigarette smoking, which confers an approximately twofold increase in risk. Pancreatic cancer is more likely to occur in patients whose pancreas received incidental radiation during radiation therapy for other malignancies, such as Hodgkin's disease or testicular cancer. Chronic relapsing pancreatitis, including that due to genetic risk factors (discussed next), is a risk factor for pancreatic cancer. The relationship between diabetes mellitus and the risk of pancreatic cancer remains a point at issue, confounded in part by the frequent development of diabetes as a result of damage to islet cells in the setting of pancreatic cancer. Nevertheless, the weight of evidence favors the view that diabetes mellitus is a risk factor. Increased body mass index could be associated with an increased risk of pancreatic cancer. Although a number of studies suggest that dietary factors such as high fat or red meat intake increase the risk of pancreatic cancer, the evidence remains inconclusive. Little evidence supports the previously held view that previous upper gastrointestinal surgery, especially for peptic ulcer disease or gallbladder disease, plays a role in the genesis of some pancreatic cancers.

Familial genetic alterations that predispose to pancreatic neoplasms include mutations in the following genes:

- p16 tumor suppressor gene
- mismatched repair genes (hMSH2 and hMLH1)
- BRCA1 gene (rare pancreatic cancers)
- BRCA2 gene
- STK11/LKB1 (Peutz-Jeghers syndrome)
- ataxia telangectasia gene
- p53 tumor suppressor gene (Li-Fraumeni syndrome)
- APC gene (familial adenomatous polyposis)
- VHL (von Hippel-Lindau) gene

Most of these changes are associated with a much greater risk for developing malignancies other than

Table 91-1 ■ Risk Factors for Pancreatic Adenocarcinoma

Smoking
Chronic pancreatitis
Diabetes mellitus
Dietary factors
Prior radiation therapy to pancreas as may occur in the therapy of Hodgkin's disease or testicular cancer
Genetic alterations (small percentage of cases)

pancreatic neoplasms. For example, individuals with p16 mutations also have an increased risk of melanoma and breast cancer, and BRCA2 mutations are associated with an increased risk of breast and ovarian cancers.

Mutations in the cationic trypsinogen gene and cystic fibrosis transmembrane regulator (CFTR) gene are associated with chronic relapsing pancreatitis and an increased risk of developing pancreatic cancer. Because these patients can be diagnosed relatively early in the disease process, they are a population for whom the development of effective screening strategies would be worthwhile. At present, the sensitivity and specificity of screening methods for other genetic abnormalities remain inadequate to help in early detection.

In a number of families, the frequency of pancreatic cancer is increased in the absence of identifiable genetic abnormalities; approximately 5% to 10% of patients with pancreatic cancer have a first-degree relative who develops pancreatic cancer.

Pathology

The major cell types within the normal pancreas include ductal cells, acinar cells, and endocrine cells. Acinar cells make up the majority of these cells, followed in number by ductal cells and then cells of endocrine origin. The pancreas also necessarily contains connective tissue support cells and endothelial cells. Malignancies can arise from any of these cell types (Table 91-2). Approximately 90% of malignancies that arise in the exocrine pancreas are derived from duct cells and are adenocarcinomas. Approximately two thirds of these arise in the head of the pancreas, one-third in the body or tail, and a small percentage are multicentric. In addition to typical ductal adenocarcinomas, other histologic subtypes of ductal origin include pleomorphic carcinomas, giant cell carcinomas, microglandular adenocarcinomas, and cystic neoplasms. Cystic neoplasms of the pancreas comprise a small but increasingly identified subgroup of pancreatic tumors. They can be divided into serous cystadenomas (usually benign) and mucinous cystadenocarcinomas. These are usually large tumors that often contain multiple cystic areas. A higher percentage of these tumors occur in middle-aged women as compared with ductal adenocarcinomas. Biologically, they appear to be divided into two groups. One of these has benign or borderline malignant cells with a good prognosis, and the other has overt carcinoma that metastasizes widely. The prognosis in the latter case is similar to that of other ductal adenocarcinomas. Noncystic mucin-producing tumors of the pancreas and papillary cystic tumors of the pancreas (which occur in women during their reproductive years) have a better-than-average prognosis after surgical excision. Acinar cell carcinomas make up 1% to 2% of pancreatic cancers. Although acinar cell tumors occur most commonly in the elderly, they can be found in young patients as well. These tumors represent a higher percentage of pancreatic tumors in children than in adults and have a clinical course similar to that of ductal adenocarcinomas.

Tumors with mixed histologies (including adenosquamous carcinomas and carcinosarcomas) occur in the pancreas as they do in other organs; the prognosis for these variants is worse than average.

Cancers arising from endocrine cells make up approximately 5% of pancreatic tumors. Although they are associated with longer survival than pancreatic adenocarcinomas, they do frequently metastasize. Their biology and treatment are discussed in the later section on pancreatic endocrine tumors.

Table 91-2 ■ Pathology of Pancreatic Neoplasms

Ductal adenocarcinomas
Mucinous noncystic carcinomas
Giant cell tumors
Signet ring cell carcinomas
Mucinous cystadenocarcinomas
Serous cystadenocarcinomas
Intraductal and invasive papillary-mucinous carcinoma
Solid pseudopapillary carcinoma
Acinar cell carcinomas and cystadenocarcinomas
Mixed histologies (adenosquamous, carcinosarcomas, mixed ductal-endocrine, mixed acinar-endocrine)
Undifferentiated
Borderline tumors
Pancreatoblastoma
Endocrine neoplasms
Sarcomas
Lymphomas
Metastatic lesions

Rare pancreatic neoplasms of uncertain histology include pancreaticoblastomas. Their cell of origin is thought to be a multipotential cell that can differentiate into mesenchymal, endocrine, or acinar cells. Pancreaticoblastomas frequently have elevated alpha-fetoprotein levels and are potentially curable when localized. Metastatic pancreaticoblastomas are responsive to chemotherapy but are usually not curable. Lymphomas, sarcomas, and other mesenchymal tumors make up only a minor proportion of pancreatic cancers. Their biology is similar to that of malignancies of like histology arising in other areas of the body on a stage-per-stage basis.

Cancers that can metastasize to the pancreas include breast, lung, melanoma, renal, and gastrointestinal neoplasms.

Biology of Pancreatic Ductal Cancer

Frequently, pancreatic ductal cancers either have invaded locally or have metastasized by the time they are initially detected. They spread directly to soft tissues around the pancreas as well as to adjacent organs. Lesions in the head of the pancreas invade the duodenum and nearby vasculature, including mesenteric vessels, portal vein, and splenic vessels. Cancers of the pancreatic tail extend out into the spleen, colon, and adrenal gland. Metastatic spread is most commonly to regional lymph nodes, liver, peritoneum, lungs, and adrenal glands, and less often to other organs (including bone and brain).

Genetic studies of pancreatic malignancies reveal variable abnormalities listed in Table 91-3. Frequent mutations have been found in proteins involved in cell-signaling pathways (K-ras) as well as in a number of tumor suppressor genes (p53, p16, and DPC4/Smad4). Mutations in the K-ras gene are found in approximately 75% to 90% of pancreatic cancers. The Ras family of proteins is involved in signal trans-

duction for a large number of cellular processes, including relaying signals downstream from activated cell-surface growth-factor receptors. Mutations in ras genes produce a partially transformed phenotype that can be altered to a fully transformed phenotype by additional mutations to provide a proliferative advantage. It is therefore reasonable to believe that mutations in the ras gene are involved in pancreatic carcinogenesis. Among the proteins whose proliferative signals to cells are mediated at least in part through Ras proteins are several families of growth factor receptors. A number of those listed in Table 91-3 are highly expressed in a variable percentage of pancreatic adenocarcinomas. Pancreatic cancers also relatively frequently have mutations in the p53, p16, and DPC4/Smad4 tumor suppressor genes. Similar to the case with Ras proteins, these genes are involved in controlling a number of processes critical for cell function and proliferation. For example, p53 is critical to those processes that ensure DNA integrity and repair, progression of cells through the cell cycle, and apoptosis. The life span of human cells is limited by the progressive shortening of telomeric DNA at the ends of chromosomes. As is true for many malignant cells, the enzyme telomerase, responsible for maintaining telomeric DNA and prolonging cell survival, is elevated in a high percentage of pancreatic ductal carcinomas.

It is less clear what role is played by other mutations found in families that have some increased risk of pancreatic cancer (e.g., BRCA2 or mismatched repair genes) in the development of nonhereditary pancreatic cancers. Mutations in these genes have been found in sporadic cases, but not at a high frequency. When BRCA2 mutations have been found in presumed sporadic cases, careful review has detected germ-line mutations in a significant percentage of cases. Tumors that have mutations in mismatched repair genes but not in Ras proteins have characteristic histopathologic changes and a better-than-average prognosis.

Table 91-3 ■ Genetic Alterations Found in Pancreatic Adenocarcinomas

K-ras mutations (oncogene)
p53 mutations (tumor suppressor gene)
p16 mutations (tumor suppressor gene)
DPC4/Smad4 mutations (tumor suppressor gene)
Growth factor receptor over-expression (e.g., epidermal growth factor receptor, Her2/Neu, and fibroblast growth factor receptor)
Increased telomerase activity (cell immortality)
CD44 variants (cell adhesion molecule)

Presenting Symptoms and Signs

Pancreatic cancers often grow to the point at which they become unresectable even before they are diagnosed; symptoms are absent early in the course of the disease and tend to be minimal and nonspecific as the disease progresses. Symptoms have been present for more than two months prior to diagnosis in the majority of patients. Tumors in the head of the pancreas, which can produce obstruction of the bile duct and jaundice as they grow, can be diagnosed at a relatively earlier stage than tumors of the body or tail. Never-

Table 91-4 ■ Presenting Signs and Symptoms of Pancreatic Adenocarcinoma

Fatigue
Weight loss
Anorexia
Nausea/vomiting
Early satiety
Abdominal pain
Back pain (cancer of the body or tail of the pancreas)
Jaundice/light stools/dark urine/pruritus (cancer of the
    pancreatic head)
Glucose intolerance
Malabsorptive symptoms
Migratory polyphlebitis
Dyspnea
Hematemesis
Ascites
Depression

theless, most cancers of the head of the pancreas are also unresectable by the time of diagnosis.

Fatigue, weight loss, anorexia (see Chapter 1), vague epigastric discomfort or pain, back pain, obstructive jaundice with light stools (see Chapter 32) and pruritus (see Chapter 3), nausea, vomiting, early satiety, dyspnea, and glucose intolerance are the most common presenting symptoms (Table 91-4). One factor involved in weight loss is malabsorption, especially of fats due to exocrine pancreatic dysfunction, which can be accompanied by diarrhea, postprandial abdominal discomfort, anorexia, and cachexia (see Chapter 1) Pain is due primarily to invasion of the mesenteric and celiac nerve plexuses; however, other mechanisms, including invasion of other organs, obstruction, and pancreatitis also can contribute to pain. The causes of the mental depression noted in a substantial proportion of affected patients are unknown. As is true of other adenocarcinomas, pancreatic cancer is associated with a relatively high incidence of venous thrombosis and thrombophlebitis. Migratory polyphlebitis is referred to as Trousseau's syndrome (see Chapter 43). Hematemesis can occur due to invasion of the duodenum or stomach, and intra-abdominal spread can present as malignant ascites (see Chapter 21).

Diagnostic Evaluation

Work-up for the diagnosis of pancreatic cancer begins with the history and physical examination (Figure 91-1). The diagnosis should be considered in individuals who present with the foregoing symptoms, especially when several symptoms are present. One should ascertain whether there is a history of cigarette smoking or other risk factors, and whether there is a family history that might suggest genetic risk factors (although the latter accounts for only a small percentage of pancreatic cancer cases). The recent onset of diabetes or of acute pancreatitis could provide clues to the diagnosis. The physical examination should assess the patient for evidence of weight loss, lymph node enlargement in the left supraclavicular area (Virchow's nodes), tumor in the umbilical area (Sister Mary Joseph nodule), jaundice, hepatomegaly, ascites, peripheral edema, and evidence of coagulopathy, such as superficial or deep venous thrombosis or symptoms suggestive of emboli. A palpable mass could be present in the right-upper quadrant of the abdomen if the tumor has grown to sufficient size. A palpable gallbladder, Courvoisier's sign, may be present. In most patients, however, findings on physical exam are nonspecific.

Laboratory Studies

Laboratory tests should include a complete blood count with differential count and liver function tests. Mild anemia is found in up to one-quarter of patients. Elevations of bilirubin as well as abnormalities in other liver function tests can be present in those with obstructing lesions of the head of the pancreas or metastases to the liver; however, laboratory studies are often normal or only mildly abnormal. The serum CA 19-9 is a useful tumor marker. It is elevated in 70% to 90% of patients with pancreatic cancer. It is not useful as a screening tool because its specificity is not high enough, but it is helpful in following a patient's response to therapy. One needs to be aware that CA 19-9 elevations can occur in patients with jaundice due to benign causes such as a common duct stone or cholangitis. Although CEA levels are less often elevated, occasional patients exhibit increased values in the face of normal CA 19-9 levels.

Imaging Studies

Once pancreatic cancer is suspected, the most important question that needs to be addressed is whether it is potentially resectable (Figure 91-2). Unless there are findings on physical exam or other radiological studies that the disease is already metastatic to the peritoneal cavity, other organs, or distant lymph nodes (which would make it unresectable), findings from computed tomography (CT) scans or magnetic resonance imaging (MRI) studies are usually the critical factor in helping to determine potential resectability.

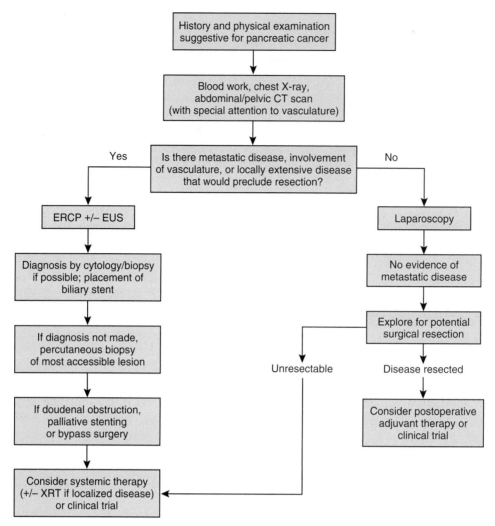

Figure 91-1 ■ Algorithm for diagnosis and treatment of pancreatic cancer. CT = computed tomography; ERCP = endoscopic retrograde cholangiopancreatography; EUS = endoscopic ultrasonography; XRT = radiation therapy.

Computed Tomography and Magnetic Resonance Imaging

Thin-sectioned, high-speed helical computed tomography scan with oral and intravenous contrast administration is the most commonly used modality for assessing the pancreatic mass itself, investigating potential vascular invasion, and determining whether the tumor has metastasized. Alternatively, magnetic resonance imaging can be utilized for this purpose, with equal efficacy. At present, the decision as to which of these to use is dependent on the specific expertise at the institution where it is being performed. Technical improvements in both of these modalities continue to be made, so the determination of which modality might be best awaits further study. Although pulmonary metastases in the absence of abdominal metastases are relatively uncommon, these certainly can occur; imaging of the chest is also impor-

tant. These studies provide a highly reliable assessment of the extent of disease and its potential for surgical resection. Unresectable lesions are those that demonstrate disease outside the pancreas, such as in the liver or peritoneum, invasion of adjacent organs such as the stomach or colon, or encasement of major arteries such as the celiac axis or superior mesenteric artery or occlusion of the portal vein or superior mesenteric vein. The accuracy of magnetic resonance imaging and computed tomography scans for this purpose obviates the need for invasive angiographic studies and reduces the likelihood of a patient going to surgery with unresectable disease.

Endoscopic Retrograde Cholangiopancreatography

Endoscopic retrograde cholangiopancreatography (ERCP) is an effective tool for the differential diagnosis of pancreatic lesions. It also provides an opportu-

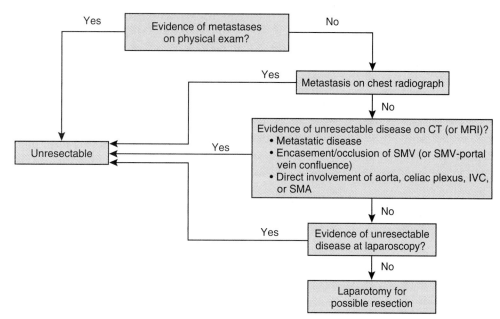

Figure 91-2 ■ Algorithm for determining whether pancreatic cancer is resectable. CT = computed tomography; MRI = magnetic resonance imaging; SMV = superior mesenteric vein; IVC = inferior vena cava; SMA = superior mesenteric artery.

nity to obtain biopsies of lesions of the pancreatic ampulla or of duodenal carcinoma. For diagnostic purposes, it has largely been replaced by computed tomography or magnetic resonance imaging, but it is occasionally useful in identifying small lesions that these other modalities cannot detect. Nevertheless, the procedure is frequently performed because it affords a means to stent the biliary tract in the case of obstructing lesions.

Endoscopic Ultrasonography

Endoscopic ultrasonography is a highly sensitive and specific test for the presence of pancreatic cancer, especially small lesions. It also can assess for local invasion and regional node involvement. Although it cannot provide information about metastatic disease, it is also useful because fine-needle aspiration biopsies for diagnosis can be performed using this technique.

Positron Emission Tomography

[18]FDG-positron emission tomography (PET) uses radiolabeled fluorodeoxyglucose to image metabolic activity. The normal pancreas does not light up, but pancreatic cancer and its metastases are usually identifiable, helping to distinguish between benign and malignant lesions in distant sites and in detecting recurrent disease after surgery.

One needs to be aware that due to inflammatory and fibrotic changes and distortion of ducts and archi-

tecture, some cases of chronic relapsing pancreatitis give an appearance on imaging studies consistent with pancreatic carcinoma.

Histologic Diagnosis and Staging
Histology

Biopsy confirmation of malignancy is required as with all cancers, no matter how suggestive the findings. For patients with unresectable disease, biopsy of the pancreas itself or of a metastatic lesion (including ascitic or pleural fluid if present) is usually obtained percutaneously under radiological guidance using ultrasound, computed tomography, or (less commonly) magnetic resonance imaging. Alternatively, biopsies of either the pancreas or nodal lesions can be obtained at the time of endoscopic ultrasound evaluation of the upper gastrointestinal tract and biliary system.

For patients with potentially resectable disease, biopsy is usually obtained during laparotomy for possible resection. Patients with a pancreatic or periampullary mass often require resection to be certain that no malignancy is present as well as to relieve symptoms, so that the surgery is necessary even if the preoperative or intraoperative fine-needle biopsy is not diagnostic. Benign tumors of the pancreas are sufficiently rare and sampling errors from biopsies (missing diagnostic tissue when a malignancy is present) high enough that surgery and open biopsy might still be required.

Table 91-5 ■ Tumor-Node-Metastasis (TNM) Staging Classification for Pancreatic Adenocarcinoma

Staging	Primary Tumor	Regional Lymph Nodes	Distant Metastasis
Stage 0	Tis	N0	M0
Stage I	T1	N0	M0
	T2	N0	M0
Stage II	T3	N0	M0
Stage III	T1	N1	M0
	T2	N1	M0
	T3	N1	M0
Stage IVA	T4	Any N	M0
Stage IVB	Any T	Any N	M1

Definitions
Primary Tumor (T)
Tis: Carcinoma in situ
T1: Tumor limited to the pancreas 2 cm or less in greatest dimension
T2: Tumor limited to the pancreas more than 2 cm in greatest dimension
T3: Tumor extends directly into any of the following: duodenum, bile duct, peripancreatic tissues
T4: Tumor extends directly into any one of the following: stomach, spleen, colon, adjacent large vessels
Regional Lymph Nodes* (N)
N0: No regional lymph node metastasis
N1: Regional lymph node metastasis
N1a: Metastasis in a single regional lymph node
N1b: Metastasis in multiple regional lymph nodes
Distant Metastasis (M)
M0: No distant metastasis
M1: Distant metastasis
*Regional lymph nodes include: peripancreatic, hepatic artery, infrapyloric, subpyloric, celiac, superior mesenteric, pancreaticolienal (body and tail tumors only), splenic (body and tail tumors only), retroperitoneal, lateral aortic

Staging

The American Joint Commission on Cancer (AJCC) staging system with the TNM format is used to group patients with pancreatic cancer into stages I–IV (Table 91-5). Although the different stages do have the expected correlation of decreasing survival with advancing stage, for purposes of treatment decisions, three groups of patients are usefully defined. These are those that have disease that is

1. potentially respectable
2. localized but unresectable or
3. metastatic.

If preliminary staging findings—including those of pancreatic protocol computed tomography scans or magnetic resonance imaging studies and/or endoscopic ultrasonography—do not indicate that the tumor is unresectable, then the next step is either laparoscopic staging or going directly to exploratory laparotomy with resection if possible. If laparoscopy is done, metastatic disease can be established by biopsy of peritoneal or other visualized lesions or detecting cancer in peritoneal washing cytologies. For example, 10% of patients (more often with tumors of the body and tail than the head of the pancreas) will be found to have positive peritoneal cytology, which is equivalent to the detection of metastatic disease. The value of laparoscopic staging in this setting is debatable. The major question is what percentage of patients who are resectable by pancreatic protocol computed tomography or magnetic resonance imaging criteria are found to be unresectable at laparoscopy and therefore spared unnecessary laparotomy. This figure is as high as 22% to 39% in some series but as low as 7% to 10% in others, depending in part on patient selection. As improvements are made in the ability of computed tomography, magnetic resonance imaging, or positron emission tomography scan imaging to detect increasingly smaller volumes of peritoneal disease, the potential added value of laparoscopic staging decreases. Thus, the frequency of staging laparoscopy varies among centers.

Therapy

Resectable Disease

Surgery

Approximately 20% to 25% of patients coming to surgery for curative excision will be found to be unresectable at laparotomy. If the disease is resectable, one of four surgical approaches is used. These are:

1. the pancreaticoduodenectomy (Whipple's procedure with various, surgeon-specific modifications);
2. total pancreatectomy;
3. regional or extended pancreatectomy; and
4. distal pancreatectomy and splenectomy.

Pancreaticoduodenectomies are the most commonly performed procedure for lesions in the head of the pancreas or periampullary lesions. This surgery includes partial resection of a number of organs, including pancreas, duodenum, stomach, bile duct, and gallbladder. The common vascular supply of the pancreatic head, distal bile duct region, and duodenum means that they must all be included in the resection. There is no agreement as to whether preservation of the pylorus as part of the procedure adds any overall benefit. The resected organs are reanastomosed through choledochojejunostomy, pancreaticojejunostomy, and gastrojejunostomy. Pancreaticoduodenectomy leaves behind a small remnant of the pancreas to provide pancreatic endocrine and exocrine function. Although this ameliorates the severity of hyperglycemia and malabsorption, the procedure carries the risk of leaving residual pancreatic cancer in patients who have multicentric disease.

Total pancreatectomy avoids the theoretical risk of residual multicentric disease, but the patient then experiences brittle diabetes and major problems with malabsorption. The data show, however, that the cure rate for patients with lesions in the pancreatic head is not improved by total pancreatectomy. Total pancreatectomy might still be necessary if resection margins are positive or if multicentric disease is found at surgery. Regional pancreatectomies include either subtotal or total pancreatectomies in combination with resection of a portion of the portal vein and en bloc resection of regional lymph nodes and adjacent soft tissue. In addition, tissues are removed from around major vessels. Extended pancreatectomies include removal of soft tissues around the pancreas and careful dissection around major blood vessels without resection of the portal vein. These surgeries allow more extensive resection of potentially involved tissues but carry higher morbidity than other approaches. Given the lack of definitive evidence that one surgical approach is better than the others, the type of surgical resection for pancreatic cancer varies by surgeon and by center.

Distal pancreatectomy and splenectomy is a fourth surgical approach used for cancers of the pancreatic tail. Diagnosis is often delayed because symptoms like back pain are nonspecific and often attributable to other causes. These lesions of the tail are usually far advanced at the time of presentation, and long-term survival is rare.

Morbidity and mortality after surgery for pancreatic cancer has declined significantly in the past decade. Currently, mortality rates are less than 5%. Potential complications include bowel paresis of varyingly long duration (the most common complication) and infections, fistulae, anastomotic leaks, and hemorrhage.

Because of enhanced ability to determine unresectability before surgery is attempted, favorable selection of patients for surgery occurs. The median survival is currently 18 months from the time of surgery, and approximately 20% of patients are alive five years later. Features that are associated with a reduced cure rate include tumor present at the margins of resection, lymph node involvement, and large tumor size. Randomized trials in the 1980s established combined adjuvant chemotherapy and postresection radiation therapy as the standard of treatment for these patients.

Palliative surgery, consisting of biliary bypass combined with gastrojejunostomy, is used to delay or prevent biliary and duodenal obstruction in patients who undergo exploration but are not resectable. Alternatively, endoscopic stent placements can be used for palliation. Stenting of the gastrointestinal tract itself remains of somewhat limited efficacy, although improvements in the stents are being made.

Adjuvant or Neoadjuvant Therapy

Clinical trials have not yet established that preoperative, intraoperative, or postoperative radiation therapy used alone without chemotherapy improves patient survival after pancreatic resection. Intraoperative radiotherapy (IORT), however, might increase the local control rate. Even when local control can be achieved with radiation therapy, the great majority of patients still die from metastatic disease.

Combined multimodality therapy has been employed to improve on these results. For example, a GI Tumor Study Group (GITSG) trial of combined postoperative external-beam radiation therapy and 5-fluorouracil chemotherapy and trials at other centers suggest that adjuvant or neoadjuvant chemotherapy and radiation therapy could lead to a longer survival than surgery alone. Studies of localized perfusion of chemotherapy have also claimed benefit from this approach compared with historical controls. It is difficult to draw a conclusion about the value of combined-modality therapy from these nonrandomized studies. When the issue was tested recently in a randomized European trial, combined chemotherapy and radiation therapy did not demonstrate a statistically significant improvement in survival. It thus remains unclear whether adjuvant chemotherapy and radiation therapy are useful on patients with pancreatic cancer who have undergone resection.

When neoadjuvant, 5-fluorouracil-based, chemotherapy combined with external-beam radiation therapy is used before surgery, 10% to 15% of localized but clinically unresectable patients became resectable. Because one cannot assess a priori before surgery what percentage of these patients would have been found to be resectable without the neoadjuvant therapy, the magnitude of the benefit cannot be defined absolutely. The role of neoadjuvant therapy therefore appears limited using current therapy.

Patients with Localized but Unresectable Disease

Radiation Therapy

Overall, only 5% to 20% of patients presenting with pancreatic cancer are deemed resectable. Radiation therapy in patients whose tumors cannot be resected can relieve symptoms, primarily pain, and perhaps slightly prolong survival. Patients receiving a total radiation therapy dose of 55 to 70 Gy experience a median survival of approximately 10 months. Addition of 5-fluorouracil-based chemotherapy provides at best only a modest improvement in survival compared with the use of radiation therapy alone. The use of additional chemotherapeutic agents, such as cisplatin, might improve on these results.

Intraoperative radiation therapy in the locally advanced setting is usually given either prior to or after external beam radiation therapy and chemotherapy. Median survival ranges from nine to 16 months, not significantly better than after external beam radiation therapy and chemotherapy used alone. Approaches using conformal 3D techniques for planning and treating patients allow enhanced radiation dose delivery to the tumor and not to surrounding normal tissues. These might enhance the effects of radiation therapy. Brachytherapy implants into the tumor using ^{125}I or ^{103}Pd isotopes also have been employed for palliation. Although they increase local control, they also are associated with local complications and do not affect metastatic disease; therefore, survival is not improved.

Chemotherapy

Chemotherapy alone has also been evaluated for patients with unresectable localized disease. Regional chemotherapy perfusion (alone or with chemofiltration) has been used in a small number of patients in an attempt to deliver high-dose therapy to the tumor (or localized metastases) without significantly increasing systemic toxicity. There is no evidence that this results in significant improvement in therapeutic index over systemic delivery of the agents. Systemic chemotherapy alone without radiation can also provide palliation for some patients with locally advanced pancreatic cancer.

Given the limited results with either modality alone, chemotherapy has been combined with radiation therapy to serve the added function of a radiation sensitizer. 5-Fluorouracil has been used for this purpose for years, but recent studies have explored two other potent radiation sensitizers—gemcitabine and paclitaxel. Phase I and II studies have defined tolerable regimens for administration of each of these agents contemporaneously with radiation therapy, but it is uncertain whether gemcitabine or paclitaxel in this setting is any more efficacious than 5-fluorouracil. Compared with either chemotherapy or radiation therapy alone, combined-modality therapy appears to be associated with a slightly longer survival and greater palliation for a proportion of patients in terms of pain relief, delayed obstructive symptoms,

improved performance status, and decreased anorexia. Combined-modality therapy has become the standard of care for these patients, providing they can tolerate the intensity of treatment and its side effects.

Stenting of the Biliary Duct

Facilitated by improved endoscopic techniques and catheter design, endoscopic stenting of the biliary system is increasingly utilized to prevent or treat biliary obstruction without resort to surgery. Metal wall stents can be placed in patients who require continued patency of the biliary system and are not surgical candidates. These permanent stents can become obstructed by tumor overgrowth. When this occurs, re-stenting with plastic stents placed inside the metal stent can be performed. For the small subset of patients who cannot be stented endoscopically, percutaneous internal stent placement under radiologic guidance sometimes can provide relief from biliary obstruction. Percutaneous transhepatic external biliary drainage might provide symptom relief for those who cannot be internally stented even by this approach.

Patients with Metastatic Pancreatic Cancer

Treatment of patients with metastatic disease remains disappointing; the median survival is only three to six months. The most active single agents achieve objective response rates in the 5% to 20% range, without improvement in two-year survival. Chemotherapy can, however, provide short-term subjective clinical benefit in quality of life for a higher fraction of patients (perhaps 25%) than those who meet the criteria for objective responses. Gemcitabine has become the standard agent for use in this setting, based on a randomized trial showing that it improved survival and provided greater clinical benefit compared with 5-fluorouracil.

Other agents with some activity against pancreatic cancer that are currently in use include 5-fluorouracil, docetaxel, camptothecins, cisplatin, epirubicin, and mitomycin C. The activity of ifosfamide, streptozotocin, nitrosoureas, and other anthracyclines is so low against pancreatic adenocarcinoma that they rarely are used. Some chemotherapy combinations might be more effective than single agent chemotherapy, but this remains to be established. Randomized studies are comparing gemcitabine alone to two-drug therapy with gemcitabine + cisplatin, gemcitabine + docetaxel, or gemcitabine + irinotecan.

Hormonal agents such as tamoxifen, progestational agents, antiandrogenic compounds, synthetic analogs of gonadotropin releasing hormone, octreotide, somatuline, and other somatostatin analogs have failed to demonstrate significant antitumor activity. Immunotherapy using cytokines, radiolabeled or toxin-linked monoclonal antibodies, or vaccines has thus far been unavailing.

Supportive Care and Symptom Management

Supportive care and the management of symptoms are vitally important in the treatment of patients with pancreatic cancer (Table 91-6). The majority of patients develop significant pain at some point in the course of their disease. Pain management with opioid analgesics, nonsteroidal agents, acetaminophen, and other analgesic agents is important. Celiac plexus blocks can be used if the pain cannot be controlled by medication. Malnutrition is a significant problem. Pancreatic enzymes can sometimes help ameliorate the malabsorption that occurs in a high percentage of patients. Although they are not always useful, they help in a sufficient percentage of patients to make an empirical trial worthwhile when malabsorption is a problem. Antacids might be useful in both enhancing the benefit of pancreatic enzymes and decreasing reflux symptoms. Megestrol acetate, dronabinol, or steroids can stimulate appetite in a percentage of patients. Megestrol has a small risk of fluid retention. It also carries an increased risk of thrombosis in this group of patients, who are already predisposed to blood-clot formation by pancreatic cancer. The use of glucocorticoids in this patient population is complicated by the frequent occurrence of glucose intolerance. If necessary, however, these can be administered with careful attention to managing glucose control.

Psychological issues are frequent problems that need attention. Depression is more frequent in these patients than in patients with other cancers. Occurring as it often does in these patients in the setting of increased anxiety, fatigue, and apathy, treatment can be difficult. The multidisciplinary approach of a dedicated palliative care team and pain service directed at physical complaints and psychological pressures is often helpful.

Pancreatic Endocrine Tumors

Islet cell tumors make up less than 10% of all pancreatic cancers. Islet cell tumors can be functional—causing symptoms related to hormone(s) that they produce—or they can be nonfunctional, not associated with hormonally related symptomatology. The islet cell tumors include insulinomas, glucagonomas, somatostatinomas, gastrinomas, VIPomas, ACTHomas, carcinoids, tumors that produce hypercalcemia, and nonfunctioning tumors. Tumors can produce more than one peptide hormone. Except for insulinomas—which have a lower risk of metastasizing—the pancreatic endocrine tumors are malignant in the majority of cases. They tend to metastasize to lymph nodes and liver. Certain of these tumors can occur as part of the familial multiple endocrine neoplasia syndrome (MEN-I). MEN-I is an autosomal-dominant trait that is associated with tumors or hyperplasia of multiple endocrine organs, often including pancreatic endocrine tumors but most commonly gastrinomas or insulinomas.

General treatment principles are similar for most of these tumors, although there are specific aspects of each that need to be addressed as well. Surgical resection should always be attempted if feasible. Even when curative surgery is not attainable, cytoreduction of the tumor mass could be of value in controlling symptoms by diminishing the amount of hormone production. This is especially useful in malignancies such as glucagonomas, somatostatinomas, and VIPomas, because medications that can block the activity of the hormones these tumors produce are not very effective.

Somatostatin analogs such as octreotide are useful in diminishing symptoms in many of these tumors. Although somatostatin analogs do not significantly increase long-term survival, they can improve quality of life markedly. A number of chemotherapeutic

---

Table 91-6 ▪ Symptom Management for Pancreatic Adenocarcinoma

Pain Relief Medications

Acetaminophen
Non-steroidal anti-inflamatory agents
Opioid analgesics
Celiac plexus block

Nutritional Support

Pancreatic enzymes
Supplements
Megestrol
Steroids
Dronabinol

Control of Malabsorption Symptoms

Pancreatic enzymes
Antidiarrheal agents (Imodium, etc.)

Control of Reflux Symptoms

Antacids/omeprazole

Control of Depression/Anxiety

Psychotherapeutic and social support
Antidepressants

agents have some limited activity against these tumors. The combination of streptozotocin and doxorubicin remains the most commonly used regimen for islet cell tumors. Interferon has also been used either alone or in combination with octreotide and/or chemotherapy to control disease for variable periods of time. Hepatic arterial embolization or chemoembolization can palliate symptoms in patients who have functional tumors and a significant tumor burden in the liver. Radiolabeled octreotide might provide a means to relatively specifically target those tumors that are positive on octreotide scan. Although responses and disease stabilization have been seen, the value of this approach is not established. Liver transplantation has been used for patients whose only apparent metastases are to the liver. It appears to have the greatest benefit in patients with metastatic carcinoid tumors but is less useful in other pancreatic endocrine histologies. It is used primarily in a setting in which the tumor has demonstrated a relatively indolent clinical course, suggesting that transplant might be beneficial.

Symptom-control measures are required for specific cancers. For gastrinomas, these include blocking gastric acid hypersecretion by agents such as H^+-K^+-ATPase inhibitors (e.g., omeprazole). For insulinomas, dietary management and diazoxide are measures used to control hypoglycemic symptoms. Glucagon, corticosteroids, and human growth hormone can also be used to try to prevent hypoglycemia, but these have limited effectiveness in the long run. Unfortunately, for most of the other tumors, specific solutions for symptoms related to elevated hormone levels are of limited efficacy.

Lymphomas and Sarcomas

Lymphomas and sarcomas arising within the pancreas are uncommon neoplasms. Multiple histologic subtypes of sarcomas can develop in the pancreas, including leiomyosarcomas, malignant fibrous histiocytomas, angiosarcomas, lymphangiosarcomas, and Kaposi's sarcoma. It is essential to establish the histologic diagnosis so that appropriate therapeutic decisions can be made. For the most part, the clinical course of these malignancies is similar to tumors of like histology arising in other organs. Localized sarcomas should certainly be resected for cure when this is possible. Those that have metastasized need to be treated with systemic therapy. Most lymphomas of the pancreas are adequately treated by means of chemotherapy and local radiation therapy, so that pancreatic resection in this circumstance is rarely necessary.

References

General Information

Aspinall RJ, Lemoine NR: Gene therapy for pancreatic and biliary malignancies. Ann Oncol 1999;10(S4):188–192.

Bouvet M, Staerkel GM, Spitz FR, et al: Primary pancreatic lymphoma. Surg 1998;123:382–390.

Brugge W, Van Dam J: Pancreatic and biliary endoscopy. N Engl J Med 1999;341:1808–1816.

Czito BG, Willett CG, Clark JW, et al: Current perspectives on locally advanced pancreatic cancer. Oncol 2000; 14:1535–1545.

DiMagno EP: Pancreatic cancer: clinical presentation, pitfalls and early clues. Ann Oncol 1999;10(S4):140–142.

Heinemann V: Present and future treatment of pancreatic cancer. Semin Oncol 2002;29(S9):23–31.

Jaffee E, Hruban RH, Biedrzycki B, et al: Novel allogeneic granulocyte-macrophage colony-stimulating factor-secreting tumor vaccine for pancreatic cancer: A phase I trial of safety and immune activation. J Clin Oncol 200;19: 145–156.

Jensen RT: Pancreatic endocrine tumors: Recent advances. Ann Oncol 1999;10(S4):170–176.

Korc M: Role of growth factors in pancreatic cancer. Surg Oncol Clin N Am 1998;7:25–41.

Krouse RS, Chu DZ, Grant M, et al: Evaluation of the quality of life (QOL) in pancreaticoduodenectomy survivors. Ann Surg 2002;235:310–311.

Lillemoe KD, Yeo CJ, Cameron JL: Pancreatic cancer: State-of-the-art care. CA Cancer J Clin 2000;50:241–268.

Passik SD: Supportive care of the patient with pancreatic cancer: Role of the psycho-oncologist. Oncol 1996;10(S):33–34.

Rosenberg L: Pancreatic cancer: A review of emerging therapies. Drugs 2000;59:1071–1089.

Rowinsky EK, Windle JJ, Von Hoff DD: Ras protein farnesyltransferase: A strategic target for anticancer therapeutic development. J Clin Oncol 1999;17:3631–3652.

Russell RC: Palliation of pain and jaundice: An overview. Ann Oncol 1999;10(S4):165–169.

Staib L, Link KH, Beger HG: Immunotherapy in pancreatic cancer—Current status and future. Langenbecks Arch Chir 1999;384:396–404.

Ulrich CD: Growth factors, receptors, and molecular alterations in pancreatic cancer. Putting it all together. Med Clin N Am 2000;84:697–705.

van den Bosch RP, van Eijk CH, Mulder PG, Jeekel J: Serum CA19-9 determination in the management of pancreatic cancer. Hepatogastroenterology 1996;43:710–713.

Warshaw AL, Fernandez-del Castillo C: Medical progress: Pancreatic carcinoma. N Engl J Med 1992;326:455–465.

Chemotherapy

Beger HG, Gansauge F, Buchler MW, Link KH: Intra-arterial adjuvant chemotherapy after pancreaticoduodenectomy for pancreatic cancer: Significant reduction in occurrence of liver metastasis. World J Surg 1999;23:946–949.

Berlin JD, Catalano P, Thomas JP, et al: Phase III study of gemcitabine in combination with fluorouracil versus gemcitabine alone inpatients with advanced pancreatic carcinoma: Eastern Cooperative Oncology Group Trial E 2297. J Clin Oncol 2002;20:3270–3275.

Blackstock AW, Bernard SA, Richards F, et al: Phase I trial of twice-weekly gemcitabine and concurrent radiation in patients with advanced pancreatic cancer. J Clin Oncol 1999;17:2208–2212.

Burris HA III, Moore MJ, Andersen J, et al: Improvements in survival and clinical benefit with gemcitabine as first-line therapy for patients with advanced pancreas cancer: A randomized trial. J Clin Oncol 1997;15:2403–2413.

Cheng PN, Saltz LB: Failure to confirm major objective antitumor activity for streptozotocin and doxorubicin in the treatment of patients with advanced islet cell carcinoma. Cancer 1999;86:944–948.

De Lange SM, van Groeningen CJ, Meijer OW, et al: Gemcitabine-radiotherapy in patients with locally advanced pancreatic cancer. Eur J Cancer 2002;38:1212–1217.

Ghaneh P, Kawesha A, Howes N, et al: Adjuvant therapy for pancreatic cancer. World J Surg 1999;23:937–945.

Hidalgo M, Castellano D, Paz-Ares L, et al: Phase I-II study of gemcitabine and fluorouracil as a continuous infusion in patients with pancreatic cancer. J Clin Oncol 1999;17:585–592.

Jessup JM, Steele G, Mayer RJ, et al: Neoadjuvant therapy for unresectable pancreatic adenocarcinoma. Arch Surg 1992;127:1335–1339.

Maisey N, Chau I, Cunningham D, et al: Multicenter randomized phase III trial comparing protracted venous infusion (PVI) fluorouracil (5-FU) with PVI 5-FU plus mitomycin in inoperable pancreatic cancer. J Clin Oncol 2002;20:3130–3136.

Ryan DP, Lynch TJ, Grossbard ML, et al: A phase I study of gemcitabine and docetaxel in patients with metastatic solid tumors. Cancer 2000;88:80–85.

Combined-Modality Therapy

Evans DB, Pisters PW, Lee JH, et al: Preoperative chemoradiation strategies for localized adenocarcinoma of the pancreas. J Hep Bil Pancr Surg 1998;5:242–250.

Foo ML, Gunderson LL: Adjuvant postoperative radiation therapy +/– 5-FU in resected carcinoma of the pancreas. Hepatogastroenterology 1998;45:613–623.

Gastrointestinal Tumor Study Group: Further evidence of effective adjuvant combined radiation and chemotherapy following curative resection of pancreatic cancer. Cancer 1987;59:2006–2010.

Klinkenbijl JH, Jeekel J, Sahmoud T, et al: Adjuvant radiotherapy and 5-fluorouracil after curative resection of cancer of the pancreas and periampullary region: Phase III trial of the EORTC Gastrointestinal Tract Cancer Cooperative Group. Ann Surg 1999;230:776–782.

Rich TA: Chemoradiation for pancreatic and biliary cancer: Current status of RTOG studies. Ann Oncol 1999;10(S4):231–233.

Safran H, Dipetrillo T, Iannitti D, et al: Gemcitabine, paclitaxel, and radiation for locally advanced pancreatic cancer. Intl J Radiat Oncol Biol Phys 2002;54:137–141.

Spitz FR, Abbruzzese JL, Lee JE, et al: Preoperative and postoperative chemoradiation strategies in patients with pancreaticoduodenectomy for adenocarcinoma of the pancreas. J Clin Oncol 1997;15:926–937.

Epidemiology

Brand RE, Lynch HT: Hereditary pancreatic adenocarcinoma. A clinical perspective. Med Clin N Am 2000;84:665–675.

DeLellis RA: The hereditary forms of pancreatic neuroendocrine tumors. Adv Anatomic Pathol 1999;6:149–153.

Gold EB, Goldin SB: Epidemiology of and risk factors for pancreatic cancer. Surg Oncol Clin N Am 1998;7:67–91.

Lowenfels AB, Maisonneuve P: Pancreatico-biliary malignancy: prevalence and risk factors. Ann Oncol 1999;10(S4):1–3.

Mack TM, Yu MC, Hanisch R, et al: Pancreas cancer and smoking, beverage consumption, and past medical history. J Natl Cancer Inst 1986;76:49–60.

Michaud DS, Liu S, Giovannucci E, et al: Dietary sugar, glycemic load, and pancreatic cancer risk in a prospective study. J Natl Cancer Inst 2002;94:1293–1300.

Silverman DT, Schiffman M, Everhart T, et al: Diabetes mellitus, other medical conditions and familial history of cancer as risk factors for pancreatic cancer. Br J Cancer 1999;80:1830–1837.

Imaging Studies

Adamek HE, Albert J, Breer H, et al: Pancreatic cancer detection with magnetic resonance cholangiopancreatography and endoscopic retrograde cholangiopancreatography: A prospective controlled study. Lancet 2000;365:190–193.

Bluemke DA, Cameron JL, Hruban RH, et al: Potentially respectable pancreatic adenocarcinoma: Spiral CT assessment with surgical and pathologic correlation. Radiology 1995;197:381–385.

Fritscher-Ravens A, Sriram PV, Krause C, et al: Detection of pancreatic metastases by EUS-guided fine-needle aspiration. Gastrointest Endosc 2001;53:65–70.

Inokama T, Tamaki N, Toizuka T, et al: Evaluation of pancreatic tumors with positron emission tomography and F-18 fluorodeoxyglucose: Comparison with CT and US. Radiology 1995;195:345–352.

Lopez Hannninen E, Amthauer H, Hosten N, et al: Prospective evaluation of pancreatic tumors: Accuracy of MR imaging with MR cholangiopancreatography and MR angiography. Radiol 2002;234:34–41.

Lu DS, Vedenthaarn S, Krassny RM, et al: Two-phase helical CT for pancreatic tumors: Pancreatic versus hepatic phase enhancement of tumor, pancreas, and vascular structures. Radiology 1996;199:697–701.

O'Malley ME, Bowland GW, Wood BJ, et al: Adenocarcinoma of the head of the pancreas: Determination of surgical unresectability with thin-section pancreatic-phase helical CT. Am J Roentgenol 1999;173:1513–1518.

Sheth S, Hruban RK, Fishman EK: Helical CT of islet cell tumors of the pancreas: Typical and atypical manifestations. Am J Roentgenol 2002;179:725–730.

Zimny M, Buell U: 18FDG-positron emission tomography in pancreatic cancer. Ann Oncol 1999;10(S4):28–32.

Pathology

Fernandez-del Castillo C, Warshaw AL: Cystic neoplasms of the pancreas. Pancreatology 2001;1:641–647.

Kern SE: Molecular genetic alterations in ductal pancreatic adenocarcinomas. Med Clin N Am 2000;84:691–695.

Pedrazzoli S, Berger MG, Obertop H, et al: A surgical and pathological based classification of resections in the treatment of pancreatic cancer. Summary of an international workshop on surgical procedures in pancreatic cancer. Dig Surg 1999;16:337–345.

Perugini RA, McDade TF, Vittemberga FJ Jr, Gallery MP: The molecular and cellular biology of pancreatic cancer. Crit Rev Eukaryot Gene Expr 1998;8:377–393.

Sakorafas GH, Tsiotou AG, Tsiotos GG: Molecular biology of pancreatic cancer; Oncogenes, tumour suppressor genes, growth factors, and their receptors from a clinical perspective. Cancer Treat Rev 2000;26:29–52.

Radiation Therapy

Bodner WR, Hilaris BS: Brachytherapy and pancreatic cancer. Semin Surg Oncol 1997;13:204–207.

Surgery

Balcom JH, Rattner DW, Warshaw, et al: Ten-year experience with 733 pancreatic resections: Changing indications, older patients, and decreasing length of hospitalization. Arch Surg 2001;136:491–498.

Forgensen J: Resected adenocarcinoma of the pancreas—616 patients: results, outcomes, and prognostic indicators. J Gastrointest Surg 2001;5:681.

Isenberg G, Gouma DJ, Pisters PW: The on-going debate about perioperative biliary drainage in jaundiced patients undergoing pancreaticoduodenectomy. Gastrointest Endosc 2002;56:310–315.

Jimenez RE, Warshaw AL, Rattner DW, et al: Impact of laparoscopic staging in the treatment of pancreatic cancer. Arch Surg 2000;135:409–414.

Koniaris LG, Lillemore KD, Yeo CJ, et al: Is there a role for surgical resection in the treatment of early-stage pancreatic lymphoma? J Am Coll Surg 2000;190:319–330.

Kwon AH, Inui H, Kamiyama Y: Preoperative laparoscopic examination using surgical manipulation and ultrasonography for pancreatic lesions. Endoscopy 2002;34:464–468.

Sohn TA, Yeo CJ, Cameron JL, et al: Resected adenocarcinoma of the pancreas in 616 patients: Results, outcomes, and prognostic indicators. J Gastrointest Surg 2000;4:567–579.

Taylor MC, McLeod RS, Langer B: Biliary stenting versus bypass surgery for the palliation of malignant distal bile duct obstruction: A meta-analysis. Liver Transpl 2000;6:302–308.

Wagner M, Dikopoulos N, Kulli C, et al: Standard surgical treatment in pancreatic cancer. Ann Oncol 1999;10(S4):247–251.

Yeo CJ, Cameron JL: Improving results of pancreaticoduodenectomy for pancreatic cancer. World J Surg 1999;23:907–912.

Chapter 92
Colorectal Cancer

Robert J. Mayer

Colorectal cancer is the fourth (after prostate, breast, and lung cancers) most common visceral malignancy and the second (after lung cancer) most frequent cause of cancer deaths in the United States. The incidence of colorectal cancer, approximately 140,000 cases annually in the United States, has not changed appreciably during the last 50 years, although the mortality of approximately 57,000 annually has decreased, especially in women.

Epidemiologic Associations

A number of congenital and acquired disorders as well as environmental influences have been associated with the development of colorectal cancer (Table 92-1).

Inherited Syndromes

As many as 20% of patients with colorectal cancer have a strong family history of the disease. Of this subset, the two best-characterized genetic syndromes that lead to colorectal cancer are familial adenomatous polyposis and hereditary nonpolyposis colon cancer.

Familial Adenomatous Polyposis

Familial adenomatous polyposis (FAP), also known as polyposis coli, accounts for approximately 1% of cases of colorectal cancer. The condition is inherited in an autosomal dominant manner, is characterized by a germline deletion of chromosome 5q21 (so-called adenomatous polyposis colon [or APC] gene), and exhibits an approximate 100% cancer penetration by age 40. Consequently, essentially all individuals who carry the gene ultimately develop colorectal cancer. Afflicted individuals have a bowel mucosa that is histologically normal but cytokinetically aberrant at the time of birth. Literally thousands of adenomatous polyps develop diffusely throughout the large bowel by age 20, eventually leading to cancer. When the presence of the diffuse polyposis is appreciated, total

colectomy with mucosal proctectomy followed by ileoanal anastomosis is the management of choice. While nonsteroidal anti-inflammatory drugs (NSAIDs) and cyclo-oxygenase-2 (COX-2) inhibitors may reduce the number and size of polyps in patients with familial adenomatous polyposis, there is no evidence that these compounds diminish the risk for cancer. Familial adenomatous polyposis may be associated with congenital hypertrophy of the retinal pigmoid epithelium, the presence of desmoid tumors, osteomas, epidermoid and sebaceous cysts, and/or periampullary cancers (known as Gardner's syndrome), or the presence of brain tumors (known as Turcot's syndrome). First-degree relatives should undergo screening proctosigmoidoscopy intermittently beginning at age 10 years; since the polyps in familial adenomatous polyposis involve the entire large bowel, colonoscopy is not required. The identification of gene carriers by means of a commercially available molecular test for the presence of the APC gene in peripheral blood mononuclear cells is being increasingly utilized as a means of making an early diagnosis, even at such a time before polyps develop.

Hereditary Nonpolyposis Colon Cancer

Hereditary nonpolyposis colon cancer, also known as Lynch syndrome, is believed to account for approximately 5% of cases of colorectal cancer. The condition is also inherited in an autosomally dominant manner and is associated with germline mutations in chromosomes 2 (h MSH2 gene) and 3 (h MLH1 gene), leading to errors in DNA replication and to DNA instability (i.e., microsatellite instability). The median age for the appearance of cancer is less than 50 years, and the developing tumors occur more frequently in the proximal colon, often associated with a lymphocytic infiltration. For as yet unknown reasons (but probably associated with the microsatellite instability), individuals with hereditary nonpolyposis colon cancer who develop a colon cancer appear to have a more favor-

Table 92-1 ■ Colorectal Cancer: Epidemiologic Associations

Hereditary syndromes: account for 10% to 15% of cases
  Polyposis coli
  Hereditary nonpolyposis colon cancer
Environment: increase in Western, urbanized societies
Diet: saturated fat, meat, calories
Associated conditions:
  Inflammatory bowel disease
  Ureterosigmoidostomy
  Streptococcus bovis septicemia
  Tobacco use
  Polyps

able prognosis than do patients who do not have hereditary nonpolyposis colon cancer who develop similar tumors. In women, the germline abnormality that characterizes hereditary nonpolyposis colon cancer is associated with an increased risk of endometrial and/or ovarian carcinomas.

Environmental Factors

Colorectal cancer occurs more frequently in Western, urbanized societies. Within a given geographic area, it is a disease of middle- and upper-class rather than lower-class individuals. The migration of succeeding generations of individuals from countries that are at lower risk for the disease to areas that are at higher risk results in the succeeding generations of immigrants adopting the risk pattern for colorectal cancer of their new environment. Consequently, it is believed that environmental factors contribute significantly to the risk for colorectal cancer. Epidemiologic studies have shown a higher rate for the development of colorectal cancer in individuals having elevated serum cholesterol levels and diets that are high in saturated fat. While the effect of diet on the development of colorectal cancer remains controversial, it does appear that the risk for developing the disease is directly related to the consumption of such high-fat meats as beef, lamb, and mutton, presumably through the development of an as yet unidentified carcinogen. Contrary to prior belief, multiple studies have failed to show any value for dietary fiber as protection against the development of colorectal cancer.

Inflammatory Bowel Disease

The presence of either ulcerative colitis or granulomatous colitis increases the risk for the subsequent development of colorectal cancer. The risk in patients with ulcerative colitis appears to correlate with the duration of active disease (Figure 92-1), the extent of involved bowel (i.e., pancolitis rather than localized colitis) and the development of mucosal dysplasia. The risk for carcinoma has been estimated to be 9% at 10 years, 20% at 20 years, and greater than 35% after 30 years; these worrisome data might reflect an overestimate because the published series reporting high cancer rates emerged from tertiary-care facilities to which the most severe patients with inflammatory bowel disease had been referred.

Total colectomy cures symptomatic ulcerative colitis and essentially eliminates the risk of subsequent carcinoma. When ileoproctostomy has been performed, thereby preserving the distal rectum and anus, a worrisome incidence of carcinoma has still been observed, despite periodic endoscopic assessments of the mucosa of the remaining distal rectum. Colectomy with mucosal proctectomy followed by an ileoanal anastomosis appears to be the procedure of choice and is probably indicated in patients with inflammatory bowel disease who remain symptomatic 15 years after their diagnosis. The proper approach to asymptomatic patients, even those with pseudopolyps on barium enema, remains unclear.

Other Epidemiologic Associations

A 5% to 10% incidence of colon cancer has been reported 15 to 30 years after performance of a ureterosigmoidostomy to correct congenital extrophy of the bladder. The tumors characteristically develop distal to the site of ureteral implantation into the

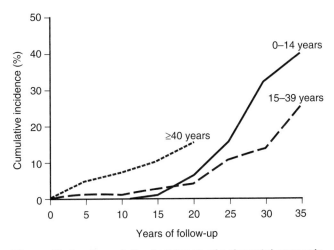

Figure 92-1 ■ Cumulative incidence of colorectal cancer in patients with pancolitis, according to age at diagnosis. (From Ekbom A, Hemick C, Zack M, Adami HO: Ulcerative colitis and colorectal cancer. N Engl J Med 1990; 323:1228–1233, with permission.)

sigmoid colon, where the colonic mucosa is chronically exposed to both urine and feces.

For uncertain reasons, individuals who are found to have *Streptococcus bovis* septicemia appear to have a higher than expected incidence of colonic neoplasms. The identification of this unusual enterococcus should prompt endoscopic or radiographic surveillance of the large bowel.

Multiple cohort studies have demonstrated a higher incidence of colorectal cancer in chronic smokers than in nonsmokers. Whether this relationship is due to a direct carcinogenic effect of a tobacco by-product on the colonic mucosa or to an indirect exposure to an associated bowel carcinogen that occurs more frequently in smokers than nonsmokers remains unknown.

Adenomatous Polyps

Regardless of etiologic cause, essentially all colorectal cancers (except possibly those developing in individuals with inflammatory bowel disease) are thought to arise from adenomatous polyps. Polyps are defined as grossly visible protrusions from the mucosal surface. They are classified pathologically as hamartomas (also known as juvenile polyps that are nonneoplastic), hyperplastic (nonneoplastic proliferation of the normal mucosa), and adenomas (which are neoplastic). Adenomatous polyps are found in the large bowels of approximately 30% of middle-aged and 50% of elderly adults. On the basis of this prevalence of adenomatous polyps and the incidence for colorectal cancer, it appears that fewer than 1% of polyps ever develop into cancers. The vast majority of polyps produce no symptoms and remain clinically undetected.

A sequence of molecular changes appears to be involved in the development of adenomatous polyps from normal mucosa and their subsequent progression to cancer (Figure 92-2). These alterations have been identified in DNA obtained from adenomatous polyps, dysplastic lesions, and polyps containing microscopic foci of tumor cells and include specific mutations in the *ras* proto-oncogene and deletions in

tumor suppressor genes in chromosomes 5, 18, and 17. On the basis of this model, it is believed that cancer develops only in those polyps in which all of these, as well as additional as yet undiscovered, events take place, whereas the presence of only one or two of such alterations might result in a polyp that spontaneously regresses. Furthermore, it has been postulated that the likelihood for multiple molecular events to occur, and for cancers to develop, is also influenced by a genetic susceptibility coupled with an exposure to environmental carcinogens. Clinically, adenomatous polyps are more likely to become malignant if they are sessile rather than pedunculated, villous rather than tubular, and greater than 1.5 cm in size.

Following the detection of an adenomatous polyp, the entire large bowel should be visualized endoscopically, since synchronous lesions (additional polyps or even occult cancers) are present in approximately 35% of cases. Colonoscopy should then be repeated intermittently, even in the absence of a previously documented cancer, since individuals with a history of polyp production have a 30% to 50% likelihood of developing another adenoma and are at higher than average risk for the development of a colorectal cancer. Adenomatous polyps are believed to require more than five years of growth before becoming clinically significant. The results of a large randomized trial, the National Polyp Study, demonstrated that such surveillance colonoscopy need not be carried out more frequently than every three or four years. A further analysis conducted as part of the National Polyp Study provided additional support for the principle that colorectal cancers emerge from polyps and that the removal of adenomatous polyps represent a highly effective means of cancer prevention (Figure 92-3). In this assessment, a comparison of the likelihood of developing colorectal cancer in this endoscopically screened cohort of polyp producers with two groups of similar polyp-producing patients from the Mayo Clinic and from St. Mark's Hospital in London who had elected not to undergo endoscopic surveillance showed that the prophylactic removal of polyps in the National Polyp Study participants reduced the colorectal cancer risk not only below that

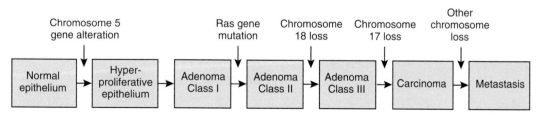

Figure 92-2 ■ Series of mutations involved in the sequential development of adenomatous polyps and their progression to cancer.

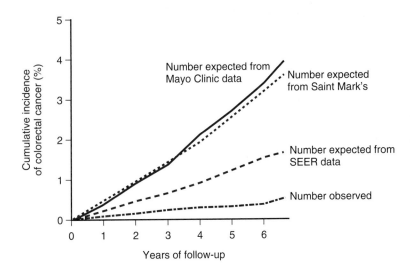

Figure 92-3 ▪ Cumulative incidence of colorectal cancer in the National Polyp Study Cohort. (From Winawer SJ, Zauber AG, Ho MN, et al: Prevention of colorectal cancer by colonoscopic polypectomy. N Engl J Med 1993;329:1977–1981, with permission.)

of the Mayo Clinic and St. Mark's groups but even below that of the general U.S. population (based on Surveillance, Epidemiology, and End Results [SEER] data of the National Cancer Institute).

Chemoprevention

Increasing evidence indicates that the incidence of adenomatous polyps can be reduced through the long-term use of a variety of chemical compounds that have been termed chemopreventative agents (Table 92-2). Nonsteroidal anti-inflammatory drugs such as aspirin or, more recently, cyclo-oxygenase-2 inhibitors have undergone the most study for this purpose. These medications are thought to inhibit cyclo-oxygenase-2 in the colonic mucosa, thereby reducing prostaglandin synthesis and retarding mucosal proliferation. Evidence that nonsteroidal anti-inflammatory drugs reduce colorectal cancer risk has emerged primarily from cohort studies in individuals who also used aspirin for at least 10 years. Emerging data, also primarily from cohort studies, suggest that dietary folic

acid supplementation (as is found in multivitamin tablets) prevents the development of colorectal cancer, particularly in individuals who have a family history of the disease, and that supplementation of dietary calcium (also supplied in multivitamin tablets) reduces the colon cancer risk (possibly through a direct inhibition of epithelial cell proliferation). Interestingly, the use of postmenopausal estrogen replacement therapy has increasingly been associated with a reduction in the appearance of colonic polyps and cancers, possibly through decreased synthesis of secondary bile acids but also, conceivably, resulting from a diminished production of insulin-like growth factor 1. Despite promising pilot data, randomized trials have failed to show that high-fiber diets or such antioxidants as ascorbic acid, beta-carotene, or vitamin E reduce the appearance of premalignant polyps.

Screening

At present, screening policies for asymptomatic individuals at standard risk for the development of colorectal cancer are controversial. Screening maneuvers that have been assessed in large groups of patients include examination of the stool for occult blood, proctosigmoidoscopy, colonoscopy, and air contrast barium enema. Such newer approaches as virtual colonoscopy (a computed tomography (CT) scan reconstruction of the large bowel lumen) and molecular screening of the stool (assessment of fecal DNA for gene mutations) hold potential promise but are not presently appropriate for routine clinical use.

Fecal Occult Blood Testing

Approximately 2% to 4% of asymptomatic adults will be found to have a positive test for the occult presence of blood in their stool utilizing the guaiac technique.

Table 92-2 ▪ Chemoprevention of Colorectal Cancer

Demonstrated Effect

Nonsteroidal anti-inflammatory drugs
Folic acid
Calcium
Estrogen (postmenopausal hormone replacement)

No Proven Effect

Increased dietary fiber
Antioxidants (ascorbic acid, beta-carotene, vitamin E)

Table 92-3 ■ Summary Data from Three Randomized Trials Assessing Fecal Occult Blood Testing

	Minnesota, 1975–1992 (NEJM, 1993)	United Kingdom, 1981–1995 (Lancet, 1996)	Denmark, 1985–1995 (Lancet, 1996)
Participants (n)	46,551	152,850	140,000
Colonoscopy rate	28% to 38%	4%	4%
Positivity rate	2% to 10%	2%	1%
Sensitivity	81% to 92%	67%	51%
Positive predictive value for colorectal cancer	2% to 6%	10% to 15%	8% to 18%
Decrease in mortality rate			
Annual screening	33%	—	—
Biennial screening	21%	15%	18%

About 60% of such individuals will have no mucosal abnormality in their bowel when further studies are conducted, implying the test to have been falsely positive. Conversely, 50% of patients with colorectal cancer (and 95% of patients with adenomatous polyps) will have a falsely negative study. Nonetheless, the use of routine guaiac testing of stool for occult blood has been shown in several large clinical trials to lead to an earlier detection of occult colorectal cancer and a subsequent enhanced likelihood of cure when these occult tumors are surgically resected. In a large study conducted in Minnesota, 46,000 asymptomatic individuals with no personal or family history for colorectal cancer were randomly assigned to undergo annual, biennial, or no testing of their stool for occult blood. The mature results of this study demonstrated a statistically meaningful reduction in the number of colorectal cancer deaths in the cohort undergoing annual testing, despite the fact that the positive predictive value of such stool guaiac evaluations was only 5.6%. Any patient who had a positive stool guaiac test was offered a colonoscopy, and 36% of the patients who were assigned to annual testing underwent at least one such endoscopic examination; interestingly, 20% fewer cancers arose in this group of patients, even though the absolute incidence of cancer should have been identical among the three study cohorts. Consequently, the question has been raised as to whether the survival benefit reported from this trial was due to guaiac testing or perhaps to polyp removal (i.e., primary prevention) associated with the endoscopic examinations. The value of fecal occult blood screening has been confirmed by experiences in 150,000 individuals from Britain and 140,000 people from Denmark, but the reduction in mortality in these two European studies was far less than that in Min-

nesota, possibly because the rate of colonoscopy in the European trials was far less than that in the American experience (Table 92-3). Consequently, it may be concluded that examination of stool for occult blood as a screening strategy for colorectal cancer is an imperfect test.

Flexible Sigmoidoscopy

Flexible sigmoidoscopy has been popularized because of its acceptable expense and its successful use by non-physicians, such as nurse practitioners. It has been proposed that flexible sigmoidoscopy performed every five years after age 50 be added to annual examinations of the stool for occult blood as a cost-effective screening strategy. The value of flexible sigmoidoscopy as a screening technique has been challenged by the publication of two reports in which the use of colonoscopy in more than 5000 asymptomatic, previously unscreened individuals revealed advanced lesions (villous or dysplastic adenomas or carcinomas) in the proximal colons of 2.1% of adults whose distal colons (which would be visible by optimal flexible sigmoidoscopy) were totally normal. A comparison of fecal occult blood testing plus flexible sigmoidoscopy to colonoscopy in a subset of this cohort revealed a sensitivity of 75%, meaning that such a screening strategy missed 25% of lesions.

Colonoscopy

Colonoscopy represents the most accurate method of screening of the large bowel for polyps and cancers. It has been shown to be clearly superior in a recent analysis to double-contrast barium enema. However, colonoscopy is expensive (presently $750 to $1000 per examination), is associated with a 0.3% to 0.5% likelihood of bowel perforation (essentially occurring only when a polypectomy is attempted), and currently can be performed only by gastroenterologists or specially trained surgeons. Performing this more accurate, albeit expensive, test on an infrequent basis (every 10 years) has been proposed as a means to optimize the balance between costs and benefit. Routine scheduled colonoscopy should commence after age 50, because initiating screening prior to age 50 does not provide additional benefit. Since essentially all colorectal cancers arise from adenomatous polyps and such polyps appear during the sixth and seventh decades, one reasonable approach might be to limit all colorectal cancer screening in standard-risk individuals to an initial colonoscopy sometime between ages 50 and 55 and, if no abnormality is noted, to repeat the study again in 10 years. Should no polyps or cancers be found at the time of the second endoscopic examination, no further screening should be undertaken. Conversely, should polyps be found during these endoscopic examinations, triennial colonoscopies would be indicated. This approach as well as several others are now being subjected to cost-efficacy analyses.

Compliance

Regardless of the above considerations, compliance with any colorectal cancer screening recommendation within the general population is currently poor; only 30% of the U.S. population receives any form of screening.

Clinical Presentation and Evaluation

Presenting symptoms of colorectal cancer vary with the anatomic site of the lesion (Table 92-4). The sole function of the large bowel is to resorb water from stool that is quite liquid as it enters the colon at the ileocecal valve and has become formed by the time it passes into the rectum. Because of the liquid nature of stool in the right colon, relatively large tumors may develop without the presence of noticeable bleeding, a change in bowel habits, or clinical obstruction. However, occult blood loss from ulcerated cancers does occur, leading to iron deficiency anemia and the development of weakness or even angina as a presenting symptom (see Chapter 24). The appearance of iron deficiency anemia in any adult (except, perhaps a menstruating woman) merits endoscopic evaluation of the large bowel, even if several stool samples test negative for occult blood. As stool passes into the transverse colon, it becomes more formed; consequently, the presence of annular tumors in the transverse colon results in crampy abdominal pain due to bowel obstruction. Such localizing symptoms often lead to an earlier diagnosis. As stool moves into the distal colon, obstructive symptoms become less frequent, since the rectum acts as a reservoir for stool and can expand proximal to a relatively large tumor. However, patients with rectosigmoid cancers frequently experience the passage of bright red blood from the rectum and such changes in bowel habits as narrowing of the stool caliber, passage of stool with increased frequency, and tenesmus. Despite the presence of bright red blood, the absolute amount of bleeding is relatively small, and anemia is uncommon. Many patients with rectosigmoid cancers may have hemorrhoids. One has to be wary of attributing bleeding to hemorrhoids until a rectosigmoid colon cancer has been ruled out. The hemorrhoids at times may be caused by the presence of a more proximally located cancer; endoscopic assessment of the distal bowel is always indicated in the presence of rectal bleeding.

In the past, the majority of colorectal cancers were thought to arise in the distal left colon or the rectosigmoid, leading to the once-held practice of utilizing rigid proctosigmoidoscopy as a screening maneuver. Recent experience, however, has indicated that an increasing percentage of such lesions are proximal to the sigmoid colon. No satisfactory explanation for this change in the natural history of colorectal cancer has been offered.

Table 92-4 ■ Colorectal Carcinoma: Presenting Symptoms by Anatomic Location

	Rectal Bleeding	Change in Bowel Habits	Obstruction	Anemia
Right colon	+	+	0-+	++
Transverse colon	+	+	++	+
Sigmoid colon	++	++	+	0-+
Rectum	+++	+++	0-+	0

The liver represents the most common site of metastatic disease in patients with colorectal cancer. Such metastases may be identified in asymptomatic patients by the presence of progressive elevation on serial studies of the plasma titer of the carcinoembryonic antigen or by their detection as an incidental finding on a computed tomography scan. When symptoms develop, fullness in the right upper quadrant leading to early satiety, a pressure sensation, and rarely pain and/jaundice may occur. As a rule, colorectal cancer does not spread to the lungs without initially involving the liver. An exception to this rule occurs occasionally in patients with rectal cancer that develops below the peritoneal reflection. In this case, disease can spread along paraspinal lymphatics, leading to pulmonary involvement in the absence of any tumor deposits in the liver.

The workup for patients with colorectal cancer is straightforward. Routine physical examination and laboratory tests look for clues to distant spread and allow assessment of general medical condition with regard to plans for therapy. A careful colonoscopy, if feasible and not performed at the time of diagnosis, is required to look for the presence of additional colonic lesions, such as carcinomas and adenomas. A computed tomography scan of the abdomen to look for disease extension or for the presence of unsuspected metastases to the liver is needed. A CEA antigen determination prior to therapy is helpful in following response to therapy and monitoring for tumor recurrence after therapy if it is known to be elevated before treatment. A computed tomography scan of the chest in search of pulmonary metastases is rarely necessary. One should be aware however, as noted previously, that although the liver is the most common initial site of metastasis, the frequency of spread to the lung (and to the pelvis) increases as the site of the cancer shifts from the right colon to the rectum, because of different patterns of venous drainage.

Staging and Prognosis

The initial staging system for colorectal cancer was developed by Dukes, who defined stage A as a superficial tumor involving the submucosa, stage B as a deeper penetrating tumor that did not involve regional lymph nodes, and stage C as a tumor with lymph node involvement. Subsequently, stage D was added to indicate distant metastatic disease. Kirklin's modification of the Dukes classification scheme for stages A, B, and C is diagrammed in Figure 92-4. More recently, the Dukes staging system has been superceded by the American Joint Committee's TNM staging of colorectal cancer; Table 92-5 shows how these two staging systems relate. In the TNM classification, the "T" reflects depth of penetration (rather than size) of the tumor. Utilizing the TNM classification system, superficial tumors that do not involve regional lymph nodes (T1N0M0 [Dukes-Kirklin A] and T2N0M0 [Dukes-Kirklin B₁]) are termed stage I, more deeply penetrating tumors that do not involve regional lymph nodes (T3N0M0 [Dukes-Kirklin B2] and T4N0M0 [Dukes-Kirklin B3]) are labeled stage II, localized tumors that involve regional lymph nodes (TxN1M0 [Dukes C]) constitute stage III, and tumors that have spread to distant sites (TxNxM1 [Dukes D]) are stage IV. Unlike the prognosis for other "solid tumors," the prognosis of colorectal cancer is not related to the size of the primary tumor.

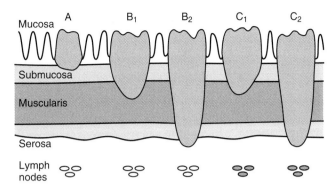

Figure 92-4 ■ Levels of bowel penetration by cancer and regional node involvement that are used in staging according to the Kirklin modification of the Dukes classification schema.

The prognosis following a surgical resection in patients with colorectal cancer depends on disease stage. Essentially all recurrences develop within five years of diagnosis, so disease-free survival after five years from diagnosis is tantamount to cure. Factors predicting for a worsening outcome include an increasing number of involved lymph nodes, lymphovascular invasion within the tumor, poorly differentiated histology, an elevated preoperative CEA titer, aneuploidy in the tumor, allelic loss (chromosome 18q ["deleted in colon cancer" {DCC} gene], or 17p [p53 gene] mutations).

The presence of microsatellite instability reflected in short sequences of tumor DNA repeated in tandem appears to predict for a more favorable prognosis, not only in patients with hereditary nonpolyposis colorectal cancer where microsatellite instability is common, but also in sporadic cases.

Overall, the anticipated five-year probability of survival is greater than 90% for patients with stage I tumors, about 75% for most patients with stage II tumors (i.e., T3N0M0 lesions), 45% to 65% for stage III tumors, and 5% for those with stage IV cancers.

Table 92-5 ■ Staging and Prognosis for Colorectal Cancer

T: Primary Tumor

TX: Cannot be assessed
T0:   Cannot be found
Tis: Is limited to carcinoma in situ (intraepithelial or intramucosal)
T1:   Invades submucosal
T2:   Invades muscularis propria
T3:   Invades through muscularis propria into subserosa, pericolic, or perirectal tissues
T4:   Invades other organs, structures, or other parts of the colon

N: Regional Lymph Nodes

NX: Cannot be assessed
N0:   Are not involved
N1:   Show involvement of 1 to 3 nodes
N2:   Show involvement of ≥4 nodes

M: Distant Metastases

M0:   Are absent
M1:   Are present

Stage Grouping

		Dukes Classification	Modified Dukes Classification	Approximate Five-year Survival Rate (%)
Stage 0	Tis N0 M0			>95
Stage I	T1 N0 M0		A	>90
		Dukes A		
	T2 N0 M0		B_1	85
Stage II	T3 N0 M0		B_2	75
		Dukes B		
	T4 N0 M0		B_3	60
Stage III	Any T, N1 M0			
		Dukes C		45–65
	Any T, N2 M0			
Stage IV	Any T, any N, M1	Dukes D		5

Postoperative Surveillance

Despite the use of regularly scheduled computed tomography scans, endoscopic procedures, and blood studies at annual or even semiannual intervals to detect recurrent disease, there is no evidence that survival is improved by the use of these extremely costly tests. Recent randomized trials, evidence-based guidelines from the American Society of Clinical Oncology, and governmental policy decisions have all concluded that most of these studies are unnecessary. Colonoscopy every three to five years is recommended to detect the early appearance of metachronous neoplasms, (i.e., new polyps or a new cancer). Such endoscopic examinations are not performed to identify intraluminal recurrences at the suture line, which are extremely uncommon. The use of serial CEA testing for surveillance remains controversial.

One suggested method of follow-up (Table 92-6) involves obtaining baseline routine blood counts and liver function tests, a CEA titer, a chest radiograph, and a postoperative computed tomography scan of the abdomen and pelvis. During the first five postoperative years, CEA levels may be measured every three months, while blood counts and liver function studies are carried out semiannually. A colonoscopy should be performed one year after the operation to be certain that no abnormalities were overlooked at the time the cancer was diagnosed; if the endoscopic examination is normal, colonoscopy should be repeated every three to four years to detect the early appearance of metachronous lesions.

Surgery for Stages I, II, and III

Surgical resection and colonic reanastomosis cures a large number of patients with early disease. The sur-

---

Table 92-6 ■ Suggested Postoperative Follow-up After "Curative" Resection of a Stage I or Stage II Colorectal Cancer

Baseline

Complete blood count and platelet count
CEA antigen level
Chest radiograph
Colonoscopy
Computed tomography scan of the abdomen and pelvis

Years 1–5

CEA antigen level every three months
Complete blood count and platelet count and liver function
 tests twice annually
Colonoscopy in year 3
Chest radiograph in year 3

Year 6 and Thereafter

CEA antigen level annually or twice annually
Complete blood count and platelet count and liver function
 tests annually
Colonoscopy in year 6 and every three years thereafter

---

gical specimen should provide at least 5-cm margins of normal tissue proximally and distally to the tumor. The supporting mesentery should be removed as well to locate and evaluate the regional draining nodes. Small, even impalpable nodes may contain cancer, and enlarged nodes may be due to lymphoid hyperplasia. Careful clearing of the specimen for all lymph nodes is essential to determine prognosis and therapy. Overall, 60% to 70% of patients undergoing resection are cured of their disease; those without regional node involvement have a cure rate of 75% to 90%. Recurrences usually become manifest within the first few years after surgery. Recurrence in colonic cancer is usually not local, as it is in rectal cancer, but metastatic to distant sites: liver, lung, and bone. No randomized study has suggested any benefit from the use of adjuvant radiation therapy in this setting, but as is discussed following, adjuvant chemotherapy has improved the results in some patient subsets.

Treatment of Advanced Disease

5-Fluorouracil

5-Fluorouracil remains the cornerstone of management of patients with metastatic disease. Its administration results in a response rate of approximately 20% and appears to prolong survival in responding patients. More than 40 years after its entry into the clinic, debate persists regarding the optimal dose schedule for 5-fluorouracil administration. Although intermittent bolus injections, given either on five consecutive days every 28 days or on a weekly basis, have been the standard intravenous schedule, interest has been rekindled concerning the delivery of the drug by means of continuous, long-term infusions. Several randomized studies have shown that this more costly method of drug delivery results in a slightly higher response rate than the bolus regimen, but differences in overall survival have been imperceptible.

Various pharmacologic strategies have been used in an attempt to biologically enhance the efficacy of 5-fluorouracil. The most promising of these has focused on the addition of leucovorin (i.e., folinic acid) to 5-fluorouracil. Leucovorin is a derivative of the reduced folate tetrahydrofolate; increasing the intracellular pool of reduced folates through pretreatment with leucovorin is thought to enhance the binding of 5-fluorouracil to its target enzyme, thymidylate synthase, thereby increasing the inhibition of DNA synthesis. 5-Fluorouracil has been compared to 5-fluorouracil/leucovorin in at least nine randomized trials in previously untreated patients with advanced colorectal cancer. A meta-analysis of these studies has shown a statistically significant increase in the likelihood of response when leucovorin has been added to 5-fluorouracil, but there has been little effect on overall survival. Several dose-schedules of 5-fluorouracil/leucovorin have been examined; none has been shown to be therapeutically superior to others.

When 5-fluorouracil was initially developed, it was given either by parenteral or oral routes. The use of oral 5-fluorouracil fell into disfavor when a randomized study showed that intravenous 5-fluorouracil led to a greater likelihood of disease regression than oral 5-fluorouracil because of the variable absorption of the oral 5-fluorouracil by the intestine. The unpredictability of drug absorption was overcome by the development of capecitabine, a prodrug of 5-fluorouracil that is given orally, absorbed intact, and metabolically activated after intestinal absorption has occurred. Randomized studies have shown oral capecitabine to have antitumor efficacy comparable to that of intravenous 5-fluorouracil/leucovorin and to be associated with diarrhea and palmar–plantar erythema in a frequency similar to that observed with continuous infusions of intravenous 5-fluorouracil.

Irinotecan

Irinotecan, also known as CPT-11, is a topoisomerase-1 inhibitor that has been associated with a 25% to 30% response rate in previously untreated patients with colorectal cancer and a 15% response rate in patients with prior exposure to 5-fluorouracil. Randomized trials documented irinotecan's efficacy in patients previously treated with 5-fluorouracil; the median survival was increased from six to nine months when irinotecan was compared to best supportive care alone and from eight months to 10 months when irinotecan was compared to 5-fluorouracil administered as a continuous intravenous infusion. Subsequently, irinotecan was added to 5-fluorouracil and leucovorin as part of initial treatment programs for patients with advanced colorectal cancer in randomized comparisons with 5-fluorouracil and leucovorin alone. The results of a North American trial utilizing weekly bolus irinotecan/5-fluorouracil/leucovorin and a European study utilizing weekly irinotecan with continuous infusional 5-fluorouracil/leucovorin provided remarkably similar outcomes; the probability of response increased from approximately 26% to approximately 44%, the median progression-free survival increased from approximately 4.5 months to 7 months, and the median survival increased from approximately 13.5 months to 16 months. These data suggest superiority for the irinotecan/5-fluorouracil leucovorin regimen. However, it remains uncertain whether sequential irinotecan and 5-fluorouracil/leucovorin might not result in the same overall survival time with less toxicity than their concomitant administration.

Oxaliplatin

Oxaliplatin is a platinum compound that acts synergistically with 5-fluorouracil in vitro against human colon cancer cell lines, possibly by reducing the expression of thymidylate synthase, thereby make the 5-fluorouracil more cytotoxic. In patients previously treated with 5-fluorouracil-containing regimens, the use of oxaliplatin/5-fluorouracil/leucovorin was associated with a 10% response rate, whereas 5-fluorouracil/leucovorin or oxaliplatin alone demonstrated no efficacy. Randomized trials from North America and Europe utilizing oxaliplatin in combination with 5-fluorouracil/leucovorin as initial therapy for patients with advanced colorectal cancer have suggested a similar response rate and survival outcome to that associated with irinotecan/5-fluorouracil/leucovorin. Studies are ongoing to assess how best to incorporate oxaliplatin into advanced disease regimens.

Targeted Therapies

The use of inhibitors of the epidermal growth factor receptor such as the moniclonal antibody cetuximab (C-225) or inhibitors of the receptor's tyrosine kinase such as Iressa or Tarceva has been the subject of considerable interest. Similarly, preliminary results utilizing a monoclonal antibody to the vascular endothelial growth factor receptor (bevacizumab) have shown activity. These targeted therapies are the focus of ongoing large-scale randomized trials.

Adjuvant Therapy

Postoperative 5-fluorouracil was compared to no postsurgical treatment to assess its possible benefit as a form of adjuvant treatment in at least five randomized trials conducted in North America during the 1970s. None of these studies showed an advantage for treatment in terms of disease-free duration or overall survival. However, little information is available regarding drug compliance in the patients who were randomized to receive 5-fluorouracil.

With the assumption that systemic 5-fluorouracil was ineffective as a means of improving operative outcome, with the appreciation that the liver is the most common site of spread for colon cancer, and with the belief that tumor cells reach the liver through the portal circulation, a series of clinical studies were initiated to determine whether a short-term infusion of 5-fluorouracil into the portal circulation during the perioperative period would reduce the likelihood of subsequently hepatic metastases. In a series of prospective trials, a catheter was placed into the portal or umbilical vein at the time of surgery, and chemotherapy was administered and completed before postoperative patients were discharged from the hospital. A meta-analysis of these studies showed that the five-year survival rate increased from approximately 60% to 65% in patients receiving the portal vein infusion, but the survival advantage occurred without a reduction in the rate of hepatic recurrences. This experience suggested that a short infusion of 5-fluorouracil enhances systemic control and that 5-fluorouracil, when given in a compliant manner, might be an effective form of adjuvant therapy.

At the same time, other investigators examined the value of levamisole, an antihelminthic compound that was believed to have some immunomodulatory capacity as a form of adjuvant immunotherapy for patients with colon cancer. A randomized trial was conducted in North America in more than 900 patients who had undergone the resection of a stage III colon cancer; these individuals were randomized to receive postoperative 5-fluorouracil combined with levamisole, levamisole alone, or no postoperative treatment. The results of this multi-institutional effort conclusively demonstrated that the 5-fluorouracil-containing program, administered to highly compliant patients, resulted in an approximate 40% reduction in recurrences and a 33% improvement in survival when compared to the outcome for the cohort of individuals assigned to levamisole alone or no postoperative

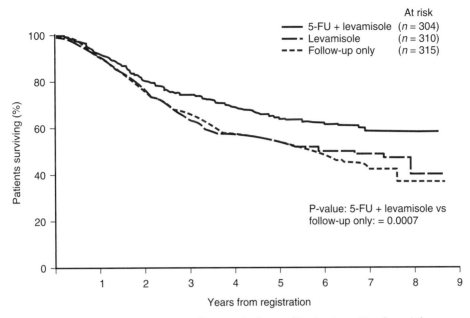

Figure 92-5 ■ Randomized trial of adjuvant therapy after surgical resection in stage III colorectal cancer, comparing observation versus levamisole alone versus the combination of 5-fluorouracil and levamisole. (From Moertel CG, Fleming TR, Macdonald JS, et al: Fluorouracil plus levamisole as effective adjuvant therapy after resection of stage III colon carcinoma: A final report. Ann Intern Med 1995; 122:321–326.)

treatment (Figure 92-5). Levamisole has subsequently been shown to be ineffective, so the study actually represented a comparison of 5-fluorouracil versus no postoperative therapy. The unequivocal benefit demonstrated in this well-conducted trial, showing more than 60% of patients to be alive and presumably cured, led to the widespread acceptance of adjuvant chemotherapy following the resection of stage III colon cancers. However, in a similar, albeit smaller, effort in 318 patients with stage II colon cancer, no reduction in recurrences or improvement in survival could be demonstrated when 5-fluorouracil combined with levamisole was compared to "follow-up only."

Similar results have emerged from three randomized trials that have shown a survival benefit for patients treated with 5-fluorouracil and leucovorin when compared to no postoperative treatment. Again, this benefit was noted in patients with stage III (Dukes C) disease but not stage II (Dukes B) disease. The value of adjuvant chemotherapy in patients with stage II colon cancers thus remains controversial with a retrospective subset analysis by the National Surgical Adjuvant Breast and Bowel Project supporting such an approach while a pooled analysis of 1016 patients with stage II disease participating in "treatment versus no treatment" trials failed to demonstrate any benefit.

More recent large cooperative group studies in the adjuvant setting of colon cancer have compared 5-fluorouracil/levamisole to 5-fluorouracil/leucovorin ± levamisole. The results of these studies indicate that six months of 5-fluorouracil/leucovorin is equivalent to 12 months of 5-FU/levamisole, that different dose schedules of 5-fluorouracil/leucovorin are similar in adjuvant efficacy but differ in toxicity profiles, and that levamisole does not add to the adjuvant effect of 5-fluorouracil/leucovorin.

The currently available data support the use of postoperative therapy in patients with stage III colon cancer. Based on prior studies, a six-month treatment course of 5-FU and leucovorin is the standard of care. Prospective data have not yet demonstrated any adjuvant benefit for patients with stage II disease. Whether such treatment will improve the prognosis for individuals having such ominous factors as aneuploidy, mutated chromosome 18q (i.e., "DCC" gene), or bowel perforation, remains to be determined.

Rectal Cancer

Rectal carcinoma is defined as a primary tumor less than 12 cm from the anal verge or any tumor characterized intraoperatively as extending below the peritoneal reflection. Lying as it does below the peritoneal reflection and surrounded by perirectal tissue, the routes of dissemination of rectal carcinoma differ from those of colonic carcinoma. The principal concern in these patients is the issue of extrarectal extension and local recurrence, because survival is curtailed and the patient is at risk for severe unrelenting pelvic pain due to infiltration of the sacral nerve plexus. Local recurrence occurs in fewer than 10% of patients with stage I (Dukes A) disease, which is associated with an

Table 92-7 ■ **Summary of Randomized Trials of Postoperative Adjuvant Therapy for Rectal Cancer**

Source	Number of patients	Five-Year Overall Survival Rate			
		Surgery	Radiation Therapy	Chemotherapy	Chemoradiation Therapy
GITSG (1985)	227	44%	52%	50%	59%
NSABP (1988)	555	43%	41%	53%	—
MRC (1996)	469	46%	52%	—	—
NSABP (2000)	694	—	—	64%	66%
NCCTG (1991)	240	—	48%	—	57%
Intergroup (1997)	1695	—	—	—	64%

approximately 80% five-year survival. The frequency of local recurrence correlates with advancing stage.

In the past, surgery required abdominoperineal resection and the establishment of a permanent colostomy. Current surgical techniques usually permit resection of the cancer and preservation of anal sphincter function and bowel continuity. Despite "curative" surgery, the incidence of local recurrences in this disease is high when conventional operative technique (blunt dissection) is carried out. In a series of 75 patients who underwent random second-look procedures, recurrences were observed in 52 patients (69%); of these 52 recurrences, 48 (92%) occurred in the pelvis. Such observations established the rationale for the use of adjuvant radiation therapy to reduce the likelihood of pelvic recurrences.

Adjuvant Radiation Therapy

Radiation therapy can be given either preoperatively or postoperatively. The results of randomized trials suggest that the use of preoperative radiation therapy utilizing standard radiation techniques (four to five weeks of daily small treatment fractions) reduces the likelihood of local recurrences but has no significant effect on overall survival. A provocative report from Sweden, however, administered higher fractions of radiation therapy on five consecutive days followed within one week by definitive rectal surgery; the outcome of this study demonstrated not only a reduction in local recurrences, but also a small yet statistically significant survival benefit for the patients who received preoperative treatment.

Surgical technique for rectal cancer has been refined, utilizing a sharp dissection of the rectum at the pelvic sidewalls (total mesorectal excision); the use of such an approach appears to reduce the likelihood of pelvic recurrence from the 20% to 25% range to approximately 10%. Yet a randomized experience in the Netherlands showed that even when a total

mesorectal excision was utilized for rectal cancer, the use of preoperative radiation therapy further reduced the likelihood of a pelvic recurrence and made a small but definite contribution to improved survival.

The use of postoperative radiation therapy alone has not been shown, in a controlled setting, to affect survival.

Combined Chemoradiation Therapy

The value of offering patients who have undergone a complete resection of a rectal cancer postoperative chemoradiation therapy has been examined in a series of randomized trials (Table 92-7). In a generally consistent manner, the results of these efforts have shown that surgery alone is associated with an approximate 45% likelihood of five-year survival; the addition of either postoperative radiation therapy or postoperative chemotherapy increases the five-year survival rate to 50% to 55%, while the use of postoperative chemoradiation therapy improves the five-year survival rate to approximately 65%. The addition of 5-fluorouracil-based chemotherapy to postoperative pelvic radiation therapy further diminishes the likelihood of a pelvic recurrence, presumably through the radiation-sensitizing effect of the 5-fluorouracil. It appears that such radiation sensitization may be maximized if the 5-fluorouracil is administered as a continuous intravenous infusion throughout the five-week time period when the pelvic radiation therapy is being given. It is currently unclear whether oral capecitabine might be satisfactorily substituted for the continuous infusion 5-FU as an effective radiation sensitizer and antitumor agent. Moreover, it is uncertain whether adding irinotecan or oxaliplatin to the chemoradiation therapy would enhance benefit.

The effectiveness of postoperative adjuvant chemoradiation therapy for patients with rectal cancer led to interest in using chemoradiation therapy preoperatively in an attempt to shrink (downstage) the primary tumor and even possibly to enhance the likelihood for curative sphincter-sparing surgery. In North America, surgical opinion has become polarized regarding the comparative merits of preoperative versus postoperative chemoradiation therapy, and attempts to compare the two strategies in randomized trials have thus far proven unsuccessful.

References

Incidence and Mortality

Jemal A, Murray T, Samuels, et al: Cancer statistics, 2002. CA Cancer J Clin 2003;53:5–26.

Troisi RJ, Freedman AN, Devesa SS: Incidence of colorectal carcinoma in the U.S.: An update of trends by gender, race, age, subsite, and stage, 1975–1994. Cancer 1999;85:1670–1676.

Heredity

Aaltonen LA, Salovaara R, Kristo P, et al: Incidence of hereditary nonpolyposis colorectal cancer and the feasibility of molecular screening for the disease. N Eng J Med 1998;338:1481–1497.

Ahsan H, Neugut AI, Garbowski GC, et al: Family history of colorectal adenomatous polyps and increased risk for colorectal cancer. Ann Intern Med 1998;128:900–905.

Fuchs CS, Giovannuci EL, Colditz GA, et al: A prospective study of family history and the risk of colorectal cancer. N Engl J Med 1994;331:1669–1674.

Giardello FM, Brensinger JD, Petersen GM, et al: The use and interpretation of commercial APC gene testing for familial adenomatous polyposis. N Engl J Med 1997;336:823–827.

Giardello FM, Yang VW, Hylind LM, et al: Primary chemoprevention of familial adenomatous polyposis with sulindar. N Engl J Med 2002;326:1054–1059.

Goss KH, Gordon J: Biology of the adenomatous polyposis coli tumor suppressor. J Clin Oncol 2000;18:1967–1979.

Hamilton SR, Liu B, Parsons RE, et al: The molecular basis of Turcot's syndrome. N Engl J Med 1995;332:839–847.

Lipkin M, Blattner WA, Gardner LJ, et al: Classification and risk assignment of individuals with familial non-polyposis, Gardner's syndrome, and familial non-polyposis colon cancer from (^{3}H) thymidine labeling patterns in colonic epithelial cells. Cancer Res 1984;44:4201–4207.

Lynch HT, Smyrk T: Hereditary nonpolyposis colorectal cancer (Lynch syndrome): An updated review. Cancer 1996;78:1149–1167.

Powell SM, Petersen GM, Krush AJ, et al: Molecular diagnosis of familial adenomatous polyposis. N Engl J Med 1993;329:1982–1987.

Rustgi AK: Hereditary gastrointestinal polyposis and nonpolyposis syndromes. N Engl J Med 1994;331:1694–1702.

Saletti P, Edwin ID, Pack K, et al: Microsatellite instability: Application in hereditary non-polyposis colorectal cancer. Ann Oncol 2001;12:151–160.

Steinbach G, Lynch PM, Phillips RKS, et al: The effect of celecoxib, a cyclooxygenase-2 inhibitor, in familial adenomatous polyposis. N Engl J Med 2000;342:1946–1952.

Syngal S, Schrag D, Falchuk M, et al: Phenotypic characteristics associated with the APC gene L1307K mutation in Askenazi Jewish patients with colorectal polyps. JAMA 2000;284:857–860.

Syngal S, Weeks JC, Schrag D, et al: Benefits of colonoscopic surveillance and prophylactic colectomy in patients with hereditary nonpolyposis colorectal cancer mutations. Ann Intern Med 1998;129:787–796.

Watson P, Lin KM, Rodriguez-Biges MA, et al: Colorectal carcinoma survival among hereditary nonpolyposis colorectal carcinoma family members. Cancer 1998;83:259–266.

Wijnen JT, Vasen HFA, Khan PM, et al: Clinical findings with implications for genetic testing in families with clustering of colorectal cancer. N Engl J Med 1998;339:511–518.

Diet

Bayerdörffer E, Mannes GA, Richter WO, et al: Decreased high-density lipoprotein cholesterol and increased low-density cholesterol levels in patients with colorectal adenomas. Ann Intern Med 1993;118:481–487.

Forman D: Meat and cancer: A relation in search of a mechanism. Lancet 1999;353:686–687.

Fuchs CS, Giovannuci EL, Colditz GA, et al: Dietary fiber and the risk of colorectal cancer and adenoma in women. N Engl J Med 1999;340:169–176.

Giovannucci E, Stampfer MJ, Colditz G, et al: Relationship of diet to risk of colorectal adenoma in men. J Natl Cancer Inst 1992;84:91–98.

Mannes GA, Maier A, Thieme C, et al: Relation between the frequency of colorectal adenoma and the serum cholesterol level. N Engl J Med 1986;315:1634–1638.

Michels KB, Giovannuci E, Joshipura KJ, et al: Prospective study of fruit and vegetable consumption and incidence of colon and rectal cancers. J Natl Cancer Inst 2000;92:1740–1752.

Tornberg SA, Holm LE, Carstenson JM, Eklund GA: Risks of cancer of the colon and rectum in relation to serum cholesterol and beta-lipoprotein. N Engl J Med 1986;315:1629–1633.

Willett WC, Stampfer MJ, Colditz GA, et al: Relation of meat, fat, and fiber intake to the risk of colon cancer in a prospective study among women. N Engl J Med 1990;323:1664–1672.

Inflammatory Bowel Disease

Bachwich DR, Lichtenstein GR, Traber PG: Cancer in inflammatory bowel disease. Med Clin N Am 1994;78:1399–1412.

Bernstein CN, Shanahan F, Weinstein WM: Are we telling patients the truth about surveillance colonoscopy in ulcerative colitis? Lancet 1994;343:71–74.

Collins RH Jr, Feldman M, Fordtran JS: Colon cancer, dysplasia, and surveillance in patients with ulcerative colitis: A critical review. N Engl J Med 1987;316:1654–1658.

Devroede GJ, Taylor WF, Sauer WG, et al: Cancer risk and life expectancy of children with ulcerative colitis. N Engl J Med 1971;285:17–21.

Ekbom A, Helmick C, Zack M, Adami HO: Ulcerative colitis and colorectal cancer. N Engl J Med 1990;323:1228–1233.

Ekbom A, Helmick C, Zack M, Adami HO: Ulcerative colitis and colorectal cancer: A population-based study. N Engl J Med 1990;323:1228–1233.

Faintuch J, Levin B, Kirshner JB: Inflammatory bowel diseases and their relationship to malignancy. Crit Rev Oncol Hematol 1985;2:323–353.

Kewenter J, Ahlman H, Hulten L: Cancer risk in extensive ulcerative colitis. Ann Surg 1978;188:824–828.

Sugita A, Greenstein AJ, Ribeiro MB, et al: Survival with colorectal cancer in ulcerative colitis: A study of 102 cases. Ann Surg 1993;218:189–195.

Other Associated Disorders

Giovannucci E: An updated review of the epidemiological evidence that cigarette smoking increases risk of colorectal cancer. Cancer Epidemiol Biomarkers Prev 2001;10:725–731.

Hossenbux K, Dale BAS, Walls ADF, Lawrence JR: Streptococcus bovis endocarditis and colonic carcinoma: A neglected association. Br Med J 1983;287:21.

Husmann DA, Spence HM: Current status of tumor of the bowel following ureterosigmoidostomy: A review. J Urol 1990;144:607–610.

Klein RS, Catalano MT, Edberg SC, et al: Streptococcus bovis septicemia and carcinoma of the colon. Ann Intern Med 1979;91:560–562.

Sheldon CA, McKinley CR, Hartig PR, Gonzalez R: Carcinoma at the site of the ureterosigmoidostomy. Dis Colon Rectum 1983;26:55–58.

Polyps

Ahsan H, Neugut AI, Garbowski GC, et al: Family history of colorectal adenomatous polyps and increased risk for colorectal cancer. Ann Intern Med 1998;128:900–905.

Cannon-Albright LA, Skolnick MH, Bishop T, et al: Common inheritance of susceptibility to colonic adenomatous polyps and associated colorectal cancers. N Engl J Med 1988;319:533–537.

Kune GA, Kune S, Watson LF: History of colorectal polypectomy and risk of subsequent colorectal cancer. Brit J Surg 1987;74:1064–1065.

Müller AD, Sonnenberg A: Prevention of colorectal cancer by flexible endoscopy and polypectomy: A case-control study of 32,702 veterans. Ann Intern Med 1995;123:904–910.

O'Brien MJ, Winawer SJ, Zauber AG, et al: The National Polyp Study: Patient and polyp characteristics associated with high-grade dysplasia in colorectal adenomas. Gastroenterology 1990;98:371–379.

Simons BD, Morrison AS, Lev R, et al: Relationship of polyps to cancer of the large intestine. J Natl Cancer Inst 1992;84:962–966.

Vatn MH, Stalsberg H: The prevalence of polyps of the large intestine in Oslo: An autopsy study. Cancer 1982;49:819–825.

Vogelstein B, Fearon ER, Hamilton SR, et al: Genetic alterations during colorectal tumor development. New Engl J Med 1988;319:525–532.

Winawer SJ, Zauber AG, Ho MN, et al: Prevention of colorectal cancer by colonoscopic polypectomy. N Engl J Med 1993;329:1977–1981.

Winawer SJ, Zauber AG, O'Brien MJ, et al: Randomized comparison of surveillance intervals after colonoscopic removal of newly diagnosed adenomatous polyps. N Engl J Med 1993;328:901–906.

Chemoprevention

Alberts DS, Martinez ME, Roe DJ, et al: Lack of effect of a high-fiber cereal supplement on the recurrence of colorectal adenomas. N Engl J Med 2000;342:1156–1162.

Baron JA, Beach M, Mandel JS, et al: Calcium supplements for the prevention of colorectal adenomas. N Engl J Med 1999;340:101–107.

Calle EE, Miracle-McMahill HL, Thun MJ, Heath CW Jr: Estrogen replacement therapy and risk of fatal colon cancer in a prospective cohort of postmenopausal women. J Natl Cancer Inst 1995;87:517–523.

Fuchs CS, Willett WC, Colditz GA, et al: The influence of folate and multivitamin use on the familial risk of colon cancer in women. Cancer Epid Biomark Prev 2002;11:227–234.

Giovannuci E, Egan KM, Hunter DJ, et al: Aspirin and the risk of colorectal cancer in women. N Engl J Med 1995;333:609–614.

Giovannucci E, Rimm EB, Stampfer MJ, et al: Aspirin use and the risk for colorectal cancer and adenoma in male health professionals. Ann Intern Med 1994;121:241–246.

Greenberg ER, Baron JA, Freeman DH, et al: Reduced risk of large-bowel adenomas among aspirin users. J Natl Cancer Inst 1993;85:912–916.

Greenberg ER, Baron JA, Tosteson TD, et al: A clinical trial of antioxidant vitamins to prevent colorectal adenoma. N Engl J Med 1994;331:141–147.

Grodstein F, Martinez E, Platz EA, et al: Postmenopausal hormone use and risk for colorectal cancer and adenoma. Ann Intern Med 1998;128:705–712.

Jänne PA, Mayer RJ: Chemoprevention of colorectal cancer. N Engl J Med 2000;342:1960–1968.

Newcomb PA, Storer BE: Postmenopausal hormone use and risk of large-bowel cancer. J Natl Cancer Inst 1995;87:1067–1071.

Schatzkin A, Lanza E, Corle D, et al: Lack of effect of a low-fat, high-fiber diet on the recurrence of colorectal adenomas. N Engl J Med 2000;342:1149–1155.

Stürmer T, Glynn RJ, Lee IM, et al: Aspirin use and colorectal cancer: Post-trial follow-up data from the Physician's Health Study. Ann Intern Med 1998;128:713–720.

Thun MJ, Namboordi MM, Heath CW Jr: Aspirin use and reduced risk of fatal colon cancer. N Engl J Med 1991;325:1593–1596.

Wu K, Willett WC, Fuchs CS, et al: Calcium intake and risk of colon cancer in women and men. J Natl Cancer Inst 2002;94:437–446.

Diagnosis, Screening, Staging, and Prognosis

Anderson WF, Guyton KZ, Hiatt RA, et al: Colorectal cancer screening for persons at average risk. J Natl Cancer Inst 2002;94:1126–1133.

Armitage NC, Ballantyne KC, Evans DF, et al: The influence of tumour cell DNA content on survival in colorectal cancer: A detailed analysis. Br J Cancer 1990;62:852–856.

Byers T, Levin B, Rothenberger D, et al: American Cancer Society guidelines for screening and surveillance for early detection of colorectal polyps and cancer: Update 1997. CA Cancer J Clin 1997;47:154–160.

Fenlon HM, Nunes DP, Schroy PC, et al: A comparison of virtual and conventional colonoscopy for the detection of colorectal polyps. N Engl J Med 1999;341:1496–1503.

Frazier AL, Colditz GA, Fuchs CS, Kuntz KM: Cost-effectiveness of screening for colorectal cancer in the general population. JAMA 2000;284:1954–1961.

Gastrointestinal Tumor Study Group: Adjuvant therapy of colon cancer: Results of a prospectively randomized trial. N Engl J Med 1984;310:737–743.

Gryfe R, Kim H, Hsieh ETK, et al: Tumor microsatellite instability and clinical outcome in young patients with colorectal cancer. N Engl J Med 2000;342:69–77.

Hardcastle JD, Chamberlain JO, Robinson MHE, et al: Randomized controlled trial of faecal-occult-blood testing for colorectal cancer. Lancet 1996;348:1472–1477.

Imperiale TF, Wagner DR, Lin CY, et al: Risk of advanced proximal neoplasms in asymptomatic adults according to the distal colorectal findings. N Engl J Med 2000;343:169–174.

Imperiale TF, Wagner DR, Lin CY, et al: Results of screening colonoscopy among persons 40–49 years of age. N Engl J Med 2002;346:1781–1785.

Jen J, Kim H, Piantadosi S, et al: Allelic loss of chromosome 18q and prognosis in colorectal cancer. N Engl J Med 1994;331:213–221.

Johnston PG, Fisher ER, Rockettem HE, et al: The role of thymidylate synthase expression in prognosis and outcome of adjuvant chemotherapy in patients with rectal cancer. J Clin Oncol 1994;12:2640–2647.

Kronborg O, Fenger C, Olsen J, et al: Randomized study of screening for colorectal cancer with faecal-occult-blood test. Lancet 1996;348:1467–1471.

Lang CA, Ransohoff DF: Fecal occult blood screening for colorectal cancer: Is mortality reduced by chance selection for screening colonoscopy? JAMA 1994;271:1011–1013.

Lieberman DA, Weiss DG: One-time screening for colorectal cancer with combined fecal occult-blood testing and examination of the distal colon. N Engl J Med 2001;345:555–560.

Lieberman DA, Weiss DG, Bond JH, et al: Use of colonoscopy to screen asymptomatic adults for colorectal cancer. N Engl J Med 2000;343:162–168.

Lieffers GJ, Cleton-Jansen AM, van de Velde CJH, et al: Micrometastases and survival in stage II colorectal cancer. N Engl J Med 1998;339:223–228.

Mandel JS, Bond JH, Church TR, et al: Reducing mortality from colorectal cancer by screening for fecal occult blood. N Eng J Med 1993;328:1367–1371.

Mandel JS, Church TR, Bond JH, et al: The effect of fecal occult blood screening on the incidence of colorectal cancer. N Engl J Med 2000;343:1603–1607.

Maule WF: Screening for colorectal cancer by nurse endoscopists. N Engl J Med 1994;330:183–187.

Ogunbiyi OA, Goodfellow PJ, Herfarth K, et al: Confirmation that chromosome 18q allelic loss in colon cancer is a prognostic indication. J Clin Oncol 1998;16:427–433.

Pignone M, Rich M, Teutsch SM, et al: Screening for colorectal cancer in adults at average risk: a summary of the evidence for the U.S. Preventative Services Task Force. Ann Intern Med 2002;137:132–141.

Ransohoff DF, Sandler RS: Screening for colorectal cancer. N Engl J Med 2002;346:40–44.

Rhodes JB, Holmes FF, Clark GM: Changing distribution of primary cancer in the large bowel. JAMA 1977;238:1641–1643.

Sonnenberg A, Delco F, Inadomi JM: Cost-effectiveness of colonoscopy in screening for colorectal cancer. Ann Intern Med 2000;133:573–584.

Traverso G, Shuber A, Levin B, et al: Detection of apc mutations in fecal DNA from patients with colorectal tumors. N Engl J Med 2002;346:311–320.

Vernon SW: Participation in colorectal cancer screening: A review. J Natl Cancer Inst 1997;89:1406–1422.

Watanabe T, Wu T-T, Catalano PJ, et al: Molecular predictors of survival after adjuvant chemotherapy for colon cancer. N Engl J Med 2001;344:1196–1205.

Winawer SJ, Stewart ET, Zauber AG, et al: A comparison of colonoscopy and double-contrast barium enema for surveillance after polypectomy. N Engl J Med 2000;342:1766–1772.

Witzig TE, Loprinzi CL, Gonchoroff NJ, et al: DNA ploidy and cell kinetic measurements as predictors of recurrence and survival in stages B_2 and C colorectal adenocarcinoma. Cancer 1991;68:879–888.

Wolmark N, Cruz I, Redmond CK, et al: Tumor size and regional lymph nodes metastasis in colorectal cancer: A preliminary analysis from the NSABP Clinical Trials. Cancer 1983;51:1315–1322.

Follow-up Surveillance

Benson AB, Desch CE, Flynn PJ, et al: 2000 Update of American Society of Clinical Oncology colorectal cancer surveillance guidelines. J Clin Oncol 2000;18:3586–3588.

Northover J: Realism or nihilism in bowel cancer follow-up? Lancet 1998;351:1074–1076.

Schoemaker D, Black R, Giles L, Toouli J: Yearly colonoscopy, liver CT, and chest radiotherapy do not influence 5-year survival of colorectal cancer patients. Gastroenterology 1998;114:7–14.

Smith TJ, Bear HD: Standard follow-up of colorectal cancer patients: Finally, we can make practice guidelines based on evidence. Gastroenterology 1998;114:211–213.

Virgo KS, Vernova AM, Longo WE, et al: Cost of patient follow-up after potentially curative colorectal cancer treatment. JAMA 1995;273:1837–1841.

Watanabe T, Wu T-T, Catalano PJ, et al: Molecular predictors of survival after adjuvant chemotherapy for colon cancer. N Engl J Med 2001;344:1196–1206.

Chemotherapy for Advanced Disease

Advanced Colorectal Cancer Meta-Analysis Project: Modulation of fluorouracil by leucovorin in patients with advanced colorectal cancer: Evidence in terms of response rate. J Clin Oncol 1992;10:896–903.

Cunningham D, Pyrhönen S, James RD, et al: Randomized trial of irinotecan plus supportive care versus supportive care alone after fluorouracil failure for patients with metastatic colorectal cancer. Lancet 1998;352:1413–1418.

De Gramont A, Figer A, Seymour M, et al: Leucovorin and fluorouracil with or without oxaliplatin as first-line treatment in advanced colorectal cancer. J Clin Oncol 2000;18:2938–2947.

Douillard JY, Cunningham D, Roth AD, et al: Irinotecan combined with fluorouracil compared with fluorouracil alone as first-line treatment for metastatic colorectal cancer: A multicenter randomised trial. Lancet 2000;355:1041–1047.

Giacchetti S, Perpoint B, Zidani R, et al: Phase III multicenter randomized trial of oxaliplatin added to chronomodulated fluorouracil-leucovorin as first-line treatment of metastatic colorectal cancer. J Clin Oncol 2000;18:136–147.

Herbst RS, Shin DM: Monoclonal antibodies to target epidermal growth factor receptor positive tumors: A new paradigm for cancer therapy. Cancer 2002;94:1593–1611.

Mayer RJ: Moving beyond fluorouracil for colorectal cancer. N Eng J Med 2000;343:963–964.

Meta-analysis Group in Cancer: Efficacy of intravenous continuous infusion of fluorouracil compared with bolus administration in advanced colorectal cancer. J Clin Oncol 1998;16:301–308.

Punt CJA: New drugs in the treatment of colorectal carcinoma. Cancer 1998;83:679–689.

Rothenberg ML, Meropol NJ, Poplin EA, et al: Mortality associated with irinotecan plus bolus fluorouracil and leucovorin: Summary findings of an independent panel. J Clin Oncol 2001;19:3801–3807.

Rougier P, van Cutsem E, Bajetta E, et al: Randomized trial of irinotecan versus fluorouracil by continuous infusion after fluorouracil failure in patients with metastatic colorectal cancer. Lancet 1998;352:1407–1412.

Saltz LB, Cox JV, Blanke C, et al: Irinotecan plus 5-fluorouracil and leucovorin for metastatic colorectal cancer. N Engl J Med 2000;343:898–904.

Tebbutt NC, Cattelll E, Midgley R, et al: Systemic treatment of colorectal cancer. Eur J Cancer 2002;38:1000–1015.

Adjuvant Therapy

Haller DG, Catalano PJ, Macdonald JS, Mayer RJ: Fluorouracil (FU), leucovorin (LV) and levamisole (LEV) adjuvant therapy for colon cancer: Five-year final report of INT-0089. Proc ASCO 1998;17:256a.

Harris JE, Ryan L, Hoover HC Jr, et al: Adjuvant active specific immunotherapy of stage II and III colon cancer with an autologous tumor cell vaccine: ECOG study E5283. J Clin Oncol 2000;18:148–157.

Hoover H, Brandhorst J, Peters L, et al: Adjuvant active specific immunotherapy for human colorectal cancer: 6.5 year median follow-up of a phase III prospectively randomized trial. J Clin Oncol 1993;11:390–399.

International Multicentre Pooled Analysis of B_2 Colon Cancer Trials (IMPACT B_2) Investigators: Efficacy of adjuvant fluorouracil and folinic acid in B_2 colon cancer. J Clin Oncol 1999;17:1356–1363.

International Multicentre Pooled Analysis of Colon Cancer Trials (IMPACT) Investigators: Efficacy of adjuvant fluorouracil and folinic acid in colon cancer. Lancet 1995;345:939–944.

Liver Infusion Meta-analysis Group: Portal vein chemotherapy for colorectal cancer: A meta-analysis of 4000 patients in 10 studies. J Natl Cancer Inst 1997;89:497–505.

Macdonald J, Astrow AB: Adjuvant therapy of colon cancer. Semin Oncol 2001;28:30–40.

Mamounas E, Wieand S, Wolmark N, et al: Comparative efficacy of adjuvant chemotherapy in patients with Dukes' B versus Dukes' C colon cancer: results from four National Surgical Adjuvant Breast and Bowel Project adjuvant studies (C-01, C-02, C-03, and C-04). J Clin Oncol 1999;17:1349–1355.

Marijnen CAM, Glimelius B: The role of radiotherapy in rectal cancer. Eur J Cancer 2002;38:943–952.

Moertel CG, Fleming TR, Macdonald JS, et al: Fluorouracil plus levamisole as effective adjuvant therapy after resection of stage III colon carcinoma: A final report. Ann Intern Med 1995;122:321–326.

Moertel CG, Fleming TR, Macdonald JS, et al: Intergroup study of fluorouracil plus levamisole as adjuvant therapy for stage II/Dukes' B2 colon cancer. J Clin Oncol 1995;13:2936–2943.

O'Connell MJ, Laurie JA, Kahn M, et al: Prospectively randomized trial of postoperative adjuvant chemotherapy in patients with high-risk colon cancers. J Clin Oncol 1998;16:295–300.

O'Connell MJ, Malliard JA, Kahn MJ, et al: Controlled trial of fluorouracil and low-dose leucovorin given for 6 months as post-operative adjuvant therapy for colon cancer. J Clin Oncol 1997;15:246–250.

O'Connell MJ: North Central Cancer Treatment Group–Mayo Clinic trials in colon cancer. Semin Oncol 2001;28(Suppl 1):4–8.

O'Dwyer PJ, Stevenson JP, Haller DG, et al: Follow-up of Stage B and C colorectal cancer in the United States and France. Semin Oncol 2001;28(Suppl 1):45–49.

Riethmüller G, Holz E, Schlimok G, et al: Monoclonal antibody therapy for resected Dukes' C colorectal cancer: Seven-year outcome of a multicenter randomized trial. J Clin Oncol 1998;16:1788–1794.

Vermorken JB, Claessen AME, van Tinteren H, et al: Active specific immunotherapy for stage II and stage III human colon cancer: A randomized trial. Lancet 1999;353:345–350.

Wolmark N, Rockette H, Mamounes EP, et al: Clinical trial to assess the relative efficacy of fluorouracil and leucovorin, fluorouracil and levamisole, and fluorouracil, leucovorin and levamisole in patients with Dukes' B and C carcinoma of the colon: Results from National Surgical Adjuvant

Breast and Bowel Project C-04. J Clin Oncol 1999;17: 3553–3559.

Radiation Therapy: Preoperative and Adjuvant

Bentzen SM, Balslev I, Pederson M, et al: A regression analysis of prognostic factors after resection of Dukes B and C carcinoma of the rectum and rectosigmoid: Does postoperative radiotherapy change the prognosis? Br J Cancer 1988;58:195–201.

Gerard A, Buyse M, Nordlinger B, et al: Preoperative radiotherapy as adjuvant treatment in rectal cancer: Final results of a randomized study of the European Organization for Research and Treatment of Cancer (EORTC). Ann Surg 1988;208:606–614.

Gunderson L, Sosin H: Areas of failure found at reoperation (second or symptomatic look) following "curative surgery" for adenocarcinoma of the rectum. Cancer 1974;34: 1278–1292.

Marijnen CAM, Glimelius B: The role of radiotherapy in rectal cancer. Eur J Cancer 2002;38:943–952.

Medical Research Council Rectal Cancer Working Party: Randomized trial of surgery alone versus surgery followed by radiotherapy for mobile cancer of the rectum. Lancet 1996;348:1610–1614.

Pahlman L, Glimeluis B: Pre- or postoperative radiotherapy in rectal and rectosigmoid carcinoma: report from a randomized multicenter trial. Ann Surg 1990;211:187–195.

Swedish Rectal Cancer Trial: Improved survival with preoperative radiotherapy in resectable rectal cancer. N Engl J Med 1997;336:980–987.

Chemoradiation Therapy (Adjuvant Treatment for Rectal Cancer)

Gastrointestinal Tumor Study Group: A controlled trial of adjuvant chemotherapy, radiation therapy, or combined chemo-radiation therapy following curative resection for rectal carcinoma. N Engl J Med 1985;312:1465–1472.

Krook JE, Moertel CG, Gunderson LL, et al: Effective surgical adjuvant therapy for high-risk rectal carcinoma. N Engl J Med 1991;324:709–715.

O'Connell MJ, Martenson JA, Wieand HS, et al: Improving adjuvant therapy for rectal cancer by continuing protracted-infusion fluorouracil with radiation therapy after curative surgery. N Engl J Med 1994;331:502–507.

Tepper JE, O'Connell MJ, Petroni GR, et al: Adjuvant postoperative fluorouracil-modulated chemotherapy combined with pelvic radiation therapy for rectal cancer: Initial results of Intergroup 0114. J Clin Oncol 1997;15: 2030–2039.

Wolmark N, Wieand HS, Hyams DM, et al: Randomized trial of postoperative adjuvant chemotherapy with or without radiotherapy for carcinoma of the rectum: National Surgical Adjuvant Breast and Bowel Project Protocol R-02. J Natl Cancer Inst 2000;92:388–396.

Chapter 93
Anal Carcinoma

David P. Ryan

Introduction

Over the last decade, a series of case-control studies and randomized studies have clarified the pathophysiology, epidemiology, and management of anal cancer. Anal cancer comprises only 1.5% of all digestive system malignancies in the United States; approximately 3000 new cases occur annually. Anal cancer can be cured, and the anal sphincter can be preserved in a majority of patients. Malignancies arising in the anus have a variety of different histologies including sarcoma, adenocarcinoma, and melanoma; however, anal carcinoma by definition refers to the most common anal malignancy, squamous cell carcinoma.

Epidemiology

In the past, anal cancer was believed to develop in areas of chronic irritation associated with benign anal conditions such as hemorrhoids, fissures, and fistulae. Case reports of anal cancer developing in patients with inflammatory bowel disease led to the assumption that anal cancer resulted from chronic inflammation, similar to the relationship between inflammatory bowel disease and colorectal neoplasia. Recent case-control studies, however, show that hemorrhoids, fistulae, fissures, and inflammatory bowel disease are not associated with an increased risk of developing anal cancer.

Viral Infection

In 80% to 90% of cases, anal cancer results from anogenital infection with human papillomavirus (HPV), analogous to the viral interaction that causes carcinoma of the uterine cervix. Risk factors for anal cancer thus include a history of multiple sexual partners, anal receptive intercourse, and prior sexually transmitted diseases (including anogenital warts). As might be expected, women with a history of cervical or vulvar carcinoma experience a four- to sixfold increase in the risk of subsequently developing anal cancer.

Human papillomavirus infection of the cervix causes a premalignant condition, called cervical intraepithelial neoplasia. The human papillomavirus can cause a similar intraepithelial neoplasia of the anus, which can be morphologically low-grade or high-grade. The lesions often are visible as polypoid condyloma acuminata (anogenital warts). Anal intraepithelial neoplasia is a precursor for anal carcinoma. Anal intraepithelial neoplasia can progress from low-grade to high-grade and exists in areas adjacent to anal squamous cell carcinoma. As in cervical cancer, human papillomavirus type 16 is most frequently isolated in anal malignancies. Its presence predicts for high-grade anal intraepithelial neoplasia and invasive cancer; other subtypes of the papilloma virus are more frequently associated with low-grade lesions.

The results of population studies on the relationship of AIDS to the incidence of anal cancer are conflicting—some reporting an increase and others no change in men with AIDS virus infection. Studies consistently show, however, that patients with AIDS are at increased risk for developing human papillomavirus infection of the anus, which tends to be a persistent infection in these patients. Immunosuppression in general increases the risk of anal cancer. For example, patients who are receiving immunosuppressant drugs for renal transplantation or who take prolonged corticosteroids for autoimmune diseases are at increased risk.

Anatomy, Histology, and Staging

The anus can be divided into the mucosa-lined anal canal and the epidermis-lined anal margin. The anal canal extends from the anal verge over a distance of approximately 4 cm. The dentate line is a macroscopic landmark in the anal canal that overlies the transition from glandular to squamous mucosa. This area is often referred to as the transitional zone. The anal margin begins approximately at the anal verge and represents the transition from the squamous mucosa to the epidermis-lined perianal skin.

Due to the variable histologic appearance and the lack of an easily identifiable landmark, there is much confusion regarding the pathological classification of tumors arising in the transitional zone of the anus. Embryologically, the transitional zone develops adjacent to the bladder, and the histology can be quite similar. Terms such as "junctional" or "cloacogenic" have been used to describe the pseudostratified epithelium with cuboidal or polygonal surface cells that closely resembles urothelium. To avoid confusion, those terms were abandoned; these cancers are now classified simply as nonkeratinizing squamous cell carcinomas. The more common anal cancers arising within the anal canal distal to the dentate line are called keratinizing squamous cell carcinomas.

Because the transitional zone can vary widely among individual patients, the critical distinction between a rectal cancer and an anal cancer depends upon the histologic findings, not the judgment of the surgeon. Adenocarcinomas arising in the transitional zone have the same natural history as other rectal adenocarcinomas and should be treated accordingly. Squamous cell carcinomas arising in the transitional zone can vary morphologically, but there are no discernible differences in biology, natural history, and treatment outcome among subtypes.

The anal margin extends from the anal verge to the perianal skin. Distinguishing between tumors of the anal canal and anal margin can be difficult clinically. Tumors of the anal margin are most often squamous cell neoplasms, but other types of cutaneous malignancies can occur in this region as well. Squamous cell cancers of the anal margin should be treated according to the same principles as squamous cell cancers of the anal canal. Tumors of the hair-bearing perianal skin should be considered skin cancers with a natural history and biology distinct from squamous cell carcinoma of the anus. Melanoma can arise in either the anal canal or the anal margin and should be treated according to the same principles commonly applied to this tumor at other sites. Bowen disease is an in situ squamous cell carcinoma that can occur on the anal margin as well as on other areas of the skin that lack sun exposure. Paget disease of the anus is an intraepithelial adenocarcinoma that is subclassified into two types: a primary cutaneous malignancy, in which the malignant cells show sweat gland differentiation; and an underlying adenocarcinoma of the rectum or perianal glands, involving the adjacent squamous epithelium by lateral intramucosal/intraepithelial spread.

Lymphatic drainage of anal cancers is dependent upon the tumor's anatomic site of origin. Above the dentate line, drainage flows to perirectal and paravertebral nodes in a manner similar to rectal adenocarcinoma. Below the dentate line, lymphatics drain to the inguinal and femoral nodes. The inguinal, femoral, and iliac nodes are the most frequent sites of nodal metastases and can help clinically to distinguish anal cancers from rectal cancers.

The American Joint Committee on Cancer and the International Union against Cancer established a TNM staging system for anal cancer (Table 93-1). At presentation, approximately 50% of patients have a superficial mass (i.e., a T1 or T2 lesion), while approximately 25% of patients have involvement of regional lymph nodes. Tumor size is the most important prognostic factor in most series. The probability of nodal spread is directly related to tumor size, occurring far more commonly in T3 and T4 lesions than in smaller tumors.

Treatment

Surgery

Prior to 1980, an abdominoperineal resection—requiring the removal of the rectum and the formation of a colostomy—represented the treatment of choice for tumors arising in the anal canal. Prior to 1980, after an abdominoperineal resection, the five-year survival was 40% to 70%, and survival was particularly poor for patients with large tumors or nodal metastases. Pilot studies demonstrated that neoadjuvant therapy with combination chemotherapy (such as 5-fluorouracil and mitomycin) combined with intermediate-dose radiation therapy (30 Gy) could produce complete clinical and pathologic responses in patients with anal canal cancers. It then became clear that the initial chemoradiation therapy could cure the majority of these patients without resort to surgery. Abdominoperineal resection was employed only in those patients who demonstrated residual microscopic tumor on biopsy after treatment.

Radiation Therapy

Radiation therapy alone as primary treatment for anal canal cancer—either by external beam or brachytherapy (i.e., direct intratumoral implantation of radioactive seeds)—results in local control and overall survival in approximately 70% to 90% of selected patients. The local control and survival rates for patients with large tumors or evidence of nodal involvement, however, is less than 50% in some series. Many clinicians consider adding chemotherapy for this group.

Table 93-1 ■ TNM Classification of Anal Canal Carcinomas

T (Primary Tumor)

TX	Primary tumor cannot be assessed
T0	No evidence of primary tumor
Tis	Carcinoma in situ
T1	Tumor 2 cm or less in greatest dimension
T2	Tumor more than 2 cm but not more than 5 cm in greatest dimension
T3	Tumor more than 5 cm in greatest dimension
T4	Tumor of any size that invades adjacent organs (invasion of sphincter muscles alone is not T4)

N (Regional Lymph Nodes)

NX	Regional lymph nodes cannot be assessed
N0	No regional lymph node metastasis
N1	Metastasis in perirectal lymph node(s)
N2	Metastasis in unilateral internal iliac and/or inguinal lymph node(s)
N3	Metastasis in perirectal and inguinal lymph nodes and/or bilateral internal iliac and/or inguinal lymph nodes

M (Distant Metastases)

MX	Distant metastasis cannot be assessed
M0	No distant metastasis
M1	Distant metastasis

Stage Grouping

Stage Grouping	T	N	M
Stage 0	Tis	N0	M0
Stage I	T1	N0	M0
Stage II	T2, T3	N0	M0
Stage IIIA	T1–T3	N1	M0
	T4	N0	M0
Stage IIIB	T4	N1	M0
	Any T	N2, N3	M0
Stage IV	Any T	Any N	M1

The optimal dose of radiation therapy in the treatment of anal cancer has been debated. Retrospective studies show that the dose of radiation is a significant prognostic indicator. Improved disease-free survival has been noted in patients receiving at least 54 Gy of external-beam radiation. But increasing radiation therapy doses show good correlation with increasing risk of later complications, such as chronic anal ulcerations, anal stenosis, and tissue necrosis. These complications have necessitated abdominoperineal resections and establishment of permanent colostomies in approximately 10% of patients who were free of disease. An attempt to reduce the toxicity by dividing a total radiation dose of 59 Gy into a "split dose" schedule (two-week delay after 36 Gy) proved unsuccessful. Currently, therefore, most investigators limit the total dose of radiation to 45 Gy, with an added boost for patients who have T3–T4 disease or node-positive disease.

Chemotherapy

Two large European trials were undertaken to explore the value of adding chemotherapy to radiation therapy. The Anal Cancer Trial Working Party of the United Kingdom Coordination Committee on Cancer Research randomized 585 patients with anal cancer to receive either radiation therapy (consisting of 45 Gy by external beam with either a 15 Gy external beam boost or a 25 Gy brachytherapy boost) or the same radiotherapy with concurrent 5-fluorouracil and mitomycin. Combined modality therapy (chemoradiation) significantly reduced the local failure rate and the death rate from anal cancer (disease-specific mortality), but overall survival remained unchanged.

The European Organization for the Research and Treatment of Cancer (EORTC) randomized 110 patients with stage II or III (T3–4, N0–3 or T1–2, N1–3) anal cancer in a nearly identical study design. The group receiving chemoradiation experienced a statistically significant improvement in pathologic complete remission rate, five-year local/regional control rate, colostomy rate, and progression-free survival. Here again, however, overall survival was not significantly improved.

These two randomized studies included mitomycin in combination chemotherapy. Mitomycin is not a radiation sensitizer, has only modest antitumor activity against squamous cell cancers, and can cause chronic toxicity to the kidneys, lungs, and probably bone marrow. The Radiation Therapy Oncology Group (RTOG) and the Eastern Cooperative Oncology Group (ECOG) randomized 310 patients with anal cancer of any tumor or nodal stage to combined-modality therapy with or without mitomycin. The addition of mitomycin resulted in a statistically significant improvement at five years in terms of the rate of locoregional failure, colostomy rate, and disease-free survival. Overall survival, disease-specific survival, and negative biopsy rate post-therapy did not differ significantly in the two arms.

The addition of chemotherapy to radiation therapy increases the frequency and degree of acute toxicity. The major toxicities include diarrhea, exfoliative dermatitis, mucositis, and myelosuppression. The results of the randomized studies discussed above also indicated that the addition of mitomycin increases the morbidity and mortality rate from acute toxicity, including fatal neutropenic sepsis. For these reasons, the wisdom of continuing to use mitomycin is questioned.

The platinum chemotherapy compounds were not available at the time the combined-modality strategy evolved for anal canal cancers. Platinum compounds are more active than mitomycin as single agents in the treatment of squamous cell carcinomas. Randomized trials are evaluating the substitution of cisplatin for mitomycin in combined modality therapy.

Although the combination of chemotherapy and radiation therapy has not improved on overall survival of patients, combined-modality therapy does have a number of intermediate-term benefits, not the least of which is a decrease in local recurrence. The task for clinical investigators is to find ways to decrease the individual and conjoint acute and chronic side effects of radiation therapy and chemotherapy while preserving efficacy. Diminution in side effects could translate into improved overall survival from combined-modality therapy for patients with anal canal cancer.

The Role of Local Excision

Whether local excision can ever be applied to the management of patients with squamous cell cancer of the anus is unresolved. Brown and colleagues reported their experience with 46 patients who underwent local excision for high-grade anal intraepithelial neoplasia. More than 40% of patients had positive surgical margins, and more than 50% of these patients had recurrent lesions after one year. Even in patients in whom complete microscopic excision was achieved, 13% developed recurrent lesions. Moreover, the morbidity of local excision was not trivial; 11% developed complications of anal stenosis and/or fecal incontinence. Anal intraepithelial neoplasia is a multifocal process due to human papillomavirus infection, and complete local excision is frequently unattainable. By extension, the same concerns apply to small or incidentally found squamous cell carcinomas of the anus. Even when local excision is combined with chemoradiation, a 20% risk of therapeutic failure is present. Therefore, local excision as sole therapy for anal cancer should be considered inadequate. More studies are needed to help define the best therapeutic options for patients with small (or incidentally found) tumors.

Treatment of Locally Recurrent Disease

Although some patients might be salvaged with surgery, persistent disease after chemoradiation and locally recurrent anal cancer is often a difficult clinical problem associated with profound morbidity and suffering. For patients with persistent disease after primary combined-modality therapy, surgical removal—either by local excision or by abdominoperineal resection—remains the treatment of choice.

Local/regional recurrences can also be cured by surgical resection. Approximately one-half of a small number of patients who underwent abdominoperineal resection for local recurrence survived for three years. The problem is that only a subset of treatment failures are candidates for salvage therapy. For example, in one series, 42 of 185 patients experienced recurrent disease after primary treatment. Only 26 of these patients were candidates for potentially curative resections. The five-year overall survival for the 42 relapsing patients was 28%, but the five-year survival for the 26 patients undergoing potentially curative resection was 44%.

Treatment of Metastatic Disease

The liver is the most frequent site of distant metastases. Few trials in metastatic disease have been published. Partial responses have been seen to single-agent 5-fluorouracil, cisplatin, and methyl-CCNU. There is little published experience in this disease with newer agents such as taxanes and irinotecan; however, phase II studies evaluating these agents in other squamous cell malignancies demonstrate promising activity.

References

General Information

Gerard JP, Chapet O, Samiei F, et al: Management of inguinal lymph node metastases in patients with carcinoma of the anal canal: Experience in a series of 270 patients treated in Lyon and review of the literature. Cancer 2001;92:77–84.

Greenall MJ, Quan SH, Urmacher C, DeCosse JJ: Treatment of epidermoid carcinoma of the anal canal. Surg Gynecol Obstet 1985;161:509–517.

Mitchell SE, Mendenhall WM, Zlotecki RA, Carroll RR: Squamous cell carcinoma of the anal canal. Intl J Radiol Oncol Biol Phys 2001;49:1007–1113.

Myerson R, Karnell LH, Menck HR: The National Cancer Data Base report on carcinoma of the anus. Cancer 1997;80:805–815.

Pintor MP, Northover JM, Nicholls RJ, et al: Squamous cell carcinoma of the anus at one hospital from 1948 to 1984. Br J Surg 1989;76:806–810.

Ryan DP, Compton CC, Mayer RJ: Carcinoma of the anal canal. N Engl J Med 2000;342:792–800.

Whiteford MH, Stevens KR Jr, Oh S, Deveney KE: The evolving treatment of anal cancer: How are we doing? Arch Surg 2002;136:886–891.

Chemotherapy and Combined Modality Therapy

Ajani JA, Carrasco CH, et al: Combination of cisplatin plus fluoropyrimidine chemotherapy is effective against liver metastases from carcinoma of the anal canal. Am J Med 1995;87:221–224.

Bartelink H, Roelofsen F, Eschwege F, et al: Concomitant radiotherapy and chemotherapy is superior to radiotherapy alone in the treatment of locally advanced anal cancer: Results of a phase III randomized trial of the European Organization for Research and Treatment of Cancer Radiotherapy and Gastrointestinal Cooperative Groups. J Clin Oncol 1997;15:2040–2049.

Doci R, Zucali R, LaMonica G, et al: Primary chemoradiation therapy with fluorouracil and cisplatin for cancer of the anus: Results in 35 consecutive patients. J Clin Oncol 1996;14:3121–3125.

Flam M, John M, Pajak TF, et al: Role of mitomycin in combination with fluorouracil and radiotherapy, and of salvage chemoradiation in the definitive nonsurgical treatment of epidermoid carcinoma of the anal canal: Results of a phase III randomized intergroup study. J Clin Oncol 1996; 14:2527–2539.

Kapp KS, Geyer E, Gebhart FH, et al: Experience with splitcourse external beam irradiation +/− chemotherapy and integrated Ir-192 high-dose brachytherapy in the treatment of primary carcinoma of the anal canal. Intl J Radiol Oncol Biol Phys 2001;49:997–1005.

Leichman L, Nigro N, Vaitkevicius VK, et al: Cancer of the anal canal. Model for preoperative adjuvant combined modality therapy. Am J Med 1985;78:211–215.

Nigro ND, Vaitkevecius VK, Considine B Jr: Combined therapy for cancer of the anal canal: A preliminary report. Dis Colon Rectum 1974;17:354–356.

Nissan A, Dangelica MI, Shoup MC, Hartley JE: Randomized clinical trials in rectal and anal cancer. Surg Clin N Am 2002;11:149–172.

UKCCCR: Epidermoid anal cancer: Results from the UKCCCR randomised trial of radiotherapy alone versus radiotherapy, 5-fluorouracil, and mitomycin. UKCCCR Anal Cancer Trial Working Party. UK Co-ordinating Committee on Cancer Research. Lancet 1996;348:1049–1054.

Epidemiology

Branum GD: Current management of perianal intraepithelial neoplasia. Obstet Gynecol 2001;28:703–710.

Chang GJ, Berry JM, Jay N, et al: Surgical treatment of highgrade intraepithelial lesions: A prospective study. Dis Colon Rectum 2002;45:453–458.

Daling JR, Weiss NS, Hislop TG, et al: Sexual practices, sexually transmitted diseases, and the incidence of anal cancer. N Engl J Med 1987;317:973–977.

Fenger C: Anal neoplasia and its precursors: Facts and controversies. Semin Diag Pathol 1991;8:90–201.

Frisch M, Glimelius B, van den Brule AJ, et al: Sexually transmitted infection as a cause of anal cancer. N Engl J Med 1997;337:1350–1358.

Frisch M, Olsen JH, Bautz A, et al: Benign anal lesions and the risk of anal cancer. N Engl J Med 1994;331:300–302.

Holly EA, Whitemore AS, Aston DA, et al: Anal cancer incidence: genital warts, anal fissure or fistula, hemorrhoids, and smoking. J Natl Cancer Inst 1989;81:1726–1731.

Kotlarewsky M, Freeman JB, Cameron W, Grimard LJ: Anal intraepithelial dysplasia and squamous carcinoma in immunosuppressed patients. Can J Surg 2001;44:450–454.

Melbye M, Spergel P: Aetiological parallel between anal cancer and cervical cancer. Lancet 1991;338:657–659.

Penn I: Cancers of the anogenital region in renal transplant recipients. Analysis of 65 cases. Cancer 1986;58:611–616.

Place RJ, Gregorcyk SG, Huber PJ, Simmang CL: Outcome analysis of HIV-positive patients with anal squamous cell carcinoma. Dis Colon Rectum 2001;44:506–512.

Sun XW, Kuhn L, Ellerbrock TV, et al: Human papilloma virus infection in women infected with the human immunodeficiency virus. N Engl J Med 1997;337:1343–1349.

Tilston P: Anal human papillomavirus and anal cancer. J Clin Pathol 1997;150:625–634.

Radiation Therapy

Allal AS, Mermillod B, Roth AD, et al: Impact of clinical and therapeutic factors on major late complications after radiotherapy with or without concomitant chemotherapy for anal carcinoma. Intl J Radiat Oncol Biol Phys 1997; 39:1099–1105.

Myerson RJ, Kong F, Birnbaum EH, et al: Radiation therapy for epidermoid carcinoma of the anal canal: Clinical and treatment factors associated with outcome. Radiother Oncol 2001;61:15–22.

Surgery

Allal AS, Laurencet FM, Reymond MA, et al: Effectiveness of surgical salvage therapy for patients with locally uncontrolled anal carcinoma after sphincter-conserving treatment. Cancer 1999;86:405–409.

Pocard M, Tiret E, Nugent K, et al: Results of salvage abdominoperineal resection for anal cancer after radiotherapy. Dis Colon Rectum 1998;41:1488–1493.

van der Wal BC, Cleffken BI, Gulec B, et al: Results of salvage abdominoperineal resection for recurrent anal carcinoma following combined chemoradiation therapy. J Gastrointest Surg 2001;5:383–387.

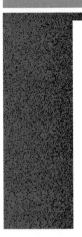

Chapter 94
Small Cell Lung Cancer

Joseph J. Merchant and Joan H. Schiller

Introduction

Small cell lung cancer (SCLC) represents a distinct and important histologic type of respiratory epithelial cancer, accounting for 16% of all patients with lung cancer. Important features of this disease are its rapid growth and tendency for early metastasis. Among the histologic types of lung cancer, five-year survival rates for patients with small cell lung cancer are the lowest; 90% of patients die within two years of diagnosis. Although the prognosis for patients with this disease remains poor, significant progress has been made in diagnosis, staging, treatment, and supportive care. In particular, the introduction of platinum-based poly-chemotherapy and effective chest radiation therapy has lengthened the survival and improved the quality of life for the majority of small cell lung cancer patients and made cure possible for a small minority of patients with limited extent of disease at diagnosis.

Epidemiology

The median age at diagnosis in several series is between 55 and 60 years. In the United States, an estimated 34,300 patients were diagnosed with this type of lung cancer in 1998. The incidence of small cell lung cancer is higher among men than women, although the gender gap has been closing because rates have increased faster for women than for men over the last 25 years.

Although lung cancer is now the leading cause of cancer death in men and women in the United States, it must be remembered that in 1900, lung cancer was a rare disease. Marked increases in the rates of cigarette smoking by men and women account for the dramatic epidemic of lung cancer witnessed over the last 100 years. Approximately 90% of all lung cancers are caused primarily by cigarette smoking or second-hand smoke exposure. Small cell lung cancer, in particular, has a strong association with cigarette smoking. More than 98% of affected patients have a history of cigarette smoking. Because of this strong association with the use of cigarettes, it is worthwhile to focus briefly on the cigarette epidemic.

Approximately 47 million—or one in four—adults smoke in the United States, with the majority smoking daily. There is an inverse correlation between the prevalence of smoking and level of education; high-school dropouts have the highest rates of smoking (41.9% and 33.7% for males and females, respectively), and college graduates have the lowest (14.3% and 13.7%). The rate of cigarette smoking has increased among high school students over the last decade (from 27.5% in 1991 to 36.4% in 1997), probably in large part due to the tobacco industry's advertising, which is specifically targeted to young people. Thus, although overall rates of smoking have declined dramatically since their peaks in the 1950s and 1960s, the recent increases among young people, if not reversed through effective smoking cessation efforts, provide a pool of individuals at high risk for the devastation of smoking-related lung cancers, including small cell lung cancer.

Pathology

Small cell lung cancer appears to originate from argyrophilic basal reserve cells that line the epithelial basement membranes of the bronchi and bronchioles. The epithelial origin of small cell lung cancer was first

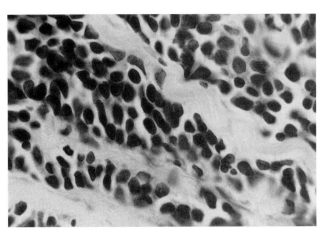

Figure 94-1 ■ 100× (original) magnification of small cell lung cancer demonstrating typical "oat cell" morphology.

proposed by Barnard in 1926. Prior to that time, this cancer had been referred to as "oat cell sarcoma of the mediastinum." Although smaller in size than non–small cell lung cancer cells, small cell cancer cells are large in relation to normal lung epithelial cells. The nuclei are often bigger in size than lymphocytes. These cells possess neuroendocrine granules similar to those of islet cells in the pancreas and Kultchitsky cells of the gastrointestinal tract. Because these cells can take up amine precursors and secrete polypeptide hormones such as adrenocorticotropic hormone (ACTH), antidiuretic hormone, and calcitonin, small cell lung cancer is associated with many hormonal paraneoplastic syndromes.

Several histologic subtypes of small cell lung cancer have been proposed over the last 75 years. In 1988, the International Association for the Study of Lung Cancer proposed dividing small cell cancer into three main groups:

1. small cell cancer or "classic"
2. intermediate or "variant"
3. combined small cell cancer

Classic small cell lung cancer consists of oval to rounded hyperchromatic cells with diffuse chromatin patterns and little or no visible cytoplasm (Figure 94-1). In a review of 628 patients in one protocol, 96% of cases were classified as "classic" small cell cancer and only 4% as "variant" type.

Recognizing this predominance, the 1999 World Health Organization revision of the histologic classification of lung tumors eliminated the variant classification. Although pathologists have a greater than 90% concordance rate in distinguishing classic small cell lung cancer from non–small cell lung cancer, the interobserver variability in determining small cell lung cancer subtype is quite high. It is also important

to recognize that it is difficult to differentiate atypical carcinoid tumor from small cell lung cancer on needle biopsy of peripheral lung nodules, making excision of such nodules imperative for accurate diagnosis and treatment. In the rare patient with combined small cell lung cancer and non–small cell lung cancer, patients are treated as if they had classic small cell lung cancer. Perhaps the most meaningful fact with regard to classification is that the histologic subtype of small cell lung cancer does not correlate with prognosis.

The growth pattern of small cell lung cancer is different from that of non–small cell lung cancer. The latter type of tumor is most often exophytic within the bronchi, presenting as a polypoid intraluminal mass. Small cell lung cancer, on the other hand, presents primarily as a submucosal growth, usually located centrally within the bronchial tree. These submucosal tumors grow centrally and compress the airway circumferentially, often causing postobstructive pneumonitis (Figure 94-2). Invasion of lymphoid and vascular channels is common, and diffuse involvement of lymphatics within the lung is often associated with pleural effusion.

Clinical Presentation

It is instructive to organize the discussion of clinical presentation according to ways in which small cell lung cancer presents similarly to non–small cell lung cancer and ways in which the presentation differs. Signs and symptoms referable to small cell lung cancer and non–small cell lung cancer can be divided into three major categories:

1. locoregional manifestations
2. metastases present at diagnosis
3. paraneoplastic syndromes

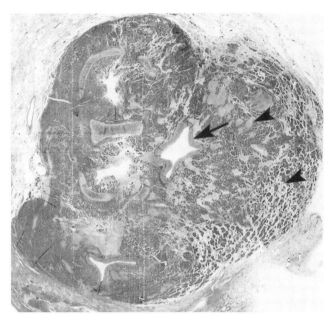

Figure 94-2 ■ Low-magnification image of a small cell lung cancer tumor showing submucosal growth pattern and tendency to compress airways by extrinsic compression (arrow). The image also demonstrates a typical pattern of small cell lung carcinoma growth in nests and cords of malignant cells (arrowheads).

With regard to the first of these categories, small cell lung cancer has many similarities with other centrally located non–small cell lung cancers at the time of presentation. More than 80% of small cell lung cancer patients have evident tumor in mainstem or lobar bronchi at diagnosis. As a result, small cell lung cancer can present with distal atelectasis or postobstructive pneumonia. The roentgenographic appearance of small cell lung cancer is that of a central tumor mass with or without mediastinal widening in 64% of cases and as a peripheral tumor with or without mediasti-

nal adenopathy in only 19%. In contrast to squamous cell cancers—in which central cavitation is noted in 10% to 20% of cases—small cell lung cancer rarely cavitates and is infrequently associated with hemoptysis.

Small cell lung cancer patients are almost always quite symptomatic at diagnosis (Table 94-1). The most common symptoms are cough (76%), chest pain (36%), dyspnea (34%), and pneumonitis (25%). Hemoptysis is noted in only 15% of cases, and obstructive pneumonia is noted in 8%. The duration of symptoms at diagnosis in small cell lung cancer is often much shorter than in non–small cell lung cancer. More than 80% of patients with small cell lung cancer have symptoms for less than three months, which contrasts with an average symptom duration of eight months in cases of non–small cell lung cancer.

Other locoregional manifestations of both small cell lung cancer and non–small cell lung cancer include superior vena cava syndrome, pleural and pericardial effusion, dysphagia due to involvement of the esophagus, and hoarseness due to impingement on the recurrent laryngeal nerve. Small cell lung cancer is the most common cause of superior vena cava syndrome, which is present in approximately 12% of cases at presentation compared with 5% at presentation of non–small cell lung cancer. Superior vena cava syndrome is almost always associated with right-sided tumors (Figure 94-3). Patients with superior vena cava syndrome have rapid onset of facial, neck, and upper extremity edema along with venous congestion and collateral vessels on the trunk. Some patients also note headache, drowsiness, and vertigo. Although once thought to be a contraindication to bronchial biopsy, superior vena cava syndrome does not appear to be associated with an excess risk of biopsy-related bleeding complications (see Chapter 17).

Hoarseness results from vocal cord paralysis due to compression of the recurrent laryngeal nerve. This

Table 94-1 ■ Signs and Symptoms of Small Cell Lung Cancer

Sign/Symptom	% Patients at Time of Diagnosis
Cough	76
Chest pain	36
Dyspnea	34
Pneumonitis	25
Pleural effusion	25
Hemoptysis	15
SVC syndrome	12
Postobstructive pneumonia	8

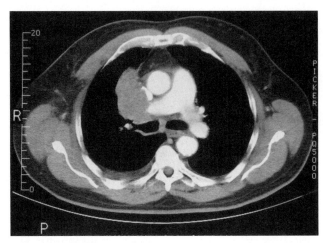

Figure 94-3 ■ Computed tomography image of patient who presented with superior vena cava syndrome (SVC), showing large right-sided mediastinal tumor compressing the SVC.

more often occurs when the tumor is on the left side of the chest because the course of the left recurrent laryngeal nerve is longer and thus more vulnerable than its counterpart on the right side. If the paralysis is only of short duration, it might be reversible after chemotherapy. Pericardial and esophageal invasion is unusual at diagnosis, although at autopsy 20% to 25% of patients exhibit cardiac metastases. Pleural effusions are present in approximately 25% of small cell lung cancer patients at diagnosis.

Small cell lung cancer has a clear tendency for early metastasis. In one autopsy study of 20 patients with limited-stage small cell lung cancer who died within 30 days of what was thought to have been a curative surgery, 12 patients (60%) had distant metastases. The most common extrathoracic sites of metastatic disease, considering patients both at initial diagnosis and at relapse, are the liver, bones, retroperitoneal lymph nodes, adrenal glands, and brain. Autopsy series have shown that more than 80% of patients have metastatic disease to the liver. Liver metastases in small cell lung cancer patients are often quite bulky, although significant abnormalities of liver function tests are uncommon. Patients with extensive liver disease often present with pronounced constitutional symptoms such as fatigue, weakness, and weight loss. Bone metastases are frequent in small cell lung cancer; despite the common involvement of bone by small cell lung cancer, hypercalcemia is uncommon. Blind bone marrow aspiration and biopsy detect metastatic disease in 10% to 20% of newly diagnosed patients.

The central nervous system is a preferential site of metastasis in small cell lung cancer. Approximately 10% of patients have brain metastases at presentation, and another 40% develop symptomatic brain metastases during or after treatment. The brain is the first site of relapse in approximately 11% and the only site

of relapse in 5% of patients. The cumulative actuarial probability of brain metastases in patients with small cell lung cancer who survive more than 1 year has been estimated at 64%; for those who survive more than two years, it is estimated at 80%. Patients with brain metastases often present with headache, altered mental status, and focal weakness, although seizures, ataxia, and aphasia also sometimes occur. Most central nervous system metastases in this disease are intracranial, although spinal cord and leptomeningeal metastases become more common with increased survival after diagnosis. Metastases to the pituitary gland are relatively common in small cell lung cancer. Lesions are usually limited to the posterior pituitary, and clinical hypopituitarism rarely occurs. Leptomeningeal metastases cause symptoms of altered mental status, headache, and focal weakness. Cerebrospinal fluid cytology is usually positive in patients with leptomeningeal disease and in 20% of patients with cranial metastases.

One series of 610 consecutive patients with small cell lung cancer found that 4% of patients had spinal cord compression due to metastases at some point during their illness. Back pain occurs in 90% of such cases and is the earliest symptom. Weakness and sensory changes commonly follow the onset of pain by days to weeks, and autonomic dysfunction is typically a late occurrence. These patients must be evaluated for leptomeningeal and intracranial disease because they are frequent concomitants of spinal cord involvement.

Paraneoplastic Syndromes

Many different paraneoplastic syndromes have been associated with small cell lung cancer. The most common and most important of these include the syndromes of inappropriate antidiuretic hormone (SIADH), ectopic adrenocorticotropic hormone secretion, Lambert-Eaton myasthenic syndrome, and paraneoplastic encephalomyelitis with its important variants, limbic encephalitis and subacute cerebellar degeneration.

Syndrome of Inappropriate Secretion of Anti-Diuretic Hormone

Small cell lung cancer is the most common cause of chronic Syndrome of Inappropriate Secretion of Anti-Diuretic Hormone (SIADH). Affected patients present with euvolemic, hypoosmolar hyponatremia, a less than maximally dilute urine, and normal kidney and adrenal function. Up to 75% of cancer-associated SIADH is due to small cell lung cancer. The cancer is the site of ectopic production of either antidiuretic hormone or atrial natriuretic factor. From 7% to 16% of small cell lung cancer patients have SIADH at diagnosis, and 40% to 60% have an abnormal response to water loading, suggesting that the majority of patients with small cell lung cancer have at least subclinical abnormalities of renal water handling. Although the degree of hyponatremia is often severe, only a minority (27% in one series) are symptomatic. When present, hyponatremia-related symptoms consist primarily of disturbances in level of consciousness, extrapyramidal signs, asterixis, and seizures.

Treatment for the syndrome itself, such as strict water restriction and demeclocycline, are effective in improving the serum sodium; however, the most effective and definitive treatment in small cell lung cancer patients is chemotherapy. Because improvement in serum sodium levels can be delayed for three to six weeks after chemotherapy begins, patients with severe hyponatremia should be continued on demeclocycline for up to two to three weeks after start of chemotherapy until serum sodium is stably within the normal range.

In patients whose SIADH responds to chemotherapy, 70% will have recurrent SIADH at the time of relapse. A minority of patients with small cell lung cancer-related SIADH will have worsening of their hyponatremia with chemotherapy. The mechanism for this is unknown, although some have postulated a tumor lysis-related dumping of ectopic hormone into the circulation after treatment.

Paraneoplastic Neurologic Syndromes

A variety of neurologic paraneoplastic syndromes have been linked to small cell lung cancer. These include paraneoplastic encephalomyelitis, sensory neuronopathy, limbic encephalitis, and opsoclonus/myoclonus. The cause of this process appears to be the production of anti-Hu antibodies that gain access to both the cerebrospinal fluid and systemic circulation and initiate autoimmune destruction of neurons in both the peripheral and central nervous systems (see Chapter 7).

The Hu antigen is expressed in the nuclei and (to a lesser extent) in the cytoplasm of most neurons of the central nervous system (including dorsal root ganglia cells) as well as in all small cell lung cancer specimens yet studied. Thus, the deleterious effects of anti-Hu antibody appear to be an "innocent bystander" effect of an antitumoral immune response. It is fascinating to note that although patients with anti-Hu antibody-related syndromes often have disabling neurologic disease, their small cell lung cancer prognosis tends to be significantly better than for those who have only low-level or absent anti-Hu antibody responses. For example, 95% of small cell lung cancer patients with anti-Hu related paraneoplastic syndromes have limited-stage disease at diagnosis, compared with 30% of all patients with small cell lung cancer.

In a definitive study of patients with anti-Hu related encephalitis, 55 of 61 patients (91%) with detectable malignancy had underlying small cell lung cancer. Signs and symptoms of these paraneoplastic neurologic syndromes precede the diagnosis of cancer in 83% of cases and appear after the diagnosis in only 12%. Detection of anti-Hu antibody in a patient presenting with a neurologic disease often prompts a search for occult malignancy. The median time from onset of neurologic symptoms to cancer diagnosis is four months, with a range of 1 to 23 months.

The most common presenting symptoms in patients with anti-Hu related syndromes are sensory changes—usually asymmetric numbness and dysesthesia affecting the proximal extremities, trunk, and/or face. Mental status changes such as confusion, memory disturbance, depression, and anxiety can occur in patients with predominantly limbic involvement. Cerebellar involvement is usually heralded by gait ataxia, which can progress to action tremor and incoordination of arm and leg. Motor weakness can occur, usually presenting as a peripheral neuronopathy with muscle wasting. Brainstem involvement has been noted, with symptoms such as diplopia, dysarthria, nystagmus, and dizziness. Autonomic neuropathy is characterized chiefly by severe orthostatic hypotension.

In 70% of patients with anti-Hu-related neurologic syndromes, symptoms develop over a period of less than eight weeks. These syndromes usually follow a progressive, unremitting pattern. Treatment of the underlying malignancy might prevent progression of neurologic dysfunction, but resolution of neurologic deficits is uncommon. In one series, the neurologic problems stabilized with treatment in 70% of patients and progressed in the other 30%. In another series of patients with paraneoplastic limbic encephalitis, 44% of patients showed clinical neurologic improvement with anticancer treatment. Other immunologic treatments, such as steroid administration or plasmapheresis, are not usually helpful in the patients who have small cell lung cancer-related paraneoplastic neurologic syndromes.

Syndrome of Ectopic Corticotropin Secretion

Ectopic production of corticotropic hormone occurs in approximately 4% of patients with small cell lung cancer. They present with increased skin pigmentation, edema, hypertension, weakness, hyperglycemia, and hypokalemic metabolic alkalosis. These processes occur relatively rapidly in these patients. The chronic manifestations of excessive adrenocorticotropic hormone production that occur in classic Cushing's syndrome (e.g., truncal obesity or moon facies) therefore do not have time to develop. The increased cortisol levels in this condition do not suppress when high-dose dexamethasone is given (cortisol suppression test). In comparison with other patients with small cell lung cancer, patients with this paraneoplastic syndrome have a far worse prognosis, a median survival of only four months with treatment. Because chemotherapy does not generally produce rapid resolution of hypercortisolism, other antiadrenal treatments such as metyrapone and/or ketoconazole could be necessary to establish initial control of the metabolic abnormalities in these patients.

Lambert-Eaton Myoclonic Syndrome

Patients with small cell lung cancer are also prone to develop antibodies targeting the P/Q type calcium channels at neuromuscular synapses. These antibodies are found in up to 28% of small cell lung cancer patients without Lambert-Eaton syndrome and in 95% of patients with this syndrome. The antibodies cause disease by impairing the presynaptic release of acetylcholine. Clinical findings include proximal muscle weakness and autonomic dysfunction. Nerve conduction studies are diagnostic, showing action potentials that are initially low but increase with exercise. Twenty-eight of 40 patients presenting with this syndrome had an underlying malignancy, and 20 of these 28 patients had small cell lung cancer. Patients with this syndrome, in contrast to those with anti-Hu-related neurologic syndromes, do respond to plasma-pheresis and immunosuppression. Symptoms also improve with effective chemotherapy.

Clinical Evaluation

Brushings and biopsy obtained through use of a flexible bronchoscope are the commonest approaches to diagnosis. Bronchial brushing is positive in 90% of patients, bronchial biopsy is positive in 65%, and a combination of the two techniques provides a diagnostic result in 94% of cases. In a patient who refuses bronchoscopy or who is too infirm for this procedure, examination of sputum cytology and/or bone marrow biopsy can be helpful. As noted previously, blind bone marrow aspiration and biopsy detects metastatic small cell lung cancer in 10% to 20% of cases.

Once a patient is diagnosed with small cell lung cancer, an attempt is made to stage the patient's cancer. In contrast to the Tumor-Node-Metastasis (TNM) system used for non–small cell lung cancer, small cell cancer is staged as either "limited" or "extensive" based on the work of the Veterans Administration Lung Cancer Study Group. This staging system evolved in the prechemotherapy era, when it became clear that the survival of patients with small cell lung cancer taken for curative resection was no longer than that of non-surgically treated patients. Thus, the main question in the treatment of small cell lung cancer before the advent of chemotherapy was whether the patient could be treated for cure with radiation therapy. Patients whose disease could be encompassed in a single radiation therapy portal were designated "limited stage;" all other patients were designated "extensive stage" (Figure 94-4).

The definition of limited-stage disease generally includes patients whose tumor is confined to one hemithorax and its regional lymph nodes, including ipsilateral supraclavicular, hilar, and mediastinal nodes. In this system, patients who have an ipsilateral pleural effusion and no other extrathoracic disease are still generally considered to have extensive stage disease, even if the pleural effusion is cytologically negative. Thus, limited-stage disease is roughly equivalent to stage I-IIIA in the TNM classification used for non–small cell lung cancer (see Chapter 95 for a discussion of TNM lung cancer staging). Extensive-stage disease refers to patients with disease outside the limits delineated previously and usually involves distant metastases.

Some investigators have characterized a third staging category termed "very limited stage," which encompasses patients with surgically resectable lesions (T1–2, N0, M0). Among patients with small cell lung cancer, 20% to 30% have limited-stage disease, and

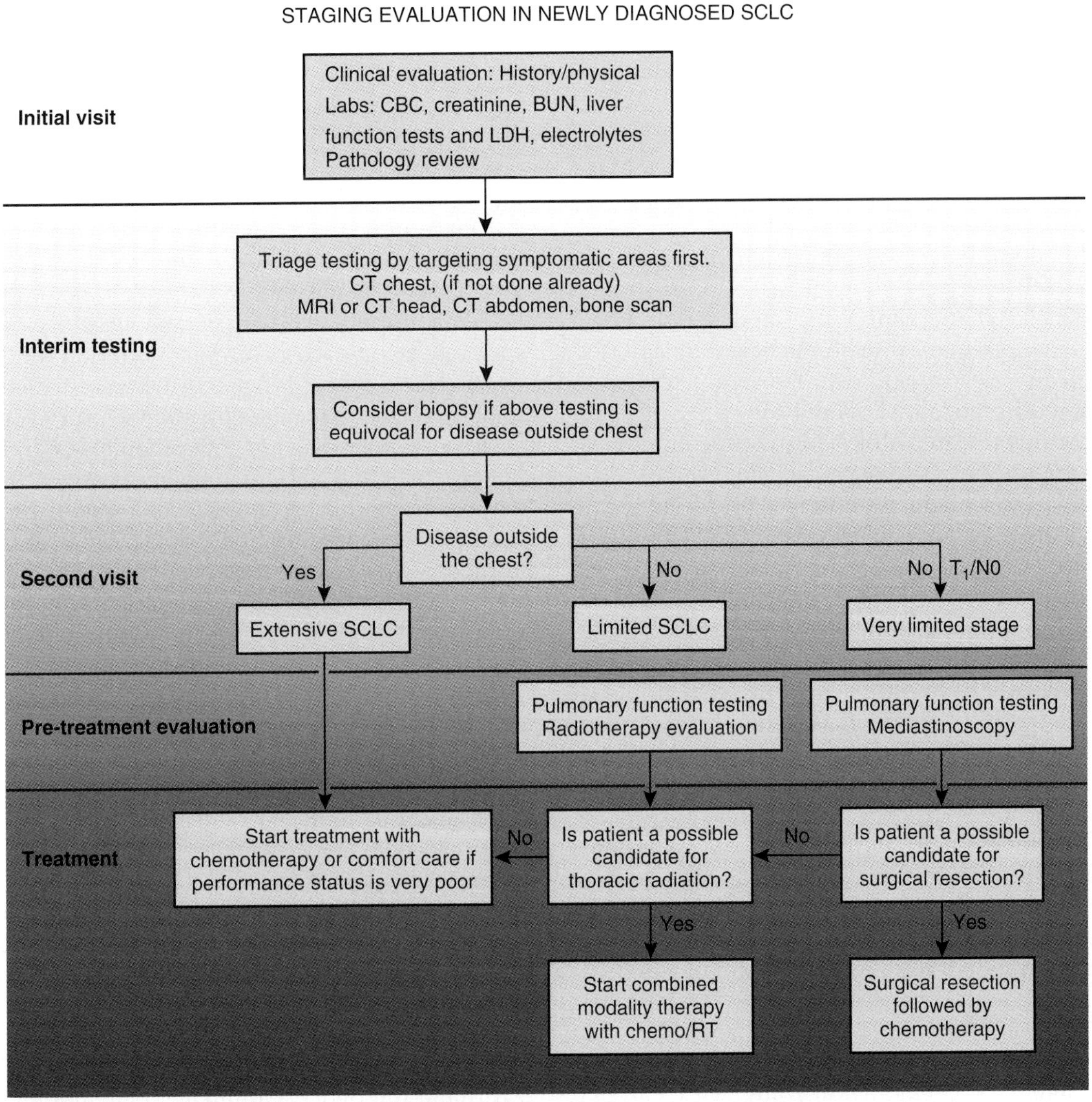

STAGING EVALUATION IN NEWLY DIAGNOSED SCLC

Figure 94-4 ■ Algorithm for staging evaluation in newly diagnosed small cell lung cancer.

70% have extensive-stage disease. Less than 5% of patients have very limited-stage disease. It has been argued that small cell lung cancer should be staged by the TNM system, at least for the purpose of clinical trials, in order to separate out subgroups of patients who might benefit from more aggressive staging procedures and/or treatment. For example, advocates of surgery recommend that all clinically T1-2, N0, M0 patients undergo complete staging as well as mediastinoscopy to identify patients with negative mediastinal nodes who should go on to surgery.

An ever-increasing array of tests is available to stage a patient with small cell lung cancer. It is crucial for the physician to determine whether the patient is a suitable candidate for aggressive chemotherapy and radiotherapy. Systems that provide a global ranking scale for fitness for treatment have been devised. These systems include measurement of performance status as a critical variable.

After a detailed history and physical examination, all patients should have laboratory assessment of basic organ function and hematologic reserve. A computed tomography (CT) scan of the chest and abdomen, extending through the level of the adrenal glands bilaterally, is a very useful staging test. Approximately 20% to 35% of patients have metastatic disease to liver at the time of diagnosis. Patients who obviously have extensive-stage disease on computed tomography scan can be spared additional staging work-up. Patients who appear to have limited-stage disease, however, should expeditiously undergo additional tests prior to starting therapy. In the past, it was customary to include bone marrow biopsy in the staging evaluation of all small cell lung cancer patients. Many physicians, however, no longer routinely include this procedure in their initial evaluation.

Technetium bone scan or magnetic resonance imaging (MRI) detects bone metastases in 30% to 45% of small cell lung cancer cases at diagnosis. Some sites of bony metastatic disease, such as skull and ribs, are difficult to evaluate by magnetic resonance imaging, so this modality has not been widely used for staging in this disease. Although it is uncommon for bone to be the only site of metastatic disease, up to 20% of patients might be upstaged from limited to extensive disease if bone imaging is included in staging work-up.

Brain magnetic resonance imaging or computed tomography is a test commonly performed in the staging of patients with small cell lung cancer because 10% of patients have central nervous system metastasis at diagnosis. In approximately one-third of these patients, the brain is the only site of central nervous system metastasis, but two-thirds have metastases in other locations as well. Two-thirds of patients with brain metastases at diagnosis had symptoms referable to central nervous system disease as their presenting complaint. It is thus unusual for a newly diagnosed patient who is neurologically asymptomatic to have brain metastases as the only site of extensive disease.

All of the effort put into staging patients accurately should yield a select minority of candidates for aggressive combination chemoradiotherapy with curative intent. Only patients with good performance status and limited stage of disease should be treated in this fashion.

Prognosis

Small cell lung cancer patients have the lowest survival rates and highest annual hazard rates among all patients with lung cancer. Without treatment, the disease is rapidly fatal within one to three months. As is true in non–small cell lung cancer, the best prognostic indicators for small cell lung cancer patients are the stage of the disease and the performance status of the patient. Patients with a good performance status of either 0 or 1 on the Eastern Cooperative Oncology Group (ECOG) scale have a one-year survival of approximately 40% to 50%, whereas patients with a performance status of either 3 or 4 have a one-year

survival of only 8% to 10%. Patients with limited-stage disease should have a median survival of 12 to 18 months, whereas extensive-disease patients will have a median survival of only eight to nine months. The rate of survival beyond five years in limited-disease patients is only 10% to 20%, and in extensive disease survival is even lower (3% to 5%). The aggressive nature of this neoplasm requires that the initial evaluation be done quickly and that therapy be initiated as soon as possible.

Patients with certain paraneoplastic syndromes, such as ectopic corticotropin secretion or SIADH, experience a worse prognosis, whereas patients with immunologically mediated paraneoplastic syndromes, such as Lambert-Eaton myasthenic syndrome, do better. The serum lactate dehydrogenase (LDH) level, derived from cell breakdown, is a useful prognostic marker. Levels are elevated in relationship to the body burden of cancer, the turnover rate of the neoplastic cells, the degree of tumor necrosis, and the infiltration of organs that are themselves rich in lactate dehydrogenase. Patients with apparently limited-stage disease who have moderate elevations of the serum lactate dehydrogenase have a high probability of occult metastatic disease and a prognosis similar to that of patients presenting with extensive disease. Small cell lung cancer patients with substantial elevations of the serum lactate dehydrogenase virtually always have extensive-stage disease.

Whether advanced age represents a negative prognostic factor in and of itself is controversial. Most studies of small cell lung cancer in the elderly show comparable results if patients are stratified for stage and performance status. Otherwise healthy, elderly patients with a good performance status appear to be able to withstand the rigors of multiagent chemotherapy and achieve responses at a rate similar to younger patients.

Treatment

The development of effective chemotherapy regimens for small cell lung cancer has dramatically increased the survival of patients with this disease. Indeed, small cell lung cancer is a potentially curable disease. Because there are notable differences in the approach to patients depending on the stage at diagnosis, therapy is discussed by stage, starting with the most common presentation—patients with extensive disease.

Treatment for Extensive-Stage Disease

A cornerstone of treatment of patients with extensive-stage small cell lung cancer is multiagent chemotherapy. The first highly effective regimen to be established

TREATMENT

Therapy of Extensive-Stage Small Cell Lung Cancer, Asymptomatic or Only Moderate Symptoms

Chemotherapy

Etoposide: 120 mg/m² intravenously days 1–3, *or* 120 mg/m² orally twice daily, days 1–3.

Cisplatin: 60–75 mg/m² intravenously day 1, following intravenous hydration with 1–2 L normal saline.

Cycles to be repeated every three weeks.

or

Carboplatin: AUC = 5 intravenously, day 1.

Etoposide: 100 mg/m² intravenously days 1–3, *or* 100 mg/m² orally twice daily, days 1–3.

Obtain chest X-ray before each cycle to ensure that there are no signs of progression.

If disease is stable following four cycles of chemotherapy: stop.

If disease is still responding following four cycles of chemotherapy: continue with another two cycles before stopping.

Dose Modifications

Weekly complete blood count and differential, platelet count.

Hold chemotherapy if absolute neutrophil count is <1000/μL or platelets <100,000/μL on day 1 until counts recover, then reduce doses 25%; if it recurs following cycle 2, start granulocyte-colony stimulating factor therapy.

Reduce doses 25% for neutropenic fevers, or an absolute neutrophil count <500/μL for seven or more days, or platelet count <50,000/μL for seven or more days.

Severe Localized Symptoms

Brain

Radiation therapy plus dexamethasone, 4–6 mg orally four times daily, then chemotherapy

Spinal Cord

Radiation therapy plus dexamethasone, 4–6 mg orally four times daily, then chemotherapy

Superior Vena Cava Syndrome or Severe Pulmonary Problems (Obstruction, Hemoptysis)

Treatment depends upon severity of symptoms. If patient has minimal or mild symptoms, initiate chemotherapy. For patients with moderate or severe symptoms, administer local radiation therapy for several days, followed by chemotherapy

as a standard for small cell lung cancer patients was cyclophosphamide, Adriamycin, and vincristine (CAV). Multiple effective chemotherapy regimens now exist for the treatment of small cell lung cancer. These include: etoposide-cisplatin (EP); etoposide-carboplatin; CAV; cyclophosphamide, doxorubicin and etoposide; and CAV alternating with EP. Randomized trials have failed to demonstrate that any one of these regimens is more efficacious than the others (Figures 94-5*A* and 94-5*B*). More recently, the Japanese Clinical Oncology group has shown a survival advantage for cisplatin plus irinotecan over cisplatin plus etoposide. The U.S. Intergroup mechanism is currently repeating this study to confirm the JCOG findings.

Etoposide-cisplatin and etoposide-carboplatin are the most commonly used regimens in the United States because they have a better toxicity profile than CAV and an equivalent efficacy when used as first-line therapy. Complete responses to chemotherapy with these regimens have been noted in 20% to 30% of cases, and the overall response rate is 50% to 70%. The median survival ranges from seven to 11 months. Carboplatin may be substituted for cisplatin in extensive-disease patients who have contraindications to cisplatin—for example, renal insufficiency.

The optimal duration of treatment seems to be four to six cycles. No advantage has been found for administering "maintenance" chemotherapy. Despite extensive efforts, no clear advantage has been established for escalating the intensity of doses of chemotherapy in small cell lung cancer. High-dose chemotherapy with autologous stem cell transplantation has been used in a small number of patients. Larger, definitive trials are necessary before any recommendation can be made regarding its application. Response rates to dose-intensive therapy have been demonstrably higher, but treatment-related mortality rates of up to 20% have canceled out any survival benefit. Alternating non–cross-resistant chemotherapy regimens is attractive conceptually, based on the hypothesis of Goldie and Coldman; however, studies of alternating regimens show no survival advantage compared with nonalternating regimens.

Patients who present with extensive disease

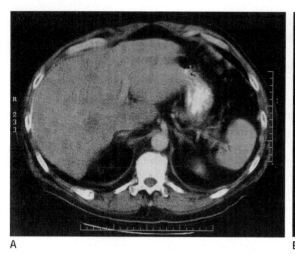
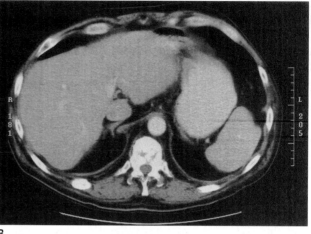

A   B

Figure 94-5 ■ *A*, Computed tomography image demonstrating significant involvement of liver with metastatic small cell lung carcinoma at the time of diagnosis. *B*, Computed tomography image demonstrating excellent response to two cycles of etoposide-cisplatin chemotherapy.

(including asymptomatic brain metastases) comprise a group deserving of special mention. Although cranial radiation and high-dose dexamethasone should be given promptly to patients with symptomatic brain metastases, many would argue that patients incidentally noted to have brain metastases on staging work-up can be treated quite successfully with chemotherapy followed by cranial radiation, particularly if the lesions are small. In some series, response of cranial metastases parallels the response of systemic disease. For example, in newly diagnosed patients who had asymptomatic brain metastases and were treated with chemotherapy alone, responses to chemotherapy, including central nervous system disease, were seen in more than 70% of patients. Giving chemotherapy initially in these patients thus treats both cranial and extracranial disease while avoiding the substantial toxicity of concurrent brain radiation therapy and systemic chemotherapy.

A similar management approach should be taken for patients with superior vena cava syndrome. Approximately 70% of these patients have extensive disease, while 30% have limited disease. Chemotherapy produces dramatic and rapid improvement in symptoms for these patients, as does radiation therapy. For patients who are markedly symptomatic, it is often helpful to initiate treatment with a few doses of radiation therapy emergently, until the rest of the staging work-up is complete and the patient is medically stable. At that point, the radiation can be stopped and the chemotherapy begun.

TREATMENT

Therapy of Limited-Stage Small Cell Lung Cancer

Evaluation for Thoracic Radiotherapy
Pulmonary function tests: Usual guidelines are FEV_1 >1.0 L in order to administer radiation therapy
Performance status 0–2

Treatment
Chemotherapy (as with extensive-stage disease) for four cycles, *except* no dose adjustments for the first two cycles
plus

Concurrent hyperfractionated thoracic radiation (45 Gy given as 1.5 Gy fractions twice daily in 30 treatments over three weeks (15 days); starting day one of cycle one of chemotherapy

Prophylactic Cranial Irradiation
Restage at completion of chemotherapy. If in complete response or "good partial response," give prophylactic cranial irradiation: 25 Gy in 2.5 Gy doses times 10 treatments

Treatment for Limited-Stage Disease

Limited-stage disease patients are treated more intensively than are patients with extensive disease. In limited-stage disease, combined modality therapy with chemotherapy and radiation therapy to the chest is superior to either treatment used alone. A Canadian study demonstrated that the strategy of early radiation therapy to the chest with chemotherapy had a substantial survival advantage over the administration of radiation therapy to the chest after completion of chemotherapy. The combination of etoposide-cisplatin chemotherapy with radiation therapy has been shown to be far less toxic for patients than Adriamycin-based regimens, which is another reason for the preference of this chemotherapy regimen in the United States.

In 1999, Turrisi et al showed a survival benefit for the combination of twice-daily radiation therapy ("hyperfractionated") with four cycles of etoposide and cisplatin for limited-stage small cell lung cancer. Patients who received hyperfractionated radiation therapy had overall two-year and five-year survival rates of 47% and 26%, whereas the two-year and five-year survival rates for patients treated with once-daily radiation therapy plus cisplatin and etoposide were 41% and 16%, respectively. Although other studies have failed to confirm a survival advantage with hyperfractionated radiotherapy, we consider the standard of care for limited-stage small cell lung cancer to be treatment with four cycles of cisplatin-based chemotherapy, giving hyperfractionated radiation therapy during the first or (if necessary) second cycle of chemotherapy.

Many investigators advocate for prophylactic cranial irradiation in patients with limited-stage disease who achieve a complete response to chemoradiotherapy. A meta-analysis of prophylactic cranial irradiation trials demonstrated a survival advantage. The rationales for prophylactic cranial irradiation are that without cranial irradiation, up to 40% of such patients relapse with brain metastases, and that survival after detection of brain metastasis is brief (less than five months). Prophylactic cranial irradiation reduces the risk of brain relapse by approximately one-half. Nonetheless, this approach remains controversial because of reports from nonrandomized retrospective series of a high rate of severe neurocognitive impairment in patients treated with whole-brain radiation therapy who had been cured of lung cancer. Identified risk factors for radiation-related brain injury include higher total radiation therapy dose and dose per fraction as well as the concurrent use of radiation therapy sensitizers. It is uncertain whether these data apply to current treatment programs, in which radiation sensitizers such as methotrexate and Adriamycin are usually avoided.

Surgery

Early studies of patients with small cell lung cancer led to the conclusion that surgery has no role in the treatment of this disease. Interest has increased recently in the potential utility of surgery as a component of therapy for patients with very limited disease. A Veterans Administration Surgical Oncology study of patients with small cell lung cancer who were treated with surgery followed by adjuvant chemotherapy found that five-year survival rates for T1N0, T1N1, and T2N0 (very limited-stage disease) patients were 60%, 31%, and 28%, respectively. Use of preoperative, neoadjuvant chemotherapy to "downstage" patients in order to make them eligible for surgery has been evaluated prospectively but appears not to improve survival.

Patients with Poor Performance Status

Approximately 25% of patients with small cell lung cancer will be more than 70 years of age at diagnosis. Patients in this age group are less likely to receive chemotherapy, in part related to poorer performance status at diagnosis and comorbid conditions. As noted, however, increasing age is not an independent predictor of worsening survival. Elderly patients with a good performance status (ECOG scale performance status 0–2) should be treated with full-dose therapy similarly to younger patients.

Patients with poor performance status (ECOG scale performance status 3–4) are at a substantially higher risk of treatment-related complications and generally have a poor outcome despite treatment efforts. Supportive measures alone might be the best option for most such patients. Two clinical studies evaluating oral etoposide as a less toxic chemotherapy alternative were discontinued prematurely when interim analyses showed worsened survival and/or quality of life for patients on the oral etoposide arm.

Relapsed and Refractory Disease

Unfortunately, most patients with small cell lung cancer relapse, even after intensive treatment. Management of such patients is best guided by the time to progression after completing primary chemotherapy. Patients with time to progression greater than three months are considered to have "chemosensitive disease" and often respond to the same regimen used in induction therapy. Patients with time to progression less than three months or progression during primary therapy are considered "refractory." The options for chemotherapy in such refractory patients are often limited by poor performance status, prior toxicity, and reduced bone marrow reserve from previous therapy. Approximately 25% of chemosensitive patients respond to second-line chemotherapy with cyclophosphamide, Adriamycin, and vincristine chemotherapy. Single-agent topotecan can produce an equivalent response rate and perhaps better symptom control in more patients than is found after CAV. For patients with poor performance status, supportive and palliative care are often the best options.

Palliative Therapy

For patients who have failed to obtain a useful response to chemotherapy or who relapse, palliative measures are available.

Palliative Radiation Therapy

Palliative radiation therapy can be helpful in controlling disease-related problems such as painful bony metastases, metastases to weight-bearing bones that threaten to cause fracture, painful liver or adrenal metastases, or severe pulmonary obstructive presentations. For patients with bronchial obstruction who have received maximum external-beam radiotherapy, the use of high-dose endobronchial irradiation could have some benefit.

Anorexia

Anorexia can be relieved in some patients by use of megestrol acetate, 800 mg in an oral suspension given daily.

Pleural Effusions

Pleural effusions that are recurrent and symptomatic can be palliated by pleurodesis. Common sclerosing agents include bleomycin, talc, and doxycycline. Bleomycin is the most expensive; talc has the disadvantage of requiring a thoracoscopy and general anesthesia for insufflation (see Chapter 15).

Toxicity

Myelosuppression

Myelosuppression and anemia represent frequent complications of the polychemotherapy regimens mentioned in preceding sections. In intensively treated patients, granulocyte-colony stimulating factor (G-CSF) decreases the incidence of neutropenic fevers,

the median duration of neutropenia, days of hospitalization, and days of antibiotic treatment. But there is no demonstrable clinical benefit to a dose-intense approach. Moreover, caution must be exercised when using colony-stimulating factors in patients receiving combined modality therapy with chemotherapy and radiation therapy. One randomized study in this group of patients observed a significant increase in thrombocytopenia compared with patients on the same regimen who did not receive granulocyte-colony stimulating factor.

Erythropoietin could be useful in the treatment of chemotherapy-related anemia. Patients with hemoglobin levels less than 10 g/dL and symptoms of anemia such as shortness of breath or fatigue may be given this growth factor as part of their comprehensive supportive care. Although there is no evidence of a survival advantage, symptoms such as fatigue do improve. This might be particularly important in many patients with small cell lung cancer who have obstructive pulmonary disease from years of smoking.

Nausea and Vomiting

These were once feared complications of cisplatin-based chemotherapy. The development of the 5-HT$_3$ receptor-blocking agents such as ondansetron revolutionized the treatment of patients receiving emetogenic chemotherapy. These agents prevent nausea and vomiting in roughly 70% of patients and have made outpatient treatment of small cell lung cancer the norm.

Neuropsychological Impairment

Neuropsychological impairment from prophylactic cranial irradiation is one of the most feared late sequelae of treatment of small cell lung cancer. Two studies prospectively evaluated the effect of prophylactic cranial irradiation on neuropsychological outcomes. A substantial proportion (24% to 60%) of the patients with small cell lung cancer had abnormalities on neuropsychological testing before the onset of treatment. The fraction of patients with abnormal findings did not differ between those who did or did not receive prophylactic cranial irradiation. Neuropsychological abnormalities in small cell lung cancer patients seem to be predominantly related to memory. This high prevalence of memory abnormalities in the screened small cell lung cancer patient population even before the use of cranial radiation therapy raises the question about whether some of these patients might have subclinical immune-mediated limbic encephalitis. Given the uncertainty about the cause of the late neurologic manifestations, we continue to recommend prophylactic cranial irradiation for limited-stage patients who achieve complete remission after primary chemotherapy and thoracic radiation therapy.

Radiation Pneumonitis

This side effect occurs in 15% of patients who receive high-dose external beam radiation therapy to the chest. Symptoms such as shortness of breath and/or nonproductive cough usually begin two to six months after completion of radiotherapy and can be severe. The risk of radiation pneumonitis directly correlates with increasing daily doses of radiation therapy and increasing lung volumes in the radiation therapy field. Patients show fibrotic changes on chest X-ray, which can progress for months after treatment. These changes are associated with a decrease in lung volume and diffusion capacity. The risk of this complication is the principal reason for obtaining pulmonary function testing in patients prior to starting radiation therapy to the chest. Patients with marginal lung function (FEV_1 <1.0 L/sec) are generally not considered to be candidates for radiation therapy because of lack of pulmonary reserve in the event that toxicity from radiation develops. Prednisone, at a dose of 1 mg/kg orally, is used to treat patients with radiation pneumonitis; doses are tapered slowly over a period of months.

Follow-up Evaluation

After completion of therapy, patients with both limited-stage and extensive-stage disease must be followed closely for evidence of relapse. The practice of these authors is to see patients every two months for the first year, every three months for the second year, and every four months for the third year. Patients who survive three years are seen every six months for two years and then annually. At each visit, in addition to history and physical examination, these authors obtain a chest X-ray, complete blood counts and platelet count, liver and renal function tests, electrolytes, and a serum lactate dehydrogenase analysis. Computed tomography scans are ordered only when indicated by symptoms or abnormal findings on physical examination or laboratory tests.

References

General

Abrams J, Doyle L, Eisner J: Staging, prognostic factors, and special considerations in small cell lung cancer. Semin Oncol 1988;15:261–277.

Elliott J, Osterlind K, Hirsch F, et al: Metastatic patterns in small cell lung cancer: Correlation of autopsy findings with clinical parameters in 537 patients. J Clin Oncol 1987;5:246–254.

Goldman J, Ash C, Souhami R, et al: Spinal cord compression in small cell lung cancer: A retrospective study of 610 patients. J. Cancer Res Clin Oncol 1989;59:591–593.

Hainsworth J, Workman R, Greco F: Management of the syndrome of inappropriate antidiuretic hormone secretion in small cell lung cancer. Cancer 1983;51:161–165.

Hirsch F, Paulson O, Hansen H, et al: Intracranial metastases in small cell carcinoma of the lung. Cancer 1983;51:529–533.

Hyde L, Hyde C: Clinical manifestations of lung cancer. Chest 1974;65:299–306.

Nugent J, Bunn P, Matthews M, et al: CNS metastases in small cell bronchogenic carcinoma. Cancer 1979;44:1885–1893.

Stokkel M, Van Eck-Smit B, Zwinderman A, et al: Pretreatment serum lactate dehydrogenase as an additional staging parameter in patients with small cell lung carcinoma. J Cancer Res Clin Oncol 1998;124:215–219.

Urban T, Lebeau B, Chastand C, et al: Superior vena cava syndrome in small cell lung cancer. Arch Intern Med 1993;153:384–387.

Wingo P, Ries L, Giovino G, et al: Annual report to the nation on the status of cancer 1973–1996, with a special section on lung cancer and tobacco smoking. J Natl Cancer Inst 1999;91:675–690.

Paraneoplastic Syndromes

Collichio F, Woolf P, Brower M: Management of patients with small cell carcinoma and the syndrome of ectopic corticotropin secretion. Cancer 1994;73:1361–1367.

Dalmau J, Graus F, Rosenblum M, et al: Anti-Hu-associated paraneoplastic encephalomyelitis/sensory neuronopathy. Med 1992;71:59–72.

Gross A, Steinberg S, Reilly J, et al: Atrial natriuretic factor and arginine vasopressin production in tumor cell lines from patients with lung cancer and their relationship to serum sodium. Cancer Res 1993;53:67–74.

Keime-Guibert F, Graus F, Broet P, et al: Clinical outcome of patients with anti-Hu-associated encephalomyelitis after treatment of the tumor. Neurology 1999;53:1719–1723.

List A, Hainsworth J, Davis B, et al: The syndrome of inappropriate secretion of antidiuretic hormone (SIADH) in small cell lung cancer. J Clin Oncol 1986;4:1191–1198.

Maddison P, Newsom-Davis J, Mills K, et al: Favorable prognosis in Lambert-Eaton myasthenic syndrome and small cell lung carcinoma. Lancet 1999;353:117–118.

Pathology

Hirsch F, Matthews M, Yesner R: Histopathologic classification of small cell carcinoma of the lung. Cancer 1982;50:1360–1366.

Hirsch F, Osterlind K, Hansen H: The prognostic significance of histopathologic subtyping of small cell carcinoma of the lung according to the classification of the World Health Organization. Cancer 1983;52:2144–2150.

Matsuda M, Horai T, Nakamura S, et al: Bronchial brushing and bronchial biopsy: comparison of diagnostic accuracy and cell typing reliability in lung cancer. Thorax 1986; 41:475–478.

Piaton E, Grillet-Ravigneaux M, Saugier B, et al: Prospective study of combined use of bronchial aspirates and biopsy specimens in diagnosis and typing of centrally located lung tumors. Br Med J 1995;310:624–627.

Twijnstra A, Thunnissen F, Lassouw G, et al: The role of the histologic subclassification of tumor cells in patients with small cell carcinoma of the lung and central nervous system metastases. Cancer 1989;65:1812–1815.

Treatment

Adjei A, Marks R, Bonner J: Current guidelines for the management of small cell lung cancer. Mayo Clin Proc 1999;74:809–816.

Arriagada R, Pignon JP, Le Chevalier T: Initial chemotherapeutic doses and long-term survival in limited small cell lung cancer. N Engl J Med 2001;345:1281–1282.

Auperin A, Arriagada R, Pignon J, et al: Prophylactic cranial irradiation for patients with small cell lung cancer in complete remission. N Engl J Med 1999;341:476–484.

Chute J, Venzon D, Hankins L, et al: Outcome of patients with small cell lung cancer during 20 years of clinical research at the U.S. National Cancer Institute. Mayo Clin Proc 1997;72:901–912.

Chute J, Chen T, Feigal E, et al: Twenty years of phase III trials for patients with extensive-stage small cell lung cancer: Perceptible progress. J Clin Oncol 1999;17:1794–1801.

Curran WJ Jr: Therapy of limited small cell lung cancer. Cancer Treat Res 2001;105:229–252.

Earl H, Rudd R, Spiro S, et al: A randomized trial of planned versus as required chemotherapy in small cell lung cancer: A Cancer Research Campaign trial. Br J Cancer 1991;64:566–572.

Evans W, Shepherd F, Feld R, et al: VP-16 and cisplatin as first-line therapy for small cell lung cancer. J Clin Oncol 1985;3:1471–1477.

Feld R, Evans W, DeBoer G, et al: Combined modality induction therapy without maintenance chemotherapy for small cell carcinoma of the lung. J Clin Oncol 1984;2:294–304.

Fukuoka M, Furuse K, Saijo N, et al: Randomized trial of cyclophosphamide, doxorubicin, and vincristine versus cisplatin and etoposide versus alternation of these regimens in small cell lung cancer. J Natl Cancer Inst 1991;83:855–861.

Giannone L, Johnson D, Hande K, et al: Favorable prognosis of brain metastases in small cell lung cancer. Ann Inter Med 1987;106:386–389.

Gridelli C, DeVivo R, Monfardini S: Management of small cell lung cancer in the elderly. Crit Rev Oncol Hematol 2002;41:79–88.

Inoue M, Miyoshi S, Yasumitsu T, et al: Surgical results for small cell lung cancer based on the new TNM staging system. Ann Thorac Surg 2000;70:1615–1619.

Inoue A, Kunitoh H, Sekine I, et al: Radiation pneumonitis in lung cancer patients: A retrospective study of risk factors and long-term prognosis. Intl J Rad Oncol Biol Phys 2001;49:649–655.

Johnson BE: NCCN. Small cell lung cancer practice guidelines panel. Cancer Cont 2001;8(S):32–43.

Kelly K: Treatment of extensive stage small cell lung cancer. Cancer Treat Res 2001;105:253–276.

Komaki R, Meyers C, Shin D, et al: Evaluation of cognitive function in patients with limited small cell lung cancer prior to and shortly following prophylactic cranial irradiation. Intl J Rad Oncol Biol Phys 1995;33:179–182.

Kotalik J, Yu E, Markman BR, et al: Practice guidelines on prophylactic cranial irradiation in small cell lung cancer. Intl J Rad Oncol Biol Phys 2001;50:309–316.

Leyvraz S, Perey L, Rosti G, et al: Multiple courses of high-dose ifosfamide, carboplatin, and etoposide with peripheral-blood progenitor cells and filgrastim for small cell lung cancer: A feasibility study by the European Group for Blood and Marrow Transplantation. J Clin Oncol 1999;17:3531–3539.

McCracken D, Janaki L, Crowley JJ, et al: Concurrent chemotherapy/radiotherapy for limited small cell lung carcinoma: A Southwest Oncology Group Study. J Clin Oncol 1990;8:892–898.

Merrill R, Henson D, Barnes M: Conditional survival among patients with carcinoma of the lung. Chest 1999;116:697–703.

Murray N, Livingston R, Shepherd F, et al: Randomized study of CODE versus alternating CAV/EP for extensive-stage small cell lung cancer: An intergroup study of the National Cancer Institute of Canada Clinical Trials Group and the Southwest Oncology Group. J Clin Oncol 1999;17:2300–2308.

Noda K, Nishiwaki Y, Saijo N, et al: Irinotecan plus cisplatin compared with etoposide plus cisplatin for extensive stage small cell lung cancer. New Engl J Med 2002;346:85–91.

Party ELCW, Mascaux C, Paesmans M, et al: A systematic review of the role of etoposide and cisplatin in the chemotherapy of small cell lung cancer with methodology assessment and meta-analysis. Lung Cancer 2000;30:23–36.

Party MRCLCW: Comparison of oral etoposide and standard intravenous multidrug chemotherapy for small cell cancer: A stopped multicentre randomized trial. Lancet 1996;348:563–566.

Postmus PE, Smit EF: Treatment of relapsed small cell lung cancer. Semin Oncol 2001;28(S4):48–52.

Rosen II, Fischer TA, Antolak JA, et al: Correlation between lung fibrosis and radiation therapy dose after concurrent radiation therapy and chemotherapy for limited small cell lung cancer. Radiol 2001;221:614–622.

Samantas E, Skaros D, Pectasides D, et al: Combination chemotherapy with low doses of weekly carboplatin and oral etoposide in poor risk small cell lung cancer. Lung Cancer 1999;29:159–168.

Sculier JP, Paesmansa M, Lecomte J, et al: A three-arm phase III randomised trial assessing, in patients with extensive-disease small cell lung cancer, accelerated chemotherapy with support of haematological growth factor or oral antibiotics. Br J Cancer 2001;85:1444–1451.

Sloan JA, Bonner JA, Hillman SL, et al: A quality-adjusted reanalysis of a phase III trial comparing once-daily thoracic radiation vs. twice-daily thoracic radiation in patients with limited-stage small cell lung cancer. Intl J Rad Oncol Biol Phys 2002;52:371–381.

Turrisi A, Kim K, Blum R, et al: Twice-daily compared with once-daily thoracic radiotherapy in limited small cell lung cancer treated concurrently with cisplatin and etoposide. N Engl J Med 1999;340:265–271.

Chapter 95
Non–Small Cell Lung Cancer

Daniel D. Karp and Robert L. Thurer

Introduction

Approximately three quarters of all lung cancers are due to non–small cell lung cancer, and adenocarcinoma and squamous cell cancer account for approximately three quarters of all of these cases. Only one in seven patients can be cured. Most of these curable patients have early-stage, resectable disease. Patients with limited lymph node involvement will suffer recurrence more than half the time after surgical resection. In the 1970s, non–small cell lung cancer was usually diagnosed with a chest X-ray, and many patients had unsuccessful surgery for what proved to be unresectable disease. Computed tomography (CT) scans and mediastinoscopy have made accurate staging possible for the great majority of patients. It is now rare for a patient to undergo surgery that results in an exploration without resection of the primary cancer.

Epidemiology

The American Cancer Society estimates that there were 169,500 cases of lung cancer in the United States in 2001, with approximately 157,400 deaths—a rise of 5400 and 500, respectively, over the 2000 projections (Table 95-1). Lung cancer death rates in the United States vary markedly not only from state to state (Figure 95-1) but even among neighborhoods. Utah consistently has the lowest lung cancer–specific mortality. These lung cancer–specific mortality estimates are clearly affected by differences in median age and ethnic variability within the populations. Nevertheless, such striking state-to-state variability also reflects differences in tobacco and alcohol use and the way people live and work. These observations support the view that appropriate interventions can lower the death rate from lung cancer.

Tobacco is now recognized as a highly addictive drug warranting Food and Drug Administration (FDA) regulation. Over 46 million individuals in the United States smoke—approximately 26% of adults—and there are about 45 million former smokers. This produces an enormous pool of people who are at risk. Lung cancer kills three times more people in the United States than any other malignancy and is now the number one cancer killer worldwide. Despite this high mortality, the long-term survival rate for lung cancer has increased from approximately 7% in the mid-1970s to over 14% today.

Ironically, former smokers now make up a large percentage of newly diagnosed cases of lung cancer, and it is becoming increasingly clear that lung cancer can develop many years after individuals stop smoking. Moreover, the small population of fortunate long-term survivors of lung cancer is estimated to have a 20% lifetime risk of developing second primary tumors. Elimination of tobacco use as primary prevention of lung cancer remains a crucial intervention for teenagers and young adults. Even though smoking produces a persistent legacy of tissue damage and potential carcinogenesis, the increased risk of lung cancer declines over time in former smokers, reaching background levels of incidence 15 years later.

Carcinogenesis of Lung Cancer

The causal pathway initiated by smoking involves multiple factors, including duration of smoking, depth of inhalation, underlying lung disease, and deposition of particulate matter in the lungs. Contribution to the genesis of lung cancer is made by chronic pulmonary inflammation, release of proteolytic enzymes and oxygen radicals, and macrophage secretion of polypeptide growth factors. Genetic susceptibility makes up a third component. Knudson, in 1985, hypothesized that the increased susceptibility to cancer in certain individuals was based on the loss or mutation of a single gene; that is, loss of heterozygosity. This circumstance then increased the likelihood that a "second hit" would occur as a result of carcinogen exposure or some other mutational stimulus. Since only 10% to 15% of smokers ultimately develop

Table 95-1 ■ Lung Cancer Causes 13% of Cancer Cases and 28% of Cancer Deaths in the United States

Cancer Incidence			Cancer Mortality	
Cancer Location	Percent	Number	Cancer Location	Percent
Prostate	16	198,100	**Lung**	**28**
Breast	15	193,700	Colon	9
Lung	**13**	**169,500**	Breast	7
Colon	8	98,200	Unknown	7
Lymphoma	4	56,200	Prostate	6
Bladder	4	54,300	Pancreas	5
Melanoma	4	51,400	Lymphoma	5
Head and neck	3	40,100	Stomach	2
Uterus	3	38,300	Ovary	3
Rectum	2	37,200	Liver	3
Unknown	2	31,400	Head and neck	2
Kidney	2	30,800	Brain	2

The total estimate for U.S. cancer cases in 2001 is 1,268,000.

lung cancer, investigators have tried to identify the genetic features that predispose to lung cancer. For example, many investigators have believed for some time that genetic polymorphisms in carcinogen metabolizing pathways were determining factors. The results of studies of a number of metabolic pathways, such as the P450 cytochrome system, have given variable results. The search for the genetic cause for the variation in susceptibility to carcinogens continues.

Multistep Carcinogenesis

Vogelstein et al established that multiple oncogene activation events are required for the development of

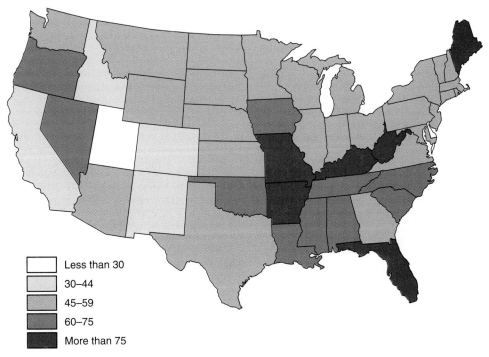

Less than 30
30–44
45–59
60–75
More than 75

Figure 95-1 ■ Marked variation in lung cancer death rates by state. Numbers of cases cited are per 100,000 population.

colon cancer, but the process of suppressor gene loss and oncogene activation in bronchogenic cancer is less well understood. It appears that abnormalities in DNA methylation, p53, and mutations of K-ras occur relatively early in the development of lung cancer. The protein encoded by the p53 gene is a key element in regulating the cell cycle and apoptosis, particularly in response to cellular damage. The region on chromosome 17 (17p13) where p53 resides is frequently deleted in lung cancer, and the remaining allele has undergone mutational inactivation in 50% to 70% of lung cancers.

Clinical Presentation

Patients with lung cancer present with a remarkable constellation of signs and symptoms, and as such, lung cancer may masquerade as many different diseases or conditions. Presenting symptoms and their relative frequency are displayed in Table 95-2. Four categories of presentation are considered

Asymptomatic Presentation

In large retrospective reviews, the number of lung cancer patients who are truly asymptomatic at the time of diagnosis is only 2% to 5%. These cases are often diagnosed by chance in patients having a chest X-ray as part of a preoperative evaluation or annual physical examination in a smoker.

Symptoms Related to Local Growth

For patients presenting with local symptoms, the extent and severity depend on the location and size of the lesion and on the involvement of the respiratory tract or invasion of adjacent structures. Peripheral lesions may cause pleural effusions or chest wall pain. Central endobronchial lesions can produce cough, dyspnea, infection, or hemoptysis. Invasion of adjacent structures, particularly within the mediastinum, may produce dysphagia, hoarseness, nerve compression, chylous pleural effusion, pericardial effusion, or superior vena cava syndrome. Tumors arising in small airways or peripherally located are usually asymptomatic. Consequently, more peripheral than central tumors are incidental findings on chest X-rays.

Pleural involvement, manifested as pleural effusions, pleural masses, or rarely pneumothorax, occurs in 8% to 15% of lung cancer patients, causing dyspnea, cough, and chest pain. Pleural effusion from lung cancer can be due either to obstruction of the lung's draining lymphatics or to direct pleural invasion by the tumor. This is an important distinction, because the small percentage of patients with pleural effusion due to lymphatic obstruction are still candidates for surgical resection. Direct pleural invasion by the tumor is diagnosed by thoracentesis, closed pleural biopsy, or pleuroscopy in order of ascending sensitivity. Chest wall pain occurs in 40% of patients presenting with lung cancer due to tumor growth into the chest wall, ribs, or vertebral bodies. Careful questioning is critical to identify those patients with peripheral tumors that are invading bony structures. Such patients usually require multimodality therapy.

Approximately 50% of lung cancers will arise from central structures and, as such, are likely to involve large airways. These will result in cough, localized wheezing, hemoptysis, focal atelectasis, dyspnea, or infections and postobstructive pneumonitis.

Cough is the most common presenting symptom in non–small cell lung cancer, affecting as many as 75% of patients at the time of diagnosis. Since chronic cough, especially in the early morning, is frequent in cigarette smokers, it often requires a change in the pattern of the cough, to persistent or unremitting for example, to bring the patient to medical attention. When cough is a dominant symptom in non–small cell lung cancer, symptomatic relief requires effective anticancer therapy.

Dyspnea is a subtle but common symptom in 40% to 60% of patients at presentation. Many smokers already have chronic shortness of breath and exercise limitations, making it difficult for them to perceive slight changes. A number of local effects contribute to the high rate of dyspnea. These include loss of

---

Table 95-2 ■ Presenting Symptoms and Signs of Lung Cancer: Approximate Percentages	
Frequent	
Cough	45–75%
Weight loss	30–70%
Dyspnea	40–60%
Chest pain	30–50%
Common	
Hemoptysis	25–35%
Skeletal pain	20–25%
Uncommon	
Clubbing, hypertrophic osteoarthropathy	10–20%
Hoarseness	10–20%
Rare	
Dysphagia	<5%
Wheezing	<5%
Pericardial effusion	<5%

alveolar space due to extensive tumor, pulmonary lymphangitic spread of cancer, pleural or pericardial effusions, atelectasis, and bronchospasm.

Pulmonary infection occurs as central tumors enlarge, obstructing airways leading to atelectasis, pneumonia, and even formation of an abscess or empyema. Persistent pneumonia on chest X-ray following a course of antibiotics is a frequent presentation. A cavitating tumor or postobstructive pneumonitis may mimic a primary infection or abscess, producing symptoms of fever, chills, and productive cough. These patients may benefit greatly from radiation therapy and/or endobronchial therapies such as laser-guided resection, photodynamic therapy, or stent placement. Initial therapy should consist of antibiotics and radiation therapy. Any chemotherapy should be delayed to avoid neutropenia until the obstructive pneumonitis has resolved.

Hemoptysis (see also Chapter 18) is a worrisome and telltale symptom, occurring in 20% to 25% of patients with non–small cell lung cancer. Many patients with chronic bronchitis and productive morning "smoker's" cough will have an occasional small amount of blood in their sputum. Indeed, although acute and chronic bronchitis are the most common causes of hemoptysis, bronchoscopic series of smokers with hemoptysis find an incidence of bronchogenic cancer of approximately 5%. Any amount of blood in the sputum warrants a chest X-ray and careful bronchoscopic evaluation for a central airway cancer.

When the tumor invades adjacent structures or spreads to the mediastinal nodes, focal symptoms occur in association with the development of fatigue, weight loss, anorexia, cachexia, and fever.

Dysphagia may result from invasion of the esophagus. The esophagus is able to function quite well in the face of extrinsic compression. Dysphagia is therefore surprisingly uncommon in patients with lung cancer despite the frequent presence of bulky lymph nodes in the mediastinum. Esophageal invasion may also produce a bronchoesophageal fistula with recurrent aspiration and pneumonia. Endoscopy is required in patients with lung cancer who have difficult or painful swallowing to rule out esophageal invasion by lung cancer and to identify other causes, such as esophagitis or concurrent esophageal or head and neck cancer.

Hoarseness can occur owing to compression of the recurrent laryngeal nerve by enlarged lymph nodes, resulting in ipsilateral vocal cord paralysis. Involvement of the recurrent laryngeal nerve classifies these tumors as at least stage 3A (see the following section on staging). Hoarseness from lung cancer usually signifies that the disease is unresectable.

Nerve compression by tumor causes variable symptomatology. Phrenic nerve entrapment in the mediastinum manifests as diaphragmatic paralysis and positional dyspnea. Tumors involving the superior sulcus at the lung apex can invade and destroy neural structures in the brachial plexus and sympathetic chain. The result is pain in the shoulder or the medial portion of the scapula, radicular pain with muscle wasting in the distribution of the ulnar nerve (T1 root) or medial forearm and hand (C8 distribution), or Horner's syndrome (ptosis, miosis, hemianhydrosis, enophthalmos). Tumors presenting in this fashion are called Pancoast's tumors, and this presentation has been labeled Pancoast's syndrome.

Superior vena cava syndrome is caused by compression of the superior vena cava, especially by tumors in the right upper lobe or by paratracheal adenopathy (see Chapter 17).

The pericardium and heart are eventually affected by lung cancers in 15% to 35% of cases. Pericardial involvement is more common than myocardial involvement. Neoplastic pericarditis causes pericardial effusions, tamponade, or arrhythmias. Its presence is suggested by an enlarging heart silhouette on chest X-ray, pulsus paradoxicus, a pericardial friction rub or Kussmaul's sign, new onset of congestive failure, or venous engorgement. The diagnosis is confirmed by echocardiography.

Extrathoracic Metastasis

Distant metastases from lung cancer have been found in virtually every organ. However, the four most common sites for metastases are adrenal, bone, brain, and liver. The frequency of metastases and specific locations vary with different histologies.

Skeletal metastases occur in up to 30% of non–small cell lung cancer patients. Patients with bone metastases often present with localized pain. However, some patients may present only with elevated calcium or elevated alkaline phosphatase on laboratory screen.

Adrenal gland metastases from lung cancer usually cause no specific signs or symptoms. Because these lesions are clinically silent, chest computed tomography scans to evaluate for lung cancer should include sections through the upper abdomen to examine the adrenals.

Central nervous system metastases are common and can cause the presenting symptoms of lung cancer (see Chapters 4, 5, and 7). Symptoms depend on the area of central nervous system involved. Brain metastases cause headaches, focal neurologic dysfunction, or seizures. Lung cancer metastatic lesions can present as solitary or multiple intracranial masses, as meningeal carcinomatosis, or with spinal cord involvement.

Liver metastases are found in 10% to 20% of non–small cell lung cancer patients. While lung cancers are a frequent cause of liver metastases, few patients have liver metastases at the time of diagnosis or as the first site of metastatic spread. Bone, brain, and adrenal metastases are more common. Patients with hepatic metastases present in one of three ways: symptoms from the lung primary with asymptomatic liver involvement discovered during evaluation; nonspecific symptoms such as weakness, fever, diaphoresis, or weight loss and liver abnormalities on blood tests or abdominal computed tomography scan; and clinical features of liver disease, including abdominal pain, ascites, or hepatomegaly.

Lymphangitic spread is most frequently seen with adenocarcinoma and is recognized by increased interstitial markings on chest imaging. The presentation can simulate congestive heart failure but is unresponsive to diuretics.

Intra-alveolar spread is most often seen with bronchioloalveolar carcinoma and results in multicentric lung involvement (an alveolar pattern on chest X-ray and computed tomography scan). Bronchorrhea is present in approximately half of the cases. This presentation is most commonly seen in women who have never smoked or who are former smokers.

Lung Cancer Presenting as Cancer of Unknown Origin

Patients presenting with lung cancer at metastatic sites due to a small, unapparent, early disseminating primary lesion in the lung may be difficult to distinguish from patients with other metastatic cancers. The location of small primary lung cancers may contribute to their concealment. For example, chest X-ray might fail to detect high apical lesions; cancers directly behind the clavicle; posterior lesions, especially those located behind the heart; and lesions in the cardiophrenic sulcus.

Paraneoplastic Syndromes

Approximately 10% of patients with lung cancer present with a paraneoplastic syndrome (Table 95-3). The pathophysiology of these syndromes is poorly understood, but many are related to ectopic hormone

Table 95-3 ■ Paraneoplastic Syndromes and Their Relative Frequency

	Endocrine	Neurologic	Musculoskeletal	Hematologic	Miscellaneous
More common	Hypercalcemia	Peripheral neuropathy	Clubbing	Anemia	Fatigue
	Hyponatremia	Lambert-Eaton myasthenic syndrome (consider mixed small cell/non–small cell cancer)	Hypertrophic pulmonary osteoarthropathy	Thrombocytosis	Cachexia
	Cushing's syndrome			Trousseau's syndrome	Fever
Less common	Gynecomastia (bHCG)	Cerebellar degeneration	Dermatomyositis	Leukocytosis	
	Hypoglycemia (insulinlike substance)	Limbic encephalitis	Polymyositis	Autoimmune hemolytic anemia	Hyperuricemia
	Acromegaly (growth hormone)	Encephalomyelitis	Myopathy	Eosinophilia	Hypertension (renin)
Rare	Hyperthyroidism (TSH)	Stiff-man syndrome		Monocytosis	Membranous nephropathy
		Opsoclonus myoclonus		Idiopathic thrombocytopenia purpura	
				Nonbacterial thrombotic endocarditis	
				Vasculitis	

production. Although the tabulation of all reported abnormalities is lengthy, only a few are common and/or clinically important.

Hypercalcemia occurs in 10% to 15% of patients with lung cancer (see Chapter 31). Bronchogenic carcinomas, especially bulky squamous cancers, can produce parathormone-like substances that can cause calcium levels to rise to dangerous levels. As a differential diagnostic point, small cell carcinoma does not cause hypercalcemia unless it is just one component of a mixed histology cancer. Destructive bone metastases, particularly if coupled to immobility, can also release sufficient calcium from bones to cause hypercalcemia. When serum calcium reaches sufficiently high levels, patients develop severe fatigue, anorexia, nausea, vomiting, dehydration, and potentially cardiac arrhythmias or death. Hypercalcemia leads to increased free water clearance by the kidneys and to dehydration. Dehydration sets up the vicious cycle of hypercalcemia, loss of free water, nausea, decreased oral intake, and worsening hypercalcemia. Proper hydration and saline diuresis with furosemide are still the mainstays of treatment, since calcium excretion by the kidney is linked to sodium excretion. Intravenous diphosphonates, such as pamidronate and zolendronate, are very effective in controlling the calcium level for most patients. It is now rarely necessary to resort to the use of plicamycin (mithramycin) to control elevated calcium.

Ectopic hormone production is most often seen in small cell lung cancer. The occurrence of endocrine syndromes in a patient with non–small cell lung cancer suggests the presence of a mixed non–small cell and small cell histology. The syndromes of inappropriate antidiuretic hormone secretion (SIADH) and of ectopic ACTH production are particularly common. Ectopic adrenocorticotropic hormone (ACTH) production causes output of high levels of glucocorticoids, marked primarily by hypokalemia and to a lesser degree by hypernatremia. Full-blown Cushing's syndrome is unusual, because patients do not often survive long enough to manifest the complete clinical syndrome.

The syndrome of inappropriate antidiuretic hormone secretion causes free water retention and hyponatremia. Despite the falling osmolality of the serum, urinary sodium excretion continues, and the net result can be profound hyponatremia. Serum sodium levels falling below 120 mEq/L place the patient at risk for seizures or cardiovascular collapse.

Neuromuscular disorders occur in 5% of patients with lung cancer. Probably the best described neurologic complication is Eaton-Lambert syndrome. This myasthenia-like syndrome differs from myasthenia gravis because motor strength improves with repetitive stimulation, whereas in myasthenia gravis, muscle strength decreases.

Joint pain in patients with lung cancer is rarely due to bone metastases. Joint pain and lower extremity (tibial) aching pain may result from hypertrophic pulmonary osteoarthropathy, which occurs in 10% to 20% of patients with non–small cell lung cancer, most commonly in patients with adenocarcinoma and large cell lung cancer. The syndrome is characterized by digital clubbing and/or periosteal elevation, demonstrable on X-rays of tubular bones, such as the distal tibia or radius. Expansion of the paronychial soft tissue around the nailbed eliminates the angle between the base of the nailbed and cuticle and produces clubbing. These findings are not necessarily indicators of metastatic disease. Bone pain from hypertrophic osteoarthropathy can regress quickly once treatment has been initiated.

Oncologic Emergencies

There are numerous explosive presentations of lung cancer that constitute true oncologic emergencies and require prompt attention and therapy. These include the following:

- Brain metastases with increased intracranial pressure or seizures
- Cardiac tamponade due to malignant pericardial effusion
- Respiratory distress due to total obstruction of a lung
- Tension pneumothorax (rare) due to a ruptured peripheral carcinoma
- Obstructive pneumonia with sepsis
- Pathologic fractures of the lower extremity
- Pulmonary embolus

Staging of Non–Small Cell Lung Cancer

Proper staging of lung cancer is the key to decision making and management. The clinical stage of disease is based on the history, physical examination, radiologic and laboratory studies, biopsy data, and data from invasive diagnostic procedures such as bronchoscopy and mediastinoscopy. Although the lung cancer staging system is initially clinical and clinical stage will determine the optimal treatment strategy, both clinical and surgical/pathologic staging are important in evaluating published data on treatment effects and outcomes. Clinical criteria and radiologic studies in surgical patients are accurate 78% of the time in determining the T stage and 47% accurate for the N stage.

The array of diagnostic tests for evaluating the extent of lung cancer includes bone, brain, and PET scanning; bronchoscopy with endobronchial and/or transbronchial biopsy; computed tomography–guided needle biopsy; mediastinoscopy to assess paratracheal and subcarinal nodes; mediastinotomy (Chamberlain procedure); and thoracoscopy. For patients with large peripheral lesions or central tumors, after computed tomography scan of the chest, surgical staging includes mediastinoscopy and mediastinotomy (for left upper lobe or left hilar lesions) to determine whether the mediastinal lymph nodes are involved. Sampling of multiple lymph node stations helps to ensure staging accuracy. For patients with gross mediastinal adenopathy, a transtracheal needle biopsy will often suffice to confirm the presence of mediastinal involvement. Since enlarged lymph nodes may be reactive and not malignant, mediastinal nodes should not be considered to contain cancer in the absence of histologic confirmation.

Non–small cell lung cancer frequently metastasizes to the adrenal glands, requiring their careful inspection on computed tomography scan. One must be wary of the fact that the enlarged adrenal glands in many patients will be due to benign adrenal adenomas rather than to metastatic disease.

Biopsy of the primary tumor confirms the presence of cancer but does not give information regarding nodal or metastatic sites that ultimately determine treatment decisions. In staging a newly diagnosed patient, it is helpful to work backward, starting from the perspective of ruling out metastatic disease. If distant spread is not apparent, then one can proceed to evaluate the extent of disease in the chest to assess whether definitive surgical therapy is feasible.

The American Joint Committee on Cancer's TNM Staging System was revised in 1997. Staging depends on assessment of the primary tumor (T), lymph node involvement (N), and presence or absence of metastatic spread (M).

T stages are defined in Figures 95-2 and 95-3. In clinical therapeutic terms, a T1 lesion should be easily resectable with an opportunity for a satisfactory surgical margin around the tumor. A T2 lesion is usually resectable, but by virtue of being large, centrally located, or penetrating the pleura, it represents a higher risk for local or distant recurrence after surgical excision. T3 lesions are adherent to important structures but are still potentially resectable by a skilled surgeon. T3 lesions that invade the superior sulcus or chest wall require more extensive resection. Radiation therapy either before or after surgery is appropriate for lesions involving the ribs, although a wide excision alone is often curative. Superior sulcus tumors should always be treated with preoperative

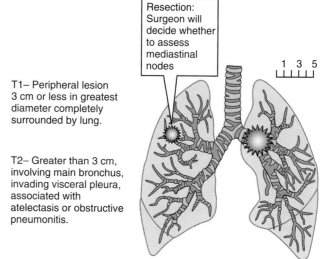

T1– Peripheral lesion 3 cm or less in greatest diameter completely surrounded by lung.

T2– Greater than 3 cm, involving main bronchus, invading visceral pleura, associated with atelectasis or obstructive pneumonitis.

Resection: Surgeon will decide whether to assess mediastinal nodes

Figure 95-2 ■ Staging of the primary tumor (T stage). Ruler is in centimeters.

radiation therapy (often with concurrent chemotherapy). The extent of resection is determined by the amount of parenchymal disease. Since chest wall tumors grow peripherally, lobectomy or even wedge resection can usually be performed. T3 lesions involving the hilum require pneumonectomy. T4 lesions, on the other hand, are usually adherent to structures in such a way that surgery is extremely difficult or impossible as the first treatment modality.

Lymph node stages are divided into N0 (no nodal involvement), N1 (intrapulmonary or hilar), N2 (ipsilateral mediastinal), and N3 (contralateral mediastinal or supraclavicular). The American Thoracic Society has developed a useful numbering system (Figures 95-4 and 95-5).

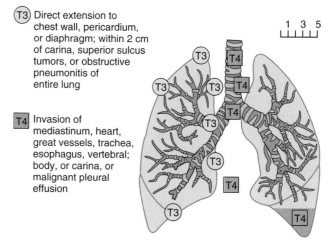

T3 Direct extension to chest wall, pericardium, or diaphragm; within 2 cm of carina, superior sulcus tumors, or obstructive pneumonitis of entire lung

T4 Invasion of mediastinum, heart, great vessels, trachea, esophagus, vertebral; body, or carina, or malignant pleural effusion

Figure 95-3 ■ Staging of the primary tumor (T stage). Ruler is in centimeters.

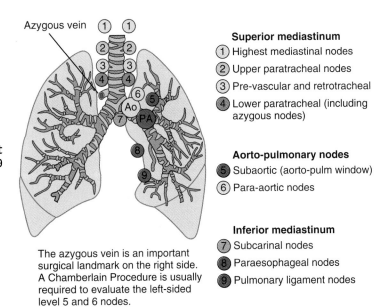

Azygous vein

Superior mediastinum
① Highest mediastinal nodes
② Upper paratracheal nodes
③ Pre-vascular and retrotracheal
④ Lower paratracheal (including azygous nodes)

Aorto-pulmonary nodes
⑤ Subaortic (aorto-pulm window)
⑥ Para-aortic nodes

Inferior mediastinum
⑦ Subcarinal nodes
⑧ Paraesophageal nodes
⑨ Pulmonary ligament nodes

Figure 95-4 ■ Mediastinal lymph nodes at different levels are numbered for staging purposes as 1 to 9 from top to bottom.

The azygous vein is an important surgical landmark on the right side. A Chamberlain Procedure is usually required to evaluate the left-sided level 5 and 6 nodes.

A staging matrix, displaying four T stages and four N stages, allows ready classification of all stages from IA through IIIB (Figure 95-6*A*, from Mountain et al.). The percentage of three-year survivors for each cell in the matrix also correlates with longer-term survival (Figure 95-6B).

Clinical Evaluation

History

Performance status is an extremely important part of the initial patient history. Besides tumor stage, patient performance status is the most critical determinant of prognosis. In 1948, David Karnofsky first pointed out that prognosis in lung cancer was closely linked to performance status and published the classification that carries his name. Patients who are fit and able to work have a median survival of nine to 12 months. Most long-term survivors are in this group. Patients with an intermediate performance status have a median survival of six to nine months and represent a small proportion of long-term survivors. Those who are unable to care for themselves (Karnofsky performance status <50) are unable to tolerate or benefit from systemic therapy. Their median survival is three to six months, and long-term survivors are rare. Gordon Zubrod adapted and simplified Karnofsky's performance scale, creating what came to be known as the ECOG (Eastern Cooperative Oncology Group) Performance Scale. The ECOG scale is a very reproducible tool, categorizing performance status in four steps from 0 (no symptoms) to 4 (completely bedridden). Careful assessment of the patient's performance status provides a powerful predictor of outcome.

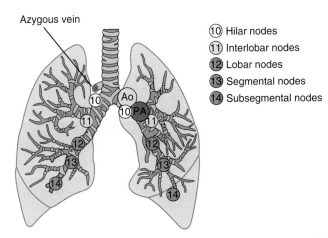

Azygous vein

⑩ Hilar nodes
⑪ Interlobar nodes
⑫ Lobar nodes
⑬ Segmental nodes
⑭ Subsegmental nodes

Figure 95-5 ■ Nodal status in the TNM classification; N1 lymph nodes are in the lung or hilum and are numbered levels 10 to 14 as shown.

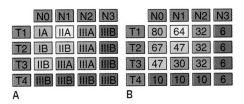

	N0	N1	N2	N3
T1	IA	IIA	IIIA	IIIB
T2	IB	IIB	IIIA	IIIB
T3	IIB	IIIA	IIIA	IIIB
T4	IIIB	IIIB	IIIB	IIIB

A

	N0	N1	N2	N3
T1	80	64	32	6
T2	67	47	32	6
T3	47	30	32	6
T4	10	10	10	6

B

Figure 95-6 ■ *A*, TNM staging matrix for non–small cell lung cancer. *B*, Three-year percentage survivorship based on pathologic (postsurgery) staging. For the T4/N3 cell, clinical staging is used owing to the low rate of surgical resection in this entity. (From Mountain CF, Dresler CM: Regional lymph node classification for lung cancer staging. Chest 1997;111:1718–1723.)

Physical Examination

Evaluation of the head and neck should include attention to eye movements to detect nystagmus or diplopia. Patients with hearing difficulty or tinnitus will be poor candidates for platinum-containing chemotherapy regimens. The oral examination should include attention to the teeth, the oral mucosa, and the patient's ability to swallow in order to exclude infection or the occasional simultaneous esophageal or head and neck cancers. Detection of lymph node metastases (confirmed by fine-needle aspiration/biopsy) in the cervical and supraclavicular area in a newly diagnosed lung cancer patient will help to avoid an unnecessary, unhelpful, or potentially even harmful surgical resection.

Careful examination of all lung zones is mandatory. Testing the oxygen saturation at rest and after a brisk walk is also important. Taking a walk with the patient and observing for pulmonary dysfunction rapidly and inexpensively provides an assessment of lung function. Many surgeons use this approach in addition to classical pulmonary function testing as a valuable component of the preoperative evaluation.

Brain metastases are present in 3% to 5% of neurologically asymptomatic newly diagnosed patients with non–small cell lung cancer. Brain involvement by cancer occurs in as many as 30% of stage III or IV patients who live more than one year after diagnosis. A thorough neurologic exam is important at each evaluation seeking suggestive evidence of brain metastases or central or peripheral nervous system abnormalities.

Imaging Studies

Chest X-ray remains the most important tool for rapidly and safely evaluating the entire thoracic cavity. The chest X-ray can reveal peripheral nodules, hilar and mediastinal changes suggestive of lymphadenopathy, and pleural effusions. Findings of subsegmental, segmental, lobar, or lung collapse will point toward an area of endobronchial obstruction. Chest X-rays are most reliable when sequential studies can be compared. The majority of peripheral lung cancer nodules can be found, in retrospect, on a previous chest X-ray.

Computed tomography scanning of the chest and upper abdomen to include the liver and adrenal glands for metastases should be obtained in any patient who is suspected of having lung cancer. The computed tomography scan will often detect a primary lesion in situations in which a chest X-ray is falsely negative. A computed tomography scan provides great detail about the extent of the primary lesion, including its size, its resectability, and the presence of pleural or chest wall involvement in the case of peripheral lesions. Both the size and shape of hilar and mediastinal lymph nodes should be determined. Mediastinal lymph nodes greater than 1.0 cm in short-axis diameter are worrisome for tumor involvement and warrant further investigation.

Benign pulmonary lesions may be detected with the current generation of computed tomography scanning devices, which can detect small subpleural nodules, even those with a diameter less than 5 mm. Many of these tiny nodules are normal subpleural lymph nodes. Others are "early" peripheral adenocarcinomas or adenomatous hyperplasia. Nodular lesions with very smooth outlines, such as hamartomas and granulomas, often have a very distinctive appearance. Hamartomas are benign and often contain fat that can be quantitated by specific Hounsfield unit analysis on computed tomography scan. Histoplasmosis is still a consideration in certain geographic locations, such as the Ohio Valley as well as other Midwest and Southwest locations.

In problem cases and for design of treatment, it is helpful to personally review the computed tomography scan with the diagnostic radiologist, thoracic surgeon, lung specialist, and pathologist and share as much clinical information as possible.

Bone scans are highly sensitive to the presence of skeletal involvement by cancer. However, solitary lesions in the ribs and spine that are identified on bone scan may represent trauma or an osteopenic compression fracture rather than metastases. Bilateral or mirror-image abnormalities, especially in the knees and wrists, are likely to be due to degenerative joint disease. Skeletal X-ray studies and/or computed tomography scans might be needed to decide whether a positive finding on bone scan is caused by a benign process.

Positron emission tomography (PET scan) is an accurate tool to demonstrate the extent of disease in patients with lung cancer. Tumors have long been known to have more rapid glucose metabolism than normal tissues—the Warburg phenomenon. Viable tumors incorporate [fluorine-18] fluoro-2-deoxy-D-glucose. The uptake signal can be displayed three-dimensionally to assess whether a particular lesion on X-ray or computed tomography scan represents viable tumor, scar, necrotic tissue, or some other process. Positron emission tomography scans are now approved for use in staging lung cancer. They are being used more widely to detect "silent" mediastinal lymph node involvement, early recurrence, or confirmation of complete response. Positron emission tomography scans currently work best for lesions that are 10 mm or greater in diameter.

DIAGNOSIS

Solitary Pulmonary Nodule

If a patient is found to have an asymptomatic lesion less than 3.0 cm in diameter without clinical evidence of metastatic disease, a chest computed tomography scan with contrast is performed that includes visualization of the liver and adrenals. If there is no evidence of lymph node enlargement (>1.0 cm in the short-axis diameter) or intra-abdominal metastasis, the patient should proceed directly to surgical wedge resection.

Lobectomy is performed during the same procedure if the biopsy is positive. A preoperative biopsy is neither necessary nor desirable. A negative percutaneous biopsy does not rule out cancer (found in one third of small solitary pulmonary nodules), so resection is appropriate even if the lesion subsequently proves to be benign.

Diagnostic Laboratory Evaluation

Sputum cytology is most sensitive for squamous carcinoma, central lesions, lower lobe lesions, and lesions that are larger than 2 cm in size. Conversely, adenocarcinoma has a lower yield. Polymerase chain reaction (PCR)-based assays are exquisitely sensitive for detecting cells containing mutations in K-ras, p53, and other genes. To date, however, there have been no prospective studies to determine the risk of lung cancer if one or more of these mutations are found in a screening study.

Obtaining an adequate biopsy with careful histologic interpretation is essential for diagnosis and treatment. Under computed tomography guidance, localized lung masses can be safely biopsied. In the fine-needle procedure, a 22- through 28-gauge needle is passed into a mass, negative pressure is applied with a syringe, and a cutting motion is used to disrupt and dislodge tumor cells. Fine-needle aspiration biopsy is very useful in many instances, but it is important to remember that even experienced pathologists might not be able to determine the histology from the limited number of malignant cells this technique provides.

Immunohistologic staining can help distinguish between non–small cell lung cancer and small cell cancer (the latter will be positive for neuron specific enolase) and can differentiate among malignant melanoma (S100 positive), Ewing's sarcoma (increased glycogen content and specific chromosome translocation), and lymphoma (positive for the leukocyte common antigen, CD30).

Invasive Procedures

Bronchoscopy is invaluable for evaluation of cancer involving the proximal airways. It can detect nodular or polypoid lesions larger than 2 mm in size and flat or superficially spreading lesions larger than 20 mm in diameter. Seventy-five percent of carcinoma in situ lesions are superficial/flat, and 25% are nodular/polypoid. Endoscopic examinations are limited to the central portions of the tracheobronchial tree; however, new ultra-thin bronchoscopes are being developed to improve visualization of the distal airways.

Other approaches may offer advantages over conventional bronchoscopy. Autofluorescence bronchoscopy is an optical endoscopic imaging method designed to localize small preinvasive lesions that are not visualized by conventional white light imaging. Autofluorescence illuminates the bronchial surface with violet or blue light (400 to 440 nm) to distinguish normal from abnormal tissues. Normal mucosa has much higher fluorescence intensity than dysplastic lesions or carcinoma in situ, especially in the green region of the emission spectrum. The light-induced fluorescence endoscopy (LIFE) device has a special light source and additional camera capability and adds only a few minutes to the autofluorescence procedure. A recent multicenter trial reported that light-induced fluorescence endoscopy improved the detection rate of early lung cancer by severalfold compared to autofluorescence bronchoscopy alone. Virtual bronchoscopy is a futuristic visualization technique in which helical computed tomography data and virtual reality computing are used to create three-dimensional endobronchial simulations. The major limitation of this technique is its inability to differentiate malignant from benign lesions.

Evaluation by mediastinoscopy of the mediastinal lymph nodes is the most accurate modality for assessing resectability in non–small cell lung cancer. A standard cervical approach allows assessment of the upper and lower paratracheal nodes (levels 1,2R, 2L, 4R, and 4L) as well as the anterior subcarinal nodes (level 7) (see Figures 95-4 and 95-5). Mediastinal sampling is 90% accurate when performed by an experienced operator and has a specificity of virtually 100%.

Thoracoscopy is a relatively easy way to evaluate pleural effusions and pleural-based nodules. Biopsies of the pleura and peripheral pulmonary nodules are

Table 95-4 ■ World Health Organization Histologic Classification of Invasive Non–Small Cell Lung Cancer (Modified)

Adenocarcinoma
Papillary
Bronchioloalveolar carcinoma (BAC)
Signet ring
Clear cell
Mixed
  Solid
  Mucinous
  Nonmucinous

Squamous cell carcinoma
Spindle cell variant
Basaloid variant
Clear cell

Adenosquamous carcinoma

Large cell carcinoma
Large cell carcinoma with neuroendocrine carcinoma

Pleomorphic carcinomas
Pleomorphic carcinoma
Spindle cell carcinoma
Giant cell carcinoma
Carcinosarcoma
Pulmonary blastoma

Carcinoid tumors
Typical carcinoid
Atypical carcinoid

Salivary gland type
Mucoepidermoid type
Adenoid cystic type

Unclassified/Non–Small Cell Carcinoma Not Otherwise Specified (NOS)

easily obtained and often reduce diagnostic confusion and the need for multiple follow-up X-rays.

Pathology

The World Health Organization (WHO) classification of invasive non-small cell cancer of the lung includes five major pathologic groups and multiple variants (Table 95-4).

Adenocarcinoma is the most common lung cancer histology in North America, accounting for approximately 40% of cases. Squamous cancer remains more common in Europe and Asia. This difference is thought to be due to variations in smoking habits, cigarette filter characteristics, and size of the particulate matter carrying the carcinogenic material. A single puff of smoke contains literally thousands of chemicals and hundreds of carcinogens. The nitrosamine 4-(methylnitrosamino)-1-(3-pyridyl)-1-butanone (NNK) and benzo[a]pyrene are the most common culprits, but many other substances contribute to the carcinogenic process. Larger particle size favors more central (squamous) cancers, whereas small particles travel more distally in the lung and are more likely to produce a peripheral adenocarcinoma. Adenocarcinoma is distinguished by the appearance of glands and mucus. Periodic acid–Schiff (PAS) staining will often be positive in these tumors.

Some adenocarcinomas of the lung have papillary features similar to those of ovarian and thyroid cancer and may even contain laminated or concentric calcification (psammoma bodies). Papillary appearance should prompt a careful pelvic exam and palpation of the neck to make sure there is no dominant mass in the ovary or thyroid. However, it is extremely uncommon for a tiny ovarian or thyroid cancer to be the source of bulky distant lung disease. Therefore, in patients with papillary adenocarcinoma involving the lung, it is usually wise to develop a treatment plan for lung cancer rather than pursuing numerous exotic diagnostic tests.

Bronchioloalveolar carcinoma produces a pattern of "fluffy" alveolar infiltrates on chest X-ray that appear to be growing on the alveolar "scaffold" in a way similar to ivy growing on a lattice. Bronchioloalveolar carcinoma often has a characteristic ground glass appearance and a biology that suggests local, and perhaps even airborne, spread within the lungs. Metastatic spread from bronchioloalveolar carcinoma is uncommon, but it is life-threatening because its local growth eventually destroys substantial amounts of lung tissue.

Squamous carcinoma of the lung, on histologic examination, exhibits keratin production and grows in a pattern of cellular bridging that lends a cobblestone appearance. As a group, squamous cancers, especially those that are well to moderately well differentiated, have lower metastatic potential than other histologic types. Large necrotic tumors in the lung, with or without a thick-walled cavity and air fluid levels, usually have a squamous cell component. Patients may develop hypercalcemia in the absence of bone metastases owing to production of parathyroidlike hormone by the tumor itself. In many, if not most, patients with squamous cell cancer of the lung, the disease remains confined to the thoracic cavity for the duration of their disease. Surgery is therefore more often considered in situations in which the tumor is locally advanced but still resectable compared to other histologic types. Brain, bone, and adrenal metastases are less common than in other histologies but certainly occur, especially in patients with poorly differentiated tumors.

Adenosquamous cancers of the lung share histologic features of both squamous cell cancer and adenocarcinomas. The cancers are prone to metastasize to the brain and carry a somewhat worse prognosis than lung cancer that is either squamous cell or adenocarcinoma.

Large cell carcinoma represents 10% to 20% of bronchogenic tumors. These tumors tend to grow rapidly and metastasize early and are strongly associated with smoking. Large cell tumors are usually large, bulky, well-circumscribed, pink-gray masses with extensive hemorrhage and necrosis. Although they commonly have central necrosis, they are less likely to cavitate.

Large cell carcinoma with neuroendocrine features has been recognized as a specific entity. Patients may present with an early-stage resectable tumor but exhibit a poor prognosis and higher than expected rate of metastatic recurrence. The relationship of this entity to peripheral small cell cancer and the role of adjuvant chemotherapy remain to be determined.

Undifferentiated tumors and carcinoma not otherwise specified (NOS) make up a subgroup of unclassifiable lung cancers. Such tumors typically lack keratin, do not form glandular structures, and do not stain positively for mucin. Undifferentiated large cell carcinomas are defined by the World Health Organization as "a malignant epithelial tumor with large nuclei, prominent nucleoli, abundant cytoplasm and usually well defined cell borders, without the characteristic features of squamous cell, small cell, or adenocarcinomas."

Pleomorphic carcinoma/giant cell carcinoma is a variant of large cell carcinoma. This subtype is particularly aggressive and carries a very poor prognosis. These tumors present as a large peripheral mass with a focal necrotic component. They do not involve the large airways, unless by direct extension. The nuclei are varied in size and shape. Although the nuclei are usually large, in some cases, multiple small nuclei occupy each cell. Immunohistochemical stains can be useful in excluding adenocarcinoma, squamous cell carcinoma, and lymphoma. These tumors are sometimes positive for human chorionic gonadotrophin (hCG) and may superficially resemble choriocarcinomas.

Adenoid cystic carcinoma is the most frequent tracheal carcinoma. Symptoms at presentation are those of bronchial obstruction, including cough, wheezing, dyspnea, and/or hemoptysis. Although these tumors may be difficult to detect by radiograph owing to their central location, they are easily biopsied by bronchoscopy. Adenoid cystic carcinomas have a slight male predominance. Grossly, adenoid cystic carcinomas present as exophytic or annular lesions of the bronchial tree. Bronchial mucosa usually covers the lesion; however, the lesion may be ulcerated or replaced with metaplastic squamous epithelium. Histologically, the tumors are composed of regular mucus-containing glands lined by epithelial and myoepithelial cells. Lymphatic and perineural invasion is frequent. The histopathologic features are identical to those of adenoid cystic carcinomas of the salivary gland and breast, and primary lesions in the lung may be difficult to differentiate from the more common metastatic lesions from these sites.

Adenoid cystic carcinomas are slowly progressive, with five- and 20-year survival rates of 85% and 20%, respectively. They are generally treated by resection if technically feasible. Patients with lesions that are not resectable are treated with radiation therapy. Postoperative radiation is usually given if the margins of resection are positive or "close." Clinical behavior cannot be accurately predicted by the histology; therefore, staging is the most important factor in predicting the clinical outcome. The role of adjuvant chemotherapy is not well defined.

Carcinoid tumors arise from neuroectodermal tissues. These tumors stain with silver stains and have a rather bland appearance. Carcinoid tumors may be either typical or atypical. The atypical form is more likely to metastasize to regional lymph nodes. Carcinoid tumors present with a single or multiple peripheral nodules or with wheezing and adult-onset asthma or recurrent pneumonias due to obstruction by a bronchial carcinoid. These tumors are treated by resection with node sampling or dissection. The role of postoperative therapy in atypical or node-positive disease is not defined.

Prognostic Factors

Performance status remains the most important prognostic factor. Other important parameters include presence of lymph node spread, degree of tumor bulk, presence of extensive pleural disease, and extent and type of metastatic spread.

Albumin levels in the blood are nonspecific indicators of overall nutrition. Albumin levels lower than 3.0 g/dL often indicate a bad prognosis.

Leukemoid reaction should be considered in patients who have increased granulocyte counts in the absence of infection (see Chapter 38). These reactions usually occur in patients who have a large tumor

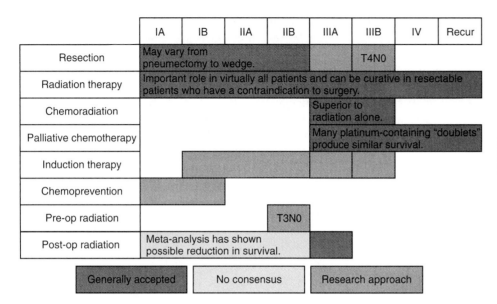

Figure 95-7 ■ Stage of non–small cell lung cancer and its relationship to treatment.

burden and necrotic tumor masses in the chest. In some cases, a leukemoid reaction can be difficult to distinguish from sepsis, empyema, or frank leukemia. Patients with non–small cell lung cancer who exhibit persistent fever and/or a leukocytosis often have a poor prognosis, even though fever and systemic symptoms might subside promptly following the institution of systemic chemotherapy.

Treatment

General Principles

In non–small cell lung cancer, the results of standard treatment are disappointing for all but the small localized and resectable lesions. Disease stage plays a major role in choosing therapy (Figure 95-7). Surgery is the major curative modality in stage I disease. Historically, surgery has been used alone or in combination with radiation and/or chemotherapy in stage II lung cancer. For stage III patients, treatment can range from palliative approaches for malignant effusion or extensive mediastinal adenopathy to aggressive multidisciplinary approaches that attempt to provide curative therapy for a small proportion of patients.

Radiation therapy can produce cures in approximately 10% of patients with localized tumors who are not candidates for surgery owing to other factors. Radiation has major palliative benefits, and approximately 80% of lung cancer patients will receive radiation therapy at some time during the course of their disease.

Chemotherapy, when compared to symptomatic care, can produce marked palliation and improve sur-vival in patients whose performance status is adequate. Chemotherapy together with radiation therapy, with or without surgery, has emerged as the standard of therapy for stage III non–small cell lung cancer and in selected stage IV patients. Unfortunately, most patients will die of their disease; therefore, one should strive to achieve a proper balance between the realistic aims of therapy and its toxicity and the quality of life.

Surgery

Lobectomy with sampling of the hilar and mediastinal lymph nodes is the generally accepted procedure for most resectable lung cancers. Lesser (segmental or wedge) resections generally result in poorer local control and decreased long-term survival. Lobectomy can be performed through a standard posterolateral thoracotomy or by muscle-sparing incisions in the application of video-assisted surgery. While the same operation can be safely performed through these less invasive methods, these approaches have not been shown to reduce postoperative morbidity or length of hospital stay.

Pneumonectomy is often required for large, proximal lung lesions. Since the right lung is larger by approximately 5% to 7%, a right pneumonectomy results in a more difficult recuperation process than a left pneumonectomy. Following removal of the entire left lung, the right lung will often compensate by expanding across the midline, whereas the left lung, constrained by the heart and other structures, does not expand as readily into the right chest. Both the tumor itself and the presence of preoperative pulmonary disease may affect the distribution of ventilation and perfusion. A preoperative quantitative ventilation and perfusion scan is helpful, when combined with pulmonary function testing, in predicting the effect of pneumonectomy in an individual patient. Patients whose FEV_1 is predicted to be less than 800 mL after surgery are at high risk for postoperative complications and chronic dependence on supplemental oxygen.

Segmental resection is an anatomically guided dissection of a specific segment or group of segments of the lung. It can be carried out in selected cases and may be especially desirable for patients with small tumors and less than optimal pulmonary reserve. Wedge resection (a lesser resection that does not necessarily follow anatomic segments) can be beneficial for elderly patients, those with very small tumors, or those with benign tumors such as carcinoids or hamartomas.

Radiation Therapy

Modern radiation therapy techniques employing sophisticated computerized treatment simulation have produced major benefits for patients with non–small cell lung cancer. Definitive radiation is usually provided to the ipsilateral hilar and mediastinal nodes. Treatment is administered in 180- to 200-cGy fractions over six to seven weeks so that the total tumor dose approaches or exceeds 6000 cGy. This treatment is often associated with esophagitis that can vary in severity depending on the age, the overall state of health and nutrition of the patient, and the length of the radiation field. Lower-lobe tumors often require a longer radiation field that may encompass the entire length of the esophagus. Patients will occasionally need a hiatus from treatment and/or parenteral hydration, although feeding tubes are usually not necessary. Supportive measures such as oral analgesics, esophageal coating agents, and topical anesthetics can be helpful in alleviating esophagitis. Occasionally, a patient develops severe radiation esophagitis and ultimately stricture formation. Nevertheless, the benefits from high-dose radiation therapy usually outweigh this vexing, and fortunately rare, side effect.

Palliative radiation can take many forms. A two-week course of radiation therapy with high fraction size (300 cGy per fraction) may be given for a small lesion involving the ribs or long bones or to the whole brain for multiple metastatic lesions. Short-course, narrow-field radiation therapy may be used for treatment of hemoptysis or an obstructed bronchus. The ability of newer conformal radiation units to accurately shape the treatment to the tumor itself spares the normal lung and mediastinal structures. Side effects are consequently diminished. Conformal or three-dimensional treatment planning can be accomplished by using computer-based radiation intensity modulation or stereotactic approaches. These techniques allow marked dose escalation as high as 8500 to 10,000 cGy total dose. Whether this will translate into increased tumor control and does not increase radiation therapy side effects, such as pneumonitis, remains uncertain.

Photodynamic Therapy

Photodynamic therapy has been used for both early and advanced superficial lung cancers since 1980. Photosensitizing hematoporphyrin derivatives are administered that, when exposed to light of the proper wavelength, form toxic oxygen radicals that result in cell death. The technique is useful for patients with lesions involving the trachea and carina and may be an alternative to surgical resection in some patients with localized endobronchial bronchogenic carcinoma, especially those with limited pulmonary function.

Chemotherapy

The modern era of systemic chemotherapy for lung cancer began in the 1970s when combinations using cyclophosphamide, Adriamycin, and cisplatin first showed meaningful tumor responses in some patients with metastatic non–small cell lung cancer. During that time, the benefits were still quite limited and lack of truly effective antiemetics made treatment a difficult hospital-based activity. With the advent of large numbers of highly trained oncology nurses, effective antiemetics, such as the HT3 antagonists ondansetron and granisetron, and better-tolerated drugs, chemotherapy is now able to be provided in an outpatient setting. Active single agents are listed in Table 95-5.

Table 95-5 ■ Single-Agent Responses in Previously Untreated Non–Small Cell Lung Cancer

	Response Rate	One-Year Survival Rate
Paclitaxel	24–26%	30–40%
Docetaxel	26%	40%
Vinorelbine	20%	24%
Gemcitabine	21%	39%
Irinotecan	27%	Not reported
Topotecan	13%	35%

Platinum Compounds

Cisplatin was a component of many of the early effective regimens in non–small cell lung cancer. The response rate as a single agent was only 10%, however. To date, treatment regimens employing doses greater than 100 mg/m^2 have not shown superiority over regimens using 60 to 80 mg/m^2. Carboplatin includes an additional ring structure and is equal in efficacy to cisplatin. Toxicity, such as nephrotoxicity and emesis, are reduced. As a result, carboplatin is used widely in combination with other agents in preference to cisplatin, particularly in elderly patients and those patients whose ECOG performance status is 2 or more.

Navelbine (Vinorelbine)

Vinorelbine is a newly developed semisynthetic vinca alkaloid. It was the first drug approved by the Food and Drug Administration specifically for lung cancer. Vinorelbine as a single agent produces response rates of approximately 20% with a one-year survival rate of 24%. The combination of vinorelbine plus cisplatin shows response rates ranging from 26% to 43%, a median survival of 32 to 40 weeks, and a one-year survival rate of 35%, substantially better than when either agent is used alone.

Taxanes

Taxol (paclitaxel) and Taxotere (docetaxel) are very active drugs in advanced non–small cell lung cancer. Paclitaxel produces response rates of 24% to 26% as a single agent with a one-year survival rate of approximately 40%. These results are much higher than those previously seen with any other single-agent drug in advanced lung cancer, and responses are increased when these agents are combined with other drugs.

Docetaxel, even when administered as second-line therapy to patients who had previously received chemotherapy, provides tumor responses in 16% to 20% of patients and a seven- to eight-month median survival. Weekly or biweekly schedules have been used in recent years. These low-dose, high-frequency regimens are well tolerated and cause predictable and tolerable degrees of myelosuppression and neurotoxicity.

Gemcitabine

Gemcitabine is an antimetabolite that the Food and Drug Administration approved for use in patients with pancreatic cancer in 1996. Early studies in non–small cell lung cancer showed definite antitumor activity when used as either a single agent or in combination with cisplatin or carboplatin. Gemcitabine may be given weekly up to three times per month with excellent patient tolerance. It has the advantage of causing very little nausea or hair loss (alopecia). Occasional patients will develop a pulmonary hypersensitivity reaction manifested by bilateral pulmonary infiltrates or fluid retention. Gemcitabine is a potent radiation sensitizer, and early studies of gemcitabine with concomitant thoracic radiation demonstrated marked mediastinal or esophageal toxicity.

Topoisomerase Inhibitors

Topotecan and irinotecan topoisomerase I inhibitors are derivatives of the camptothecin plant. The camptothecins are finding their way into treatment regimens as a substitute for vinca alkaloids or as a third agent. Topotecan has been used as a third-line agent and seems to have beneficial effects in controlling brain metastases in some patients when radiation therapy is not an option.

Combined Method Therapy

The combined use of thoracic radiation and chemotherapy is an appealing strategy for patients with locally advanced non–small cell lung cancer. This approach potentially provides both the hope of rapid control of local symptoms and inhibition of metastases. The chemotherapy may also serve as a radiation potentiator, adding to regional disease control. The theoretical advantages of combined method therapy include the following:

1. enhancement of the radiation therapy dose-response curve
2. decreased opportunity for the cancer cell to repair lethal or sublethal damage
3. increased proportion of tumor cells in a sensitive phase of the cell cycle
4. immediate decrease in tumor bulk leading to improved blood supply and higher proportion of oxygenated cells, which will be more sensitive to radiation
5. decrease in the risk of tumor cell repopulation and resistance, which is seen when radiation is given weeks to months after the initiation of chemotherapy.

A number of pilot studies used induction, or neoadjuvant, chemotherapy plus radiation therapy, reporting median survival ranging from 9 to 16 months and two-year survival rates as high as 40%.

A Cancer and Leukemia Group B (CALGB) randomized trial compared cisplatin plus vinblastine and thoracic radiation therapy to thoracic radiation therapy alone. The combined modality therapy group experienced one-year and two-year survival rates of 54% and 26%, respectively, versus 40% and 13%, respectively, for patients receiving radiation therapy alone. This benefit from combined modality therapy was confirmed in another randomized trial. One needs to be aware that the Cancer and Leukemia Group B trial excluded any patient with supraclavicular node involvement, poor performance status, or weight loss of over 5%. Many patients in clinical practice will have one or more of the above adverse predictors; therefore, these results cannot be expected to apply to all stage III patients presenting outside of the clinical trial setting. Nevertheless, combined modality therapy makes long-term survival possible for a group of patients with local but advanced non–small cell lung cancer.

Although surgery remains the most effective mode of local control and intuitively should offer a survival advantage for patients with marginally resectable lung cancers that become resectable following chemoradiation, large prospective confirmatory studies have been lacking to date. Nevertheless, there appears to be a growing number of long-term surviving patients who have participated in aggressive multimodality programs employing combination chemotherapy, radiation, and surgery.

Radiation Therapy Considerations

Historically, most combined modality studies employed a schedule of chemotherapy followed by radiation therapy to decrease the radiation side effects, particularly esophagitis. However, several recent studies have suggested an advantage for concomitant chemoradiation. Caution is required because many patients will not tolerate combined chemoradiation owing to logistical problems, poor performance status, or altered quality-of-life factors.

Local control in non–small cell lung cancer remains an elusive goal even with combined modality therapy. Despite older reports, local control may be as low as 20% for patients receiving a radiation dose of 6500 cGy. New approaches to improve local control include the use of radiation-sensitizing drugs and radio-protective agents; conformal or three-dimensional treatment planning to deliver higher doses of radiation to the tumor while sparing the heart, mediastinal structures, and spinal cord; altered fractionation schemes, using twice- and even three-times-daily schedules; and finally, resection following aggressive chemotherapy.

A number of chemotherapeutic agents, including cisplatin, mitomycin, Taxol, Taxotere, and gemcitabine, are radiation sensitizers. A prospective randomized three-arm European study compared radiation therapy plus either concurrent low-dose daily or weekly cisplatin to radiation therapy alone. The two-year survival rate for patients receiving radiation therapy plus either daily or weekly cisplatin was 30% ± 6% versus 19% ± 5% for radiation therapy alone, confirming the benefit of the combined modality approach.

Altered radiation fractionation schemes have been employed for many years to improve the therapeutic ratio and spare normal tissues. A British study of three daily fractions, continuous hyperfractionated accelerated radiotherapy (CHART), administered a total of 5400 cGy over 12 consecutive days with no break for weekends. This approach provided a statistically significant superior survival rate when compared to traditional once-daily radiotherapy. Benefits appeared to accrue purely from local control of tumor, with squamous cancer patients benefiting the most. The hyperfractionation of radiation therapy is logistically difficult for radiation therapy centers and patients, however, and pulmonary fibrosis developed more commonly than in patients who were treated with conventional fractionation of doses.

Treatment by Disease Stage

Carcinoma in Situ

Carcinoma in situ (Tis) is also known as stage 0 non–small cell lung cancer and denotes microscopic squamous cell carcinoma, usually discovered during the course of bronchoscopy. The in situ designation ordinarily refers to the squamous cell type only and does not apply to the other tumor histologies. Occult lung cancer (Tx), on the other hand, denotes a patient whose sputum or bronchial washings contain malignant cells although tumor is not visualized on imaging studies or by bronchoscopy. Most patients with Tx cancer are smokers who are being evaluated for a productive cough or hemoptysis. Histologically, in situ squamous carcinomas range from thickening erythema, and loss of the normal bronchial mucosal longitudinal ridges to ulceration and full-thickness atypia of the squamous epithelium. The multistage model assumes that atypical squamous metaplasia and dysplasia precede the development of in situ carcinoma, which in turn evolves to invasive cancer. Carcinoma in situ and occult lung cancers are noninvasive by definition and, if localized, should be curable with surgical resection. Patients with positive sputum cytology should have a full medical examination, including a careful otolaryngology evaluation and a chest X-ray and chest computed tomography scan. Selective bronchoscopy with brushings and washings of the individual lobes should be the next step. Autofluorescence bronchoscopy may be of value in finding occult lesions. If a localized unequivocally malignant area is identified, resection should be curative. If any question remains regarding the degree of dysplasia, a waiting period followed by repeat bronchoscopy may be a valuable maneuver. During this period, the patient should absolutely refrain from smoking. In the event that no localizing cytology is obtained, the patient should stop smoking and have careful follow-up with history and physical exam and repeat bronchoscopy.

Stage IA

Surgical resection is the treatment of choice for patients with stage IA disease. Patients with satisfactory pulmonary reserve should undergo a lobectomy. If pulmonary function is limited or there are other comorbidities, a segmental or wedge resection can be done to preserve postoperative pulmonary function. Surgical mortality for lobectomy or a lesser resection in modern series is 3% to 5%. Older studies suggest that the local recurrence rate for segmental or wedge resection is 10% to 20% higher than that for lobectomy. Emerging evidence indicates that lesions less than 15 mm in diameter have a cure rate in the range of 90%, whereas those closer to 30 mm have a long-term survival rate in the 80% to 85% range. For the smaller lesions, less extensive surgery such as segmental or wedge resection may be adequate in some patients, although lobectomy remains the standard. For patients with stage I non–small cell lung cancer who are medically inoperable, two retrospective studies have reported five-year survival rates of 10% and 27% for primary thoracic radiation, consisting of 6000 cGy. Stage IA patients are a very important target for smoking cessation and chemoprevention efforts, since second primary tumors or complications of smoking are a major cause of morbidity and mortality in this group.

Stage IB

Although the tumors are larger in stage IB than in stage IA and may involve the visceral pleura, surgery is nonetheless the mainstay of treatment. Resection should be by lobectomy. Pneumonectomy is rarely necessary. Adjuvant chemotherapy and chemoprevention may help to reduce the risk of recurrence as well as prevent second primary tumors. The long-term survival rate for this group of patients is in the 60% to 70% range.

Stage IIA

Surgery is the treatment of choice for patients with stage IIA non–small cell lung cancer. These patients may have limited (N1) lymph node involvement at the time of surgery. The surgical cure rate for this group is approximately 50% to 60%. For patients with hilar or intrapulmonary lymph node involvement at surgery, the appropriate postoperative adjuvant therapy continues to be controversial.

A meta-analysis of nine randomized trials evaluating postoperative radiation therapy versus surgery alone in 2128 patients showed a 21% relative increase in the risk of death associated with radiation therapy. These data suggest that postoperative radiation therapy should not be considered standard therapy in patients with early-stage, completely resected non–small cell lung cancer.

Stage IIB

Tumors involving the chest wall or the superior sulcus (T3N0) often require a combination of radiation therapy and chemotherapy in conjunction with aggressive surgery. Long-term survival is still possible. Despite their large size and local invasiveness, these tumors often present prior to regional or metastatic spread. Larger, but resectable, tumors involving the hilar lymph nodes (T2N1) often require a complete pneumonectomy or, alternatively, a complex bronchial resection and anastomosis (sleeve resection) to save a portion of the lung. These patients are at high risk for both local and distant failure. An ECOG trial randomizing patients to postoperative radiation therapy alone or with added cisplatin and etoposide showed no benefit to the addition of chemotherapy.

Stage IIIA

Stage III lung cancer comprises a wide spectrum of disease presentations. Some patients who have a peripheral tumor and no mediastinal adenopathy on chest computed tomography scan are nevertheless found to have a low volume of mediastinal lymph node involvement with no extracapsular spread. The long-term survival rate for this group of patients following complete resection ranges from 18% to 30% with surgery alone in single institution series.

For patients who have clinically detectable mediastinal involvement with an obviously abnormal chest computed tomography or a positive biopsy at mediastinoscopy or transbronchial biopsy, the five-year survival rate is only 2% to 5%. Surgery as the initial treatment for clinically apparent stage IIIA disease will usually result in an incomplete resection. Long-term survival in this circumstance is very uncommon. Patients must recover from a suboptimal operation and, as a consequence, are less capable of tolerating aggressive chemotherapy or radiation treatment. Radiation therapy at a dose of 6000 cGy with standard fractionation can produce substantial palliation and is associated with a long-term survival rate of 5% to 6% in this subset of patients.

The use of preoperative (neoadjuvant) chemotherapy with or without concurrent radiation therapy can produce long-term survival in some patients with stage IIIA disease. The Southwest Oncology Group evaluated combined-modality therapy with neoadjuvant chemoradiation prior to surgery in 126 patients with stage IIIA and stage IIIB non–small cell lung cancer. Patients received two cycles of cisplatin and etoposide plus 4500 cGy prior to surgery. The objective response rate to induction chemotherapy was 59% (29% had stable disease). Over 80% of patients were candidates for definitive surgery. The three-year survival rate for the subset of patients who underwent surgery was approximately 25%. Predictors of long-term survival after thoracotomy included stages T4N0, N1, or T1N2 disease and/or the absence of viable tumor in the mediastinal nodes at surgery.

Consequently, combined-modality therapy utilizing neoadjuvant chemotherapy, radiation therapy, and surgery appears to be a worthwhile strategy in some patients with adequate performance status who have stage IIIA non–small cell lung cancer. The value of induction neoadjuvant therapy prior to surgery is not well established. Even so, surgical resection should not be the initial treatment modality in these patients. Careful preoperative staging is essential to avoid inappropriate surgery for these patients.

Stage IIIB

Owing to invasion of the mediastinum, heart, or other central structures, T4 non–small cell lung cancer is almost always unresectable. The outcome for most patients with stage IIIB non–small cell lung cancer is similar to that of patients with stage IV disease.

For patients with symptomatic pleural effusions, the pulmonary specialist and/or the thoracic surgeon should be consulted early on with regard to treatment. Malignant effusions can often (in 60% of patients) be controlled by local therapy. Talc, doxycycline, or bleomycin may be introduced into the pleural space by thoracoscopic insufflation or through an indwelling chest tube to reduce or prevent fluid reaccumulation. Unfortunately, if repeated pleural taps are needed, control may become difficult owing to the formation of multiple discrete collections (loculations), which impede external drainage. Pleurodesis may be beneficial in some patients but is disappointing in many others.

Adenocarcinomas may cause not only malignant pleural effusions but also extensive pleural implants that cause pleural fibrosis and lung entrapment. The pleura sometimes takes on the appearance of a thick circumferential rind. Dyspnea at rest results from limitations in lung expansion and chest wall compliance. This mesothelioma-like syndrome is particularly difficult to treat and is associated with few long-term survivors.

Stage IV

The type and duration of chemotherapy in advanced or metastatic non–small cell lung cancer should be based on the patient's medical condition, life circumstances, and willingness to pursue aggressive or research-based therapy (Table 95-6). For most patients under age 75 years with good performance status, the best first approach is double-agent chemotherapy utilizing carboplatin plus a second agent, usually paclitaxel, gemcitabine, or docetaxel. Benefits are usually apparent within the first six to eight weeks. An imaging study to confirm response should then be done before continuing treatment. Most patients achieve maximal benefits after four to six cycles. Indeed, several studies have shown that only limited benefit accrues to the patient who received seven or more cycles of combination chemotherapy.

In contrast, single agents can be given weekly or twice monthly with less toxicity and excellent stabilization for many patients, even those over age 80 years. For second-line therapy, or patients who are

---

Table 95-6 ■ An Approach to Chemotherapy for Metastatic Non–Small Cell Lung Cancer

First-Line Therapy

Patients with good performance status should be encouraged to participate in a clinical research protocol

Patients ineligible or unable to participate in a clinical trial

Taxol/carboplatinum

Gemcitabine/platinum

Carboplatinum/navelbine is useful in elderly patients

Other non-platinum-containing doubles are being tested

Second-Line Therapy

Try another chemotherapy doublet if performance status remains good

Sequential single agents can be very effective

Taxotere: Weekly therapy is gaining acceptance

Gemcitabine: Twice monthly can be well tolerated

Navelbine: Rarely produces major response in taxane-resistant patients

TREATMENT

An Approach to Therapy of Advanced Non–Small Cell Lung Cancer

Because there is a great need to improve the therapy of advanced non–small cell lung cancer, patients with stage IIIB or stage IV disease should be considered for participation in clinical trials. For nonresearch patients, the authors treat with one of the two following combination chemotherapy regimens:

Paclitaxel: 175 to 200 mg/m^2 plus carboplatin (area under the curve (AUC) of 5 to 6) Gemcitabine: 1000 mg/m^2 plus (cisplatin 75 mg/m^2 or carboplatin (AUC = 5 to 6)).

Treatment cycles are repeated every 21 days. Evaluation of response is determined by chest X-ray, physical examination, or computed tomography scan after two cycles. For patients who tolerate the treatment and have stable or improving clinical status, therapy is continued for a maximum of six cycles even though studies have not demonstrated that six cycles of therapy are clearly superior to four cycles. For patients who find the toxicity unacceptable or who have minimal or no objective response, therapy is changed to single-agent Taxotere (if the patients had been receiving the gemcitabine combination) or gemcitabine (if the patients had been receiving the paclitaxel combination).

elderly or frail, weekly docetaxel, gemcitabine, or navelbine have produced some gratifying results. Of note, navelbine rarely produces a major objective response in a patient who is resistant to initial combination therapy.

Patients who have an ECOG performance status of 0 or 1 seem to benefit most from the combination of a platinum agent, either cisplatin or carboplatin, and a second agent. To discover the most effective combination, the Eastern Cooperative Oncology Group conducted ECOG study 1594, which randomized patients with stage IIIB or IV disease to receive one of the four two-drug combinations shown in Figure 95-8. Patients with performance status 2 were excluded from further participation early on in the trial when an excessive mortality rate was observed in the first 60 patients. This highlights a caution in choosing a regimen from a clinical trial outside of that setting and emphasizes the importance of performance status in determining who can tolerate treatment.

Overall, documented major tumor responses occurred in approximately 20% of the patients, the median time to progression was 3.3 to 4.5 months, and the median survival was eight to nine months. There was no difference in outcome among any of the four-treatment combinations (Figure 95-9). Although the study failed to identify a superior combination, it did serve as a comparative benchmark for future studies. Regardless of treatment selection, very few of these patients live longer than three years.

Prevention

Prevention has three different aims depending on the setting. These are primary prevention, secondary prevention, and prevention of second primary tumors in

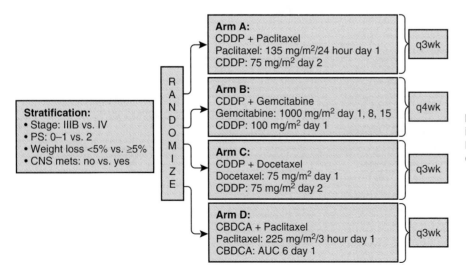

Figure 95-8 ▪ ECOG clinical trial 1594 in patients with stage IIIB and stage IV non–small cell lung cancer. CDDP = cisplatin; CBDCA = carboplatin.

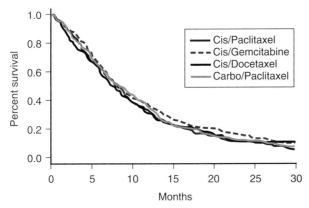

Figure 95-9 ■ Overall survival for patients with advanced non–small cell lung cancer treated on ECOG study 1594. Cis = cisplatin; Carbo = carboplatin.

those who have had successful treatment for a previous cancer. Interventions include behavior modification, drugs to deal with addictive behavior, diet, and chemopreventive agents.

Primary Prevention

The elimination of smoking must be considered the highest priority in preventing lung cancer. Children and teenagers must be taught to avoid starting to smoke. This would be the most effective preventive measure one could employ. Even if the number of smokers declines, however, the legacy of decades of smoking means that millions of individuals will remain at high risk for lung cancer well into the current century.

Secondary Prevention

Former smokers and those with occupational exposure and a strong family history of genetic risk are important target groups for prevention programs. Tobacco is an even more harmful carcinogen than was first thought. Studies from the University of Minnesota documented that toxic carcinogenic metabolites of tobacco are measurable in the urine of smokers

for months after they stop using tobacco. One can infer from this that there is a chronic ongoing exposure in people who smoke sporadically. Dysplasia of the tracheobronchial tree has been shown to improve if smoking ceases. Several new drugs are available to aid in smoking cessation, including psychotropic agents and various forms of nicotine.

Prevention of Second Primary Tumors After Successful Initial Therapy

Apart from smoking cessation, a number of substances have been proposed as chemopreventive agents to reduce the risk of a second lung cancer. Chemoprevention is the use of natural or biologically occurring nontoxic agents to retard the development of cancer in individuals at risk. The focus of chemoprevention is on the process of carcinogenesis rather than the cancer itself. To date, there is no evidence that supplementation with any of the proposed chemopreventive agents or other dietary manipulations can decrease the risk of lung cancer. The most thoroughly evaluated agents are described below.

Retinoids

Retinoids are derivatives of vitamin A. They are potent regulators of gene expression and work through an elaborate family of cytoplasmic retinoic acid binding proteins as well as intranuclear retinoic acid receptors. Loss of detectable beta subunit of this receptor RAR-β has been associated with lung cancer and has been found in lung cancer cell lines.

Pastorino reported a study of 307 patients with resected stage I non–small cell lung cancer who were randomized to receive 300,000 units of retinol palmitate daily or placebo for 12 months. There was no statistically significant difference in second primary tumors or estimated five-year survival between the two groups. The Intergroup study number 91025 randomized 1295 patients with stage I (T1N0M0 or T2N0M0) resected non–small cell lung cancer to 13-cis retinoic acid 30 mg daily orally versus placebo.

TREATMENT

Smoking Cessation

Smoking cessation is important to any patient's care. To determine whether the patient has stopped smoking, don't ask, "Have you quit smoking?" The expected answer is implicit in this setting. Most patients will feel obliged to answer, "Yes," even if they decided to quit only when the physician walked into the exam room. A more fruitful approach is to inquire, "When was your last cigarette?" The patient's response is more likely to be truthful to this second question than to the first. This allows the clinician to reinforce the importance of smoking cessation if necessary.

Table 95-7 ■ Chest X-Ray Screening Programs Did Not Lower Lung Cancer Mortality*

Institution	Number (Subset) of Participants	Chest X-Ray Interval	Cases Detected Versus Controls (Lung Cancer Deaths)	Comments
Mayo Clinic	9211 (1-pack-a-day smokers)	Every four months	206 versus 160 (122 versus 115)	No benefit for screening
Czech Project	6346 (age 40–64)	Six months	108 versus 82 (85 versus 67)	No benefit for screening
Memorial SKCC	10,040 ("high risk")	Six months	144 versus 144	Five-year survival rate >30% for screened cases detected
Johns Hopkins	10,387	Six months	194 versus 202	Five-year survival rate >30% for screened cases detected

*They increased five-year survival rate but did not lower lung cancer specific mortality.

Yearly endpoint analysis has been consistent with the expected rate of 2% to 3% new second primary tumors per year in this patient population. Preliminary analysis does not show significant benefit in the major prevention endpoint between the two groups.

Beta-Carotene

Beta-carotene is a dimer of the active moiety retinol. It has been extensively studied as a primary chemoprotective agent over the past decade. Three large studies showed no benefit in chemoprevention of lung cancer, and the results in two studies even suggested that overall death rate and deaths from lung cancer are higher in smokers who take pharmacologic doses of beta-carotene. Consequently, smokers should not take beta-carotene supplements.

Vitamin E

Vitamin E is a naturally occurring antioxidant. Epidemiologic and dietary studies have suggested that there is an inverse relationship between vitamin E intake and the incidence of lung cancer. It remains uncertain what role, if any, vitamin E (α-tocopherol) has on its own or as a modulator of other drug effects in the prevention of lung cancer.

Selenium

Selenium, an essential trace element, was first associated with cancer protection in the 1960s on the basis of epidemiologic evidence suggesting that it prevented the development of human cancers. A randomized controlled trial consisting of 1312 normal participants suggested that L-selenomethionine supplementation (200 μg/day) in the form of selenized yeast reduced the risk of developing lung and prostate cancer. The

original primary endpoint had been the risk of developing nonmelanoma skin cancers, for which no protection was observed. Further analysis of the data revealed a significant (39%) reduction in overall cancer incidence (77 versus 119 in controls) and a 48% reduction in mortality (29 deaths versus 57 in controls). Proposed mechanisms of selenomethionine activity include stimulation of glutathione peroxidase, alterations in carcinogen metabolism, production of cytotoxic metabolites, and inhibition of protein synthesis. Large prospective randomized trials need to be performed to confirm these results in lung and prostate cancer before formal public health recommendations regarding selenium supplementation can be made.

Screening Programs for Lung Cancer

Studies carried out at the Mayo Clinic, Memorial Sloan-Kettering Cancer Center, the Johns Hopkins Cancer Center, and the Czechoslovakia/National Cancer Institute Collaborative Screening Program did not show a benefit for chest X-ray and sputum cytology collections in lowering long-term lung cancer-specific mortality (Table 95-7). With chest X-ray detection of lung cancer, two thirds of the patients are nevertheless diagnosed with regionally advanced disease. As a result, chest X-ray screening is not recommended for large population groups.

New-generation spiral and helical computed tomography scanners acquire more data with less radiation exposure than prior machines. Shorter scan times overcome respiratory motion artifact and allow a larger number of studies to be performed with each machine. Henschke at al recently reported their experience using low-dose spiral computed tomography and chest radiography. They screened a group of 1000 asymptomatic individuals age 60 years or older with a minimum of 10 pack years of smoking. A total of 233 (23%) of the patients were found to have between one and six lesions on spiral computed tomography scan. An algorithm for the evaluation of noncalcified pulmonary nodules was developed on the basis of nodule size. Nodules less than 5 mm were followed with serial computed tomography scans at 3, 6, 12, and 24 months to assess for interval growth. Nodules 5 to 10 mm in diameter were either followed or biopsied. Nodules greater than 10 mm in diameter were biopsied or resected. Overall, 27 (2.7%) of 1000 subjects were found to have lung cancer detected by spiral computed tomography detection versus seven (0.7%) by chest X-ray. Of those detected by computed tomography, 26 (96%) were resectable and 23 (85%) were stage I neoplasms. By contrast, only four tumors detected by chest X-ray were stage I. For the 19 individuals with a solitary noncalcified nodule detected on computed tomography, there was a strong correlation between lesion size and risk of malignancy. One has to be wary of the potential hazard of this approach. Many more lesions that are not malignant than are malignant will be found, generating unnecessary and potentially morbid invasive procedures (pulmonary resections) for benign disease.

References

Screening and Early-Stage Disease

Bunn PA Jr, Mault J, Kelly K: Adjuvant and neoadjuvant chemotherapy for non–small cell lung cancer: A time for reassessment? Chest 2000;117(4, Suppl 1):S119–S122.

Cox G, Jones JL, Andi A, et al: A biological staging model for operable non–small cell lung cancer. Thorax 2001;56:561–566.

Henschke CI: Early lung cancer action project: Overall design and findings from baseline screening. Cancer 2000;89:2474–2482.

Henschke CI, McCauley DI, Yankelevitz DF, et al: Early lung cancer action project: A summary of the findings on baseline screening. Oncologist 2001;6:147–152.

Khuri FR, Lotan R, Kemp BL, et al: Retinoic acid receptor-beta as a prognostic indicator in stage I non–small cell lung cancer. J Clin Oncol 2000;18:2798–2804.

Lippman SM, Lee JJ, Karp DD, et al: Randomized phase III intergroup trial of isotretinoin to prevent second primary tumors in stage I non–small cell lung cancer. J Natl Cancer Inst 2001;93:605–618.

Pisters KM: The role of chemotherapy in early-stage (stage I and II) resectable non–small cell lung cancer. Semin Radiat Oncol 2000;10:274–279.

Sugarbaker DJ, Strauss GM: Extent of surgery and survival in early lung carcinoma: Implications for overdiagnosis in stage IA non–small cell lung carcinoma. Cancer 2000;89:2432–2437.

Wagner H Jr: Postoperative adjuvant therapy for patients with resected non–small cell lung cancer: Still controversial after all these years. Chest 2000;117(4, Suppl 1):S110–S118.

Walsh GL, Pisters KM, Stevens C: Treatment of stage I lung cancer. Chest Surg Clin N Am 2001;11:17–38.

Diagnosis and Staging

Boiselle PM, Ernst A, Karp DD: Lung cancer detection in the 21st century: Potential contributions and challenges of emerging technologies. Am J Roentgenol 2000;175:1215–1221.

Bragg DG: The diagnosis and staging of primary lung cancer. Radiol Clin North Am 1994;32:1–14.

Daly BD, Mueller JD, Faling LJ, et al: N2 lung cancer: Outcome in patients with false-negative computed tomographic scans of the chest. J Thorac Cardiovasc Surg 1993;105:904–910.

Garpestad E, Goldberg S, Herth F, et al: CT fluoroscopy guidance for transbronchial needle aspiration: An experience in 35 patients. Chest 2001;119:329–332.

Mountain CF: The international system for staging lung cancer. Semin Surg Oncol 2000;18:106–115.

Mountain CF, Dresler CM: Regional lymph node classification for lung cancer staging. Chest 1997;111:1718–1723.

Long-Term Survival

Albain KS, Crowley JJ, LeBlanc M, et al: Survival determinants in extensive-stage non–small cell lung cancer: The Southwest Oncology Group experience. J Clin Oncol 1991;9:1618–1626.

Julien S, Jacoulet P, Dubiez A, et al: Non–small cell lung cancer: A study of long-term survival after vinorelbine monotherapy. Oncologist 2000;5:115–119.

Langer CJ, Curran WJ, Keller SM, et al: Ten-year survival results for patients with locally advanced, initially unresectable non–small cell lung cancer treated with aggressive concurrent chemoradiation. Cancer J Sci Am 1996;2:99.

Le Chevalier T, Brisgand D, Soria JC, et al: Long-term analysis of survival in the European randomized trial comparing vinorelbine/cisplatin to vindesine/cisplatin and vinorelbine alone in advanced non–small cell lung cancer. Oncologist 2001;6(Suppl 1):8–11.

Martini N, Bains MS, Burt ME, et al: Incidence of local recurrence and second primary tumors in resected stage I lung cancer. J Thorac Cardiovasc Surg 1995;109:120–129.

Quddus AM, Kerr GR, Price A, Gregor A: Long-term survival in patients with non–small cell lung cancer treated with palliative radiotherapy. Clin Oncol (R Coll Radiol) 2001;13:95–98.

Sculier JP, Paesmans M, Libert P, et al: Long-term survival after chemotherapy containing platinum derivatives in patients with advanced unresectable non–small cell lung cancer. European Lung Cancer Working Party. Eur J Cancer 1994;30:1342–1347.

Shahidi H, Kvale PA: Long-term survival following surgical treatment of solitary brain metastasis in non–small cell lung cancer. Chest 1996;109:271–276.

Wagner W, Striehn E, Klinke F, et al: Analysis of long-term survival in patients with locally advanced non–small cell lung cancer. Oncol Rep 1998;5:1547–1550.

Biologic Markers

Graziano SL, Tatum AH, Gonchoroff NJ, et al: Blood group antigen A and flow cytometric analysis in resected early-stage non–small cell lung cancer. Clin Cancer Res 1997;3:87–93.

Greenwald HP, Polissar NL, Borgatta EF, et al: Social factors, treatment, and survival in early-stage non–small cell lung cancer. Am J Public Health 1998;88:1681–1684.

Veale D, Kerr N, Gibson GJ, et al: The relationship of quantitative epidermal growth factor receptor expression in non–small cell lung cancer to long-term survival. Br J Cancer 1993;68:162–165.

Stage I Disease

Ginsberg RJ, Rubinstein LV: Randomized trial of lobectomy versus limited resection for T1N0 non–small cell lung cancer. Ann Thor Surg 1995;60:615–623.

Noordijk EM, Clement EP, Hermans J, et al: Radiotherapy as an alternative to surgery in elderly patients with resectable lung cancer. Radiother Oncol 1988;13:83–89.

PORT Meta-analysis Trialists Group: Postoperative radiotherapy in non–small cell lung cancer: Systematic review and meta-analysis of individual patient data from nine randomized controlled trials. Lancet 1998;2:257–263.

Shennib HA, Landreneau R, Mulder DS, et al: Video-assisted thoracoscopic wedge resection of T1 lung cancer in high-risk patients. Ann Surg 1993;218:555–560.

Warren WH, Faber LP: Segmentectomy versus lobectomy in patients with stage I pulmonary carcinoma. J Thorac Cardiovasc Surg 1994;107:1087–1094.

Stage II Disease

Allen MS, Jett JR, Kozelsky TF: Stage II (T3) lung cancer. Chest Surg Clin N Am 2001;11:61–67.

Baldini EH, DeCamp MM Jr, Katz MS, et al: Patterns of recurrence and outcome for patients with clinical stage II non–small cell lung cancer. Am J Clin Oncol 1999;22:8–14.

Choy O, Jahan T, Roach M 3rd, You L, Jablons D: Stage II (N1) lung cancer. Chest Surg Clin N Am 2001;11:39–59.

Dumont P, Gasser B, Rouge C, et al: Bronchoalveolar carcinoma: Histopathologic study of evolution in a series of 105 surgically treated patients. Chest 1998;113:391–395.

Keller SM, Adak S, Wagner H, et al: A randomized trial of postoperative adjuvant therapy in patients with completely resected stage II or IIIA non–small cell lung cancer: Eastern Cooperative Oncology Group. N Engl J Med. 2000;343:1217–1222.

Martini N, Burt ME, Bains MS, et al: Survival after resection of stage II non–small cell lung cancer. Ann Thorac Surg 1992;54:460–465; discussion 466.

Martini N, Rusch VW, Bains MS, et al: Factors influencing ten-year survival in resected stages I to IIIa non–small cell lung cancer. J Thorac Cardiovasc Surg 1999;117:32–36; discussion 37–38.

Naruke T, Tsuchiya R, Kondo H, et al: Implications of staging in lung cancer. Chest 1997;112(Suppl):S242–S248.

Park JH, Shim YM, Baek HJ, et al: Postoperative adjuvant therapy for stage II non–small cell lung cancer. Ann Thorac Surg 1999;68:1821–1826.

Robnett TJ, Machtay M, Stevenson JP, et al: Factors affecting the risk of brain metastases after definitive chemoradiation for locally advanced non–small cell lung carcinoma. J Clin Oncol 2001;19:1344–1349.

Tyldesley S, Boyd C, Schulze K, et al: Estimating the need for radiotherapy for lung cancer: An evidence-based, epidemiologic approach. Int J Radiat Oncol Biol Phys 2001;49:973–985.

Stage III Disease

Albain KS, Rusch VW, Crowley JJ, et al: Concurrent cisplatin/etoposide plus chest radiotherapy followed by surgery for stages IIIA (N2) and IIIB non–small cell lung cancer: Mature results of Southwest Oncology Group phase II study 8805. J Clin Oncol 1995;13:1880–1892.

Evans WK, Will BP, Berthelot JM, Earle CC: Cost of combined modality interventions for stage III non–small cell lung cancer. J Clin Oncol 1997;15:3038–3048.

Friedberg JS: Clinical presentation of stage IIIA (N2) non–small cell lung cancer: Role of multimodality therapy. Chest 1999;116(6, Suppl):S497–S499.

Gandara DR, Leigh B, Vallieres E, Albain KS: Preoperative chemotherapy in stage III non–small cell lung cancer: Long-term outcome. Lung Cancer 1999;26:3–6.

Garland L, Robinson LA, Wagner H: Evaluation and management of patients with stage IIIA (N2) non–small cell lung cancer. Chest Surg Clin N Am 2001;11:69–100.

Gaspar LE: Optimizing chemoradiation therapy approaches to unresectable stage III non–small cell lung cancer. Curr Opin Oncol 2001;13:110–115.

Jeremic B, Shibamoto Y, Acimovic L, et al: Second cancers occurring in patients with early stage non–small cell lung cancer treated with chest radiation therapy alone. J Clin Oncol 2001;19:1056–1063.

Mac Manus MP, Hicks RJ, Matthews JP, et al: High rate of detection of unsuspected distant metastases by PET in apparent Stage III non–small cell lung cancer: Implications for radical radiation therapy. Int J Radiat Oncol Biol Phys 2001;50:287–293.

Rendina EA, Venuta F, De Giacomo T, et al: Stage IIIB non–small cell lung cancer. Chest Surg Clin N Am 2001;11:101–119.

Rosell R, Gomez-Codina J, Camps C, et al: A randomized trial comparing preoperative chemotherapy plus surgery with surgery alone in patients with non–small cell lung cancer. N Engl J Med 1994;330:153–158.

Rosell R, Green M, Gumerlock P: Advances in the treatment of non–small cell lung cancer: Molecular markers take the stage. Semin Oncol 2001;28(1, Suppl 3):28–34.

Roth JA, Atkinson EN, Fossella F, et al: Long-term follow-up of patients enrolled in a randomized trial comparing perioperative chemotherapy and surgery with surgery alone in resectable stage IIIA non–small cell lung cancer. Lung Cancer 1998;21:1–6.

Rusch VW: Surgery for stage III non–small cell lung cancer. Cancer Control 1994;1:455–466.

Tombolini V, Bonanni A, Donato V, et al: Radiotherapy alone in elderly patients with medically inoperable stage IIIA and IIIB non–small cell lung cancer. Anticancer Res 2000;20:4829–4833.

Chemotherapy and Advanced Disease

Fossella FV, DeVore R, Kerr RN, et al: Randomized phase III trial of docetaxel versus vinorelbine or ifosfamide in patients with advanced non–small cell lung cancer previously treated with platinum-containing chemotherapy regimens: The TAX 320 Non–small Cell Lung Cancer Study Group. J Clin Oncol 2000;18:2354–2362.

Gandara DR, Vokes E, Green M, et al: Activity of docetaxel in platinum-treated non–small cell lung cancer: results of a phase II multicenter trial. J Clin Oncol 2000;18:131–135.

Manegold C: Chemotherapy for advanced non–small cell lung cancer. Semin Oncol 2001;28(Suppl 7):1–6.

Miller VA, Kris MG: Docetaxel (Taxotere) as a single agent and in combination chemotherapy for the treatment of patients with advanced non–small cell lung cancer. Semin Oncol 2000;27(Suppl 3):3–10.

Shepherd FA: Chemotherapy for advanced non–small cell lung cancer: Modest progress, many choices. J Clin Oncol 2000;18:S35–S8.

Smith IE, O'Brien ME, Talbot DC, et al: Duration of chemotherapy in advanced non–small cell lung cancer: A randomized trial of three versus six courses of mitomycin, vinblastine, and cisplatin. J Clin Oncol 2001;19:1336–1343.

Brain Metastases

Alexander E, Moriarty TM, Davis RB, et al: Stereotactic radiosurgery for the definitive, noninvasive treatment of brain metastases. J Natl Cancer Inst 1995;87:34–40.

Bonnette P, Puyo P, Gabriel C, et al: Surgical management of non–small cell lung cancer with synchronous brain metastases. Chest 2001;119:1469–1475.

Kelly K, Bunn PA Jr: Is it time to reevaluate our approach to the treatment of brain metastases in patients with non–small cell lung cancer? Lung Cancer 1998;20:85–91.

Lee JS, Pisters KM, Komaki R, et al: Paclitaxel/carboplatin chemotherapy as primary treatment of brain metastases in non–small cell lung cancer: A preliminary report. Semin Oncol 1997;24(4, Suppl 12):S12-52–S12-55.

Patchell RA, Tibbs PA, Walsh JW, et al: A randomized trial of surgery in the treatment of single metastases to the brain. N Engl J Med 1990;322:494–500.

Rodrigues P, de Brouwer P, Raaymakers E: Brain metastases and non–small cell lung cancer. Prognostic factors and correlation with survival after irradiation. Lung Cancer 2001;32:129–136.

Symptom Control and Supportive Care

Earle CC, Evans WK: A comparison of the costs of paclitaxel and best supportive care in stage IV non–small cell lung cancer. Cancer Prev Control 1997;1:282–288.

Ellis PA, Smith IE, Hardy JR, et al: Symptom relief with MVP (mitomycin C, vinblastine, and cisplatin) chemotherapy in advanced non–small cell lung cancer. Br J Cancer 1995;71:366–370.

Hopwood P, Stephens RJ: Depression in patients with lung cancer: Prevalence and risk factors derived from quality-of-life data. J Clin Oncol 2000;18:893–903.

Schroen AT, Detterbeck FC, Crawford R, et al: Beliefs among pulmonologists and thoracic surgeons in the therapeutic approach to non–small cell lung cancer. Chest 2000;118:129–137.

Shepherd FA, Dancey J, Ramlau R, et al: Prospective randomized trial of docetaxel versus best supportive care in patients with non–small cell lung cancer previously treated with platinum-based chemotherapy. J Clin Oncol 2000;18:2095–103.

Sollner W, DeVries A, Steixner E, et al: How successful are oncologists in identifying patient distress, perceived social support, and need for psychosocial counseling? Br J Cancer 2001;84:179–185.

Prevention

Battey JF, Brown PH, Gritz ER, et al: Primary and secondary prevention of lung cancer: An International Association for the Study of Lung Cancer workshop. Lung Cancer 1995;12:91–103.

Hong WK: Chemoprevention of lung cancer. Oncol 1999;13(10, Suppl 5):135–141.

Karp DD: Lung cancer chemoprevention and management of carcinoma in situ. Semin Oncol 1997;24:402–410.

Khuri FR, Lippman SM: Lung cancer chemoprevention. Semin Surg Oncol 2000;18:100–105.

McLarty JW, Holiday DB, Girard WM, et al: Beta-carotene, vitamin A, and lung cancer chemoprevention: Results of an intermediate endpoint study. Am J Clin Nutr 1995;62(6, Suppl):S1431–S1438.

Omenn GS, Goodman G, Thornquist M, et al: Chemoprevention of lung cancer: The beta-Carotene and Retinol Efficacy Trial (CARET) in high-risk smokers and asbestos exposed workers. IARC Sci Publ 1996;136:67–85.

Pastorino U, Infante M, Maioli M, et al: Adjuvant treatment of stage I lung cancer with high-dose vitamin A. J Clin Oncol 1993;11:1216–1222.

Pastorino U, Soresi E, Clerici M, et al: Lung cancer chemoprevention with retinol palmitate: Preliminary data from a randomized trial on stage I non–small cell lung cancer. Acta Oncol 1988;27:773–782.

Rioux N, Castonguay A: Induction of COX expression by a tobacco carcinogen: Implication in lung cancer chemoprevention. Inflamm Res 1999;48(Suppl 2):S136–S137.

Tockman MS: Lung cancer: Chemoprevention and intermediate effect markers. IARC Sci Publ 2001;154:257–270.

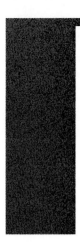

Chapter 96
Thymoma

Patrick J. Loehrer Sr.

The thymus gland serves a critical role in the differentiation and maturation of lymphocytes. Malignant tumors of the thymus are rare but constitute the most common malignancy in the anterior mediastinum. The Surveillance, Epidemiology and End Results (SEER) section of the National Cancer Institute reports the incidence of thymomas to be 0.13 case per 100,000 population. The histologic differences between benign and malignant thymomas are blurred, and the true incidence of malignant thymoma may be underreported. The separation of thymomas into benign and malignant categories can be made clinically according to whether the disease is resectable and cured or recurs and/or is invasive of other tissues at presentation.

Thymomas and thymic carcinomas usually occur in patients between the ages of 40 and 60 but have been reported in patients in the first and ninth decades of life. There is no specific gender predominance, although women have a peak incidence of thymomas approximately one decade later than that of men.

The risk factors for developing thymic cancer are poorly defined. An increased association of Epstein-Barr viral infection has been associated with lymphoepithelioma-type thymic carcinoma. Radiation exposure may also be a predisposing factor. Several cases of familial thymoma have also been reported. Although some investigators report recurrent patterns of reciprocal translocations of chromosomes 15 and 19, no consistent genetic abnormalities have been identified.

Clinical Presentation

Patients with newly diagnosed thymoma are evenly distributed between those with no symptoms (incidental findings), local symptoms, infections, or paraneoplastic syndromes such as myasthenia gravis. A paraneoplastic syndrome or an unexplained rare infection can be the presenting manifestation of the disease. Approximately 80% of patients with incidentally discovered thymomas have noninvasive disease.

Signs and symptoms of local progression include cough, chest pain, dysphagia, dysphonia, dyspnea, hemoptysis, cardiac arrhythmias, and fatigue. Physical examination may reveal signs of superior vena caval syndrome, supraclavicular lymphadenopathy, or Horner's syndrome. As many patients with advanced thymoma develop pleural or pericardial metastases, clinical evaluation may also reveal dullness to percussion of the hemithorax, respiratory lag (as a result of pleural metastases), pulsus paradoxus, or Ewart's sign (consistent with a pericardial effusion).

Paraneoplastic Syndromes

Myasthenia Gravis

Thymoma is associated with a variety of paraneoplastic syndromes (Table 96-1); the most common of these is myasthenia gravis, which occurs in 30% to 50% of patients with thymoma. In contrast, only 10% to 12% of patients with myasthenia gravis have thymoma. The relationship of myasthenia gravis with thymoma and thymic hyperplasia has long been recognized. Myasthenia gravis results from the production within the thymomas of autoantibodies to acetylcholine receptors. Although most patients with myasthenia gravis will have some pathology within the thymus (hyperplasia or neoplasia), a favorable response to thymectomy is more frequently observed in patients with hyperplasia. Other neurologic entities occurring in patients with thymoma include the Lambert-Eaton syndrome (see Chapter 94), limbic encephalopathy, peripheral neuropathy, and Isaac's syndrome (painful myalgias with fasciculations). The diagnosis of myasthenia gravis is based upon the clinical findings and laboratory confirmation. These include administration of an anticholinesterase drug such as edrophonium (Tensilon), repetitive nerve stimulation (looking for rapid reduction in amplitude of evoked muscle action potential), and the finding of acetylcholine receptor antibodies.

Table 96-1 ■ Paraneoplastic Syndromes Associated with Thymomas

Acute pericarditis	Pernicious anemia
Addison's disease	Polymyositis
Agranulocytosis	Red blood cell aplasia
Alopecia areata	Rheumatoid arthritis
Cushing's syndrome	Sarcoidosis
Hemolytic anemia	Scleroderma
Hypogammaglobulinemia	Sensorimotor radiculopathy
Limbic encephalopathy	Stiff-man syndrome
Myasthenia gravis	Systemic lupus erythematosus
Myocarditis	Thyroiditis
Nephrotic syndrome	Ulcerative colitis
Panhypopituitarism	

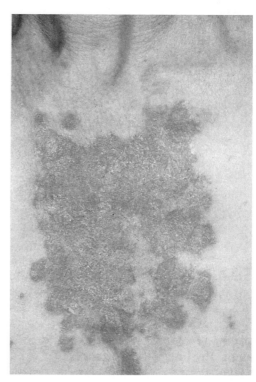

Figure 96-1 ■ Rash that developed during treatment in a 69-year-old patient with cortical-type thymoma. This is a typical rash that has been associated with patients with thymoma. (From du Vivier A: Atlas of Clinical Dermatology, 3rd ed. London, Churchill Livingstone, 2002.)

Several options exist for the treatment of myasthenia gravis. These include systemic therapy, for example, anticholinesterase drugs such as pyridostigmine, immunosuppressants, and immunotherapy, such as plasmapheresis and intravenous immunoglobin. Thymectomy is employed for patients with either thymoma or thymic hyperplasia. Most patients with thymic hyperplasia respond favorably to thymectomy, whereas only approximately 30% of patients with thymoma improve. In some patients with thymoma, exacerbation of myasthenia gravis may occur immediately following thymectomy.

Pure Red Cell Aplasia

Approximately 5% of patients with thymoma will have pure red cell aplasia, and approximately 50% of patients with red cell aplasia have a thymoma. Nearly all patients who are affected by this autoimmune disorder are more than 40 years old. Many patients with pure red cell aplasia have associated deficiencies in other hematologic lineages (thrombocytopenia and/or leukopenia) as well as low serum gamma globulin levels. In affected patients, bone marrow aspiration and biopsy will reveal an absence of erythroid precursors. Thymectomy improves the red cell aplasia in approximately 40% of patients.

Hypogammaglobulinemia

Hypogammaglobulinemia is observed in approximately 5% to 10% of patients with thymoma. Most of these thymomas have spindle cell histology. This association was first recognized by Good in 1954, who noted a syndrome of repetitive infections, diarrhea, and lymphadenopathy. Thymectomy rarely resolves the findings in this disorder.

Autoimmune Disease

Thymoma is associated with a myriad of other autoimmune disorders, including rheumatoid arthritis, dermatomyositis, systemic lupus erythematosus, progressive systemic sclerosis, and giant cell myocarditis. A variety of dermatologic disorders, such as a macular papular rash, herpetiform reaction, or a frank purpuric vasculitis, have also been observed (Figure 96-1).

Second Malignancies

Cancer of nonthymic origin may occur in up to 20% of patients with thymoma. In many patients, the cancer may antedate the diagnosis of thymoma. The spectrum of malignancies is wide ranging and includes colon cancer, lung cancer, leukemia, and lymphoma. The cause of this association is unclear, but altered immunosurveillance mechanisms have been postulated.

Infections

Several unusual infections have been reported in treated and untreated patients with thymoma. These infections usually represent those typically associated with defects in cell-mediated immunity such as disseminated herpes, candida, and listeria infections; cryptococcal meningitis; and progressive multifocal leukoencephalopathy. Fever is generally not associated with thymoma in the absence of infection.

Clinical Evaluation

A chest radiograph will demonstrate an abnormal mass in the majority of patients with thymoma. In the case of a small thymoma, the posteroanterior film might appear normal, but the lateral film will show a mass in what should be the clear portion of the retrosternal, anterior mediastinal space. Typically, a mass is noted that projects over one of the hila of the lung. The tumor is usually well defined (rounded or lobulated) and might be mistaken for the heart border or pulmonary outflow tract (Figure 96-2). Comparison with previous films is useful. In more advanced disease, pleural-based metastases occur commonly and are a hallmark of metastatic disease.

Computed tomography (CT) of the chest and upper abdomen is used to confirm the presence of the mediastinal mass and determine invasiveness. Calcification may be observed in up to 10% of the cases. Computed tomography scans can identify pleural and pericardial metastases, which are the most common sites of initial spread. Although distant metastases to, for example, liver, kidney, bone, brain, and skin occur, extensive radiographs or radionuclide imaging is unnecessary in the absence of signs or symptoms of metastases. Magnetic resonance imaging (MRI) may be useful in some cases to determine the degree of vascular involvement of the tumor. Radionuclide imaging using gallium scans or, more recently, octreotide scans can identify areas of disease.

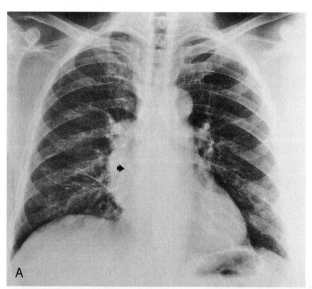

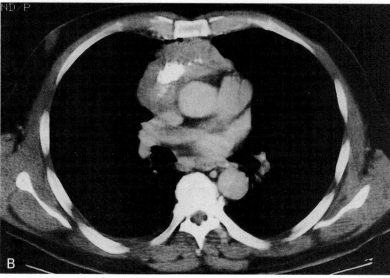

Figure 96-2 ■ A computed tomography scan of chest in a patient with stage IIIB thymoma. Note the anterior mediastinal mass that falls predominantly to the right hemithorax. Pleural-based metastases characteristic of metastatic thymoma (not seen here) are the typical site of metastasis. (From Bragg DG, Rubin P, Hricak H [eds]: Oncologic Imaging, 2nd ed. Philadelphia, WB Saunders, 2002, p 337.)

Routine blood studies should include a complete blood count looking for signs of aplasia or hypoplasia in the erythroid or other blood cell lineages. Lymphocytosis has been reported in some patients with thymoma. For patients with signs of myasthenia gravis, acetylcholine receptor antibodies are appropriate. A serum protein electrophoresis and/or quantitative immunoglobulin level determination should be obtained, especially in patients with unexplained infections, to test for hypogammaglobulinemia.

Staging

Histologic Staging

Several different histologic staging systems that are correlated with long-term survivals have been proposed without general agreement about a common standard formulation (Table 96-2). One of the earliest staging systems divided thymoma into four categories depending on the predominance of lymphocytes or epithelial cells: lymphocyte predominant (greater than 66% lymphocytes), epithelial predominant (greater than 66% of epithelial cells), mixed lymphoepithelial (34% to 66% epithelial cells), and spindle cell. A variant classification utilizes the predominant cell type to distinguish four different categories. Thymic carcinoma is considered to be at one end of the spectrum of thymic neoplasms. These tumors differ from thymomas because they lack associated paraneoplastic syndromes and typically present with advanced disease. Thymic carcinoma lacks the encapsulation or

Table 96-2 ■ Histology of Thymomas

Classification Schema	Subgroups	Percentage
Verley, Silbert, Hollman, et al.	Type I: spindle and oval cell	30%
	Type II: lymphocyte rich	30%
	Type III: differentiated epithelial-rich	33%
	Type IV: undifferentiated, epithelial-rich (equivalent to thymic carcinoma)	7%
Lewis, Wick, Scheithauer, et al.	Predominantly lymphocytic (>66% lymphocytes)	25%
	Mixed lymphoepithelial (33–66% lymphocytes)	43%
	Predominantly epithelial (<33% lymphocytes)	25%
	Spindle cell (predominantly epithelial cells with prominent fusiform cells)	6%

Table 96-3 ■ Histologic Types of Thymic Carcinoma

Squamous cell carcinoma
  Basaloid
  Keratinizing
  Nonkeratinizing
  Lymphoepithelioma-like
Adenosquamous and mucoepidermoid carcinoma
Clear cell carcinoma
Primary adenocarcinoma
Sarcomatoid carcinoma
Carcinoid

fibrous septae of the thymus; on gross examination, it appears as white-gray tissue with frequent areas of hemorrhage and necrosis. Histologically, some thymic carcinomas resemble metastatic tumors from either the lung or the esophagus. Various histologic classifications for thymic carcinoma are shown in Table 96-3. The low-grade histologic types of thymic carcinoma include the keratinizing squamous, basaloid squamous, and mucoepidermoid variants. Median survival of the low-grade types is twice as long as that in the high-grade histologies: 25 months versus 11 months, respectively.

Special stains such as keratin, leukocyte common antigen, and epithelial membrane antigen are useful to distinguish thymic carcinoma from lymphoma. Neuroendocrine markers or a distinctive pattern of intracellular filament expression suggests a thymic carcinoid. CD-5 expression by the epithelial cells is typically seen only in carcinoma of the thymus; it is absent in metastatic or other mediastinal tumors.

Clinical Staging

Different staging systems, shown in Table 96-4, have been proposed for patients with thymoma. A TNM system exists but is little used. The most commonly used clinical staging systems are those of Masaoka and colleagues. Some of the earliest attempts at clinical staging failed to take into account the propensity for pleural metastases to appear early in the progression of thymomas. Most reports included too few patients with stage IV disease to identify distinct prognostic factors. The Masaoka Staging System incorporates pleural metastases; however, the stage IVB category does not define whether lymphatic metastases are intrathoracic or extrathoracic. One additional problem with the Masaoka Staging System is the omission of the significance of capsular invasion into mediastinal fat, which may be a prime predictor of local recurrence after initial therapy.

Table 96-4 ■ Staging Systems for Thymomas

Masaoka Staging

I	Macroscopically completely encapsulated and microscopically no capsular invasion
II	(1) Macroscopic invasion into surrounding fatty tissue, mediastinal pleura or both
	(2) Microscopic invasion into capsule
III	Macroscopic invasion into neighboring organ, such as pericardium, great vessels, or lung
IVa	Pleural or pericardial dissemination
IVb	Lymphatic or hematogenous metastasis

GETT Classification

Stage I	
IA	Encapsulated tumor, totally resected
IB	Macroscopically encapsulated tumor, totally resected, but the surgeon suspects mediastinal adhesions and potential capsular invasion
Stage II	Invasive tumor, totally resected
Stage III	
IIIA	Invasive tumor subtotally resected
IIIB	Invasive tumor, biopsy
Stage IV	
IVA	Supraclavicular metastasis or distant pleural implants
IVB	Distant metastasis

The Groupe d'Etudes des Tumeurs Thymiques (GETT) classification is based on operative findings and provides more specific details than the Masaoka Staging System. Some authors have simply classified patients as limited or extensive in a manner similar to that for small cell lung cancer. Patients with disease confined to a single radiation therapy portal (locally advanced, unresectable thymoma) are labeled limited disease, while those patients who have distant spread are classified as having extensive thymoma. This classification is useful because it segregates by treatment options: single modality for limited thymoma and combined modality for extensive thymoma. The estimated five- and 10-year survival rates by stage are listed in Table 96-5.

Treatment

In light of the rarity of the tumor, no prospective randomized trial has defined the standard of therapy. Most of the therapeutic data are derived from historical series and Phase II trials. An outline of the management of this cancer is provided in Figure 96-3.

Thymic Carcinoma

Virtually all patients with thymic carcinoma present with locally advanced (stage III) or metastatic (stage

Table 96-5 ■ Survival Rates in Patients with Thymoma and Thymic Carcinoma

Disease	Three-Year Survival Rate (%)	Five-Year Survival Rate (%)	10-Year Survival Rate (%)
Thymoma			
Stage I		85	75
Stage II		70	65
Stage III		70	50
Stage IV		25–50	10–30
Thymic carcinoma	45	35	

Adopted from Sweeney CJ, Wick MR, Loehrer PJ: Thymoma and thymic carcinoma. In Raghavan D, Brecher ML, Johnson DH, et al (eds): Textbook of Uncommon Cancer. New York, Wiley, 1999, pp 485–504.

IV) disease. For patients with resectable disease, surgical extirpation of the mass is warranted with postoperative radiation therapy for those patients with involved margins. For patients with stage IV disease, systemic therapy is given. In patients with advanced disease, chemotherapeutic regimens with documented antitumor activity include cisplatin, doxorubicin, and cyclophosphamide; etoposide, ifosfamide, and cisplatin (VIP); and 5-fluorouracil plus leucovorin. Initial treatment options also include those directed against non–small cell lung cancer (see Chapter 95).

Thymoma

Noninvasive (Masaoka or GETT Stage I)

Surgical removal of the tumor is sufficient therapy for patients with stage I thymoma. Numerous surgical series have reported five-year survival rates exceeding 90% with a 10-year survival rate of approximately 80%. Radiation therapy is not recommended in resectable patients, given their good overall prognosis.

Locally Invasive Disease (Masaoka Stage II and III or GETT Stage III)

Surgery remains the mainstay of treatment for patients with locally invasive thymoma. Several surgeons have logically concluded that survival is significantly better for patients who are able to undergo a complete resection than for those who undergo debulking only. The complete resectability rates vary with the extent of disease. Complete resection rates are approximately 100% for stage II, 50% to 60% for stage III, but rare for stage IVA disease.

Historical data support postoperative radiotherapy for these patients after complete resection is attempted. In one series, eight of 21 patients (38%) with completely resected thymoma (18 stage II, 3 stage III) treated with surgery alone had mediastinal

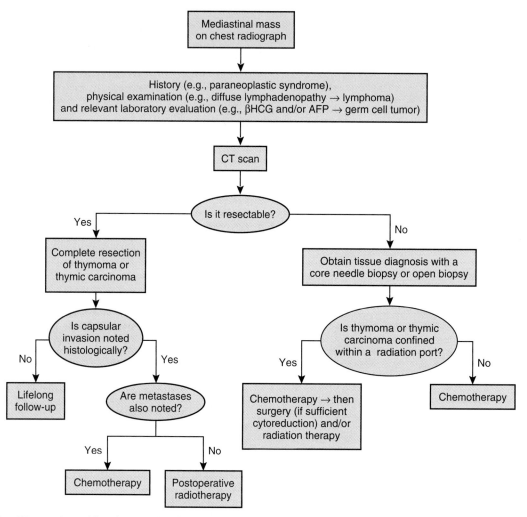

Figure 96-3 ■ Diagnosis and treatment algorithm for a finding of mediastinal mass on chest X-ray.

recurrence and an actual five-year relapse-free survival rate of 47%. This compares with no relapses in five patients (one stage II, four stage III) who received postoperative radiotherapy during the same time period. Pooled data from multiple series of patients with completely resected stage II and stage III thymoma show relapse rates of 28% and 5% for those receiving or not receiving postoperative radiation therapy, respectively.

Unresectable/Locally Advanced Disease

The Masaoka and the TNM staging systems define stage III disease as that in which the tumor macroscopically invades neighboring organs such as the pericardium, lung, or great vessels. In contrast, the GETT System is clinically oriented, separating patients with invasive disease from those with subtotally resected (stage IIIA) or biopsy-only documented involvement of adjacent organs (stage IIIB). However, even this subclassification includes a varied patient population in stage IIIA, because the degree of subtotal resection can range from 10% to slightly less than 100% of the initial tumor volume.

The amount of residual carcinoma following surgery influences the likelihood of local and systemic relapse. The relapse-free rates for patients with complete resection, partial resection, or biopsy for diagnosis only were 97%, 45%, and 16%, respectively, and the five-year survival rates were 80%, 64%, and 37%, respectively. Patients with incompletely resected locally advanced disease should receive postoperative radiation therapy. The optimal dosage of radiation therapy is uncertain, but 40 to 50 Gy in conventional 1.8- to 2.0-Gy fractions per day is given for adjuvant therapy. The higher total dose is used in patients with unresectable or gross residual disease. Several combination chemotherapy regimens have been employed in patients with locally advanced or metastatic thymoma. Some of these trials are outlined in Table

Table 96-6 ▪ Combination Chemotherapeutic Regimens in Thymoma

Authors	Regimen	Number of Patients	Complete Response	Partial Response	Complete Response + Partial Response (%)	Median Survival Time (years)	Comments
Loehrer et al.	PAC	30	3	12	50	3.2	Extensive disease
Loehrer et al.	PAC + XRT	23			70	5	Limited disease
Fornasiero et al.	ADOC	32	15	14	90	1.25	—
Giaccone et al.	PE	16	5	4	56	4.3	—
Shin et al.	PACP	12	3	8	92	NR	Limited disease
Loehrer et al.	VIP	28	0	9	32	2.5	Two-year survival rate: 70%*

NR = not reached; PAC = cisplatin, doxorubicin, and cyclophosphamide; ADOC = doxorubicin, cisplatin, vincristine, cyclophosphamide; PACP = PAC plus prednisone; PEpE = cisplatin, epirubicin, etoposide; VIP = etoposide, ifosfamide, and cisplatin.
*Projected two-year survival rate.

96-6. Although not directly compared, the weight of data from these studies suggests that anthracycline-based regimens are associated with improved survival when compared to other treatment regimens.

The Southeastern Cancer Study Group initiated the first prospective trial of combination chemotherapy in thymomas, using cisplatin, doxorubicin, and cyclophosphamide (PAC). Use of corticosteroids was specifically discouraged in these patients because of their lympholytic effect and an uncertain impact on the malignant epithelial cells. For patients with locally advanced disease (GETT stage IIIA or IIIB), treatment consisted of two to four cycles of chemotherapy followed by radiation therapy. In 23 patients with limited unresectable disease, chemotherapy achieved a 70% objective response rate and a 50% five-year survival rate. On the basis of this outcome and initial responsiveness, the strategy of choice in these patients is to first give chemotherapy to reduce the mass of tumor, followed by surgical resection and postoperative chemotherapy and/or radiation therapy.

Chemotherapy or Recurrent Advanced (Stage IV) Disease

Only a few prospective Phase II trials have been conducted in patients with advanced or recurrent thymoma. These include studies of single agents such as cisplatin (two partial responses in 21 patients), ifosfamide (seven complete and partial responses in 14 patients), and interleukin-2 (no responses in 14 patients). The combination chemotherapy regimens listed in Table 96-6 improve on single-agent response rates.

Numerous drugs have produced objective responses in patients with recurrent thymoma. These drugs include 5-fluorouracil, paclitaxel, gallium nitrate, daily oral etoposide, and octreotide. It is not uncommon to have objective responses in patients who have received multiple prior chemotherapeutic regimens and meaningful remissions that may last for years with second-line therapy. Because of the indolent nature of this disease and the fact that cure in advanced, recurrent disease is not feasible, chemotherapy should be administered only to patients whose disease is progressing rather than to patients with persistent but relatively stable disease.

Follow-up Care

Most, but not all, thymomas have an indolent course. Chest X-rays and physical examination are recommended every two to three months during the first year, every four to six months during the second and third years, every six months thereafter until the five-year anniversary, and thereafter on an annual basis. Chest computed tomography scans can be performed to better evaluate the extent of pleural-based metastases. Recurrences of tumor after 20 years or more have been observed following surgical resection.

Late Sequelae

Data on late sequelae of treatment are sparse. Combined-modality therapy including anthracyclines and radiation to the chest can be expected to cause damage to the heart and pericardium. Second malignancies are common in patients with thymoma. They may antedate the diagnosis of thymoma or occur later, but they probably relate to the altered immunologic function in these patients rather than the impact of treatment.

The immunologic derangement that is associated with thymoma can be manifested by the appearance of paraneoplastic syndromes many years after the primary treatment of thymoma.

References

General Information

Drachman DB: Myasthenia gravis. N Engl J Med 1994;330: 1797–1810.

Hoffacker V, Schultz A, Tiesinga JJ, et al: Thymomas alter the T cell subset composition in the blood: A potential mechanism for thymoma-associated disease. Blood 2000;96: 3872–3879.

Johnson SB, Eng TY, Giacone G, Thomas CR Jr: Thymoma: Update for the new millennium. Oncologist 2001;6: 239–246.

Loehrer PJ Sr, Wick MR: Thymic malignancies. Cancer Treat Res 2001;105:277–302.

Palmieri G, Lastoria S, Calao A, et al: Successful treatment of a patient with a thymoma and pure red cell aplasia with octreotide and prednisone. N Engl J Med 1997;336: 263–265.

Sweeney CJ, Wick MR, Loehrer PJ: Thymoma and thymic carcinoma. In Rhagavan D, Brecher ML, Johnson DH, et al: Textbook of Uncommon Cancer. New York, Wiley, 1999, pp 485–504.

Tarr PE, Lucey DR: Good's syndrome: The association of thymoma with immunodeficiency. Clin Infect Dis 2001;33: 585–586.

Thomas CR, Wright CD, Loehrer PJ: Thymoma: State of the art. J Clin Oncol 1999;17:2280–2289.

Tomiyama N, Muller NL, Ellis SJ, et al: Invasive and non-invasive thymoma: Distinctive CT features. J Comput Assist Tomog 2001;25:388–393.

Chemotherapy

Bonomi PD, Finkelstein D, Aisner S, et al: EST 2582 phase II trial of cisplatin in metastatic or recurrent thymoma. Am J Clin Oncol 1993;16:342–345.

Fornasiero A, Daniele O, Ghiotto C, et al: Chemotherapy for invasive thymoma: A 13 year experience. Cancer 1991; 68:30–33.

Giaccone G, Ardizzoni A, Kirkpatrick A, et al: Cisplatin and etoposide combination chemotherapy for locally advanced or metastatic thymoma: A phase II study of the European Organization for Research and Treatment of Cancer Lung Cancer Cooperative Group. J Clin Oncol 1996;14:814–820.

Loehrer PJ Sr, Chen M, Kim K, et al. Cisplatin, doxorubicin, and cyclophosphamide plus thoracic radiation therapy for limited stage, unresectable thymoma: An intergroup trial. J Clin Oncol 1997;15:3093–3099.

Loehrer PJ Sr, Kim K, Aisner SC, et al: Cisplatin plus doxorubicin plus cyclophosphamide in metastatic or recurrent thymoma: Final results of an intergroup trial. J Clin Oncol 1994;12:1164–1168.

Shin DM, Walsh GL, Komaki R, et al: Induction chemotherapy (IC) followed by surgical resection (SR), radiotherapy and consolidative chemotherapy may cure the advanced stages of unresectable invasive thymoma. Ann Intern Med 1998;129:100–104.

Pathology and Prognosis

Bernatz PE, Harrison EG Jr, Clagett OT: Thymoma: A clinico-pathologic study. J Thorac Cardiovasc Surg 1961;42:424–444.

Bernatz PE, Khonsari S, Harrison EG, et al: Thymoma: Factors influencing prognosis. Surg Clin North Am 1973;53:885–893.

LeQuaglie C, Giudice G, Brega Massone PP, et al: Clinical and pathologic predictors of survival in thymic tumors. J Cardiovasc Surg 2002;43:269–274.

Lewis JE, Wick MR, Scheithauer BW, et al: Thymoma: A clinicopathologic review. Cancer 1987;60:2727–2743.

Marino M, Muller-Hermelink HK: Thymoma and thymic carcinoma: Relation of thymoma epithelial cells to the cortical and medullary differentiation of thymus. Virchows Arch 1985;407:119–149.

Masaoka A, Monden Y, Nakahara K, et al: Follow-up study of thymomas with special reference to their clinical stages. Cancer 1981;48:2485–2492.

Pan CC, Chen WY, Chiang H: Spindle cell and mixed spindle/lymphocytic thymomas: An integrated clinico-pathologic and immunohistochemical study of 81 cases. Am J Surg Pathol 2001;25:111–120.

Quintanilla-Martinez L, Wilkins EW Jr, Ferry JA, et al: Thymoma: Morphologic subclassification correlates with invasiveness and immunohistologic features—A study of 122 cases. Hum Pathol 1993;24:958–969.

Verley JM, Silbert D, Hollmann KH, et al: Histopathology and prognosis of thymomas. Rev Maladies Respir 1988;5:179–185.

Radiation Therapy

Curran WJ, Kornstein MJ, Brooks JJ, et al: Invasive thymoma: The role of mediastinal irradiation following complete or incomplete surgical resection. J Clin Oncol 1977; 6:1722–1727.

Dziuba SJ, Curran WJ Jr: The radiotherapeutic management of invasive thymomas. Chest Surg Clin N Am 2001;11:457–466.

Mornex F, Resbeut M, Richard P, et al: Radiotherapy and chemotherapy for invasive thymoma: A multicentric retrospective review of 90 cases. Int J Radiat Oncol Biol Phys 1995;32:651–659.

Ogawa K, Uno T, Toita T, et al: Postoperative radiotherapy for patients with completely resected thymoma: A multi-institutional, retrospective review of 103 patients. Cancer 2002;94:1405–1413.

Chapter 97
Mesothelioma

Joseph Aisner

Introduction

Malignant mesothelioma is a rare disease that is unique because of its association with workplace asbestos exposure. Mesothelioma also arises on other mesothelial surfaces such as the pericardium, peritoneum, and tunica vaginalis testes. While there are case reports of mesotheliomas associated with irradiation and thoratrast injection, most mesotheliomas of the pleura and peritoneum are associated with asbestos exposure. The association often depends on the thoroughness of the occupational history evaluation and the recognition of asbestos-contaminated products, such as the old wallboard spackle. As a reflection of the asbestos workplace exposure, malignant mesothelioma occurs more frequently in men than in women. However, mesothelioma has also been reported as a consequence of secondary exposure among family members of asbestos workers, such as the wives who washed their husband's work clothes, and in young adults as a consequence of other household or neighborhood exposure. These secondary exposure cases suggest that even relatively mild exposure to asbestos increases the risk of mesothelioma. Most cases occur late in life, with a median age at presentation in excess of 65. This reflects the very long period of latency from exposure to disease of up to 40 years or more.

Clinical Presentation

Mesotheliomas tend to grow and invade locally until late in their natural history. In thoracic presentations, dysphagia, chest pain, cord compression, plexopathy, Horner's syndrome, or superior vena cava syndromes can arise from extension into the esophagus, ribs, vertebrae, nerves, and superior vena cava. The tumor also tends to grow along drainage and needle tracts and out thoracotomy scars. Extension into the pulmonary parenchyma, chest wall, mediastinum, and diaphragm are common as the disease progresses. Mediastinal and cervical lymph nodes may also become involved. As the disease advances, the patient typically complains of fatigue and dyspnea out of proportion to chest X-ray findings owing to the shunting of poorly aerated blood in the trapped lung. The disease occurs more frequently in men than in women and more commonly on the right than on the left side.

Clinical Evaluation

Imaging studies are critical to the evaluation of mesothelioma. Chest X-rays are usually obtained after the patient first presents with shortness of breath or chest pain. Typically, a pleural effusion is found, prompting additional studies. Pleural plaque or calcifications in the diaphragm may be seen and denote asbestos exposure, but these are found in fewer than 20% of patients with mesothelioma. These radiologic findings are thus sufficient although not necessary to define asbestos exposure.

Computed tomography (CT) scans can provide details of the extent of disease as it progressively encircles and traps the lung (Figures 97-1 and 97-2), extends into the fissures and along the pericardium, and invades into the chest wall, diaphragm, and mediastinal structures. The computed tomography scan can also define enlarged mediastinal lymph nodes, a circumstance that carries an adverse prognosis.

Magnetic resonance imaging (MRI) can theoretically improve differentiation between tumor and surrounding normal tissue. This is of particular value in the evaluation of the penetration into the mediastinal structures, chest wall, and diaphragm. However, staging information derived from computed tomography and magnetic resonance imaging offer approximately equivalent information. Positron emission tomography (PET) offers the ability to identify tumors on the basis of their metabolism of 18-F fluorodeoxyglucose and to locate malignant lesions. Positron emission tomography scanning may become a valuable adjunct to computed tomography or magnetic resonance imaging scanning.

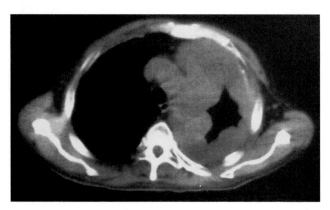

Figure 97-1 ■ Computed tomography scan of thorax demonstrating regionally advanced pleural mesothelioma on the left side. The disease has encircled and trapped the lung, extended into the mediastinum, and invaded the chest wall, producing pain. Note the beginning asymmetry of the left chest as the left lung collapses.

Prognosis and Staging

Median survival depends on histologic subtype and stage but is generally less than a year without treatment. Adverse prognostic factors include chest pain, male gender, weight loss, impaired performance status, a high lactate dehydrogenase (LDH) level, leukocytosis, and thrombocytosis.

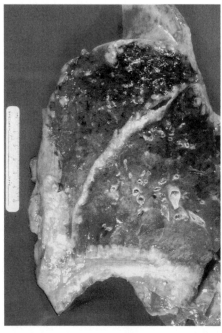

Figure 97-2 ■ Surgical extrapleural pneumonectomy specimen demonstrating the growth and spread of malignant pleural mesothelioma. The major bulk of disease involves the diaphragmatic and lateral pleural surfaces in contiguity. Note the disease involvement of the fissure and the parenchymal invasion from the areas of bulk pleural involvement as well as the nodular invasion from the apical pleura. (Photo courtesy of S.C. Aisner, MD.)

A TNM classification schema has been modified to account for very early disease found on pleuroscopy. This staging revision was recently incorporated into Version 6 of the American Joint Committee on Cancer (AJCC) staging manual (Table 97-1).

Diagnosis/Pathology

Three histologically defined subtypes of mesothelioma are recognized: epithelial, sarcomatous (spindle cell, fibrosarcomatous, etc.), and mixed (epithelial and sarcomatous). The latter two histologic subtypes are usually easily defined, while the epithelial subtype still remains somewhat challenging in the need to distinguish it from adenocarcinoma. Special histochemistry sometimes helps to define the diagnosis. The reference standard remains the characteristic electron microscopic findings of elongated long, thin, branched microvillae; absent mucin granules; and no myelin figures. Standard histochemistry includes positive Alcian blue staining with diastase digestion. In recent years, immunohistochemistry (Table 97-2) has provided considerable aide in establishing the diagnosis even in cytopathologic material. The combination of positive cytokeratin, negative CEA, and negative Leu-M1 staining on immunohistochemistry argues very strongly for mesothelioma. In fact, this immunohistochemical staining has replaced other techniques of diagnosis.

Treatment

Early Intervention

Early disease often involves the parietal pleura first. Instillation of γ-interferon into the pleural cavity causes regression of the pleural nodules as demonstrated on repeat pleuroscopy. Patients who have only parietal pleural involvement experience a high response and a prolonged disease-free survival with this approach, while those with disease beyond the confines of parietal pleura do not have a favorable outcome; nearly all of the patients with more advanced disease experience disease progression.

Surgical Options

Pleuroscopy/Pleuradesis

The use of fiber-optic instruments has allowed investigation into various closed spaces and less invasive surgical procedures. The adaptation of this instrumentation into the thorax allows for investigation of the pleural cavity. As such, it permits inspection of the pleura and the acquisition of sufficient material to make histologic diagnosis. This approach can also be

Table 97-1 ■ AJCC Staging of Malignant Mesothelioma

T (Primary Tumor)

Tx: Primary tumor cannot be assessed.

T0:   No evidence of primary tumor.

  T1a: Primary tumor limited to ipsilateral parietal pleura.

  T1b: Tumor foci involving ipsilateral visceral pleura.

T2:   Tumor involves ipsilateral pleural surfaces and invades any of the following: ipsilateral lung, diaphragm, or pericardium (locally advanced, resectable).

T3:   Tumor invades any of the following: ipsilateral chest wall muscle, endothoracic fascia, ribs, mediastinal organs or tissues (locally advanced, unresectable).

T4:   Tumor extends to any of the following: contralateral pleura or lung by direct extension, peritoneum or intra-abdominal organs by direct extension, direct extension to the spine.

N (Lymph Nodes)

Nx: Regional lymph nodes cannot be assessed.

N0:   No regional lymph node metastases.

N1:   Metastases in ipsilateral bronchopulmonary or hilar lymph nodes.

N2:   Metastases in subcarinal or ipsilateral mediastinal or internal mammary lymph nodes.

N3:   Metastases in contralateral mediastinal, supraclavicular, or scalene lymph nodes.

M (Metastases)

Mx: Presence of distant metastases cannot be assessed.

M0:   No (known) distant metastases.

M1:   Distant metastasis present.

Stage Grouping

Stage IA   T1aN0M0

Stage IB   T1bN0M0

Stage II   T1N1M0

            T2N1M0

Stage III   T1N2M0

            T2N2M0

            T3N0M0

            T3N1M0

            T3N2M0

Stage IV   anyT N3M0

            T4 anyN M0

            anyT anyN M1

*Staging solely on clinical measures is designated cTNM. Staging following pathologic information is designated as pTNM.

Table 97-2 ■ Immunohistochemistry of Malignant Mesothelioma

Stain	Mesothelioma, Percent Positive	Adenocarcinoma, Percent Positive
Cytokeratins	100	100
CEA	10	95
Leu-M1	5	90
EMA	90	100

increasing solid tumor within the pleural cavity, forming a ring of tumor as the pleural space disappears. On the other hand, early pleuradesis tends to obscure the disease, at least until it progresses, and complicates performance of other surgical procedures. While this approach is quite popular, it offers very little palliative benefit, and its use in otherwise healthy individuals with good performance greatly compromises surgical options.

Pleurectomy

Since the disease involves the pleura, one surgical approach is to remove or rather "strip off" the visceral and parietal pleura on the lung and chest wall. With pleurectomy, the pleura are stripped along with the pericardium from the apex of the lung to the diaphragm. This approach has been used to control effusions, including cases of pleuradesis failure, and has achieved control of effusions in over 80% of cases. Pleurectomy with decortication is a more aggressive technique that produces a far greater degree of tumor volume reduction, although this more aggressive approach is usually not warranted for mere palliation. Pleurectomy has been performed with relatively few complications, including air leaks (10%), subcutaneous emphysema (2%), empyema (2%), bronchopleural fistulae (1%), and hemorrhage (1%). The 30-day mortality rate is less than 2%. The outcomes for pleurectomy alone in early, minimal-bulk tumors demonstrate median survival ranging from about six to 20 months, with few patients alive beyond two years. Unfortunately, as the tumor grows from the pleura into adjacent tissues and lung, a clean separation of lung and visceral pleura is often difficult to achieve (Figure 97-3), and therefore some pleura and tumor are necessarily left behind. For this reason, some investigators added postoperative radiotherapy to the chest and chest wall or postoperative intrapleural and systemic chemotherapy. The median survival for this combined approach ranges from 11 to 21 months, and few patients live beyond two or three years. The median survival duration for the epithelial subtype is two to three times greater than that for the

used to insufflate talc to achieve pleuradesis, the goal of which is to reduce the frequency of thoracentesis. By insufflating two to five grams of asbestos-free, sterile talc, the pleural effusions can be controlled in about 90% of cases. However, the need for thoracentesis usually decreases as the disease progresses with

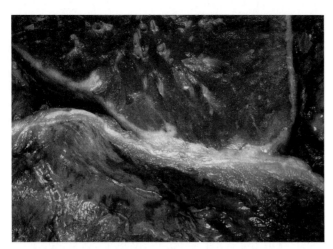

Figure 97-3 ■ Surgical extrapleural pneumonectomy specimen demonstrating parenchymal invasion from the involved diaphragmatic pleura surface. (Photo courtesy of S.C. Aisner, MD)

sarcomatous form, and the mixed subtype shows an intermediate survival. In addition, virtually all the long-term survivors beyond three years have the epithelial form. While there are no studies that directly compare the various surgical approaches, the median survival for pleurectomy appears similar to the median survival reported with even more aggressive surgical approaches.

Extrapleural Pneumonectomy

This approach is a more extensive extirpative procedure in which the parietal and visceral pleura, the contained lung, pericardium, and diaphragm, are resected en bloc. To avoid herniation of the abdominal contents into the chest or the heart through the pericardial defect, fenestrated prosthetic patches are inserted into the diaphragm and pericardium, respectively. With increasing experience, studies have seen a reduction in the operative and postoperative mortality rate to about 5%, similar to that of a pneumonectomy. Serious complications are seen in up to 25% of patients and include bronchial leaks, empyema, vocal cord paralysis, subcutaneous emphysema, hemorrhage, chylothorax, arrhythmias, and respiratory insufficiency.

In view of the extensive nature of the surgery and the relatively older age of the population, careful preoperative staging is needed to ensure adequate pulmonary, cardiac, and renal functions. With the use of such vigorous preoperative screening and accumulated experience, the rate of these postoperative complications has significantly decreased to 5% or less. The median duration of survival for extrapleural pneumonectomy ranges from four months to 21 months, similar to that for pleurectomy. Given the difficulties with this procedure, the complication rate, and the lack of clear differences, many thoracic surgeons are reluctant to undertake extrapleural pneumonectomy. Extrapleural pneumonectomy does, however, offer the opportunity of additional therapies and the unique opportunities afforded by an empty chest cavity with maximal debulking. Another potential advantage of extrapleural pneumonectomy is that arteriovenous shunts resulting from a trapped lung do not occur when disease returns locally; thus, patients who previously underwent extrapleural pneumonectomy may have less end-stage respiratory distress.

Surgical Prognostic Factors

Subhistologies, preoperative tumor bulk, mediastinal lymph node involvement, resection margins, and invasion beyond the pleural envelope have important prognostic impact on the survival of malignant pleural mesothelioma. Patients with the sarcomatous and mixed forms of mesothelioma have a significantly worse outcome than those with the epithelial form of the disease. Therefore, patients with the sarcomatous and mixed subhistologies should be offered palliative therapies and be spared the operative consequences of aggressive surgical procedures. Similarly, nodal involvement carries an adverse prognosis. Since patients with mediastinal lymph node involvement have a significantly inferior survival compared to those without such involvement, preoperative staging should now assess the mediastinum. This is traditionally done with a preoperative mediastinal exploration; however, newer imaging techniques such as fluorodeoxyglucose positron emission tomography scanning may provide a less invasive substitute for surgical mediastinal exploration. Other factors that predict survival include diaphragmatic penetration or other extracapsular extension as well as preoperative tumor volume. An alternative functional staging system is shown in Table 97-3.

Radiation Therapy

The role of radiation therapy in the definitive treatment of malignant pleural mesothelioma remains uncertain. Radiation therapy alone for unresected disease produces inconsistent results, with some anecdotal reports of long-term survival following external beam irradiation or intracavitary instillation of radioisotopes. Given the large area of potential involvement (pleural space), tumoricidal doses of irradiation are limited by the extent of the disease and organ toxicity to the lung, the heart, and possibly the

Table 97-3 ■ Revised Postoperative Brigham/DFCI Staging System

Stage	Definitions
I	Disease completely resected within the capsule of the parietal pleura without adenopathy; ipsilateral pleura, lung, diaphragm, or chest wall. Disease limited to prior biopsy sites.
II	All of stage I but with positive resection margins or intrapleural adenopathy.
III	Local extension into the chest wall or mediastinum; into the heart or through the diaphragm; or into the peritoneum; or with extrapleural lymph node involvement.
IV	Distant metastatic disease.

Table 97-4 ■ Single Agents Active for Malignant Pleura Mesothelioma*

Agent	Number Evaluable	Percent Responding
Cisplatin	73	18%
Carboplatin	88	11%
Doxorubicin	35	26%
High-dose methotrexate	60	36%
Trimetrexate	51	12%
Edatrexate + folinic acid	40	15%
Gemcitabine	57	12%
Vinorelbine	57	20%

*Derived from trials in which adequate numbers of patients were enrolled in the individual trial.

liver. Nevertheless, radiation therapy is frequently used for palliation of local pain. Greater palliation is achieved with doses of 40 Gy or more. With the advent of conformal therapy and the ability to deliver higher doses to more defined irradiation portals, it is likely that radiation therapy will provide better palliation than it did in the past.

Radiation therapy has been added to surgical series to reduce the high incidence of local recurrence. Because of the propensity of this tumor to grow out the needle tracts, pleuroscopy wounds, and thoracotomy scars, radiation therapy has been used successfully to prevent chest wall wound growths. Thus, radiation therapy has the potential to reduce the high incidence of local failures following pleurectomy to improve local control following extrapleural pneumonectomy.

Chemotherapy

Single Agents

Table 97-4 shows the various active single chemotherapy agents according to trials with adequate numbers to define some level of response. None of the single agents show significant activity, and only the antifolate antimetabolites have shown consistent activity as a group. High-dose methotrexate showed one of the highest reported single-agent activities, and the consistent response with other agents in this class confirms this activity. The platinum analogs cisplatin and carboplatin also show consistent, albeit small, response frequencies.

Combination Chemotherapy

One study of doxorubicin plus cyclophosphamide ± DTIC showed a response rate of only 7%. A large study of doxorubicin plus cisplatin showed only a 13% response rate. Doxorubicin, cyclophosphamide, and cisplatin showed a response rate of 26% in one small study. With the identification of several new active single agents, new combinations are now under study, with promising early results (Table 97-5). A prospectively randomized, double-blind study was conducted comparing pemetrexed plus cisplatin to cisplatin alone. The group receiving the pemetrexed had a significantly greater response rate, time to progression, and survival rate. This combination represents a new standard of treatment for this otherwise very difficult disease.

Intracavitary Therapies

Since mesotheliomas develop and grow superficially along the pleural surface of the thoracic cavity, intrapleural chemotherapy, radionuclides, or biologics could potentially treat early superficial disease. However, intrapleural therapy is necessarily limited

Table 97-5 ■ Combination Chemotherapy for Malignant Pleural Mesothelioma

Combination	Number in Study	Percent Responding
Doxorubicin + cisplatin	59	16%
Mitomycin C + cisplatin	35	26%
Gemcitabine + cisplatin	140	31%
Pemetrexed + cisplatin	226	41%
Pemetrexed + carboplatin	27	32%
Raltitrexed + oxaliplatin	89	27%
Vinorelbine + oxaliplatin	26	23%

to early disease, since the pleural space progressively disappears as the disease advances. In addition, intrapleural therapy is limited by the penetration of the therapy into the tumor, which is usually only a few millimeters. Cisplatin has been extensively studied for intrapleural therapy; unfortunately, this approach has not met with the same degree of success as has been seen with intraperitoneal administration of cisplatin for peritoneal mesothelioma.

Biologic and Targeted Therapies

Another approach to the treatment of malignant pleural mesothelioma has been the use of biological agents, including the interferons, other cytokines such as IL-2, gene therapy, and vaccines. In addition, the identification of growth regulatory pathways has opened new vistas and targets for therapeutic intervention such as the inhibition of the vascular proliferation and various cell growth signals. Indeed, these therapeutic approaches offer the opportunity of developing more individualized therapies.

Biologic Therapies

The interferons (IFNs) offer the possibility of augmenting the immune recognition of the tumor by the host immune system. Preclinical studies showed that malignant mesothelioma cell lines were susceptible to IFN-α alone and enhanced in combination with other cytokines such as IFN-γ and tumor necrosis factor (TNF) as well as chemotherapy. Both IFN-β and IFN-γ also showed in vitro activity. These data served as the rationale for clinical trials with the IFNs (Table 97-6). The trial of intrapleural IFN-γ in asbestos-exposed individuals involved pleuroscopy at the earliest sign of effusion. When tumor was identified, IFN-γ was instilled via the pleuroscope, and the procedure was repeated for subsequent evaluation. While the overall response was 20%, patients with stage IA disease had a 45% response, with eight confirmed complete responses, and a prolonged disease-free survival. The interferons produced considerable sys-

temic toxicities, including fever, nausea, vomiting, chill, myalgias, and anorexia. Intrapleural therapy also produced some empyema.

Interleukin-2 (IL-2) stimulates activated lymphocytes and has an antiproliferative effect on mesothelioma cell lines. Intrapleural interleukin-2 in mesothelioma has met with variable results (see Table 97-6) and considerable systemic toxicities. The combination of tumor necrosis factor + IFN-γ was toxic and without efficacy.

Combinations of chemotherapy and immunotherapy have been evaluated. The majority of these trials combined chemotherapy with IFN-α (Table 97-7). The combination of doxorubicin plus IFN-α produces a modest response with unacceptable toxicity. IFN-α at two different doses plus cisplatin produces a composite response of 33%, but the toxicities, including nausea, vomiting, fever, anorexia, and asthenia, were unacceptable. IFN-α plus mitomycin and cisplatin produces a 23% response rate but does not appear to produce a survival benefit when compared to a group who refused therapy and produced a response similar to that of mitomycin and cisplatin chemotherapy alone in other studies. The combination of high-dose methotrexate and systemic IFN-α and IFN-γ produced a 29% response rate, similar to that seen for high-dose methotrexate alone.

Table 97-6 ■ Clinical Trials of Interferons and Other Cytokines in Malignant Mesothelioma

Agent	Route	Number Entered	Percent Responding
IFN-α	Systemic	38	11%
IFN-γ	Intrapleural	89	20%
IL-2	Intrapleural infusion	37	55%
IL-2	Intrapleural	21	19%
TNF + IFN-γ	Intramuscularly	36	3%

Table 97-7 ■ Chemoimmunotherapy for Malignant Mesothelioma

Chemotherapy	Immunotherapy	Number Entered	Percent Responding
Doxorubicin	IFN-α	25	16%
Cisplatin	IFN-α	55	33%
Cisplatin + mitomycin	IFN-α	43	14%
High-dose methotrexate	IFN-α + γ	24	29%

Postoperative Therapies

Despite the lack of clearly defined useful combinations and combined modality therapies, chemotherapy and radiotherapy have been added to surgical extirpation and stripping procedures. There have been no randomized trials to validate this approach. Most decortication techniques added radiotherapy to enhance local control. In contrast, both radiotherapy and chemotherapy have been applied in series of extrapleural pneumonectomy.

Neoadjuvant Therapies

Given the complexity of the surgical choices, any therapies that produce a consistent response that might downstage disease, make the surgical planes more easily achieved, or control microscopic disease could prove very useful. Unfortunately, the number of effective regimens remains relatively sparse.

References

Aisner J: Diagnosis, staging, and natural history of pleural mesothelioma. In Aisner J, Arriagada R, Green MR, Martini N, Perry MC (eds): Comprehensive Textbook of Thoracic Oncology. Baltimore: Williams and Wilkins, 1996, pp 786–798.

Aversa SML, Favaretto AG: Carboplatin and gemcitabine chemotherapy for malignant pleural mesothelioma: A phase II study of the GSTPV. Clin Lung Cancer 1999;1:73–75.

Benard F, Sterman D, Smith RJ, et al: Metabolic imaging of malignant pleural mesothelioma with fluorodeoxyglucose positron emission tomography. Chest 1998;114:713–722.

Bissett D, Macbeth FR, Cram I: The role of palliative radiotherapy in malignant mesothelioma of the pleura. Clin Oncol 1991;3:315.

Boutin C, Nussbaum E, Monnet I, et al: Intrapleural treatment with recombinant gamma interferon in early stage malignant pleural mesothelioma. Cancer 1994;74:2460–2467.

Boutin C, Rey F: Thoracoscopy in pleural malignant mesothelioma: A prospective study of 188 patients. Part 1: Diagnosis. Cancer 1993;72:389–393.

Boutin C, Rey F, Gouvernet J, et al: Thoracoscopy in pleural malignant mesothelioma: A prospective study of 188 consecutive patients. Part 2: Prognosis and staging. Cancer 1993;72:394–404.

Boutin C, Rey F, Viallat JR: Prevention of malignant seeding after invasive diagnostic procedures in patients with pleural mesothelioma: A randomized trial of local radiotherapy. Chest 1995;108:754–758.

Byrne MJ, Davidson JA, Musk AW, et al: Cisplatin and gemcitabine for malignant mesothelioma: A phase II study. J Clin Oncol. 1999;17:25–30.

Corson J, Renshaw AA: Pathology of mesothelioma. In Aisner J, Arriagada R, Green MR, Martini N, Perry MC (eds): Comprehensive Textbook of Thoracic Oncology. Baltimore: Williams and Wilkins, 1996, pp 757–778.

Fry DW: Inhibition of the epidermal growth factor receptor family of the tyrosine kinases as an approach to cancer chemotherapy: Progression from reversible to irreversible inhibitors. Pharmacol Ther 1999;82:207–218.

Heelan RT, Rusch VW, Begg CB, et al: Staging of malignant pleural mesothelioma: Comparison of CT and MR imaging. Am J Roentgenol 1999;172:1039–1047.

Kindler H, Belani CP, Herndon J, et al: Edatrexate (10-ethyl—deaza-aminopterin) (NSC:626715) with or without leukovorin rescue for malignant mesothelioma: Sequential phase II trials by the CALGB. Cancer 1999;86:1985–1991.

Kindler HL, Millard F, Herndon JE II, et al: Gemcitabine for malignant mesothelioma: A phase II trial by the Cancer and Leukemia Group B. Lung Cancer 2001;31:311–317.

Maasilta P: Deterioration in lung function following hemithorax irradiation for pleural mesothelioma. Int J Radiat Oncol Biol Phys 1991;20:433–438.

McDonald IC, McDonald AD: The epidemiology of mesothelioma in historical context. Eur Respir J 1992;9:1932–1942.

Nowak AK, Lake RA, Kindler HL, et al: New approaches for mesothelioma: Biologics, vaccines, gene therapy, and other novel agents. Semin Oncol 2002;29:82–96.

Ong ST, Vogelzang NJ: Chemotherapy in malignant pleural mesothelioma: A review. J Clin Oncol 1996;14:1007–1017.

Peto J, Decarli A, La Vecchia C, et al: The European mesothelioma epidemic. Br J Cancer 1999;79:666–672.

Pogrebniak HW, Lubensky IA, Pass HI: Differential expression of platelet-derived growth growth factor-beta in malignant mesothelioma: A clue to future therapies? Surg Oncol 1993;2:235–240.

Risberg B, Nickels J, Wagermark J: Familial clustering of malignant mesothelioma. Cancer 1980;45:2422.

Rusch VW, Godwin JD, Shuman WP: The role of computed tomography scanning in the initial assessment and follow-up of malignant pleural mesothelioma. J Thorac Cardiovasc Surg 1988;96:171–177.

Rusch VW, Ventkatraman ES: Important prognostic factors in patients with malignant pleural mesothelioma, managed surgically. Ann Thorac Surg 1999;68:1799–1804.

Shin DM, Scagliotti G, Kindler H, et al: A phase II trial of pemetrexed in malignant pleural mesothelioma (MPM) patients: Clinical outcome, role of vitamin supplementation, respiratory symptoms, and lung function. Proc Am Soc Clin Oncol 2002;21:294a.

Solheim OP, Saeter G, Finnanger AM, Stenwig AE: High dose methotrexate in the treatment of malignant mesothelioma of the pleura. Br J Cancer 1992;65:956–996.

Steele JPC, Shamash J, Evans MT, et al: Phase II study of vinorelbine in patients with malignant pleural mesothelioma. J Clin Oncol 2000;3912–3918.

Sterman DH, Kaiser LR, Albelda SM: Advances in the treatment of malignant pleural mesothelioma. Chest 1999;116:504–520.

Strizzi L, Catalano A, Vianale G, et al: Vascular endothelial growth factor is an autocrine growth factor in human malignant mesothelioma. J Pathol 2001;193:468–475.

Sugarbaker DJ, Flores R, Jacklitsch M, et al: Resection margins, extrapleural nodal status, and cell type determine postoperative long-term survival in trimodality therapy of malignant pleural mesothelioma. J Thorac Cardiovasc Surg 1999;117:54–65.

Vogelzang NJ, Weissman LB, Herndon JE, et al: Trimetrexate in malignant mesothelioma: A CALGB phase II study. J Clin Oncol 1994;12:1436–1442.

Wanebo HJ, Martini N, Melamed MR, et al: Pleural mesothelioma. Cancer 1986;38:2481–2488.

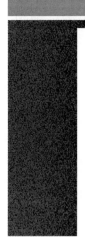

Head and Neck Cancer

Chapter 98
Primary Head and Neck Cancer

Fadlo R. Khuri and Edward S. Kim

Introduction

Head and neck cancers are among the major causes of cancer-related death. In the United States alone, head and neck cancers are the fifth most common cancer, with more than 40,000 new cases and 14,000 deaths annually. Worldwide, more than 500,000 cases of head and neck cancers are diagnosed annually. Despite substantial progress that has been made in the areas of surgery, concomitant chemoradiotherapy, and intensity-modulated radiation therapy over the past few decades, the five-year survival rate has improved only slightly over the last 40 years. The high mortality rate makes head and neck cancers a worldwide public health menace.

Head and neck cancers also cause considerable morbidity. They can result in devastating effects on speech, swallowing, and cosmetic appearance, all of which contribute to impaired self-esteem and depression. Second or metachronous primary cancers are a common problem in this patient group (see Chapter 99). Even those patients who are fortunate enough to be cured of this illness often succumb to a second, smoking-related cancer. The development of second malignancies is in large part responsible for the failure to improve overall survival, despite improvements in control of primary tumors.

Many different anatomic sites constitute the upper aerodigestive tract where cancer can develop. Cancer in each location has some distinctive features. This chapter discusses the major sites of head and neck cancers, namely cancers of the larynx, hypopharynx, cervical esophagus, oropharynx, oral cavity, and nasopharynx, emphasizing the principles common to the staging and evaluation of all head and neck cancers and elaborating on therapy of the individual disorders.

Epidemiology

The major risk factors in the development of head and neck cancers are alcohol abuse and smoking. In 1953, Slaughter et al reported that upper aerodigestive tract carcinogenesis involves a process of "field cancerization." Repeated exposure of the entire mucosal lining of the upper aerodigestive tract (the field) to carcinogenic agents—for example, human papillomavirus, tobacco, and alcohol—creates a risk for the development of multiple independent premalignant and malignant foci. Oral mucosal lesions, such as leukoplakia, can appear as a result. Injury to the upper aerodigestive tract produces genetic changes, including loss of heterozygosity at the chromosomal loci 9p21 and 3p14. Mucosal samples taken from patients with known leukoplakia were studied. Of 19 patients with loss of heterozygosity, seven (37%) subsequently developed squamous cell carcinoma, whereas only one of 18 patients (6%) without such changes developed head and neck cancer (P = 0.005). Although such clonal genetic alterations can precede overt cancer, no phase of leukoplakia or erythroplakia is observed in most patients who develop head and neck cancer. The ability to screen for head and neck cancer development is thus limited and made more difficult by the fact that most patients at risk also are poorly compliant with screening programs, in part due to inadequate social support systems and reduced access to routine health care. Although careful visual examination of the oral cavity and palpation of the intraoral surfaces are part of routine physical examinations, the detection of unsuspected asymptomatic cases is exceedingly rare. Routine screening for sporadic cases of head and neck cancer even among populations at risk is not cost effective. Moreover, the determination of which screening studies (such as panendoscopy) would be useful remains unclear. The best opportunity for early detection is, in fact, during routine dental care.

Clinical Evaluation of Head and Neck Cancers

Head and neck cancers generally present because of local symptoms and/or because the patient becomes aware of an enlarged cervical lymph node. The clinician needs to take a comprehensive history and perform a careful physical examination with special regard for medical conditions associated with tobacco and alcohol abuse, such as concurrent cardiac and liver disease. Routine laboratory studies (e.g., liver function tests) are used to determine the degree of organ involvement by concurrent medical conditions. Many of these patients have varyingly severe chronic obstructive pulmonary disease from years of smoking. A general nutritional assessment is also warranted, for these patients are not infrequently undernourished. Understanding the patient's general medical status is essential to treatment planning in order to determine the intensity of therapy that can be administered safely.

Otolaryngologists usually are responsible for the diagnosis of a specific site of disease and evaluation of the extent of disease. Diagnosis is obtained by biopsy of the affected area. In the case of isolated cervical node enlargement, biopsy of the cervical lymph node to determine whether metastatic cancer is present is usually necessary before a search for the primary site is made. One needs to be aware of the possibility that enlarged cervical lymph nodes can be due to a hematologic malignancy, an inflammatory process, or infection. Metastases to lower cervical lymph nodes or supraclavicular nodes are usually from lung cancer or gastrointestinal (GI) malignancies, whereas metastases to high cervical lymph nodes are usually from cancers of the head and neck.

Magnetic resonance imaging and/or computed tomography scans are used to evaluate the local extent of disease fully for staging purposes. The information they offer is complementary. Magnetic resonance imaging is especially useful in defining the limits of the primary tumor and detecting extension into soft tissues, whereas computed tomography is better at detecting metastases and bone destruction. The cervi-

cal lymph nodes might be mildly enlarged due to non-malignant disease, such as gum infections. For this reason, the results of computed tomography scans of the cervical lymph nodes are not included in staging considerations. Categorization of the extent of lymph node involvement is based on clinical data from the physical examination and, if necessary, from biopsy. Apart from regional lymph node involvement, the next most common site of metastasis is the lung. Chest X-ray is a routine part of the initial evaluation, and many clinicians include a computed tomography scan of the chest as well.

Once the diagnosis is established, the patient should have full dental evaluation, because these patients often have periodontal disease, dental abscesses, and dental caries. These should be corrected prior to definitive therapy to prevent later complications.

Panendoscopy, which includes bronchoscopy, esophagoscopy, and laryngoscopy, is advocated by some as essential to the evaluation of patients with a documented head and neck cancer. The intent is to search for second primary malignancies in the aerodigestive tract. These are so rarely detected at the time of diagnosis of the initial primary tumor, however, that most clinicians do not perform panendoscopy unless the patient's symptoms direct attention to other potential areas of disease.

Pathology

Nearly all malignant tumors of the head and neck arise from the surface epithelium; squamous cell carcinoma occurs in more than 90% of cases. Uncommon variants of squamous cell carcinomas include

- verrucous carcinomas, which have a more favorable prognosis and are considered a low-grade malignancy;
- basaloid squamous carcinomas, which are a more aggressive variant of squamous cell carcinoma; and
- sarcomatoid carcinoma, an aggressive spindle cell variant of squamous cell carcinoma with an often infiltrative and rapid growth pattern. The mean survival time of sarcomatoid carcinoma is less than two years from diagnosis.

Spindle cell carcinoma and salivary gland tumors such as adenoid cystic carcinoma, mucoepidermoid carcinoma, and acinar cell carcinoma are much less common. Together, cartilaginous tumors (e.g., chondroma or chondrosarcoma) and neuroendocrine tumors (including paraganglioma, large cell, and small cell neuroendocrine tumors) represent less than 5% of all head and neck cancers. Squamous cell carcinomas with lymphoid stroma (lymphoepithe-liomas) and non-Hodgkin's lymphomas account for a small fraction of cases.

Staging of Head and Neck Cancers

An outline of the approach to staging head and neck cancer by the TNM classification appears in Table 98-1. The system for classifying cancers of the oral cavity or oropharynx, the hypopharynx, nasopharynx, and various levels of involvement of the larynx is shown.

Although other, less frequent sites of head and neck cancer use somewhat different T classification parameters, Table 98-1 provides a useful framework for interpreting staging information.

Some general considerations are listed below.

- The M classification for the presence of metastases is the same for all head and neck cancers.
- The N classification of cervical lymph node involvement is the same for all head and neck cancers.

Table 98-1 ■ The TNM Classification of Head and Neck Cancers

M Classification

| M0 | No metastases |
| M1 | Distant metastases |

N Classification

N0	No regional lymph nodes involved
N1	Single ipsilateral lymph node measuring ≤3 cm in diameter
N2	Single ipsilateral lymph node measuring >3 cm and ≤6 cm in diameter or multiple lymph nodes, all ≤6 cm in diameter or bilateral or contralateral lymph nodes ≤6 cm in diameter
N3	Any regional lymph node measuring >6 cm in diameter

T Classification for Common Oropharyngeal Cancers

Site	Oral Cavity or Oropharynx	Hypopharynx	Nasopharynx
T1	Tumor ≤2 cm in diameter	Tumor ≤2 cm in diameter	Confined to single site in nasopharynx
T2	Tumor >2 cm but ≤4 cm in diameter	Tumor >2 cm, but ≤4 cm or > one site	Extends to oropharynx or to nasal fossa
T3	Tumor >4 cm in diameter	Tumor >4 cm or larynx is fixed	Invades bones or sinuses
T4	Tumor invades adjacent structures	Tumor invades adjacent structures	Intracranial extension

T Classification for Cancer of the Larynx

Site	Supraglottic	Glottic	Infraglottic
T1	Confined to a single site, normal vocal cord mobility	Confined to a single site, normal vocal cord mobility	Confined to a single site, normal vocal cord mobility
T2	More than one adjacent area involved	Extends to supra- or subglottis, vocal cord mobility impaired	Extends to vocal cords, normal or impaired cord mobility
T3	Limited to larynx + fixed vocal cord or invades outside immediate area	Limited to larynx, vocal cord fixed	Limited to larynx, vocal cord fixed
T4	Extends through cricoid or thyroid cartilage or into soft tissues of the neck or the esophagus	Extends through cricoid or thyroid cartilage or into soft tissues of the neck or esophagus	Extends through cricoid or thyroid cartilage or into soft tissues of the neck or the esophagus

Stage of Disease Based on TNM Classification Groupings

Stage	TNM Classification
I	T1, N0, M0
II	T2, N0, M0
II	T1/T2, N1, M0
	T3, N0/N1, M0
IV	T4, N0/N1, M0
	Any T, N2/N3, M0
	Any T, Any N, M1

Slight variations from these groupings in stages II and IV occur in the different head and neck cancers; these are aggregated here for simplification of the discussion in the text. Consult staging manuals for a more detailed presentation of TNM stage groupings.

■ The T classification is based on the size of the primary tumor for oropharyngeal or hypopharyngeal cancers or, in the case of nasopharyngeal and laryngeal carcinomas, on the degree of extension to other sites.

■ Once clinical lymph node involvement occurs, the patient has advanced disease (stage III or IV)

■ Patients whose tumors invade adjacent structures, regardless of lymph node involvement, or who have even a single lymph node measuring more than 3 cm in diameter, regardless of tumor size, have a prognosis similar to that of patients who have distant metastases (M1).

Cancer of the Larynx

Laryngeal cancer accounts for 2% of all cancers in the United States, affecting approximately 11,000 patients newly diagnosed each year and 4000 patients who die annually. Men are four times more likely to be affected than females. The frequency of sites of laryngeal cancer—supraglottic, glottic, or infraglottic—varies by country. The anatomic geographic variation in primary site suggests that some undefined factors play a role in carcinogenesis. Seventy-five percent of laryngeal cancers in the United States occur on the vocal folds (glottic region). At the time of diagnosis, 65% of cases are localized; only 5% of cases present with distant metastases. Although the major contributing factors are cigarette smoking and alcoholism, human papillomavirus has been implicated in verrucous carcinoma and oropharyngeal cancers occurring in nonsmokers.

Clinical Presentation

Patients with early glottic laryngeal cancer present with hoarseness. Patients with more locally advanced disease can present with odynophagia (painful swallowing), otalgia (ear pain), laryngeal pain, and stridor. On the other hand, supraglottic laryngeal cancers typically present with odynophagia, dysphagia, change in voice quality, a mass in the neck, or otalgia. Advanced supraglottic laryngeal cancer usually is associated with weight loss, malodorous breath, aspiration, and stridor. Finally, subglottic laryngeal cancers typically present with hoarseness in their early stages and with dyspnea, stridor, and airway obstruction when they are advanced.

Therapy

The primary goals of laryngeal cancer therapy are cure of the cancer and preservation of function, including voice quality and phonation. Patient compliance with follow-up and rehabilitation efforts substantially affects functional outcomes. Radiation therapy is the preferred treatment option for patients with early (T1–2, N0) glottic carcinoma, with local control and survival ranging from 70% to 90%. Multimodality therapy, which includes radiation therapy, chemotherapy, and surgery, is required for advanced laryngeal cancers.

Radiation Therapy for Laryngeal Cancer

Radiation therapy is typically delivered with Cobalt-60 gamma-rays or six MV X-rays, frequently in combination with six to 12 MeV electron beams. The choice of the beam type and the energy is based on the geometric parameters of the target volume. Brachytherapy has no role in the treatment of laryngeal cancer. The initial target volume for T1–2, N0, M0 glottic carcinomas is the larynx proper. Treatment of supraglottic carcinomas (even T1, N0, M0 tumors) targets the larynx as well as the subdigastric lymph nodes and midjugular lymph nodes. For T3, N0 glottic carcinomas and T2–3, N0 supraglottic carcinomas, the target volume is extended to include the larynx, the subdigastric lymph nodes, and the mid- and low-jugular nodes. Any abnormal lymphadenopathy, regardless of T-stage, necessitates treatment of the larynx and all cervical nodes. Frequently, a boost to the primary tumor (and to the involved nodes when these are present) is administered with 1 to 2 cm margins.

Recommended radiation doses for T1, N0 lesions are 50 GY to the initial target volume followed by a 16 GY boost to the primary tumor, delivered in 2-Gy fractions five times per week. More advanced tumors receive a larger boost or hyperfractionated, twice daily, radiation therapy in 1.2 GY fractions at six-hour intervals. The field is usually adjusted after 40 to 45 GY to spare the spinal cord. Involved nodes receive the same dose as the primary lesions.

Surgery for Laryngeal Cancer

Although radiation therapy is the preferred modality for treatment of early-stage laryngeal cancer, selective function-preserving laryngeal surgery can be performed. Surgical procedures include partial horizontal supraglottic laryngectomy, supra-cricoid laryngectomy, and vertical partial laryngectomy. Partial horizontal supraglottic laryngectomy can be performed for lesions of the epiglottis, ariepiglottic folds, and false cords, particularly when extension of the tumor into the base of the tongue is less than 10 mm. This procedure requires that the anterior glottic commissure be free of tumor and the hypopharyngeal mucosa have only minimal involvement. Partial horizontal supraglottic laryngectomy should be capable of achieving total gross tumor removal with salvage of at least one arytenoid.

Supra-cricoid laryngectomy with cricohyoidopexy

or cricohyoidalepiglottopexy could be suitable for glottic cancers with unilateral or bilateral involvement and minimal subglottic extension. This procedure could also be suitable for lesions of the epiglottis, false cords, anterior portion of the larynx, or the laryngeal ventricle. Supra-cricoid laryngectomy requires that subglottic extension be less than 10 mm at the anterior commissure and that the base of the tongue be free of tumor. It may be done in selected patients whose disease has recurred or persisted after radiation therapy. Although the epiglottis can be preserved, aspiration remains a major morbidity associated with this procedure.

Vertical partial laryngectomy is an elegant procedure developed for glottic cancer. This procedure requires that subglottic extension be confined to 10 mm anteriorly and 5 mm at the level of the arytenoid. It may be used in selected T2–3 stage cancers or for patients who relapse after radiation therapy. Again, it is necessary to preserve at least one arytenoid and the posterior two-thirds of the less affected vocal cord. Two problems associated with this procedure are aspiration pneumonia and formation of strictures at the level of the glottic/arytenoid mucosa.

Multimodality Therapy of Advanced Laryngeal Cancer

Multimodality therapy is the preferred approach for T3 or T4 tumors or any node-positive laryngeal cancer. Early trials demonstrated that total laryngectomy was superior to radiotherapy in terms of survival for patients with advanced laryngeal cancers, particularly T4 lesions with involvement of the cricoid or thyroid cartilage. Radiation therapy, however, resulted in a superior quality of life. Chemotherapy was therefore considered as a way to possibly preserve the larynx in patients with advanced laryngeal cancer. The results of multiple studies in advanced laryngeal and other advanced head and neck cancers are outlined in Table 98-2. Early studies showed that combinations of cisplatin and 5-fluorouracil induced a pathologic

complete response in approximately 30% to 35% of patients. These patients, when treated with subsequent radiation therapy, had a superior survival compared with patients who achieved only a partial pathologic response. Moreover, tumor sensitivity to radiation therapy correlated directly with sensitivity to chemotherapy. Preservation of the larynx is possible in advanced laryngeal cancer with combined chemotherapy and radiation therapy. A VA trial randomized 332 patients with T2–4, N0–3 squamous cell carcinoma of the larynx to one of two approaches: either surgery (generally a total laryngectomy) followed by postoperative radiation therapy, or initial cytoreductive chemotherapy with cisplatin and 5-fluorouracil for two to three cycles (depending on the response) followed by definitive radiation therapy. Individuals who failed to achieve at least a partial response to the first two cycles of chemotherapy were treated with total laryngectomy and postoperative radiotherapy.

Results showed equivalent survival extending out beyond 10 years. Local and regional failures were more common in patients receiving chemotherapy, whereas distant metastatic failures were more frequent among patients undergoing total laryngectomy and postoperative radiation therapy. Approximately two-thirds of patients who received induction chemotherapy responded sufficiently well to avoid laryngectomy over long-term follow-up. The survival of the 15% of patients who did not respond to chemotherapy and underwent delayed total laryngectomy and postoperative radiation therapy was identical to the patients who were randomized to this therapy initially. Thus, induction chemotherapy followed by radiation therapy is an effective approach for most patients with advanced laryngeal cancer, and the attempt at organ preservation does not prejudice their long-term survival. The results of combined-modality therapy can be improved by the administration of radiation therapy concurrently rather than sequen-

Table 98-2 ■ Randomized Trials of Combined Chemotherapy and Radiation Therapy versus Radiation Therapy in Advanced Head and Neck Cancer

Author	N	Chemotherapy	Radiation Therapy	Regional Control Chemotherapy + Radiation Versus Radiation	Survival Chemotherapy + Radiation Versus Radiation
Merlano	157	Cisplatin, 5-FU	60–70 Gy	64% vs. 32% (P = 0.038)	24% vs. 10% (P = 0.01) at five years
Wendt	270	Cisplatin, 5-FU	70 Gy, split	36% vs. 17% (P = < 0.004)	48% vs. 24% (P = 0.0003) at three years
Calais	226	Carbo, 5-FU	70 Gy	66% vs. 42% (P = 0.03)	51% vs. 31% (P = 0.02) at three years
Adelstein	295	Cisplatin	70 Gy		37% vs. 20% (P = 0.016) at three years

Carbo = carboplatin; 5-FU = 5-fluorouracil; MMC = mitomycin C; ChemoRad = chemotherapy and radiation therapy; Rad = radiation therapy.

tially after chemotherapy, without significant worsening of toxicity. Such therapy has become the standard of care in patients with advanced laryngeal cancer who, because they do not have bilateral cervical lymph node metastases, are not at high risk of distant metastases.

Recurrent or Metastatic Laryngeal Cancer

The results of treatment of recurrent or metastatic laryngeal cancer are the same as for other recurrent or metastatic squamous cell cancers of the head and neck. Overall response rates for recurrent or metastatic laryngeal cancer to frontline chemotherapy regimens (such as 5-fluorouracil and cisplatin) are 35% to 40%, and median survivals are approximately six months. Single-institution phase II studies of three-drug regimens containing a taxane and a platinum compound (such as paclitaxel), ifosfamide, and cisplatin or the combination of docetaxel, cisplatin, and 5-fluorouracil, reported increased response rates compared with two-drug regimens, and median survivals of eight to 10 months. Favorable patient selection of patients able to tolerate the increased toxicity, however, might explain the perceived benefit. The issue of toxicity is a factor in treatment selection for those patients with a limited projected survival. For example, the combination of paclitaxel and cisplatin is less toxic than cisplatin and 5-fluorouracil, while being equally efficacious.

Cancer of the Hypopharynx and Cervical Esophagus

Although microvascular reconstruction has improved the local management of patients with hypopharyngeal and cervical esophageal cancer, it has contributed little to lengthening their survival. The management of these patients requires a multidisciplinary team of head and neck surgeons, reconstructive surgeons, thoracic surgeons, radiation oncologists, medical oncologists, speech therapists, nutritionists, diagnostic radiologists, pathologists, and specialty nurses. This multidisciplinary approach increases the likelihood of organ preservation and improves quality of life.

Clinical Presentation and Patterns of Spread

The hypopharynx and cervical esophagus drain extensively into the subdigastric, upper, middle, and inferior jugular nodes, and the lateral and retropharyngeal lymphatic basins. Metastases to the paratracheal lymph nodes or superior mediastinum often presage distant metastases. Progression of the cancer is most often initially by submucosal extension. This should be anticipated in every hypopharyngeal and cervical

esophageal cancer. Paraneural extension along cervical sympathetics, vagus, and glossopharyngeal nerves is also common. Medial extension of cancers arising in the piriform sinus can fixate the larynx, and extension into the subglottic area causes stridor and impaired phonation. Lateral extension of piriform sinus cancers through the thyrohyoid membrane and the thyroid cartilage is frequently observed, resulting in invasion of the parathyroid and thyroid glands. Extension substantially increases the likelihood of lymph node metastases, which complicate the therapy of these tumors. The vast majority of affected patients present with T3–T4 tumors and at least one lymph node that is more than 3 cm—i.e., at least stage N2 according to the TNM classification.

Treatment of Early-Stage Hypopharyngeal Cancer

The detection of early-stage (T1–T2) hypopharyngeal cancers without nodal involvement is extremely rare. The preferred treatment for such patients is definitive radiation therapy to the primary site of cancer and to the draining lymphatic basin. This approach provides adequate organ preservation, providing the regional lymph nodes are included in the radiation therapy field.

With surgery, on the other hand, laryngeal conservation is possible in only about one-half of the early-stage patients, although surgical resection can be effective in controlling primary disease. Surgical approaches include transoral/microlaryngeal laser-assisted approaches, lateral pharyngectomy, and suprahyoid/infrahyoid laryngectomy, mandibulotomy, and/or glossotomy. Radical lymph node dissection is required at the time of surgery due to the high incidence of occult metastases.

Treatment of Advanced-Stage Hypopharyngeal Cancer

More than 80% of patients with hypopharyngeal tumors present with T3–T4 primaries and/or clinical evidence of nodal disease. Surgical therapy includes total laryngectomy with a partial or total pharyngectomy followed by postoperative irradiation, especially if lymph node metastases are present. Piriform sinus primary tumors also undergo unilateral thyroidectomy and bilateral paratracheal lymph node dissections.

Equivalent survivals were noted in stages III and IV hypopharyngeal cancer in randomized trials comparing chemotherapy plus radiation therapy with total laryngectomy plus radiation therapy.

One needs to be aware of the fact that even with organ-preserving therapy, some compromise of function is likely to occur, and many of these patients will still require tracheostomy and gastric feeding tubes. Moreover, regardless of the approach to therapy, the survival rates of patients with stage III or IV hypopharyngeal cancer are dismal. The five-year survival is less than 20%, and surgical salvage for recurrent disease is feasible in less than 15%. These results compare unfavorably with most other squamous cell cancers of the head and neck.

Selection of Therapy in Hypopharyngeal Cancer

The choice of surgery or radiation therapy depends on the site of the primary tumor. Patients with hypopharyngeal wall involvement require radiation therapy alone for early-stage disease and have a 47% survival at three years. Surgery can be used as salvage for patients with residual disease after radiation therapy or combined chemotherapy and radiation therapy, resulting in a 41% survival at two years. Surgical salvage of patients with advanced hypopharyngeal or cervical esophageal cancer who have failed to respond to primary chemotherapy, radiation therapy, or initial surgery, however, results in poor long-term survival; only 15% of such patients survive for five years. Finally, although esophagectomy is not necessary in hypopharyngeal cancers with minimal cervicoesophageal extension, it is generally necessary in the patients presenting with more advanced disease.

Cancer of the Oropharynx

The oropharynx is one of the most common sites of head and neck cancers in the United States. Within the oropharynx, the sites of involvement by cancer, in order of decreasing frequency, are

- the tonsillar region
- the base of the tongue
- the soft palate
- the pharyngeal wall

The base of the tongue plays a crucial role in swallowing, as it propels the food bolus from the oropharynx into the hypopharynx. The soft palate must close off the oropharynx from the nasopharynx during swallowing to prevent nasopharyngeal regurgitation of food. The soft palate and base of the tongue also have important functions in phonation. Cancers in these various areas can disrupt normal function significantly.

Clinical Presentation and Pattern of Spread

Early base of tongue tumors grow either in an exophytic or (more typically) according to a submucosal infiltrative pattern, invading the intrinsic tongue muscles. With progression, tongue-based tumors can extend anteroinferiorly through the intrinsic tongue muscles and involve the extrinsic muscles, spreading laterally via the glossopharyngeal sulcus to the tonsillar fossa and pharyngeal wall and then inferiorly into the preepiglottic space, hypopharynx, and larynx. Very advanced tumors can extend into the soft tissues of the neck. Invasion can extend all the way through the mandibular cortex in rare instances. Conversely, tumors originating in the tonsillar fossa can grow as exophytic masses extending into the oropharyngeal airspace, or spreading into the tonsillar pillar or medially along the soft palate. Such tumors can also spread across the glossopharyngeal sulcus into the tongue base or posteriorly to the posterior tonsillar pillar and lateral pharyngeal wall. More advanced tonsillar fossa tumors can extend laterally into the pterygoid muscles, superiorly into the nasopharynx, and inferiorly into the piriform sinus. Invasion of the extrinsic muscles of the root of the tongue can impair tongue mobility, and significant infiltration of the pterygoid muscles can cause trismus (clenched jaw due to spasm of the masseter muscles).

Soft palate tumors almost always arise on the oral surface and grow superficially along the mucosal surfaces, with advanced tumors spreading down the interior tonsillar pillars into the tonsillar fossa and pharyngeal wall. Most of these tumors present with odynophagia, trismus, and dysphagia. The frequency of nodal involvement at diagnosis in patients with soft-palate carcinoma is approximately 40%.

Treatment of Early-Stage Oropharyngeal Cancer

Oropharyngeal tumors—particularly cancers of the tonsil and tonsillar pillar—are usually sensitive to both chemotherapy and radiation therapy. High local control rates can be achieved with radiation therapy to both the primary tumor and the neck nodes. Well lateralized tonsillar carcinoma with limited neck disease can occasionally be treated with radiation therapy alone to the primary site and ipsilateral lymph nodes. Excellent functional outcome can be achieved. Whether they are treated with radiation therapy alone or with combined-modality therapy, however, some patients later develop problems with swallowing function.

High local control rates are also achieved by surgery of early-stage oropharynx cancer; radiation therapy, however, is the preferred primary modality for T1, N2, M0 disease, for several reasons:

1. Postoperative radiotherapy is required for patients with positive resection margins, perineural inva-

sion, involvement of more than one lymph node, or extracapsular nodal extension.

2. Resection of the soft palate and base of tongue leads to substantial functional losses resulting in nasal regurgitation, speech and swallowing deficits, and dysphagia, which inevitably require a prolonged and difficult period of rehabilitation.

3. Other complex surgical procedures also result in substantial morbidity.

Treatment of Advanced-Stage Oropharyngeal Cancer

Concomitant chemotherapy and radiation therapy is the optimal approach for patients with advanced cancer of the oropharynx (T3–T4, N2–N3), as this approach improves both local control and survival compared with radiation therapy alone (see Table 98-2). A phase III trial in patients with advanced-stage oropharyngeal carcinoma compared radiation therapy with or without concurrent chemotherapy using three cycles of carboplatin and 5-fluorouracil. The local recurrence rates were 51% for patients receiving radiation therapy alone but only 33% in the patients who received chemoradiation. Three-year actuarial survival was 51% in the combined-modality arm vs. 31% in the radiotherapy arm (P = 0.02). Other studies have confirmed these data, making concomitant chemoradiotherapy of advanced oropharynx cancer the standard of care. Intensified chemotherapy treatment programs combined with standard or intensified radiation therapy regimens can achieve pathologic complete remissions in patients with advanced disease, but these have so far proved to be too toxic, impairing the quality of life.

Although response rates to chemotherapy for metastatic tumors of oropharyngeal origin tend to be higher than for tumors of hypopharyngeal or oral cavity origin, the role of chemotherapy for recurrent or metastatic oropharynx cancer remains palliative.

Oral Cavity Cancer

Cancer of the oral cavity is the most prevalent tumor of the upper aerodigestive tract, with 22,000 new cases in the United States annually; it is the cause of death in 6000 individuals each year. Primary site locations include the lips, tongue, floor of mouth, buccal mucosa, alveolar ridge, retromolar trigone, and hard palate. Sun exposure is a risk factor for the development of lip cancer. Cigarettes, smokeless tobacco products, exposure to second-hand smoke, alcohol consumption, and chewing of betel nuts are all carcinogenic. Although certain genetic polymorphisms and dietary and nutritional syndromes (such as Plummer-Vinson syndrome) can also be associated with this disease, oral cavity cancer remains largely a disease of chronically inhaled or smokeless tobacco exposure.

Clinical Presentation and Pattern of Spread

Oral cavity cancer frequently presents with pain related to the site of disease, local invasion of pain-sensitive structures, ulceration, and local infection. Disease extension can include mandibular spread from the lips, floor of the mouth, buccal mucosa, mandibular alveolus, and retromolar trigone; maxillary spread

---

TREATMENT

Selection of Patients with Advanced Oropharyngeal Cancer and Bulky Neck Disease for Neck Dissection

Patients who present with locally advanced disease of the oropharynx or with bulky neck nodal disease should be considered for concurrent chemoradiation therapy. Several randomized trials established that concurrent chemoradiation is superior to radiation alone in terms of local control, time to progression, and most importantly, overall survival. Nevertheless, although concurrent treatment is highly effective in achieving local control, survival is not improved, and quality of life diminishes markedly during and immediately following chemoradiation therapy. Careful consideration needs to be given to the balance between the increase in toxicity of initial therapy and the benefit of decreasing local recurrence, with its distressing (and often overwhelming) symptomatology.

In patients undergoing concurrent chemoradiation therapy, a neck dissection could be appropriate if the following criteria are met:

- radiographic or clinical evidence of residual disease in the neck
- residual disease no longer responding to radiation therapy
- performance status of the patient adequate to undertake the neck dissection
- complete resection of the residual neck mass feasible
- no active infection or comorbid condition

from hard and soft palate cancer; and bony invasion from affected mucosa overlying the bone such as the gingiva, hard palate, or retromolar trigone. Bone invasion is also common with squamous cell cancers located in the floor of the mouth or the tongue and indicates highly aggressive disease. Other locoregional problems include perineural invasion of the lingual nerve, hypoglossal nerve, omental nerve, and mandibular nerve. These patients often present with ear pain (otalgia) due to referred pain from cranial nerves V, IX, and X; other presentations can include perioral ulcers, white or reddish plaques, bleeding lesions in the mouth, masses, or throat pain. Patients also can present with a primary neck mass, halitosis, trismus, or speech impairment. In advanced disease, systemic symptoms—including anorexia, weight loss, fatigue, weakness, and malaise—often develop.

Therapy for Early-Stage Oral Cavity Cancer

Treatment of early oral cavity cancer varies according to site. Lip cancer has the best survival, with five-year disease-free survival rates for squamous cell cancers of the lower lip ranging from 70% to 90% and of the upper lip from 40% to 60%. Although surgery is the dominant initial therapy for early- to intermediate-stage oral cancer, generally involving the transoral approach for most anterior lesions of the tongue and a mandibulotomy approach for more posterior lesions, the goal is to avoid a total glossectomy for all but the most extensive tumors. Total glossectomies often can require laryngectomies to diminish the risk of chronic aspiration. Occult neck node metastases are present in up to 40% of patients. Elective neck dissections are performed in clinically node-negative patients who have T3–T4 primary lesions or tumors with depths greater than 4 mm. Patients with small primary tumors might require only supraomahyoid neck dissections. Early-stage tumors have excellent five-year locoregional control rates of 91% and survival rates of 55–62% with local therapy. Advanced-stage tumors have a three-year survival of only 40% to 50%, even with multimodality therapy.

Treatment of Advanced-Stage Oral Cavity Cancer

Multimodality therapy has become the standard approach for advanced oral cavity cancer. For advanced disease—namely, lip lesions greater than 2 cm or those involving the commissure—combined surgery and postoperative radiation therapy is the preferred approach. Such combinations provide a primary tumor control rate of at least 85%, depending on the size and the presence of nodal disease. Better surgical reconstructive techniques have resulted in preserva-tion of function. Primary radiation therapy is recommended only for patients at high risk for complications from prolonged anesthesia, as several studies have indicated that surgery yields a superior survival and substantial local control advantages. An exception could be T1–T2 tumors within the retromolar trigone or anterior fossa pillar, where good results can be obtained with external beam radiotherapy, even when it is administered through lateral ports to preserve salivary function.

Postoperative radiation therapy is always given to patients with close or positive surgical resection margins. Adjuvant postoperative nodal irradiation is indicated with larger primary tumors (T3–T4) or when perineural spread is documented. The presence of cervical node metastasis is the most reliable predictor of poor outcome for squamous cell cancers of the oral cavity. Particularly poor prognostic signs are the presence of extracapsular spread and involvement of multiple cervical lymph nodes. A supraomahyoid neck dissection is recommended for all lesions except a small T1 primary. A modified neck dissection should be performed in patients who have a greater than T1 primary tumor, or who have evidence of lymph node involvement on physical examination or CT scan evidence for nodal disease. Postoperative radiation therapy to the neck is warranted in patients who have more than one lymph node involved or evidence of extracapsular spread.

Chemotherapy in Oral Cavity Cancers

Chemotherapy—particularly neoadjuvant chemotherapy prior to surgery—provides disappointing results in cancer of the oral cavity. Concurrent chemotherapy and radiation, however, appears to offer better locoregional control and modest survival advantages over neoadjuvant chemotherapy followed by radiation therapy or radiation therapy alone. Cisplatin at a dose of 100 mg/m^2 at three-week intervals is a commonly used regimen.

Therapy of Recurrent or Metastatic Squamous Cell Carcinoma of the Head and Neck

Single-agent response rates in metastatic or recurrent squamous cell carcinoma of the head and neck are shown in Table 98-3. Combination chemotherapy regimens improve the response rate without improving survival. Thus, although the combination of cisplatin and 5-fluorouracil remains the most frequently used regimen, in the absence of a meaningful survival advantage, no single regimen can be considered as the established treatment standard.

The most extensively studied newer agents are the taxanes (paclitaxel and docetaxel), which are among

Table 98-3 ■ Activity of Single Agents in Recurrent and Metastatic Head and Neck Squamous Cell Carcinoma

Chemotherapy	Number of Patients	Response Rate
Methotrexate	988	31%
Bleomycin	347	21%
Cisplatin	288	28%
Carboplatin	169	22%
5-Fluorouracil	118	15%
Ifosfamide	120	23%
Vinorelbine	102	18%
Paclitaxel in mg/m² (duration of administration):		
250 (24 hours)	73	40%
175 (24 hours)	41	20%
175 (3 hours)	60	15%
Docetaxel in mg/m²/hr:		
100	89	33%
60	23	30%
Gemcitabine	54	3%
Topotecan	43	14%

Table 98-4 ■ Biological Targets in the Therapy of Squamous Cell Carcinoma of the Head and Neck

Target	Class of Agent	Agent	Phase of Trials
Epidermal growth factor receptor	Monoclonal antibody	IMC225	II/III
Epidermal growth factor receptor	Tyrosine kinase inhibitor	ZD1839 051-774	II/III II/IV
RAS	Farnesyl transferase inhibitor	SCH66336 R115777	I/II
P53	Replication-selective adenovirus	ONYX-015	III
P53	Tumor suppressor gene-containing adenovirus	Adp53	III

that are responsible for continued proliferation of the transformed cells (Table 98-4).

Cancer of the Nasopharynx

Epidemiology

The epidemiology of nasopharyngeal cancer differs from that of other head and neck cancers. The incidence of cancer of the nasopharynx is highest in Southern China and Hong Kong but is also increasing in Saudi Arabia, Kuwait, Alaska, and North Africa. The people in these regions eat salt-cured foods. The cooking of these foods leads to dispersal of volatile carcinogenic nitrosamines on the nasal mucosa. The endemic nature of the disease in these areas might also be based on genetic susceptibility of these populations.

Pathology

Histologically, squamous cell carcinomas of the nasopharynx can be keratinizing, nonkeratinizing, or undifferentiated; the latter is the most common variant. The cancer has been called lymphoepithelioma because of the frequent admixture and infiltration of the tumor by lymphoid cells.

Clinical Presentation and Pattern of Spread

Nasopharyngeal carcinoma has the highest metastatic potential of all head and neck cancers; distant metastases occur in 40% to 70% of patients who have locally advanced disease, and regional lymph node metastases are present in more than 50%. The anatomy of the nasopharynx puts a number of

the most active single agents in head and neck cancer. A number of paclitaxel- and cisplatin-based combination chemotherapy regimens have been evaluated in squamous cell cancers of the head and neck. Small phase I/II trials using paclitaxel as part of a cisplatin-containing regimen report improved response rates and survival duration in comparison with historical controls treated with cisplatin and 5-fluorouracil. In an effort to reduce the substantial nephrotoxicity, neurotoxicity, ototoxicity, and GI toxicity that occur with cisplatin-containing combination therapy, carboplatin has been substituted in clinical trials. In a trial of the combination of paclitaxel, ifosfamide, and carboplatin, the overall response rate was 58%, median survival was nine months, and two-year survival was 18%. This regimen was surprisingly well tolerated with minimal rates of serious toxicity, except for neutropenic fever in 30% of patients.

A number of docetaxel-based combination regimens have also been studied; the most active of these appear to be the three-agent combination of docetaxel, cisplatin, and 5-fluorouracil, with favorable results. It is likely that taxane-containing regimens will become the standard of care for patients with advanced disease and an important investigational tool in the neoadjuvant setting.

A number of molecularly targeted treatment strategies are under investigation for cancers of the head and neck. The targets are those genes that play a role in carcinogenesis of head and neck cancers or oronasal structures at risk for injury. Presenting symptoms are diverse. For example, blockage of the eustachian tube leads to unilaterally diminished hearing and middle-ear infections, whereas extension along vascular channels or growth into the base of the brain can cause cranial nerve palsies. Nevertheless, the most common presentation, due to the high frequency of cervical lymph node metastases, is of an asymptomatic mass in the neck.

Therapy of Nasopharyngeal Cancer

Radiation therapy in doses of 6500 to 7000 cGy as the sole modality of treatment is highly effective in early stage T1 or T2 disease, achieving local control rates of 85% to 90%. The rate of local control shrinks to 66% in more advanced lesions. The precision of radiation therapy in achieving local control at the primary site and at neck node metastases has been enhanced by use of computed tomography-guided treatment planning, the purpose of which is to shape the field of therapy to encompass the occult full extent of the primary cancer. Improvements in radiation therapy techniques—for example, by means of conformal radiation therapy—have facilitated protection of vital structures (such as the spinal cord) from toxicity.

Given the unfavorable results of patients with locally advanced disease and/or cervical lymph node metastases, chemotherapy either administered concurrently or after radiation therapy is a reasonable consideration. But the timing and value of the addition of chemotherapy to radiation therapy remains controversial.

Several small studies from Asia and the Middle East failed to demonstrate benefit from added chemotherapy. In contrast, a United States Intergroup study demonstrated a survival advantage for combination chemoradiation when compared with radiation therapy alone. Cisplatin was given concurrently at 100 mg/m^2 every three weeks with 70 Gy of radiation therapy in seven weeks, followed by three cycles of cisplatin and 5-fluorouracil in patients receiving chemoradiation. Overall survival at three years was 78% for the chemoradiation arm, compared with 47% when radiation therapy was used alone. Highly significant local control and survival differences between the two treatments led to early termination of this trial. The results of this study have been questioned, however, because the control arm had a 24% three-year disease free survival rate, far lower than what had been published previously in the smaller Asian studies. Moreover, three randomized trials from Hong Kong, Asia, and North Africa showed no improvement in local control or survival when the added chemotherapy consisted of combinations of bleomycin, epirubicin, and cisplatin, cisplatin and 5-fluorouracil, or cisplatin and epirubicin. The cause of the difference in results remains unclear. It is conceivable that either inexperience with various chemotherapy regimens or differences in radiation techniques could have compromised the ability to generalize the U.S. results with chemotherapy to other countries.

TREATMENT

Treatment of Patients with Locally Advanced Nasopharyngeal Cancer

North American and Asian physicians continue to disagree about the management of locally advanced nasopharyngeal cancer. The Intergroup study by Al-Sarraf and others convinced North American clinicians that concurrent chemoradiation therapy using cisplatin at 100 mg/m^2 and 70 Gy radiation therapy was the optimal management strategy for patients with locally advanced nasopharyngeal cancer. Chemoradiation therapy is supposed to be followed by three cycles of cisplatin and 5-fluorouracil; however, toxicity often interferes with full dosage delivery. At MD Anderson, patients are treated with three cycles of cisplatin and 5-fluorouracil initially, followed by either radiation therapy alone or concurrent chemoradiotherapy.

In contrast, several trials of nasopharyngeal cancer from Asia and Europe have shown no benefit when chemotherapy treatment is added to radiation therapy.

In these studies, chemotherapy was associated with excessive toxicity and/or the delivered dose has been less than that used in United States trials.

The difference in perspective on appropriate therapy could be related to one or more of the following factors:

- ineffective chemotherapy dosing in the Asian and European trials
- inadequate expertise in the management of the toxicity of bleomycin and cisplatin-containing chemotherapy (one study showed an unacceptably high 8% to 10% toxic death rate)
- superior expertise in Hong Kong, Mainland China and other areas in the administration of radiation therapy by external beam and brachytherapy

Therapy for Recurrent or Metastatic Nasopharyngeal Cancer

Cisplatin-based combination chemotherapy is highly active in patients with recurrent or metastatic nasopharyngeal cancer. These regimens achieve overall response rates of 50% to 70% and complete response rates of 15% to 20%, even in patients with distant metastases. Median survivals approximating 12 months have been observed in recent phase II trials, including those in which new combinations of taxanes and platinum have been used. Patients with metastatic disease who respond completely to therapy can experience long-term disease-free remissions. In some instances, patients have been cured. In general, long-term favorable responses have been limited to patients with undifferentiated carcinoma and those with metastases to bone or lung rather than to the liver.

References

General Information

Beltrami CA, Desinan L, Rubini C: Prognostic factors in squamous cell carcinoma of the oral cavity. A retrospective study of 80 cases. Pathol Res Pract 1992;188:510–516.

Cooper JS, Pajak TF, Rubin P, et al: Second malignancies in patients who have head and neck cancer: Incidence, effect on survival and implications based on the RTOG experience. Int J Radiat Oncol Biol Phys 1989;17:449–456.

Khuri FR, Nemunaitis J, Ganly I, et al: A controlled trial of intratumoral ONYX-015, a selectively-replicating adenovirus, in combination with cisplatin and 5-fluorouracil in patients with recurrent head and neck cancer. Nat Med 2000;6:879–885.

Khuri FR, Shin DM, Glisson BS, et al: Treatment of patients with recurrent or metastatic squamous cell carcinoma of the head and neck: Current status and future directions. Semin Oncol 2000;27:25–33.

Laccourreye O, Gutierrez-Fonseca R, Garcia D, et al: Local recurrence after vertical partial laryngectomy, a conservative modality of treatment for patients with stage I–II squamous cell carcinoma of the glottis. Cancer 1999;85:2549–2556.

Mashberg A, Samit AM: Early detection, diagnosis, and management of oral and oropharyngeal cancer. CA Cancer J Clin 1989;39:67–88.

Schwartz LH, Ozsahin M, Zhang GN, et al: Synchronous and metachronous head and neck carcinomas. Cancer 1994;74:1933–1938.

Vikram B: Changing patterns of failure in advanced head and neck cancer. Arch Otolaryngol 1984;110:564–565.

Vokes EE, Weichselbaum RR, Lippman SM, Hong WK: Head and neck cancer. N. Engl J Med 1993;28:184–193.

Chemotherapy

El-Sayed S, Nelson N: Adjuvant and adjunctive chemotherapy in the management of squamous cell carcinoma of the head and neck region: A meta-analysis of prospective and randomized trials. J Clin Oncol 1996;14:838–847.

Forastiere AA, Metch B, Schuller DE, et al: Randomized comparison of cisplatin plus fluorouracil and carboplatin plus fluorouracil versus methotrexate in advanced squamous cell carcinoma of the head and neck: a Southwest Oncology Group study. J Clin Oncol 1992;10:1245–1251.

Jacobs C, Lyman G, Velez-Garcia E, et al: A phase III randomized study comparing cisplatin and fluorouracil as single agents and in combination for advanced squamous cell carcinoma of the head and neck. J Clin Oncol 1992;10:257–263.

Paredes J, Hong WK, Felder TB, et al: Prospective randomized trial of high-dose cisplatin and fluorouracil infusion with or without sodium diethyldithiocarbamate in recurrent and/or metastatic squamous cell carcinoma of the head and neck. J Clin Oncol 1988;6:955–962.

Shin DM, Glisson BS, Khuri FR, et al: Phase II trial of paclitaxel, ifosfamide, and cisplatin in patients with recurrent head and neck squamous cell carcinoma. J Clin Oncol 1998;16:1325–1330.

Shin DM, Glisson BS, Khuri FR, et al: Role of paclitaxel, ifosfamide, and cisplatin in patients with recurrent or metastatic squamous cell carcinoma of the head and neck. Semin Oncol 1998;25:40–44.

Taylor SG, Murthy AK, Vannetzel JM, et al: Randomized comparison of neoadjuvant cisplatin and fluorouracil infusion followed by radiation versus concomitant treatment in advanced head and neck cancer. J Clin Oncol 1994;12:385–395.

Combined-Modality Therapy

Adelstein DJ, Saxton JP, Lavertu P, et al: A phase III randomized trial comparing concurrent chemotherapy and radiotherapy with radiotherapy alone in resectable stage III and IV squamous cell head and neck cancer: Preliminary results. Head Neck 1997;19:567–575.

Adelstein DJ: Oropharyngeal cancer: the role of the medical oncologist in organ-function conservation. In Perry MC (ed): American Society of Clinical Oncology Educational Book. Baltimore, Md, Lippincott Williams and Wilkins, 1999, pp 544–550.

Al-Sarraf M, LeBlanc M, Giri PG, et al: Chemoradiotherapy versus radiotherapy in patients with advanced nasopharyngeal cancer: Phase III randomized intergroup study 0099. J Clin Oncol 1998;16:1310–1317.

Brizel DM, Albers ME, Fisher SR, et al: Hyperfractionated irradiation with or without concurrent chemotherapy for locally advanced head and neck cancer. N Engl J Med 1998;338:1798–1804.

Calais G, Alfonsi M, Bardet E, et al: Randomized trial of radiation therapy versus concomitant chemotherapy and radiation therapy for advanced-stage oropharynx carcinoma. J Natl Cancer Inst 1998;91:2081–2086.

Dimery IW, Hong WK: Overview of combined modality therapies for head and neck cancer. J Natl Cancer Inst 1993;85:95–111.

Forastiere AA, Trotti A: Radiotherapy and concurrent chemotherapy: A strategy that improves locoregional control and survival in oropharyngeal cancer. J Natl Cancer Inst 1999;91:2065–2066.

Hong WK, Lippman SM, Wolf GT: Recent advances in head and neck cancer-larynx preservation and cancer chemoprevention: the seventeenth annual Richard and Hinda Rosenthal Foundation Award Lecture. Cancer Res 1993;53:1513–1520.

Jeremic B, Shibamoto Y, Stanisavljevic B, et al: Radiation therapy alone or with concurrent low-dose daily either cisplatin or carboplatin in locally advanced unresectable squamous cell carcinoma of the head and neck: A prospective randomized trial. Radiother Oncol 1997;43:29–37.

Jeremic B, Shibamoto Y, Milicic B, et al: Hyperfractionated radiation therapy with or without concurrent low-dose daily cisplatin in locally advanced squamous cell carcinoma of the head and neck: A prospective randomized trial. J Clin Oncol 2000;18:1458–1464.

Kies MS, Haraf DJ, Athanasiadis I, et al: Induction chemotherapy followed by concurrent chemoradiation for advanced head and neck cancer: Improved disease control and survival. J Clin Oncol 1998;16:2715–2721.

Kies MS, Haraf DJ, Rosen F, et al: Concomitant infusional paclitaxel and fluorouracil, oral hydroxyurea, and hyperfractionated radiation for locally advanced squamous head and neck cancer. J Clin Oncol 2001;19:1961–1996.

Lefebvre JL, Chevalier D, Luboinski B, et al: Larynx preservation in pyriform sinus cancer: Preliminary results of a European Organization for Research and Treatment of Cancer phase III trial. J Natl Cancer Inst 1996;88:890–899.

List MA, Siston A, Haraf D, et al: Quality of life and performance in advanced head and neck cancer patients on concomitant chemoradiotherapy: A prospective examination. J Clin Oncol 1999;17:1020–1028.

Merlano M, Banasso M, Corvo R: Five-year update of a randomized trial of alternating radiotherapy with chemotherapy compared with radiotherapy alone in treatment of unresectable squamous cell carcinoma of the head and neck. J Natl Cancer Inst 1996;88:583–589.

Merlano M, Vitale V, Rosso R, et al: Treatment of advanced squamous cell carcinoma of the head and neck with alternating chemotherapy and radiotherapy. N Engl J Med 1992;327:1115–1121.

Pignon JP, Bourhis J, Domenge C, Designe L: Chemotherapy added to locoregional treatment for head and neck squamous cell carcinoma: Three meta-analyses of updated individual data. MACH-NC Collaborative Group. Meta-analysis of chemotherapy in head and neck cancer. Lancet 2000;355:949–955.

Vokes E, Kies MS, Haraf D, et al: Concomitant chemoradiotherapy as primary therapy for locoregionally advanced head and neck cancer. J Clin Oncol 2000;18:1652–1661.

Wendt TG, Grabenhauer GG, Rodel GM, et al: Simultaneous radiochemotherapy versus radiotherapy alone in advanced head and neck cancer: A randomized multicenter study. J Clin Oncol 1998;16:1318–1324.

Epidemiology

Califano J, van der Riet P, Westra W, et al: A genetic progression model for head and neck cancer; implications for field cancerization. Cancer Res 1996;56:2488–2492.

Castigliano SG: Influence of continued smoking on the incidence of second primary cancers involving mouth, pharynx, and larynx. J Am Dent Assoc 1968;77:580–585.

Greenlee RT, Hill-Harmon MB, Murray T, Thun M: Cancer statistics, 2001. CA Cancer J Clin 2001;51:15–25.

Licciardello JT, Spitz MR, Hong WK: Multiple primary cancers in patients with cancer of the head and neck: Second cancer of the head and neck, esophagus and lung. Int J Radiat Oncol Biol Phys 1989;17:467–476.

Mao L, Lee JS, Fan YH, et al: Frequent microsatellite alterations at chromosomes 9p21 and 3p14 in oral premalignant lesions and their value in cancer risk assessment. Nat Med 1996;2:682–685.

Moore C: Cigarette smoking and cancer of the mouth, pharynx, and larynx: A continuing study. JAMA 1971;218:553–558.

Russo A, Crosignani P, Berrino F: Tobacco smoking, alcohol drinking and dietary factors as determinants of new primaries among male laryngeal cancer patients: A case-cohort study. Tumori 1996;82:519–525.

Silverman S Jr., Gorsky M, Greenspan D: Tobacco usage in patients with head and neck carcinomas: A follow-up study on habit changes and second primary oral/oropharyngeal cancers. J Am Dent Assoc 1983;106:33–35.

Slaughter DP, Southwick HW, Smejkal LW: Field cancerization in oral stratified squamous epithelium. Cancer 1953;6:963–968.

Neoadjuvant Therapy

Coleves AD, Norris CM, Tishler RB, et al: Phase II trial of docetaxel, cisplatin, fluorouracil, and leucovorin as induction for squamous cell carcinoma of the head and neck. J Clin Oncol 1999;17:3503–3511.

Coleves AD, Busse PM, Norris CM, et al: Induction chemotherapy with docetaxel, cisplatin, fluorouracil, and leucovorin for squamous cell carcinoma of the head and neck: a phase I/II trial. J Clin Oncol 1999;16:1331–1339.

Dimery IW, Peters LJ, Goepfert H, et al: Effectiveness of combined induction chemotherapy and radiotherapy in advanced nasopharyngeal carcinoma. J Clin Oncol 1993;11:1919–1928.

Forastiere AA: Another look at induction chemotherapy for organ preservation in patients with head and neck cancer. J Natl Cancer Inst 1996;88:855–856.

Glisson BS, Hong WK: Primary chemotherapy of advanced head and neck cancer: Where do we go from here? J Natl Cancer Inst 1996;88:567–568.

Jacobs C, Goffinet DR, Goffinet L, et al: Chemotherapy as a substitute for surgery in the treatment of advanced resectable head and neck cancer. A report from the Northern California Oncology Group. Cancer 1987;60:1178–1183.

Kies MS, Gordon LI, Hauck WW, et al: Analysis of complete responders after initial treatment with chemotherapy in head and neck cancer. Otolaryngol Head Neck Surg 1985;93:199–205.

Paccagnella A, Orlando A, Marchiori C, et al: Phase III trial of initial chemotherapy in stage III–IV head and neck cancers; a study in the Gruppo di Studio sui Tumori della Testa e del Collo. J Natl Cancer Inst 1994;86:265–272.

Wolf GT, Hong WK: Induction chemotherapy for organ preservation in advanced laryngeal cancer: Is there a role? Head Neck 1995;17:279–283.

Chapter 99
Second Primary Cancers of the Head and Neck

Fadlo R. Khuri

A substantial majority of patients with squamous cell carcinoma of the head and neck present with stage III or IV disease, which carries a 30% to 40% five-year survival. Extensive advances in the treatment of locally advanced head and neck cancer, such as concurrent chemoradiation therapy and improved surgical techniques coupled with postoperative radiation, have improved local disease control greatly. The appearance of second, metachronous primary cancers in this high-risk group continues to be a problem. Second primary cancers are the major determinants of overall prognosis in patients who are definitively treated and free of primary tumor recurrence two years after treatment. These additional primary cancers ultimately limit the patient's survival from the primary cancer.

A Question of Clonality

The origin of the clonal malignancies in metachronous (later) or synchronous (simultaneous) primary cancers remains uncertain. The question is whether other primary cancers of the head and neck are derived from the same or a different clone from that causing the primary cancer. For example, genetic studies on serial biopsies of premalignant lesions have shown that the subsequently developing primary squamous cell cancer of the head and neck might demonstrate the same clonal abnormality as the premalignant lesions, evolution to a secondary clone, or the appearance of a new clone. In one study of patients who had a primary head and neck cancer and then developed a solitary squamous cell cancer of the lung, both cancers were examined for loss of heterozygosity at chromosomal arms 3p and 9p. These alterations are often found during neoplastic transformation of the respiratory tract epithelium. The paired tumors from 10 patients had concordant patterns of loss at all chromosomal loci, suggesting metastatic spread, whereas three paired tumors had discordant patterns at all assayed chromosomal loci, suggesting

an independent tumor origin. The investigators concluded that most cases of squamous cell cancer of the lung developing after head and neck cancer were likely to be metastases from the primary cancer rather than metachronous, second primary cancers.

Similar studies in patients with second primary squamous cell cancers arising in the esophagus yielded different results. Sixteen patients with head and neck cancer and a second squamous cell carcinoma of the esophagus were evaluated for patterns of loss of heterozygosity for chromosomal arms 3p, 9p, and 17p. In 14 patients, the paired tumors had discordant patterns of allelic loss, suggesting that these tumors were not clonally related. In the other two patients, the paired tumors had identical genetic alterations, suggesting a common clonal origin. One of these two pairs involved spread from the hypopharynx into the cervical esophagus, and the other from the tonsil to the distal esophagus. Based on the small number of patients studied, most second primary esophageal cancers after head and neck cancer arise as independent neoplasms.

The Potential Value of Molecular Markers

Genetic changes have been documented to occur during tumor progression in squamous cell carcinoma. Loss of chromosome 18 appears to confer an adverse prognosis, because deaths from head and neck cancer occurred in 80% of patients in this group compared with a death rate of 33% among patients whose cancers lacked this abnormality. Overexpression of p53 in the primary tumor might also be a useful marker, but conflicting data have been presented regarding its relationship to the likelihood of local recurrence, incidence of second primary tumors, and overall survival.

The development of a molecular model that could augment clinical-pathologic data in order to predict the likelihood of developing second primary tumors would be invaluable not only in identifying those individuals at highest risk but also in individualizing therapy.

Chemoprevention of Upper Aerodigestive Tract Cancers

The concept of field cancerization provides the rationale for the chemoprevention of aerodigestive tract epithelial cancers. Field cancerization is the term that is used to explain the development of diffuse premalignant lesions, which lead to synchronous and metachronous cancers scattered throughout the tobacco carcinogen-damaged aerodigestive tract. Chemoprevention encompasses the use of specific natural or synthetic chemical agents to reverse, suppress, or prevent premalignant lesions from progressing to invasive cancers.

Upper Aerodigestive Tract Premalignant Lesions

Table 99-1 summarizes the active chemoprevention trials utilizing retinoids in the reversal of premalignant lesions of the head and neck. Oral premalignant lesions include both leukoplakia and erythroplakia. Small hyperplastic leukoplakia lesions have approximately a 30% to 40% spontaneous regression rate and a less than 5% risk of malignant transformation. On the other hand, erythroleukoplakia and dysplastic leukoplakia lesions have a less than 5% rate of spontaneous regression and a 30% to 40% risk of developing into oral cancer. Retinoids are far more effective in the chemoprevention of early to intermediate premalignancy than they are in the reversal of advanced premalignant lesions of the larynx or oral cavity. After the initial trial by Hong et al in 1986 using high-dose 13-cis-retinoic acid (13cRA) at 1 to 2 mg/kg/day for three months vs. placebo demonstrated a 67% response rate for the retinoid versus 10% for placebo ($P = 0.002$), several other randomized trials confirmed the activity of retinoids in the reversal of premalignant lesions.

Advanced Premalignant Lesions

Papadimitrakopoulou et al demonstrated significant and differential efficacy for a biochemoprevention combination of α-interferon (3 million units/m^2 three times per week subcutaneously) with 13-cis-retinoic acid (50 mg/m^2/daily orally) and α-tocopherol (1200 IU daily orally) in the reversal of advanced premalignant lesions of the larynx as opposed to those found in the oral cavity. In this trial of 36 patients with advanced premalignant lesions of the larynx and oral cavity (which were defined as either moderate or severe dysplasia or carcinoma-in-situ), durable complete responses were seen in approximately 50% of

Table 99-1 ■ Selected Chemoprevention Trials in Oral Premalignancy

Author	Year	Agent(s)	Number of Patients	Responses
Hong et al	1986	13-cis-retinoic acid (1–2 mg/kg/d) for three months versus placebo	44	67% (P = .0002) 10%
Stich et al	1988	β-carotene + retinol (100,000 IU/wk) versus placebo	103	28% (P < .001) 3%
Han et al	1990	4-HCR versus placebo	61	87% (P < .01) 17%
Chiesa et al, Costa et al	1993, 1994	4-HPR versus placebo	153	6% failure (P < .05) 30%
Papadimitrakopoulou et al	1999	13-cis-retinoic acid (50 mg/m²/d), α-interferon (3 million units/m² three times weekly), α-tocopherol 1200 IU/day)	36	50% pathologic complete remission in advanced laryngeal premalignant lesions versus none in advanced oral cavity premalignant lesions (P = 0.02)

4-HCR = 4(hydroxycarbophenyl)retinamide; 4-HPR = 4-N-(4-hydroxyphenyl)retinamide.

the laryngeal premalignancy patients. Several of these patients had durable complete responses for several months after discontinuation of therapy. Although this regimen was effective in causing complete phenotypic reversion, the genetic abnormalities associated with carcinogenesis persisted. In contrast, none of the 12 patients with oral cavity premalignant lesions had a durable complete response, and disease progression commonly occurred. A randomized trial now studies advanced premalignant lesions of the larynx. Patients receive α-interferon, 13-cis-retinoic acid, and α-tocopherol initially for one year and then are randomized to maintenance therapy with 4-N-4-hydroxyphenyl retinamide or placebo.

Second Primary Tumors

Patients with prior laryngeal cancers have a lifetime risk of second primary cancers of 25% to 40% (Table 99-2). Hong et al conducted a randomized, double-blind, placebo-controlled trial of high-dose 13-cis-retinoic acid versus placebo in adjuvant therapy following curative surgery and/or radiation therapy for a primary head and neck cancer. Second primary tumors developed in significantly fewer 13-cis-retinoic acid-treated patients (14%) than in patients receiving placebo (31%) ($P = 0.042$). The difference was all the more striking in the frequency of second primary tumors developing in the tobacco-exposed field of the

upper aerodigestive track and lungs. In this location, second primary tumors occurred in 6% of the 13-cis-retinoic acid-treated patients compared with 26% of the patients receiving placebo ($P = 0.008$). The chemo-preventive effect of 13-cis-retinoic acid persisted for only two years after the completion of therapy; subsequently, the incidence of second primary tumors increased rapidly and by three years did not differ from that of placebo-treated patients. Substantial toxicity of high-dose 13-cis-retinoic acid led one-third of the retinoid-treated patients to use a lower dose or discontinue the treatment. The data did show that continued smoking increased the likelihood of second primary tumor development in these patients, reinforcing the importance of smoking cessation efforts.

The European Organization for Research and Treatment of Cancer (EORTC) randomized 2600 patients (60% with stage I–III head and neck squamous cell cancer and 40% with non–small cell lung cancer) to receive one of the following regimens:

1. retinyl palmitate, 300,000 IU daily for one year followed by 150,000 IU daily for a second year;
2. N-acetyl-cysteine, 600 mg daily for two years;
3. both compounds; or
4. no intervention.

No statistically significant difference was observed in overall survival or event-free survival between those patients who received either agent, both agents, or

Table 99-2 ▪ Chemoprevention in Patients with Aerodigestive Tumors to Prevent Second Primary Tumors

Author	Year	Patient Population	N	Median Follow-Up, Months	Agent(s)	Frequency of Second Primary Tumors
Hong et al, Benner et al	1990, 1994	HNSCC	103	54	13-cis-retinoic acid (50–100 mg/m^2) for 12 months	14%
					versus	(P = .042)
					placebo	31%
Pastorino et al	1993	NSCLC	307	46	retinyl palmitate (300,000 IU) for 12 months	9%
					versus	(P = .05)
					placebo	19%
Bolla et al	1994	HNSCC	316	41	etretinate (50 mg/day) for one month; 25 mg/day for 24 months	25%
					versus	N.S.
					placebo	25%
EORTC (van Zandwijk et al)	2000	HNSCC/ NSCLC	2592	49	retinyl palmitate vs. N-acetylcysteine versus both versus placebo	No difference

NSCC = head and neck squamous cell carcinoma; NSCLC = non–small cell lung cancer; N.S. = not significant placebo. Surprisingly, second primary tumors were less common in the no-intervention arm, although the difference was not statistically significant. This raised the question of whether certain supplements given after squamous cell cancer of the head and neck, as was noted in a trial of vitamin C after lung cancer therapy, might adversely affect the incidence of second primary cancers.

The efficacy of retinoids in the chemoprevention of head and neck cancers remains controversial. Although retinoids in leukoplakia are effective in reversing early to intermediate premalignant lesions up to the stage of early dysplasia, they are of benefit for only 30% to 40% of the patients who have advanced premalignant lesions of the oral cavity. Moreover, the responses are not durable. The frequency of responses is directly correlated with the intensity of the dose of retinoids. At high doses, such toxicity is often prohibitive for patients who do not have active invasive cancer. Low doses are better tolerated but are less effective. The differences noted in the results of the trial by Hong et al and the European Organization for Research and Treatment of Cancer are now being evaluated in a large randomized U.S. trial comparing 13-cis-retinoic acid to placebo. Until these results are known, it remains unclear whether retinoic acid or derivatives can prevent the appearance of secondary primary cancers reliably.

The combination of alpha-tocopherol and alpha-interferon is highly effective, not only in the reversal of premalignant lesions of the larynx, but also as a bioadjuvant approach in patients previously treated for a locally advanced head and neck cancer. A phase II trial by Shin et al showed that 84% of patients (all of whom had stage III or IV disease) were disease-free at two years. This effective regimen could prove useful in chemoprevention or as adjuvant therapy. However, Vokes et al noted that after initial treatment of patients with an aggressive regimen that combined hyperfractionated radiation therapy with hydroxyurea, cisplatin, and 5-fluorouracil, few patients were able to tolerate treatment with 13-cis-retinoic acid and alpha-interferon.

References

Ahrendt SA, Sidransky D: The potential of molecular screening. Surg Oncol Clin N Am 1999;8:641–656.

Baselga J, Herbst R, LoRusso P, et al: Continuous administration of ZD1839 (Iressa), a novel oral epidermal growth factor receptor tyrosine kinase inhibitor (EFGR-TK1), in patients with five selected tumor types: Evidence of activity and good tolerability. Proc Am Soc Clin Oncol 2000;19:177a.

Baselga J, Rischin D, Ranson M, et al: Phase I safety, pharmacokinetic, and pharmacodynamic trial of ZD 1839, a selective epidermal growth factor receptor tyrosine kinase inhibitor, in patients with five selected solid tumor types. J Clin Oncol 2002;20:4292–4302.

Bedi GC, Westra WH, Gabrielson E, et al: Multiple head and neck tumors: Evidence for a common clinical origin. Cancer Res 1996;56:2484–2487.

Benner SE, Pajak TF, Lippman SM, et al: Prevention of second primary tumors with isotretinoin in patients with squamous cell carcinoma of the head and neck: Long-term follow-up. J Natl Cancer Inst 1994;86:140–141.

Bolla M, Lefur R, Ton Van J, et al: Prevention of second primary tumours with etretinate in squamous cell carcinoma of the oral cavity and oropharynx. Results of a multicentric double-blind randomized study. Eur J Cancer 1994; 30A:767–772.

Bradford CR, Zhu S, Wolf GT: Overexpression of p53 predicts organ preservation using induction chemotherapy and radiation in patients with advanced laryngeal cancer. Otolaryngol Head Neck Surg 1995;113:408–412.

Califano J, Leong PL, Koch WM, et al: Second esophageal tumors in patients with head and neck squamous cell carcinoma: An assessment of clonal relationships. Clin Cancer Res 1999;5:1862–1867.

Califano J, van der Riet P, Westra W, et al: Genetic progression model for head and neck cancer: Implications for field cancerization. Cancer Res 1996;56:2488–2492.

Carey TE, Frank CJ, Raval JR, et al: Identifying genetic changes associated with tumor progression in squamous cell carcinoma. Acta Otolaryngol 1997;529:229–232.

Chan G, Boyle JO, Yang EK, et al: Cyclooxygenase-2 expression is up-regulated in squamous cell carcinoma of the head and neck. Cancer Res 1999;59:991–994.

Chiesa F, Tradan N, Mazzara M, et al: Fenretinide (4-HPR) in chemoprevention of oral leukoplakia. J Cell Biochem 1993;17(Suppl):255–261.

Cooper JS, Pajak TF, Rubin P, et al: Second malignancies in patients who have head and neck cancer: Incidence, effect on survival and implications based on the RTOG experience. Int J Rad Oncol Biol Phys 1989;17:449–456.

Costa A, Formelli F, Decensi A, et al: Prospects of chemoprevention of human cancers with the synthetic retinoid fenretinide. Cancer Res 1994;54(7 Suppl):2032s–2037s.

Gao X, Fisher SG, Mohideen N, et al: Second primary cancers in patients with laryngeal cancer: A population-based study. Proc Am Soc Clin Oncol 2001;19:414a.

Gasparotto D, Maestro R, Barzan L, et al: Recurrences and second primary tumours in the head and neck region: differentiation by p53 mutation analysis. Ann Oncol 1995; 6:933–939.

Han J, Jiao L, Lu Y, et al: Evaluation of N-4 hydroxycarbophenyl retinamide as a cancer prevention agent and as a cancer therapeutic agent. In Vivo 1990;4:153–160.

Hong W, Endicott J, Itri LM, et al: 13-cis-retinoic acid in the treatment of oral leukoplakia. N Engl J Med 1986; 315:1501–1505.

Hong WK, Lippman SM, Itri LM, et al: Prevention of second primary tumors with isotretinoin in squamous cell carcinoma of the head and neck. N Engl J Med 1990; 323:795–801.

Khuri FR, Kim ES, Lee JJ, et al: The impact of smoking status, disease stage, and index tumor site on second primary tumor incidence and tumor recurrence in the head and neck retinoid chemoprevention trial. Cancer Epidemiol Biomarkers Prev 2001;10:823–829.

Khuri FR, Lee JJ, Winn RJ, et al: Interim analysis of randomized chemoprevention trial of HNSCC. Proc Am Soc Clin Oncol 1999;18:389a.

Khuri FR, Lippman SM, Spitz MR, et al: Molecular epidemiology and retinoid chemoprevention of head and neck cancer. J Natl Cancer Inst 1997;89:199–211.

Kim ES, Khuri FR, Lee JJ, et al: Second primary tumor incidence related to primary index tumor and smoking status in a randomized chemoprevention study of head and neck squamous cell carcinoma. Proc Am Soc Clin Oncol 2000; 19:416a.

Koch WM, Brennan JA, Zahurak M, et al: p53 mutation and locoregional treatment failure in head and neck squamous cell carcinoma. J Natl Cancer Inst 1996;88:1580–1586.

Leong PP, Rezai B, Koch WM, et al: Distinguishing second primary tumors from lung metastases in patients with head and neck squamous cell carcinoma. J Natl Cancer Inst 1998;90:972–977.

Mao L, El-Naggar AK, Papadimitrakopoulou VA, et al: Molecular paradox of complete phenotypic response of advanced head and neck premalignancies to biochemoprevention. J Natl Cancer Inst 1998;90:1545–1551.

Papadimitrakopoulou VA, Hong WK, Lee JS, et al: Low-dose isotretinoin versus β-carotene to prevent oral carcinogenesis: Long-term follow-up. J Natl Cancer Inst 1997;89:257–258.

Papadimitrakopoulou VA, Clayman GL, Shin DM, et al: Biochemoprevention for dysplastic lesions of the upper aerodigestive tract. Arch Otolaryngol Head Neck Surg 1999;125:1083–1089.

Pastorino U, Infante M, Maioli M, et al: Adjuvant treatment of stage I lung cancer with high-dose vitamin A. J Clin Oncol 1993;11:1216–1222.

Richardson GE, Tucker MA, Venzon DJ, et al: Smoking cessation after successful treatment of small cell lung cancer is associated with fewer smoking-related second primary cancers. Ann Intern Med 1993;119:383–390.

Russo A, Crosignani P, Berrino F: Tobacco smoking, alcohol drinking and dietary factors as determinants of new primaries among male laryngeal cancer patients: A case-cohort study. Tumori 1996;82:519–525.

Schwartz LH, Ozsahin M, Zhang GN, et al: Synchronous and metachronous head and neck carcinomas. Cancer 1994;74: 1933–1938.

Shin DM, Khuri FR, Murphy B, et al: Combined interferon-alfa, 13-cis-retinoic acid, and alpha-tocopherol in locally advanced head and neck squamous cell carcinoma: Novel bioadjuvant phase II trial. J Clin Oncol 2001;19:3010–3017.

Shin DM, Lee JS, Lippman SM, et al: p53 expression: predicting recurrence and second primary tumors in head and neck squamous cell carcinoma. J Natl Cancer Inst 1996;88: 519–529.

Slaugher DP, Southwich HW, Smejkal W: "Field cancerization" in oral stratified squamous epithelium: Clinical implications of multicentric origin. Cancer 1953;6:963–968.

Stich HF, Hornby AP, Matthew B, et al: Response of oral leukoplakias to the administration of vitamin A. Cancer Lett 1988;30:93–101.

Stich HF, Rosin MP, Hornby AP, et al: Remission of oral leukoplakias and micronuclei in tobacco/betel chewers treated with beto-carotene plus vitamin A. Intl J Cancer 1988;42:195–199.

Tucker MA, Murray N, Shaw EG, et al: Second primary cancers related to smoking and treatment of small cell lung cancer. J Natl Cancer Inst 1997;89:1782–1788.

Van Zandwijk N, Dalesio O, Pastorino U, et al: EUROSCAN, a randomized trial of vitamin A and N-acetylcysteine in patients with head and neck cancer or lung cancer. J Natl Cancer Inst 2000;92:977–986.

Vokes EE, Weichselbaum RR, Lippman SM, et al: Head and neck cancer. N Engl J Med 1993;328:184–194.

Chapter 100
Salivary Gland Carcinoma

Roy B. Sessions and Douglas K. Frank

Introduction

For the treating physician, salivary gland malignancies are a fascinating but frustrating group of epithelial neoplasms. Although uncommon (less than 5% of all head and neck cancers), these malignancies demonstrate a myriad of histologic patterns and clinical behavior; for this reason, their infrequency contributes to the difficulties that confront physicians charged with their management. Some histologic subtypes of salivary malignancies behave in a nonaggressive fashion and are amenable to cure, but other variants can demonstrate an extremely aggressive natural history that leads to a relatively rapid patient demise. Other variants are characterized by apparent cure, only to relapse many years later.

The head and neck region contains both major and minor salivary glands. The three paired major glands are the parotid, the submandibular, and the sublingual; and approximately 1000 minor glands are distributed for the most part in the oral cavity and oropharynx. A small number of minor salivary glands exist in the remainder of the aerodigestive sites—specifically, in the paranasal sinuses, hypopharynx, larynx, and trachea. Common to all salivary glands is the duct-acinus unit. The typical duct is composed of three different types of specialized lining epithelia that are involved in the modification and ultimate excretion of the saliva produced in the acinus. Smooth-muscle myoepithelial cells surround these unique secretory acinar cells. The cellular complexity of the salivary duct-acinus unit leads to the development of multiple malignant histologic variants of carcinoma.

The common variants of primary salivary gland carcinoma are shown in Table 100-1.

Because intraglandular lymph nodes exist within the parotid gland, lymphomas also can occur as primary tumors within this organ.

Any discussion of salivary gland tumors would be incomplete without some mention of nonmalignant lesions. The varied cellular architecture of salivary tissue also lends itself to a wide array of benign neoplasms that are not necessarily predecessors to or counterparts of the malignant tumors. The one exception to this is the pleomorphic adenoma, commonly known as benign mixed tumor. This lesion is one of the few salivary gland benign neoplasms that undergoes malignant metamorphosis; thus its name, carcinoma ex-pleomorphic adenoma. Although the incidence of this conversion is small, it occurs often enough to justify a wary appraisal to any salivary gland lesion that exhibits accelerated growth.

Epidemiology

Malignancies of the salivary glands are uncommon relative to the overall frequency of other cancers, develop mostly in adults, and fail to demonstrate gender predominance across all sites. These cancers are rare in children and young adults; less than 10% of salivary gland cancers occur in this population.

Because the parotid glands constitute the largest volume of salivary tissue, the greatest proportion of salivary neoplasms occurs in this organ. In tumors of the salivary glands, the chances of finding a malignancy rather than a benign lesion varies by site—for example, 1:4 in the parotid, 1:1 in the submandibular gland, and 4:1 in the sublingual and minor glands. A minor salivary gland tumor, therefore, is far more worrisome than is one located in the parotid gland.

Interestingly, the various histologic subtypes of salivary neoplasia do not occur with the same relative frequency at different sites. The most common malignancies of the parotid gland, for example, are mucoepidermoid carcinoma and adenocarcinoma. In the submandibular and minor salivary glands, on the other hand, adenoid cystic carcinoma is prevalent. Whereas mucoepidermoid carcinoma is the second most common cancer of submandibular gland origin,

Table 100-1 ■ Histologic Variants of Salivary Gland Carcinomas of the Head and Neck

Mucoepidermoid carcinoma (low-, intermediate-, and high-grade)
Adenocarcinoma (low- and high-grade)
Low-grade polymorphous adenocarcinoma
Carcinoma ex-pleomorphic adenoma
Undifferentiated carcinoma
Adenoid cystic carcinoma
Acinic cell carcinoma
Squamous cell carcinoma

this type occurs less often in cancers of the sublingual and minor salivary glands.

Risk Factors

Although no consistent racial distribution has been demonstrated, there seems to be a clustering of lymphoepitheliomas (undifferentiated squamous cell carcinoma) of the major glands in certain Eskimo populations. As is the case in all patients with nasopharyngeal carcinoma, there could be an association of the salivary cancers with the Epstein-Barr virus in Eskimo populations. Otherwise, no clear environmental or hereditary risk factors are known for the development of carcinoma of the major salivary glands. One potential exception, reported in the British literature, is the development of sinonasal adenocarcinoma in wood workers who have inhaled particulate wood dust. The consistent carcinogenic role of alcohol and tobacco, so obvious in other head and neck cancers, is not present in salivary cancer.

Clinical Presentation (Table 100-2)

Common Presentations of Salivary Cancer

Major Salivary Glands

Most major salivary gland carcinomas present as painless, mobile masses. Parotid and submandibular gland cancers are usually appreciated by palpation in the respective subcutaneous locations. Sublingual carcinomas typically present as a painless floor-of-mouth prominence. When pain is present, however, either spontaneously or following palpation, malignancy is strongly suggested. This is especially true when the pain is radicular in nature. Moreover, pain often signals ominous, aggressive tumor biology.

Minor Salivary Glands

The wide distribution of minor salivary gland tissue throughout the upper aerodigestive tract causes

Table 100-2 ■ Common and Uncommon Presentations of Salivary Gland Carcinomas in the Head and Neck

Common Presentations
Major Salivary Glands

Painless mass
Nasal obstruction
Sinusitis
Epistaxis
Dysphagia
Aspiration
Hoarseness
Respiratory difficulty

Uncommon Presentations
Major and Minor Salivary Glands

Soft palate bulge
Cranial nerve weakness

Minor Salivary Glands (Anatomic Subsite Dependent)

Anosmia
Cerebrospinal fluid leak
Diplopia
Epiphora
Proptosis
Visual compromise

considerable variation in the presentation of these cancers. A high percentage occurs in the mucosa covering the hard palate of the oral cavity, and are only incidentally found during routine oral examinations. The dental community bears critical responsibility if one is to detect these tumors at an early stage. Regardless of location, minor salivary gland cancers are usually submucosal, and early cancers are rarely ulcerated and usually painless. Sinonasal cancers most often present with nasal obstruction, sinusitis, or epistaxis. Pharyngeal and laryngeal tumors cause dysphagia, aspiration, hoarseness, and respiratory difficulty.

Uncommon Presentations of Salivary Cancer

Major Salivary Glands

Because the deep lobe of the parotid gland is located adjacent to the oropharyngeal constrictor muscles, a bulge in the soft palate can be the only sign of a tumor in that part of that organ. This finding is often discovered on routine oral examination or during an examination for dysphagia, snoring, or sleep apnea–related symptoms. In this latter group of patients, the alteration of the oropharyngeal anatomy leads to noisy breathing and sleep problems. Fortunately, the majority of deep-lobe parotid tumors are benign, but in any given mass of this area, the burden is on the physician to rule out the possibility of cancer. Even benign parotid tumors located deep in the lobe of the gland should be resected. One needs to be wary of accelerated growth of a preexisting salivary gland mass, because it can represent malignant metamorphosis.

The parotid, submandibular, and sublingual glands are intimately related to major cranial nerves. Even a small parotid malignancy can present with partial or total facial nerve palsy, while submandibular and sublingual cancers can present with deficits of the marginal branch of the facial nerve or of the lingual, hypoglossal, or inferior alveolar nerves. Such presentations, although unusual, can be a manifestation of a small but particularly neurotropic tumor, such as adenoid cystic carcinoma. Alternatively, a locally advanced and highly aggressive cancer can surround and invade major nerves. In either case, the presentation of salivary gland cancer with one of these neurologic deficits usually occurs in the presence of an obvious mass and some degree of pain.

Neurotropic tumors (such as adenoid cystic carcinoma) also can present with seemingly unrelated or out-of-field trigeminal nerve anesthesia. The tumor can invade and travel along distal branches of the fifth cranial nerve in a retrograde fashion (perineural spread) back to the skull base and Meckel's cave, where the trigeminal ganglion is located. Once in the ganglion, any part of the widely distributed trigeminal nerve can be affected. Finally, due to the anatomic proximity of the parotid, the submandibular, and the sublingual gland to the distal branches of the trigeminal nerve itself, tumors in these areas occasionally can produce the same result.

Although cervical lymphatic metastases are not infrequent in the high-grade malignancies—for example, high-grade adenocarcinoma, squamous cell carcinoma, and high-grade mucoepidermoid carcinoma—cancers of the major salivary glands rarely present with clinically positive nodes. Cervical metastasis usually occurs in the context of obvious disease at the primary major salivary gland site.

Minor Salivary Glands

Because they often are located in such concealed anatomic locations as the nose, paranasal sinuses, or upper pharynx, minor salivary gland cancers can grow to considerable size before causing symptoms that lead to discovery. For example, a sinonasal carcinoma could cause anosmia or even anterior invasion of the base of the skull and a cerebrospinal fluid leak before it becomes clinically apparent. Other minor salivary

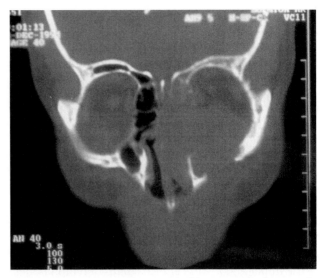

Figure 100-1 ■ Coronal computed tomography image of a patient with an adenoid cystic carcinoma that arose in a minor salivary gland of the left ethmoid-maxillary region. The tumor completely obstructs the left nasal cavity and is invading the left inferior-medial orbit. This patient presented with diplopia, nasal obstruction, and intermittent epistaxis.

gland cancers can invade the orbit, presenting with diplopia, epiphora, proptosis, or visual compromise (Figure 100-1). A minor salivary gland cancer of the maxillary sinus can go undetected until anterior bony wall destruction occurs, leading to what would appear to be a cheek mass or even anesthesia in the distribution of the second division of the fifth cranial nerve (infraorbital nerve), which is located in the area. These presentations are associated with poor survival.

Clinical Evaluation

Physical Examination

The physical examination is the cornerstone of the evaluation of the patient with salivary gland cancer. For both major and minor salivary gland lesions, the examination yields important information about the extent of the tumor that is important for purposes of staging and treatment. Malignancy must always be ruled out, regardless of the location of the mass. Physical findings that frequently indicate a malignancy include

■ fixation to surrounding structures
■ pain
■ regional motor or sensory cranial nerve deficit
■ ulceration of surrounding soft tissues

The primary site of disease must be evaluated carefully and the greatest tumor dimension measured for staging. Because of the neurotropism of some salivary gland cancers, a complete cranial nerve examination is essential.

Palpation of the regional cervicofacial lymph nodes is very useful. Cancers originating in the parotid gland can spread to the intraparotid lymph nodes as well as to the nodes of the upper and lower internal jugular chain. Submandibular and sublingual carcinomas can involve submental, submandibular, and internal jugular chain lymph nodes, either high or low in the neck. In much the same manner as cancers of the upper aerodigestive tract, cancers originating in a minor salivary gland in this area usually metastasize to the cervical lymphatic nodes in patterns consistent with their anatomic site of origin. For example, spread from minor salivary gland cancers of the oral tongue can be expected to be to the submandibular as well as to the upper and lower cervical chains of lymph nodes. Tumors of the tongue base, oropharyngeal walls, hypopharyngeal walls, and larynx typically spread directly to the jugular chain of nodes. Minor salivary gland cancers of the hard palate and sinonasal region, particularly when diagnosed at an early stage, seem to have fewer propensities for spread to the regional cervical lymph nodes.

Rigid and flexible fiberoptic scopes assist with the evaluation of known or suspected lesions in the sinonasal region, oropharynx, hypopharynx, and larynx. Such an evaluation can document impending airway compromise in the rarely encountered tracheal lesions, most of which are adenoid cystic carcinoma.

Histologic Evaluation

Histologic confirmation of the diagnosis of salivary gland cancer is essential. Options for obtaining tissue include either fine-needle aspiration and cytologic evaluation, or excision of the lesion. When possible, the former is preferred. Because the diagnostic possibilities include inflammatory disorders, embryologic abnormalities, and neoplasms, the information provided by the cytologist can, at the minimum, help the treating physician to categorize the mass; in most neoplasms, this information can give a definitive diagnosis. This technology can be particularly helpful in the evaluation of a patient with a major salivary gland tumor or a mass in the regional lymph node basin.

Needle aspiration and biopsies are performed in accessible minor salivary gland sites in the oral cavity, nasal cavity, and oropharynx. These procedures can frequently be accomplished in the physician's office. On the other hand, caudal lesions such as those in the larynx, hypopharynx, or trachea are more appropriately biopsied in the operating room. Particular caution must be exercised in biopsies of lesions in the

superior nasal cavity. Such masses can be intimately associated with the skull base and even the brain. Appropriate imaging studies can help in evaluating the safety of performing such procedures in the office setting.

Imaging Studies

Computed tomography (CT) and magnetic resonance imaging (MRI) allow accurate staging of salivary gland cancers. These studies are usually ordered after a diagnosis of carcinoma has already been established by physical examination and biopsy. Computed tomography with intravenous contrast (from the base of the skull base to the clavicles) is usually the initial study of choice (Figure 100-2). It can reasonably determine the local extent of disease and is an excellent modality to detect the presence of subclinical cervical lymph node metastases. A salivary gland cancer (particularly one of high-grade histology) that is locoregionally advanced at presentation or recurrence also requires computed tomography imaging to rule out distant metastatic disease or direct extension into other tissues. This can entail imaging of the brain, chest, and abdomen. If pain suggests spread to the bony skeleton, a bone scan is indicated.

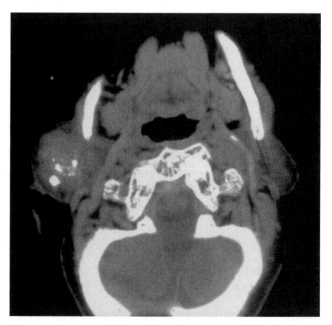

Figure 100-2 ▪ Axial computed tomography image of a right parotid adenoid cystic carcinoma. Note how nicely computed tomography delineates the relatively superficial nature of this large tumor—it does not extend into the parapharyngeal space. Intratumoral calcifications, not necessarily a regular feature of adenoid cystic carcinoma, are demonstrated.

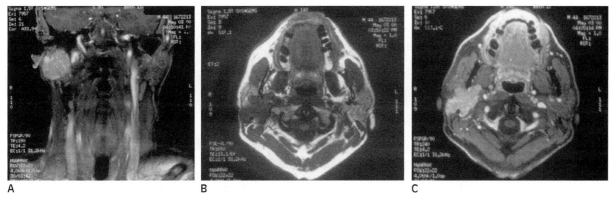

A   B   C

Figure 100-3 ■ Serial magnetic resonance images of a patient with carcinoma ex-pleomorphic adenoma of the right parotid gland. All images are T1 weighted, with image A performed in the coronal plane and images B and C in the axial plane. Images A and C are fat suppressed and intravenous gadolinium contrast enhanced. Note how MRI demonstrates the soft tissue extent of the tumor into the parapharyngeal space on image C, delineating it from the surrounding muscle. Computed tomography imaging is not capable of such sharp soft tissue demarcation.

Under certain circumstances, magnetic resonance imaging can present diagnostic advantages over computed tomography (Figure 100-3). The former can often detect the extent of major cranial nerve involvement, particularly in patients with adenoid cystic carcinoma. Because of its superior ability to contrast soft tissues, magnetic resonance imaging also can help differentiate carcinoma in the sinonasal region from such non-neoplastic conditions as obstructive secretions.

Staging, Prognostic Features, and Outcomes

The American Joint Committee on Cancer (AJCC) has devised a tumor, node, and metastasis (TNM) system to stage salivary gland cancers. This staging system applies only to malignancies of the major salivary glands, such as the parotid and submandibular glands (Table 100-3). Minor salivary gland cancer TNM staging adheres to the AJCC system for all epithelial malignancies in upper aerodigestive tract locations. Thus, the criteria for local tumor (T) staging of a minor salivary gland cancer of the oral cavity are different from those for the same tumor in the hypopharynx or paranasal sinuses. Because this staging system was developed largely for the staging of squamous cell carcinomas of the upper aerodigestive tract, there are inherent problems in applying it to salivary tumors.

The varied types of histology and different grades of salivary malignancies further complicate the issue of TNM staging. The American Joint Committee on Cancer has tried to account for tumor factors such as major nerve invasion and extraglandular extension in its staging system of major salivary gland cancer; thus, the current staging system correlates reasonably well with prognosis. The extent of treatment in some circumstances, however, is dictated by specific tumor histology. For example, even a relatively small high-grade mucoepidermoid carcinoma is best treated aggressively, despite the designation of a low stage by the TNM criteria. Generally speaking, however, advanced stage is more predictive of ominous prognosis than is histology.

The presence of pain, male gender, and recurrent disease are additional factors that seem to portend a worse prognosis for all salivary cancers. The location of a salivary gland cancer also seems to affect prognosis. In the major salivary glands, submandibular tumors can fare worse than those of the parotid. For carcinomas of minor salivary gland origin, those located in the larynx and paranasal sinuses have a worse prognosis in terms of survival than those located in the oral cavity. In general, minor salivary gland cancers have a worse prognosis than those found in the major salivary glands.

As indicated earlier, salivary cancers are rare. Individual institutions generally accrue too few patients of each histologic type of salivary gland cancer who are followed long enough to define firmly the survival statistics for each of the varying presentations. Nonetheless, a retrospective review of patients over 35 years at Memorial Sloan Kettering Cancer Center provides some frequently referenced information on patient survival. These data show that acinic cell carcinoma and all types of mucoepidermoid carcinoma have a better survival rate (80% and 70%, respectively at 10 years) compared with adenocarcinoma, carcinoma ex-pleomorphic adenoma, squamous cell

Table 100-3 ■ AJCC Tumor, Nodes, Metastases (TNM) Staging of Major Salivary Gland Carcinomas in the Head and Neck

Tumor (T)

TX	Primary tumor cannot be assessed
T0	No evidence of primary tumor
T1	Tumor ≤2 cm in greatest dimension without extraparenchymal extension
T2	Tumor >2 cm and ≤4 cm in greatest dimension without extraparenchymal extension
T3	Tumor >4 cm and ≤6 cm in greatest dimension and/or tumor with extraparenchymal extension without seventh cranial nerve involvement
T4	Tumor >6 cm in greatest dimension and/or invades base of skull or seventh cranial nerve.

Nodes (N)

NX	Regional lymph nodes cannot be assessed
N0	No regional lymph node metastases
N1	Single ipsilateral lymph node metastasis ≤3 cm in greatest dimension
N2A	Single ipsilateral lymph node metastasis >3 cm and ≤6 cm in greatest dimension
N2B	Multiple ipsilateral lymph node metastases, none greater than 6 cm in greatest dimension
N2C	Bilateral or contralateral lymph node metastases, none greater than 6 cm in greatest dimension
N3	Lymph node greater than 6 cm in greatest dimension

Metastases (T)

MX	Distant metastasis cannot be assessed
M0	No evidence of distant metastases
M1	Distant metastases present

Stage Groupings

Stage I	T1/T2, N0, M0
Stage II	T3, N0, M0
Stage III	T1/T2, N1, M0
Stage IV	any T, N2/N3, M0
	any T, any N, M1
	T4, N0, M0
	T3/T4, N1, M0

carcinoma, or adenoid cystic carcinoma, which carry, respectively, a 45%, 48%, 32%, and 50% survival at 10 years. Overall, however, high-grade lesions have a shorter survival than low-grade lesions.

Treatment

General Treatment Principles (Figure 100-4)

The treatment of all histologic subtypes of salivary gland cancer involves an initial adequate surgical resection. To date, chemotherapy has not found consistent practical use in the management of most salivary gland carcinomas.

Adjuvant postoperative radiation therapy to total doses usually greater than 5000 cGy offers a survival advantage as well as an improvement in local control of disease in patients with high-grade and locoregionally advanced (stage III and IV) carcinomas in the major salivary glands. Both survival and local control rates five years after treatment exceed 50% using combined surgery and radiation therapy, compared with 20% when only surgical resection is employed. Despite limited data, most clinicians treat advanced minor salivary gland cancers with a similar strategy. A small, localized tumor that has spread to the regional lymphatics carries a high-stage classification and thus should be managed with aggressive multimodality treatment.

The high-grade salivary gland cancers include high-grade mucoepidermoid carcinoma, high-grade adenocarcinoma, carcinoma ex-pleomorphic adenoma, adenoid cystic carcinoma, squamous cell carcinoma, and undifferentiated carcinoma. Postoperative radiation therapy is used, even in early stage tumors. Early-stage, low-grade tumors (low-grade mucoepidermoid carcinoma, low-grade adenocarcinoma, low-grade polymorphous adenocarcinoma, acinic cell carcinoma) are generally treated with surgical resection alone. When microscopic residual disease is believed to be present after gross surgical resection of an early stage, low-grade tumor, however, strong consideration is given to adjuvant radiation. Postoperative radiation is less effective in the management of gross disease left after surgical resection; hence the importance of ensuring an adequate surgical excision.

When neural involvement is documented, it is important to resect the involved nerve along the primary lesion and to follow the nerve proximally until a clear margin can be obtained, if possible. Involvement of a major nerve by carcinoma is associated with a compromised survival, even when postoperative external beam radiation therapy is utilized. Because of the morbidity associated with sacrifice of the facial nerve during parotid tumor extirpation, surgeons may be inclined to attempt to preserve this structure at the expense of increasing the likelihood of local recurrence. Attempts to preserve the facial nerve should not be made in instances of gross neural invasion despite the fact that the muscles supplied by the facial nerve may have been functioning normally before surgery. Attempting to "peel" the facial nerve off of a very adherent tumor is not recommended. In this instance, gross residual disease can be left behind and neural function is often compromised in any case.

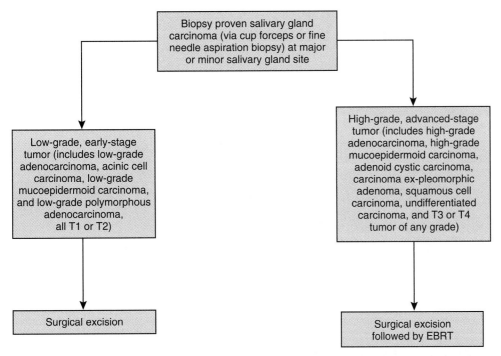

Figure 100-4 ■ Management of the primary site in salivary gland carcinoma. (EBRT = External beam radiation therapy.)

The facial nerve, however, often can be dissected free of deep-lobe parotid cancers that do not involve the nerve. In rare instances, a small tumor might involve only one of the two main divisions of the facial nerve. It is reasonable to attempt preservation of the uninvolved portion of the nerve under these circumstances.

Extraordinary radiation therapy techniques have been employed successfully in special clinical circumstances with salivary gland cancer. Brachytherapy (interstitial radiation therapy) is effective in the retreatment of patients with local recurrence who have previously been treated with surgery and external beam radiation therapy; local control and survival at five years are approximately 60% and 50%, respectively. For the management of unresectable disease (i.e., that situation in which complete gross tumor resection is not possible), fast neutron radiation therapy seems to be beneficial. Experience with this methodology is limited, however, and there are few treatment facilities that have this technology.

Treatment of the Cervical Lymphatics
(Figure 100-5)

Clinically obvious cervical lymph node metastases are treated with neck dissection, the extent of which is tai-

lored to address the particular volume and location of cervical disease. The classic radical neck dissection is reserved for the very uncommon circumstance in which bulky neck disease involves the internal jugular vein, the sternocleidomastoid muscle, or the spinal accessory nerve. In most cases of cervical lymph node enlargement, selective neck dissection is performed by means of which specific lymph node groups are harvested without sacrificing major muscles, nerves, or veins. In general, cervical lymphadenectomy for clinically positive lymph nodes in the neck is followed by adjuvant external beam radiation therapy. This enhances regional control, but its effect on distant metastasis and therefore on survival is uncertain.

The management of the neck in the setting in which there is no clinically obvious disease is somewhat complicated. Salivary gland cancers of the nose and paranasal sinuses, regardless of size or histologic subtype, do not readily drain to the regional lymph nodes, and in these lesions neck dissection is performed only when there is clinically apparent disease. Tumors of the other upper aerodigestive tract subsites (oral cavity, pharynx, larynx) as well as those of the major salivary glands tend to metastasize to the lymph nodes in the neck. It is generally accepted that high-grade tumors at these latter upper aerodigestive tract and major salivary gland subsites have a rate of occult cervical lymphatic metastases approximating 50%; in

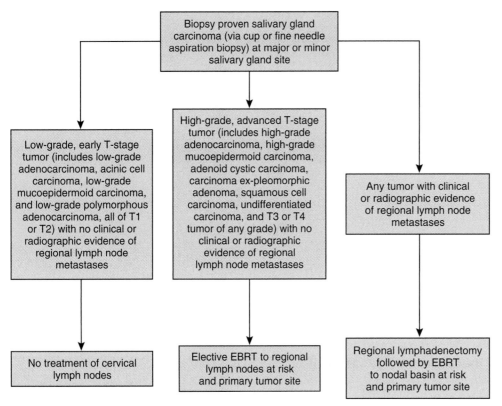

Figure 100-5 ■ Management of the regional cervical lymph nodes in salivary gland carcinoma. (EBRT = External beam radiation therapy.)

these circumstances, radiation therapy to the neck is often recommended. Because high-grade malignancies typically are treated with adjuvant external beam radiation therapy after resection at the primary site, including the at-risk cervical lymph nodes in the radiation field is readily accomplished. A similar treatment strategy is recommended for low-grade but locally advanced (T3 and T4) tumors—even though the neck is clinically negative for disease, such tumors are associated with a relatively high incidence of occult cervical metastases.

Complications of Surgical Treatment

Adverse sequelae associated with surgical treatment of salivary malignancies depend on the location of the tumor and the extent of the operation. Relatively small, low-grade tumors of the major salivary glands are usually excised without significant morbidity. Parotidectomy or submandibular gland resection results in minimal morbidity and minimal cosmetic or functional consequences. Gustatory sweating (Frye's syndrome) follows a significant percentage of parotidectomies. The inappropriate reinnervation of sweat glands results in cutaneous moisture in the operative site associated with eating. This can be severe and embarrassing but is most commonly mild and of no social consequence. Facial numbness is always present immediately after the parotid operation, but this is usually short-lived. In most patients, skin sensation returns within several months. Parotidectomy is followed by a very low but consistent incidence of facial palsy; this is usually temporary but can be permanent. The incidence of facial nerve dysfunction following parotidectomy is directly related to the proximity of the tumor to the facial nerve. Nerve dysfunction is usually related to nerve bruising or compression caused by adjacent tissue secondary to swelling of the tissues from the surgery. This state of affairs is known as neuropraxia. By contrast, the permanent condition of neurodegeneration (in which axons are anatomically interrupted) is much less common.

Occasionally, part of or all of the facial nerve is sacrificed during a radical parotidectomy. This results in significant functional as well as cosmetic morbidity. Rehabilitation with nerve grafts (dynamic procedures) or muscle/fascial slings (static procedures) is possible. Radical tumor extirpation in the submandibular triangle can result in sacrifice of one or multiple nerves, including the hypoglossal, lingual, and/or inferior alveolar nerve. Specific procedures designed to reha-bilitate these nerves are yet to be defined.

Follow-up Evaluation

The post-treatment evaluation of salivary gland cancer patients generally follows the same timetable as other types of head and neck cancers. Patients are seen monthly during the first post-treatment year, bimonthly during the second post-treatment year, every three months during the third post-treatment year, and every six to 12 months every year thereafter. The clinician might find it helpful to use computed tomography or magnetic resonance imaging to assist with the clinical evaluation of locoregional disease during follow-up. This is particularly true when following high-grade or locally advanced tumors post-treatment. Tumors excised from areas (such as the paranasal sinuses) that are difficult to evaluate clinically, extensively reconstructed treatment fields, and/or irradiated treatment fields are often followed via periodic imaging. Imaging at least twice a year during the first three post-treatment years, with annual imaging thereafter, is a reasonable policy. Periodic chest X-ray (or a higher-sensitivity study such as computed tomography scanning with contrast) done on the same time scale as imaging of the primary site in the follow-up of high-grade tumors is performed to evaluate for distant metastases, which most frequently are to the lung. Certain salivary gland cancers, particularly adenoid cystic carcinomas, are capable of developing pulmonary metastases many years after diagnosis and supposedly successful management of the primary tumor.

References

General Information

Hamilton-Dutoit SJ, Therlkildsen MH, Nielsen NH, et al: Undifferentiated carcinoma of the salivary gland in Greenlandic Eskimos—Demonstration of Epstein-Barr virus DNA by in situ nucleic acid hybridization. Hum Pathol 1991;22:811–815.

Sobin LH, Wittekind C (eds): TNM Classification of Malignant Tumors, 5th ed. New York, Wiley-Liss, 1997, pp 43–46.

Sun EC, Curtis R, Melbye M, Goedert JJ: Salivary gland cancer in the United States. Cancer Epidemiol, Biomarkers Prev 1999;8:1095–1100.

Combined Modality Therapy

Avery CM, Moody AB, McKinna FE, et al: Combined treatment of adenoid cystic carcinoma of the salivary glands. Int J Oral Maxillofac Surg 2000;29:277–279.

Garden AS, Weber RS, Morrison WH, et al: The influence of positive margins and nerve invasion in adenoid cystic carcinoma of the head and neck treated with surgery and radiation. Intl J Radiat Oncol Biol Phys 1995;32:619–626.

Jackson GL, Luna MS, Byers RM: Results of surgery alone and surgery combined with postoperative radiotherapy in the treatment of cancer of the parotid gland. Am J Surg 1983;146:497–500.

Diagnosis

Batsakis JG, Sneige N, El-Naggar AK: Fine needle aspiration of salivary glands: Its utility and tissue effects. Ann Otol Rhinol Laryngol 1992;101:185–188.

Imaging

Rabinov JD: Imaging of salivary gland pathology. Radiol Clin N Am 2000;38:1047–1057.

Browne RF, Golding SJ, Watt-Smith SR: The role of MRI in facial swelling due to presumed salivary gland disease. Br J Radiol 2001;74:127–133.

Pathology

Evans HL, Luna MA: Polymorphous low-grade adenocarcinoma: A study of 40 cases with long-term follow-up and an evaluation of the importance of papillary areas. Am J Surg Pathol 2000;24:1319–1328.

Spiro RH, Huvos AG, Strong EW: Adenoid cystic carcinoma of salivary origin: A clinicopathologic study of 242 cases. Am J Surg 1974;128:512–520.

Spiro RH, Koss LG, Hajdu SI, et al: Tumors of minor salivary gland origin: A clinicopathologic study of 492 cases. Cancer 1973;31:117–129.

Prognosis

Calearo C, Pastore A, Storchi OF, Polli G: Parotid gland carcinoma: Analysis of prognostic factors. Ann Otorhinolaryngol 1998;107:969–973.

Fordice J, Kershaw C, El-Naggar A, et al: Adenoid cystic carcinoma of the head and neck: Predictors of morbidity and mortality. Arch Otolaryngol Head Neck Surg 1999;125:149–152.

Spiro RH: Salivary neoplasms: Overview of a 35-year experience with 2,807 patients. Head Neck Surg 1986;8:177–184.

Vander Poorten VL, Balm AJ, Hilgers FJ, et al: Stage as major long-term outcome predictor in minor salivary gland carcinoma. Cancer 2000;89:1195–1204.

Radiation Therapy

Armstrong JG, Harrison LB, Spiro RH, et al: Brachytherapy for malignant tumors of salivary gland origin. Endocurie Hypertherm Oncol 1990;6:19–23.

Douglas JG, Lee S, Laramore GE, et al: Neutron radiotherapy for the treatment of locally advanced major salivary gland tumors. Head Neck 1999;21:255–263.

Douglas JG, Einck J, Austin-Seymour M, et al: Neutron radiotherapy for recurrent pleomorphic adenomas of the major salivary glands. Head Neck 2001;23:1037–1042.

Epstein JB, Robertson M, Emerton S, et al: Quality of life and oral function in patients treated with radiation therapy for head and neck cancer. Head Neck 2001;23:389–398.

Harrison LB, Armstrong JG, Spiro RH, et al: Postoperative radiation therapy for major salivary gland malignancies. J Surg Oncol 1990;45:52–55.

Le QT, Birdwell S, Terris DJ, et al: Postoperative irradiation of minor salivary gland malignancies of the head and neck. Radiother Oncol 1999;52:165–171.

Surgery

Armstrong JG, Harrison LB, Spiro RH, et al: Malignant tumors of major salivary gland origin. Arch Otolaryngol Head Neck Surg 1990;116:290–293.

Armstrong JG, Harrison LB, Thaler HT, et al: The indications for elective treatment of the neck in cancer of the major salivary glands. Cancer 1992;69:615–619.

Callender DL, Frankenthaler RA, Luna MA, et al: Salivary gland neoplasms in children. Arch Otolaryngol Head Neck Surg 1992;118:472–476.

Goepfert H, Luna MA, Tortoledo E, et al: Malignant salivary gland tumors of the paranasal sinuses and nasal cavity. Arch Otolaryngol 1983;109:662–668.

Robbins KT: Indications for selective neck dissection, when, how, and why. Oncol 2000;14:1455–1469.

Sinha UK, Ng M: Surgery of the salivary glands. Otolaryngol Clin N Am 1999;32:887–906.

Chapter 101
Bone Sarcomas

Shreyaskumar R. Patel and Robert S. Benjamin

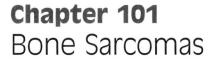

Sarcomas are tumors of mesenchymal origin. The incidence of primary bone sarcomas in the United States in 2003 will be approximately 2400 new cases. In addition to being rare, these tumors are very heterogeneous and include more than 50 different subtypes. The most common subtypes of bone sarcomas include osteosarcoma, chondrosarcoma, Ewing's sarcoma, and malignant fibrous histiocytoma. Some other rare variants include unclassified sarcoma of bone and angiosarcoma. The presenting symptoms of most bone sarcomas are nonspecific and include pain and swelling overlying the involved bone. Plain radiographs are the simplest and most informative tool and can frequently be diagnostic in expert hands, precluding need for further invasive evaluations. The plain radiographic information can be complemented by appropriate cross-sectional imaging for better bone and soft-tissue details. Laboratory parameters are usually not very helpful in the diagnostic process. Histologic confirmation of radiographic differential diagnosis is usually accomplished with radiology-guided multiple-core needle biopsies performed by expert interventional radiologists. In the majority of cases, this provides enough tissue for differentiation between benign and malignant lesions and appropriate classification of malignant tumors. In rare situations in which more tissue is necessary, a small open biopsy performed by the orthopedic oncologist with specific attention to eventual limb-sparing and function-preserving surgery is appropriate.

The vast majority of primary bone tumors are histologically and biologically benign. When asymptomatic and diagnosed incidentally, these can be managed with careful observation. When symptomatic, they are treated with limited surgery where appropriate for local control or managed symptomatically. There are, however, some primary bone tumors that have a benign histologic appearance by conventional criteria but occasionally can manifest a biologically malignant behavior. The classic example of this entity is a giant cell tumor of bone, which has benign histologic characteristics but is locally aggressive and occasionally can metastasize to lungs without any obvious de-differentiation or malignant transformation. Careful long-term follow-up is necessary in this situation.

Bone tumors are classified based on their cell or tissue of origin (Table 101-1). Many of them have well-defined benign entities corresponding to their malignant counterparts. New onset of pain, recent history of more rapid growth, or signs of inflammation overlying the preexisting lesion are indicators of possible de-differentiation into a malignant process.

The staging systems are based on the important pretreatment prognostic factors, including the grade and size (local extent) of the primary tumor and the presence or absence of distant metastases. Two different staging systems have been used. The surgical staging is based predominantly on the grade of the tumor and its confinement to the compartment of origin (Table 101-2). The American Joint Committee on Cancer (AJCC) classification based on the tumor characteristics, nodes, and metastases is listed in Table 101-3. This latter system is currently being revised to incorporate some additional prognostic factors.

Table 101-1 ▪ Classification of Bone Tumors (Simplified)

Cell/Tissue of Origin	Benign Lesion	Malignant Lesion
Osseous	Osteoma, osteoblastoma	Osteosarcoma
Cartilaginous	Enchondroma Osteochondroma	Chondrosarcoma
Fibrohistiocytic	Desmoid	Malignant fibrous histiocytoma
	Chondroblastoma Chondromyxoid fibroma	
Unknown	Giant cell tumor	Giant cell tumor Ewing's sarcoma
Notochordal		Chordoma
Vascular	(Hem/Lymph)angioma	Angiosarcoma

Osteosarcoma

Clinical Features

Osteosarcoma is the most common primary bone sarcoma (Table 101-4). It is a spindle cell malignancy arising in bone with the ability to make bone. It accounts for 20% to 45% of all malignant bone tumors. Its incidence has a bimodal peak, with the most common group affected in the second decade of life. There is a slight male preponderance. The etiology of these primary/de novo osteosarcomas in teenagers is unknown; however, some associations have been established. For example, deletion of the retinoblastoma gene is found in many of these tumors. The second peak affects older patients in the sixth to eighth decades of life. The tumors in this group are comprised primarily of osteosarcomas secondary to some preexisting condition (e.g., radiation therapy) or prior benign bone lesions with de-differentiation. Patients with osteosarcoma typically present with pain

Table 101-2 ▪ Surgical Staging of Bone Sarcomas

Stage	Grade	Site
IA	Low (G1)	Intracompartmental (T1)
IB	Low (G1)	Extracompartmental (T2)
IIA	High (G2)	Intracompartmental (T1)
IIB	High (G2)	Extracompartmental (T2)
III	Any G, regional or distant metastasis (M1)	Any (T)

G = grade; G1 = any low-grade tumor; G2 = any high-grade tumor; T = site; T1 = intracompartmental location of tumor (confined to bone); T2 = extracompartmental location of tumor. M = regional or distal metastases; M0 = no metastases; M1 = any metastases.

Table 101-3 ▪ TNM Staging System for Bone Tumors

Primary Tumor (T)

TX	Primary tumor cannot be assessed
T0	No evidence of primary tumor
T1	Tumor (maximum dimension) ≤8 cm
T2	Tumor (maximum dimension) >8 cm

Regional Lymph Nodes (N)

NX	Regional lymph nodes cannot be assessed
N0	No regional lymph node metastasis
N1	Regional lymph node metastasis to be considered equivalent to distant metastatic disease (see M_{1b} below)*

Distant Metastasis (M)

MX	Distant metastasis cannot be assessed	
M0	No distant metastasis	
M1	Distant metastasis	
	M1a	Lung-only metastases
	M1b	All other distant metastases including lymph nodes

Histopathologic Grade (G)

GX	Grade cannot be assessed
G1	Well differentiated—low grade
G2	Moderately differentiated—low grade
G3	Poorly differentiated—high grade
G4	Undifferentiated—high grade[†]

Stage Grouping

Stage IA	G1,2	T1	N0	M0
Stage IB	G1,2	T2	N0	M0
Stage IIA	G3,4	T1	N0	M0
Stage IIB	G3,4	T2	N0	M0
Stage III	Not defined			
Stage IVA	Any G	Any T	N0	M1a
Stage IVB	Any G	Any T	N0/N1	M1b

*Because of the rarity of lymph node involvement in sarcomas, the designation NX might not be appropriate and could be considered N0 if no clinical involvement is evident.
[†]Ewing's sarcoma is classified as G4.

and swelling. Occasionally, a pathologic fracture is the presenting feature.

Primary osteosarcoma of bone typically affects the metaphyses of long bones, with distal femur being the most common site, followed by proximal tibia and proximal humerus. Rarely, it can affect the axial skeleton, but when it does it carries a worse prognosis. The classic radiographic appearance follows the definition of osteosarcoma. This manifests as a destructive lesion arising within the bone with cortical interruption, periosteal reaction, and a soft-tissue mass with poorly organized calcification. The pattern of calcification and

Table 101-4 ■ Clinical Presentation of Common Bone Tumors

Type	Frequency	Age Group (Yrs)	Sex	Site	Symptoms and Signs	Pathologic Features
Osteosarcoma	45%	10–20	M > F	Metaphyses	Pain/swelling	Spindle cells, osteoid matrix
Chondrosarcoma	22%	20–80	M > F	Pelvic/shoulder girdles	Pain/swelling	Lobules, chondroid matrix
Ewing's/primitive neuroectodermal tumors	15%	10–20	M > F	Diaphyses/flat bones	Pain/swelling	Small round blue cells
Malignant fibrous histiocytoma	8%	20–80	M > F	Long bones	Pain/swelling	Pleomorphic spindle cells, storiform pattern, no osteoid

matrix can frequently be diagnostic of the subtype of primary bone tumor. Typical osteosarcoma calcifications are described as having a sunburst appearance (Figure 101-1). This radiographic appearance and clinical presentation are diagnostic of osteosarcoma. The degree of soft-tissue calcification varies depending on the specific histologic subtype. Osteoblastic osteosarcomas typically show dense calcifications when compared with chondroblastic and fibroblastic subtypes. Diagnosis of a telangiectatic osteosarcoma requires, by definition, a purely lytic radiographic appearance. It is otherwise nondescript and indistinguishable on radiographic appearance from other malignancies like malignant fibrous histiocytoma or carcinomatous metastasis. For other subtypes, however, the association of histology and radiographic appearance is not absolute. For example, osteoblastic osteosarcomas can be purely lytic, and fibroblastic osteosarcomas can be densely blastic.

Histologic diagnosis is usually accomplished by core needle biopsies taken, where possible, from the soft-tissue component of the tumor. Occasionally, a hole needs to be drilled in the bone to allow access of the biopsy needle to the intramedullary component of the tumor. Osteosarcomas frequently show the presence of multiple subtypes within the same tumor—including osteoblastic, chondroblastic, fibroblastic, or malignant fibrous histiocytoma-like patterns—and are classified based on the predominant subtype. A simplified classification useful for the clinician is outlined in Table 101-5.

Prognostic Factors

Several pretreatment prognostic factors have been identified. These include grade and size of the primary tumor, morphology, site, extent of disease, duration of

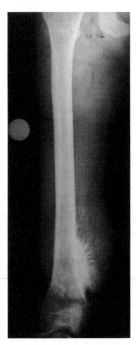

Figure 101-1 ■ Radiograph showing osteosarcoma.

Table 101-5 ■ Classification of Osteosarcomas

High-Grade Intramedullary Osteosarcoma

Conventional/classic (osteoblastic, chondroblastic, fibroblastic)
Others (small cell, telangiectatic, epithelioid, giant cell rich)

Low-Grade Intramedullary Osteosarcoma (Well Differentiated)
Surface/Juxtacortical Osteosarcoma

High-grade surface
Periosteal—Low to intermediate-grade chondroblastic
Parosteal—Low-grade fibroblastic

Secondary Osteosarcomas

Radiation-associated
Paget's sarcoma
De-differentiated osteosarcoma (from preexisting bone lesion)

symptoms, weight loss greater than 4.5 kg, swelling at the primary site, and lytic appearance. In a multivariate model, the histologic response to preoperative chemotherapy is the single most important predictor of long-term survival.

Staging

The metastatic pattern of this disease is very predictable, with the first and most common site of involvement being the lungs. The second most common site is the bony skeleton. Other sites are rarely involved at an early stage but frequently can follow the more common sites of involvement. Lymph node involvement is extremely rare; when encountered, it is frequently a late phenomenon appearing after or in conjunction with other sites of metastasis. The staging work-up for a patient with osteosarcoma, therefore, should include appropriate imaging of the primary tumor, the lungs, and the bony skeleton. The primary tumor is best imaged by a plain radiograph of the entire bone. Cross-sectional imaging with computed tomography (CT) scans yields good details of cortical and bony skeleton areas, while magnetic resonance imaging (MRI) provides better soft-tissue and intramedullary details. These tests, therefore, should be viewed as complementary. Plain radiographs and computed tomography scans of the chest give adequate information about the chest cavity, and a bone scan is appropriate to rule out any distant bone metastases or an occasional skip metastasis. The utility of the new high-resolution positron emission tomography (PET) scans in the staging of bone tumors remains to be determined. These metabolic scans, including radionuclide tumor localization scans with thallium or sestamibi, are sometimes helpful in assessing viability of tumor after therapy. The positive-predictive values of these tests are greater than 90%; however, the negative-predictive values favor positron emission tomography over other metabolic scans (90% vs. 50%).

Treatment

Osteosarcoma is the prototypical bone sarcoma. The strategy of multidisciplinary management, using all effective therapeutic options early on, has improved outcomes in these patients and has been used to treat other bone sarcomas. Osteosarcoma is a systemic disease at presentation, with micrometastases in the vast majority of patients. This reality explains the poor long-term survival (less than 20%) in patients treated with radical surgery alone in historical series. It also emphasizes the fact that "cure" of a given patient with cancer depends on how effectively one can control the distant micrometastases in addition to local control of the tumor. With the use of aggressive combination

chemotherapy as the primary modality along with adjuvant surgery for adequate local control, approximately 70% of patients with localized, conventional extremity osteosarcoma can be cured. In addition to improving the cure fraction, the effective use of chemotherapy prior to surgery facilitates limb-sparing surgery, which in turn improves the functional outcome for the patient, thereby providing a better quality of life. The current standard of care for this type of tumor, therefore, is primary chemotherapy tailored to best response, combined with appropriate limb-sparing surgery and followed by postoperative chemotherapy (Figure 101-2).

Randomized trials have compared surgery alone with surgery plus postoperative chemotherapy. Vincristine and high-dose methotrexate as the chemotherapy regimen failed to show any significant advantage in either disease-free or overall survival. In contrast, doxorubicin, cisplatin, high-dose methotrexate, and BCD (bleomycin, cyclophosphamide, and dactinomycin) showed a significant difference in relapse-free survival favoring adjuvant chemotherapy at two years but no difference in overall survival. A combination regimen of doxorubicin, methotrexate, and vincristine along with radiation therapy yielded a significant difference in both relapse-free survival and overall survival. Based on these data, adjuvant chemotherapy is now the standard of care for patients with osteosarcoma.

The rationales for administering the chemother-

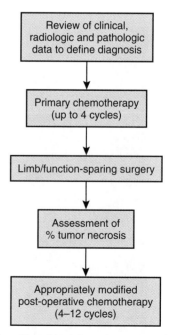

Figure 101-2 ■ Algorithm for management of osteosarcoma, malignant fibrous histiocytoma, and de-differentiated chondrosarcoma.

apy before surgery include the benefits of early initiation of systemic therapy and tumor response that might facilitate limb-sparing surgery. Doxorubicin, cisplatin, ifosfamide, and high-dose methotrexate are the four most active chemotherapy drugs available for the treatment of a patient with osteosarcoma.

For high-grade extremity osteosarcoma, the authors' preoperative chemotherapy consists of doxorubicin and cisplatin, repeated for four cycles prior to limb-sparing surgery in the vast majority of patients. Response to therapy judged by the percentage of tumor necrosis is the single most important predictor of long-term disease-free and overall survival. Postoperative chemotherapy consists of Adriamycin-based regimens with the addition of high-dose methotrexate or ifosfamide. Patients with 90% or greater necrosis to preoperative chemotherapy have a five-year disease-free survival rate of 79%. The five-year disease-free survival rate of patients with chondroblastic osteosarcoma is 75%, for fibroblastic osteosarcoma 49%, and for osteoblastic osteosarcoma 62%. The 10-year disease-free survival and overall survival rate for all patients with 90% or greater necrosis is 75%, compared with about 25% for patients with less than 90% necrosis. Recently, routine incorporation of postoperative ifosfamide in addition to high-dose methotrexate in these patients with less than 90% necrosis has resulted in a five-year disease-free survival rate of 67%.

In a separate study (Meyers et al.), patients were randomized to receive either high-dose methotrexate and BCD preoperatively plus Adriamycin or cisplatin postoperatively, or a more intensified preoperative regimen consisting of Adriamycin and cisplatin in addition to high-dose methotrexate and BCD. The percentage of patients showing a good histologic response was greater for the more intensive regimen, but the five-year event-free survival was comparable for both regimens at about 75%.

Bocci et al. preoperatively treated patients with single-agent high-dose methotrexate followed by one cycle of two-drug combinations, namely cisplatin and ifosfamide, cisplatin and Adriamycin, or Adriamycin and ifosfamide. All four drugs were used as single agents postoperatively. The limb salvage rate was 94%, and 32% of the patients achieved total tumor necrosis. At 6.5 years, the five-year event-free survival and overall survival were 56% and 71% for patients with localized disease and 17% and 24% for patients with metastatic disease at diagnosis.

A randomized trial of preoperative versus postoperative chemotherapy in patients with primary extremity osteosarcoma demonstrated five-year event-free survival and overall survival rates of 61% and 76%, respectively, for the preoperative arm, compared with 69% and 79% event-free and overall survival rates for the postoperative arm. No significant difference was noted between the two arms for any other parameter, such as complication rates and quality-of-life assessments.

The standard of care for a patient with a conventional high-grade extremity osteosarcoma consists of preoperative chemotherapy, followed by limb-sparing surgery, followed by postoperative chemotherapy based on the knowledge of the extent of necrosis accomplished with preoperative chemotherapy. Patients with high-grade osteosarcomas of other sites except the jaw (for example, the axial skeleton) are also managed in a similar fashion. Their overall outcome, however, appears to be poorer than that of patients with extremity tumors, due in part to decreased sensitivity to the same chemotherapy agents and in part to difficulties in accomplishing a margin-negative surgical resection because of anatomic constraints. Patients with low-grade osteosarcomas—for example, well-differentiated intramedullary osteosarcoma or parosteal osteosarcoma, or the biologically unique jaw osteosarcoma that typically arises in the mandible (which has a lower tendency to distant metastases)—are best managed with a margin-negative surgical excision alone, without routine use of adjuvant chemotherapy. If margin-negative surgical excision cannot be achieved, preoperative chemotherapy should be considered for patients with osteosarcoma of the jaw and for patients with intermediate-grade periosteal osteosarcoma; postoperative therapy should be adjusted based on response to preoperative therapy.

Patients with Metastatic Disease

Patients presenting with synchronous primary tumor and resectable lung metastases are treated with curative intent using primary chemotherapy and surgical resection of all disease, either at the same time or as staged operations. These patients have a 15% to 30% probability of long-term disease-free survival or even cure. On the other hand, patients presenting with multiple bone metastases have a much poorer prognosis and are incurable. Therapy is directed at palliation and prolongation of the natural history of the disease, keeping in mind issues related to quality of life.

Patients with metachronous metastases are also approached much the same way. Their systemic therapy options might be limited, depending on their prior exposure to chemotherapy. Surgical resection of lung metastases is recommended, as it results in three- to five-year disease-free intervals in about 15% to 20% of patients.

Follow-up

Long-term follow-up is essential for curable tumors like osteosarcoma. The use of effective chemotherapy has changed the history of the disease, with increased cure fractions. Patients should be monitored with frequent chest radiographs to detect lung metastases and with plain films of the primary tumor-bearing area to detect local recurrence or complications related to the prosthesis (e.g., loosening) or allograft (e.g., nonunion, malunion, or infection). Patients should be seen and examined every two to three months for the first two years, every three to four months for the next two years, every four to six months for years five to six, and subsequently on a yearly basis. Late side effects of chemotherapy are rare, but need to be monitored. The incidence of cardiomyopathy varies with the cumulative dose and duration of infusion of doxorubicin. Ifosfamide nephrotoxicity can also manifest weeks to months after discontinuation of the drug, especially if patients have received nonsteroidal anti-inflammatory drugs or other nephrotoxic drugs as well. Sensory neuropathy secondary to cisplatin is usually seen in almost all patients receiving more than $300\,mg/m^2$ of cumulative dose. This condition is usually self-limiting, although it can persist for several months to years after discontinuation of the drug. It can also be potentiated by ifosfamide, especially at high doses (greater than $12\,g/m^2$ total dose per cycle). The incidence of secondary malignancies (e.g, leukemias) is also very low, but clinicians need to be aware of this potentially lethal sequela.

Malignant Fibrous Histiocytoma

Clinical Features

Malignant fibrous histiocytoma of bone is a recently recognized entity comprising approximately 5% of all bone tumors. The age distribution is variable, patients are generally older than those with osteosarcoma, and there seems to be a slight predilection for males (see Table 101-4). The skeletal distribution is also variable, with a predilection for the metaphyses of long bones. Radiologically, it manifests as an aggressive radiolucent defect with ill-defined margins, often with an associated soft-tissue mass. Histologically, it shows striking resemblance to malignant fibrous histiocytoma arising in soft tissues (see Chapter 102). Not infrequently, malignant fibrous histiocytoma appears to constitute the high-grade component of a dedifferentiated chondrosarcoma. In addition, malignant fibrous histiocytoma often can be a component of osteosarcomas. Histologically, the only major difference between a fibroblastic osteosarcoma and a malignant fibrous histiocytoma is the presence or absence of osteoid. Malignant fibrous histiocytoma of bone, therefore, could well be part of a spectrum of osteosarcomas in which the spindle cells do not produce osteoid visible by light microscopy. Instances have been documented in which pathologic diagnosis of the primary tumor was believed to be a malignant fibrous histiocytoma, whereas the subsequent metastases unequivocally demonstrated osteoid, thus lending credence to the hypothesis that malignant fibrous histiocytoma of bone could indeed be a variant of fibroblastic osteosarcoma. The natural histories of malignant fibrous histiocytoma of bone and fibroblastic osteosarcoma, including the overall survival rates, are comparable.

Staging

Malignant fibrous histiocytoma of bone also exhibits a lung-dominant metastatic pattern similar to that of osteosarcoma. The staging studies, therefore, are identical to those described for osteosarcoma.

Treatment

Malignant fibrous histiocytoma of bone is managed under the same guiding principles as osteosarcoma (see Figure 101-2). Patients are treated with primary chemotherapy followed by surgical resection and postoperative chemotherapy, which is formulated based on the knowledge of patient response to preoperative therapy.

Patients at M.D. Anderson who received surgery plus a postoperative adjuvant chemotherapy regimen consisting of cyclophosphamide, Adriamycin, and dacarbazine were compared to control patients undergoing surgery alone, showing superior results (median disease-free survival 24 vs. 8 months and overall survival not reached vs. 19 months) for postoperative chemotherapy. Preoperative Adriamycin and cisplatin in patients with localized malignant fibrous histiocytoma caused 90% or greater necrosis. Survival data computed based on Kaplan Meier Life Table analysis revealed that the median disease-free survival for all patients was 19 months and the median survival was 23 months. The median disease-free survival for patients achieving 90% or greater necrosis was 43 months, and the median survival was 66 months. In a separate study, patients with primary extremity bone malignant fibrous histiocytoma were treated with Adriamycin and cisplatin preoperatively and with additional cycles postoperatively. Forty-two percent of patients achieved a 90% or greater tumor necrosis, and 80% underwent limb-sparing surgery. The five-year progression-free survival and overall survival were 56% and 59%, respectively. Patients with a good histologic response experienced a more prolonged time to progression and better overall survival compared with poor responders.

Follow-up

Patients should be monitored as outlined in the section on osteosarcoma.

Chondrosarcoma

Clinical Features

Chondrosarcoma is the second most common bone sarcoma, comprising up to 20% of all bone tumors. It is usually a tumor of older individuals, with a peak incidence in the fifth decade of life (see Table 101-4). There is slight male preponderance. The tumor typically involves long or flat bones. It has a characteristic chondroid matrix with annular ringlet-like calcifications seen on plain films or computed tomography scans (Figure 101-3). The exact etiology is unknown. Patients typically present with a painful mass with some signs of local inflammation. Preexisting benign cartilaginous lesions—for example, an enchondroma or an osteochondroma—can transform into a malignant lesion such as chondrosarcoma. Patients with this clinical syndrome present with a long-standing history of an asymptomatic mass that recently started growing at a faster pace and is associated with pain and signs of local inflammation. Plain radiographs suggest an aggressive bone lesion with

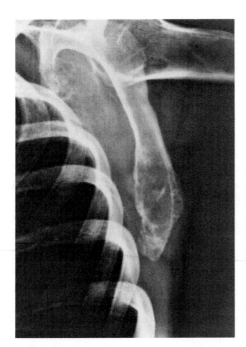

Figure 101-3 ■ Radiograph showing chondrosarcoma.

Table 101-6 ■ Classification of Chondrosarcomas

Intramedullary Chondrosarcoma
Conventional/classic (low/intermediate/high-grade)
Clear cell
De-differentiated
Mesenchymal

Surface/Juxtacortical

some destruction, typically with endosteal scalloping of the bony cortex and a chondroid matrix. Diagnosis and subclassification are confirmed by a core needle biopsy or after surgical resection of the tumor.

Classification

Like osteosarcoma, chondrosarcoma is a heterogeneous tumor with various subtypes. A simplified classification is outlined in Table 101-6.

Prognostic Factors

The most common subtype is that of conventional chondrosarcoma. In this subtype, grade is of prognostic significance. Low-grade chondrosarcomas can exhibit highly indolent biologic behavior and usually have a low probability of distant metastases. Intermediate-grade chondrosarcomas have a higher likelihood of local recurrence but still carry a low risk of metastasis. High-grade chondrosarcomas can have a more rapid rate of growth and frequently produce distant metastases. The two variants, which include mesenchymal chondrosarcoma and de-differentiated chondrosarcoma, have specific prognostic and therapeutic implications discussed in the following sections.

Staging

The metastatic pattern follows the general trend for osteosarcomas; lungs are the most common site, and involvement of other bones is rare. Patients are therefore staged as outlined for osteosarcoma. Low-grade chondrosarcomas do not need extensive metastatic work-up.

Treatment

Conventional chondrosarcoma is refractory to most standard chemotherapeutic drugs and is thus treated primarily with surgery regardless of the grade of the tumor. Exceptions to this practice are two specific rare variants, namely mesenchymal chondrosarcoma and de-differentiated chondrosarcoma.

The natural history of a de-differentiated chondrosarcoma is very aggressive, characterized universally by metastases within approximately 12 months from diagnosis and almost certain death from disease within 24 months from diagnosis. The median disease-free interval and overall survival are about four months and six months, respectively. The use of preoperative Adriamycin and cisplatin in those patients with localized, resectable de-differentiated chondrosarcoma has resulted in a five-year continuous relapse-free survival of 51%.

Ewing's Sarcoma

Clinical Features

Ewing's sarcoma is a small round cell tumor; it belongs to a group of systemic diseases that include the closely related primitive neuroectodermal tumors (PNET) and are referred to generically as small cell sarcomas (see Table 101-4). These small cell sarcomas need to be distinguished from other small round cell tumors such as neuroblastomas, lymphomas, small cell osteosarcomas, and an occasional eosinophilic granuloma or chronic osteomyelitis. The peak incidence for Ewing's sarcoma is in the second decade of life, and the median age is lower than for any other bone tumor. A male preponderance is noted. Typically, Ewing's sarcoma involves the diaphysis of long bones or flat bones of the pelvic girdle and ribs. Pain and swelling are the most common presenting features. Most patients have a palpable warm, tender mass. Occasionally, this is associated with fever, anemia, and elevated erythrocyte sedimentation rate and serum lactate dehydrogenase. Radiographically, it manifests as a lytic lesion with a large soft-tissue component (Figure 101-4).

Staging

The metastatic pattern includes lungs, other bones, and occasionally bone marrow. Radiologic work-up, therefore, should include a plain film and a magnetic resonance imaging scan of the entire bone, which together provide information about the extent of soft-tissue and intramedullary involvement. A bone scan helps rule out bone metastases, and a chest X-ray or computed tomography scan of the chest can exclude lung metastases. Patients with no distant metastases on either a bone scan or computed tomography scan of the chest can undergo a bone marrow aspirate and biopsy; however, in the absence of peripheral blood count or blood smear evidence of a myelophthisic (leukoerythroblastic) picture, the yield is small. A more effective, less invasive way to assess bone marrow involvement is a magnetic resonance imaging

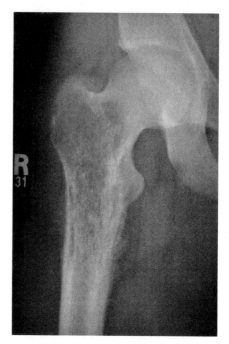

Figure 101-4 ▪ Radiograph showing Ewing's sarcoma.

screening of the spine and pelvis. This can detect areas of bone marrow replacement, even when a bone scan is negative. The role of metabolic scans (including positron emission tomography scans) in the staging of this tumor remains to be defined.

Prognostic Factors

Patients who are older than 20 years, who have a central or unresectable tumor, pelvic lesions, or obvious metastatic disease have a poor prognosis, especially when bone metastases are present. Histologic response to chemotherapy is also of prognostic significance; as with osteosarcoma, complete tumor necrosis predicts a better outcome. Ewing's sarcomas are characterized by a balanced translocation between chromosomes 11 and 22, resulting in the EWS-FLI 1 gene product. The type 1 translocation, which codes for a weaker transactivator, has a better prognosis than the others. Tumors expressing the p53 gene or with a deletion of INK4A have been associated with poor outcome.

Treatment

Systemic therapy is the mainstay of treatment. These tumors respond well to chemotherapy regimens that include one or more of the following drugs: Adriamycin, actinomycin-D, ifosfamide, cyclophosphamide, vincristine, or VP16. The popular standard regimens for the treatment of Ewing's sarcoma are vincristine-Adriamycin-cyclophosphamide or vincristine-actinomycin D-cyclophosphamide, ifos-famide-VP16, and vincristine-Adriamycin-ifosfamide. These chemotherapy regimens form the backbone of initial therapy. Consolidation local therapy can be accomplished by surgical resection, where this is possible with low morbidity. Alternatively, primary radiation therapy can be used for consolidation when the tumor is unresectable or morbidity of resection is unacceptable. With aggressive combined-modality treatment, cure rates of greater than 50% can be achieved. A strategy of myeloablative chemotherapy with autologous bone-marrow transplant has been tried in the past, with disappointing results in duration of response and cure.

The Cooperative Ewing's Sarcoma Study (Paulussen et al.) experience included patients with high-risk and standard-risk factors. All patients were treated with vincristine, Adriamycin, actinomycin-D, and either cyclophosphamide or ifosfamide. Local therapy varied between surgery, radiation, or the combination of the two. The 10-year event-free survival of the entire group was 52% without any difference between the two risk groups. Good histologic response and inclusion of ifosfamide predicted for a favorable outcome. In a separate study, patients with localized Ewing's sarcoma of bones excluding the pelvis were randomized to receive vincristine, Adriamycin, cyclophosphamide, and actinomycin-D either intermittently at high dose or continuously at moderate dose (Burgert et al.). At a median follow-up of 5.6 years, 68% of patients on the high-dose arm were disease-free, and 77% were still alive. These results were significantly better than in patients receiving the moderate-dose regimen. Comparable results were obtained in a study using intensified chemotherapy that included ifosfamide and etoposide in addition to vincristine, actinomycin-D, Adriamycin, and cyclophosphamide; the three-year event-free survival and overall survival were 78% and 84%, respectively.

Patients with Metastatic Disease

Managing patients with Ewing's sarcoma is dependent on the disease stage (Figure 101-5). Patients with concurrent metastatic disease to lungs are treated with curative intent. In younger children, cure can be accomplished in up to one-third of these patients. Long-term survival is more difficult to accomplish in patients with bone or bone-marrow metastases.

With intensification of chemotherapy, the time-to-progression curves seem to have been pushed towards the right. Late relapses between years four and six and even later relapses at or beyond 10 years

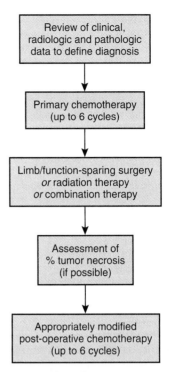

Figure 101-5 ■ Algorithm for management of Ewing's sarcoma, primitive neuroectodermal tumors, and mesenchymal chondrosarcoma.

have been documented. A retrial of appropriate systemic therapy and surgical resection if feasible is the therapeutic strategy of choice in patients who relapse after primary therapy.

Chordoma

Chordoma, a tumor developing in the remnants of the primitive notochord, is a locally aggressive tumor with an indolent biology. Rarely, it can metastasize on its own or after de-differentiation to a frank sarcoma. It has a predilection for the two ends of the spinal column, shows male preponderance, and commonly affects young adults. Sacrococcygeal chordomas present with pain with or without mechanical symptoms of pressure such as constipation or plexopathy. Sphenooccipital chordomas present with pain with or without cranial nerve palsies and symptoms of intracranial extension. Radiologic evaluation reveals a mass. Biopsy is necessary to confirm the characteristic histologic features. Treatment is usually surgical resection where feasible. Unresectable tumors are treated with radiation therapy with long-term control but do run the risk of late recurrences, de-differentiation, or a radiation-associated sarcoma. Chemotherapy is of little value except for de-differentiated tumors.

Giant Cell Tumors of Bone

This is a tumor characterized by osteoclast-like giant cells that has a predilection for females and is most common in the third decade of life. It usually involves the epiphyses of long bones but has been documented at other central sites. Pain, swelling, and limitation of range of motion are the common presenting symptoms. Radiographs usually show an expansile lytic area located eccentrically in the epiphysis of a long bone (Figure 101-6). Pathologic fractures are not uncommon. Histologically, this is a "benign" lesion; however, it can recur in up to 50% of patients. Over a period of many years, it can undergo a "malignant" change in its biologic behavior without obvious change in the cellular characteristics of the giant cells; however, the stromal cells show malignant transformation. These tumors can metastasize to the lungs with typical sarcoma-like lung metastases. Local recurrences or metastatic lesions need to be biopsied to differentiate between metastatic giant cell tumor and metastatic sarcoma (de-differentiated giant cell tumor) or metastatic radiation-associated sarcoma. Up to 10% of these patients can have a sarcomatous de-differentiation that requires aggressive multimodality therapy.

Treatment

The majority of giant cell tumors are treated with intralesional curettage and cementation. Occasionally, complete resection is feasible and necessary for good local control. Effective local control can also be accomplished by single or multiple embolizations of all feeding arteries in patients with unresectable disease or disease recurring after curettage. Alternatives include radiation therapy, which is also effective for local control; however, this strategy runs a small risk of late complications, especially de-differentiation or a radiation-associated sarcoma.

Because giant cell tumors are extremely vascular, anti-angiogenic therapy could theoretically provide benefit. To test this hypothesis, in an M.D. Anderson pilot study, 10 patients with locally advanced, recurrent, or metastatic giant cell tumor of bone were treated between 1991 and 1999 with interferon alpha 2b, an agent whose activities include anti-angiogenesis. After receiving 10 million U/m^2 of interferon alpha 2b subcutaneously three times a week for a period of 6 to 12 months, 5 patients achieved a major response, including three patients with pulmonary metastases. Responses occurred gradually and continued even after therapy was discontinued. One patient had continued increase in size of the tumor for 6 months and then started to regress, suggesting that prolonged exposure to the drug is necessary. Additional trials are warranted to confirm this observation.

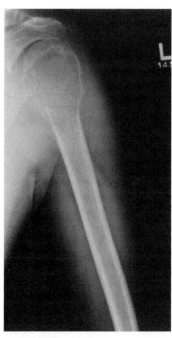

Figure 101-6 ▪ Radiograph showing giant cell tumor.

References

De-Differentiated Chondrosarcoma

Benjamin RS, Chu P, Patel SR, et al: De-differentiated chondrosarcoma—A treatable disease. Proc Am Assoc Cancer Res 1995;36:243.

Johnson S, Tetu B, Ayala A, Chawla SP: Chondrosarcoma with additional mesenchymal component (de-differentiated chondrosarcoma). A clinicopathologic study of 26 cases. Cancer 1986;58:278–286.

Mercuri M, Picci P, Campanacci M, Rulli E: De-differentiated chondrosarcoma. Skeletal Radiol 1995;24:409–416.

Ewing's Sarcoma

Burgert EO, Nesbit ME, Garnsey LA, et al: Multimodal therapy for the management of nonpelvic, localized Ewing's sarcoma of bone: Intergroup study IESS-II. J Clin Oncol 1990;8:1514–1524.

Craft A, Cotterill S, Malcolm A, et al: Ifosfamide-containing chemotherapy in Ewing's sarcoma: The second UK Children's Cancer Study Group and the MRC Ewing's tumor study. J Clin Oncol 1998;16:3628–3633.

Evans RG, Nesbit ME, Gehan EA, et al: Multimodal therapy for the management of localized Ewing's sarcoma of pelvic and sacral bones: A report from the second intergroup study. J Clin Oncol 1991;9:1173–1180.

Paulussen M, Ahrens S, Dunst J, et al: Localized Ewing tumor of bone: Final results of the cooperative Ewing's Sarcoma Study CESS 86. J Clin Oncol 2001;19:1818–1829.

Rosito P, Mancini AF, Rondelli R, et al: Italian cooperative study for the treatment of children and young adults with localized Ewing's sarcoma of bone: A preliminary report of 6 years of experience. Cancer 1999;86:421–428.

Giant Cell Tumor of Bone

Benjamin RS, Patel SR, Gutterman JU, et al: Interferon alpha-2b as anti-angiogenesis therapy of giant cell tumor of bone: Implications for the study of newer angiogenesis-inhibitors. Proc Am Soc Clin Oncol 1999;18:548a.

Malignant Fibrous Histiocytoma

Bacci G, Ferrari S, Bertoni F, et al: Neoadjuvant chemotherapy for osseous malignant fibrous histiocytoma of the extremity: Results in 18 cases and comparison with 112 contemporary osteosarcoma patients treated with the same chemotherapy regimen. J Chemother 1997;9:293–299.

Bacci G, Picci P, Mercuri M, et al: Neoadjuvant chemotherapy for high-grade malignant fibrous histiocytoma of bone. Clin Orthop 1997;346:178–189.

Bramwell VHC, Steward WP, Nooij M, et al: Neoadjuvant chemotherapy with doxorubicin and cisplatin in malignant fibrous histiocytoma of bone: An EOI study. J Clin Oncol 1999;17:3260–3269.

Chawla SP, Benjamin RS, Abdul-Karim F, et al: Adjuvant chemotherapy of primary malignant fibrous histiocytoma of bone—Prolongation of disease-free and overall survival. In Jones SE, Salmon SE (eds): Adjuvant Therapy of Cancer IV. New York: Grune and Stratton, 1984, pp 621–629.

Patel SR, Armen T, Carrasco CH, et al: Primary chemotherapy in malignant fibrous histiocytoma of bone—Updated U.T.M.D.Anderson Cancer Center Experience. In Banzet P,

Holland J, Khayat D, Weil M (eds): Cancer Treatment—An Update. Paris, Springer Verlag, 1994, pp 577–580.

Osteosarcoma

Bacci G, Briccali A, Ferrari S, et al: Neoadjuvant chemotherapy for osteosarcoma of the extremity: Long-term results of the Rizzoli's 4th protocol. Eur J Cancer 2001;37:2030–2039.

Benjamin RS, Patel SR, Armen T, et al: The value of ifosfamide in postoperative neoadjuvant chemotherapy of osteosarcoma. Proc Am Soc Clin Oncol 1995;14:516.

Edmonson JH, Green SJ, Ivins JC, et al: A controlled pilot study of high dose methotrexate as postsurgical adjuvant treatment for primary osteosarcoma. J Clin Oncol 1984;2:152–156.

Eilber F, Giuliano A, Eckardt J, et al: Adjuvant chemotherapy for osteosarcoma: A randomized prospective trial. J Clin Oncol 1987;5:21–26.

Enneking WF, Spanier SS, Goodman MA: A system for the surgical staging of musculoskeletal sarcoma. Clin Orthop 1980;153:106–120.

Jaffe N, Patel SR, Benjamin RS: Chemotherapy in osteosarcomas. Hematol Oncol Clin N Am 1995;9:825–846.

Link MP, Goorin AM, Miser AW, et al: The effect of adjuvant chemotherapy on relapse-free survival in patients with osteosarcoma of the extremity. N Engl J Med 1986;314:1600–1602.

Meyers P, Gorlick R, Heller G, et al: Intensification of preoperative chemotherapy for osteogenic sarcoma: Results of the Memorial Sloan-Kettering (T12) protocol. J Clin Oncol 1998;16:2452–2458.

Chapter 102
Soft-Tissue Sarcomas

Pasquale Benedetto

Soft-tissue sarcomas are a heterogeneous group of malignancies that derive from the supporting structures of tissue and organs. Thus, these tumors can occur in any location and can arise as a malignant transformation of benign supporting tissue such as muscle, nerve, blood vessel, fat cell, and so on. The names for these tumors are generally derived from the cell of origin. For example, a malignant fat cell tumor is called a liposarcoma, and a malignant tumor derived from smooth muscle cells is called a leiomyosarcoma. The cells of origin of some histologic subtypes are unclear or unknown; one such example is malignant fibrous histiocytoma (MFH). In another example, synovial cell sarcoma is derived not from the synovium of joints, but rather from the aponeurosis of a tendon.

These tumors invade local tissues and spread both hematogenously and via lymphatics. The issues in patient care relate to preventing local recurrences and distant dissemination. Treatment varies by institution because the incidence of these cancers is relatively low and because few randomized studies have been conducted to establish definitive standards of care. Treatment recommendations in this chapter represent the author's interpretation of what constitutes optimal care based on his own studies, experience, and the best evidence from the literature. Pediatric soft-tissue tumors are not discussed in detail here; other chapters provide information about the diagnosis and management of osteosarcomas (see Chapter 101), Kaposi's sarcoma (see Chapter 113), and mesothelioma (see Chapter 97).

Pathology

A full listing of all of the histologic diagnoses applied by pathologists to soft-tissue sarcomas would be quite lengthy. The diagnosis of the specific type of soft-tissue sarcoma can be difficult despite the expertise of the pathologist and the use of a number of special procedures on the tissue biopsy. Table 102-1 lists only the most common histologies noted in adult soft-tissue sarcomas. The frequencies of each subtype are approximations because they vary remarkably among reported series due to differences in referral patterns and in categorization among pathologists. An alternate approach to defining the histologic categories is to consider whether the soft-tissue sarcoma is one of two general types—namely, spindle cell or small cell neoplasm. This dichotomy has clinical merit because the management of patients with spindle cell neoplasms and small cell neoplasms differs, regardless of the specification of their subtype.

Round Cell Neoplasms

From the pathologist's perspective, the differential diagnosis of small cell tumors is broad and can include such disparate entities as lymphoma, neuroendocrine tumors (e.g., carcinoids), melanoma, small cell carcinoma of the lung, embryonal rhabdomyosarcoma, neuroblastoma, or Ewing's sarcoma. Ancillary testing to distinguish among these various types of neoplasms includes the use of immunoperoxidase staining to detect the presence of surface and cytoplasmic markers, nuclear protein analysis, or cytogenetic analysis. The leukocyte common antigen (LCA or CD45) is a lymphocytic cell marker; its presence supports the diagnosis of lymphoma. S-100 staining suggests a diagnosis of neuroendocrine or neuroectodermal histiogenesis, which when associated with HMB45 positivity points to a diagnosis of melanoma. Synaptophysin or chromogranin positivity identifies a tumor (e.g., carcinoid) that is derived from neuroendocrine tissues. Cytokeratin expression establishes the tumor as epithelial in origin, as would be seen in small cell carcinoma, whether pulmonary or extrapulmonary in origin. Desmin and/or myogenin staining establishes muscle differentiation. The marker CD99 (myc-2) is associated with the Ewing's and primitive neuroectodermal tumor (PNET) family of tumors.

Most childhood sarcomas are in the category of small blue round cell tumors. Small cell tumors occur

Table 102-1 ■ Common Subtypes and Their Frequency* in Adult Soft-Tissue Sarcoma

Subtype (Cell of Origin)	Frequency
Malignant fibrous histiocytoma (unknown)	20%
Liposarcoma (adipose tissue)	15%
Fibrosarcoma (fibrous connective tissue)	15%
Synoviosarcoma (tendon sheath)	10%
Rhabdomyosarcoma (striated, voluntary muscle)	10%
Leiomyosarcoma (smooth, involuntary muscle)	5%
Neurofibrosarcoma, schwannoma (neural sheath)	5%
Angiosarcoma (blood or lymphatic vessels)	5%
Other/unclassified	15%

*Frequencies are approximate and rounded off to the nearest 5%.

in extrapulmonary sites in adults but are rare aside from metastases from small cell cancer of the lung.

Spindle Cell Tumors

This histology of spindle cell tumors is most characteristic of adult types of sarcoma. The major differential diagnosis to exclude would be spindle cell carcinoma. The presence of cytokeratin staining can help distinguish between these entities. Although sarcomas do not generally express the epithelial marker keratin, synovial cell sarcomas are unique among soft-tissue tumors because within a biphasic histologic pattern, they can exhibit both a spindle cell and an epithelial cell–appearing component. Within the spindle cell sarcomas, one might be able to distinguish the cell of origin by supportive immunoperoxidase staining, to include Factor VIII and CD31 (angiosarcoma), human caldesmon or desmin (leiomyosarcoma), c-kit and CD34 (gastrointestinal stromal tumor, GIST), or S100 (malignant peripheral nerve sheath tumor). The cell of origin of malignant fibrous histiocytoma, the most common adult soft-tissue sarcoma, is unknown. Whether this category is biologically homogeneous or a heterogeneous collection of sarcomas whose degree of differentiation provides no clues to the etiology remains uncertain.

Tumor Grade

The histologic grading of biologic aggressiveness of sarcomas is the single most important prognostic factor at the time of diagnosis and contributes to decisions about treatment planning. Histologically, these tumors are described as low-, intermediate-, or high-grade (G1, G2, and G3, respectively). In some centers, the designation of intermediate-grade is coalesced with the high-grade category, leaving only two prognostic subgroups of patients—favorable and unfavor-

able. Advancing tumor grade is judged based on decreased evidence of tumor cell differentiation, increased mitotic rate, increased extent of pleomorphism, and increasing areas of cellular necrosis. Because the grading of aggressiveness is based on numerous criteria that require separate judgments of the degree of abnormality over a continuous spectrum of morphologic changes, concordance about grading among pathologists is at times problematic. Moreover, these tumors are often heterogeneous in appearance, and sampling errors can affect the diagnosis rendered. Because of these concerns about establishing the biologic characteristics of a given tumor, open biopsy might be preferred to needle biopsy in order to ensure that an adequately representative tissue sample has been obtained from large tumors.

Tumor grade does correlate to some extent with the specific histologic subtype of sarcoma. For example, rhabdomyosarcoma, extraosseous Ewing's sarcoma/primitive neuroectodermal tumor, angiosarcoma, malignant peripheral nerve sheath tumor, and pleomorphic liposarcoma are all high-grade malignancies, whereas myxoid liposarcoma is virtually always low-grade. That histologic tumor grade carries greater prognostic import than individual histologic subtyping is evident in the variable histology of liposarcomas, which can be described as well differentiated, myxoid, round cell, or pleomorphic. The first two are low-grade tumors with a five-year survival rate as high as 80%, whereas the latter two subtypes are higher grade, carrying a much more unfavorable prognosis; in these types, the five-year survival rate is only 20%.

Histology and Correlations with Patient Age and Tumor Location

Unlike organ-specific tumors, soft-tissue sarcomas, taken as a group, occur across the entire age spectrum; they do not have a propensity to occur with increasing frequency at any specific age. The incidence of the specific histologic subtypes of soft-tissue sarcomas does, however, vary with the age of the patient. Most childhood forms are small blue round cell tumors; whereas most adult sarcomas are spindle cell neoplasms. The pattern that emerges is of rhabdomyosarcoma being more common in the young population (particularly among children), synovial cell sarcoma and neurogenic tumors increasing in frequency in young adults, and liposarcoma and malignant fibrous histiocytoma in the older adult. Rhabdomyosarcoma and the neural derived tumors that predominate in the young population typically involve the head and neck region, genitourinary tract, and (less commonly) the extremities.

In the adult, the most common histology is malignant fibrous histiocytoma. The most common site for a soft-tissue tumor is the extremity. The lower extremity predominates over the upper; proximal sites are more frequent than distal. Thus, the common presentation of an adult with a soft-tissue sarcoma is a thigh mass. Truncal, retroperitoneal, and visceral sarcomas are the other usual locations. It is rare for an adult to have a tumor arising in the head and neck region. When this does occur, frequently the histology is that which would be expected in the childhood disease, i.e., embryonal rhabdomyosarcoma.

Retroperitoneal tumors are most commonly liposarcomas or leiomyosarcomas. Less commonly, neurogenic tumors can arise in this location, especially in association with neurofibromatosis. These tumors represent a difficult therapeutic dilemma because of their frequent large size at presentation and the limitations of surgical intervention and radiation therapy in this location. Most visceral sarcomas are leiomyosarcomas; the largest group arising from the myometrium of the uterus. Tumors of the bowel wall are infrequent but important entities. Although all of these lesions were previously considered to be leiomyosarcomas, a subset, called gastrointestinal stromal tumor (GIST) is now recognized as a distinct clinical entity. These tumors arise from the pacemaker cells in the wall of the gastrointestinal tract (most commonly the stomach) and are identified by a specific immunohistochemical pattern that involves expression of CD34 and c-kit (CD117) genes, which code for an enzyme that is a molecular target for treatment (see the discussion that follows).

Epidemiology

The risk factors for the development of soft-tissue sarcomas depend on the age of the patient. Childhood tumors most frequently demonstrate a genetic predisposition. For example, malignant nerve sheath tumors are associated with neurofibromatosis and the NF-1 gene, while retinoblastomas and the Rb-1 gene are associated with the development of osteogenic sarcoma and soft tissue sarcomas. The Li-Fraumeni syndrome involves a p53 mutation, resulting in an increased risk of multiple types of cancers, including soft tissue and bone sarcomas. Soft-tissue sarcomas are also increased in incidence in other inherited genetic disorders such as the following:

- tuberous sclerosis (rhabdomyosarcoma)
- Gardner's disease (fibrosarcoma and its aggressive variant, the desmoid tumor)
- basal cell nevus syndrome (fibrosarcoma and rhabdomyosarcoma)

Acquired genetic mutations, such as translocations involving chromosome 22, are consistently found in the Ewing's/primitive neuroectodermal tumors family of tumors.

The etiology of sarcomas is unknown. There are, however, specific carcinogens that might induce sarcomas—for example, thoratrast, a radiologic contrast medium; polyvinyl chloride; arsenic; viruses such as Rous sarcoma virus and HIV; and ionizing radiation therapy. Despite these potential predisposing factors, most sarcomas appear sporadically rather than endemically.

The incidence of soft-tissue sarcomas is low relative to other tumor types. The annual incidence of adult soft-tissue sarcomas is approximately 6000, and approximately 3500 patients die of disease-related causes annually. Relative to the incidence of epithelial tumors such as breast, lung, colorectal, or prostate cancers, these tumors are infrequent. Because of the age distribution, however, sarcomas do represent a potentially serious health risk for youngsters and young adults and must be considered in the differential diagnosis of mass lesions in any location in these populations.

Clinical Presentation

The presentation of patients with soft-tissue sarcomas depends on the location of the tumor. Because these tumors can occur anywhere in the body, presenting symptoms and findings are highly variable. In adults who have soft-tissue sarcomas, because of the propensity for disease in the extremity, the cancers tend to present with an enlarging mass in the deep tissues. In these sites, the tumor can grow to a very large size before detection because of the lack of specific symptomatology in the early phases of development and the substantial expansile capacity of the surrounding tissues. On occasion, these tumors can appear in more superficial locations and be confused with benign lesions such as lipoma, ganglion, baker's cyst, or sebaceous cyst. It is important to remember that a superficial presentation does not preclude that a malignant lesion is present. Truncal lesions also cause symptoms based on mass effects. Both truncal and extremity tumors do not cause pain unless they are associated with local hemorrhage that produces rapid expansion of the mass or compression of an adjacent structure, such as a nerve or nerve root.

Retroperitoneal tumors can grow to be enormous and at times are diagnosed only by the palpation of a large abdominal mass or the recognition of increasing abdominal girth. Less frequently, the tumors present with back pain, sciatica secondary to nerve root compression, renal dysfunction, or alterations of digestive function such as early satiety, gastric outlet obstruction, constipation, gastrointestinal bleeding, or jaundice. Uterine sarcomas can present with a large mass interpreted as a fibroid or can be found when a previously diagnosed uterine fibroid suddenly increases in size, which might be a clue to malignant degeneration. Less commonly, the tumor can cause vaginal bleeding. Tumors arising from the gastrointestinal tract in general present with symptoms of gastrointestinal bleeding or intestinal obstruction.

In children, the most common location of a soft-tissue tumor is in the head and neck region. The most common presentation is proptosis, diplopia, and/or impaired extraocular movements. A neck mass might be evident due to regional node metastases from an orbital rhabdomyosarcoma. These tumors also can arise in the sinuses causing nasal obstruction, epistaxis, facial pain, and cranial nerve palsies. The genitourinary tract in children gives rise to soft-tissue tumors in paratesticular sites and in the prostate of boys and the vagina of girls; the latter is often termed sarcoma botryoides because its gross appearance is similar to a cluster of grapes. Retinoblastoma comes to diagnosis when there is evidence of visual impairment or when abnormal findings are noted on routine ophthalmologic exam.

Angiosarcomas are very rare tumors that have four common patterns of presentation: 1) as erythematous infiltrative or nodular lesions that usually involve the scalp but are occasionally located at other cutaneous sites in a predominantly elderly patient population; 2) as primary breast tumors; 3) as deep-seated soft-tissue tumors; and 4) as superficial skin lesions associated with chronic lymphedema.

Imaging a Soft-Tissue Mass

The evaluation of a soft-tissue mass requires that one always consider that the lesion could be malignant. Special attention is required when a preexisting lesion undergoes a rapid increase in size, such as might occur in the nodules of patients with neurofibromatosis or in other, previously benign, soft-tissue mass. In such a case, an imaging study should be obtained to evaluate the true extent of the lesion and the anatomic proximity to surrounding structures. The most helpful imaging study for an extremity lesion is magnetic resonance imaging (MRI). It provides better resolution than does computed tomography (CT) in defining the lesion in relation to other anatomic structures, especially with regard to the adjacent neurovascular bundles in extremity lesions. Magnetic resonance imaging, because it uses enhancement with contrast material and analysis of the change in signal on T1- and T2-weighted images, also permits assess-

ment of the internal characteristics of the mass. Tumors characteristically demonstrate gadolinium contrast enhancement and heterogeneity of signal on the T2 images.

Diagnostic Biopsy Considerations

The most frequent error made in the evaluation of a soft-tissue mass involves the lack of preoperative planning because the diagnosis was not considered prior to biopsy. Failure to plan in advance for the possibility that a lesion is in fact a sarcoma can have devastating long-term consequences for the patient because of increased morbidity, poor cosmesis, or increased risk of local recurrence when definitive therapy is ultimately attempted. In the case of extremity or truncal lesions, the operator performing a biopsy should plan the surgical incision in such a way that a future definitive procedure is not compromised or complicated by the first procedure. The surgical incision should be oriented along the vertical axis, which facilitates the removal of the scar and an ellipse of tissue in the definitive wide excision necessary for the surgical management of a sarcoma. In some centers, large-bore needle biopsies can be employed to obtain sufficient tissue for diagnosis. The biopsy tract should avoid proximity to the neurovascular bundle because of the hazards involved. Similarly, biopsy should be discouraged, unless unavoidable, especially if the lesion is hypervascular. This creates the potential for development of a hematoma, resulting in contamination of the surrounding tissue with tumor cells.

Although surgery is the definitive therapy for adult-type sarcomas, this is not true for childhood tumors, most of which fall into the category of small blue round cell neoplasms. Notably, these tumors are highly chemosensitive; therefore, chemotherapy, not surgery, forms the basis for therapy, with or without radiation therapy and/or surgery. In the case of childhood tumors, particularly those in the head and neck region, complete surgical resection is neither feasible nor contemplated, and an incisional biopsy usually suffices for diagnosis.

Staging and Prognosis

The staging system for adult soft-tissue sarcoma (Table 102-2) is described by a TNM classification based primarily on the size and grade of the tumor. Soft-tissue sarcomas are divided by size into two groups: those that are ≤5 cm (T1) or >5 cm (T2). More recently, the location of the tumor, defined as either superficial (a tumor that is situated exclusively above the fascia, without penetrating it) or deep, has been added to the staging in recognition that the prognosis differs

Table 102-2 ▪ American Joint Committee Staging System for Sarcomas

T (Primary Tumor)

T1	≤5 cm in diameter (a = superficial lesion; b = deep lesion)
T2	>5 cm in diameter (a = superficial lesion; b = deep lesion)

G (Histologic Grade)

G1	Low
G2	Intermediate
G3	High

N (Regional Lymph Nodes)

N0	No histologically verified involved nodes
N1	Histologically verified lymph node involvement

M (Distant Metastases)

M0	Not found
M1	Present

Stage Groupings	G	T	N	M	Approximate Five-Year Survival
I	G1	T1a, 1b, 2a, 2b	N0	M0	80%
II	G2/3	T1a, 1b, 2a	N0	M0	70%
III	G2/3	T2b	N0	M0	50%
			N1	M0	
IV	any G	any T	N1	M0	20%
			N0	M1	

between superficial and deep high-grade tumors. Tumors of visceral, intra-abdominal, or intrathoracic sites are considered deep by convention. The presence of metastatic disease either to distant sites or to regional lymph nodes is uncommon at presentation of a primary soft-tissue sarcoma but is increased in incidence when disease recurs. Stage IV metastatic disease is seen in circumstances in which the primary lesion is unusually large or the diagnosis has been delayed for a long period of time. It is also more likely to occur in association with particular histologies, such as rhabdomyosarcoma, synovial cell sarcoma, and epithelioid sarcoma. The stage groupings highlight the prognostic import of tumor grade.

The most common method of tumor spread for sarcomas is hematogenous (via the bloodstream). For extremity lesions, the first site of metastasis is the lung, and not infrequently this site remains the only apparent site of disease at the time of death from disease. For visceral lesions, the portal circulation can be the avenue of tumor dissemination; therefore, the liver can be a site of metastatic spread. Less frequently, these tumors spread to bone or brain.

The prognostic factors that have independent predictive value for survival outcome are listed in

Table 102-3. Apart from tumor grade, these include the size and depth of the primary lesion, the location, and the presence of regional dissemination. After surgical excision, the presence of tumor at the margins of the specimen adversely affects disease-related morbidity (local recurrence) and mortality, in comparison with patients who have a margin of surrounding normal tissue. A retrospective review of patients with

Table 102-3 ▪ Favorable versus Unfavorable Prognostic Factors for Survival in Patients with Soft-Tissue Sarcomas

	Favorable	Unfavorable
Tumor grade	Low	Intermediate or high
Size of primary tumor	Small	Large
Site	Proximal	Distal
	Extremity	Trunk
Regional lymph node involvement	Absent	Present
Tumor depth	Superficial	Deep

unfavorable (high-grade, deep, or ≥5 cm) primary sarcomas of the extremity at Memorial Sloan-Kettering Cancer Center showed, as expected, that the incidence of microscopically positive margins was 8% after amputation versus 28% in patients who had a limb-sparing surgical procedure. The latter patients also received postoperative radiation therapy, and the number of local recurrences were the same in both groups. No difference in survival or frequency of distant metastases was noted. Although not a prospective study, this led to the conclusion that a limb-sparing surgical procedure was the treatment of choice in patients with biologically aggressive tumors whenever possible, because the disability imposed by amputation was not balanced by any improvement in outcome. Thus, at least in aggressive tumors, the intrinsic tumor biology was a greater determinant of the likelihood of distant spread than whether clean surgical margins had been achieved.

In patients with metastatic or recurrent disease, independent favorable prognostic factors for survival include the following:

- good performance status
- young age
- absence of liver metastases
- low-grade histology
- prolonged time from initial diagnosis to advanced disease

Staging Evaluation

The studies needed to clinically stage a patient with newly diagnosed soft-tissue sarcoma depend on the location and histology of the tumor and the presence of unexplained symptoms. For extremity lesions in the adult, chest imaging by computed tomography scan is essentially the only test required because the lung is overwhelmingly the most likely site of initial distant spread. For intra-abdominal sites, an imaging study of the abdomen with emphasis on the liver is necessary. Bone scan and brain imaging are not required components of the metastatic evaluation unless there is a clinical suspicion of disease involvement based on neurologic symptoms, bone pain, or an elevated alkaline phosphatase.

For childhood tumors—in particular, for rhabdomyosarcoma, which comprises the largest histologic group—the assessment of the extent of disease is more complicated than in adults, because metastatic disease is more common, disease more readily disseminates by dual pathways (both lymphatic and hematogenous), and the disease is more often inaccessible to surgical excision, especially in the head and neck region. For these reasons, the evaluation of childhood sarcoma includes a bone scan, bone marrow aspirate and biopsy, and, in cases of parameningeal location, lumbar puncture for cerebrospinal fluid cytology. The staging system for childhood rhabdomyosarcoma is modified to take into account the local extent of the tumor and its location and the amount of residual disease after biopsy or resection, which can result in complete removal, microscopic residual disease, or gross disease.

Overview of Therapeutic Modalities for Adult Soft-Tissue Sarcomas

The two chief concerns in the treatment of soft-tissue sarcomas are ensuring local control and preventing distant metastases. The dimensions of the problem in cutting patients are substantial. In primary sarcomas of the extremity, after initial therapy 33% of patients experience disease recurrence. In approximately half of these patients, the first recurrence is local, and it is metastatic in the other half. In retroperitoneal sarcomas, approximately 25% of patients are alive and disease-free at five years; however, 40% of these five-year disease-free survivors will have relapsed by 10 years. Long-term assessments of the outcome of treatment are needed in patients with soft-tissue sarcomas.

Surgery

The primary treatment for adult soft-tissue sarcomas is surgery, which can be curative. As mentioned previously, cure requires that the initial biopsy procedure be planned carefully with subsequent therapy in mind. Otherwise, en bloc biopsy scar excision can be difficult, tissue planes can be disrupted, and cancer cells can spread through the tissues. These issues can lead to an increase in volume of tissue removed, with impairment of function and a requirement for skin grafting to close the wound. Moreover, lack of planning could make amputation necessary in extremity lesions, whereas a limb-sparing procedure could have sufficed. Although surgical therapy is the primary modality of treatment in adult sarcomas, therapy is multidisciplinary in most instances, requiring the expertise of the orthopedic or surgical oncologist, the medical oncologist, and the radiation oncologist. The tumor grade of the lesion does not alter the surgical approach to soft-tissue sarcomas.

Extremity Lesions

The definitive surgical procedure for extremity sarcomas involves amputation, en bloc compartment resection, or wide excision. Marginal resections—"shelling" out a tumor that appears to be encapsulated with a limited margin—is not an optimal surgical procedure, because local recurrence is sure to follow. Amputation is rarely required to remove an extremity tumor adequately except in the most distal aspects of the anatomy, namely, the foot, ankle, hand, and distal forearm. In these sites, the functional result with amputation and prosthesis is superior to the functional deficits of radical surgery and reduces the inherent risk of local recurrence due to limited margins. Compartment resection—the removal of the entire muscle compartment from origin to insertion—results in significant functional disability. Wide excision—resection of the tumor with a surrounding rim of at least 2 cm of noninvolved tissue—is the preferred approach. This leads to substantial preservation of function, which is balanced by an acceptable risk of local relapse (less than 20%).

Intrathoracic and Intra-Abdominal Sites

In the case of intra-abdominal or intrathoracic masses, quite frequently the exact nature of the lesion is unknown preoperatively despite evaluation by a computed tomography scan. Complete surgical excision is the contemplated procedure. In any situation in which complete resection is problematic, biopsy for disease documentation followed by multimodality treatment is used. Retroperitoneal sarcomas represent a difficult management problem. The completeness of the excision is a major determinant of outcome of the patient after surgery. Surgical intervention in this area is difficult. The surgeon is frequently unable to establish a clearly adequate margin of normal tissue because of the need to avoid damage to adjacent organs and the tendency of these tumors to infiltrate into the surrounding musculature of the abdominal wall or to abut adjacent vascular, neural, or osseous elements.

Truncal lesions by definition are treated by wide radical excision due to the anatomic limitations of the location. Visceral lesions of gastrointestinal and genitourinary sites are treated by the surgical procedures appropriate for the location.

Radiation Therapy

Radiation therapy is most frequently used as adjuvant therapy after wide tumor excision. Some centers do advocate preoperative radiation therapy for high-grade lesions. In the preoperative setting, the volume of irradiated normal tissue is less, and the treatment might be effective in generating an apparent capsule around the tumor, allowing for the development of clearly defined, clean surgical margins. Although the addition of radiation therapy to surgery decreases the risk of local recurrence, there is no affect on the rate of systemic relapse.

Chemotherapy in Advanced Disease

Few chemotherapeutic agents demonstrate reproducible activity in adult-type sarcomas. The most effective drugs are doxorubicin (single-agent response rate is 30%) and ifosfamide; other active drugs include cyclophosphamide, dacarbazine, cisplatinum, topotecan, and gemcitabine. In laboratory studies, the dose-response curve for these drugs (particularly for doxorubicin) is steep. This means that small increments in dosage yield larger increments in tumor cell killing and suggests that dosage reductions during treatment are to be avoided whenever possible. At the same time, the doses of the drugs needed to achieve a treatment response are associated with substantial toxicity. If treatment is administered with curative intent, it might be acceptable to ask the patient to tolerate the toxicity. In patients with metastatic disease, however, treatment is very rarely curative, and the median survival is only one year. In this setting, the toxicity mitigates against the application of these drugs in many patients. Despite a steep dose-response curve demonstrable in vitro, studies of chemotherapy dose escalation in advanced disease show an increase in response rate but no increase in survival. Moreover, trials of high-dose chemotherapy with autologous hematopoietic stem cell transplantation have not improved survival in patients with advanced disease, even though these patients are preselected for chemoresponsiveness to standard doses. Because of the limitations of current therapy in metastatic disease, patients should be enrolled in investigative clinical trials whenever feasible.

Clinical trials frequently include multiple types of sarcomas because the number of total cases available for study is small. Because the subtypes vary remarkably in terms of their chemosensitivity, the results of a clinical trial continuing heterogeneous subtypes might not accurately reflect the therapeutic efficacy against individual subtypes. Leiomyosarcomas and angiosarcomas respond poorly to chemotherapy, while synovial cell sarcomas are responsive. Malignant peripheral nerve sheath tumors do not respond to doxorubicin but are responsive to ifosfamide. Gastrointestinal stromal tumors are essentially chemoresistant, but the c-kit mutation activates the expression of a tyrosine kinase that is sensitive to blockade by imatinib mesylate (Gleevec), the drug that is used regularly in the treatment of chronic myeloid leukemia (see Chapter 71). With this agent, responses occur in more than 50% of patients who have gastrointestinal stromal tumors with minimal toxicity, although complete regression is rare.

Treatment of Specific Subsets of Sarcoma

Adult Low-Grade Sarcomas

Low-grade lesions, depending on the size, margins of resection, and the location of the tumor, are treated by definitive surgical resection followed by radiation therapy. This approach applies to low-grade malignancies, such as dermatofibrosarcoma protuberans, fibromatosis, and desmoid tumors. Adjuvant radiation therapy does decrease the risk of local recurrence but does not improve survival.

Adult High-Grade Sarcomas

Radiation therapy is generally included in the postoperative management of patients with high-grade lesions treated by wide excision to reduce the likelihood of local recurrence. High-grade tumors have a significant risk of distant disease relapse, however. Patients with large (>5 cm), grade 3 tumors have an approximately 50% risk of distant disease relapse. These relapses are usually at multiple sites in the lung. Although treatment with thoracotomy and chemotherapy salvages some patients for cure, the great majority of those who relapse will die of disease. For this reason, chemotherapy has become an integral part of the initial treatment of adult patients with extremity lesions.

Neoadjuvant Chemotherapy

Preoperative chemotherapy has been used in high-risk patients with localized disease in the hope that outcomes will be improved, as was shown for bone tumors. Such neoadjuvant therapy can cause substantial preoperative tumor regression, thereby facilitating surgical excision and reducing the tissue volumes that need to be removed. Moreover, a small fraction of the responding patients have no detectable viable cancer cells based on examination of the surgical resection specimen; this represents a pathologic complete remission reflected in the finding that >95% of the tumor cells are necrotic. Although it is uncertain that neoadjuvant therapy improves overall survival, the degree of response correlates directly with the duration of survival. The data on patients with advanced stage sarcoma of multiple histologic types treated at a single institution (Pisters et al., M.D. Anderson) with varying neoadjuvant chemotherapy programs were analyzed retrospectively. The authors believed that the results were no better than those achieved in other trials of postoperative chemotherapy. This kind of analysis is inconclusive, and at the University of Miami, the author favors the use of this admittedly controversial approach for the following reasons. Surgical excision is made easier in responding patients, and the prognostic information thus obtained is useful in deciding whether to use other treatment approaches postoperatively. Moreover, the histologic and clinical response at the time of definitive surgery allows individualization of therapy postoperatively, especially for those patients who have a poor response to neoadjuvant therapy. This in vivo assessment of chemosensitivity is patient- and tumor-specific and usefully applied to considerations of additional postoperative therapy.

Adjuvant Chemotherapy

Some investigators have reported prolonged survival, but no increase in the cure rate, after adjuvant chemotherapy, whereas others have concluded that chemotherapy has no demonstrable long-term survival benefit. The value of this approach remains uncertain. The failure to date to demonstrate the utility of adjuvant chemotherapy is due, in large part, to the inclusion of all sarcoma histologies in clinical trials, despite significant differences in chemosensitivity of various subtypes that make it difficult to compare the results across studies. Because of the relative rarity of each tumor subtype, most sarcoma trials have been underpowered (including too few patients with any one subtype) to demonstrate a statistically significant clinical benefit for adjuvant therapy compared with control patients who were treated with surgery alone.

Childhood Sarcomas

Most childhood sarcomas, rhabdomyosarcomas, or Ewing's/ primitive neuroectodermal tumor family of tumors are high-grade. Although Ewing's sarcoma (see Chapter 101) and primitive neuroectodermal tumor do not look similar histologically, they are combined for treatment strategies because they share a similar genetic translocation, implying similar biology and clinical behavior. These tumors are chemosensitive, and the primary therapy is multiagent drug therapy. Radiation therapy with or without surgery is used as needed after chemotherapy.

References

General Information

Antman KH: New biology and therapies in soft-tissue sarcomas. Biomed Pharmacother 2001;55:553–557.

Cormier JN, Patel SR, Herzog CE, et al: Concurrent ifosfamide-based chemotherapy and irradiation. Analysis of treatment-related toxicity in 43 patients with sarcoma. Cancer 2001;92:1550–1555.

Lewis JJ, Leung D, Heslin M, et al: Association of local recurrence with subsequent survival in extremity soft-tissue sarcoma. J Clin Oncol 1997;15:646–652.

Maki RG: Multidisciplinary management of soft-tissue sarcomas. Cancer Invest 2002;20:818–824.

McCarter MD, Jaques DP, Brennan MF: Randomized clinical trials in soft-tissue sarcoma. Surg Oncol Clin North Am 2002;11:11–22.

Pirayesh A, Chee Y, Helliwell TR, et al: The management of retroperitoneal soft-tissue sarcoma: A single institution experience with a review of the literature. Eur J Surg Oncol 2001;27:491–497.

Sandberg AA, Bridge JA: Updates on the cytogenetics and molecular genetics of bone and soft-tissue tumors. Desmoplastic small round cell tumors. Cancer Genetics Cytogen 2002;138:1–10.

Siegel MJ: Magnetic resonance imaging of musculoskeletal soft-tissue masses. Radiol Clin North Am 2001;39:701–720.

Wickerham DL, Fisher B, Wolmark N, et al: Association of tamoxifen and uterine sarcoma. J Clin Oncol 2002; 20:2758–2760.

Adjuvant and Neoadjuvant Chemotherapy

Eilber FC, Rosen G, Eckardt J, et al: Treatment-induced pathologic necrosis: A predictor of local recurrence and survival in patients receiving neoadjuvant therapy for high-grade extremity soft-tissue sarcomas. J Clin Oncol 2001;19: 3203–3209.

Frustaci S, Gherlinzoni F, De Paoli A, et al: Adjuvant chemotherapy for adult soft-tissue sarcomas of the extremities and girdles: Results of the Italian randomized cooperative trial. J Clin Oncol 2001;19:1238–1247.

Meric F, Milas M, Hunt KK, et al: Impact of neoadjuvant chemotherapy on postoperative morbidity in soft-tissue sarcomas. J Clin Oncol 2000;18:3378–3383.

Pisters PW, Patel SR, Varma DG, et al: Preoperative chemotherapy for stage IIIB extremity soft-tissue sarcoma: Long-term results from a single institution. J Clinical Oncol 1997;15: 3481–3487.

Wendtner CM, Abdel-Rahman S, Krych M, et al: Response to neoadjuvant chemotherapy combined with regional hyperthermia predicts long-term survival for adult patients with retroperitoneal and visceral high-risk soft-tissue sarcomas. J Clin Oncol 2002;20:3156–3164.

Chemotherapy for Advanced Disease

Le Cesne A, Judson I, Crowther D, et al: Randomized phase III study comparing conventional-dose doxorubicin plus ifosfamide versus high-dose doxorubicin plus ifosfamide plus recombinant human granulocyte-macrophage colony-stimulating factor in advanced soft-tissue sarcomas: A trial of the European Organization for Research and Treatment of Cancer/Soft-Tissue and Bone Sarcoma Group. J Clin Oncol 2000;18:2676–2684.

Patel SR, Vadhan-Raj S, Papadopolous N, et al: High-dose ifosfamide in bone and soft-tissue sarcomas: Results of phase II and pilot studies–dose-response and schedule dependence. J Clin Oncol 1997;15:2378–2384.

Patel SR, Gandhi V, Jenkins J, et al: Phase II clinical investigation of gemcitabine in advanced soft-tissue sarcomas and window evaluation of dose rate on gemcitabine triphosphate accumulation. J Clin Oncol 2001;19:3483–3489.

Reichardt P, Tilgner J, Hohenberger P, Dorken B: Dose-intensive chemotherapy with ifosfamide, epirubicin, and filgrastim for adult patients with metastatic or locally advanced soft-tissue sarcoma: A phase II study. J Clin Oncol 1998;16:1438–1443.

Verweij J, Lee SM, Ruka W, et al: Randomized phase II study of docetaxel versus doxorubicin in first- and second-line chemotherapy for locally advanced or metastatic soft-tissue sarcomas in adults: A study of the European Organization for Research and Treatment of Cancer soft-tissue and bone sarcoma group. J Clin Oncol 2000;18:2081–2086.

High-Dose Chemotherapy and Hematopoietic Stem Cell Transplantation

Blay JY, Bouhour D, Ray-Coquard I, et al: High-dose chemotherapy with autologous hematopoietic stem cell transplantation for advanced soft-tissue sarcoma in adults. J Clin Oncol 2000;18:3643–3650.

Lopez M, Vici P, Di Lauro L, Carpano S: Increasing single epirubicin doses in advanced soft-tissue sarcomas. J Clin Oncol 2002;20:1329–1334.

Nachman JB, Sieger L, Wadman J, Gorlick RG: High-dose melphalan, etoposide, total-body irradiation, and autologous stem cell reconstitution as consolidation therapy for high-risk Ewing's sarcoma does not improve prognosis. J Clin Oncol 2001;19:2812–2820.

Reichardt P: High-dose chemotherapy in adult soft-tissue sarcoma. Crit Rev Oncol Hematol 2002;41:157–167.

Pediatric Soft-Tissue Sarcomas

Paulussen M, Ahrens S, Dunst J, et al: Localized Ewing tumor of bone: Final results of the cooperative Ewing's Sarcoma Study CESS 86. J Clin Oncol 2001;19:1818–1829.

Raney RB: Soft-tissue sarcoma in childhood and adolescence. Curr Oncol Repts 2002;4:291–298.

Saylors RL 3rd, Stine KC, Sullivan J, et al: Cyclophosphamide plus topotecan in children with recurrent or refractory solid tumors: A Pediatric Oncology Group phase II study. J Clin Oncol 2001;19:3463–3469.

Wolden SL, Anderson JR, Crist WM, et al: Indications for radiotherapy and chemotherapy after complete resection in rhabdomyosarcoma: A report from the Intergroup Rhabdomyosarcoma Studies I to III. J Clin Oncol 1999;17: 3468–3475.

Prognosis

Coindre JM, Terrier P, Bui NB, et al: Prognostic factors in adult patients with locally controlled soft-tissue sarcoma. A study of 546 patients from the French Federation of Cancer Centers Sarcoma Group. J Clin Oncol 1996;14:869–877.

Fleming JB, Berman RS, Cheng SC, et al: Long-term outcome of patients with American Joint Committee on Cancer stage IIB extremity soft-tissue sarcomas. J Clin Oncol 1999;17:2772–2780.

Fletcher CD, Gustafson P, Rydholm A, et al: Clinicopathologic re-evaluation of 100 malignant fibrous histiocytomas: Prognostic relevance of subclassification. J Clin Oncol 2001;19:3045–3050.

Heslin MJ, Lewis JJ, Nadler E, et al: Prognostic factors associated with long-term survival for retroperitoneal sarcoma: Implications for management. J Clin Oncol 1997;15:2832–2839.

Heslin MJ, Woodruff J, Brennan MF: Prognostic significance of a positive microscopic margin in high-risk extremity soft-tissue sarcoma: Implications for management. J Clin Oncol 1996;14:473–478.

Levine EA, Holzmayer T, Bacus S, et al: Evaluation of newer prognostic markers for adult soft-tissue sarcomas. J Clin Oncol 1997;15:3249–3257.

Pisters PW, Leung DH, Woodruff J, et al: Analysis of prognostic factors in 1,041 patients with localized soft-tissue sarcomas of the extremities. J Clin Oncol 1996;14:1679–1689.

Spillane AJ, Ahern R, Judson IR, et al: Synovial sarcoma: A clinicopathologic, staging, and prognostic assessment. J Clin Oncol 2000;18:3794–3803.

Stojadinovic A, Leung DH, Allen P, et al: Primary adult soft-tissue sarcoma: Time-dependent influence of prognostic variables. J Clin Oncol 2002;20:4344–4352.

Trassard M, Le Doussal V, Hacene K, et al: Prognostic factors in localized primary synovial sarcoma: a multicenter study of 128 adult patients. J Clin Oncol 2001;19:525–534.

Van Glabbeke M, van Oosterom AT, Oosterhuis JW, et al: Prognostic factors for the outcome of chemotherapy in advanced soft-tissue sarcoma: An analysis of 2,185 patients treated with anthracycline-containing first-line regimens—a European Organization for Research and Treatment of Cancer Soft-Tissue and Bone Sarcoma Group Study. J Clin Oncol 1999;17:150–157.

Radiation Therapy

Alektiar KM, Leung D, Zelefsky MJ, Brennan MF: Adjuvant radiation for stage II-B soft-tissue sarcoma of the extremity. J Clin Oncol 2002;20:1643–1650.

Baldini EH, Goldberg J, Jenner C, et al: Long-term outcomes after function-sparing surgery without radiotherapy for soft-tissue sarcoma of the extremities and trunk. J Clin Oncol 1999;17:3252–3259.

Neuro-Oncology

Chapter 103
Primary Brain Tumors

Stuart A. Grossman

Primary brain tumors are second only to strokes as a cause of death from neurologic illness in adults. It is estimated that 17,000 new cases occur in the United States annually, resulting in 13,000 deaths. These tumors account for 1.4% of all cancers and 2.4% of all cancer deaths. In children, nearly one-quarter of all pediatric cancers are brain tumors. Approximately 60% of all primary brain tumors are high-grade gliomas (glioblastoma multiforme, anaplastic astrocytoma, anaplastic oligodendroglioma). The remainder are meningiomas (18%), low-grade astrocytomas (12%), medulloblastomas (2%), oligodendrogliomas (2%), ependymoma (2%), mixed oligoastrocytomas (2%), or other tumors (2%). The most common type of brain tumor differs between adults and children. More than 50% of all adult primary brain tumors are high-grade astrocytomas, whereas medulloblastomas and ependymomas account for only 3.6% of the total. In children, medulloblastomas and ependymomas account for 20% and 13% of the total, respectively, while glioblastoma multiforme accounts for only 12% of the pediatric brain tumor population. The incidence of primary brain tumors is greatly overshadowed by the incidence of metastatic brain tumors that occur in approximately 20% of all patients dying of cancer (see Chapter 104)

Ionizing radiation therapy is a known risk factor. Children who received cranial irradiation for tinea capitis or to prevent central nervous system leukemia have a significantly higher risk of developing a primary brain tumor. Certain chemical exposures from working in synthetic rubber production or from polyvinyl chloride also appear to predispose individuals to develop these tumors. In addition, there are several genetically transmitted disorders that are commonly associated with an increased risk of primary brain tumors. These include neurofibromatosis type 1 (von Recklinghausen's neurofibromatosis), neurofibromatosis type 2, tuberous sclerosis, and the Li-Fraumeni syndrome, which is an autosomal dominant aggregation of osteosarcomas, soft tissue sarcomas, breast cancers, and occasionally gliomas. Affected individuals with Turcot syndrome have an inherited adenomatous polyposis coli associated with astrocytomas and medulloblastomas (see Chapter 92).

Clinical Presentation

The clinical presentation of patients with primary brain tumors can be extremely variable. The signs and symptoms that initiate an evaluation, however, generally result from either increased intracranial pressure or focal neurologic abnormalities related to the location of the tumor.

The most common signs and symptoms of increased intracranial pressure include headache, nausea, vomiting, seizures, and changes in mental status. As primary brain tumors grow, they invade and compress normal tissue. As the brain is confined by the rigid structures of the skull, this growth can be sufficient to elevate intracranial pressure. Several other factors, however, can contribute to further rises in intracranial pressure (Table 103-1). Occasionally, these tumors are associated with enlarging cysts. Normal intracranial blood vessels are characterized by an intact blood-brain barrier that inhibits extravasation of large or water-soluble compounds into brain parenchyma. The blood vessels supplying aggressive

Table 103-1 ■ Causes of Increased Intracranial Pressure in Patients with Primary Brain Tumors

Expanding mass of tumor
Cyst associated with tumor
Peritumoral edema
Bleeding into tumor bed
Obstructive hydrocephalus

Table 103-2 ■ Conditions Causing Progressive Neurologic Deficits and/or Increased Intracranial Pressure

Neoplastic

Primary brain tumors
Metastatic brain tumors
Leptomeningeal metastases

Nonneoplastic

Subdural hematomas
Hydrocephalus
Brain abscesses
Multiple sclerosis
Progressive multifocal leukoencephalopathy
Vasculitis
Vascular malformations
Cerebral infarctions or bleeds
Cysts
Benign intracranial hypertension
Degenerative diseases
Congenital anomalies

brain tumors frequently have a disrupted blood-brain barrier. This disruption allows plasma proteins to extravasate into adjacent brain parenchyma, and water osmotically accompanies these proteins. In contrast to other organs in the body, the brain does not have a typical lymphatic system to clear extracellular fluid rapidly. As a result, peritumoral edema accumulates, generating additional mass effect in the region of the tumor. In addition, the blood vessels supplying these tumors may be friable. Occasionally, one of these vessels will bleed, further elevating intracranial pressure. Finally, the tumor mass and the peritumoral edema can compress normal cerebrospinal fluid flow pathways, causing obstructive hydrocephalus.

Patients also present with focal signs and symptoms related to the sites of their tumors. Thus, tumors or peritumoral edema compressing or involving the optic tracts or occipital lobe can present with visual disturbances. Parietal lobe lesions can cause motor or sensory symptoms or difficulty with speech. Temporal lobe lesions can be associated with memory problems, and frontal lesions can be relatively asymptomatic. Some of these tumors irritate the cerebral cortex sufficiently to trigger focal or generalized seizures.

Clinical Evaluation

Adults who present with a change in mental status, seizures, focal neurologic findings, or symptoms of increased intracranial pressure must be evaluated thoroughly. A complete history and physical examination are essential, as the differential diagnosis is extensive (Table 103-2). Many of these conditions are readily identifiable with appropriate neuroimaging studies; however, certain intracranial lesions—for example, an abscess, a hematoma, or an inflammatory, demyelinating, or congenital lesion—could be difficult to distinguish radiologically from a neoplasm. As a result, pathologic tissue sampling is required to reach a definitive diagnosis. Tissue is also routinely obtained from lesions that are highly likely to be tumors to determine the exact histology and grade, as these factors are critical to determining the prognosis and therapy.

Neuroimaging techniques are improving rapidly. Skull radiographs, tomography, and angiography have largely been replaced by computed tomography (CT) and magnetic resonance imaging (MRI). Magnetic resonance imaging has played an increasingly important role in the evaluation and clinical management of patients with primary brain tumors. It is more sensitive than computed tomography, providing better detail in the posterior fossa, skull base, and brain stem. In addition, magnetic resonance angiography (MRA) provides accurate information on blood vessels, and magnetic resonance spectroscopy permits novel information on tumor metabolism. Single-photon emission computed tomography (S-PECT) and positron emission tomography (PET) have limited roles in the initial evaluation of patients with primary brain tumors.

With modern neuroimaging and neurosurgical techniques, other laboratory studies are rarely required. Cerebrospinal fluid (CSF) examinations are potentially dangerous in patients with intracranial mass lesions and contribute little except to evaluate leptomeningeal involvement in patients with primary central nervous system lymphomas, medulloblastomas, or primitive neuroectodermal tumors. Biologic markers in the cerebrospinal fluid can be helpful in germ cell tumors of the pineal region. Visual field examinations and audiometry can provide important baseline values to supplement sequential magnetic resonance imaging results. Electroencephalography provides little in the diagnostic evaluation of these patients that is not already apparent from history,

Table 103-3 ■ Glioma Grading and Outcome

Histology	Median Survival
Pilocytic astrocytoma	>20 years
Astrocytoma (grade II)	Five to eight years
Anaplastic astrocytoma (grade II)	Three to five years
Glioblastoma multiforme (grade IV)	One year
Oligodendroglioma	Six to ten years
Anaplastic oligodendroglioma	Three to five years

physical examination, and a magnetic resonance imaging scan.

Staging, Prognostic Features, and Outcomes

The tumor, node, metastases (TNM) classification system is of little assistance in the management of primary brain tumors. The central nervous system does not contain lymph nodes, and tumors rarely disseminate to other organs. The most commonly used grading systems for the gliomas and the associated survival information are provided in Table 103-3.

Treatment

Corticosteroids, neurosurgery, and radiation therapy remain the principal treatment modalities for most patients with primary brain tumors. Corticosteroids reduce peritumoral brain edema, thereby reducing swelling in areas adjacent to the tumor and intracranial pressure. Reduction of swelling in turn often results in dramatic improvement in symptoms such as headaches, nausea, vomiting, altered mental status, or abnormalities of speech, balance, and motor strength. In addition, the reduction of intracranial pressure enables surgery to be performed more safely. Surgery is indicated to obtain diagnostic tissue and to remove as much tumor as possible without impairing the patient's functional status. Many tumors involve the deep structures of the brain, extend bilaterally or diffusely within a hemisphere, or infiltrate eloquent areas of the brain. In these situations, a stereotactic or open biopsy might be the best surgical option. Other tumors in a favorable location might lend themselves to a gross total resection. Frequently, these malignancies are associated with extensive mass effect, and a partial debulking of the tumor can provide diagnostic tissue as well as a marked functional improvement in the postoperative patient. Most malignant primary brain tumors are invasive and extend considerable dis-

tances into "normal" brain at the time of diagnosis. As a result, surgical cure is impossible. Radiation therapy is administered postoperatively to treat residual macroscopic or microscopic tumor. Chemotherapy plays a far less important role in most adult brain tumors, as these tumors are not very responsive to this treatment modality. In many childhood brain tumors and in primary central nervous system lymphomas, however, chemotherapy adds significantly to survival time.

Low-Grade Gliomas

Low-grade gliomas comprise approximately 15% of primary brain tumors in adults and a higher percentage in children. This heterogeneous group of tumors includes the astrocytomas, oligodendrogliomas, oligoastrocytomas, and gangliogliomas. They are most common in patients from age 20 to 40 years. The median survival for patients with these tumors is five to eight years, and only a few patients are cured. Most patients present with seizures, headaches, change in memory or personality, or focal neurologic signs. On computed tomography and magnetic resonance imaging scans, these tumors appear as nonenhancing masses and are often difficult to distinguish from infarctions, encephalomalacia, demyelination, inflammation, or infection (Figure 103-1). Only the pilocytic astrocytomas have a unique radiological appearance, with a cystic mass and an enhancing mural nodule. Patients with large, symptomatic, and growing lesions require surgery. There is considerable controversy, however, regarding the best therapy for patients who present with seizures or other mild symptoms that can be managed medically. Although pilocytic astrocytomas can be cured surgically, surgery is rarely curative for patients with the infiltrative astrocytomas, oligodendrogliomas, or oligoastrocytomas. Thus, the surgical options include initial debulking surgery or careful observation plus surgical debulking when the tumor clearly changes in size. The data concerning when to employ radiation therapy are similarly in transition. Unfortunately, radiation therapy is not curative and is associated with neuropsychological and neuroendocrine dysfunction, which become increasingly severe the longer the patient survives. Because current data suggest that there is no survival advantage to radiating these tumors early, most radiation oncologists treat these patients only when they have evidence of progressive disease. As a general rule, chemotherapy is most effective in patients with rapidly growing neoplasms and would not be expected to be very active for the low-grade gliomas. Nevertheless, occasional responses have been noted in oligodendrogliomas and oligoas-

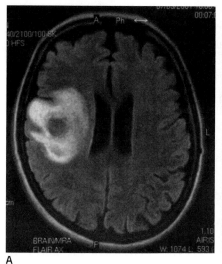
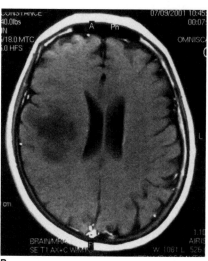

A   B

Figure 103-1 ▪ A 62-year old woman presented with the gradual onset of slurred speech. *A*, T2 flair magnetic resonance imaging demonstrating a right parietal lesion associated with little mass effect. *B*, T1-weighted magnetic resonance imaging with contrast revealing an abnormal hypodense area with no contrast enhancement. A needle biopsy was diagnostic for a low-grade astrocytoma.

trocytomas. Clinical trials are being conducted using a combination of procarbazine, CCNU, and vincristine in this patient population. The results of these efforts, however, are difficult to quantify because determining radiographic "responses" in these nonenhancing lesions can be difficult and because these tumors often remain stable for months or years without therapy. In addition, there is a significant risk of myelodysplasia and leukemia five years after treatment with nitrosoureas. For these reasons, chemotherapy is gen-

erally limited to patients with progressive disease after surgery and radiation therapy when other therapeutic options are limited.

High-Grade Gliomas

Malignant gliomas account for more than 50% of all primary brain tumors. Approximately 60% are glioblastomas, 30% are anaplastic astrocytomas, and the remainder are anaplastic oligodendrogliomas,

---

TREATMENT

Low-Grade Gliomas

Low-grade gliomas are most common in patients between 20 and 40 years of age. The median survival for patients with these tumors is five to eight years, and few are curable. Most patients present with seizures, headaches, changes in memory or personality, or focal neurologic signs.

Radiology

▪ Magnetic resonance imaging is the preferred imaging modality and usually reveals a nonenhancing mass with considerable T2 abnormality and a variable amount of mass effect.

Preoperative Interventions and Work-up

▪ Dexamethasone is prescribed if needed to reduce intracranial pressure and local edema.
▪ Anticonvulsants are prescribed if the patient has had a seizure.
▪ A careful history and physical examination are performed to narrow the differential diagnosis. These tumors can be difficult to differentiate from some benign conditions.

Neurosurgical Consultation

▪ Surgical options include initial debulking or careful observation and surgical debulking when the tumor clearly changes in size. Patients with large, symptomatic, and growing lesions require surgery.

Radiotherapy Consultation

▪ Because current data suggests there is no survival advantage to early radiation in these tumors, most radiation oncologists treat patients only when they have evidence of progressive disease.

Neuro-Oncology Consultation

▪ Chemotherapy with BCNU, PCV (procarbazine, CCNU, and vincristine), or temozolomide provide modest benefit in these tumors. No available data documents a survival advantage using these agents. In general, they are best used when there are no reasonable surgical or radiotherapy options.

Figure 103-2 ■ A 43-year-old man presented with headaches, worsening memory, and visual changes. *A,* His T2 flair magnetic resonance imaging demonstrated a large abnormal region in the left parietooccipital region with compression of the ipsilateral ventricle, loss of cortical sulci, and signal abnormality crossing the posterior corpus callosum into the contralateral hemisphere. *B,* The T1-weighted magnetic resonance imaging with contrast revealed extensive extravasation of contrast into the lesion, an area of central necrosis, and the presence of adjacent small enhancing areas. Debulking surgery was diagnostic for a glioblastoma multiforme.

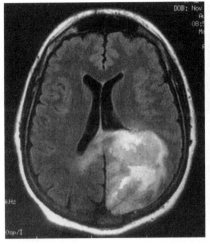

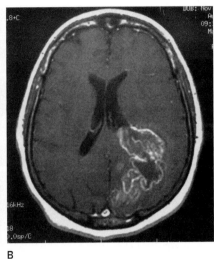

A

B

anaplastic oligoastrocytomas, and anaplastic ependymomas. The incidence of anaplastic astrocytomas peaks between the ages of 30 and 50, while glioblastomas are most common in patients over 50 years of age. The presenting symptoms are similar to those of other brain tumors. Neuroimaging studies typically reveal a central hypodense area of necrosis surrounded by a contrast-enhancing tumor with extensive edema and mass effect. Tumor cells are demonstrable as a T2 signal on magnetic resonance imaging and frequently cross the corpus callosum and extend to distant regions of the brain along white matter tracts (Figure 103-2 *A, B*). Longer survival is correlated with young age, high performance status, and anaplastic astrocytoma rather than glioblastoma. Standard therapy for the high-grade astrocytomas has changed little during the past several decades. Surgical resection of as much of the tumor as is safe and involved-field radiation therapy are the mainstays of therapy. Higher doses of radiation, novel fractionation schedules, and newer techniques that allow high doses of radiation to be deposited with accuracy (i.e., seed implants, stereotactic radiosurgery, gamma knife, etc.) have been explored. So far, these have yet to yield significant improvements in survival. Three chemotherapeutic agents have some efficacy in the treatment of high-grade astrocytomas: the nitrosoureas (BCNU or CCNU), procarbazine, and temozolomide. BCNU provides a small survival benefit early on, but its benefits are no longer apparent 24 months later. Procarbazine and temozolomide have limited activity in glioblastoma multiforme. During the past decade, there has been enthusiasm for the use of the procarbazine, CCNU, and vincristine (PCV) regimen in patients with anaplastic astrocytoma; however, recent reviews of the RTOG database and a large randomized prospective study from Great Britain suggest that any benefit from this regimen in anaplas-

tic astrocytomas or glioblastoma multiforme is modest. In patients with recurrent high-grade astrocytomas who are undergoing surgery, placement of biodegradable polymers containing BCNU into the resection bed confers a modest survival advantage when compared with placement of a placebo polymer. Preliminary findings on patients with newly diagnosed high-grade gliomas suggest a small survival advantage in this population as well.

Primary Central Nervous System Lymphoma

Primary central nervous system lymphoma (PCNSL) is a very uncommon brain tumor that is associated with congenital or acquired immunodeficiency states. Before active antiretroviral agents became available, approximately 2% to 6% of all patients with AIDS developed primary central nervous system lymphoma (see Chapter 113). This disease is also increasing in frequency in immunocompetent patients for unknown reasons. The peak incidence in immunocompetent patients is in the sixth and seventh decades of life. Primary central nervous system lymphoma is a rapidly growing tumor, and patients typically present with progressive symptoms that have been present for only weeks. Headache, symptoms of increased intracranial pressure, focal neurologic symptoms, and cognitive or personality changes are most common. This type of tumor usually involves the deep structures of the brain, is frequently multifocal at diagnosis, and can also involve the spinal fluid, spinal cord, and eyes. Computed tomography scan and magnetic resonance imaging are critical for diagnosis (Figure 103-3). Pathologically, this tumor appears identical to a systemic, aggressive, large cell, diffuse, B cell lymphoma. As these tumor cells are sensitive to glucocorticoids, early administration of corticosteroids with the intent of decreasing peritumoral edema in a patient with a

TREATMENT

High-Grade Gliomas

Patients with glioblastoma multiforme, anaplastic astrocytoma, or anaplastic oligodendroglioma often present with headaches, seizures, and/or progressive neurologic deficits.

Radiology

- Magnetic resonance imaging is the preferred imaging modality and usually reveals a contrast-enhancing mass with considerable edema and mass effect.

Preoperative Interventions and Work-Up

- Dexamethasone is prescribed to reduce intracranial pressure and local edema.
- Anticonvulsants are prescribed if the patient has had a seizure.
- A careful history and physical examination are performed to narrow the differential diagnosis. It is important to remember that brain metastases are much more common than primary brain tumors.

Neurosurgical Consultation

- If the magnetic resonance imaging scan suggests primary central nervous system lymphoma, glucocorticoids should be withheld, and stereotactic biopsy should be considered.
- If the magnetic resonance imaging scan suggests high-grade glioma, a maximal safe resection should be done if feasible; otherwise, a stereotactic biopsy should be performed.

Radiotherapy Consultation

- Involved field radiation is prescribed to a margin around the region of T2 abnormality on the magnetic resonance imaging scan. As the tumor cells are present considerable distances from the visible tumor, techniques that deliver focused radiation to small areas (e.g., gamma knife, stereotactic radiation) are not likely to be of much benefit.

Neuro-Oncology Consultation

- Chemotherapy consisting of BCNU, PCV (procarbazine, CCNU, and vincristine), or temozolomide provide little benefit in the adjuvant setting. For high-grade gliomas (unlike breast or colon cancer), these agents do not provide patients with a chance for cure.
- Clinical trials are a reasonable option for patients with high-grade gliomas, as results with available therapies are unsatisfactory. Trials for newly diagnosed patients must be considered immediately after surgery, as initiating radiation or chemotherapy could render them ineligible for a clinical trial until they have obvious tumor recurrence.

Careful Follow-up with Examinations and Scans Every Two Months

- Standard approaches or clinical trials should be considered when there is progressive tumor. Standard options might include chemotherapy or additional surgery or radiation.

---

mass lesion can cause the tumor to shrink or even disappear. This can lead to a false negative brain biopsy or cerebral spinal fluid cytology. Without treatment, this neoplasm is fatal within approximately three months. Surgical resection contributes little to survival, as this is a diffuse, multifocal disease. Radiation has been the mainstay of therapy. Whole-brain radiotherapy prolongs survival to 12 months, but the tumor rapidly recurs. The five-year survival is approximately 3%, and the few survivors are usually devastated by the long-term consequences of whole-brain radiation. Chemotherapy regimens effective in systemic lymphomas produce brief remissions but no increase in overall survival. In the 1980s, Neuwelt initiated a treatment program using osmotic blood-brain barrier disruption followed by intra-arterial methotrexate and intravenous cyclophosphamide, procarbazine, and dexamethasone. Radiation was used only if patients failed to respond. The median survival was 44 months. Shortly thereafter, DeAngelis and colleagues used high-dose intravenous methotrexate ($1 \, g/m^2$), intrathecal methotrexate, radiation therapy, and high-dose cytarabine and obtained a median survival of 31 months. Severe cognitive deficits were noted, especially in the older patients treated with this regimen. More recently, high doses of methotrexate ($8 \, gm/m^2$) given every two weeks followed by monthly maintenance methotrexate have been explored. Radiation was withheld unless the patients failed to respond or relapsed. The median survival of these patients is approximately three years, and thus far there does not appear to be appreciable neurotoxicity from the therapy. High doses of systemically administered methotrexate might also provide adequate treatment of the leptomeninges and vitreous in responsive patients.

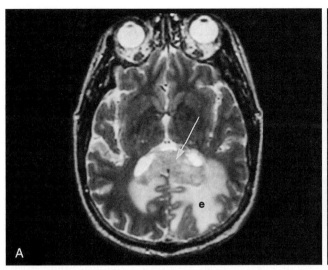
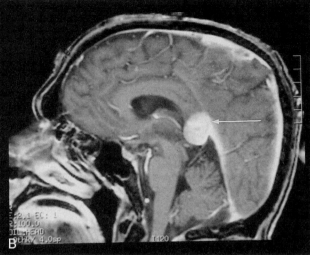

Figure 103-3 ■ Magnetic resonance imaging of central nervous system lymphoma. *A*, The mass is of low signal intensity (at arrow), and the surrounding edema shows high signal intensity. *B*, The sagittal view shows the enhancing tumor (arrow) in the splenium of the corpus callosum. (From Grainger RG, Allison DJ: *Diagnostic Radiology: A Textbook of Medical Imaging*. New York: Churchill Livingstone, 1998, p 2085.)

Meningiomas

Meningiomas account for about 20% of all brain tumors. They are the second most common brain tumor and the most common benign brain tumor. The incidence of meningioma peaks in the sixth to seventh decade, and these tumors are more common in women than men. Many meningiomas are completely asymptomatic. Approximately 90% of meningiomas are supratentorial, and the most common locations are in the falx and parasagittal regions, convexity, and sphenoid wing. Convexity meningiomas often remain asymptomatic until they reach a large size and then present with seizures, focal deficits, or headaches. Falx and parasagittal lesions present similarly but often involve the sagittal sinus, making resection more difficult. The parasagittal lesions can cause bilateral leg weakness. Sphenoid ridge meningiomas can involve the cavernous sinus and carotid arteries and can produce occulomotor palsies and facial numbness. These lesions are easily appreciated on modern neuroimaging studies. On computed tomography scan, they appear as well-defined hyperdense masses with calcification and a broad dural base (Figure 103-4). They enhance brightly and homogeneously with contrast. The primary therapy for meningiomas is surgery. Complete removal of the tumor is associated with 10% to 20% recurrence rate at 10 years, whereas recurrence rates for subtotal resections are 30% to 55%. Radiation is often suggested for patients with residual or recurrent disease when another surgical resection is ill advised. Patients with small menin-

giomas who are asymptomatic or who have medically controlled seizures and without associated brain edema are commonly observed with serial imaging studies. Malignant meningiomas are a small but important subset of meningiomas. They have a high recurrence rate after surgery and usually respond poorly to radiation or chemotherapy. Approximately one-quarter of these patients develop systemic metastases, usually to lung and bone.

Medulloblastoma

Medulloblastoma is the most common malignant brain tumor in children and accounts for about one-quarter of all brain tumors in patients under the age of 15 years. It occurs most frequently in children between the ages of 5 and 9 and usually arises in the cerebellum. Patients usually present with signs and symptoms of increased intracranial pressure and cerebellar findings. Imaging studies reveal a contrast-enhancing lesion distorting the fourth ventricle and invading the cerebellum, its peduncles, and (less commonly) the brain stem. Staging of the spinal subarachnoid space is required, and a bone scan is commonly performed. Surgical resection, radiation therapy, and chemotherapy all play a significant role in the management of this tumor.

Ependymomas

Ependymomas arise from the ependymal cells surrounding the ventricles and central canal of the spinal

TREATMENT

Primary Central Nervous System Lymphoma

Central nervous system lymphoma is a rare tumor but one that might be curable with high-dose methotrexate-based chemotherapy regimens.

Radiology

■ Magnetic resonance imaging is the preferred imaging modality. These tumors homogeneously enhance with contrast and are often deep, periventricular, bilateral, and multifocal at the time of presentation. They often shrink dramatically after treatment with dexamethasone administered to control increased intracranial pressure.

Preoperative Interventions and Work-Up

■ If the patient's clinical condition permits, dexamethasone should be withheld until after the biopsy is performed.
■ Anticonvulsants are prescribed if the patient has had a seizure.
■ Slit lamp exam of eyes, cerebral spinal fluid cytology (if this can be done safely), and human immunodeficiency virus (HIV) test should be performed. Systemic lymphoma with central nervous system metastases usually presents with leptomeningeal disease without diffuse intraparenchymal involvement. Computed tomography scan of chest and abdomen can be considered if systemic lymphoma is a concern.

Neurosurgical Consultation

■ If diagnostic tissue is not available from the cerebral spinal fluid or the eye, a stereotactic biopsy should be performed.

Radiotherapy Consultation

■ Although whole-brain radiation was the standard of care 10 years ago, it is now frequently prescribed either with a high-dose methotrexate-based regimen or when a patient progresses after chemotherapy.

Neuro-Oncologic Consultation

■ A high-dose methotrexate-based regimen is the treatment of choice. The dose (3.5–8.0 g/m^2) is modified based on the creatinine clearance. Hydration, alkylinization, methotrexate levels, and high-dose leukovorin rescue are required. Methotrexate is repeated at intervals as frequent as every two weeks, with scans repeated every month. Treatments are continued using the same dose and frequency for one month after complete response occurs, and then maintenance therapy once per month is suggested. The optimal duration of maintenance therapy is unknown but can last as long as one year.
■ Enrollment in a clinical trial is strongly recommended, as progress is being made in this rare tumor and there are many important clinical questions to answer.
■ The combination of glucocorticoids, methotrexate, and radiation therapy is immunosuppressive. As a result, prophylaxis for *Pneumocystis carinii* pneumonia (PCP) is highly recommended. Extreme caution is required, as many of the agents commonly used for PCP prophylaxis (e.g., Bactrim) interfere with methotrexate excretion or are antifolates.
■ If the eyes or cerebrospinal fluid is involved, they must be followed carefully to ensure that these sites are also responding to methotrexate. Radiation to the eyes or intrathecal chemotherapy can be considered if needed.
■ Clinical trials are a reasonable option for patients.

Careful Follow-up with Examinations and Scans Every Two Months

■ Retreatment with high-dose methotrexate, whole-brain radiation (if not already administered), or therapy with other chemotherapy drugs can be considered if the tumor recurs.

---

cord. These represent about 10% of brain tumors in children and less than 5% of gliomas in adults. The median age at diagnosis is 6 years. The most common location for these tumors is in the fourth ventricle, where they frequently lead to obstructive hydrocephalus or invasion or compression of the brain stem. Spinal cord ependymomas are more common in adults than in children. Surgical resection and radiation are the primary therapies for this tumor. A gross total resection is associated with higher sur-

vival rates. Chemotherapy is of little benefit in these tumors. Tumor can disseminate in the cerebrospinal fluid, especially in patients with higher-grade ependymomas.

Brain Stem Gliomas

Primary tumors of the brain stem comprise less than 5% of gliomas in adults and 10% to 15% of primary brain tumors in children. In children, the median age at diagnosis is 5 to 7 years. Because of their location,

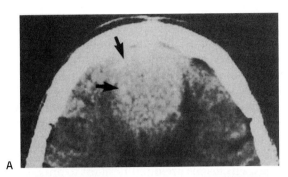

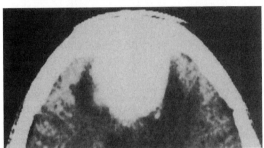

Figure 103-4 ■ Meningioma; computed tomography. Before (*A*) and after (*B*) intravenous contrast medium: a large, rounded lesion, denser than the surrounding brain, lies in the midline anteriorly. It has small foci of calcification within it (arrows). After contrast medium, there is typical marked homogenous enhancement. The tumor arises in relation to the anterior part of the falx cerebri. (From Bragg DG, Rubin P, Youker JE (eds): Oncologic Imaging. New York, Elsevier Science, 1985, p 868.)

intrinsic lesions of the brain stem are not surgically accessible. An open or stereotactic biopsy is considered when the diagnosis is in doubt. Exophytic lesions are usually approached surgically for both diagnosis and resection. Ependymoma and medulloblastoma can be in the differential diagnosis of these lesions. The primary therapy for these patients is radiation, but even with radiation the median survival for the most common subtypes is less than one year.

Important Management Issues

The optimal management of patients with primary brain tumors involves more than providing excellent surgery, radiation therapy, and chemotherapy. In fact, the care of these patients is accompanied by an assortment of challenges unique in the field of oncology:

- Responses are often difficult to assess.
- Anticonvulsants dramatically affect the pharmacology of chemotherapy drugs.
- The chronic use of glucocorticoids predispose patients to serious and debilitating side effects.
- Thromboembolic disease is common.

- Patients often have difficulty meeting eligibility criteria for clinical trials.

Furthermore, the psychosocial impact on patients and families that accompanies the loss of independence and cognitive ability, and the special issues that arise in caring for patients dying of brain tumors, require careful attention.

Judging the Efficacy of Therapy

Determining the efficacy of therapy is more difficult in patients with brain tumors than in patients with systemic malignancies. Clinical signs and symptoms are unreliable indicators of response, as damage to the nervous system from tumor, surgical intervention, or increased intracranial pressure can be irreversible. As a result, a patient's signs and symptoms might not improve, even if the tumor has dramatically regressed. Conversely, clinical improvement can be due to a reduction in edema following the administration of glucocorticoids or improved seizure control, even if the tumor has not changed in size. Computed tomography and magnetic resonance imaging studies can be similarly misleading. Responses are generally determined by measuring the size of the contrast-enhancing lesion and the amount of mass effect and peritumoral edema. These are all a function of blood-brain barrier integrity. Thus, glucocorticoid therapy can diminish the amount of contrast leaking into the tumor and reduce the amount of mass effect and peritumoral edema without affecting the actual size of the tumor. Likewise, radiation therapy, which can increase disruption of the blood-brain barrier for months, makes the tumor, mass effect, and edema appear to increase. In addition, necrosis from radiation therapy is indistinguishable from progressive tumor by magnetic resonance imaging or computed tomography scan. Positron emission tomography, magnetic resonance imaging spectroscopy, or a repeat tissue biopsy are often required to distinguish dead tissue from progressive tumor.

Anticonvulsants

Most patients with primary brain tumors are treated with anticonvulsants because they present with or are believed to be at high risk for seizures. In addition, neurosurgeons routinely place patients on these agents prior to surgery. As a result, anticonvulsant use is common, and many patients continue therapy for the remainder of their lives, even though current data suggest that prophylactic anticonvulsants provide little benefit. These agents can significantly complicate the care of patients with primary brain tumors in many ways. Allergic reactions are relatively frequent and can be severe. Carbamazepine is myelosuppressive and makes it more difficult to administer full doses of chemotherapy. Anticonvulsants that are hepatic P450 system inducers, such as phenytoin, phenobarbital, and carbamazepine, can dramatically affect the pharmacology of many chemotherapeutic agents. Due to the concomitant use of such anticonvulsants, these antineoplastic agents are metabolized by the liver much more rapidly than normal, resulting in subtherapeutic levels reaching the tumor. In addition, some chemotherapeutic agents can alter the pharmacology of the anticonvulsants. For example, cisplatin can reduce phenytoin levels and make it more likely for susceptible patients to have seizures. Some patients might require as much as twice the amount of phenytoin to maintain therapeutic levels shortly after receiving cisplatin.

Glucocorticoids

Glucocorticoids are essential to reversing neurological signs and symptoms caused by peritumoral edema. The highest doses of these agents are usually administered in the perioperative period, during radiation therapy, and at the time of tumor recurrence; however, many patients remain dependent on glucocorticoids. The side effects associated with these agents are often more troublesome than those that accompany antineoplastic therapies. The toxicities most likely to affect patient survival relate to the immunosuppressive and antipyretic effects of these agents. These predispose patients to infection and make it more difficult to recognize a serious infection when it occurs. Special care must be exercised in neutropenic patients taking glucocorticoids, as they can be septic without rigors, fevers, or localizing signs of infection. *Pneumocystis carinii* pneumonia also occurs in these patients as glucocorticoids are tapered. This often begins with fever and dyspnea and rapidly progresses to hypoxia and respiratory failure. It is associated with a mortality rate that approaches 50%. Other glucocorticoid toxicities severely affect quality of life in these patients. Patients note a voracious appetite, weight gain, fluid retention, and the typical changes in body habitus associated with Cushing's disease. In addition, emotional lability, sleep disturbances, hyperglycemia, gastric hyperacidity, osteoporosis, skin and capillary fragility, joint pains, visual changes, and an acneform rash are common. One of the most disabling consequences is a proximal myopathy that usually begins with the proximal muscles of the lower and upper extremities but can spread to the pelvic and respiratory muscles. Early symptoms include difficulty rising from a low chair. This commonly progresses to unexpected falls and inactivity.

Thromboembolic Disease

Clinically apparent thromboembolic events occur in approximately one-quarter of all patients with high-grade astrocytomas and represent a major cause of morbidity and mortality. The incidence is likely to be even higher in elderly, immobile patients with multiple medical problems. Administration of chemotherapy to these patients probably further increases the incidence of thromboembolic events, as it does in other malignancies. Physicians are often hesitant to anticoagulate patients with primary brain tumors for fear of an intracranial bleed. Fortunately, the use of conservative heparin loading doses followed by warfarin and careful monitoring is usually well tolerated by these patients. Drugs commonly prescribed to patients with brain tumors are known to potentiate (phenytoin) or diminish (glucocorticoids, phenobarbital, carbamazepine) the anticoagulant effect of warfarin. The platelet count should be kept above 50,000/μL while anticoagulants are administered, and aspirin-containing drugs and nonsteroidal anti-inflammatory agents should be avoided. Thrombolytics are contraindicated, and vena caval filters are rarely required.

Psychosocial Issues (See Chapter 120)

The rapid and relentless natural history of most brain tumors heralds devastating changes for patients and their families. Seizures or motor or visual deficits can render patients unable to drive a car from the time they present with this illness. Others cannot dress, walk, eat, or bathe independently. Cognitive deficits, expressive or receptive aphasias, or poor short-term memory can make it impossible for patients to remain unsupervised even for short periods. The sudden and extreme dependence on family and friends, along with the potential loss of mental function and communicative capacity, place great stresses on both patients and their families. In addition, alopecia from radiation and the changes in body habitus, acne, and proximal myopathy that occur with glucocorticoids cause further damage to patients' self-image. Patients are frequently unable to return to work, and caregivers often need to adjust their work schedules to provide care. These circumstances often add significant financial stress to the situation. Issues of competence, guardianship, power of attorney, and wills need to be addressed. Care must be taken to ensure that the patient and family have access to a broad range of medical and social support services.

Care of the Dying Patient (See Chapter 122)

Most patients with malignant brain tumors cannot be cured with currently available therapies. Thus, ensuring that the patients have maximal quality of life and die comfortably and with dignity are important goals. The end of life can be difficult for this patient population. Patients might be physically unable to communicate their needs or feelings. Progressive confusion, disorientation, and somnolence are common, and many patients are distraught by their extraordinary dependence. Many patients become increasingly lethargic and die peacefully; however, headaches, nausea and vomiting from increased intracranial pressure, seizures, bedsores, and candida mucositis or esophagitis are not uncommon. Controlling the symptoms of increased intracranial pressure and preventing seizures are paramount during this phase of the illness. Increasing doses of glucocorticoids might transiently reduce intracranial pressure but could also prolong the illness. Alternatively, opioids can be administered to reduce the intensity of the headaches. As the patient develops increasing difficulty with oral medications, however, glucocorticoids, opioids, and anticonvulsants might have to be administered rectally, parenterally, transdermally, or via a small, flexible nasogastric feeding tube. Many of these changes must be made thoughtfully; converting a patient with a known seizure disorder to a new anticonvulsant or a new route of administration is hazardous and can precipitate seizure activity.

Follow-up Evaluation

The follow-up evaluation of patients with primary brain tumors is highly dependent on the nature of the tumor. For example, a patient with a complete surgical resection of a meningioma or a pilocytic astrocytoma is likely to be cured. A follow-up examination and magnetic resonance imaging scan would occur in the postoperative period and then again about six months later. If no evidence of recurrence is found, this patient could probably be seen annually for several years. At the other end of the spectrum is the follow-up for a patient with a glioblastoma multiforme. This tumor in this patient is virtually guaranteed to recur; the disease is highly likely to have a complicated course; and the patient will probably die of this disease within one to two years of diagnosis. These patients are usually seen in follow-up, examined, and scanned every two to three months. Alternate therapies are considered with evidence of progressive disease. Patients with low-grade astrocytomas are usually seen, examined, and imaged at four- to six-month intervals. Follow-up visits for patients with any primary brain tumor must also be used to consider possible complications from surgery (infection), radiation (edema, necrosis, or long-term sequelae), chemotherapy (neutropenia, thrombocytopenia,

anemia, neuropathy), and the supportive care medications the patient is taking (e.g., glucocorticoids, anticonvulsants, and/or anticoagulants).

References

Epidemiology

Inskip PD, Linet MS, Heineman EF: Etiology of brain tumors in adults. Epidemiol Rev 1995;17:382–414.

Legler JM, Ries LA, Smith MA, et al: Brain and other central nervous system cancers: recent trends in incidence and mortality. J Natl Cancer Inst 1999;91:1382–1390.

Walter AW, Hancock ML, Pui CH, et al: Secondary brain tumors in children treated for acute lymphoblastic leukemia at St Jude Children's Research Hospital. J Clin Oncol 1998;16:3761–3767.

Radiologic and Histologic Evaluation

Burger PC: Revising the World Health Organization (WHO) Blue Book "Histological typing of tumours of the central nervous system." J Neurooncol 1995;24:3–7.

Pomper MG, Port JD: New techniques in MR imaging of brain tumors. Magn Reson Imaging Clin N Am 2000;8:691–713.

General Brain Tumor and Treatment Reviews

De Angelis LM : Brain tumors. N Eng J Med 2001;344:114–123.

Grossman SA, Levin V, Sawaya R, et al: National Comprehensive Cancer Network adult brain tumor practice guidelines. Oncology 1997;11:237–277.

Low-Grade Gliomas

Henderson KH, Shaw EG: Randomized trials of radiation therapy in adult low-grade gliomas. Semin Radiat Oncol 2001;11:145–151.

Karim AB, Afra D, Cornu P, et al: Randomized trial on the efficacy of radiotherapy for cerebral low-grade glioma in the adult: European Organization for Research and Treatment of Cancer Study 22845 with the Medical Research Council study BRO4: An interim analysis. Int J Radiat Oncol Biol Phys 2002;52:316–324.

Karim AB, Maat B, Hatlevoll R, et al: A randomized trial on dose response in radiation therapy of low-grade cerebral glioma: European Organization for Research and Treatment of Cancer (EORTC 2284). Int J Radiat Oncol Biol Phys 1996;36:549–556.

Kiebert GM, Curran D, Aaronson NK, et al: Quality of life after radiation therapy of cerebral low-grade gliomas of the adult: Results of a randomized phase III trial on dose response (EORTC trial 2284). Eur J Cancer 1998;34:1902–1909.

Recht LD, Lew R, Smith TW: Suspected low-grade glioma: Is deferring treatment safe? Ann Neurol 2000;31:431–436.

Shaw E, Arusell R, Scheithauer B, et al: Prospective randomized trial of low versus high-dose radiation therapy in adults with suprtentorial low-grade glioma: Initial report of a North Central Cancer Treatment Group / Radiation

Therapy Oncology Group / Eastern Cooperative Oncology Group study. J Clin Oncol 2002;20:2267–2276.

Tatter SB: Neurosurgical management of low- and intermediate-grade gliomas. Semin Radiat Oncol 2001;11: 113–123.

High-Grade Gliomas

Brem H, Piantadosi S, Burger PC, et al: Placebo-controlled trial of safety and efficacy of intraoperative controlled delivery by biodegradable polymers of chemotherapy for recurrent gliomas. Lancet 1995;345:1008–1012.

Curran WJ, Scott CB, Horton J, et al: Recursive partitioning analysis of prognostic factors in three Radiation Therapy Oncology Group malignant glioma trials. J Natl Cancer Inst 1993;85:704–710.

Fine HA, Dear BG, Loeffler JS, et al: Meta-analysis of radiation therapy with and without adjuvant chemotherapy for malignant gliomas in adults. Cancer 1993;71:2285–2297.

Galanis E, Buckner JC: Chemotherapy of brain tumors. Curr Opin Neurol 2000;13:619–625.

Medical Research Council Brain Tumor Working Party: Randomized trial of procarbazine, lomustine, and vincristine in the adjuvant treatment of high-grade astrocytoma: A Medical Research Council trial. J Clin Oncol 2001;19: 509–518.

Prados MD, Scott C, Curran WJ Jr, et al: Procarbazine, lomustine, and vincristine (PCV) chemotherapy for anaplastic astrocytoma: A retrospective review of radiation therapy oncology group protocols comparing survival with carmustine or PCV adjuvant chemotherapy. J Clin Oncol 1999;17:3389–3395.

Walker MD, Green SB, Byar DP: Randomized comparisons of radiotherapy and nitrosoureas for the treatment of malignant glioma after surgery. N Engl J Med 1980;303: 1323–1329.

Yung WK, Prados MD, Yaga-Tur R, et al: Multicenter phase II trial of temozolamide in patients with anaplastic astrocytoma or anaplastic oligoastrocytoma at first relapse. Temodal Brain Tumor Group. J Clin Oncol 1999;17: 2762–2771.

Oligodendroglioma

Bigner SH, Rasheed K, Wiltshire RN, McLendon R: Morphologic and molecular genetic aspects of oligodendroglial neoplasms. Neurooncol 1999;1:52–60.

Cairncross JG, Ueki K, Zlatescu MC, et al: Specific genetic predictors of chemotherapeutic response and survival in patients with anaplastic oligodendrogliomas. J Natl Cancer Inst 1998;90:1473–1479.

Fortin D, Cairncross GJ, Hammond RR: Oligodendroglioma: An appraisal of recent data pertaining to diagnosis and treatment. Neurosurgery 1999;45:1279–1291.

Primary Central Nervous System Lymphomas

Abrey LE, Yahalom J, DeAngelis LM: Treatment for primary CNS lymphoma: The next step. J Clin Oncol 2000;18: 3144–3150.

Bataille B, Dewail V, Menet E, et al: Primary intracerebral malignant lymphoma: Report of 248 cases. J Neurosurg 2000;92:261–266.

Batchelor T, Carson K, O'Neill A, et al: Treatment of primary CNS lymphoma with methotrexate and deferred radiotherapy: A Report of NABTT 96-07. J Clin Oncol 2003;21:1044–1049.

Blay JY, Conroy T, Chevreau C, et al: High-dose methotrexate for the treatment of primary cerebral lymphomas: Analysis of survival and late neurologic toxicity in a retrospective series. J Clin Oncol 1998;16:864–871.

Buhring U, Herrlinger U, Krings T, et al: MRI features of primary central nervous system lymphomas at presentation. Neurology 2001;57:393–396.

DeAngelis LM: Primary central nervous system lymphoma. Curr Opin Neurol 1999;12:687–691.

DeAngelis LM, Seiferheld W, Schold SC, et al: Combination chemotherapy and radiotherapy for primary central nervous system lymphoma: Radiation Therapy Oncology Group Study 93-10. J Clin Oncol 2002;20:4643–4648.

McAllister LD, Doolittle ND, Guastadisegni PE, et al: Cognitive outcomes and long-term follow-up results after enhanced chemotherapy delivery for primary central nervous lymphoma. Neurosurgery 2000;46:51–60.

Nasir S, De Angelis LM: Update on the management of primary CNS lymphoma. Oncology 2000;14:228–234.

Schabet M: Epidemiology of primary CNS lymphoma. J Neurooncol 1999;43:199–201.

Schultz C, Scott C, DeAngelis L, et al: Radiation therapy alone vs. pre-RT chemotherapy for the treatment of primary cns lymphoma: aged matched survival analysis of RTOG 83-15 and RTOG 93-10. Proc Am Soc Clin Oncol 2000;19:159a.

Meningiomas

Bondy M, Ligon BL: Epidemiology and etiology of intracranial meningiomas: A review. J Neurooncol 1996;29:197–205.

Braunstein JB, Vick NA: Meningiomas: The decision not to operate. Neurology 197;48:1459–1462.

Chamberlain MC: Meningiomas. Curr Treat Options Neurol 2001;3:67–76.

Go RS, Taylor BV, Kimmel DW: The natural history of asymptomatic meiningiomas in Olmsted County, Minnesota. Neurology 1998;51:1718–1720.

Maire JP, Caudry M, Geurin J, et al: Fractionated radiation therapy in the treatment of intracranial meningiomas: Local control, functional efficacy and tolerance in 91 patients. Int J Radiat Oncol Biol Phys 1995;33:315–321.

Medulloblastoma

Chintagumpala M, Berg S, Blaney SM: Treatment controversies in medulloblastoma. Curr Opin Oncol 2001;13:154–159.

Neuwelt EA, Hill SA, Frenkel EP: Osmotic blood-brain barrier modification and combination chemotherapy: Concurrent tumor regression in areas of barrier opening and progression in brain regions distant to barrier opening. Neurosurg 1984;15:362–366.

Ependymoma

Smyth MD, Horn BN, Russo C, Berger MS: Intracranial ependymomas of childhood: Current management strategies. Pediatr Neurosurg 2000;33:138–150.

Brainstem Glioma

Walker DA, Punt JAG, Sokal M: Clinical management of brain stem glioma. Arch Dis Child 1999;80:558–564.

Supportive Care Issues

Fetell MR, Grossman SA, Fisher J, et al: Pre-irradiation paclitaxel in glioblastoma multiforme: Efficacy, pharmacology, and drug interactions. J Clin Oncol 1997;15:3121–3128.

Grossman SA, Hochberg F, Fisher JD, et al: Increased 9-aminocamptothecin requirements in patients on anticonvulsants. Cancer Chemother Pharmacol 1998;42:118–126.

Grossman SA, Sheidler VR, Gilbert MR: Decreased phenytoin levels in patients receiving chemotherapy: Report of a series and a review of the literature. Am J Med 1989;87:505–510.

Grossman SA, Zeltzman M: Practical considerations in the management of patients with primary brain tumors. Neurologist 1996;2:130–138.

Marras LC, Geerts WH, Perry JR: The risk of venous thromboembolism is increased throughout the course of glioma: An evidence-based review. Cancer 2000;89:640–646.

Weissman DE: Glucocorticoid treatment for brain metastases and epidural cord compressions. A review. J. Clin Oncol 1988;6:543–551.

Chapter 104
Brain Metastases

Minesh P. Mehta and Ivo Tremont-Lukats

Brain metastases are a common consequence of systemic cancer. They represent the most common intracranial tumor and are an important cause of morbidity and mortality in patients with cancer. The incidence of brain metastases in the United States is 150,000 to 170,000 cases per year, but these figures could be conservative. Large autopsy series have found that one-quarter of patients who died of cancer had intracranial metastases. The most common primary tumors causing brain metastases in adults, in decreasing order of frequency, are melanoma lung, breast, melanoma, renal, and colon cancers (Figure 104-1). The peak age group for brain metastases is 55 to 65 years. Lung cancer is the most common source of brain metastases in men, whereas breast cancer is the most frequent source in women. In terms of risk, patients with melanoma are most likely to develop brain metastases, with an eventual lifetime risk of one in two patients with stage IV melanoma developing brain metastases. Rarely, sarcoma, testicular, uterine, ovarian, prostate, bladder, and thyroid cancers also metastasize to the brain. The most common tumors responsible for brain metastases in the pediatric age group include Ewing's sarcoma, rhabdomyosarcoma, neuroblastoma, and osteosarcoma. About 80% of brain metastases are located in the arterial border zones of the cerebral hemispheres, 3% to 5% in the basal nuclei and brain stem, and 15% to 17% in the cerebellum.

Clinical Presentation

Up to 33% of brain metastases are asymptomatic and are discovered incidentally during staging of malignancies such as small cell lung cancer (SCLC), non–small cell lung cancer, or melanoma. Most brain metastases, however, are detected due to symptoms of increased intracranial pressure. Although brain metastases can sometimes be the first clinical manifestation of cancer in some patients, in most cases these lesions are identified metachronously, several months after the initial diagnosis of cancer. In most large clinical trials, the median time from diagnosis of the primary tumor to the development of clinically evident brain metastases is approximately eight months.

The number and severity of symptoms depend on the size, number, and location of metastatic lesions. Signs and symptoms can be focal or generalized and depend on the predominant pathophysiologic mechanism (Figure 104-2). The clinical manifestations of brain metastases usually have a gradual onset, with an evolution over days or weeks that can be intermittent or steadily progressive. In some cases, symptoms can be acute, such as seizures (15%) or intratumoral bleeding masquerading as a cerebrovascular accident (less than 10% of cases).

Generalized Symptoms

Headache
Headache is one of the most common presenting symptoms of brain metastases (26% to 57% of cases). It can mimic any type of headache and be misdiagnosed as sinusitis, tension-type headaches, chronic daily headaches, and even migraine. In most cases, it is diffuse or bilateral. When the headache is unilateral, it can have a localizing value, but this is the exception rather than the rule. The intensity of pain also varies but in most cases is mild or moderate. Pain might or might not respond to analgesics. Its lack of specificity makes the diagnosis of an intracranial mass based only on headache difficult unless there are other symptoms or signs and there is a known history of cancer. Of all cancer patients presenting with headache, brain metastases are found in approximately 20%. The causes of headaches in the remainder of this patient population include fever, migraine, skull-base metastases, intracranial hemorrhage, and miscellaneous conditions (see Chapter 4).

Changes in Mental Status
Mental and behavioral symptoms are also very common presenting features in patients with brain

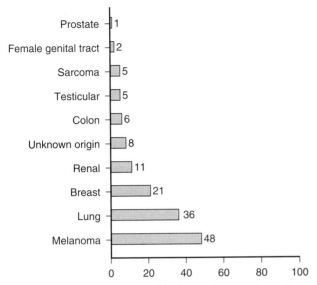

Figure 104-1 ■ Frequency of brain metastases by primary tumor in adults. Data labels represent the percentage of patients developing brain metastases with stage IV of a given disease. (Data from Greenberg HS, Chandler WF, Sandler HM: Brain metastases. In Greenberg HS, Chandler WF, Sandler HM [eds]: Brain Tumors, 1st ed. New York: Oxford University Press; 1999, pp 299–317; Posner JB. Intracranial metastases. In: Posner JB [ed]: Neurological Complications of Cancer. Philadelphia: FA Davis, 1995, pp 77–110; and Sawaya R, Bindal RK: Metastatic brain tumors. In Kaye AH, Laws ER Jr, [eds]: Brain Tumors: An Encyclopedic Approach. Edinburgh: Churchill Livingstone, 1995, pp 923–946).

metastasis (22% to 80%). These symptoms are frequently reported by friends or family members and are due to metastatic disease in about 15% of cancer patients with changes in mental status as an initial complaint. The most common cause of severe cognitive impairment in cancer patients is toxic-metabolic encephalopathy (60%), a term that encompasses a wide array of conditions such as sepsis, hypoxia, electrolyte disturbance, drug side effects, hypoglycemia, and renal or liver failure. Finally, an intracranial hemorrhage can explain cognitive derangement in approximately 5% of cancer patients. The onset of symptoms can be subtle or dramatic and can include an altered sleep pattern, forgetfulness, apathy, irritability, confusion, difficulty in concentration, and impaired judgment. It is extremely important to obtain or confirm these symptoms with other reliable sources of information, as patients sometimes do not have full insight into their own symptoms (see Chapter 7).

Focal Symptoms

Focal symptoms include weakness, deficits of higher cortical function, and seizures.

Weakness

Focal weakness overlaps with headache as one of the most common symptoms in published case series. Its presentation ranges from mild monoparesis of slow, gradual onset to acute hemiparesis resembling an acute cerebrovascular accident (CVA). It has localizing value, but its ability to precisely delineate the location of the lesion is limited by the surrounding peritumoral edema, which frequently can be far more extensive than the tumor itself.

Deficits of Higher Cortical Function

Deficits of higher cortical function suggest a focal cortical or subcortical lesion. Such deficits include

- visual field cuts
- visual neglect if the lesion is in the nondominant hemisphere

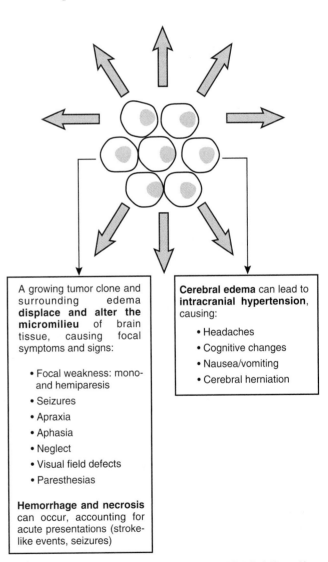

Figure 104-2 ■ Schematic illustration highlighting the pathophysiology of symptoms in patients with brain metastases.

- aphasia in any of its varieties
- impaired comprehension, reading, or calculation
- difficulty performing motor tasks such as dressing or writing

These complaints are less frequent relative to other types of symptoms (6% to 12%), but they justify a careful assessment for the presence of brain metastases. The onset can be gradual, insidious, and intermittent but sometimes can be acute. These symptoms of higher cortical dysfunction can be isolated or combined with more diffuse, nonlocalizing changes in mental status.

Seizures

Between 5% and 20% of patients present with seizures, either partial simple or partial complex and with or without secondary generalization. It is important to obtain the fullest possible description of the seizure from witnesses. Such a description should include the following details:

- onset
- premonitory symptoms (aura)
- description of the convulsive episode
- eye and head deviation
- changes in skin color
- postictal behavior
- duration of the postictal period

It is also important to approximate the duration and frequency of seizures if the patient has had more than one seizure.

The classic example of a partial simple seizure is the focal motor convulsion that starts in the face or in the arm and remains focal or spreads sequentially to the rest of the motor cortex. Partial complex seizures—that is, focal convulsive activity with impairment of consciousness—usually indicate a lesion in the temporal lobe. This presentation occurs rarely from metastases and is due far more frequently to mesial hippocampal sclerosis, cortical dysplasia, or a primary brain tumor. In some instances of secondary generalization, the spread of the seizure is so fast that localization based on seizure semiology is difficult. The presence of postictal hemiparesis (Todd's paralysis) suggests focality and at times can be confounded with a cerebrovascular accident. This motor deficit can last from minutes to days but is usually transient and is followed by full recovery.

Regardless of type, the presence of seizures generally suggests multiple parenchymal metastases, leptomeningeal metastases, or both. Melanoma and choriocarcinoma are among the most epileptogenic metastases, given their propensity to seed in the cerebral cortex and to bleed locally. Although uncommon,

a convulsive epileptic status is possible. If seizures are partial sensory causing paresthesias (tingling and numbness), transient ischemic attacks (TIAs) and migraines should be in the differential diagnosis, especially in patients with risk factors for cerebrovascular disease or with a history of migraine.

Other Symptoms

Paresthesias, sensory deficits, and unsteady gait are relatively infrequent complaints. Hemichorea and hemiballismus due to metastases to the basal nuclei are exceptional but have been reported. Diplopia, ptosis, ataxia, postural hypotension, and hiccups can be presenting symptoms in infratentorial metastases located in the brain stem or in the posterior fossa. Finally, some patients present with episodic, transient behavioral spells that last several hours and then resolve completely. Symptoms during these spells include dizziness, visual obscurations, extracorporeal sensations, and confusion. The anatomical location of these symptoms is unclear, but some authorities regard and treat them as seizures, whereas others consider them symptoms of increased intracranial pressure.

Clinical Evaluation

Physical Examination

A thorough general physical exam should never be ignored, and this principle applies particularly to the patient with de novo brain metastases without a known primary tumor or to those patients with a history of cancer who have been disease-free or in apparent remission from treatment for some time. The initial interview as well as the physical exam will help the clinician to establish a global assessment of the patient's performance status. This assessment of well-being can be quantitated with the Karnofsky Performance Score. Despite its limitations (subjectiveness, inter- and intraobserver variability), the Karnofsky Performance Score is useful because it is a robust predictor of survival and functional quality of life in patients with brain metastases.

Careful attention should be paid to palpation of cervical, supraclavicular, and axillary lymph nodes; palpation of the thyroid gland; auscultation of lungs; an abdominal and pelvic examination, including a testicular exam in men and a rectal exam. Inspection of the skin is crucial to detect cutaneous melanoma. Bony tenderness, especially spinal, should be explored on physical exam, as bone and brain metastases frequently occur together.

A careful neurologic evaluation often reveals deficits that the patient was unaware of or had little insight about, especially focal weakness and mental status changes. Some patients report symptoms that seem to be disproportionate to the actual findings on examination. It is frequently possible to document cerebellar ataxia, dysmetria, or incoordination in patients with symptoms suggestive of cerebellar metastasis.

An evaluation of all cranial nerves should follow, searching for localizing signs such as cranial nerve palsies, cortical localizing signs such as visual field deficits or visual neglect, or signs of increased intracranial pressure such as papilledema or uni- or bilateral cranial nerve VI palsy. Fewer than 25% of patients with brain metastases develop papilledema; an isolated cranial nerve VI palsy can be a false localizing sign when it is due in fact to intracranial hypertension, and a cranial neuropathy (particularly multiple) could be the result not only of brain stem metastases but also of leptomeningeal and skull-base metastatic disease.

An exam of the motor system, including muscle tone, bulk, and power, is performed mainly to detect a motor deficit. When the deficit is acute or subacute, the extremity is weak with varying degrees of hypotonia. Myotatic reflexes can be absent, hypoactive, normal, or hyperactive compared with those on the contralateral side. These findings depend on the magnitude, the acuteness, and the evolution of the deficit. Asking the patient to mimic or carry out motor tasks such as saluting, combing, brushing teeth, and so forth, takes only a few seconds and can unveil surprising degrees of ideomotor apraxia.

A sensory exam can reveal deficits not noted by the patient, such as astereognosis and agraphesthesia due to lesions located in the parietal lobes or tactile neglect from the nondominant parietal lesions. Cerebellar metastases can be evidenced from the finger-to-nose and heel-to-knee tests, rapid alternating movements, tremor, and gait ataxia, with the caveat that some patients with unsteady gait have surprisingly little or no signs of cerebellar dysfunction. The plantar extensor response should always be sought, as it can be the sole sign of a metastasis affecting the corticospinal tract.

Any validated tool to evaluate the mental status is of enormous importance when brain metastases are suspected. The mini-mental state exam (MMSE) is one of such tools; it is easy to administer, takes about 10 minutes or less to carry out, is reproducible, and is accurate enough to evaluate mental status in patients with brain metastases (Table 104-1). An additional advantage of the mini-mental state exam is that it permits an evaluation of speech output and language, screening for aphasias of fluent or nonfluent type.

Table 104-1 ■ The Mini-Mental State Exam (MMSE)

Inquiry	Maximum Score
Orientation[1]	
What is the (year) (season) (date) (day) (month)?	5
Where are we: (state) (county) (town or city) (hospital) (floor)?	5
Registration[2]	
Name three common objects ("apple, table, penny")	3
Attention and Calculation[3]	
Count backwards in multiples of 7 serially Alternatively, spell "world" backwards	5
Instant Recall[4]	
Ask the patient to repeat the three objects named above	3
Language[5]	
Name a pencil and a watch	2
Repeat: "No ifs, ands, or buts"	1
Follow a three-step command: "Take this paper with your right hand, fold it in half, and put it on the floor."	3
Read and obey the following: "Close your eyes"	1
Write a sentence	1
Copy a design	1
Maximum Total	**30**
Total Score	

[1]Some patients might not know details like county, floor, or hospital area if they live elsewhere or have a baseline cognitive dysfunction. One point for each correct response.
[2]Count trials and record. Words can be simple but need to be unrelated to each other. Note whether patient remembers words after cueing.
[3]One point for each correct response. If both choices are evaluated, take the worst score.
[4]One point for each correct response.
[5]Other examples for naming, repetition, and three-stage commands are acceptable. If patient has limitations in completing the test—for example, if the patient is blind, cannot write, or cannot draw—take the total number of points that were scored over the total number of points that were actually tested.

Imaging

Magnetic resonance imaging (MRI) is the imaging method of choice for the diagnosis of brain metastases. Contrast-enhanced T1- as well as T2-weighted images are obtained. Peritumoral edema is hypointense, and the metastatic core is hyperintense on T1, particularly after gadolinium injection. T2-weighted images offer the opposite picture and are best for assessing edema. (Figure 104-3) The typical magnetic resonance

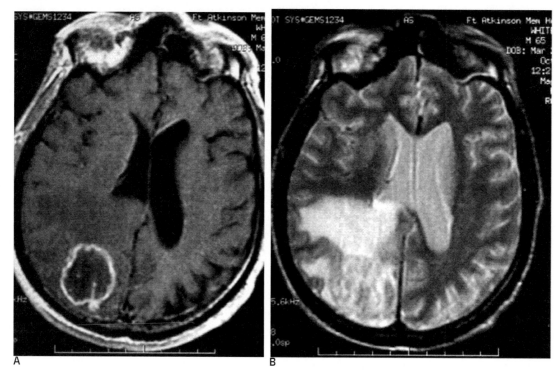

Figure 104-3 ■ Magnetic resonance imaging scans demonstrating an enhancing metastatic lesion surrounded by extensive vasogenic edema with mass effect. *A*, T1 contrast-enhanced magnetic resonance scan demonstrates a centrally necrotic lesion with ring enhancement. *B*, T2-weighted magnetic resonance scan shows vasogenic edema.

imaging appearance of a brain metastasis is that of a spherical or quasispherical lesion, well demarcated from adjacent brain, with marked surrounding edema, and peripherally located at the junction between gray and white matter. With larger tumors, peripheral enhancement with a nonenhancing core that represents tumor necrosis is often noted. With magnetic resonance imaging, it is apparent that between 65% and 80% of brain metastases are multiple, in contrast to previous computed tomography (CT) scan-based observations, in which nearly 50% of brain metastases were reported to be solitary.

For patients who cannot undergo a magnetic resonance imaging scan, a contrast-enhanced computed tomography scan is the alternative procedure; however, computed tomography scans with contrast can miss smaller lesions, especially those in the brain stem and cerebellum. A metastatic lesion appears on computed tomography scans as hypo- or isodense without contrast, although melanoma, colon lesions, and choriocarcinoma can appear hyperdense. Most lesions turn hyperdense after contrast injection. (Figure 104-4). The sensitivity of computed tomography scans in detecting brain metastases can be enhanced by injecting a higher dose of contrast and decreasing the slice thickness.

Laboratory Studies

Cytologic analysis of cerebrospinal fluid (CSF) has a very low yield in brain metastases unless there is concomitant leptomeningeal disease. This is important in patients with no known primary tumor. Known tumor markers such as

- CA-125 for ovarian cancer
- carcinoembriogenic antigen (CEA) for lung, breast, or colon cancer
- beta human chorionic gonadotropin for choriocarcinoma
- prostate-specific antigen for prostate cancer
- alpha-fetoprotein for non-seminomatous germ cell tumors

should be ordered when patients with a history of those cancers present with metastatic lesions to the brain. Liver function tests are commonly ordered to rule out concomitant liver metastases.

Staging, Prognostic Features, and Outcomes

In the patient with known cancer and multiple brain lesions, the history and the imaging studies estab-

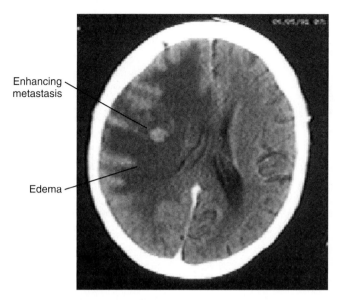

Figure 104-4 ■ Contrast-enhanced computed tomography scan demonstrating an enhancing metastatic lesion surrounded by extensive vasogenic edema with mass effect.

lish the diagnosis with relative certainty. In the patient with known cancer and a single metastatic lesion or in those without history of systemic cancer, a tissue diagnosis must be obtained. In these circumstances, a stereotactic needle biopsy or an open craniotomy is warranted. The differential diagnoses include

- a primary brain tumor (meningioma, glial tumor, lymphoma, vestibular schwannoma);
- brain abscess (bacterial, fungal, toxoplasma);
- granuloma (tuberculosis, sarcoidosis);
- a cerebrovascular accident in the subacute stage;
- multiple sclerosis; and
- radiation necrosis if the patient has had radiation therapy.

Although, by convention, cancer patients are staged at initial diagnosis and the subsequent clinical course does not result in restaging, patients with brain metastases either present at initial diagnosis or subsequently are generally considered to be stage IV.

The median survival of untreated brain metastases is approximately one month; two months if steroids are added; four to six months after whole-brain irradiation; and eight to nine months if surgery or radiosurgery is utilized. The ability of whole brain irradiation, surgery, radiosurgery, chemotherapy, or any other treatment modality to control metastatic brain disease, however, will largely depend on patient- and disease-dependent covariates that bear prognostic value. Common prognostic factors with predictive value are listed in Table 104-2. The Radiation Therapy Oncology Group has

identified three prognostic subgroups with different survival outcomes (Figure 104-5):

1. Class I includes patients 65 years or younger with a Karnofsky Performance Score of 70 or more, a controlled primary tumor, and absence of extracranial metastases. This is a select group of patients that constitutes less than 20% of all patients with brain metastases.
2. Class III includes patients with a Karnofsky Performance Score of less than 70 regardless of other prognostic factors.
3. Class II includes all other patients.

Table 104-2 ■ **Common Prognostic Factors in Brain Metastases and Their Impact on Outcome**

Factor	Impact on Outcome
Age*	Older patients do worse
Karnofsky Performance Score (KPS)	Survival is better with higher KPS
Controlled primary tumor	Superior survival
Extracranial metastases	Worse outcome
Multiple brain metastases	Worse than single metastases
Time from diagnosis of primary tumor to brain metastases	The longer the better

*Age: Most studies have found that age greater than 65 has a negative effect on prognosis.

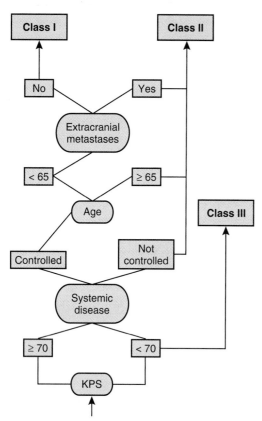

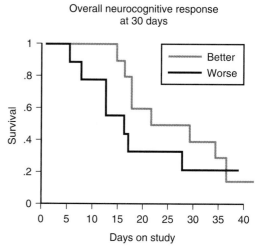

Figure 104-7 ■ Survival of patients with brain metastases by change in neurocognitive status.

Figure 104-5 ■ The RTOG Recursive Partitioning Tree. From a practical perspective, start at the bottom (KPS box) and work upward, addressing the patient's status for the four parameters in the ovals, to determine RPA class (bold type). KPS = Karnofsky Performance Score. (From Gaspar LE, Scott C, Murray K, Curran W: Validation of the RTOG recursive partitioning analysis [RPA] classification for brain metastases. Int J Radiat Oncol Biol Phys 2000;47:1001–1006.)

This prognostic classification for brain metastases has been validated, showing statistically significant median survival rates among the different groups. As illustrated in Figure 104-6, patients in Class I have a median survival of 7.1 months, whereas those in Class

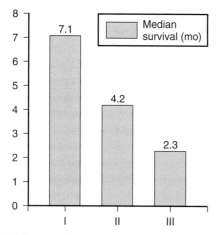

Figure 104-6 ■ Median survival of patients with brain metastases, stratified by RPA class.

III have a median survival of only 2.3 months. The intermediate group, Class II, has a median survival of 4.2 months.

Brief instruments of cognition such as the mini-mental state exam and other neurocognitive tests such as Trail Making A and B are independent prognostic tools, and there seems to be a reciprocal correlation between median survival and number of tests showing impairment. In addition, early improvement in neurocognitive status following whole-brain radiation therapy (WBRT) predicts for improved survival (Figure 104-7). An improvement of mini-mental state exam score of greater than 23 has been associated with long-term survival. Decisions based on management, treatment, or treatment sequence are largely dependent on a careful consideration of these prognostic factors and can have an important effect on individual cases.

Treatment

The decision to treat and how to treat is best taken with a multidisciplinary approach, according to which (ideally) the patient or relatives understand the benefits and risks of every method being considered. In the last decade, there has been progress and refinement of some modalities in the treatment of metastatic brain tumors.

The Unstable Patient

The unstable patient is a significant challenge and is characterized by uncontrolled intracranial pressure, seizures, or both.

The neurologically unstable patient has

- uncontrolled intracranial pressure with symptoms suggesting ongoing or impending brain herniation,
- epileptic status, or
- both.

Patients needing ventilatory assistance should be intubated and hyperventilated to keep pCO$_2$ in the range of 25–30 mmHg. The advantage of this approach is that it is possible both to maintain adequate ventilatory support and to have a rapid effect on lowering intracranial pressure. This measure is temporary, however, because it loses effectiveness within one hour. Simultaneously, give mannitol intravenously (1 g/kg) and dexamethasone intravenously in boluses of 32–64 mg. Mannitol can be given at 0.5–g/kg, and dexamethasone can be given at higher doses (40–100 mg/kg). The maintenance doses of mannitol and dexamethasone are 0.5 g/kg intravenously, four times within one to two hours, and 40–100 mg/day divided in 4 doses, respectively. The authors rarely use mannitol after 48 hours and do not use diuretics.

Seizures worsen intracranial hypertension, sub-jecting the patient to cerebral hypoxia and ischemia, so prompt and aggressive treatment is indicated. If the patient is seizing, give lorazepam 1–4 mg intravenously, followed by fosphenytoin 20 mg/kg intravenously as a loading dose, with a maintenance dose of 5 mg/kg/day of phenytoin, either intravenously or orally. If seizures recur, reload for a second time with 10 mg/kg fosphenytoin. After one hour, phenytoin levels should be in the target range of 25–35 mcg/mL. An electroencephalogram (EEG) should be obtained after loading with fosphenytoin, to rule out nonconvulsive status epilepticus. If there are no clinical seizures or nonconvulsive status epilepticus, no further treatment other than maintenance phenytoin is necessary. If clinical or subclinical convulsive activity continues, use propofol at 2–5 mg/kg intravenously with a maintenance dose of 0.1–0.2 mg/kg/min intravenously. If this drug is ineffective in terminating seizure activity and if high intracranial pressure is a major concern or if hypotension cannot be controlled, start pentobarbital at 5 mg/kg, followed by a continuous infusion of 1 mg/kg hourly, with titration up to 3 mg/kg hourly to obtain burst suppression by electroencephalogram with no electroencephalographic seizures.

The Stable Patient

For all other patients who are stable enough to receive specific treatment, the following therapeutic considerations apply:

Symptomatic Treatment

Many patients eventually need to be on steroids, anticonvulsant therapy, or both.

Anticonvulsants

After an exhaustive analysis of the best available evidence, the American Academy of Neurology concluded that anticonvulsants were ineffective in preventing new-onset seizures in patients with brain tumors. The current standard of care is that anticonvulsants are indicated only in those patients who already have had seizures, and treatment should begin after the first convulsive episode. Anticonvulsants should be tapered and discontinued one week after craniotomy in those patients who are seizure-free, who are medically stable, or who have substantial side effects from the anticonvulsant drugs.

Phenytoin and carbamazepine are the most commonly used anticonvulsants, although valproic acid and phenobarbital are also used. It is unclear whether newer anticonvulsants such as lamotrigine, topiramate, tiagabine, and zonisamide are more effective than the traditional anticonvulsant drugs, but each one of them can be used in cases in which a second drug is needed or when intolerance or side effects to traditional anticonvulsants is a problem. It is also unclear whether a subset of patients at high risk for seizures (such as those with metastatic melanoma) could benefit from prophylaxis. There are no clear-cut rules concerning when anticonvulsants should be stopped in patients with well documented seizure activity related to brain metastases. If the metastastic lesion has been treated and there is no evidence of intracranial disease, anticonvulsants may be tapered after two years in long-term survivors. Recurrence of metastases does not necessarily indicate that seizures will recur. Therefore, the decision of seizure prophylaxis in this particular situation depends on clinical judgment and the patient's wishes.

Glucocorticoids

Dexamethasone is the most commonly used glucocorticoid to decrease peritumoral edema and its associated symptoms for two reasons: It has less mineralocorticoid effect and is less protein binding than prednisone. The reduction of vasogenic edema and consequential clinical improvement can usually be seen within one to two days. The conventional approach in symptomatic patients is to start with a high initial dose (16–32 mg given intravenously or intramuscularly), followed by 4 to 8 mg intravenously or by mouth, four times daily, if the patient tolerates the oral route. Recent data suggest that lower doses (2 to 4 mg) given twice a day are equally effective with fewer side effects, and this is the preferred approach of the authors. The twice-a-day schedule is more appropriate and rational because dexamethasone has a very long half-life (24 to 36 hours). There is good evidence that in stable but symptomatic patients without significant intracranial hypertension, 4 mg, four times daily, is sufficient. Once the patient is clinically stable, a slow tapering should be initiated, with the aim of discontinuing steroids altogether or achieving the lowest effective dose. We taper by 2 mg every five to seven days.

Radiation Therapy

Whole-brain radiation therapy is the conventional treatment for most patients with brain metastases. No specific dose or radiation schedule has been found to be superior. The addition of radiation sensitizers (such as bromodeoxyuridine or misonidazole) has not yielded better results. The most commonly used schedule uses 10 fractions of 3 Gy each for a total dose of 30 Gy over a period of two weeks. This schedule has been associated with a greater than 10% risk of significant neurocognitive impairment in long-term survivors (typically more than nine months). In consequence, potentially safer schedules using more prolonged administration times (such as three to four

weeks) with a concomitant decrease in dose per fraction are used for patients with a likelihood of surviving more than nine months.

The acute side effects of whole-brain radiation therapy include alopecia, grade 1 to 2 dermatitis, otitis externa, serous otitis media, and rarely, a somnolence syndrome a few weeks after completion of treatment. Late side effects can include neurocognitive impairment, cerebellar dysfunction, cataracts, and rarely, blindness. Table 104-3 presents a summary of some of these side effects.

Whole-brain radiation therapy is most effective in the treatment of small metastases (less than 3 cm) not previously irradiated, although recurrent metastases can still respond to reirradiation for a brief duration. Whole-brain radiation therapy is frequently the best option for patients in Classes II and III.

Approximately 50% of patients with brain metastases treated with whole-brain radiation therapy die of neurologic causes, whereas the other half succumb to uncontrolled systemic disease. This observation suggests that if it were possible to identify patients likely to die from neurologic causes and achieve superior intracranial disease control in these patients, survival could be enhanced. Patients in Classes I and II could constitute such a subgroup. As a consequence, strategies to improve local control by escalating the radiation dose to the metastatic tumor(s) in these patients have been developed and tested. These strategies include accelerated hyperfractionated radiation therapy, brachytherapy, fractionated stereotactic radiosurgery, and stereotactic radiosurgery. The latter has been used actively in the last decade. The objective is to deliver a large dose of radiation in a single fraction to a small intracranial target, with minimal

---

TREATMENT

Steroid Therapy

It is crucial to remember that prolonged use of steroids is associated with a very high frequency of side effects, including oral candidiasis, gastric acid hypersecretion and peptic ulcer disease, opportunistic infections, glucose intolerance or overt diabetes, hypertension, cushingoid changes, sleep and personality disturbances, osteoporosis, avascular necrosis, increased risk of deep venous thrombosis, and so forth. Therefore, it is imperative to be extremely judicious when using these agents. The authors' practice applies the following principles:

■ Do not use steroids for patients who do not need them—i.e., patients who are asymptomatic or

minimally symptomatic and have no significant edema or mass effect on magnetic resonance imaging.

■ Taper down to the lowest possible clinically needed dose within two to four weeks of completion of treatment.

■ Use prophylactic H2 blockers and candida prophylaxis if patients are using more than 4 mg/day of dexamethasone.

■ Prevent *Pneumocystis carinii* using trimethoprim-sulfamethoxazole (TMP-SMX) orally, twice daily on weekends for patients who are on prolonged high doses of dexamethasone, are immunocompromised, or have significant pulmonary disease.

Table 104-3 ■ Radiation-Related Neurotoxicity

Toxicity (Time of Presentation)	Findings	Outcome
Acute (days)	Headache, vomiting, fatigue	Good. Recovery is the rule; steroids might be useful
Early onset (one to three months)	Somnolence, fatigue, focal signs	Good. Recovery is the rule; steroids may be useful
Late (months to years)		
Necrosis	Magnetic resonance imaging and MRS useful, PET/SPECT used at times Focal signs; cognitive problems	Variable. Steroids of minor value—help reduce edema. Hyperbaric oxygen is controversial; anticoagulation has been attempted
Atrophy	Dementia, gait ataxia, MR/computed tomography atrophy, leukoencephalopathy	Bad. VP shunt might help in a few cases
Infarction	Focal	Variable
Hemorrhage	Focal	Variable
Secondary tumor	Focal	Bad unless it is benign (e.g., meningioma.)

MRS = Magentic resonance spectroscopy; PET = Positron emission tomography; SPECT = Single photon emission computed tomography; VP shunt = ventriculoperitoneal shunt.

dose to surrounding normal brain. Several techniques have been developed to achieve this end. Most require patient immobilization with an invasive headframe, similar to those used for stereotactic intracranial biopsy. These frames also provide a rigid fiducial system that permits precise targeting. Recently, noninvasive methods have also been described. The radiation is delivered using proton beams, gamma rays, or high-energy X-rays from specially modified linear accelerators.

Regardless of the technique used, radiosurgery can treat relatively small lesions (3 cm or smaller) quite effectively. In addition, multiple, recurrent, and even surgically inaccessible lesions can be targeted. A compilation of studies found a mean local control rate of 81% with a response rate of 69%. This figure represents an approximate 20% improvement over whole-brain radiation therapy alone. In one small trial of whole-brain radiation therapy plus radiosurgery versus whole-brain irradiation alone, significant survival advantage accrued to patients undergoing radiosurgery. In a larger trial, survival was not prolonged for patients with two to three metastases treated with radiosurgery; however, local control was enhanced, Karnofsky Performance Score was improved, and steroid dependence was diminished. In other trials, patients treated with radiosurgery alone with whole-brain irradiation deferred for salvage appear to do as well as (and in some cases, even better than) those who receive radiosurgery and whole-brain radiation therapy together. The precise role, application, and sequencing of radiosurgery, therefore, remains controversial and subject to considerable variation among institutions.

Surgery

The surgical treatment of brain metastases is still evolving. Clear indications for resection include situations in which the diagnosis is in doubt and patients for whom removal of the tumor mass is likely to provide immediate palliation. Such considerations lead to a very high level of selectivity in surgical series. It is common practice in some institutions to select for surgical resection those patients with single brain metastases who are otherwise clinically stable. The goals of surgery are mainly twofold:

- complete eradication of the brain metastasis and
- the effective and prompt relief of symptoms.

Surgical resection followed by whole-brain radiation therapy can result in useful and prolonged survival ranging from a median of 16 to 26 months.

In studies intended to establish whether improved intracranial control would reduce morbidity, improve the quality of life, prolong survival, and alter mortality patterns, surgical resection in addition to whole-brain radiation therapy was found to be better than whole-brain irradiation alone in terms of median survival and functional independence, especially for patients younger than 65 years with a Karnofsky Performance Score greater than 70 and controlled systemic disease. These trials validated the concept that superior intracranial control can improve survival; however, another trial found no advantage by adding surgery to whole-brain irradiation. These divergent results are likely due to different selection criteria (Table 104-4).

Surgical removal of brain metastasis without whole-brain radiation therapy has also been evalu-

Table 104-4 ■ Randomized Controlled Trials of Whole-Brain Radiation Therapy Alone versus Surgery Plus Whole-Brain Radiation Therapy for Single Brain Metastases

Author	Treatment (N)	Radiation Dose (Total)	Outcomes	Results	Comments
Patchell et al (1990)	Bx + WBRT (23) vs. surgery + WBRT (25)	3 Gy in four daily fractions, 10 days (30 Gy)	OS, LR, FI, mortality	Surgery group had longer median OS (40 vs. 15 wk, P < 0.01); less LR (20% vs. 52%, P < 0.02), and better FI (median 38 wk vs. 8 wk., P < 0.005)	Randomization method described. Estimation of power and sample size were given. 11% percent of initally eligible patients excluded because of nonmetastatic lesions.
Vecht et al (1993)	Surgery + WBRT (32) vs. WBRT (31)	2 Gy twice daily, 10 days (40 Gy)	Survival, FI (WHO Scale ≤1 and Neurological Disability Scale ≤1)	Surgery group had longer median OS (10 vs. 6 months, P < 0.04); longer FI (P = 0.06). Age and extracranial disease were important predictors	Randomization method described. No statistical power with small sample size. 31% of patients had progressive systemic disease.
Mintz et al (1996)	Surgery + WBRT (41) vs. WBRT (43)	3 Gy in four daily fractions, 10 days (30 Gy)	Survival, functional status (KPS), QOL (Spitzer QOL Score)	No difference in median OS (5.6 vs. 6.3 mo, P = 0.24), KPS or QOL	Randomization method described; Estimation of sample size with power of 80%. 18 of 84 patients (21%) had a KPS = 50–60; a higher proportion of patients with systemic disease (45%) than in other trials

N = Number of participants; Bx = Biopsy; WBRT = Whole brain radiation therapy; Gy = Gray; OS = Overall survival; LR = Local recurrence; FI = Functional independence; WHO = World Health Organization; KPS = Karnofsky Performance Score; QOL = Quality of Life; Wk = Weeks

ated. These studies found high relapse rates (up to 85%) for those patients who did not receive whole-brain radiation therapy. Patchell tested the hypothesis that the addition of postoperative whole brain radiation therapy was better than surgery alone in patients with single brain metastases. In this randomized trial, patients were allocated to surgery alone or to surgery plus whole-brain radiation therapy. After approximately one year, local recurrences were significantly fewer (18% vs. 70%); the median length of time to tumor recurrence was significantly longer (226 vs. 38 weeks); and deaths due to neurological causes were significantly reduced (14% vs. 44%) for patients receiving surgery plus whole-brain irradiation. On the other hand, median survival and the ability to function independently were not significantly different between the two groups, a finding that highlights the importance of adequate control of systemic cancer.

For all the foregoing reasons, the combination of surgery and whole-brain irradiation for patients under the age of 65 who have a Karnofsky Performance Score greater than 70, a single brain metastasis, and no minimal and stable extracranial disease is considered at present to be the best treatment option.

Surgical resection of multiple brain metastases (two to three) has recently been explored. The standard of care for patients with two or more metastatic lesions is whole-brain radiation therapy only (although radiosurgery is increasingly being used in these patients). Evidence from nonrandomized studies also suggest that resection of two to three brain metastases in some patients is feasible, yielding increased local control, a rate of recurrence similar to that for single metastases, and reduction of deaths from neurologic causes. In this regard, a study from the M.D. Anderson Cancer Center compared patients with two to three metastases who underwent resection with patients having single metastases who were treated similarly. Local and distant recurrence rates were similar for both groups. It is likely that the best candidates for surgical resection of multiple metastases are those in RPA class I, although some in RPA class II might also benefit, especially those with controlled systemic disease. With good surgical experience, the one-month mortality rate is 2% or less. This mortality is due to herniation, hemorrhage in the operative site, uncontrolled systemic cancer, and thromboembolic complications. The rate of postoperative neurologic deficits averages 6%.

Chemotherapy

Chemotherapy has been disappointing in the management of brain metastases in patients with known, advanced cancer who have received cytotoxic drugs previously. Reasons for this lack of effectiveness include the poor permeability of the blood-brain barrier, the relative chemoresistance of metastatic clones, and the presence of multiple other foci of metastatic disease that contribute to early death. Despite the fact that the blood-brain barrier is disrupted in virtually all patients with brain metastases, water-soluble cytotoxic agents cannot penetrate brain tissue optimally to achieve therapeutic concentrations.

Patients with brain metastases from chemosensitive tumors such as breast cancer, small cell lung cancer, and testicular cancer might respond to chemotherapy.

In clinical practice, patients most likely to respond are chemotherapy-naïve patients in Class I and some in Class II. Chemotherapy is recommended if there is active systemic disease with or without extracranial metastases. If whole-brain radiation therapy is withheld, these patients will need close follow-up and, at the earliest suggestion of intracranial progression, chemotherapy should be discontinued and whole-brain irradiation instituted. Specific examples in which chemotherapy may play a role include lung cancer, breast cancer, melanoma, and testicular cancer.

Lung Cancer

The overall response of brain metastases in patients with untreated small cell lung cancer with chemotherapy alone is between 70% to 80% with a median survival of approximately 8 months, comparable to the rates for whole-brain irradiation. In previously treated patients presenting with central nervous system metastases, the response rate is lower (40%) and the duration of response is shorter. The most commonly used regimens include various combinations of cisplatin, etoposide, teniposide, CCNU, vincristine, cyclophosphamide, 5-fluorouracil, doxorubicin, and topotecan. The median duration of response appears to be longer with combination chemotherapy, but survival does not differ significantly for single or combination regimens.

Teniposide alone was compared with teniposide plus whole-brain irradiation in patients with brain metastases from small cell lung cancer to test the hypothesis whether single-agent chemotherapy was as effective as combined-modality treatment. Patients had histologic evidence of small cell lung cancer, brain metastases confirmed by contrast-enhanced computed tomography scan, evidence of systemic disease, and no prior treatment with chemo- or radiotherapy for brain metastases, and they were younger than 76 years. Patients treated with teniposide plus whole-brain irradiation had a statistically significant improvement in tumor response rate (57% vs. 22%) with longer time to progression in the brain. There were no differences in clinical response, time to extracranial progression, or overall survival; median survival was 3.5 months in the combined-modality arm and 3.2 months in the teniposide arm. The addition of whole-brain irradiation did not prolong survival despite higher intracranial tumor control, because most patients died from extracranial progression.

For patients with non–small cell lung cancer, multiple drug regimens using etoposide, cisplatin, carboplatin, fotemustine, and ifosfamide yield overall response rates of 8% to 10%, and a median duration of response and survival of five months. A trial with patients having brain metastases from non–small cell lung cancer allocated to whole-brain radiation therapy; whole-brain radiation therapy plus chloroethylnitrosoureas; and whole-brain radiation therapy plus dichloroethylnitrosoureas and tegafur found higher tumor response rates (up to 74%) but similar median survival across treatment arms.

Chemotherapy as first-line treatment for brain metastases in non–small cell lung cancer has also been attempted. The Italian Oncology Group treated patients with non–small cell lung cancer and brain metastases that were not amenable to surgery and that had not previously been treated with radiation or chemotherapy. The regimen used was cisplatin plus etoposide. Fifty-four percent of patients had extracranial disease, 45% had multiple metastases, and 90% had an Eastern Cooperative Oncology Group (ECOG) performance status of 0–2. The overall response rate was 30%, with a median time to progression of four months and a median survival of eight months. The one-year survival rate was 25%.

Newly diagnosed, previously untreated small cell lung cancer patients with brain metastases could be treated effectively with chemotherapy. For all other patients, whole-brain radiation therapy remains the standard of care.

Breast Cancer

Studies have found an overall response rate of 50%, a median survival of 5.5 to 14 months, and a one-year survival of 31% in patients with breast cancer and brain metastases. The chemotherapy regimens used included various combinations of cyclophosphamide,

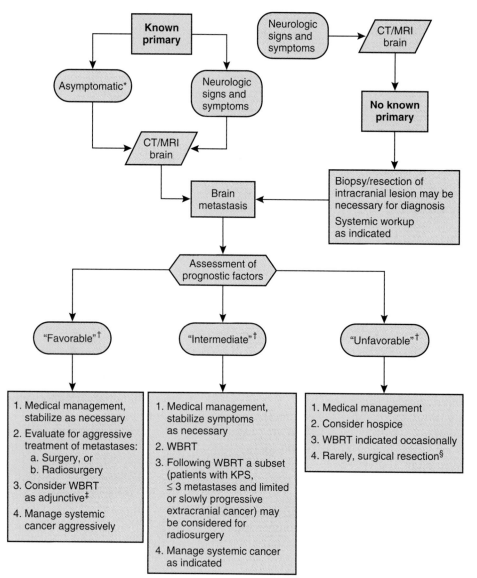

Figure 104-8 ▪ Algorithm for management of newly diagnosed brain metastasis. (CT = computed tomography; MRI = magnetic resonance imaging; WBRT = whole-brain radiation therapy; CVA = cerebrovascular accident; KPS = Karnosky Performance Score; RPA = recursive partitioning analysis.)

* Brain metastases found incidentally in asymptomatic cancer patients during staging or when imaging has been done for a different reason, such as head trauma or investigation of a CVA.

† "Favorable": These patients have a good KPS (≥ 70%), are usually RPA Class I but sometimes Class II, with no or minimal extracranial metastatic disease, a well-controlled primary tumor and have little intracranial disease burden, usually 1 or < 3 metastases. "Intermediate": These patients are usually RPA Class II and have features that exclude them from being categorized as "favorable." "Unfavorable": These patients have a poor KPS, are usually RPA Class III, generally have substantial extracranial disease, and often have a large number of brain metastases.

‡ Some investigators withhold WBRT until intracranial progression after radiosurgery or resection.

§ If the patient is "unfavorable" specifically because a single, large intracranial metastasis is causing significant mass effect, this lesion could be resected to improve the patient's status.

methotrexate, doxorubicin, 5-fluorouracil, vincristine, prednisone, etoposide, and cisplatinum. Front-line chemotherapy with cisplatinum and etoposide was also used in a cohort study of patients with breast cancer and brain metastases. The overall response rate was 38%, and the one-year survival rate was 31%. Patients with multiple brain metastases from breast

and lung cancer and active extracranial disease with good performance status can potentially be treated with chemotherapy.

Melanoma

Although metastatic melanoma to the brain has been found to respond to interferon, dacarbazine, and fote-

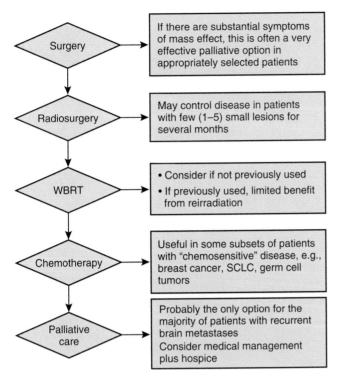

| Surgery | → | If there are substantial symptoms of mass effect, this is often a very effective palliative option in appropriately selected patients |

| Radiosurgery | → | May control disease in patients with few (1–5) small lesions for several months |

| WBRT | → | • Consider if not previously used
• If previously used, limited benefit from reirradiation |

| Chemotherapy | → | Useful in some subsets of patients with "chemosensitive" disease, e.g., breast cancer, SCLC, germ cell tumors |

| Palliative care | → | Probably the only option for the majority of patients with recurrent brain metastases
Consider medical management plus hospice |

Figure 104-9 ■ Suggested approach for the management of recurrent brain metastases. (WBRT = whole-brain radiation therapy; SCLC = small cell lung cancer).

mustine, these responses are rare, partial, and short-lived.

Testicular Cancer

Patients with testicular cancer who present with brain metastases at initial diagnosis have a high response rate to cisplatin-based chemotherapy, with a five-year survival rate of 45%. However, in patients who develop metastatic disease following chemotherapy, the response rate is low, with a five-year survival rate of 12%. Survival is increased, however, with surgery and radiation therapy if patients have an isolated recurrence in the central nervous system.

Figures 104-8 and 104-9 summarize a practical decision tree that could be used in the management of these patients. An approach to this clinical problem based on a prognostic three-tiered system is outlined in Figure 104-8. For patients with recurrent disease, retreatment is a viable option in certain situations, as outlined in Figure 104-9.

Follow-up

There are no absolute guidelines regarding the need for follow-up imaging in patients with brain metas-

tases. If patients are stable, they can be evaluated clinically once a month for three months after treatment. Most patients will require follow-up for their primary malignancy as well as for other potential sites of metastases. Central nervous system imaging is repeated only if it will yield information that would influence the clinical management.

References

Fosså SD, Bokemeyer C, Gerl A, et al: Treatment outcome of patients with brain metastases from malignant germ cell tumors. Cancer 1999;85:988–997.

Franciosi V, Cocconi G, Michiara M, et al: Front-line chemotherapy with cisplatin and etoposide for patients with brain metastases from breast carcinoma, non–small cell lung carcinoma, or malignant melanoma: a prospective study. Cancer 1999;85:1599–1605.

Gaspar LE, Scott C, Murray K, Curran W: Validation of the RTOG recursive partitioning analysis (RPA) classification for brain metastases. Int J Radiat Oncol Biol Phys 2000;47:1001–1006.

Greenberg HS, Chandler WF, Sandler HM: Brain metastases. In Greenberg HS, Chandler WF, Sandler HM (eds): Brain Tumors, 1st ed. New York: Oxford University Press; 1999, pp 299–317.

Mintz AH, Kestle J, Rathbone MP, et al: A randomized trial to assess the efficacy of surgery in addition to radiotherapy in patients with a single cerebral metastasis. Cancer 1996;78:1470–1476.

Murray KJ, Scott C, Zachariah B, et al: Importance of the mini-mental status examination in the treatment of patients with brain metastases: A report from the Radiation Therapy Oncology Group protocol 91–04. Int J Radiat Oncol Biol Phys 2000;48:59–64.

Patchell RA, Tibbs PA, Regine WF, et al: Postoperative radiotherapy in the treatment of single metastases to the brain: A randomized trial. JAMA 1998;280:1485–1489.

Patchell RA, Tibbs PA, Walsh JW, et al: A randomized trial of surgery in the treatment of single metastases to the brain. N Engl J Med 1990;322:494–500.

Posner JB: Intracranial metastases. In: Posner JB (ed): Neurological Complications of Cancer. Philadelphia: FA Davis, 1995, pp 77–110.

Postmus PE, Haaxma-Reiche H, Smit EF, et al: Treatment of brain metastases of small cell lung cancer: comparing teniposide and teniposide with whole-brain radiotherapy. A phase III study of the European Organization for the Research and Treatment of Cancer Lung Cancer Cooperative Group. J Clin Oncol 2000;18:3400–3408.

Postmus PE, Smit EF: Chemotherapy for brain metastases of lung cancer: A review. Ann Oncol 1999;10:753–759.

Sawaya R, Bindal RK: Metastatic brain tumors. In Kaye AH, Laws ER Jr, (eds): Brain Tumors: An Encyclopedic

Approach. Edinburgh: Churchill Livingstone, 1995, pp 923–946.

Schiff D, Batchelor T, Wen PY: Neurologic emergencies in cancer patients. Neurol Clin North Am 1998;16:449–454.

Ushio Y, Arita N, Hayakawa T, et al: Chemotherapy of brain metastases from lung carcinoma: A controlled randomized study. Neurosurgery 1991;28:201–205.

Vecht CJ, Haaxma-Reiche H, Noordijk EM, et al: Treatment of single brain metastasis: Radiotherapy alone or combined with neurosurgery? Ann Neurol 1993;33:583–590.

Chapter 105
Epidural Tumors and Spinal Cord Compression

Fred Hochberg

Epidemiology

Epidural tumors are the most frequent cause of spinal cord compression. Fewer than one third begin in the vertebral bodies or the brain and spinal cord. The rest are metastatic from other primary sites. When tumors arise from the vertebral column or its supporting structures, they are of bone origin (multiple myeloma, osteogenic sarcoma, chordoma, Ewing's sarcoma) or are derived from connective tissue (vascular, fibrous, hematopoietic, lipomatous, and undifferentiated mesenchymal elements). Rarely, subarachnoid deposits of brain tumors (primitive neuroectodermal tumors, lymphoma, or ependymoma) seed the dura. In general, metastatic cancer that spreads to bone does not enter brain or subarachnoid space. This is generally true for epidural deposits from previously diagnosed cancer of the breast, lymphoma, kidney cancer, myeloma, melanoma, female reproductive tract tumors, and gastrointestinal tract tumors. Lung and prostate cancers may first appear with spinal cord compression, although sarcoma and neuroblastoma are most common in children. In the magnetic resonance imaging (MRI) era, the true incidence of epidural cancer has been found to peak at age 50 to 70 years.

Anatomic Implications

Vascular Supply

Spinal cord compression is one of the major mechanisms of damage from epidural cancer. Equally significant is the morbidity produced by congestion of the spinal cord veins as well as the loss of stability of the vertebral bodies, which then compress the spinal cord or its nerve roots. Both problems can be immediately addressed by treatment. Venous congestion results in cord edema and axonal swelling, and myelopathy ensues. Unlike other organs, in which veins and arteries course in a common vascular bundle, the spinal cord has fewer veins than arteries. Tumor compresses the posterior vein that drains the sensory fiber tracts or the small anterior veins draining the motor fibers. These empty into the ventral vein that runs parallel to the artery. The midthoracic cord is particularly vulnerable. The spinal cord circulation is usually resistant to arterial compromise—thus the rarity of strokes involving the cord. Tumors lying anteriorly or posteriorly to the cord reduce its radicular blood flow and cause swelling. Most vulnerable to compression is the single anterior spinal artery, which delivers 80% of the blood supply. Less important are the two smaller posterior spinal arteries and feeders entering the cord at varying levels. Spinal cord edema, leg weakness, and pain may be improved by the administration of corticosteroids. Otherwise, uncontrolled spinal cord edema further reduces blood flow and damages both myelin tracks and neurons.

Spinal Stability

Epidural tumors can coexist with other bony lesions, including hypertrophic growth of bone and ligament, dorsal osteophytes, and herniated cervical discs. The clinician is urged to ask a single question: "Is the spine stable?" An unstable spine can damage the cord and compress vessels or nerve roots. Three columns support the cord (Figure 105-1). The middle and anterior columns are the most often affected in the thoracolumbar spine, as most epidural deposits lie in the anterior vertebral body or emerge out of the retropleural or retroperitoneal spaces. The anterior column comprises the anterior ligament, the anterior vertebral body, and the anterior disc substance. The posterior longitudinal ligament, the posterior vertebral body, and the posterior disc material form the middle column. The posterior column is made up of posterior bone such as the posterior facet joint and its capsule, part of the bony neural arch, the ligaments between the vertebral bodies, and the ligamentum flavum.

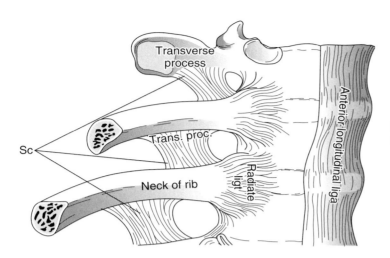

Figure 105-1 ■ The three columns that support the spinal cord.

Primary and Metastatic Epidural Tumors

The vertebral venous system has no valves and is a low-pressure system. Rising abdominal pressure from coughing, sneezing, and straining allows venous effluent from the breast, intrathoracic, intra-abdominal, and pelvic organs to enter and move unimpeded up or down the veins. Epidural metastases occur in the bony spinal vertebra, the paravertebral soft tissues, or the epidural space itself. A tumor in any of these locations may impinge on the nerve roots to produce "electrical sensations" of pain. Although epidural cancer commonly deforms the vertebral body or pedicles, renal cell cancer, Pancoast's syndrome, neuroblastoma, and lymphoma compress nerves without involving bone. Thus, an unremarkable plain radiograph of the spine does not exclude epidural tumor. Computed tomography (CT) with iodine contrast and magnetic resonance imaging provide more accurate depiction of these areas and are the imaging modalities of choice. Even then, epidural tumor as the sole manifestation of cancer is rare. A general rule is that the spinal cord is involved in proximity to the primary cancer. The most frequent thoracic spine lesions (68%) reflect lung cancer, breast cancer, or lymphoma, whereas cervical involvement (16%) appears in the setting of head and neck cancers as well as bone tumors of the skull base. Colon cancer and adenocarcinoma of the prostate predispose to lumbosacral spinal (15%) involvement.

Clinical Manifestations

A single rule should define the clinician's approval to urgent evaluation: Back or thoracic pain with a change in gait heralds most epidural tumors. In cancer patients, back or neck or radicular pain must be immediately evaluated by radiologic and clinical examinations to exclude spinal metastatic disease. Pain usually has a radiating quality reflecting compression of sensory fibers. Tingling sensations resembling heat or electricity may travel down an extremity in over three quarters of cervical epidural tumors or circumscribe the chest or abdominal walls in half of thoracic appearances. Patients complain of a "constrictive band" or tightness in the absence of weakness. The diagnosis of epidural cancer at this stage is associated with a high likelihood of preserved ambulation. To touch or palpation, the vertebrae are tender in almost one third of afflicted patients, leaving the remainder without bone tenderness, but epidural pain can be worsened by Valsalva's maneuver, neck flexion, and tests of straight-leg raising. Often, pain of spinal cord compression is confounded by arthritic complaints or masked by opiates. Not uncommonly, months go by before diagnosis.

Proximal weakness of the legs is the second most common symptom of epidural tumor. Even patients with cervical cord compression develop leg weakness before arm difficulties. For rapid evaluation, the patient is asked to walk, climb stairs, and stand on one leg. Any difficulty in the performance of these simple tasks is highly suspicious for cord compression. Several features of the examination serve as clues. The reflexes of the knees and ankles are more active than those of the arms. There is often weakness of the thigh-flexing muscles and dorsiflexor plantar responses. The only exception occurs in the setting of metastasis to the cauda equina or meninges, which reduces the leg reflexes. Diagnosis and prompt treatment are likely to preserve gait. Sensory loss, such as numbness and paresthesia, is experienced by half of patients. Several bedside tests may aid in identifying the level or levels of compression: Patients should be asked to identify the location on their back at which pin sensation changes from 100% to something less. Similarly, clinicians may identify the location at which a pin scratch over the torso elicits a less obvious local wheal and flare reaction or at which the upward or downward movement of skin is not appreciated. Autonomic disturbance, male impotence, constipation, and bladder incontinence or urgency are the most common complaints. Sweating is decreased below the lesion level and increased above it. The patient exhibits a wide-based gait.

Spinal Fluid Studies

Spinal fluid evaluation offers little benefit and carries potential risk in the setting of epidural cancer. As epidural cancer seldom breaks through the dural barrier, the cerebrospinal fluid (CSF) is usually without tumor cells. Removal of fluid may actually increase the compression of the spinal cord, resulting in transformation of subtle symptoms into plegia of the legs. Lumbar puncture is best performed in the course of myelography or to assess for concomitant meningeal cancer or infection after radiographic delineation of the site(s) of epidural involvement. The protein content is typically increased by as much as twentyfold, as cerebrospinal fluid does not flow beneath a blockage (Froin's syndrome). However, the cell count is normal.

Imaging

Magnetic Resonance Imaging

Magnetic resonance imaging provides the most specific and sensitive identification of epidural cancer. This modality is superior to myelography, computed tomography, and standard radiography. The integrity and stability of the bony spine are visualized in addition to the extent of compression and damage of the spinal cord and its roots. Most centers provide epidural protocols of magnetic resonance imaging (T1, T2, or FLAIR images before and after gadolinium administration), which assess the entire sagittal spinal canal from the foramen magnum to sacral roots. The neurologic examination cannot replace the magnetic resonance images, as epidural disease is often present at multiple levels. Sagittal images localize the level of epidural disease, whereas axial studies define the anterior or posterior displacement of the cord and its roots and provide a measure of cord damage (as T2

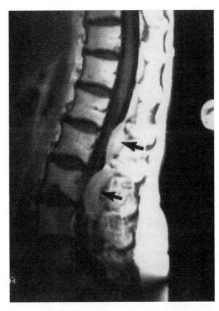

Figure 105-2 ■ Sagittal T1-W magnetic resonance imaging following gadolinium injection demonstrates a plaque of enhancing epidural lymphoma (*arrows*) extending posterior to the theca from L1 to L4. Tumor tissue penetrated the neural foramen of L2. (From MacVicar D, Husband JE: Reticuloendothelial disorders: Lymphoma. In Grainger RG, Alison DJ [eds]: Diagnostic Radiology: A Textbook of Medical Imaging, 3rd ed. CD-ROM. Philadelphic, WB Saunders, 1999.)

changes within the white matter) (Figures 105-2 and 105-3). Seldom can radiation fields or operative plans be created without these studies. Rules emerge that will aid the clinician: (1) All epidural cancer is a potential emergency, so magnetic resonance imaging is an emergency procedure; (2) the entire spine should be imaged after the injection of gadolinium contrast; and (3) the radiologist should assess the number and location of epidural lesions, the anterior-posterior location of the mass, the stability of the spine, and any changes within the spinal cord. Plain radiographs are of limited value, as one quarter of epidural lesions have little bone destruction and at least 50% of bone must be destroyed before changes are visualized. The collapse of the vertebral bodies and pedicle destruction are better characterized by computed tomography scan. Computed tomography studies are now available reformatted in coronal and sagittal planes to provide inexpensive and rapid vertebral evaluation.

Magnetic resonance imaging scans also provide the basis for separation of epidural metastasis from other processes, including multiple sclerosis, paraneoplastic myelopathy, osteoporotic bone disease, and leptomeningeal cancer. One needs to be aware of nonmalignant causes of spinal damage in patients with cancer, such as:

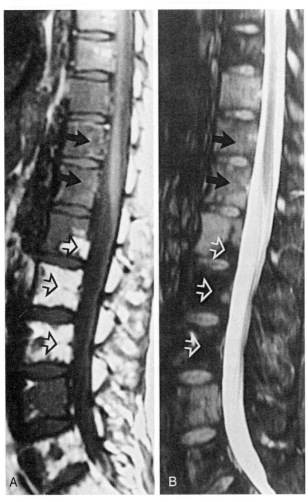

Figure 105-3 ■ Neuroblastoma. **A,** Sagittal lumbar T1-weighted magnetic resonance image shows widespread metastatic disease replacing the normal high-signal intensity of fatty marrow (*open arrows*) with intermediate-signal intensity (*solid arrows*). There is no epidural spread. **B,** Sagittal lumbar T2-weighted magnetic resonance image with fat suppression. The areas of infiltrated marrow appear as high-signal intensity (*solid arrows*), indicating the relatively higher water content of the neoplastic marrow, whereas areas of normal fatty marrow are markedly low-signal intensity (*open arrows*) with suppression of the fat signal. (From Andrews C, Hynes P: Metastatic bone disease. In Bragg, Rubin, Hricak, eds: Oncological Imaging, 2nd ed. Phildelphia, WB Saunders, 2002, p 695.)

1. Herniated discs commonly afflict cervical and lumbar sites rather than thoracic ones. The radicular pain can be relieved by bed rest. Magnetic resonance imaging findings are diagnostic and do not cross disc spaces.
2. Epidural abscess of bacterial origin in immunosuppressed patients can produce both localized pain and erosive bone changes that cross the disc space to involve contiguous vertebral bodies. The proliferative infection, especially tuberculosis, is not easily separated from cancer. Magnetic resonance imaging scanning should be followed by needle biopsy in the febrile patient.
3. Epidural hemorrhage can suddenly produce back pain and paresis in the cancer patient with thrombocytopenia or coagulopathy. The echo gradient-weighted magnetic resonance imaging or computed tomography scan provides evidence of bleeding. Although epidural cancers can bleed, such occurrence is rare for melanoma or neoplasms of renal or lung origin.
4. Spinal cord damage can occur after radiation therapy or as a slowly evolving syndrome of weakness (inflammatory neuropathy or Guillain-Barré syndrome or anterior horn cell disease or inflammatory myelopathy). These do not produce epidural deposits.

Computed Tomography

Computed tomography is more sensitive and specific than radionuclide bone scan or plain radiographs for identifying neoplasms of the vertebral column and paravertebral structures. In patients with retropleural or retroperitoneal cancer extending to vertebrae, computed tomography may be the initial diagnostic study. With parenteral contrast material, computed tomography can delineate the extension of tumor from vertebrae and paravertebral structures to the epidural space and provide images of direct extension of metastasis in adjacent vertebra, extension from tumor arising in vertebrae at the rostral or caudal levels, and epidural extension from paravertebral tissues through the intervertebral foramina. Spinal computed tomography provides excellent bone detail except in the setting of either severe ankylosis or osteoporosis, with associated indistinct cortical margins.

Other Imaging Formats

Myelography has been replaced by less invasive and more informative magnetic resonance imaging scans. For patients with pacemakers or metallic implants who cannot undergo magnetic resonance imaging, myelography with computed tomography scans remains the procedure of choice, although with the risk of further decompensating spinal fluid dynamics. When myelographic computed tomography is performed, the entire spinal axis should be examined. Thus, the rostral and caudal extent of the compression can be visualized, and smaller, asymptomatic lesions can be identified. Radiation therapy portals and surgical approaches depend on this information.

Radionuclide bone scanning is the most sensitive radiologic technique for the visualization of skeletal metastases. However, this exceptional sensitivity is gained at the expense of low specificity. The scans identify metastatic deposits without definition of the anatomy of the skeletal changes or distinction from other bone diseases, including degenerative joint diseases.

Approach to Management

Patients can be segregated into two groups according to the following scheme: (1) those with back or neck pain radiating into the chest or abdomen or an extremity but who lack leg weakness and (2) those with leg weakness. Because the outcome of therapy is so much more favorable in the first group, physicians must recognize patients with spinal metastases before irreversible neurologic abnormalities arise. In cancer patients with pain and no weakness whose examination of reflexes and sensation is normal, most physicians obtain a radionuclide bone scan and plain spine radiograph. A magnetic resonance imaging scan should be performed irrespective of the preliminary results. In patients with any evidence of spinal cord compression or with leg weakness, a total spine magnetic resonance imaging must be performed. Often the separation between groups rests on a simple test of leg weakness (e.g., whether the patient can walk up stairs or can stand on one leg with the knee slightly bent). Patients lacking weakness have a better outcome after treatment; thus, early intervention is always advisable. Suspected epidural cancer is always a neurologic and therapeutic emergency.

Treatment

Even prompt administration of radiation therapy or surgery will not improve neurologic damage if the veins and arteries are obstructed or if there is spinal cord edema or ischemia. For this reason, immediate treatment with high-dose steroids and hyperosmolar agents is indicated. Lacking the results of a randomized trial of radiation or surgical decompression, physicians can be guided by certain rules of therapy: (1) Radiation therapy is definitive, provided that the tumor is radiosensitive; (2) patients should be operated on if the tumor is radioresistant or if paraplegia has occurred; and (3) systemic chemotherapy is reserved for epidural leukemia or lymphoma.

Corticosteroids

Prompt administration of steroids provides three benefits. Within one hour, the patient experiences pain relief, reduced spinal cord edema, and an oncolytic effect on cancer of lymphoma or breast origin. A randomized trial of dexamethasone, using 96 mg daily compared to placebo demonstrated improved neurologic outcome. However, no benefit has been seen with 100 mg of dexamethasone compared to a 10-mg initial bolus followed by 16 mg daily. Pain control, ambulation, and bladder function were not different. Dexamethasone is most commonly provided as an intravenous bolus of 20 to 100 mg followed by 8 to 20 mg every eight hours for the next several days. The maintenance dose depends on functional level and the existence of comorbidities such as diabetes mellitus, infection, disorders of mentation, or heart failure. There is no edema rebound with this medication, and short-term steroids do not produce significant suppression of endogenous production. However, use over weeks induces weakness of proximal leg muscles, hypertension, cataracts, and glaucoma.

Mannitol

Mannitol, a nonmetabolized sugar, is a mainstay of short-term control of brain and spinal edema. Lacking a metabolic contraindication, intravenous injection of 40 grams over one hour is followed by 20 grams every six hours to achieve a serum osmolality in excess of 300 milliosmols.

Radiation Therapy

Most patients, after steroids, receive radiation therapy. Several considerations govern the use of radiation:

1. Epidural cancer is a medical emergency for which radiation therapy must be started as soon as possible.
2. The radiation fields, based on magnetic resonance imaging or computed tomography images, must include all of the metastatic tissue plus a margin. Any paravertebral mass should be included in treatment. Although it is mandatory to irradiate at least the epidural symptomatic deposit, most therapists will treat all potentially significant spinal lesions at the same time.
3. There is no convincing difference between the benefits of commonly used doses and fraction sizes (e.g., 3000 cGy in 10 sessions of 300-cGy fractions, 4000 cGy in 20 sessions of 200-cGy fractions, or 2500 cGy in five sessions of 500-cGy fractions).
4. Radiation-induced myelopathy and radiculopathy can be avoided by staying within the above doses and fractions and limiting concomitant chemotherapy (including gemcitabine and Taxol in gynecologic tumors and cisplatin in lung cancers) and the use of radiosensitizers.

The benefits of radiation therapy are improved for the following patients:

1. Those without motor deficits at the start of radiation. They will likely remain ambulatory. Those with moderate paraparesis at the start have a 50% chance of gait recovery.

2. Those with slowly progressive paraplegia in comparison to rapidly progressive onset.

3. Of those who ambulate at the end of radiation, 75% are likely to preserve this function six months later and 50% 12 months later.

4. Those with any gait retention at the end of radiation. Patients who have not reachieved ambulation likely will remain paraplegic and survive no more than a few months.

Because epidural metastases may occur at multiple levels, the entire rostrocaudal spinal axis is usually imaged with magnetic resonance imaging to provide the design of radiotherapy ports that include adjacent asymptomatic metastatic epidural deposits. If these adjacent epidural metastases are not included in the original treatment field and later require radiotherapy, the amount of radiation tolerated may be limited by overlapping spinal radiotherapy ports. Postradiation prognosis depends on the preradiation neurologic function and the extent of spinal involvement as well as spine stability. The goal of therapy is to avoid progressive neurologic morbidity and a "neurologic death."

Surgery

In the absence of randomized studies comparing surgery with radiation therapy across all tumor types and levels of preoperative morbidity, several indications exist for surgical decompression:

1. For patients with presumed epidural cancer without a previously known primary tumor, decompression or stereotactic biopsy may provide definitive diagnosis of cancer histology or infectious origin absent significant neurologic morbidity.

2. Operative decompression may be the only means of preserving gait in the setting of radiation-resistant epidural cancer (undifferentiated carcinoma of the lung, sarcoma, melanoma, hemorrhagic metastasis, or infection in proximity to metastatic deposit) that has caused acutely evolving paresis or plegia.

3. Surgical resection may be the only option for patients with relapse in a previously irradiated area or clinical deterioration during irradiation or those with a potential contraindication to irradiation (preexisting myelopathy or radiculopathy, inadequate bone marrow reserve, inability to tolerate radiation positioning or planning).

4. For centers with dedicated spine surgery, operative intervention is commonly used with good outcome for the treatment of metastatic tumor involving one vertebral body. This lesion can likely be cured. In patients with multilevel spinal instability on magnetic resonance imaging or computed tomography study, because radiation therapy is not likely to improve spine stability, operative decompression is followed by the placement of metallic rods across the decompressed area.

Surgery has several theoretical limitations. Decompressive laminectomy is often followed by radiation therapy. Laminectomy followed by radiation therapy is not superior to radiation therapy alone. Moreover, surgeons are reluctant to operate on the anterior component of tumor, as the procedure requires a transthoracic or transabdominal approach. Posterior resection followed by stabilization offers the benefit of providing room for the cord to swell but does not truly address the actual tumor deposit. In posterior or posteriolateral laminectomy, the surgeon removes the posterior ligaments. The spinal cord is free to move into a portion of the operative space, relieving the compression produced by the anterior mass, which is untouched. In anterior resection procedures, the vertebral body is removed along with contiguous retropleural or retroperitoneal tumor tissue. The spine must then be stabilized with bone or metal. If the metastasis involves several contiguous vertebral bodies, the stabilization cannot be performed, and the procedure is not possible.

The estimated morbidity from both procedures is a 4% risk of significant wound infection, epidural bleeding, or accidental spinal cord damage. To these must be added the two-week delay in provision of radiation therapy after operation.

Chemotherapy

Chemotherapy is occasionally used as first-line treatment in patients with metastatic breast carcinoma, for non-Hodgkin's lymphoma, and for Hodgkin's disease and germ cell tumors. Chemotherapy is restricted to patients with minimal gait or bladder symptoms and those for whom radiation or surgery is contraindicated. Combined chemotherapy and radiation or surgery are recommended for treatment of widespread bone and systemic metastases that also involve the spine.

Other Medical Care

Bed rest and braces are prescribed for spinal instability. Symptomatic involvement of the cervical spine obligates the use of a firm (Thomas, Philadelphia, or similar) collar during ambulation. Pain medication is commonly provided by radicular blockade of afflicted roots, but intradural or extradural infusions are contraindicated.

Specific Tumor Types

Epidural Lymphoma

The thoracic spine is the most frequent area of involvement, but coincident involvement can exist in the cervical and lumbar vertebrae, subarachnoid space, nerve roots, eye, and brain parenchyma. Back pain occurs in more than 80% of patients, often months prior to weakness in the lower extremities. For both non-Hodgkin's lymphoma and Hodgkin's disease, nervous system involvement can occur in as many as 10% of patients. A minority of patients present with parenchymal brain or cord invasion, with anecdotal reports of primary tumors in epidural spinal and calvarial locations, most complications being seen in the setting of diffuse systemic disease. Therapy is based on radiation to the area of symptomatic affliction with surgery reserved if tissue diagnosis is required. Radiation approaches involve fractionated photons at varying schedules, of which 3000 cGy in daily fractions of 180 cGy are commonly used. After treatment, over 50% of patients are ambulatory, but paraplegics do not regain ambulation. Three different radiation schemes have been used without prognostic differences: 500 cGy per fraction for five or six fractions, 300 cGy for 10 fractions, and 200 cGy per fraction for 18 to 20 fractions. In general, more protracted schemes with low fraction size protect the spinal cord and thus may be selected for good prognosis patients. Little value is achieved by escalating total dose above cord tolerance of 4000 cGy. Epidural calvarial lymphoma can be approached with electron beam irradiation. Chemotherapy has provided sporadic complete or partial response of spinal cord compression in Hodgkin's disease. The combination of radiation and chemotherapy (with methotrexate, vinca alkaloids, or Taxol) poses unacceptable risks of spinal cord or nerve root damage.

Leukemia

Epidural involvement occurs in fewer than 0.5 percent of patients with acute leukemia. Granulocytic sarcomas or chloromas are destructive masses formed by collections of immature myeloid cells in the setting of acute or chronic myeloproliferative disease. Patients with acute myeloid leukemia with t(8;21) or chromosome 16 rearrangement are at highest risk of developing these masses in the brain parenchyma, or epidural skull, orbits, or spine. The thoracic spine is most commonly involved with pain at the level of the compression followed by weakness. In patients with acute lymphocytic leukemia, the treatment of choice is high-dose intravenous dexamethasone and systemic chemotherapy. In acute myeloid leukemia, radiation therapy is frequently provided because chemotherapy may provide only a slow response.

References

Aabo K, Walbom-Jorgensen S: Central nervous system complications by malignant lymphomas: Radiation schedule and treatment results. Int J Radiat Oncol Biol Phys 1986;12: 197–202.

Buch PA, Grossman SA: Treatment of epidural cord compression from Hodgkin's disease with chemotherapy. Am J Med 1988;84:555–558.

Mullins GM, Flynn JPG, El-Mahdi AH, McQueen D, Owens AH: Malignant lymphoma of the spinal epidural space. Ann Intern Med 1971;74:416–423.

Perry JR, Deodhare SS, Bilbao JM, Murray D, Muller P: The significance of the spinal cord compression as the initial manifestation of lymphoma. Neurosurgery 1993;32:157–162.

Peschel RE, Mai D, Dowling S, Knowlton A, Farber L, Fischer JJ: Pathology stage I and II Hodgkin's disease: Long-term results from three Connecticut hospitals. Conn Med 1991;55:449–453.

Sapoznick MD, Kaplan HS: Intracranial Hodgkin's disease. Cancer 1983;52:1301–1307.

Vecht CJ, Haaxma-Reiche H, van Putten WLJ, de Visser M, Vries EP, Twijinstra A: Initial bolus of conventional versus high-dose dexamethasone in metastatic spinal cord compression. Neurology 1989;39:1255–1257.

Chapter 106
Melanoma

Lawrence E. Flaherty and Jared A. Gollob

Incidence, Epidemiology, and Genetics

Incidence

The incidence of malignant melanoma in the United States is increasing faster than any other malignancy. Over a 15-year period from 1973 to 1987, an 83% increase in incidence was noted, associated with a nearly 30% increase in mortality. In the year 2002, an estimated 51,000 new melanomas and 7300 melanoma-related deaths were anticipated in the United States. The median age of diagnosis of melanoma is in the low fifties. This is a young age relative to other tumors and means that melanoma accounts for a disproportionate number of productive years of life lost.

Epidemiology

Melanoma occurs predominantly in Caucasian populations, with a significantly lower risk in individuals of Hispanic or Asian descent. African Americans make up approximately 1% of individuals diagnosed with melanoma in the United States, primary lesions typically occurring in nonpigmented areas of the body. Men have a slightly higher incidence of melanoma than do women. Men are also more likely to develop a melanoma on a truncal location, while women more often have melanomas develop on their extremities.

The dramatic increase in the incidence of melanoma has largely been attributed to an increase in sun-related ultraviolet B (UVB) irradiation exposure, although ultraviolet A (UVA) exposure may play a role as well. This increased exposure is likely due to both changes in the earth's atmosphere and increased recreational sun exposure. Melanoma is particularly common in Caucasian populations that have migrated to more equatorial locations.

Five-year survival rates for patients with melanoma have increased steadily over time. The largest factor in this improvement in survival has been early detection. Both patients and physicians have become more familiar with the clinical A, B, C, D features of melanoma (Table 106-1); consequently, skin lesions that are suspicious for melanoma (see Chapter 45) are being identified and biopsied at an earlier stage.

Cutaneous melanomas do not occur only on sun-exposed areas of the body, a finding suggesting that factors beyond cumulative lifetime sun exposure have a role. These include intermittent intense sun exposure, blistering sunburns, increased sun exposure during childhood, and phenotypic features such as skin type, hair color, mole count, and number of atypical moles. In addition, genetic factors appear to play a role.

A large number of studies have identified the individuals who are at greatest risk of developing melanoma. Risk factors include the following:

1. Fair complexion, a tendency to freckle or sunburn, or a history of severe sunburns, particularly at a young age
2. Atypical nevi, nevi on sun-unexposed areas, large numbers of nevi, or raised nevi
3. A history of dysplastic nevi or a family history of melanoma
4. A personal history of nonmelanoma skin cancer
5. A personal history of melanoma

Table 106-1 ▪ Melanoma Identification

A	Asymmetry
B	Border Irregularity
C	Color Change
D	Diameter (≥6 mm)

Individuals in the last group have an estimated 4% to 30% risk of developing another melanoma over their lifetime. Consequently, it is recommended that they receive lifelong dermatologic follow-up.

Genetics

Approximately 10% of patients diagnosed with melanoma have a family member with a history of melanoma, a finding suggesting a possible genetic susceptibility. While some of this familial concordance can be explained by nonspecific factors such as skin type or similar sun exposure history, in 10% to 20% of these affected families, a germline mutation or deletion in the CDKN2A tumor suppressor gene has been identified. Mutations of this tumor suppressor gene, found on chromosomal region 9p21, have been identified in other human cancers and may be one of the more frequently affected genes. This tumor suppressor gene encodes a protein, p16, which acts as an inhibitor of cyclin-dependent kinases, leading to cell cycle arrest. Recent studies have identified an increased risk of pancreas and breast cancers in affected kindred as well (see Chapter 118). The incidence of this gene deletion in sporadic forms of melanoma is less than 10%. A commercial test for mutations of p16/CDKN2A is available; because neither a positive nor a negative test alter the recommendations for close patient follow-up and screening of family members, this test has not been accepted as a standard tool for assessing patients with either familial or sporadic melanoma.

Clinical Presentation

Cutaneous Melanoma

Most primary melanomas present as a changing or new mole on the skin. Any pigmented lesion that demonstrates a change in one or more of the features listed in Table 106-1 should be considered for an excisional biopsy (see Chapter 45 for more details). In addition, moles that bleed, become pruritic, or develop a depigmented or erythematous halo at the periphery are also highly suspicious and should be considered for biopsy. However, not all melanomas express pigment.

Those that are amelanotic may be confused with warts, calluses, seborrheic keratoses, or other benign skin lesions or may mimic the appearance of basal cell cancers or actinic keratoses and, as a consequence, may be particularly difficult to diagnose early. About 5% of patients present with isolated metastases in draining lymph nodes without an identifiable cutaneous primary. It is presumed in these situations that the primary tumor has regressed spontaneously but not before allowing some cells to travel to the regional nodes. These patients are treated as stage III disease.

Noncutaneous Primary Melanoma

A small number of melanomas arise from mucosal surfaces. Mucosal melanomas can arise from the sinuses, oral mucosa, vagina, vulva, and anorectal area. Because these locations may be difficult to visualize, mucosal melanomas are often not identified until they have become large enough to produce symptoms. As a consequence, mucosal melanomas have a poorer prognosis. Mucosal, subungual, and acral melanomas are the most common sites for melanoma in African-American populations.

Metastatic Disease

The emphasis on early detection has resulted in fewer melanoma patients having clinically overt metastatic disease at the time of diagnosis. In patients who do present with metastatic disease, this will usually involve locoregional sites, including dermal deposits close to the primary lesion (satellites) or in lymphatics between the primary lesion and one or more draining nodal basins (in-transit disease) and/or regional lymphadenopathy. Satellite and in-transit metastases may be pigmented or may be amelanotic even if the primary lesion was pigmented. Lymphadenopathy is usually painless at first but may subsequently cause pain as it enlarges. Unilateral lower extremity edema can also be the first sign of deep inguinal/iliac lymph node metastases. Patients with primary lesions on the scalp may present with occipital, cervical, submandibular, or parotid swelling, heralding metastases to those nodal basins.

Following treatment for primary or regional disease, the most common sites for first recurrence are the skin, subcutaneous tissues, and lymph nodes (Figure 106-1A). While wide local excision scars and skin grafts can normally develop areas of pigmentation and irregular thickening, the appearance of pigmented or amelanotic cutaneous or subcutaneous nodules in the vicinity of a previously resected primary lesion is often a sign of local recurrence or in-transit metastases. The most common distant site for first relapse is the lung; the liver, brain,

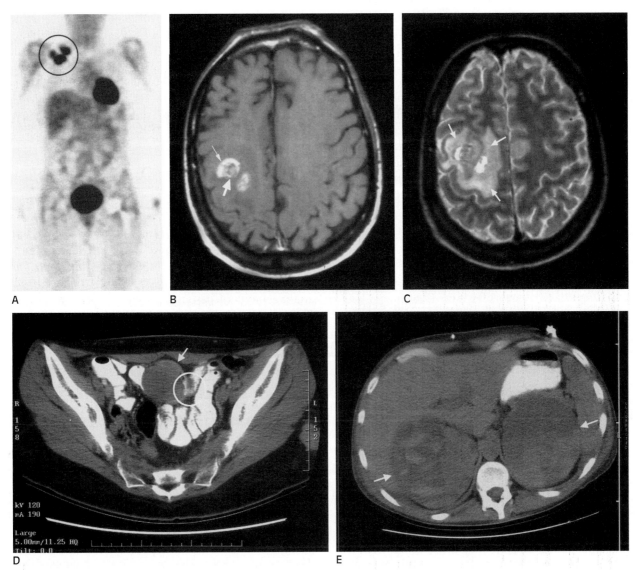

Figure 106-1 ■ Presentations of metastatic disease. *A*, PET scan (SPECT images of torso following IV injection of ¹⁸F-fluorodeoxyglucose (FDG)) showing areas of intense uptake in right axillary and right supraclavicular regions (circled area) in a patient with lymph node metastases. *B, C*, Magnetic resonance imaging images of brain metastasis (*B*, thick arrow) with associated hemorrhage (*B*, thin arrow) and surrounding edema (*C*, thin arrows). *D*, Abdominal metastasis (arrow) with involvement of serosal surface of bowel (circled area). *E*, Bilateral renal metastases (arrows) with massive renal enlargement due to tumor hemorrhage.

and bone are also frequent sites of recurrence. As a consequence of the radiologic surveillance applied to patients who are at high risk for recurrence, liver and lung metastases are usually discovered on computed tomography (CT) scan or chest X-ray before they have caused symptoms. However, patients with more advanced metastatic disease in these organs may present with painful hepatomegaly, abnormal liver function tests, chest pain/cough, and/or elevation of the serum lactate dehydrogenase (LDH) level. Bone metastases from melanoma have a predilection for the spine, and patients can present with back pain and neurologic symptoms due to spinal cord or nerve root compression. The development of brain metastases may be heralded by a seizure or focal motor weakness but may also be discovered in asymptomatic patients with metastases to other sites who are undergoing routine imaging of the brain with computed tomography or magnetic resonance imaging (MRI) prior to starting systemic therapy. Hemorrhage into brain metastases is seen more often with melanoma than with any other metastatic tumor, occurring in 30% to 50% of patients with central nervous system (CNS) melanoma (Figures 106-1*B* and 106-1*C*). The gastrointestinal (GI) tract is another common site of metastasis for melanoma (Figure 106-1*D*), and disease in this area may cause intermittent cramping abdominal pain, bowel obstruction due to intussusception, occult or acute gastrointestinal bleeding, or bowel perforation. Metastases to the kidney or adrenal glands may present as abdominal or costovertebral angle pain, especially when these lesions hemorrhage (Figure 106-1*E*). In rare cases, patients with extensive metastatic disease may present with generalized cutaneous melanosis in which the skin has a gray or blue-black appearance due to deposition of melanin in the dermis and/or melanituria in which the urine turns black in color due to excretion of circulating melanin.

Clinical Evaluation

The cornerstone of a clinical evaluation for patients who have been diagnosed with malignant melanoma is a thorough history and physical examination. Patients should undergo a thorough skin exam to detect second primary melanomas and to detect satellite and in-transit lesions between the original primary melanoma and regional nodal basin(s).

Recently, the National Institutes of Health have provided consensus guidelines for melanomas diagnosed with a depth of 1 mm or less. According to these guidelines, neither a chest X-ray nor routine laboratory tests aimed at identifying distant metastases are necessary in this patient population owing to the low risk of recurrence.

Patients diagnosed with a melanoma that is either greater than 1 mm thick, Clark level IV, or ulcerated are usually considered candidates for a sentinel lymph node biopsy. In the absence of sentinel lymph node involvement, an additional evaluation including baseline chest X-ray, complete blood count and liver chemistries, including a serum lactate dehydrogenase, are appropriate, but these tests are rarely helpful in detecting occult metastatic disease. A computed tomography scan to evaluate regional lymph nodes may be appropriate for patients who have a difficult clinical exam, although the yield is likely to be low.

Patients with palpable regional nodes (clinical stage III) either at the time of presentation or later should have tissue confirmation of melanoma by either a fine-needle aspiration or excisional biopsy followed by staging procedures. Staging should include a chest X-ray; computed tomography scans of the head, abdomen, and pelvis; and complete blood count (CBC), serum lactate dehydrogenase, albumin, and liver chemistries.

Patients with presumptive stage IV disease should have biopsy confirmation of initial recurrence. This is especially true for those with a suspected solitary metastasis. Additional evaluation should include routine CBC, chemistries, a chest X-ray, and computed tomography scans of the abdomen and pelvis. Routine chest computed tomography scans are not mandatory and may be omitted in asymptomatic patients who do not wish to receive therapy. For patients receiving treatment it may be worthwhile to obtain a head computed tomography scan with contrast as the identification of central nervous system metastases will significantly influence the clinical management approach.

Pathologic Assessment, Staging, and Prognosis

Melanomas are classified into several histologic categories, which have little prognostic significance (Table 106-2). An accurate pathologic assessment and a complete pathology report are essential to the appropriate management of patients presenting with melanoma. The following information should be included in every report:

1. Melanoma diagnosis (including subtype)
2. Breslow's thickness and Clark's level
3. Presence or absence of ulceration
4. Presence or absence of microscopic satellites
5. Surgical margin status: free or involved (identify location)

Additional elements of interest include lymphocytic infiltration, mitotic activity, tumor regression, tumor diameter, and radial and vertical growth phase patterns.

Staging and Prognostic Factors

The overall prognosis for patients diagnosed with melanoma is related to the following major features: the thickness of the lesion (Breslow's depth), presence or absence of ulceration, existence of regional lymph node involvement, and evidence of distant spread.

Table 106-2 ■ Melanoma: Pathologic Subtypes

Name	Incidence	Feature
Superficial spreading	70%	Most common, may arise in preexisting nevi, initially flat and irregular.
Nodular	10–15%	Raised or domed, more symmetric, deeply pigmented.
Lentigo maligna	5–10%	Larger, often slow growing in older individuals in sun-exposed areas, especially the face.
Acral-lentiginous	2–8%	Arise in palms, soles, subungual locations.

Few individuals who are initially diagnosed with melanoma have clinically apparent regional nodal involvement, and fewer than 5% will have evidence of distant metastases. Thus, factors related to the primary tumor (T stage) are most important in assessing initial prognosis and determining initial clinical management. A recent compilation and review of several large melanoma patient databases with long-term follow-up has identified the most important risk factors for melanoma recurrence and has prompted a change in the American Joint Committee on Cancer (AJCC) staging system for melanoma (Tables 106-3 and 106-4).

T (Tumor) Classification

Numerous tumor features have been evaluated for melanoma, including tumor thickness or depth of invasion (Breslow's thickness), level of invasion (Clark's level), ulceration, gender, anatomic site, growth patterns, tumor-infiltrating lymphocytes, and mitotic index. Although many are independent prognostic features, the strongest predictors of outcome

Table 106-3 ■ New TNM Classification

Classification

T Classification: Use modifier a. if no ulceration or b. if ulcerated or level IV or V penetration.

T1	≤1.0 mm
T2	1.01–2.0 mm
T3	2.01–4.0 mm
T4	>4.0 mm

N Classification

N1	One lymph node	a: micrometastasis*
		b: macrometastasis†
N2	Two or three lymph nodes	a: micrometastasis*
		b: macrometastasis†
		c: in-transit metastases without metastatic lymph nodes
N3	Four or more metastatic lymph nodes, matted lymph nodes, or combinations of in-transit metastases satellite(s), or ulcerated melanoma and metastatic lymph node(s)	

M Classification

M0	No distant metastases
M1	Systemic metastases
	a. distant skin, soft tissue, or nodes
	b. pulmonary
	c. any other visceral involvement and/or elevated LDH

Mets = metastases.
*Micrometastases are diagnosed after elective or sentinel lymphadenectomy.
†Macrometastases are defined as clinically detectable lymph node metastases confirmed by therapeutic lymphadenectomy or when any lymph node metastasis exhibits gross extracapsular extension.

Table 106-4 ■ New AJCC Stage Groupings for Cutaneous Melanoma

	T	N	M
Clinical Staging*			
0	Tis	N0	M0
IA	T1a	N0	M0
IB	T1b	N0	M0
	T2a	N0	M0
IIA	T2b	N0	M0
	T3a	N0	M0
IIB	T3b	N0	M0
	T4a	N0	M0
IIC	T4b	N0	M0
IIIA	T1–4a	N1b	M0
IIIB	T1–4a	N2b	M0
IIIC	Any T	N2c	M0
	Any T	N3	M0
IV	Any T	Any N	Any M
Pathologic Staging†			
0	Tis	N0	M0
IA	T1a	N0	M0
IB	T1b	N0	M0
	T2a	N0	M0
IIA	T2b	N0	M0
	T3a	N0	M0
IIB	T3b	N0	M0
	T4a	N0	M0
IIC	T4b	N0	M0
IIIA	T1–4a	N1a	M0
IIIB	T1–4a	N1b	M0
	T1–4a	N2a	M0
	T1–4a/b	N2c	M0
IIIC	Any T	N2b	M0
	Any T	N3	M0
IV	Any T	Any N	M1

*Clinical staging includes microstaging of the primary melanoma and clinical/radiologic evaluation for metastases; by convention, it should be used after complete excision of the primary melanoma with clinical assessment for regional and distant metastases.
†Pathologic staging includes microstaging of the primary melanoma and pathologic information about the regional lymph nodes after partial or complete lymphadenectomy, except for pathologic Stage 0 or Stage 1A patients, who do not need pathologic evaluation of their lymph nodes.

were depth of invasion (thickness) and ulceration. These two features have been incorporated into the new T classification for melanoma.

Melanoma thickness is determined with the aid of an ocular micrometer. Thickness measures the total vertical height of a melanoma, from the granular layer of the skin to the area of deepest penetration. Clark's level assesses the depth of penetration into the dermal layers and subcutaneous fat (i.e., levels I to V). Though useful, particularly for thin melanomas, Clark's level is subject to more interobserver variability. Tumor thickness has therefore become the preferred microstaging technique for assessing the primary tumor. Tumor thickness is a continuous variable for which there are no apparent natural breakpoints. In the present staging criteria, simple whole-integer increments (i.e., 1.0, 2.0, 4.0 mm) have been chosen for practical reasons. However, a patient with a stage IIA, T3a melanoma that is 2.05 mm and nonulcerated has virtually the same prognosis as a patient with a stage IB, T2a melanoma that is 1.95 mm and nonulcerated, even though they are in different stage categories.

Ulceration is the second most important prognostic variable discernible from the pathologic examination of the primary tumor. Ulceration is based on the microscopic assessment of the histologic sections and is defined as the absence of an intact epidermis overlying a portion of the primary melanoma. The presence of ulceration predicts a worse prognosis, raising the risk of melanoma recurrence to that of the next thickness category (Table 106-5).

N (Nodal) Classification

Lymph node involvement in melanoma is an important prognostic feature and frequently influences therapeutic decisions. Recent analyses show that the number of lymph nodes that are involved with melanoma and whether the metastases are microscopic or macroscopic are important determinants of risk. The new AJCC staging system incorporates both of these features into nodal (N) staging. Subgroupings for one, two, or three, and four or more nodes are denoted by N1, N2, and N3, respectively, and as either Na for occult (microscopic) or Nb for palpable (macroscopic) metastases.

The advent of intraoperative lymphatic mapping for identification of the draining or "sentinel" node and selective lymphadenectomy of the sentinel node has increased the number of patients undergoing surgical lymph node assessment and has increased the proportion of patients diagnosed with microscopic regional nodal involvement. There are significant differences in prognosis for patients who have had only clinical staging of their lymph nodes compared to those with additional pathologic staging. Pathologic staging of patients who are clinically node-negative will improve their prognosis for survival by up to 10% if their nodes are free of tumor or will decrease anticipated survival by 15% to 30% if their nodes contain melanoma.

Patients with in-transit metastasis or microscopic satellites, defined as "a nest of tumor cells measuring 0.05 mm or greater, that is present in the section in which the maximum thickness measurement has been made and is distinctly separate from the main tumor mass," have been identified to have prognoses similar to patients with lymph node involvement. Therefore, both of these features have been incorporated into the N classification (N2c, see Table 106-3). Finally, ulceration of the primary melanoma has also been identified to have a negative influence on prognosis even in patients with lymph node involvement (Table 106-6). For this reason, individuals with an ulcerated primary melanoma and lymph node involvement are upstaged by one staging category.

M (Metastasis) Classification

The identification of melanoma metastasis, defined as the presence of disease beyond the regional lymph node basin(s), is a poor prognostic factor. The specific organs involved, the number of organs involved, the patient's performance status, disease-free interval, and the serum lactate dehydrogenase level have been identified to have a significant influence on median survival for this group of patients. The recent AJCC classification recognizes a better prognostic group, M1a, consisting of patients with skin, soft-tissue, and lymph node involvement who have a normal serum lactate dehydrogenase. An intermediate-risk group, M1b, is defined as having lung involvement with a normal serum lactate dehydrogenase. The highest-risk group, M1c, comprises those patients with either

Table 106-5 ▪ Impact of Ulceration on Prognosis

Depth	Ulceration	Five Year	Ten Year
≤1.0 mm	No	95	88
≤1.0 mm	Yes	91	83
1.01–2.0 mm	No	89	79
1.01–2.0 mm	Yes	77	64
2.01–4.0 mm	No	79	64
2.01–4.0 mm	Yes	63	51
>4.0 mm	No	67	54
>4.0 mm	Yes	45	

Table 106-6 ▪ Impact of Nodal Status and Ulceration of Primary on Five-Year Survival

Number of Nodes	Ulceration	Micro	Macro
1	No	70	59
1	Yes	53	29
2–3	No	63	46
2–3	Yes	50	24
≥4	No/yes	27	27

Micro-microscopic lymph node involvement; macro-clinically palpable lymph node involvement.

an elevated serum lactate dehydrogenase level or evidence of other visceral involvement. Median survival figures range from 12 months for M1a patients to four to five months for M1c patients.

Therapy

Surgery

Primary Melanoma: Wide Local Excision

The definitive local management of a biopsy-confirmed melanoma is the complete removal of the melanoma along with a margin of normal tissue, referred to as a wide local excision. The recommended margins of tissue removal have decreased over the past several decades, representing an important advance in the surgical management of melanoma. Previously, resections with 3- to 5-cm margins were advocated, necessitating a split thickness skin graft and prolonged hospitalization. Several recent trials have adequately demonstrated that narrower margins provide adequate local control and equivalent survival and allow primary surgical closure without necessitating grafting in most cases.

For example, the World Health Organization (WHO) surgical trial randomized patients with melanomas less than 2 mm in thickness to surgical margins of either 1 or 3 cm. In patients with a thickness of 1 mm or less, there were no local recurrences in either group. In patients with melanomas greater than 1 mm, however, there was a 3% incidence of local recurrence in the 1-cm-margin group compared to a 1% recurrence rate in the 3-cm-margin group. Disease-free and overall survival was similar at eight years of follow-up.

On the basis of these multiple trials, surgery with 1-cm margins for primary melanomas less than or equal to 1 mm in thickness and 2-cm margins for primary lesions that are greater than 1 mm thick is recommended. In recognition that ulceration increases as thickness increases and that both thickness and ulceration increase the risk of local recurrence, a surgical margin of at least 2 cm for any melanoma greater than 4 mm is recommended.

The margin recommendations (Table 106-7) are based on clinical assessment at the time of surgery and should be clearly described in the operative report. The pathologic margin might not correspond well with the measured margin that is obtained at the time of surgery, as tissue elasticity can result in margin shrinkage of the excised specimen by as much as one third in some instances.

Minor compromises in the excision margins that allow for a primary closure rather than a skin graft may be worthwhile, particularly in cosmetically sen-

Table 106-7 ■ Suggested Guidelines for Surgical Margins

Lesion	Surgical Margin
Dysplastic nevus	Complete excision
Melanoma in situ	5-mm margins
Melanoma ≤ 1.0 mm	1.0-cm margins
Melanoma > 1.0 mm	2.0-cm margins
Melanoma > 4.0 mm	≥2.0-cm margins

sitive areas such as the face, hands, and feet, and should be discussed with patients prior to surgery. Facial lesions might not permit the usual 1- or 2-cm margins; thus, margins are left to the judgment of the physician. Subungual melanomas and melanomas on the skin of the digits also require special consideration. Melanomas of the toe usually require an amputation at the metatarsal-phalangeal joint. Lesions on the fingers are frequently managed by amputation at the middle interphalangeal joint and proximal to the distal joint of the thumb. Lesions involving the sole of the foot are generally managed to preserve as much of the heel or ball as possible to maintain weight-bearing function. Regardless of the recommended margins, a histologically negative margin is necessary. Therefore, if after a wide local excision, a margin is found to be positive for melanoma cells or for an atypical melanocytic proliferation, further excision is warranted.

Clinically Palpable or Radiographically Enlarged Lymph Nodes

A regional lymph node dissection is the appropriate management for a patient presenting with palpable or radiographically apparent regional lymph nodes. A fine-needle aspiration of a suspicious palpable mass is often the most expeditious way to obtain an initial diagnosis and enable further treatment planning. A regional nodal dissection performed under these circumstances is referred to as a "therapeutic" regional lymph node dissection. This procedure should not be confused with either "selective" or "elective" lymph node dissections, which refer to surgical procedures performed on clinically negative regional nodal basins. Patients who present after a simple surgical excision of involved nodes should undergo a "completion" node dissection performed using the guidelines for that anatomic nodal region. A completion node dissection provides several important benefits, including the elimination of residual disease, identification of important prognostic features such as the number of nodes involved with tumor or the presence of extracapsular disease, and the identification of candidates for aggressive adjuvant treatment approaches.

Clinically Nonpalpable and/or Radiographically Normal Lymph Nodes

The role of an elective regional nodal dissection—the removal of all nodes in a clinically or radiographically negative regional nodal basin—is controversial. Retrospective surgical series and prospective randomized trials have produced conflicting results. For example, the Mayo Clinic randomized patients into three cohorts: (1) no node dissection, (2) an immediate elective node dissection at the time of the wide local excision, and (3) a delayed elective node dissection between 30 and 60 days after the wide local excision. No survival advantage was identified for groups that underwent elective node dissections. A number of other randomized studies failed to demonstrate that elective regional node dissection improved overall survival.

Despite the absence of a survival benefit, the results of subset analyses have continued to justify this procedure for some clinicians. They point out that up to 80% of patients undergoing elective regional node dissections are found to have no pathologic evidence of melanoma in their nodes. It is concezent that the large proportion of patients that receive no benefit from this procedure obscures any benefit that might accrue to the small proportion of patients with subclinical disease in their regional lymph nodes as a result of earlier detection and treatment.

The advent of preoperative and intraoperative lymph node mapping and selective sentinel lymph node biopsy has rendered this debate largely moot. The sentinel lymph node biopsy procedure has enabled the restriction of completion node dissections to patients with microscopically positive nodes, who are most likely to obtain some benefit from this procedure.

Lymphatic mapping studies have demonstrated that the lymphatics from the skin drain to a limited number of specific regional lymph nodes. Some melanoma sites have less predictable drainage patterns or drain to more than one regional nodal basin. This is particularly true of primaries found near the midline or midsection regions of the trunk or anywhere on the head and neck.

The first step in the selective lymphadenectomy procedure involves the preoperative identification of all the regional lymph node drainage basins for a given primary melanoma site through lymphoscintigraphy. Lymphoscintigraphy can also help to identify the first, or sentinel, lymph node(s) draining the region of the primary melanoma (Figure 106-2*A*). This approach involves the intradermal injection of technetium-labeled radioactive sulfur colloid around the site of a primary melanoma at the time of the wide local excision. This is often complemented by the intradermal injection of isosulfan blue dye. A surgical incision is then made over the sentinel lymph node area that is identified either by lymphoscintigraphy or by an intraoperative handheld gamma counter. Selec-

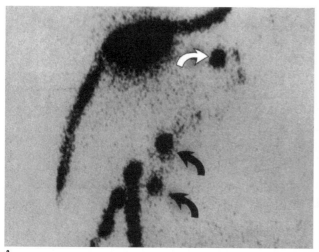
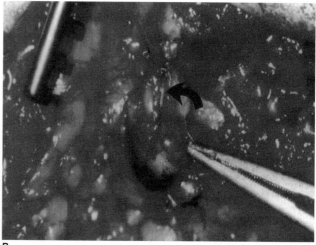

A   B

Figure 106-2 ■ Sentinel lymph node biopsy. *A,* Lymphoscintigraphy following injection around primary lesion on right shoulder (large area of activity to left of white arrow) with ^{99m}Tc-sulfur colloid shows drainage to sentinel nodes in the right axilla (black arrows) and the posterior triangle of the right neck (white arrow). Linear areas of increased activity were made by a hot marker used to outline the right arm, chest, and neck areas for orientation. *B,* Intraoperative lymphatic mapping with a vital blue dye in a patient with a right scapular melanoma. The dye was injected around the primary site. After 10 minutes, an axillary incision was made, and a blue-staining afferent lymphatic was identified (arrow) draining into a blue-staining node (the sentinel lymph node). This node contained a 5-mm focus of metastatic melanoma and was the only site of disease in the basin (original magnification × 10). (See Color Plate 20.)

tive removal of these first, or sentinel, draining nodes (Figure 106-2B) can then be performed. In the original study of this technique, Morton et al removed the sentinel node as well as all the remaining lymph nodes in the regional nodal basin. Among the 194 complete lymphadenectomy specimens from patients in whom no melanoma was detected within the sentinel lymph node, an additional 3079 lymph nodes were removed, of which only two were identified to contain melanoma, for a false-negative rate of less than 1%. This information provided confidence that this technique could successfully identify individuals who were free of involvement of their lymph nodes by melanoma and who would therefore be unlikely to benefit from completion lymph node dissections. Subsequently, the use of intradermally injected ^{99m}Tc-sulfur colloid and the use of a nuclear probe, along with the isosulfan blue dye, has enhanced the ability to identify the sentinel lymph node(s) to well over 95% and has made this technique easier and more widely applicable.

This technique requires the coordinated efforts of surgeons, nuclear medicine physicians, and pathologists. The sentinel lymph node should be subjected to a detailed pathologic examination with multiple sections examined by hematoxylin and eosin staining as well as by immunohistochemistry. Currently, most decisions regarding further surgery and/or adjuvant therapy are based on whether the sentinel lymph node is positive either on initial stain or by subsequent immunohistochemistry. Patients who are identified to have positive sentinel lymph nodes are appropriate candidates for a completion node dissection of the involved regional nodal basin or basins. Although data to support a survival advantage for such aggressive surgery are still lacking, completion node dissections identify additional nodes involved by tumor in up to 20% of patients. This additional information will affect staging and prognosis. It is also possible that performing a completion node dissection will prevent disease recurrence in the affected nodal basin and thereby improve overall survival.

The majority of patients (over 80%) have a negative sentinel node biopsy and consequently have an improvement in their prognosis and require no additional surgical management. In contrast, patients who have a positive sentinel lymph node biopsy have a substantially worse prognosis with a five-year survival rate ranging from 50% to 60%. Such patients should be managed with appropriate completion lymph node dissection and are candidates for adjuvant therapy with either interferon alpha or for participation in clinical trials of adjuvant therapy for patients with stage III disease. This combination of critical prognostic information and the identification of patients who may benefit from additional surgery followed by adjuvant therapy, obtained from a minimally invasive outpatient surgical procedure, has made the sentinel

DIAGNOSIS

Candidates for Sentinel Lymph Node Biopsy

Most centers in the United States consider individuals with a 10% or greater risk of having nodal involvement as candidates for a sentinel lymph node biopsy. This includes individuals in the following categories:

1. Patients with a melanoma >1 mm in depth
2. Patients with a melanoma ≤1 mm in depth that either is ulcerated or invades to Clark's level IV or V
3. Patients with a melanoma the depth of which cannot be accurately ascertained
4. Patients with a pigmented lesion of undefined malignant potential

The sentinel lymph node biopsy should be done prior to or concomitant with wide local excision of the primary lesion. For truncal and head/neck lesions in particular, lymphatic mapping is more likely to be inaccurate if the wide excision has already been performed. For extremity lesions, this is less of an issue, as most lesions in these locations will drain to the ipsilateral axillary or inguinal lymph node basins. In patients who have not had a prior sentinel lymph node biopsy and who develop a local or in-transit recurrence following excision of the primary, it is reasonable to perform a sentinel lymph node biopsy by injecting around the site of recurrence.

Patients with a positive sentinel lymph node biopsy should undergo a completion lymph node dissection. Their preoperative evaluation should include a thorough physical examination, complete blood count, liver chemistries, and a chest X-ray. In asymptomatic individuals with no X-ray or laboratory abnormalities, computed tomography scans of the head, chest, abdomen, and pelvis are optional but should be considered if additional positive nodes are found following full completion lymphadenectomy. Patients with a positive sentinel node, regardless of whether additional positive nodes are found following full node dissection, should receive up to one year of high-dose adjuvant IFN-α or consider treatment with an IFN-α-containing regimen on a clinical study. Local radiation therapy may be considered prior to IFN-α therapy for patients whose lymph node metastases exhibit grossly visible extracapsular extension.

Patients with a negative sentinel node should not undergo further surgical lymph node management.

lymph node biopsy an important new tool in the management of patients with melanoma.

Local Recurrence and In-Transit Metastasis

A local recurrence is defined as tumor that recurs within 5 cm of the surgical scar from a previously resected primary melanoma. The development of a local recurrence in a patient whose primary lesion was excised with inadequate surgical margins is not as ominous as a local recurrence following adequate wide excision. Although the risk of local recurrence is generally low (3.2% in one large series), certain features increase the risk, including tumor thickness greater than 4 mm (13%), ulceration (12%), microsatellites, inadequate surgical margins, and primaries located on the hands, feet, scalp, or face. A local recurrence is a frequent harbinger of distant metastasis. In one series, the 10-year survival rate was only 20%.

In-transit metastases are palpable metastases that arise in the skin or subcutaneous tissue between the primary site and the regional lymph node basin(s). In-transit metastases are presumed to be due to cells trapped in lymphatic channels. Although they are an uncommon manifestation of recurrent melanoma, they pose distinct problems. In-transit metastasis have been grouped in the current AJCC staging system as stage IIIB (N2c) because they convey a risk of death similar to that attributable to lymph node involvement.

Surgical excision is the most common approach to a local recurrence when a single lesion is present. Generally, resection with margins of 1 to 2 cm or more where technically feasible are considered appropriate. In-transit metastasis, when solitary or few in number, can be considered for surgical resection as above. Given that local recurrence and in-transit metastases are strongly associated with lymphatic disease, it may be appropriate to perform either an elective or sentinel lymph node dissection in patients with a local recurrence and no evidence of distant metastatic disease. Patients who are rendered disease-free by surgical management should be considered candidates for adjuvant interferon.

The majority of patients presenting with in-transit metastasis have multiple lesions, a situation that often makes surgical resection impractical. Individuals with extremity melanomas are appropriate candidates for isolated limb perfusion. Isolated limb perfusion requires the isolation of the arterial supply for the involved limb. This enables the perfusion of high doses of chemotherapy agents, which are then retrieved via the limb's venous system. Melphalan has been the most frequently used perfusate. It has been used alone and in combination with tumor necrosis factor (rTNF-

α) and interferon-gamma. Response rates of 90% to 100% with complete responses in 50% to 60% of patients have been reported in selected series. Limb perfusion is usually considered only in patients who have no distant metastatic disease. It can be combined with a regional lymph node dissection for patients who present with concomitant palpable regional nodal involvement. Isolated limb perfusion is occasionally considered as palliative therapy for patients who have regionally dominant disease that is painful, bleeding, or debilitating in the presence of minimal and asymptomatic distant metastases.

Adjuvant Therapy

Numerous therapies including chemotherapies such as DTIC and immunologic agents such as BCG, various vaccines, or interferon-alpha (IFN-α) have been evaluated in an attempt to improve relapse-free and overall survival for patients who have been diagnosed with high-risk primary stage IIB, IIC, and III melanoma. Only IFN-α has reproducibly shown improvement in therapeutic outcomes in large-scale Phase III trials.

High-Risk Melanoma (>4 mm Thick or Positive Nodes)

In one trial, patients with high-risk primary melanomas were randomly assigned to either observation or IFN-α (20 million IU/m² intravenously) for four weeks, then 10 million IU/m² subcutaneously three times each week for an additional 48 weeks. Interferon increased median relapse-free survival by nine months and provided a 42% improvement in the five-year relapse-free survival rate, from 26% to 37%. Median overall survival also improved by one year with a 24% improvement in the five-year overall survival rate, from 37% to 46%. The greatest benefit was seen in patients with lymph node metastases, especially those with one positive node. As a consequence of this trial, this high-dose adjuvant IFN-α regimen was approved as standard therapy for patients with high-risk melanoma.

A second IFN-α adjuvant trial attempted to confirm these results by enrolling patients of similar risk to randomly receive (1) observation, (2) high-dose IFN-α, or (3) low-dose IFN-α, administered at a dose of 3 MU subcutaneously three times per week for two years. This trial demonstrated a relapse-free survival advantage for the high-dose IFN-α arm relative to observation but no overall survival advantage. The low-dose IFN-α arm demonstrated neither a relapse-free nor an overall survival advantage relative to patients in the observation arm.

A third trial evaluating the role of high-dose IFN-α assigned patients with either T4N0 or stage III melanoma to either high-dose IFN-α or GM2-KLH-

QS-21 vaccine. This ganglioside vaccine had been shown to induce IgM and IgG antibodies in the majority of patients with melanoma and possibly to delay disease recurrence. Patients who were assigned to high-dose IFN-α therapy demonstrated both a relapse-free survival advantage and an overall-survival advantage relative to patients who received the vaccine. Two European trials of adjuvant low-dose IFN-α detected no relapse-free or survival advantage.

Although benefit for various patient subsets was inconsistent among the various trials, overall benefit was seen equally across all risk strata providing high-dose IFN-α was used. Hence, patients with sufficient risk of recurrence (greater than 30%) should be considered candidates for IFN-α therapy. Risk reduction by approximately one third can be anticipated for IFN-α use. Furthermore, high-dose IFN-α should remain the appropriate control arm for future clinical research trials for this group of patients.

Currently, many patients undergo sentinel lymph node staging. As a consequence, more patients demonstrate microscopic involvement of one or more lymph nodes at the time of initial diagnosis. These stage IIIA patients have a 40% risk of relapse over five to 10 years. Although this population was underrepresented in the adjuvant trials described previously, there is no reason to assume that these patients would benefit less well from adjuvant high-dose IFN-α administration.

The recent AJCC staging reclassification has also determined that patients with ulcerated 2- to 4-mm-thick melanomas (stage T3b, N0) have a prognosis similar to that of patients with microscopic regional node disease. Therefore, these patients, even if the sentinel lymph node is tumor free, could still be considered at sufficient risk to warrant adjuvant high-dose IFN-α treatment.

Intermediate-Risk Melanoma (1 to 4 mm and Negative Nodes)

European trials have evaluated low-dose IFN-α (3 million IU subcutaneously three times weekly) administered for either 18 or 12 months in patients with melanomas that were deeper than 1.4 or 1.5 mm, respectively, and clinically or pathologically negative nodes. A small disease-free survival advantage but no overall survival advantage was identified in both studies. At the present time, low-dose IFN-α treatment is not recommended in this intermediate-risk melanoma population.

Alternative Adjuvant Therapies

Patients with thick primary melanomas were randomized to wide local excision followed by either observation or isolated limb perfusion with melphalan and hyperthermia. Although perfusion achieved a lower incidence of local and regional recurrence, the overall and relapse-free survival rates were similar. There is no confirmed role for isolated limb perfusion in the adjuvant therapy of primary melanoma.

The role of adjuvant radiation therapy in patients with high-risk local or regional melanoma has not been clearly defined. Patients with head and neck primary melanomas, divided into three groups, were evaluated: those with intermediate-thickness melanoma (1.5 to 4.0 mm) with clinically negative lymph nodes and no regional nodal dissection, those who at presentation had clinically involved regional lymph nodes with subsequent pathological confirmation, and those who had recurrent regional nodal involvement and underwent a regional lymph node dissection. All groups received radiation therapy. Local control rates were excellent (86% to 92% at five years) compared with historical controls (40% risk of local or regional relapse). The number of involved lymph nodes or presence of extracapsular extension did not appear to influence the local control rate. At present, the decision to administer adjuvant radiation therapy to patients with either narrow margins around the primary tumor or extensive regional nodal disease (extracapsular extension, more than four nodes) should be based on individual patient issues. Surgical management of either the primary site or regional nodes remains the paramount means of control.

Metastatic Melanoma: Stage IV

Metastatic melanoma has a bleak outcome. It tends to metastasize widely (Table 106-8), and median survival is only six to nine months, with few patients (2%) surviving five years.

Table 106-8 ■ Common Distant Sites of Metastatic Melanoma

Site	Clinical Series* (%)	Autopsy Series* (%)
Skin, subcutaneous, lymph nodes	42–59	50–75
Lungs	18–36	70–87
Liver	14–20	54–77
Brain	12–20	36–54
Bone	11–17	23–49
Gastrointestinal tract	<1	26–58
Heart	<1	40–45
Pancreas	<1	38–53
Adrenals	<1	36–54
Kidneys	<1	35–48
Thyroid	<1	25–39

Adapted from Balch CM, Milton GW: Diagnosis of metastatic melanoma at distant sites. In Balch CM, Milton GW (eds): Cutaneous Melanoma: Clinical Management and Treatment Results Worldwide. Philadelphia: JB Lippincott, 1985, p 221.

Management of Patients Receiving Adjuvant High-Dose Interferon-Alpha

Successful use of high-dose adjuvant IFN-α 2b (Intron A) requires the appropriate management of toxicities to optimize the amount of interferon that can be safely delivered. There are two phases of therapy, referred to as induction and maintenance.

Dose

Induction: 20 million U/m² IV daily, Monday through Friday for 4 weeks, followed by
Maintenance: 10 million U/m² SC t.i.w. for 48 weeks

It is important to note that missed doses of interferon during the induction and maintenance period are not replaced. Patients should begin the maintenance phase of therapy on day 29 from the start of treatment. The maintenance phase begins at full dose regardless of any dose reductions that may have been required during the induction phase. Dosing is based on the actual weight and body surface area.

Treatment Monitoring

Patients need to be carefully monitored during the induction period and during the first few months of the maintenance period to minimize toxicity and make proper adjustments in dosing. The following schedule is recommended:

	Evaluation	Laboratory	Interval
Induction	History/physical	CBC/LFTs*	Weekly
Maintenance	History/physical	CBC/LFTs*	q 2 weeks†

*LFTs should include bilirubin, alkaline phosphatase, SGOT, SGPT, and lactate dehydrogenase.
†Until clinically stable (usually four to eight weeks), then every six to 12 weeks until the completion of therapy.

Dose Adjustments for Toxicity

Any toxicity that reaches grade 3 (severe) in the NCI Common Toxicity Criteria is sufficient to interrupt therapy. Because transient neutropenia is common during IFN therapy, treatment is usually not held until neutropenia reaches grade 4. Doses of IFN-α are held for a white blood cell count of <2000/μL. In addition, prolonged grade 2 toxicity of a constitutional, gastrointestinal, or neuropsychiatric nature may occur and often requires interruption of therapy. When toxicity occurs, treatment should be held. Treatment can be resumed with a 33% dose reduction once toxicity has resolved to grade 1 or less. If the same or another significant toxicity occurs, a second 33% dose reduction is permitted after the toxicity resolves. If IFN-α needs to be held a third time for toxicity, treatment is permanently dis-

continued. The following are the most common laboratory toxicities of concern:

Parameter	Value Requiring Reduction	Recommended Dose Modification
Leukocytes	<2000 cells/μL	33% after return to grade 1 or normal
Platelets	<50,000 /μL	33% after return to grade 1 or normal
SGPT/SGOT	>5 X ULN	33% after return to <2.5 X ULN
Bilirubin	>2 X ULN	33% after return to normal

ULN-upper limit of normal.

Supportive Care

A variety of constitutional side effects are seen during IFN therapy and can be reduced by simple management strategies. They include the following:

1. Acetaminophen*: 325 mg po should be administered prior to IFN and repeated in four hours to reduce or control fever.
2. Nonsteroidals* (NSAIDs): Indocin 25 to 50 mg, Motrin 400 to 800 mg, or Naprosyn 375 mg po should be administered prior to IFN and may be repeated daily to reduce fevers or chills.
3. Ranitidine*: 150 mg po twice daily should be given as long as an NSAID (above) is administered as prophylaxis against gastrointestinal irritation.
4. Prochlorperazine 10 mg po every four hours or Ondansetron 8 mg po every eight hours should be administered to patients who develop nausea, vomiting, or severe anorexia.
5. Diphenhydramine: 25 to 50 mg po or Atarax 25 mg po may be used for erythematous skin rash and/or pruritus.
6. Hydration: Adequate hydration minimizes many of the constitutional symptoms from IFN therapy. Patients should be encouraged to drink 2 liters of fluids each day. Some patients may benefit from the routine administration of IV fluids 250 to 1000 cc each day during the induction phase of treatment.
7. Celexa for depression.

Corticosteroids and immunosuppressive medications are contraindicated.

*Note: Many of these routinely administered medications may be reduced or omitted after the first few months of therapy in patients who are experiencing few acute constitutional side effects.

TREATMENT

Surgery in Metastatic Melanoma

Surgery has an important role in the management of some patients with metastatic melanoma. Surgery has been documented to provide effective disease control for patients who present with an isolated metastasis. In this subset of patients, the benefit can be long lasting. In four large series involving over 250 patients, the two-year survival ranged from 15% to 31%. Some biases in these series may exist and include selection of patients for referral, the surgeon's decision to perform surgery on selected patients, and the inclusion of some stage III patients as well as stage IV patients who received subsequent systemic therapy. Sites that are frequently considered for this approach include skin, soft tissue, distant lymph nodes, lung, brain, and gastrointestinal tract. Patients with solitary liver involvement have generally been excluded. This approach can also be important in excluding the possibility of a second primary tumor (e.g., lung cancer, central nervous system primary, or lymphoma) in a setting in which a fine-needle aspiration is not performed prior to surgical excision.

The role of adjuvant systemic therapy for patients who have been rendered disease-free by the surgical resection of isolated metastatic disease has yet to be defined. The standard of care is close observation. The small number of patients in this group and their heterogeneous sites of metastasis have been obstacles to the development of phase III trials. Because of the benefit of high-dose adjuvant interferon in patients with high-risk stage III melanoma, it is not unreasonable to discuss such therapy in this group of patients.

Surgical management may also be appropriate to provide local symptomatic control (e.g., bleeding or obstructing gastrointestinal metastasis, painful regional adenopathy, spinal cord/nerve root metastasis causing pain and/or neurologic symptoms) when there is a modest disease burden elsewhere in a patient whose projected survival warrants the intervention for a longer anticipated survival. Surgery can also be considered to render disease-free those patients who have had an excellent response to systemic therapy but who have isolated and relatively accessible residual radiologic abnormalities.

Single-Agent Therapy

Single-agent chemotherapy produces response rates in the 10% to 20% range; fewer than 5% of patients experience a complete remission. Most responses to chemotherapy are short-lived, with median response durations of three to four months.

Interleukin-2 (IL-2) and IFN-α have been the most extensively evaluated immunomodulatory drugs, with IL-2 receiving FDA approval for use in patients with stage IV melanoma in 1998. Both agents have response rates in the 10% to 20% range, although most responses to IFN-α are partial and of short duration. While low-dose IL-2 is ineffective as a single agent in melanoma, high-dose bolus IV IL-2 appears to be unique in its ability to induce durable remissions in select patients with metastatic melanoma. The high-dose bolus intravenous regimen consists of 600,000 to 720,000 IU/kg/dose administered IV every eight hours on days 1 through 5 and again on days 15 through 19, with a maximum of 28 doses per course. Patients treated with high-dose bolus IL-2 showed a response rate of 16%, including 6% complete remissions and 10% partial remissions. About 60% of the complete remission patients remained progression-free at five years, with no relapses observed after 24 months (Figure 106-3). Although responses are seen in patients with large tumor burdens and visceral metastases, patients with subcutaneous and/or cutaneous metastases are more likely to respond to IL-2 than are patients with disease at other sites. The development of vitiligo (Figure 106-4) and thyroid function test abnormalities following IL-2 therapy has been associated with response to high-dose IL-2.

High-dose bolus IL-2 is associated with significant toxicities, including hypotension requiring fluid and pressors, renal and hepatic dysfunction, cardiac arrhythmias, nausea/vomiting and diarrhea, and mental status changes. However, when administered in a closely monitored setting by physicians and nurses who are experienced with managing these side effects, high-dose IL-2 can be given safely with no long-term complications. As high-dose IL-2 is one of the few therapies that has been shown to induce durable remissions in metastatic melanoma, it should be considered as a first-line therapy in good-performance status patients with subcutaneous/cutaneous or lung metastases. The addition of IFN-α, activated peripheral blood lymphocytes (LAK cells), or autologous tumor infiltrating lymphocytes to high-dose bolus IL-2 has not been shown to be superior to IL-2 alone.

Multiagent Chemotherapy Combinations

Many drug combinations, including the "Dartmouth" regimen consisting of DTIC, cisplatin, BCNU, and tamoxifen, have been built around dacarbazine

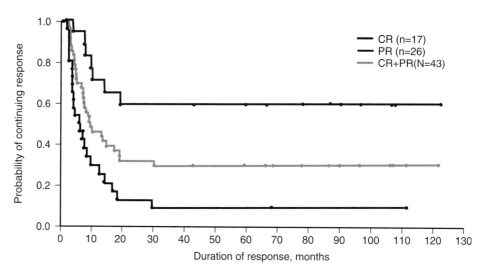

Figure 106-3 ■ Durability of responses to high-dose IL-2. Shown are progression-free survival (PFS) curves for patients with metastatic melanoma who achieved either a CR (uppermost curve) or PR (lowest curve) following treatment with high-dose bolus IV IL-2. The middle curve shows PFS for both groups (CR + PR). CR-complete response; PR-partial response.

(DTIC) and/or cisplatin. These regimens demonstrated response rates in the 20% to 50% range in single-institution studies. The response rates have been lower, however, when these regimens have been used in multi-institutional or cooperative group trials. For example, only a 15% response rate and median survival of nine months were observed for patients treated with the Dartmouth regimen in a phase II Southwest Oncology Group trial, and this regimen was found to be no better than DTIC alone in a large-scale phase III Eastern Cooperative Oncology Group Trial. The Dartmouth regimen should no longer be used in the routine therapy of patients with metastatic melanoma. Although initial reports suggested that the addition of tamoxifen improved chemotherapy results, this was not confirmed in randomized trials. Similarly, a suggested benefit from adding IFN-α to DTIC was not confirmed in a large multi-institutional Phase III trial, compared with 16% for the non-IFN-containing arms. No overall survival advantage and no improvement in time to treatment failure were attributable to the addition of IFN-α. It also became clear that high dose IFN-α in combination with chemotherapy is associated with substantial toxicity and makes the addition of other agents to that combination difficult.

IL-2-Based Biochemotherapy Regimens

Combinations of IL-2- and cisplatin-based chemotherapy (so-called biochemotherapy) have been characterized by impressive individual responses, particularly in visceral organs (Figures 106-5A and 106-5B). Meta-analyses comparing results of therapy with either IL-2 alone, IL-2 plus IFN-α, IL-2 plus chemotherapy, and IL-2 plus IFN-α and chemotherapy indicate that the IL-2, IFN-α, and chemotherapy combination produced the highest response rate (45%) and the longest median survival duration (11.4 months), and a five-year survival rate of 12%. Biochemotherapy combinations showed the greatest benefit in regimens in which the chemotherapy was given either prior to or concurrent with the IL-2.

Several trials evaluated the role of biochemotherapy relative to either chemotherapy or immunotherapy alone with mixed results. In one trial patients were randomized to either CVD (cisplatin, Velban, and DTIC) or to CVD with continuous infusion IL-2 and IFN-α administered after the chemotherapy regimen. A response rate of 48% was observed in the group receiving biochemotherapy compared with 25% for the chemotherapy-alone population. The time to treatment failure (4.9 vs. 2.4 months) and the median survival (11.9 vs. 9.2 months) also favored the biochemotherapy arm.

Other trials showed equal improvement in response rate for biochemotherapy versus chemotherapy alone or IL-2/IFN-α alone but no improvement in overall survival. Although biochemotherapy regimens

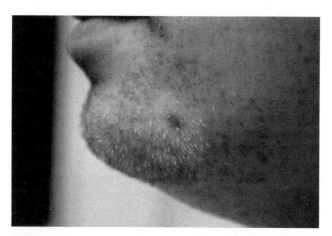

Figure 106-4 ■ Vitiligo in a melanoma patient responding to high-dose IL-2. A halo of depigmentation developed around cutaneous metastases in this patient with metastatic melanoma who exhibited tumor regression in response to high-dose bolus intravenous IL-2.

Brain Metastasis

Patients with metastatic melanoma frequently develop brain metastasis. Brain metastasis is associated with poor prognosis and a median survival of one to four months in most series. Patients with central nervous system metastasis have been excluded from many clinical trials in recent years, as most systemic therapies do not penetrate into the central nervous system.

Solitary Brain Metastasis

Patients who have solitary metastatic lesions by computed tomography scan should have this confirmed by magnetic resonance imaging if surgical intervention is planned. Solitary brain lesions can be removed surgically with good long-term benefit in many circumstances. Favorable circumstances include (1) no other systemic disease, (2) systemic disease that has responded to therapy, and (3) systemic disease of low volume that has yet to be treated. Alternatives to resection include stereotactic radiosurgical approaches, including gamma knife. Many physicians commonly recommend whole-brain radiation therapy following surgery or radiosurgery, though trials in melanoma supporting the benefit of whole-brain irradiation are limited. Stereotactic radiosurgery may also be given to the surgical bed following resection to diminish the risk of local recurrence.

Multiple Brain Metastasis

Patients more frequently present with multiple brain metastases. Historically, whole-brain irradiation has been the recommended treatment, along with corticosteroids to reduce edema and symptoms. However, major responses to whole-brain irradiation are infrequent. Patients with two or three lesions less than 1 to 2 cm in diameter may benefit from radiosurgery. This has the advantage of shorter treatment time, increased dose to the involved areas, and reduced dose to uninvolved brain parenchyma.

Therapies

Systemic therapies have generally been viewed as ineffective. Cytokine therapies have not been shown to be effective for disease in the central nervous system, and the increased vascular permeability that often ensues during cytokine therapy has been shown to cause or exacerbate cerebral edema around metastases. While chemotherapy drugs such as BCNU and CCNU can penetrate the central nervous system, they have not been shown to be effective in melanoma patients with central nervous system metastases. Temozolomide, an oral derivative of DTIC, has a response rate equivalent to that of DTIC and has the added advantage of penetrating into the central nervous system. However, in a recent phase II trial of WBXRT plus temozolomide in melanoma patients with central nervous system metastases, the response rate was <10%. A new trial is exploring the activity of thalidomide combined with temozolomide and WBXRT in central nervous system melanoma. At present, temozolomide remains a reasonable adjunct to XRT in melanoma patients with multiple central nervous system metastases and disease outside the central nervous system.

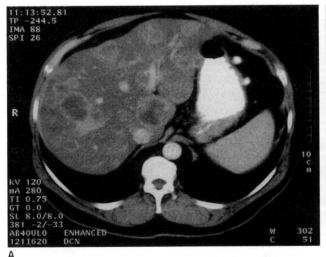 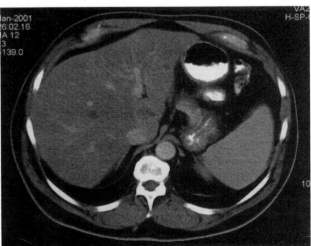

Figure 106-5 ■ Response of liver metastases to biochemotherapy. This patient with extensive liver involvement by metastatic melanoma (A) demonstrated a complete response (B) to biochemotherapy.

Table 106-9 ■ **Recommended Follow-up Schedule By Stage**

Stage	Description	Follow-up	Duration
IA	<1.0 mm without ulceration	History and physical every six months	1–2 years
		History and physical yearly	Indefinite
IB–IIC	<1.0 mm with ulceration	History and physical every 3–6 months	3 years
	>1.0 mm without ulceration	History and physical every 6–12 months	2 years
	>1.0 mm with ulceration	History and physical yearly; chest X-ray, liver tests every 6–12 months (optional)	Indefinite
III	Lymph node involvement	History and physical every six weeks to three months	3 years
	In-transit metastatis	History and physical every 4–12 months	2 years
		History and physical yearly; chest X-ray, liver tests, CBC every 3–12 months optional)	Indefinite

have been widely used, establishment of their value as a standard of care awaits the completion of a large-scale confirmatory intergroup trial.

Follow-up Evaluation

The utility of follow-up tests and examinations for detecting a recurrence of melanoma has been the subject of debate. In intermediate- to high-risk melanomas (≥1.69 mm), almost all recurrences are identified by the history and physical examination. Only 6% of recurrences are identified from chest radiographs, and none were picked up from routine laboratory evaluation. The first recurrence is in regional lymph nodes in about half of cases. Although no clear standards exist for follow-up procedures, reasonable guidelines are described below and summarized in Table 106-9.

History and Physical Examination

Since the majority of recurrences of melanoma have been discovered during an office examination, this remains a critical component of standard follow-up. In the absence of routine laboratory and radiologic testing, new symptoms in a patient's history become critical, and it is important to fully evaluate those symptoms with appropriate laboratory tests and X-rays. Symptoms suggesting possible metastasis may include new skin lesions or soft-tissue masses, headaches, facial weakness or sensory changes, new bone pain, persistent cough, dyspnea, abdominal pain, weight loss, change in bowel habits, gastrointestinal bleeding, or generalized weakness and fatigue. During the examination, special attention should be given to the primary site, lymphatic drainage pathways, and regional lymph node basins. The area around the primary site should be thoroughly examined for the detection of a local recurrence or satellite/in-transit

metastasis. In addition, it is important to perform a thorough skin examination, including evaluation of the scalp, nailbeds, palms, soles, and perineum, to detect new primary melanomas.

X-Rays and Laboratory Tests

There is no information that suggests that routine laboratory evaluations or X-rays done routinely are of value. A recent consensus from the National Comprehensive Cancer Network recommended that chest X-ray, liver function tests, and complete blood count be considered optional in the follow-up of the asymptomatic patient. Computed tomography scans and bone scans are probably unnecessary in asymptomatic individuals. However, patients who develop symptoms or display new physical findings, abnormal lactate dehydrogenase or anemia, or abnormalities on chest X-ray during their follow-up should have these thoroughly evaluated to exclude metastatic disease as the cause.

Patient Education

An important component of follow-up is the instruction of patients in self-examination. Skin self-examination should be taught, and literature with color photographs of melanomas should be provided. In addition, instruction in self-examination of regional lymph nodes is important, since it is the most frequent site of first metastasis.

References

General Information

Greelee RT, Murry T, Bolden S, Wingo PA: Cancer statistics, 2000. CA Cancer J Clin 2000;50:7–33.

NCCN Melanoma Practice Guidelines. NCCN Proceedings 1998;3(Oncology 7):153–177.

NIH Consensus conference: Diagnosis and treatment of early melanoma. JAMA 1992;268:1314.

Patel JK, Didolkar MS, Pickren JW, Moore RH: Metastatic pattern of malignant melanoma: A study of 216 autopsy cases. Am J Surg 1978;135:807.

Quinn MJ, Crotty KA, Thompson JF, et al: Desmoplastic and desmoplastic neurotropic melanoma: Experience with 280 patients. Cancer 1998;83:1128.

Weiss M, Loprinzi CL, Creagan ET, et al: Utility of follow-up tests for detecting recurrent disease in patients with malignant melanomas. JAMA 1995;274(21):1703–1705.

Adjuvant Therapy

Ang KK, Byers RM, Peters LJ, et al: Regional radiotherapy as adjuvant treatment for head and neck malignancy melanoma. Arch Otolaryngol Head Neck Surg 1990;116: 169.

Cole BF, Gelber RD, Kirkwood JM, et al: Quality-of-life adjusted survival analysis of interferon alfa-2b adjuvant treatment of high-risk resected cutaneous melanoma: An Eastern Cooperative Oncology Group Study. J Clin Oncol 1996;14:2666.

Creagan ET, Dalton RJ, Ahmann DL, et al: Randomized, surgical adjuvant clinical trial of recombinant interferon alfa-2a in selected patients with malignant melanoma. J Clin Oncol 1995;13:2776.

Grob JJ, Dreno B, de la Salmoniere P, et al: Randomised trial of interferon alpha-2a as adjuvant therapy in resected primary melanoma thicker than 1.5 mm without clinically detectable node metastases: French Cooperative Group on Melanoma. Lancet 1998;351:1905.

Hillner BE, Kirkwood JM, Atkins MB, et al: Economic analysis of adjuvant interferon alfa-2b in high-risk melanoma based on projections from Eastern Cooperative Oncology Group 1684. J Clin Oncol 1997;15: 2351.

Kirkwood JM, Ibrahim JG, Sondak VK, et al: High and low dose interferon alfa-2b in high risk melanoma: First analysis of Intergroup Trial E1690/S9111/C9190. J Clin Oncol 2000;18:2444–2458.

Kirkwood JM, Ibrahim JG, Sosman JA, et al: High-dose interferon alfa-2b significantly prolongs relapse-free and overall survival compared with the GM2-KLH/QS-21 vaccine in patients with resected stage IIB-III melanoma: Results of Intergroup Trial E1694/S9512/C509801. J Clin Oncol 2001;19:2370–2380.

Kirkwood JM, Strawderman MH, Ernstoff MS, et al: Interferon alpha-2b adjuvant therapy of high risk resected cutaneous melanoma: The Eastern Cooperative Oncology Group trial EST-1684. J Clin Oncol 1996;14:7–17.

Livingston PO, Wong GYC, Adluri S: A randomized trial of adjuvant vaccination with BCG versus BCG plus the melanoma ganglioside GM2 in patients with AJCC stage III melanoma. J Clin Oncol 1994;12:1036.

Pehamberger H, Soyer HP, Steiner A, et al: Adjuvant interferon alfa-2a treatment in resected primary stage II cutaneous melanoma: Austrian Malignant Melanoma Cooperative Group. J Clin Oncol 1998;16:1425.

Sondak VK, Wolfe JA: Adjuvant therapy for melanoma. Curr Opin Oncol 1997;9:189–204.

Chemotherapy

Chapman PB, Einhorn LH, Meyers ML, et al: Phase III multi-center randomized trial of the Dartmouth regimen versus dacarbazine in patients with metastatic melanoma. J Clin Oncol 1999;17:2745– 2751.

Cocconi G, Bella M, Calabresi F, et al: Treatment of metastatic melanoma with dacarbazine plus tamoxifen. N Engl J Med 1992;327(8):516–523.

DelPrete SA, Maurer LH, O'Donnel J, et al: Combination chemotherapy with cisplatin, carmustine, dacarbazine, and tamoxifen in metastatic melanoma. Cancer Treat Rep 1984;68:1403–1405.

Falkson CI, Falkson G, Falkson HC: Improved results with the addition of interferon alfa-2a to dacarbazine in the treatment of patients with malignant melanoma. J Clin Oncol 1991;9:1403.

Falkson CI, Ibrahim J, Kirkwood JM, et al: Phase III trial of dacarbazine versus dacarbazine with interferon α-2b versus dacarbazine with tamoxifen versus dacarbazine with interferon α-2b and tamoxifen in patients with metastatic melanoma: An Eastern Cooperative Oncology Group study. J Clin Oncol 1998;16:1743–1751.

Legha SS, Ring S, Eton O, et al: Development and results of biochemotherapy in metastatic melanoma: The University of Texas M.D. Anderson Cancer Center experience. Cancer J Sci Am 1997;3(Suppl 1):S9–S15.

Legha SS, Ring S, Eton O, et al: Development of a biochemotherapy regimen with concurrent administration of cisplatin, vinblastine, dacarbazine, interferon alfa, and interleukin-2 for patients with metastatic melanoma. J Clin Oncol 1998;16:1752–1759.

McClay EF, Mastrangelo MJ, Sprandio JD, et al: The importance of tamoxifen to a cisplatin-containing regimen in the treatment of metastatic melanoma. Cancer 1989;63: 1292.

Richards JM, Ramming K, Bitran JD, et al: Combination of chemotherapy and biologic therapy for the treatment of melanoma. Clin Res 1990;38:844A.

Rosenberg SA, Yang JC, Schwartzentruber DJ, et al: Prospective randomized trial of the treatment of patients with metastatic melanoma using chemotherapy with cisplatin, dacarbazine, and tamoxifen alone or in a combination with interleukin-2 and interferon alfa-2b. J Clin Oncol 1999;17:968.

Epidemiology

After treatment of early melanoma, should patients and family members be followed? Why and how? NIH Consent Statement 1992;10:1–26.

Clark WH Jr, From L, Bermardino EA, et al: The histogenesis and biologic behavior of primary human malignant melanomas of the skin. Cancer Res 1969;29:705–727.

Clark WH, Reimer RR, Greene M, et al. Origin of familial malignant melanomas from heritable melanocytic lesions: The B-K mole syndrome. Arch Dermatol 1978;114:732.

Elder DE, Goldman LI, Goldman SC, et al: Dysplastic nevus syndrome: A phenotypic association of sporadic cutaneous melanoma. Cancer 1980;46:1787.

Friedman RJ, Rigel DS, Kopf AW: Early detection of malignant melanoma: the role of physician examination and self-examination of the skin. CA Cancer J Clin 1985;35: 130.

Greene MH: The genetics of hereditary melanoma and nevi: 1998 update. Cancer 1999;86:1644.

Greene MH, Clark WH Jr, Tucker MA, et al: High risk of malignant melanoma in melanoma-prone families with dysplastic nevi. Ann Intern Med 1985;102:458.

Holman CD, Armstrong BK, Heenan PJ: Relationship of cutaneous malignant melanoma to individual sunlight-exposure habits. J Natl Cancer Inst 1986;76:403.

Koh HK: Cutaneous melanoma. N Engl J Med 1991;325: 171.

Koh HK, Miller DR, Geller AC, et al: Who discovers melanoma? Patterns from a population-based survey. J Am Acad Dermatol 1992;26:914.

Koh HK, Norton LA, Geller AC, et al: Evaluation of the American Academy of Dermatology's National Skin Cancer Early Detection and Screening Program. J Am Acad Dermatol 1996;34:971.

Rigel DA, Friedman R, Kopf A, et al: Importance of complete skin exam for the detection of malignant melanoma. J Am Acad Dermatol 1986;14:857.

Immunotherapy

Allen I, Kupelnick B, Kumashiro M: Efficacy of interleukin-2 in the treatment of metastatic melanoma: Systemic review and metastasis-analysis. Cancer Therapeutics 1998; 1:168–173.

Atkins MB, Lotze MT, Dutcher JP, et al: High-dose recombinant interleukin 2 therapy for patients with metastatic melanoma: Analysis of 270 patients treated between 1985 and 1993. J Clin Oncol 1999;17:2105–2116.

Berd D, Maguire HC Jr, Mastrangelo MJ: Treatment of human melanoma with a hapten-modified antologous vaccine. Ann NY Acad Sci 1993;690:147.

Berd D, Maguire HC Jr, McCue P, Mastrangelo MJ: Treatment of metastatic melanoma with an autologous tumor cell vaccine: Clinical and immunologic results in 64 patients. J Clin Oncol 1990;8:1858.

Bystryn JC, Oratz R, Harris MN, et al: Immunogenicity of a polyvalent melanoma antigen vaccine in humans. Cancer 1988;61:1065.

DiFronzo LA, Morton DL: Melanoma vaccines: Current status of clinical trials. Adv Oncol 2000;16:16–29.

Hersey P: Evaluation of vaccinia viral lysates as therapeutic vaccines in the treatment of melanoma. Ann NY Acad Sci 1993;690:167.

Hersey P, Edwards A, Coates A, et al: Evidence that treatment with vaccinia melanoma cell lysates (VMCL) may improve survival of patients with stage II melanoma. Cancer Immunol Immunother 1987;25:257.

Keilholz U, Conradt C, Legha SS, et al: Results of interleukin-2-based treatment in advanced melanoma: A case record-based analysis of 631 patients. J Clin Oncol 1998;16:2921–2929.

Legha SS, Gianan MA, Plager C, et al: Evaluation of interleukin-2 administered by continuous infusion in patients with metastatic melanoma. Cancer 1996;77:89.

Mitchell MS: Perspective on allogeneic melanoma lysates in active specific immunotherapy. Semin Oncol 1998;25:623–635.

Morton DL, Foshag LJ, Hoon DS, et al: Prolongation of survival in melanoma after active specific immunotherapy with a new polyvalent melanoma vaccine. Ann Surg 1992;16: 463–482.

Musselman DL, Lawson DH, Gumnick JF, et al: Paroxetine for the prevention of depression induced by high-dose interferon alfa. New Engl J Med 2001;344:961–966.

Restifo NP, Rosenberg SA: Developing recombinant and synthetic vaccines for the treatment of melanoma. Curr Opin Oncol 1999;11:50.

Rosenberg SA, Lotze MT, Muul LM, et al: Special report: observations on the systemic administration of autologous lymphokine-activated killer cells and recombinant interleukin-2 to patients with metastatic cancer. N Engl J Med 1985;313:1485.

Rosenberg SA, Yang JC, Schwartzentruber DJ, et al: Immunologic and therapeutic evaluation of a synthetic peptide vaccine for the treatment of patients with metastatic melanoma. Nat Med 1998;4:321.

Rosenberg SA, Yang JC, Topalian SL: The treatment of 283 consecutive patients with metastatic melanoma or renal cell cancer using high-dose bolus interleukin-2. JAMA 1994;271:945.

Rosenberg SA, Yang JC, Topalian SL, et al: Treatment of 283 consecutive patients with metastatic melanoma or renal cell cancer using high-dose bolus interleukin-2. JAMA 1994;271:907–913.

Sparano JA, Fisher RI, Sunderland M: Randomized phase III trial of treatment with high-dose interleukin-2 either alone or in combination with interferon-alfa-2a in patients with advanced melanoma. J Clin Oncol 1993;11: 1969.

Wallack MK, Sivanandham M, Balch CM, et al: A phase II randomized, double-blind, multi-institutional trial of vaccinia melanoma oncolysate-active specific immunotherapy for patients with stage II melanoma. Cancer 1995;75: 34.

Limb Perfusion

Alexander HR Jr, Fraker DL, Bartlett DL: Isolated limb perfusion for malignant melanoma. Semin Surg Oncol 1996;12:416.

Fraker DL, Alexander HR, Andrich M, Rosenberg S: Treatment of extremity melanoma with hyperthermic isolated limb perfusion with melphalan, tumor necrosis factor and interferon-gamma: Results of TNF dose escalation study. J Clin Oncol 1996;14:479.

Koops HS, Vaglini M, Suciu S, et al: Prophylactic isolated limb perfusion for localized, high-risk limb melanoma: Results of a multicenter randomized phase III trial. J Clin Oncol 1998;16:2906–2912.

Prognosis

Amer MH, Al-Sarraf M, Vaitkevicius VK: Clinical presentation, natural history and prognostic factors in advanced melanoma. Surg Gynecol Obstet 1979;149:687.

Balch CM, Buzaid AC, Alkins MB, et al: A new AJCC staging system for cutaneous melanoma. Cancer 2000;88:1484–1491.

Balch CM, Wilkerson JA, Murad TM, et al: The prognostic significance of ulceration of cutaneous melanoma. Cancer 1980;45:3012.

Breslow A: Thickness cross-sectional areas and depth of invasion in the prognosis of cutaneous melanoma. Ann Surg 1970;172:902.

Chang AE, Karnell LH, Menck HR: The National Cancer Data Base report on cutaneous and noncutaneous melanoma: A summary of 84,836 cases from the past decade. The American College of Surgeons Commission on Cancer and the American Cancer Society. Cancer 1988;83:1664.

Curry BJ, Myers K, Hersey P: Polymerase chain reaction detection of melanoma cells in the circulation: Relation to clinical stage, surgical treatment, and recurrence from melanoma. J Clin Oncol 1998;16:1760.

Gershenwald JE, Colome MI, Lee JE, et al: Patterns of recurrence following a negative sentinel lymph node biopsy in 243 patients with stage I or II melanoma. J Clin Oncol 1998;16:2253.

Gershenwald JE, Thompson W, Mansfield PF, et al: Multi-institutional melanoma lymphatic mapping experience: The prognostic value of sentinel lymph node status in 612 stage I or II melanoma patients. J Clin Oncol 1999;17:976.

MacKie RM: Pregnancy and exogenous hormones in patients with cutaneous malignant melanoma. Curr Opin Oncol 1999;11:129.

MacKie RM, Bufalino R, Morabito A, et al: Lack of effect of pregnancy on outcome of melanoma: For The World Health Organisation Melanoma Programme. Lancet 1991;337:653.

Sutherland CM, Chmiel JS, Bieligk S, et al: Patient characteristics, treatment, and outcome of unknown primary melanoma in the United States for the years 1981 and 1987. Am Surg 1996;62:400.

Radiation Therapy

Ang KK, Peters LJ, Weber RS, et al: Postoperative radiotherapy for cutaneous melanoma of the head and neck region. Int J Radiat Oncol Biol Phys 1994;30:795.

Hagen NA, Cirrincione C, Thaler HT, DeAngelis LM: The role of radiation therapy following resection of single brain metastasis from melanoma. Neurology 1990;40:158.

Kondziolka D, Patel A, Lunsford LD, et al: Stereotactic radiosurgery plus whole brain radiotherapy versus radiotherapy alone for patients with multiple brain metastases. Int J Radiat Oncol Biol Phys 1999;45:427.

Seegenschmiedt MH, Keilholz L, Altendorf-Hofmann A, et al: Palliative radiotherapy for recurrent and metastatic malignant melanoma: Prognostic factors for tumor response and long-term outcome: A 20-year experience. Int J Radiat Oncol Biol Phys 1999;44:607.

Vlock DR, Kirkwood JM, Leutzinger C, et al: High-dose fraction radiation therapy for intracranial metastases of malignant melanoma: A comparison with low-dose fraction therapy. Cancer 1982;49:2289.

Surgery

Alex JC, Weaver DL, Fairbank JT, et al: Gamma-probe-guided lymph node localization in malignant melanoma. Surg Oncol 1993;2:303.

Balch CM, Soong SJ, Bartolucci AA, et al: Efficacy of an elective regional lymph node dissection of 1 to 4 mm thick melanomas for patients 60 years of age and younger. Ann Surg 1996;224:255–266.

Balch CM, Urist MM, Karakousis CP, et al: Efficacy of 2-cm surgical margins for intermediate-thickness melanomas (1 to 4 mm): Results of a multi-institutional randomized surgical trial. Ann Surg 1993;218(3):262–269.

Cascinelli N, Morabito A, Santinami M, et al: Immediate or delayed dissection of regional nodes in patients with melanoma of the trunk: A randomized trial. Lancet 1998;351:793–796.

Karakousis CP: Therapeutic node dissections in malignant melanoma. Semin Surg Oncol 1998;14:291.

Morton DL, Thompson JF, Essner R, et al: Validation of the accuracy of intraoperative lymphatic mapping and sentinel lymphadenectomy for early-stage melanoma. Ann Surg 1999;230:453.

Morton DL, Wen DR, Wong JH, et al: Technical details of intraoperative lymphatic mapping for early stage melanoma. Arch Surg 1992;27:392.

Reintgen D: Lymphatic mapping and sentinel node harvest for malignant melanoma. J Surg Oncol 1997;66:277.

Sherry RM, Pass HI, Rosenberg SA, Yang JC: Surgical resection of metastatic renal cell carcinoma and melanoma after response to interleukin-2-based immunotherapy. Cancer 1992;69:1850.

Sim FH, Taylor WF, Pritchard DJ, Soule EH: Lymphadenectomy in the management of stage I malignant melanoma: A prospective randomized study. Mayo Clin Proc 1986;61:697.

Veronesi U, Adams J, Bandiera DC, et al: Delayed regional lymph node dissection in stage I melanoma of the skin of the lower extremities. Cancer 1982;49:2420.

Veronesi U, Cascinelli N: Narrow excision (1-cm margin): A safe procedure for thin cutaneous melanoma. Arch Surg 1991;126:438-441.

Veronesi U, Cascinelli N, Adamus J, et al: Thin stage 1 primary cutaneous malignant melanoma: Comparison of excision with margins of 1 or 3 cm. N Engl J Med 1988;318:1159–1162. (Published erratum appears in N Engl J Med 1991;25:325–(4):292.)

Chapter 107
Nonmelanoma Skin Cancer

Reed E. Drews and Lara Kelley

Nonmelanoma skin cancers occur nearly as frequently as all other cancers combined, affecting an estimated 900,000 to 1.2 million Americans each year. Since nonmelanoma skin cancers are not generally reported to central tumor registries, accurate incidence rates are difficult to assess. However, trends indicate that these numbers are rising, largely owing to changes in sun exposure patterns over the past several decades.

Basal cell carcinoma and squamous cell carcinoma are the two most common forms of nonmelanoma skin cancer. Like melanoma, they are sun-related. Other, less common nonmelanoma skin cancers are listed in Table 107-1. With the possible exception of Merkel cell carcinoma, most of these other non–melanoma skin cancers are not sun-related. Basal cell carcinomas arise from basal cells in the epidermis, while squamous cell carcinomas arise from epidermal keratinocytes. Merkel cell carcinomas arise from neuroendocrine cells of the skin. Malignant tumors can also arise from the skin appendages (e.g., apocrine glands, eccrine glands, and sebaceous glands). The histology is typically that of an adenocarcinoma, making differentiation from a metastatic adenocarcinoma difficult. Various lymphomas can involve the skin, either primarily without evidence of systemic lymphoma or secondarily from systemic disease. Sarcomas can also arise entirely within skin. In addition to Kaposi's sarcoma, examples of skin sarcomas include dermatofibrosarcoma protuberans, leiomyosarcoma, angiosarcoma, and malignant fibrous histiocytoma.

Epidemiology

Incidence rates for basal cell carcinoma and squamous cell carcinoma rise even more sharply by age than that for melanoma. Although numbers vary by latitude, overall basal cell carcinoma incidence rates outnumber those for squamous cell carcinoma by 4:1. Males have a larger proportion of lesions than females. Chronic sun exposure is the most significant risk factor for developing basal cell carcinoma and squamous cell carcinoma, in contrast to most cases of melanoma, in which intermittent sun exposure appears to be important. Accordingly, the majority of basal cell carcinomas and squamous cell carcinomas arise on chronically sun-exposed skin sites (e.g., head, neck, hands, and forearms). These observations pertain primarily to fair-skinned individuals who have a tendency to burn rather than tan. In individuals with more intensely colored skin (e.g., blacks, Asians, and Hispanics), age-adjusted incidences of skin cancers are only 1% of that seen in whites.

Incidence rates for Merkel cell carcinoma are substantially less than those for basal cell carcinoma and squamous cell carcinoma. While Merkel cell carcinoma may develop in patients of all ages, the majority of Merkel cell carcinomas arise in the sixth or seventh decade of life. As with basal cell carcinoma and squamous cell carcinoma, sun exposure likely plays a role in pathogenesis. Hence, the majority of lesions are found on sun-exposed skin sites.

Pathogenesis

A role for ultraviolet light in the development of basal cell carcinomas and squamous cell carcinomas is well recognized. In addition to causing mutations in cellular DNA, ultraviolet light has profound suppressive effects on the cutaneous immune system. Genetic alterations induced by ultraviolet light lead to unchecked cell growth and impaired programmed cell death pathways. In addition, ultraviolet light suppresses the cutaneous immune system, preventing tumor rejection. In patients receiving long-term psoralen and ultraviolet light therapy, the incidence of squamous cell carcinoma in particular is significantly increased. Exposure to ionizing radiation is also associated with an increased risk of nonmelanoma skin cancer. For example, uranium miners and individuals treated with X-rays in childhood for tinea capitis or for thymic enlargement have increased incident rates of nonmelanoma skin cancer. With therapeutic radia-

Table 107-1 ■ Nonmelanoma Skin Cancers

Basal cell carcinoma
Squamous cell carcinoma
Merkel cell carcinoma
Microcystic adnexal carcinoma
Sebaceous carcinoma
Atypical fibroxanthoma
Malignant fibrous histiocytoma
Dermatofibrosarcoma protuberans
Angiosarcoma
Kaposi's sarcoma
Extramammary Paget's disease
Primary mucinous carcinoma
Primary cutaneous lymphomas

tion, basal cell carcinomas are the most commonly encountered secondary malignancy. Other risk factors for nonmelanoma skin cancer are exposure to chimney soot in chimney sweeps, burn scars, chronic wounds, chronic inflammatory disorders, and arsenic ingestion.

Tumor suppressor gene inactivation and oncogene activation have been implicated in nonmelanoma skin cancer pathogenesis. For example, mutations in the tumor-suppressor patched (PTCH) gene system are present in the vast majority of basal cell carcinomas, while almost all tumors without PTCH mutations have activating mutations in the PTCH partner, smoothened (SMO). Additionally, a large proportion of basal cell carcinomas and the vast majority of squamous cell carcinomas harbor mutations in the tumor suppressor p53. In squamous cell carcinoma, mutations in p53 appear to be an early event, since p53 mutations have been detected in actinic keratoses (precursors to squamous cell carcinoma) as well as normal skin from sun-exposed sites in patients with skin cancer. Oncogenes that have been found to be mutated in nonmelanoma skin cancers include *ras* and *fos*. However, specific roles for these mutations in relation to those involving SMO and the tumor suppressors PTCH and p53 are less clear.

Inherited genetic syndromes also predispose affected individuals to nonmelanoma skin cancer formation. For example, nonmelanoma skin cancers commonly arise in patients with albinism, in which skin pigment is absent, and in patients with xeroderma pigmentosum, in which DNA repair of ultraviolet-light-induced DNA damage is defective. Another genetic syndrome causing nonmelanoma skin cancer is basal cell nevus syndrome. Basal cell nevus syndrome is caused by mutations in the PTCH gene and is characterized clinically by numerous basal cell carcinomas, pits of the palms and soles, and cysts of the jaw.

Rates of nonmelanoma skin cancer development are also markedly increased in immunosuppressed patients, particularly patients on immunosuppression following organ transplantation. Squamous cell carcinoma is 65 times as likely to develop in transplant recipients as in age-matched control subjects. These carcinomas usually take two to four years to arise and increase over time. In posttransplant immunosuppressed patients, the incidence ratio of squamous cell carcinoma to basal cell carcinoma is reversed, in contrast to patients infected with human immunodeficiency virus (HIV) who, like immunocompetent individuals, have an incidence rate of basal cell carcinoma exceeding that of squamous cell carcinomas.

While the pathogenesis of Merkel cell carcinoma is not completely characterized, indirect evidence suggests that ultraviolet light exposure likely plays a role. For example, the majority of Merkel cell carcinoma lesions are found on sun-exposed areas. Mixed Merkel cell carcinoma/squamous cell carcinoma and Merkel cell carcinoma/basal cell carcinoma lesions have been reported, suggesting a shared pathogenetic origin. Further, the incidence of Merkel cell carcinoma in patients treated with ultraviolet light is about 100 times higher than that expected in the general population. Additional potential contributors to Merkel cell carcinoma development include immunosuppression and arsenic-induced Bowen's disease.

Basal Cell Carcinoma

Clinical Presentation

Basal cell carcinoma, the most common of the nonmelanoma skin cancers, derives its name from its origin in the basal cell layer of the epidermis. Some differentiation toward squamous epithelium can occur. However, most basal cell carcinomas retain a histologic resemblance to basal cells. There are three major types of basal cell carcinoma, with varying treatment and prognostic implications: nodular basal cell carcinoma, sclerosing basal cell carcinoma, and superficial basal cell carcinoma.

Nodular basal cell carcinoma is the most common form, occurring predominantly on the head and neck. Typically, it presents as a well-circumscribed nodule with translucent and pearly appearance and telangiectasias that is best appreciated with a magnifying lens. Friability and bleeding may occur with minor trauma. In large tumors that outgrow vascular blood supply, central ulceration and necrosis may occur, leaving a raised rim of tumor. Histologically, tumor cells can extend from the dermal-epidermal junction into the deep dermis and subcutaneous fat. However, the collections of cells tend to be well defined and circumscribed, and the cells are almost always round and well differentiated.

Pigmented basal cell carcinoma is a variant of nodular basal cell carcinoma that has importance because its appearance may lead to confusion with nodular melanoma.

Sclerosing basal cell carcinoma, also known as morpheaform basal cell carcinoma, has a higher rate of recurrence than other basal cell carcinoma forms owing to its aggressive growth characteristics and subclinical histologic spread. It presents as a whitish firm plaque with fibrosis or sclerosis by palpation and indistinct margins by inspection. Histologically, small collections of tumor and spindle-shaped cells infiltrate the dermis, resulting in the use of terms such as "micronodular basal cell carcinoma" and "infiltrative basal cell carcinoma." Sclerosing basal cell carcinoma is the most likely subtype of basal cell carcinoma to be incompletely removed by conventional excision.

Superficial basal cell carcinoma occurs most commonly on the back. It presents as a patch of erythema and scaling, which may be confused with dermatitis. However, close inspection reveals a threadlike rim of border that demarcates tumor from surrounding skin. Histologically, numerous small nodular collections of tumor cells appear to bud from the basal layer of the epidermis, giving rise to the term "multifocal superficial basal cell carcinoma."

Presentations of nonmelanoma skin cancer differ in individuals with more intensely colored skin. For example, basal cell carcinomas, which are usually nonpigmented in whites, are almost always pigmented in black, Hispanic, and Asian patients.

Metastasis in basal cell carcinoma is rare and is suspected only in very large ulcerating tumors (Figure 107-1). Lung, lymph nodes, esophagus, oral cavity, and skin are reported sites of metastasis.

Clinical Evaluation

While basal cell carcinoma is often suspected by clinical exam alone, diagnosis usually requires histologic confirmation (see Figure 107-1). Punch biopsies are preferred over shave biopsies, providing more accurate pathologic results, since shave biopsies can miss important histologic features in deeper dermal components. By identifying the depth of involvement, the histologic type of basal cell carcinoma, and the presence of "aggressive" histologic features, biopsies help to direct treatment. All patients should have complete skin examination to exclude other skin lesions requiring biopsy.

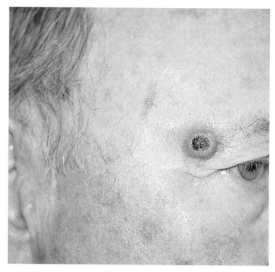

Figure 107-1 ■ Basal cell carcinoma that has become an ulcerating tumor. (From Callen JP, Paller AS, Greer KE, Swinyer LJ: Color Atlas of Dermatology, 2nd ed. Philadelphia: WB Saunders, 2000.) (See Color Plate 20.)

Staging, Prognostic Features, and Outcomes

Staging for nonmelanoma skin cancers is summarized in Table 107-2. Factors defining low-risk versus high-risk basal cell carcinoma are listed in Table 107-3. Patients with depressed cellular immunity secondary to human immunodeficiency virus (HIV) infection show a higher frequency of infiltrative basal cell carcinoma. Although perineural involvement also predicts for a higher likelihood of recurrence, this is a feature that is more likely to be seen in squamous cell carcinoma than in basal cell carcinoma.

Basal cell carcinoma has a tendency to grow along paths of least resistance. Embryonic fusion planes represent sites of little resistance for tumor migration. Migration of invasive basal cell carcinoma can occur along perichondrium, periosteum, fascia, and tarsal plate. This feature of basal cell carcinoma accounts for higher recurrence rates in tumors involving eyelid, nose, scalp, inner canthus, philtrum, middle to lower chin, nasolabial groove, preauricular area, and retroauricular sulcus.

Depending on the treatment modality and factors influencing risk of recurrence, cure rates for localized basal cell carcinoma are high, ranging between 90% and 99%. Although survival with metastatic basal cell carcinoma may be long, prognosis is generally poor, with median overall survival of only eight to 10 months.

Treatment

Surgery

The most widely used treatment for basal cell carcinoma is surgical excision with primary closure and

Table 107-2 ■ Staging for Nonmelanoma Skin Cancer

Primary Tumor (T)

TX	Primary tumor cannot be assessed
Tis	No evidence of primary tumor
T1	Carcinoma in situ
T2	Tumor 2 cm or less in greatest dimension
T3	Tumor more than 2 cm but no more than 5 cm in greatest dimension
T4	Tumor invades deep extradermal structures, e.g., cartilage, skeletal muscle, or bone
	Note: In the case of multiple simultaneous tumors, the tumor with the highest T category is classified and the number of separate tumors is indicated in parentheses, e.g., T2 (5).

Regional Lymph Nodes (N)

NX	Regional lymph nodes cannot be assessed
N0	No regional lymph node metastasis
N1	Regional lymph node metastasis

Distant Metastasis (M)

MX	Distant metastasis cannot be assessed
M0	No distant metastasis
M1	Distant metastasis

Stage Grouping

Stage 0	Tis	N0	M0
Stage I	T1	N0	M0
Stage II	T2	N0	M0
	T3	N0	M0
Stage III	T4	N0	M0
	Any T	N1	M0
Stage IV	Any T	Any N	M1

Adapted with permission from Fleming ID, Cooper JS, Henson DE, et al (eds): AJCC Cancer Staging Manual, 5th ed. Philadelphia: Lippincott-Raven, 1997.

postoperative margin assessment (Figure 107-2). With suitable margins (at least 4 mm), this approach is generally curative for subtypes of basal cell carcinoma that are at low risk for recurrence, such as nodular and superficial basal cell carcinoma. Postoperative margin assessment is typically done by a "breadloaf" technique that examines only a small fraction of the actual tumor margin. For basal cell carcinoma subtypes with more aggressive growth patterns (i.e., sclerosing basal cell carcinoma) or other characteristics predicting high risk for recurrence (see Table 107-3), Mohs surgery (excision with complete circumferential peripheral and deep-margin intraoperative frozen section assessment) is preferable, since it examines 100% of the peripheral margin. If surgical excision with postoperative margin assessment is performed on high-risk lesions, wider margins (at least 10 mm) should be

obtained. Tumors with positive margins after conventional excision should be referred for Mohs surgery or radiation therapy. Occasionally, basal cell carcinoma will appear to have been removed completely by biopsy alone. Mohs surgery, however, following biopsy in such cases frequently will reveal residual cancer. This finding appears to be unrelated to age, site of lesion, histologic subtype, or extent of surrounding inflammation. Thus, small basal cell carcinomas that appear to have been completely removed by initial biopsy may be at risk for recurrence if not treated further.

Curettage followed by electrodesiccation is a treatment option for low-risk tumors involving non-hair-bearing areas. However, if subcutaneous fat is reached during the curettaging, surgical excision must be performed.

Radiation Therapy

Primary superficial radiation therapy is an option in cases in which surgical access is difficult or there is a contraindication to surgery. With radiation therapy alone, long-term cure rates are high (nearly identical to those with surgical excision), and cosmetic outcomes are good to excellent. In contrast, radiation therapy for recurrent basal cell carcinoma yields poor outcomes, with control rates of only 56% at five years for such lesions compared with 95% control rates for primary basal cell carcinoma treated by radiation therapy. Adjuvant radiation therapy plays a role in the management of high-risk lesions, particularly lesions with extensive perineural involvement. In tumors less than 20 mm in size, radiation field margins should be 5 to 10 mm, and a total of 4500 to 5400 cGy should be administered in 250- to 300-cGy fractions. In tumors equal to or greater than 20 mm in size, radiation field margins should be 15 to 20 mm, and a total of at least 6600 cGy should be administered in fractions of 200 cGy. The risk of induction of secondary cancers, although rare, should be discussed with the patient, especially a young patient.

Chemotherapy

Intralesional injection of 5-fluorouracil or interferon-alpha may yield beneficial effects in select cases, with complete resolution of tumor on follow-up pathologic evaluation. Imiquimod is another chemotherapeutic agent that has been shown to be very effective for superficial basal cell carcinomas. It clears the tumors by local induction of cytokines, including interferon-alpha.

Follow-up Evaluation

The likelihood of basal cell carcinoma recurrence, as determined by prognostic features summarized in

Table 107-3 ▪ National Comprehensive Cancer Network Guidelines: Risk Factors for Recurrence of Basal Cell Carcinoma and Squamous Cell Carcinoma

Clinical Risk Factors in Both Basal Cell Carcinoma and Squamous Cell Carcinoma	Low Risk	High Risk
Location/size*	Area L < 20 mm	Area L ≥ 20 mm
	Area M < 10 mm	Area M ≥ 10 mm
	Area H < 6 mm	Area H ≥ 6 mm
Borders	Well defined	Poorly defined
Primary versus recurrent	Primary	Recurrent
Immunosuppression	Negative	Positive
Tumor at site of prior radiotherapy	Negative	Positive
Clinical Risk Factors in Squamous Cell Carcinoma Only		
Tumor at site of chronic inflammatory process	Negative	Positive
Rapidly growing tumor	Negative	Positive
Neurologic symptoms: pain, paresthesia, paralysis	Negative	Positive
Pathology in Basal Cell Carcinoma		
Subtype	Nodular, superficial	Aggressive growth pattern†
Perineural involvement	Negative	Positive
Pathology in Squamous Cell Carcinoma		
Degree of differentiation	Well differentiated	Moderately or poorly differentiated
Adenoid (acantholytic), adenosquamous (showing mucin production) or desmoplastic subtypes	Negative	Positive
Depth: Clark level or thickness‡	I, II, III, or < 4 mm	IV, V, or ≥4 mm
Perineural or vascular involvement	Negative	Positive

Area H = high risk for recurrence: mask areas of face (central face, eyelids, eyebrows, periorbital, nose, lips (cutaneous and vermillion), chin, mandible, preauricular and postauricular skin/sulci, temple, ear), genitalia, hands, and feet; area M = middle risk for recurrence: cheeks, forehead, neck, scalp; area L = low risk for recurrence: trunk, extremities.
*Must include peripheral rim of erythema in squamous cell carcinoma lesions.
†Having morpheaform (or desmoplastic), sclerosing, mixed infiltrative, or micronodular features in any portion of the tumor.
‡A modified Breslow measurement should exclude parakeratosis or scale/crust and be made from base of ulcer if present.
Adapted with permission from Miller S: NCCN practice guidelines for nonmelanoma skin cancer. Oncology 1999;13:529–549.

Table 107-3, helps to guide frequency of follow-up evaluation. Irrespective of recurrence risk, however, up to 40% of patients will develop another non-melanoma skin cancer during a three-year follow-up period. For this reason, patients should continue to be evaluated periodically by a dermatologist at least once yearly for occurrence of new lesions.

Squamous Cell Carcinoma

Clinical Presentation

Squamous cell carcinomas are the second most common nonmelanoma skin cancer, arising from malignant keratinocytes within the epidermis. Up to 60% of squamous cell carcinomas are thought to develop from actinic keratoses. Representing clonal collections of abnormal epidermal squamous cells that harbor genetic alterations induced by ultraviolet light, actinic keratoses transform to squamous cell carcinoma at a rate of 1 in 1000 annually.

Actinic keratoses appear as patches of hyperkeratosis, often surrounded by a rim of erythema. Because of their relationship to ultraviolet light, they are almost always found on sun-exposed areas of the head, neck, forearms, hands, and upper back. Erythema surrounding the base of the lesion is a common feature that helps distinguish actinic keratoses from seborrheic keratoses. Further, the hyperkeratosis of actinic keratoses is usually hard or spinelike and irregular, while that of seborrheic keratoses is soft and smooth.

Cutaneous squamous cell carcinoma usually presents as an asymptomatic hyperkeratotic papule, nodule, or plaque that grows slowly over months to years (Figure 107-3). Hyperkeratosis distinguishes these lesions from basal cell carcinomas. Lesions that are tender or painful raise concern for perineural invasion. Variants of squamous cell carcinoma include Bowen's disease (squamous cell carcinoma in situ), keratoacanthoma, and cutaneous horns. Bowen's

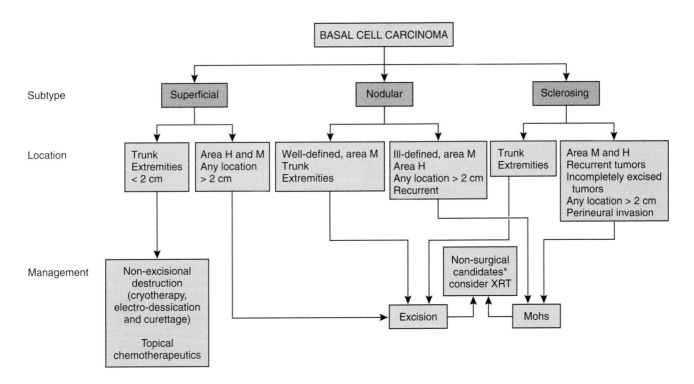

BASAL CELL CARCINOMA

Subtype
- Superficial
- Nodular
- Sclerosing

Location

| Trunk Extremities < 2 cm | Area H and M Any location > 2 cm | Well-defined, area M Trunk Extremities | Ill-defined, area M Area H Any location > 2 cm Recurrent | Trunk Extremities | Area M and H Recurrent tumors Incompletely excised tumors Any location > 2 cm Perineural invasion |

Management

- Non-excisional destruction (cryotherapy, electro-dessication and curettage)

  Topical chemotherapeutics
- Excision
- Non-surgical candidates* consider XRT
- Mohs

Area H = High risk for recurrence: "mask areas" of the face (central face, eyelids, eyebrows, periorbital, nose, lips, chin, mandible, preauricular and postauricular skin/sulci, temple, ear), genitalia, hands and feet
Area M = Middle risk for recurrence: cheeks, forehead, neck, scalp

***Non-surgical candidates** = Infirmed, extremity with vascular compromise (this option is rarely recommended)

Figure 107-2 ■ Algorithm for the management of basal cell carcinoma. Areas designated as "H" are at high risk for recurrence: mask areas of the face (central face, eyelids, eyebrows, periorbital region, nose, lips, chin, mandible, preauricular and postauricular skin/sulci, temple, ear), genitalia, hands, and feet. Areas designated as "M" are at medium risk for recurrence: cheeks, forehead, neck, and scalp. Nonsurgical candidates are the infirm and those with a vascularly compromised extremity; this option is rarely recommended. XRT = Radiation therapy.

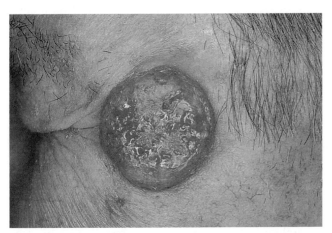

Figure 107-3 ■ Squamous cell carcinoma. (From Callen JP, Paller AS, Greer KE, Swinyer LJ: Color Atlas of Dermatology, 2nd ed. Philadelphia: WB Saunders, 2000.) (See Color Plate 21.)

disease characteristically presents as a red plaque with variable hyperkeratosis. "Bowenoid" papulosis, another form of squamous cell carcinoma in situ, appears as small hyperpigmented papules and is often associated with human papillomavirus 16 and 18. Keratoacanthomas typically present as hyperkeratotic, dome-shaped nodules with central keratin plugs (Figure 107-4). In contrast to squamous cell carcinomas, keratoacanthomas grow quickly over weeks, often regressing spontaneously and leaving scars. Cutaneous horns present as columns of hyperkeratosis on an erythematous base.

Presentations of nonmelanoma skin cancer differ in individuals with more intensely colored skin. For example, in blacks, squamous cell carcinomas appear most commonly on less sun-exposed skin areas such as the legs.

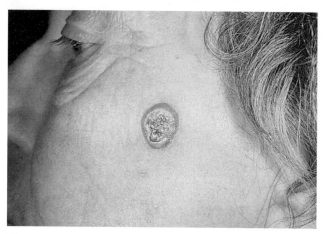

Figure 107-4 ▪ Keratoacanthoma. (From Callen JP, Paller AS, Greer KE, Swinyer LJ: Color Atlas of Dermatology, 2nd ed. Philadelphia: WB Saunders, 2000.) (See Color Plate 21.)

Clinical Evaluation

Although usually suspected on the basis of appearance, diagnosis of squamous cell carcinoma requires histologic confirmation. Since cutaneous horns may develop in actinic keratoses and verrucae as well as squamous cell carcinomas, histologic confirmation is necessary. Punch biopsies are preferred over shave biopsies, providing more accurate pathologic results, since shave biopsies can miss important histologic features in deeper dermal components. By identifying the depth of involvement, the histologic type of squamous cell carcinoma, and the presence of "aggressive" histologic features, biopsies help to direct treatment. Rapidly growing tumors require immediate surgical removal.

All patients with squamous cell carcinoma should have a complete review of systems and physical exam, with palpation of lymph nodes and internal organs. Patients with palpable lymph nodes should have fine-needle aspiration or open biopsy and frozen sections if fine-needle aspiration is negative. Patients with lymph nodes that are positive for metastasis should undergo staging with torso computed tomography. While the benefits of sentinel lymph node biopsy are uncertain, this procedure should be considered in patients who have squamous cell carcinoma features predicting high rates of regional lymph node metastasis.

Staging, Prognostic Features, and Outcomes

Staging for nonmelanoma skin cancer is summarized in Table 107-2. Overall, the risk of squamous cell carcinoma recurrence ranges from 1% to more than 20% and is predicted by clinical risk factors and pathology as listed in Table 107-3. With regard to lesion size, various size divisions have been used to distinguish recurrence risks in different studies. However, 2 cm probably represents the most common size division. In one meta-analysis, lesions less than 2 cm in diameter were associated with a regional recurrence rate of 7.4% at five years compared with 15.2% for tumors greater than 2 cm in diameter. With regard to other factors influencing risk of regional recurrence in this same meta-analysis, lesions less than 4 mm thick had a recurrence rate of 5.3% at five years compared with 17.2% for lesions greater than 4 mm in thickness. Poorly differentiated tumors had recurrence rates twofold higher than for well-differentiated tumors. Perineural invasion, regardless of squamous cell carcinoma subtype, predicted for high local recurrence rates of up to 47.2% when treated by surgical excision alone. Recurrent tumors, regardless of histopathologic characteristics in the original primary, had associated high risks of second recurrence (20%) when treated with surgery alone. Tumors recurring within a previously irradiated field were particularly aggressive in their locoregional behavior. All squamous cell carcinomas arising in immunosuppressed patients had potential for more aggressive behavior, warranting treatment as high-risk lesions. Finally, any symptom (e.g., pain) suggesting neurologic involvement in the region of squamous cell carcinoma places that tumor in a high-risk category.

Squamous cell carcinoma in situ carries no risk of metastasis, while invasive squamous cell carcinoma has the potential to metastasize. Five-year metastatic rates range from 3% or less for low-risk squamous cell carcinomas to as high as 35% to 45% for high-risk tumors such as those arising in inflammatory lesions (chronic wounds or infections), large tumors, or those having perineural invasion. The most common site of metastasis is the regional lymph node, occurring in 85% of cases with metastases. However, distant sites can be involved, including lungs and bones. Squamous cell carcinoma features predicting metastasis are similar to those predicting regional recurrence. For example, metastasis from lesions involving the external ear and lip occurred in 11% and 14% of cases, respectively, at five years. Primary tumors less than 2 cm in size had one third the metastatic rate of tumors greater than 2 cm in size; 7% of patients with primary tumors less than 4 mm thick had metastasis, while 46% of patients with primary tumors greater than 4 mm had metastasis. Well-differentiated tumors had one third the metastatic rate of poorly differentiated tumors (9% vs. 33%, respectively). Tumors with perineural invasion gave rise to metastasis in 47% of cases at five years. In immunosuppressed patients, the likelihood of metastasis following resection of the primary lesion was 12.5%.

Certain histologic variants of squamous cell carcinoma, regardless of size or depth, may have particularly aggressive behaviors and should be treated as high risk. These high-risk squamous cell carcinoma variants include the spindle cell variant of squamous cell carcinoma, clear cell squamous cell carcinoma, adenoid (or acantholytic) and adenosquamous (or mucin-producing) squamous cell carcinoma, and desmoplastic squamous cell carcinoma. The spindle cell and clear cell variants of squamous cell carcinoma have increased propensities for perineural invasion, which may explain their high local and distant recurrence rates of 25% at five years. Adenoid and adenosquamous squamous cell carcinomas are composed of neoplastic keratinocytes that form glandular or adenoidlike structures and acantholytic cells. These tumors arise most commonly on the neck and other sun-exposed areas but may also occur on the vulva, lip, and oral mucosa. Acantholytic squamous cell cancers greater than 1.5 cm in size have a metastatic risk of 14%.

Patients with metastatic squamous cell carcinoma have low five-year survival rates (34%), with more than 1500 deaths per year in the United States attributed to cutaneous squamous cell carcinoma. Hence, the goal of management is to identify high-risk lesions and treat them properly and promptly.

Treatment

Actinic Keratoses

Treatment of actinic keratoses depends on lesion size and number. Small lesions can be treated with liquid nitrogen cryotherapy, while larger lesions require shave removal or curettage. Because of their low risk for transformation, the decision to treat actinic keratoses varies among clinicians. Some clinicians treat all actinic keratoses; others treat only those that are enlarging. If the histologic diagnosis is in doubt, however, biopsy is required.

In patients with multiple actinic keratoses, topical 5-fluorouracil (1% or 2% on the face, 5% elsewhere), applied twice daily for three to four weeks, has been used with good success. Inflammatory changes of erythema, blistering, and necrosis with superficial ulceration generally take place. Low-potency topical corticosteroid cream helps to reduce inflammation until complete re-epithelialization occurs, generally four to six weeks after treatment onset. Concomitant use of topical 5-fluorouracil and corticosteroid cream applied 15 minutes after 5-fluorouracil may also be used to produce less inflammation. Dermabrasion, laser resurfacing, and chemical peels (e.g., Jessner's/30% TCA) are other treatment options.

Keratoacanthomas

Since some keratoacanthomas are invasive, with potential for metastasis, this tumor should be treated like squamous cell carcinoma.

Low-Risk Squamous Cell Carcinoma

The majority of squamous cell carcinomas are low-risk lesions arising as small, well-differentiated tumors on low-risk anatomic sites in immunocompetent patients. Hence, most squamous cell carcinomas can be treated with simple surgical excision and postoperative margin assessment (Figure 107-5). Four- to 6-mm margins are advocated. Any peripheral rim of erythema around a squamous cell cancer should be included in the surgical resection.

Simple surgical excision yields cure rates of about 90%, while Mohs surgery yields cure rates closer to 97%. Radiation therapy as a primary treatment modality has slightly lower cure rates than those for basal cell carcinoma but is useful in cases in which surgery is not an option or in patients older than age 55 years whose lesions are small and involve cosmetically sensitive areas of the head or neck. A competing concern regarding use of radiation as primary therapy of squamous cell carcinoma is the risk of nonmelanoma skin cancers secondary to the radiation. Since nonmelanoma skin cancers secondary to radiation therapy typically arise after 10 to 20 years, patients' ages should influence use of radiation as primary therapy. Finally, radiation should not be used to treat verrucous carcinomas, since several reports in the literature document increased metastatic risk in patients with this generally low-risk malignancy following treatment with radiation.

High-Risk Squamous Cell Carcinoma

High-risk squamous cell carcinomas require more aggressive management strategies to prevent locoregional and distant recurrences. For tumors with high-risk features other than size, Mohs surgery to obtain 100% microscopically controlled margins is the treatment of choice. Excision with postoperative margin assessment may be considered if size is the only factor determining high risk and the lesion is located on the trunk or extremities and can be excised with 10-mm margins and primary repair. Radiotherapy as primary treatment of high-risk squamous cell carcinomas should be considered only if surgery is contraindicated or not desired.

When high-risk features such as perineural involvement are present, excision of an extra 4- to 6-mm margin of tissue should be considered following tumor clearance by Mohs technique. In addition, adjuvant radiotherapy should be considered to sterilize undetectable in-transit metastatic disease that may

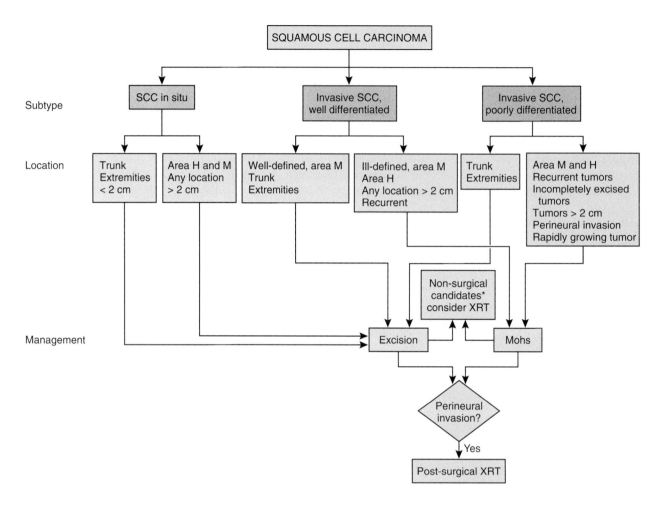

Area H = High risk for recurrence: "mask areas" of the face (central face, eyelids, eyebrows, periorbital, nose, lips, chin, mandible, preauricular and postauricular skin/sulci, temple, ear), genitalia, hands, and feet
Area M = Middle risk for recurrence: cheeks, forehead, neck, scalp

*Non-surgical candidates = Infirmed, extremity with vascular compromise (this option is rarely recommended)

Figure 107-5 ■ Algorithm for the management of squamous cell carcinoma (SCC). Areas designated as "H" are at high risk for recurrence: mask areas of the face (central face, eyelids, eyebrows, periorbital region, nose, lips, chin, mandible, preauricular and postauricular skin/sulci, temple, ear), genitalia, hands, and feet. Areas designated as "M" are at medium risk for recurrence: cheeks, forehead, neck, and scalp. XRT = Radiation therapy.

be present in such lesions beyond the margins of surgery. Guidelines for radiation therapy are the same as those detailed for basal cell carcinoma.

In patients with positive lymph nodes and no evidence of distant metastatic disease, regional lymph node dissection should be performed, followed by adjuvant radiotherapy to the regional nodal basin, particularly if tumor involves more than one lymph node or extends beyond the lymph node capsule. In patients with a palpable intraparotid mass, superficial parotidectomy should be performed.

Chemotherapy

Retinoids and interferon-alpha (IFN-α) are regulators of malignant cell differentiation and proliferation with immunomodulatory and antiangiogenesis activities. Both have been used in squamous cell carcinoma. In one study, combination therapy with oral 13-*cis*-retinoic acid and subcutaneous recombinant human IFN-α-2a yielded responses (68% overall responders, 25% complete remissions) in patients with heavily pretreated, advanced inoperable cutaneous squamous cell carcinoma. However, responses were more likely to occur in patients with less extensive disease. Cisplatin-based chemotherapy has yielded similar response rates.

There is no proven role for adjuvant chemotherapy in preventing recurrence of high-risk primary lesions or distant metastasis in cases with regional nodal disease. Patients with squamous cell carcinoma metastatic to distant sites may respond to platinum-based chemotherapy regimens, such as those used in treating squamous cell carcinomas arising from other organs such as lung, head, neck, and cervix. Other active antineoplastic agents include 5-fluorouracil, bleomycin, and doxorubicin. Where applicable, surgery and radiation should be offered in combination with chemotherapy, since complete remissions (up to 30%) are more likely with multimodality approaches. Remission durations vary, ranging from 3 to 81 months, with a median of 15 months.

Follow-up Evaluation

The median time to recurrence or development of a new squamous cell carcinoma is 12 to 15 months. For high-risk squamous cell carcinoma, recommended follow-up intervals following definitive treatment are every three months during the first year, every six months during the second year, and annually thereafter. Evaluation should include examination of the entire skin and palpation of draining lymph nodes. In uncomplicated cutaneous squamous cell carcinoma, there is no role for routine imaging, either by computed tomography (CT) or magnetic resonance imaging (MRI).

Merkel Cell Carcinoma

Clinical Presentation

Merkel cell carcinoma is a malignant tumor derived from cutaneous neuroendocrine cells demonstrating epithelial differentiation. On physical exam, Merkel cell carcinomas appear as small, asymptomatic, rapidly growing, red to deep purple nodules with shiny surfaces and telangiectasias (Figure 107-6). Most tumors

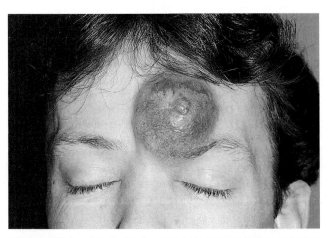

Figure 107-6 ■ Merkel cell carcinoma. (From Callen JP, Paller AS, Greer KE, Swinyer LJ: Color Atlas of Dermatology, 2nd ed. Philadelphia: WB Saunders, 2000.) (See Color Plate 21.)

are less than 2 cm in diameter at the time of diagnosis. Fifty percent to 55% of Merkel cell carcinomas involve the head and neck, 40% arise on the extremities, and 5% involve the trunk.

There are three histologic subtypes of Merkel cell carcinoma, and all three subtypes may be seen in a single tumor. The trabecular variant is well differentiated and is seen in fewer than 25% of patients. The intermediate cell variant is the most common subtype. The small cell variant has the most aggressive behavior. Tumors with vascular or lymphatic invasion or a high mitotic index also behave more aggressively.

Merkel cell carcinoma is an aggressive tumor with spread from the initial skin site to regional lymph nodes and distant organs. Symptoms and signs of regional and distant metastatic disease may be evident at time of presentation. Common sites of metastasis are liver, bone, brain, lung, and skin.

Clinical Evaluation

Diagnosis of Merkel cell carcinoma requires histologic confirmation. Punch biopsies are preferred over shave biopsies, providing more accurate pathologic results, since Merkel cell carcinomas are dermally based masses and shave biopsies can miss important histologic features in deeper dermal components.

All patients with Merkel cell carcinoma should have a complete review of systems and physical exam, with palpation of lymph nodes and internal organs. Chest radiograph and liver function tests should be obtained to assess possible metastatic disease. Patients with palpable lymph nodes should have fine-needle aspiration or open biopsy and frozen sections if fine-needle aspiration is negative. Patients with lymph nodes that are positive for metastasis should undergo torso staging with computed tomography. While the benefits of sentinel lymph node biopsy are uncertain, this procedure should be considered because of high rates of regional lymph node metastasis in Merkel cell carcinoma.

Staging, Prognostic Features, and Outcomes

Staging for nonmelanoma skin cancer is shown in Table 107-2. Features that predict high risk for recurrence as well as for metastasis and death include tumor location, patient gender and age, local or nodal or systemic disease, and histologic characteristics such as perineural and vascular or lymphatic invasion. Mortality is greatest for tumors presenting on the head, neck, and trunk and lowest for tumors presenting on the extremities. Younger patients have higher associated mortality, with as many as 60% of patients below the age of 40 dying of their disease. Men do less well than women. Patients with lymph node involvement, which occurs in 20% of Merkel cell carcinoma cases at initial presentation and up to one half to two thirds of patients at some point in the disease course, have higher mortality compared with patients who do not have lymph node involvement. Recurrent tumors are associated with high mortality, and nearly all patients with systemic metastasis die from their disease. Overall survival rates decline from 88% at one year to 55% at three years. Three-year survival rates are 17% for patients with metastatic disease and 35% for those with locally advanced disease.

Treatment

Wide surgical excision with 2.5- to 3-cm margins is indicated for treatment of the primary lesion. If postoperative margins are involved by tumor, Mohs surgery should be considered. Mohs surgery is useful to determine the subclinical extent of the tumor. If possible anatomically, a 2-cm margin outside a clear Mohs margin is advocated. Lymph node dissection should be performed if lymphadenopathy is detected. While sentinel lymph node biopsy remains unproven, it may be a useful adjunct.

Adjuvant postsurgical radiation therapy to the primary site and draining lymphatics should be administered to decrease regional recurrence and prolong survival. With adjuvant regional radiotherapy, local recurrence rates are 22%, compared with 39% to 65% when radiotherapy is not administered. While unproven, adjuvant chemotherapy, using regimens administered for treatment of metastatic disease, should be considered in patients whose primary lesions exhibit vascular or lymphatic invasion or spread to regional lymph nodes.

The most common regimens used in treating metastatic disease are cyclophosphamide, doxorubicin, and vincristine or cisplatin and etoposide. The overall response rate to first-line chemotherapy is 61%, with a 57% response rate in metastatic disease and a 69% response rate in locally advanced disease.

Follow-up Evaluation

In view of the aggressive behavior of Merkel cell carcinoma, post-treatment follow-up examinations should be given monthly for six months, every three months for two years, and every six to 12 months thereafter. Follow-up examination should include review of systems, complete physical examination, liver function testing, and chest radiograph.

References

General

Allen PJ, Zhang ZF, Coit DG: Surgical management of Merkel cell carcinoma. Ann Surg 1999;229:97–105.

Demetrius RW, Randle HW: High-risk nonmelanoma skin cancers. Dermatol Surg 1998;24:1272–1292.

Evans GR, Williams JZ, Ainslie NB: Cutaneous nasal malignancies: Is primary reconstruction safe? Head Neck 1997;19: 182–187.

Grossman D, Leffell DJ: The molecular basis of nonmelanoma skin cancer: New understanding. Arch Dermatol 1997;133: 1263–1270.

Guthrie TH, Porubsky ES, Luxenberg MN, et al: Cisplatin-based chemotherapy in advanced basal and squamous cell carcinomas of the skin: Results of 28 patients including 13 patients receiving multimodality therapy. J Clin Oncol 1990;8:342–346.

Karagas MR, McDonald JA, Greenberg ER, et al: Risk of basal cell and squamous cell skin cancers after ionizing radiation therapy: For the Skin Cancer Prevention Study Group. J Natl Cancer Inst 1996;88:1848–1853.

Karagas MR, Stukel TA, Greenberg ER, et al: Risk of subsequent basal cell carcinoma and squamous cell carcinoma of the skin among patients with prior skin cancer. Skin Cancer Prevention Study Group. JAMA 1992;267:3305–3310.

Lobo DV, Chu P, Grekin RC, Berger TG: Nonmelanoma skin cancers and infection with the human immunodeficiency virus. Arch Dermatol 1992;128:623–627.

Miller DL, Weinstock MA: Nonmelanoma skin cancer in the United States: Incidence. J Am Acad Dermatol 1994;30: 774–778.

Miller SJ: NCCN practice guidelines for nonmelanoma skin cancer. Oncology 1999;13:529–549.

Penn I: The changing patterns of posttransplant malignancies. Transplant Proc 1991;23:1101–1103.

Pierceall WE, Goldberg LH, Ananthaswamy HN: Presence of human papillomavirus type 16 DNA sequences in human nonmelanoma skin cancers. J Invest Dermatol 1991;97: 880–884.

Salgarello M, Seccia A, Sturla M, et al: Analysis of infiltrating epitheliomas of the nose examined from 1986 to 1995. J Otolaryngol 1998;27:288–292.

Stern RS, Liebman EJ, Vakeva L: Oral psoralen and ultraviolet-A light (PUVA) treatment of psoriasis and persistent risk of nonmelanoma skin cancer: PUVA follow-up study. J Natl Cancer Inst 1998;90:1278–1284.

Terashi H, Kurata S, Tadokoro T, et al: Perineural and neural involvement in skin cancers. Dermatol Surg 1997;23: 259–264.

Ziegler A, Jonason AS, Leffell DJ, et al: Sunburn and p53 in the onset of skin cancer. Nature 1994;372:773–776.

Squamous Cell Carcinoma

Alam M, Ratner D: Cutaneous squamous cell carcinoma. N Engl J Med 2001;344:975–983.

Banks ER, Cooper PH: Adenosquamous carcinoma of the skin: A report of 10 cases. J Cutan Pathol 1991;18:227–234.

Bernstein SC, Lim KK, Brodland DG, Heidelberg KA: The many faces of squamous cell carcinoma. Dermatol Surg 1996;22: 243–264.

Breuninger H, Schaumburg-Lever G, Holzschuh J, et al: Desmoplastic squamous cell carcinoma of skin and vermilion surface: A highly malignant subtype of skin cancer. Cancer 1997;79:915–919.

Brodland DG, Zitelli JA: Surgical margins for excision of primary cutaneous squamous cell carcinoma. J Am Acad Dermatol 1992;27:241–248.

Edwards MH, Hirsch RM, Broadwater JR, et al: Squamous cell carcinoma arising in previously burned or irradiated skin. Arch Surg 1989;124:115–117.

Geohas J, Roholt NS, Robinson JK: Adjuvant radiotherapy after excision of cutaneous squamous cell carcinoma. J Am Acad Dermatol 1994;30:633–636.

Lippman SM, Parkinson DR, Itri LM, et al: 13-*cis*-retinoic acid and interferon alpha-2a: Effective combination therapy for advanced squamous cell carcinoma of the skin. J Natl Cancer Inst 1992;84:235–241.

Marks R, Rennie G, Selwood TS: Malignant transformation of solar keratoses to squamous cell carcinoma. Lancet 1988;1:795–797.

Nappi O, Pettinato G, Wick MR: Adenoid (acantholytic) squamous cell carcinoma of the skin. J Cutan Pathol 1989;16:114–121.

Rowe DE, Carroll RJ, Day CL Jr: Prognostic factors for local recurrence, metastasis and survival rates in squamous cell carcinoma of the skin, ear, and lip: Implications for treatment modality selection. J Am Acad Dermatol 1992;26:976–990.

Basal Cell Carcinoma

Arlette JP, Carruthers A, Threlfall WJ, Warshawski LM: Basal cell carcinoma of the periocular region. J Cutan Med Surg 1998;2:205–208.

Childers BJ, Goldwyn RM, Ramos D, et al: Long-term results of irradiation for basal cell carcinoma of the skin of the nose. Plast Reconstr Surg 1994;93:1169–1173.

Gailani MR, Bale AE: Developmental genes and cancer: Role of patched in basal cell carcinoma of the skin. J Natl Cancer Inst 1997;89:1103–1109.

Glied M, Berg D, Witterick I: Basal cell carcinoma of the conchal bowl: Interdisciplinary approach to treatment. J Otolaryngol 1998;27:322–326.

Holmkvist KA, Rogers GS, Dahl PR: Incidence of residual basal cell carcinoma in patients who appear tumor free after biopsy. J Am Acad Dermatol 1999;41:600–605.

Miller BH, Shavin JS, Cognetta A, et al: Nonsurgical treatment of basal cell carcinomas with intralesional 5-fluorouracil/epinephrine injectable gel. J Am Acad Dermatol 1997;36:72–77.

Miller SJ: Biology of basal cell carcinoma (part I). J Am Acad Dermatol 1991;24:1–13.

Miller SJ: Biology of basal cell carcinoma (part II). J Am Acad Dermatol 1991;24:161–175.

Moeholt K, Aagaard H, Pfeiffer P, Hansen O: Platinum-based cytotoxic therapy in basal cell carcinoma: A review of the literature. Acta Oncol 1996;35:677–682.

Rowe DE, Carroll RJ, Day CL Jr: Long-term recurrence rates in previously untreated (primary) basal cell carcinoma: Implications for patient follow-up. J Dermatol Surg Oncol 1989;15:315–328.

Silverman MK, Kopf AW, Grin CM, et al: Recurrence rates of treated basal cell carcinomas. Part 2: Curettage-electrodesiccation. J Dermatol Surg Oncol 1991;17:720–726.

Wilder RB, Kittelson JM, Shimm DS: Basal cell carcinoma treated with radiation therapy. Cancer 1991;68:2134–2137.

Wolf DJ, Zitelli JA: Surgical margins for basal cell carcinoma. Arch Dermatol 1987;123:340–344.

Xie J, Murone M, Luoh SM, et al: Activating smoothened mutations in sporadic basal cell carcinoma. Nature 1998;391:90–92.

Merkel Cell Carcinoma

Haag ML, Glass LF, Fenske NA: Merkel cell carcinoma: Diagnosis and treatment. Dermatol Surg 1995;21:669–683.

Hill AD, Brady MS, Coit DG: Intraoperative lymphatic mapping and sentinel lymph node biopsy for Merkel cell carcinoma. Br J Surg 1999;86:518.

Kokoska ER, Kokoska MS, Collins BT, et al: Early aggressive treatment for Merkel cell carcinoma improves outcome. Am J Surg 1997;174:688–693.

Lunder EJ, Stern RS: Merkel cell carcinomas in patients treated with methoxsalen and ultraviolet A radiation. N Engl J Med 1998;339:1247–1248.

Messina JL, Reintgen DS, Cruse CW, et al: Selective lymphadenectomy in patients with Merkel cell (cutaneous neuroendocrine) carcinoma. Ann Surg Oncol 1997;4:389–395.

Miller RW, Rabkin CS: Merkel cell carcinoma and melanoma: Etiological similarities and differences. Cancer Epidemiol Biomarkers Prev 1999;8:153–158. (Published erratum appears in Cancer Epidemiol Biomarkers Prev 1999;8:485.)

Ott MJ, Tanabe KK, Gadd MA, et al: Multimodality management of Merkel cell carcinoma. Arch Surg 1999;134:388–393.

Tai PTH, Yu E, Winquist E, et al: Chemotherapy in neuroendocrine/Merkel cell carcinoma of the skin: Case series and review of 204 cases. J Clin Oncol 2000;18:2493–2499.

Tsuruta D, Hamada T, Mochida K, et al: Merkel cell carcinoma, Bowen's disease and chronic occupational arsenic poisoning. Br J Dermatol 1998;139:291–294.

Voog E, Biron P, Martin JP, Blay JY: Chemotherapy for patients with locally advanced or metastatic Merkel cell carcinoma. Cancer 1999;85:2589–2595.

Williams RH, Morgan MB, Mathieson IM, Rabb H: Merkel cell carcinoma in a renal transplant patient: Increased incidence? Transplantation 1998;65:1396–1397.

Chapter 108
Thyroid Cancer

Robert D. Utiger

There are five major types of thyroid carcinoma: papillary carcinoma, follicular carcinoma, anaplastic carcinoma, medullary carcinoma, and lymphoma. Among them, papillary carcinoma is the most frequent, accounting for over 70% of cases (Table 108-1). The estimated number of new cases in the United States in 2001 was 19,500, of whom 14,900 were women and 4600 were men.

Clinical Presentation

Most thyroid carcinomas are identified in the course of evaluation of a patient who has a palpable nodule of the thyroid gland. The nodule might have been noticed first by the patient, a relative, or a friend; during a routine physical examination; or on an imaging of study of the neck. Thyroid nodules greater than 1 cm in diameter can be detected in approximately 5% of adults by physical examination and in many more by ultrasonography. However, only 5% to 8% of thyroid nodules of this size are thyroid carcinomas. The other, much more numerous causes, consist of thyroid adenomas, dominant nodules of a multinodular (adenomatous) goiter, and rarely thyroid cysts or localized regions of thyroiditis. In a few patients, the presenting manifestation of thyroid carcinoma is an enlarged cervical lymph node or metastasis elsewhere or a rapidly enlarging nodule in a multinodular goiter.

Among patients with thyroid nodules, some symptoms and physical findings are clues that the nodule might be a carcinoma, but none is sensitive or specific (Table 108-2). The patients are virtually always euthyroid; the presence of hyperthyroidism is strong evidence that a nodule is not a carcinoma but is instead an autonomously functioning thyroid adenoma. Both benign thyroid nodules and thyroid carcinomas are more common in women than in men, but the proportion of nodules that are carcinomas is higher among men.

Evaluation of Patients with Thyroid Nodules

Biochemical Studies

Serum thyrotropin (TSH) should be measured in all patients with thyroid nodules. Virtually all patients with thyroid carcinomas have normal values. Low values indicate the presence of an autonomously functioning thyroid adenoma or toxic multinodular goiter, and high values indicate the presence of chronic autoimmune thyroiditis. Serum calcitonin should be measured in patients who are suspected to have a medullary carcinoma of the thyroid.

Imaging Studies

Patients with thyroid nodules may be evaluated by ultrasonography (Figure 108-1), radionuclide imaging, or, rarely, other imaging tests. However, none of these tests distinguish between benign thyroid nodules and thyroid carcinomas, with the exception that imaging with iodine-123 or iodine-131 may reveal an autonomously functioning thyroid adenoma. Iodine-123 is preferred for diagnostic imaging because it is safer and the quality of the images is higher. Ultrasonography often detects nodules in addition to the one that was palpated and

Table 108-1 ▪ Thyroid Carcinoma in the United States, 1973–1991

Carcinoma	Percentage
Papillary carcinoma	76%
Follicular carcinoma	17%
Anaplastic carcinoma	2%
Medullary carcinoma	3%
Other (lymphoma, metastatic carcinoma)	2%

From Gilliland FD, Hunt WC, Morris DM, Key CR: Prognostic factors for thyroid carcinoma: A population-based study of 15,598 cases from the Surveillance, Epidemiology and End Results (SEER) Program 1973–1991. Cancer 1997;79:564–573.

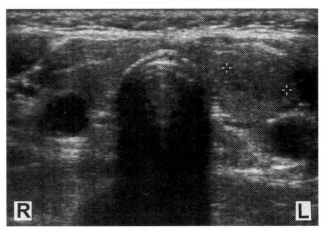

Figure 108-1 ▪ Transverse ultrasound image of the thyroid gland showing a solid nodule in the left lobe of the gland. The nodule is slightly hypoechogenic, compared with the right lobe of the gland. The midline structure is the trachea, the carotid arteries are posterolateral to the thyroid lobes, and the jugular veins are lateral to the thyroid lobes. The nodule proved to be a papillary thyroid carcinoma, but benign nodules have the same appearance.

will distinguish between nodules that are solid and nodules that are partially or completely cystic, but these distinctions have little diagnostic importance. In particular, partially cystic nodules are as likely to be carcinomas as are solid nodules.

Thyroid Biopsy

The key step in the evaluation of patients with a thyroid nodule is fine-needle aspiration biopsy. This is usually done with local anesthesia using a 22- to 25-gauge needle to obtain thyroid follicular cells and follicles for cytological examination. The biopsy may be guided by palpation, but guidance by ultrasonography is preferable, especially if the nodule is relatively small or partially cystic, so that a region of solid tissue can be biopsied. Nodules that are less than 1 cm in diameter are not usually biopsied.

Fine-needle aspiration biopsy is simple and safe. The nodule should be aspirated several times; the cellular material obtained may be applied directly to microscope slides or placed in fluid and then concentrated by filtration. A common criterion for adequacy of biopsy is that at least six groups of 10 to 15 well-preserved thyroid follicular cells are seen on each of at least two slides. A commonly used system for reporting the results of biopsies is as follows: benign follicu-

lar cells, papillary carcinoma, follicular tumor or neoplasm, and inadequate specimen. These categories may be subdivided according to cell type and probability of carcinoma. The category of follicular tumor or neoplasm reflects the fact that there are no cytologic differences between follicular carcinomas and follicular adenomas. They are distinguished by the presence or absence of capsular and especially vascular invasion in permanent histologic sections. Follicular carcinomas tend to be larger than follicular adenomas, and affected patients are older and more likely to be men, but these associations are not strong. Papillary carcinomas (and the rare medullary carcinomas) can be identified on the basis of well-defined cytologic criteria.

Among large groups of patients undergoing biopsy, the biopsy results are benign nodule in approximately 70%, carcinoma in 5%, follicular tumor in 10%, and inadequate for diagnosis in 15%. False-negative and false-positive results are rare. Among follicular tumors, 10% to 25% prove to be follicular carcinomas. Patients in whom the biopsy is inadequate should have a second biopsy.

Benign Thyroid Nodules

Patients with a benign nodule may be treated surgically—by excision of the nodule or thyroid lobectomy—if the nodule is a cosmetic problem or causes local symptoms. Hyperthyroid patients with autonomously functioning thyroid adenomas should be treated with iodine-131 or surgery. Otherwise, periodic follow-up is indicated. Thyroxine may be given if the patient desires treatment, but in most

Table 108-2 ▪ Factors Associated with Moderate or High Likelihood of Carcinoma in Patients with a Thyroid Nodule

Age <20 or >60 years
Male sex
History of head and neck irradiation
Rapid growth of nodule
Firm nodule, fixed to adjacent structures
Nodule >4 cm in diameter
Enlarged cervical lymph node(s)
Nodule is partially cystic

controlled studies thyroxine was little more effective than placebo in reducing nodule size. A nodule that enlarges during follow-up should be biopsied again. Nodules that on biopsy are called follicular tumors may be autonomously functioning adenomas. These nodules can be identified as such by radionuclide imaging.

Thyroid Cysts

Fewer than 5% of solitary thyroid nodules are completely cystic. If a cyst is encountered during a fine-needle aspiration biopsy in a patient with a thyroid nodule, as much fluid as possible should be withdrawn and the cells should be examined cytologically to be sure the nodule is not a cystic thyroid carcinoma. Aspiration usually results in substantial regression or disappearance of the cyst. If fluid reaccumulates, the cyst may be aspirated again or excised.

Thyroid Carcinoma

There are three types of carcinoma of thyroid follicular cells: papillary carcinoma, follicular carcinoma, and anaplastic carcinoma. Tumor-node-metastasis (TNM) staging of these carcinomas is shown in Table 108-3.

Papillary and Follicular (Differentiated) Carcinoma

Papillary carcinomas and follicular carcinomas (including Hurthle cell carcinomas) are often grouped together as differentiated thyroid carcinomas. These carcinomas account for about 90% of all thyroid carcinomas (see Table 108-1). The two types of carcinoma differ in some clinical and histologic respects (Table 108-4), but the differences are not large, and each type of carcinoma may have histologic and clinical features

Table 108-3 ■ TNM Staging of Thyroid Carcinomas

Primary Tumor

T1	Tumor ≤1 cm in diameter
T2	Tumor >1 cm but ≤4 cm in diameter
T3	Tumor >4 cm in diameter
T4	Tumor of any size extending beyond the thyroid capsule

Regional Lymph Nodes

N0	No regional lymph node metastasis
N1	Regional lymph node metastasis

Distant Metastasis

M0	No distant metastasis
M1	Distant metastasis

Stage Grouping

Papillary or follicular carcinoma

Stage I	<45 years	Any T, any N, M0
Stage I	≥45 years	T1, N0, M0
Stage II	Any T, any N, M1	T2 or T3, N0, M0
Stage III		T4, N0, M0
		Any T, N1, M0
Stage IV		Any T, any N, M1

Anaplastic carcinoma

All cases are stage IV	Any T, any N, any M

Medullary carcinoma

Stage I	T1, N0, M0
Stage II	T2–T4, N0, M0
Stage III	Any T, N1, M0
Stage IV	Any T, any N, M1

From AJCC Cancer Staging Handbook: Philadelphia: Lippincott-Raven 1998, pp 62–63.

Table 108-4 ■ Characteristics of Papillary and Follicular Carcinomas of the Thyroid

Characteristic	Papillary Carcinoma	Follicular Carcinoma
Peak ages (years)	30 to 50	40 to 60
Women/men	W > M	W > M
Risk factors	Head and neck irradiation	
Primary tumor	Solitary nodule	Solitary nodule
Usual size of primary tumor	1–3 cm	2–5 cm
Recurrence		
Cervical lymph nodes	20–40%	5–10%
Distant metastases	2–5%	15–20%
Pattern of spread	Via lymphatics	Via bloodstream
Sites of metastasis	Cervical lymph nodes, lungs, bone	Lungs, bone, brain

of the other. Patients with follicular carcinoma are usually considered to have a poorer prognosis, but among patients of the same age and sex with the same stage of disease, the prognosis and outcome are similar.

Most papillary and follicular carcinomas have little capacity to transport, oxidize, and organify iodide, compared with normal thyroid tissue. When all normal thyroid tissue has been removed or destroyed and serum thyrotropin concentrations are high, approximately 75% of differentiated carcinomas take up enough iodide to be detected by radioiodine imaging, and 90% to 95% synthesize and secrete thyroglobulin. Measurements of serum thyroglobulin are therefore very useful for detecting persistent or recurrent tumor in these patients. Hyperthyroidism is extremely rare and occurs only in patients with very large burdens of tumor.

Papillary Carcinoma

Papillary carcinomas are the most common thyroid carcinomas (see Table 108-1). They occur in children and adolescents as well as adults of all ages and are more common in women than in men (2:1 to 3:1). The most important risk factor for papillary carcinoma is radiation of the thyroid gland. This takes several forms: low doses of external radiation given to shrink enlarged tonsils, adenoids, or thymus in infants and to treat acne in adolescents (these practices were abandoned in the 1960s); high doses of external radiation given to treat Hodgkin's disease in children, adolescents, and adults; and inhalation or ingestion of radioiodine, as exemplified by the marked increase in thyroid carcinoma in infants and children in Belarus, Russia, and Ukraine after the explosion of the nuclear power plant at Chernobyl in 1986. The risk of thyroid carcinoma in people who receive radiation is lifelong. Rearrangements of the *ret* oncogene, which codes for a tyrosine kinase, that result in activation of the kinase have been found in from 10% to 40% of papillary carcinomas, especially those related to radiation. Papillary carcinoma may occur in several rare inherited syndromes, including Gardner's syndrome, Cowden's disease, and familial adenomatous polyposis, and it alone has been described in several kindreds.

Papillary carcinomas are poorly encapsulated masses of thyroid follicular cells arranged in papillae or cords (Figure 108-2). The nuclei of the cells are large, irregularly shaped or folded, and clear or empty; they often have grooves and pseudo-inclusions; and the chromatin is clumped along the nuclear membrane. There are several subtypes of papillary carcinoma, all characterized by nuclei with a similar appearance. They include the follicular variant of papillary carcinoma, in which the cells are arranged in a microfollicular pattern or sheets; tall or columnar cell carcinoma; and sclerosing or fibrous carcinoma.

Follicular Carcinoma

Follicular carcinomas are considerably less common than papillary carcinomas (see Table 108-1). These tumors are rare in children and adolescents, and the patients tend to be older than patients with papillary carcinoma. The tumors are encapsulated masses of thyroid follicular cells arranged in microfollicles or sheets. The nuclei contain more chromatin than is present in papillary carcinomas and resemble those of normal thyroid follicular cells. Hurthle cell carcino-

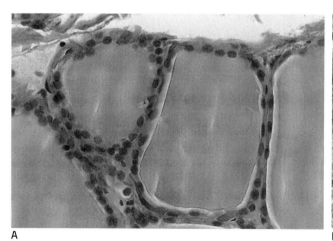
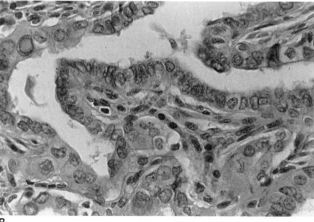

A   B

Figure 108-2 ■ Microscopic sections of normal thyroid tissue (*A*) and papillary carcinoma of the thyroid (*B*). In the normal thyroid, the follicular cells are arranged in follicles, and the cells have hyperchromatic nuclei. In the carcinoma, the cells are crowded together, and the nuclei overlap, are pale-staining, and have grooves and pseudo-inclusions. (Hematoxylin and eosin, original magnification ×400.) (See Color Plate 22.)

mas are follicular carcinomas in which the cells have an eosinophilic granular cytoplasm, which is caused by the presence of many mitochondria. Some thyroid adenomas are composed of Hurthle cells (also called oxyphil or oncocytic cells), and scattered Hurthle cells are found in some hyperplastic nodules and in chronic autoimmune thyroiditis. Hurthle cell carcinomas account for 20% to 40% of follicular carcinomas, their biologic characteristics are similar to those of follicular carcinomas, and treatment and prognosis are similar.

The distinction between a follicular carcinoma and adenoma (or a Hurthle cell carcinoma and adenoma) is based on identification of invasion of tumor cells through the capsule or into blood vessels. These carcinomas are often subdivided into minimally and markedly invasive subgroups, according to whether just one or two foci or many foci of invasion, especially blood vessel invasion, are seen. The prognosis of patients with minimally invasive carcinomas is excellent, whereas that of patients with markedly invasive follicular carcinomas is poor. The overall frequency of follicular carcinoma seems to be decreasing, probably because follicular carcinomas in which the nuclei of some cells have the features of papillary carcinoma are more often diagnosed as follicular variants of papillary carcinoma than in the past.

Staging and Prognosis of Differentiated Thyroid Carcinoma

Patients with a thyroid nodule that is found to be a differentiated thyroid carcinoma on fine-needle aspiration biopsy, which in practice means a papillary carcinoma because of the difficulty of identifying follicular carcinomas in biopsy specimens, need little preoperative evaluation. Some have palpable cervical lymph nodes, and enlarged nodes may be detected by ultrasonography at the time of biopsy in others, but a search for abnormal lymph nodes or distant metastases in asymptomatic patients is not indicated. Patients with symptoms or signs suggesting that the tumor is locally invasive should undergo direct laryngoscopy and computed tomography (CT) of the neck, primarily to aid the surgeon in planning for thyroidectomy.

The TNM staging system for differentiated thyroid carcinoma (see Table 108-3) is based on age, but not sex, and pathologic findings. In this system, patients are divided into four stages, with progressively poorer survival with increasing stage. In several studies, the 20-year survival rate varied from nearly 100% in patients with stage I tumors to approximately 25% in patients with stage IV tumors. The recurrence rates range from 0% to 20% in patients with stage I tumors and 10% to 30% in patients with stage II tumors to 65% to 80% in those with stage IV tumors. Note that the presence of tumor in cervical lymph nodes in young patients does not change the stage (see Table 108-3). Other staging systems that include factors such as tumor histology, the completeness of resection, and the number of foci of tumor within the thyroid in addition to the basic components of the TNM system have been devised, but none has proven superior to the TNM system for predicting outcome.

Factors associated with higher recurrence and mortality rates in patients with differentiated thyroid carcinoma are age greater than 40 years and male sex, local tumor invasion, large tumor size, no iodine-131 therapy, and thyroid lobectomy (versus more than lobectomy). Nevertheless, some patients with stage IV tumors with metastases that cannot be destroyed with radioiodine or resected survive for prolonged periods.

Treatment of Differentiated Thyroid Carcinoma

The key treatments for patients with differentiated thyroid carcinoma are surgery and iodine-131.

Surgery

For patients with small (1 cm or smaller) papillary carcinomas and no evidence of extrathyroidal tumor, thyroid lobectomy, including removal of the isthmus of the thyroid, is adequate treatment. These microcarcinomas are often discovered incidentally in a patient who is undergoing surgery for another, larger benign nodule or a multinodular goiter. The prognosis for patients with a microcarcinoma is excellent.

For patients with larger papillary carcinomas or any evidence of extrathyroidal tumor, the most appropriate operation is total thyroidectomy, or, more precisely, near-total thyroidectomy, in which a small portion of the posterior capsule of the contralateral lobe of the thyroid is left to minimize the likelihood of hypoparathyroidism and laryngeal dysfunction. In practice, some ipsilateral thyroid tissue is often left as well, on the basis of postoperative radioiodine imaging studies. There are two reasons to remove so much thyroid tissue. First, many carcinomas are multifocal (which may represent intrathyroidal spread of the main tumor or another tumor), and therefore some patients—as many as 50% in some studies—who undergo lobectomy have recurrence only in the contralateral lobe. Second, more extensive surgery facilitates postoperative iodine-131 therapy, because it is difficult to destroy a large amount of normal thyroid tissue with iodine-131. Near-total thyroidectomy should be done even in patients with obvious metastatic disease because of the need to remove normal thyroid tissue to facilitate radioiodine therapy.

In most studies, near-total thyroidectomy was associated with lower rates of local and regional recur-

TREATMENT

Therapy for Papillary Thyroid Carcinoma

Most patients with thyroid carcinoma present with a thyroid nodule that is at least 1 cm in diameter and usually larger. The first step in evaluation should be fine-needle aspiration biopsy. This is a reliable way to identify whether the nodule is a thyroid carcinoma or a benign nodule. When the biopsy reveals papillary thyroid carcinoma, the most common type of thyroid carcinoma, the cytologic diagnosis is almost always confirmed at surgery.

The questions that need to be considered are as follows:

What is the most appropriate therapy? For most patients, it is near total thyroidectomy, care being taken not to remove any parathyroid glands or injure the recurrent laryngeal nerves. Cervical lymph nodes should be sampled, but neck dissection is not indicated unless the nodes are positive. This operation minimizes the likelihood of recurrence in the thyroid gland and the likelihood of postoperative complications.

What postoperative therapy is indicated? Patients with tumors greater than 1 cm should be treated with iodine-131 while hypothyroid if they have any uptake on a diagnostic iodine-123 scan, whether that uptake is in the thyroid bed or outside of it. Patients with uptake only in the thyroid bed should be given 50 or 100 mCi; those with uptake outside the thyroid bed should be given higher doses, up to 300 mCi, depending on the extent of the disease. All patients, including those who are not given iodine-131, should be treated with thyroxine in a dose that is sufficient to lower serum thyrotropin concentrations to below normal.

What is the prognosis? The prognosis is very good for all patients except those with metastatic disease at the time of diagnosis. Twenty-year survival rates vary from nearly 100% for patients with small tumors confined to the thyroid to approximately 25% for patients with metastatic disease.

How should the patient be followed? Patients with papillary thyroid carcinoma should be followed initially at six-month intervals with physical examination, ultrasonography of the neck, and measurements of serum thyrotropin and thyroglobulin. If there is evidence of persistent or recurrent tumor, for example, a high serum thyroglobulin concentration, iodine-123 imaging and, if uptake is detected, iodine-131 treatment are indicated. The frequency of follow-up can be reduced after five years.

---

rence and mortality, compared with lobectomy or lobectomy and partial contralateral lobectomy, yet low rates of hypoparathyroidism and recurrent laryngeal nerve damage (less than 5%). At the same time, any visibly abnormal regional lymph nodes should be removed, and if they contain tumor, a regional neck dissection should be performed. The resection should be more extensive if the tumor extends into the soft tissue adjacent to the thyroid or invades the esophagus, trachea, or strap muscles.

Patients with follicular tumors are often treated with lobectomy; contralateral lobectomy (completion thyroidectomy) is then advised if the follicular tumor proves on pathologic examination to be a follicular carcinoma (this diagnosis cannot be made by frozen section). Near-total thyroidectomy is indicated if the tumor is large or if local invasion is seen at surgery. From 10% to 25% of follicular tumors prove to be follicular carcinomas.

Radioiodine Therapy

The most important nonsurgical treatment for patients with differentiated thyroid carcinoma is radioiodine in the form of iodine-131. It is a beta- and gamma-emitter; its destructive effects result primarily from the former, which have a path length of 1 to 2 mm. Iodine-131 is initially administered to patients with thyroid carcinoma to destroy any remaining normal thyroid tissue, called remnant ablation, and to destroy carcinoma tissue. Destruction of any remaining normal thyroid tissue should result in the destruction of any microscopic foci of carcinoma within the remnant, and it facilitates treatment of carcinoma elsewhere.

Radioiodine treatment is indicated for all patients with differentiated thyroid carcinoma except those with stage I tumors. Single doses of iodine-131 reduce the frequency of recurrence and metastases in patients with stage II tumors, and single or repeated doses reduce the frequency of recurrence and mortality in patients with stage III and IV tumors. Survival may be greatly prolonged even in patients with metastatic disease.

Patients to be treated with iodine-131 should have serum thyrotropin concentrations of 25 mU/L or higher, to facilitate iodine-131 uptake by normal and abnormal thyroid tissue. These concentrations are given three to four weeks after surgery or cessation of thyroid hormone therapy. Alternatively, thyroid hormone therapy can be continued and remnant or tumor uptake of iodine-131 stimulated by administration of thyrotropin for several days. Patients to be treated with iodine-131 should eat an iodine-deficient diet for a week before treatment (and avoid iodine-containing medications for at least that period). Before treatment, a diagnostic whole-body scan should be done six or 24 hours after oral administration of 1.5 to 2 mCi iodine-123. If no uptake is seen, iodine-131 treatment is not needed. If uptake is limited to the thyroid bed, 50 to 100 mCi of iodine-131 should be given. Patients with uptake in the neck outside the thyroid bed should be given 100 to 200 mCi, and those with distant metastases should be given 200 to 300 mCi. A whole-body scan should be done five to seven days later; this scan may reveal regions of uptake not seen on the diagnostic scan that need to be monitored during follow-up. The latter doses are also appropriate for patients found during follow-up to have persistent or recurrent carcinoma. Most patients can be treated as outpatients, but in some states, patients who are given a high dose of iodine-131 must be hospitalized for a few days, and it may be prudent to hospitalize those who live in very confined spaces or have very young children at home. Acute complications of iodine-131 treatment include radiation sialadenitis, radiation thyroiditis, and tumor hemorrhage or edema. Later complications include transient menstrual dysfunction, testicular damage, and pulmonary fibrosis in patients with diffuse pulmonary metastases.

Thyroid Hormone Therapy

All patients with differentiated thyroid carcinoma should be treated with thyroxine, whether they were treated with iodine-131 or not, in doses that reduce thyrotropin secretion to below normal. This goal is based on the presumption that thyrotropin is a growth factor for thyroid carcinoma, as it is for normal thyroid cells, and the benefit of suppression of thyrotropin secretion is supported by some clinical observations. The limiting factor is induction of clinical manifestations of hyperthyroidism, but even doses that induce subclinical hyperthyroidism may cause cardiac dysfunction, including atrial fibrillation or osteoporosis. Therefore, the dose of thyroxine and degree of suppression of thyrotropin secretion should be varied according to tumor stage and patient age. For example, patients with stage I tumors should be given thyroxine in doses that lower their serum thyrotropin concentrations to the lower end of the normal range, whereas those with stage III tumors should be given enough thyroxine to lower the concentrations to

well below normal (0.05 mU/L if the normal range is 0.5 to 5.0 mU/L). Patients who remain disease-free for five years can be given lower doses.

External-Beam Radiation Therapy

Radiation therapy, in doses of 40 to 60 Gy, may be beneficial for palliation in patients with differentiated thyroid carcinoma but in most studies has not been associated with improved survival. The patients who are most likely to benefit are those with locally invasive tumors that could not be removed surgically or that recur locally in the neck and cannot be resected and those with metastatic disease, especially bone metastases, that cannot be destroyed by iodine-131 or do not concentrate iodine-131.

Chemotherapy

There are no effective chemotherapy regimens for patients with differentiated thyroid carcinoma. In patients with skeletal metastases, pamidronate may reduce bone pain and improve quality of life.

Follow-up of Patients with Differentiated Thyroid Carcinoma

Most recurrences of differentiated thyroid carcinoma occur in the first five years after initial treatment, but they can occur later, even decades later. After initial treatment, whether surgery alone or surgery plus iodine-131, thyroxine should be given immediately and maintained as described previously. Follow-up evaluations should include physical examination and measurements of serum thyrotropin and thyroglobulin and may include ultrasonography, X-rays, computed tomography, and iodine-123 or other radionuclide scans.

Measurements of Serum Thyroglobulin

Thyroglobulin is a unique thyroid protein, and its presence in serum indicates the presence of normal or abnormal thyroid tissue. Therefore, its presence in the serum of patients with differentiated thyroid carcinoma who have little or no normal thyroid tissue indicates the presence of carcinoma. After initial surgical and iodine-131 treatment, the serum thyroglobulin concentration should be very low (less than 1 to 3 ng/mL), both during thyroxine therapy and after it is discontinued. A value of 5 ng/mL or higher while the patient is taking thyroxine and has a low serum thyrotropin concentration suggests that tumor is present and more extensive evaluation is indicated. However, 5% to 10% of patients with tumor recurrences do not have increases in serum thyroglobulin concentrations, even after cessation of thyroxine therapy. Serum thyroglobulin cannot be measured accurately in serum containing antithyroglobulin antibodies. Approximately 25% of patients with thyroid carcinoma have high serum concentrations of these antibodies initially, but the proportion falls with time.

Imaging

The key imaging procedures for following patients with differentiated thyroid carcinoma are ultrasonography of the neck and iodine-123 scans. The latter necessitates that thyroxine therapy be withdrawn. In patients with evidence of recurrent carcinoma—for example, patients with high serum thyroglobulin concentrations who have negative iodine-123 scans—fluorodeoxyglucose (FDG) positron emission tomography (PET) scanning may identify tumor that can be resected.

Initial Follow-up (One to Five Years)

Clinical examination and measurements of serum thyrotropin and thyroglobulin should be done every six months, and neck ultrasonography should be done every six to 12 months. Thyroxine therapy should be stopped and serum thyroglobulin measured and iodine-123 imaging performed at six or 12 months in high-risk patients. Among patients with recurrent tumor, some have high serum thyroglobulin concentrations only after cessation of thyroxine therapy, and the results of serum thyroglobulin measurements and iodine-123 imaging may be discordant, so the presence of tumor might be missed if both are not done.

Later Follow-up (More Than Five Years)

Clinical examination and measurements of serum thyrotropin and thyroglobulin should be done annually, with ultrasonography or iodine-123 scanning if there is any evidence of recurrence.

Detection and Treatment of Recurrent Carcinoma

Recurrent tumor in the neck may be detected by clinical examination, ultrasonography, or rising serum thyroglobulin concentrations. Primary therapy should be surgical resection for metastases larger than 1 cm in cervical lymph nodes, followed by diagnostic iodine-123 imaging and, if possible, iodine-131 therapy. Recurrence within the thyroid bed may be associated with soft tissue, laryngeal, tracheal, or esophageal invasion and may require more extensive resection. After surgery, iodine-131 therapy or perhaps external-beam radiation therapy should be given. Recurrences elsewhere should be treated with high doses of iodine-131 if tumor uptake is demonstrable on a diagnostic scan. If the diagnostic scan is negative, a high dose of iodine-131 can still be given, on the assumption that some iodine-131 will be taken

up if the dose is very high. This often happens, as is demonstrated by post-treatment imaging. Alternatively, external-beam radiation or surgery may be indicated. Repeated high doses of iodine-131 can be given if necessary, but doses of 1000 mCi (37,000 MBq) or more have been associated with acute leukemia and other tumors.

Anaplastic Thyroid Carcinoma

Anaplastic thyroid carcinomas are undifferentiated tumors of the thyroid follicular cells. In contrast to differentiated thyroid carcinomas, they are very aggressive tumors; the median survival is three to five months, and the one-year survival rate is less than 10%. The patients are usually 50 to 80 years old, many have a long-standing history of a multinodular goiter, and approximately 25% have a history of differentiated thyroid carcinoma or a coexisting differentiated carcinoma, usually a papillary carcinoma.

Clinical Presentation and Evaluation

Most patients with anaplastic thyroid carcinomas present with an enlarging, sometimes rapidly enlarging, thyroid mass, and approximately 80% have regional disease and 50% have distant disease at the time of diagnosis. The thyroid mass is often painful and tender, and many patients have hoarseness, dyspnea, cough, or dysphagia, indicative of compression (or invasion) of the upper aerodigestive tract. The patients also may have constitutional symptoms such as fatigue, anorexia, and weight loss.

Physical examination reveals bilateral but asymmetric thyroid enlargement with a dominant mass that is hard and tender, but there may be only a solitary nodule. The tumor is usually at least 5 cm in diameter, but its borders are often indistinct. Approximately 50% of patients have enlarged cervical lymph nodes. Other findings of local extension of the disease include stridor, tracheal deviation, and vocal cord paralysis due to compression or invasion of the trachea; and venous dilatation and superior vena cava syndrome due to compression of the jugular vein. Most patients have normal serum thyroxine and thyrotropin concentrations.

The diagnosis of anaplastic carcinoma is usually established by cytologic examination of cells obtained by fine-needle aspiration biopsy or of sections of tissue obtained by large-needle or open biopsy. Ultrasonography of the neck provides information about the extent of thyroid enlargement, extrathyroidal tumor extension, and lymph node involvement. Computed tomography provides information about the extent of disease not only in the neck, but also in the mediastinum and lungs.

Treatment

There is no effective treatment for patients with anaplastic carcinoma. Patients with tumors that seem to be localized to the thyroid should be treated by thyroidectomy, because a few patients do survive for long periods, and surgery may be indicated in others for palliative debulking. External-beam radiation therapy or chemotherapy is of little benefit, although occasional patients have had temporary responses to combined radiation and chemotherapy or chemotherapy (doxorubicin, paclitaxel) alone.

Medullary Thyroid Carcinoma

Medullary thyroid carcinomas are relatively slow-growing tumors of the parafollicular, calcitonin-secreting cells (C cells) of the thyroid gland. Most of these tumors occur sporadically, but approximately 25% occur as part of one of three familial tumor syndromes: familial medullary thyroid carcinoma; multiple endocrine neoplasia (MEN) type 2A, consisting of medullary thyroid carcinoma, pheochromocytoma and primary hyperparathyroidism, and, in some families, cutaneous lichen amyloidosis; and multiple endocrine neoplasia type 2B, consisting of medullary thyroid carcinoma, pheochromocytoma, and mucosal neuromas. These familial syndromes are characterized by activating germline mutations in the *ret* proto-oncogene on chromosome 10 that codes for a tyrosine kinase. The inheritance is autosomal dominant.

Sporadic Medullary Carcinoma

Patients with sporadic medullary carcinoma are typically in their forties or fifties and present with a solitary thyroid nodule; approximately 50% have lymph node metastases at the time of diagnosis. The diagnosis of medullary carcinoma can be made on the basis of fine-needle aspiration biopsy. The characteristic findings are masses of oval or spindle-shaped cells, and the cells stain with anticalcitonin antibodies. Virtually all patients have high serum calcitonin concentrations, which have no effect on serum calcium concentrations. Once the diagnosis is confirmed, the patients should be tested for germline *ret* mutations and screened for pheochromocytoma. If a *ret* mutation is detected, their first-degree relatives, especially young relatives, should be tested for the same mutation. In studies of patients with apparently sporadic medullary carcinoma, from 5% to 20% had germline *ret* mutations.

As in patients with differentiated thyroid carcinoma, factors that indicate a poor prognosis are older age, male sex, larger size of the primary tumor, more extensive disease, and inadequate initial surgery. The overall 10- and 20-year survival rates are approximately 60% and 50%, respectively.

Familial Medullary Carcinoma and Multiple Endocrine Neoplasia Type 2

Among patients with either of these syndromes, the penetrance of medullary carcinoma, which is often multifocal, approaches 50% by age 15 years and 100% by age 30 years; carcinoma has been detected in 5-year-old children with multiple endocrine neoplasia type 2A and 1-year-old children with multiple endocrine neoplasia type 2B. The carcinomas are preceded by C cell hyperplasia, which itself is often associated with high serum calcitonin concentrations. Total thyroidectomy is curative in nearly all patients with C cell hyperplasia and in most of those with one or more microscopic medullary carcinomas.

Like patients with apparently sporadic medullary carcinoma, any patient with medullary carcinoma and pheochromocytoma should be tested for *ret* mutations. If a mutation is detected, all first-degree relatives should be tested for that mutation. In kindreds with multiple endocrine neoplasia type 2A or multiple endocrine neoplasia type 2B, the penetrance of pheochromocytoma is approximately 50%, and in multiple endocrine neoplasia type 2A kindreds, the penetrance of primary hyperparathyroidism is approximately 25%. Testing for pheochromocytoma—by measurements of blood pressure, plasma metanephrines or catecholamines, or urinary metanephrines or catecholamines—should begin before thyroidectomy and should be done annually thereafter. Primary hyperparathyroidism can be screened for adequately by periodic measurements of serum calcium.

Staging and Prognosis of Medullary Carcinoma

Patients with a thyroid nodule that is a medullary carcinoma on fine-needle aspiration biopsy should have a measurement of serum calcitonin and ultrasonography or computed tomography of the neck to look for tumor in cervical lymph nodes. If there is any evidence of extrathyroidal disease or the serum calcitonin concentration is very high, chest computed tomography should be done. Patients with inherited medullary carcinoma or those with germline mutations but no palpable thyroid abnormalities should undergo the same preoperative evaluation.

Medullary carcinomas are bilateral in approximately 25% of patients with sporadic medullary carcinoma and virtually all patients with inherited medullary carcinoma, and all the latter patients have

C cell hyperplasia. The carcinomas spread by local invasion and metastasis to cervical lymph nodes and distant sites, usually the lungs. Staging for medullary carcinoma is based on tumor size, the presence or absence of extrathyroidal invasion, and local and distant metastases (see Table 108-3). Among patients treated by total thyroidectomy, the five-year survival rate is 100% in those with stage I tumors, 85% to 90% in those with stage II tumors, 40% to 60% in those with stage III tumors, and 0% to 20% in those with stage IV tumors.

The most important prognostic factor unrelated to stage is age at the time of diagnosis. The five- and ten-year survival rates are higher among patients 40 years old or younger, compared with patients older than 40 years. Among patients of the same age, the prognosis of patients with familial medullary carcinoma and multiple endocrine neoplasia type 2A and that of patients with sporadic medullary carcinoma is similar. In contrast, in patients with multiple endocrine neoplasia type 2B, medullary carcinoma may be more aggressive, and their prognosis is poorer.

Treatment

The only effective treatment for medullary carcinoma is surgery, and cure is possible only by complete resection of the thyroid tumor and any local and regional metastases. The operation should be a total thyroidectomy, not near-total thyroidectomy as is done for patients with differentiated thyroid carcinoma, because of the C cell hyperplasia and high frequency of multifocal medullary carcinoma. The surgery should include dissection of adjacent nodal tissue in the central compartment from the hyoid bone to the innominate veins and medial to the jugular veins. One or more lateral cervical and mediastinal nodes should be excised and examined by frozen section, followed by cervical or mediastinal node dissection if the nodes contain tumor. In families with multiple endocrine neoplasia type 2A or 2B or familial medullary carcinoma, gene carriers should undergo thyroidectomy by age 5 years in families with multiple endocrine neoplasia type 2A and familial medullary carcinoma and by age 1 year in those with multiple endocrine neoplasia type 2B.

Postoperatively, patients should be followed closely for the development of hypoparathyroidism or recurrent or superior laryngeal nerve injury. Thyroxine therapy should be started immediately after surgery. The goal of thyroxine therapy is replacement, not overtreatment as is the goal for patients with differentiated carcinoma, because there is no evidence that medullary carcinomas are thyrotropin-dependent.

Follow-up and Treatment of Patients with Persistent or Recurrent Medullary Carcinoma

Patients with medullary carcinoma who have been operated on should be followed by periodic examination of the neck and measurements of serum calcitonin. Serum calcitonin concentrations should fall after surgery, but in some patients, the fall is slow, and the nadir is not reached for several months. Patients who have serum calcitonin concentrations less than 10 pg/mL six months after surgery are considered cured, whereas a higher value suggests the presence of persistent tumor.

Patients with high serum calcitonin concentrations six months or more after surgery should be evaluated for resectable disease in the neck or the presence of distant metastases. In addition to physical examination, this evaluation should include ultrasonography of the neck and computed tomography of the neck, chest, and abdomen (liver). Some medullary carcinomas have somatostatin receptors and therefore may be detected by imaging with indium-111-pentetreotide.

Patients who have no clinical or biochemical evidence of recurrence should be evaluated at six-month intervals for five years and less often thereafter. Patients with slightly high serum calcitonin concentrations in whom no tumor can be detected by imaging should be followed in the same way. In patients with persistent or recurrent tumor limited to the neck or upper mediastinum, thorough dissection and removal of all lymph nodes may result in cure.

External-beam radiation therapy, in doses of 40 to 50 Gy, may prolong the interval until disease progression or recurrence in patients with medullary carcinoma in the neck and elsewhere. Radiotherapy also can be given for palliation in patients with painful bone metastases.

Systemic chemotherapy can also be tried. Regimens that include doxorubicin, dacarbazine, or cyclophosphamide have resulted in transient objective benefit in up to 50% of patients.

Thyroid Lymphoma

Primary lymphomas of the thyroid gland account for fewer than 1% of thyroid carcinomas and fewer than 2% of extranodal lymphomas. Nearly all are non-Hodgkin's lymphomas of B cell lineage, mostly of intermediate grade. Most patients are older women who present with a rapidly enlarging goiter or, less often, a solitary nodule, the latter often superimposed on a diffuse or multinodular goiter. The majority of patients have underlying chronic autoimmune thyroiditis.

Large cell lymphomas can be identified by fine-needle aspiration biopsy. Small cell lymphomas can be difficult to distinguish from chronic autoimmune thyroiditis. Immunohistochemical studies for surface markers can be done on biopsy specimens, but it is often best to confirm the diagnosis by open biopsy. Diagnosis should be followed by staging, to determine whether the tumor is limited to the thyroid (approximately 50% of cases) or is more extensive and therefore should be treated with external-beam radiation alone or combined with chemotherapy. Combined therapy is more effective than radiation therapy alone both for patients with tumor confined to the thyroid and for those with extrathyroidal tumor, 10-year survival rates ranging from 50% to 95% in different studies (see also Chapter 68).

References

Ain KB: Anaplastic thyroid carcinoma: Behavior, biology, and therapeutic approaches. Thyroid 1998;8:715–726.

Baloch ZW, Fleischer S, LiVolsi V, Gupta PK: Diagnosis of "follicular neoplasm": A gray zone in thyroid fine-needle aspiration cytology. Diagn Cytopathol 2002;26:41–44.

Brennan MD, Bergstralh EJ, van Heerden JA, McConahey WM: Follicular thyroid cancer treated at the Mayo Clinic, 1946 through 1970: Initial manifestations, pathologic findings, and outcome. Mayo Clin Proc 1991;66:11–22.

Brierley JD, Tsang RW: External-beam radiation therapy in the treatment of differentiated thyroid cancer. Semin Surg Oncol 1999;16:42–49.

Cailleux AF, Baudin E, Travagli JP, et al: Is diagnostic iodine-131 scanning useful after total thyroid ablation for differentiated thyroid cancer? J Clin Endocrinol Metab 2000; 85:175–178.

Dottorini ME, Assi A, Sironi M, et al: Multivariate analysis of patients with medullary thyroid carcinoma: Prognostic significance and impact on treatment of clinical and pathologic variables. Cancer 1996;77:1556–1565.

Gilliland FD, Hunt WC, Morris DM, Key CR: Prognostic factors for thyroid carcinoma: A population-based study of 15,698 cases from the Surveillance, Epidemiology and End Results (SEER) program, 1973–1991. Cancer 1997;79:564–573.

Ha CS, Shadle KM, Medeiros LJ, et al: Localized non-Hodgkin's involving the thyroid gland. Cancer 2001;91:629–635.

Hay ID, Grant CS, Bergstralh EJ, et al: Unilateral total lobectomy: Is it sufficient surgical treatment for patients with AMES low-risk papillary thyroid carcinoma? Surgery 1998; 124:958–966.

Hundahl SA, Cady B, Cunningham MP, et al: Initial results from a prospective cohort study of 5583 cases of thyroid carcinoma treated in the United States during 1996: An American College of Surgeons Commission on Cancer Patient Care Evaluation Study. Cancer 2000;89:202–217.

Hundahl SA, Fleming ID, Fremgen AM, et al: A National Cancer Data Base Report on 53,856 cases of thyroid carcinoma treated in the United States, 1985–1995. Cancer 1998;83: 2638–2648.

Kitamura Y, Shimizu K, Nagahama M, et al: Immediate causes of death in thyroid carcinoma: Clinicopathological analysis of 161 fatal cases. J Clin Endocrinol Metab 1999;84:4043–4049.

Ladenson PW, Braverman LE, Mazzaferri EL, et al: Comparison of administration of recombinant human thyrotropin with withdrawal of thyroid hormone in patients with thyroid carcinoma. N Engl J Med 1997;337:888–896.

Loh K-C, Greenspan FS, Gee L, et al: Pathological tumor-node-metastasis (pTNM) staging for papillary and follicular thyroid carcinomas: A retrospective analysis of 700 patients. J Clin Endocrinol Metab 1997;82:3553–3562.

Mazzaferri E: NCCN thyroid carcinoma practice guidelines. Oncology (NCCN Proceedings) 1999;13:391–442.

Mazzaferri EL, Kloos RT: Current approaches to primary therapy for papillary and follicular thyroid cancer. J Clin Endocrinol Metab 2001;86:1447–1463.

McIver B, Hay ID, Giuffrida DF, et al: Anaplastic thyroid carcinoma: A 50-year experience at a single institution. Surgery 2001;130:1020–1034.

Pujol P, Daures JP, Nsakala N, et al: Degree of thyrotropin suppression as a prognostic determinant in differentiated thyroid cancer. J Clin Endocrinol Metab 1996;81:4318–4323.

Puxeddu E, Fagin JA: Genetic markers in thyroid neoplasia. Endocrinol Metab Clin North Am 2001;30:493–513.

Ravetto C, Columbo L, Dottorini ME: Usefulness of fine-needle aspiration in the diagnosis of thyroid carcinoma: A retrospective study in 37,895 patients. Cancer (Cancer Cytopathol) 2000;90:357–363.

Schlumberger MJ: Papillary and follicular thyroid carcinoma. N Engl J Med 1998;338:297–306.

Schlumberger MJ, Tubiana M, de Vathaire F, et al: Long-term results of treatment of 283 patients with lung and bone metastases from differentiated thyroid cancer. J Clin Endocrinol Metab 1986;63:960–967.

Scopsi L, Sampietro G, Boracchi P, et al: Multivariate analysis of prognostic factors in sporadic medullary carcinoma of the thyroid. Cancer 1996;78:2173–2183.

Sherman SI, Brierley JD, Sperling M, et al: Prospective multicenter study of thyroid carcinoma treatment: Initial analysis of staging and outcome. Cancer 1998;83:1012–1021.

Taylor T, Specker B, Robbins J, et al: Outcome after treatment of high-risk papillary and non–Hurthle cell follicular thyroid carcinoma. Ann Intern Med 1998;129:622–627.

Thieblemont C, Mayer A, Dumontet Y, et al: Primary thyroid lymphoma is a heterogeneous disease. J Clin Endocrinol Metab 2002;87:105–111.

Wang W, Larson SM, Fazzari M, et al: Prognostic value of [18F]fluorodeoxyglucose positron emission tomographic scanning in patients with thyroid cancer. J Clin Endocrinol Metab 2000;85:1107–1113.

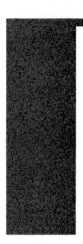

Chapter 109
Adrenal Cancer

William K. Oh

Cancers of the adrenal cortex are extremely rare, with an annual incidence estimated at 0.5 to 2 cases per million. They account for only 0.2% of all cancer deaths in the United States. There is a slight preponderance of diagnoses in women, and although adrenocortical cancers have been described in children, most cases have been described in adults aged 30 to 50 years. Patients with adrenocortical cancers may present with symptoms of hormonal excess or mass effect in the abdomen. Most are diagnosed at a late stage, at which point cancer is often surgically unresectable and the prognosis poor. The etiology of adrenocortical carcinomas is unknown, though mutations in tumor suppressor genes such as p53 and rb have been found in some adrenocortical cancers.

Clinical Presentation

Signs and Symptoms

About one half of the patients who are diagnosed present with hormonally functional tumors. This may be manifest as Cushing's syndrome, virilization in women, feminization in men, primary aldosteronism, or some combination. Most commonly, patients present with a several-month history of progressive cortisol excess, including weight gain, fatigue, easy bruisability, weakness, and irritability. Frequently, women also will complain of concomitant virilization, with hirsutism, male pattern hair loss, and irregular menses, symptoms suggesting an excess of sex steroids. Similarly, estrogen-producing tumors in men may cause feminizing symptoms such as gynecomastia, although this is less common. Excess production of aldosterone is rare but can lead to hypertension and hypokalemia. Nonfunctional tumors usually present with symptoms of local tumor growth, including abdominal or back pain, weight loss, or a palpable mass. Some nonfunctional tumors are detected incidentally during the course of unrelated radiographic studies.

Laboratory Testing

Biochemical evaluation typically demonstrates elevated levels of free cortisol and/or 17-ketosteroids in a 24-hour urine collection. Serum cortisol, testosterone, estradiol, andrenal androgens (androstenedione, DHEA-S), and aldosterone levels may be elevated in the appropriate clinical setting. Characteristically, these elevated steroid levels are not suppressed by the administration of low doses or high doses of dexamethasone.

Radiographic Findings

Adrenocortical masses are among the most common in humans. However, the vast majority has no clinical significance, and fewer than 1% are malignant. Though the management of incidentally discovered sized adrenal masses remains controversial, several guidelines are generally accepted. If hormonally active, an adrenal mass of any size should be resected, though the majority of these will not be malignant. Any nonfunctional adrenal mass under 3 cm can be monitored with serial computed tomography (CT) scans, while tumors over 6 cm should be resected, since the risk of carcinoma increases with size. Controversy exists about the optimal management for masses between 3 and 6 cm in size.

Contrast-enhanced computed tomography scans of the abdomen usually can distinguish between adenomas and cancers. In general, carcinomas are large, inhomogeneous with areas of necrosis and sometimes demonstrate invasion into the kidney, liver, or inferior vena cava. Metastatic disease may be evident on computed tomography scan, involving liver, lymph nodes, lung, and bone. In one study, patients with symptomatic nonfunctioning cancers presented with masses whose mean diameter was 17 cm.

Magnetic resonance imaging (MRI) offers some advantages over computed tomography scanning, including an enhanced ability to visualize invasion of adjacent blood vessels and other organs. This is of particular value in planning the surgical approach. Other studies have shown that magnetic resonance imaging is accurate in distinguishing carcinomas from adenomas. Other imaging techniques, including ultrasound and iodocholesterol scintigraphy, have a less established role.

Pathology and Staging

Pathology

Pathologic distinction between adrenocortical adenomas and carcinomas can be difficult. Features such as a high mitotic rate, atypical mitotic features, necrosis, high nuclear grade, and venous or capsular penetration can usually distinguish the two (Weiss criteria), but sufficient pathologic material is necessary for this distinction to be made. A high mitotic rate may also signify a poor prognosis.

Staging

The most commonly used staging system, the modified Macfarlane classification, is based on tumor size and extent of disease. Patients with stage I disease have tumors less than 5 cm and no evidence of lymph node or distant metastases, while stage II tumors are greater than 5 cm. Stage III disease includes patients with local or regional involvement of any size, and stage IV disease includes patients with distant metastases. Patients historically presented with stage III or IV disease in over two thirds of cases, but recent series suggest that as many as one half of new presentations are organ-confined at diagnosis.

Treatment

Surgery

Surgical resection remains the principal treatment for stage I to III disease. Even in patients for whom complete resection is not possible, surgical debulking should be strongly considered for palliation of hormonal and local symptoms, as well as to optimize the likelihood of a systemic treatment response. Cases of patients with prolonged disease-free periods after aggressive surgical resection of metastases have been reported.

Radiation

Though no recent studies have evaluated its efficacy, adrenocortical carcinomas are considered relatively radioresistant.

Chemotherapy

The standard of care for the medical management of metastatic or locally advanced adrenocortical carcinoma is mitotane. Also known as o,p-DDD, mitotane is related to the insecticide DDT. The mechanism of action of mitotane is unknown, but it has been shown to inhibit adrenocorticol function and is cytotoxic to the adrenal cortex. In patients treated with mitotane, 35% had at least a partial response in measurable lesions. The duration of response was extremely variable, but was generally less than one year. However, some long-term responders have been reported. Also, mitotane can decrease urinary steroid levels in up to 75% of patients. It is not known whether mitotane improves survival. Its value as adjuvant therapy after surgical resection in high-risk patients has also never been assessed.

Mitotane causes significant toxicity. Nearly all patients develop adrenal insufficiency and require replacement steroids. Anorexia, nausea, vomiting, and diarrhea are common, occurring in 80% of patients. Neurologic toxicity, including lethargy and dizziness, occurs in 40%, and skin rash occurs in 15%. The optimal dosing of mitotane is controversial. Initially, 1 to 6 grams orally per day in three or four divided doses is prescribed. Patients are often started at a lower dose and escalated to the maximum tolerated dose, which ranges from 2 to 16 grams per day. Several groups have recommended mitotane dosing based on serum levels rather than on toxicity. In one patient series, serum mitotane levels over 14 µg/mL were associated with an objective response in seven of eight patients, while only one of 20 patients had regression with mitotane levels below 14 µg/mL. Another group recently suggested that low doses of mitotane (2 to 3 grams per day) could achieve serum levels of 14 µg/mL within three months, though others have suggested that at least 6 grams per day is necessary to achieve this level.

Cytotoxic chemotherapy has modest benefit in the treatment of advanced adrenocortical carcinoma. Patients treated with cisplatin plus mitotane, along with replacement cortisone and fludrocortisone, had objective responses in 30%. Response duration was nearly eight months, and median survival was 12 months. Moderate to severe gastrointestinal, renal, and neurologic toxicity was seen. Another trial evaluated cisplatin and etoposide followed by mitotane. At progression, patients who had previously not been treated with mitotane were eligible to receive mitotane. Only 11% responded to cisplatin plus etoposide, and median survival was 10 months. Of patients who had not received prior mitotane therapy, 13% responded. Toxicity of the regimen was signifi-

TREATMENT

Mitotane Therapy

Mitotane is best begun by administering it as an escalating dose on a weekly basis. The patient is given 1 gm orally twice daily initially, and then the dose increased by 1 gm daily each succeeding week, as long as toxicity does not supervene. Thus, by the beginning of the fourth week, the patient will be taking 4 gm daily. An attempt should be made to use the highest tolerable dose, but most patients are not able to tolerate more than 6 to 8 gm per day. Routine testing of serum mitotane levels may be useful in monitoring for acceptable levels. Frequent consultation with an endocrinologist and surgeon is invaluable.

Because single agent mitotane is of limited benefit, combination therapy is worth attempting in patients with metastatic disease if it can be safely given. Based on limited phase II clinical trial data, the combination of etoposide, cisplatin, doxorubicin, and mitotane may be more useful than mitotane alone.

cant, including two treatment-related deaths. Cisplatin plus etoposide had low activity through the concurrent use of mitotane might increase response rates.

Two recent trials have evaluated mitotane given concurrently with combination chemotherapy. Patients were treated with cisplatin and etoposide initially, and mitotane treatment was maintained during chemotherapy. The total response rate was 33%. Patients who were treated with doxorubicin and cisplatin and etoposide plus daily mitotane had a response rate of 53%. Time to progression was 24 months. Treatment was well tolerated, with mostly mild to moderate gastrointestinal, neurologic, and hematologic toxicity. This latter regimen is among the most promising combinations available.

Supportive Care Issues

Mitotane is adrenolytic, and therefore treatment eventually will require the use of replacement physiologic cortisol (hydrocortisone 25 to 40 mg daily) and, with higher mitotane doses, replacement mineralocorticoid, fludrocortisone acetate 0.1 mg daily. Replacement therapy should usually be initiated as urinary free cortisol levels begin to decrease with mitotane. Treatment of hormonal excess can also be accomplished by the use of adrenal steroid inhibitors, including ketoconazole and aminoglutethimide. Both can decrease steroid production by the adrenal gland and can rapidly diminish the symptoms of steroid excess. Ketoconazole is used in doses of 200 mg 1 to 3 times per day and can cause nausea, vomiting, diarrhea, and abdominal pain. Adrenal insufficiency is uncommon at such doses. Aminoglutethimide is used in doses of 500 to 2000 mg/day and often requires cortisol replacement. Side effects include nausea, vomiting, lethargy, and skin rash.

Prognosis

The overall survival rate for adrenocortical carcinomas remains poor, ranging between 25% and 50% at five years. Outcomes for patients with stage I and II disease are significantly better than for those with stage III or IV disease. In one series, the five-year actuarial survival rate for stage I and II disease was 54%, that for stage III was 21%, and that for stage IV was 6.5%. Median survival for patients with metastatic disease is approximately one year.

Follow-up Recommendations

Recurrence after resection of the primary adrenocortical tumor is common. Over 70% of patients recur after a median follow-up of 17 months. Though the majority recur in multiple distant sites, some patients have had isolated recurrences in the liver or lung. Subsequent surgical resection of metastases led to long-term remissions. Because further surgery may influence survival, frequent follow-up visits after surgical resection are warranted, with 24-hour urinary free cortisol and 17-ketosteroid levels and computed tomography or magnetic resonance imaging scans of the chest and abdomen repeated every three to four months in the first two years. After that point, scans and hormonal evaluations can be gradually decreased in frequency but are generally continued even beyond five years.

References

Barzon L, Fallo F, Sonino N, Daniele O, Boscaro M: Adrenocortical carcinoma: Experience in 45 patients. Oncology 1997;54:490–496.

Bellantone R, Ferrante A, Boscherini M, et al: Role of reoperation in recurrence of adrenal cortical carcinoma: Results from 188 cases collected in the Italian National Registry for

Adrenal Cortical Carcinoma. Surgery 1997;122:1212–1218.

Berruti A, Terzolo M, Pia A, Angeli A, Dogliotti L: Mitotane associated with etoposide, doxorubicin, and cisplatin in the treatment of advanced adrenocortical carcinoma: Italian Group for the Study of Adrenal Cancer. Cancer 1998;83:2194–2200.

Bonacci R, Gigliotti A, Baudin E, et al: Cytotoxic therapy with etoposide and cisplatin in advanced adrenocortical carcinoma: Reseau Comete INSERM. Br J Cancer 1998;78:546–549.

Bornstein SR, Stratakis CA, Chrousos GP: Adrenocortical tumors: Recent advances in basic concepts and clinical management. Ann Intern Med 1999;130:759–771.

Brennan MF: Adrenocortical carcinoma. CA Cancer J Clin 1987;37:348–365.

Bukowski RM, Wolfe M, Levine HS, et al: Phase II trial of mitotane and cisplatin in patients with adrenal carcinoma: A Southwest Oncology Group study. J Clin Oncol 1993;11:161–165.

Crucitti F, Bellantone R, Ferrante A, et al: The Italian Registry for Adrenal Cortical Carcinoma: Analysis of a multi-institutional series of 129 patients. The ACC Italian Registry Study Group. Surgery 1996;119:161–170.

Dickstein G, Shechner C, Arad E, et al: Is there a role for low doses of mitotane (o,p′-DDD) as adjuvant therapy in adrenocortical carcinoma? J Clin Endocrinol Metab 1998;83:3100–3103.

Evans HL, Vassilopoulou-Sellin R: Adrenal cortical neoplasms: A study of 56 cases. Am J Clin Pathol 1996;105:76–86.

Haak HR, Hermans J, van de Velde CJ, et al: Optimal treatment of adrenocortical carcinoma with mitotane: Results in a consecutive series of 96 patients. Br J Cancer 1994;69:947–951.

Jensen JC, Pass HI, Sindelar WF, Norton JA: Recurrent or metastatic disease in select patients with adrenocortical carcinoma: Aggressive resection vs chemotherapy. Arch Surg 1991;126:457–461.

Kasperlik-Zaluska AA, Migdalska BM, Zgliczynski S, Makowska AM: Adrenocortical carcinoma: A clinical study and treatment results of 52 patients. Cancer 1995;75:2587–2591.

Kendrick ML, Lloyd R, Erickson L, et al: Adrenocortical carcinoma: Surgical progress or status quo? Arch Surg 2001;136:543–549.

Luton JP, Cerdas S, Billaud L, et al: Clinical features of adrenocortical carcinoma, prognostic factors, and the effect of mitotane therapy. N Engl J Med 1990;322:1195–1201.

Prinz RA, Brooks MH, Churchill R, et al: Incidental asymptomatic adrenal masses detected by computed tomographic scanning: Is operation required? JAMA 1982;248:701–704.

Ross NS, Aron DC: Hormonal evaluation of the patient with an incidentally discovered adrenal mass. N Engl J Med 1990;323:1401–1405.

Schulick RD, Brennan MF: Long-term survival after complete resection and repeat resection in patients with adrenocortical carcinoma. Ann Surg Oncol 1999;6:719–726.

Schulick RD, Brennan MF: Adrenocortical carcinoma. World J Urol 1999;17:26–34.

Sullivan M, Boileau M, Hodges CV: Adrenal cortical carcinoma. J Urol 1978;120:660–665.

Terzolo M, Pia A, Berruti A, et al: Low-dose monitored mitotane treatment achieves the therapeutic range with manageable side effects in patients with adrenocortical cancer. J Clin Endocrinol Metab 2000;85:2234–2238.

Wajchenberg BL, Albergaria Pereira MA, Medonca BB, et al: Adrenocortical carcinoma: Clinical and laboratory observations. Cancer 2000;88:711–736.

Weiss LM, Medeiros LJ, Vickery AL, Jr: Pathologic features of prognostic significance in adrenocortical carcinoma. Am J Surg Pathol 1989;13:202–206.

Williamson SK, Lew D, Miller GJ, et al: Phase II evaluation of cisplatin and etoposide followed by mitotane at disease progression in patients with locally advanced or metastatic adrenocortical carcinoma: A Southwest Oncology Group Study. Cancer 2000;88:1159–1165.

Wooten MD, King DK: Adrenal cortical carcinoma: Epidemiology and treatment with mitotane and a review of the literature. Cancer 1993;72:3145–3155.

Chapter 110
Neuroendocrine Cancer

Matthew H. Kulke

Neuroendocrine tumors are generally classified into two groups: carcinoid tumors and pancreatic endocrine tumors. Both tumor types are thought to arise from neuroendocrine cells, and they are often histologically indistinguishable. These tumors are typically composed of small cells containing regular, well-rounded nuclei. The cytoplasm of these cells contains numerous membrane-bound neurosecretory granules, which contain a variety of hormones and biogenic amines. The release of these substances into the systemic circulation results in the unique systemic syndromes associated with neuroendocrine tumors. Differences in these systemic syndromes, as well as differences in the location of the primary tumor, account for the diverse clinical presentations of patients with carcinoid and pancreatic endocrine tumors.

Carcinoid Tumors

Carcinoid tumors occur in one to two individuals per 100,000 per year. They may originate anywhere in the body but most commonly develop in the bronchi, stomach, small intestine, appendix, or rectum. The clinical and biologic characteristics of the tumors may vary considerably depending on their site of origin. A commonly used classification scheme groups carcinoid tumors according to their presumed embryonic site of origin: foregut (bronchial and gastric carcinoids), midgut (small intestine and appendiceal carcinoids), and hindgut (rectal carcinoids) (Table 110-1).

Bronchial Carcinoid Tumors

Bronchial carcinoids comprise approximately 2% of primary lung tumors and most commonly occur in individuals in the fifth decade of life. They often arise in the proximal bronchi and consequently may be associated with symptoms of cough, hemoptysis, or recurrent pneumonia. Neuroendocrine manifestations are relatively uncommon. When present, these man-ifestations may include ectopic secretion of corticotropin, resulting in Cushing's syndrome. Bronchial carcinoid tumors can usually be successfully treated with conservative procedures such as wedge or segmental resection. These procedures are associated with low rates of local recurrence and excellent long-term survival rates.

Approximately one third of bronchial carcinoid tumors have atypical histologic features. In comparison to typical carcinoid tumors, these tumors have increased nuclear pleomorphism and higher mitotic activity and may contain areas of necrosis. More aggressive surgical procedures have been advocated for such atypical tumors. Despite such procedures, distant recurrence is common, and the five-year survival rate following resection is only approximately 50%.

Gastric Carcinoid Tumors

Gastric carcinoid tumors make up fewer than 1% of gastric neoplasms. They can be classified into three distinct groups: those associated with chronic atrophic gastritis type A (CAG-A), those associated with Zollinger-Ellison syndrome, and sporadic gastric carcinoids. Both type I (chronic atrophic gastritis type A–associated gastric carcinoids) and type II (Zollinger-Ellison syndrome–associated gastric carcinoids) are associated with hypergastrinemia. High levels of gastrin are thought to result in hyperplasia of enterochromaffinlike cells in the gastric mucosa; these areas of hyperplasia may ultimately develop into carcinoid tumors. Both type I and type II gastric carcinoids are often small and multifocal. Lesions measuring less than 1 cm in diameter can be treated with endoscopic resection followed by close endoscopic surveillance. Gastric carcinoids associated with hypergastrinemia tend to follow an indolent course, and metastatic spread of disease is extremely rare. For larger lesions, antrectomy and treatment with somatostatin analogs results in tumor regression in selected cases.

Table 110-1 ■ Neuroendocrine Tumors: Clinical Presentation

Carcinoid Tumors

Foregut

Bronchial carcinoids	Cough, hemoptysis, postobstructive pneumonia, Cushing's syndrome. Carcinoid syndrome rare.
Gastric carcinoids	Usually asymptomatic and found incidentally.

Midgut

Small intestine carcinoids	Intermittent bowel obstruction or mesenteric ischemia. Carcinoid syndrome common when metastatic.
Appendiceal carcinoids	Usually found incidentally. May cause carcinoid syndrome when metastatic.

Hindgut

Rectal carcinoids	Either found incidentally or discovered due to bleeding, pain, and constipation. Rarely cause hormonal symptoms, even when metastatic.

Pancreatic Endocrine Tumors

Insulinoma	Symptoms of hypoglycemia: intermittent confusion, sweating, weakness, nausea.
Glucagonoma	Necrotizing migratory erythema, cachexia, diabetes.
VIPoma	Secretory diarrhea, electrolyte disturbances.
Gastrinoma	Acid hypersecretion: peptic ulcer disease, esophageal reflux, diarrhea.
Somatostatinoma	Diabetes, diarrhea, cholelithiasis.
PPoma	"Nonfunctioning"; may be first diagnosed owing to mass effect.

In contrast to type I and type II gastric carcinoids, sporadic (type III) gastric carcinoids develop in the absence of hypergastrinemia and tend to pursue an aggressive clinical course. These lesions are usually solitary and often measure more than 1 cm in diameter. The majority of these tumors are metastatic at the time of presentation. Those that remain localized should be treated with radical gastrectomy.

Carcinoid Tumors of the Small Intestine

Small bowel carcinoid tumors make up approximately one third of all small bowel tumors. They are classically multicentric and located in the distal ileum. Patients with small bowel carcinoids may present with a long history of abdominal pain or intermittent small bowel obstruction, often initially attributed to irritable bowel syndrome. Because of their submucosal location, standard imaging techniques such as computed

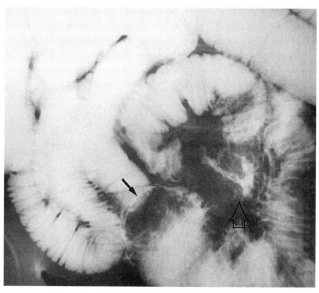

Figure 110-1 ■ Ileal carcinoid. Enteroclysis shows luminal narrowing and marked distortion of the bowel contour (*open arrow*). A carcinoid tumor is depicted as a circular mass defect (*arrow*). (From Lappas JC, Maglinte DDT: Small bowel cancer. In Bragg DG, Rubin P, Hricak H [eds]: Oncologic Imaging, 2nd ed. Philadelphia: WB Saunders, 2002, pp 419–433.)

tomography (CT) scan, endoscopy, and small bowel follow-through often fail to detect these lesions (Figure 110-1). At the time they are detected, they are frequently associated with extensive mesenteric fibrosis and metastases to local lymph nodes or liver (Figure 110-2). Small bowel resection is usually

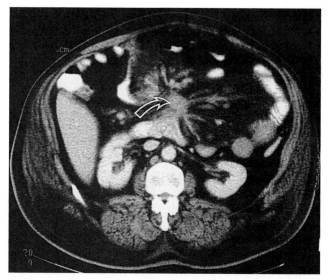

Figure 110-2 ■ Metastatic carcinoid. Computed tomography shows a mesenteric mass (*arrow*) with fibrotic strands extending from the mass that represent the typical desmoplastic response. (From Lappas JC, Maglinte DDT: Small bowel cancer. In Bragg DG, Rubin P, Hricak H [eds]): Oncologic Imaging, 2nd ed. Philadelphia: WB Saunders, 2002, pp 419–433.)

undertaken, even in the presence of metastatic disease, for palliative purposes.

Appendiceal Carcinoid Tumors

Carcinoid tumors are the most common cancers of the appendix. They are often diagnosed in younger individuals, in the fourth or fifth decade of life, and are usually found incidentally during appendectomy for other reasons. Tumor size is the best predictor of prognosis in patients with appendiceal carcinoid tumors. The vast majority of appendiceal carcinoid tumors measure less than 2 cm in diameter. Metastases are extraordinarily uncommon in such tumors, and simple appendectomy is nearly always curative. In contrast, approximately one third of patients with appendiceal carcinoids greater than 2 cm in diameter have nodal or even distant metastases. Most patients with tumors measuring more than 2 cm are treated with right hemicolectomy.

Rectal Carcinoid Tumors

Rectal carcinoid tumors make up 1% to 2% of all rectal tumors. Approximately 50% are asymptomatic and are found during routine endosocopy; patients who have symptoms usually experience rectal bleeding, pain, or constipation. As with appendiceal carcinoids, size is an accurate predictor of prognosis in patients with rectal carcinoids. Patients with tumors measuring less than 2 cm in diameter can be successfully treated with local excision, which is nearly always curative. Tumors measuring more than 2 cm in diameter are generally treated with either low anterior resection or abdominoperineal resection. Despite the use of radical resection in such cases, distant metastases occur in the majority of patients, and the prognosis for such patients is poor.

Pancreatic Endocrine Tumors

Pancreatic endocrine tumors occur in three to four individuals per million per year. These tumors may arise sporadically or, less commonly, in patients with multiple endocrine neoplasia type I (MEN I). This autosomal-dominant inherited syndrome is associated with loss of chromosome 11q13 and is characterized by a high incidence of pancreatic endocrine tumors, as well as tumors involving the pituitary and parathyroid glands. The clinical presentations of pancreatic endocrine tumors are diverse and most often related to symptoms of hormonal hypersecretion (Table 110-2). The best-characterized of these syndromes are those associated with insulinoma, glucagonoma, VIPoma, and gastrinoma.

Table 110-2 ■ Hormone Levels in Neuroendocrine Tumors

Tumor	Typical Hormone Level
Carcinoid tumor	24-hour urinary 5HIAA > 24 mg/dL*
Insulinoma	Fasting insulin $\geq$ 6 µU/mL
Glucagonoma	Fasting glucagon $\geq$ 50 pmol/L
VIPoma	Fasting VIP > 200 pg/mL
Gastrinoma	Fasting gastrin > 100 pg/mL
Somatostatinoma	Somatostatin > 100 pg/mL

*24-hour urinary 5HIAA is most commonly elevated in patients with metastatic small bowel or appendiceal carcinoids and only rarely elevated in patients with bronchial, gastric, or rectal carcinoids.

One of the first described patients with insulinoma is said to have "resembled an acute alcoholic—great motor activity, dancing and talking, squinting and frowning, apparently having hallucinations of sight and hearing, negativistic, and difficult to control." These symptoms are the classic manifestations of hypoglycemia, which typically can cause not only central nervous system dysfunction but also autonomic symptoms such as sweating, weakness, and nausea. The combination of symptoms of hypoglycemia, a documented blood glucose level of less than 50 mg/dL, and relief of symptoms with administration of glucose constitutes *Whipple's triad,* first described in 1935 and still useful in the diagnosis of insulinoma.

Although glucagonomas may be associated with diabetes mellitus, clinically significant hyperglycemia occurs in just over half of such patients. Patients with glucagonomas are in fact most frequently diagnosed by a dermatologist after presenting with necrolytic migratory erythema. This rash, characterized by raised erythematous patches beginning in the perineum and subsequently involving the trunk and extremities, is found in nearly 75% of all patients. Patients with the glucagonoma syndrome may also experience profound cachexia. A tendency for patients with glucagonoma to develop venous thrombosis makes perioperative anticoagulation mandatory.

Pancreatic tumors that secrete vasoactive intestinal peptide (VIPomas) classically cause a syndrome characterized by watery diarrhea, hypokalemia, hypochlorhydria, and acidosis, hence the occasionally used acronym *WDHA syndrome.* Others have referred to this syndrome as *pancreatic cholera.* Like the cholera toxin, VIP causes intracellular elevation of cyclic AMP, resulting in inhibition of electrolyte absorption and profound secretory diarrhea.

The gastrinoma syndrome is characterized by gastric hypersecretion. Gastrin, which is normally secreted by the G cells in the gastric antrum, not only stimulates acid secretion in parietal cells, but also acts as a trophic factor, causing parietal cell hyperplasia. The net effect is an increase in both basal and maximal acid output. The profound acid hypersecretion associated with gastrinomas typically causes abdominal pain due to peptic ulcer disease or reflux esophagitis. Diarrhea also occurs in more than half of patients.

In contrast to other pancreatic endocrine tumors, gastrinomas occur more commonly outside the pancreas than within it. The overwhelming majority of gastrinomas are found in the *gastrinoma triangle*, an area bounded by the cystic and common bile ducts, the duodenum, and the pancreas. Recent surgical series have found that within this area, over half of gastrinomas are found in the duodenum.

Two other types of pancreatic endocrine tumor have been somewhat less well characterized. The first of these, somatostatinomas, may be associated with diabetes, hypochlorhydria, and diarrhea. PPomas are pancreatic neuroendocrine tumors associated with high serum levels of pancreatic polypeptide. Secretion of pancreatic polypeptide is not associated with any clinical syndrome; these tumors are therefore generally classified as *nonfunctioning* pancreatic endocrine tumors. They are usually first diagnosed when they grow large enough to cause symptoms from tumor bulk.

The initial medical management of pancreatic endocrine tumors centers on control of the symptoms of hormonal hypersecretion (Table 110-3). Administration of somatostatin analogs such as octreotide is often highly effective in controlling the symptoms of VIPoma as well as glucagonoma. Its efficacy is somewhat less predictable in the treatment of patients with insulinomas and gastrinomas. Patients with insulinomas more reliably benefit from administration of car-

bohydrates and the use of diazoxide, which directly inhibits the release of insulin from insulinoma cells. Patients with gastrinomas often achieve excellent symptomatic relief simply with the use of proton pump inhibitors.

The localization of pancreatic endocrine tumors often presents a clinical challenge, since these tumors may be physically small yet still cause profound hormonal symptoms. Invasive studies such as angiography and portal venous sampling are highly sensitive but have more recently been largely replaced with other, less invasive imaging techniques. In cases in which conventional modalities such as computed tomography scan and magnetic resonance imaging (MRI) fail, endoscopic ultrasound, with a reported sensitivity in excess of 80%, may be useful. Somatostatin scintigraphy detects 70% of pancreatic endocrine tumors and may detect not only occult primary tumors, but also previously unsuspected metastatic disease. Once localized, pancreatic endocrine tumors are usually successfully treated with either enucleation (in the case of smaller tumors), pancreaticoduodenectomy (for tumors in the pancreatic head), or distal pancreatectomy (for tumors in the tail of the pancreas).

Metastatic Neuroendocrine Tumors

The clinical course of patients with metastatic neuroendocrine tumors is highly variable, and some patients with indolent tumors may remain free of symptoms for years. Asymptomatic patients with metastatic neuroendocrine tumors can occasionally be followed for years without treatment. In most cases, metastatic lesions can easily be followed by conventional computed tomography scan. In patients with metastatic carcinoid tumors, measurements of the serotonin metabolite 5-HIAA in 24-hour urine collections may also be useful in confirming the diagnosis and in the subsequent monitoring of patients.

It is not uncommon for patients with metastatic disease to first become symptomatic from symptoms of hormonal hypersecretion rather than from symptoms related to tumor bulk. This is especially true for patients with small bowel or appendiceal carcinoid tumors, who generally do not experience systemic symptoms unless metastases to the liver are present. In these patients, the secretion of serotonin and other vasoactive substances into the systemic circulation results in the carcinoid syndrome, which is manifested by episodic flushing, wheezing, and diarrhea and the eventual development of carcinoid heart disease.

The carcinoid syndrome can often be well controlled with somatostatin analogs. In an initial study, subcutaneous administration of octreotide at a dosage

Table 110-3 ▪ Medical Management of Hormonal Symptoms in Patients with Neuroendocrine Tumors

Symptom	Treatment
Carcinoid syndrome	Somatostatin analogs, interferon-alpha
Insulinoma	Diazoxide, administration of carbohydrates, somatostatin analogs (benefit less predictable)
Glucagonoma	Somatostatin analogs, amino acid infusion
VIPoma	Somatostatin analogs, administration of IV fluids
Gastrinoma	Proton pump inhibitors, somatostatin analogs (benefit less predictable)
Somatostatinoma	Not available

of 150 μg three times a day improved symptoms of the carcinoid syndrome in 88% of patients. A long-acting depot form of octreotide, which can be administered on a monthly basis, is now commonly used to manage symptoms of hormonal secretion associated with both carcinoid and pancreatic endocrine tumors.

The successful use of somatostatin analogs to control the carcinoid syndrome has led to increased interest in the management of carcinoid heart disease. Carcinoid heart disease occurs in two thirds of patients with the carcinoid syndrome and is characterized by the development of plaquelike endocardial thickening involving the right side of the heart. Tricuspid regurgitation is a nearly universal finding and, when severe, may lead to right-sided heart failure. Valvular replacement should be considered in patients who have significant symptoms from their valvular disease and in whom the other manifestations of hormonal hypersecretion are well controlled.

Interferon-alpha (IFN-α) has been reported to result in improved symptoms of hormonal hypersecretion in 40% to 50% of patients with the carcinoid syndrome and in tumor regression in approximately 15% of patients. The addition of IFN-α to therapy with somatostatin analogs has also been effective in controlling the symptoms of patients whose symptoms are resistant to somatostatin analogs. A high rate of side effects, which may include fever, fatigue, anorexia, weight loss, and depression, has limited the routine use of IFN-α in this setting.

The surgical resection of liver metastases may be of benefit to patients with limited hepatic metastases from either carcinoid or pancreatic endocrine tumors. Such surgery has resulted in the long-term relief of symptoms and prolonged survival in highly selected patients. Hepatic arterial embolization is an alternative for patients who are not candidates for hepatic resection. Unfortunately, the duration of response following hepatic artery embolization is often short. In one study of patients with metastatic pancreatic endocrine or carcinoid tumors, objective regressions were observed in 60% of patients, but the duration of response was only four months.

Cytotoxic therapy has played only a limited role in the management of patients with metastatic neuroendocrine tumors. Cytotoxic therapy appears to be most useful in patients with more aggressive, atypical neuroendocrine tumors. In one study, a combination of cisplatin and etoposide produced a 67% response rate in such patients. Cytotoxic therapy also appears to be beneficial in the treatment of pancreatic endocrine tumors. In an initial randomized study involving patients with metastatic pancreatic endocrine tumors, the combination of streptozotocin and 5-fluorouracil was shown to be superior to streptozotocin alone, with response rates of 36% and 33%, respectively. A subsequent study demonstrated that the combination of streptozotocin and doxorubicin resulted in a response rate of 69%, whereas the combination of streptozotocin and 5-fluorouracil resulted in responses in only 45% of patients. An analysis of patients with pancreatic endocrine tumors treated with a combination of streptozotocin and doxorubicin found a true radiologic response rate of less than 10%.

Trials have shown only minor activity associated with cytotoxic chemotherapy in the treatment of patients with metastatic carcinoid tumors. Patients with metastatic carcinoid tumors assigned to receive either streptozotocin combined with 5-fluorouracil or streptozotocin combined with cyclophosphamide had response rates, measured by either tumor regression or a decrease in urinary 5-HIAA levels, of 33% for streptozotocin/5-fluorouracil and 26% for streptozotocin/cyclophosphamide. There was no difference in survival between the two treatment groups.

References

Arnold R, Frank M: Gastrointestinal endocrine tumors: Medical management. Baillieres Clin Gastroenterol 1996;10:737–759.

Cheng P, Saltz L: Failure to confirm major objective antitumor activity for streptozocin and doxorubicin in the treatment of patients with advanced islet cell carcinoma. Cancer 1999;86:944–948.

Engstrom PF, Lavin PT, Moertel CG, et al: Streptozocin plus fluorouracil versus doxorubicin therapy for metastatic carcinoid tumor. J Clin Oncol 1984;2: 125–129.

Frankton S, Bloom SR: Glucagonomas. Baillieres Clin Gastroenterol 1996;10:697–705.

Grant C: Insulinoma. Baillieres Clin Gastroenterol 1996;10:645–672.

Harpole DH, Feldman JM, Buchanan S, et al: Bronchial carcinoid tumors: A retrospective analysis of 126 patients. Ann Thorac Surg 1992;54:50–55.

Jensen RT: Gastrinoma. Baillieres Clin Gastroenterol 1996;10: 603–644.

Jetmore AB, Ray JE, Gathright JB, et al: Rectal carcinoids: The most frequent carcinoid tumor. Dis Colon Rectum 1992;35:717–725.

Kulke MH, Mayer RJ: Carcinoid tumors. N Engl J Med 1999;340:858–868.

Kvols LK, Moertel CG, O'Connell MJ, et al: Treatment of the malignant carcinoid syndrome: Evaluation of a long-acting somatostatin analog. N Engl J Med 1986;315:663–666.

LeTreut YP, Delpero JR, Dousset B, et al: Results of liver transplantation in the treatment of metastatic neuroendocrine tumors: A 31-case French multicentric report. Ann Surg 1997;225:355–364.

Modlin I, Sandor A: An analysis of 8305 cases of carcinoid tumors. Cancer 1997;79:813–829.

Modlin I, Tang L: Approaches to the diagnosis of gut neuroendocrine tumors: The last word (today). Gastroenterology 1997;112:583–590.

Moertel CG, Hanley JA: Combination chemotherapy trials in metastatic carcinoid tumor and the malignant carcinoid syndrome. Cancer Clin Trials 1979;2:327–334.

Moertel CG, Hanley JA, Johnson LA: Streptozocin alone compared with streptozocin plus fluorouracil in the treatment of advanced islet cell carcinoma. N Engl J Med 1980;303:1189–1194.

Moertel CG, Johnson CM, McKusick MA, et al: The management of patients with advanced carcinoid tumors and islet cell carcinomas. Ann Intern Med 1994;120:302–309.

Moertel CG, Kvols LK, O'Connell MJ, Rubin J: Treatment of neuroendocrine carcinomas with combined etoposide and cisplatin: Evidence of major activity in the anaplastic variants of these neoplasms. Cancer 1991;68:227–232.

Moertel CG, Lefkopoulo M, Lipsitz S, et al: Streptozocin-doxorubicin, streptozocin-fluorouracil, or chlorozotocin in the treatment of advanced islet cell carcinoma. N Engl J Med 1992;326:519–523.

Moertel CG, Weiland LH, Nagorney DM, Dockerty MB: Carcinoid tumor of the appendix: Treatment and prognosis. N Engl J Med 1987;317:1699–1701.

Oberg K, Eriksson B: The role of interferons in the management of carcinoid tumors. Acta Oncol 1991;30:519–522.

Park SK, O'Dorisio MS, O'Dorisio TM: Vasoactive intestinal polypeptide secreting tumors: Biology and therapy. Baillieres Clin Gastroenterol 1996;10:673–696.

Que FG, Nagorney DM, Batts KP, et al: Hepatic resection for neuroendocrine carcinomas. Am J Surg 1995;169:36–43.

Rindi G, Bordi C, Rappel S, et al: Gastric carcinoids and neuroendocrine carcinomas: Pathogenesis, pathology, and behavior. World J Surg 1996;20:168–172.

Rubin J, Ajani J, Shchirmer W, et al: Octreotide acetate long-acting formulation versus open-label subcutaneous octreotide acetate in malignant carcinoid syndrome. J Clin Oncol 1999;17:600–606.

Chapter 111
Pituitary Tumors

Robert D. Utiger

Pituitary tumors are identified because the patient has symptoms of a pituitary mass, clinical manifestations of pituitary hormone excess or deficiency, or both. Among patients with a pituitary mass, approximately 90% have a pituitary adenoma, 8% have a craniopharyngioma or other cell-rest tumor (Rathke's pouch cyst, epidermoid cyst), and 2% have other masses, including metastatic tumors, aneurysms, and inflammatory masses.

Pituitary Adenoma

Pituitary adenomas are benign, slow-growing monoclonal adenomas of the different types of cells present in the normal anterior pituitary gland. They are rare, occurring with an estimated frequency of 10 cases per 1,000,000 people per year, mostly in older adults. Genetic abnormalities in signal transduction systems or the receptors for the hormones that inhibit the production and secretion of particular pituitary hormones have been identified in some adenomas. Pituitary adenomas occur in approximately 40% of patients with multiple endocrine neoplasia type 1; the other components are parathyroid adenomas and pancreatic islet cell adenomas. Small, incidental pituitary adenomas are found in up to 10% of people at autopsy.

Clinical Presentations

Pituitary adenomas are classified according to size—as microadenomas (tumor diameter less than 1 cm) or macroadenomas (tumor diameter 1 cm or greater)—and according to their secretory products.

Nonsecretory Microadenomas

Nonsecretory microadenomas do not cause symptoms and rarely cause hormonal deficiencies. They are usually detected incidentally by imaging in patients who are being evaluated for unrelated problems.

Nonsecretory Macroadenomas

Nonsecretory macroadenomas may also be detected incidentally, but they can cause mass effects as they enlarge and extend superiorly from the sella turcica toward the hypothalamus or laterally toward the cavernous sinuses. The major symptoms are headaches and visual difficulties. The headaches may be frontal, bitemporal, or occipital and are often relieved by minor analgesic drugs. The characteristic visual abnormality is bitemporal hemianopsia, but some patients have quadrant defects, decreased visual acuity, scotomas, or third or sixth nerve palsies.

Nonsecretory macroadenomas may cause deficiency of any pituitary hormone, including vasopressin. The most common deficiency is that of gonadotropins (follicle-stimulating hormone [FSH] and luteinizing hormone [LH]), which is present in approximately 80% of patients, followed by growth hormone (GH) deficiency (60%), thyrotropin (TSH) deficiency (40%), corticotropin (ACTH) deficiency (25%), and vasopressin deficiency (5%). Any of these can occur as an isolated deficiency or as one of multiple deficiencies.

The hypogonadism that results from gonadotropin deficiency is easily detected in young women by the presence of amenorrhea, but it is not as easily detected in men because of the unwillingness of many men to describe loss of libido and other symptoms of hypogonadism (or the unwillingness of the physician to ask). Many of the symptoms of growth hormone, thyrotropin, and corticotropin deficiency are nonspecific, for example, muscle weakness, mental fatigue, and anorexia, and the presence of more specific symptoms, such as cold intolerance and weight loss, may go unnoticed because their onset is so gradual.

Some nonsecretory macroadenomas produce and secrete no hormones or hormonal components, but many produce the common alpha subunit of follicle-stimulating hormone and luteinizing hormone (and thyrotropin), the beta subunits of follicle-stimulating hormone or luteinizing hormone, or intact follicle-stimulating hormone or luteinizing hormone, as detected by mRNA and immunohistochemical analyses of tumor tissue. These tumors often secrete one or both subunits, which lack biologic activity, but only rarely do they secrete excess amounts of intact follicle-stimulating hormone or luteinizing hormone. Therefore, they are in fact gonadotroph adenomas.

Secretory Microadenomas and Macroadenomas

The majority of secretory pituitary adenomas are microadenomas.

Among the secretory tumors, lactotroph adenomas (prolactinomas) are the most common (Table 111-1). In young women, even moderate hyperprolactinemia inhibits pituitary-gonadal function, causing infertility, oligomenorrhea or amenorrhea, and, less often, galactorrhea. Most of these women have microadenomas. In contrast, postmenopausal women and men usually present with headaches or visual problems and have macroadenomas. Hyperprolactinemia also inhibits pituitary-gonadal function in men, causing hypogonadism and rarely galactorrhea. Hyperprolactinemia does not necessarily indicate the presence of a lactotroph adenoma. It also can result from loss of tonic hypothalamic inhibition of prolactin secretion, for example, by interruption of hypothalamic-pituitary blood flow.

Somatotroph adenomas cause acromegaly, with acral enlargement, macroglossia, skin thickening, excessive perspiration, arthralgia, sleep apnea, hypertension, and cardiomyopathy. Somatotroph adenomas are extremely slow-growing tumors. At the time of diagnosis, many patients have had changes attributable to growth hormone excess for many years, and the majority have macroadenomas. Many somatotroph adenomas also hypersecrete prolactin.

Corticotroph adenomas cause Cushing's disease and account for approximately 70% of cases of Cushing's syndrome. The major clinical findings are moon facies, plethora, central obesity, hypertension, myopathy, psychological disturbances, and osteoporo-sis. Most of the tumors are microadenomas, and in some patients, the tumor is so small that it cannot be detected by imaging.

Thyrotroph adenomas are rare and are far less common than Graves' disease, nodular goiter, and thyroiditis as a cause of hyperthyroidism. In addition to hyperthyroidism, the patients have a diffuse goiter, but they do not have Graves' ophthalmopathy. Most of the adenomas are macroadenomas, and approximately 40% secrete prolactin or other pituitary hormones.

Gonadotroph adenomas may secrete sufficient follicle-stimulating hormone or luteinizing hormone to have clinical effects. In young women, follicle-stimulating hormone hypersecretion can cause ovarian hyperstimulation with multiple ovarian cysts and oligomenorrhea or amenorrhea. In men, excess luteinizing hormone secretion causes high serum testosterone concentrations, but this has little clinical effect in normal men. The adenomas are nearly always macroadenomas.

Pituitary Apoplexy

Occasional patients, most of whom have macroadenomas, present with pituitary apoplexy. It is characterized by the sudden onset of severe headache; visual field deficits; third, fourth, or sixth cranial nerve palsies; nausea and vomiting; and decline in mental status. It is caused by hemorrhagic infarction of the adenoma.

Clinical Evaluation

All patients who are suspected of having a pituitary adenoma or other pituitary disease should undergo magnetic resonance imaging (MRI), with special attention given to the region of the sella turcica (Figure 111-1). Magnetic resonance imaging provides better resolution of the anatomy of this region and reveals more microadenomas than does computed tomography. Visual field testing should be done if there is clinical or radiologic evidence of compression of the optic chiasm or optic tracts.

Hormonal Deficiencies

The possible deficiency of corticotropin, follicle-stimulating hormone and luteinizing hormone, or thyrotropin in a patient with a pituitary tumor should be assessed by simultaneous measurements of the particular pituitary hormone and its respective target gland hormone (cortisol, estradiol or testosterone, or thyroxine) in serum (Table 111-2). Pituitary hormone deficiency is characterized by a normal or low serum pituitary hormone concentration in the presence of a low serum concentration of the target gland hormone.

Table 111-1 ■ Types and Relative Frequency of Pituitary Adenomas

Type of Adenoma	Frequency
Nonsecretory adenoma	35%
Lactotroph (prolactinoma) adenoma	30%
Somatotroph (GH-secreting) adenoma	15%
Corticotroph (ACTH-secreting) adenoma	15%
Other (thyrotroph [TSH-secreting] adenoma, gonadotroph [FSH- or LH-secreting]) adenoma	<5%

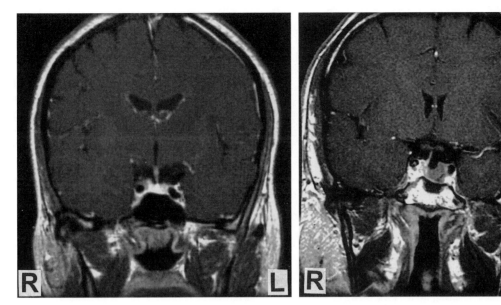

Figure 111-1 ■ Coronal magnetic resonance images of the head (contrast-enhanced) of a patient with a normal pituitary gland (*left*) and a patient with a pituitary macroadenoma (*right*). The macroadenoma fills the left side of the sella turcica and is hypodense relative to the normal pituitary gland, and it has displaced the pituitary stalk to the right.

Growth hormone secretion need not be assessed. Many stimulation tests have been devised to determine whether secretion of pituitary hormones can be raised, but these tests add little and are rarely indicated.

Hormonal Excesses

Excess hormonal secretion also can be assessed adequately in most patients by serum measurements of both the pituitary and target gland hormones or the pituitary hormone alone (see Table 111-2), but demonstration of failure of target hormones or other substances to inhibit pituitary hormone secretion is important in some patients. In patients with Cushing's disease, many of whom do not have a radiologically identifiable pituitary tumor, petrosal sinus cannulation and measurements of plasma corticotropin before and after intravenous administration of corticotropin-releasing hormone that reveal high petrosal; peripheral plasma ratios of corticotropin provide strong evidence for the presence of a corticotroph adenoma.

Treatment

Patients with nonsecretory microadenomas need no treatment but should have repeat magnetic resonance imaging and basal hormone measurements in six and 12 months and then at longer intervals to be sure the adenoma is not enlarging. These adenomas do not often change during follow-up.

Patients with nonsecretory macroadenomas and most patients with secretory microadenomas or macroadenomas should be treated by transsphenoidal resection of the tumor, but drug therapy is appropriate for some patients with secretory adenomas (Table 111-3). Among patients treated by transsphenoidal surgery, the success rate depends on the size of the tumor. Patients with microadenomas are considerably more likely to be cured than are those with macroadenomas (60% to 90% versus 30% to 50%). The operative mortality is very low (less than 1%). Postoperatively, fewer than 20% of patients have new anterior pituitary hormone deficiencies or diabetes insipidus (usually transient), and approximately 1% have bleeding or vascular occlusion, new visual loss, meningitis, sinusitis, third and sixth cranial nerve palsies, or hyponatremia.

Drug therapy, in the form of dopaminergic agonist drugs, is the preferred initial treatment for patients with a prolactinoma, including those with visual impairment. These drugs not only decrease prolactin secretion, but also reduce tumor size. Similarly, long-acting somatostatin analogs are gaining favor as initial treatment for patients with acromegaly.

Patients with pituitary adenomas who are not cured by surgery or do not respond well to drugs may be treated with external-beam radiation, usually in a dose of 50 Gy. This is effective therapy, but its effect is slow; serum hormone concentrations usually fall at a rate of 10% to 20% per year, and it eventually causes

Table 111-2 ■ Hormonal Findings in Patients with Pituitary Adenomas

Hormonal Deficiency

Corticotropin Deficiency

Normal or low plasma corticotropin and low serum cortisol concentrations (measured at 8 or 9 A.M.)

Gonadotropin (Follicle-Stimulating Hormone [FSH] and Luteinizing Hormone [LH]) Deficiency

Young women with normal menstrual cycles: no tests needed
Young women with amenorrhea: normal or low serum follicle-stimulating and luteinizing hormone and low serum estradiol concentrations
Postmenopausal women: serum follicle-stimulating hormone and luteinizing hormone concentrations low for age
Men: normal or low serum follicle-stimulating hormone and luteinizing hormone and low serum testosterone concentrations
All these abnormalities may be caused by hyperprolactinemia, rather than destruction of gonadotrophs

Growth Hormone

No tests needed, unless growth hormone treatment is contemplated

Prolactin

Low serum prolactin concentration (prolactin deficiency not clinically important except in women who wish to lactate)

Thyrotropin

Normal or low serum thyrotropin and low serum free thyroxine concentrations

Vasopressin

24-hour urine volume > 2000 mL
Ratio of urine:plasma osmolality < 2 after water restriction for six hours or longer

Hormonal Excess

Corticotropin Excess (Cushing's Disease)

Screening tests: high 24-hour urine cortisol excretion, or serum cortisol concentration >5 μg/dL at 8 or 9 A.M. after administration of 1 mg dexamethasone at midnight
Diagnosis: normal or high plasma ACTH and high serum cortisol concentrations (measured at 8 or 9 A.M.)

Gonadotropin Excess

High serum follicle-stimulating hormone or luteinizing hormone and high serum estradiol or testosterone concentrations

Growth Hormone Excess (Acromegaly)

High serum growth hormone concentration two hours after ingestion of 75 g glucose
High serum insulin-like growth factor I concentration

Prolactin Excess

High serum prolactin concentration (value may be high because of prolactinoma, or because another pituitary tumor blocks hypothalamic inhibition of prolactin secretion)

Hyperthyroidism

Normal or high serum thyrotropin and high serum free thyroxine concentrations

hypopituitarism in most patients. It also has been associated with psychological dysfunction and rarely extrapituitary brain tumors. Stereotactic radiosurgery using the gamma knife, in which high doses of radiation can be delivered to small regions with little radiation of adjacent tissue, results in more rapid reduction in hormonal secretion and adenoma size than external-beam radiation and is likely safer. So far, it has been used mostly in patients with persistent or recurrent adenomas.

Post-treatment care depends on the type and extent of the tumor and its secretory products. Many patients need treatment for one or more pituitary hormone deficiencies, those with hormonal hypersecretion need to be monitored periodically for hormonal recurrence, and those with macroadenomas need periodic monitoring for regrowth of the adenoma.

Craniopharyngioma

Craniopharyngiomas arise from rests of squamous cells derived from Rathke's pouch, the diverticulum of the roof of the embryonic oral cavity that gives rise to the anterior pituitary. They originate within the sella turcica or, more often, in the suprasellar region. The

Table 111-3 ■ Treatment of Pituitary Adenomas

Type of Adenoma	Treatment*†
Nonsecretory microadenoma	No treatment
Nonsecretory macroadenoma	Surgery
Corticotroph adenoma	Surgery*
	Inhibitors of adrenal hormone synthesis (ketoconazole, metyrapone, mitotane)
Gonadotroph adenoma	Surgery
Lactotroph adenoma	Dopamine agonist drugs (bromocriptine, caberogoline)
	Surgery
Somatotroph adenoma	Surgery
	Long-acting somatostatin analogs
	Dopamine agonist drugs
	Growth hormone receptor antagonist drugs (pegvisomant)
Thyrotropin-secreting adenoma	Surgery
	Long-acting somatostatin analogs
	Dopamine agonist drugs

*Treatments are listed in usual order of preference.
†Patients with any type of macroadenoma (or persistent or recurrent adenoma) may be treated with external beam radiation therapy or gamma knife radiation therapy.

Therapy Considerations for Pituitary Tumor

Patients with a pituitary tumor present because they have symptoms and signs that suggest the presence of a pituitary mass lesion, deficiency of one or more pituitary hormones, or an excess of a pituitary hormone.

The questions that need to be considered are as follows:

Is there a pituitary mass lesion? This is best answered by magnetic resonance imaging.

Does the patient have any pituitary hormone deficiency or excess? A deficiency might be suspected on clinical grounds, but the symptoms and signs may be vague and nonspecific. Hormonal status can usually be accurately assessed by measurements in serum of the pituitary hormone and the hormone(s) produced by target glands.

What treatment is indicated? Patients with a pituitary macroadenoma may need transsphenoidal resection of the tumor. Patients with pituitary deficiencies are usually treated with a target gland hormone, but administration of the pituitary hormone may on occasion be indicated. Patients with hormonal excess may be treated surgically or with one of several drugs, depending on the type of tumor.

---

incidence is bimodal, with peaks in late childhood and adolescence and in the sixth decade; craniopharyngiomas are the most common tumors of the hypothalamic-pituitary region in children. The major clinical manifestations are headache, visual abnormalities, growth hormone deficiency, follicle-stimulating hormone and luteinizing hormone deficiency, and diabetes insipidus. Many patients have hyperprolactinemia. Magnetic resonance imaging usually reveals a large cystic mass, which may be calcified. Most patients should be treated with transsphenoidal or transfrontal surgery, depending on the location of the tumor, and external-beam radiation. The tumors are often difficult to resect completely, and the recurrence rate is reduced by postoperative radiation therapy.

References

Ben-Shlomo A, Melmed S: Acromegaly. Endocrinol Metab Clin North Am 2001;30:565–583.

Ciric I, Ragin A, Baumgartner C, Pierce D: Complications of transsphenoidal surgery: Results of a national survey, review of the literature, and personal experience. Neurosurgery 1997;40:225–236.

Donovan LE, Corenblum B: The natural history of the pituitary incidentaloma. Arch Intern Med 1995;155:181–183.

Invitti C, Giraldi FP, De Martin M, et al: Diagnosis and management of Cushing's syndrome: Results of an Italian multicentre study. J Clin Endocrinol Metab 1999;84:440–448.

Jackson IM, Noren G: Gamma knife radiosurgery for pituitary tumors. Baillieres Best Pract Res Clin Endocrinol 1999;13:461–469.

Laws ER Jr, Thapar K: Pituitary surgery. Endocrinol Metab Clin North Am 1999;28:119–131.

Molitch ME: Disorders of prolactin secretion. Endocrinol Metab Clin North Am 2001;30:585–610.

Nilsson B, Gustavsson-Kadaka E, Bengtsson B-A, Jonsson B: Pituitary adenomas in Sweden between 1958 and 1991: Incidence, survival, and mortality. J Clin Endocrinol Metab 2000;85:1420–1425.

Pinzone JJ, Katznelson L, Danila DC, et al: Primary medical therapy of micro- and macroprolactinomas in men. J Clin Endocrinol Metab 2000;85:3053–3057.

Shin JL, Asa SL, Woodhouse LJ, et al: Cystic lesions of the pituitary: Clinicopathological features distinguishing craniopharyngioma, Rathke's cleft cyst, and arachnoid cyst. J Clin Endocrinol Metab 1999;84:3972–3982.

Swearingen B, Barker FG II, Katznelson L, et al: Long-term mortality after transsphenoidal surgery and adjunctive therapy for acromegaly. J Clin Endocrinol Metab 1998;83:3419–3426.

Verhelst J, Abs R, Maiter D, et al: Cabergoline in the treatment of hyperprolactinemia: A study in 455 patients. J Clin Endocrinol Metab 1999;84:2518–2522.

Section IV
Special Considerations in the Treatment of Patients with Cancer

Chapter 112
Cancer of Unknown Primary

Melanie B. Thomas and James L. Abbruzzese

Epidemiology

Oncologists are frequently asked to evaluate and treat a subset of patients with metastatic cancer for whom, despite the wide array of diagnostic tools available to establish the diagnosis of human malignancy, detailed investigations fail to identify a primary anatomic site of disease (see also Chapter 46). The reported prevalence of unknown primary carcinoma varies with the practice setting and the definition used but ranges between 0.5% and 9% of all patients diagnosed with cancer. The histology is read as adenocarcinoma (50% to 60%), poorly differentiated carcinomas or poorly differentiated adenocarcinomas (30% to 40%), squamous cell carcinomas (5% to 8%), and undifferentiated malignancies (2% to 5%).

Since identifying the origin of the primary tumor forms the basis for predicting the behavior of and assigning appropriate therapy for malignant diseases, the absence of a primary tumor poses a major challenge. Considerable controversy surrounds the optimal evaluation of patients with unknown primary carcinoma. Many authors have outlined arguments in favor of an extensive versus a directed evaluation of patients. The overall goal of the evaluation is to rapidly identify the treatable patient subsets through a rational, calculated approach. The demographics of this patient population mirror those of the general population of patients referred to a large cancer center, except that the proportion of men is higher among patients with unknown primary carcinoma.

Pathology

The pathologist is usually able to confirm that the lesion is neoplastic and may be able to judge whether the lesion is primary or metastatic. However, in some situations, it is impossible to determine whether the tumor has arisen from the organ site at which the biopsy was performed. This problem often complicates the cytologic evaluation of fine-needle aspirate speci-

mens (i.e., in cases in which information on tissue architecture is unavailable).

The initial assessment of the biopsy material is usually performed via light microscopic examination of paraffin sections stained with hematoxylin and eosin. Using established cytologic criteria, pathologists can usually categorize tumors as either carcinoma, sarcoma, or lymphoma. Additionally, many carcinomas are immediately recognized as manifesting at least some glandular differentiation, indicating an adenocarcinoma. Patients with unknown primary carcinoma whose tumors do not show glandular differentiation are frequently diagnosed as poorly differentiated carcinoma or undifferentiated carcinoma. Other specimens lack any distinguishing cytologic features; such cases are diagnosed as undifferentiated malignancy. It is in groups of patients with poorly differentiated carcinoma, undifferentiated carcinoma, or undifferentiated malignancy that additional studies, including histochemistry, immunohistochemistry, and electron microscopy, are most frequently and productively employed. Only a few of the vast array of tissue markers are regularly used. Increasingly, pathologists user cytokeratin immunohistochemical stains to distinguish neoplasms of epithelial origin. Since many centers do not routinely perform special stains unless there is a reasonable belief that such studies will contribute to an accurate diagnosis, direct discussions between the pathologist and the clinician are critical to ensure optimal histologic characterization. Every effort should be made to identify patients with lymphoma, since these neoplasms are curable with appropriate therapy.

Biologic Features

It is uncertain whether unknown primary carcinoma represents an entity with specific biologic characteristics or is merely a clinical presentation of metastases among patients in whom the primary tumor remains undetected. Is the biology of unknown primary carcinoma fundamentally different from that of known primary cancer with systemic metastases? It appears that no significant differences in the patterns of metastases occurs, although the overall survival rate for patients with unknown primary carcinoma is inferior to that of patients in whom the primary tumor is known.

Why the primary organ site in patients with unknown primary carcinoma is difficult to diagnose is uncertain. Investigators have speculated that in such cases, the tumor size is below the limits of clinical or radiographic detection or that the tumor spontaneously regressed before the metastatic sites presented. Another possibility is that a phase of a clinically detectable primary never appeared owing to specific genetic changes that support metastatic rather than local growth.

Chromosomal Abnormalities

Investigators have performed relatively few studies on the chromosomal abnormalities in unknown primary carcinomas. Abnormalities of chromosome 1, including deletion of 1 p, translocations, isochromosome 1 q, and evidence of gene amplification, are the ones most commonly detected. Motzer used karyotyping to determine the frequency of specific abnormalities of chromosome 12, a chromosomal marker characterizing germ cell tumors. Twelve patients (30%) had an increased 12 p copy number or deletion of the long arm of chromosome 12, which proved to be predictive for tumor response. Objective responses to cisplatin-based therapy were achieved in 75% of these patients, compared with 17% of patients without these aberrations. In patients with undifferentiated carcinoma, isochromosome 12 p [i(12 p)] correlated with a good response to platinum-based chemotherapy, though lack of i(12 p) did not exclude a small percentage of responses. Because i(12 p) occurs in over 80% of the germ cell tumors and only sparsely in a few other malignancies (acute leukemia, embryonal rhabdomyosarcoma, and neuroepithelioma), determination of the presence or absence of i(12 p) can help to diagnose extragonadal germ cell tumors in patients with unknown primary carcinoma.

Aneuploidy

Aneuploidy is a well-recognized phenomenon, occurring in most solid tumors. In many carcinomas, such as breast, prostate, and colorectal cancers, a diploid DNA content is associated with a better prognosis. Aneuploidy is also found in the biopsy specimens of 70% of the patients with unknown primary carcinoma. In these patients, aneuploidy is equally distributed among men and women, and its presence does not correlate with any particular pattern of metastatic involvement. In unknown primary carcinoma, the median survival of patients with diploid tumors is 4.2 months, whereas it is 4.8 months for patients with aneuploid tumors. The incidence of aneuploidy in this heterogeneous group of patients is similar to that reported for metastatic carcinomas with a known primary site. Why diploid metastatic adenocarcinomas of unknown primary origin do not also exhibit a more favorable prognosis than those that are aneuploid is unexplained.

Oncogenes

As in many other solid tumors, unknown primary carcinomas exhibit overexpression of c-myc (96%), ras (92%), and c-erB-2 (65%). The overexpression of these oncogenes does not correlate with histologic or clinical features or provide diagnostic or prognostic information. Bcl-2 is expressed to lesser degree, but the level of expression has no prognostic value. Approximately 10% of the carcinomas of unknown primary site that are poorly differentiated overexpress the Her-2 protein, but this does not correlate, as it does in breast cancer, with the likelihood of a chemotherapy response.

Tumor Suppressor Genes

Mutations of p53 tumor suppression genes are common, occurring in about 55% of all human cancers. Although qualitative immunohistochemical studies of unknown primary carcinoma also show the expected high frequency of p53 overexpression, a search for specific mutations in the p53 coding revealed abnormalities in only six of 23 (26%) patients. Thus, although unknown primary carcinomas are, by definition, highly metastatic tumors, the frequency of p53 mutations was low in comparison with that in other human malignancies. It appears from this limited study that p53 mutations might not play a major role in the development and progression of unknown primary carcinoma.

Microvessel Density

In solid tumors, measurement of angiogenesis by assessing microvessel density correlates with the incidence of metastastic disease. In unknown primary carcinoma, as in other solid tumors, high micro vessel density correlated with short survival in both univariate and multivariate analyses. However, the microvessel density in hepatic metastases from unknown primary carcinomas was similar to that in metastases developing from carcinomas of a known primary site.

Table 112-1 ■ Major Sites of Tumor Involvement and Identified Histologic Diagnoses in 1196 Patients with Unknown Primary Carcinoma

Parameter	Patients	Percentage
Histologic Diagnosis		
Adenocarcinoma	706	59.0
Carcinoma	335	28.0
Squamous carcinoma	75	6.3
Neuroendocrine carcinoma	54	4.5
Unknown/other*	26	2.2
Major Metastatic Sites[†]		
Lymph nodes	519	43.4
Liver	404	33.8
Bone	334	27.9
Lung	315	26.3
Pleura/pleural space	129	10.8
Peritoneum	118	9.9
Brain	84	7.0
Adrenal	71	5.9
Skin	41	3.4

*Includes patients with malignant neoplasm (5) and unknown pathology (21).
[†]Some patients had more than one major metastatic site.

Clinical Presentation

The clinical presentation varies markedly, and categorization of patient subgroups is difficult. Investigators have begun to subclassify patients with unknown primary carcinoma largely on the basis of clinicopathologic criteria, including histology, involved organ sites, and responsiveness to therapy. Such a composite analysis allows definition of well-characterized patient subsets that are clinically relevant therapeutically. Unfortunately, most patients present with solitary or multiple areas of involvement in diverse visceral sites and do not fit neatly into any of these therapeutic categories.

The median age of patients presenting with unknown primary carcinoma is approximately 60 years. Other family members frequently have a history of cancers of established primary origin; however, no clearly familial instances of unknown primary carcinoma have been reported. Table 112-1 shows the distribution of metastatic sites and histologic classification in a series of 1196 patients.

Clinical Evaluation

A thorough history, including detailed social, occupational, and family history and complete physical examination, form the basis of evaluating patients with suspected unknown primary carcinoma. The physical examination should include breast and pelvic examinations for women, testicular and prostate examinations for men, and digital rectal examination for both genders. Routine additional baseline studies should include serum chemistry, liver and kidney function tests, complete blood count, chest radiography, and mammography in women. Depending on the clinical situation, additional studies might include sputum cytology, computed tomography of the chest, breast ultrasonography, or gastrointestinal endoscopy. Extensive testing for the numerous serum markers now available (e.g., CEA, CA125, CA19-9, and AFP) is generally not warranted, because none of these are pathognomonic for a particular neoplasm. Other studies are dictated by the physician's clinical judgment (see Chapter 46). Computed tomography of the pelvis is indicated routinely in women because of a potential gynecologic origin of a metastatic adenocarcinoma but does not seem warranted in men without specific symptoms.

Several studies suggested that 2-[^{18}F]fluoro-2-deoxy-D-glucose (FDG) positron emission tomography (PET) contributes to the diagnostic evaluation of unknown primary carcinoma. The studies had a small number of patients who principally presented with cervical or supraclavicular lymphadenopathy. Since patients with metastatic lymph nodes in these regions often are treated empirically with extensive radiation therapy for a primary head and neck tumor or, conversely, may be eligible for radical neck dissection, this subset in particular may benefit from identifying the primary tumor. But in patients with presumed head and neck cancer, the positron emission tomography scan did not improve on the detection of the primary site provided by panendoscopy (endoscopic examination of the nasopharynx, larynx, and esophagus). The positron emission tomography scan's discriminatory power is limited because of a true-positive rate of 38% to 47% and a false-positive rate as high as 20%. The variability in test results is probably due to differences in tissue-specific tracer uptake rates as well as in interindividual glucose metabolism. Moreover, although the positron emission tomography scan is a promising diagnostic modality, it is not clear whether identification of the primary tumor and thus potentially more directed therapy will lead to improved survival rates for patients with unknown primary carcinoma.

Prognostic Features and Outcome

Unknown primary carcinomas are a heterogeneous group of tumors with widely varying natural histories. Overall unknown primary carcinomas are aggressive neoplasms with a median survival of 9 to 11 months.

Table 112-2 ■ Multivariate Survival Analysis in Patients with Unknown Primary Carcinoma

Variable	Relative Risk*	P†	Effect on Survival
Male sex	1.39	.0007	Deleterious
Increasing number of organ sites	1.23	<.0001	Deleterious
Involved organ sites			
Liver	1.33	.0064	Deleterious
Lymph nodes (all sites)	0.46	<.0001	Advantageous
Supraclavicular	1.56	.013	Deleterious
Peritoneum	0.59	.0099	Advantageous
Histology			
Adenocarcinoma	1.46	.0001	Deleterious
Neuroendocrine carcinoma	0.30	.0005	Advantageous

*Calculated from the Cox proportional hazards regression.
†Log rank test.
Adapted from Abbruzzese JL et al., J Clin Oncol 1995;13:2094–2103, with permission.

The survival rates for the four most frequently encountered histologic subtypes of unknown primary carcinoma differ considerably. The median survival for patients with squamous cell carcinoma (exclusive of patients with mid or high cervical adenopathy) is 13 months, compared to six months for adenocarcinoma, 11 months for carcinoma, and 27 months for neuroendocrine carcinoma.

The degree of differentiation or mucin production does not significantly influence the poor survival rate of patients with adenocarcinoma. The influence of multiple clinical-pathologic features such as age, histology, and organ site involvement on the survival of patients with unknown primary carcinoma was examined. After multivariate analysis, the several variables listed in Table 112-2 emerged as significant.

Treatment

While most of these patients are treated with systemic chemotherapy, the careful integration of surgery, radiation therapy, and even periods of observation are important in the overall management of many of these patients. Careful observation in follow-up is particularly important for patients with single sites of disease that have received adequate local therapy.

The most common difficult-to-treat cases of unknown primary carcinoma are those with progressive metastatic carcinoma or adenocarcinoma involving two or more organ sites. Table 112-3 outlines the results from a series of recent trials of various treatment regimens. All of these trials produce similar results in terms of responses and median survivals. It is therefore difficult to recommend one regimen over the other in these patients with poor-prognosis disease. The outcomes of these patients should be contrasted with the results and approaches to therapy of patients who present with a relatively favorable prognosis. Although these favorable groups represent only a small proportion of patients, it is important to recognize them, since specific treatment may significantly extend their survival.

Table 112-3 ■ Selected Chemotherapeutic Trials in Unknown Primary Carcinoma

Author	Chemotherapy Regimen	Number of Patients	Responses		Median Survival (months)
			N	(%)	
Hainsworth et al. (1997)	Paclitaxel/carboplatin/etoposide	53	25	(47)	13.4
Greco et al. (2000)	Docetaxel + cisplatin	23	6	(25)	8
	Docetaxel + carboplatin	47	8	(22)	12
Greco et al. (2002)	Gemcitabine, carboplatin, paclitaxel	120	28	(25)	9
Briasoulis (1998)	Carboplatin, etoposide epirubicin	62	23	(37)	8 (visceral) 10 (nodal)
Briasoulis (2000)	Carboplatin, paclitaxel	77	30	(39)	13

TREATMENT

Unfavorable Clinical Subsets of Unknown Primary Carcinoma: Patients with Adenocarcinoma or Carcinoma of Unknown Origin

Background

Two thirds of patients with unknown primary carcinoma have metastatic adenocarcinoma with involvement of two or more visceral sites, usually some combination of liver, lung, lymph nodes, or bone. Many men and women with poorly differentiated carcinoma or poorly differentiated adenocarcinoma have no clinically favorable features and respond poorly to chemotherapy. Even in series showing promising results for selected patients with poorly differentiated carcinoma or poorly differentiated adenocarcinoma, the overall median survival remains poor. For unselected patients, numerous empiric chemotherapy combinations have been used. Many have been based on Adriamycin, 5-fluorouracil, or cisplatin. In a recent study of carboplatin, paclitaxel, and etoposide, 47% (25 of 53 patients) had objective responses. In this series, seven patients (13%) experienced complete responses. However, the actuarial median survival for the entire group was 13.4 months. The disappointing aspect of this survival statistic is that it is not substantially different from the 11-month median survival reported in large series of consecutively treated patients. Response rates to most combination regimens generally range from 20% to 30%; however, most responses are partial and brief and therefore have little or no impact on the median survival. Although newer regimens continue to be tested, there has been no substantial progress in the treatment of these patients to date.

Recommended Therapy

Cisplatin 20 mg/m^2 IV daily for five days + etoposide 100 mg/m^2 IV daily for three to five days or cisplatin 100 mg/m^2 IV on day 1 + etoposide 100 mg/m^2 IV daily for three days; repeat courses administered every three to four weeks

Or

Paclitaxel 200 mg/m^2 by one-hour IV infusion on day 1, carboplatin calculated to achieve AUC = 6 IV on day 1, etoposide 50 mg alternated with 100 mg p.o. on days 1 to 10; repeat courses administered every 21 days

Or

Cisplatin 75 mg/m^2 iv on day 1, folinic acid 500 mg/m^2 in 200 mL normal saline IV over two hours on days 1 through 5, 5-FU 375 mg/m^2 IV after one hour of folinic acid on days 1 through 5; repeat courses administered every 28 days.

TREATMENT

Favorable Clinical Subsets of Unknown Primary Carcinoma: Squamous Cell Carcinoma Involving Mid- to High Cervical Lymph Nodes

Background

High cervical adenopathy with squamous cell carcinoma is an important clinical subset because of its well-defined natural history and responsiveness to therapy. With appropriate evaluation, including direct visualization of the hypopharynx, nasopharynx, larynx, and upper esophagus, an occult primary lesion will frequently be identified. When no primary is found, aggressive local therapy is applied to the involved neck. Five-year survival rates of 30% to 50% have been reported with radical neck surgery, high-dose radiation therapy, or a combination of both modalities. A potential advantage of radiation therapy is that the suspected primary anatomic sites (nasopharynx, oropharynx, and hypopharynx) can be included in the radiation port. Recent studies suggest that the eventual appearance of the primary site adversely affects the prognosis. The role of chemotherapy in the treatment of these patients is unclear. However, one randomized study suggested that in comparison with radiation therapy alone, chemotherapy with cisplatin and 5-fluorouracil (5-FU) improved the response rate and median survival.

Compared with other patient groups, patients with adenocarcinoma involving mid- to high cervical nodes and patients with lower cervical or supraclavicular adenopathy of any histology have a much poorer prognosis. These patients either are managed with local measures (usually radiation therapy) or may be candidates for systemic chemotherapy protocols.

Recommended Therapy*

1. Low N stage (NX, N1, or N2A): Surgery followed by radiation therapy (>50 Gy) or radiation therapy alone (minimum 50 Gy) alone to ipsilateral neck +/– naso-oropharynx.
2. High N stage (N2B, N3A, or N3B) or poorly differentiated tumors: Cisplatin 100 mg/m^2 IV on days 1, 22, and 43, with concurrent radiation therapy

Or

Cisplatin 100 mg/m^2 IV on day 1 + 5-FU 1000 mg/m^2 IV daily by continuous infusion on days 1 to 5. Repeat courses of cisplatin and 5-FU every three to four weeks times three courses followed by radiation therapy.

*See Chapter 98, regarding N stages of head an neck cancer.

TREATMENT

Favorable Clinical Subsets of Unknown Primary Carcinoma: Women with Isolated Axillary Adenopathy

Background

Isolated axillary adenopathy secondary to metastatic adenocarcinoma usually occurs in women and has unique clinical features. Many women with these tumors have occult breast primary tumors that can be identified in 40% to 70% of these patients who undergo mastectomy. In this setting, performing another biopsy of involved axillary nodes to determine estrogen and progesterone levels should be considered, in view of the influence of this information on diagnosis and management. Management is based on the treatment of stage II breast cancer and should include both local and systemic therapies. Prognosis following treatment is comparable to that for women with stage II breast cancer. Older series have advocated modified radical mastectomy and axillary dissection for primary treatment. However, the results of a series of 42 patients suggested that the survival time for patients receiving systemic chemotherapy was superior to that for patients treated with surgery alone and that local control was improved by irradiating the breast and axilla. The actuarial disease-free survival rates in this study were 71% at five years and 65% at 10 years.

Patients with axillary adenopathy and involvement of additional sites (usually liver, bone, or both) or with a histology not indicative of adenocarcinoma constitute a much more heterogeneous group composed of equal numbers of men and women as well as a broader histologic spectrum, with poorly differentiated carcinomas and neuroendocrine carcinomas represented in addition to adenocarcinoma. The survival rate for patients with adenopathy in the axillary nodes and in other involved organ sites is between that of the overall population of patients with unknown primary carcinoma and that of women with isolated axillary adenopathy.

The management of patients with involvement of the axilla as well as other sites or with nonadenocarcinoma histology is less certain. Such cases are generally managed by using a combination of local and systemic modalities, and these patients may be good candidates for novel systemic chemotherapy protocols.

Recommended Therapy

General principles are based on the management of women with stage II or III breast cancer. Tamoxifen is added to systemic therapy for patients with estrogen-receptor-positive neoplasms.

Modified radical mastectomy with axillary nodal dissection followed by systemic chemotherapy with 5-FU, doxorubicin, cyclophosphamide, or similar regimen for six courses

Or

Chemotherapy with 5-FU, doxorubicin, cyclophosphamide, or a similar regimen for six to eight months (courses) followed by irradiation of the ipsilateral breast and axillary nodes. (Axillary dissection before chemotherapy can be considered to assess receptor status and complete nodal staging but will increase the risk of arm edema following radiation therapy.)

TREATMENT

Favorable Clinical Subsets of Unknown Primary Carcinoma: Poorly Differentiated Neuroendocrine Carcinoma

Background

Poorly differentiated (anaplastic) neuroendocrine carcinoma is an emerging clinicopathologic entity that is recognized primarily for its responsiveness to therapy. There is probably considerable overlap with extrapulmonary small cell carcinomas, anaplastic carcinoid, anaplastic islet cell tumors, Merkel cell tumors, and paragangliomas. Histologically, these tumors are very poorly differentiated, but histochemical stains are positive for chromogranin or neuron-specific enolase. Patients with these tumors often present with diffuse hepatic or bone metastases but do not have the indolent histologic or clinical features of typical carcinoid tumors, islet cell tumors, or paragangliomas, and therefore observation might not be appropriate. These tumors are also highly responsive to cisplatin-based chemotherapy.

Recommended Therapy

Etoposide 130 mg/m^2 IV daily for three days + cisplatin 45 mg/m^2 IV on days 2 and 3; courses repeated every four weeks.

Favorable Clinical Subsets of Unknown Primary Carcinoma: Women with Peritoneal Carcinomatosis

Background

Women with diffuse peritoneal carcinomatosis with adenocarcinoma make up another recently recognized subset. These patients form a distinctive subset because of their clinical similarities to patients with typical ovarian carcinoma. Often, papillary histology and elevations in CA-125 will be found, but exploratory laparotomy fails to document a primary tumor. Other workers have also recognized this patient subset, terming this syndrome "peritoneal papillary serous carcinoma" or "multifocal extraovarian serous carcinoma." Patients with these tumors frequently respond to platinum-based chemotherapy. Many patients in these series also underwent exploratory laparotomy with surgical debulking followed by chemotherapy. The reported median survival rates range from 16 months to two years.

The natural history of disease in men with isolated peritoneal carcinomatosis or in patients with disease histology inconsistent with that of ovarian carcinoma (e.g., mucin-positive adenocarcinoma) or additional metastatic sites are much more poorly characterized, and the overall survival rate, even with therapy, is poor.

Recommended Therapy

Papillary serous carcinoma of the peritoneum: Surgical debulking followed by systemic chemotherapy with carboplatin AUC = 6 on day 1 + paclitaxel 175 mg/m^2 IV on day 1, both intravenous; repeat every three to four weeks.

Adenocarcinoma of the peritoneum: Systemic chemotherapy using cisplatin 75 mg/m^2 IV on day 1, folinic acid 500 mg/m^2 in 200 mL of normal saline IV over two hours on days 1 through 5, 5-FU 375 mg/m^2 IV after one hour of folinic acid on days 1 through 5, or carboplatin AUC = 6 on day 1 + paclitaxel 175 mg/m^2 on day 1, both IV; repeat every three to four weeks.

Favorable Clinical Subsets of Unknown Primary Carcinoma: Poorly Differentiated or Undifferentiated Carcinoma

Background

Approximately one third of patients with unknown primary carcinoma have poorly differentiated or undifferentiated carcinoma on histologic testing. In this subset, detailed histochemical or immunohistochemical studies may identify highly treatment-responsive patients with lymphoma (leukocyte common antigen), germ cell (B-HCG, AFP), or neuroendocrine (neuron-specific enolase, chromogranin) neoplasms. Greco and colleagues have identified a group of patients with poorly differentiated carcinoma or poorly differentiated adenocarcinoma that are responsive to platinum-based chemotherapy. However, other investigators conclude that these highly responsive patients are infrequently encountered. On diagnosis, most of these patients had clinical features typical of the extragonadal germ syndrome (i.e., young age, mediastinal and retroperitoneal involvement, and rapid growth). Many of these patients are male and have elevated B-HCG or AFP, although the usefulness of these serum tumor markers in predicting response is in question. In a group of male patients with poorly differentiated carcinoma involving midline structures, Motzer and coworkers identified chromosome 12 abnormalities specific for germ cell neoplasms, confirming the germ cell origin of these tumors.

Combination chemotherapy regimens specific for germ cell carcinoma of testicular origin have usually been employed in the treatment of these patients These regimens have produced documented complete responses and an actual 10-year disease-free survival rate of 16%.

Recommended Therapy

Cisplatin 20 mg/m^2 IV per day for five days + etoposide 100 mg/m^2 IV per day for three to five days +/– bleomycin i.m. 30 U/week. Assess response after two courses of therapy; total of four to six courses for responding patients. Alternative approaches include IV carboplatin AUC = 6 + paclitaxel 200 mg/m^2 by one-hour IV infusion + oral etoposide 50 mg alternating with 100 mg p.o. on days 1 to 10, or cisplatin 75 mg/m^2 IV on day 1, folinic acid 500 mg/m^2 in 200 mL of normal saline IV over two hours on days 1 through 5, 5-FU 375 mg/m^2 IV after one hour of folinic acid on days 1 through 5.

References

Abbruzzese JL, Abbruzzese MC, Hess KR, et al: Unknown primary carcinoma: Natural history and prognostic factors in 657 consecutive patients. J Clin Oncol 1994;12:1272–1280.

Abbruzzese JL, Abbruzzese MC, Lenzi R, et al: Analysis of a diagnostic strategy for patients with suspected tumors of unknown origin. J Clin Oncol 1995;13:2094–2103.

Assar OS, Fischbein NJ, Caputo GR, et al: Metastatic head and neck cancer: Role and usefulness of FDG PET in locating occult primary tumors. Radiology 1999;210:177–181.

Atkin NB: Chromosome 1 aberrations in cancer. Cancer Genet Cytogenet 1986;21:279–285.

Bar-Eli M, Abbruzzese JL, Lee-Jackson D, et al: p53 gene mutation spectrum in human unknown primary tumors. Anticancer Res 1993;13:1619–1623.

Bell CW, S Pathak, P Frost: Unknown primary tumors: Establishment of cell lines, identification of chromosomal abnormalities, and implications for a second type of tumor progression. Cancer Res 1989;49:4311–3215.

Briasoulis E, Kalofonos H, Bafaloukos D, et al: Carboplatin plus paclitaxel in unknown primary carcinoma: A phase II Hellenic Cooperative Oncology Group study. J Clin Oncology 2000;18:3101–3107.

Briasoulis E, Tsavaris N, Fountzilas G, et al: Combination regimen with carboplatin, epirubicin and etoposide in metastatic carcinomas of unknown primary site: A Hellenic Cooperative Oncology Group Phase II study. Oncology 1998;55:426–430.

Briasoulis E, Tsokos M, Fountzilas G, et al: Bcl2 and p53 protein expression in metastatic carcinoma of unknown primary origin: biological and clinical implications: A Hellenic Cooperative Oncology Group study. Anticancer Res 1998;18:1907–1914.

de Campos ES, Menuice LP, Radford J, et al: Metastatic carcinoma of uncertain primary site: A retrospective review of 57 patients treated with vincristine, doxorubicin, cyclophosphamide (VAC) or VAC alternating with cisplatin and etoposide (VAC/PE). Cancer 1994;73:470–475.

Gamble AR, Bell JA, Roman JE, et al: Use of tumor marker immunoreactivity to identify primary site of metastatic cancer. Br Med J 1993;306:295–298.

Greco FA, Burris HA 3rd, Litchy S, et al: Gemcitabine, carboplatin, and paclitaxel for patients with carcinoma of unknown primary site: A Minnie Pearl Cancer Research Network study. J Clin Oncol 2002;20:1651–1656.

Greco FA, Erland JB, Morissey LH, et al: Carcinoma of unknown primary site: Phase II trial with docetaxel plus cisplatin or carboplatin. Ann Oncol 2000;11:211–215.

Hainsworth JD, Erland JB, Kalman LA, et al: Carcinoma of unknown primary site: Treatment with 1-hour paclitaxel, carboplatin, and extended-schedule etoposide. J Clin Oncol 1997;15:2385–2393.

Hainsworth JD, Greco FA: Treatment of patients with cancer of an unknown primary site. N Engl J Med 1993;329:257–263.

Hainsworth JD, Johnson DH, Greco FA: Cisplatin-based combination chemotherapy in the treatment of poorly differentiated carcinoma and poorly differentiated adenocarcinoma of unknown primary site: Results of a 12-year experience. J Clin Oncol 1992;10:912–922.

Hainsworth JD, Lennington WJ, Greco FA: Overexpression of Her-2 in patients with poorly differentiated carcinoma or poorly differentiated adenocarcinoma of unknown primary site. J Clin Oncol 2000;18:632–635.

Henry-Tillman RS, Haines SE, Westbrook KC, et al: Role of breast magnetic resonance imaging in determining breast as a source of unknown metastatic lymphadenopathy. Am J Surg 1999;178:496–500.

Hess KR, Abbruzzese MC, Lenzi R, et al: Classification and regression tree analysis of 1000 consecutive patients with unknown primary carcinoma. Clin Cancer Res 1999;5:3403–3410.

Ilson DH, Motzer RJ, Rodriguez E, et al: Genetic analysis in the diagnosis of neoplasms of unknown primary tumor site. Semin Oncol 1993;20:229–237.

Jackson B, Scott-Conner C, Moulder J: Axillary metastasis from occult breast carcinoma: diagnosis and management. Am Surg 1995;61:431–434.

Karsell PR, Sheedy PF 2nd, O'Connell MJ: Computed tomography in search of cancer of unknown origin. JAMA 1982;248:340–343.

Kole AC, Nieweg OE, Pruim J, et al: Detection of unknown occult primary tumors using positron emission tomography. Cancer 1998;82:1160–1166.

Lassen U, Daugaard G, Eigtved A, et al: 18F-FDG whole body positron emission tomography (PET) in patients with unknown primary tumours (UPT). Eur J Cancer 1999;35:1076–1082.

Lenzi R, Hess KR, Abbruzzese MC, et al: Poorly differentiated carcinoma and poorly differentiated adenocarcinoma of unknown origin: Favorable subsets of patients with unknown primary carcinoma? J Clin Oncol 1997;15:2056–2066.

Motzer RJ, Rodriguez E, Reuter VE, et al: Genetic analysis as an aid in diagnosis for patients with midline carcinomas of uncertain histologies. J Natl Cancer Inst 1991;83:341–346.

Motzer RJ, Rodriguez E, Reuter VE, et al: Molecular and cytogenetic studies in the diagnosis of patients with poorly differentiated carcinomas of unknown primary site. J Clin Oncol 1995;13:274–282.

Orel SG, Weinstein SP, Schnall MD, et al: Breast MR imaging in patients with axillary node metastases and unknown primary malignancy. Radiol 1999;212:543–549.

Raber MN, Abbruzzese JL, Frost P: Unknown primary tumors. Curr Opin Oncol 1992;4:3–9.

Chapter 113
Cancer and the Immunocompromised Host

David T. Scadden and Jonathan W. Friedberg

Like opportunistic infections, opportunistic neoplasms can develop in the setting of T cell immunodeficiency, whether due to congenital immunologic dyscrasias, immunosuppressive therapy given after organ transplantation, or AIDS. Although each of these circumstances has unique characteristics, common among them is an association with secondary infectious events predisposing to tumorigenesis. The spectrum of tumor types is therefore quite narrow, with lymphoma and cutaneous neoplasms predominating. In the setting of human immunodeficiency virus (HIV) infection, the spectrum of secondary tumors is broader but is not associated with an increase in otherwise common epithelial malignancies. This chapter discusses the predominant immunodeficiency states encountered by physicians who treat adult patients—namely, HIV infection and post-transplantation immunosuppression—and focuses on the common tumor types that develop.

Epidemiology of AIDS-Related Malignancies

The risk of developing a cancer in the context of HIV-1 infection varies among different subsets of individuals, based on the risk factor operant for HIV transmission, the genotype of the host, and the epidemiology of concurrent oncogenic viruses. The frequency and types of these tumors have been affected substantially by the advent of combination, highly active, antiretroviral therapy (HAART). The introduction of combination anti-HIV therapy with protease inhibitors in 1996 heralded a virtual revolution in the AIDS epidemic, rapidly changing the morbidity and mortality of HIV infection. Among individuals with access to HAART, opportunistic disease of all types diminished, a change that has been readily apparent among subsets of opportunistic malignancies.

Kaposi's sarcoma was an early harbinger of the AIDS epidemic and became an early indicator of the changes wrought by the use of HAART in HIV disease. Although the incidence of Kaposi's was already declining prior to the availability of HIV protease inhibitor therapy, HAART made what was once the most common HIV-associated neoplasm a relative rarity. The incidence of new cases of Kaposi's sarcoma has declined by almost 80-fold. Moreover, existing Kaposi's lesions regress in the majority of patients in whom HAART successfully suppresses HIV replication.

The incidence of some, but not all, non–Hodgkin's lymphomas has also been altered, especially in the case of primary central nervous system (CNS) lymphomas. This complication of far-advanced HIV disease has always been much less common than Kaposi's sarcoma. The decline in incidence of primary central nervous system lymphomas is, therefore, much more difficult to document. Major AIDS centers in the United States now a fraction of the number of new cases previously seen annually. Primary central nervous system lymphoma is an agonal manifestation of AIDS, and, like post-transplant lymphoproliferative disease (PTLPD), it is almost uniformly associated with the presence of Epstein-Barr virus in the tumor tissue. In both settings, the profile of Epstein-Barr virus latent gene expression includes expression of Epstein-Barr antigens in a pattern of markers that is seen when Epstein-Barr virus is used to transform B cells in vitro. Among these Epstein-Barr gene products are those that are readily targeted by cytotoxic T lymphocytes (CTL). The availability of these antitumor cells in those patients who achieve successful control of HIV-induced immune destruction by HAART could account for the marked reduction in incidence of primary central nervous system lymphoma among successfully treated patients who have AIDS. It is also true, however, that such Epstein-Barr–specific cytotoxic lymphocytes can be dysfunctional, and they can be detectable in patients who develop Epstein-Barr virus–induced lymphoproliferative disease.

Whether systemic lymphomas are also reduced in incidence in patients with AIDS who are receiving

HAART is uncertain. The current consensus is that the incidence of these lymphomas, like the incidence of central nervous system lymphomas, is diminished, but the reduction is less dramatic than that observed for Kaposi's sarcoma.

Non-Hodgkin's Lymphoma

Pathophysiology

The lack of a proportionate reduction in systemic lymphomas could reflect a more complex pathophysiology involved in the genesis of these tumors than is the case with Kaposi's sarcoma. In systemic lymphomas, control of the HIV virus might be insufficient to reverse B lymphocyte proliferation. AIDS-related primary central nervous system lymphomas have a relatively straightforward mechanism of tumorigenesis. Epstein-Barr virus is present in the tumor cells, resulting in expression of latent genes that deregulate cell growth and cause autonomous proliferation of B lymphocytes. In contrast, in AIDS-related systemic lymphomas, the pattern of gene expression in the Epstein-Barr virus-containing cells differs (in one-third to two-thirds of cases) from that seen in the primary central nervous system lymphomas. In AIDS-related systemic lymphomas, a number of genetic abnormalities that are found in B cell malignancies of nonimmunodeficient patients—for example, the Bcl-6 rearrangement, c-myc rearrangement, and p53 mutations that are commonly seen in large cell lymphomas—have been detected. As one example, in AIDS-related lymphomas of the small cell histology (Burkitt's and Burkitt's-like), c-myc rearrangements (but not Bcl-6 rearrangements) are common, whereas p53 mutations are rare. The rearrangements of c-myc seen in AIDS-related lymphomas juxtapose c-myc with the immunoglobulin gene heavy-chain switch region that indicates rearrangement occurring at the time of class switching. There is no clear link between Epstein-Barr virus and any specific genetic mutation.

The HIV itself contributes antigenic stimulation that drives the proliferation of B cells, and the HIV envelope glycoprotein could enhance B cell activation directly. HIV envelope protein interaction with chemokine receptors might participate in events that mediate growth stimulation. Perturbation of the T cell compartment and release of B cell stimulating factors (interleukins) further augment proliferation. The hypergammaglobulinemia that accompanies HIV infection reflects one aspect of B-lineage stimulation, and control of HIV with HAART gradually decreases total serum immunoglobulin levels. The relationship

of stimulus to production of proliferative factors by the host could well depend upon host-specific characteristics, which are only beginning to be explored. For example, individuals with AIDS who have variant regulatory regions in the chemokine gene SDF-1 or the encoding regions of the chemokine receptor gene, CCR-5, alter the predisposition to the development of lymphomas. Genomic analysis of the host and contributory pathogens is an area rich with possibility for understanding why some individuals are more predisposed than others to AIDS-related lymphomas, despite the fact that HIV and Epstein-Barr virus are present in all those who are affected.

Clinical Presentation

Systemic AIDS-related lymphomas present with a wide range of symptoms due to the propensity for disease outside the confines of the lymphatic system, with particular predilection for gastrointestinal tract, bone marrow, central nervous system, liver, and soft tissues. Predominant sites of involvement vary depending on the histology of the lymphoma. Large cell lymphomas preferentially involve the gastrointestinal tract, whereas small cell lymphomas tend to invade the bone marrow and meninges. The presentation of AIDS-related lymphoma does not appear to be appreciably affected by HAART, although one study has suggested a decline in the frequency of the small cell lymphoma subtypes.

Primary effusion lymphoma is an uncommon form of lymphoma that has distinct clinicopathologic characteristics. It is unique among lymphomas because it is a liquid-phase hematologic malignancy that rarely involves the blood or lymph nodes. The tumor presents with body cavity effusions with large anaplastic or immunoblastic appearing cells that mark for CD45 (common leukocyte antigen) on the cell surface, in the absence of either B lymphocyte- (CD19 or CD20) or T lymphocyte- (CD3) specific markers. Southern blotting of the immunoglobulin locus demonstrates VDJ rearrangement verifying their B cell origin. Viral genome analyses show a consistent association with Kaposi's sarcoma herpes virus and frequent coassociation with Epstein-Barr virus. This kind of lymphoma also appears in immunodeficiency disorders other than AIDS.

Clinical Evaluation

Evaluation of patients with AIDS-related lymphoma should follow guidelines for lymphomas contracted outside the setting of HIV. The clinician should obtain a careful history of "B" symptoms (fever, night sweats, weight loss), radiographic imaging studies, complete blood and platelet count and differential, and a chemistry panel for liver and renal function tests, uric acid, calcium, lactate dehydrogenase, and bone marrow aspiration and biopsy. Work-up also involves determination of specific parameters for patients with AIDS, such as CD4+ cell counts and HIV RNA. Patients who present with fever must have a careful microbiologic assessment to exclude concurrent opportunistic infections that could complicate therapy.

The incidence of central nervous system involvement in patients with AIDS-related systemic lymphoma has been estimated to be as high as 20%. Thus, all HIV-positive patients presenting with systemic non-Hodgkin's lymphoma should undergo careful assessment of the central nervous system, generally by both radiographic imaging and lumbar puncture. Particular vigilance is required for those patients whose lymphoma carries the Epstein-Barr virus, for they have a substantially increased risk of central nervous system disease, either at diagnosis or later. Central nervous system prophylaxis with intrathecal chemotherapy should be targeted to those who have Epstein-Barr virus in the tumor tissue or extranodal involvement of high-risk sites such as the bone marrow, testis, or paranasal sinus.

Staging, Prognostic Features, and Outcome

Prognosis in patients with AIDS-related lymphomas was previously bleak. With overall improvement in general health status among patients successfully treated with HAART, chemotherapy is better tolerated than it was in the past. Treatment with curative intent should now be pursued in such patients with the expectation of an improved outcome. Adverse prognostic factors in the era of HAART are not yet well established. In a pre-HAART trial of chemotherapy regimens involving patients with AIDS-related lymphomas, multivariate analysis revealed the following negative indicators of prognosis:

- CD4 count less than 100 cells/μL,
- age greater than 35 years,
- intravenous drug use, and
- stage III/IV disease.

When one or none of these factors was present, the median survival was 46 weeks, whereas it declined to 44 weeks when two factors were present, and to 18 weeks when three or four factors were present.

The International Prognostic Index (IPI) used effectively for non–AIDS-related lymphomas is also likely to prove useful for AIDS-related lymphomas, but it has only been evaluated in a small number of patients without a selective examination of the different histologic subsets.

Treatment

Treatment options for AIDS-related lymphomas are beginning to expand as the impact of HAART makes aggressive therapies that previously were considered untenable in the AIDS population both tolerable and testable. Because of the risks of overwhelming opportunistic and other infections after chemotherapy, initial studies of chemotherapy focused on reducing toxicity by reducing the doses of conventional therapeutic regimens used for patients with lymphomas who did not have HIV infection. For example, half-standard dose m-BACOD (methotrexate, bleomycin, Adriamycin, cyclophosphamide, Oncovin) proved to be useful in patients with advanced HIV disease. Administering antilymphoma drugs by continuous infusion, rather than by intravenous bolus, also appears to moderate the toxicity without diminishing the response, as was shown in the studies of CDE (cyclophosphamide, hydroxydaunorubicin [Adriamycin] etoposide) by the National Cancer Institute and the Eastern Cooperative Oncology Group. Recent trials, appropriately, have shifted in emphasis from tolerability of drugs to curability of tumor. The improvement in outcome in intermediate-grade lymphomas by adding rituximab to CHOP (cyclophosphamide, hydroxydaunorubicin, Oncovin, and prednisone) is also under study in a nearly completed trial in the AIDS-related lymphoma population. A trial using EPOCH (etoposide, prednisone, oncovin, cyclophosphamide, hydroxydanorubicin, [Adriamycin]) by the National Cancer Institute has been enconraging. Currently, however, the treatment of choice for AIDS-related intermediate grade lymphomas is CHOP in standard doses.

Whether high-dose regimens requiring autologous stem cell rescue or nonmyeloablative allogeneic stem cell transplants have a role in AIDS-related lymphomas is a subject of considerable interest. Scattered case reports indicate reasonable tolerance and no difficulty with engraftment in the autologous setting. Tolerability in the allogeneic setting is yet untested in patients whose HIV infection is controlled by HAART. The issue of whether to continue HAART or other combinations of anti-HIV medication during the course of cytotoxic chemotherapy remains unresolved. Concurrent antiretroviral combinations (stavudine, lamivudine, and indinivir) combined with CHOP chemotherapy did not result in untoward or unexpected toxicities. In the presence of these antiretroviral drugs, pharmacokinetics was little changed, except for a 50% reduction in the clearance of cyclophosphamide. In contrast, in the study by the National Cancer Institute, all antiretroviral drugs were discontinued during treatment with EPOCH. This resulted in a rise in HIV viral load and a decline in CD4 counts, but both parameters became normal following reintroduction of medications at the end of tumor therapy. Weighing the relative risks and benefits in the absence of determining data, it would seem appropriate to either discontinue all antiretroviral therapy or continue with combination antiretroviral treatment. Half-measures—that is, giving a single agent or markedly reduced doses of drugs—are to be avoided to forestall the development of drug resistance by HIV.

Additional supportive care is generally necessary for the patient with AIDS-related lymphoma. Given the underlying immunocompromise and the likelihood of further impairment secondary to the cytotoxic therapy, use of prophylactic antibiotics is suggested for all patients and is essential for those patients with CD4+ cells less than 200/µL. Trimethoprim/sulfamethoxazole is the preferred agent to protect from *Pneumocystis carinii*, toxoplasmosis, and bacterial disease. Other agents, such as dapsone, atovoquone, and aerosolized pentamadine, are also available to protect patients from pneumocystis infection. Bone marrow reserve is commonly decreased in these patients who have been heavily treated with HAART, and growth factor support is often required to diminish the degree and duration of neutropenia from chemotherapy.

Kaposi's Sarcoma

Epidemiology

Kaposi's sarcoma is associated with subsets of HIV-positive patients whose risk for HIV infection is predominantly men having sex with men. The disproportionate risk for this tumor within this select immunodeficient population presented an intriguing epidemiologic scenario strongly suggesting the activity of a secondary infectious agent. This was finally identified by comparative genetic analysis in 1994 as a member of the gammaherpesvirus family, a group containing at least two other viruses capable of transforming human cells (Epstein-Barr virus and *Herpesvirus saimiri*). Kaposi's sarcoma herpesvirus is a 165 kb double-stranded DNA virus that is present in patients prior to tumor formation; it has a high seroprevalence in populations with a high incidence of Kaposi's sarcoma, and, if present, infects those cells composing the tumors. Although it does not formally fulfill Koch's criteria to document an agent as causative of a specific disease, these features make a compelling argument for Kaposi's sarcoma herpesvirus as the viral pathogen necessary for the induction of Kaposi's sarcoma.

Seroepidemiologic studies of Kaposi's sarcoma herpesvirus infection provide varying results depending on the assay used for its detection. The ORF73 gene product provides a serodominant antigen whose reactivity demonstrates high specificity, although the sensitivity is only approximately 80% in HIV-infected individuals who have Kaposi's sarcoma. Using this method, the prevalence of Kaposi's sarcoma herpesvirus infection has been estimated to be at least 1% to 2% in the U.S. blood donor population, 2% in patients with hemophilia, 3% to 4% in HIV-positive women, and 25% to 30% in HIV-positive homosexual men. In contrast, a whole-virus lysate assay provides increased sensitivity, detecting viral reactivity in 92% of patients with Kaposi's sarcoma (regardless of HIV status) and in 11% of healthy blood donors. Although a single standard assay system has not yet been adopted, the epidemiology of the Kaposi's sarcoma herpesvirus in North American and Northern European populations more closely resembles that of the herpes simplex virus than the Epstein-Barr virus. In contrast, areas of sub-Saharan Africa and the Mediterranean basin have prevalence rates exceeding 40%.

The Kaposi's sarcoma herpesvirus mechanisms of transmission are only partly understood. A longitudinal study of men followed over a ten-year period demonstrated that male homosexual activity correlated with Kaposi's sarcoma herpesvirus seroconversion. The risk was linearly related to the number of sexual intercourse contacts. In men who had more than 250 sexual partners in the preceding two years, the seropositivity rate was 65%. Other populations, however, are clearly infected by other means. In particular, the prevalence of the virus in populations of young children in Africa suggests that vertical or paravertical transmission can occur. In this regard, the recent finding of Kaposi's sarcoma herpesvirus in saliva suggests that an oral route of spread is a possible, if inefficient, mode of transmission.

Pathology and Pathogenesis

Infection with Kaposi's sarcoma herpesvirus is a necessary condition for the development of Kaposi's sarcoma. The virus is found in Kaposi's sarcoma lesions regardless of whether the setting is HIV disease, organ transplantation, or endemic Kaposi's sarcoma. The specific mechanism by which the virus participates in tumor generation is unclear and does not conform to the established paradigms for other virus-related neoplastic diseases. The latent genes implicated in Epstein-Barr virus-induced transformation do not have homologues in Kaposi's sarcoma herpesvirus.

The closely related *Herpesvirus saimiri*, which is capable of transforming human cells, encodes a transforming gene product with homology to Kaposi's sarcoma herpesvirus, but only in the lytic, not the latent, phase of the viral life cycle. Other genes that are homologous to genes with transforming capability in other systems are active in the lytic phase as well. Moreover, mice transgenic for the chemokine receptor encoding lytic phase gene develop a tumor that is histologically similar to human Kaposi's sarcoma. The hypothesis that lytic phase genes participate in tumorigenesis draws indirect support from retrospective studies, which disclose an association between the use of antiherpesvirus medication (ganciclovir and foscarnet) and a decreased incidence of Kaposi's sarcoma.

Clinical Presentation

Kaposi's sarcoma most often presents as a violaceous or salmon-colored macule on mucocutaneous surfaces. It can be singular or multiple and has no orderly pattern of progression. Lesions can be flat and plaquelike or nodular, and small or extensive enough to encase a limb. The absence of Kaposi's sarcoma on the skin, however, does not mean that occult disease sites are not present. Lymph node involvement is relatively common and could be the exclusive site of disease, particularly in pediatric populations. Visceral disease most often includes mucous membranes such as the gastrointestinal tract or airway, but involvement of liver, lung parenchyma, or spleen is also frequent. The presence of mucous membrane lesions does not necessarily indicate deep tissue involvement because bronchial Kaposi's sarcoma can exist without parenchymal infiltration. The presence of mucosal disease can predispose to local complications—such as gingival hypertrophy or cough or bleeding—that can be extensive and life threatening, but mucous membrane involvement is most often asymptomatic and is not by itself an indication to proceed with aggressive therapy.

After cutaneous lesions, the next most common presentation of Kaposi's sarcoma is edema. Kaposi's sarcoma is composed of ectatic blood vessels whose abnormal permeability is manifested by the presence of red cells in the interstitium. The accompanying plasma protein accumulation can create particularly troubling problems because lymphatic drainage is impaired. Due to the increased load on the lymphatics and their reduced capacity, local accumulations of fluid can be extensive. Peculiar sites of edema occur in the periorbital or peripubic tissue, as well as in the more common site of the lower extremities.

Clinical Evaluation

When assessing a patient with hyperpigmented lesions suspicious for Kaposi's sarcoma, a biopsy is recommended, even though the Communicable Disease Center's formal definition does not require histologic confirmation if an experienced observer makes the diagnosis clinically. In the immunocompromised host, however, one must be especially wary of missing the diagnosis of cutaneous bacillary angiomatosis (detected by silver stain of the biopsy), which can be treated successfully with antibiotics.

Patients with Kaposi's sarcoma should have studies performed to define their immunologic status (e.g., CD4+ T cell count), routine examination with particular attention to emerging edema, and a chest radiogram to exclude cryptic parenchymal lung involvement. Extensive staging radiographically with computed tomography (CT) scans or visually by endoscopy is not warranted except when indicated for specific signs or symptoms. Diagrammatic recording of the location, size, and palpability of lesions (flat vs. raised) is a useful means of following patients. Ancillary serial photographic documentation should be employed whenever possible.

Staging, Prognostic Features, and Outcome

Staging criteria have been established and validated by clinical outcomes (Table 113-1). Those features that

Table 113-1 ■ Proposed Revised Staging System for AIDS-Associated Kaposi's Sarcoma

Stage	CD4 Count	Tumor Risk Group	Median Survival (months)
I	≥150/μL (I_0)	Good (T_0): KS confined to skin, lymph nodes, or flat palate lesions; no tumor-associated edema or visceral Kaposi's sarcoma	NR*
II	≥150/μL (I_0)	Poor (T_1): Any visceral Kaposi's sarcoma, nodular oral Kaposi's sarcoma, or tumor-associated edema	35
III	<150/μL (I_1)	Any	13

NR = median not reached; Severe immunodeficiency absent (I_0) or present (I_1); T_0 or T_1 = tumor sites as defined in the table. From Krown SE, Testa MA, Huang J: AIDS-related Kaposi's sarcoma: prospective validation of the AIDS Clinical Trials Group staging classification. AIDS Clinical Trials Group Oncology Committee. J Clin Oncol 15:3085–3092, 1997.

predict for likelihood of a response to changes in anti-HIV therapy are not well defined. It is clear, however, that immunologic function plays a central role in the evolution of Kaposi's sarcoma. The issue of how to achieve the best balance between minimizing immunologic impairment and blocking tumor progression is beginning to be explored as cytotoxic T cell epitopes are being defined and correlations of reactivity to disease state are characterized.

Treatment

The presence of Kaposi's sarcoma is not by itself an indication to treat, because disease progression is so variable. Kaposi's sarcoma can remain as an indolent, limited cutaneous disease for considerable periods of time, and cosmesis could be the primary determinant of whether to treat. Some individuals, however, will have aggressive, life-threatening symptomatic disease, necessitating immediate cytotoxic therapy.

In all patients, treatment of the underlying HIV disease is an essential component of Kaposi's sarcoma therapy. Those patients who have no prior anti-HIV treatment have a tumor response rate from anti-HIV medications that is comparable to that achieved by chemotherapy. The anti-HIV therapy does not act directly on the Kaposi's sarcoma herpesvirus but rather affects the immunologic background of the host, which is critical for control of the virus. Response in Kaposi's sarcoma to anti-HIV medications can be quite durable. For example, in one report only six of 39 patients required any therapy beyond that of anti-HIV medications 24 months after the initiation of HAART. Time to response varies, but most patients who will respond to HAART note improvement by four to eight weeks. If no response occurs within 12 weeks of treatment, alternative therapy should be initiated.

Local or systemic therapy can be employed for the tumor collections of Kaposi's sarcoma. Local therapy for cutaneous disease consists either of liquid nitrogen, intralesional vinblastine, or radiation therapy, each of which is associated with some local discomfort. Such treatment is thus generally reserved for patients whose cutaneous lesions are small in size and number. Topical 9-*cis*-retinoic acid cream is also effective. Skin sensitivity can limit its usefulness, and patients must be particularly careful to avoid applying the cream beyond the margins of the tumor lesions.

Cytotoxic chemotherapy is appropriate for patients who have edema, extensive mucocutaneous disease, or symptomatic pulmonary or gastrointestinal involvement. Responses to systemic chemotherapy are common, although precise definition of responses has varied in many studies. A skin lesion can regress histologically yet leave a pigmented hemosiderin stain whose diameter is unchanged from that noted prior to treatment. A set of criteria specific for Kaposi's sarcoma for gauging responses was recently defined in the United States and is now used widely. Using the variable response criteria of previous trials, a wide range (57% to 88%) of response rates was reported after chemotherapy with bleomycin and vincristine or the combination of doxorubicin, bleomycin, and vincristine. In part because of their side effects, these drugs have been superceded by liposomal anthracyclines and paclitaxel. The leaky vasculature of Kaposi's sarcoma predisposes to deposition of the drug within lesions in concentrations almost an order of magnitude higher than is found in non-involved tissue. Two phase III trials demonstrated the superior toxicity profile of liposomal doxorubicin or liposomal daunorubicin compared with either bleomycin plus vincristine or that combination plus Adriamycin. The response rate with liposomal doxorubicin appeared to be higher than with liposomal daunorubicin, but these drugs have not been compared directly in a randomized study. Because the superiority of liposomal doxorubicin has not been established, knowledgeable clinicians in the field use the drugs interchangeably.

The taxane tubulin stabilizer, paclitaxel, is a highly active and generally well tolerated agent for Kaposi's sarcoma. In a phase I trial involving heavily pretreated, anthracycline-treated patients, 70% achieved a major response to paclitaxel therapy. Another trial showed a 60% major response rate, with a longer duration of response than had been observed before with other agents. Patients can tolerate very prolonged use of this agent at low doses (100 mg/m^2 every two weeks) with minimal side effects and excellent tumor control.

No therapy for Kaposi's sarcoma is curative. If control of HIV infection is lost and immune impairment recurs, Kaposi's sarcoma will reappear even in patients who have had prolonged regression of their disease. Discontinuing chemotherapy in responding patients leads to gradual recurrence of the lesions. For some patients, however, the interval to recurrence can be long if effective anti-HIV therapy is given. Among patients who do recur after a drug "holiday," resuming the same medications is generally effective. It is therefore a common practice to achieve a desired extent of tumor regression, after which the interval between cytotoxic treatments is gradually extended, administering chemotherapy as infrequently as possible while trying to maintain the response. Guidelines for such an approach are not well delineated, requiring individualization of therapy for each patient.

Due to the highly vascular nature of Kaposi's sarcoma, a number of antiangiogenesis agents have been tested in this disease. Thalidomide, the dipeptide IM862, and the metalloproteinase inhibitor col-3, all have shown encouraging activity in early trials. One or more of these might eventually emerge as a first-line therapy for those with limited disease or as maintenance therapy after a response to chemotherapy has been achieved.

Post-Transplant Lymphoproliferative Disease (PTLPD)

Epidemiology and Risk Factors

The immunosuppressive regimen used to prevent organ rejection diminishes the immune response, permitting uncontrolled lymphoid proliferation under the stimulus of the Epstein-Barr virus. This post-transplant lymphoproliferative disease is a significant cause of morbidity and mortality following organ transplantation and the most common malignancy that occurs in this setting. A multicenter, collaborative project quantified the risk of post-transplant lymphoproliferative disease occurring after kidney or heart transplantation in more than 50,000 patients. The risk of non-Hodgkin's lymphoma is higher after heart transplant than after kidney transplant, probably due to the more intensive immunoppression employed after heart transplants. During the first post-transplant year, 1.2% of heart transplant patients develop non-Hodgkin's lymphoma. The incidence decreases in subsequent years, to a rate of 0.3% per year. With long-term follow-up after heart transplant, the cumulative risk of development of post-transplant lymphoproliferative disease exceeds 5%.

The incidence of post-transplantation non-Hodgkin's lymphoma is higher in the United States compared with Europe, probably due to the use of more aggressive immunosuppressive regimens after transplantation in the United States. Antithymocyte globulin or OKT3 (the antibody directed at T cells), both of which are used commonly after heart transplants, increases the incidence compared with patients not receiving either of these agents. Similarly, the risk increases when immunosuppressive therapy consists of the combination of cyclosporine and azathioprine rather than cyclosporine, used alone or with corticosteroids. Patients who are seronegative for Epstein-Barr virus have a 24-fold higher risk of post-transplant lymphoproliferative disease than patients who are seropositive, and mismatch between donor and recipient in cytomegalovirus seropositivity further increases the risk. The two major risk factors for the development of post-transplant lymphoproliferative disease after cardiac transplantation are negative Epstein-Barr serology in the recipient pretransplant and the intensity of post-transplant immunosuppression.

Clinical Presentation

Post-transplant lymphoproliferative disease after solid organ transplantation has several unique features that differentiate it from non-Hodgkin's lymphoma in the immunocompetent host. Most patients present with lymphadenopathy or a mass; however, extranodal involvement, a poor prognostic indicator, is often present. In some series, isolated extranodal disease is the most common presentation of post-transplant lymphoproliferative disease and, as is true in AIDS-related lymphoma, in only a minority of patients is the disease confined to the lymphatic system. Central nervous system involvement occurs in more than 20% of patients with post-transplant lymphoproliferative disease, and other common extranodal sites include the lung and gastrointestinal tract, which could be associated with a better prognosis. Involvement of the allografted organ itself is not common but has been noted in approximately 20% of patients with post-transplant lymphoproliferative disease after heart, lung, and liver transplants. Lymphoid infiltration of these organs can be confused with organ rejection, a circumstance that emphasizes the importance of having an experienced hematopathologist evaluate biopsies of transplanted organs.

Pathology

In general, post-transplant lymphoproliferative diseases are classified using the World Health Organization's non-Hodgkin's lymphoma classification. This spectrum of Epstein-Barr virus-driven proliferation has been difficult to categorize beyond simple clonality studies. Biopsies can reveal polyclonal or monoclonal proliferation. Why this variation exists among patients with post-transplant lymphoproliferative disease is unknown. Polymorphic post-transplant lymphoproliferative disorder with Epstein-Barr Nuclear Antigen-2 expression, however, does not occur in normal individuals and therefore is a separate classification. The classification schema is summarized in Table 113-2. Rare cases of indolent B cell malignancies and Hodgkin's disease have been reported after organ transplantation. These are not considered as post-transplant lymphoproliferative diseases at the present time and should be treated as disease in the nonimmunosuppressed host.

In addition to standard histologic evaluation, studies for CD20 expression might add information useful in the choice of therapy. Clonality can be assessed by flow cytometry. The Epstein-Barr virus

Table 113-2 ■ Categories of Posttransplant Lymphoproliferative Disorders (PTLPD)

Reactive plasmacytic hyperplasia

Polymorphic post-transplant lymphoproliferative disorders
  Polyclonal/oligoclonal
  Monoclonal

Monomorphic post-transplant lymphoproliferative disorders (as per classification of non-Hodgkin's lymphoma)
  B cell lymphomas
  Diffuse large cell lymphoma (most common), including immunoblastic
  Burkitt's/Burkitt's-like
  Multiple myeloma

T cell lymphomas

status of the malignancy should be determined using in situ assays or immunostaining for Epstein-Barr latent membrane protein-1 or small nuclear RNAs. Quantitative Epstein-Barr virus assay by polymerase chain reaction technology is emerging as an approach to allow early, reliable diagnosis, but additional study is required before clinical use becomes routine.

Clinical Evaluation

Evaluation of patients with post-transplant lymphoproliferative disease should follow guidelines for aggressive lymphomas outside the setting of immunodeficiency. The evaluation should include

- a careful history for "B" symptoms (fever, night sweats, weight loss)
- radiographic imaging (chest X-ray, computed tomography of chest, pelvis, and abdomen as a baseline, obtaining other studies based on signs and symptoms)
- complete blood count, differential, and platelet count
- chemistry panel, including liver and renal function tests, uric acid, calcium, and lactate dehydrogenase.

Careful examination should be performed with documentation of the size of abnormal nodes, liver, and spleen, and attention should be paid to abnormalities on neurologic examination. A low threshold for studies of the central nervous system by radiographic imaging (e.g., magnetic resonance imaging [MRI] scan of the brain with gadolinium enhancement) and lumbar puncture for cerebrospinal fluid sampling are appropriate, given the high frequency of central nervous system involvement. All patients should undergo bone marrow biopsy and aspiration. Staging evaluation uses the standard Ann Arbor criteria for non-Hodgkin's lymphoma (see Chapter 67).

Gallium imaging or fluoro-deoxyglucose-positron emission tomography (FDG-PET) scanning could be useful in patients who have bulky disease that is difficult to assess by serial computed tomography alone.

TREATMENT

The AIDS Patient with a Suspicious Brain Lesion

In the setting of profound immunosuppression, mass lesions in the brain can have a number of different etiologies with highly distinct implications. Lymphoma, toxoplasmosis, mycobacterial or other bacterial abscess, and progressive multifocal leukoencephalopathy are the major diagnostic considerations. Definitive stereotactic biopsy is clearly preferred, but in many cases it is difficult to obtain. Features suggestive of lymphoma are radiographic lesions that are paraventricular or multicentric in location or cross the midline, the active use of trimethoprim-sulfamethoxazole prophylaxis, negative toxoplasma serology, and a positive signal by SPECT-thallium or positron emission technology (PET) scanning.

Perhaps the most powerful non-histologic tool, however, is cerebrospinal fluid analysis for Epstein-Barr virus by polymerase chain reaction. Virtually all primary CNS lymphomas in AIDS are associated with Epstein-Barr virus in the tumor tissue. Detection of the Epstein-Barr virus by polymerase chain reaction has an estimated sensitivity of 80% to 100% and a specificity of 98% to 100%. It is highly reliable and should be used whenever possible. While diagnostic studies are underway, it is reasonable to initiate empiric antitoxoplasma therapy. In patients with a tissue diagnosis of lymphoma, positive studies for Epstein-Barr virus in the spinal fluid, and suggestive scans of the brain, radiation therapy is usually the primary approach to therapy. Participation of patients in clinical studies is highly encouraged, given the lack of satisfactory therapy for this disease. Corticosteroids can be used judiciously with the intent to prescribe a rapid taper in these already highly immunosuppressed individuals. Antiretroviral therapy should be maximized in patients with central nervous system lymphoma. Prolonged remissions in central nervous system lymphoma have occurred after improved immunologic function induced by control of HIV-1 replication.

Patients who present with fever must have a careful microbiologic assessment to exclude concurrent opportunistic infections that could complicate therapy.

Therapy

Reduction or discontinuation of immunosuppression is the initial therapeutic intervention for patients who have post-transplant lymphoproliferative disease. It might result in complete regression of localized disease, often without subsequent rejection of the graft. The optimal approach to reducing immunosuppressive treatment remains unclear. Most studies support the elimination of azathioprine and mycophenolate mofetil and a 50% reduction in the dose of cyclosporine or tacrolimus whenever possible. Prednisone should also be tapered as tolerated. For patients who are critically ill from post-transplant lymphoproliferative disease, complete discontinuation of all immunosuppressives should be considered, and prednisone should be tapered rapidly to a maintenance dose of 5 to 10 mg/day. Polyclonal disease and post-transplant lymphoproliferative disease occurring early after transplantation are more likely to respond to modulation of immunosuppressive therapy than monoclonal and/or late onset disease.

Acyclovir inhibits viral DNA polymerase and has been shown to decrease oropharyngeal shedding of Epstein-Barr virus; many algorithms for initial treatment of post-transplant lymphoproliferative disease include antiviral therapy in an attempt to control Epstein-Barr virus infection. Ganciclovir, according to anecdotal reports, has resulted in disease control, primarily in polyclonal disease. Plasmacytic hyperplasia and aggressive mononucleosis-like syndromes after transplant might respond to antiviral therapy. Although foscarnet has activity against post-transplant lymphoproliferative disease, because of lesser toxicities, most centers continue instead to use either acyclovir or gancyclovir with decreased immunosuppression and other therapies.

Interferon-alpha is a cytokine that has been shown to decrease Epstein-Barr virus-induced B cell proliferation. Although anecdotal responses have been noted, the use of interferon after transplantation has been associated with organ rejection, particularly in renal allografts. Because this drug is also associated with other toxicities, further study is necessary before recommending its incorporation in standard therapy.

Complete surgical resection followed by radiation therapy has been recommended for the rare case of localized, accessible post-transplant lymphoproliferative disease, in conjunction with other treatments such as reduction in immunosuppression; however, there are no controlled studies to support this approach. Cranial radiation, with or without addi-

---

TREATMENT

The Sequential Approach to Therapy

Most centers currently employ a sequential approach to therapy of Epstein-Barr virus-associated post-transplant lymphoproliferative disease. If immunosuppression withdrawal with or without antiviral therapy, immunoglobulin, or interferon does not induce a remission within 14 to 21 days, then chemotherapy is considered. Although data are limited, the promising results and low toxicity associated with monoclonal antibody therapy suggest an early role for this evolving modality. Studies in the immunocompetent host setting have suggested a role for combining immunotherapy with chemotherapy. The treatment of Epstein-Barr virus-negative post-transplant lymphoproliferative disease is less defined, but the general principle of sequential therapy is valid.

The authors' current approach to therapy of post-transplant lymphoproliferative disease is summarized as follows:

■ All patients: Taper immunosuppression.* Consider intravenous immunoglobulin, interferon, antiviral therapy.

■ Localized, accessible disease: Consider surgery and localized radiation therapy.
■ Diffuse disease, if no response in 14 to 21 days: If the patient is clinical stable, clinical trial (preferred); monoclonal antibody (rituximab) therapy, if patient is CD20 positive; combination chemotherapy (if no response to rituximab, or if patient is CD20 negative). If the patient has rapidly progressing disease, use combination chemotherapy, with or without monoclonal antibody therapy.

*A standard immunosuppressive taper schedule is outlined here and should be attempted in all patients unless there is evidence of ongoing allograft rejection. For non-critically ill patients: Eliminate azathioprine and mycophenolate mofetil; reduce cyclosporine or tacrolimus by 50%; taper prednisone by 50% or as tolerated. For critically ill patients: Eliminate all immunosuppressive agents; maintenance dose of prednisone 5–10 mg/day.

tional therapy, is the most effective treatment of post-transplant lymphoproliferative disease of the central nervous system.

Rituxan (rituximab, IDEC-C2B8) is an anti-CD20 chimeric monoclonal antibody that is active in B cell lymphoma. Initial reports of rituximab therapy for post-transplant lymphoproliferative disease that is CD20 positive are promising, and this approach is becoming the standard first-line therapy with a response ratio of approximately 60%. Radiolabeled conjugated antibodies directed against B cell antigens expressed in post-transplant lymphoproliferative disease might also be helpful. Advantages include lack of susceptibility to multidrug resistance mechanisms and the ability to kill adjacent tumor cells (whether or not they express the target antigen) by conjugation with beta-emitting isotopes.

High mortality and failure rates are associated with combination cytotoxic chemotherapy in post-transplant lymphoproliferative disease, compared with nonimmunosuppressed patients. Small series of patients treated in noncontrolled studies suggest that responses can be seen in anthracycline-based chemotherapy regimens, such as CHOP. The optimal cytotoxic therapy for patients with post-transplant lymphoproliferative disease remains undefined.

The most important defense mechanism against the growth of Epstein-Barr virus-infected B cells is Epstein-Barr virus-specific cytotoxic T-lymphocytes, the CD8+ atypical lymphocytes that are found in infectious mononucleosis and that serve to control the infection. Such Epstein-Barr virus-specific cytotoxic lymphocytes, selected and expanded ex vivo, have controlled some cases of post-transplant lymphoproliferative disease developing after allogeneic bone marrow transplantation. Application of this approach to solid organ transplant post-transplant lymphoproliferative disease is limited, however, by the difficulty of obtaining cells from the donor and the lack of expandable cells from the recipient.

Prevention of Post-transplant Lymphoproliferative Disease after Solid Organ Transplantation

Elimination of identified risk factors, when possible, should lead to a reduction in post-transplant lymphoproliferative disease. The benefit of prophylactic antiviral therapy noted initially in uncontrolled reports has not been substantiated in randomized clinical trials.

As a general rule, immunosuppression should be minimized in all patients. The use of OKT3 and anti-lymphocyte preparations is discouraged, and prolonged use of azathioprine and mycophenolate mofetil should be avoided whenever possible. Further study

is needed to determine whether new immunosuppressive drugs like tacrolimus will be associated with a lower risk of post-transplant lymphoproliferative disease than other cyclosporine-based immunosuppressive regimens.

Data from mouse models suggest that concomitant immunoglobulin infusion with transplant could limit subsequent development of lymphoma. In the setting of allogeneic bone marrow transplantation, gamma-globulin infusion has been shown to decrease the incidence of bacterial infection and cytomegalovirus infection, but there has been no effect on survival rates, Epstein-Barr virus infection, or the incidence of post-transplant lymphoproliferative disease.

Serial measurement of Epstein-Barr viral load using quantitative polymerase chain reaction technology might allow early intervention by modulation of immunosuppressive therapy before symptomatic post-transplant lymphoproliferative disease develops. This technique can also be used to evaluate response to therapy. In a study of liver transplant recipients, clearance of the Epstein-Barr viral load from the peripheral blood correlated with restoration of the host's immune response, reflected in the regression of the post-transplant lymphoproliferative disease and the onset of rejection.

References

Bais C, Santomasso B, Coso O, et al: G-protein-coupled receptor of Kaposi's sarcoma–associated herpesvirus is a viral oncogene and angiogenesis activator. Nature 1998;391:86–89.

Ballerini P, Gaidano G, Gong JZ, et al: Multiple genetic lesions in acquired immunodeficiency syndrome-related non-Hodgkin's lymphoma. Blood 1993;81:166–176.

Benkerrou M, Jais JP, Leblond V, et al: Anti-B cell monoclonal antibody treatment of severe post-transplant B-lymphoproliferative disorder: Prognostic factors and long-term outcome. Blood 1998;92:3137–3147.

Brander C, O'Connor P, Suscovich T, et al: Definition of an optimal cytotoxic T lymphocyte epitope in the latently expressed Kaposi's sarcoma–associated herpesvirus kaposin protein. J Infect Dis 2001;184:119–126.

Cesarman E, Chang Y, Moore PS, et al: Kaposi's sarcoma–associated herpesvirus-like DNA sequences in AIDS-related body-cavity-based lymphomas. N Engl J Med 1995;332:1186–1191.

Chang Y, Cesarman E, Pessin MS, et al: Identification of herpesvirus-like DNA sequences in AIDS-associated Kaposi's sarcoma. Science 1994;266:1865–1869.

Cingolani A, Gastaldi R, Fassone L, et al: Epstein-barr virus infection is predictive of CNS involvement in systemic AIDS-related non-Hodgkin's lymphomas. J Clin Oncol 2000;18:3325–3330.

Cook RC, Connors JM, Gascoyne RD, et al: Treatment of post-transplant lymphoproliferative disease with rituximab monoclonal antibody after lung transplantation [letter]. Lancet 1999;354:1698–1699.

Gill P, Tulpule A, Espina B, et al: Paclitaxel is safe and effective in the treatment of advanced AIDS-related Kaposi's sarcoma. J Clin Oncol 1999;17:1876–1883.

Gill PS, Levine AM, Meyer PR, et al: Primary central nervous system lymphoma in homosexual men. Clinical, immunologic, and pathologic features. Am J Med 1985;78:742–748.

Gill PS, Wernz J, Scadden DT, et al: Randomized phase III trial of liposomal daunorubicin versus doxorubicin, bleomycin, and vincristine in AIDS-related Kaposi's sarcoma. J Clin Oncol 1996;14:2353–2364.

Grulich AE: AIDS-associated non-Hodgkin's lymphoma in the era of highly active antiretroviral therapy. J Acquir Immune Defic Syndr 1999;21(S1):27–30.

Grulich AE, Li Y, McDonald AM, et al: Decreasing rates of Kaposi's sarcoma and non-Hodgkin's lymphoma in the era of potent combination anti-retroviral therapy. AIDS 2001;15:629–633.

Hamilton-Dutoit SJ, Pallesen G, Franzmann MB, et al: AIDS-related lymphoma. Histopathology, immunophenotype, and association with Epstein-Barr virus as demonstrated by in situ nucleic acid hybridization. Am J Pathol 1991;138:149–163.

Kaplan LD, Straus DJ, Testa MA, et al: Low-dose compared with standard-dose m-BACOD chemotherapy for non-Hodgkin's lymphoma associated with human immunodeficiency virus infection. National Institute of Allergy and Infectious Diseases AIDS Clinical Trials Group. N Engl J Med 1997;336:1641–1648.

Karcher DS, Alkan S: Human herpesvirus-8-associated body cavity-based lymphoma in human immunodeficiency virus-infected patients: A unique B cell neoplasm. Hum Pathol 1997;28:801–808.

Kedes DH, Operskalski E, Busch M, et al: The seroepidemiology of human herpesvirus 8 (Kaposi's sarcoma-associated herpesvirus): Distribution of infection in KS risk groups and evidence for sexual transmission. Nat Med 1996;2:918–924.

Kohn DB, Bauer G, Rice CR, et al: A clinical trial of retroviral-mediated transfer of a rev-responsive element decoy gene into CD34(+) cells from the bone marrow of human immunodeficiency virus-1-infected children. Blood 1999;94:368–371.

Krown SE, Testa MA, Huang J: AIDS-related Kaposi's sarcoma: Prospective validation of the AIDS Clinical Trials Group staging classification. AIDS Clinical Trials Group Oncology Committee. J Clin Oncol 1997;15:3085–3092.

Levine AM, Seneviratne L, Espina BM, et al: Evolving characteristics of AIDS-related lymphoma. Blood 2000;96:4084–4090.

Martin JN, Ganem DE, Osmond DH, et al: Sexual transmission and the natural history of human herpesvirus 8 infection. N Engl J Med 1998;338:948–954.

Matthews GV, Bower M, Mandalia S, et al: Changes in acquired immunodeficiency syndrome–related lymphoma since the introduction of highly active antiretroviral therapy. Blood 2000;96:2730–2734.

Northfelt DW, Dezube BJ, Thommes JA, et al: Pegylated-liposomal doxorubicin versus doxorubicin, bleomycin, and vincristine in the treatment of AIDS-related Kaposi's

sarcoma: Results of a randomized phase III clinical trial. J Clin Oncol 1998;16:2445–2451.

Opelz G, Henderson R: Incidence of non-Hodgkin's lymphoma in kidney and heart transplant recipients. Lancet 1993;342:1514–1516.

Pauk J, Huang ML, Brodie SJ, et al: Mucosal shedding of human herpesvirus 8 in men. N Engl J Med 2000;343:1369–1377.

Paya CV, Fung JJ, Nalesnik MA, et al: Epstein-Barr virus–induced post-transplant lymphoproliferative disorders. ASTS/ASTP EBV-PTLD Task Force and The Mayo Clinic Organized International Consensus Development Meeting. Transplantation 1999;68:1517–1525.

Penn I: Incidence and treatment of neoplasia after transplantation. J Heart Lung Transplant 1993;12:S328–S336.

Rabkin CS: AIDS and cancer in the era of highly active antiretroviral therapy (HAART). Eur J Cancer 2000;37:1316–1319.

Rabkin CS, Yang Q, Goedert JJ, et al: Chemokine and chemokine receptor gene variants and risk of non-Hodgkin's lymphoma in human immunodeficiency virus-1-infected individuals. Blood 1999;93:1838–1842.

Ratner L, Lee J, Tang S, et al: Chemotherapy for human immunodeficiency virus-associated non-Hodgkin's lymphoma in combination with highly active antiretroviral therapy. J Clin Oncol 2001;19:2171–2178.

Rooney CM: Use of gene-modified virus-specific T lymphocytes to control Epstein-Barr virus-related lymphoproliferation. Lancet 1995;345:9–13.

Stewart S, Jablonowski H, Goebel FD, et al: Randomized comparative trial of pegylated liposomal doxorubicin versus bleomycin and vincristine in the treatment of AIDS-related Kaposi's sarcoma. International Pegylated Liposomal Doxorubicin Study Group. J Clin Oncol 1998;16:683–691.

Straus DJ, Huang J, Testa MA, et al: Prognostic factors in the treatment of human immunodeficiency virus-associated non-Hodgkin's lymphoma: Analysis of AIDS Clinical Trials Group protocol 142—low-dose versus standard-dose m-BACOD plus granulocyte-macrophage colony-stimulating factor. National Institute of Allergy and Infectious Diseases. J Clin Oncol 1998;16:3601–3606.

Swinnen LJ, Mullen GM, Carr TJ, et al: Aggressive treatment for postcardiac transplant lymphoproliferation. Blood 1995;86:3333–3340.

Tulpule A, Scadden DT, Espina BM, et al: Results of a randomized study of IM862 nasal solution in the treatment of AIDS-related Kaposi's sarcoma. J Clin Oncol 2000;18:716–723.

Tulpule A, Yung RC, Wernz J, et al: Phase II trial of liposomal daunorubicin in the treatment of AIDS-related pulmonary Kaposi's sarcoma. J Clin Oncol 1998;16:3369–3374.

Walker RC, Marshall WF, Strickler JG, et al: Pretransplantation assessment of the risk of lymphoproliferative disorder. Clin Infect Dis 195;20:1346–1353.

Welles L, Saville MW, Lietzau J, et al: Phase II trial with dose titration of paclitaxel for the therapy of human immunodeficiency virus-associated Kaposi's sarcoma. J Clin Oncol 1998;16:1112–1121.

Yang TY, Chen SC, Leach MW, et al: Transgenic expression of the chemokine receptor encoded by human herpesvirus 8 induces an angioproliferative disease resembling Kaposi's sarcoma. J Exp Med 2000;191:445–454.

Chapter 114
Hematologic Manifestations of Cancer

John K. Erban

Introduction

Cancer causes protean hematologic manifestations that are often the initial or presenting signs of the disease. For this reason, proper interpretation of simple, inexpensive laboratory studies such as the complete blood count (CBC) and red blood cell indices, prothrombin time, and partial thromboplastin time can lead to the diagnosis of early-stage or asymptomatic advanced disease. Some manifestations of cancer, such as iron deficiency anemia, are crucial to allow a diagnosis of cancer at a curable stage. Others, such as the presence of a paraprotein, do not specify a diagnosis but might explain potentially life-threatening symptoms. As the biology of tumor growth and spread has become better understood, clinicians can now predict secondary effects of cancer on tissues such as the bone marrow and the blood. For all these reasons, the ability to interpret and respond to abnormal hematologic values is most important for the internist.

Abnormalities of Red Blood Cells

Anemia

Anemia is a cardinal manifestation of chronic disease, and cancer is not an exception to this rule. A low hemoglobin level and low hematocrit in an otherwise asymptomatic patient require explanation, for the answer is most often found in an undiagnosed disease such as cancer. Once anemia has been identified, the mean corpuscular volume (MCV) remains a key to proper interpretation of the cause of anemia. In the absence of a history of hemoglobinopathy such as thalassemia, anemia with a low mean corpuscular volume indicates iron deficiency until proven otherwise. Tracking the mean corpuscular volume back in time and proving that it has fallen is another clue to iron deficiency. Unlike other types of anemia that are often later manifestations of cancer, iron deficiency betrays the primary lesion at a time when it may be otherwise occult and often curable. A low mean corpuscular volume coupled with iron deficiency, as manifested by a low ferritin and iron saturation, is an indication to evaluate the gastrointestinal tract for occult blood loss. Occult blood loss is a manifestation of adenocarcinoma of the colon, colonic polyps, or, less commonly, tumors of upper gastrointestinal organs. Lack of pathology explaining iron loss in the colon, or a history of chronic dysphagia, chronic ethanol excess, or tobacco user; or gastric reflux indicate a need for upper endoscopy to exclude the diagnosis of esophageal carcinoma. Less commonly, the discovery of a low mean corpuscular volume and iron deficiency is not the result of blood loss in the stool. In this circumstance, chronic iron loss should be sought in the urine from a urologic lesion or may arise from a lesion in the female reproductive organs, such as a uterine cancer, which is otherwise occult.

Anemia in the absence of iron deficiency may be a presenting sign of systemic illness. Cancer that is disseminated commonly results in the anemia of chronic disease. The hematocrit and hemoglobin level are rarely significantly depressed, and the mean corpuscular volume remains normal or is low normal. Anemia of chronic disease rarely, if ever, is a presenting sign of localized cancer.

Other than direct blood loss and subsequent iron loss, or through the suppression of erythropoiesis via the anemia of chronic disease, cancer may cause anemia through several other mechanisms. Bone marrow involvement from metastasis is common in breast and prostate cancers. Even at the time of diagnosis, asymptomatic micrometastasis in bone marrow from patients with node-negative breast cancer can be identified by immunocytochemistry or clonogenic assays. They may predict for worse outcome if present following completion of adjuvant therapy. Extensive marrow involvement will commonly result in a myelophthisic picture with a leukoerythroblastic blood smear. Teardrop-shaped red blood cells are a

DIAGNOSIS

Hematologic Manifestations of Cancer

Virtually all of the major hematologic manifestations of cancer can be identified through highly reproducible, low-cost, and readily available tests, which should be included as of any initial assessment of a patient who is suspected of having a malignancy. These include the following:

- Automated complete blood count with red blood cell and platelet indices, especially the mean red cell volume (MCV).
- Reticulocyte count in patients who manifest anemia, especially when the mean red cell volume is increased.
- Peripheral blood smear.
- Iron, total iron-binding capacity, and ferritin studies for patients who may be clinically well with microcytic red blood cell indices.
- Oximetry for patients who manifest erythrocytosis.
- Prothrombin time and partial thromboplastin time.
- Fibrinogen and fibrin degradation product levels where applicable.

- Two-hour mixing study for patients who have significantly prolonged prothrombin time or partial thromboplastin time and a history of bleeding.
- Euglobulin clot lysis time.
- Total protein level.
- Whole-blood or serum viscosity.

These simple studies will uncover all of the likely manifestations of cancer that may present as abnormalities of the cellular elements, clotting cascade, or rheology of the blood.

While initial studies may be normal, manifestations may change at any time in the course of active disease. Therefore, careful attention to symptoms of the patients may indicate the need for retesting at any time.

Among the most important signs to interpret correctly are the red blood cell indices. Lack of attention to a falling mean red cell volume and hemoglobin, however subtle, in an otherwise healthy patient may be the difference between detecting an occult gastrointestinal cancer and delay in diagnosis of a year or more.

---

common finding when cancer involves the bone marrow (Figure 114-1). Other cancers such as lung cancer, colon cancer, renal cell carcinoma, and cancer of the upper gastrointestinal tract less commonly involve the bone marrow. Significant marrow involvement is a poor prognostic finding and results in fibrosis and pancytopenia. The mechanism of anemia is largely through marrow replacement, but cytokine-induced suppression of erythropoiesis may play a role as well.

Pure red cell aplasia in the absence of other hematologic abnormalities has been reported with specific neoplastic disorders of the immune system. Most commonly, benign or malignant thymoma has been associated with severe red cell aplasia. Resection may be curative.

All of the above cancer-related anemias are characterized by suppression of erythropoiesis and low erythrocyte production, a low reticulocyte count, and diminished iron transport. Anemia that accompanies chronic disseminated intravascular coagulation (DIC) and intravascular hemolysis leads to an increased reticulocyte count as the bone marrow compensates for red cell destruction. This syndrome is seen mainly in patients who have and are being treated for mucin-producing metastatic adenocarcinoma. The reticulo-

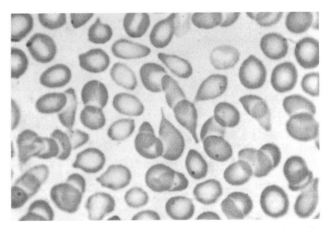

Figure 114-1 ■ Teardrop cells are seen most prominently in thalassemias and diseases involving bone marrow infiltration by fibrosis or malignancy. Erythrocytes are distorted as they travel through the vasculature of an abnormal bone marrow or spleen. Pointed ends may be sharp or blunt. (From Tkachuk DC, Hirschmann JV, McArthur JR: Atlas of Clinical Hematology. Philadelphia: WB Saunders, 2002.) (See Color Plate 22.)

cyte and lactate dehydrogenase (LDH) levels are elevated as intravascular fibrin leads to red cell fragmentation, hemolysis, and anemia. The outcome of patients who present with disseminated intravascular coagulation is frequently poor. Rarely, there is resolution with successful treatment of the underlying cancer. A second cause of anemia from hemolysis involves immune-mediated red cell destruction from the production of autoantibodies directed against the red blood cells. Immune hemolysis occur with some regularity in non-Hodgkin's lymphoma or chronic lymphocytic leukemia. Warm reactive IgG type antibodies are most commonly identified. The autoimmune hemolytic anemia occurs most frequently in the later stages of these diseases. Its presence signifies a general immune dysregulation and is not the result of associated paraproteins produced by the malignant cells. Rather, immune hemolysis is caused by polytypic autoantibodies. Examination of the blood smear demonstrates spherocytes, the hallmark of immune-mediated hemolytic anemia (Figure 114-2). Cold agglutinins of the IgM subtype are less frequently associated with lymphoproliferative disorders, and these may mediate hemolysis through complement activation on the red cell membrane. Complement fixation following IgM antibody deposition may induce both intravascular and extravascular hemolysis.

Polycythemia (see Chapter 40)

Acquired secondary polycythemia may rarely be a presentation of cancer. In the absence of chronic hypoxia, such as in patients with pulmonary disease and lung cancer or carbon monoxide exposure from smoking, ectopic sources of erythropoietin should be sought. Although renal cell carcinoma presents more commonly with anemia, this disease may cause elevations in the hemoglobin level and hematocrit. Other tumors may present with polycythemia, including hepatocel-

lular carcinoma and cerebellar tumors, Wilms' tumor, and even benign tumors such as atrial myxoma. These neoplasms should be specifically considered and sought when searching for secondary causes of polycythemia. Often, the presenting symptoms are related to circulatory insufficiency resulting in unstable angina, exertional shortness of breath, claudication, or transient ischemic events.

Effects on White Blood Cells

Primary effects on the white blood cell count are unusual. When changes do occur, they signify disseminated disease. Mild leukemoid reactions can be associated with cancer and are usually of no clinical significance. Neutrophilia is common, but less commonly, solid tumors or hematologic malignancies may induce elevations of other cells such as monocytes, basophils, or eosinophils. Monocytosis frequently accompanies neoplasia of the lymphoid system and may be seen in a variety of lymphoid malignancies, including Hodgkin's disease. While not usually a cause of symptoms, mild eosinophilia is commonly associated with underlying malignancy. It is one of the six major categories of disease associated with unexplained eosinophilia. Leukocyte function is usually normal.

Depression of the leukocyte count is uncommon in the absence of direct marrow infiltration, secondary splenomegaly, or myelofibrosis from chemotherapy or sclerosing tumors. The isolated depression of the leukocyte count does not indicate a need for bone marrow biopsy. However, the concomitant depression of platelets and red blood cells in the context of a cancer diagnosis strongly suggests bone marrow infiltration or suppression from chemotherapy. Bone marrow biopsy should be considered for any patient in whom two or more blood cell lines are suppressed in the absence of chemotherapy or when immature myeloid and erythroid cells are present in the peripheral blood (leukoerythroblastosis) in the absence of hematopoietic growth factors.

Commonly used agents in cancer treatment that are not chemotherapeutic drugs may also cause reversible leukopenia. For example, tamoxifen used in adjuvant breast cancer therapy and carbamazepine used in seizure prophylaxis with brain tumors cause leukopenia in a minority of patients. Hematologic toxicities of chemotherapeutic agents are important manifestations because prolonged use of certain agents such as carbamazepine can lead to aplastic anemia. Common classes of drugs used in cancer therapy that induce clinically significant leukopenia are shown in Table 114-1.

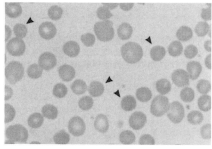

Figure 114-2 ■ Spherocytes in immune-mediated hemolytic anemia. (From Hoffman R, Benz EJ Jr, Shattil SJ, et al [eds]: Hematology: Basic Principles and Practice, 3rd ed. New York: Churchill Livingstone, 2000.) (See Color Plate 22.)

Table 114-1 ■ Common Drug Effects from Cancer-Related Treatment

Chemotherapy

The rules are changing. Chemotherapy schedules were originally designed to be dose limiting on the basis of toxicity, usually myeloid. Thus, schedules administering chemotherapy every three to six weeks were established with predictable nadir leukocyte and platelet counts and more chronic anemia. Now some schedules of weekly or even daily therapy are being employed that have significant anticancer activity while reducing myeloid toxicity. Many chemotherapeutics are relatively sparing of platelets. Anthracyclines, such as doxorubicin, and alkylating agents, such as cyclophosphamide, are exceptions.

Hormonal Agents

Hormonal agents are more than antihormones. Tamoxifen may induce leukopenia as well as thrombocytopenia. Effects on cytokines such as TGF-β have been recognized. Monitoring is recommended.

Immunologic Agents

Antibodies to Her-2/neu (Herceptin) for breast cancer, CD20 (Rituxin) for lymphoma, CD52 (CAMPATH-1h) for chronic lymphocytic leukemia, and other antibodies have been shown to be effective. Allergic responses, eosinophilia, neutropenia, lymphopenia, and susceptibility to infection have been reported. Interferons may cause leukopenia and thrombocytopenia.

Anticonvulsants for brain metastases or primary tumors can have significant toxicities that require monitoring. Dilantin and Depakote may induce thrombocytopenia and leukopenia, and Tegretol may induce leukopenia, agranulocytosis, and even aplasia. Anemia is usually not a limiting problem. Newer agents such as Neurontin may be associated with a lower frequency of hematologic side effects.

Antiulcer/H_2 blockers such as Tagamet, Zantac, and Axid have been associated with thrombocytopenia.

Heparin exposure for indwelling catheter flushes or anticoagulation should be considered as a cause of thrombocytopenia whenever platelets fall without obvious explanation.

Growth factors such as G-CSF, GM-CSF, erythropoietin, and interleukin 11 have been licensed for use for stimulation of recovery of neutrophils, red blood cells, and platelets, respectively. Bone pain and low-grade fever may accompany use of cytokines to stimulate neutrophil production.

Thrombocytosis and Thrombocytopenia

One cause of asymptomatic elevations in the platelet count is the presence of an underlying malignancy. The mechanism of these elevations is uncertain but is likely to be cytokine- and inflammation-related. Secondary elevations in the platelet count associated with malignancy are usually below 1,000,000/μL, but higher levels can be seen. The spleen is normal in size, and platelet function is nearly always normal. There is no need to treat modest elevations in the platelet count in the vast majority of cases. Rather, treatment should focus on the underlying disorder and elevations in the setting of cancer usually signify disseminated disease and poorer prognosis. In contrast, major elevations over 1,000,000 to as high as 3,000,000/μL of blood may be seen in myeloproliferative syndromes, including chronic myeloid leukemia, polycythemia vera, and essential thrombocythemia. Platelet function is often abnormal.

Platelet counts may be depressed to abnormal levels by a number of mechanisms. Tumor may infiltrate the bone marrow and diminish megakaryocyte production and hematopoiesis. Platelet counts are rarely below 10,000/μL but may be severe enough to

risk spontaneous bleeding. The peripheral blood smear often shows a number of changes suggestive of marrow infiltration with tumor, such as nucleated red blood cells, misshapen red cells including teardrop-shaped cells, and large platelets. Prognosis is poor in these situations. Severe platelet depressions may signify reversible, drug-induced thrombocytopenia. All agents, including the heparin utilized for port flushes, must be considered. In contrast to marrow infiltration, drug-induced thrombocytopenia does not alter red blood cell morphology. As such, the peripheral smear may give clues to the mechanism of suppression of the platelet count. Drug-induced platelet suppression may be due to direct suppression of megakaryocytopoiesis, in which case platelet size is uniformly normal. By contrast, immune-mediated drug-induced thrombocytopenia causes increased platelet turnover, and the mean platelet volume increases with increased distribution of platelet size, as a result of increased platelet production.

Thrombocytopenia may be caused by autoimmune mechanisms induced by malignancies of the lymphatic system. Immune thrombocytopenia has been associated both with chronic lymphocytic leukemia and with non-Hodgkin's lymphoma. The clinical stage of chronic lymphocytic leukemia, and therefore the prognosis, is determined by the platelet count only if the mechanism of thrombocytopenia does not involve immune-mediated suppression.

Mechanisms other than direct suppression of thrombopoiesis or immune-mediated peripheral destruction can lower the platelet count. Disseminated intravascular coagulation occurs in neoplastic diseases and results in consumptive thrombocytopenia. Low-grade disseminated intravascular coagulation results in relatively modest increases in the prothrombin time, partial thromboplastin time, and fibrin degradation products. Fibrinogen may be low but is commonly normal or even elevated; its absolute level should not be relied on to exclude the diagnosis. The fibrinogen level depends on both the rate of consumption and the rate of synthesis often increased by cancer and inflammation. Some patients with cancer may have an elevation in fibrinogen levels that fall to normal at the onset of disseminated intravascular coagulation. Fragmentation of red blood cells occurs as a result of intravascular shearing. The absence of occasional helmet cells on repeated examinations of the peripheral blood smear should eliminate the diagnosis.

Tumor cells may generate a prothrombotic state and increase the frequency of thromboembolic events. Bleeding may be due to excessive fibrinogenolysis or fibrinolysis through high levels of plasmin activity. Bleeding may be common, especially from mucosal sites of disease. Clotting times may be normal, or they may be prolonged through decrease in fibrinogen levels. Suspicion of excessive clot lysis can be confirmed through the euglobulin clot lysis time.

Unusual Hematologic Manifestations of Malignancy

Hypereosinophilic Syndrome

The idiopathic hypereosinophilic syndrome (HES) is an unusual cause of absolute eosinophilia but is a disorder that causes profound organ dysfunction as a result of infiltration of eosinophils. Newly identified eosinophilia should suggest a differential diagnosis that includes underlying neoplasia, allergy (atopic, medication-induced, or known allergen), asthma, Addison's disease, collagen vascular disorders, and parasitic diseases. Hypereosinophilic syndrome is characterized by a marked eosinophilia, organomegaly, cardiac dysfunction, and bone marrow findings often showing atypia characteristic of a myeloproliferative syndrome. Distinction from other causes of eosinophilia is made by the number of circulating eosinophils (usually more than 1500/μL), the appearance of the bone marrow, and the degree of tissue infiltration and organ dysfunction. The disease is aggressive and is often fatal without successful treatment.

Cold Agglutinins and Cryoglobulinemia

Cold agglutinins and cryoglobulins are distinct entities that can appear in patients with malignancy. They are rarely found in the same individual, and even more rarely associated with the same molecule. Cold agglutinins are autoreactive antibodies directed against red cells that cause agglutination, both in vitro and in vivo. The thermal amplitude of the antibody is the temperature at which binding and hemolysis occur, and generally antibodies that bind at a high thermal amplitude (near body temperature) will induce hemolysis. As a rule, cold agglutinins that are associated with malignancy occur mainly in patients over age 50, primarily in women, and cause hemolysis when present in high titer (greater than 1:1000). Cold agglutinins may herald the onset of a lymphoproliferative disorder, such as chronic lymphocytic leukemia, or lymphoma. While each of these disorders may be associated with a monoclonal gammopathy, it is uncommon for these monoclonal proteins to have the capacity to act as a cold agglutinin. Cold agglutinins of the chronic idiopathic type are rarely monoclonal IgM proteins, often of kappa subtype, that have specificity for a red cell antigen, usually the I antigen.

Because cold agglutinins are almost always IgM immunoglobulins, they fix complement readily. Thus, the clinical picture is often of immune hemolysis induced by cold temperatures. Signs and symptoms are associated with acral cyanosis and ischemia of cooler parts of the body and with vascular insufficiency. Diagnosis is made by obtaining a blood sample at 37° and detecting agglutination on cooling in vitro. The demonstration of agglutination can be done at the bedside by observing a small amount of anticoagulated blood for flocculation. Blood smears show characteristic features (Figure 114-3).

In contrast, cryoglobulins are antibodies that bind and precipitate other immunoglobulins when incubated at cold temperatures. Cryoglobulinemia may be subclassified into types I, II, and III, depending on whether the autoreactive antibodies are a mixture of monoclonal and polyclonal antibodies (I), purely monoclonal (II), or purely polyclonal (III). The serum electrophoresis will demonstrate a monoclonal gammopathy in cases of type I or type II cryoglobulinemia. Acral cyanosis and palpable purpura, as well as glomerulonephritic lesions, are hallmarks of the disease. Quantification of cryoglobulins involves measurement of cold protein precipitation and immunoelectrophoresis to determine the pattern of antibody. Type III cryoglobulinemia is most often associated with

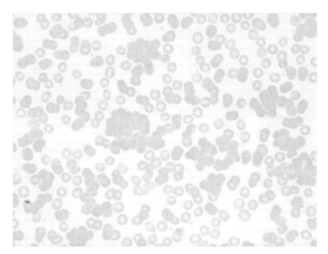

Figure 114-3 ■ Agglutination of red cells in a patient with cold agglutinins (original magnification ×40). (See Color Plate 6, same as Fig. 42-3. courtesy of Cabello Inchausti B: Chapter 42 of this book.)

chronic viral hepatitis, such as hepatitis B or C, or autoimmune diseases.

Monoclonal Gammopathies

Identifying the source of a monoclonal gammopathy, or M-spike, often presents a clinical challenge, as they are relatively common, especially in the elderly, and are often asymptomatic. Many times, the M-protein is detected by finding an elevated total protein as part of a routine chemistry panel. Serum protein electrophoresis is diagnostic and reveals the presence of a protein spike in the gamma region (Figure 114-4). Further characterization involves the following analysis: (1) quantification, (2) immunofixation to determine heavy chain subtype and light chain restriction (kappa or lambda), and (3) determination of whether the monoclonal protein or its light chain subunit is excreted in the urine (24-hour urine for urine protein electrophoresis and protein quantification).

When found in isolation, a small M-spike is most often a benign monoclonal gammopathy. These will remain stable for up to 50% of patients; the other half will progress to frank multiple myeloma or plasmacytoma. Before diagnosing a benign gammopathy, in addition to the serum protein electrophoresis, urine protein electrophoresis, and serum immunoelectrophoresis, patients should undergo skeletal X-ray survey of all bones, computed tomography (CT) scans to eliminate occult adenopathy, complete blood count to evaluate for chronic lymphocytic leukemia, and bone marrow biopsy to quantitate plasma cell number. The M-spike should be quantified every six to 12 months. A significant change should warrant reassessment for conversion to a malignant monoclonal gammopathy.

M-spikes that are not due to benign gammopathy are most commonly due to multiple myeloma, Waldenström's macroglobulinemia, chronic lympho-

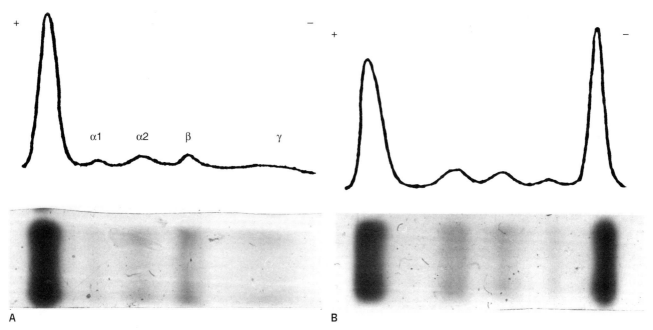

A   B

Figure 114-4 ■ Zone electrophoresis on cellulose acetate with densitometric scans. *A*, Normal human serum. *B*, Serum with large monoclonal spike in the mid γ-globulin area. (From Leddy JP: Electrophoretic and immunochemical analysis of human immunoglobulins. In Hoffman R, Benz EJ Jr, Shattil SJ, et al [eds]: Hematology: Basic Principles and Practice, 3rd ed. New York: Churchill Livingstone, 2000, p 2505.)

cytic leukemia, or B cell lymphomas. The size of the spike is usually larger than that for benign gammopathies. The presence of free light chain or heavy chain rules out benign gammopathy as well. In any patient who presents with anemia, bone pain, hypercalcemia, or constitutional symptoms, the search for a malignant clone must include a skeletal survey and a bone marrow biopsy and, if multiple myeloma or a plasma cell disorder is not identified, computed tomography scans of the body to search for lymphoma. Rarely, the search will lead to the identification of an isolated plasmacytoma of bone or an extraosseous plasmacytoma that is treated by surgical excision and/or radiation therapy.

Hyperviscosity

Polycythemia is only one way in which viscosity of the blood may increase. Macroglobulinemia results in increased plasma viscosity as a result of excessive serum IgM. Waldenström's macroglobulinemia is a disease characterized by splenomegaly, hyperviscosity, excessive bruising, and infiltration of the bone marrow with clonal plasmacytoid lymphocytes. While Waldenström's macroglobulinemia is the most common cause of hyperviscosity secondary to a monoclonal gammopathy, excessive IgM may also be secreted by other malignant lymphomas. In this setting, the circulatory symptoms are identical, but the clinical presentation of adenopathy without primary marrow involvement is a differentiating factor.

Inhibitors of Coagulation

Acquired inhibitors of factor VIII or von Willebrand's factor may cause spontaneous bleeding. Diagnosis is made in the appropriate clinical setting by identification of an abnormal prothrombin time, partial thromboplastin time, or both in conjunction with a circulating anticoagulant assay that demonstrates that normal plasma fails to correct the defect after prolonged incubation with patient's plasma. The induction of autoimmune inhibitors to coagulation factors is unusual but important to recognize, as the risks to the patient are extreme and the treatment is complex (see Chapter 58).

References

Arkel YS: Thrombosis and cancer. Semin Oncol 2000;27:362–374.

Begley CG, Basser RL: Biologic and structural differences of thrombopoietic growth factors. Semin Hematol 2000;37(2, Suppl 4):19–27.

Erslev AJ: Erythropoietin and anemia of cancer. Eur J Haematol 2000;64:353–358.

Gouin-Thibault I, Samama MM: Laboratory diagnosis of the thrombophilic state in cancer patients. Semin Thromb Hemost 1999;25:167–172.

Grima KM: Therapeutic apheresis in hematological and oncological diseases. J Clin Apheresis 2000;15:28–52.

Kuter DJ: Future directions with platelet growth factors. Semin Hematol 2000;37(2, Suppl 4):41–49.

Kwaan HC, Bongu A: The hyperviscosity syndromes. Semin Thromb Hemost 1999;25:199–208.

Levi M, de Jonge E: Current management of disseminated intravascular coagulation. Hosp Pract 2000;35:59–66.

Mauro FR, Foa R, Cerretti R, Giannarelli D, Coluzzi S, Mandelli F, Girelli G: Autoimmune hemolytic anemia in chronic lymphocytic leukemia: Clinical, therapeutic, and prognostic features. Blood 2000;95:2786–2792.

McNicholl FP: Clinical syndromes associated with cold agglutinins. Transfus Sci 2000;22:125–133.

Mercadante S, Gebbia V, Marrazzo A, Filosto S: Anaemia in cancer: pathophysiology and treatment. Cancer Treat Rev 2000;26:303–311.

Rockey DC: Gastrointestinal tract evaluation in patients with iron deficiency anemia. Semin Gastrointest Dis 1999;10:53–64.

Wazny LD, Ariano RE: Evaluation and management of drug-induced thrombocytopenia in the acutely ill patient. Pharmacotherapy 2000;20:292–307.

Webb IJ, Anderson KC: Risks, costs, and alternatives to platelet transfusions. Leuk Lymphoma 1999;34:71–84.

Chapter 115
Febrile Neutropenia

Joel T. Katz and Lindsey R. Baden

Introduction

Forty years ago, infections—particularly gram-negative infections—accounted for most of the mortality in people with cancer. In the intervening years, well-designed epidemiological and clinical studies have established the role of neutropenia as a risk factor for cancer death and the value of empiric antimicrobial therapy in this population. In addition, new diagnostic methods and treatment options have greatly improved the prognosis of these patients. Currently, fewer than one-third of cancer deaths are caused by infections.

With progress, however, new problems have inevitably arisen. Widespread empiric antimicrobial use has resulted in bacteria with diminished susceptibility to standard antibiotics. In addition, advances in chemotherapy (particularly stem cell transplantation) have increased the number of patients surviving with prolonged and profound immunosuppression. Many of these patients are further immunosuppressed by chronic administration of medications targeting specific host mechanisms. Previously unrecognized pathogens, including angioinvasive fungi and viruses, have taken on increasing importance.

The foundation for the initial approach to a febrile neutropenic patient is well grounded in controlled trials. Astute clinicians must also be able to evaluate their patients' specific epidemiological risks, exposures, and host integrity in determining the need for further targeted diagnostics and more aggressive therapy.

Epidemiology

A review of deaths on the leukemia service at the National Cancer Institute (NCI) between 1954 and 1963 showed that 70% of the mortality was attributable to infection, most commonly due to gram-negative bacterial sepsis. Follow-up studies demonstrated the inverse relationship between the patient's circulating granulocyte level and both infections and death (Figure 115-1). Based on this observation and subsequent controlled trials, the prevailing dogma of the day—that antibiotics should be started when an infection was identified—was soon replaced with a model of empiric antibiotic use for all febrile patients at high risk, defined by a low granulocyte count. Currently, infections account for fewer than 30% of deaths in leukemia patients, and even fewer for patients with solid tumors.

The spectrum of pathogens responsible for infections in cancer patients has changed in the past three decades as well. In the setting of empiric antibiotic therapy for febrile neutropenia, a specific microbiologic diagnosis is the exception rather than the rule. Early studies implicated gram-negative rods most frequently, including *Pseudomonas aeruginosa*, *Escherichia coli*, and *Klebsiella pneumoniae* (Figure 115-2). Recent studies show that gram-positive infections are increasingly common but rarely fatal. Pathogens causing such infections include *Staphylococcus epidermidis*, *Staphylococcus aureus*, and *Enterococcus* species, and these are often associated with the near-ubiquitous use of long-term in-dwelling percutaneous catheters. Although bacterial infections account for the majority of early fevers, as patients remain neutropenic for longer periods, environmental fungi such as *Aspergillus* species emerge as the most important pathogens (Figures 115-3 and 115-4).

Latent viruses of the *Herpes* family and seasonal respiratory viruses cause symptomatic disease in cancer patients at higher rates than for the general population; these should be considered in the appropriate epidemiological situation, particularly after stem cell transplantation.

Definitions

Fever is defined as a single oral temperature of 38.4°C (101.4°F), or a sustained temperature of 38°C (100.4°F) for more than one hour.

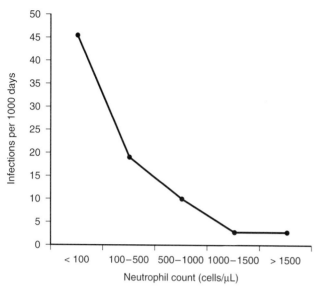

Figure 115-1 ■ Relation between granulocyte count and infection. (From Bodey GP, Buckley M, Sathe YS, et al: Quantitative relationships between circulating leukocytes and infection in patients with acute leukemia. Ann Intern Med 1966;64:328–340.)

Neutropenia is defined as a neutrophil count of less than 500 cells/μL^3, or less than 1000 cells/μL^3 with an anticipated nadir of less than 500 cells/μL^3.

Risk Factors

The risks of serious infection and death in cancer patients is most closely related to both the degree and

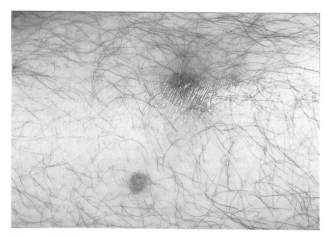

Figure 115-2 ■ Cutaneous manifestation of pseudomonas sepsis. A 28-year-old man with acute myeloid leukemia developed a fever and these palpable skin lesions on his arms and legs five days after receiving chemotherapy. Biopsy confirmed a necrotizing vasculitis with thrombosis, characteristic of ecthyma gangrenosum. Both skin biopsy and blood cultures grew *Pseudomonas aeruginosa*. (See Color Plate 23.)

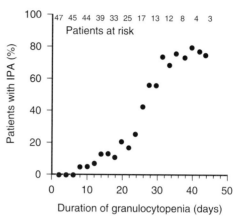

Figure 115-3 ■ Relationship between invasive pulmonary aspergillosis (IPA) and duration of neutropenia.

duration of neutropenia. Additional risk factors include host immune status, the nature of the underlying disease, mucosal integrity, the presence of in-dwelling catheters, and immunomodulatory treatments such as corticosteroids or antithymocyte globulin. Risk stratification based on history and routine laboratory studies can separate low-risk from high-risk patients, who might qualify for oral outpatient management of febrile neutropenia.

Host Factors

Patients with acute myeloid leukemia (AML) are particularly susceptible to extracellular bacteria (e.g., *Pseudomonas*) and environmental fungi (e.g., *Aspergillus*), due to granulocytopenias and mucosal breakdown. Leukemic patients with chronic neutropenia or myelodysplastic syndromes are at especially high risk for invasive fungal infections, which can arise from sinus colonization or be newly acquired though inhalation. Patients with acute lymphocytic leukemia (ALL) and lymphoma have specific defects in cell-mediated immunity, raising their risk for *Pneumocysitis carinii* pneumonia, tuberculosis, cryptococcus, and intracellular bacteria (e.g., *Listeria* or *Salmonella* species). Patients with chronic lymphocytic leukemia (CLL) and multiple myeloma often present with infections related to hypogammaglobulinemia, such as pneumococcus, *Staphylococcus aureus*, and *Haemophilus influenza* infections.

In addition to the risk posed by chemotherapy-induced granulocytopenia, patients with solid tumors are predisposed to infections at the sites of their underlying malignancy. For example, lung cancers cause postobstructive pneumonias, and colon cancers are associated with sepsis from colonic flora, such as *Streptococcus bovis* and *Clostridium septicum*. Tumors involving the skin and its appendages often result in

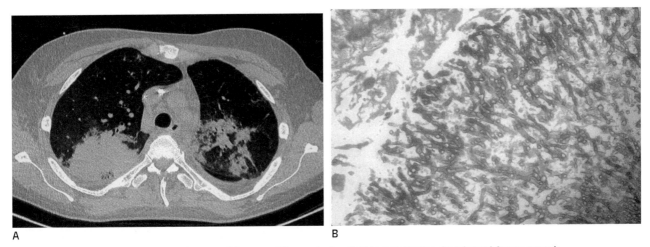

Figure 115-4 ■ Aspergillosis. A 48-year-old man with myelodysplastic syndrome developed fever, cough, and pleuritic chest pain 12 days after receiving chemotherapy. His neutrophil count was 0.02/μL³, and chest radiograph showed a peripheral cavitary infiltrate (*A*). Video-assisted thoracoscopic biopsy revealed branching invasive hyphae characteristic of invasive pulmonary aspergillosis (*B*). (See Color Plate 23.)

cellulitis that is particularly difficult to eradicate due to local skin breakdown and obstructed lymphatic drainage. Patients whose treatment has required splenectomy are at high risk of developing sepsis if they become infected with either encapsulated organisms (e.g., pneumococcus, *Haemophilus influenza, Nisseria meningitides,* and *Capnocytophaga* species) or erythrocytic parasites (e.g., babesiosis and malaria).

Treatment Factors

Cytotoxic agents are, by design, lethal to granulocyte progenitors and are the most potent predisposing agents for neutropenia and its complication. In addition, these agents affect the rapidly dividing intestinal cells that act as a major defense to the translocation of enteric gram-negative bacteria and fungi. By impairing granulocyte migration and killing, corticosteroid use should alert clinicians to the possibility of an increased rate of infections, including herpes virus infections, thrush, cryptococcosis, aspergillosis, listeriosis, and reactivation of latent tuberculosis. Stem cell transplantation carries its own specific pattern of infections, which can be predicted based on time since transplant and degree of graft-versus-host disease (GVHD). Graft-versus-host disease, with its interruption of gut mucosa, is an additional important risk factor for sepsis from enteric flora.

Evaluation

Evaluation of febrile cancer patients should include a careful history and physical examination. Sepsis can present with hypothermia or with isolated hypoten-

sion, especially in elderly patients or in those receiving corticosteroids. In addition, certain pathogens (such as *Clostridium septicum* and *Listeria monocytogenes*) are less likely to present with fever.

Review of prior infections, pathogens, and their antimicrobial susceptibility patterns is crucial. Particular attention should be paid to the skin, oropharynx, sinuses, lungs, abdomen, perirectal area, surgical sites, and vascular catheter access sites. Due to impaired inflammatory response, signs of infection (e.g., purulence, fluctuance, erythema) might be muted in neutropenic patients. Pain might be the only clue to localizing an infection. One should search for noninfectious causes of fevers, including cutaneous drug eruptions, erythema multiforme/Stevens-Johnson syndrome, neutrophilic dermatoses, transfusion reactions, and graft-versus-host disease.

Laboratory studies should include two sets of blood cultures obtained under sterile conditions by peripheral venipuncture from distinct sites. If the patient remains febrile, follow-up blood cultures should be repeated every 48 to 72 hours, or daily if the clinical situation changes. Very little additional useful information is obtained from routine cultures of the nares, throat, or rectum without specific signs of local infection. Diarrheal stools might be useful in identifying infections due to *Clostridium difficile,* rotavirus, and certain protozoa. In patients whose diarrhea began after chemotherapy, repeat stool cultures and evaluations for ova and parasites are not required due to low diagnostic yield. Additional laboratory studies should be directed by the history and examination and can include liver function tests, amylase, and electrolytes. A chest radiograph should be obtained at the onset of fever and repeated only for new or worsening respiratory symptoms, cough, dyspnea, or new lung findings.

If the source of a worsening pulmonary infection cannot be established with routine microbiologic studies, early bronchoscopy should be strongly considered. Respiratory infections that do not respond to antibacterial agents for neutropenia should raise consideration of seasonal respiratory viruses (influenza, parainfluenza, respiratory syncytial virus), *Pneumocystis carinii,* non–*Pneumophilia legionella* species, or invasive pulmonary apergillosis. Noninvasive methods for diagnosing fungal infections in their early stages are currently inadequate. Serum markers for invasive aspergillosis, such as measurement of galactomannan and quantitative polymerase chain reaction (PCR), remain experimental.

Treatment

Empiric antibiotics should be initiated with the onset of fever in neutropenic patients and continued until the patient is no longer neutropenic. Identification of a specific pathogen does not obviate the need for continued broad-spectrum coverage.

Effective initial antibiotic choices include duotherapy (antipseudomonal beta lactam such as piperacillin, plus an aminoglycoside) or monotherapy (ceftazidime, imipenem, meropenem, or cefepime). The choice of initial antibiotics should be informed by both local antimicrobial susceptibility patterns and the patient's history of previous infections and adverse drug reactions. Patients with severe beta lactam/cephalosporin allergies can be treated with two of the following antibiotics: aztreonam, a fluoroquinolone (e.g., levofloxacin), and/or an aminoglycoside (e.g., gentamicin). If a regimen is chosen with pure aerobic gram-negative rod coverage (e.g., aztreonam and gentamicin), consideration of empiric gram-positive coverage is warranted given the potential role of some *Streptococcus* species in the morbidity associated with febrile neutropenia.

Empiric addition of vancomycin or metronidazole are not of proven benefit and should be considered only when there are clinical data suggesting a gram-positive or anaerobic infection, respectively. In addition, indiscriminant antibiotic use can encourage the emergence of highly resistant bacteria, and routine use in this setting should be discouraged.

If fever persists beyond four to five days or recur later in the course of febrile neutropenia, the empiric addition of amphotericin B is indicated. Patients at highest risk for invasive fungal infections—such as those with long-standing chronic neutropenia or with a history of prior fungal infections—could require earlier initiation of amphotericin. Alternative choices for antifungal therapy with significant activity against *Aspergillus* species include liposomal preparations of amphotericin, extended-spectrum azoles (e.g., voriconazole), and echincandins (e.g., caspofungin). Combined therapy with two or more of these classes could have a role in documented disseminated disease such as central nervous system and other deep-seated fungal disease.

Outpatient Management of Febrile Neutropenia

Randomized trials of low-risk patients have demonstrated that some patients with febrile neutropenia can be managed safely at home (Table 115-1, p. 1178). The suggested regimen in adults is ciprofloxacin and augmentin.

TREATMENT

Spiraling Empiricism

Fevers in neutropenic patients should precipitate a vigilant, cost-effective evaluation for the source, relying particularly on careful physical examination. Antibiotic therapy should be added sequentially, based on the results from large randomized trials.

Not all fevers are caused by infections, and failure to identify the cause of a persistent fever does not always necessitate "more powerful" or "broader" antibiotics. Spiraling empiricism (i.e., frequently altering and escalating the antimicrobial regimen in response to uncertainty rather than clinical change) might be appropriate in critically ill or unstable patients, but in most instances this approach clouds the picture rather than clarifying it. In addition, frequent antibiotic changes lead to increased antimicrobial resistance, antibiotic-associated diarrhea, and confusion over true adverse drug associations for future prescribing.

Fevers in stable cancer patients are not necessarily untreated infections. Avoid spiraling empiricism.

TREATMENT

Fungi Unresponsive to Amphotericin

Although the vast majority of fungal pathogens infecting cancer patients are responsive to amphotericin, clinicians should be aware of a few important exceptions, for which early suspicion and recognition can be life saving.

Candida lusitaniae, an emerging yeast that can infect in-dwelling catheters, is often resistant to amphotericin preparations. *Pseudalleschieria boydii* and *Scedosporium prolificans* are important invasive molds that clinically resemble *Apergillus* infection, with vascular invasion in leukemic patients (particularly those on cortico-steroids). Unlike *Aspergillus* species, they are relatively easily grown in tissue culture and do not respond to amphotericin therapy. Recovery of neutrophils (with stem cell growth factors or white blood cell [WBC] transfusions) and possible surgical debridement are the only known effective interventions. Voriconazole might have some benefit. Although invasive *Mucormycosis* and related species might be modestly responsive to amphotericin, high doses (1.5 to 2 mg/kg/day) and surgical resection are required (Figure 115-5).

TREATMENT

Fevers After Neutrophil Recovery

Enigmatic fevers that persist beyond neutrophil recovery occur occasionally. Infectious considerations include *Clostridium difficile* colitis, chronic viral infections (especially *Herpes simplex* and *Herpes zoster*), and invasive, deep-seated fungal infections. When the fevers flare with the recovery of neutrophils, hepatosplenic candidiasis should be suspected. This diagnosis is best excluded via liver-spleen magnetic resonance imaging (MRI).

Not all fevers in recovering neutropenia are infectious; these less dangerous fevers include drug fever and recurrence of the underlying cancer. Graft-versus-host disease in stem cell transplant recipients can present with fevers in the setting of immune recovery.

Once the neutrophil count is greater than $500/\mu L^3$ on two consecutive days, antibiotics can generally be stopped safely in clinically stable patients, as the risk of overwhelming sepsis has been reduced significantly. Once the patient is off antibiotics, an assessment of possible drug fever or a search for occult infections can be performed. Patients with documented bacterial or fungal infections during periods of neutropenia will require continuation of antibiotics beyond neutrophil recovery.

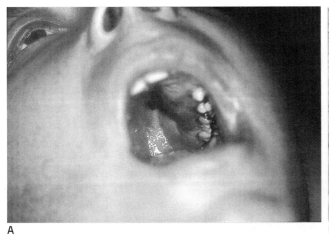
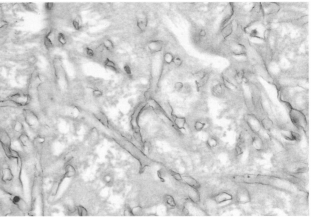

A   B

Figure 115-5 ■ Mucormycosis. This rapidly evolving oral lesion occurred in a patient with chronic lymphocytic leukemia in the setting of fever to 101.0° F and chemotherapy-induced neutropenia (*A*). Autopsy results (*B*) and postmortem cultures demonstrated mucormycosis, a largely fatal complication of advanced cancer. Prompt surgical evaluation is required in patients with suspected mucormycosis. (See Color Plate 23.)

Table 115-1 ■ Requirements in Order to Consider Outpatient Management of Febrile Neutropenia

Anticipated duration of neutropenia <7 days
Granulocyte nadir ≥10 days after chemotherapy
Solid tumor malignancy
No major comorbidities
Adequate oral intake
Adequate social support
Malignancy responding to current chemotherapy

Prevention of Infection in Neutropenic Patients

Although many strategies have been investigated to prevent fevers in cancer patients with neutropenia, few have gained widespread acceptance. Selective gut decontamination with oral, nonabsorbed antibiotics (polymixin and/or bacitracin) is not recommended, except for patients undergoing non–T cell depleted stem cell transplantation, in whom it might decrease rates of graft-versus-host disease. In the absence of antiviral therapy, reactivation of herpes simplex virus and varicella-zoster virus is common; thus, acyclovir, 400 mg orally three times daily, preemptive therapy is recommended for all patients with a history of previous zoster or recurrent herpes labialis and in all stem cell transplant recipients. Oral fluconazole prophylaxis is recommended only for allogeneic stem cell recipients, in whom it has been shown to decrease infections and prevent mortality. This effect on mortality is likely due to the role that gut inflammation plays in the initiation of graft-versus-host disease, a clear risk factor for death.

Prophylactic antibacterial agents (trimethoprim/sulfamethoxazole or fluoroquinolones) are effective in preventing infections but not in reducing mortality. Routine use is not recommended due to induction of antibiotic resistance, antibiotic-associated diarrhea, and other drug side effects.

References

Bodey GP, Buckley M, Sathe YS, et al: Quantitative relationships between circulating leukocytes and infection in patients with acute leukemia. Ann Intern Med 1966:64:328–340.

Dykewicz CA: Summary of the guidelines for preventing opportunistic infections among hematopoietic stem cell transplant recipients. Clin Inf Dis 2001:33:139–144.

Feld R: Vancomycin as part of initial empirical antibiotic therapy for febrile neutropenia in patients with cancer: Pros and cons. Clin Inf Dis 1999;29:503–507.

Finberg R, Talcott J: Fever and netropenia—How to use a new treatment strategy. New Engl J Med 1999;341:362–363.

Freifeld A, Marchigiani D, Walsh T, et al: A double-blind comparison of empirical oral and intravenous antibiotic therapy for low-risk febrile patients with neutropenia during cancer chemotherapy. New Engl J Med 1999;341:305–311.

Hersh EM, Brody GP, Niles BA, et al: A ten year study of 414 patients from 1954–1963. JAMA 1965;193:105–109.

Hughes WT, et al: 1997 guidelines for the use of antimicrobial agents in neutropenic patients with unexplained fever. Clin Inf Dis 1997;25:551–573.

Momin F, Chandrasekar P: Antimicrobial prophylaxis in bone marrow transplantation. Ann Intern Med 1995;123:205–215.

Pizzo P: Fever in immunocompromised patients. New Engl J Med 1999;341:893–900.

Quadri TL, Brown AE: Infectious complications in the critically ill patient with cancer. Semin Oncol 2000;27:335–346.

Chapter 116
Thromboembolic Manifestations of Cancer

James D. Levine

Introduction

Compared with the general population, patients with cancer are at an increased risk to develop thromboembolic disorders. Trousseau first described patients with pancreatic cancer, migratory peripheral thrombophlebitis, and deep venous thrombosis (DVT) in 1872. Between 15% and 25% of patients who are diagnosed with either deep venous thrombosis or pulmonary embolism (PE) have a malignancy. There have been many explanations for this increase in thromboembolic phenomenon, including

- procoagulant factors produced by the tumor
- surgical procedures
- immobility
- decreased inhibitors of coagulation such as protein C, protein S, and antithrombin
- the concomitant use of chemotherapy and endocrine therapy
- the use of indwelling venous access devices and catheters

In addition to the factors associated with the cancer, these patients might also have the added risk factors associated with genetic predispositions to thromboembolic disease.

With these procoagulant forces operant, the cancer patient could also be at increased risk for bleeding. Bleeding could be due to necrosis of the tumor either from growth pressure or therapy. Thrombocytopenia or coagulopathies secondary to the tumor or the treatment are also important. This double jeopardy of increased risk for both thromboembolic and bleeding complications makes the management of cancer patients with or at risk for thrombosis a challenge for the physician.

Etiology and Natural History

Patients with cancer who develop thromboembolic complications exhibit the same risk factors as patients without cancer. Superimposed on these risks, cancer also adds some factors that are not clearly understood. Patients with cancer are often immobile or at bed rest—circumstances that are known risk factors for the development of both deep venous thrombosis and pulmonary embolism. In addition, these patients frequently have concomitant infections or have been given drugs known to increase the incidence of thrombosis. Excess expression of cytokines such as tumor necrosis factor (TNF) and interleukins by tumor cells (or by normal cells stimulated by tumor cells) have been implicated in the etiology of cancer-related thromboembolic phenomena. Increased levels of factor VIII, von Willebrand factor, and factor VII have been found in patients diagnosed with cancer and either deep venous thrombosis or pulmonary embolism.

Tumors that produce mucin, such as adenocarcinomas of the bowel, lung, and pancreas, increase a patient's risk for the development of thromboembolic events. A cysteine protease that has been isolated from human tumors such as pancreas, lung, bowel, kidney, and breast has been found capable of activating factor X without tissue factor or factor VII.

Monocytes and many tumor cells produce tissue factor. The prototype cell that produces tissue factor is the promyelocyte found in patients with acute promyelocytic leukemia. This subtype of leukemia is frequently associated with disseminated intravascular coagulation, and patients can have bleeding complications, thrombotic complications, or both. Many other tumors have been shown to increase the expression of tissue factor. Pancreatic cancer cells, sarcoma cells, melanoma cells, brain tumor cells, and lymphoma cells are associated with increased tissue factor expression and thus result in an increased risk of thromboembolic phenomena.

An episode of pulmonary embolism or deep venous thrombosis in patients without known risk factors sometimes leads to a diagnosis of cancer. Studies of large cancer registries have demonstrated an increased risk of cancer in patients less than 60 years of age diagnosed with deep venous thrombosis or pulmonary embolism, suggesting that cancer has a role in the development of thromboembolic events. This raises questions as to how extensive a search for malignancy should be in a patient with a thromboembolic event and no other risk factors.

Studies addressing this question suggest that the use of extensive diagnostic procedures to diagnose an occult malignancy is not warranted. Most cancers (breast, prostate, lung, or colon) found in patients with thromboembolic events were discovered in the first year after the event and for the most part could have been found with routine screening maneuvers. Outcomes are probably not impacted by making the diagnosis at the time of the pulmonary embolism or deep venous thrombosis, as many of the tumors found were metastatic. Recent observations show that a diagnosis of cancer made within one year of an episode of deep venous thrombosis or pulmonary embolism is associated with a poorer prognosis or more advanced disease than a diagnosis of cancer made without a previous diagnosis of thromboembolic disease. Survival rates for patients in whom cancer was diagnosed at the same time as the venous thromboembolism were only 12% at one year, compared with 36% in the patients diagnosed with cancer without concomitant venous thromboembolism. Sorensen et al found that if the cancer was diagnosed within one year of an episode of venous thromboembolism, the one-year survival was 38%, compared with 47% in patients with no previous thromboembolic diagnosis. Thus, it appears that thromboembolic events associated with cancer predict for a poor outcome. In a curious and unexpected twist in another cancer registry study, investigators found that after two years, the risk of newly diagnosed cancer was lower in patients with an antecedent pulmonary embolism or deep venous thrombosis who had previously been treated with oral anticoagulants for at least six months.

Drugs, Cancer, and Thromboembolic Phenomena

Drugs administered to patients as an element of their cancer treatment also can increase the risk of thromboembolic disorders. The agents implicated most often are hormones used to treat breast and prostate cancer. Of these, tamoxifen is most important because of the number of women exposed to this agent for both adjuvant and primary therapy. The use of tamoxifen increases the number of thromboembolic events compared with patients not receiving the drug; this finding is true regardless of whether tamoxifen treatment is for metastatic disease or in the adjuvant setting. Patients who are given chemotherapy in addition to tamoxifen have a higher incidence of thromboembolic disease. The risk of thromboembolic events also increases in patients over age 50.

There are other drugs used by oncologists in the treatment of cancer that also have been associated with an increase in thromboembolic events. These include estrogen compounds such as diethylstilbestrol (previously used to treat men with metastatic prostate cancer), platinum, L-asparaginase, and the vinca alkaloids.

Thromboembolic Phenomena and High-dose Chemotherapy

A specific thromboembolic complication of high-dose chemotherapy is venoocclusive disease of the liver or (less commonly) the lung. This disorder is usually seen in the setting of bone marrow or peripheral blood stem cell transplant, although it has been reported occasionally in patients receiving standard doses of chemotherapy. The hallmarks of venoocclusive disease are sudden weight gain, ascites formation, a rise in the serum bilirubin, and tender hepatomegaly, with only minimal increase in liver enzymes without any other obvious cause. The diagnosis is usually made on clinical grounds because clinical circumstances usually prohibit liver biopsy. Greyscale and Doppler ultrasound of the liver could be efficacious in differentiating hepatic venoocclusive disease from graft-versus-host disease of the liver. Hepatic venoocclusive disease is a potentially fatal condition with few effective treatment options. As opposed to Budd-Chiari syndrome, there is a conspicuous absence of thrombi in the central, sublobular, and hepatic veins. In spite of the lack of thrombi in biopsy and autopsy specimens, some of the most effective treatments and preventative measures involve either anticoagulation or fibrinolytic therapy. Anticoagulants have been tested as both prophylaxis and treatment. A study of low-dose heparin and low-molecular-weight heparin were both shown to be efficacious at preventing hepatic venoocclusive disease. Fibrinolytic therapy, such as tissue plasminogen activator, also has demonstrated some efficacy but is associated with increased bleeding. Defibrotide is an agent that affects fibrinolysis but does not have a systemic anticoagulant effect; it has been used to treat patients with severe hepatic venoocclusive disease successfully without the concomitant bleeding that often is seen with anticoagulant or fibrinolytic therapy. At present, there are no universally accepted therapies for hepatic venoocclusive disease. Supportive maneuvers (e.g., saline and volume control) along with careful diuresis to avoid volume depletion are beneficial in early disease. Once severe venoocclusive disease occurs, however, one of the therapeutic options just discussed should be considered.

Clinical Presentation and Diagnosis of Venous Thromboembolic Events

Because of the potential impact of therapy on quality of life, other therapeutic modalities, and the demonstrated increased risk of bleeding and rethrombosis in patients with cancer, an objective diagnosis of thrombosis is imperative. The diagnosis is often not entertained because many of the signs and symptoms of thromboembolic disease are similar to those caused by the patient's malignancy. For example, cancer patients often have edema and swelling of lower extremities because of extrinsic compression of vessels by tumor or lymph nodes. A large intra-abdominal mass can compress the abdominal blood vessels, resulting in edema or swelling of the lower extremity. This in turn leads to development of thrombus because of decreased flow. Upper-extremity edema can be secondary to axillary lymphadenopathy, tumor mass, superior vena cava syndrome, or axillary vein or subclavian vein thrombosis (Figure 116–1). Shortness of breath and pleuritic chest pain can be secondary to the patient's primary malignancy, metastasis, pulmonary embolism, or all three. The clinician needs to have a high level of suspicion when dealing with patients who have known malignancy and should be alert to

the fact that both tumor and thrombus can present simultaneously and cause symptoms.

The modalities used for the diagnosis of thromboembolism are not different from those used to establish the diagnosis in patients without cancer; these have been reviewed in Chapter 59. The tests used to make the diagnosis depend on the expertise and availability at individual institutions. Patients with a known history of cancer are viewed with increased suspicion because of their increased risk. Noninvasive tests are frequently preferred in patients with cancer. Invasive tests such as contrast venography are often not possible because of the inability to cannulate blood vessels and the physician's desire to decrease the possible morbidity caused by procedures. Therefore, tests such as duplex ultrasound, spiral or helical computed tomography (CT) angiogram, and magnetic resonance imaging (MRI) often take precedence over intravenous dye studies.

The D-dimer assay is a test that has demonstrated modest utility in diagnosing venous thrombosis. D-dimer is the result of proteolytic cleavage by plasmin on crosslinked fibrin or the stabilized fibrin clot. Elevated D-dimer implies fibrinolysis, which is associated with clot formation. When used to evaluate outpatients in emergency rooms, the D-dimer has a sensitivity and specificity approaching 95% and 60% to 90%, respectively. If the D-dimer is not elevated, the diagnosis of deep venous thrombosis or pulmonary embolism can be excluded. Unfortunately, when used for patients with malignancy, the D-dimer assay is not specific, and a significant number of false positives

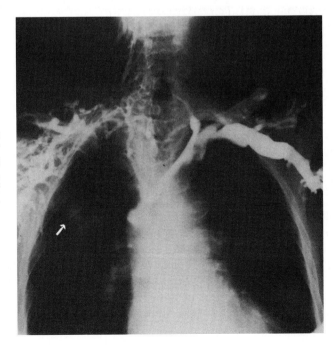

Figure 116-1 ■ Obstruction of the superior vena cava and brachiocephalic veins by mediastinal tumor deposits. Arrow indicates multiple collateral vessels and the primary bronchial tumor. (From Grainger RG, Allison D [eds]: Diagnostic Radiology: A Textbook of Medical Imaging, 3rd ed. London, Churchill Livingstone, 1997, p 2429.)

occur. Patients with cancer but with no other objective evidence for thromboembolism often have positive or high titers of D-dimer. Studies have found a 97% negative predictive value in noncancer patients but only a 79% negative predictive value in cancer patients. Thus, a negative D-dimer assay should not be used to exclude the diagnosis of deep venous thrombosis or pulmonary embolism in patients with known malignancy.

Patients with indwelling catheters—for example, tunneled venous lines and reservoir catheters that insert into the jugular, subclavian, or antecubital fossa—often have pain in the arm, neck, or shoulder as their first sign of thrombosis. Occasionally, difficulty swallowing or sore throat is the only complaint. Once the clot has occluded the vessel, swelling is often observed in the proximal drainage site. If enough time has elapsed, one might find collateral vessels, often across the anterior chest. If the catheter tip has been inserted into the superior vena cava and the clot is occluding, the signs and symptoms of superior vena cava syndrome—dyspnea, facial or arm swelling, head fullness, cough, chest pain, sore throat or dysphagia—might be present. Patients who have superior vena cava syndrome secondary to extrinsic compression of the superior vena cava often also have clot within the vessel. This clot might be composed of pure fibrin or of a combination of fibrin and tumor that has either infiltrated or metastasized to the area. Studies have shown that about a third of all upper-extremity clots are associated with the presence of an intravenous catheter, and a third are associated with a cancer diagnosis.

Treatment of Thromboembolic Phenomena

Studies regarding anticoagulation treatment for deep venous thrombosis or pulmonary embolism have documented a threefold increase in recurrent thrombosis in cancer patients over noncancer patients and a similar increase in major bleeding events when cancer patients are compared with noncancer patients. A subset of patients have an increased incidence of recurrence of thrombosis in spite of adequate intensity of oral anticoagulation, and this subset often consists of patients with malignancy. Indeed, cancer patients treated with oral anticoagulants for thrombosis have an increased relapse rate and warfarin resistance. Several treatment strategies have been proposed for this group of patients. One is to substitute oral anticoagulation with unfractionated heparin or low-molecular-weight heparin for all patients with thrombosis and malignancy. The other strategy is to use vena cava interruption devices. The advantages of

warfarin are that it is an oral preparation, less expensive than low-molecular-weight heparin, and easier to administer than infusional or subcutaneous unfractionated heparin. Warfarin requires, however, frequent monitoring and dosing adjustments. Low-molecular-weight heparin must be given subcutaneously by the patient, nursing staff, or family. A stated advantage of low-molecular-weight heparin is that it supposedly does not require monitoring; however, as clinicians use low-molecular-weight heparin more frequently, an increase in bleeding has been noted. This usually occurs because of reliance on weight-based dosing of low-molecular-weight heparin in patients with renal insufficiency. Patients with renal insufficiency should have their low-molecular-weight heparin monitored and adjusted by using an assay to measure anti-Xa activity. This requirement might negate some of the advantages over warfarin.

Oral anticoagulation is efficacious in reducing the risk of recurrent thromboembolic events in patients with cancer. Cancer patients with deep venous thrombosis maintained on oral anticoagulation at a subtherapeutic international normalized ratio (INR) have a much higher incidence of recurrence than those maintained at a target international normalized ratio between 2 and 3. Thus, full-intensity warfarin therapy can be effective in patients with malignancy.

Thrombosis and Central Venous Catheters

The advent of the semipermanent in-dwelling catheter has permitted the efficacious administration of chemotherapeutic agents, blood products, antibiotics, and fluids. The use of these devices might also be responsible for the increased incidence of upper-extremity thrombosis seen in patients with cancer. Anywhere between 5% and 50% of patients with central venous catheters develop thrombosis, usually of the subclavian or axillary vein. Many of these events are asymptomatic initially, but if left untreated they cause pain, swelling, embolic events, or catheter failure.

The most common complaint seen in catheter-associated thrombosis is pain or swelling in the extremity or distal to the obstruction. Hand swelling, neck or shoulder pain, or even difficulty swallowing and sore throat all have been associated with catheter-related thrombosis. In addition, problems with catheter function, such as difficulty withdrawing blood or infusing fluids, could be the first sign of thrombosis in patients without symptoms. The new onset of dyspnea or chest pain could be the first signs of emboli from catheter-associated clot. The clinician must have a high degree of suspicion and pay attention to and elicit what otherwise could be considered trivial complaints. Many of the complaints and symptoms of these patients could also be caused by the underlying tumor. On inspection, there could be evidence of distal swelling or edema. The presence of collateral vessels can be observed across the anterior chest and could be an indication of thrombosis in the subclavian vein or superior vena cava.

Thrombi in vessels of the upper extremity and chest might embolize to the lung and result in morbidity and mortality in ways parallel to clots from the lower extremity or pelvic veins. If the patient also has a patent foramen ovale or septal defect, there is risk for arterial thrombosis.

Diagnosis of Thrombosis in Patients with Central Venous Catheters

Making the diagnosis of thrombosis by objective methods is important; a catheter that has no venous return should not be presumed to be clotted, as it might well be obstructed because of a mechanical kink (often seen in catheters that tunnel under the clavicle) or because of a tip that is occluded against the vessel wall. If Valsalva or other positional maneuvers do not result in a venous return or improvement in infusion, thrombosis should be evaluated by contrast venogram (Figure 116–2). Unfortunately, the very reason for central line placement often precludes the use of venography; placement of a peripheral intravenous catheter, and infusion of contrast dye—procedures

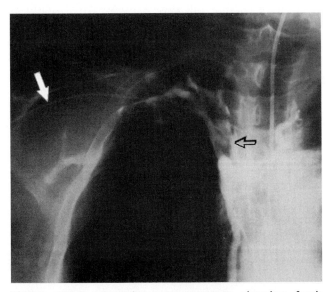

Figure 116-2 ■ Superior venacavogram showing fresh thrombus in the innominate vein and superior vena cava (*hatched arrow*), which has occurred following the insertion of a central feeding line (*white arrow*) for parenteral nutrition. (From Grainger RG, Allison D [eds]: Diagnostic Radiology: A Textbook of Medical Imaging, 3rd ed. London, Churchill Livingstone, 1997, p 2430.)

that might not be possible in a patient with a swollen edematous arm. Ultrasound techniques such as duplex, B-mode, or color Doppler are both sensitive and specific; however, when the sternum, clavicle, or ribs are overlying the vessel under study, these techniques are less likely to be diagnostic, and other diagnostic modalities need to be considered. Computed tomography and magnetic resonance imaging are other methods that can be used to establish a diagnosis.

Clot Prevention in Patients with Central Venous Catheters

Several studies of venous catheters used for delivery of chemotherapy have demonstrated that low doses of warfarin or a fixed dose of low-molecular-weight heparin are effective in preventing clot from forming on and around intravenous catheters. Warfarin (1 mg/day) can decrease the catheter thrombosis rate from 37% in untreated patients to 10%. There is no increase in bleeding in the anticoagulated group. Patients with poor nutritional status or who require systemic antibiotics should be monitored regularly while on warfarin, as even the small doses used for prophylaxis can prolong the prothrombin time to standard intensity or supratherapeutic ranges, resulting in a bleeding diathesis.

Low-molecular-weight heparin is used as prophylaxis in patients with central venous catheters. The major advantage of this form of prophylaxis is that monitoring is not required. The disadvantages of using low-molecular-weight heparin involve patient compliance issues because this therapy requires self-injection of a subcutaneous dose of heparin. In addition, even low doses of low-molecular-weight heparin used for prophylaxis can result in overanticoagulation in patients with renal insufficiency or renal failure. The clinician in these circumstances needs to monitor the degree of anticoagulation by assaying anti-factor Xa activity.

Some manufacturers have designed catheters with heparin bonded to the catheter material in an effort to make a catheter that would not promote clot formation. To date, none of these devices appears to be of benefit for long-term catheter use.

Lysing Clots in Central Venous Catheters

Catheters used for delivery of chemotherapy develop thrombi in spite of prophylactic anticoagulation. The best method to differentiate thrombus occlusion from mechanical occlusion is by radiographic study. Fluoroscopy using a small infusion of radiographic contrast instilled into the catheter is usually sufficient to diagnose clot when there is a question of mechanical obstruction versus thrombus. If left untreated, the clot could extend and the patient could become symptomatic. When a fibrin sheath or ball clot at the end of a catheter occurs, urokinase or streptokinase is used. Tissue plasminogen activator has also been used in these situations. The lysis of the attachment point of the clot to the catheter resulting in embolism of the thrombus is a rare or clinically insignificant phenomenon.

A volume of urokinase containing 5000 U to 10,000 U (slightly over the void volume of the catheter) is instilled. This is to avoid systemic instillation of the lytic agent and the resultant systemic lytic state. The urokinase is allowed to remain in the catheter for 15 to 30 minutes, after which the solution is withdrawn. Two attempts are usually made to clear the catheter. If this is unsuccessful and the catheter cannot be replaced, a six- to 10-hour infusion of urokinase at 40,000 units/hour is administered through the catheter. If function is not established, removal and replacement of the catheter is considered. Some clinicians have recommended the use of tissue plasminogen activator (t-PA) when urokinase fails, or cannot be obtained. The dose of t-PA is 1 mg to 2 mg instilled into the catheter with a dwell time of one to two hours followed by aspiration. If aspiration is not successful, this procedure can be repeated once with a dwell time of up to 10 hours before aspiration.

Treatment of Catheter-Associated Upper Extremity, Axillary Vein, and Subclavian Vein Thrombosis

If the catheter is no longer used, or if other means are available to gain venous access, the best approach is to remove the catheter. If this is not an acceptable option, lytic therapy can reestablish function, followed by administration of heparin and warfarin. If the catheter is to remain in place and there are no contraindications to anticoagulation, long-term anticoagulation is reasonable. If the catheter can be removed, anticoagulation should be continued until one or two months after removal. A clot in one catheter does not necessarily predict that the replacement catheter will also cause thrombosis.

Superficial Thrombophlebitis and Cancer

Migratory superficial thrombophlebitis associated with cancer was originally described by Trousseau in 1865. The syndrome that now has his name is often loosely applied to any thromboembolic phenomenon in a patient with cancer or who subsequently develops cancer. Most patients with true superficial thrombophlebitis are females in the early postpartum period. The events that occur in the lower extremities in these patients usually respond to conservative therapy consisting of heat, elevation, and nonsteroidal anti-inflammatory agents.

The most serious complication of superficial thrombophlebitis is the possible extension of superficial clot into the veins of the deep system and the resultant increased risk of fatal pulmonary embolism. The risk of this occurrence is between 5% and 30%. It is more likely in patients with a cancer diagnosis and in patients with superficial thrombophlebitis involving the lower extremity—in particular, events above the knee involving the saphenous vein. Management of cancer patients with superficial thrombophlebitis in light of the significant risk of extension into the deep venous system requires demonstration that extension into the deep venous system has not occurred in cases of lower-extremity superficial thrombophlebitis. These patients can be treated conservatively with heat and nonsteroidal anti-inflammatory agents, with frequent noninvasive monitoring and early intervention with anticoagulation at the first sign of extension of clot into the deep venous system. If there are no contraindications to anticoagulation, prophylaxis with low-molecular-weight heparin or low-dose warfarin to prevent extension into the deep venous system may be employed.

Patients with malignancy who develop superficial thrombophlebitis often have had an intravenous catheter in one of the veins of the upper extremity. Direct irritation by certain chemotherapy agents might be associated with superficial thrombophlebitis. These agents include vinca alkaloids, the taxanes, and anthracyclines. Treatment should provide symptomatic relief, nonsteroidal anti-inflammatory agents if not otherwise contraindicated, and avoidance of further instillation of chemotherapy into the vessels involved.

L-asparaginase is also associated with both superficial thrombophlebitis and deep venous thrombosis and pulmonary embolism. This agent causes significant suppression of protein synthesis, leading to decreases in protein S, protein C, and antithrombin.

Interruption of the Inferior Vena Cava

Interruption of the vena cava with transvenous devices inserted via the vascular system purport to allow maximal blood flow while preventing emboli from traveling beyond the device to the lungs. When used both with and without anticoagulation, fewer patients in whom the device is placed have pulmonary embolism within two weeks of insertion. There is, however, no difference in long-term mortality, and at two years, patients who had a device placed were more likely to have had additional deep venous thrombotic events than those who did not have placement of a device.

The indications for the use of vena caval interruption devices are to prevent pulmonary embolism in patients with deep venous thrombosis who have contraindications to anticoagulation: active bleeding, recent stroke, recent surgery, or hemorrhagic pericarditis. A relative contraindication is brain metastasis; anticoagulation of patients with brain metastasis must be risked on an individual basis. The risk of subsequent bleeding might be overestimated, however, and anticoagulation is usually safe unless a brain computed tomography or magnetic resonance imaging study shows blood associated with the metastatic lesion. The complications of a vena caval interruption device include protrusion of the anchoring legs through the vena cava, migration of the device (including embolization to the right heart), or thrombosis of the device itself, resulting in massive lower-extremity edema. Fortunately, these complications are rare. Placement of inferior vena cava (IVC) devices in patients with cancer remains controversial.

Monitoring Anticoagulation

Patients with cancer require more frequent monitoring of oral anticoagulation to keep the international normalized ratio within a therapeutic range. Many patients with cancer also have central venous catheters placed to allow more effective administration of chemotherapy and more comfortable venous blood sampling. Blood samples used for anticoagulation monitoring should not be drawn through these catheters, especially if they have been heparinized. Samples drawn through these lines do not yield accurate measurements of coagulation and should be drawn through peripheral venipuncture if they are to be used to measure prothrombin times, partial thromboplastin times, or other coagulation-based tests.

References

Anticoagulation

Bona RD, Sivjee KY, Hickey AD, et al: The efficacy and safety of oral anticoagulation in patients with cancer. Thromb Haemost 1995;74:1055.

Bona RD, Hickey AD, Wallace DM: Efficacy and safety of oral anticoagulation in patients with cancer. Thromb Haemost 1997;78:137.

Hutten BA, Prins MH, Gent M, et al: Incidence of recurrent thromboembolic and bleeding complications among patients with venous thromboembolism in relation to both malignancy and achieved international normalized ratio: A retrospective analysis. J Clin Oncol 2000;18:3078.

Monreal M, Alastrue A, Rull M, et al: Upper extremity deep venous thrombosis in cancer patients with venous access devices—Prophylaxis with a low-molecular-weight heparin (Fragmin). Thromb Haemost 1996;75:251.

Schulman S, Lindmarker P: Incidence of cancer after prophylaxis with warfarin against recurrent venous thromboembolism. Duration of anticoagulation trial. N Engl J Med 2000;342:1953.

Zacharski LR, Henderson WG, Rickles FR, et al: Effect of warfarin anticoagulation on survival in carcinoma of the lung, colon, head and neck, and prostate. Final report of VA Cooperative Study #75. Cancer 1984;53:2046.

Cancer Therapy

Castaman G, Rodeghiero F, Dini E: Thrombotic complications during L-asparaginase treatment for acute lymphocytic leukemia. Haematologica 1990;75:567.

Fisher B, Costantino JP, Wickerham DL, et al: Tamoxifen for prevention of breast cancer: report of the National Surgical Adjuvant Breast and Bowel Project P-1 Study. J Natl Cancer Inst 1998;90:1371.

Gugliotta L, D'Angelo A, Mattioli Belmonte M, et al: Hypercoagulability during L-asparaginase treatment: the effect of antithrombin III supplementation in vivo. Br J Haematol 1990;74:465.

Pritchard KI, Paterson AH, Paul NA, et al: Increased thromboembolic complications with concurrent tamoxifen and chemotherapy in a randomized trial of adjuvant therapy for women with breast cancer. National Cancer Institute of Canada Clinical Trials Group Breast Cancer Site Group. J Clin Oncol 1996;14:2731.

Semeraro N, Montemurro P, Giordano P, et al: Unbalanced coagulation-fibrinolysis potential during L-asparaginase therapy in children with acute lymphoblastic leukaemia. Thromb Haemost 1990;64:38.

Tallman MS: The thrombophilic state in acute promyelocytic leukemia. Semin Thromb Hemost 1999;25:209.

Catheter Thrombosis

Bern MM, Lokich JJ, Wallach SR, et al: Very low doses of warfarin can prevent thrombosis in central venous catheters. A randomized prospective trial. Ann Intern Med 1990;112:423.

Bissett D, Kaye SB, Baxter G, et al: Successful thrombolysis of SVC thrombosis associated with Hickman lines and continuous infusion chemotherapy. Clin Oncol 1996;8:247.

Carr KM, Rabinowitz I: Physician compliance with warfarin prophylaxis for central venous catheters in patients with solid tumors. J Clin Oncol 2000;18:3665.

Goldhaber SZ, Nagel JS, Theard M, et al: Treatment of right atrial thrombus with urokinase. Am Heart J 1988;115:894.

Haire WD, Atkinson JB, Stephens LC, et al: Urokinase versus recombinant tissue plasminogen activator in thrombosed central venous catheters: a double-blinded, randomized trial. Thromb Haemost 1994;72:543.

Moss JF, Wagman LD, Riihimaki DU, et al: Central venous thrombosis related to the silastic Hickman-Broviac catheter in an oncologic population. J Parenteral Nutr 1989;13:397.

Pinto KM: Accuracy of coagulation values obtained from a heparinized central venous catheter. Oncol Nurs Forum 1994;21:573.

Diagnosis

Anderson DR, Wells PS: Improvements in the diagnostic approach for patients with suspected deep vein thrombosis or pulmonary embolism. Thromb Haemost 1999;82:878.

Freyburger G, Trillaud H, Labrouche S, et al: D-dimer strategy in thrombosis exclusion—A gold standard study in 100 patients suspected of deep venous thrombosis or pulmonary embolism: 8 DD methods compared. Thromb Haemost 1998;79:32.

Lee AY, Julian JA, Levine MN, et al: Clinical utility of a rapid whole-blood D-dimer assay in patients with cancer who present with suspected acute deep venous thrombosis. Ann Intern Med 1999;131:417.

van der Graaf F, van den Borne H, van der Kolk M, et al: Exclusion of deep venous thrombosis with D-dimer testing—Comparison of 13 D-dimer methods in 99 outpatients suspected of deep venous thrombosis using venography as reference standard. Thromb Haemost 2000;83: 191.

Etiology

Baron JA, Gridley G, Weiderpass E, et al: Venous thromboembolism and cancer. Lancet 1998;351:1077.

Bastounis EA, Karayiannakis AJ, Makri GG, et al: The incidence of occult cancer in patients with deep venous thrombosis: A prospective study. J Intern Med 1996;239:153.

Bevilacqua MP, Pober JS, Majeau GR, et al: Recombinant tumor necrosis factor induces procoagulant activity in cultured human vascular endothelium: Characterization and comparison with the actions of interleukin 1. Proc Natl Acad Sci USA 1986;83:4533.

Gordon SG, Cross BA: A factor X-activating cysteine protease from malignant tissue. J Clin Invest 1981;67:1665.

Prandoni P, Lensing AW, Buller HR, et al: Deep-vein thrombosis and the incidence of subsequent symptomatic cancer. N Engl J Med 1992;327:1128.

General Information

Burihan E, de Figueiredo LF, Francisco Junior J, et al: Upper-extremity deep venous thrombosis: Analysis of 52 cases. Cardiovasc Surg 1993;1:19.

Sorensen HT, Mellemkjaer L, Olsen JH, et al: Prognosis of cancers associated with venous thromboembolism. N Engl J Med 2000;343:1846.

Sorensen HT, Mellemkjaer L, Steffensen FH, et al: The risk of a diagnosis of cancer after primary deep venous thrombosis or pulmonary embolism. N Engl J Med 1998;338: 1169.

Verlato F, Zucchetta P, Prandoni P, et al: An unexpectedly high rate of pulmonary embolism in patients with superficial thrombophlebitis of the thigh. J Vasc Surg 1999;30: 1113.

Vena Cava Filters

Athanasoulis CA, Kaufman JA, Halpern EF, et al: Inferior vena caval filters: review of a 26-year single-center clinical experience. Radiology 2000;216:54.

Decousus H, Leizorovicz A, Parent F, et al: A clinical trial of vena caval filters in the prevention of pulmonary embolism in patients with proximal deep-vein thrombosis. Prevention du Risque d'Embolie Pulmonaire par Interruption Cave Study Group. N Engl J Med 1998;338:409.

Rosen MP, Porter DH, Kim D: Reassessment of vena caval filter use in patients with cancer. J Vasc Interv Radiol 1994;5:501.

Schwarz RE, Marrero AM, Conlon KC, et al: Inferior vena cava filters in cancer patients: Indications and outcome. J Clin Oncol 1996;14:652.

Venoocclusive Disease of the Liver

Attal M, Huguet F, Rubie H, et al: Prevention of hepatic veno-occlusive disease after bone marrow transplantation by continuous infusion of low-dose heparin: A prospective, randomized trial. Blood 1992;79:2834.

Bearman SI, Lee JL, Baron AE, et al: Treatment of hepatic venoocclusive disease with recombinant human tissue plasminogen activator and heparin in 42 marrow transplant patients. Blood 1997;89:1501.

Bearman SI, Shuhart MC, Hinds MS, et al: Recombinant human tissue plasminogen activator for the treatment of established severe venoocclusive disease of the liver after bone marrow transplantation. Blood 1992;80:2458.

Hagglund H, Ringden O, Ljungman P, et al: No beneficial effects, but severe side effects caused by recombinant human tissue plasminogen activator for treatment of hepatic venoocclusive disease after allogeneic bone marrow transplantation. Transplant Proc 1995;27:3535.

Laporte JP, Lesage S, Tilleul P, et al: Alteplase for hepatic veno-occlusive disease complicating bone-marrow transplantation [letter]. 1992;339:1057.

Lassau N, Leclere J, Auperin A, et al: Hepatic veno-occlusive disease after myeloablative treatment and bone marrow transplantation: Value of gray-scale and Doppler US in 100 patients. Radiology 1997;204:545.

Or R, Nagler A, Shpilberg O, et al: Low-molecular-weight heparin for the prevention of veno-occlusive disease of the liver in bone marrow transplantation patients. Transplantation 1996;61:1067.

Richardson P, Guinan E: The pathology, diagnosis, and treatment of hepatic veno-occlusive disease: Current status and novel approaches. Br J Haematol 1999;107:485.

Richardson PG, Elias AD, Krishnan A, et al: Treatment of severe veno-occlusive disease with defibrotide: Compassionate use results in response without significant toxicity in a high-risk population. Blood 1998;92:737.

Rosti G, Bandini G, Belardinelli A, et al: Alteplase for hepatic veno-occlusive disease after bone-marrow transplantation [letter; comment]. Lancet 1992;339:1481.

Chapter 117
Tumor Lysis Syndrome

Daniel J. De Angelo

Tumor lysis syndrome occurs as a result of the rapid release of intracellular contents into the bloodstream following the death of a significant number of cells. Hyperuricemia, hyperkalemia, hyperphosphatemia, and hypocalcemia characterize the syndrome. Metabolic acidosis and acute renal failure can occur as well (Table 117-1). The release into the bloodstream of intracellular potassium and organic as well as inorganic phosphates from killed cells results in the development of hyperkalemia and hyperphosphatemia, respectively. Hyperphosphatemia can result in the development of hypocalcemia. The rapid breakdown of nucleic acids leads to hyperuricemia. Tumor lysis syndrome can develop prior to the administration of chemotherapy in patients with rapidly proliferating hematologic neoplasms; however, it is typically triggered after the administration of high doses of chemotherapy and rapid destruction of tumor cells.

Patients with large tumor burdens are at an increased risk for tumor lysis syndrome, especially if the neoplasm is sensitive to chemotherapy (Table 117-2). These disorders typically include acute myelogenous and lymphoblastic leukemias (Table 117-3). In addition, tumor lysis syndrome is commonly seen in patients with acute lymphoblastic lymphomas and Burkitt's or other high-grade lymphoproliferative disorders. Significant destruction of solid tumors also places patients at risk for tumor lysis syndrome. Elevated lactate dehydrogenase levels are markers of cell lysis. Commonly observed in patients with aggressive hematologic malignancies, the syndrome has also been described after the use of myelosuppressive agents such as α-interferon or hormonal therapy for breast cancer. The risk of developing tumor lysis syndrome is greater in patients with renal insufficiency. These patients have a lower glomerular filtration rate and are more susceptible to electrolyte disturbances than patients with normal renal function. In addition, patients with preexisting renal insufficiency are more likely to develop acute renal failure.

Hyperuricemia

Xanthine oxidase catalyzes the breakdown of hypoxanthine and xanthine to uric acid. The pK_a of uric acid is approximately 5.4. In the blood, where the pH is higher, uric acid is present in the ionized, acid-soluble form. In the acidic environment of the renal tubules, uric acid is present in a nonionized, less soluble form. Hyperuricemia can be present as an isolated abnormality without the other characteristic metabolic findings associated with tumor lysis syndrome. Renal insufficiency develops when uric acid crystals precipitate in the renal tubules and distal renal collecting system. In addition to uric acid stones, patients with hyperuricemia can develop gouty arthritis, nausea, vomiting, diarrhea, and anorexia. As renal function declines, patients develop edema and lethargy. Certain medications—namely, diuretics such as thiazides and furosemide as well as antituberculous drugs and certain cytotoxic agents—can aggravate hyperuricemia.

Patients with the potential to develop tumor lysis syndrome need to be recognized prospectively so that appropriate prophylactic measures can be initiated. Drugs that elevate serum uric acid levels should be discontinued. Intravenous hydration should be initiated. When the patient's urinary outflow increases, the serum concentration of uric acid decreases substantially. Alkalinization of the urine, with a concomitant increase in uric acid solubility, is obtained with the addition of sodium bicarbonate (50 to 100 mEq/L) to the intravenous fluids. Although furosemide increases the renal tubular reabsorption of uric acid, this is offset by the preservation of increased urinary flow rates. Therefore, furosemide can be used safely to maintain a proper total body fluid balance.

Allopurinol is the standard medical treatment for both the prevention and treatment of hyperuricemia. Allopurinol is an inhibitor of xanthine oxidase and is well tolerated; the most common adverse reaction is a hypersensitivity erythematous skin rash. This reac-

Table 117-1 ■ Findings in Tumor Lysis Syndrome

Metabolic complications
  Hyperuricemia
  Hyperkalemia
  Hyperphosphatemia
  Hypocalcemia
  Metabolic acidosis
Acute renal failure

Table 117-3 ■ Risk for Tumor Lysis Syndrome by Tumor Type

Frequently Associated

Acute myelogenous leukemia
Acute lymphoblastic leukemia or lymphoma
Burkitt's and other high-grade lymphomas

Less Frequently Associated

Diffuse large B cell lymphoma
Chronic myelogenous leukemia
Low-grade lymphoma
Small cell lung cancer
Breast cancer
Germ cell tumor
Nonseminoma, seminoma, mediastinal, ovarian cancers

tion is usually delayed for several days after the onset of therapy, and allopurinol can be given safely during the period of highest risk of tumor lysis. Allopurinol increases the serum levels of both hypoxanthine and xanthine, but neither is commonly associated with the development of acute renal failure. Allopurinol is administered orally once or twice daily at doses typically ranging from 300 to 600 mg/day. Allopurinol is cleared by the kidney, so the dose should be adjusted in older patients or patients with chronic renal failure. Allopurinol is now available intravenously. 6-Mercaptopurine is metabolized by xanthine oxidase; therefore, the dose of this agent must be reduced during treatment with allopurinol.

Patients who develop oliguria or acute renal failure should be evaluated with ultrasonography or computed tomography in order to rule out ureteral obstruction due to uric acid stones. Intravenous contrast agents should be avoided due to the risk of acute tubular necrosis. Hemodialysis and continuous venous-venous hemofiltration are both effective in reversing severe uric acid nephropathy.

Hyperkalemia

Hyperkalemia is the principal life-threatening electrolyte abnormality that develops during tumor lysis syndrome. Hyperkalemia, defined as a serum concen-

Table 117-2 ■ Risk Factors for Tumor Lysis Syndrome

Large tumor burden
  Acute leukemias and lymphomas
  High-grade lymphomas
  Bulky solid tumors
High tumor growth fraction
Tumors highly sensitive to chemotherapy
Markedly elevated lactate dehydrogenase
Baseline renal insufficiency

tration greater than 5.0 mEq/L, is a result of the release of intracellular potassium due to cell lysis during chemotherapy. Iatrogenic causes, such as the administration of potassium, should be excluded. Pseudohyperkalemia can result from poor phlebotomy technique, hemolysis, marked leukocytosis, or thrombocytosis. The latter two causes are due to the release of intracellular potassium in the test tube sample following clot formation. Measurement of the plasma potassium using heparin as anticoagulant can minimize confusion when an elevated serum potassium has been obtained.

Hyperkalemia causes a partial depolarization of the resting membrane potential. Prolonged depolarization eventually leads to impaired excitability, resulting in muscular weakness, which can progress to flaccid paralysis. The most serious and life-threatening manifestation of hyperkalemia is cardiac toxicity; however, cardiac toxicity does not necessarily correlate with the magnitude of hyperkalemia. The initial electrocardiographic abnormalities include increased amplitude of the T-waves or peaked T-waves. Subsequent changes include prolongation of the PR and QRS intervals, atrioventricular conduction blocks, and flattening of the P waves. The QRS complex can merge with the T wave, resulting in a sine-wave pattern that often terminates in ventricular fibrillation or asystole. Fatal hyperkalemia rarely occurs at a plasma potassium concentration less than 7.5 mEq/L.

The treatment of hyperkalemia is dependent on the serum potassium concentration. All patients with hyperkalemia, regardless of the degree of elevation, require an immediate electrocardiogram. Furthermore, medications that interfere with potassium metabolism (e.g., nonsteroidal anti-inflammatory drugs [NSAIDs] and angiotensin-converting enzyme inhibitors) should be discontinued. Oral cation-exchange resins promote the exchange of potassium and sodium ions within the lumen of the gastrointestinal tract. This is an effective initial strategy for patients with mild asymptomatic hyperkalemia. A dose of 15 to 30 gm of sodium polystyrene sulfonate (Kayexalate) generally lowers the serum potassium concentration by 0.5 to 1.0 mEq/L within one to two hours and has a duration of action of about four hours.

Severe hyperkalemia requires more emergent treatment. Calcium gluconate, 10 mL of a 10% solution administered over the course of one to three minutes, should be given to decrease membrane excitability. The effect can be observed rapidly but is short lived. The administration of insulin (10 to 20 units of regular insulin) with glucose (25 to 50 gm) shifts potassium into cells. This technique typically results in reduction of the serum potassium concentration by 0.5 to 1.5 mEq/L, which lasts for several hours. Glucose should be avoided if the patient is severely hyperglycemic. Alkalinization of the blood with bicarbonate also leads to a shift of potassium into cells. Hemodialysis and continuous venous-venous hemofiltration are the most effective methods for rapidly lowering the serum potassium levels, especially for patients with either preexisting or acute renal failure. Peritoneal dialysis is not as effective as hemodialysis in lowering the serum potassium level and should be avoided in patients receiving chemotherapy.

Hyperphosphatemia

Hyperphosphatemia results from the release of intracellular phosphate into the serum following cell lysis. Hyperphosphatemia is defined as a serum phosphate level above 5.0 mg/dL. Spurious hyperphosphatemia can occur in patients with a marked thrombocytosis, and the phosphorus levels should be confirmed in heparinized plasma. Paraproteins with a net positive charge, as in plasma cell dyscrasias, can cause marked elevations in the serum phosphate levels.

Hyperphosphatemia is a dangerous condition due to the potential of extraosseous calcification. A calcium-phosphorus product {serum Ca (mg/dL) × serum P (mg/dL)} greater than 70 suggests a potential risk of metastatic calcification. Hyperphosphatemia eventually results in lowering of the serum calcium levels. Except for those patients with renal failure, the initial treatment of hyperphosphatemia includes volume expansion, with a resultant increase in the fractional clearance of phosphorus by the kidney. Aluminum-based antacids bind to phosphorus in the gut and prevent further absorption. Although the

chronic use of these agents can lead to aluminum toxicity, they are safe and effective for short-term use. Other phosphate binders, such as calcium acetate (PhosLo) may also be used. The treatment of hyperphosphatemia in the setting of renal failure often requires hemodialysis.

Hypocalcemia

Hypocalcemia is a direct manifestation of hyperphosphatemia. Many cancer patients have hypocalcemia, defined as a serum calcium level less than 8.5 mg/dL; however, only 10% of these patients have a reduction in ionized calcium. Thus, most of these patients with hypocalcemia actually are normocalcemic, as only the ionized calcium is biologically active. Hypoalbuminemia is the principal cause of a reduced total serum calcium level in severely ill patients. Excessive alkalinization of the serum increases the binding of calcium to proteins and results in a further reduction of the serum calcium level. In these cases, an ionized calcium level should be measured. Transient hypocalcemia also can arise from repeated transfusions of blood products due to the citrate anticoagulant. Although parathyroid hormone regulates serum calcium levels, its effect is overwhelmed in patients with tumor lysis syndrome due to the excessive loss of calcium from the extracellular fluid. Transient hypocalcemia is seldom clinically significant, but if it is of long standing, it can lead to several serious clinical manifestations (Table 117-4). These include muscle spasms, carpopedal spasms, and in severe cases tetany, laryngeal spasms, or convulsions. The QT interval on the EKG can become prolonged, which might lead to ventricular arrhythmias. Rarely, patients

Table 117-4 ■ Signs and Symptoms of Tumor Lysis Syndrome

Laboratory Abnormality	Clinical Symptoms
Hyperuricemia	Nausea, vomiting, diarrhea, joint pain, oliguria, anuria, azotemia, flank pain, hematuria, crystalluria
Hyperkalemia	Muscle cramps, nausea, weakness, paresthesias, paralysis, EKG changes, bradyarrhythmias, tachyarrhythmias, cardiac arrest
Hyperphosphatemia	Oliguria, anuria, azotemia, renal failure
Hypocalcemia	Muscle twitching, tetany, laryngospasm, paresthesias, hypotension, ventricular arrhythmias, heart block

become irritable, depressed, or psychotic due to prolonged hypocalcemia.

The principal focus on correcting the hypocalcemia of tumor lysis syndrome revolves around the treatment of the hyperphosphatemia. Calcium supplementation with oral calcium or calcium gluconate in severe symptomatic cases must be taken with caution, especially if the calcium-phosphate solubility product is greater than 70. In general, calcium should not be given, as this might precipitate calcium phosphate deposition. The correction of serum phosphate levels usually improves the serum calcium levels. For patients who have persistent hypocalcemia, calcitrol may be used until the serum calcium level normalizes.

References

Abramson E, Gajardo H, Kukreja SC: Hypocalcemia in cancer. Bone Miner 1990;10:161–169.

Arrambide K, Toto R: Tumor lysis syndrome. Semin Nephrol 1993;13:273–280.

Barton J: Tumor lysis syndrome in nonhematopoietic neoplasms. Cancer 1989;64:738–740.

Boccia R, Longo D, Lieher M, et al: Multiple recurrences of acute tumor lysis syndrome in an indolent non-Hodgkin's lymphoma. Cancer 1985;56:2295–2297.

Cech P, Block JB, Cone LA, et al: Tumor lysis syndrome after tamoxifen flare. N Engl J Med 1986;315:263–264.

Cohen LF, Balow JE, Magrath IT, et al: Acute tumor lysis syndrome. A review of 37 patients with Burkitt's lymphoma. Am J Med 1980;68:486–491.

Conger JD, Falk SA: Intrarenal dynamics in the pathogenesis and prevention of acute urate nephropathy. J Clin Invest 1977;59:786–793.

DeFronzo R, Smith J: Clinical Disorders of Hyperkalemia, 5th ed. New York: McGraw-Hill, 1994, pp 697–754.

Drakos P, Bar-Ziv J, Catane R: Tumor lysis syndrome in nonhematologic malignancies. Am J Clin Oncol 1994;17:502–505.

Dunlay RW, Camp MA, Allon M, et al: Calcitriol in prolonged hypocalcemia due to the tumor lysis syndrome. Ann Intern Med 1989;110:162–164.

Fer M, Bottino G, Sherwin S, et al: Atypical tumor lysis syndrome in a patient's T cell lymphoma treated with recombinant leukocyte interferon. Am J Med 1984;77:953–956.

Fleming D, Doukas M: Acute tumor lysis syndrome in hematologic malignancies. Leuk Lymphoma 1992;8:315–318.

Flomenbaum C: Metabolic emergencies in the cancer patient. Semin Oncol 2000;27:322–334.

Hande KR, Hixson CV, Chabner BA: Postchemotherapy purine excretion in lymphoma patients receiving allopurinol. Cancer Res 1981;41:2273–2279.

Hogan D, Rosenthal L: Oncologic emergencies in the patient with lymphoma. Semin Oncol Nurs 1998;14:312–320.

Holick M, Krane S: Introduction to Bone and Mineral Metabolism, 15th ed. New York: McGraw-Hill, 2001, pp 2192–2205.

Jones D, Mahmoud H, Chesney R: Tumor lysis syndrome: pathogenesis and management. Pediatr Nephrol 1995;9:206–212.

Klinenberg JR, Kippen I, Bluestone R: Hyperuricemic nephropathy: pathologic features and factors influencing urate deposition. Nephron 1975;14:88–98.

Mandell GA, Swacus JR, Rosenstock J, et al: Danger of urography in hyperuricemic children with Burkitt's lymphoma. J Can Assoc Radiol 1983;34:273–277.

Potts J: Diseases of the Parathyroid Gland and Other Hyper- and Hypocalcemic Disorders, 15th ed. New York: McGraw-Hill, 2001, pp 2205–2226.

Razis E, Arlin Z, Ahmed T, et al: Incidence and treatment of tumor lysis syndrome in patients with acute leukemia. Acta Haematol 1994;91:171–174.

Smalley RV, Guaspari A, Haase-Statz S, et al: Allopurinol: intravenous use for prevention and treatment of hyperuricemia. J Clin Oncol 2000;18:1758–1763.

Steinberg SM, Galen MA, Lazarus JM, et al: Hemodialysis for acute anuric uric acid nephropathy. Am J Dis Child 1975;129:956–958.

Tsokos G, Balow J, Spiegel R, et al: Renal and metabolic complications of undifferentiated and lymphoblastic lymphomas. Medicine 1981;60:218–229.

Section V
Supportive Care of the Patient with Cancer

Chapter 118
Screening and Genetic Counseling for the Patient with Cancer

Jeffrey N. Weitzel

Introduction

Advances in our understanding of the genetic basis for cancer have led to the development of new technologies and tools for genetic cancer risk assessment. All cancer is genetic in origin at the cellular level. Mutations of the genetic blueprint in the lineage of a cell may all be acquired during an individual's lifetime, as is the case for the vast majority of genetic lesions identified in tumor cells, or in some cases may start with a mutation in the germline that is inherited from a parental gamete. Oncologists are in an important position to recognize hereditary cancer patterns and often have the opportunity to advise patients and family members regarding the potential need for genetic cancer risk assessment. Genetic cancer risk assessment is an emerging standard of care for numerous hereditary cancer syndromes, and algorithms for referral and management of patients with increased risk are being developed.

While inherited forms of cancer are rare, representing approximately 5% of many types of adult-onset cancers, the magnitude of risk conferred by cancer susceptibility genes is significant. For example, the cumulative risk of developing breast or ovarian cancer in the hereditary breast/ovarian cancer syndrome may be as high as 90% over a woman's lifetime. This is in contrast to the lifetime risk of 11% for sporadic occurrence of breast cancer in the general population. Since earlier age at onset is typical of the inherited form of this disease, screening guidelines geared for the general population are not adequate. Identification of persons who are at increased risk for cancer allows for application of potentially life-saving surveillance or preventive measures.

Genetic cancer risk assessment is an attempt to predict the future, to quantify the probability that an individual will develop cancer. Hereditary cancer risk assessment, counseling, and management strategies need to consider several dynamic domains: (1) state of cancer genetics knowledge, (2) state of mind (e.g., previous cancer experience within the family), (3) state of technology, and (4) state of the art in terms of management.

State of Cancer Genetics Knowledge

A small proportion of common cancers (e.g., breast, ovarian, colorectal, and endometrial) are caused by highly penetrant autosomal-dominant genes. Recognizing potentially hereditary patterns of cancer in families is challenging when the sporadic form of the disease is common (e.g., breast or colon cancer). The key features of hereditary cancer are listed in Table 118-1.

There are now over 50 cancer-associated syndromes for which the genetic basis is known, and several new genes are reported every year. Table 118-2 lists hereditary syndromes and their respective genetic loci.

Germline Versus Somatic or Acquired

Knudson introduced a new paradigm of tumor suppressor genes and offered clinical insights from the now-proven pathogenetic mechanisms of hereditary retinoblastoma tumorigenesis in 1971. In his two-hit hypothesis, Knudson theorized that one mutated copy of the *RB1* gene is inherited in the germline and the other copy becomes inactivated through an acquired mutation in the somatic cell. Most hereditary cancer syndromes involve mutations in putative tumor suppressor genes. However, the types of genes that are involved in cancer predisposition have expanded to include proto-oncogenes and genes involved in maintaining the fidelity of the genome. Vogelstein and colleagues documented the multistep nature of acquired (somatic) mutations that are necessary for cancer development, using colorectal tumorigenesis as their model. Complex somatic genetic alterations are characteristic of all adult-onset carcinomas. It is currently believed that at least five different critical gene muta-

Table 118-1 ■ Hallmarks of Familial Cancer

Occurrence of cancer at an unusually young age or in the less usually affected gender

Vertical transmission of cancer within a family over multiple generations

Multifocal disease or bilateral disease in paired organs

Multiple primary cancers in an individual

Clustering of unusual or rare cancers in a family

tions are required for a given clonal expansion of cells to acquire a full cancerous phenotype. Some molecular markers, such as loss of the long (q) arm of chromosome 18 in colorectal cancer and amplification of Her2/neu in breast cancer, have proven to have prognostic significance and have led to novel targeted therapeutics.

Microsatellite instability is now recognized as a somatic molecular marker for colon tumors in patients with the inherited mismatch repair gene defects that characterize hereditary nonpolyposis colorectal cancer syndrome. More recently, the presence of microsatel-

lite instability in colorectal cancer was found to be associated with better survival in patients treated with adjuvant chemotherapy. Thus, a somatic marker can have both etiologic and prognostic implications. Identification of both germline and inherited genetic changes will likely prove useful for prognostication in the future.

There is emerging knowledge about gene-gene and gene-environment interactions. The recognition of the importance of moderate risk genes, those that may influence an individual's response to a given carcinogenic exposure or the efficacy of a therapeutic intervention, has led to the development of the field of pharmacogenetics.

Another level of complexity in genetic cancer risk assessment is that different genes may cause a similar phenotype, a phenomenon called genetic heterogeneity. For example, both *BRCA1* and *BRCA2* may cause hereditary breast and ovarian cancer syndrome, while hereditary breast cancer may also be the primary manifestation of Cowden disease or Li-Fraumeni syndrome, caused by germline mutation in the *PTEN* or *TP53* genes, respectively. Knowledge about differentiating clinical features is important for identifying the

Table 118-2 ■ Hereditary Cancer Syndromes and Involved Gene

Hereditary Tumor or Syndrome	Candidate Gene or Locus	Chromosomal Location
Familial adenomatous polyposis (FAP)	APC	5q21
Hereditary nonpolyposis colon cancer (HNPCC) (mismatch repair gene family)	MSH2	2p16
	MLH1	3p21
	PMS1	2q31
	PMS2	7p22
	MSH6	2p18
Hereditary diffuse gastric cancer	CDH1	16q22
Hereditary breast/ovarian cancer (HBOC)	BRCA1	17q21
	BRCA2	13q12
Li-Fraumeni syndrome (LFS)	p53	17p13
Cowden disease (hamartomas, breast cancer)	PTEN	10q22
Multiple endocrine neoplasia		
Type I	MEN I	11q13
Type II (A & B)	RET	10q11.2
Familial retinoblastoma	RB1	13q14
Neurofibromatosis		
Type I	NF1	17q11
Type II	NF2	22q12
von Hippel-Lindau (VHL) disease	VHL	3p25
Wilms' tumor associated with WAGR	WT1	11p13
Hereditary papillary renal cancer	c-MET	7q31.1
Familial melanoma	p16 / CDKN2A	9p21
Dysplastic nevus syndrome	CMM/DN	1p32
Nevoid basal cell carcinoma syndrome (Gorlin's syndrome)	PTC	9q22
Ataxia telangiectasia (radiation sensitivity, cancer)	ATM	11q22

Table 118-3 ■ Features That Indicate an Increased Likelihood of Having *BRCA* Gene Mutations

Multiple cases of early onset breast cancer
Ovarian cancer with family history of breast or ovarian cancer
Breast and ovarian cancer in the same woman
Bilateral breast cancer
Ashkenazi Jewish heritage
Male breast cancer

correct syndrome and underscores the need for both a thorough family history and physical examination.

Major Hereditary Cancer Syndromes

Breast Cancer Susceptibility

Breast cancer is the most common malignant disease and the second most common killer of women in the United States, with more than 184,000 new cases and 46,000 deaths each year. An estimated 5% to 10% of breast cancer and ovarian cancer cases occur as part of heritable syndromes due to mutations in highly penetrant genes. Several separate syndromes are thought to exist. Indicators of possible hereditary breast cancer are listed in Table 118-3. Genetic segregation studies of breast cancer suggest that among women with breast cancer that is diagnosed before age 30, approximately one third might have their disease because of an inherited susceptibility.

Hereditary breast and ovarian cancer syndrome is a highly penetrant disease. Hall et al first mapped a locus for hereditary breast and ovarian cancer (*BRCA1*) to chromosome 17q. An international effort was culminated in 1994 by the cloning of *BRCA1*, the same year that a second locus, *BRCA2*, was mapped to chromosome 13q. These two genes accounted for the majority of the highly selected families in the Breast Cancer Linkage Consortium (BCLC) cohort that was used for these studies. More than 500 different mutations have been discovered in each *BRCA* gene. Mutations are inherited in an autosomal-dominant fashion and are associated primarily with an increased risk for breast and ovarian cancer. The lifetime risk of developing breast cancer ranges from 56% to 85% in women with *BRCA1* mutations. *BRCA1* mutations also confer a 40% to 60% lifetime risk for epithelial ovarian cancer, though earlier onset is not a characteristic feature. Alterations in *BRCA2* have been associated with an increased incidence of breast cancer in both women and men (6% lifetime risk). An increased risk for ovarian cancer (5% to 28% lifetime risk), pancreatic cancer, and melanoma (less than 10% lifetime risk) have also been reported.

Figure 118-1 shows how the age-specific penetrance estimates (with wide 95% confidence intervals) for inherited breast cancer susceptibility mutations may vary depending on the populations being examined. Note especially the 20% risk of breast cancer by age 40 and the 33% to 59% risk by age 50. A population-based study by Streuwing et al of over 5000 individuals with Ashkenazi Jewish ancestry was pos-

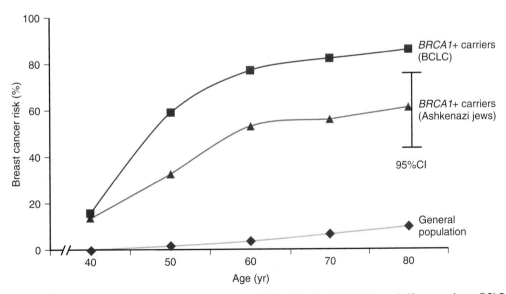

Figure 118-1 ■ Comparison of breast cancer risk estimates in *BRCA* mutation carriers. BCLC = Breast Cancer Linkage Consortium; CI = confidence interval. (Modified with permission from American Society of Clinical Oncology.)

sible because three founder mutations (185delAG and 5382insC in *BRCA1* and 6174delT in *BRCA2*) account for over 90% of mutant *BRCA* carriers in this ethnic group. Figure 118-2 shows the position and prevalence of the three founder mutations on a representation of the *BRCA* genes. One in 40 Ashkenazi Jews bear one of these three mutations. Breast cancer occurrence under age 55 or any combination of breast and/or ovarian cancer in a woman of Jewish ancestry indicates a greater than 10% probability that a *BRCA* gene mutation is responsible for the disease. Thus, directed screening for these founder mutations can be a cost-efficient approach to genotyping in individuals with this ancestry.

Models for estimating the probability of a detectable *BRCA* gene mutation have been developed from genotyping experience. Couch et al derived tables for estimating the probability that a detectable *BRCA1* mutation is present given the average age of onset for breast cancer cases, the presence of ovarian cancer within the family, and ethnicity (Ashkenazi Jewish ancestry). The highest probability for *BRCA1* mutation in a family was associated with the occurrence of both breast cancer and ovarian cancer in an individual. An algorithm uses first- and second-degree family history of breast or ovarian cancer to calculate the probabilities that either a *BRCA1* or a *BRCA2* mutation is responsible for the disease. Data from sequence analysis of the *BRCA* genes have been used to derive simple tables for estimating the probability of a detectable mutation given various combinations of personal and family cancer history.

Although analysis of *BRCA1* and *BRCA2* by sequencing is very sensitive, 5% to 8% of high-risk families without detectable mutations in these assays will have large genomic rearrangements such as deletions, duplications, or mutations of the regulatory region that are detectable only by Southern blot analysis or other methods. Therefore, the significance of a "negative" test result must be interpreted in the context of the personal and family history.

Table 118-4 ▪ Risk Management Options for *BRCA* Mutation Carriers*

Recommended for Breast Cancer Detection or Prevention

Monthly self-examination of the breasts beginning in late teen years
Beginning at age 25–35 or at least 10 years before the earliest-onset cancer in the kindred:
  Clinician breast exam every six months
  Annual mammography
Discussed as options for risk reduction:
  Bilateral prophylactic mastectomy (simple or skin-sparing)
  Chemoprevention clinical trial participation (i.e., STAR) or tamoxifen off study

Recommended for Ovarian Cancer Detection or Prevention

Pelvic examination and PAP smear annually
Serum CA125 every 6 to 12 months
Transvaginal ultrasound every 6 to 12 months
Discussed as options for risk reduction:
  Prophylactic salpingo-oophorectomy upon completion of childbearing
  Oral contraceptive use (may be associated with increased breast cancer risk)
  Reproductive counseling (? earlier childbearing)

*Also offered to women at increased risk because of their position in families with a history of breast and/or ovarian cancer, but for whom genotypic information is not available. Derived from Burke et al. Recommendations for follow-up care of individuals with an inherited predisposition to cancer. JAMA 277:997–1003, 1997.

Risk management guidelines for *BRCA* gene mutation carriers are summarized in Table 118-4. Breast tissue density in younger women limits the usefulness of mammography as a surveillance tool. Consequently, about half of the women who are determined to be at high risk for breast cancer choose to undergo bilateral prophylactic mastectomy. Recent retrospective data suggest that bilateral prophylactic mastectomy significantly decreases by approximately 90% the risk of developing breast cancer in women who

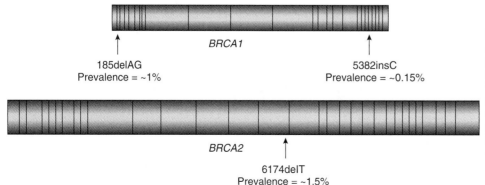

Figure 118-2 ▪ *BRCA1* and *BRCA2* mutations in the Ashkenazi Jewish population. The position and prevalence of the three founder mutations are shown here on a representation of the *BRCA* genes. Vertical lines in the figure indicate the complex exon structure of these relatively large genes.

have a family history of the disease. The recommended surgical technique for breast cancer risk reduction is simple mastectomy, including the removal of the nipple and areola, with immediate reconstruction.

There are no proven methods of screening for ovarian cancer. Although elevated CA125 levels are seen in 80% of advanced-stage epithelial ovarian cancer cases, CA125 is elevated in only 50% of stage I ovarian cancers. Moreover, false-positive elevations can be seen in benign disorders such as endometriosis, uterine fibroids, and pelvic inflammatory disease. Transvaginal ultrasound examination can often detect subtle alterations in ovarian architecture. However, false-positive scans are problematic, especially for premenopausal women, in whom the detection of functional ovarian cysts may necessitate a period of heightened surveillance with follow-up scans at short intervals or even surgical evaluation. Consideration of prophylactic bilateral salpingo-oophorectomy is warranted in women with *BRCA* gene mutations because of the limited efficacy of screening methods and the poor prognosis for patients with advanced disease, in spite of the fact that the lifetime risk for ovarian cancer is usually less than 50% and that there is still a residual risk for primary peritoneal cancer after such surgery. Rebbeck et al recently reported that prophylactic bilateral salpingo-oophorectomy may result in breast cancer risk reduction in women with *BRCA1* mutations, implicating a beneficial effect from reduction in ovarian hormone exposure.

Li-Fraumeni syndrome, a rare autosomal dominant cancer syndrome caused by germline *TP53* mutations, is associated with very early onset breast cancer. The classic constellation of cancers in Li-Fraumeni syndrome includes breast cancer, sarcomas, brain tumors, leukemia, adrenocorticocarcinoma, and other solid tumors and is marked by multiple primary cancer risk. Lifetime penetrance estimates range from 70% to 90% for males and females, respectively. Cancer risk is as high as 50% by age 30. Testing for germline mutations has been undertaken in these rare families, modeled after the experience with genetic testing for Huntington disease. Increased surveillance or prophylactic mastectomy for prevention of breast cancer is generally recommended for women in Li-Fraumeni syndrome families. However, the efficacy of surveillance programs for the other malignancies seen in this syndrome is uncertain.

Cowden disease (multiple hamartoma syndrome) is a cancer-associated autosomal-dominant genodermatosis with characteristic mucocutaneous findings including multiple smooth facial papules (cutaneous tricholemmomas), acral keratosis, and multiple oral papillomas. Central nervous system manifestations of Cowden disease may include megalencephaly, epilepsy, and dysplastic gangliocytomas of the cerebellum (Lhermitte Duclos disease). Other associated lesions include benign and malignant disease of the thyroid, intestinal polyps, and genitourinary abnormalities. Expression of the disease is variable, and penetrance of the dermatologic lesions is thought to be complete by age 20. Identification of the characteristic skin features should raise a suspicion of Cowden disease. Early diagnosis is important, since females with Cowden disease have a high frequency of breast carcinoma in early middle age. The incidence of breast cancer in affected females ranges from 22% to 50%. Recent observations of early-onset breast cancer among women with only subtle cutaneous manifesta-

---

TREATMENT

Genetic Cancer Risk Status May Influence Management of Newly Diagnosed Breast Cancer

The data from the Breast Cancer Linkage Consortium suggest that the cumulative risk of developing a contralateral second primary breast cancer is approximately 5% per year (up to 65% by age 70) among *BRCA1* mutation carriers who have already had a breast cancer. Breast conservation therapy (lumpectomy) plus regional radiotherapy for initial management of breast cancer appears to be equally efficacious at the five-year time point with respect to locoregional recurrence in both the hereditary and sporadic circumstances. However, a few studies with longer follow-up indicate that the incidence of late ipsilateral breast tumor recurrence, likely representing new primary breast cancers, is increased in individuals with hereditary breast cancer (22% to 48% at 10 years). Therefore, although breast conservation therapy is still considered an option for hereditary cancer cases, many women may choose bilateral mastectomy as initial treatment as both a therapeutic and a preventive procedure. Thus, knowledge of genetic status for a young woman with newly diagnosed breast cancer might influence the initial surgical approach, and urgent genetic cancer risk assessment should be considered for anyone with a greater than 10% probability of having a *BRCA* gene mutation.

tions of the disease raise concern that the syndrome may be unrecognized in many cases. The gene for Cowden disease was localized to chromosome 10q22–23 by linkage analysis and was subsequently demonstrated to be the *PTEN* gene. DNA-based predictive testing is available as a research tool. Management of increased breast cancer risk in these patients is similar to that for patients with hereditary breast and ovarian cancer syndrome. However, surveillance for thyroid cancer overshadows ovarian surveillance, since Cowden disease is not associated with increased ovarian cancer risk.

Ataxia telangiectasia is a rare (1:40,000 to 1:100,000) autosomal-recessive disorder with developmental abnormalities, telangiectasias, truncal ataxia, and a significant risk (38%) for cancer, predominantly lymphoproliferative, and a lesser risk for other types of solid tumors. Ataxia telangiectasia is associated with germline mutations in the *ATM* gene, which normally mediates cell cycle arrest after ionizing radiation damage. Swift et al previously reported that breast cancer was increased among presumed heterozygous *ATM* mutation carriers in families with a child affected by ataxia telangiectasia. Carriers were postulated to have an intermediate degree of radiation sensitivity, posing issues for routine mammography and increasing the risk of adverse reactions to therapeutic radiation. Discovery of the *ATM* gene led to examinations of the relationship between heterozygosity at the locus and breast cancer risk. Most studies employing genotyping for *ATM* have not found any significant association between *ATM* mutations and early-onset breast cancer. In general, any family history of breast cancer in association with ataxia telangiectasia is an indication for increased surveillance.

Multiple Endocrine Neoplasia Syndromes

Multiple endocrine neoplasia (MEN) is characterized by the occurrence of tumors in two or more endocrine glands in a single patient or in close relatives. There are two clinically and genetically distinct multiple endocrine neoplasia syndromes: MEN1 and MEN2.

Multiple endocrine neoplasia type 1 (MEN1) (incidence 1:10,000 to 1:100,000) is an autosomal-dominant predisposition to tumors of the parathyroid glands (more than 90% of cases), the pituitary gland (44%), and the pancreatic islet cells (73%), with rare involvement of the thyroid gland and adrenal cortex (16%). Typical clinical manifestations may include unexplained hypercalcemia (hyperparathyroidism, nephrolithiasis) or symptoms related to the endocrine pancreas (e.g., peptic ulcer disease resulting from hypergastrinemia, also known as Zollinger-Ellison syndrome, or diarrhea resulting from vasoactive

intestinal peptide-secreting tumors) or the pituitary. Pituitary findings include local pressure effects, amenorrhea or impotence, or acromegaly resulting from functioning tumors. Germline mutations in the *MEN1* gene, on chromosome 11q13, are responsible for this disease. Genetic testing is available on a research basis. More than 80% of *MEN1* gene mutation carriers will have a detectable manifestation by age 50 years. Although expression of the disorder may vary between different MEN1 families, there is significant intrafamilial consistency. Clinical surveillance or screening for mutation carriers or at-risk individuals (older than age 15 years) usually includes annual measurement of serum calcium, glucose, cortisol, prolactin, and phosphorus levels, as well as levels of parathyroid hormone, 5-hydroxyindoleacetic acid, urinary metanephrine, and pancreatic hormones (gastrin, pancreatic polypeptide, IGF-1, insulin, proinsulin, and glucagon), every one to two years. Magnetic resonance imaging (MRI) of the pituitary and pancreas should be considered every three to five years. Treatments are tumor-specific and are often directed at symptoms or metabolic consequences.

Multiple Endocrine Neoplasia Types 2A and 2B (MEN2A, MEN2B) and Familial Medullary Thyroid Carcinoma (FMTC)

Medullary thyroid carcinoma, derived from the calcitonin-producing C cells of the thyroid, represents 10% of all thyroid cancers, and 25% of these are hereditary in nature owing to germline mutations in the *RET* gene on chromosome 10q11.2. Multifocal medullary thyroid carcinoma is the hallmark of MEN2, a syndrome with three distinct subsets: MEN2A (90%), MEN2B (5%), and familial medullary thyroid carcinoma (5%). Distinguishing clinical features are described in Table 118-5.

In sporadic medullary thyroid carcinoma, tumors typically develop in the fifth or sixth decade of life and are unilateral and unifocal, with no family history or

Table 118-5 ■ Clinical Presentation of Medullary Thyroid Carcinoma

Type	Distribution	Familial Pattern	Associated Abnormalities
Sporadic	Unilateral	No	None
MEN 2A	Bilateral	Yes	Pheochromocytomas Hyperparathyroidism
MEN 2B	Bilateral	Yes/no	Pheochromocytomas Mucosal neuromas Ganglioneuromas Characteristic phenotype
FMTC	Bilateral	Yes	None

associated abnormalities. In MEN2A, tumors are bilateral and multifocal with an onset often in the first two decades. There is a family history of related disease, and associated pheochromocytomas and/or hyperparathyroidism occurs. Although penetrance is incomplete, the lifetime risk for the development of medullary thyroid carcinoma is 100%, that for pheochromocytoma is 50%, and that for hyperparathyroidism is 30% among those who actually develop clinical manifestations of MEN2A. MEN2B is characterized by early age at onset and a more clinically aggressive course of disease. Parathyroid lesions are absent, but developmental abnormalities (mucosal neuromas, intestinal ganglioneuromatosis, megacolon, and a marfanoid body habitus) are the rule. Up to one half of MEN2B cases result from de novo germline mutations; therefore, family history may be absent. In familial medullary thyroid carcinoma, tumors are bilateral and multifocal, and there is a family history, but there are no other associated endocrine abnormalities, tumors, or developmental abnormalities.

Genetic testing for at-risk individuals is an established clinical procedure. Unlike most other cancer susceptibility genes, *RET* is a proto-oncogene rather than a tumor suppressor gene, and is the exclusive cause of hereditary predisposition to medullary thyroid carcinoma. To date, all described mutations are point mutations leading to amino acid substitution (missense mutations). Further, particular clinical manifestations are associated with mutations clustered in specific regions of the gene. Almost all MEN2A families with both pheochromocytoma and parathyroid involvement carry mutations in codon 634. Point mutations in codon 918 resulting in a substitution of threonine for methionine, which alters the function of the second intracellular tyrosine kinase domain, are found in 95% of MEN2B cases. Testing for *RET* mutations is highly predictive and of modest cost, though approximately 12% of familial medullary thyroid carcinoma families do not have a detectable *RET* mutation.

Overall, *RET* mutation testing is more effective and accurate than biochemical screening in unaffected individuals. Before the advent of genetic testing, biochemical screening with provocative studies (pentagastrin- and calcium-stimulated calcitonin levels) was used in individuals at risk for MEN2 on an annual basis starting at age 5 and continuing until age 45. Although elevated calcium-stimulated calcitonin levels in at-risk individuals correlated with the presence of C cell hyperplasia and/or medullary thyroid carcinoma, 10% of cases had metastatic disease at the time of thyroidectomy. Consequently, molecular diagnostic testing for *RET* mutations is considered the standard of care in affected families, as well as in patients with apparently sporadic medullary thyroid carcinoma. Up to 7% of the latter group will have a detectable mutation. Calcitonin testing is still used to screen for residual medullary thyroid carcinoma following prophylactic thyroidectomy in carriers of *RET* mutations. Once the diagnosis of hereditary medullary thyroid carcinoma is established in a patient, additional screening for pheochromocytomas and hyperparathyroidism is initiated. Biochemical screening for pheochromocytomas remains extremely important because of the potential for fatal hypertension associated with increased catecholamines during general anesthesia or childbirth.

For unaffected family members who test positive for *RET* mutations, prophylactic thryoidectomy is recommended to prevent the development of medullary thyroid carcinoma. The current guidelines call for prophylactic thyroidectomy, whereas parathyroid glands may be conserved in situ or autotransplanted to the forearm. Surgery should be performed between the ages of 5 and 10 years in individuals from MEN2A families and in infancy in MEN2B families. Although genetic testing is the standard of care in families with MEN2 syndromes, genetic counseling and informed consent remain essential to the testing process and should include age-appropriate education and counseling for pediatric patients. Delayed intervention may be reasonable in familial medullary thyroid carcinoma, in which onset of disease is often later and the disease has a more indolent course. By identifying individuals from affected families who do not carry mutations, *RET* testing also eliminates the need for screening in those that are not at risk.

Hereditary Colorectal Cancer

Colorectal cancer accounts for about 9% of all cancers, with an estimated 131,200 new cases each year. Approximately 5% to 10% occur in the setting of hereditary nonpolyposis colorectal cancer syndrome, while familial adenomatous polyposis accounts for fewer than 1% of colorectal cancer (see also Chapter 92).

Familial adenomatous polyposis is a rare autosomal-dominant syndrome (1:5000) caused by germline mutations in the APC gene on chromosome 5q21. De novo mutations occurring in a parental gamete account for approximately 30% of cases, so family history can be unrevealing. Consequently, the first manifestation in a family may be development of colorectal cancer onset in the third or fourth decade in an individual with concomitant polyposis on endoscopy. Adenomas may appear during adolescence, and penetrance is virtually complete by age 40. Additional clues to the diagnosis include a number of extracolonic manifestations (e.g., congenital hypertrophy of the retinal pigment epithelium, a benign marker that may be present in childhood) and both benign (desmoids) and malignant tumors (e.g., hepatoblastoma in childhood and upper gastrointestinal (GI) cancers in adulthood). Surgical management involves a total colectomy, which is also offered as effective prophylaxis to carriers of *APC* gene mutations at or prior to the onset of polyposis. A subset of patients have a distinctive variant of familial adenomatous polyposis called Gardner's syndrome, which is characterized by epidermal cysts in the skin; osteomas in the long bones, mandible, and skull; and supernumerary teeth, in addition to the typical features of familial adenomatous polyposis. Genetic testing is considered standard of care in familial adenomatous polyposis and is offered by the age of 10 to 12 years, just prior to the age of regular annual endoscopic surveillance in at-risk individuals. The strategy is to test the affected individual first to identify the familial mutation. *APC* mutations are detectable in approximately 80% of cases by available commercial assays. Once the familial mutation is identified, the efficacy of carrier detection is nearly absolute, and noncarriers may be spared the need for invasive surveillance. Mutations at either the beginning or at the end of the APC gene may result in an attenuated phenotype characterized by oligopolyposis (30 to 100 polyps) and moderate propensity to develop colorectal cancer, which tends be of later onset. The distinctive phenotype of classic familial adenomatous polyposis, with early-onset florid polyposis and virtually 100% risk of subsequent colorectal cancer if left untreated, marks this as an important genetic condition to recognize, given that prophylactic surgical intervention has a major impact on morbidity and mortality. Gastroscopy is recommended every two to three years for *APC* gene mutation carriers because of concomitant risk for gastric, duodenal, and ampullary polyps. Upper gastrointestinal carcinoma is the major residual cause of cancer-related mortality (10%) in familial adenomatous polyposis patients who have undergone prophylactic colectomy. Further, the Food and Drug Administration (FDA) recently approved Celecoxib, a Cox-2 inhibitor, as a chemopreventive agent for patients with familial adenomatous polyposis.

Hereditary nonpolyposis colorectal cancer, also known as Lynch syndrome, is inherited in an autosomal-dominant manner. The clinical characteristics of hereditary nonpolyposis colorectal cancer syndrome include early onset of colorectal cancer (average age at diagnosis: 45 years), an increased proportion of proximal colon cancers, and a propensity to develop extracolonic malignancies, predominantly cancer of the endometrium, ovary, stomach, urinary tract, small bowel, and bile duct. The lifetime risk of colorectal cancer is up to 80%. The risk of a metachronous new primary colorectal cancer is 30% at 10 years after a limited resection and up to 50% at 15 years. Endometrial adenocarcinoma is the second most common tumor, with the average age at diagnosis of 45 years. The lifetime risk of endometrial adenocarcinoma is 30% to 60% in different studies.

Although hereditary nonpolyposis colorectal cancer was first described clinically over 100 years ago, its genetic basis was elucidated only recently with the discovery of microsatellite instability in 1993, leading to the recognition of the role of mismatch repair genes in the pathogenesis of the disorder. Microsatellite instability is a somatic genetic change that produces a distinctive pattern of small insertion and deletion mutations in short repetitive sequences that are detectable in tumors. High-frequency microsatellite instability is present in greater than 90% of hereditary nonpolyposis colorectal cancer–related tumors and is circumstantial evidence that a mismatch repair gene defect was responsible for the disease. However, up to 10% of apparently sporadic colorectal cancer may manifest microsatellite instability, so this laboratory finding alone is not diagnostic. To date, five genes involved in the mismatch repair pathway have been implicated in hereditary nonpolyposis colorectal cancer: *MLH1* at 3p21.3, *MSH2* at 2p22-p21, *PMS1* at 2pq31-q31, *PMS2* at 7p22, and *MSH6* at 2p16. The products of these five genes all participate in a multimeric DNA mismatch repair complex. Other genes also participate in this complex, but germline mutations in those genes have not yet been reported. Once again genetic heterogeneity adds a layer of complexity to genetic cancer risk assessment in these patients. Diagnostic strategies include pedigree analysis and often a two-stage laboratory approach: microsatellite instability analysis of a tumor from an affected individual followed by genotyping for the two most commonly implicated mismatch repair genes if the microsatellite instability score is high or indeterminate. *MLH1* and *MSH2* account for more than 90% of the germline mutations in hereditary nonpolyposis colorectal cancer families studied to date. Immunohistochemistry demonstrating loss of expression of a mismatch repair gene in a tumor is also used as an indicator for genotyping in some centers. Mutation analysis is now available on a clinical basis, although the current assays are costly and the sensitivity is estimated at only 70%. Unfortunately, the histologic appearance of the tumors is nondiagnostic.

In an effort to define the diverse picture of hereditary nonpolyposis colorectal cancer, the Amsterdam criteria were developed: (1) three cases of colon cancer in which two of the affected individuals are first-degree relatives of the third, (2) colon cancers occurring in two generations, (3) one colon cancer diagnosed before age 50 years, and (4) no evidence of familial adenomatous polyposis in the family. These criteria are generally recognized to be overly restrictive for clinical purposes, because up to 20% of true hereditary nonpolyposis colorectal cancer families (as determined by germline mutation identification) do not meet these criteria. Commonly, this is because of limitations in a given family structure and incomplete penetrance.

The Bethesda guidelines (Rodriguez-Bigas et al, 1997) to broaden the scope of clinical features that should prompt consideration for evaluation for possible hereditary nonpolyposis colorectal cancer are listed in Table 118-6.

Hereditary nonpolyposis colorectal cancer–related variants include Muir-Torre syndrome, an association of sebaceous neoplasia (benign or malignant sebaceous skin tumors) with internal cancer. Linkage and mutational analyses of both *hMSH2* and *hMLH1* have demonstrated that Muir-Torre syndrome is a form of hereditary nonpolyposis colorectal cancer syndrome. Glioblastoma multiforme may be associated with hereditary nonpolyposis colorectal cancer syndrome. The glioblastoma appear at an early age (typically younger than 20 years) and demonstrate microsatellite instability. In contrast, patients with familial adenomatous polyposis display an increased risk of medulloblastoma. A brain tumor in combination with colorectal tumors, whether familial adenomatous polyposis or hereditary nonpolyposis colorectal cancer, is called Turcot's syndrome.

Management guidelines for hereditary nonpolyposis colorectal cancer families are evolving. The Cancer Studies Consortium Task Force on Preventive Recommendations published a consensus statement in 1997 for the care of individuals with hereditary nonpolyposis colorectal cancer. For asymptomatic, suspected, or known mutation carriers, the following two recommendations were made: (1) full colonoscopy to the cecum every one to three years beginning at age 20 to 25 years and (2) annual screening for endometrial cancer with transvaginal ultrasound beginning at age 25 to 35 years. Prophylactic hysterectomy and oophorectomy after childbearing is completed may be considered. Prophylactic subtotal colectomy can be considered, but the proven efficacy of colonoscopy and reports of more favorable prognosis disease make this option less palatable in unaffected individuals. The incidence of colorectal cancer was reduced 62% in hereditary nonpolyposis colorectal cancer families with intensive colonoscopic surveillance, presumably because of polypectomies, and when colorectal cancer did occur, the tumor stage was more favorable. However, because of the high risk of subsequent new primary tumors (up to 50% lifetime risk), subtotal colectomy is a reasonable initial surgical approach for a hereditary nonpolyposis colorectal cancer patient with newly diagnosed colorectal cancer. We make the following additional recommendations: (1) periodic (every four years) upper gastrointestinal endoscopy starting at age 35 and for Muir Torre families, (2) annual urinalysis and cytologic examination beginning at age 25, and (3) annual skin surveillance.

Hereditary Diffuse Gastric Cancer

Hereditary diffuse gastric cancer is a rare highly penetrant autosomal-dominant cancer syndrome associated with germline *E-cadherin* mutations and marked by susceptibility to the diffuse variant of gastric cancer. Linkage to *CDH1* (E-cadherin) on chromosome 16q22.1 was recently identified in three Maori families, and germline mutations account for approximately 25% of hereditary diffuse gastric cancer families worldwide. Families with two or more first-degree relatives with gastric adenocarcinoma should be considered for genetic cancer risk assessment. The majority of reported cases occurred in individuals under the age of 40, the youngest subject being 14 years of age. In contrast, 80% of gastric carcinomas in the general population occur after the age of 60 years.

Intestinal metaplasia of the gastric mucosa may be a precursor lesion for sporadic gastric cancer.

Table 118-6 ■ Bethesda Guidelines for Hereditary Nonpolyposis Colorectal Cancer (HNPCC)

Individuals with:

1. Cancer in families that meet the Amsterdam criteria
2. Two HNPCC-related cancers, including synchronous and metachronous colorectal cancers or associated extracolonic cancers (defined as endometrial, ovarian, gastric, hepatobiliary, small bowel, or transitional cell carcinoma of the renal pelvis or ureter)
3. Colorectal cancer and a first-degree relative with colorectal cancer and/or HNPCC-related extracolonic cancer and/or a colorectal adenoma with one of the cancers diagnosed before age 45 years and the adenoma diagnosed before age 40 years
4. Colorectal cancer or endometrial cancer diagnosed before age 45 years
5. Right-sided colorectal cancer having an undifferentiated pattern (solid/cribriform) on histopathologic diagnosis before age 45 years
6. Signet-ring cell-type colorectal cancer diagnosed before age 45 years
7. Adenomas diagnosed before age 40 years

However, a high prevalence of frank in situ gastric cancer was observed in prophylactic gastrectomy specimens from asymptomatic individuals with E-cadherin germline mutations despite normal gastroscopy and negative surveillance biopsies. Undoubtedly, the failure of surveillance in hereditary diffuse gastric cancer families reflects the submucosal spread that is seen with the diffuse gastric cancer subtype. Gastric cancer appears to be part of the tumor spectrum of hereditary nonpolyposis colorectal cancer and familial adenomatous polyposis, so these possibilities should be considered as well in any family with two or more cases of gastric cancer. The intestinal subtype of gastric cancer is more typical in hereditary nonpolyposis colorectal cancer-associated disease, so surveillance with gastroscopy is appropriate. We recommend gastroscopy every three to four years, beginning at an age that is 5 to 10 years younger than the age at diagnosis for the youngest individual with reported gastric cancer in the family. Finally, case-control studies suggest that family members of probands with gastric adenocarcinoma have a twofold to threefold increased empiric risk to develop gastric cancer themselves. A similar screening interval may be applied to these patients.

Hereditary Cutaneous Melanoma/Dysplastic Nevus Syndrome

Familial melanoma is genetically and etiologically heterogeneous, and both environmental factors (e.g., sun exposure) and constitutional factors (e.g., fair skin and light eyes) play a significant role in the disease. The most important clues to an hereditary etiology include a family history of melanoma and/or dysplastic nevi. Ten percent of melanoma patients have at least one affected first-degree relative, while 1% of melanomas occur in families with multiple affected members. Familial melanomas tend to occur at an earlier age: median 35 years versus 54 years in sporadic cases. Dysplastic nevi are often associated with familial melanomas, though they may also be seen in 30% to 50% of sporadic cases. Individuals with dysplastic nevi have a 7% lifetime risk for melanoma. The cumulative probability of developing melanoma in high-risk families is approximately 9% by age 20, rising to 49% by age 50 and 82% by age 70. A subset of melanoma-prone families and some individuals with multiple primary melanomas have been shown to carry mutations in the *CDKN2A* gene (also known as *p16* or *MTS1*). Pancreatic cancer risk is also elevated in *CDKN2A*-associated disease. Germline mutations in *CDKN2A* on chromosome 9 account for approximately 25% of melanoma-prone families, and mutations were observed in *CDK4* on chromosome 9 in rare families. Other regions of the genome have been impli-

cated in unlinked families. At this point, testing for *CDKN2A* mutations has only modest potential to alter care of families with a genetic predisposition because of incomplete penetrance and genetic complexity. All children in melanoma-prone families should be protected from sunburn. Comprehensive annual skin examinations should begin by age 10 and continue through puberty, when dysplastic nevi may change. For all at-risk family members, sun exposure should be minimized, monthly skin self-examinations should be performed, and skin examination by a trained clinician is recommended every six to 12 months and should include photodocumentation. Suspicious lesions should be removed by excisional biopsy, but prophylactic removal of nonchanging dysplastic nevi is not recommended.

Nevoid Basal Cell Carcinoma Syndrome (Gorlin's Syndrome)

Nevoid basal cell carcinoma syndrome is an autosomal-dominant developmental syndrome characterized by multiple basal cell carcinomas, reported in 90% of affected individuals by age 40 years. Nevoid basal cell carcinoma syndrome accounts for approximately 0.5% of adults with a history of basal cell carcinomas. The incidence of nevoid basal cell carcinoma syndrome is 20% among individuals under age 19 who develop basal cell carcinoma. Medulloblastoma (5%), ovarian carcinomas and fibrosarcomas, seminomas, and nasopharyngeal carcinomas are also reported in these patients. Associated nonmalignant features include palmar and plantar pits (65%), mandibular cysts (90% by age 40), tall stature, large head with frontal bossing, ocular hypertelorism and other benign ocular abnormalities, broad nasal root, enlarged jaw, long fingers with short fourth metacarpals, hypogonadotrophic hypogonadism, cleft lip and/or palate (5%), skeletal malformation of the spine and ribs, hydrocephalus, sellar bridging, and mental retardation (1% to 10%). While nevoid basal cell carcinoma syndrome is fully penetrant, there is considerable variation in expressivity of these features.

Nevoid basal cell carcinoma syndrome is associated with germline mutations in the *PTC* gene on 9q22.3, a human homologue of the *Drosophila* patched gene, which encodes a transmembrane protein controlling cell fate, patterning, and growth in numerous tissues. Up to 40% of affected individuals have a de novo germline mutation. Most mutations are nonsense point mutations leading to premature stops or frameshift mutations leading to a truncated protein. Genetic testing by direct analysis or linkage is available. Although nevoid basal cell carcinoma syndrome is associated with only 0.5% of all basal cell carcinoma, the fact that basal cell carcinoma is one of the most common malignancies in the world means that there are a significant number of hereditary cases. Individuals with this condition have extreme sensitivity to radiation, so it is critical that oncologists recognize the diagnostic features of this disease. Diagnosis of nevoid basal cell carcinoma syndrome should be considered when two major or one major and two minor criteria are fulfilled. Major criteria include (1) multiple (more than two) basal cell carcinomas, one basal cell carcinoma before 30 years of age, or more than 10 basal cell nevi; (2) any odontogenic keratocyst or polyostotic bone cyst; (3) palmer or planter pits (three or more); (4) ectopic calcification, lamellar or early (less than age 20 years) falx calcification; and (5) a family history of basal cell nevus syndrome. Minor criteria include (1) congenital skeletal anomaly: bifid, fused, splayed, or missing rib or bifid, wedged, or fused vertebra; (2) head circumference greater than 97th percentile, with frontal bossing; (3) cardiac or ovarian fibroma; (4) medulloblastoma; (5) lymphomesenteric cysts; and (6) congenital malformation: cleft lip and/or palate, polydactyly, or eye anomaly (cataract, coloboma, or microphthalmia).

Basal cell carcinomas in the syndrome seldom occur before puberty. Annual screening by an experienced dermatologist is suggested, beginning at puberty. Use of sunscreen is essential. Careful gynecologic examination should be conducted annually in adulthood. Clinicians should be aware of the possibility of medulloblastoma in affected children.

Hereditary Prostate Cancer

Hereditary prostate cancer has been linked to loci on chromosome 1 (*HPC1*, *PCAP*, *CAPB*), chromosome 20 (*HPC20*), and the X chromosome (*HPCX*). *ELAC2* was recently identified on chromosome 17 and is implicated in a few high-risk families. A moderate risk alteration in *ELAC2* was reported as well. Moderate risk associated with polymorphisms in genes for the androgen receptor and 5-alpha-reductase 2 has also been reported. Genetic analysis is still a research tool in this disease. If there is a family history of prostate cancer, the primary recommendation is for all at-risk men to initiate annual surveillance with prostate-specific antigen (PSA) and digital rectal exam by age 50 or at least 10 years prior to the earliest diagnosis in the family. Ancillary surveillance techniques such as transrectal ultrasound or random prostate biopsies are investigational at present.

Retinoblastoma

Retinoblastoma is the most common ocular tumor of childhood. Over 90% of retinoblastoma tumors present before age 5. Approximately 40% of individuals with retinoblastoma have an inherited or de novo germline mutation of the *RB1* gene. The pattern of inheritance is autosomal-dominant. These individuals usually present in infancy (mean age: 8 months) with bilateral, multifocal disease, and 2% may develop a benign retinal lesion (retinoma) or, more rarely, both bilateral retinoblastoma and a tumor of the pineal gland. This scenario is referred to as trilateral retinoblastoma. Individuals with a germline mutation are at risk for secondary mesenchymal tumors, especially osteosarcoma and soft-tissue sarcomas, malignant melanoma, and brain tumors, which can be exacerbated by exposure to radiotherapy. Sporadic retinoblastoma presents later in childhood (mean age: 25 months) with unilateral, unifocal disease. Individuals with sporadic retinoblastoma do not have an increased risk for secondary tumors; therefore, radiation therapy is not considered a potential risk for these patients. Risk of occurrence in offspring of individuals with sporadic retinoblastoma is 4% to 6%.

Von Hippel-Lindau Disease

Von Hippel-Lindau (VHL) disease is an autosomal-dominant syndrome with an incidence of about one in 30,000. The responsible *VHL* gene on chromosome band 3p25.5 encodes a protein that interacts with and suppresses the function of elongin complexes that regulate transcriptional elongation by RNA polymerase II.

Although the manifestations of this disease are myriad, the most common are retinal angiomas; cerebellar, spinal, and medullary hemangioblastomas; pheochromocytoma (3% to 17%, often bilateral); and renal cell carcinoma (35% to 75%). Pancreatic cystadenocarcinoma or islet cell tumors are seen in some von Hippel-Lindau families (7% to 25%).

Genetic testing is considered standard of care and is relatively straightforward because the *VHL* gene is relatively small, spanning only three exons. Common genetic abnormalities in this gene are truncations or missense mutations. Molecular diagnosis has important clinical implications because there are complex screening regimens recommended for von Hippel-Lindau patients.

Genetic Cancer Risk Assessment Process

It is important to understand the epidemiology and natural history of common cancers, since sporadic cancer cases are more common than the hereditary cases. Insight into standard treatments and diagnostic techniques will assist in counseling patients about options for management. The process begins with assessment of perceived risk and the impact of cancer on the patient and his or her family. This information forms the counseling framework. Detailed information regarding personal, reproductive, and hormonal risk factors is noted. Family history, including age at disease onset, types of cancer, and current age or age at death, is obtained for all family members in at least three generations. Documentation of cancer cases is crucial to accurate risk estimation. Pathology reports, medical record notes, and death certificates may be useful for confirming the exact diagnosis. The family pedigree is then analyzed to determine whether a pattern of cancer in the family is consistent with genetic disease. Sometimes small family structure or lack of family information limits assessment. Empiric cancer risk estimates are derived from the information gathered, as well as an estimate of the likelihood that a detectable mutation is responsible for the disease in the family. Information on the application of genetic testing (appropriateness, limitations, advantages, and disadvantages) is provided to the patient. All of the elements of genetic counseling, patient education, and informed consent are addressed before genetic testing is offered to a family (Table 118-7). Finally, delineation of a management plan with the goal of prevention or early detection of malignancy is formulated within the context of an individual's personal preferences and degree of risk.

Quantifying Cancer Risk

There are several ways of calculating and expressing cancer risk. Relative risk or odds ratios have been determined for common cancers and reflect the contribution of family history at a population level. A 1.5-fold to threefold increased risk for colorectal cancer or breast cancer can be assigned for the presence of a first-degree relative with the same malignancy. However, the confidence intervals for such measures are often wide, and these moderate figures clearly underestimate risk in families with known suscepti-

---

Table 118-7 ■ Components of a Genetic Cancer Risk Assessment Service

Comprehensive personal and family history
Pedigree construction and evaluation
Documentation of cancer history
Individualized risk assessment
Education about principles of genetics and hereditary cancer
  patterns
Genetic counseling and testing (if appropriate) after informed
  consent
Results disclosure and interpretation
Customized screening and prevention recommendations,
  follow-up care, and support

---

bility mutations. Absolute risk estimates, both age-specific and cumulative, are generally more useful in counseling patients.

Risk Assessment Models

Working empiric risk assessment models may utilize personal risk factors and/or family history information. For example, Gail et al used data from the Breast Cancer Detection and Demonstration Project to develop a formula for estimating the chance that a woman with a given age and risk factors will develop breast cancer over a specified interval. The Gail model served as the risk stratification tool for the NSABP (P1) Breast Cancer Prevention Trial. The model does not take age at onset of cancer into account; nor does it consider paternal inheritance, since only first-degree relatives (mother or sister) are counted. Therefore, the model is not appropriate for women whose families fit the profile of hereditary breast and ovarian cancer syndrome. Claus et al determined useful age-specific breast cancer risk estimates based on the number and age of first-degree relatives with breast cancer from analysis of epidemiologic data from the Cancer and Steroid Hormone study. One can use pedigree analysis and clinical tools such as these to help fit individuals into broad risk categories: low (baseline population risk), moderate, and high risk. It is important to scrutinize at least a three-generation, validated pedigree with an eye for features suggestive of hereditary cancer or the possibility of masked paternal inheritance if expression of the cancer is sex-limited. Injudicious use of empiric risk models (e.g., in families with features suggestive of hereditary disease) may lead to significant underestimation of risk and false reassurance.

Genetic testing has the potential to provide more accurate risk estimation than any of the empiric risk assessment tools. The magnitude of risk that is conferred by a deleterious mutation in either *BRCA1* or *BRCA2* is greater than the highest empiric risk estimates, even allowing for variations in penetrance estimates. However, genetic testing has significant costs and potential adverse consequences. The assays have technical limitations, and consequently, the value of a negative test result in an unaffected person is limited when the familial mutation is not known. The optimal strategy is to test an affected family member to establish the familial mutation, followed by specific testing of at-risk relatives. Mendelian risk is the most straightforward calculation in the setting of a known familial mutation (50% for first-degree relatives, 25% for second, etc.). A more sophisticated approach takes into account age-specific penetrance estimates in a Bayesian modification of risk. In short, if a person is unaffected at age 80 years, then the probability that this person or any of his or her offspring is a carrier of a highly penetrant gene mutation is diminished. Bayesian calculations can also be employed to gauge the significance of a negative result in an unaffected individual if the family diagnosis is certain (but mutation unknown) and the sensitivity of the genetic test is well established. In general, discovery of an inactivating or deleterious mutation of a cancer susceptibility gene such as *BRCA1* is indicative of a high probability of developing cancer. One of the greatest challenges is the interpretation of "variants of unknown significance"—typically missense mutations in which there is a substitution of a single amino acid. The variant is more likely to be of significance if the mutation is located in an evolutionarily conserved or functionally critical region of the protein. However, they are most often ultimately reclassified as a rare polymorphism once adequate data accumulate and there is an absence of a clear disease association. Given all of the complex information that is delivered in the counseling session, it is not surprising that patients can confuse estimates of the probability of carrying a mutation with estimates of the probability of developing cancer.

Counseling Issues

State of Mind

Complex issues arise in genetic predisposition testing. Previous cancer experience within the family will strongly influence an individual's state of mind. This, in turn, may affect risk perception and risk tolerance. A woman who helped to care for her mother with cancer through the complicated end stages of the disease might perceive a modestly increased risk estimate (e.g., 5%) as intolerable, even though it might be less than the average risk for breast cancer in the general population. Both the patient and the practitioner might be affected by their experience with death and dying. An oncologist has significant experience in terminal care and support for grieving families and therefore might be better equipped to develop empathy for a fearful patient. It is important to appreciate the motivations of a patient who is seeking cancer risk assessment. Timing of the request often follows life events such as the birth of a child. Indeed, concern for offspring is one of the most commonly cited motivations; reaching the same age as a relative was when he or she was first diagnosed with cancer is another commonly cited reason. A family's previous experience with the medical system or personal cancer experience can influence their level of trust in physicians' recommendations. A patient's state of mind and

willingness to undergo the genetic testing process may also be influenced by the patient's fear about adverse effects on insurability. Many individuals who are deemed appropriate for genetic testing decline to be tested because of fears about insurance discrimination, despite counseling about emerging state and federal legal protections that are available. Concerns about subject confidentiality in research registries may be addressed in part by obtaining a certificate of confidentiality from the NIH Office for Protection of Research Risks for Investigational Research Board–approved investigations.

State of Technology

Technologic innovation in the Human Genome Project has also resulted in new tools for genetic analysis in patients. Practitioners need to be aware of the rapid changes and limitations in genetic testing tools. A variety of techniques and strategies for detecting mutations in cancer genes have been adopted by different researchers and commercial vendors. These include methods for gene scanning or heteroduplex analysis, assays designed to detect only specific mutations, functional assays such as the protein truncation test, and complete sequencing of coding exons and flanking splice junction sequences in PCR-amplified genomic DNA. Virtually all these techniques will miss deleterious mutations in the upstream regulatory sequences of genes and may miss large deletions. No single method can identify all disease-causing mutations in a given gene. Very few studies have directly compared sensitivity and specificity of available methods for detecting gene mutations. For now, clinicians must decide on testing options on a gene-by-gene and lab-by-lab basis. One must also understand the difference between research laboratory-based testing and commercial vendors. A genetic testing laboratory that is used for clinical service should have a Board of Medical Genetics–certified Director, and the laboratory should be CLIA (Clinical Laboratory Improvement Amendments of 1988)-approved.

State of the Art: Management

General guidelines for evaluation and management of genetic cancer risk may be drawn from clinical expertise, review of the literature, professional society position statements, and working group recommendations. Clinical options for the management of inherited susceptibility to cancer are often extrapolated from intervention studies in the general population or are based simply on expert opinion when there is a void of data. The most definitive approach to risk reduction is often surgical, but the consequences of the procedures with respect to quality of life have yet to be characterized. Continued clinical research on genetically defined individuals is critically needed to develop viable therapeutics and less invasive preventive measures.

The American Society of Clinical Oncology recommends that cancer predisposition testing be offered when (1) the person has a strong family history of cancer or very early age of onset of disease, (2) the test can be adequately interpreted, and (3) the results will influence the medical management of the patient or family member. Table 118-8 lists American Society of Clinical Oncology guidelines for cancer predisposition testing. As a practical matter, a probability of greater than 5% to 10% that a detectable mutation caused the disease in a family is commonly the threshold for offering genetic testing. The evaluation by a health care professional experienced in cancer genetics should be relied upon in making interpretations of pedigree information and determinations of the appropriateness of genetic testing.

Genetic Testing Service Models

Cancer risk assessment services are delivered in a broad range of clinical settings. Any clinician may order commercial analysis of several cancer-associated genes. However, given the aforementioned complexities of the genetic testing process, there is a significant potential for misinterpretation of results by clinicians and provision of misinformation to patients. In the

Table 118-8 ■ ASCO Guidelines for Cancer Predisposition Testing

Group 1: Genetic Test Result Will Change Medical Care and Is Standard Management

Examples	Gene(s)
Familial adenomatous polyposis	*APC*
Multiple endocrine neoplasia 2	*RET*
Multiple endocrine neoplasia 1	*MEN1*
Retinoblastoma	*RB1*
Von Hippel-Lindau disease	*VHL*

Group 2: Possible Medical Benefit in the Identification of a Germline Mutation

Hereditary nonpolyposis colorectal cancer*	*MLH1, MSH2, MSH6, PMS1, PMS2*
Hereditary breast and ovarian cancer*	*BRCA1, BRCA2*
Li-Fraumeni syndrome	*TP53*
Cowden disease	*PTEN*

*Emerging as standard management.
Modified from ASCO Statement. J Clin Oncol 14:1730, 1996; updated statement, 2003.

research/academic model, there is usually a multidisciplinary subspecialty clinic for genetic cancer risk assessment services. Thorough pretest and post-test counseling is carried out. International Review Board (IRB)-approved protocols are the rule, and certificate of confidentiality protection is sought for research sub-

---

DIAGNOSIS

General Guideline for Genetic Cancer Risk Assessment Referral

Most patients have family histories that do not suggest an inherited increased risk for cancer. Cancer screening for these patients should be based on clinical practice guidelines and recommendations of national organizations. All patients should be asked about their extended family history. Family structure may limit the usefulness of immediate family history. Generations may be skipped if the cancer expression is sex-limited.

Step 1

Obtain an accurate family history, and construct a pedigree. Collect information on cancer in the patient, offspring, siblings, parents, aunts, uncles, and grandparents.

For gender-specific cancers such as breast, ovarian, and prostate cancer, one might need to collect cancer histories on more distant relatives.

Determine the number of relatives with cancer, biological relationships, and types of cancer in the family.

Step 2

Is there a first-degree relative with cancer? (parent, sibling, offspring)

Are there two or more second-degree relatives with cancer? (aunts, uncles, grandparents)

Are there two or more relatives with the same type of cancer?

Consider referral for comprehensive risk assessment for any two positive responses.

Step 3

For affected relatives, determine age at cancer diagnosis and the occurrence of synchronous or metachronous tumors.

Is the age of onset unusually early? (e.g., breast cancer < age 40 or colon cancer < age 45)

Does one of the relatives have multiple primary malignancies?

Consider referral for comprehensive risk assessment for one positive response in both steps 2 and 3.

jects. Many academic centers have a registry or other mechanism for tracking outcomes. Members of the staff are often cross-trained in oncology and cancer genetics. Most of the major centers are directed by a board-certified oncologist with focused training in cancer genetics. Other centers use a board-certified clinical or clinical molecular geneticist in this role. Additional members of the team should include certified genetic counselors with cancer genetics experience and/or advanced practice nurses with master's-level training in genetics and oncology and experience in primary counseling roles. Other support staff may include clinical social workers and mental health professionals.

References

General

ASCO: Resource document for curriculum development in cancer genetics education. J Clin Oncol 1997;15:2157–2169.

ASCO: Statement of the American Society of Clinical Oncology: Genetic testing for cancer susceptibility. J Clin Oncol 1996;14:1730–1736.

Daly M: NCCN practice guidelines: Genetics/familial high-risk cancer screening. Oncology 1999;13:161–183.

Greenlee RT, et al: Cancer statistics, 2000. CA Cancer J Clin 2000;50:7–33.

Hodgson SV, Maher ER: A practical guide to human cancer genetics. Cambridge, England: Press Syndicate of the University of Cambridge, 1993, p 240.

Li FP, et al: Recommendations on predictive testing for germline p53 mutations among cancer-prone individuals. J Natl Cancer Inst 1992;84:1156–1160.

Lindor NM, Greene MH: The concise handbook of family cancer syndromes: Mayo Familial Cancer Program. J Natl Cancer Inst 1998;90:1039–1071.

Malkin D, et al: Germ line p53 mutations in a familial syndrome of breast cancer, sarcomas, and other neoplasms. Science 1990;250:1233–1237.

Offit K: Clinical Cancer Genetics: Risk Counseling and Management. New York: Wiley-Liss, 1998, p 419.

Savitsky K, et al: A single ataxia telangiectasia gene with a product similar to PI-3 kinase. Science 1995;268:1749–1753.

Secretary's Advisory Committee on Genetic Testing, Enhancing the Oversight of Genetic Tests: Recommendations of the SACGT. 2000;1–33.

Swift M, et al: Incidence of cancer in 161 families affected by ataxia-telangiectasia. N Engl J Med 1991;325:1831–1836.

Weitzel JN: Genetic cancer risk assessment: Putting it all together. Cancer 1999;86:2483–2492.

Colorectal Cancer

Burke W, et al: Recommendations for follow-up care of individuals with an inherited predisposition to cancer. I: Hereditary nonpolyposis colon cancer. JAMA 1997;277:915–919.

Giardiello FM: Genetic testing in hereditary colorectal cancer. JAMA 1997;278:1278–1281.

Gryfe R, et al: Tumor microsatellite instability and clinical outcome in young patients with colorectal cancer. N Engl J Med 2000;342:69–77.

Jarvinen HJ, Mecklin J-P, and Sistonen P: Screening reduces colorectal cancer rate in families with hereditary nonpolyposis colorectal cancer. Gastroenterology 1995;108:1405–1411.

Jen J, et al: Allelic loss of chromosome 18q and prognosis in colorectal cancer. New Engl J Med 1994;331:213–221.

Lynch HT, et al: Genetics, natural history, tumor spectrum, and pathology of hereditary nonpolyposis colorectal cancer: An updated review. Gastroenterology 1993;104:1535–1549.

Rodrignez-Bigos MA, Boland CR, Hamilton SR, et al: A National Cancer Institute Workshop on Hereditary Nonpolyposis Colorectal Cancer Syndrome: Meeting highlights and Bethesda guidelines. J Natl Cancer Inst 1997;89:1758–1762.

Breast/Ovarian Cancer

Burke W, et al: Recommendations for follow-up care of individuals with an inherited predisposition to cancer. II: BRCA1 and BRCA2. JAMA 1997;277:997–1003.

Claus EB, Risch R, Thompson WD: Autosomal dominant inheritance of early-onset breast cancer: Implications for risk prediction. Cancer 1994;73:643–651.

Couch F, et al: BRCA1 mutations in women attending clinics that evaluate the risk of breast cancer. N Engl J Med 1997;336:1409–1415.

Easton DF, et al: Breast and ovarian cancer incidence in BRCA1-mutation carriers. Am J Hum Genet 1995;56:265–271.

Ford D, et al: Genetic heterogeneity and penetrance analysis of the BRCA1 and BRCA2 genes in breast cancer families. Am J Hum Genet 1998;62:676–689.

Frank TS, et al: Sequence analysis of BRCA1 and BRCA2: Correlation of mutations with family history and ovarian cancer risk. J Clin Oncol 1998;16:2417–2425.

Gail MH, et al: Projecting individualized probabilities of developing breast cancer for white females who are being examined annually. J Natl Cancer Inst 1989;81:1879–1886.

Giardiello FM, et al: The use and interpretation of commercial APC gene testing for familial adenomatous polyposis. N Engl J Med 1997;336:823–827.

Hall JM, et al: Linkage of early-onset familial breast cancer to chromosome 17q21. Science 1990;250:1684–1689.

Hartmann LC, et al: Efficacy of bilateral prophylactic mastectomy in women with a family history of breast cancer. N Engl J Med 1999;340:77–84.

Johannsson OT, et al: Survival of BRCA1 breast and ovarian cancer patients: A population-based study from southern Sweden. J Clin Oncol 1998;16:397–404.

Miki Y, et al: A strong candidate for the breast and ovarian susceptibility gene BRCA1. Science 1994;266:66–71.

Narod SA, et al: An evaluation of genetic heterogeneity in 145 breast-ovarian cancer families. Amn J Hum Genet 1995;56:254–264.

Parmigiani G, Berry DA, Agiular O: Determining carrier probabilities for breast cancer susceptibility genes BRCA1 and BRCA2. Hum Genet 1998;62:145–158.

Rebbeck TR, et al: Breast cancer risk after bilateral prophylactic oophorectomy in BRCA1 mutation carriers. J Natl Cancer Inst 1999;91:1475–1479.

Robson M, et al: Breast conservation therapy for invasive breast cancer in Ashkenazi women with BRCA gene founder mutations. J Natl Cancer Inst 1999;91:2112–2117.

Slamon DJ, et al: Studies of the HER-2/neu proto-oncogene in human breast and ovarian cancer. Science 1989;244:707–712.

Struewing JP, et al: The risk of cancer associated with specific mutations of BRCA1 and BRCA2 among Ashkenazi Jews. New Engl J Med 1997;336:1401–1408.

Weber BL: Genetic testing for breast cancer. Sci Am Sci Med 1996;12–21.

Weitzel JN: Genetic testing for breast cancer predisposition. In Jatoi I (ed): Breast Cancer Screening. Austin, Texas: RG Landes, 1997, pp 155–178.

Wooster R, et al: Localization of a breast cancer susceptibility gene, BRCA2, to chromosome 13q12-13. Science 1994;265:2088–2090.

Cowden Disease

Albrecht S, et al: Cowden syndrome and Lhermitte-Duclos disease. Cancer 1992;70:869–876.

Eng C: Will the real Cowden syndrome please stand up: Revised diagnostic criteria. J Med Genet 2000;37:828–830.

Liaw D et al: Germline mutations of the PTEN gene in Cowden disease, an inherited breast and thyroid cancer syndrome. Nat Genet 1997;16:64–67.

Nelen MR, et al: Localization of the gene for Cowden disease to chromosome 1Oq22-23. Nat Genet 1996;13:114–116.

Starink TM, et al: The Cowden syndrome: A clinical and genetic study in 21 patients. Clin Genet 1986;29:222–233.

Chapter 119
Unorthodox Approaches to Cancer Therapy

Brent A. Bauer and Charles L. Loprinzi

Introduction

Unorthodox:

1. Not conforming to established doctrine
2. Unconventional
   —*Webster's New Collegiate Dictionary*

Perhaps at no other time in history has the patient with cancer been so overwhelmed with information. A brief survey of the Internet quickly reveals a daunting array of choices for someone interested in learning more about cancer and its treatment. Unfortunately, quantity is not necessarily a marker for quality. Thanks to modern technology, misinformation—both well intended and mercenary—can be disseminated to literally millions of people with a few keystrokes. Helping patients navigate this overwhelming sea of products and agents increasingly requires the expertise of a physician. Patients need their physicians to be advocates for them, to know enough about the unorthodox treatments and to be able to provide counsel regarding the potential risks and benefits of such treatments. The clinician requires knowledge of unorthodox treatments, along with specific information about some commonly encountered treatments. Armed with this information, physicians can discuss these issues with their patients in an honest and open manner. Unless patients feel comfortable coming to their physician and exploring all concerns in such an open and nonjudgmental fashion, physicians run the risk of driving them closer to the unorthodox realm.

What Is an "Unorthodox" Treatment?

Even the question "What is an unorthodox treatment?" is a difficult one to answer. Almost any attempt to define the concept inflames someone's sensibilities—either the terminology is derogatory or the language is too accepting. Hence, terms such as "alternative" or "unconventional" have been derided as being too harsh or too exclusionary. On the other hand, "complementary" and "integrative" are terms that conventional practitioners view as implying blanket acceptance or endorsement. Furthermore, the concept is a dynamic, not a static, one. Modalities that begin in the unorthodox realm can be tested and found to be efficacious, and then cross over to the mainstream or orthodox realm (e.g., acupuncture for certain pain syndromes). In fact, most treatments or modalities exist on a continuum, ranging from those that have been thoroughly tested in a scientifically rigorous fashion to those that have claims for efficacy based on anecdotes or on the unsubstantiated claims of a few practitioners. Thus, it has been suggested that one of the distinguishing features between orthodox and unorthodox medicine might be the level of evidence that proponents require before endorsing a particular therapy.

Academic medicine has clearly struggled with how to define unorthodox therapies. Currently, the rubric of Complementary and Alternative Medicine (CAM) is most widely employed when conventional medicine groups discuss this realm. The questions surrounding unorthodox therapies were brought into sharp focus in 1992 with legislation establishing the Office of Alternative Medicine at the National Institutes of Health (NIH). This was in response to constituent cries for more research and information on nonconventional treatments that were becoming increasingly popular. Because of this burgeoning interest in CAM, the Office grew to become a full-fledged Center—the National Center for Complementary and Alternative Medicine (NCCAM)—by 1998.

Unorthodox cancer treatments can be considered to be any therapy that has not been rigorously tested and proven to be of benefit and is not an integral part of conventional medicine. This definition allows categorization without necessarily judging the quality of the therapy. Where evidence exists, informed recommendations can be made. Where evidence is scanty or of poor quality, this can be stated simply.

Why Do Patients Seek Unorthodox Treatments?

The early history of America is replete with images of "quack" doctors, riding from town to town in a horse-drawn wagon, selling nostrums that were ineffective at best and dangerous at worst, often containing mind-altering, alarming quantities of alcohol, opium, and other substances. We tend to laugh at the "unsophisticated" folk who succumbed to high-pressure sales pitches from traveling medicine shows. Yet it is instructive for us to consider why these purveyors of patent medicine did such a thriving business. The period of time from the late 1700s until the late 1800s is a period when conventional medicine often had little to offer patients. Physicians were poorly trained, and what training they did receive was often in the "heroic" tradition, a school of thought that emphasized dramatic results such as those achieved via bloodletting, purgatives, and emetics. Mercury was a commonly employed treatment, leading one contemporary to observe, "Physicians learned nothing about the true nature of medicines they prescribed, except . . . how much poison could be given without causing death" (Samuel Thompson). Thus, in the past, patients often sought alternative treatments when mainstream medicine had little to offer them. Now, in the twenty-first century, those with illnesses not readily cured (e.g., arthritis, obesity, chronic pain syndromes, cancer, etc.) are likewise increasingly willing to explore unorthodox treatments.

Furthermore, chemotherapy and radiation therapy frequently cause significant toxicity. Mention the word "chemotherapy" to lay people who have not personally experienced chemotherapy, and they will still identify hair loss, nausea, vomiting, and weight loss as "inevitable" side effects of the treatment. Unorthodox treatments are portrayed as natural, less toxic, and less expensive. Thus, the realities of conventional treatment, balanced against the implied (or explicit) promises of unorthodox therapies, in part explain the allure of such therapies.

Another possible contributing factor is the perception that conventional medicine has become too technical, too "cold," and too impersonal. Certainly, there is a ring of truth to these charges, especially in the era of managed care and cost containment strategies. Providers of unorthodox treatments are often not constrained to a significant degree with regard to the time that they can spend with patients. Conventional physicians are increasingly painted as being focused on disease, while unorthodox practitioners are portrayed as caring about the whole person. It has been claimed that conventional physicians "focus on disease" while unorthodox practitioners "promote wellness."

Finally, paternalism in medicine has been fully discarded for a paradigm that emphasizes patient autonomy. Patients want to be more informed about their treatments and the options they have. Again, the information explosion enables patients to quickly locate information specific to their types of cancer, staging, etc. Ready access to a variety of unorthodox treatments, combined with increasing patient autonomy, probably accounts for much of the popularity of such treatments.

Risks of Unorthodox Treatments

The image of the "quack" purveyor of nostrums and potions is well ingrained in the American memory. Though they promised cures for everything and rarely did more than relieve ailing individuals of their money, "quacks" now have a quaint and almost romantic aura about them. Perhaps this is because they operated in a time when conventional medicine did not have much else to offer either. The situation today, however, is much different. Contemporary medicine usually has something to offer almost any patient. Thus, the concern with "unorthodox" treatments is not only that they might not be effective but also that they might divert patients who could be helped by available treatments. When there is discussion about unorthodox treatments and the potential risks they pose, therefore, there are really five categories into which these therapies may fall:

1. *Potentially beneficial:* Almost all current treatments of contemporary medicine were at some point considered "unorthodox"—that is, they were introduced as potentially new treatments, subjected to testing, and eventually judged to be helpful in some regard. For this reason, it would be unwise to dismiss all "unorthodox" treatments categorically. Those that have promise (i.e., long history of use, *in vitro* data, and so on) should be investigated with the same rigor and attention that any new therapy receives.

2. *Benign:* Many "treatments," although unlikely to affect cancer significantly, are also unlikely to cause any harm. For example, patients who supplement their radiation therapy with some extra vitamin C are likely to cause neither significant harm nor benefit.

3. *Potentially harmful:* Some unorthodox treatments that have been touted as cures actually have great potential to cause harm (e.g., intravenous ozone, Laetrile, etc.). Others, because they are produced and sold outside of the usual regulatory spheres, can be impure, can be contaminated with bacteria or viruses, or can contain adulterants, for example.

4. *Potentially interactive:* Although some agents seem to pose little risk in and of themselves, they might interact with conventional medicine in a detrimental fashion. For example, St. John's wort (a popular herbal treatment for depression) has recently been discovered to dramatically alter drug levels of certain antiretrovirals, digoxin, and cyclosporine. In the latter example, two heart transplant patients experienced rejection when the herb reduced systemic levels of cyclosporine.

5. *Diversionary:* The final category is one that tends to receive less attention but could be one of the greatest threats posed by unorthodox treatments. Patients often fear the side effects and toxicity of some conventional treatments. Others believe that "natural" therapies are less toxic and more in tune with natural healing concepts. For whatever reason, some patients choose to use an unorthodox approach to the exclusion of conventional therapy. Thus, a new risk is interposed—that of missing a treatable stage of the disease while the patient tries an alternative approach. By the time the patient determines that the alternative approach has not yielded optimal results and returns to conventional practice, the disease might have progressed from a potentially curable stage to one that is not.

How to Approach a Patient Interested in Using Unorthodox Treatments

How should a practitioner approach the patient who is considering using (or is already using) an unorthodox treatment? To dismiss all inquiries regarding unorthodox treatment out of hand will be dissatisfying to the patient and the physician alike. This approach simply encourages the patient to use the treatments in a surreptitious fashion, with the result that potential interactions or contraindications with conventional therapy will not be identified. By the same token, openly embracing every new "cure" that pops up on a Web site is intellectually dishonest and is not in the best interest of the patient. The middle ground (neither total skeptic not total believer) is perhaps the high ground. Sifting claims and evaluating them in a scientific manner will allow physicians to pass information to their patients and enable them to make informed decisions.

Basic Information

Herbs

The use of herbal medicine in the United States has been increasing for over a decade. Although the consumption of herbal therapies is no longer increasing as rapidly as a few years ago, it still remains at a high level. Approximately $5 billion annually is being spent on herbal supplements alone. Herbal supplements continue to receive increasing exposure through national media, in lay journals, and more recently, in the scientific press. Thus, it is unlikely that the use of herbs by patients is going to cease in the foreseeable future.

Interest in herbal medicine, as with all unorthodox treatments, has been facilitated by multiple factors, including the perception that pharmaceutical medications are expensive, overprescribed, and often dangerous. Alternatively, herbal medicines are often perceived as being "natural" and therefore considered safe. Because herbal therapies constitute a significant portion of the unorthodox therapies that are currently popular, it is important for physicians to have some basic knowledge regarding herbs in order to navigate the often murky realm of unorthodox therapies successfully.

By strict botanical definition, an herb is "a seed-producing annual, biennial, or perennial that does not develop persistent woody tissue but dies down at the end of a growing season." Of course, patients and consumers do not adhere to this strict classical definition when they inquire about, or use, "herbal" products. Webster's dictionary also defines *herb* as a "plant or plant part valued for its medicinal, savory, or aromatic qualities." This broader definition probably comes closer to what most people mean when they discuss herbal medicines. For example, gingko is a very popular "herb," but, strictly speaking, it is actually from a tree. To avoid semantic confusion, some authorities prefer the term "botanical," which encompasses any plant-derived product used for a medicinal or health purpose.

Finally, it is important to remember that herbs are chemically complex entities, often containing hundreds of compounds and chemical constituents. Conventional "Western" science generally takes a "reductionistic" approach (i.e., an attempt to isolate a single active ingredient), whereas traditional herbalists and healers generally use whole plants or combinations of plants. They theorize that herb constituents other than the main "active ingredient" might be just as important, modifying effects of the "active ingredient" in beneficial ways. Carrying this argument further, whereas the "active ingredient" in isolation might produce a harsh or unpleasant effect, the sum of the constituents acting in concert (with some of the secondary or "non-active ingredients" affecting both agonist and antagonist receptors) is quite different. The final effect might be a milder one, slower in onset and with fewer side effects than the purified isolated "active ingredient." This possibility complicates research in the botanical realm tremendously and is one of the reasons why there is so much controversy regarding the efficacy of herbal therapies. If one is constrained to using whole plant compounds, one is then faced with the variations in components that occur within plant species, in different growing locations, and even within the same plant depending on season of year, rainfall, and other factors.

Dietary Supplements

Further complicating the study of unorthodox treatments is the fact that many of them fall into the classification of "dietary supplements." The Dietary Supplement Health Education Act of 1994 (DSHEA) governs the regulation of dietary supplements and places them in a truly unique category. Thus, any discussion of unorthodox therapies requires an understanding of this classification and its regulatory implications.

What Is a Dietary Supplement?

For the purposes of the DSHEA, a dietary supplement

- is a product (other than tobacco) that is intended to supplement the diet that bears or contains one or more of the following dietary ingredients: a vitamin, a mineral, an herb or other botanical, or an amino acid
- is intended for ingestion in a pill, capsule, tablet, or liquid form
- is not represented for use as a conventional food or as the sole item of a meal or diet
- is labeled as a "dietary supplement"

The classification of "dietary supplement" is specifically separate from "food" or "drug" categories and, as such, lies outside the jurisdiction of many of the safety and regulatory rules that cover these categories.

This definition came about as the result of several interesting events. First, by the late 1980s, concern was growing regarding the safety of the herbs and other supplements that Americans were consuming in ever-increasing amounts. In response, in the early 1990s, the Food and Drug Administration (FDA) set forth a proposal to begin to increase the regulatory oversight of this type of product. Herbal manufacturers and many consumers, however, saw this as the first step toward eliminating access to dietary supplements. An unusually effective campaign flooded members of congress with pleas to preserve access to, and availability of, herbs and other supplements. Congress responded by passing the DSHEA, an act

that in many respects had the effect opposite to what the Food and Drug Administration had been proposing.

First, the DSHEA specifically states that, unlike pharmaceutical preparations, dietary supplements can be marketed without proving either safety or efficacy. Thus, the onus of proving that the product is harmful falls on the Food and Drug Administration. The Food and Drug Administration can restrict the sale of an herbal product only if well-documented health problems have occurred.

Furthermore, for the first time, the DSHEA allowed herbal preparations to carry suggested dosages on the label. Prior to this act, herbal preparations could not suggest a dosage without risking classification as a drug and the tighter regulatory oversight that would occur.

Although the DSHEA precludes manufacturers from making specific medical claims (e.g., "saw palmetto reduces the frequency of urination"), it does allow "structure or function" claims. These include descriptions of the supplements' effect on the physiology of an organ or system. Thus, a claim that "saw palmetto promotes healthy prostate functioning" is acceptable. The distinction between medical claims and "structure or function" claims is often a fine one, and many manufacturers have tested the limits of this restriction.

The act also mandates the following disclaimer—"This statement has not been evaluated by the Food and Drug Administration. This product is not intended to diagnose, treat, cure, or prevent any disease."—be present on each product label. Much like warnings on cigarette packages, however, this disclaimer seems to go unnoticed by most consumers. The common misperception is that because the herb or supplement is in a sealed, plastic container on a shelf next to other products (such as over-the-counter drugs that are FDA-approved), herbs must also be FDA-approved.

It is within this relative "no-man's land" of limited regulatory oversight that many unorthodox products thrive. As long as direct medical claims are not made and as long as significant injuries from a product are not reported, the likelihood of savvy promoters having their products pulled from the shelves is low. Hence, few Web sites make direct claims for their products' ability to actually cure cancer. Many state that their product "supports the body" or "strengthens the immune system," then provide testimonials from customers who have been "cured." Knowing at least the basics of the current regulatory milieu surrounding dietary supplements allows both physicians and their patients to evaluate the myriad claims more competently.

Table 119-1 ■ Classification of Unorthodox Therapies

Dietary supplements
  Herbs
  Herbal mixtures
  Vitamins and minerals
Pharmacologic and biologic therapies
Nutritional/metabolic therapies
Miscellaneous

Types of Unorthodox Therapies

There are probably as many ways to categorize unorthodox therapies as there are unorthodox therapies. Table 119-1 provides a somewhat arbitrary classification of different unorthodox therapies. Table 119-2 and the rest of the tables in this chapter provide specific examples of common therapies within each category.

For illustrative purposes, detailed discussions of a few selected therapies are provided in the following pages. Dosages or treatment descriptions included in the discussion of each therapy are not intended to endorse or encourage use of any of the therapies. Dosage and treatment plan information is generally taken directly from proponent Web sites or literature and is included only to allow the reader to see what information patients are likely to encounter regarding each therapy.

Cat's Claw

History

Una de gato or cat's claw (*Uncaria tomentosa*) is a large woody vine found in Peru and other tropical areas of South and Central America. Hooklike thorns that grow along the vine are said to resemble the claw of a cat, hence its name. *Uncaria guianensis* is a closely related species, but most of the medicinal interest has focused on *U. tomentosa*. Traditional uses found in some Peruvian Indian tribes include treatment of asthma, arthritis, gastric ulcers, and cancer.

Table 119-2 ■ Herbal Therapies

Herbs	Also Known As	Primary Claim	Secondary Claim	Origin/Proponent	Studies	Toxicity
Aloe (*Aloe vera*)		S	T, P	Traditional use	Insufficient studies	Low
Cat's claw (*Uncaria tomentosa*)	Una de Gato	S	T	South and Central America, especially Peru Traditional use	Potentially beneficial	Low
Chaparral (*Larrea divericata*)	Creosote bush, Greasewood	S	T, P	Southwestern United States Native American traditional use	Potentially harmful	Medium to high
Garlic (*Allium sativum*)		P	S	Traditional use	Potentially beneficial	Low
Green tea (*Camellia sinesis*)		P	S	Traditional use	Potentially beneficial	Low
Pau d'arco (*Tabebuia impetiginosa*)	Lapacho, Taheebo, Trumpet Bush	S	T	South and Central America, especially Brazil and Argentina Traditional use	Mixed results	Medium
Mistletoe (*Viscum album*)	Iscador, Helixor, Eurixor, Isorel	T	S	Rudolf Steiner, Ph.D. (1861–1925) Anthroposophical medicine treatment	Neutral to potentially beneficial	Medium

S = Supportive (recommended to support the body systems while undergoing cancer treatment); **T** = Treatment (recommended as a primary treatment of cancer); **P** = Prevention (recommended to prevent cancer).
Studies = Authors' assessment of the available studies with regard to the primary claim.
Toxicity = Authors' assessment of available literature regarding toxicity.

Theory/Proposed Mechanism of Action

One of the leading proponents of cat's claw is Austrian scientist Klaus Keplinger. He holds two U.S. patents for his process of isolating six oxindole alkaloids from the root of *Uncaria tomentosa* and for the finding that these alkaloids are "suitable for the unspecific stimulation of the immunologic system." According to Keplinger's research, these six alkaloids have been shown to enhance phagocytosis. Thus, most advertising for cat's claw emphasizes its role as an "immune enhancer."

Evidence/Clinical Trials

A few animal and in vitro studies do suggest that cat's claw could have a significant influence on host immunity and some antimutagenic activity as well. Keplinger's company has published case reports of several patients with brain tumors who were reputed to have improved while taking cat's claw; however, no peer-reviewed clinical studies evaluating cat's claw as a treatment for cancer have been published.

Treatment/Dose

Varying doses are suggested, depending on the manufacturer or Web site consulted. Most suggest an average of 1000 mg three times daily, although some sites recommend between six and 20 gm per day, the latter dose primarily in advanced cancers.

Interestingly, the key alkaloids are supposedly bound to tannins, which prevents significant absorption or activation until the complexes are split by the acidic milieu of the stomach. For this reason, several Web sites caution against giving cat's claw concomitantly with antacids or H2-blockers.

Toxicity

Available studies suggest very limited toxicity, even at high doses. Some concern has been raised that it might have a contraceptive effect and thus use by pregnant women or women planning to conceive should be avoided. The authors are aware of one local case in which the ingestion of cat's claw was terminally associated with a 10-fold increase in serum glutamic-oxaloacetic transaminase (SGOT), suggesting liver toxicity.

Essiac

History

Essiac is an herbal mixture, widely used in Canada for over half a century, with an interesting and colorful history. Over the past 75 years, it has received a great deal of media attention and is the subject of numerous books and articles as well as of radio and TV programs. Rene N. Caisse (1888–1978), a nurse who developed the treatment while working in a medical clinic in rural Ontario, claimed to have received the remedy from a patient. That patient told Caisse that her breast cancer had been cured 20 years earlier using a tonic provided by an Ojibwa medicine man. Caisse obtained the tonic recipe, called it "Essiac" (her surname spelled backwards), and began treating cancer patients in 1924 (Table 119-3). Anecdotally, she claimed to have cured several "hopeless" cases of cancer, and her reputation grew among the Canadian public. She kept the recipe a secret during most of her life, however, and she never published any peer-reviewed studies of her experience treating hundreds of patients. Stiff opposition from conventional medicine mounted even as she treated patients into the late 1970s. Shortly before her death, Caisse assigned the formula and the right to use the Essiac name to the Resperin Corporation of Ontario. The formula is now manufactured as Essiac by Essiac Products in New Brunswick. Another Canadian product—Flor-Essence—contains an additional four herbs that are said to enhance the effectiveness of the original formula. It is manufactured in British Columbia.

The Resperin formula contains burdock root (*Arctium lappa*), sheep sorrel (*Rumex acetosella*),

Table 119-3 ■ Herbal Mixtures

Mixture	Also Known As	Primary Claim	Secondary Claim	Origin/Proponent	Studies	Toxicity
Essiac	Flor-Essence	S	T	Rene Caisse (1888–1978)	Insufficient data	Low
Hoxsey		T		Harry Hoxsey (1901–1974) Mildred Nelson RN (1919–1999)	Insufficient data	Low to medium
PC-SPES		P	T	Sophie Chen Ph.D.	Potentially beneficial	Low to medium

S = Supportive (recommended to support the body systems while undergoing cancer treatment); **T** = Treatment (recommended as a primary treatment of cancer); **P** = Prevention (recommended to prevent cancer).
Studies = Authors' assessment of the available studies with regard to the primary claim.
Toxicity = Authors' assessment of available literature regarding toxicity.

slippery elm (*Ulmus fulva*), and Indian rhubarb root (*Rheum officinale*). Flor-Essence also contains watercress (*Nasturtium officinale*), blessed thistle (*Cnicus benedictus*), red clover (*Trifolium pratense*), and kelp (*Laminaria digitata*).

Theory/Proposed Mechanism of Action

Proponents of Essiac claim that it strengthens the immune system, improves appetite, relieves pain, and improves overall quality of life. Others claim that it could reduce tumor size and prolong the lives of people with many types of cancer. Caisse gave her version of how Essiac works in a magazine interview (Homemakers) in 1977: "Often patients would report an enlarging and hardening of the tumor after a few treatments; then the tumor would begin to soften and if it was located in any body system with a route to the exterior, the patient would report discharging large amounts of pus and fleshy material. After this, the tumor would be gone." Caisse believed that Essiac induced the cancerous cells to return to the site of the original tumor, shrink, and then be discharged. In a letter to the Deputy Ministry of Health in Canada, she further stated: "My treatment consists of an intramuscular injection of herbs which causes the growth to localize. If there are secondaries, they recede into the primary growth, causing it to become larger, until it is all localized; then the mass starts to reduce in size."

Evidence/Clinical Trials

Except for sheep sorrel, the herbs found in the original formula have a long history of use as folk medicines and have been touted as laxatives, promoters of wound healing, and folk remedies for cancer. All four of the herbs have been studied individually to assess their antitumor activity. Both burdock and Indian rhubarb were shown to have some antitumor activity in selected animal tumor systems. Slippery elm contains beta-sitosterol, which has also been reported to have antitumor activity in animal tumor models. Little information is available regarding sorrel. A few isolated compounds from sorrel have demonstrated some weak antitumor activity.

Actual clinical trials of the complete Essiac formula have been limited. In 1938, the Royal Cancer Commission examined, via interviews, 49 patients whom Caisse had claimed to have cured; however, review of the clinical records brought the original diagnosis of cancer into question for several of these patients. Others had received conventional treatment prior to the use of Essiac. Ultimately, the Commission concluded that only two possible cures or improvements could be actually attributed to the herbal therapy.

In 1959, Caisse and the Science Research Institute of New York did collaborate on mouse studies of Essiac. Favorable pathological changes were apparently noted at necropsy of several of the mice, but further research was hampered by Caisse's unwillingness to disclose the formula. Further mice experiments were conducted through the mid-1970s, but the earlier preliminary positive findings were not duplicated. Caisse charged that this was due to improper handling of the herbs.

In 1978, a new trial in terminal cancer patients was undertaken. This was terminated prematurely as questions surfaced regarding both the study design and the quality controls used in the manufacture of Essiac.

There appear to be no completed, published case-control studies or randomized controlled clinical trials of Essiac. Many of the anecdotal observations or limited reviews that are available do not reliably distinguish between the effects of Essiac and the conventional therapies that patients already had received.

Treatment/Dose

Currently, the Resperin Web site lists a 1.5 ounce bottle of powdered Essiac for $35.95. One unit (1.5 ounces of herbs) makes "72 liquid ounces (2 L) of Nurse Rene Caisse's famous decoction. This is an 18-day supply using two ounces every 12 hours" (http://www.essiac-resperin.com/faq.html). Another Web site selling a similar formula states that the tea might need to be taken one to three times a day.

Toxicity

The Resperin Company Web site states "Essiac is natural, safe and non-toxic. It can be taken without any adverse side effects. Indian Rhubarb Root is known to occasionally produce more frequent bowel movements. Should this occur, reduce your dosage and consult your healthcare practitioner, if it persists" (http://www.essiac-resperin.com/faq.html). No published reports of adverse effects associated with the use of Essiac have been reported.

Vitamin C

History

Vitamin C, a water-soluble vitamin, is found in many fruits (e.g., oranges, grapefruit, strawberries, raspberries, and kiwi fruit), and in some vegetables (e.g. cabbage, tomatoes, and bell peppers). Humans cannot manufacture vitamin C and must therefore obtain it from dietary sources. Vitamin C is necessary for the synthesis of collagen, for wound healing, and as a participant in numerous immunologic and biochemical reactions. It is also an excellent antioxidant. Recent studies have suggested that vitamin C might also help promote cell differentiation.

Vitamin C deficiency, which results in scurvy, is rare in people who are able to eat a well-balanced diet; however, there seems to be increasing support for the concept that there is an increased need for vitamin C during periods of physical or chemical stress. This belief has helped contribute to the widespread use of vitamin C supplements.

The most famous proponent of vitamin C was Linus Pauling. In 1976 and 1978, he and a Scottish surgeon, Ewan Cameron, reported that patients treated with high doses of vitamin C had survived three to four times longer than similar patients who did not receive vitamin C supplements.

Cameron and Pauling collaborated and theorized that an increased intake of vitamin C could stimulate the synthesis of more collagen fibrils, thereby strengthening collagen, which in turn would help restrain malignant cells from invading surrounding tissue. This would then increase the body's natural resistance to cancer. Both scientists advocated the use of high-dose vitamin C as a supportive measure, not as a replacement for conventional therapy.

Theory/Proposed Mechanism of Action

Epidemiological evidence suggests that high dietary intake of vitamin C reduces the risk of some types of cancer, particularly stomach cancer (Table 119-4). Whether these effects are due to the antioxidant function of the vitamin or its ability to block the formation of N-nitrosamines is still a matter of some debate. Regardless, most proponents view vitamin C as an adjunct to conventional therapy to help promote the patient's natural defenses against the tumor, rather than as a primary treatment in and of itself.

Evidence/Clinical Studies

The original case series reported by Cameron was subsequently reviewed and called into serious question. For example, the patient groups were not shown to be comparable. Cameron treated all of the patients receiving vitamin C, while other physicians treated the "controls." No data have been published to demonstrate that the patients had been matched by stage of their disease, functional ability, weight loss, and so on. Cameron decided when a patient was "untreatable," and it has been shown subsequently that Cameron's patients were labeled untreatable much earlier in the course of their disease than were the control subjects.

Despite this negative review, Pauling and Cameron were successful in bringing vitamin C to the attention of the public. Continued interest in the therapy eventually necessitated several clinical trials. Mayo Clinic-based investigators conducted two double-blind studies involving patients with advanced cancer. Both studies found that patients given 10 g of vitamin C daily did no better than those given a placebo.

Pauling and others vocally criticized the studies, claiming that vitamin C had not been administered appropriately. Hence, a third study was undertaken, this time in a multicenter trial involving Mayo and several other sites. Again the results were negative, despite addressing the concerns raised against the first two studies. Thus, three prospectively randomized, placebo-controlled studies involving 367 patients documented no consistent benefit from vitamin C among cancer patients with advanced disease.

Anecdotally, both Pauling and his wife died of cancer, despite years of high-dose vitamin C therapy.

Table 119-4 ■ Vitamins and Minerals

Agent	Also Known As	Primary Claim	Secondary Claim	Origin/Proponent	Studies	Toxicity
Coenzyme Q-10	Ubiquinone	P	S	Karl Folkers, M.D. (1906–2000)	Potentially beneficial	Low
Selenium		P	S	Epidemiological studies Emmanuel Revici (1896–1998)	Potentially beneficial	Medium to high
Vitamin A		P		Epidemiological studies	Neutral	Low to medium
Vitamin C		P	T, S	Epidemiological studies Linus Pauling, Ph.D. (1901–1994) Ewan Cameron, MB, ChB (1922–1991)	Potentially beneficial	Low
Vitamin E		P	S	Epidemiological studies	Potentially beneficial	Low

S = Supportive (recommended to support the body systems while undergoing cancer treatment); **T** = Treatment (recommended as a primary treatment of cancer); **P** = Prevention (recommended to prevent cancer).
Studies = Authors' assessment of the available studies with regard to the primary claim.
Toxicity = Authors' assessment of available literature regarding toxicity.

Treatment/Dose

The recommended daily allowance for vitamin C had been 45 mg per day but was recently changed to 75 mg per day for women and 90 mg daily for men. Smokers are advised to obtain an additional 35 mg per day. Its use in unconventional cancer treatment, however, usually involves doses of up to 10 gm per day or more, administered either intravenously or orally. Some proponents advocate 20 gm per day or more.

Toxicity

Most clinical studies have found very minimal side effects, even from very large doses of vitamin C. Nonetheless, stomach irritation, heartburn, nausea, vomiting, drowsiness, headaches, and rash have all been reported. That high-dose vitamin C might increase the risk of kidney stones has been suggested, but documentation in the literature appears to be lacking.

Antineoplastons

History

Stanislaw R. Burzynski coined the term "antineoplastons" to identify substances that he claims can "normalize" cancer cells that are constantly being produced within the body (Table 119-5). Antineoplastons are naturally occurring peptides that he discovered during his graduate research. He noted that electrophoretic gels of urine samples from healthy individuals had a streak that was not present in gels of urine samples from cancer patients. He then isolated peptides in the blood of normal subjects that were not present in cancer patients. These he identified as "antineoplastons." In 1980, Burzynski synthesized the antineoplaston compounds, which he has divided into two groups: compounds with broad-spectrum activity and compounds with selective activity.

Burzynski has been the subject of considerable legal activity. He was eventually indicted on 75 counts,

Table 119-5 ■ Pharmacologic and Biologic Therapies

Therapy	Also Known As	Primary Claim	Secondary Claim	Origin/Proponent	Studies	Toxicity
Antineoplastons		T		Stanislaw R. Burzynski, MD (1943–)	Negative	Low
Cancell	Entelev, Cantron	T		James V. Sheridan (1912–2001) Edward Sopcak	Negative	None reported
Cellular treatment	Live cell therapy, glandular therapy, embryonic cell therapy, organotherapy	S	T	Paul Niehans, MD (1882–1971)	Insufficient studies	Medium to high
Coley toxins	Mixed bacterial vaccines (MBV)	T		William B. Coley, MD (1862–1936)	Mostly negative	Low to medium
Dimethyl sulfoxide	DMSO	T	S	Popular tradition	Negative	Low (topical), High (intravenous)
Hydrazine sulfate		S	T	Joseph Gold, MD (1930–)	Negative	Low to medium
Immuno-augmentative therapy		T		Lawrence Burton, PhD (1927–1993)	Insufficient studies	Medium to high
Laetrile	Amygdalin, "Vitamin B17"	T		Ernst Krebs Sr., MD (1877–1970) Ernst Krebs Jr	Negative	Medium to high
Livingston-Wheeler regimen		S		Virginia C. Livingston (1902–1990)	Negative	Varies as treatment plan varies
Shark cartilage		T	S	John F. Prudden, MD William Lane, Ph.D.	Negative	Low
714-X		T		Gaston Naessons (1924–)	Insufficient studies	None reported

S = Supportive (recommended to support the body systems while undergoing cancer treatment); T = Treatment (recommended as a primary treatment of cancer); P = Prevention (recommended to prevent cancer.
Studies = Authors' assessment of the available studies with regard to the primary claim.
Toxicity = Authors' assessment of available literature regarding toxicity.

including fraud, but a federal judge overturned this verdict in 1977. In 1995, a federal grand jury indicted Burzynski for mail fraud and marketing an unapproved drug. The indictment charged that he had billed insurance companies using procedure codes for chemotherapy, even though his treatment was not chemotherapy. He was tried in 1997 but not convicted.

In 1998, the Texas Attorney General secured a consent agreement stating that Burzynski.

- cannot distribute unapproved drugs in Texas;
- can distribute "antineoplastons" only to patients enrolled in FDA-approved clinical trials, unless the Food and Drug Administration approves his drugs for sale;
- cannot advertise "antineoplastons" for the treatment of cancer; and
- must place a disclaimer that the safety and effectiveness of "antineoplastons" have not been established.

Theory/Proposed Mechanism of Action

Burzynski's theory holds that antineoplastons are a part of the body's "natural biochemical defense system." Antineoplastons work by causing cancer cells to differentiate appropriately. He postulates that a wide variety of antineoplastons exist in a healthy body but that cancer patients excrete antineoplastons excessively in the urine, resulting in low plasma levels. Burzynski claims that "controlling neoplastic growth by a naturally occurring biochemical defense mechanism (i.e. directing the cancer cell into normal channels of differentiation) seems to be the ideal approach to tumor therapy."

Evidence/Clinical Trials

In the early 1980s, the National Cancer Institute (NCI) conducted several animal studies that showed no benefit. The NCI also reviewed the clinical records of several patients who had been treated with antineoplastons and found no evidence of benefit from the treatment. In 1985, the Canadian Bureau of Prescription Drugs reviewed the records of 36 Canadian patients who had been treated by Dr. Burzynski. Of 36 patients, 32 were found to have not benefited from the treatment and had died. Of the remaining four, two died within one year and two were alive but with widespread disease.

In 1991, a review of Dr. Burzynski's best cases was conducted by the National Cancer Institute. Seven patients with incurable brain cancer were felt to have possibly benefited from antineoplastons treatment. A formal clinical trial was then proposed to fully assess the safety and efficacy of antineoplaston therapy.

Though the study began in 1993, it was closed in 1995 because of disagreements between the National Cancer Institute and Burzynski regarding patient accrual. The report from this study did not suggest that antineoplastons were helpful.

Treatment/Dose

It is claimed that "antineoplaston therapy is unlike traditional chemotherapy because it is safe enough to be given to patients 24 hours a day. Antineoplastons are delivered intravenously through a catheter inserted in a central venous line. A pump infuses the medications at scheduled intervals. The dose and dosing schedule depends on the type of cancer. The pump and the antineoplaston bags are small and light enough to be carried around by a young child.

"The length of treatment depends on the patient's response. When patients achieve a complete response of long duration, intravenous therapy is discontinued. Patients then take antineoplastons in capsule form." (http://www.burzynskipatientgroup.org/mission.htm)

Patients on intravenous treatments are further instructed to plan a two- to four-week stay in Houston.

Toxicity

Dr. Burzynski has claimed that antineoplastons are not toxic and that they have few side effects. Brochures from the Burzynski Research Institute, however, suggest that side effects could include "excessive gas in the stomach, slight skin rash, slightly increased blood pressure, chills and fever." Reversible moderate to marked neurologic toxicity (transient somnolence, confusion, and exacerbation of an existing seizure disorder) was noted in five of nine patients treated.

Hydrazine Sulfate

History

Hydrazine sulfate, probably most readily recognized as a component of rocket fuel, has been championed as a cancer treatment by Joseph Gold. Dr. Gold was influenced by the research of Dr. Otto Warburg, a 1931 Nobel Prize laureate whose work revealed that cancer cells preferentially metabolize glucose anaerobically. Believing that cachexia in cancer patients was due to glycolysis in tumor cells resulting in increased gluconeogenesis in the liver, he sought to break this "energy-losing cycle" via several different agents. He eventually decided that hydrazine sulfate served this role. During animal studies of this effect, he also noted that hydrazine sulfate also seemed to have antitumor effects and also potentiated the effectiveness of certain chemotherapeutic agents. Gold initially recommended hydrazine sulfate for patients with breast cancer, sarcomas, and lymphomas, but he now reportedly recommends its use for all cancers.

Theory/Proposed Mechanism of Action

Gold postulated that excessive gluconeogenesis, (necessitated by the body's need to reconstitute the tumor's anaerobic metabolites into glucose) was a major determinant of cancer-related cachexia. He next determined that the enzyme phosphoenol pyruvate carboxykinase (PEP-CK) played a key role in gluco-neogenesis. Thus, he theorized that blocking the activity of PEP-CK would impede gluconeogenesis and reduce the severity of cachexia. Gold then tested several substances before deciding that hydrazine sulfate was the best agent for inhibiting this enzyme. It was during his studies of its effects on cachexia in rats with transplanted tumors that Gold surmised that hydrazine sulfate also inhibited tumor growth and increased survival. He was unable to explain a mechanism for this.

Evidence/Clinical Trials

In clinical studies published in the 1970s and early 1980s, Gold reported that the use of hydrazine sulfate resulted in improved appetite and reduced weight loss in cancer patients. In terms of improving outcomes for patients with cancer, studies conducted in the mid-1970s, including work from the Soviet Union, reported mixed results. In the 1980s, Chlebowski et al published the report of a clinical trial from UCLA. This placebo-controlled trial did not show any overall benefit for hydrazine sulfate compared with placebo in patients with non–small cell lung cancer who were receiving concomitant chemotherapy. Nonetheless, Chlebowski et al reported that there was a trend for improvement in the good performance status of patients who were randomized to hydrazine sulfate versus placebo. An accompanying editorial in the journal issue titled "The hazards of small clinical trials" warned against making any strong conclusions based on subsets of small clinical trials. In response to Dr. Chlebowski's study, the National Cancer Institute did support three randomized placebo-controlled clinical trials. These trials were reported in 1994 concluding that there was no advantage for hydrazine sulfate over placebo. Stimulated by controversy generated by the proponents of hydrazine sulfate, a review of these studies was performed by the United States General Accounting Office (GAO). This federal agency confirmed the integrity of these trials, with the title page of its report stating "Contrary to allegation, NIH hydrazine sulfate studies were not flawed." It is interesting that a current Web page for the proponents draws attention to the fact that there was a question regarding the integrity of these hydrazine sulfate studies, but the Web page does not disclose the findings of the General Accounting Office report.

Treatment/Dose

One Web site contains the following recommendations: "Hydrazine sulfate is usually administered orally, with food or immediately before eating. It may also be given by injection. The usual cycle of treatment is 60 mg 3 times daily for 30 to 45 days followed by a rest period of 2 to 6 weeks. The cycle can be repeated as many times as desired. Each 60 mg dose is available in capsule form or in 15-mL vials for injection."

The use of alcohol, barbiturates, and tranquilizers (particularly benzodiazepines) is strictly contraindicated according to Gold, as combining these agents with hydrazine sulfate can increase toxicity and decrease efficacy. He also cautions that because hydrazine and hydrazine sulfate are monoamine oxidase (MAO) inhibitors, people using hydrazine sulfate should avoid foods that are rich in tyramine (for example, certain aged cheeses).

Toxicity

Reports of toxicity have been limited but include mild nausea, pruritus, dizziness, drowsiness, excitation, and peripheral neuropathies (motor and sensory), occurring in 5% to 10% of patients. A recent case report, however, suggests the possibility of severe hepatic injury resulting in death.

Laetrile

History

Laetrile, which achieved great notoriety during the 1970s and early 1980s, is the trade name for a synthetic relative of amygdalin, a chemical derived primarily from apricot pits. It is sometimes also referred to as vitamin B_{17}, although there has never been any scientific support for its designation as a vitamin. Laetrile was developed by Ernst Krebs, Sr. and Ernst Krebs, Jr. and was first used to treat cancer patients in California in the early 1950s. It became increasingly popular and controversial during the 1970s.

In 1975, a class action suit was filed to stop the Food and Drug Administration from interfering with the sale and distribution of Laetrile. Early in the case, a federal district court judge in Oklahoma issued orders allowing cancer patients to import a six-month supply of Laetrile for personal use if they could obtain a physician's affidavit that they were "terminal." In 1979, the United States Supreme Court ruled that it is not possible to be certain who is terminal and that even if it were possible, both terminally ill patients and the general public deserve protection from fraudulent cures. In 1987, after further appeals were denied, the district judge (a strong proponent of Laetrile) finally yielded to the higher courts and terminated the affidavit system. Few sources of Laetrile are now available within the United States, but it still is utilized at a few Mexican clinics.

Theory/Proposed Mechanism of Action

According to proponents, Laetrile kills tumor cells selectively while leaving normal cells unharmed. Some proponents claim cancer is actually a deficiency caused by a lack of Laetrile ("vitamin B_{17}").

Krebs theorized that enzymatic breakdown of Laetrile yields three chemicals: glucose, benzaldehyde, and hydrogen cyanide. He believed that normal cells were able to metabolize the cyanide to thiocyanate using an enzyme (rhodanese); however, Krebs also believed that cancer cells lack this second enzyme, allowing the unmetabolized cyanide to destroy the cancer cells.

Evidence/Clinical Trials

In the 1970s, the National Cancer Institute tested Laetrile in laboratory animals and did not find significant evidence that it was effective against animal cancers. In 1978, because of public interest and the increasing use by patients, the National Cancer Institute sent nearly a half million letters to physicians, health professionals, and Laetrile support groups requesting documented case histories of patients who had had a positive response to Laetrile. Despite this unprecedented effort, only 230 patients were identified. Of the 230, only 93 gave permission for their records to be reviewed. Of the 93, 26 were found to have insufficient information to permit a meaningful review. The 67 remaining case histories failed to show any significant benefit from the Laetrile treatment.

In response to political pressure, the Mayo Clinic and three other U.S. cancer centers under National Cancer Institute sponsorship began a clinical trial in 1982. Laetrile and "metabolic therapy" were administered as recommended by their promoters, and 178 patients with advanced cancers were enrolled. Approximately one-third of the patients had colorectal cancer, with lung cancer, breast cancer, and melanoma being the next largest categories. It is important to note that almost one-third of the patients had not received chemotherapy prior to receiving Laetrile therapy. This eliminated a previous contention that Laetrile loses its effectiveness in patients whose immune systems have already been "damaged" by conventional chemotherapy. Of the 178 patients, not one was cured or stabilized, nor did any appear to experience an improvement in quality of life. Several patients experienced symptoms of cyanide toxicity or had blood levels of cyanide approaching the lethal range.

Toxicity

Laetrile is approximately 6% cyanide by weight, thus making cyanide toxicity a distinct possibility. Beta-glucosidase is present in several common foods such as raw almonds, certain nuts, bean and alfalfa sprouts, peaches, lettuce, celery, and mushrooms. Increased consumption of beta-glucosidase along with consumption of Laetrile could result in toxic levels of cyanide being released. Other common side effects noted in clinical studies included nausea, vomiting, headache, and dizziness. There also have been case reports in the literature of cyanide poisoning secondary to consumption of Laetrile.

Shark Cartilage

History

John Prudden, a surgeon at Columbia Presbyterian Medical Center in the early 1950s, used bovine cartilage to promote wound healing in surgical patients. He later used powdered cartilage to treat an ulcerated breast cancer and reported a dramatic response. Renewed interest came in the early 1990s, when I. William Lane published a book called *Sharks Don't Get Cancer*, claiming cartilage was a cancer cure. Public interest was further raised by a 1993 television episode of *60 Minutes* promoting the book. The program showed several "terminal" cancer patients from a Cuban study who were "improved" by treatment with shark cartilage. A National Cancer Institute review of the Cuban data found the study to be "incomplete and unimpressive."

Much of this early excitement centered around the erroneous concept that sharks do not get cancer, and preliminary findings that showed a modest antiangiogenic effect in laboratory experiments.

Theory/Proposed Mechanism of Action

While studies have demonstrated some antiangiogenic effects of shark cartilage in laboratory studies, no evidence so far exists that any specific antiangiogenic effect occurs in cancer patients who consume shark cartilage. Prudden and other proponents have suggested that its anticancer effect could actually be through enhancement of the immune system.

Evidence/Clinical Trials

Animal studies in the late 1970s and 1980s suggested that immune stimulation could occur from factors within the cartilage. Early clinical results provided by Prudden were encouraging; however, subsequent clinical trials were generally disappointing. In one

Table 119-6 ■ Nutritional Metabolic Therapy

Therapy	Also Known As	Primary Claim	Secondary Claim	Origin/Proponent	Studies	Toxicity
Gerson therapy		S	T	Max B. Gerson, MD (1881–1959)	Insufficient studies	Low
Macrobiotics		S	T	Michio Kasha (1926–)	Insufficient studies	Low
Revici therapy	Lipid therapy, biologically guided chemotherapy	T	S	Emanuel Revici, MD (1896–1998)	Mostly negative	None reported

S = Supportive (recommended to support the body systems while undergoing cancer treatment); **T** = Treatment (recommended as a primary treatment of cancer); **P** = Prevention (recommended to prevent cancer).
Studies = Authors' assessment of the available studies with regard to the primary claim.
Toxicity = Authors' assessment of available literature regarding toxicity.

study, 58 patients with advanced cancer were followed for 12 weeks. Four patients had to discontinue treatment because of toxicity, five had died, and none achieved a complete or partial response to the shark cartilage treatment. The researchers concluded: "Shark cartilage was inactive in patients with advanced stages of cancer, specifically in breast, colon, lung, and prostate cancer."

Treatment/Dose

Shark cartilage is available as a food supplement in capsule and powder form. Some people take cartilage by enema because the recommended dosage by the major proponents is very high (60 to 90 gm a day) and because the substance has a bad taste and can cause nausea and diarrhea.

Toxicity

The main identified toxicity is gastrointestinal intolerance, and many patients stop the shark cartilage as a consequence (Tables 119-6 and 119-7).

Table 119-7 ■ Miscellaneous Complementary and Alternative Medicine Therapies

Therapy	Also Known As	Primary Claim	Secondary Claim	Origin/Proponent	Studies	Toxicity
Chelation therapy		T	S	American College for Advancement in Medicine (ACAM)	Negative	High
Detoxification enemas	Colonic hydrotherapy, high colonic therapy	P	S, T	Traditional	Insufficient studies	Medium
Detoxification-fasting		P	S	Traditional	Insufficient studies	Low to medium
Homeopathy		S		Samuel Hahnemann (1755–1843)	Insufficient studies	Low
Oxygen treatments	Hyperoxygenation therapy, bio-oxidative therapy, oxidative therapy, oxymedicine, oxydology	T		Various	Negative	High

S = Supportive (recommended to support the body systems while undergoing cancer treatment); **T** = Treatment (recommended as a primary treatment of cancer); **P** = Prevention (recommended to prevent cancer).
Studies = Authors' assessment of the available studies with regard to the primary claim.
Toxicity = Authors' assessment of available literature regarding toxicity.

Conclusion

Whether one is reading broadsides and tracts from a quack peddler of the 1800s or perusing the innumerable and current unorthodox cancer treatment Web sites, one cannot help but be struck by the similarity of the two approaches. In fact, across the ages, it seems as if the "pitch" has almost become formulaic. Today, it seems as if almost all unorthodox cancer treatment proponents are following this same formula, regardless of how divergent the products themselves might be:

1. *Treatment "X" is the result of unique knowledge or science:* Almost all of the unorthodox Web sites and literature reviewed make some claim to a special or unique knowledge regarding cancer or its treatment. Many of these claims seem laughable from a professional and scientific perspective but can be strongly appealing to a more naïve lay readership. Other theories appear to be quite well thought-out and plausible enough to make even a savvy reader take a second look. The appeal of a new and exciting approach to a dreaded disease cannot be underestimated.
2. *The unique knowledge is being suppressed:* From the quacks of the 1800s to the most sophisticated current Web sites, almost all unorthodox treatment proponents claim that their discovery/cure is being withheld from the ailing public by a mercenary medical profession. Physicians (or the American Medical Association, pharmaceutical companies, etc.) suppress information about the unorthodox cure because they "prefer to make money by keeping people sick." This suppression is usually characterized as the result of a well-organized conspiracy motivated primarily by monetary concerns, but also because physicians and scientists are too proud to admit that something from outside the bounds of conventional medicine might be effective.
3. *Use treatment "X" or else:* Especially in the realm of cancer, unorthodox treatment proponents are quick to point out the toxicities of conventional chemotherapy and radiation therapy. According to the proponents, the reward for enduring such side effects is a dismally poor prognosis. Yet, because of the new knowledge being extolled in the form of treatment "X," the patient has a choice. Hence, most proponents exhort patients to exert their autonomy, throw off the yoke of the mercenary or shortsighted medical profession, and reap the miraculous benefits of treatment "X." Such entreaties take on an evangelistic quality. Especially to a severely ill patient who feels that "modern medicine" has failed them, the pitch can be persuasive. Web sites are replete with testimonials from fellow sufferers who now have been cured through the wonderful effects of treatment "X."

Hence, desperate patients, learning of a wonderful new treatment (wrongly and selfishly hidden from the world by a greedy cabal of physicians and pharmaceutical companies) cannot be faulted for their interest. Invariably, treatment "X" is promised to be "natural," "safe," or "nontoxic." Not only will treatment "X" cure cancer but it also is promised to "promote health," "strengthen the immune system," and/or "support the body" while doing so. Thus, whether patients have untreatable cancer and feel "let down" by conventional medicine, or whether they have eminently treatable tumors but unrealistically fear conventional forms of treatment, the promise put forth by most of the unorthodox proponents can be a siren song hard to resist.

To successfully sort their way through the tangled web of information and misinformation, cancer patients need an advocate—not someone who will disdainfully dismiss all questions about unorthodox therapies, but rather somebody who will address their questions carefully, in an honest and compassionate manner. Patients clinging to fragile (but desperately sought) hopes need to be heard. Carefully listening to what the patient thinks the unorthodox treatment might offer is a valuable clue as to what it is that the patient wants but has not found in conventional treatment. Recognizing the unmet need might allow the physician to adapt his/her approach to the patient.

The cancer patient's advocate needs to know at least something about the most commonly encountered unorthodox therapies, or where to go to find out more. Learning about unorthodox treatments does not imply endorsement. But having that basic knowledge to share with the patient using (or contemplating using) an unorthodox therapy can help guide them to a truly informed decision. Enabling patients to distinguish between the categories previously mentioned (i.e., potentially beneficial, benign, potentially harmful, potentially interactive, and diversionary) increases the chance that patients will make a good decision regarding the use of an unorthodox therapy.

Thus, keeping communication open could be one of the most important things a physician can do for their patients with cancer who potentially are interested in unorthodox therapy. Patients who feel that they will be ridiculed for bringing this interest to the attention of their physician will not do so. Their "facts" will come from well-intentioned friends, neighbors, or the Internet, unfiltered through the knowledge of their physician. Ultimately, by being available to answer questions for patients with cancer, physicians can help steer these often-desperate individuals through the relatively uncharted waters of unorthodox therapies. By being neither dismissive nor all-embracing, but adhering to time-tested scientific principles, physicians who share their knowledge in a collaborative fashion with their patients have the best chance of navigating their patients safely through the maze of unorthodox therapies.

References

Buckner J, Malkin M, Reed E, et al: Phase II study of antineoplastons A10 (NSC 648539) and AS2-1 (NSC 620261) in patients with recurrent glioma. Mayo Clin Proc 1999;74:137–145.

Cameron E, Pauling L: Supplemental ascorbate in the supportive treatment of cancer: Prolongation of survival times in terminal human cancer. Proc Natl Acad Sci U S A 1976;73:3685–3689.

Chlebowski RT, Bulcavage L, Grosvenor M, et al: Hydrazine sulfate influence on nutritional status and survival in non–small cell lung cancer. J Clin Oncol 1990;8:9–15.

Chlebowski RT, Heber D, Richardson B, et al: Influence of hydrazine sulfate on abnormal carbohydrate metabolism in cancer patients with weight loss. Cancer Res 1984;44:857–861.

Creagan ET, Moertel CG, O'Fallon JR, et al: Failure of high-dose vitamin C (ascorbic acid) therapy to benefit patients with advanced cancer. A controlled trial. New Engl J Med 1979;301:687–690.

DeWys WD: How to evaluate a new treatment for cancer. Your Patient and Cancer. 1982;2:31–36.

Ellison NM, Byar DP, Newell GR: Special report on Laetrile: the NCI Laetrile review. Results of the National Cancer Institute's retrospective Laetrile analysis. New Engl J Med 1978;299:549–552.

Gold J: Proposed treatment of cancer by inhibition of gluconeogenesis. Oncology 1968;22:185–207.

Gold J: Inhibition of gluconeogenesis at the phosphoenolpyruvate carboxykinase and pyruvate carboxylase reactions, as a means of cancer chemotherapy. Oncology 1974;29:74–89.

Gold J: Use of hydrazine sulfate in terminal and preterminal cancer patients: Results of investigational new drug (IND) study in 84 evaluable patients. Oncology 1975;32:1–10.

Gold J: Anabolic profiles in late-stage cancer patients responsive to hydrazine sulfate. Nutr Cancer 1981;3:13–19.

Hainer M, Tsai N, Komura S, et al: Fatal hepatorenal failure associated with hydrazine sulfate. Ann Intern Med 2000;133:877–880.

"herb". In Mish FC (ed): Merriam Webster's Collegiate Dictionary, 10th ed. Springfield, Library of Congress Cataloging, 1993, p 542.

Kosty MP, Fleishman SB, Herndon JE, et al: Cisplatin, vinblastine, and hydrazine sulfate in advanced, non–small cell lung cancer: A randomized placebo-controlled, double-blind phase III study of the Cancer and Leukemia Group B. J Clin Oncol 1994;12:1113–1120.

Loprinzi CL, Kuross SA, O'Fallon JR, et al: Randomized placebo-controlled evaluation of hydrazine sulfate in patients with advanced colorectal cancer. J Clin Oncol 1994;12:1121–1125.

Loprinzi CL, Goldberg RM, Su JQ, et al: Placebo-controlled trial of hydrazine sulfate in patients with newly diagnosed non-small cell lung cancer. J Clin Oncol 1994;12:1126–1129.

Merill A, Foltz A, McCormick D: Vitamins and cancer. In Alfin-Slater R, Kritchevsky D (eds): Cancer and Nutrition. New York, Plenum Press, 1991, pp 261–320.

Miller DR, Anderson GT, Stark JJ, et al: Phase I/II trial of the safety and efficacy of shark cartilage in the treatment of advanced cancer. J Clin Oncol 1997;16:3649–3655.

Moertel CG, Fleming TR, Creagan ET, et al: High-dose vitamin C versus placebo in the treatment of patients with advanced cancer who have had no prior chemotherapy. A randomized double-blind comparison. New Engl J Med 1985;312:137–141.

Moertel CG, Fleming TR, Rubin J, et al: A clinical trial of amygdalin (Laetrile) in the treatment of human cancer. New Engl J Med 1982;306:201–206.

Ontario Breast Cancer Information Exchange Project: A Guide to Unconventional Cancer Therapies. Aurora Ontario, R&R Bookbar, 1994, pp 278–280.

Rizzi R, Re F, Bianchi A, et al: Mutagenic and antimutagenic activities of *Uncaria tomentosa* and its extracts. J Ethnopharmacol 1993;38:63–77.

Ruschitzka F, Meier PJ, Turina M, et al: Acute heart transplant rejection due to Saint John's wort [letter]. Lancet 2000;355:548–549.

Straus SE: Complementary and alternative medicine: challenges and opportunities for American medicine. Acad Med 2000;75:572–573.

US Department of Health, Education, and Welfare, Public Health Service, Food and Drug Administration: Laetrile. Commissioner's decision on status. Federal Reg 1977;42:39768–39806.

Warburg O: On the origin of cancer cells. Science 1956;123:309–314.

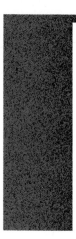

Chapter 120
Psychosocial Issues

Elizabeth M. Thomas, Carlos J. Sandoval, and Sharlene M. Weiss

Over the past 40 years, interest in the psychosocial issues of cancer patients has developed into a subspecialty of oncology known as psycho-oncology. Psycho-oncology has concerned itself with identifying and treating the psychological and social variables of cancer patients to enhance their quality of life.

Psychological Distress

The diagnosis of cancer evokes great emotion. For most people, the word "cancer" conjures up gruesome images of disfigurement, suffering, and death. An emotional response is a normal and expected reaction to a stressor of this magnitude. To recognize the normalcy of a psychological response to the cancer experience, many researchers and clinicians have adopted the term *distress* when talking about the various emotions that cancer patients experience. However, distress exists along a continuum, from common feelings of sadness and fearfulness to clinically diagnosable distress, such as depression or panic.

Adjustment to a Cancer Diagnosis

Holland and Massie at Memorial Sloan-Kettering Cancer Center have provided a general framework for understanding the emotional process by which people respond to the diagnosis of cancer. They have divided the diagnostic crisis period into three stages; disbelief, turmoil, and adaptation. When individuals receive a cancer diagnosis, they tend to experience an initial period of disbelief or shock. Patients and accompanying family members report hearing only several key words or phrases voiced by the physician, such as "cancer," "chemotherapy," or "radiation." Patients might think, "I've never been sick in my life, this makes no sense"; "I don't feel sick, so I can't possibly have cancer"; or "This is the wrong diagnosis. The doctor must have made a mistake." These types of thoughts represent a normal and healthy psychological defense against a potentially life-threatening event.

Life as patients know it has come to an abrupt halt, and the reality of having cancer takes some time to digest, typically about one week or less.

This initial shock is followed by a period of confusion as the person attempts to integrate this life-altering information. Feelings of anxiety, depression, irritability, anger, and guilt may surface. Many people report a sense of being out of control, of being helpless against a disease that has invaded their bodies. Disruptions in sleep, appetite, concentration, and the ability to carry out a normal routine may occur. Thoughts may now be exclusively focused on the cancer: "How did I get cancer when I've always taken such good care of myself?" "There's no history of cancer in my family, why me?" As patients contemplate such existential issues, they describe a sense of isolation and separateness from the rest of the world, which continues to move forward as if nothing has changed. Generally, these symptoms begin to resolve themselves within several weeks as patients adapt and mobilize themselves for treatment. Over the course of medical therapy, however, individuals may experience a resurgence of these intense feelings, particularly at different crisis points (e.g., recurrence, cancer has spread, treatment is not working).

Depressive and Anxiety Disorders

For some patients, high levels of distress continue beyond this adjustment period. Available data suggest that one third to one half of cancer patients experience persistent and clinically significant levels of distress that interfere with daily functioning and potentially affect the ability to actively engage in medical treatment. Across subjects, psychiatric disorders involving depression and anxiety tend to be the most commonly observed conditions. Within any particular individual, symptoms of both depression and anxiety may be present, although one syndrome may dominate the clinical picture.

In regard to depression, there are a number of

DIAGNOSIS

Stages of Emotional Adjustment

Stages of emotional adjustment to a cancer diagnosis are as follows:

- *Disbelief*: shock over cancer diagnosis; lasts one week or less
- *Turmoil*: may experience intense feelings of anxiety, depression, irritability, anger, guilt over the course of several weeks
- *Adaptation*: resolution of overwhelming feelings and engagement in treatment

From Massie MJ, Holland JC: Overview of normal reactions and prevalence of psychiatric disorders. In: Holland JC, Rowland JH (eds): Handbook of Psychooncology. Psychological Care of the Patient with Cancer. New York: Oxford University Press, 1989, pp 273–282.

factors that appear to place certain individuals at risk. Being young, elderly, or female; having advanced disease; and receiving treatment of either a palliative or an active nature, as opposed to medical follow-up, appear to increase vulnerability to depression. Those who have a greater level of disability or discomfort are also at risk, including individuals who are not fully ambulatory and those who have uncontrollable pain. Other risk variables include a lack of social support, a generally pessimistic outlook on life, substance abuse, recent losses, and a personal or family history of mood disorders.

Psychiatric disorders and their symptoms are classified in the Diagnostic and Statistical Manual of Mental Disorders of the American Psychiatric Association (DSM-IV). For an individual to fulfill diagnostic criteria for a clinical depression, the patient must experience feelings of depression and/or anhedonia (i.e., loss of interest or pleasure), more often than not, for at least two weeks. Once this initial criterion has been met, a patient should have at least four of the following symptoms (or three if the patient has both depression and anhedonia): appetite or weight change, sleep disturbance, psychomotor retardation or agitation, fatigue, feelings of worthlessness or guilt, inadequate concentration or indecisiveness, and suicidal ideation.

Diagnosing depression in cancer patients can be challenging, as several of the symptoms of depression can actually be caused by the illness (e.g., pancreatic cancer) or by the treatment itself (e.g., corticosteroids). For clinical purposes, most mental health professionals tend to utilize an inclusive diagnostic approach. That is, they consider all symptoms of depression as diagnostic indicators, including loss of appetite and fatigue, which are two of the most highly controversial symptoms in the diagnosis of depression in cancer patients. But the value of symptoms is weighed against larger issues such as cancer site, type of treatment, and clinical course. An inclusive diagnostic approach ensures maximum sensitivity and avoids disregarding a patient who is in need of mental health services.

Notably, admission of suicidal thoughts should always be taken seriously and assessed fully. Although relatively few cancer patients actually commit suicide, the risk of suicide in cancer patients is generally twice that of the general population. Individuals with oral, pharyngeal, lung, and brain tumors are at increased risk of suicide in comparison to patients with other cancers. Cancer at these sites is generally associated with excessive and prolonged alcohol and tobacco usage, suggesting more potential for disinhibition of impulses and perhaps a history of inadequate coping abilities. Second, treatment of these cancers may have a substantial impact on body integrity, resulting in disfigurement and impaired functioning of basic abilities such as talking or eating. Similarly, patients with advanced disease, a poor prognosis, or inadequately controlled pain are at increased risk of suicide, as are individuals with premorbid psychopathology who may have attempted suicide in the past and those with a family history of suicide. In assessing suicidal risk, depression might or might not be a factor. While the presence of depression increases risk for suicide, only one half of suicides suffer from clinical depression. Instead, other factors such as hopelessness about the future and helplessness in overcoming obstacles come into play. Indeed, hopelessness is a larger predictor for suicide than is depression. Proper assessment includes inquiring about relevant risk and vulnerability factors, the nature of the suicidal ideation (i.e., a fleeting versus a dwelling thought), the presence and lethality of a plan for committing suicide, means to carry out the plan (e.g., possession of a gun in the home, pill stockpiling), and intent.

When patients fulfill the DSM-IV criteria for clinical depression, they are considered to have a major depressive disorder. Studies indicate that approximately 10% of cancer patients with elevated distress levels will be diagnosed with major depression. Individuals who do not fully meet these criteria but continue to experience marked distress or deficits in at least one area of life functioning are generally labeled with the subthreshold diagnosis of adjustment disorder with depressed mood. Adjustment disorders may also occur with anxiety or with mixed anxiety and depressed mood. Adjustment disorders represent a stress-related psychiatric disorder and are a bridge between normal and pathologic responses. Diagnosis with an adjustment disorder is generally the predominant diagnosis given to individuals who are struggling with their reactions to the cancer experience, representing about 70% of those with heightened distress.

While most psychiatric disorders involving an anxiety component develop after the onset of cancer and therefore receive the diagnosis of adjustment disorder, a subpopulation of people with significant anxiety possess preexisting anxiety conditions. This constitutes about 5% of those who are experiencing elevated distress levels. Even if individuals do not possess a preexisting anxiety disorder, a tendency to become anxious when confronted with a stressor, a desire for control, and obsessive personality traits appear to predispose people to the development of a clinical or subclinical anxiety disorder. Other risk factors for anxiety include advanced-stage illness, active or palliative care status, and poorly controlled pain.

The experience of anxiety is characterized by excessive worry and fear and apprehensive expectation for the future. Thinking tends to be global (e.g., "I can't stand going to the doctor."), catastrophic (e.g., "If I go to the doctor, I'm going to be tortured by having to get all kinds of tests."), and irreversible (e.g., "I'm just unable to handle these situations."). Individuals experience these thoughts as intrusive and difficult to control. Feelings of anxiety may affect motor functions, causing physical restlessness, tension, and subsequent muscle soreness and aches. Patients with elevated anxiety levels generally report becoming easily fatigued. Increased arousal and vigilance may be present. Patients may report feeling keyed up, on edge, or irritable; having difficulty concentrating; or having their mind go blank. In addition, a sleep disturbance may be present. Sleep problems that have an anxiety component tend to be expressed as difficulties in falling or staying asleep. In contrast, a sleep disturbance characterized by early morning awakening is more indicative of a depressive state.

For individuals who have long-standing anxiety disturbances, the cancer experience may reactivate or exacerbate these disorders. Patients with a history of panic disorder are vulnerable to experiencing discrete attacks of anxiety. Panic attacks are characterized by sudden, intense bursts of terror in which autonomic activity increases rapidly over a short period of time and sympathetic responses such as an accelerated heart rate, shortness of breath, chest discomfort, sweating, trembling, dizziness, parasthesias, and chills or hot flashes are produced. These attacks are typically accompanied by a sense of imminent danger and fears that one will die, become insane, or lose control. As a consequence, patients seek to flee the situation attached to this experience and for this reason might abruptly leave a treatment situation. Agoraphobic individuals are another group who may experience difficulties. These patients fear being away from the home, an environment that provides an impression of safety and security. Such a fear can severely impair their ability to successfully carry out a treatment regime. Individuals with post-traumatic stress disorder (PTSD) are a third vulnerable subpopulation. Typically, this diagnosis is associated with war veterans, although this type of anxiety disorder can arise from any life-threatening trauma. These individuals experience extreme anxiety and avoidant behavior when exposed to events that resemble or symbolize any aspect of the original trauma experience, including sounds, sensations, or images. Because the treatment of cancer can cause discomfort, treatment situations may trigger old memories or feelings, and behavior in this group may become erratic. Finally, simple phobias, especially those related to blood, needles, or a fear of closed spaces (i.e., claustropho-

---

DIAGNOSIS

Psychological Disorders

Roughly one third to one half of patients experience persistent and elevated distress that may necessitate medical and/or psychological intervention, including the following:

- 10%: major depressive disorder
- 70%: adjustment disorders
  - A subclinical and stress-related disorder
  - Subtypes: with depressed mood, with anxious mood, or with mixed anxiety and depressed mood

- 5%: preexisting anxiety disorder
  - May be reactivated or exacerbated by cancer experience
  - Includes such diagnoses as panic disorder, agoraphobia, post-traumatic stress disorder, phobias
- 15%: assorted diagnoses, including the following:
  - Major mental illness (e.g., psychotic disorders, bipolar disorder)
  - Delirium
  - Personality disorders (i.e., "the difficult patient")

Adapted from Derogatis LR, Morrow GR, Felting J: The prevalence of psychiatric disorder among cancer patients. JAMA 1983;249:751–757.

bia), may interfere with procedures that cancer patients are asked to perform routinely as part of their treatment

Medication Options for Psychiatric Conditions

Numerous medications are available for the treatment of depression. The first-line treatments are the serotonergic agents such as fluoxetine, sertraline, and paroxetine. These may initially cause insomnia, and a hypnotic may need to be added. Nefazodone has both anxiolytic and sedating properties. Mirtazapine not only has sedating effects, but also increases appetite in many patients and is therefore useful in those who suffer from anorexia. Finally, psychostimulants such as methylphenidate can be utilized as an adjuvant to antidepressants to combat the fatigue and anergy of advanced illness as well as the somnolence of opioids.

Treatment of anxiety disorders consists of the judi-

TREATMENT

Common Psychiatric Medications Used with Cancer Patients

Disorder	Medication(s)
Major depressive disorder	Fluoxetine (Prozac): 10–80 mg Sertraline (Zoloft): 25–200 mg Paroxetine (Paxil): 10–50 mg Citalopram (Celexa): 10–40 mg Nefazodone (Serzone): 200–600 mg in divided doses Mirtazapine: 15–45 mg Buproprion (Wellbutrin-SR): 50–300 mg in divided doses
Illness-related fatigue, apathy, and withdrawal states	Methylphenidate (Ritalin): 10–80 mg in divided doses
Anxiety disorders (also PTSD)	Alprazolam (Xanax): 1–4 mg in divided doses Lorazepam (Ativan): 1–6 mg in divided doses Clonazepam (Klonopin): 1–4 mg in divided doses Buspirone (Buspar): 30–60 mg in divided doses Hydroxyzine (Vistaril): 100–400 mg in divided doses Sertraline (Zoloft): 25–200 mg Paroxetine (Paxil): 10–50 mg
Panic attacks	Paroxetine (Paxil): 10–40 mg Sertraline (Zoloft): 25–200 mg Imipramine (Tofranil): 25–200 mg Alprazolam (Xanax): 1.5–4 mg in divided doses Lorazepam (Ativan): 3–6 mg in divided doses Clonazepam (Klonopin): 1–4 mg in divided doses
Insomnia	Triazolam (Halcion): 0.25–0.5 mg Temazepam (Restoril): 15–60 mg Zolpidem (Ambien): 5–10 mg Trazodone (Desyrel): 50–100 mg Diphenhydramine: 25–100 mg
Delirium and psychotic smptoms (also PTSD)	Olanzapine (Zyprexa): 2.5–20 mg Risperidone (Risperdal): 0.5–6 mg Quetiapine (Seroquel): 50–600 mg Haloperidol (Haldol): 0.5–10 mg, IV for agitated delirium
Bipolar mood disorder	Lithium carbonate: 600–1800 mg titrated by blood levels (0.6–1.0 mEq/L) Valproic acid (Depakene): 500–2000 mg, titrated by blood levels (50–100 mg/mL) Carbamazepine (Tegretol): 200–1800 mg in divided doses
Alcohol withdrawal	Lorazepam (Ativan): 0.5—2 mg q 4 hour doses while awake and not lethargic, decreased over a three-day period

Adapted from Kobayashi J: Psychiatric issues. In Anderson J (ed): A Guide to the Clinical Care of Women with HIV. Washington, DC: USDHHS/HSRA, 2001, p 307.

DIAGNOSIS

Familial Issues

Approximately one third of families experience emotional distress and psychosocial disruption. Risk factors for caregiver distress include the following:

- Site of patient's cancer: Caregivers of patients with lung or brain cancer are more likely to experience high distress.
- High demands: Caregivers who have multiple tasks or roles may experience elevated distress.
- Prognosis and stage: Caregivers of patients with a poor prognosis or advanced disease may exhibit elevated distress; distress levels peak in terminal stage.

- Gender: Female caregivers are more likely to exhibit increased distress.
- Socioeconomic status: Lower-status individuals have fewer resources and may suffer more distress from overload.
- Development life stage: Younger caregivers are more emotionally distressed; elderly caregivers are more physically distressed, fatigued from caregiving.
- Communication: Rigid or closed style may hinder crucial cancer related discussions in family.
- Social support: Lack of social support increases likelihood of distress.

Adapted from Sales E, Schulz R, Biegel D. Predictors of strain in families of cancer patients: A review of the literature. J Psychosoc Onc 1992;10:1–26.

cious use of anxiolytics, such as the benzodiazepines, alprazolam, and lorazepam for short-term treatment or certain antihistamines such as hydroxyzine. Chronic anxiety can be treated with the benzodiazepine clonazepam or with the serotonergic antidepressants sertraline and paroxetine. Buspirone may also be useful in mild to moderate anxiety but takes several weeks to become effective.

The Family of the Cancer Patient

Cancer affects the constellation of a patient's world. Central to this is life with family members. Family members experience many of the same emotions as the patients themselves, including feelings of depression and anxiety. In addition, family members may exhibit feelings of anger, resentment, and guilt over the illness and the subsequent reorganization that occurs in the family as it accommodates to the cancer experience. Distress in family members likely contributes to that of the patient and may require medical or psychological attention in its own right.

The stress and demands that families face are numerous. Because of economic pressures, much of the care given to patients has shifted from medical personnel to the families. Today, patients have shorter hospital stays, and outpatient centers for the cancer patient have greatly expanded. Ambulatory care services now routinely provide adjuvant cancer treatment, and even procedures such as a bone marrow transplant, traditionally done during an in-patient hospitalization, are performed with greater frequency on an outpatient basis. Community and nursing care resources have diminished, putting much of the burden on the family for coordinating care. Because spouses and adult daughters tend to be the primary

caretakers, they are faced with the task of accommodating to the patient's treatment needs while meeting the demands of their own daily routines. Despite these constraints, most families genuinely desire and are motivated to care for their ill relative and manage to marshal a robust response. However, roughly one third of families struggle with less success and will experience clinically significant levels of emotional distress and psychosocial disruption.

The Caregiver

A number of factors related to the patient's illness appear to increase the risk of caretaker maladjustment. For example, the site of a patient's cancer appears to be related to caregiver distress. Caretakers of a patient who has lung or brain cancer appear to be most emotionally distressed, likely because of the severity of symptoms (e.g., shortness of breath, confusion), which may engender feelings of fear and helplessness within the caregiver and alienation from the patient. High demands, of either an instrumental or an emotional nature, placed on the caregiver owing to a decrease in the patient's performance status also appear to contribute to elevated distress levels. In fact, as caregiver demands increase, distress levels appear to rise, making periods of active or terminal care the most highly stressful periods. Caregivers of patients with a poor prognosis or advanced disease also reveal greater distress levels, distress peaking in the terminal stage of a patient's disease process. Overall, patient and caregiver distress levels generally tend to be moderately related to one another. Patients who show increased levels of emotional distress in regard to their diagnosis or their treatment may have caregivers who are experiencing elevated distress levels themselves.

There are also a number of family contextual variables that predict increased distress. Chief among these is gender, female caregivers tending to be more emotionally distressed than male caregivers. However, some mental health professionals assert that the gap between gender distress reactions may be smaller than is believed, as men may be hiding their feelings to protect their partners and perhaps themselves from the emotional nature of the experience. Another factor related to distress levels is socioeconomic status. Caregivers of lower socioeconomic levels appear to have elevated levels of distress, as they tend to have less knowledge of or access to resources that might relieve some of the caretaking burden.

An additional component related to adjustment is the family's developmental life stage. In this domain, younger couples appear to be most at risk for elevated distress levels. Younger couples that have recently separated from their primary families and begun developing a life with their partner may exhibit difficulties in altering family roles. Younger couples have less security in newly defined roles and are more threatened by change. They experience increased disruption from assistance and contributions of others outside of the dyad. Others, including members of the partner's family of origin, may easily usurp problem solving and decision making by the partner. In addition, financial concerns may affect the young couples' ability to maintain their level of independence.

During the middle stages of partnership, members are more established in their familial roles and are actively cultivating their professional and personal lives. In addition, couples often have the additional nurturing and financial obligations of children. Couples who experience cancer at this stage are at an increased risk of role overload. Families with rigid or traditional roles may experience particular disruption as they have difficulty utilizing flexible role assignment and a reallocation of responsibilities to meet the needs of the cancer situation.

Older couples tend to be easily overwhelmed and fatigued by the addition of partner caretaking responsibilities. Elderly spouses often feel burdened by the physical demands of care and perceive themselves as having limited personal resources. They may also be dealing with problems associated with their own aging process. In fact, one of the moderating variables in the distress of the elderly is the health status of the caretaker. While couples that are older likely have adult children, the physical proximity and developmental life stage of the children may override their ability to provide meaningful secondary support. Thus, many of the caretaking responsibilities tend to fall on the spouse, who may be hindered by limited physical, social, and financial resources.

Within each family system, the quality of the patient–partner relationship and the communication between the couple may facilitate or obstruct the adjustment process. Families with open styles of communication are more likely to share feelings and are able to talk explicitly about the challenges of cancer. They are better able to negotiate illness-induced roles and share in decision making. Although cancer concerns appear to be best resolved through active and open communication between partners, the ability to utilize and tolerate this type of communication depends on the premorbid style of relating. For example, couples that are more comfortable communicating through nonverbal methods are unlikely to deviate greatly from this pattern in the face of cancer and may require professional assistance if this style interferes with effective functioning.

As with patients, the caretaker's use of a social support network may assist in tempering the level of emotional distress. This is an often neglected area, as family, friends, and professionals frequently call on the partner to be the central source of social support for the patient, without consideration being given to validating or augmenting their own social needs. In addition, caregivers frequently lack the time to develop or take advantage of potentially supportive relationships. In this domain, men, whether as patients or partners, are unlikely to turn to other people as a method of coping with illness-related concerns. Men tend to derive their primary support from their female partners. Women, however, whether as patient or partner, tend to seek outside support and to turn to other women for comfort. Thus, men as well as women tend to rely on and benefit most from women as their means of social support.

The Children

The ages and reactions of children in the home can also contribute to the adjustment of the family. Children are exquisitely sensitive to the reactions of others, in large part because they are dependent on others to have their needs met. As a consequence, children can sense when parents are worried or preoccupied with something other than themselves. They can easily misinterpret this parental behavior and may misbehave. Children also have fertile imaginations and, if not informed about the cancer and the effects of treatment on the parent, may imagine that things are worse than they actually are.

Very young children under the age of 2 have little verbal skill with which to articulate or comprehend what is going on around them. They tend to thrive on routine and are focused on how things make them feel and how to control things that happen around them.

They are afraid of separation from their parents and benefit from continued closeness and attention.

Generally, children between the ages of 2 and 6 are better able to understand illness but may think of it in terms of being contagious, like the flu or a cold. Children at this age are egocentric, meaning that they tend to view things only from their own perspective. They are unable to grasp the concept that things occur in life that have nothing to do with them. They tend to link events to themselves and to one particular event. Children at this age may believe that they did something to cause their parent's illness and that they are being punished for their transgressions. Reassuring children that nothing they or anyone else did has caused the cancer is important at this age. In addition, informing children that cancer is a serious and noncontagious disease is helpful, as children might worry that they or the healthy parent will also contract the illness. Simple explanations about the disease and treatment are useful, such as conveying the situation in terms of a fight between good and bad cells.

Children between the ages of 7 and 12 are less likely to believe that the illness has something to do with them. They are better able to see a perspective other than their own and thus can see relationships between things. They can handle information about the cancer and treatment that is more sophisticated. Children in this age range also begin to think about death and dying and understand that death is irreversible. They may harbor fears that the ailing parent will die. Parents with a child of this age might need to prepare themselves to discuss death. An open and honest approach is best, and if cure is not a reasonable expectation, then an acknowledgment of the possibility of death should be tempered by optimism and hope through treatment.

Children age 12 and beyond have abstract reasoning skills and are able to understand complex relationships. At this age, children are beginning to move away from the family toward their peers in an effort to gain independence and a separate identity. Cancer in a parent at this age may disrupt this developmental stage and create a conflict between dependence and auton-omy. Children at this age are vulnerable to becoming overly involved with the ill parent or, conversely, becoming avoidant and/or acting out. Maintaining a balance between spending time with the family and spending time with friends is crucial.

Ethnic and Cultural Issues

Ongoing demographic changes in the U.S. population make it mandatory that attention be paid to cultural issues in dealing with cancer patients. A patient's ethnic and cultural background and subsequent identification play a critical role in how the patient and his or her family interpret and respond to the illness experience and the health care provider.

The Hispanic population is the fastest-growing minority population in the United States, although there is great diversity in the subgroups that make up this population. Regardless of country of origin, Marin has identified cultural values that are shared by most Hispanics:

- *Familismo*: the importance of the family to the individual
- *Colectivismo*: the importance of friends and extended family members such as godmothers (madrinas) and godfathers (padrinos)
- *Simpatia*: the act of being polite and respectful, not confrontational
- *Personalismo*: the preference to be with other persons of the same ethnic group
- *Respeto*: the act of upholding one's own integrity without damaging another person

For the Hispanic cancer patient, illness is not an individual issue, but one that affects the extended family and the community. Within that larger familial and communal system, status and hierarchy are of significance. In many Hispanic families, even those that appear to be well acculturated, the husband and other senior members of the extended family might still make decisions for all members of the family. In dealing with cancer, this might translate into demanding that the patient not be informed of a cancer diagnosis, making treatment or no-treatment decisions for female and

---

DIAGNOSIS

Children's Issues with Illness

- 0–2 years: Fearful of separation from parents; limited ability to profit from discussion; benefit from continued attention and physical closeness
- 2–6 years: May believe they caused cancer in parent; may believe cancer is contagious; are concrete in thinking and benefit from simple explanations
- 7–12 years: Think about death and dying; under-stand that death is irreversible; parent may need to balance doubt (e.g., acknowledgment of death) with optimism (e.g., hope through treatment)
- 12 and beyond: May develop conflict between dependence on family and desire for autonomy; encourage balance between world of family and world of friends

younger members of the family, and not allowing the patient to meet alone with the physician. A common error made by health care team members in interacting with non–English-speaking Hispanic patients is asking children in the family to translate health-related information. The result is that information provided to the patient is often diluted or incorrect, and senior family members might perceive the health care provider as lacking in respect for involving the children in important decisions. It is critical for health care providers to understand and integrate these core Hispanic beliefs into their interpersonal style in order to develop communication patterns and therapeutic practices that will be of benefit to patients.

Another large minority group are African-Americans. Their core values have historical roots in Africa and have been defined by Sudarkasa as follows:

- *Respect*: the respect of others toward elders or leaders in the community
- *Responsibility*: being accountable for self and for those less fortunate in the extended family and community
- *Reciprocity*: giving back to family and community in return for what has been given (mutual assistance)
- *Restraint*: giving due consideration to the family or community/group when making decisions
- *Reverence*: deep awe and respect first toward God, toward the ancestors, and toward many things in nature
- *Reason*: taking a reasoned approach to settling disputes within the family or the community
- *Reconciliation*: the art of settling differences; that is, putting a matter to rest between two parties

Spirituality is a strong cultural value among African-Americans, and the church has been the single most important organization advocating for improvements in health and education among this ethnic group. Within the church, these core values become actualized. For example, pastors and other church members are often part of the extended family and are key supporters for patients, becoming involved in health care decisions and visiting patients regularly in the hospital. Many African-Americans share a distrust of the health care system based on past negative experiences or related to historical events such as the Tuskegee experiment. Therefore, trust in the health care team becomes an integral component in their response and adherence to a treatment regime.

Tools for a Good Physician–Patient Working Relationship

Physicians spend many years studying the practice of medicine. Inherent in this educational process is a focus on the technical aspects of disease and treatment that aims to eradicate or control illness. Yet illness occurs within the context of the person, whose well-being and quality of life are also affected. Unfortunately, studies indicate that physicians provide limited consideration to quality-of-life issues, frequently overlooking the emotional distress of their patients and underestimating their psychosocial needs. Because of this, a broader picture of the patient within the medical model has come to the foreground, and increasing attention to the nature and quality of the patient–physician relationship has emerged as a means to achieve optimal patient care.

Physicians can begin to attend to patients' psychosocial issues by enhancing their own style of communication within the therapeutic relationship. Good communication begins with the creation of an environment that is conducive to its practice. In speaking with patients, privacy and minimal stimulation should be attempted. Nonverbal behavior should also be monitored, as it imparts basic information to a patient. For example, good eye contact conveys respect and suggests genuine attention to what is being communicated. Similarly, sitting down with the patient, in close proximity and at eye level, projects an atmosphere of mutual cooperation and concern. To demonstrate the importance of these simple behaviors, studies suggest that doctors who pull up a chair to talk with patients are perceived by patients as more concerned and having spent a longer time talking with them than doctors who stand while talking.

When bad news must be imparted to patients, it is best that these conversations take place face to face. Although it might be easier to do otherwise, consider that this is a sensitive discussion that is likely to generate significant emotion. This warrants attention on the physician's part. In addition, this discussion may herald the beginning of a working relationship with a patient, and a therapeutic encounter requires that a physician take the time to talk with a patient. Certainly, patients can be impatient, wanting "the news" as soon as it becomes available. However, if bad news is to be given, consider firing a warning shot on the phone and asking the patient to come into the office. For example, physicians may preliminarily indicate that "the situation is serious and needs to be discussed in person." Such an approach assists in preparing the patient for the ensuing office discussion. Moreover, in the initial meeting, physicians may choose to broach the cancer discussion by first providing a broad explanation of diagnosis and treatment. This provides the patient the opportunity to absorb the cancer diagnosis. A follow-up appointment can then be scheduled to further discuss treatment options and develop a management plan.

Even when patients understand that they have

DIAGNOSIS

Physician–Patient Communication

When giving bad news to patients, the physician should do the following:

- Fire a warning shot on the telephone
- Attempt to talk face-to-face
- Consider breaking up discussion of diagnosis and management plan
- Provide written information about medical treatment and resources

- Engage in shared decision making
- Address feeling states:
  - Reflect or validate affect in the conversation
  - Normalize feelings of distress
  - Inquire directly about the presence of depression and anxiety
- Encourage parents of young children to talk with the children about the cancer and its treatment

---

cancer, they tend to experience anxiety during consultations with physicians and easily forget what has been communicated. In fact, estimates suggest that cancer patients who see their doctors remember only about 25% of what has been discussed. To combat this problem, patients can be encouraged to use strategies that strengthen memory. For example, patients can be told to bring someone with them to the consultations. Another ear at the visit can enhance subsequent retrieval of information and assist in flushing out the needs and problems of the patient in the office visit. Patients can be prompted to tape-record the session so that they can listen to the consultation again at their leisure, although not every physician will feel comfortable with this option. In lieu of this, patients can write down questions prior to an appointment and then write down the answers that are provided in the office visit.

Despite these types of safeguards, patients frequently leave the physician's office uncertain about their diagnosis and prognosis, unclear about the management plan, and confused about the therapeutic intent of treatment. To supplement verbal discussions with patients, physicians might consider providing written information to patients. Pamphlets are available from numerous organizations at reasonable fees that provide basic information about different types of cancers and the treatments employed. There are also some very good books, as well as Internet Web sites, from reputable authorities that discuss general and/or specific cancer issues. Physicians might wish to maintain a listing of educational and psychological resources that can be given to patients to direct them appropriately. Written materials and resource lists have the advantage of being available to patients when they leave the office and can be read when their anxiety level is reduced. While there is individual variability among peoples' informational needs and these needs may vary over time, written information is often unthreatening, as patients can choose when and how much of the material to review. Additionally, family members have something they may also utilize. The general population has little knowledge about biology and medical terminology. Much of what people know comes from the media, which may be misleading or inaccurate. Patients who wish to know more appreciate any direction and screening of resources that physicians can give them.

Similar to the individual variation that occurs in informational needs is that of participation in medical decisions. In this regard, Fallowfield et al have written about the concept of shared decision making between the patient and the physician. In one study, physicians working with breast cancer patients recommended mastectomies, another group recommended lumpectomy and radiation, and a third group offered a choice, discussing the pros and cons of each alternative. Patients who had doctors that discussed both options and allowed the patient to choose were more psychologically adjusted over the year follow-up. This finding suggests that patients benefit from being given some control over their treatment. In considering this approach however, be aware that taking an active role in treatment decisions can be affected by variables such as culture, socioeconomic status, and age. That is, certain cultures, patients of lower socioeconomic status, and the elderly might be more comfortable with and predisposed to allowing the physician to take charge. Whatever the case, each patient benefits from options and reasons for treatment, whether as a means to involve them in decision making or to help them to understand the physician's decisions.

Because physicians receive very little education in counseling, one of the most confusing and awkward situations can be addressing the emotions and psychosocial needs of cancer patients. Physicians might wish to begin these types of discussions with open-ended questions (e.g., "How are you feeling?"). When patients respond, avoid the temptation to address the first thing that the patient says, which might not be the primary concern. Instead, use statements that are facilitative or encouraging to get sufficient information. Think about what emotion the patient might be expressing, and comment on it (e.g., "You sound nervous about the surgery."). Reflecting feelings indicates that you are able to see things from the patient's perspective. Another technique is to validate the existence of a particular feeling. For example, when a patient cries, a comment such as "I know this is difficult. It's okay to cry." allows the patient to feel appreciated for what he or she might be experiencing. Yet another strategy is normalizing the existence of emotions. This helps patients to feel as if they are not alone or abnormal in their feelings (e.g., "Many people have a difficult time coping with the loss of a breast. It takes time to adjust."). Overall, the goal when talking about feelings is not to solve a problem. Feelings are not solved; they are handled, usually slowly and over time. As such, physicians might choose to follow up these types of conversations about emotions with reassuring statements that indicate partnership and support through the treatment process.

When discussing feelings of distress, inquire directly about clinical levels of depression and anxiety (e.g., "Are you feeling depressed most of the time?" "Are you bothered by feelings of intense anxiety?"). Assess accordingly, and consider whether medication and/or mental health assistance is warranted. Sometimes, patients resist when physicians suggest a mental health referral, worrying that the doctor believes they are abnormal or is giving up on them. Therefore, framing these types of referrals as useful adjuncts to adjustment and coping will assist in allaying patient fears.

Finally, when patients have young children, encourage them to talk with the children about the cancer. In general, it is best to tell children about the situation sometime after the diagnosis, as children recognize a change in routine and sense that something is wrong. Age-appropriate information about cancer and treatment should be provided. Furthermore, all children benefit from being prepared for the effects of treatment on the parent, such as hair loss and fatigue, which might limit the parent's involvement in activities. Children also profit from being reminded or informed what specific people are available to them for what purpose (e.g., grandmother will make dinner during this time). At the same time, children should be given the opportunity to assist the ill parent so that they feel part of the process but are not overburdened with responsibility. Small tasks, such as bringing the ill parent an afternoon sandwich, allow the child to feel helpful.

References

Aranda-Naranjo B, Davis R: Psychosocial and cultural considerations. In Anderson J (ed): A Guide to the Clinical Care of Women with HIV. Washington, DC, USDHHS/HSRA, 2001, pp 280–282.

American Psychiatric Association: Diagnostic and Statistical Manual of Mental Disorders, 4th ed. Washington, DC, American Psychiatric Association, 1994.

Antoni MH, Lehman JM, Kilbourn KM, et al: Cognitive-behavioral stress management intervention decreases the prevalence of depression and enhances benefit finding among women under treatment for early-stage breast cancer. Health Psychol 2001;20:20–32.

Baider L, Kaufman B, Peretz T, et al: Mutuality of fate: Adaptation and psychological distress in cancer patients and their partners. In Baider I, Cooper CI, Kaplan De-Nour A (eds): Cancer and the Family. New York, John Wiley, 1996, pp 173–186.

Carver CS, Pozo C, Harris SD, et al: How coping mediates the effect of optimism on distress: A study of women with early stage breast cancer. J Pers Soc Psychol 1993;65:375–390.

Carver CS, Pozo-Kaderman C, Harris SD, et al: Optimism versus pessimism predicts the quality of women's adjustment to early stage breast cancer. Cancer 1994;73:1213–1220.

Cull A, Stewart M, Altman DG: Assessment of and intervention for psychosocial problems in routine oncology practice. Br J Cancer 1995;72:229–235.

Derogatis LR, Morrow GR, Felting J. The prevalence of psychiatric disorder among cancer patients. JAMA 1983;249:751–757.

Fallowfield L, Hall A, Maguire G, Baum M: Psychological outcomes of different treatment policies in women with early stage breast cancer outside a clinical trial. Br Med J 1991;301:575–580.

Fallowfield L, Jenkins V: Effective communication skills are the key to good cancer care. Eur J Cancer 1999;35:1592–1597.

Ford S, Fallowfield L, Lewis S: Doctor–patient interactions in oncology. Social Sci Med 1996;42:1511–1519.

Geffen J: The Journey Through Cancer: An Oncologist's Seven-Level Program for Healing and Transforming the Whole Person. New York, Crown, 2000.

Keller M, Henrich G, Sellschopp A, Beutel M: Between distress and support: Spouses of cancer patients. In Baider I, Cooper CI, Kaplan De-Nour A (eds): Cancer and the Family. New York, John Wiley, 1996, pp 187–223.

Kobayashi J: Psychiatric issues. In Anderson J (ed): A Guide to the Clinical Care of Women with HIV. Washington, DC: USDHHS/HSRA, 2001, p 307.

Lederberg MS, Massie MJ: Psychosocial and ethical issues in the care of cancer patients. In DeVita VT, Hellman S, Rosenberg SA (eds): Cancer: Principles and Practice of Oncology, 4th ed. Philadelphia, JB Lippincott, 1993, p 2448.

Lowenstein A, Gilbar O: The perception of caregiving burden on the part of elderly cancer patients, spouses and adult children. Families Syst Health 2000;18:337–346.

McDaniel JS, Musselman DL, Porter MR, et al: Depression in patients with cancer: Diagnosis, biology and treatment. Arch Gen Psychiatry 1995;52:89–99.

Marin G: AIDS prevention among hispanics: Needs, risk behaviors and cultural values. Public Health Rep 1989;104:411–415.

Massie MJ, Holland JC: Overview of normal reactions and prevalence of psychiatric disorders. In: Holland JC, Rowland JH (eds): Handbook of Psychooncology. Psychological Care of the Patient with Cancer. New York: Oxford University Press, 1989, pp 273–282.

Massie MJ, Krivo S: Depressive disorders. In Holland JC (ed): Psycho-Oncology. New York, Oxford University Press, 1998, pp 518–540.

Noyes R Jr, Holt CS, Massie MJ: Anxiety disorders. In Holland JC (ed): Psycho-Oncology. New York, Oxford University Press, 1998, pp 548–563.

Roter D, Fallowfield L: Principles of training medical staff in psychosocial and communication skills. In Holland JC (ed): Psycho-Oncology. New York, Oxford University Press, 1998, pp 1074–1082.

Sales E, Schulz R, Biegel D: Predictors of strain in families of cancer patients: A review of the literature. J Psychosoc Oncol 1992;10:1–26.

Spencer SM, Carver CS, Price AA: Psychological and social factors in adaptation. In Holland JC (ed): Psycho-Oncology. New York: Oxford University Press, 1998, pp 211–222.

Spiegel D: Living Beyond Limits: New Hope and Help for Facing Life-Threatening Illness. New York, Random House, 1993.

Stewart MA: Effective physician–patient communication and health outcomes: A review. Can Med Assoc J 1996;152:1423–1433.

Sudarkasa N: The Strength of our Mothers. African and African American Families: Essays and Speeches. Trenton, N.J., Africa World Press, 1996.

Chapter 121
Male Sexual Dysfunction

Abraham Morgentaler

Sexual function is a key component of quality of life for most men. In the not-so-distant past, loss of libido and erectile dysfunction were not considered medically important issues in general and even less so for the patient with cancer. There were several reasons for this, including widespread awkwardness regarding sexuality in health care providers and patients alike. A common but misguided notion prevailed that sexuality was of particularly limited importance for the cancer patient. Although the debilitating effects of cancer and its treatment may reduce sexual desire or pleasure for some individuals, many cancer patients continue to desire sexual activity. Indeed, within any stable, loving relationship, sex may be one of the most gratifying and relationship-enhancing activities that couples enjoy together, and this continues to be true even when one partner is afflicted with cancer.

Advances in cancer treatment, in terms of both prognosis and reduced morbidity, have made it even more important that sexual issues be addressed for the patient and, where appropriate, for the patient's partner. As men live longer following treatment, it becomes essential to address quality-of-life issues, including sexual function. This is particularly true for younger individuals but applies to many otherwise vigorous men of a certain maturity as well. A good example is the young man in his early twenties who is cured of testis cancer following retroperitoneal lymph node dissection. An inability to achieve antegrade ejaculation directly affects his hopes to have a family. The clinician must therefore be cognizant of the range of sexual dysfunction that can occur in men, whether or not these effects are associated with cancer therapy, and the options for treatment.

Classification of Male Sexual Dysfunction

There are several types of sexual dysfunction in men. Erectile dysfunction refers to the inability of the penis to achieve or maintain sufficient rigidity for satisfac-

tory intercourse. Ejaculatory dysfunction may refer to either the timing of ejaculation or an abnormality in the actual process of emitting seminal fluid. Altered libido refers to the subjective experience of sexual desire. This may be a change in how often an individual experiences desire, a reduced overall level of desire, or a diminished ability to experience sexual pleasure. Reduced libido can be a primary symptom but also commonly occurs in men when other aspects of their sexuality are impaired.

Evaluation

When a man presents with sexual dysfunction, it is critical to define the exact problem. Table 121-1 lists the common causes of sexual dysfunction and their frequency. Many men and women are uncomfortable talking about sex and the pertinent body parts and functions. This applies to health providers as well. The details of the problem might thus be lost in a misleading discussion that relies on euphemisms. Using proper terminology in a matter-of-fact, nonjudgmental manner frees the patient to use similar language. It is enormously useful to ask directly the question "What happens when you try to have sex?" The answers to this question are usually quite specific, for example "My penis doesn't become hard enough for intercourse" or "I don't try anymore because I just don't have the interest," directing the clinician toward the appropriate type of problem.

Once the problem has been identified, the history focuses on possible causes. When did the problem begin? Was the onset sudden, or has it been a gradual process? What events, medical or personal, might have occurred around the time of onset of difficulties and might therefore be contributory? In particular, were any new medications or treatments initiated around the time the problem began? Risk factors for erectile dysfunction include diabetes; hypertension; smoking; elevated cholesterol and lipid levels; coronary or peripheral vascular disease; obesity; radiation

Table 121-1 ■ Etiology of Male Sexual Dysfunction

Psychogenic	15%
Neurologic	5%
Arterial	5%
Veno-occlusive dysfunction	60%
Hormonal	15%

therapy to the abdomen or pelvis; chemotherapy; hormonal therapy; certain kinds of pelvic surgery, such as radical prostatectomy, radical cystoprostatectomy, abdominoperineal resections, and low colectomies; and vascular procedures involving the internal iliac arteries. Renal and hepatic failure and various neuropathies are also associated with erectile dysfunction.

Medications are a frequent contributor to sexual dysfunction. Many cancer patients take antidepressants, which can have a major effect on several aspects of male sexuality. The serotonin reuptake inhibitors are associated with diminished libido and delayed or absent ejaculation, with erectile dysfunction as an isolated complaint occurring less frequently. Many antihypertensive medications contribute to erectile dysfunction and/or diminished desire, the beta-blocker class being most prominent among these. Hormonal therapy for prostate cancer produces castrate levels of testosterone, resulting in greatly diminished libido and erectile dysfunction in a majority of cases. The list of other medications associated with sexual dysfunction is long. However, just because a man takes a medication that is known to cause sexual dysfunction in some cases does not necessarily mean that the medication is the culprit. For instance, if a man develops new erectile dysfunction while having taken a stable dose of a beta-blocker for 10 years, he should not be diagnosed as having medication-induced erectile dysfunction. To attribute causality to the medication, there must be a temporal relationship between starting a new medication or increasing the dose of an existing medication and the onset of the problem.

Evaluation of Sexual Dysfunction in a Cancer Patient

What about cancer itself as a cause of sexual dysfunction? Erectile dysfunction and diminished libido frequently occur in men during any major illness, especially those causing diminished vigor. Direct impact on male sexual function can also result from any aspect of cancer that affects the brain, the vascular system, the endocrine system, or the spinal cord and peripheral nerves. Anemia may contribute to

erectile dysfunction. Spinal cord compression by tumor or vertebral fractures may contribute to erectile dysfunction but will also generally be associated with bladder or bowel function abnormalities, since those structures share innervation via S2–4 roots.

Cancer treatments can directly cause sexual dysfunction. Bone marrow transplant recipients appear vulnerable to erectile dysfunction, presumably owing to radiation effect to the pelvis. Neurotoxicity from chemotherapeutic agents can cause erectile dysfunction as well as reduced penile sensation, the latter resulting in difficulty achieving orgasm.

Treatments of genitourinary malignancies are associated with a high rate of sexual dysfunction owing to the close relationship of affected structures with male reproductive anatomy and physiology. The nerves controlling erection run adjacent to the prostate and are therefore frequently injured during radical prostatectomy and cystoprostatectomy, even when a surgical attempt is made to spare the nerves (see Chapter 87). The result is loss of rigidity. However, the vast majority of these men are still able to achieve an orgasm, albeit with a soft penis, and penile sensitivity, libido, and intensity of the orgasm usually remain intact. Radiation therapy for prostate or bladder cancer is also associated with a high rate of erectile dysfunction, although the onset may be delayed for 12 to 24 months. Brachytherapy, with implantation of radioactive seeds into the prostate, was lauded as a potentially less morbid treatment, but recent data indicate that there is still a significant rate of erectile dysfunction with this treatment. Antihormonal therapy is a common treatment for metastatic prostate cancer, and since it reduces testosterone to castrate or near-castrate levels, treated men note reduced libido, difficulty achieving orgasm, and erectile dysfunction. Retroperitoneal lymph node dissection performed for testis cancer can cause damage to the sympathetic nerves controlling ejaculation. The absence of an ejaculate with orgasm may reflect retrograde ejaculation, with semen going into the bladder, or absence of seminal emission, in which there is failure to deposit seminal fluid within the prostatic urethra.

Physical Examination

The examination of the man who is complaining of sexual dysfunction is straightforward. It is useful to obtain an overall sense of the patient's general health and vitality. The presence of gynecomastia may indicate an endocrinopathy. The phallus is examined for firm subcutaneous nodules signifying Peyronie's disease. Soft, small testes indicate testicular insufficiency and probable diminished serum testosterone

DIAGNOSIS

Diagnostic Approach to Male Sexual Dysfunction

Diagnostic Studies Can Be Performed for the Following Reasons:

1. To identify modifiable risk factors, such as hypercholesterolemia
2. To determine etiology
3. To aid in choice of treatment
4. For "need to know" by patient

The following algorithm is used for diagnostic studies:

Level 1: Blood tests only: Glucose, hematocrit, cholesterol, prolactin testosterone and free testosterone (if low, check gonadotrophins)

If low gonadotrophins or high prolactin, obtain pituitary MRI

Level 2: For Viagra failures, young age, possible psychogenic etiology, legal cases, or "need to know"
   Nocturnal penile tumescence and rigidity monitoring
   Penile sensation versus biothesiometry
   Penile brachial index
   Penile ultrasound with pharmacologic injection

Level 3: Pelvic arteriogram for highly selected, young individuals who are candidates for penile revascularization secondary to traumatic arterial injury

levels, although this may also occur with palpably normal testes. Femoral and peripheral pulses provide information regarding the arterial tree, but it must be emphasized that the specific arteries involved in erection cannot be directly assessed by physical examination. Anal tone, as well as the bulbocavernosus reflex, reflects the integrity of the S2–4 nerves, which are involved in erection.

Evaluation

Testing is tailored to the individual and his circumstances. For example, a presentation of diminished libido or anorgasmia following initiation of antidepressant therapy requires no studies at all. It is to be expected that these symptoms will resolve with change of medication or when such treatment is no longer needed. Minimal to no testing is required also for clear-cut situations, such as loss of erections following radical prostatectomy, in which injury to the erection-inducing nerves is common and the etiology is not in question.

Often, however, the history is less clear, and a basic evaluation should be performed. This should include blood tests for complete blood count (CBC), serum glucose, lipids, total and free testosterone, and prolactin. In some instances, it may be useful to obtain liver and renal function tests, as well as levels of luteinizing hormone.

Further studies are indicated in selected cases. Nocturnal erections can be measured on an ambulatory basis by a portable device that provides a computer printout revealing the duration and rigidity of erections that occur in association with REM (rapid eyeball movement) sleep. These studies are helpful to determine whether erectile dysfunction is psychogenic or organic, since the patient is unaware of the presence of erections during sleep. A complaint of erectile dysfunction with normal sleep erections suggests a psychogenic etiology, for example. Penile blood pressure and sensation can be determined in the office with appropriate instrumentation. Finally, in some men, it may be worthwhile to perform penile ultrasound in combination with injection of vasoactive medication to determine the integrity of arterial blood flow during a pharmacologically induced erection.

Treatment

Not all men with sexual dysfunction desire treatment. Some men are curious about their condition and are interested only in an explanation. Others are worried that the onset of a problem such as erectile dysfunction indicates a more serious medical condition. Some may have a desire to be treated but are not yet prepared to proceed with treatment because of personal circumstances, such as having an ill partner at home.

If an offending cause can be identified, for example, a specific medication, it is best to remove this cause as the initial treatment if this can be done safely. However, many men must continue with their medication regimen for general health considerations, such as hypertension or coronary disease, and treatment of sexual dysfunction must be considered in light of the individual's overall medical condition.

First-line therapy for men with erectile dysfunction is the oral medication sildenafil. Sildenafil is effective in approximately 45% to 80% of men, depending on etiology and medical condition. It must be taken at least 30 to 60 minutes prior to sexual activity and works best if taken on an empty stomach. Side effects include headache, nasal congestion, dyspepsia, flush-

TREATMENT

Management of Erectile Dysfunction

1. Sildenafil unless contraindicated by nitrate use
2. If sildenafil ineffective or contraindicated:
   Penile injection therapy with vasoactive medications
   Intraurethral alprostadil
   Vacuum erection device
3. Penile prosthesis

ing, and transient changes in color vision. The only absolute contraindication to sildenafil use is concurrent use of nitrates owing to the hypotensive effect of this combination. This includes men who carry nitroglycerin but use it sparingly or not at all, since sexual activity may precipitate angina. Caution should be exercised in prescribing sildenafil to men who have significant heart failure or are on complex antihypertensive regimens.

Sildenafil works only if the nerves controlling erection are intact. Therefore, there is little hope of success in men who have undergone a non–nerve-sparing radical prostatectomy (Figure 121-1).

For those in whom sildenafil fails or in whom it is contraindicated, second-line therapy consists of vacuum erection devices, penile injections, or intraurethral suppositories. Vacuum devices consist of a plastic cylinder positioned over the penis with a pump that creates a partial vacuum, thus drawing blood into the penis until it is engorged and reasonably firm. A band is then placed over the base of the penis, trapping blood in the penis and thus maintaining rigidity. The cylinder is removed, and the man engages in intercourse with the band on the base of the penis. This treatment is noninvasive and is successful in a majority of cases of erectile dysfunction, regardless of etiology. However, many men and their partners find the treatment cumbersome and the quality of the erection suboptimal.

Penile injections of a vasoactive medication, usually alprostadil, is well tolerated and highly effective in producing firm, enduring erections. Erections last 0.5 to 3 hours, depending on individual response to the drug. The medication is injected by the patient into the side of the penis, delivering medication into one of the corpora cavernosa. A firm erection is obtained within 10 minutes in approximately 75% to 80% of men. Disadvantages include patient awkwardness regarding self-injections and medication-related pain, which occurs in 20% of men. A small percentage of men develop fibrotic nodules at the site of injection. Priapism can occur if too much medication is used. Many men are initially reluctant to consider penile injections but quickly become pleased with the treatment after an initial office injection demonstrates that little or no discomfort is involved. Alprostadil is also available as a urethral suppository. This treatment is less effective than injections but may be useful for the individual who is needle-phobic.

The penile prosthesis is an excellent and underused treatment for selected individuals with erectile dysfunction. Hollow cylinders filled with saline are placed within the paired corpora cavernosa, and a pump is placed within the scrotum. The man initiates the erection by squeezing the pump, transferring saline into the penile cylinders. This mimics a normal erection, with fluid under pressure within the proper chambers. Squeezing a different area restores flaccidity. Satisfaction rates exceed 90% for men and their partners. The cosmetic appearance with inflatable devices is quite normal, allowing men to shower at the gym, for instance, without the implant being noticeable. Furthermore, the risks of infection and mechanical failure are low.

Men with diminished libido in association with low testosterone are best served by testosterone sup-

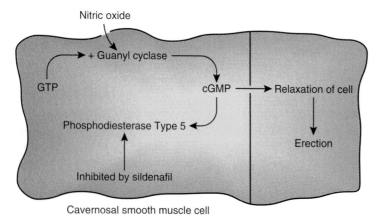

Figure 121-1 ■ Biochemical mechanism of action of sildenafil.

plementation, since this may restore all aspects of sexuality rather than only the rigidity issue addressed by sildenafil. However, testosterone therapy is contraindicated in men with a history of prostate cancer. In some cases, the combination of testosterone for libido with some other treatment for erectile dysfunction, such as sildenafil, provides the best treatment.

Men with retrograde ejaculation or failure of seminal emission require treatment for attempts at achieving a pregnancy with their partners. Alpha-adrenergic medications such as pseudoephedrine are taken one hour prior to sexual activity. Vibratory stimulation may be useful for men unable to achieve orgasm, usually due to neurologic injury or disease. Surgical extraction of sperm is possible for men who do not respond to these treatments.

Conclusions

Sexuality is important to men, women, and their relationships, regardless of whether an individual has been diagnosed with cancer. Patients appreciate the willingness of their physicians to listen to their sexual problems and are grateful for any help that can be offered to improve their quality of life in this regard. The compassionate clinician should therefore inquire about sexual function and initiate an evaluation and treatment when indicated.

References

Feldman HA, Goldstein I, Hatzichristou DG, et al: Impotence and its medical and psychosocial correlates: Results of the Massachusetts male aging study. J Urol 1994;151:54–61.

Goldstein I, Lue TF, Padma-Nathan H, et al: Oral sildenafil in the treatment of erectile dysfunction. N Engl J Med 1998;338:1397–1404.

Karacan I: Clinical value of nocturnal erection in the prognosis and diagnosis of impotence. Med Aspects Hum Sex 1970;4:227–234.

Khoudary K, DeWolf WC, Bruning CO III, Morgentaler A: Immediate sexual rehabilitation in radical prostatectomy patients by simultaneous placement of penile prosthesis: Initial results in 50 patients. Urology 1997;50:395–399.

Laumann EO, Paik A, Rosen RC: Sexual dysfunction in the United States: Prevalence and predictors. JAMA 1999;281:537–544.

Morgentaler A: Male impotence. Lancet 1999;354:1713–1718.

Morgentaler A, Bruning CO III: Iatrogenic male sexual dysfunction. American Urological Association Update Series 1996;15:70–76.

NIH Consensus Development Panel on Impotence: JAMA 1998;270:83–90.

Schramek P, Dorninger R, Waldhauser M, et al: Prostaglandin E1 in erectile dysfunction: Efficiency and incidence of priapism. Br J Urol 990;65:68–71.

Chapter 122
Symptom Management

Janet L. Abrahm

Introduction

Symptom management is crucial to the success of any program of care of patients with cancer or hematologic diseases. Symptoms must be controlled if these patients are to undergo staging procedures, endure treatment, and die in comfort. Symptoms must be controlled to enable patients to fulfill their familial and community roles, achieve their goals, and prepare their legacies—and they can be. With appropriate assessment and management, often utilizing home health or hospice teams, pain, for example, can be controlled for over 90% of patients using only oral or transdermal medications. The assessment and management of many of the most common symptoms experienced by patients with hematologic and oncologic disorders during active treatment and as the last days approach, as well as the role of hospice in patients with advanced cancer, will also be reviewed.

Pain Assessment

Pain assessment is the cornerstone of pain management. All the basic elements are included in the 1994 Agency for Health Care Policy and Research (AHCPR) guideline, "Management of Cancer Pain."

AHCPR Guideline

Health professionals should *ask* about the pain, and *the patient's self-report* should be the primary source of assessment.

Patients, their families, and their health care providers continue to underestimate pain. These differences in perception can obstruct clinicians' pain relief efforts. Cancer patients and patients with painful hematologic conditions such as hemophilia or sickle cell anemia might be reluctant to report their pain to providers because they suspect that they will not be believed. They might be reluctant to admit that they need a stronger opioid to relieve their pain because they fear that they will be treated as though they are drug addicts. Providers might also harbor cultural stereotypes that affect how they interpret patients' pain complaints. Black and Hispanic cancer patients, patients with a history of drug abuse, women, the elderly, and the cognitively impaired are more likely to have their pain underestimated and undertreated.

Patients with acute pain are usually believed because they appear uncomfortable and anxious and are often sweating. But patients with chronic pain do not "look like" they are in pain. Their complaints often seem out of proportion to the amount of disease that can be documented by physical exam or X-rays. Patients with severe arthritis or bone pain from sickle cell disease, hemophilia, or metastatic breast cancer, for example, have a normal pulse and blood pressure but usually guard the parts that hurt and have a generalized lack of spontaneous movement. They might appear anxious or depressed, withdrawn, or angry and might have difficulty relating to others, sleeping, concentrating, or eating. Relieving the pain will eliminate these functional and behavioral changes and produce profound changes in the life of these patients' quality of life.

Clinicians should assess pain with easily administered rating scales and should document the efficacy of pain relief at regular intervals after starting or changing treatment. Documentation forms should be readily accessible to all clinicians involved in the patient's care.

Patient reports of pain before and after treatment are consistent, reproducible, and reliable. Pain rating scales are subjective, not objective, but are still accurate, and they provide a number that represents the intensity of the patient's pain. Physicians and other health care professionals can judge the patient's response to pain therapy by noting how the pain intensity number changes.

Equally important, they can ask patients whether that degree of pain relief is satisfactory to them. For some patients, a pain rating of 5 on a scale from 0 (no pain) to 10 (the worst pain) is satisfactory. These

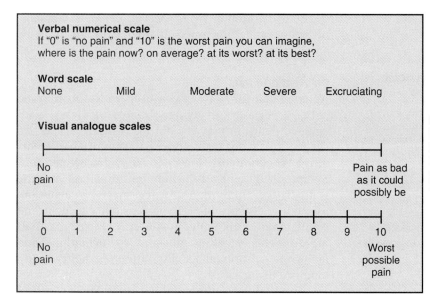

Verbal numerical scale
If "0" is "no pain" and "10" is the worst pain you can imagine, where is the pain now? on average? at its worst? at its best?

Word scale
None   Mild   Moderate   Severe   Excruciating

Visual analogue scales

No pain ———————————————————— Pain as bad as it could possibly be

0   1   2   3   4   5   6   7   8   9   10
No pain   Worst possible pain

Figure 122-1 ■ Samples of validated pain intensity scales to be used in assessing patients' pain. (From Abrahm JL: Management of pain and spinal cord compression in patients with advanced cancer. Ann Intern Med 1999;131:37–46.)

patients can tolerate the pain better than they can the side effects caused by higher doses of analgesic. For others, a level of 2 or 3 must be achieved.

A visual analog scale, either ruled or unruled, is a common pain assessment tool. It is a 10-cm horizontal or vertical unruled line anchored by numbers or words describing the two extremes of a symptom. In the case of pain, for example, one end would be labeled either "0" or "No pain," and the other would be labeled "10" or "Worst pain" (Figure 122-1). Patients usually need instruction in using the scales, but they can be taught to use them to determine the average, worst, and mildest pain intensity over the preceding few weeks and to measure the effectiveness both of drugs and of nonpharmacologic therapies.

Patients who cannot tell you whether their pain number has changed or cannot give you a word to describe it report changes in their functional levels that indicate the efficacy of the treatment. Common pain-induced alterations include changes in physical activity, mood, walking ability, relationships with others, sleep, and enjoyment of life.

Pain diaries are sometimes needed to assess patients who have so-called breakthrough pains, which are moderate to excruciating acute pains that occur intermittently, often with a background of well-controlled chronic pain. There are three types of breakthrough pains: (1) end-of-dose pain, which is pain that recurs before the next regularly scheduled dose of medication is due; (2) incident pain, which is directly related to an activity (such as turning over in bed); and (3) spontaneous pain, which occurs unpredictably. If the pain recurs four hours before the next sustained-release morphine pill is due (i.e., is end-of-dose pain), for example, the dosing interval can be

decreased from 12 hours to eight hours. Or if a patient's pain reliably exacerbates with movement (i.e., incident pain), an immediate- or short-acting medication can be given before the scheduled activity.

Clinicians should teach patients and their families to use assessment tools in their homes in order to promote continuity of effective pain management across all settings.

The initial evaluation of the pain should include:

- A detailed history, including an assessment of pain intensity and characteristics
- A physical examination
- A psychological and social assessment
- A diagnostic evaluation of signs and symptoms associated with the common cancer pain syndromes

An Assessment of Pain Intensity and Characteristics

To assess pain intensity and characteristics, both the temporal aspects of the pain (Is it acute, chronic, or a breakthrough pain?) and its quality (Is it somatic, visceral, or neuropathic?) must be explored. The quality of cancer pain is often helpful in identifying the site of tissue injury because somatic, visceral and neuropathic pains all have characteristic presentations. Table 122-1 indicates the characteristics that can help to distinguish among these types of pain.

Psychological and Social Assessment

Anxiety and depression can exacerbate pain, but it can be difficult to discern which patients with uncontrolled pain due to advanced cancer or disabling hematologic disease are depressed. Many of the usual somatic signs (e.g., anorexia, sleep disturbances,

Table 122-1 ■ Quality of Pain from Varying Sources

Pain Type	Example of Source	Pain Character
Nociceptive		
Somatic	Arthritis, bone metastases	Well-localized, constant, dull, aching, increased by movement
Visceral	Myocardial ischemia Liver metastases	Poorly localized, deep, aching, cramping, twisting, tearing
Neuropathic	Postherpetic neuralgia Brachial, lumbar plexus metastases	Burning, shooting, tingling, electrical, shocklike, lancinating

fatigue, or weight loss) are not helpful because they may be due to the underlying illness. Depressed patients, however, will also feel sad, will cry, might be unable to get pleasure from any activity, or might feel worthless, guilty, hopeless, or helpless.

Social workers can help to discern whether concerns about financial matters or unresolved family issues are troublesome to the patient. In addition, they can help to identify cultural and religious aspects that affect patient and family attitudes toward pain and their ability to communicate their distress. Other social sources of distress arise from the disruptions that occur in a person's normal family structure and in his place in the community when the disease advances.

Social workers can also advise physicians as to which families or patients need more intensive psychological support. They may themselves be able to provide the needed counseling and education in coping skills. If the disease later progresses, the social worker can continue to provide patients and family members with psychological and social assessments, along with intensive counseling or assistance in coping with impending death.

Spiritual Assessment

Patients with chronic moderate to severe pain are in special need of assessment for spiritual or existential distress. As we learned as children, if we are bad, we are punished. Patients who are in pain, therefore, might seek to understand what they are being punished for: "If I hurt this much, I must have done something awful." As a form of atonement, patients might even resist taking pain medication. As one patient reported, "I'd rather burn here than burn there!" Patients such as these might benefit from

spiritual counseling from specially trained chaplains or priests and forgiveness if their suffering is to be ameliorated.

Delirium and Pain

Agitated delirium can be confused with uncontrolled pain, especially in dying patients. Patients with agitated delirium may cry out, be restless, pick at bed sheets, and constantly appear uncomfortable. Delirium has been reported in up to 80% of dying patients. Symptoms of delirium include insomnia and daytime somnolence, nightmares, restlessness or agitation, irritability, distractibility, hypersensitivity to light and sound, anxiety, difficulty in concentrating or marshaling thoughts, fleeting illusions, hallucinations and delusions, emotional liability, attention deficits, and memory disturbances.

The etiology is often multifactorial. Medical causes of delirium include metabolic abnormalities (hypercalcemia, hyperglycemia, and uremia), malnutrition, dehydration, hypoxia, fever, infection, uncontrolled pain or hepatic failure, primary brain tumor, and brain metastases. Medications, especially opioids, nonsteroidal anti-inflammatory drugs (NSAIDs), and high-dose corticosteroids, often contribute to delirium. A comprehensive psychiatric evaluation can detect the presence of delirium and exclude other disorders such as anxiety, minor depression, anger, dementia, or psychosis.

Clinicians should be aware of common pain syndromes; this prompt recognition may hasten therapy and minimize the morbidity of unrelieved pain.

Cancer-related pain syndromes are most often caused by nerve damage either from the cancer therapy or from the cancer itself.

Therapy-Related Pain

Peripheral neuropathies and the postmastectomy, post-thoracotomy, and postradical neck dissection syndromes are the result of therapy for the tumor. Neurotoxic chemotherapy agents such as cisplatin, vinca alkaloids, and the taxanes often induce painful peripheral neuropathies requiring combinations of opioids and neuropathic adjuvants to moderate the pain.

Postmastectomy syndrome occurs in 4% to 10% of all women who have undergone breast surgery, including lumpectomy and more extensive procedures. It can present immediately after the procedure or up to six months later. Patients complain of a burning, constricting feeling in the anterior chest, axilla, and back of the arm, often made worse by movement. A similar syndrome may occur from Port-a-Cath placement in the upper chest area. The pathology is thought to be a neuroma of the T1–T2 intercostobrachial nerve.

Post-thoracotomy pain presents along the incision with tenderness to touch and sensory loss caused by an injury of the intercostal nerve during retraction. Postradical neck syndrome is particularly troublesome when it occurs. It is associated with both sharp, shooting pain and burning and tightness in the area of sensory loss and is due to cervical nerve and plexus injury during surgery.

Unless patients are treated early by anesthesia pain specialists, the pain and the cancer it recalls will remain long after the tumor itself has been removed. The pain can often be eliminated up to six months after the surgery, but if treatment is delayed, the injury to the nerve will affect the central nervous system in such a way that the pain will be much more difficult to ameliorate or eradicate. Prompt, accurate diagnosis and referral are the key to avoiding a lifetime of suffering.

Cancer-Related Pain

In cancer-related syndromes, the cancer usually has spread to the bone or tissue adjacent to the nerve, and as it grows, it compresses the nerve or its blood supply, causing neuropathic pain and eventual nerve death. Recognizing neuropathic pain, therefore, is crucial to identifying patients with lesions of (1) cranial nerves as they exit the skull, (2) nerve plexi (cervical, brachial, and lumbosacral), (3) peripheral nerves, and, (4) most dangerously, the spinal cord (from tumors in vertebral bodies and the epidural space). Rarely, metastases may cause only referred pain, with no localizing findings to the vertebra itself, but if untreated, they will progress to cord compression. Patients with C7 metastases, for example, may present with pain between the scapulae, and those with T12 lesions can present with isolated hip pain.

However, epidural involvement with cancer usually does not cause a unique pain syndrome. It presents most commonly as back pain in the area of the vertebral metastasis, with or without radiation in the distribution of the spinal nerves exiting at that level from the spinal cord. Its very similarity, therefore, to the pain of benign disc disease is a source of dangerous diagnostic confusion. Cancer patients with back pain, abnormal plain films of the spine, and a totally normal neurologic exam have a 70% chance of epidural metastases. A related radiculopathy raises the probability to 90%. A magnetic resonance image (MRI) of the entire spine should be obtained immediately.

Epidural metastatic disease must be diagnosed and treated before any neurologic findings develop because once they appear, they are often irreversible. Only 10% of patients who lose their ability to walk because cancer is compressing their spinal cord will ever walk again. In contrast, 90% of those who are treated while still ambulatory will remain so.

Changes in pain patterns or the development of new pain should trigger a diagnostic evaluation and modification of the treatment plan.

Pain Management

Always consider attempting to reverse the underlying cause of the pain. Recurrent cancer, for example, may still be responsive to surgery, chemotherapy, or radiation therapy. However, during diagnostic testing to define the cause, during specific therapy, or after all disease-related therapies are exhausted, pain can be relieved.

Diagnostic Testing

The frequent diagnostic tests that patients with cancer or hematologic diseases undergo are a common source of distress. Some of that distress can be prevented entirely if the physician anticipates the patient's predictable fears and concerns, provides clear explanations of the nature of the scheduled test, and reports the results promptly. A day's fear of widespread cancer can be averted by warning the elderly patient with a breast lump and extensive arthritis to expect a number of X-rays after a positive staging bone scan and that in all probability, the films will simply reveal her arthritis. A week's delay in telling the patient that the ultrasound showed his computed tomography (CT) discovered "kidney lesion" to be a simple cyst is a week of unnecessary suffering for him and his family. The claustrophobia from magnetic resonance imaging or computed tomography scanners can be approached with hypnotic techniques, special audiotapes, and/or antianxiety agents.

If painful procedures such as venipunctures, puncturing of the skin over implanted ports, intramuscular injections, lumbar punctures, or bone marrows are repeatedly needed, the physician should consider developing a plan with the patient to minimize the associated discomfort. Topical EMLA cream, applied in a mound over the area of skin at least one hour before the planned puncture, can eliminate the pain of the skin puncture. Conscious sedation can be used in the inpatient or outpatient setting for repeated bone marrow aspirations or lumbar punctures.

Nonpharmacologic Therapies

While they do not replace drug therapies, nonpharmacologic techniques are valuable adjuncts and can be very effectively incorporated into symptom management strategies. Although these therapies are most commonly used to manage pain, they are also helpful adjuncts in controlling nausea, vomiting, insomnia, and dyspnea. They require skilled practitioners such as physical and occupational therapists, psychiatrists, and mental health care providers. Because properly trained laypeople can perform many of the techniques, the practitioners often serve both as therapist and as teacher.

Physical techniques include cutaneous interventions such as heat and cold, massage, acupuncture/auriculotherapy, and transcutaneous electrical nerve stimulation (TENS), as well as positioning and exercise.

Cognitive-behavioral interventions are effective in ameliorating a wide range of symptoms, especially pain, anxiety, depression, mild delirium, anorexia, nausea, and dyspnea. If we can change the way a patient views his or her disease or pain, we can lessen the patient's suffering. Education and reassurance of patients and families relieve a great deal of fear and correct potentially harmful misconceptions. Diversion of attention with music, videos, visitors, progressive muscle relaxation and imagery, and hypnosis help patients to escape the problem or to think in alternative ways about it. Biofeedback teaches patients techniques to relieve their own pain by modifying certain physiologic functions. Music therapy offers diversion, distraction, and enhanced relaxation. Psychological counseling and cognitive behavioral training offer support, education, and help in developing coping skills and diminish the anxiety, depression, or delirium that may exacerbate the symptoms. Therapists can help patients feel comfortable relinquishing the "good patient" role and retaining their sense of control and self-esteem even in the hospital setting. Spiritual counseling relieves hidden concerns, reestablishes hope and meaning, and, in the terminal setting, enables patients to resolve issues that might prevent a peaceful death.

Of the cognitive-behavioral therapies, the efficacy of relaxation, hypnosis, and psychological counseling are well established. The physical technique of transcutaneous electrical nerve stimulation has documented utility in nonmalignant pain syndromes, but its effectiveness has not been demonstrated in patients with cancer pain. And much less data support the efficacy of the other nonpharmacologic therapies in relieving cancer pain. Much of the data that are available, such as those on acupuncture and biofeedback, are contradictory.

Pharmacologic Pain Therapy

The WHO Analgesic Ladder

The World Health Organization (WHO) analgesic ladder is an effective, validated tool for providing pain relief for patients with mild, moderate, or severe pain. It suggests using nonopioids such as aspirin, acetaminophen, or nonsteroidal anti-inflammatory drugs for mild pain (Step 1); low-dose oxycodone or the weaker opioids codeine or hydrocodone, used alone or combined with Step 1 agents, or tramadol for moderate pain (Step 2); and potent opioids such as morphine, oxycodone, hydromorphone, fentanyl, or methadone for patients with severe pain (Step 3).

Nonsteroidal Anti-Inflammatory Drugs

Nonsteroidal anti-inflammatory drugs (NSAIDs) are very useful for patients whose pain has an inflammatory component (Table 122-2). Indomethacin is excellent for pleuritis and pericarditis pain and for acute inflammatory arthritides. Other nonsteroidal anti-inflammatory drugs are helpful against bone pain from infarcts or metastases. Ketorolac tromethamine (Toradol) is a particularly useful nonsteroidal anti-inflammatory drug in relieving moderate to severe acute pain. An intramuscular dose of 30 mg ketorolac equals the pain-relieving potency of 12 mg intramuscular morphine; however, ketorolac has all the side effects of the nonsteroidal anti-inflammatory drugs and is not recommended for long-term use. If that degree of pain relief is needed chronically, an opioid agent should be substituted.

Patients with low platelets or defects in platelet function or patients who are receiving systemic anticoagulation can be given either acetaminophen, a cyclooxygenase-2 (Cox-2) selective agent such as celecoxib (Celebrex) or rofecoxib (Vioxx), or a nonacetylating salicylate such as trilisate or disalcid. Because the salicylates are highly albumin bound, patients on Coumadin should be monitored initially for downward dose adjustment.

Patients on nonselective nonsteroidal anti-inflammatory drugs may develop gastrointestinal bleeding, dizziness, confusion, and excessive salt and water retention. To minimize gastrointestinal (GI) toxicity, use acetaminophen or one of the nonsteroidal anti-inflammatory drugs that is selective for Cox-2 (e.g., etodolac, meloxicam, celecoxib, and rofecoxib). These drugs do not cause gastrointestinal toxicity or inhibit platelet function with the same frequency as nonselective nonsteroidal anti-inflammatory drugs. For patients over 70 whose pain is well controlled only by a nonsteroidal anti-inflammatory drug that has a higher risk of inducing gastrointestinal toxicity, consider adding omeprazole 20 mg or misoprostol at 200 µg q.i.d. as tolerated. If clinically appropriate, monitor patients periodically with occult blood testing. Since nonsteroidal anti-inflammatory drugs may exacerbate hypertension and can induce significant hyperkalemia and renal toxicity, electrolytes and renal

Table 122-2 ■ Nonsteroidal Anti-Inflammatory Drugs (NSAIDs)

Chemical Class	Generic Name	Interval	Initial Dose*	Maximum 24-Hour Dose
p-Aminophenol	Acetaminophen	q 4–6 h	650 mg	6000 mg
Salicylates	Aspirin†	q 4–6 h	650 mg	6000 mg
	Choline magnesium salicylate	q 12 h	750–1000 mg	4500 mg
	Salsalate	q 12 h	500–1000 mg	4000 mg
	Diflunisol	q 12 h	500 mg	n/a
Propionic acids	Ibuprofen	q 6 h	400 mg	2400 mg
	Fenoprofen	q 6 h	200 mg	3200 mg
	Ketoprofen	q 6 h	25 mg	300 mg
	Naproxen†	q 12 h	250 mg	1500 mg
	Flurbiprofen	q 12 h	100 mg	300 mg
Acetic acids	Indomethacin†	q 8 h	25 mg	200 mg
	Tolmetin	q 8 h	200 mg	2000 mg
	Diclofenac	q 8 h	25 mg	200 mg
	Sulindac	q 12 h	150 mg	400 mg
	Ketorolac	q 6 h	30–60 mg IM load 15–30 mg IM q 6 h (p.o.: 10 mg q 6 h)	150 mg day 1, 120 mg day 2–7 (po: 40 mg)

*In elderly and in patients with renal insufficiency, start at half to two thirds of these doses.
†Available in suppository form.
Modified from Coyle N, et al: Pharmacologic management in cancer pain. In McGuire DB, Yarbro CH, Ferrell BR (eds): Cancer Pain Management, 2nd ed. Boston: Jones and Bartlett, 1995.

function should be checked within two weeks after a nonsteroidal anti-inflammatory drug is started.

Opioids

Opioids are the mainstay of therapy for patients with pain of moderate or greater intensity. But many patients will be reluctant to accept a prescription for opioids even for severe pain. They and their families might harbor a number of misconceptions about opioids: becoming an addict, "feeling high," "using up" the effective agents and having nothing left if the pain gets worse, and developing refractory constipation. To explore their fears and enhance compliance, they must understand (1) the distinction between tolerance, physical dependence, and psychological addiction; (2) the fact that their chances of addiction are less than 1%; (3) that they will not "feel high" on effective doses; (4) that a feeling of euphoria does not imply that they are misusing medications; and (5) that they will be able to achieve relief using higher doses if the pain worsens.

Step 2 Agents

Codeine, hydrocodone, or oxycodone (5 or 10 mg) combined with acetaminophen, aspirin, or a nonsteroidal anti-inflammatory drug, and tramadol is used for moderate pain. Codeine use, however, may be problematic. Doses over 1.5 mg/kg are not well tolerated, and codeine requires activation by hepatic enzymes that are not present in some patients and that can be inactivated by inhibitors such as cimetidine, quinidine, or fluoxetine.

Tramadol is a nonopioid that binds μ opiate receptors. At recommended doses (not to exceed 400 mg a day), it is safe and as well tolerated as acetaminophen or aspirin plus codeine. Slow titration (i.e., 50 mg increases every three days) minimizes development of nausea, vomiting, dizziness, and vertigo.

Step 3 Agents

For moderate pain that does not respond to Step 2 agents or for severe pain, the Step 3 opioids are indicated (Table 122-3). When using opioids in pain management, (1) use the WHO analgesic ladder, advancing up the ladder if pain persists; (2) prescribe doses high enough to relieve the pain, and give them frequently enough to prevent pain recurrence; (3) provide a rescue dose of a short-acting opioid for unexpected pain exacerbations, using 10% of the total daily opioid dose; and (4) prescribe a scheduled laxative, not a "prn" laxative.

Sustained-release preparations of morphine, oxycodone, or transdermal fentanyl are used to control baseline, continuous pain. Morphine is available in sustained-release pellets in capsules that can be sprinkled on food or suspended in liquid and placed into feeding tubes. A pellet formulation of sustained-release hydromorphone will soon be available. Trans-

Table 122-3 ■ Commonly Used Step 3 Opioids: Preparations Available

Name	Initial Dose (mg)* Oral	Initial Dose (mg)* IM/IV	Dose Interval (hours)	Dose Adjustments Needed	Preparations Available†
				Transdermal, transmucosal	IM/IV, SQ, IR, SR, rectal, liq, liq conc;
Morphine	30	10	3–4	Renal failure	IM/IV/SQ, IR, rectal, liquid, liq conc
Morphine, SR 60	n/a		8–12	Renal/hepatic failure	SR
Morphine, SR 120	n/a		24	Renal/hepatic failure	SR
Hydromorphone	6	1.5	4	Hepatic failure	IM/IV/SQ, IR, rectal
Oxycodone	10	n/a	3–4	Renal failure	IR, liq, liq conc
Oxycodone, SR	20	n/a	12	Renal/hepatic failure	SR
Fentanyl	n/a	50 µg/h	72	Hepatic failure	Transdermal
Methadone	20	10	6–8	Renal/hepatic failure	IM/IV/SQ, IR, liq
Levorphanol	4	2	6–8	Renal/hepatic failure	IM/IV, IR
Oxymorphone	n/a	1	3–4	Renal failure	IM/IV/SQ, rectal
Demerol‡	N/R	100	3	Renal failure	IM/IV, IR

*For patients weighing over 110 pounds who have moderate to severe pain (from AHCPR 94-0593: Management of Cancer Pain: Adults).
†IM/IV: parenteral—suitable for intravenous or intramuscular use; SQ: subcutaneous; IR: oral, immediate release; SR: oral, sustained release; liq: liquid; liq conc: concentrated liquid solution; comb: oral combination preparation with an NSAID (e.g., acetaminophen, aspirin, ibuprofen).
‡Not recommended for use other than for a limited time. See text.
From Abrahm JL: Promoting symptom control in palliative care. Semin Oncol Nürs 1998;14:95–109.

dermal fentanyl diffuses into a skin reservoir, from which it enters the bloodstream. This causes a 12- to 24-hour delay in onset of pain relief and, should toxicity occur, a similar delay in its resolution. Because of this, immediate-release opioids are routinely required for opioid-naive patients who are beginning therapy with transdermal fentanyl.

Immediate-release morphine, oxycodone, or hydromorphone preparations are needed to treat breakthrough pain. Morphine and oxycodone are available in concentrated liquid preparations (20 mg/mL) for oral or sublingual administration. Morphine is offered as a controlled-release suppository and in a topical preparation. These opioid rescue doses start at 10% of the total daily opioid dose, given every one to two hours as needed. The dose of the oral transmucosal fentanyl lozenge must be individually determined.

Methadone, the least expensive opioid, is as safe as sustained-release morphine for advanced cancer patients with normal renal and hepatic function and no cognitive impairment who are cared for by skilled palliative care teams making frequent home visits. The equianalgesic dose of morphine to methadone, however, varies as the dose of morphine increases. Dose ratios vary from 4 : 1 at morphine doses of 30 to 90 mg to 6 : 1 at 90 to 300 mg morphine and 8 : 1 at doses of more than 300 mg morphine.

Meperidine is not indicated for repeated dosing in patients with chronic severe pain. It has poor oral bioavailability and a short therapeutic half-life. Toxic levels of its metabolite, normeperidine, accumulate with repeat dosing or renal insufficiency and can cause dysphoria, myoclonic jerks, and seizures.

Patients with Opioid Addiction

Drug requirements may be significantly higher and dosing intervals shorter in a patient with current or past opioid addiction. In patients on methadone maintenance, therapeutic dosing must be provided over and above their baseline dose. In all cases, the goal should be to deliver adequate medication to relieve the pain. The physician should always work from a written treatment plan; one physician should prescribe all psychotropic medication; and information about the patient's drug use should be obtained from sources in addition to the patient. When the question of "addiction" first arises, consultation should be obtained from an addiction medicine specialist. If opioids are needed, patients should be given limited quantities of long-acting medications on a scheduled basis.

Opioid Administration in Elderly Patients

It is safest to "start low; go slow" and reassess elderly patients frequently. Initial doses are 25% to 50% lower than those for younger adults. Rescue doses, which are about 10% of the total daily opioid dose in younger patients, are initially no more than 5% in the elderly. Rescue medication should be taken no more often than every four hours, rather than the every two hours recommended for younger patients. If par-

TREATMENT

Examples of Opioid Conversions

Changing from Oral to Parenteral Opioids

A 45-year-old woman taking 6 mg p.o. q 4 h hydromorphone (e.g., Dilaudid) for sickle cell crisis at home is admitted for parenteral pain relief. Intravenous access is limited. To use subcutaneous hydromorphone, determine the equianalgesic dose of parenteral hydromorphone for the initial basal rate. The oral:parenteral ratio for hydromorphone is 5:1.

  36 mg oral hydromorphone ~ 7 mg parenteral hydromorphone (5:1 ratio)
  7 mg/24 h = 0.3 mg/h basal rate of subcutaneous hydromorphone

If she were taking morphine for her pain, a different oral:parenteral ratio (3:1) would be needed.
    For a dose of 60 mg of oral sustained-release morphine q12h:

120 mg of oral morphine = 40 mg parenteral morphine (3:1 ratio)
40 mg/24 hours ≈ 1.7 mg/h basal rate of subcutaneous morphine

Changing from Fentanyl to Morphine at the Equianalgesic Dose

A 64-year-old woman with well-controlled pain from metastatic breast cancer uses a 150 μg/h transdermal fentanyl patch. She plans a cruise and wishes to switch to sustained-release tablets so that she can swim and sunbathe without embarrassment.

150 μg/h fentanyl = 331 to 390 mg of oral morphine/ 24 hours
New prescription: 150 to 200 mg sustained-release morphine q 12 h + 30 to 40 mg IR morphine q 4 h; clinical circumstances will guide the choice of high or low end of the range.

---

enteral opioids are needed, avoid bolus injections because of the enhanced toxicity associated with peak effects. Continuous infusion via subcutaneous or intravenous routes is preferred. Intraspinal opioids can also be given safely.

Changing Opioid Agent or Route of Administration

It is often necessary to exchange one opioid agent or route of administration for another. Patients might develop difficulty swallowing or an opioid-induced side effect or might prefer a different route. A small proportion of actively dying patients will require subcutaneous or intravenous opioid infusions to maintain pain control. To convert to another opioid safely while maintaining pain control, do the following:

- Know the equianalgesic dose of the new agent (Table 122-4).
- Decrease the calculated dose by one third to allow for incomplete cross-tolerance to side effects (e.g., respiratory depression, sedation) between opioids.
- Provide appropriate rescue dosing (i.e., 5% to 10% of the total 24-hour opioid dose).

Management of Opioid-Induced Side Effects

Opioid-induced side effects are often barriers to effective pain relief. To prevent constipation, most patients must start a prophylactic bowel regimen along with opioid therapy. Senna BID to TID plus/minus lactulose at bedtime is often used; fiber should be discouraged

because it can exacerbate opioid-induced constipation in patients with poor oral intake.

Urinary retention, which occurs most often in patients with prostatic hypertrophy or patients who are taking other drugs with anticholinergic side effects, usually resolves in one to two days, but rare patients will require either a trial of finasteride or an agent that produces smooth muscle relaxation, such as terazocin (1 mg PO at bedtime, which is increased gradually to 2 to 5 mg as tolerated and as needed).

Table 122-4 ▪ Opioid Equianalgesic Doses

Drug	PO/PR (mg)	SQ/IV (mg)
Morphine	30	10
Hydromorphone	7.5	1.5
Oxycodone-SR	20	n/a
Oxycodone-IR	20–30	
Levorphanol	4	2
Meperidine*	300	100

Fentanyl (μg/hr)	Morphine (mg/24 hours)	
	PO	IM/IV
25	30–90	10–30
50	91–150	31–50
75	151–210	51–70
100	211–270	71–90
125	271–330	91–110
150	331–390	111–130

*Not recommended.
PR = per rectum.

Table 122-5 ■ Delirium*

Drug	Dose	Comment
Haloperidol	0.5–5 mg po, IM, SQ, IV[†]; repeat q 2–12 h as needed.	Do not exceed 20 mg in 24 hours; maintain the patient on the effective dose (divided into a bid dose) for three to four days then taper over 1 week, as tolerated.
Chlorpromazine	25–50 mg po/IV/pr q 6–8 h	Sedating; may give q 1 h til sedation occurs in very agitated patients.
Lorazepam	0.5–2 mg q 1–4 h	Add to haloperidol for patients with an agitated delirium; tablets can be used p.r. for terminal delirium.
Diazepam	10–30 mg	Useful pr for patients unable to take oral medication.
Clonazepam	0.5–6 mg tid	Tablets have been used p.r. for terminal delirium. Do not exceed 20 mg in 24 hours.
Midazolam	30–100 mg over 24 hours	Intravenous drip or subcutaneous infusion for terminal delirium.

*In delirious patients, first attempt to identify the underlying cause and begin to correct it as you give the agents listed; make the patient's surroundings as familiar as possible; have a family member or friend sit with the patient.
[†]Oral doses are half as potent as parenteral doses.
From Abrahm JL: Promoting symptom control in palliative care. Semin Oncol Nurs 1998;14:95–109.

Nausea and vomiting also usually resolve in two to three days but may require prochlorperazine for up to one week. Continued opioid-induced nausea often responds to a change of opioid agent.

Opioid-related sedation is most severe in the first few days after the opioid is initiated or the dose is escalated. Naloxone (Narcan) should not be used in opioid-tolerant patients. It will precipitate opioid withdrawal symptoms and reverse the analgesia. If a patient develops significant respiratory depression, the standard 0.4 mg of naloxone should be diluted in 10 mL of saline, and only enough should be given to reverse this but not to awaken the patient. If sedation persists, other causes should be sought, other sedating medications should be discontinued, a different opioid should be substituted, and the patient should be advised to increase caffeine intake, if not contraindicated.

If sedation persists despite these measures, consider adding more potent psychostimulants. Significant decreases in opioid-induced sedation have been reported with methylphenidate or dextroamphetamine beginning at 2.5 to 5 mg in the morning and repeated, if needed, at noon. Doses can be increased as needed. Patients with hypertension, glaucoma, or symptomatic cardiac disease should not receive psychostimulants, but brain tumors or a history of seizures is not a contraindication.

Mild opioid-induced cognitive disturbances (e.g., nightmares and hallucinations) often resolve when the opioid is replaced by another agent. Patients with opioid-induced delirium should be hospitalized for evaluation and treatment unless the clinical condition warrants symptomatic treatment at home. Haloperidol (Haldol) and chlorpromazine are the agents of choice for patients who are suffering from an agitated delirium (Table 122-5). Initial dose of haloperidol is 0.5 to 1 mg IV/SQ or 1 to 2 mg orally, followed by 0.5 to 2 mg at 45- to 60-minute intervals as needed. Chlorpromazine (Thorazine) can be used if sedation is desired, though hypotension can be a serious side effect. Doses are 25 to 50 mg PO or PR every 6 to 8 hours, though it can be given hourly if agitation is severe, unless the patient becomes sedated.

A short-acting benzodiazepine such as lorazepam (Ativan) may also be added if agitation is prominent or if the patient has developed akathisia from the haloperidol. It is unlikely to be effective alone, however, and may paradoxically exacerbate the agitation. Diphenhydramine (Benadryl) or Cogentin may be required to reverse the extrapyramidal side effects of high doses of haloperidol.

Adjuvant Pain Relievers

Adjuvant agents are often needed for patients with neuropathic pain. The anticonvulsant gabapentin (Neurontin) has the fewest side effects and is very effective for patients with neuropathic pain from tumor, peripheral neuropathy from tumor or treatment, and postherpetic neuralgia. To minimize sedation, doses should be low at first (e.g., 100 mg TID) and should be raised as tolerated every three to five days until pain is relieved satisfactorily or a total of 2700 to 3000 mg are given. Other anticonvulsants (phenytoin, carbamazepine) and tricyclic antidepressants are also useful for neuropathic pain (Table 122-6).

Corticosteroids are useful for both nerve and bone pain (see Table 122-6). They act quickly and can provide pain relief while doses of gabapentin or a tricyclic antidepressant are being titrated upward. Treatment can be initiated with dexamethasone at 4 to 8

Table 122-6 ■ Adjuvants for Neuropathic Pain

Class	Agent	Dose
Anticonvulsants	Gabapentin	Initial dose: 100 mg bid–tid; increase by 100 tid to 900–3600 mg po/day
	Carbamazepine	200 mg po hs, increase q 3 d
	Phenytoin	1000-mg load; 200–300 mg q d
Tricyclic antidepressants	Amitriptyline, imipramine, doxepin, clomipramine, desipramine, nortriptyline	Begin at 10–25 mg p.o. hs; increase to therapeutic dose (50–150 mg in divided doses)
Corticosteroids	Prednisone	40–60 mg in divided doses; taper to qod as tolerated.
	Dexamethasone	10–100 mg bolus; 6 mg po/IV qid; taper as tolerated
Alpha-2 agonist	Clonidine	0.1–0.3 mg patch

From Abrahm JL: Advances in pain management for older adult patients. Clin Geriatr Med 2000;6:269–311.

mg twice a day, for example, along with 100 mg of gabapentin TID and an opioid if appropriate. If pain relief is achieved, the dose of dexamethasone can be lowered gradually as the dose of gabapentin is raised, thus maintaining good pain relief while minimizing sedation.

Radiation Therapy
Patients with localized pain from a bone metastasis, even those with far-advanced disease, may benefit from radiation to the painful lesion. Numerous randomized trials support the efficacy of single doses of 8 Gy in relieving pain.

Bisphosphonates
In osteolytic bony lesions from breast cancer or multiple myeloma, oral agents are not useful, but intravenous bisphosphonates such as pamidronate (Aredia) are very effective in relieving bone pain even in patients with refractory disease.

Radiopharmaceuticals
In patients with diffuse pain from bone metastases who do not respond to pamidronate and who cannot tolerate the side effects of opioid therapy or whose pain is not well controlled by opioid therapy with or without nonsteroidal anti-inflammatory drugs, radio-

pharmaceuticals may provide significant relief. Both ^{89}strontium and samarium-153-lexidronam showed documented efficacy in relieving the pain of bony metastases in phase III double-blind placebo-controlled trials. Ten percent to 30% of patients obtained complete pain relief, and pain was significantly improved in 70% to 80%. For both agents, relief begins in one to two weeks and lasts for a median of three to six months. The cost is significant: approximately $2000 per treatment of ^{89}strontium. A nuclear medicine specialist administers these agents.

Anesthetic/Neurolytic Techniques
Selected patients with advanced disease may benefit from techniques offered by anesthesia pain specialists. These include spinal (epidural or intrathecal) delivery of opioids, anesthetics such as bupivicaine, and other analgesic agents (e.g., clonidine); blocks/lysis of peripheral nerves causing postherpetic neuralgia and the postmastectomy and post-thoracotomy pain syndromes; and blocks/lysis of ganglia-mediating pain syndromes, such as the trigeminal ganglia (relieving the pain of tic doloureux), or the celiac ganglia (mediating the upper abdominal pain typical of pancreatic and gastric carcinomas). Indications for and application of these procedures are well described.

Other Common Problems
Oral

Oral discomfort in patients with cancer arises from poor oral hygiene, mucositis, *Candida* infections, or dry mouth caused by mouth breathing, previous radiation therapy, or medications for pain or other symptoms. General measures for oral comfort include presenting food at moderate temperatures; avoiding dry, acidic, or highly spiced foods; and minimizing alcohol and tobacco use.

Oral hygiene should not be neglected, even in very debilitated patients. Patients should be urged to continue daily brushing using a soft-bristle brush, flossing with unwaxed floss, and rinsing with a non–alcohol-containing antibacterial mouthwash or a solution of bicarbonate in water (e.g., 1 teaspoon in a cup of water). They should be monitored closely for the development of mucositis, infection, and xerostomia, and each should be treated promptly.

Mucositis occurs in 40% of patients receiving standard chemotherapy, about 75% of those undergoing transplant, and virtually all patients undergoing radiation therapy to the head and neck. A thorough dental examination including inspection and removal of all prosthesis is mandatory prior to beginning therapy. Clinical approaches to prophylaxis usually include ice, chlorhexidine gluconate, rinses with saline or bicarbonate, and antimicrobials (amphotericin, acyclovir). General topical regimens include a combination of local anesthetic, Maalox or Mylanta, and diphenhydramine. Sucralfate has also been used to treat chemotherapy- and radiation therapy-induced mucositis, but trials are contradictory concerning its benefit. Antiprostaglandins have been studied for radiation-induced mucositis. Good results have been seen with benzydamine but not with prostglandin E_2. Capsaicin and oral cryotherapy have also been shown to be of benefit. Amifostine, however, is not recommended to prevent radiation therapy-associated mucositis. Patient-controlled (opioid) analgesia is usually needed for pain relief for patients with grade 3 or 4 mucositis.

Candida presents as a burning tongue or pain when eating or swallowing; white plaques (which are easily wiped off but bleed) along the sides of the tongue or cheeks, on the gums, or on the roof of the mouth; angular chelitis; or, in denture wearers, red, edematous areas. Even in immunosuppressed patients, such as the severely malnourished or those receiving steroids, mucositis from *Candida* can be effectively treated with fluconazole or topical antifungal agents such as clotrimazole troches. Topical agents do not prevent esophageal candidiasis. It usually presents as a delayed pain that occurs after swallowing, located anywhere from the throat to the sternum. Fluconazole therapy usually provides relief in 24 to 48 hours.

Xerostomia should be addressed, as saliva is important to oral health. Saliva is a lubricant that helps to control plaque; protects teeth from dissolution and the mouth from bacterial, fungal, or viral infection; and enhances taste and the ability to swallow food. Mild xerostomia may respond to sugar-free sour lemon drops or other sugar-free hard candy. For those without cardiac contraindications, pilocarpine (5 mg) can be given an hour before meals; it is especially helpful for patients who have undergone radiation to the oral cavity or neck. Amifostine use may be considered to decrease the incidence of acute and later xerostomia in certain patients undergoing fractionated radiation therapy in the head and neck region.

Nausea and Vomiting

Pathophysiology of Chemotherapy-Induced Vomiting

The means by which chemotherapy agents induce vomiting are still incompletely understood but are thought to include stimulation of the chemoreceptor trigger zone (CTZ), which is probably the most common mechanism; gastrointestinal injury; stimulation of the cerebral cortex; inner ear processes; and changes in taste and smell. Higher centers in the brain, such as the cortex, are also thought to be involved in producing anticipatory nausea and vomiting. A past history of alcohol intake of more than five alcoholic drinks per day (more than 100 g of alcohol) is protective. Such patients have a lower incidence of chemotherapy-induced nausea and vomiting.

Anticipatory Nausea and Vomiting

Anticipatory nausea and vomiting are thought to be a classic conditioned response. Chemotherapy administration (the unconditioned stimulus) results in nausea and vomiting (the unconditioned response). Clinic sights, smells, and sounds are the conditioned stimulus. After frequent pairings of chemotherapy administration and the clinic sights, smells, and sounds, the response (nausea and vomiting) can be triggered in the absence of any chemotherapy by clinic sights, smells, or sounds or simply by seeing clinic personnel, even at a location distant from the site of treatment.

Patients in whom post-treatment nausea or vomiting never develops do not develop anticipatory nausea and vomiting. Of those who do experience post-treatment nausea and vomiting, the risk of developing anticipatory nausea and vomiting increases with the increasing frequency, severity, and duration of the symptoms. Other possible predisposing factors include susceptibility to motion sickness, awareness of tastes or odors during infusions, younger age, lengthier infusions, greater autonomic sensitivity, and general anxiety or emotional distress.

Both clonidine (five days before chemotherapy) and alprazolam (given the night before, the morning of, and just before chemotherapy and then QID for two days after therapy) significantly reduce anticipatory nausea and vomiting compared with placebo. For patients with refractory symptoms, a trial of hypnosis, progressive muscle relaxation with guided imagery, systemic desensitization, or distraction is warranted.

Antiemetic Prophylaxis for Chemotherapy-Induced Emesis

Guidelines for antiemetic prophylaxis in patients receiving chemotherapy or radiation therapy recommend tailoring the antiemetic to the emetogenic potential of the treatment or the agents being used (Table 122-7). Antianxiety and amnesic agents are included in the regimens because of the cortical inputs into nausea and vomiting. Cannabinoids (e.g., dronabinol) are not listed because their side effects (ataxia, dry mouth, orthostatic hypotension and dizziness, euphoria or dysphoria, and a feeling of being "high") are poorly tolerated by all but the adolescent and young adult population.

Table 122-7 ■ Antiemetic Therapy Recommendations*

Emetic Agent	Therapy
Highly/moderately to highly emetogenic chemotherapy or radiation therapy, daily low-dose platinum, high-dose chemotherapy, radiation therapy	5-HT antagonist + dexamethasone
Delayed emesis: platinum	Add metoclopramide
Delayed emesis: other	Dexamethasone ± 5HT antagonist
Refractory emesis after prophylaxis	5-HT antagonist + dexamethasone + metopimazine
Anticipatory emesis	Alprazolam; cognitive Rx (e.g., hypnosis)
Radiation: moderately emetogenic	5-HT antagonist

Emetogenic Potential of Chemotherapeutic Agents

High (>90%)
  Carmustine: >250 mg/m²
  Cisplatin: >50 mg/m²
  Cyclophosphamide: >1500 mg/m²
  DTIC
  Mechlorethamine
Moderately high (60–90%)
  Carboplatin
  Carmustine: <250 mg/m²
  Cisplatin: <50 mg/m²
  Cyclophosphamide: >750–1500 mg/m²
  CytarabineL >1000 mg/m²
  Doxorubicin
  Epirubicin
  Ifosfamide
  Irinotecan
  Methotrexate: >250 mg/m²
  Mitoxantrone
  Procarbazine
  Topotecan

From Antiemetic Subcommittee of the Multinational Association of Supportive Care. Ann Oncol 1998;9:811–819.

5-HT₃ receptor antagonists have essentially replaced regimens containing high-dose metoclopramide and diphenhydramine because the latter regimen was associated with a high incidence of akathisias and acute dystonic reactions in young patients and a high risk of extrapyramidal side effects and anticholinergic and sedating side effects in elderly patients.

The 5-HT₃ receptor antagonists ondansetron, granisetron, dolasetron, and tropisetron along with dexamethasone can control acute nausea and emesis in about 90% of patients receiving moderate to highly emetogenic chemotherapy, including that given for stem cell or bone marrow transplant. Delayed emesis remains a problem despite combination prophylactic therapy, but addition of other agents is often helpful. The 5-HT₃ antagonists and dexamethasone are both effective in preventing emesis induced by single- or multiple-fraction radiotherapy and total body irradiation (TBI). Patients chronically receiving ondansetron or granisetron may develop symptomatic severe constipation that can be prevented by prophylactic laxatives. The efficacy of the new neurokinin-1 receptor antagonists, however, suggests that substance P is the major mediator of delayed emesis. When combined with 5-HT₃ antagonists and dexamethasone, these agents are effective in preventing delayed vomiting due to cisplatin.

The benzodiazepine lorazepam has only mild antiemetic activity on its own, but the dose-related memory loss and sedation that it induces can be helpful adjuncts for selected patients.

Other agents that are more active than placebo include the butyrophenones haloperidol and droperidol and the phenothiazine prochlorperazine. These agents are less effective drugs than the agents mentioned above, and all but prochlorperazine are associated with significant side effects. All cause sedation. In addition, the butyrophenones produce dystonic reactions, akathisia, and occasionally hypotension.

Nausea and Vomiting Unrelated to Chemotherapy or Radiation Therapy

Other common etiologies of nausea and vomiting in this population include pain, opioids, constipation, gastritis or gastric ulcer disease, gastric outlet or bowel obstruction, hypercalcemia, hyponatremia, hepatic or renal failure, or disease of the central nervous system (CNS). Reversing the underlying problem is usually effective and is worth pursuing even in patients with far-advanced disease. For some patients, frequent, small feedings of cold foods that have less odor and acupuncture or hypnosis may alleviate the nausea.

Pharmacologic recommendations for nausea from any of these etiologies and for bowel obstruction that cannot be treated surgically are reviewed in Table 122-8.

Respiratory

Cough

Cough, which is present in about 40% of patients with advanced cancer, is caused by postnasal drip, infection,

Table 122-8 ■ Antiemetics*

Etiology of Nausea	Drug	Dose
Initiation or escalation of opioid therapy	Prochlorperazine (Compazine)	10 mg po or 25 mg pr bid or tid
	Olanzepine	2.5–10 mg once daily
Emetogenic chemotherapy or radiation	Ondansetron	4–8 mg po tid or bid; 8 mg IV or 24 mg p.o.; highly emetogenic
	Granisetron	2 mg p.o. q d or bid; 10 µg/kg or 2 mg p.o.; highly emetogenic
	Tropisetron	5 mg IV; highly emetogenic
	Dolasetron	100–200 mg po q d; 1.8 mg/kg IV or 200 mg po; highly emetogenic
Metabolic stimulation of chemoreceptor trigger zone (e.g., liver failure)	Haloperidol	1.5–5 mg po tid to qid, 2–10 mg IM bid to tid
	Prochlorperazine (Compazine)	10 mg po or 25 mg pr bid or tid.
	Methotrimeprazine	2–6.25 mg IM tid or 6–25 mg over 24 hours
Delayed gastric emptying	Metoclopramide	10–20 mg bid to qid or 1–3 mg/h IV
Vertigo	Hyoscyamine	0.125–0.25 mg tid po or SQ
	Scopolamine	Transdermal Patch
	Meclizine (Bonine, Antivert)	50 mg tid po or 25–50 mg IM
Bowel obstruction†	Octreotide	50–100 µg SQ bid to tid or 300–600 µg over 24 hours SQ
Increased intracranial pressure	Dexamethasone	4–8 mg bid or tid po

*For nausea, initial steps should be: (1) treat cause, if identified; (2) consider changing to a different opiate agent (see text); and (3) use adjuvants to decrease opiate dose.
†For symptomatic therapy when surgery is not possible.
Modified from Abrahm JL: Promoting symptom control in palliative care. Semin Oncol Nurs 1998;74:95–109.

heart failure, asthma/COPD, esophageal reflux, ACE inhibitors, obstruction of the airway, or disorders of swallowing. Nonspecific therapy includes oral opioids or sweet elixirs containing dextromethorphan or one of the opioids used for mild pain; methadone syrup, if available, can be very effective. For more resistant coughs, higher doses of oral or nebulized opioids (morphine or hydromorphone often combined with dexamethasone every 4 hours through a nebulizer using room air or oxygen through an open facemask) may be helpful. In addition, nebulized anesthetics (e.g., 2 mL of 2% lidocaine in 1 mL of normal saline for 10 minutes) can be given up to three times a day. For patients who cough from tenacious mucous, nebulized saline, albuterol (0.5 mg in 2.5 mg normal saline) and terbutaline have been helpful, while expectorants and mucolytics have not. Since ipatroprium worsens this problem, it is discontinued when possible.

Hiccups

Hiccups are embarrassing and exhausting and interfere with a patient's ability to eat, drink, and sleep. In patients with cancer, they are most commonly caused by gastric compression, injury to vagus or phrenic nerves, uremia, hyponatremia, hypocalcemia, benzodiazepines, barbiturates, intravenous corticosteroids, or rarely ear infections, pharyngitis, esophagitis, or pneumonia. If the underlying cause cannot be reversed, metoclopramide is usually very effective. Chlorpromazine is also effective but causes significant postural hypotension. Baclofen and haloperidol are probably equally effective and safer in older patients. If none of these work and sedation is not a concern, methotrimeprazine or midazolam is often administered.

Fungating Lesions and Pressure Sores

Fungating lesions from cancers growing out through the skin, frequently malodorous, can cause a profound loss of self-esteem and lead to patient isolation. They occur in patients with primary skin cancers, cancers of the head and neck that are refractory to chemotherapy and radiation, metastatic breast cancer, renal cancer, and rarely other cancers. Surgery, chemotherapy, and radiation are all considered when the metastases first appear.

Symptomatic treatment is often needed. General treatment principles include the following:

- Prevent contamination and minimize shear forces. Use polyurethane films or hydrocolloid dressings (e.g., Tegaderm, Omniderm, Duoderm, and Granuflex).
- Protect the wound and promote healing. If it is infected or necrotic, use normal saline irrigation and enzymatic agents (Elase, Travase, and streptokinase) to remove eschar. Use hydrocolloid dressings or alginate dressings (Kaltocarb, Kaltostat).
- Eliminate or control infection and debride (Debrisan).
- Control odor with a charcoal dressing (Actisorb).

Insomnia

Insomnia is present in one third to one half of patients with advanced cancer. Patients usually do not report difficulty falling asleep, but they have trouble staying asleep. The sleeplessness can often be more troublesome to the patients' families than it is to the patient, but sleep deprivation can exacerbate their pain and increase the probability of developing depression.

Causes of insomnia in the cancer population include pain, depression, anxiety, delirium, dyspnea, nausea and vomiting, pruritus, and drugs (e.g., caffeine, alcohol, or corticosteroids). Restless-leg syndrome may awaken patients who are severely anemic or uremic, are on tricyclic medications, or have a peripheral neuropathy.

Insomnia may be treated either nonpharmacologically or with medications. Psychological, financial, and spiritual counseling may be of help, as may the techniques developed by sleep experts for patients without cancer. Patients should be encouraged not to nap during the day, to remain out of bed as long as possible, to go to bed and get up at set times, and, if they do not fall asleep within 30 minutes, to get out of bed and do some relaxing activity or do that activity in bed. Progressive muscle relaxation or other forms of relaxation therapy, biofeedback, and hypnosis using imagery have been shown to be helpful as components of short-term management of insomnia.

Data from controlled trials indicate that benzodiazepines, antidepressants, zolpidem (Ambien), and, in one trial, melatonin are effective medications. Temazepam (Restoril) (15 to 30 mg) might not induce sleep, but it has been shown to help people stay asleep. Triazolam (Halcion) has a shorter half-life (two to three hours) and can be used in patients with hepatic dysfunction or in those needing sublingual medications. Initial doses should be low in the elderly or the cachectic or in those taking the medication sublingually, as blood levels are higher when the drug is taken by this route. Some elderly patients develop paradoxical agitation from benzodiazepines and may do well with either a sedating tricyclic agent such as doxepin (12.5 to 25 mg PO), or chloral hydrate (500 mg PO).

For patients who develop nighttime delirium that presents as insomnia, oral haloperidol (e.g., Haldol) (beginning at 0.5 to 2 mg PO and increasing as needed to 5 mg), given in the late afternoon before the onset of the agitation and repeated if needed during the night, is usually very effective. Clonazepam (Klonopin) (0.5 to 1 mg) is used for patients with restless-leg syndrome.

Weakness and Fatigue

Validated fatigue assessment tools have revealed that almost all patients who are receiving chemotherapy or radiation therapy (96%) or who enter the terminal phases of cancer suffer from fatigue, but its pathophysiology, etiology, and effective therapies remain to be defined.

Identifiable and even sometimes reversible causes can be found for some patients. Pain and insomnia, discussed above, and anemia, anorexia with weight loss, anxiety, cancer-related metabolic abnormalities (hypercalcemia, hypomagnesemia, hyponatremia, hypokalemia, and hyperglycemia and hypoglycemia), and depression are important causes of generalized weakness and fatigue. Drug side effects; pulmonary, renal, hepatic, or cardiac failure; infection; and certain neurologic problems can all present as generalized weakness, and the weakness may resolve if these problems can be reversed. Plasmapheresis and agents that promote neurotransmitter release such as guanidine hydrochloride (125 to 500 mg PO TID) have been helpful for lung cancer patients with the Eaton-Lambert syndrome.

When the weakness is not reversible, it is useful to give the patient and his or her family some strategies for dealing with it. Patients might mistakenly think that going to bed for a period of time will help them regain their normal strength, but they should actually minimize the time they spend in bed so as to maximize their remaining strength. In fact, exercise effectively reduces fatigue in breast cancer patients who are undergoing chemotherapy. Selected patients may benefit from physical therapy consultation.

In addition, counsel patients to plan for short rest periods during the day, limit trips, and delegate exhausting chores. It is often hard for people to relinquish these tasks, especially if the tasks helped to define their role in the family. Assist patients in identifying which of these tasks are most important to them and which they could delegate. For those who are bedridden, sensory, intellectual, or interpersonal stimulation is still important. Listening to music or books on tape, reading, drawing, playing games, or reminiscing should be encouraged.

To help them maintain mobility, patients are likely to benefit from walkers, wheelchairs, lift-chairs, electric hospital beds, tray-tables, and commodes or shower chairs. Many insurance companies cover rental of such equipment, and eligible veterans can have use of them free of charge.

Common Physical Problems in the Last Days of Life

In the last days to weeks of life, patients may experience problems of a physical, social, psychological, or spiritual nature.

Symptom Complex of Dying Patients

Data are somewhat conflicting about the frequency of the various symptoms that occur in the last days to week before death. Up to 70% of patients with advanced cancer have pain that requires ongoing therapy until death. Noisy or moist breathing, urinary incontinence or retention, or restlessness and agitation are seen in almost half of the patients who are "actively dying." One in five patients will be short of breath, and about one in 10 will have nausea and vomiting or manifestations of delirium such as sweat-

ing, confusion, jerking, twitching, or plucking at bed sheets. Patients may also experience fatigue, and many exhibit signs of existential or spiritual distress. As the patient is in the process of dying, his or her arms and legs may cool, and when the patient's pulse and blood pressure decrease, the skin may become pale or mottled. Some patients may develop fecal incontinence as they die.

Commonly Required Medications

Most of the problems experienced by dying patients can be controlled by using a limited number of medications given by the rectal, transdermal, or rarely parenteral route (Table 122-9).

Using WHO guidelines for cancer pain relief, 50% of cancer patients who are near death will have no pain, 25% will have mild to moderate pain, and only 3% will have severe pain. Patients require close monitoring, and both opioids and nonopioid adjuvants are usually required. If the patient is unable to take pills, buccal, sublingual, rectal, or transdermal opioids are usually effective. In some cases, however, subcutaneous or, when intravenous access is available, intravenous infusions will be needed. Concentrated morphine or oxycodone oral solutions (20 to 40 mg/mL) can be given hourly or every two hours and are often satisfactory. Rectal administration of sustained-release opioid preparations are not FDA

Table 122-9 ■ Treatment of Problems That Are Common in the Final Days

Problem	Agent	Dose
Baseline pain	Morphine/hydromorphone sl, sq	Individualized
	Fentanyl transdermal	
Breakthrough pain	Concentrated morphine solution	Individualized
	Fentanyl transmucosal	
Death rattle	Scopolamine	Gel; Transdermal 1–3 patches q 3 d; 0.1–2.4 mg/24 h SQ/IV
	Hycosamine (Levsin SL)	0.125 mg SL tid to qid
	Atropine (A) + morphine (M) + dexamethasone (D)	2 mg (A) + 2.5 mg (M) + 2 mg (D) by nebulizer
	Atropine + Lasix	Atropine 1–2 mg IM + Lasix 20–40 mg IV
Anxiety	Lorazepam or alprazolam	1 mg po or sublingual q 2 h
Delirium	Haloperidol	2–4 mg po, SC, IM, IV q 30 min prn to total 20 mg/24 h
	Methotrimeprazine	12.5–50 mg po/IM q 4–8 h
	Chlorpromazine	25–50 mg po q 4–12 h or 25 mg q 4–12 h pr; preferred for dyspnea
	Midazolam	2–3 mg load; 0.5–1 mg/h SC or IV; increase prn to 100 mg/24 h
	Barbiturates	
Dyspnea from anxiety/panic	Midazolam	5–10 mg IV slowly or 0.1–1.25 mg/h SQ
	Morphine	5–10 mg IV or by nebulizer
	Chlorpromazine	25 mg po/pr q 4–12 h; or 12.5 mg IV q 4–12 h

approved, but studies indicate that morphine absorption from a sustained-release preparation placed in the rectal vault is equivalent to that from oral administration. If pain is a new problem and the patient is opioid-naive, institute therapy with 15 to 30 mg sustained-release morphine over 12 hours.

Adjuvants to opioids can also be given rectally or subcutaneously. Patients who previously benefited from oral nonsteroidal anti-inflammatory drugs can receive rectal indomethacin; patients on a stable glucocorticoid dose for bone or nerve pain can receive subcutaneous dexamethasone. Rectal doxepin can replace oral tricyclic antidepressants.

As many as one half of patients need an increase in opioid dose during their last days. If the calculated opioid dose is too large to be delivered by sublingual, transdermal, or rectal routes, if pain relief does not seem to be satisfactory using any of these routes, or if the routes are unacceptable to the patient or his or her caregiver, use a subcutaneous or intravenous opioid infusion.

While pain relief is the goal in dying patients, the family is sometimes concerned that the opioid is killing the patient. If the respiratory rate of the patient declines, the family might mistakenly think that the patient is oversedated. Unlike patients who are in less advanced stages of their illness, the normal respiratory rate in terminal patients is about six to 12 breaths a minute. If the rate falls to fewer than six, reducing the dose of the opioid by 25% is usually effective; naloxone is almost never indicated in such situations.

Death Rattle

Patients are usually unaware of these loud respirations, but they can be very distressing for families. They occur in 60% to 90% of dying patients. Reposition the patient to a lateral recumbent position and, if needed, add hycosamine (Levsin SL) or scopolamine in a transdermal patch. Scopolamine has been reported to be efficacious in as many as 70% of patients.

Terminal Restlessness

Almost one half of the patients who are actively dying of cancer show signs of restlessness and agitation. They may toss and turn, moan, have muscle twitching or spasm, and only intermittently be awake. Even though patients might appear not to be in contact with the external world, they often seem to be reassured by familiar voices or by being touched.

The agitation is sometimes due to reversible physical problems, such as a full bladder, fecal impaction, pain, nausea, or trouble breathing due to hypoxia or poorly cleared secretions. In others, unresolved spiri-

tual, psychological, or social problems induce the distress. Therapies include lorazepam (e.g., Ativan) or alprazolam (e.g., Xanax) (1 mg PO or SL every 2 hours), spiritual reassurance, a visit from an estranged family member or friend, or family permission to "let go."

Other agitated patients are delirious and need haloperidol (e.g., Haldol, 2 mg PO, SQ, IV every 30 min as needed; double dose every 30 to 60 minutes as needed), or chlorpromazine (25 to 50 mg IV or PR, as often as every hour until sedated). Chlorpromazine should be used if both dyspnea and delirium are present. For more severe delirium, give haloperidol or chlorpromazine plus midazolam (Versed) by subcutaneous infusion (e.g., haloperidol 10 to 20 mg/24 hours + midazolam 1.25 mg/hour). Larger doses of midazolam (i.e., up to 100 mg/24 hours) may be needed if there is a great deal of myoclonus.

Dyspnea

Dying patients with dyspnea benefit from the same symptomatic therapies recommended for patients with less advanced disease. Aggressive treatment of panic due to perceived breathlessness includes oral morphine (5 to 10 mg PO), chlorpromazine, or, for refractory panic, midazolam.

Hydration

Although patients are unlikely to be thirsty or hungry, they might have a dry mouth caused by opioids. Rehydration is not indicated to relieve this symptom because there is no difference in the reports of thirst or dry mouth between dehydrated and normally hydrated dying patients, and no controlled studies have shown that rehydration is effective. Providing parenteral hydration increases distress by increasing urine output, inducing pulmonary or peripheral edema, or increasing ascites, pulmonary secretions, or nausea and vomiting from increased gastric secretions. Moistening the mouth with gauze soaked in ice water or offering sips of water, ice chips, or fruit-flavored ice pops is usually sufficient.

Massive Hemoptysis (or Other Bleed)

Massive hemoptysis is rare, but if the patient is likely to develop either a massive bleed or massive hemoptysis, recommend that the family purchase dark-colored sheets, towels, and blankets to mask the blood. Because emergency intravenous access might be needed for patient sedation, consider insertion of a PICC line in patients without an in-dwelling venous access device.

If the patient is enrolled in hospice, the nurse can

provide instruction for administering prefilled syringes of morphine, to be given intravenously when possible, and a benzodiazepine. Midazolam (Versed) can be given intramuscularly or intravenously; diazepam or lorazepam (e.g., Ativan) can be given rectally. When the event occurs, the patient is placed bleeding side down, in the Trendelenburg position, and the above medications are given. If the nurse arrives in time, he or she can start continuous infusions of morphine and/or midazolam if necessary.

Miscellaneous

Lidocaine can be added to saline bladder irrigation for patients with catheters who are experiencing dysuria. For patients with nausea or vomiting due to bowel obstruction, use octreotide (150 to 300 µg twice a day or by continuous subcutaneous infusion); for nausea or vomiting from other causes, metoclopramide 30 mg + haloperidol (e.g. Haldol) 1.5 mg + promethazine (Phenergan) 6.25 mg can be safely infused subcutaneously or intravenously over 24 hours. Famotidine can be converted to a subcutaneous infusion if the patient had been using it for relief from gastrointestinal symptoms. Myoclonus responds to midazolam (5-mg load, then 10 to 100 mg/24 hours).

Sedation for Refractory Symptoms

Sedation is considered when, despite expert evaluation and management, a patient who is near death continues to experience intolerable physical, psychological, or spiritual/existential symptoms. Most often, desires for terminal sedation arise when psychological or spiritual/existential concerns coexist with physical problems. Expert palliative care and pastoral consultation should be undertaken before sedation is administered.

If the doses of opioid, neuroleptic, or benzodiazepine needed to control severe pain, cough, dyspnea, seizures, or agitation sedate the patient, discussions are needed among the health care team, the patient, and the family members. Most often, all concerned reach a consensus on the need for and the acceptability of sedation as a means of achieving symptom control. Obtaining formal informed consent either from the patient or from the health care proxy is recommended. In addition, attempt to ensure that families will not regret their decision after the patient dies. Ask them to imagine that several months after the death, they are recalling the events immediately preceding it and asking themselves whether they feel anything should have been done differently.

If neither the therapies described above for specific syndromes nor opioid infusions effectively relieve the distressing symptom, intravenous benzodiazepines, or

Table 122-10 ■ Sedation for Refractory Pain Dosage

Drug	Dosage
Midazolam	Bolus 0.5 mg; then 0.5 to 1.5 mg/h
Lorazepam	0.5 to 1 mg/h
Phenobarbital	130 mg q 30 min to 1000 mg/24 h
Pentobarbital	3.3 mg/kg load, then 1 to 2 mg/kg/h
Thiopental	5 to 7 mg/kg/h

subcutaneous or intravenous barbiturates can be used and will work (Table 122-10). The benzodiazepine midazolam, while quite effective, is also quite costly.

Hospice

Hospice nurses and medical directors, who are present in both rural and urban communities, are valuable sources of expertise in pain and palliative medicine for patients with uncontrolled symptoms at any stage of their disease. They are especially valuable as partners in caring for patients who are dying from hematologic diseases or cancer. Through their efforts and those of the other team members, hospices ensure that patients and family suffering is ameliorated, whatever its cause.

History of the Modern Hospice Movement

In 1899, Calvary Hospital in New York City was founded as an inpatient facility for those who were incurable or dying. In Great Britain, Canada, and the United States, the modern hospice movement began in the late 1960s and early 1970s. In 1975, coincident with the publication and popularity of *On Death and Dying* by Dr. Elisabeth Kübler-Ross, the hospice movement spread widely in the United States. Hospices were working to counter an active euthanasia movement, as well as "the loneliness, isolation, lack of family involvement and unrelieved pain that came to be synonymous with individuals dying in acute care hospitals." The Medicare Hospice Benefit was established in 1982. By 1997, the National Hospice Organization (NHO) estimated that there were almost 3000 operational hospice programs in the United States that served about 450,000 patients per year, or about 17% of all patients who die each year. The majority of hospice patients are white cancer patients over 65 years of age.

Hospice seeks neither to prolong life nor to hasten death. The focus of care is on providing comfort and dignity and enhancing the quality of the life remaining. Hospice supports both the patient and family, helps them to identify their remaining hopes and goals, and assists them in realizing them. In the United States, most hospice care takes place in the home, though increasingly, hospice is involved in the care of inpatients and of nursing home residents. Hospice also prepares families for their losses and offers continued assistance through bereavement programs after the death.

The services provided by hospice are listed in Table 122-11. Hospice provides 95% of the cost of prescription drugs related to the terminal diagnosis and necessary for its palliative treatment (and many waive the other 5% if there is no insurance coverage). Hospice provides all durable medical equipment, supplies, and oxygen for needs related to the terminal diagnosis; laboratory and diagnostic procedures related to the terminal diagnosis; and transportation when medically necessary for changes in the patient's level of care.

Hospices provide a continuum of care, from home to the inpatient setting. While most patients are cared for in their homes, as stated in the 1983 federal regulations, all Medicare-certified hospices are required to provide four levels of care: routine, continuous, respite, and inpatient (Table 122-12). By law, 80% of days of patient care must take place in the home. Respite or inpatient care cannot exceed 20% of the days of care delivered each year.

The Medicare Hospice Benefit was established in 1982 as part of the Tax Equity and Fiscal Responsibility Act. Then, as now, both the attending physician and the hospice medical director were required to certify that the patient was terminally ill with a prognosis of six months or less if the disease follows its usual course. There are no other mandated criteria for cancer patients. Patients with non-oncologic diagnoses must meet the 1997 Health Care Financing Administration (HCFA) criteria. These criteria were originally guidelines developed by the National Hospice Organization in 1996, and they have never been validated.

Table 122-11 ■ Hospice Services

Personnel

Medical director, nurses, social workers, home health aides, chaplains, volunteers, administrative personnel, medical consultations, occupational therapy, physical therapy, speech therapy, bereavement counseling

Items Needed for Palliation of Terminal Illness

Prescription medications
Durable medical equipment and supplies
Oxygen
Radiation and chemotherapy
Laboratory and diagnostic procedures

Other

Transportation when medically necessary for changes in level of care
When needed, continuous care at home or in a skilled nursing facility or inpatient setting
Respite care (care in a nursing facility that provides a respite for the caregivers)

Table 122-12 ■ Levels of Clinical Care Provided

	Routine	Continuous*	Inpatient[†]	Respite[‡]
24-hour on-call				
HHA	≥2 hr/day			
RN visits	~3/wk + prn			
Social worker visits	q 2 wks			
Chaplain visits	q 2–4 wks			
Volunteer	2–4 hr/wk			
M.D.	prn			
OT/PT/RT	prn			
Continuous nursing		≥8 hours RN/day		
Inpatient care			prn	
Respite care				5 days/month

*Continuous home care: Patients with, for example, refractory cough, dyspnea, pain, or delirium can receive 24-hour nursing and home health aide services.
[†]Inpatient care. Rarely utilized. For refractory symptoms that cannot be controlled at home, even with continuous care. The referring physician admits the patient and may bill for his/her services under Medicare Part B.
[‡]Respite care. The goal of the respite (in a community skilled or intermediate nursing facility) is either to provide a rest for the caregiver or to remove the patient to an adequate facility when the home is temporarily inadequate to meet the patient care needs.

Hospice coverage is offered by only 80% of large and medium-sized employers, and hospice coverage for those who are not eligible for Medicare or Medicaid varies enormously in terms of what services and providers are covered and with what limitations (e.g., exclusions for preexisting conditions). For those who are eligible, the Medicare hospice benefit is a managed care, capitated reimbursement program that reimburses a hospice a per diem based on the patient's level of care (about $100/day for routine or respite care and about $400 per day for inpatient acute care). Aggressive palliation, including expensive palliative radiation and chemotherapeutic or hematopoietic agents, is often prohibitively expensive for small to moderately sized hospices, given this reimbursement schedule.

Common Misconceptions

The following are some common misconceptions about hospice:

- *Misconception: Patients enrolling in hospice must choose not to be resuscitated.* Patients do not have to relinquish resuscitation to enroll in hospice. Most commonly, patients elect not to be resuscitated once they or their families fully understand the implications of the resuscitation after thorough explanations by hospice personnel.
- *Misconception: Patients enrolled in hospice lose their primary physicians.* The referring attending physician continues to direct and approve all of the patient's care, from the initial certification of terminal prognosis to the medication and durable medical equipment orders, approves the frequency of home health aide visits and consultations, and certifies the resuscitation status. If the patient requires either inpatient hospice admission for symptom control or routine admission for a diagnosis unrelated to the terminal illness, the physician may bill Medicare under Part B for any visits.
- *Misconception: Hospice patients cannot be hospitalized and remain enrolled in hospice.* Hospices are required to offer admission to an acute, inpatient level of care if that is needed to control a distressing symptom.
- *Misconception: Hospice patients cannot participate in research projects while enrolled in hospice.* They can participate in research as long as the project is consistent with the mission of hospice.
- *Misconception: Hospice nursing personnel do not provide sophisticated care.* Hospice personnel provide expert palliative care. They do not simply hold patients' hands, place cool washcloths on their foreheads, and change the linen. The palliative care that they deliver requires astute assessment and expert intervention tailored to the patient and family goals. Even tube feedings, intravenous hydration, or intravenous medications to control symptoms may be provided, depending on the clinical status of the patient.
- *Misconception: Patients can use up their hospice eligibility, so it is important not to enroll them too soon.* Patients who live longer than six months will continue to receive services as long as they continue to meet eligibility criteria for hospice care. And patients who choose to revoke the hospice benefit to seek life-prolonging therapies may choose to re-enroll if their goals change.
- *Misconception: Patients must have a live-in caregiver to enroll in hospice.* Many hospices care for "live-alone" patients, employing special protocols to enhance their safety. Medical alert devices worn around the neck, lock-boxes to provide access in an emergency, and daily patient contact are some measures that are used.

Patient and Family Education, Support, and Counsel

In addition to assessing and managing the patient's physical problems, the hospice team is a source of patient and family education, support, and counseling. The hospice nurse provides the family with suggestions for answering patient questions. When requested or when appropriate, the nurse reviews the dying process with written materials that explain how the family or the personnel in inpatient or long-term care facilities can determine that death is imminent. He or she also describes the signs and symptoms of dying, instructs the family in emergency procedures, and is available for support while the patient dies.

The social workers assess the social and financial needs of the dying patient and family and identify those who are at risk for a particularly painful bereavement period. They offer support and family counseling and, often working with the chaplain, facilitate family reconciliation. Social workers engage the patient and family in advance care and funeral planning, help in completion of living wills and durable powers of attorney, provide applications for financial aid or waivers, and help to identify financing for additional home health care. They assist patients in making plans for their survivors (e.g., guardianship for children) and in completing life reviews.

Chaplains provide support both for the traditionally religious and for those who have spiritual or existential sources of distress (e.g., loss of hope, loss of connection or of love, a need for forgiveness or to forgive, or a need to identify the meaning of their lives).

Volunteers do any number of tasks, depending on what the family needs. These might include sitting with the patient to enable the caregiver to go to church, driving the patient or caregiver to doctor appointments, shopping, or picking up supplies. Volunteers provide phone support and are especially vital for hospice patients who live alone.

Bereavement counselors can provide support for family members who are experiencing anticipatory grief prior to the patient's death and routinely communicate with the bereaved for the year after the death. Survivors receive letters containing advice and expressing concern and are invited to memorial services and to participate in drop-in support groups or groups designed to meet special needs (e.g., parents who have lost young children, teenagers who have lost a parent).

References

Pain

Abrahm JL: Management of pain and spinal cord compression in patients with advanced cancer. Ann Intern Med 1999;131:37–46.

Abrahm JL: A Physician's Guide to Pain and Symptom Management in Cancer Patients. Baltimore, MD: Johns Hopkins University Press, 2000.

Ad Hoc Committee on Cancer Pain, American Society of Clinical Oncology: Cancer pain assessment and treatment curriculum guidelines. J Clin Oncol 1992;10:1976.

Body JJ, Bartl R, Burckhardt P, et al: Current use of bisphosphonates in oncology. J Clin Oncol 1998;16:3890.

Cassileth BR, Chapman CC: Alternative cancer medicine: A ten-year update. Cancer Invest 1996;14:396–404.

Donner B, Zena M, Tryba M, et al: Direct conversion from oral morphine to transdermal fentanyl: A multicenter study in patients with cancer pain. Pain 1996;64:527.

Eisenberg E, Berkey CS, Carr DB, et al: Efficacy and safety of nonsteroidal anti-inflammatory drugs for cancer pain: A meta-analysis. J Clin Oncol 1994;12:2756.

Fitchett G, Handzo G: Spiritual assessment, screening, and intervention. In Holland J (ed): Psycho-Oncology. New York: Oxford University Press, 1998.

Forman WB: Opioid analgesics drugs in the elderly. Clin Geriatr Med 1996;12:489.

Hawkey CJ: Cox-2 inhibitors. Lancet 1999;353:307.

Jacox A, Carr DB, Payne R, et al: Management of Cancer Pain: Clinical Practice Guideline No 9. UPHS, AHCPR. 1994. AHCPR publication 94-0592.

Janjan NA: Radiation for bone metastases: Conventional techniques and the role of systemic radiopharmaceuticals. Cancer 1997;80:1628.

Kaiko RF, Foley KM, Grabinski PY, et al: Central nervous system excitatory effects of meperidine in cancer patients. Ann Int Med 1983;13:180.

Levy MH: Pharmacologic treatment of cancer pain. N Engl J Med 1996;335:1124.

Loblaw DA, Lapierre NJ: Emergency treatment of malignant extradural spinal cord compression: An evidence-based guideline. J Clin Oncol 1998;16:1613.

Manfredi PL, Ribeiro S, Chandler SW, et al: Inappropriate use of naloxone in cancer patients with pain. J Pain Symptom Manage 1996;11:131.

McCaffery M, Wolff M: Pain relief using cutaneous modalities, positioning, and movement. Hospice J 1992;8:121–154.

McEwan AJB: Unsealed source therapy of painful bone metastases: an update. Sem Nucl Med 1997;27:165.

Mercadante S, Casuccio A, Agnello A, et al: Morphine versus methadone in the pain treatment of advanced-cancer patients followed up at home. J Clin Oncol 1998;16:3656.

Meyers CA, Weitzner MA, Valentine AD, et al: Methylphenidate therapy improves cognition, mood and function of brain tumor patients. J Clin Oncol 1998;16:2522.

Patt RB, Ellison NM: Breakthrough pain in cancer patients: Characteristics, prevalence, and treatment. Oncology 1998;12:1035.

Ripamonti C, Groff L, Brunelli C, et al: Switching from morphine to oral methadone in treating cancer pain: What is the equianalgesic dose ratio? J Clin Oncol 1998;16:3216.

Syrjala KL, Donaldson GW, Davis MW, Kippes ME, Carr JE: Relaxation and imagery and cognitive-behavioral training reduce pain during cancer treatment: A controlled clinical trial. Pain 1995;63:189–198.

Watanabe S, Bruera E: Corticosteroids as adjuvant analgesics. J Pain Symptom Manage 1994;9:442.

Zech D, Grond S, Lynch J, et al: Validation of World Health Organization Guidelines for cancer pain relief: A 10 year prospective study. Pain 1995;63:65.

Delirium

Breitbart W, Marotta R, Platt MM, et al: A double-blind trial of haloperidol, chlorpromazine, and lorazepam in the treatment of delirium in hospitalized AIDS patients. Am J Psychiatry 1996;153:231.

Mucositis

Hensleyml ML, Schuchter LM, Lindley C, Meropol NJ, Cohen GI, et al. ASCO clinical practice guidelines for the use of chemotherapy and radiotherapy and protectants. J Clin Oncol 1999;17:3333–3335.

Johnson JT, Ferretti GA, Nethery WJ, et al: Oral pilocarpine for post-irradiation xerostomia in patients with head and neck cancer. N Engl J Med 1993;329:390–395.

Loprinzi CL, Ghosh C, Camoriano J, Sloan J, et al: Phase III controlled evaluation of sucralfate to alleviate stomatitis in patients receiving fluorouracil-based chemotherapy. J Clin Oncol 1997;15:1235–1238.

Toth BB, Chambers MS, Fleming TJ, Lemon JC, Martin JW: Minimizing oral complications of cancer treatment. Oncology 1995;9:851–8585.

Antiemetics

Abrahm JL: Pain management and antiemetic therapy in hematologic disorders. In Hoffman R, Benz EJ, Shattil S, Furie B, Cohen HJ, Silberstein LE, McGlave P (eds): Hematology: Basic Principles and Practice, 3rd ed. New York: Churchill Livingston, 1999, pp 1522–1534.

Anti-emetic Subcommittee of the Multinational Association of Supportive Care in Cancer. Ann Oncol 1998;9:811–819.

Baines M: Nausea and vomiting in the patient with advanced cancer. J Pain Symptom Manage 1988;3:81.

Currow DC, Coughlan M, Fardell B, Cooney NJ: Use of ondansetron in palliative medicine. J Pain Symptom Manage 1997;13:302–307.

Mercadante S: The role of octreotide in palliative care. J Pain Symptom Manage 1994;9:406–411.

Navari RM, Reinhardt RR, Gralla RJ, Kris MG, Hesketh PJ, Khojasteh A, Kindler H, Grote TH, Pendergrass K, Grunberg SM, Carides AD, Gertz BJ: NCCN antiemesis practice guidelines. Oncology 1997;11:57–89.

Navari RM, Reinhardt RR, Gralla RJ, et al: Reduction of cisplatin-induced emesis by a selective neurokinin-1-receptor antagonist: L-754,030 Antiemetic Trials Group. N Engl J Med 1999;340(3):190–195.

Skin Ulcers

Clinical practice guidelines on "Pressure ulcers in adults: prediction and prevention." AHCPR Publications Clearing House, PO Box 8547, Silver Spring, MD 20907, 1992.

Symptoms in the Last Days

Cherny NI, Portenoy RK: Sedation in the management of refractory symptoms: Guidelines for evaluation and treatment. J Palliative Care 1994;10:31–38.

Coyle N, Adelhardt J, Foley KM, Portenoy RK: Character of terminal illness in the advanced cancer patient: Pain and other symptoms during the last four weeks of life. J Pain Symptom Manage 1990;5:83–93.

Ellershaw JE, Sutcliffe JM, Saunders CM: Dehydration and the dying patient. J Pain Symptom Manage 1995;10:192–197.

McCann RM, Hall WJ, Groth-Junker A: Comfort care for terminally ill patients: The appropriate use of nutrition and hydration. JAMA 1994;272:1263–1266.

McIver B, Walsh D, Nelson K: The use of chlorpromazine for symptom control in dying cancer patients. J Pain Symptom Manage 1994;9:341–345.

Truog RD, Berde CB, Mitchell C, Grier HE: Barbiturates in the care of the terminally ill. N Engl J Med 1992;327:1678–1682.

Hospice

42 Codes of Federal Regulations, Part 418, 1993. Medicare Hospice Regulations.

Kinzbrunner BM: Hospice: 15 years and beyond in the care of the dying. J Palliative Med 1998;1:127–137.

Index

Note: Page numbers followed by f indicate figures; those followed by t indicate tables; those followed by b indicate boxed material.

A

Abdominal adenopathy, 217
Abdominal catastrophe, 146
Abdominal ultrasound, for erythrocytosis, 259–260, 260f, 261f
Abdominoperitoneal resection, for anal carcinoma, 939
Abducens nerve deficit, 29t
ABL gene, 678–679, 679f, 680
ABO groups
    and platelet transfusions, 436, 452
    and red blood cell transfusions, 432, 433, 435f
    with stem cell transfusions, 438, 438t
Abscess, epidural, 159, 161, 1080
Absolute neutrophil count (ANC), 241, 244
ABVD regimen, for Hodgkin's disease, 623, 624t, 625, 626
ABX-EGF, 387
Acanthocytes, 276, 277f
Acanthoma, endometrial, 788t
Accelerated fractionation, 327
Accessory nerve deficit, 30t
Acetaminophen
    for pain, 1244, 1245t
    with interferon-alpha therapy of melanoma, 1096b
Acetic acids, for pain, 1245t
Achalasia, 141
Acidified serum lysis test, 469
Acinar-cell carcinoma, of pancreas, 909
Aclarubicin, for acute myeloid leukemia, 533
Acquired immunodeficiency syndrome (AIDS). See Human immunodeficiency virus (HIV).
Acral plantar lesions, 310
Acromegaly, due to pituitary adenoma, 1142t
ACTH (adrenocorticotropic hormone), ectopic production of, 963
Actinic keratoses, 1108, 1111
Actinomycin-D (dactinomycin), 338t
    for Ewing's sarcoma, 1034–1035
    for gestational trophoblastic tumor, 810, 810t
Activated protein C resistance, 289b
Acute chest syndrome, in sickle-cell disease, 465
Acute lymphoblastic leukemia (ALL), 549–564
    Burkitt cell, 550, 552, 559t, 561, 562t
    classification of, 551–552
    clinical and laboratory evaluation of, 551–555, 553t, 554t
    clinical presentation of, 551
    CNS involvement in, 551, 559–561, 563b
    cranial neuropathies due to, 28t
    epidemiology of, 549, 550t
    etiology of, 549–551
    follow-up evaluation for, 563–564
    hematopoietic stem cell transplantation for, 408–409, 409f
    immunophenotyping of, 552–553, 553t
    in children vs. adults, 549, 550t
    morphology and cytochemistry of, 552
    Philadelphia chromosome–positive, 561–562

precursor B-cell, 601–602
precursor T-cell, 601–602
progenitor B cell with t(4:11), 562–563
prognostic factors for, 555
relapse of, 563–564, 563b
treatment of, 555–561
    CNS prophylaxis in, 557t, 559–561
    cranial irradiation in, 557t, 560
    induction therapy in, 556–558, 557t–559t
    maintenance therapy in, 557t, 558–559
    overview of, 555–556
    remission consolidation, 557t, 558
    rescue, 563–564
    stem cell transplantation in, 559
    terminology used in, 556t
Acute lymphocytic leukemia, 280, 281f
    febrile neutropenia in, 1174
    headache with, 21t
    myeloid growth factors for, 424–425, 425t
Acute myelogenous leukemia. See Acute myeloid leukemia (AML).
Acute myeloid leukemia (AML), 521–546
    aberrant expression of lymphoid markers in, 530
    anemia in, 532t
    Auer rods in, 280, 280f, 530
    blood transfusions with, 531
    cell differentiation in, 521, 522f
    classification systems for, 523, 524t, 525t
    clinical evaluation of, 530
    clinical presentation of, 528–531, 529f
    cranial neuropathies due to, 28t
    cytogenetics and molecular genetics of, 523–528, 526t–528t, 527f
    cytologic findings in, 530
    defined, 521
    disseminated intravascular coagulation in, 529–530, 529f, 532t
    due to multiple myeloma treatment, 585
    epidemiology of, 521–523, 522f, 523f
    etiology of, 521
    extramedullary disease in, 528–529, 529f
    febrile neutropenia in, 1174
    genetic factors in, 522, 524, 526t
    hyperleukocytosis and leukostasis in, 529, 532t
    immunophenotype findings in, 530
    in older adults
        prognosis for, 528
        treatment of, 540–541
    metabolic abnormalities with, 530, 532
    neutropenia in, 532, 532t
    prior chemotherapy exposure and, 522–523, 522f, 523f
    prognostic markers for, 525–528, 525t–527t, 527f
    risk factors for, 522–523, 522f, 523f
    routine follow-up in remission for, 546
    secondary, 521, 528
    surface antigen expression in, 530–531
    thrombocytopenia in, 532t, 533
    treatment of, 531–543

anthracyclines for, 533–534, 535t
cytarabine for, 533, 534–536, 534t–536t, 537f, 541–542, 542t
    for relapsed or refractory disease, 540–543, 541f, 542t
gemtuzumab for, 346, 542–543
hematopoietic stem cell transplantation for, 405–408, 406f–407f, 536–540, 538t–540t
in older adults, 540
induction therapy for, 531t, 533–534, 535t
intensive consolidation chemotherapy for, 534–536, 536t, 537f, 539–540, 540t
myeloid growth factors for, 421–424, 421t–425t, 426b
overview of, 531, 531t
postremission therapy in, 531t, 534–540
supportive care in, 531–533, 532t
treatment-related, 521, 528
tumor lysis syndrome in, 530, 532, 532t
vascular access in, 532t
Acute promyelocytic leukemia
    all-trans retinoic acid for, 344, 543, 544t, 545b
    arsenic trioxide for, 544–545, 545t
    hematopoietic stem cell transplantation for, 405–408, 406f–407f
    relapsed or refractory, 543–544
    treatment of, 543–545, 543t–545t, 545b
    unique biologic features of, 543, 543t
Acute pulmonary embolectomy, 514t, 519
Acyclovir, for Epstein-Barr virus, 1163
Adamantinoma, 154, 154f
Adaptation, 1224, 1225b
Adenocarcinoma
    of cervix, 770
    of lung, 968, 968t
    of peritoneum, 1153b
    of unknown primary, 314, 1151b
    pancreatic. See Pancreatic cancer.
Adenoid cystic carcinoma, of trachea, 969
Adenoma(s)
    adrenal, 169, 170, 170f
    hepatocellular, 125–126, 125f
    pituitary. See Pituitary adenoma.
    thyroid, 1117, 1121
Adenomatous polyp(s)
    and colorectal cancer, 923–924, 923f, 924f
    and gastric cancer, 889
Adenomatous polyposis, familial, 1199–1200
    and colorectal cancer, 921, 1199–1200
    genetic basis for, 1194t
    prophylactic surgery for, 371–372
Adenopathy. See Lymphadenopathy.
Adenosine triphosphate, for cachexia, 7–8
Adenosquamous carcinoma
    endometrial, 788–789, 788t
    of lung, 969
Adenovirus vectors, for gene therapy, 383, 383t
Adhesion molecules, in multiple myeloma, 582

Adjustment, to cancer diagnosis, 1224, 1225b
Adjustment disorders, 1224–1226, 1226b
    medication options for, 1227–1228, 1227b
Adjuvant pain relievers, 1248–1249, 1249t
Adjuvant therapy
    for bladder cancer, 855, 855b
    for colorectal cancer, 930–932, 931f, 932t
    for gastric cancer, 896–897, 897f, 897t
    for melanoma, 1094–1095, 1096b
    for pancreatic cancer, 915
    for soft tissue sarcoma, 1045
Adolescents, vaginal bleeding in, 187
ADR-529 (dexrazoxane), with doxorubicin, 351
Adrenal adenoma, 169, 170, 170f
Adrenal carcinoma, 1129–1131
    clinical presentation of, 170, 171f,
        1129–1130
    epidemiology of, 1129
    follow-up for, 1131
    pathology of, 1130
    prognosis for, 1131
    staging of, 1130
    treatment for, 1130–1131, 1131b
Adrenal function abnormalities, after
        hematopoietic stem cell
        transplantation, 404
Adrenal hyperplasia, 169
Adrenal masses
    classification of, 169t
    diagnosis of, 168–171, 169f–171f, 1129–1130
    incidence of, 165
    signs and symptoms of, 165
Adrenal metastasis
    of melanoma, 1088
    of non–small cell lung cancer, 961, 964
Adrenal myelolipoma, 170, 170f
Adrenal-spleen signal ratio (ASR), 170
Adrenocortical carcinoma, 1129–1131
    clinical presentation of, 170–171, 170f,
        1129–1130
    epidemiology of, 1129
    follow-up for, 1131
    pathology of, 1130
    prognosis for, 1131
    staging of, 1130
    treatment for, 1130–1131, 1131b
Adrenocorticotropic hormone (ACTH), ectopic
        production of, 963
Adriamycin. See Doxorubicin (Adriamycin).
Adult T-cell leukemia-lymphoma (ATLL), 248,
        550, 672–675, 673t
African-Americans
    breast cancer in, 724
    cancer in, 1231
    neutropenia in, 246
Agammaglobulinemia, congenital, 551
Age. See also Older adults.
    and breast cancer, 724
Agency for Health Care Policy and Research
        (AHCPR) guideline, for pain
        assessment, 1240–1242
Agitation, in final days, 1255
Agoraphobia, 1226
Agranulocytosis, 245
AIDS. See Human immunodeficiency virus (HIV).
AIHA. See Autoimmune hemolytic anemia
        (AIHA).
AIPC (androgen-independent prostate cancer),
        871–873
Akt, 387
Albinism, and skin cancer, 1105
ALCL (anaplastic large-cell lymphoma), 608f,
        609, 612, 655–656, 668
Alcohol use
    and esophageal cancer, 875
    and head and neck cancer, 999
    pancytopenia due to, 252
Alcohol withdrawal, 1227b
ALG (antilymphocyte globulin), for acute severe
        aplastic anemia, 445
Alkaline phosphatase, in reactive leukocytosis,
        242, 243f
Alkyl sulfonates, 332t, 333t
Alkylating agents, 332t–334t, 348
    for chronic lymphocytic leukemia, 692–693
    myelodysplasia due to, 569, 569t
ALL. See Acute lymphoblastic leukemia (ALL).
Allergic drug reactions, pruritus due to, 15

Allergic granulomatosis, 249
Allium sativum, 1213t
Allogeneic blood donations, 431
Allogeneic hematopoietic stem cell
        transplantation, 391, 392–397
    advantages and disadvantages of, 394, 398t
    autologous vs., 398t
    conditioning regimens for, 393, 394–396,
        395t, 396t
    for chronic myeloid leukemia, 683–684
    for Hodgkin's disease, 627
    for leukemia
        acute lymphoblastic, 559
        acute myeloid, 536, 537–539, 538t,
            540t
        chronic lymphocytic, 696
        chronic myeloid, 683–684
    for multiple myeloma, 592
    for myelodysplastic syndrome, 575b, 578
    for non-Hodgkin's lymphoma, 643–644
    graft-versus-host disease due to, 391, 396–
        397
    graft-versus-tumor effect in, 394
    identification of donor for, 392–393
    nonmyeloablative, 394
    principles underlying, 393–394
    sources of cells for, 391–392, 392t
Alloimmune hemolysis, 470t
Alloimmunization, due to transfusion, 440, 452
Allopurinol, for hyperuricemia, 1187–1188
All-trans retinoic acid (ATRA, Tretinoin,
        Vesanoid), 344
    for acute promyelocytic leukemia, 543, 544t,
        545b
Aloe (Aloe vera), 1213t
Alpha-2 agonists, for neuropathic pain, 1249t
Alphanate SD/HT, for von Willebrand's disease,
        506
Alpha-tocopherol
    and head and neck cancer, 1013–1014,
        1013t, 1015
    and prostate cancer, 861
Alprazolam (Xanax)
    for agitation, 1255
    for anticipatory nausea and vomiting, 1250
    for anxiety, 1227, 1227b, 1254t
Alprostadil, for erectile dysfunction, 1238
Alternative therapies. See Unorthodox
        treatment(s).
Alum, for hematuria, 177
Ambien (zolpidem), 1227b
American Society of Clinical Oncology (ASCO),
        cancer predisposition testing
        guidelines of, 1206, 1206t
Amines, secondary, and gastric cancer, 889
Aminoglutethimide, 341t, 347
    for adrenal cancer, 1131
D-Aminophenol, for pain, 1245t
Amitriptyline, for neuropathic pain, 1249t
AML. See Acute myeloid leukemia (AML).
Amphotericin B, for febrile neutropenia, 1176,
        1177b, 1177f
Amygdalin, 1217t, 1219–1220
Amyloidosis, 595–596
    immunoglobulin abnormalities due to, 205,
        205b
    vascular cutaneous manifestations of, 297,
        297f
    with multiple myeloma, 582, 596
Anagrelide, for essential thrombocythemia, 712
Anal carcinoma, 938–941
    anatomy of, 938–939
    chemotherapy for, 940–941
    epidemiology of, 938
    histology of, 939
    human papillomavirus and, 938
    local excision for, 941
    locally recurrent, 941
    metastatic, 941
    radiation therapy for, 939–941
    staging of, 939, 940t
    surgery for, 939, 941–942
Analgesic(s), for back pain, 162
Analgesic ladder, 1244–1246
Anaphylactoid reaction, to paclitaxel and
        carboplatin, 798
Anaplastic large-cell lymphoma (ALCL), 608f,
        609, 612, 655–656, 668

Anastrozole (Arimidex), 341t, 347
    for breast cancer
        locally invasive, 741
        metastatic, 753t, 754, 754t
ANC (absolute neutrophil count), 241, 244
Androgen(s)
    and prostate cancer, 860–861
    for Fanconi's anemia, 450
    for refractory severe aplastic anemia, 448
Androgen ablation, for prostate cancer, 867,
        869–871, 872
Androgen receptor antagonists, 332t, 341t, 344
Androgen-independent prostate cancer (AIPC),
        871–873
Anemia, 232–240
    aplastic, 443–448
        acute severe, 444–446, 444t
            hematopoietic stem cell transplantation
                for, 395, 395t, 413–414, 413t
            infections with, 452
        moderate, 446–448
        pancytopenia in, 253, 255, 255f
        refractory severe, 448
        reticulocyte count in, 240, 240b
        transfusions for, 451
    bone marrow aspirate and biopsy for, 234b
    defined, 232
    diagnostic approach to, 235–240, 240b
    Diamond-Blackfan, 451
    due to cancer, 1166–1168, 1167f, 1168f
    due to myelodysplasia, 569, 569t, 575b
    due to therapy for small cell lung cancer, 954
    dyspnea due to, 79
    Fanconi's, 450
        leukemia in, 551
        myelodysplasia in, 568
        pancytopenia in, 253
    hemolytic, 238–240, 239f, 240b, 240f
        due to cancer, 1167–1168, 1168f
        immune-mediated, 233t, 238, 276, 276f,
            1168, 1168f
        in sickle-cell disease, 464t
        microangiopathic, 238–240, 492, 492f
        nonimmune-mediated, 238
        transfusion support of, 434b
        warm autoimmune, 470–471, 470t, 472f,
            473b
    history of, 232, 233t
    hypochromic microcytic, 234, 234b, 235t,
        236–238, 276–277
    in acute lymphoblastic leukemia, 551
    in acute myeloid leukemia, 532t
    in idiopathic myelofibrosis, 706–707, 708
    in myelodysplasia, 428b
    iron deficiency. See Iron deficiency.
    laboratory diagnosis of, 233–237, 235f, 235t,
        236t, 237f
    macrocytic, 234, 234b, 235t, 238, 277
    megaloblastic
        hyperbilirubinemia due to, 197–198
        mean corpuscular volume in, 235
    normocytic normochromic, 234, 234b, 235t,
        238–240, 239f, 240f, 276
    of chronic disease, 233t, 457–458
    of prematurity, 420–421
    of renal failure, 419–420
    pathophysiology of, 232, 235–236
    peripheral blood smear for, 235, 236t, 237f
    pernicious, 233t, 455–457
        and gastric cancer, 888
    physical examination for, 232–233, 233t
    red blood cell abnormalities in, 272b,
        276–277, 277f
    red blood cell indices in, 234–235, 235f, 235t
    refractory, 253
    reticulocyte count in, 235
        increased, 238–240, 239f, 240f
        reduced, 240
    reticulocyte(s) in, 235, 237f, 238f
    sickle cell. See Sickle-cell disease.
    sideroblastic, 276
Anesthetic techniques, for pain, 1249
Aneuploidy, with cancer of unknown primary,
        1148
Aneurysm bleed, headache due to, 20t
Aneurysmal bone cysts, 153–154
Angiocentric lymphoma, 669
Angiodysplasia, GI bleeding due to, 144

Angiogenesis
    in cancer of unknown primary, 1148
    in multiple myeloma, 582
    tumor, 384–385, 384t
Angiography
    computed tomography pulmonary, 288–289,
        289f
    magnetic resonance
        of brain tumor, 1050
        of neck mass, 46–47
    pulmonary contrast, 287
Angioimmunoblastic T-cell lymphoma, 668
Angiokeratoma corporis diffusum, 296, 296f
Angiomata, spider, 297
Angiomyolipoma, renal, 167, 168f
Angiosarcoma, 1039t, 1041
Angiostatin, 384
Angular cheilitis, 232
Anhedonia, 1225
Anisocytosis, 235, 274
Anisopoikilocytosis, 571f
Ann Arbor staging system, for lymphomas,
    638–639, 638t, 650, 650t
Anorexia
    in small cell lung cancer, 954
    pathogenesis of, 3
    therapy for, 5–6, 5t
Anorexia nervosa, pancytopenia due to, 252
Antacids
    for hyperphosphatemia, 1189
    for pancreatic cancer, 917
Anthracenediones, 332t, 338t, 351
Anthracyclines, 332t, 337t, 350–351, 351f, 356t
    for acute myeloid leukemia, 533–534, 535t
    for acute promyelocytic leukemia, 545b
    for locally invasive breast cancer, 739, 742
Antiandrogens, 332t, 341t, 344
    for prostate cancer, 870–871, 872
Antiangiogenic therapy, 384–385, 384t
    for giant cell tumors of bone, 1036
Antibiotic prophylaxis
    for aplastic anemia, 452
    for chronic lymphocytic leukemia, 689
    for febrile neutropenia, 1176, 1176b
    for Hodgkin's disease, 622
    for multiple myeloma, 592
Anticardiolipin antibodies, 289b
Anticipatory nausea and vomiting, 1250
Anticoagulant therapy
    complications of, 517–518, 518f
    for superior vena cava syndrome, 104
    for venous thromboembolism, 514–517,
        514t, 515t, 516f, 1182
    monitoring of, 1185
Anticonvulsants, 25, 25t, 26b
    for brain metastases, 1069, 1069b
    for brain tumors, 1057–1058
    for neuropathic pain, 1248, 1249t
Anti-D immune globulin, for idiopathic
    thrombocytopenic purpura, 489
Antidepressants, tricyclic, for neuropathic pain,
    1248, 1249t
Antidiuretic hormone, syndrome of
    inappropriate secretion of, in lung
    cancer
    non–small cell, 963
    small cell, 947
Antiemetics, 1250–1251, 1251t, 1252t
Antiepileptic drugs, 25, 25t, 26b
Antiestrogens, 340t–341t
Antihuman immune globulin, 433, 471t
Anti-idiotypic antibodies, 379, 381
Anti-inflammatory agents, for cachexia, 8
Antilymphocyte globulin (ALG), for acute severe
    aplastic anemia, 445
Antimetabolites, 332t
Antimicrotubule agents, 340t, 352–353
Antimitotic drugs, 332t, 352
Antineoplastic agents, encephalopathy due to, 35
Antineoplastons, 1217–1218, 1217t
Antiphospholipid antibodies, 289, 289b
Antiphospholipid syndrome, cutaneous
    manifestations of, 303
Antiplatelet agents, for thrombotic
    thrombocytopenic purpura, 493
Antiplatelet antibody testing, 224
Antiseizure medications. See Anticonvulsants.
Antisense oligonucleotides, 383

Anti-Tac, for adult T-cell leukemia/lymphoma,
    675
Antithrombin assay, 289, 289b
Antithymocyte globulin (ATG)
    for aplastic anemia
        acute severe, 445–446
        moderate, 446–447
        refractory severe, 448
    for Diamond-Blackfan anemia, 451
    for graft-versus-host disease, 396
    for paroxysmal nocturnal hemoglobinuria,
        449
    for pure red cell aplasia, 450
    in conditioning regimen for hematopoietic
        stem cell transplantation, 395,
        395f
Antivert (meclizine), for nausea and vomiting,
    1252t
Anxiety disorders, 1226, 1226b, 1254t
    medications for, 1227–1228, 1227b
Anxiolytics, 1227–1228, 1227b
APC gene, 1200
Apheresis platelets, 431n, 432t
Aplastic anemia, 443–448
    acute severe, 444–446, 444t
        hematopoietic stem cell transplantation for,
            395, 395t, 413–414, 413t
        infections with, 452
    moderate, 446–448
    pancytopenia in, 253, 255, 255f
    refractory severe, 448
    reticulocyte count in, 240, 240b
    transfusions for, 451
Apoptosis, in radiation therapy, 323
Appendiceal carcinoid tumors, 1134t, 1135
Aquagenic pruritus, 15
    in polycythemia vera, 705
Arctium lappa, 1214, 1215
Aredia. See Pamidronate (Aredia).
Argatroban, for heparin-induced
    thrombocytopenia, 487–488, 488t
Arginine desmopressin (DDAVP)
    for acquired platelet function disorders, 495
    for hemophilia A, 499, 500b
    for surgery with chronic renal failure, 509b
    for von Willebrand's disease, 506
Arimidex. See Anastrozole (Arimidex).
Aromasin (exemestane), 341t, 347
    for metastatic breast cancer, 753t, 754, 754t
Aromatase, 347
Aromatase inhibitors, 332t, 341t, 347
    for breast cancer
        locally invasive, 741
        metastatic, 752, 753t, 754–755, 754t,
            755f
Arsenic trioxide
    for acute promyelocytic leukemia, 544–545,
        545t
    for adult T-cell leukemia/lymphoma, 674
    for multiple myeloma, 591
Arterial thrombosis
    due to essential thrombocythemia, 711
    due to polycythemia vera, 702
Arteritis, temporal, 20t
Arthrodesis, for joint disease in hemophilia A,
    502b
Arthroplasties, for joint disease in hemophilia A,
    502b
Arytenoid dislocation, 51t
Ascites, 128–134
    asymptomatic, 130–131
    bloody, 146
    chylous, 129t, 131
    defined, 128
    diagnosis of, 128–131, 130t
    due to lymphadenopathy, 217
    due to ovarian carcinoma, 792, 792f
    malignant
        as presenting sign of disease, 133
        causes of, 128, 129t
        diagnosis of, 129–130, 130t, 131–132
        treatment for, 132–133, 132f, 132t, 133f
    nonmalignant
        causes of, 128, 129t
        diagnosis of, 130
        treatment for, 131
    pathophysiology and pathogenesis of, 128
    tumor types associated with, 128, 129f, 129t

ASCO (American Society of Clinical Oncology),
    cancer predisposition testing
    guidelines of, 1206, 1206t
Ascorbic acid, for Chèdiak-Higashi syndrome,
    479
ASCUS (atypical squamous cells of
    undetermined significance), and
    cervical cancer, 770
Ashkenazi Jewish population, hereditary breast
    cancer in, 1195–1196, 1196f
L-Asparaginase
    for acute lymphoblastic leukemia, 557t
    superficial thrombophlebitis with, 1184
Aspergillus infection
    febrile neutropenia due to, 1173, 1174f,
        1175f, 1176
    fever of unknown origin due to, 11
    in chronic granulomatous disease, 481,
        482–483
    with hematopoietic stem cell transplantation,
        400–401
Aspirin
    bleeding disorder due to, 265, 270
    for pain, 1245t
    for prevention of colorectal cancer, 924
    for thrombotic thrombocytopenic purpura,
        493
Asplenia, 243
ASR (adrenal-spleen signal ratio), 170
Astrocytomas, 1051, 1052f
    anaplastic, 1052, 1053
    pilocytic, 1051
    seizures due to, 23
    temozolomide for, 348
    thromboembolic events due to, 1058
Atarax, with interferon-alpha therapy of
    melanoma, 1096b
Ataxia telangiectasia
    cutaneous manifestations of, 296
    genetic basis for, 1194t, 1198
    leukemia in, 551
    myelodysplasia in, 568
ATG. See Antithymocyte globulin (ATG).
Atheroemboli, cutaneous manifestations of, 303
Ativan. See Lorazepam (Ativan).
ATLL (adult T-cell leukemia-lymphoma), 248,
    550, 672–675, 673t
ATM gene, 1198
ATRA (all-trans retinoic acid), 344
    for acute promyelocytic leukemia, 543, 544t,
        545b
Atrial myxoma, fever due to, 9
Atropine, for death rattle, 1254t, 1255
Atypical squamous cells of undetermined
    significance (ASCUS), and
    cervical cancer, 770
Auer rods, 280, 280f, 530
Auras, 23
Autoerythrocyte sensitization, 300, 300f
Autofluorescence bronchoscopy, for non–small
    cell lung cancer, 967
Autoimmune disorders
    after hematopoietic stem cell transplantation,
        403–404
    due to thymoma, 984, 984f
    in chronic lymphocytic leukemia, 689–690
    vascular cutaneous manifestations of, 299
Autoimmune hemolytic anemia (AIHA), 233t,
    469–472
    classification of, 469, 470t
    cold, 470t, 471–472, 472f
    diagnosis of, 238, 456t, 469–470, 471f
    due to cancer, 1168, 1168f
    in chronic lymphocytic leukemia, 689
    red blood cell abnormalities in, 276, 276f,
        469, 470f
    signs and symptoms of, 469
Autoimmune thrombocytopenic purpura,
    488–492, 490f
Autologous blood donations, 431
Autologous hematopoietic stem cell
    transplantation, 391, 397–398,
    399t
    for Hodgkin's disease, 627
    for leukemia
        acute lymphoblastic, 559
        acute myeloid, 536, 539, 539t, 540t
        chronic myeloid, 684

Autologous hematopoietic stem cell
   transplantation, *(Continued)*
   for multiple myeloma, 589b, 591–592
   for non-Hodgkin's lymphoma, 642
      intermediate-grade, 652
Autologous tumor proteins, in vaccine therapy,
   380–381
Automated dose optimization, for radiation
   therapy, 326
Autonomic neuropathy, 37
Avascular necrosis, after hematopoietic stem cell
   transplantation, 404
Axillary adenopathy, 215t, 216, 217
   isolated, 1152b
Axillary lymph node involvement, in breast
   cancer, 718, 719, 720t
Axillary vein thrombosis, catheter-associated, 1184
Axonal neuropathy, 36–37
5-Azacytidine, for myelodysplasia, 576
Azathioprine, for idiopathic thrombocytopenic
   purpura, 491
Azygos veins, 98, 99f

B
BAC (bronchoalveolar carcinoma), 968
Bacille Calmette-Guèerin (BCG) vaccine, for
   superficial bladder cancer, 846,
   847b, 848b
Back pain, 156–163
   as medical emergency, 158b
   differential diagnosis of, 159–162, 159t, 160f
   due to bacterial infection, 158–159, 159t,
      161–162, 162t
   due to degenerative disease of spine, 159t,
      160–161, 162t
   due to epidural compression by metastasis,
      159–160, 159t, 160f, 162t
   due to herpes zoster, 159t, 161, 162, 162t
   due to meningismus, 157, 159t, 161, 162t
   due to vertebral compression fracture, 159t,
      160, 162t
   evaluation of, 156–159, 157f
   in myeloma, 582
   location of, 156
   management of, 162–163, 162t
   natural history of malignancy with, 158
   neuroimaging of, 158–159
   neurologic signs and symptoms with,
      157–158, 162–163
   quality of, 156
   temporal pattern of, 156–157
Bacterial inclusions, 281f, 282
Bacterial infection(s)
   back pain due to, 158–159, 159t, 161–162,
      162t
   in multiple myeloma, 582, 584, 592
   with hematopoietic stem cell transplantation,
      400
Barbiturates, for delirium, 1254t
Barium esophagram, 876, 876f
Barium swallow
   for dysphagia, 140, 141f
   for hoarseness, 54
Barrel cervix, 773b
Barrett's esophagus, 140, 875, 876, 889
Basal cell carcinoma, 1105–1108
   clinical evaluation of, 1106, 1106f
   clinical presentation of, 1105–1106
   follow-up evaluation of, 1107–1108
   low-risk *vs.* high-risk, 1106, 1108t
   metastatic, 1106
   nevoid, 1194t, 1202–1203
   nodular, 1105–1106
   of vulva, 778
   pathogenesis of, 1104–1105
   pigmented, 308t, 1106
   recurrence of, 1107–1108, 1108t
      risk factors for, 1106, 1108t
   sclerosing, 1106
   staging of, 1106, 1107t
   superficial, 1106
   treatment for, 1106–1107, 1109f
   ulcerated, 1106f
Basal cell nevus syndrome, 1040, 1105
Basaloid squamous carcinomas, of head and
   neck, 1000
Basket cells, 279
Basophilic stippling, 237f, 277, 278f

Bayesian modification of risk, 1204–1205
B-cell leukemia
   chronic lymphocytic, 602–604, 604f, 604t
   precursor (acute) lymphoblastic, 601–602
   prolymphocytic, 696–697
B-cell lymphoma
   diffuse large, 604f, 608
   marginal zone, 604f, 605–606
   precursor lymphoblastic, 601–602
   rituximab for, 345–346
   small lymphocytic, 603–604, 604f, 604t, 612
   types of, 602–603
BCG (bacille Calmette-Guèrin) vaccine, for
   superficial bladder cancer, 846,
   847b, 848b
Bcl-2, in cancer of unknown primary, 1148
BCMVP regimen, for multiple myeloma, 589
BCNU. *See* Carmustine (BCNU).
BCR gene, 678, 679f, 680
BEACOPP regimen, for Hodgkin's disease, 624t,
   625
Beam arrangement, for radiation therapy,
   325–326, 325f, 326f
Beam-shaping devices, for radiation therapy,
   321–322, 322f
Bellini duct carcinoma, 826, 826t, 827f
Benadryl (diphenhydramine), 1227b
   with haloperidol, 1248
   with interferon-alpha therapy of melanoma,
      1096b
Bence-Jones protein, in multiple myeloma, 587
Benzodiazepines
   for anxiety, 1227–1228, 1227b
   for delirium, 1248, 1248t
   for nausea and vomiting, 1251
Bereavement counselors, 1259
Bernard-Soulier syndrome, 270, 494
Beta-2 microglobulin, in multiple myeloma, 588
Beta-carotene
   for head and neck cancer, 1013t
   for lung cancer, 978
Bexarotene (Targretin), 344–345
Bexxar (tositumomab), for non-Hodgkin's
   lymphoma, intermediate-grade,
   653
BFU-E (burst-forming unit erythroid) assays,
   261–262
Bicalutamide (Casodex), 341t, 344
   for prostate cancer, 870
Biliary cancer, 903–905, 905b
Biliary cystadenoma, 123, 125f
Biliary drainage, for biliary cancer, 905b
Biliary duct stenting
   for biliary cancer, 905b
   for pancreatic cancer, 916
Biliary tract obstruction
   hyperbilirubinemia due to, 198
   pruritus due to, 14
Bilirubin
   direct (conjugated), 196, 198–199
   elevated. *See* Hyperbilirubinemia.
   in hemolytic anemia, 240b
   indirect (unconjugated), 196, 197–198
   serum, 196
   sources of, 196
Billroth I gastrectomy, 362
Binet system, for chronic lymphocytic leukemia,
   692, 692t
Biofeedback, for pain management, 1244
Biologic behavior, of cancer of unknown origin,
   315
Biologic therapy, 376–388
   antiangiogenic, 384–385, 384t
   cell signaling in, 385–387
   cytokines in, 376–377, 377t
   for head and neck cancer, 1008t
   for melanoma, 1094–1095, 1096b,
      1097–1100, 1098f, 1099f
   for mesothelioma, 996–997
   gene therapy as, 382–384, 382t, 383t
   monoclonal antibodies in, 377–379, 378t
   vaccine therapy as, 379–382, 380t
Biologically guided chemotherapy, 1221t
Bio-oxidative therapy, 1221t
Biopsy
   bone marrow
      for acute lymphoblastic leukemia, 551
      for anemia, 234b

for erythrocytosis, 261, 262f
   for multiple myeloma, 587, 587f
   for myelodysplasia, 570, 570t, 571f, 572t
   for pancytopenia, 254–255, 254t, 255f
   for splenomegaly, 137–138
   for thrombocytopenia, 224, 224f, 226b
   for Waldenström's macroglobulinemia,
      598
   endometrial, 186, 783–784
   for bladder cancer, 851
   for breast cancer, 61, 63–64
   for cancer of unknown primary, 314–315,
      315t, 1147
   for hilar and mediastinal adenopathy, 96,
      97b
   for hoarseness, 55, 56b
   for lung cancer
      non–small cell, 967, 967b
      small cell, 948
   for pancreatic cancer, 913
   for peripheral neuropathy, 37, 39t
   for salivary gland carcinoma, 1020
   for splenomegaly, 137–138
   for superficial bladder cancer, 846–847
   lymph node, 218–219, 219b
   of breast mass, 63–64
   of neck mass, 47, 48
   of pigmented skin lesions, 308, 311–312
   of pleural effusion, 89
   of soft-tissue mass, 1041
   of solitary pulmonary nodule, 85–86
   of vulva, 776b, 776f, 777f
   sentinel lymph node
      for breast cancer, 718
      for gastrointestinal cancer, 366
      for melanoma, 1092–1094, 1092f, 1093b
   testicular, 182
   thyroid, 1118
Bioreductive alkylating agents, 334t
Bipolar mood disorder, 1227b
BI-RADS (Breast Imaging Reporting Data
   System), 65, 66t
Bispecific antibodies, 379
Bisphosphonates
   for hypercalcemia, 193–194, 194t
      in metastatic breast cancer, 760–761
   for pain, 1249
   for skeletal complications of multiple
      myeloma, 592–593
Bite cells, 275, 276
Blackledge staging system, for gastrointestinal
   non-Hodgkin's lymphomas, 654,
   654t
Bladder cancer
   cigarette smoking and, 842, 850
   epidemiology of, 842
   familial clustering of, 842, 851
   hematuria due to, 173
   histologic subtypes of, 842
   muscle-invasive, 850–856
      chemotherapy for, 853–856
      clinical presentation and initial
         evaluation of, 851
      epidemiology of, 850–851
      histologic subtypes of, 850
      locally advanced, 855b
      metastatic, 853, 855b
      radical cystectomy for, 851–853
      risk factors for, 850
      staging and prognostic factors for, 851,
         852b, 852t
   superficial, 842–848
      clinical presentation and evaluation of,
         842–843, 843f
      cystoscopy of, 844, 844f
      cytology of, 843, 845b
      defined, 842
      follow-up evaluation for, 846–848, 847b,
         848b
      radiographic appearance of, 843, 843f
      recurrence of, 844, 845t
      staging, prognostic features, and
         outcomes for, 843–844, 843f,
         844t, 845b, 845t
      treatment of, 844–846
Bladder irrigation, for hematuria, 176–177
Blast crisis, in chronic myeloid leukemia, 677b,
   678, 682–683

Bleeding
  elevated platelet count after, 229
  epidural, 1080
  gastrointestinal. *See* Gastrointestinal (GI)
      bleeding.
  in dying patient, 1255–1256
  in myelodysplasia, 575b
  in surgical patient, 510
  intramuscular, 499
  subarachnoid, 157–158, 159
  subcutaneous, 295, 295f
  vaginal. *See* Vaginal bleeding.
Bleeding disorder(s), 265–271
  acquired, 267–270, 269b
  coagulation disorders as, 266–267, 267t
  concurrent disease with, 265
  congenital, 265–266, 270–271
  cutaneous manifestations of. *See* Cutaneous
      manifestations, of bleeding and
      thromboembolic disorders.
  diagnosis of, 267–271
  drug-related, 265
  due to platelet function abnormalities, 267
  familial, 265–266
  fibrolytic, 267
  history of, 265–266
  indications for evaluation of, 266b
  presentation of, 265
  spectrum of, 265–267
  von Willebrand's disease as, 267
Bleeding risk, of thrombocytopenia, 221
Bleomycin, 339t, 355t
  for cervical cancer, 775t
  for esophageal cancer, 878t
  for germ-cell tumors, 818, 819b, 820b, 822
  for head and neck cancer, 1008t
  for Kaposi's sarcoma, 1160
  for pleural effusion, 92
  pulmonary complications of, 78t, 630
Blessed thistle, 1215
Blindness, due to cranial neuropathy, 29t
Blood collection, 431
Blood components. *See* Blood product(s).
Blood donations, 431
Blood loss, iron deficiency due to, 210
Blood product(s), 431–438, 432t
  cryoprecipitate as, 432t, 437
  hematopoietic progenitor cells as, 437–438,
      438t
  plasma as, 432t, 436–437, 437t
  platelets as, 432t, 434–436
  red blood cells as, 431–433, 432t, 433f, 434b,
      435f
Blood tests
  for encephalopathy, 33–34
  for peripheral neuropathy, 39t
Blood transfusions, 431–440
  adverse consequences of, 438–440, 439t
  blood collection for, 431
  blood products for, 431–438, 432t
  for acute myeloid leukemia, 531
  for myelodysplasia, 575b
  for sickle-cell disease, 464b
  for thalassemia, 460b
  for warm antibody autoimmune hemolytic
      anemia, 473b
  of cryoprecipitate, 432t, 437
  of granulocytes
      for bone marrow failure syndrome, 452
      for chronic granulomatous disease, 481
  of hematopoietic progenitor cells. *See*
      Hematopoietic stem cell
      transplantation (HSCT).
  of plasma, 432t, 436–437, 437t
  of platelets, 432t, 434–436
      for acquired platelet function disorders,
          495
      for acute myeloid leukemia, 533
      for bone marrow failure syndrome,
          451–452
      for idiopathic thrombocytopenic purpura,
          491
      for myelodysplasia, 575b
      for thrombocytopenia, 486
  of red blood cells, 431–433, 432t, 433f, 434b,
      435f
      for bone marrow failure syndrome, 451
      for myelodysplasia, 575b

Blood vessels, of tumor, 354
Bloody ascites, 146
Bloom syndrome
  leukemia in, 551
  myelodysplasia in, 568
Blue nevus, 308t
"Blue-gray veil," 305–306
Blumer's shelf, 890
Body position, and headache, 21b
Bone cysts, 153–154
Bone destruction, in multiple myeloma, 583–
      584
Bone marrow aspiration and biopsy
  for acute lymphoblastic leukemia, 551
  for anemia, 234b
  for erythrocytosis, 261, 262f
  for multiple myeloma, 587, 587f
  for myelodysplasia, 570, 570t, 571f, 572t
  for pancytopenia, 254–255, 254t, 255f
  for splenomegaly, 137–138
  for thrombocytopenia, 224, 224f, 226b
  for Waldenström's macroglobulinemia,
      598
Bone marrow dysplasia, in myelodysplasia,
      571f, 572t
Bone marrow failure syndrome(s), 443–452
  acquired aplastic anemia as, 443–448
      acute severe, 444–446, 444t
      moderate, 446–448
      refractory severe, 448
  Diamond-Blackfan anemia as, 451
  due to myelodysplasia, 567
  due to parvovirus infection, 451
  Fanconi's anemia as, 450
  paroxysmal nocturnal hemoglobinuria as,
      448–450
  pure red cell aplasia as, 450–451
  pure white cell aplasia as, 451
  supportive treatment in, 451–452
Bone marrow findings, in chronic myeloid
      leukemia, 677
Bone marrow transplantation. *See also*
      Hematopoietic stem cell
      transplantation.
  fever of unknown origin due to, 11–13,
      12b
  for aplastic anemia
      acute severe, 444, 444t, 446t
      moderate, 447–448
      refractory severe, 448
  for chronic granulomatous disease, 481
  for Diamond-Blackfan anemia, 451
  for Fanconi's anemia, 450
Bone metastasis
  of breast cancer, 151f, 155f, 255f, 751t,
      760–761
  of lung cancer
      non–small cell, 961, 966
      small cell, 946
  of melanoma, 1087
  of multiple myeloma, 582, 585, 592–593
  pancytopenia due to, 253
  pathologic fractures due to. *See* Pathologic
      fractures.
Bone pain
  due to multiple myeloma, 582
  due to pathologic fracture, 150
Bone sarcoma(s), 1027–1036
  chondro-, 1029t, 1033–1034, 1033f, 1033t
  classification of, 1027, 1028t
  diagnosis of, 1027
  Ewing's, 154, 315, 1029t, 1034–1035, 1034f,
      1035f
  incidence of, 1027
  malignant fibrous histiocytoma as, 1029t,
      1032–1033
  osteo-, 1028–1032, 1029f, 1029t, 1030f
  staging of, 1027, 1028t
Bone scans
  for back pain, 159
  for non–small cell lung cancer, 966
Bone tumor(s)
  benign, 1027
  chordoma as, 1035
  classification of, 1027, 1028t
  giant-cell, 1036, 1036f
  pathologic fractures due to. *See* Pathologic
      fractures.

Bonine (meclizine), for nausea and vomiting,
      1252t
Bosniak classification, of renal cysts, 166, 166t
Bowel injury, radiation-induced, 371
Bowel obstruction, 109–113
  differential diagnosis of, 109–110, 110f, 110t
  due to colorectal cancer, 926, 926t
  gastric outlet or duodenal, 109, 110t, 111,
      112
  in Ogilvie's syndrome, 110
  in patients with history of malignancy, 111
  initial evaluation and management of,
      111–112, 111f
  large, 109–110, 110t, 111–113
  operative management of, 112–113, 370–
      371
  small, 109, 110t, 111, 112
Bowel preparation, mechanical, 112
"Bowenoid" papulosis, 1109
Bowen's disease, 1108–1109
Brachytherapy, 321, 322
  for prostate cancer, 868
Brain metastasis, 1062–1075
  clinical evaluation of, 1064–1066, 1065t,
      1066f, 1067f
  clinical presentation of, 1062–1064, 1063f
  differential diagnosis of, 1067
  encephalopathy due to, 35
  epidemiology of, 1062, 1063f
  follow-up for, 1075
  headache due to, 1062
  mental status changes due to, 1062–1063,
      1065, 1065t
  newly diagnosed, 1074f
  of breast cancer, 751t, 1073–1074
  of germ-cell tumors, 822b
  of lung cancer, 1073
      non–small cell, 961–962, 966
      small cell, 946, 952
  of melanoma, 1074–1075, 1087–1088, 1088t,
      1100b
  of testicular cancer, 1075
  of unknown origin, 316
  recurrent, 1075f
  seizures due to, 1064
  staging, prognostic features, and outcome of,
      1066–1068, 1067t, 1068f
  treatment of, 1068–1075
      anticonvulsants for, 1069
      chemotherapy for, 1073–1075, 1074f,
          1075f
      glucocorticoids for, 1069–1070, 1070b
      in stable patient, 1069–1075
      in unstable patient, 1068, 1069b
      radiation therapy for, 1070–1071, 1071t
      surgery for, 1071–1073, 1072t
      symptomatic, 1069–1070, 1070b
  weakness due to, 1063
Brain tumor(s), 1049–1059
  anticonvulsants for, 1057–1058
  care of dying patient with, 1058–1059
  clinical evaluation of, 1050–1051, 1050t
  clinical presentation of, 1049–1050, 1050t
  encephalopathy due to, 32, 34t
  ependymomas as, 1056
  epidemiology of, 1049
  follow-up evaluation for, 1059
  gliomas as
      brainstem, 1056–1057
      high-grade, 1052–1053, 1053f, 1054b
      low-grade, 1051–1052, 1052b, 1052f
  glucocorticoids for, 1058
  headache due to, 19, 20t, 21, 21t, 22t
  in children, 1049
  management issues for, 1057–1059
  medulloblastoma as, 1055
  meningiomas as, 1055, 1057f
  primary central nervous system lymphoma
      as, 1053–1054, 1055f, 1056b
  psychosocial issues with, 1058
  risk factors for, 1049
  seizures due to, 23, 24–25, 24f, 1058
  staging, prognostic features, and outcomes
      of, 1051, 1051t
  temozolomide for, 348
  thromboembolic disease due to, 1058
  treatment for, 1051–1057
Brainstem gliomas, 1056–1057

BRCA1 and BRCA2 genes, 765, 1194,
    1195–1196, 1196f, 1196t, 1204
Breakthrough pain, 1241
Breast cancer
    axillary lymph node involvement in, 718,
        719, 720t
    biologic therapy for, 378
    biopsy for, 61, 63–64, 66–70
    capecitabine for, 348
    cranial neuropathies due to, 28t
    disease-free interval in, 750
    ductal
        in situ. See Ductal carcinoma in situ
            (DCIS).
        infiltrating, 61, 62f, 67f, 69f
            calcifications with, 68f
    epidemiology of, 1195
    genetic basis for, 1195–1198
        age-specific penetrance with, 1195, 1195f
        conditions associated with, 1197–1198
        epidemiology of, 1195
        genes involved in, 1194, 1194t, 1195
        in Ashkenazi Jewish population,
            1195–1196, 1196f
        indicators of, 1195, 1195t
        initial management with, 1197b
        models for evaluating, 1196
        risk management guidelines with, 1196t,
            1197
    genetic testing for, 765
    headache with, 21t
    hematopoietic stem cell transplantation for,
        414
    history taking for, 59
    hormone replacement therapy after, 765,
        766b
    hypercalcemia due to, 191, 194
    imaging studies of, 59–60, 61f, 62f, 65–66,
        67f–69f
    in pregnant or lactating women, 62–63
    in situ
        ductal. See Ductal carcinoma in situ
            (DCIS).
        lobular, 726, 733–735, 734f
    inflammatory, 67f, 717
    isolated tumor cells in, 717–718
    lifestyle and dietary changes for, 765–767
    lobular, in situ, 726, 733–735, 734f
    locally invasive, 737–749
        follow-up of, 747, 747t
        incidence of, 737
        initial evaluation of, 737, 738f
        pathology report for, 737, 738t
        prognostic factors for, 745–746, 746t
        recurrence of, 743, 747
        therapy for
            breast-conserving, 737–738
            chemohormonal, 742
            chemotherapy as, 738–740, 742, 743t
            endocrine, 740–742
            radiation, 737–738, 743t
            selection of, 742–747, 744f, 745f
            tamoxifen as, 739, 740–741, 742,
                743t
            ten-year survival after, 743–745, 746t
            toxicity of, 742, 743t
    lymphedema after, 763
    malpractice litigation on, 60b
    mammography of, 62f, 65, 67f–69f
    medical surveillance after, 764, 764b
    medullary, 67f
    menopausal symptoms and health with, 765,
        766b
    metastatic, 750–762
        approach to solitary sites of, 761b
        chemotherapy for, 756–760, 756t
            high-dose, 758
            in older women, 758
            suggested approach to, 759–760,
                759f
            vs. hormonal therapy, 755
            with capecitabine, 756t, 758
            with doxorubicin and taxanes,
                756–758, 756t, 757t
            with trastuzumab, 756t, 758
        clinical trials for, 761–762
        factors in management of, 750, 751f
        future of treatment of, 762

hormonal treatment of, 751–756, 753t,
    754t, 755f
incidence of, 750
micro-, 717–718
    in ductal carcinoma in situ, 726–727
natural history of, 750
of unknown origin, 316
presentation of, 750, 751t
prognostic and predictive factors in,
    750–751, 752t
psychosocial aspects and symptom
    management for, 761
pure estrogen antagonist for, 754
spinal cord compression due to, 160f,
    751t, 760
to axillary lymph nodes, 718, 719, 720t
to bone, 151f, 155f, 255f, 751t, 760
to brain, 751t, 1073–1074
to nonaxillary lymph nodes, 718–719
MRI of, 65–66, 66f, 69f
nipple discharge due to, 71, 72–73
noninvasive, 726–735
Paget's disease as, 73–74
physical examination for, 59
pleural effusion due to, 87, 91f
prognostic factor(s) in, 719–724, 720t
    age as, 724
    axillary lymph node involvement as, 719,
        720t
    clinical use of, 723b
    ethnicity as, 724
    flow cytometry for DNA ploidy and S-
        phase fraction as, 722
    for ductal in situ carcinoma, 728–729,
        729t
    gene expression profiling as, 723
    growth factors and receptors as, 721–722,
        722f
    histopathologic subtype as, 719, 723b
    hormone receptor status as, 721, 723b
    Ki-67 as, 722
    lymphatic/vascular invasion as, 720–721
    mitotic index as, 722
    patient characteristics as, 724
    plasminogen activators and inhibitors as,
        723
    proliferative indices as, 722–723
    thymidine-labeling index as, 723
    tumor grade as, 719–720, 721f
    tumor size as, 719, 720f, 723b
psychosocial aspects of, 761, 767, 767t
reconstructive surgery after, 763–764
recurrences of, 764
risk factors for, 59
screening for, 62f, 65, 67f–69f, 1196t
second malignancies with, 764
sentinel lymph node dissection in, 718
staging of, 715–719, 716t, 717t
    primary tumor in, 715–717, 716t
    regional lymph nodes in, 716t, 717–719,
        717t
superior vena cava syndrome in, 99
supportive measures and follow-up care for,
    763–767
tamoxifen for, 331–343
trastuzumab for, 345
tumor size in, 715–717, 719, 720f, 723b
ultrasonography of, 62f, 65, 69f
with vague thickening or nodularity, 61–62
Breast cysts, 60–61, 60f, 60t
Breast Imaging Reporting Data System (BI-
    RADS), 65, 66t
Breast lymphoma, 663
Breast mass(es), 59–64
    additional diagnostic imaging studies for,
        65–66, 68f, 69f
    biopsy of, 61, 63–64, 66–70
    cystic, 60–61, 60f, 60t, 61f
    discrete palpable, 59, 60–61, 60t, 61f
    due to Paget's disease, 73–74
    evaluation of, 59–60
    in pregnant or lactating women, 62–63
    mammography of, 61f, 62f, 65, 67f–69f
    management of, 60–65
    MRI of, 65–66, 66f, 69f
    nuclear medicine studies of, 66
    short-interval follow-up for, 66
    solid, 60t, 61, 61f, 62f

ultrasonography of, 61f, 62f, 65, 69f
vaguely thickened or nodular, 59, 60t, 61–62
wire localization of, 70
Breast reconstructive surgery, 763–764
Breast-conserving surgery
    for ductal carcinoma in situ, 729–731, 730b,
        731t
    for locally invasive breast cancer, 737–738
Breast-feeding, breast masses during, 62–63
Breslow's thickness, for melanoma, 1088, 1089
Brodifacoum, coagulation disorders due to, 265,
    268, 507, 507t
Bronchial carcinoid tumors, 1133, 1134t
Bronchiolitis obliterans, after hematopoietic stem
    cell transplantation, 403
Bronchoalveolar carcinoma (BAC), 968
Bronchogenic carcinoma, diagnosis of solitary
    pulmonary nodule as. See Solitary
    pulmonary nodule.
Bronchoscopy
    for hemoptysis, 107
    for non–small cell lung cancer, 967
    for solitary pulmonary nodule, 86
Bronchus sign, positive, 83, 83f
Bruising, 265, 266b, 295
Bruton's hypogammaglobulinemia, 202
BU. See Busulfan (BU).
Budd-Chiari syndrome
    due to polycythemia vera, 702
    due to renal cell cancer, 828
Bulky bleeds, 499
Bupropion (Wellbutrin-SR), 1227b
Burdock root, 1214, 1215
Burkitt's leukemia, 550, 552, 559t, 561, 562t
Burkitt's lymphoma, 656–657
    diagnosis of, 552, 604f, 606–607, 612
    etiology of, 550
    treatment for, 562t
Burkitt's-like lymphoma, 656–657
Burr cells, 274, 276
Burst-forming unit erythroid (BFU-E) assays,
    261–262
Burton, Lawrence, 1217t
Burzynski, Stanislaw, 1217–1218, 1217t
Buserelin, 341t
Buspirone (Buspar), 1227b
Busulfan (BU), 333t
    for chronic myeloid leukemia, 680–681
    in conditioning regimen for hematopoietic
        stem cell transplantation
        allogeneic, 394–395, 395t, 396t
        autologous, 399t
    toxicities of, 396t
Butyrophenones, for nausea and vomiting, 1251

C

C cell hyperplasia, 1125
C-225 (cetuximab), 387
    for colorectal cancer, 930
CA-125
    in endometrial cancer, 784
    in ovarian cancer, 796, 799–801, 800b, 1197
    with pelvic mass, 189
Cachexia, 3–8
    defined, 3
    differential diagnosis of, 4b
    metabolic changes in, 3–5, 4t
    pathogenesis of, 3–5, 4b, 4t
    therapy for, 5–8, 5t, 7t
    vs. starvation, 3–4, 4t
Café-au-lait macule, 308t
Caisse, Rene N., 1214, 1215
Calcifications
    in breast cancer, 728, 728f, 730
        ductal, 68f
    in solitary pulmonary nodule, 81, 83b, 84,
        84f
Calcitonin, for hypercalcemia, 194, 194t
Calcitriol, for hypocalcemia, 1190
Calcium
    for hypocalcemia, 1190
    for prevention of colorectal cancer, 924
    measurement of plasma, 192
Calcium acetate (PhosLo), for
    hyperphosphatemia, 1189
Calcium gluconate
    for hyperkalemia, 1189
    for hypocalcemia, 1190

Calcium homeostasis, 192
Calvarial metastasis, headache due to, 21, 21t, 22, 22t
CAM (Complementary and Alternative Medicine), 1209. *See also* Unorthodox treatment(s).
Camellia sinensis, 1213t
Cameron, Ewan, 1216
CAMPATH-1H, for chronic lymphocytic leukemia, 696
Camptosar. *See* Irinotecan (Camptosar, CPT-11).
Camptothecins, 339t, 352
Cancell, 1217t
Cancer diagnosis, adjustment to, 1224, 1225b
Cancer of unknown primary, 313–316, 1147–1153
    adenocarcinoma as, 1151b
    aneuploidy in, 1148
    biological features of, 315, 1147–1148
    chromosomal abnormalities in, 1148
    clinical evaluation of, 313–314, 1149
    clinical presentation of, 1149, 1149t
    defined, 313
    epidemiology of, 1147
    lung cancer as, 962
    major sites and histologic types of, 1149, 1149t
    microvessel density in, 1148
    oncogenes in, 1148
    pathology of, 314–315, 315t, 1147
    peritoneal carcinomatosis as, 1153b
    poorly differentiated or undifferentiated, 1153b
        neuroendocrine, 1152b
    prognostic features and outcome for, 1149–1150, 1150t, 1151b–1153b
    squamous cell carcinoma with high cervical adenopathy as, 1151b
    treatment for, 316, 316b, 1150, 1150t
    tumor suppressor genes in, 1148
    with isolated axillary adenopathy, 1152b
Cancer risk, quantification of, 1204
Cancer vaccines, 331f, 379–382, 380t
Candida infection
    fever of unknown origin due to, 11
    oral discomfort due to, 1250
    with hematopoietic stem cell transplantation, 400–401
Candida lusitaniae, febrile neutropenia due to, 1177b
Cannabinoids, for chemotherapy-induced emesis, 1250
Cantron, 1217t
Capecitabine (Xeloda), 335t, 348–349
    for metastatic breast cancer, 756t, 757t, 758
Capnocytophaga spp, febrile neutropenia due to, 1175
Carbamazepine (Tegretol, Carbatrol), 1227b
    for brain metastases, 1069
    for neuropathic pain, 1248, 1249t
    for seizures, 25t, 26b
Carboplatin, 335t, 348, 355t
    for cancer of unknown primary, 1150t, 1151b, 1153b
    for esophageal cancer, 878
    for germ-cell tumors, 818, 821b
    for head and neck cancer, 1008t
    for laryngeal cancer, 1003t
    for lung cancer
        non–small cell, 972, 976b, 976f, 977f
        small cell, 951, 951b
    for mesothelioma, 995t, 996t
    for oropharyngeal cancer, 1006
    for ovarian cancer, 796–799, 797b, 801
    for prostate cancer, 873t
    for renal cell cancer, 834t
    side effects of, 798–799
Carboxyhemoglobin, cigarette smoking and, 258, 259
Carcinoembryonic antigen (CEA), 378
    in colorectal cancer, 927, 928
    in gastric cancer, 891
Carcinoid tumors, 1133–1135
    appendiceal, 1134t, 1135
    bronchial, 1133, 1134t
    clinical presentation of, 1134t
    gastric, 1133–1134, 1134t
    hormone levels in, 1135t

liver metastasis from, 120f
    metastatic, 1134, 1134f, 1137
    of lung, 969
    of small intestine, 1134–1135, 1134f, 1134t
    rectal, 1134t, 1135
    treatment for, 1136–1137, 1136t
Carcinoma
    adrenal, 1129–1131
        clinical presentation of, 170, 171f, 1129–1130
        epidemiology of, 1129
        follow-up for, 1131
        pathology of, 1130
        prognosis for, 1131
        staging of, 1130
        treatment for, 1130–1131, 1131b
    breast. *See* Breast cancer.
    hepatocellular, 119–120, 120t, 121f
        GI bleeding due to, 144–145, 146
        intrahepatic cholangio-, 120–122, 121f, 122f
    of parotid gland, 46f
    of unknown origin, 314, 315
    parotid gland, 46f, 1018–1019, 1020f, 1021f
    pigmented basal cell, 308t
    squamous cell. *See* Squamous cell carcinoma.
Carcinoma in situ (CIS)
    of bladder, 842, 843, 844, 845b
    of lung, 973–974
    of vulva, 776b, 777f
Carcinomatosis, large bowel obstruction due to, 113
Carcinomatous meningitis, due to metastatic breast cancer, 751t
Cardiac risk, perioperative, 362–364, 363t, 364t
Cardiac toxicity, of anthracyclines, 350–351, 351f
Cardiomyopathy, congestive, due to anthracyclines, 350
Cardiovascular complications, of Hodgkin's disease, 629–630
Caregiver, 1228–1229
Carmustine (BCNU), 333t
    for gastric cancer, 895t
    for high-grade gliomas, 1053, 1054b
    for melanoma, 1097–1098
    in conditioning regimen for autologous hematopoietic stem cell transplantation, 399t
    toxicities of, 396t
        pulmonary, 78t
Carotid sinus syndrome, due to cranial neuropathy, 30t
Carpal tunnel syndrome, in multiple myeloma, 582
Casodex (bicalutamide), 341t, 344
    for prostate cancer, 870
Castleman's disease, hilar and mediastinal adenopathy in, 95, 96f
Cataracts, after hematopoietic stem cell transplantation, 404
Catharanthine, 353
Catheter(s)
    chronic indwelling pleural, 92–93, 92f
    thromboembolic disease with, 1182–1184, 1183f
Cat's claw, 1213–1214, 1213t
CAV regimen, for small cell lung cancer, 951
Cavernous hemangiomas, in Kassabach-Merritt syndrome, 295–296, 296f
CBC (complete blood count), in erythrocytosis, 256, 258
CBF (core binding factor) leukemias, 525, 528t
CCA (choriocarcinoma), 807
    phantom, 811
CCI (count increment), for platelet transfusions, 434
CCNU (lomustine), 334t
    for high-grade gliomas, 1053, 1054b
CD-20 antigen, 345
CD-30–positive lymphoma, 609
CD-33 antigen, 346
CDH-1 gene, in hereditary diffuse gastric cancer, 1201
CDK4 gene, in familial melanoma, 1201
CDKN2A gene, in familial melanoma, 1201
CDKs (cyclin-dependent kinases), in cell signaling, 386

CEA (carcinoembryonic antigen), 378
    in colorectal cancer, 927, 928
    in gastric cancer, 891
CeaVAC, 381
Celecoxib (Celebrex), for pain, 1244
Celexa (citalopram), 1227b
Celiac disease, and peripheral T-cell lymphoma, 668
Celiac plexus blocks, for pancreatic cancer, 917
Cell death, in radiation therapy, 322–323
Cell membrane, in radiation therapy, 323
Cell membrane receptors, 386
Cell signaling, biologic therapy using, 385–387
Cell surface antigens, in acute myeloid leukemia, 530–531
Cellular treatment, 1217t
Cellulitis, eosinophilic granulomatous, 249
Centigray (cGy), 321
Central nervous system (CNS) effects, pruritus due to, 15
Central nervous system (CNS) infections, encephalopathy due to, 34t
Central nervous system (CNS) involvement
    in acute lymphoblastic leukemia, 551, 557t, 559–561, 563b
    in acute myeloid leukemia, 529
    in non-Hodgkin's lymphoma, 652
Central nervous system (CNS) lymphoma, 655, 662, 662b, 1053–1054, 1055f, 1056b
Central nervous system (CNS) metastasis
    of non–small cell lung cancer, 961–962
    of small cell lung cancer, 946
Central venous catheters
    superior vena cava syndrome due to, 100
    thromboembolic disease with, 1182–1184, 1183f
c-erbB-2 gene
    in cancer of unknown primary, 1148
    in locally invasive breast cancer, 745–747
Cerebellar degeneration, due to ovarian carcinoma, 792
Cerebral hemorrhage, encephalopathy due to, 35
Cerebral infarction, encephalopathy due to, 35
Cerebrospinal fluid (CSF)
    in epidural cancer, 1079
    in Epstein-Barr virus, 1162b
Cerebrovascular disorders, encephalopathy due to, 34t, 35
Cerrobend block, 322f
Cervical adenopathy, 214–216, 215t
    with squamous cell cancer of unknown origin, 1151b
Cervical cancer, 769–775
    adenocarcinoma form of, 770
    advanced
        chemotherapy and radiation therapy for, 773t
        in elderly woman, 774b
        locally, 772, 773t
        regionally, 772
        single-agent chemotherapy for, 775t
    bulky, 772, 773b, 773t
    chemotherapy for
        combination, 775t
        single-agent, 775t
        with radiation therapy, 773t
    cytology of, 770
    epidemiology of, 770
    follow-up evaluation for, 774
    invasive, 772, 772f, 774f
    melanoma form of, 778
    metastatic, 774–775, 774t, 775t
    microscopic, 772
    neuroendocrine, 770–771
    pathogenesis of, 770
    pathology of, 770–771, 770f
    presentation of, 770
    prognostic factors for, 774
    radiation therapy for, 772, 773b, 773t
    radical hysterectomy for, 772, 773b, 774f
    recurrent, 774–775, 775t
    squamous cell, 770, 770f, 774–775
    staging of, 771–772, 771t
    treatment of, 772–773
    verrucous, 770
Cervical dysplasia, 769

Cervical esophageal cancer, 1004–1005
Cervical intraepithelial neoplasia (CIN), 769
Cervical lymph node(s), in head and neck cancer, 1000
Cervical lymph node metastasis, of salivary gland carcinoma, 1019, 1020, 1023–1024, 1024f
Cervical neuritis, headache due to, 20t
Cervical spondylosis, 161
Cervix
    as source of vaginal bleeding, 185, 185t
    barrel, 773b
Cetuximab (C-225), 387
    for colorectal cancer, 930
cGy (centigray), 321
Chaparral, 1213t
Chaplains, 1258
CHART (continuous hyperfractionated accelerated radiotherapy), for non–small cell lung cancer, 973
Chédiak-Higashi syndrome, 279, 479–480, 480f
Chelation therapy, 1221t
    for thalassemia, 460b, 462b
Chemicals, acute lymphoblastic leukemia due to, 550
Chemoembolization
    for hepatocellular carcinoma, 902–903
    for islet cell tumors, 918
Chemohormonal therapy, for locally invasive breast cancer, 742
Chemoprevention
    of colorectal cancer, 924, 924t
    of non–small cell lung cancer, 970f, 977–978
    of upper aerodigestive tract cancers, 1013–1015, 1013t, 1014t
Chemoreceptor trigger zone (CTZ), 1250
Chemotherapy, 330–356
    adjuvant
        for bladder cancer, 855, 855b
        for gastric cancer, 896–897, 897f, 897t
        for non–small cell lung cancer, 975
    as conditioning regimen for hematopoietic stem cell transplantation
        allogeneic, 395t
        autologous, 399t
    biological basis of, 330, 331f
    biologically guided, 1221t
    classification of, 332t–342t
    drug modification guidelines for, 354, 355t, 356t
    encephalopathy due to, 35
    for adrenal cancer, 1130–1131, 1131b
    for anal carcinoma, 940–941
    for basal cell carcinoma, 1107
    for biliary cancer, 904–905
    for brain metastases, 1073–1075
    for breast cancer
        locally invasive, 738–740, 742, 743t
        metastatic, 756–760, 756t
            high-dose, 758
            in older women, 758
            suggested approach to, 759–760, 759f
            vs. hormonal therapy, 755
            with capecitabine, 756t, 758
            with doxorubicin and taxanes, 756–758, 756t, 757t
            with trastuzumab, 756t, 758
    for cancer of unknown primary, 1150, 1150t
    for cervical cancer
        combination, 775t
        recurrent or advanced, 774–775, 775t
        single-agent, 775t
        with radiation therapy, 773t
    for chondrosarcoma, 1034
    for colorectal cancer, 929–931, 931f, 932–933, 932t
    for endometrial cancer, 787–788
    for epidural cancer, 1082
    for esophageal cancer, 878–879, 878f
        locally advanced, 884b
        neoadjuvant, 879–880, 881f, 881t
        palliative, 879
        preoperative, 879, 880–883, 881f, 881t
        vs. surgery, 884
        with radiation, 881–883, 883f, 884
    for Ewing's sarcoma, 1034–1035
    for gastric cancer, 895, 895t–897t, 896–897

for germ-cell tumors
    advanced, 817–818, 818b
    extragonadal, 822b
    follow-up after, 819t
    good-risk, 819b
    high-dose, 818
    intermediate- and poor-risk, 820b
    low-stage, 815–817
    relapsed, 820–821
    salvage, 820
    sequelae of, 821–823
    surgery after, 818–819
    with brain metastases, 822b
for gestational trophoblastic tumor, 809–811, 810t
for gliomas
    high-grade, 1053, 1054b
    low-grade, 1051–1052, 1052b
for head and neck cancer, 1008t
for hepatocellular carcinoma, 902–903
for Hodgkin's disease, 621b, 622–626, 624t
for islet cell tumors, 917–918
for Kaposi's sarcoma, 1160
for laryngeal cancer, 1003–1004, 1003t
for leukemia
    adult T-cell, 674
    chronic myeloid, 680–681
for lung cancer
    non–small cell
        by stage, 970f, 974, 975–976
        general principles of, 970, 970f
        metastatic, 975t, 976b, 976f, 977f
        single-agent, 971–972, 971t
        with radiation therapy, 972–973
    small cell, 950–951, 951b, 952b, 952f, 953
for lymphoma
    adult T-cell, 674
    AIDS-related, 1157–1158
    CNS, 1054, 1056b
    peripheral T-cell, 670
for malignant fibrous histiocytoma, 1032
for melanoma, 1097–1100, 1099b, 1099f
for Merkel cell carcinoma, 1114
for mesothelioma, 995, 995t
for mycosis fungoides and Sézary syndrome, 667
for nasopharyngeal cancer, 1009–1010, 1009b
for neuroendocrine tumors, 1137
for non-Hodgkin's lymphoma
    intermediate-grade, 651–652, 651t
    low-grade, 641, 642t, 643, 643t
for oral cavity cancer, 1007
for oropharyngeal cancer, 1006, 1006b
for osteosarcoma, 1030–1031
for ovarian cancer, 796–799, 797b, 801–802
    intraperitoneal, 796
for pancreatic cancer, 915, 916
for prostate cancer, 872–873, 873t
for renal cell cancer, 834, 834t
for soft tissue sarcoma, 1044–1045
for squamous cell carcinoma, 1112–1113
for superficial bladder cancer, 844–846
for superior vena cava syndrome, 103
for thymoma, 989, 989t
for thyroid carcinoma
    differentiated, 1123
    medullary, 1126
future of, 356
GI bleeding due to, 147–148
intraperitoneal
    for ascites, 132
    for gastric cancer, 897–898
    for ovarian cancer, 796
neoadjuvant
    for bladder cancer, 854–855, 855b
    for esophageal cancer, 879–880, 881t
    for gastric cancer, 897
    for soft tissue sarcoma, 1045
neutropenia due to, 245
pancytopenia due to, 253
peripheral neuropathy due to, 40
peritoneal, 368–369
principles of drug dosing for, 353–354
pulmonary toxicity due to, 76–77, 78t
rational drug selection based on pharmacogenomics for, 354–356

    thromboembolic phenomena with, 1180–1181
    with alkyl sulfonates, 332t, 333t
    with alkylating agents, 332t–334t, 348
        bioreductive, 334t
    with all-trans retinoic acid (Tretinoin, Vesanoid), 344
    with aminoglutethimide, 341t, 347
    with anastrozole, 341t, 347
    with androgen receptor antagonists (antiandrogens), 332t, 341t, 344
    with anthracenediones, 332t, 338t, 351
    with anthracyclines, 332t, 337t, 350–351, 351f, 356t
    with antiestrogens, 340t–341t
    with antimetabolites, 332t
    with antimicrotubule agents, 340t, 352–353
    with antimitotic drugs, 332t, 352
    with aromatase inhibitors, 332t, 341t, 347
    with bexarotene (Targretin), 344–345
    with bicalutamide (Casodex), 341t, 344
    with bleomycin, 339t, 355t
    with buserelin, 341t
    with busulfan, 333t
    with camptothecins, 339t, 352
    with capecitabine (Xeloda), 335t, 348–349
    with carboplatin, 335t, 348, 355t
    with carmustine (BCNU), 333t
    with catharanthine, 353
    with chlorambucil, 333t
    with cisplatin, 335t, 348, 355t
    with cladribine (2-chlorodeoxyadenosine), 336t
    with cyclophosphamide, 333t, 355t
    with cytarabine (cytosine arabinoside), 335t
    with dacarbazine (DTIC), 334t
    with dactinomycin (actinomycin-D), 338t
    with daunorubicin, 350
    with denileukin diftitox (DAB389IL-2, Ontak), 342t, 346–347
    with DNA topoisomerase inhibitors, 332t, 337t–339t, 349–352, 349f, 351f
    with docetaxel, 340t, 353, 356t
    with doxorubicin, 337t, 350, 351, 351f
        liposomal (Doxil), 350
    with drugs that affect growth factor/receptor interactions, 331–345, 332t
    with drugs that decrease circulating growth factors, 332t, 347
    with epidermal growth factor (EGF)/EGF receptor (EGFR)–family antagonists, 332t, 345–347
    with epipodophyllotoxins, 332t, 338t–339t
    with epirubicin (Ellence), 337t, 350
    with estrogen receptor modulators (ERMs), 331–343, 331f, 332t, 340t
        selective (SERMs), 340t–341t, 343–344
    with ethylenimines, 332t, 333t
    with etoposide, 338t, 350, 355t, 356t
    with exemestane, 341t, 347
    with floxuridine (fluorodeoxyuridine, FUDR), 335t, 369–370
    with fludarabine, 336t, 355t
    with 5-fluorouracil, 335t, 370
    with flutamide (Eulexin), 341t, 344
    with folate antagonists (folate analogues), 332t, 335t
    with gemcitabine (Gemzar), 335t, 349
    with gemtuzumab ozogomicin (Mylotarg), 342t, 346
    with gonadotropin-releasing agents, 341t–342t
    with hepatic dysfunction, 356t
    with hexamethylmelamine, 333t
    with hydroxyurea, 336t, 355t
    with idarubicin, 337t, 350
    with ifosfamide, 333t, 355t
    with imidazotetrazines, 332t
    with intracellular receptors, 331
    with invasion/metastasis inhibitors, 331f
    with irinotecan (Camptosar, CPT-11), 339t, 352
    with letrozole, 341t, 347
    with leuprolide, 341t
    with lomustine (CCNU), 334t
    with luteinizing hormone–releasing hormone (LHRH), 332t
    with mechlorethamine, 332t

Chemotherapy, (*Continued*)
with megestrol acetate, 342t
with melphalan, 333t
with membrane receptors, 342t, 345–347
with mercaptopurine, 336t
with methotrexate, 335t, 355t
with methylmelamines, 333t
with mitomycin-C, 334t
with mitoxantrone, 338t, 351
with monoclonal antibodies, 342t, 345–347
with nilutamide (Nilandron), 341t, 344
with nitrogen mustards, 332t, 333t, 348
with nitrosoureas, 332t, 333t–334t
with nucleic acid synthesis inhibitors, 332t, 335t–336t, 347–350
with oxaliplatin, 335t, 348
with paclitaxel, 340t, 352–353, 356t
with pentostatin (2-deoxycoformycin), 336t, 355t
with platinating agents (platinum analogues), 332t, 335t, 348
with progestins, 342t
with purine analogues, 332t, 336t
with pyrimidine analogues, 332t, 335t
with raloxifene (Evista), 341t, 344
with renal dysfunction, 355t
with retinoic acid receptor modulators, 332t, 344–345
with rituximab (Rituxan), 342t, 345–346
with selective tyrosine kinase inhibitors, 331f
with semustine (methyl-CCNU), 334t
with signal transduction modulators, 340t–342t
with STI 571, 356
with streptozocin, 334t, 355t
with tamoxifen (Nolvadex), 331–343, 340t
with taxanes, 332t, 340t, 352–353
with temozolomide, 334t, 348
with teniposide, 338t, 350
with thioguanine, 336t
with thiotepa, 333t, 356t
with topotecan (Hycamtin), 339t, 351–352, 355t
with toremifene (Fareston), 340t, 343–344
with trastuzumab (Herceptin), 331f, 342t, 345
with triazenes, 332t, 334t
with tumor vaccines, 331f
with vinblastine, 340t, 353, 356t
with vinca alkaloids, 332t, 340t, 353, 356t
with vincristine, 340t, 353, 356t
with vindoline, 353
with vinorelbine, 340t, 353, 356t
Chemotherapy-induced neutropenia, 245
myeloid growth factors for, 428
Chest tube, for pleural effusion, 90–91
Chest x-rays
of mesothelioma, 991
of non–small cell lung cancer, 966, 978, 978t
of pleural effusion, 88
of solitary pulmonary nodule, 81, 83b
of superior vena cava syndrome, 101, 101f
of thymoma, 985, 985f
Children
acute lymphoblastic leukemia in, 549, 550t
brain tumors in, 1049
hematopoietic stem cell transplantation in, 400
of cancer patient, 1229–1230, 1230b, 1233
pelvic mass in, 187, 190
soft tissue sarcomas in, 1038, 1039, 1040, 1041, 1042, 1043
superior vena cava syndrome in, 100
testicular mass in, 179, 180b
vaginal bleeding in, 186–187
Chloral hydrate, for insomnia, 1253
Chlorambucil, 333t
for chronic lymphocytic leukemia, 692–693, 694f, 695, 695f
for Waldenström's macroglobulinemia, 598
2-Chlorodeoxyadenosine (Cladribine), 336t
for hairy cell leukemia, 698
Chloromas, orbital, 529, 529f
Chlorpromazine (Thorazine)
for delirium, 1248, 1248t, 1254t, 1255
for dyspnea, 1254t

Cholangiocarcinoma
intrahepatic, 120–122, 121f, 122f
peripheral, 122f, 904
Cholangiography, percutaneous transhepatic, 903, 905b
Cholangiopancreatography, endoscopic retrograde, 903, 905b, 912–913
Choledochojejunostomy, 905b
Cholera, pancreatic, 1135
Cholestasis, hyperbilirubinemia due to, 198–199
Cholesterol emboli, cutaneous manifestations of, 303, 303f
Choline magnesium salicylate, for pain, 1245t
Chondrosarcoma, 1033–1034
classification of, 1033, 1033t
clinical features of, 1029t, 1033, 1033f
de-differentiated, 1034
mesenchymal, 1034
pathologic fractures due to, 154, 154f
prognostic factors for, 1033
staging of, 1033
treatment for, 1033–1034
CHOP regimen, for non-Hodgkin's lymphoma
AIDS-related, 1157
intermediate-grade, 651, 651t
low-grade, 641
Chordoma, 1035
Choriocarcinoma (CCA), 807
phantom, 811
Chromophobe renal cell cancer, 825–826, 826t, 827f, 831
Chromosomal abnormalities
in acute myeloid leukemia, 523–528, 526t–528t, 527f
in anaplastic large-cell lymphoma, 609
in cancer of unknown primary, 1148
in chronic lymphocytic leukemia, 688
in essential thrombocythemia, 709–710
in multiple myeloma, 581–582
in myelodysplasia, 568, 568t, 573, 573t
Chronic disease, anemia of, 233t, 457–458
Chronic granulomatous disease, 480–483, 482t, 483t
Chronic lymphocytic leukemia (CLL), 688–696
aggressive transformation in, 689
autoimmunity in, 689–690
B-cell, 603–604, 604f, 604t
clinical evaluation of, 690–691, 690f, 691f, 691t
clinical features of, 689–690
clinical presentation of, 688–689, 691b
cytogenetics of, 688
diagnosis of, 247–248, 248f, 697t
differential diagnosis of, 690, 691f
epidemiology of, 688
febrile neutropenia in, 1174
follow-up evaluation for, 696
infections in, 689
molecular biology of, 688
prognosis for, 691–692, 692t
second malignancies in, 690
staging of, 691–692, 692t
therapy of, 692–696
algorithm for, 693t
allogeneic stem cell transplantation for, 696
CAMPATH-1H for, 696
chlorambucil for, 692–693, 694f, 695f
combination chemotherapy for, 694–695
corticosteroids for, 689, 693
erythropoietin for, 696
fludarabine for, 693–694, 694f, 695, 695f
initial, 692–695, 693b
interferon for, 696
intravenous immunoglobulins for, 689
new approaches in, 695–696, 697t
rituximab for, 345–346, 690, 696
second-line, 695
splenectomy for, 690, 696
white blood cell abnormalities in, 279–280, 279f
Chronic myeloid leukemia (CML), 676–685
accelerated phase of, 678
blast phase of, 677b, 678, 682–683
bone marrow findings in, 677

chronic phase of, 676, 678
clinical and hematologic characteristics of, 676–677, 677b
differential diagnosis of, 677–678
epidemiology of, 676
etiology of, 676
fluorescence in situ hybridization test for, 679–680
molecular biology of, 678–679, 679f
natural history of, 678
peripheral blood findings in, 280, 280f, 676–677
Philadelphia chromosome-positive (Ph-positive), 243–244
treatment of, 680–685
chemotherapy for, 680–681
hematopoietic stem cell transplantation for, 409–410, 683–684
imatinib mesylate for, 409, 684–685, 685b
in blast crisis, 682–683
interferon for, 681–682
white blood cell count in, 676–677, 677b
Chronic myelomonocytic leukemia (CMML), 570, 572, 576
Chronic neutrophilic leukemia, 244
Chronic renal disease, pruritus due to, 14–15
Chylous ascites, 129t, 131
Cigarette smoking
and bladder cancer, 842, 850
and colorectal cancer, 923
and endometrial cancer, 783
and esophageal cancer, 875
and gastric cancer, 889
and head and neck cancer, 999
and lung cancer, 943, 958–959, 968, 977, 977b
and pancreatic cancer, 908
and renal cell cancer, 825
erythrocytosis due to, 258, 259
leukocytosis due to, 243
CIN (cervical intraepithelial neoplasia), 769
CIS. *See* Carcinoma in situ (CIS).
Cisplatin, 335t, 348, 355t
for anal carcinoma, 941
for bladder cancer, 853, 854
for cancer of unknown primary, 1150t, 1151b–1153b
for cervical cancer, 775t
for esophageal cancer, 878–879, 878t
preoperative, 881, 881t, 882
with radiation therapy, 881t, 882, 883
for gastric cancer, 895, 895t, 896t
for germ-cell tumors, 817, 818, 819b, 820, 820b, 821–822, 821b
for head and neck cancer, 1008t
for laryngeal cancer, 1003, 1003t
for lung cancer
non–small cell, 972, 973, 976f, 977f
small cell, 951, 951b, 953
for melanoma, 1097–1098
for mesothelioma, 995, 995t, 996, 996t
for neuroendocrine tumors, 1137
for oral cavity cancer, 1007
for osteosarcoma, 1031
for renal cell cancer, 834t
for soft tissue sarcoma, 1044
for thymoma, 989, 989t
intraperitoneal, for ascites, 132
Cis-retinoic acid, for renal cell cancer, 836
Citalopram (Celexa), 1227b
Cladribine (2-chlorodeoxyadenosine), 336t
for hairy cell leukemia, 698
Clark's level, for melanoma, 1089
Clear-cell carcinoma
endometrial, 788, 788t
of cervix, 771
of vagina, 779
ovarian, 795–796, 795t
renal cell, 825, 826, 826t, 827f
Clinical target volume (CTV), 324
Clinical Trials Support Unit (CTSU), 761–762
CLL. *See* Chronic lymphocytic leukemia (CLL).
Clomipramine, for neuropathic pain, 1249t
Clonal lymphocyte disorders, 247–248, 247t, 248f
Clonal malignancies, in head and neck cancer, 1012

Clonazepam (Klonopin), 1227b, 1228
　for delirium, 1248t
　for restless leg syndrome, 1253
　for seizures, 25t
Clonidine
　for anticipatory nausea and vomiting, 1250
　for neuropathic pain, 1249t
Clorazepate (Tranxene), for seizures, 25t
Clostridium difficile, febrile neutropenia due to,
　　1177b
Clostridium septicum, febrile neutropenia due to,
　　1174, 1175
Clotting factors, 267
"Cloverleaf" cells, in adult T-cell
　　leukemia/lymphoma, 674
Cluster headache, 20t
CML. See Chronic myeloid leukemia (CML).
CMML (chronic myelomonocytic leukemia),
　　570, 572, 576
c-mpl, in erythrocytosis, 262
CMV (cytomegalovirus), with hematopoietic
　　stem cell transplantation,
　　401–402
c-myc, in cancer of unknown primary, 1148
Cnicus benedictus, 1215
CNS. See Central nervous system (CNS).
Coagulation
　disseminated intravascular. See Disseminated
　　intravascular coagulation (DIC).
　pathways of, 268f
Coagulation disorder(s), 498–510
　disseminated intravascular coagulation as,
　　508–510, 509f
　　due to liver disease, 507–508
　　due to renal disease, 508, 509b
　　due to warfarin ingestion, 506–507, 507f,
　　　508b
　hemophilia A (factor VIII deficiency) as,
　　498–501, 499f, 500b, 501f, 502b
　　with factor VIII alloantibody inhibitors,
　　　501–504, 503b, 503f
　hemophilia B (factor IX deficiency) as, 504
　hemophilia C (factor XI deficiency) as,
　　504–505, 505b
　in acute myeloid leukemia, 529–530, 529f
　in surgical patient, 510
　of liver disease, 269, 507–508
　partial thromboplastin time and prothrombin
　　time in, 266–267, 267t
　vaginal bleeding due to, 184, 186b
　von Willebrand's disease as, 505–506
Coagulopathy(ies). See Coagulation disorder(s).
Cobalamin deficiency, 455–457, 456t
Cobalt machines, for radiation therapy, 321
Cochlear nerve deficit, 30t
Codeine
　for pain, 1245
　pruritus due to, 15
Coenzyme Q-10, 1216t
Cogentin, with haloperidol, 1248
Cognitive disturbances, opioid-induced, 1248,
　　1248t
Cognitive-behavioral interventions, for pain
　　management, 1244
Cold agglutinin disease, 273f, 470t, 471–472,
　　472f
　due to cancer, 1170, 1171f
　in Waldenström's macroglobulinemia, 597
Cold antibody autoimmune hemolytic anemia,
　　470t, 471–472, 472f
Colectivismo, 1230
Colectomy, for ulcerative colitis, 922
Coley, William B., 1217t
Coley toxins, 1217t
Colitis
　granulomatous, and colorectal cancer, 922
　ulcerative
　　and colorectal cancer, 922, 922f
　　prophylactic surgery for, 372
Collecting duct carcinoma, 826, 826t, 827–828,
　　827f
Colonic hydrotherapy, 1221t
Colonic obstruction, 109–110, 110t
Colonic polyps, 145
Colonoscopy
　for colorectal cancer, 923–924, 924f, 925–926
　for rectal bleeding, 146–147
　virtual, 146–147

Colorectal cancer, 921–932
　adenomatous polyps and, 923–924, 923f,
　　924f
　adjuvant chemotherapy for, 930–931,
　　931f
　adjuvant radiation therapy for, 932
　advanced, 929–930
　and endometrial cancer, 783
　capecitabine for, 348–349
　chemoprevention of, 924, 924t
　chemotherapy for, 929–930
　clinical presentation and evaluation of,
　　926–927, 926t
　combination chemoradiation therapy for,
　　932–933, 932t
　cranial neuropathies due to, 28t
　early, 928–929
　environmental factors in, 922
　epidemiology of, 921–923, 922f, 922t, 1199
　familial adenomatous polyposis and, 921,
　　1199–1200
　genetic basis for, 921–922, 1199–1201, 1201t
　GI bleeding due to, 145
　hereditary nonpolyposis, 921–922,
　　1200–1201
　　Amsterdam criteria for, 1200–1201
　　and endometrial cancer, 783
　　Bethesda guidelines for, 1201, 1201t
　　clinical characteristics of, 1200
　　epidemiology of, 921
　　genetic basis of, 921, 1194, 1194t, 1200
　　management of, 1201
　　prognosis for, 921–922
　　prophylactic surgery for, 371–372
　　variants of, 1201
　inflammatory bowel disease and, 922, 922f
　irinotecan for, 352
　large bowel obstruction due to, 109–110,
　　112–113
　liver metastasis from, 118f, 927
　postoperative surveillance for, 928, 929t
　screening for, 924–926, 925t
　staging and prognosis for, 927, 927f, 928t
　surgery for, 928–929
Colposcopy, for cervical cancer, 770
COMLA regimen, for non-Hodgkin's lymphoma,
　　651t
Common variable immunodeficiency,
　　hypogammaglobulinemia in,
　　202–203
Communication, physician-patient, 1231–1233,
　　1232b
Compazine (prochlorperazine), for nausea and
　　vomiting, 1251, 1252t
Complementary and Alternative Medicine
　　(CAM), 1209. See also
　　Unorthodox treatment(s).
Complete blood count (CBC), in erythrocytosis,
　　256, 258
Compound nevus, 307f, 308t
Compression fractures, vertebral, 160, 162t
　in multiple myeloma, 582, 585, 592–593
Compression neuropathies, 40
Compression ultrasound venous imaging, 287,
　　287f, 288, 511
Compression views, of breast, 65, 68f
Compton effect, 321
Computed tomography (CT)
　for back pain, 159
　for cranial neuropathy, 28
　for dysphagia, 141
　for encephalopathy, 34
　for erythrocytosis, 260, 260f, 261f
　for hematuria, 175–176, 175f
　for hoarseness, 54
　for seizures, 24–25
　of adrenocortical masses, 170f, 171f, 1129
　of brain metastases, 1066, 1067f
　of endometrial cancer, 784, 785f
　of epidural cancer, 1080
　of esophageal cancer, 876, 877f
　of germ-cell tumors, 814
　of head and neck cancer, 1000
　of hilar and mediastinal adenopathy, 94–95,
　　95f, 96f
　of liver, 115, 116, 117, 118f–120t
　of mesothelioma, 991, 992f
　of multiple myeloma, 588

　of neck mass, 46–47
　of non–small cell lung cancer, 966, 978–979
　of pancreatic cancer, 912
　of pleural effusion, 88
　of renal cell cancer, 828–829, 829f, 830
　of salivary gland carcinoma, 1019f, 1020,
　　1020f
　of solid renal masses, 167
　of solitary pulmonary nodule, 81–84, 83t,
　　84t
　　enhanced, 84–85
　of superior vena cava syndrome, 101, 101f
　of thymoma, 985, 985f
　pulmonary angiogram, 288–289, 289f
　spiral, 288–289, 289f
　　of liver, 115
Computed tomography (CT) simulator, in
　　radiation therapy, 324
Conditioning regimen, for hematopoietic stem
　　cell transplantation
　allogeneic, 393, 394–396, 395t, 396t
　autologous, 397, 399t
Congestive cardiomyopathy
　due to anthracyclines, 350, 351, 351f
　pleural effusion due to, 87
Conjunctival melanoma, 310–311
Connective tissue disorders, cutaneous
　　manifestations of, 296
Constipation, due to opioids, 1247
Continuation therapy, defined, 556t
Continuous hyperfractionated accelerated
　　radiotherapy (CHART), for
　　non–small cell lung cancer, 973
Contrast materials, for liver imaging, 115, 117
Contrast venography, for deep vein thrombosis,
　　287
Convulsions. See Seizures.
Coombs' reagent, 433
Coombs' test
　direct, 433, 433f, 469–470, 471f
　indirect, 470, 471f
COP regimen, for low-grade non-Hodgkin's
　　lymphoma, 641
COPP regimen, for intermediate-grade non-
　　Hodgkin's lymphoma, 651t
Cord compression. See Spinal cord compression.
Core binding factor (CBF) leukemias, 525, 528t
Core needle biopsy
　of breast mass, 63, 66–70
　of lymph nodes, 219
Corneal damage, due to facial nerve palsy, 31
Corticosteroid(s)
　for aplastic anemia, 445
　for brain metastases, 1069–1070, 1069b, 1070b
　for brain tumors, 1051
　for cachexia, 7, 7t
　for chronic granulomatous disease, 481–482
　for chronic lymphocytic leukemia, 689, 693
　for Diamond-Blackfan anemia, 451
　for epidural cancer, 1081
　for graft-versus-host disease, 396–397
　for hypercalcemia, 194, 194t
　for idiopathic thrombocytopenic purpura,
　　489, 490f, 491, 492
　for lymphadenopathy, 218–219
　for neuropathic pain, 1248–1249, 1249t
　for paroxysmal nocturnal hemoglobinuria,
　　449
　for pure red cell aplasia, 450
　for superior vena cava syndrome, 104
　for thrombotic thrombocytopenic purpura,
　　493
　for warm antibody autoimmune hemolytic
　　anemia, 473b
　neutrophilia due to, 243
Corticosteroid excess, purpura due to, 296
Corticotropin deficiency, due to pituitary
　　adenoma, 1142t
Corticotropin excess, due to pituitary adenoma,
　　1142t
Corticotropin secretion, ectopic, in small cell
　　lung cancer, 948
Cotswolds Staging Classification, of Hodgkin's
　　disease, 619, 619t
Cough, 1251–1252
　due to lung cancer, 960
Count increment (CCI), for platelet transfusions,
　　434

Cowden's disease, 1194, 1194t, 1197–1198
CPT-11. *See* Irinotecan (Camptosar, CPT-11).
Cranial irradiation
    for acute lymphoblastic leukemia, 557t, 560, 561
    for Burkitt's leukemia/lymphoma, 562t
    for small cell lung cancer, 953, 954–955
Cranial nerve palsy, in acute myeloid leukemia, 529
Cranial neuropathy(ies), 27–31
    due to brain metastases, 1065
    evaluation of, 27, 28, 28f, 31b
    management of, 28–31
    metastatic pattern of malignancies causing, 28t
    pathophysiology of, 27
    presentation of, 27–28
    types of, 29t–30t
Craniopharyngioma, 1142–1143
Crenated cells, 274, 276
Creosote bush, 1213t
CREST syndrome, telangiectasia in, 297, 298f
Crigler-Majjar syndrome, hyperbilirubinemia due to, 198
Cryoglobulinemia
    due to cancer, 1170–1171
    in Waldenström's macroglobulinemia, 597
    vascular cutaneous manifestations of, 298–299, 298f, 303
Cryoprecipitate transfusions, 432t, 437
Cryotherapy, for hepatocellular carcinoma, 902
Cryptococcus infection, febrile neutropenia due to, 1174
Cryptorchidism, and testicular cancer, 179–180
CSF (cerebrospinal fluid)
    in epidural cancer, 1079
    in Epstein-Barr virus, 1162b
CT. *See* Computed tomography (CT).
CTCL. *See* Cutaneous T-cell lymphoma (CTCL).
CTSU (Clinical Trials Support Unit), 761–762
CTV (clinical target volume), 324
CTZ (chemoreceptor trigger zone), 1250
Cultural issues, 1230–1231
Cushing's disease/syndrome
    due to pituitary adenoma, 1142t
    purpura due to, 296
Cutaneous horns, 1109
Cutaneous lesions, pigmented. *See* Pigmented skin lesions.
Cutaneous manifestations
    of acute bacterial endocarditis, 298f
    of amyloidosis, 297, 297f
    of antiphospholipid antibody syndrome, 303
    of ataxia telangiectasia, 296
    of atheroemboli, 303
    of autoerythrocyte sensitization, 300, 300f
    of bleeding and thrombotic disorders, 293–303
        ecchymoses as, 294–295
        history of, 293–294
        petechiae as, 294, 294f
        physical examination of, 294–295, 294f, 295f
        purpura as, 294, 294f
            Gaugerot-Blum, 300
            "glove and socks" papular, 300
            Henoch-Schönlein, 298
            hypergammaglobulinemic, 299, 300f
            perifollicular, 296, 297f
            psychogenic, 300, 300f
            senile, 296–297, 297f, 298f
            stasis, 301, 301f
        spider angiomata as, 297
        subcutaneous hemorrhage as, 295, 295f
        without hemostatic defects, 300–301, 300f, 301f
    of cholesterol emboli, 303, 303f
    of CREST syndrome, 297, 298f
    of cryoglobulinemia, 298–299, 298f, 303
    of disseminated intravascular coagulation, 294f, 301, 301f
    of Fabry's disease, 296, 296f
    of fat embolism, 303
    of Gardner-Diamond syndrome, 300, 300f
    of heparin-induced thrombocytopenia, 303
    of hereditary connective tissue disorders, 296

of hereditary hemorrhagic telangiectasia, 295, 295f
of iron deficiency, 232, 233t
of Kaposi's sarcoma, 301, 301f
of Kassabach-Merritt syndrome, 295–296, 296f
of lichen aureus, 300, 301f
of Majocchi's pigmented purpuric eruption, 300, 300f
of meningococcemia, 297f
of primary purpura fulminans, 301–302, 302f
of primary vascular disorders
    acquired
        with vasculitis, 298–299, 298f–300f
        without vasculitis, 296–297, 297f, 298f
    hereditary, 295–296, 295f, 296f
of Rocky Mountain spotted fever, 298f
of Schaumberg's progressive pigmentary dermatosis, 300, 300f
of scurvy, 296, 297f
of systemic autoimmune disorders, 299, 299f
of thromboembolic disorders, 301–303, 301f–303f
of vasculitis(itides), 298–299, 298f–300f
of venous limb gangrene, 302–303
of warfarin skin necrosis, 302, 302f, 518, 518f
of Wegener's granulomatosis, 299f
Cutaneous T-cell lymphoma (CTCL), 664–667
    anaplastic, 668
    clinical presentation of, 665, 665f, 666f
    epidemiology of, 664
    pathophysiology of, 664–665
    staging and prognosis of, 665–666
    treatment for, 666–667
        bexarotene in, 344–345
        denileukin in, 347
Cyclic neutropenia, 477
Cyclin-dependent kinases (CDKs), in cell signaling, 386
Cyclo-oxygenase-2 inhibitors, for prevention of colorectal cancer, 924
Cyclophosphamide (CY, Cytoxan), 333t, 355t
    for acute lymphoblastic leukemia, 556, 557t, 558t
    for aplastic anemia, 448
    for breast cancer, 739, 740, 742, 756t
    for Burkitt's leukemia/lymphoma, 562t
    for cancer of unknown origin, 1152b
    for Ewing's sarcoma, 1034–1035
    for Fanconi's anemia, 450
    for germ-cell tumors, 821b
    for mesothelioma, 995
    for renal cell cancer, 834t
    for small cell lung cancer, 951
    for soft tissue sarcoma, 1044
    for thymoma, 989, 989t
    in conditioning regimen for hematopoietic stem cell transplantation
        allogeneic, 395, 395f, 396f
        autologous, 399t
    toxicities of, 396t
Cyclosporine
    for aplastic anemia
        acute severe, 445, 446
        moderate, 446
    for Diamond-Blackfan anemia, 451
    for graft-*versus*-host disease, 396, 397
    for paroxysmal nocturnal hemoglobinuria, 449
    for pure red cell aplasia, 450
Cyproheptadine, for cachexia, 8
Cyst(s)
    bone, 153–154
    breast, 60–61, 60f, 69f
    epididymal, 180, 182
    liver, 122–123, 123f
    mesenteric, 189t
    ovarian, 793, 793f
    renal, 165–166, 166f, 166t
    thyroid, 1119
Cystadenocarcinoma
    of pancreas, 909
    ovarian papillary serous, 795, 795f, 795t
Cystadenoma
    biliary, 123, 125f
    ovarian serous, 793, 793f

Cystectomy, for muscle-invasive bladder cancer, 851–853
Cystic renal lesions, 165–166, 166f, 166t
Cystitis
    hematuria due to, 173, 174t, 176, 177
    hemorrhagic, 173, 176, 177
    radiation, 173, 176, 177
Cystoscopy
    for hematuria, 176, 177f
    for superficial bladder cancer, 844, 844f, 847
Cytarabine (cytosine arabinoside), 335t
    for acute lymphoblastic leukemia, 556, 557t, 558t, 560, 561t
    for acute myeloid leukemia
        induction therapy with, 533, 534, 535t
        postremission therapy with, 535–536, 536t, 537f
        relapsed or refractory, 541, 542t
    for Burkitt's leukemia/lymphoma, 562t
    for CNS lymphoma, 1054
    for myelodysplasia, 578
    in conditioning regimen for autologous hematopoietic stem cell transplantation, 399t
    pulmonary toxicity due to, 78t
Cytogenetic complete remission, defined, 556t
Cytogenetics
    defined, 556t
    for cancer of unknown origin, 314–315, 315t
Cytokine(s). *See also* Growth factor(s).
    biologic therapy with, 376–377, 377t
    for multiple myeloma, 582
    for renal cell cancer, 834–838, 835t, 836t, 837f, 838f, 838t
    in cachexia, 4–5, 4t
    in gene therapy, 383
Cytokine receptors, 376–377
Cytomegalovirus (CMV), with hematopoietic stem cell transplantation, 401–402
Cytoreductive surgery, 368–369
Cytosine arabinoside. *See* Cytarabine (cytosine arabinoside).
Cytotoxic therapy
    for ovarian cancer, 801–802
    pulmonary toxicity due to, 76–77, 78t
Cytoxan. *See* Cyclophosphamide (CY, Cytoxan).

D
DAB389IL-2 (denileukin diftitox), 342t, 346–347
Dacarbazine (DTIC), 334t
    for melanoma, 1097–1098
    for mesothelioma, 995
    for soft tissue sarcoma, 1044
Dacryocytes, 274, 274f, 707f
Dactinomycin (actinomycin-D), 338t
    for Ewing's sarcoma, 1034–1035
    for gestational trophoblastic tumor, 810, 810t
Dalteparin, for venous thromboembolism, 515t
Danaparoid, for heparin-induced thrombocytopenia, 487–488, 488t
Danazol
    for aplastic anemia, 448
    for idiopathic thrombocytopenic purpura, 490–491
Dapsone, for idiopathic thrombocytopenic purpura, 491
Dartmouth regimen, for melanoma, 1097–1098
DAT (direct antiglobulin test), 433, 433f, 469–470, 471f
Daunorubicin, 350
    for Kaposi's sarcoma, 1160
    for leukemia
        acute lymphoblastic, 557t
        acute myeloid, 533, 534, 534t, 535t
        acute promyelocytic, 545b
D&C (dilation and curettage), for vaginal bleeding, 186
DCIS. *See* Ductal carcinoma in situ (DCIS).
DDAVP. *See* Arginine desmopressin (DDAVP).
D-dimers, in venous thromboembolic disease, 285–286, 511, 1181–1182
Death rattle, 1254t, 1255
Decaduralin, for aplastic anemia, 448
Decompressive laminectomy, for epidural cancer, 1082
Decortication, for pleural effusion, 93

Deep vein thrombosis (DVT)
　clinical assessment for, 283–284
　clinical features predicting probability of, 283, 284t, 511
　diagnosis of
　　algorithm for, 284f, 512f
　　differential, 283
　　laboratory testing for, 285–287
　　objective tests for, 287–289, 287f, 511–512, 512f
　inherited and acquired causes of, 290t
　prothrombic risk factors with, 289–290, 289b
　recurrent, 512
Deferoxamine therapy, for thalassemia, 462b
Degenerative disease, of spine, 159t, 160–161, 162t
Delirium, 1227b, 1242, 1248, 1248t, 1254t
Demerol, for pain, 1246t
4-Demethoxy-daunorubicin (idarubicin), 337t, 350
　for acute myeloid leukemia, 533, 535t
Dendritic cell vaccines, 381
Denileukin diftitox (DAB389IL-2, Ontak), 342t, 346–347
Denver shunt, for ascites, 131, 133, 133t
2-Deoxycoformycin (Pentostatin), 336t, 355t
　for hairy cell leukemia, 698
Depakene (valproate), 1227b
　for seizures, 25t, 26b
Depakote (valproate), 1227b
　for seizures, 25t, 26b
Depo-Provera (medroxyprogesterone acetate), for cachexia, 6–7
Depression
　in cancer patient, 1224–1225, 1226b, 1233b
　　medications for, 1227, 1227b
　leukocytosis due to, 243
　with seizures, 26
Dermatofibroma, pigmented, 308t
Dermatologic lesions, pigmented. See Pigmented skin lesions.
Dermatologic manifestations, of bleeding and thromboembolic disorders. See Cutaneous manifestations, of bleeding and thromboembolic disorders.
DES (diethylstilbestrol)
　and cervical cancer, 771
　and vaginal cancer, 779
　for prostate cancer, 869, 870
Desipramine, for neuropathic pain, 1249t
Desmoid tumor, 1040
Desmoplasia, 216
Desyrel (trazodone), 1227b
Detorubicin, for mesothelioma, 995t
Detoxification enemas, 1221t
Detoxification-fasting, 1221t
Dexamethasone
　for acute lymphoblastic leukemia, 557t, 558t
　for acute promyelocytic leukemia, 545b
　for brain metastases, 1069–1070, 1069b
　for Burkitt's leukemia/lymphoma, 562t
　for cachexia, 7, 7t
　for cranial neuropathy, 31
　for epidural cancer, 1081
　for idiopathic thrombocytopenic purpura, 491
　for multiple myeloma, 588–589, 589b, 590
　for nausea and vomiting, 1251, 1252t
　for neuropathic pain, 1249t
　for small cell lung cancer, 951b, 952
Dexrazoxane, for breast cancer, 756–757
Dexrazoxane (ADR-529), with doxorubicin, 351
Dextroamphetamine, for opioid-related sedation, 1248
DHT (dihydrotestosterone), and prostate cancer, 860
Diabetes mellitus, and pancreatic cancer, 908
Diacyl-glycerol, in cell signaling, 386
Diagnostic and Statistical Manual of Mental Disorders (DSM-IV), 1225
Diamond-Blackfan anemia, 451
Diarrhea, due to irinotecan, 352
Diazepam, for delirium, 1248t
DIC. See Disseminated intravascular coagulation (DIC).
Diclofenac, for pain, 1245t

Diet
　and breast cancer, 766–767
　and colorectal cancer, 924
　and gastric cancer, 889
　and pancreatic cancer, 908
　and prostate cancer, 860
　for cachexia, 5–6
　pancytopenia due to, 252
Dietary Supplement Health Education Act (DSHEA), 1212
Dietary supplements, 1212, 1213–1217, 1213t, 1214t, 1216t
Diethylstilbestrol (DES)
　and cervical cancer, 771
　and vaginal cancer, 779
　for prostate cancer, 869, 870
Diflunisal, for pain, 1245t
Dihydro-5-azacytidine, for mesothelioma, 995t
Dihydrofolate reductase gene, in gene therapy, 383–384
Dihydrotestosterone (DHT), and prostate cancer, 860
Dilation and curettage (D&C), for vaginal bleeding, 186
Dilaudid (hydromorphone), for pain, 1245, 1246, 1246t, 1247b, 1247t, 1254t
Dimethyl sulfoxide (DMSO), 1217t
Diphenhydramine (Benadryl), 1227b
　with haloperidol, 1248
　with interferon-alpha therapy of melanoma, 1096b
Direct antiglobulin test (DAT), 433, 433f, 469–470, 471f
Direct Coombs' test, 433, 433f
Directed blood donations, 431
Disalcid, for pain, 1244
Disbelief, 1224, 1225b
Disease-free interval, in breast cancer, 750
Disk herniation, 160–161, 1080
Diskitis, 161–162
Disseminated intravascular coagulation (DIC), 508–510
　acute, 268–269
　anemia due to, 239, 1167–1168
　chronic, 268, 269
　clinical manifestations of, 509
　cutaneous manifestations of, 294f, 301, 301f
　encephalopathy due to, 34t
　etiology of, 508–509
　forms of, 268–269
　fulminate, 268
　in acute myeloid leukemia, 529–530, 529f, 532t
　in pregnancy, 493–494
　laboratory evaluation of, 509, 509f
　management of, 509–510
　venous thromboembolic disease with, 286–287
Diuretics
　for ascites, 131
　for hypercalcemia, 193, 194t
Diversion, for pain management, 1244
Diverticulum, Zenker's, 140
DMSO (dimethyl sulfoxide), 1217t
DNA analysis, of lymphoma, 603b
DNA double-strand break, in radiation therapy, 322–323
DNA ploidy, in breast cancer, 722
DNA topoisomerase inhibitors, 332t, 337t–339t, 349–352, 349f, 351f
Docetaxel (Taxotere), 340t, 353, 356t
　for cancer of unknown primary, 1150t
　for gastric cancer, 895t, 896t
　for head and neck cancer, 1008t
　for metastatic breast cancer, 756t, 757–758, 757t
　for non–small cell lung cancer, 971t, 972, 976f, 977f
　for oral cavity cancer, 1008
　for prostate cancer, 872, 873t
　for renal cell cancer, 834t
Döhle bodies, in neutrophilic leukocytosis, 242, 242f
Dolasetron, for nausea and vomiting, 1251, 1252t
Dopaminergic agonist drugs, for pituitary adenoma, 1141

Dose distribution, for radiation therapy, 325–326, 326f
Dose optimization, automated, for radiation therapy, 326
Dose volume histogram (DVH), 326, 326f
Dose-density approach, 740
Double vision, due to cranial neuropathy, 29t, 31
Down syndrome, leukemia in, 551
Doxepin
　for insomnia, 1253
　for neuropathic pain, 1249t
Doxil (liposomal doxorubicin), 350
Doxil (pegylated doxorubicin), for multiple myeloma, 590
Doxorubicin (Adriamycin), 337t, 350, 351, 351f
　for bladder cancer, 853
　　superficial, 844
　for breast cancer
　　locally invasive, 739, 740, 742
　　metastatic, 756–758, 756t, 757t
　for Burkitt's leukemia/lymphoma, 562t
　for cancer of unknown origin, 1152b
　for esophageal cancer, 878
　for Ewing's sarcoma, 1034–1035
　for gastric cancer, 895t, 896t
　for Kaposi's sarcoma, 1160
　for leukemia
　　acute lymphoblastic, 557t, 558t
　　acute myeloid, 533
　for mesothelioma, 995, 996, 996t
　for multiple myeloma, 588–589, 589b, 590
　for neuroendocrine tumors, 1137
　for osteosarcoma, 1030, 1031
　for renal cell cancer, 834t
　for small cell lung cancer, 951
　for soft tissue sarcoma, 1044
　for thymoma, 989, 989t
　liposomal (Doxil), 350
　　for ovarian cancer, 802
Doxycycline, for pleural effusion, 92
Dronabinol, for cachexia, 8
Droperidol, for nausea and vomiting, 1251
Drug(s), neuropathies due to, 36–37
Drug reactions, pruritus due to, 15
Drug-induced eosinophilia, 249
Drug-induced immune hemolysis, 417, 470t, 472t
Drug-induced lymphocytosis, 247
Drug-induced neutropenia, 245
　myeloid growth factors for, 428
Drug-induced pancytopenia, 252
Drug-induced pulmonary toxicity, dyspnea due to, 76–77, 78t
Drug-induced thrombocytopenia, 222, 487–488, 488t
Drug-related bleeding disorders, 265
Drug-related leukocytosis, 243
Drug-related myelodysplasia, 568–569, 569t
DSHEA (Dietary Supplement Health Education Act), 1212
DSM-IV (Diagnostic and Statistical Manual of Mental Disorders), 1225
DTIC. See Dacarbazine (DTIC).
Duct ectasia, 74
Duct excision, 72–73
Duct lavage, 72
Ductal carcinoma, 61, 62f
Ductal carcinoma in situ (DCIS), 726–733
　calcifications in, 430, 728, 728f
　classification of, 727–729, 727f
　comedo-type, 727–728, 727f, 729t
　cribriform, 727, 727f
　differential diagnosis of, 729
　incidence of, 726
　lymph node sampling for, 730b
　mammography of, 730b
　micropapillary, 727, 727f
　nipple discharge in, 73, 726
　nuclear grading of, 728, 728f, 729t
　papillary, 727, 727f
　pathologic and mammographic features of, 727–728, 727f, 728f
　presentation of, 726–727
　prognostic correlation for, 728–729, 729t, 730b
　risk factors for, 727

Ductal carcinoma in situ *(Continued)*,
    solid, 727, 727f
    therapy for, 729–733
        breast-conserving surgery as, 729–731,
            730b, 731t
        lumpectomy as, 731, 732f
        mastectomy as, 729
        options of, 729–732
        overview of, 730b
        radiation, 730b, 731–732, 731f, 732t
        salvage, 732, 732f
        selection of, 733
        systemic, 732–733, 733f
        tamoxifen as, 733, 733f
        wide excision as, 730–731, 731t
Ductography, 72
Ductoscopy, 72
Duodenal obstruction, 109
Durie-Salmon staging system, for multiple
        myeloma, 583, 583t
DVH (dose volume histogram), 326, 326f
DVT. *See* Deep vein thrombosis (DVT).
Dying patient
    physical problems in, 1254–1256, 1254t
    with brain tumor, 1058–1059
Dynamic equilibrium, 352
Dysembryopathic neuroepithelial tumors,
        seizures due to, 23
Dysfunctional bleeding, vaginal, 184
Dysphagia, 139–143
    defined, 139
    diagnostic tests for, 140–141, 141f
    due to esophageal cancer, 140, 141–143,
        141f, 879, 880b
    due to hilar and mediastinal adenopathy, 94,
        95f
    initial assessment of, 139–140
    management of, 141–143, 142f
    oropharyngeal, 139–140
    pathophysiology of, 139
Dysphonia
    defined, 50
    functional, 51t
    muscle tension, 51t
    physical examination for, 53
    spasmodic, 51t
Dysplastic nevus syndrome, 1194t, 1202
Dyspnea, 75–79
    causes of, 75–77, 76t
    defined, 75
    due to anemia, 79
    due to drug-induced pulmonary toxicity,
        76–77, 78t
    due to lung cancer, 960–961
    due to pericardial effusion, 76
    due to pleural effusion, 75–76, 77, 79
    due to pulmonary embolism, 284
    evaluation of, 77
    in dying patient, 1254t, 1255
    therapy for, 77–79
Dysuria, 1256

E

EACA (ε-aminocaproic acid)
    for platelet function defects, 494
    for thrombocytopenia, 486–487
Eastern Cooperative Oncology Group (ECOG)
        Performance Scale, 965
Eaton-Lambert syndrome, in non–small cell lung
        cancer, 963
EBV. *See* Epstein-Barr virus (EBV).
E-cadherin mutations, in hereditary diffuse
        gastric cancer, 1201
Ecchymoses, 294–295
Echinocytes, 274
Ectopic corticotropin secretion, in small cell lung
        cancer, 948
Ectopic hormone production, in non–small cell
        lung cancer, 963
Ectopic pregnancy, pelvic mass due to, 188
Edatrexate, for mesothelioma, 995t
Edema
    due to superior vena cava syndrome, 100, 100f
    Reinke's, 51t
EGFR. *See* Epidermal growth factor receptor
        (EGFR).
Ehlers-Danlos disease, cutaneous manifestations
        of, 296

Eicosapentaenoic acid (EPA), for cachexia, 7
Ejaculatory dysfunction, 1235
ELAC2 gene, in prostate cancer, 1203
Elderly. *See* Older adults.
Electroencephalogram (EEG)
    for encephalopathy, 34
    of seizures, 24
Electroglottography, 54–55
Electromyography (EMG)
    for hoarseness, 54–55
    for peripheral neuropathy, 39t
Electrons, in radiation therapy, 321
Electrophoresis, for immunoglobulin
        abnormalities, 205, 206f
Ellence. *See* Epirubicin (Ellence).
Elliptocytes, 276, 276f
Elliptocytosis, 276
    hereditary, 468
ELM (epiluminescence microscopy), 305–306,
        310f
EMAP-II (endothelial monocyte activating
        polypeptide-2), in antiangiogenic
        therapy, 385
Embolectomy, acute pulmonary, 514t, 519
Embryonic cell therapy, 1217t
Emesis, chemotherapy-induced, 1250–1251,
        1251t, 1252t
Emotional adjustment, to cancer diagnosis, 1224,
        1225b
Encephalitis
    in small cell lung cancer, 947
    paraneoplastic limbic, 34t, 35
Encephalopathy, 32–35
    causes of, 32, 33t, 34t, 35
    defined, 32
    differential diagnosis of, 32
    evaluation of, 32–34, 34t
    management of, 35b
    metabolic, 32, 34t
    toxic-metabolic, 1063
    Wernicke's, 35b
Endarterectomy, pulmonary, 514t, 519
Endocarditis, acute bacterial, vascular cutaneous
        manifestations of, 298f
Endocervical curettage, 783
Endocrine therapy, for locally invasive breast
        cancer, 740–742
Endocrine tumors. *See* Neuroendocrine tumors.
Endolymphatic stromal myosis, 789
Endometrial biopsy, 783–784
    for vaginal bleeding, 186
Endometrial cancer, 782–789
    chemotherapy for, 787–788
    clinical presentation of, 783
    diagnostic methods for, 783–784
    discovered at hysterectomy, 789
    epidemiology of, 782
    estrogen replacement therapy and, 782, 789
    follow-up care for, 789
    high-risk histologic types of, 788–789, 788t
    metastatic, 786t
    precursor lesions for, 783
    preoperative imaging of, 784, 785f
    progestins for, 786, 787–788
    radiation therapy for, 787
    recurrent, 787–788, 788f
    risk factors for, 782–783
    surgical staging of, 784–786, 785t–787t
    vaginal bleeding due to, 186, 783
    with ovarian neoplasms, 789
Endometrial hyperplasia, 783
Endometrioid ovarian cancer, 795, 795t
Endoscopic retrograde cholangiopancreatography
        (ERCP)
    for biliary cancer, 903, 905b
    for pancreatic cancer, 912–913
Endoscopic ultrasonography (EUS)
    of esophageal cancer, 876, 877f
    of pancreatic cancer, 913
Endoscopy
    for dysphagia, 140, 141, 141f
    for gastric cancer, 891
    for hoarseness, 55, 56b
    for upper GI bleeding, 145
Endostatin, 384
Endothelial monocyte activating polypeptide-2
        (EMAP-II), in antiangiogenic
        therapy, 385

Enoxaparin, for venous thromboembolism, 515t
Entelev, 1217t
Enteral feedings, for cachexia, 6
Enteritis, radiation-induced, 371
Enterococcus, febrile neutropenia due to, 1173
Enteropathy-type intestinal T-cell lymphoma,
        669, 670
Environmental factors
    in colorectal cancer, 922
    in gastric cancer, 888t, 889
Enzyme-linked cell-surface receptors, 386
Eosinophilia, 249–250
    due to cancer, 1168
Eosinophilic fasciitis, 249
Eosinophilic granulomatous cellulitis, 249
Eosinophilic syndrome, 249–250
EP regimen, for small cell lung cancer, 951, 953
EPA (eicosapentaenoic acid), for cachexia, 7
Ependymomas, 1052–1053, 1056
Epidermal growth factor receptor (EGFR)
    in breast cancer, 721–722
    in head and neck cancer, 1008t
Epidermal growth factor receptor (EGFR)–family
        antagonists, 332t, 345–347
Epidermal growth factor receptor (EGFR)
        inhibitors, for colorectal cancer,
        930
Epidermal growth factor receptor (EGFR)
        pathway, 387
Epididymal cysts, 180, 182
Epididymitis, 180, 182
Epidural abscess, 159, 161, 1080
Epidural hemorrhage, 1080
Epidural leukemia, 1083
Epidural lymphoma, 1079f, 1083
Epidural metastasis, pain due to, 1243
Epidural tumor(s), 1077–1083
    approach to management of, 1081
    clinical manifestations of, 1078–1079
    epidemiology of, 1077
    imaging of, 1079–1081, 1079f, 1080f
    leukemia as, 1083
    lymphoma as, 1083
    pathology of, 1077, 1078f
    primary *vs.* metastatic, 1077, 1078
    spinal fluid studies for, 1079
    spinal stability and, 1077, 1078f
    treatment of, 1081–1083
    vascular supply to, 1077
Epilepsy. *See* Seizures.
Epiluminescence microscopy (ELM), 305–306,
        310f
Epipodophyllotoxins, 332t, 338t–339t
Epirubicin (Ellence), 337t, 350
    for cancer of unknown primary, 1150t
    for esophageal cancer, 878
    for gastric cancer, 895, 895t, 896t
    for locally invasive breast cancer, 739
    for superficial bladder cancer, 844
    for thymoma, 989t
Epistaxis, 265, 266b
Epitrochlear adenopathy, 215t
EPO. *See* Erythropoietin (EPO).
EPOCH regimen, for AIDS-related non-Hodgkin's
        lymphoma, 1157
ε-aminocaproic acid (EACA)
    for platelet function defects, 494
    for thrombocytopenia, 486–487
Epstein-Barr virus (EBV)
    and Hodgkin's disease, 616
    and non-Hodgkin's lymphoma, 648–649,
        1155–1156
    and peripheral T-cell lymphoma, 667
    and posttransplant lymphoproliferative
        disease, 1161–1162, 1163, 1164
    Burkitt's leukemia/lymphoma due to, 550
    cerebrospinal fluid analysis of, 1162b
    lymphocytosis due to, 247
Equianalgesic doses, 1247t
ERCP (endoscopic retrograde
        cholangiopancreatography)
    for biliary cancer, 903, 905b
    for pancreatic cancer, 912–913
Erectile dysfunction, 1235, 1237–1238, 1238b
ERMs (estrogen receptor modulators), 331–343,
        331f, 332t, 340t, 752–754, 753t
    selective (SERMs), 340t–341t, 343–344, 740
Erythrocytes. *See* Red blood cell(s) (RBCs).

Erythrocytosis, 256–264
  abdominal ultrasound for, 259–260, 260f,
      261f
  absolute
      classification of, 257, 257t
      defined, 256
      evaluation of, 258–263, 260t
      in polycythemia vera, 703, 703t
      vs. apparent, 256
  acquired, 257, 257t, 1168
  apparent, 256, 263
  bone marrow aspiration and biopsy for, 261,
      262f
  burst-forming unit erythroid assays for,
      261–262
  c-mpl in, 262
  complete blood count in, 256, 258
  computed tomography for, 260, 260f, 261f
  congenital, 257, 257t
  defined, 256
  diagnostic criteria for, 259t
  diagnostic studies for, 258–263, 260t
  ferritin and vitamin B_{12} in, 259
  history and physical examination for,
      257–258
  idiopathic, 257, 263
  in polycythemia vera, 702, 703
  marrow karyotype studies for, 261
  oxygen dissociation curve in, 263
  oxygen saturation in, 258–259
  pathogenesis of, 256
  primary, 257, 257t
  PRV-1 expression in, 262–263
  relative, 263–264
      in polycythemia vera, 703, 703t
  renal and liver function tests for, 259
  secondary, 257, 257t
  serum erythropoietin in, 260
  signs and symptoms of, 257–258, 258f, 258t,
      259f
  truncation of erythropoietin receptor in, 263
Erythroderma, in Sézary syndrome, 665, 666f
Erythromelalgia, 227, 228
  in essential thrombocythemia, 710, 711
  in polycythemia vera, 702, 705
Erythropoiesis
  in myelodysplasia, 571f
  ineffective, hyperbilirubinemia due to,
      197–198
  iron deficiency, 207–208
Erythropoietic growth factors, 419–421, 420t
Erythropoietin (EPO)
  for anemia of chronic disease, 457–458
  for chemotherapy-related myelosuppression,
      954
  for chronic lymphocytic leukemia, 696
  for myelodysplasia, 576, 577f
  serum, 260
  therapeutic uses of, 419–421, 420t, 428b
Erythropoietin receptor, truncation of, 263
Escherichia coli
  febrile neutropenia due to, 1173
  white blood cell inclusion of, 281f
Esophageal cancer, 875–885
  cervical, 1004–1005
  chemoradiotherapy for
      concurrent, without surgery for, 883,
          883f
      intensification of, 884
      preoperative, 881–883
  chemotherapy for, 878–879, 878t
      preoperative, 879, 880–881, 881f, 881t
  diagnosis of, 876, 876f, 877f
  dysphagia due to, 140, 141–143, 141f, 879,
      880b
  epidemiology of, 875
  locally advanced, 876, 884b
  management of, 883–884, 884b
  neoadjuvant therapy for, 879–880
  nonsurgical vs. surgical therapy for, 884
  palliation for, 879, 880b
  small cell carcinoma form of, 885
  staging of, 876–877, 876f, 877f, 884b
  surgery or radiation alone for, 877–878
  surgical salvage for, 884b
  tumorigenesis of, 875–876
Esophageal reflux. See Gastroesophageal reflux
      disease.

Esophageal stents, 142–143
Esophageal stricture, 140
Esophageal varices, GI bleeding due to, 144
Esophagobronchial fistulae, 143
Esophagram, barium, of esophageal cancer, 876,
      876f
Esophagus, Barrett's, 140, 875, 876, 889
Essential thrombocythemia, 709–712
  chromosomal abnormalities in, 709–710
  clinical evaluation of, 710–711
  clinical presentation of, 710
  diagnostic criteria for, 710t
  differential diagnosis of, 709, 709t
  epidemiology of, 709
  follow-up evaluation for, 712
  in pregnancy, 712
  platelet count in, 227, 229, 281f
  staging, prognostic features, and outcomes
      for, 711
  treatment for, 711–712
Essiac, 1214–1215, 1214t
Estramustine, for prostate cancer, 872–873, 873t
Estrogen antagonists, pure, for metastatic breast
      cancer, 754
Estrogen receptor(s), in breast cancer, 721
Estrogen receptor modulators (ERMs), 331–343,
          331f, 332t, 340t, 752–754, 753t
      selective (SERMs), 340t–341t, 343–344, 740
      for hot flashes, 766b
Estrogen replacement therapy
  after breast cancer, 765, 766b
  and endometrial cancer, 782, 789
  for prevention of colorectal cancer, 924
Ethnic issues, 1230–1231
"Ethnic" neutropenia, 246
Ethnicity, and breast cancer, 724
Ethoglucid, for superficial bladder cancer, 844
Ethosuximide (Zarontin), for seizures, 25t
Ethylenimines, 332t, 333t
Etodolac, for pain, 1244
Etoposide (VP-16), 338t, 350, 355t, 356t
  for acute myeloid leukemia, 535t
  for Burkitt's leukemia/lymphoma, 562t
  for cancer of unknown primary, 1150t,
      1151b–1153b
  for esophageal cancer, 878t
  for Ewing's sarcoma, 1035
  for gastric cancer, 895t, 896t
  for germ-cell tumors, 818, 819b, 820b, 821b,
      822, 823
  for gestational trophoblastic tumor, 810–811,
      810t
  for myelodysplasia, 576
  for neuroendocrine tumors, 1137
  for prostate cancer, 873t
  for small cell lung cancer, 951, 951b, 953
  for thymoma, 989t
  in conditioning regimen for hematopoietic
      stem cell transplantation
      allogeneic, 395t, 396t
      autologous, 399t
  toxicities of, 396t
Etretinate, for head and neck cancer, 1014t
Euglobulin lysis time, 267
Eulexin (flutamide), 341t, 344
  for prostate cancer, 870
Eurixor, 1213t
EUS (endoscopic ultrasonography)
  of esophageal cancer, 876, 877f
  of pancreatic cancer, 913
Evanescent pulmonary eosinophilic infiltrates,
      249
Evista (raloxifene), 341t, 344
Ewing's sarcoma, 1034–1035
  clinical features of, 1029t, 1034, 1034f
  cytogenetics of, 315, 1040
  epidemiology of, 1034
  metastatic, 1035, 1035f
  pathologic fractures due to, 154
  prognostic factors for, 1034
  staging of, 1034
  treatment of, 1034–1035, 1045
Excisional biopsy, of neck mass, 47
Exemestane (Aromasin), 341t, 347
  for metastatic breast cancer, 753t, 754, 754t
Exercise, hematuria due to, 174
Expectant management, for prostate cancer,
      863b, 868–869

Extended field, 622
Extended mantle field, 622
External-beam radiation therapy, for thyroid
      carcinoma
      differentiated, 1123
      medullary, 1126
Extracorporeal photophoresis, for Sézary
      syndrome, 666–667
Extragonadal germ-cell tumors, 822b
Extramedullary disease
  in acute lymphoblastic leukemia, 563t
  in acute myeloid leukemia, 528–529, 529f
Extranodal marginal zone lymphoma, 604f
Extranodal NK/T-cell lymphoma, nasal type, 669
Extrapleural pneumonectomy, for mesothelioma,
      991f, 994, 994f
Eydrocortisone, for prostate cancer, 873t

F
FAB Classification. See French-American-British
      (FAB) Classification.
FAB classification, of leukemia, 280
Fabry's disease, cutaneous manifestations of,
      296, 296f
Facial nerve, in salivary gland carcinoma,
      1022–1023, 1024
Facial nerve deficit, 30t
Facial nerve palsy, 31
Facial numbness, due to cranial neuropathy, 29t
Facial pain, due to cranial neuropathy, 29t
Facial weakness, due to cranial neuropathy, 30t
Factor VII deficiency, 267, 268, 270
Factor VIII, for hemophilia A, 499–501, 500b,
      501f
Factor VIII alloantibody inhibitors, hemophilia A
      with, 501–504, 503b, 503f
Factor VIII assay, 289b
Factor VIII deficiency. See Hemophilia A.
Factor IX, for hemophilia B, 504
Factor IX deficiency, 266, 267, 268, 270, 504
Factor X deficiency, 267, 268, 270
Factor XI deficiency, 267, 268, 270, 504–505, 505b
Factor XII deficiency, 271
Factor V Leiden, 289, 289b
Familial adenomatous polyposis (FAP),
      1199–1200
  and colorectal cancer, 921, 1199–1200
  genetic basis for, 1194t
  prophylactic surgery for, 371–372
Familial medullary thyroid carcinoma,
      1198–1199, 1198t
Familial melanoma, 1194t, 1202
Familial neutrophilia, 243
Familial retinoblastoma, 1194t
Familial thrombocytosis, 230
Familismo, 1230
Family, of cancer patient, 1228–1230, 1228b
Famotidine, for nausea and vomiting, 1256
Fanconi's anemia, 450
  leukemia in, 551
  myelodysplasia in, 568
  pancytopenia in, 253
FAP. See Familial adenomatous polyposis (FAP).
Fareston (toremifene), 340t, 343–344
Farnesyl transferase, 386–387
Farnesyl transferase inhibitors, 387
Fasciitis, eosinophilic, 249
Faslodex (fulvestrant), for metastatic breast
      cancer, 754
Fat embolism, cutaneous manifestations of, 303
Fatigue, management of, 1253–1254
Febrile neutropenia, 1173–1178
  after neutrophil recovery, 1177b
  defined, 1173–1174
  epidemiology of, 1173, 1174f
  evaluation of, 1175–1176
  pathogenesis of, 1173, 1174f, 1175f
  prevention of, 1178
  risk factors for, 1174–1175
  treatment for, 1176–1178
      choice of, 11, 12b
      considerations in, 1175
      empiric, 245, 1176, 1176b
      for fungi unresponsive to amphotericin,
          1177b, 1177f
      outpatient, 245, 1178t
Febrile nonhemolytic transfusion reactions, 439
Fecal occult blood testing, 924–925, 925t

Felbamate (Felbatol), for seizures, 25t
Felty's syndrome, 136t, 253
Femara (letrozole), 341t, 347
    for metastatic breast cancer, 753t, 754–755,
        754t
Fenoprofen, for pain, 1245t
Fentanyl, transdermal, for pain, 1245–1246,
        1246t, 1254t
Ferritin
    in erythrocytosis, 259
    serum, 208–210, 209t, 211b, 237
Ferrous gluconate (Ferrlecit), 456b
Ferumoxides, for liver imaging, 117
Fetal platelet counts, 491–492
Fever
    defined, 1173
    with neutropenia. See Febrile neutropenia.
Fever of unknown origin, 9–13
    causes of, 9–10, 10t
    defined, 9
    due to cancer, 9
    due to common infections, 9, 11
    due to fungal infections, 11
    general considerations with, 10
    in splenectomized patient, 10, 10b
    initial approach to, 9b
    life-threatening emergencies with, 10
    predisposing factors for, 11
    urgent therapy for, 10b
    with bone marrow (stem cell)
        transplantation, 11–13, 12b
    with neutropenia, 11, 12b
Fibroadenoma, 61f
Fibrolytic disorders, 267
Fibroma, 154
Fibrosarcoma, 1039t, 1040
Fibrous histiocytoma, malignant, 154, 1029t,
        1032–1033, 1039t, 1040
Filgrastim. See Granulocyte colony-stimulating
        factor (G-CSF, lenograstim,
        Filgrastim).
Fine needle aspiration biopsy
    of breast mass, 63
    of lymph nodes, 219
    of neck mass, 47
    of thyroid nodule, 1118
FISH (fluorescence in situ hybridization)
    for acute myeloid leukemia, 524–525
    for chronic myeloid leukemia, 679–680
"Flare reactions," to anthracyclines, 350
Flexible sigmoidoscopy, for colorectal cancer, 925
Flor-Essence, 1214–1215, 1214t
Flow cytometry
    for breast cancer, 722
    for lymphoma, 603b
"Flower" cells, in adult T-cell
        leukemia/lymphoma, 674
Floxuridine (fluorodeoxyuridine, FUDR), 335t,
        369–370
    for renal cell cancer, 834, 834t
Fludarabine, 336t, 355t
    for chronic lymphocytic leukemia, 693–694,
        694f, 695f
    in conditioning regimen for hematopoietic
        stem cell transplantation, 395,
        395t, 396t
    toxicities of, 396t
Fluid volume expansion, for hypercalcemia, 193,
        194t
Fluorescence in situ hybridization (FISH)
    for acute myeloid leukemia, 524–525
    for chronic myeloid leukemia, 679–680
Fluorodeoxyuridine, 335t, 369–370
    for renal cell cancer, 834, 834t
5-Fluorouracil (5-FU), 335t, 370
    for actinic keratoses, 1111
    for anal carcinoma, 940
    for basal cell carcinoma, 1107
    for cancer of unknown origin, 1151b–1153b
    for cervical cancer, 775t
    for colorectal cancer, 929, 930–931, 931f, 932
    for esophageal cancer, 878–879, 878t
        preoperative, 881, 881t, 882
        with radiation therapy, 881t, 882, 883
    for gastric cancer, 895, 895t, 896t, 897f
    for head and neck cancer, 1008t
    for laryngeal cancer, 1003, 1003t
    for locally invasive breast cancer, 739, 742

    for neuroendocrine tumors, 1137
    for oral cavity cancer, 1007
    for oropharyngeal cancer, 1006
    for pancreatic cancer, 915, 916
    for renal cell cancer, 834, 834t, 837–838
Fluoxetine (Prozac), 1227, 1227b
    for hot flashes, 766b
Flurbiprofen, for pain, 1245t
Flutamide (Eulexin), 341t, 344
    for prostate cancer, 870
Focal nodular hyperplasia (FNH), 124–125, 125f
Folate, for paroxysmal nocturnal
        hemoglobinuria, 449
Folate antagonists (folate analogues), 332t, 335t
Folate deficiency, 233t, 238, 277, 455–457, 456b
Folic acid, for prevention of colorectal cancer, 924
Folinic acid. See Leucovorin.
Follicle-stimulating hormone (FSH) deficiency,
        due to pituitary adenoma, 1142t
Follicular lymphoma, 248, 248f, 607, 608f
    low-grade, 636–637, 637t
Formalin, for hematuria, 177–178
Fosphenytoin, for brain metastases, 1069b
Fractionated total body irradiation (FTBI), as
        conditioning regimen for
        hematopoietic stem cell
        transplantation
    allogeneic, 395, 395t, 396t
    autologous, 399t
Fractionation, 323, 326, 327
Fractures, pathologic, 149–155
    causes of, 150–152, 151f
    clinical evaluation of, 149b, 152–153, 152b,
        152f
    definitive treatment of, 153–154, 154f, 155f
    issues to explore with, 149–150
    presenting features of, 150, 150f, 151f
    primary management of, 153
French-American-British (FAB) Classification
    for acute lymphoblastic leukemia, 551–552
    for acute myeloid leukemia, 523, 524t
    for myelodysplasia, 566, 572–573, 572t
Frye's syndrome, 1024
FSH (follicle-stimulating hormone) deficiency,
        due to pituitary adenoma, 1142t
FTBI. See Fractionated total body irradiation
        (FTBI).
5-FU. See 5-Fluorouracil (5-FU).
FUDR (fluorodeoxyuridine), 335t, 369–370
    for renal cell cancer, 834, 834t
Fulvestrant (Faslodex), for metastatic breast
        cancer, 754
Fumagillin, in antiangiogenic therapy, 385
Functional classification of physical status, 363t
Fungal infections
    fever of unknown origin due to, 11
    with hematopoietic stem cell transplantation,
        400–401
Fungating lesions, 1252–1253
Furosemide (Lasix)
    for death rattle, 1254t, 1255
    for hypercalcemia, 193, 194t
    for hyperuricemia, 1187

G

G-6-PD (glucose-6-phosphate dehydrogenase)
        deficiency, 456t, 466–468, 466f,
        467f, 467t
Gabapentin (Neurontin)
    for neuropathic pain, 1248, 1249t
    for seizures, 25t
Gabitril (tiagabine), for seizures, 25t
Gabobenate dimeglumine, for liver imaging, 117
Gadolinium chelates, for liver imaging, 117
Galactography, 72
Galactorrhea, 71
Gallbladder cancer, 905–906
Gallium nitrate, for hypercalcemia, 194
Gamma globulin, for warm antibody
        autoimmune hemolytic anemia,
        473b
Gammopathy(ies). See also Immunoglobulin
        abnormalities.
    monoclonal
        differential diagnosis of, 202t, 203–205,
            203b
        due to amyloidosis, 205, 205b
        due to multiple myeloma, 203, 204–205

    due to plasmacytoma, 205
    due to Waldenström's
        macroglobulinemia, 205
    hypogammaglobulinemia due to, 203
    of undetermined significance, 203–204
    peripheral neuropathy due to, 36, 40
    serum protein electrophoresis of, 200, 201f
    polyclonal, 200–202, 201f, 202t
Ganciclovir, for Epstein-Barr virus, 1163
Ganglogliomas, seizures due to, 23
Gangliomas, 1051
Gangrene, venous limb, 302–303
Gardner-Diamond syndrome, 300, 300f
Gardner's disease, 1040
Gardner's syndrome, 921, 1200
Garlic, 1213t
Gastrectomy
    Billroth I, 362
    distal, and gastric cancer, 889
    for gastric cancer, 892, 893–894, 893t, 894t
Gastric cancer, 887–898
    adjuvant therapy for, 896–897, 897f, 897t
    advanced, treatment vs. supportive care for,
        895–896, 896t
    chemotherapy for, 895, 895t–897t, 896–897
    clinical presentation of, 890, 890t
    diagnostic studies of, 890–892
    environmental factors in, 888t, 889
    epidemiology of, 887
    genetic factors in, 888t, 889–890, 1194t,
        1201–1202
    hereditary diffuse, 1194t, 1201–1202
    intraperitoneal therapy for, 897–898
    neoadjuvant therapy for, 897
    palliative surgery and endoscopic procedures
        for, 894
    pathogenesis of, 888–890, 888t
    pathology of, 887–888
    precursor conditions for, 888–889, 888t
    radiation therapy for, 894–895, 896–897,
        897f, 897t
    risk factors for, 888–890, 888t
    screening for, 891–892
    staging and prognosis of, 892–893, 892t, 893t
    surgery with curative intent for, 893–894,
        894t
Gastric carcinoid tumors, 1133–1134, 1134t
Gastric lymphomas, 654–655, 654t
Gastric outlet obstruction, 109, 110t, 111, 112
Gastric varices, 144
Gastrinoma, 1134t, 1135–1136, 1136t
Gastrinoma triangle, 1136
Gastritis, chronic atrophic, 888
Gastroesophageal reflux disease
    and esophageal cancer, 875
    hoarseness due to, 50
Gastrointestinal (GI) bleeding, 144–148
    acute lower, 145–146, 145t
    acute upper, 144–145, 145t
    as complication of cancer treatment, 147–148
    as complication of known cancer, 147
    chronic, 146–147
    due to colorectal cancer, 926, 926t
    hemobilia as, 146
    hemoperitoneum as, 146
Gastrointestinal (GI) cancer
    metastases of unknown origin due to, 316
    sentinel nodes in, 366
    staging of, 365–366
Gastrointestinal (GI) lymphomas, 654–655, 654t,
        662
Gastrointestinal (GI) oncologic surgery, 362–372
    extent of resection of primary tumor in, 367
    for bowel obstruction, 370–371
    for complications of radiation therapy, 371
    history of, 362
    laparoscopic resection as, 368
    molecular characterization of tumors in, 367,
        367t
    nutritional assessment for, 364–365, 364t
    prophylactic, 371–372
    radioimmune-guided, 366–367
    risk assessment for, 362–364, 363t, 364t
    sentinel nodes in, 366
    staging laparoscopy as, 365–366
    with hepatic artery infusion, 369–370
    with intraoperative radiation therapy, 368
        and peritoneal chemotherapy, 368–369

Gastrointestinal stromal tumor (GIST), 1040, 1044–1045
Gastrointestinal (GI) tract metastases, of melanoma, 1087–1088, 1087f
Gastropathy, hypertrophic, and gastric cancer, 889
Gaucher's disease, pancytopenia due to, 253
Gaugerot-Blum purpura, 300
G-CSF. *See* Granulocyte colony-stimulating factor (G-CSF, lenograstim, Filgrastim).
GCTs. *See* Germ-cell tumors (GCTs).
Gemcitabine (Gemzar), 335t, 349
    for bladder cancer, 854
    for cancer of unknown primary, 1150t
    for gastric cancer, 895t, 896t
    for head and neck cancer, 1008t
    for mesothelioma, 995t
    for metastatic breast cancer, 756t
    for non–small cell lung cancer, 971t, 972, 976b, 976f, 977f
    for renal cell cancer, 834, 834t
    for soft tissue sarcoma, 1044
    pulmonary toxicity due to, 78t
Gemtuzumab ozogomicin (Mylotarg), 342t, 346
    for acute myeloid leukemia, 346, 542
Gene expression profiling, in breast cancer, 723
Gene therapy, 382–384, 382t, 383t
Genetic basis, 1193–1203
    for acute lymphoblastic leukemia, 551
    for acute myeloid leukemia, 522, 524, 526t
    for breast cancer, 1195–1198
        age-specific penetrance with, 1195, 1195f
        conditions associated with, 1197–1198
        epidemiology of, 1195
        genes involved in, 1194, 1194t, 1195
        in Ashkenazi Jewish population, 1195–1196, 1196f
        indicators of, 1195, 1195t
        initial management with, 1197b
        models for evaluating, 1196
        risk management guidelines with, 1196t, 1197
    for colorectal cancer, 921–922, 1199–1201, 1201t
    for dysplastic nevus syndrome, 1194t, 1202
    for gastric cancer, 888t, 889–890, 1201–1202
    for medullary thyroid carcinoma, 1198–1199, 1198t
    for melanoma, 1086, 1202
    for multiple endocrine neoplasia syndromes, 1194t, 1198–1199
    for nevoid basal cell carcinoma syndrome (Gorlin syndrome), 1194t, 1202–1203
    for pancreatic cancer, 908–909, 910, 910t
    for pancreatic endocrine tumors, 1135
    for prostate cancer, 860, 1203
    for renal cell cancer, 826–828
    for retinoblastoma, 1193, 1194t, 1203
    for skin cancer, 1105
    for von Hippel–Lindau disease, 1194t, 1203
    mechanisms of, 1193–1195
Genetic cancer risk assessment, 1203–1205, 1204t
Genetic counseling, 1205–1207
Genetic heterogeneity, 1194–1195
Genetic testing, 1204–1205
    for breast cancer, 765
    for familial adenomatous polyposis, 1200
    for familial medullary thyroid carcinoma, 1199
    for hereditary nonpolyposis colorectal cancer, 1201
    for iron overload disorders, 210–211, 211b
    for ovarian cancer, 791–792
    recommendations for, 1206–1207, 1206b, 1206t
Genitalia, pigmented lesions of, 311
Germ-cell tumors (GCTs), 813–823
    clinical evaluation of, 180, 813–814, 814f
    clinical presentation of, 813
    cranial neuropathies due to, 28t
    cryptorchidism and, 179–180
    extragonadal, 822b
    headache with, 21t
    imaging of, 814
    management of, 815–821

for advanced metastatic disease, 817–821, 819b, 819t, 820b–822b
    for low-stage germ-cell tumors, 815–817, 817t, 818b
    for metastatic disease, 817–821, 819b, 819t, 820b–822b
    for nonseminoma, 815–817, 817t, 818b
    for relapse, 821b
    for seminoma, 815, 817t
    initial, 814b
    postchemotherapy surgery in, 818–819
    salvage chemotherapy for, 820
    sequelae of, 821–823
    surgery in salvage setting for, 820–821
    with good-risk disease, 818, 819b
    with intermediate- and poor-risk disease, 818, 820b
metastatic
    management of, 817–821, 819b, 819t, 820b–822b
    pattern of nodal spread for, 814, 814f
occult extragonadal, 316
pathology of, 814–815, 815t
pelvic mass in, 187–188
staging of, 815, 816t
Germline mutations, 1193–1194
Gerson therapy, 1221t
Gestational trophoblastic tumors (GTT), 804–812
    epidemiology of, 804
    long-term follow-up after, 811
    molar pregnancy (hydatidiform moles) as, 804–806, 805t, 807, 807b, 811
    persistent, 807–811
        clinical presentation of, 807
        diagnosis and staging of, 807–809, 808t, 809t
        metastatic, 807–808, 808t, 810–811
        molar pregnancy and, 807b
        nonmetastatic, 809–810, 809f, 810t
        treatment for, 809–811, 809f, 810t
    placental site, 807, 811
    subsequent pregnancy experience after, 811
    surveillance following chemotherapy for, 811
    terminology for, 804
    vaginal bleeding due to, 184–185, 185f
    vs. phantom hCG syndrome, 811–812
GETT (Groupe d'Etudes des Tumeurs Thymiques) classification, for thymoma, 987, 987t
GI. *See* Gastrointestinal (GI).
Giant cell tumors, of bone, 1036, 1036f
    pathologic fractures due to, 153f, 154
Gilbert syndrome, hyperbilirubinemia due to, 198
Gilman, Alfred, 348
Gingival hyperplasia, in acute myeloid leukemia, 528–529, 529f
GIST (gastrointestinal stromal tumor), 1040, 1044–1045
Glandular therapy, 1217t
Glanzmann's thrombasthenia, 270, 494
Gleevec (imatinib mesylate), 356
    for chronic myeloid leukemia, 410, 685, 685b
    for gastrointestinal stomal tumors, 1044–1045
Glioblastoma(s), 1052, 1053, 1053f
Glioblastoma multiforme, 1053, 1053f
    seizures due to, 23
    with hereditary nonpolyposis colorectal cancer, 1201
Glioma(s)
    grading of, 1051t
    headache with, 21t
    high-grade, 1052–1053, 1053f, 1054b
    low-grade, 1051–1052, 1052b, 1052f
    MRI of, 24f
    seizures due to, 23
Glossitis, 232
Glossopharyngeal nerve deficit, 30t
"Glove and socks" papular purpura, 300
Glucagonoma, 1134t, 1135, 1136t
Glucocorticoids
    for brain metastases, 1069–1070, 1069b, 1070b
    for brain tumors, 1058
    for cachexia, 7, 7t
    for multiple myeloma, 589b

Glucose, for hyperkalemia, 1189
Glucose-6-phosphate dehydrogenase (G-6-PD) deficiency, 456t, 466–468, 466f, 467f, 467t
Glucuronide, defective conjugation of, 198
Glycoprotein IbIX, 485
GM-CSF. *See* Granulocyte-macrophage colony-stimulating factor (GM-CSF, sargramostim, molgramostim).
GnRH (gonadotropin-releasing hormone) agonist, for breast cancer, 755
Gold, Joseph, 1217t, 1218–1219
Goldman classification, of physical status, 363t
Goldman's cardiac risk index, 363t
Gonadal function abnormalities, after hematopoietic stem cell transplantation, 404
Gonadotropin deficiency, due to pituitary adenoma, 1142t
Gonadotropin excess, due to pituitary adenoma, 1142t
Gonadotropin-releasing agents, 341t–342t
Gonadotropin-releasing hormone (GnRH) agonist, for breast cancer, 755
Goodman, Louis, 348
Gorlin syndrome, 1194t, 1202–1203
Goserelin acetate (Zoladex)
    for breast cancer
        locally invasive, 741–742
        metastatic, 753t
    for prostate cancer, 870
G-protein receptors, 386
Graft-*versus*-host disease (GVHD), 391, 396–397, 438, 439
Graft-*versus*-tumor effect, 394
Grand mal seizures, 23
Granisetron, for nausea and vomiting, 1252t
Granular lymphocytes, 246, 246f
Granulocyte colony-stimulating factor (G-CSF, lenograstim, Filgrastim). *See also* Myeloid growth factors.
    for aplastic anemia
        acute severe, 445
        refractory severe, 448
    for chemotherapy-related myelosuppression, 954
    for cyclic neutropenia, 477
    for leukemia
        acute lymphoblastic, 558t
        acute lymphocytic, 425, 425t
        acute myeloid, 426b, 532
    for myelodysplasia, 427, 428b, 576, 577f
    for severe congenital neutropenia, 475–477
    recruitment of cells into S-phase with, 424, 425t
    reduced periods of neutropenia with, 422t, 423t
    with stem cell transplantation, 425–426, 426t
Granulocyte count, and infection, 1173, 1174f
Granulocyte transfusions
    for bone marrow failure syndrome, 452
    for chronic granulomatous disease, 481
Granulocyte-macrophage colony-stimulating factor (GM-CSF, sargramostim, molgramostim). *See also* Myeloid growth factors.
    enhanced antimicrobial function with, 423–424, 424t
    for aplastic anemia, 448
    for leukemia
        acute lymphocytic, 425
        acute myeloid, 426b, 532
    for mesothelioma, 996t
    for myelodysplasia, 427, 576
    recruitment of cells into S-phase with, 424, 425t
    reduced periods of neutropenia with, 422t, 423t
    with stem cell transplantation, 425–426, 426t
Granulocytic sarcomas, in acute myeloid leukemia, 529, 529f
Granulocytopenia, and fever of unknown origin, 11
Granulomas, of lung, 966
Granulomatosis, allergic, 249
Granulomatous colitis, and colorectal cancer, 922
Granulomatous disease, chronic, 480–483, 482t, 483t

Gray (Gy), 321
Gray platelet syndrome, 270
Greasewood, 1213t
Green tea, 1213t
Gross tumor volume (GTV), 323–324
Groupe d'Etudes des Tumeurs Thymiques (GETT) classification, for thymoma, 987, 987t
Growth factor(s), 419–429
    biologic therapy using, 376, 377t
    drugs that decrease circulating, 332t, 347
    erythropoietic, 419–421, 420t
    for myelodysplasia, 576
    in breast cancer, 721–722
    myeloid, 421–428
        enhanced antimicrobial function with, 423–424, 424t
        for chemotherapy-induced neutropenia, 428
        for leukemia
            acute lymphocytic, 424–425, 425t
            acute myeloid, 421–424, 421t–425t, 426b
        for myelodysplasia, 427–428, 428b
        recruitment of cells into S-phase of cell cycle with, 424, 425t
        reduced period of neutropenia with, 421–423, 422t, 423t, 425–426, 426t
        uses of, 421, 421t
        with stem cell transplantation, 425–427, 426t, 427t
    thrombopoietic, 429
Growth factor/receptor interactions, drugs that affect, 331–345, 332t
Growth hormone deficiency, due to pituitary adenoma, 1142t
Growth hormone excess, due to pituitary adenoma, 1142t
GTT. See Gestational trophoblastic tumors (GTT).
GTV (gross tumor volume), 323–324
Guaiac testing, for colorectal cancer, 924–925, 925t
Gustatory sweating, 1024
GVHD (graft-versus-host disease), 391, 396–397, 438, 439
Gy (gray), 321

H

H cells, 608f, 611
HAART (highly active antiretroviral therapy), 1155
    and Kaposi's sarcoma, 1160
    and non-Hodgkin's lymphoma, 1155, 1156, 1157, 1158
Haemophilus influenzae, febrile neutropenia due to, 1174, 1175
HAI (hepatic artery infusion), 369–370
    for hepatocellular carcinoma, 902–903
    for islet cell tumors, 918
Hairy cell leukemia, 248, 248f, 253, 697–698, 698b
Halcion (triazolam), 1227b
    for insomnia, 1253
Halo nevus, 309f
Haloperidol (Haldol)
    for delirium and psychotic symptoms, 1227b, 1248, 1248t, 1254t, 1255
    for insomnia, 1253
    for nausea and vomiting, 1251, 1252t, 1256
HAM (HTLV-1–associated myelopathy), 673
Ham test, 469
HAMA (human anti-mouse antibodies), 379
Hamartoma(s)
    multiple, 1194, 1194t, 1197–1198
    of lung, 966
    seizures due to, 23
Haploidentical transplantation, 392t, 393
    for acute myeloid leukemia, 538
Hb H disease, 456t, 459, 459t, 460, 460b
Hb S (hemoglobin S), 275, 275f, 462
HBOC (hereditary breast/ovarian cancer), 1194, 1194t, 1195, 1197
HBV (hepatitis B virus), and hepatocellular carcinoma, 899, 903
HCC. See Hepatocellular carcinoma (HCC).
β-hCG (β-human chorionic gonadotropin)
    in gestational trophoblastic tumors, 810, 811–812
    in molar pregnancy, 806

HCV (hepatitis C virus)
    and hepatocellular carcinoma, 899
    with hemophilia A, 500b
HD. See Hodgkin's disease (HD).
Head and neck cancer, 999–1010
    biologic targets in therapy of, 1008t
    clinical evaluation of, 1000
    combined chemotherapy and radiation therapy vs. radiation therapy alone in, 1003t
    epidemiology of, 999–1000
    of hypopharynx and cervical esophagus, 1004–1005
    of larynx, 1002–1004, 1003t
    of nasopharynx, 1008–1010, 1009b
    of oral cavity, 1006–1008, 1008t
    of oropharynx, 1005–1006, 1006b
    pathology of, 1000–1001
    recurrent and metastatic, single-agent chemotherapy for, 1008t
    risk factors for, 999
    screening for, 999–1000
    second primary, 1012–1015, 1013t, 1014t
    squamous cell, 999–1010
    staging of, 1001–1002, 1001t
Headache(s), 19–22
    after seizures, 23, 24f
    body position and, 21b
    changes in characteristics of, 21b
    cluster, 20t
    due to aneurysm bleed, 20t
    due to brain metastases, 1062
    due to brain tumor, 19, 20t, 21, 21t, 22t
    due to calvarial metastasis, 21, 21t, 22, 22t
    due to cervical neuritis, 20t
    due to hydrocephalus, 20t, 21, 21t
    due to hyperviscosity, 21t, 22, 22t
    due to meningitis, 20t
    due to temporal arteritis, 20t
    intrathoracic pressure and, 21b
    management of, 21–22, 22t
    migraine, 20t
    neuroimaging for, 20f, 21, 21b
    nocturnal, 21, 21b
    presentation and evaluation of, 19–21, 20f, 20t
    with neurologic signs, 21b
    worst, 21b
Hearing loss, due to cranial neuropathy, 30t
Heart failure, congestive
    due to anthracyclines, 350, 351, 351f
    pleural effusion due to, 87
Heat shock proteins (HSPs), in vaccine therapy, 381
Hegar's sign, 188
Heinz bodies, 277, 278f
Helicobacter pylori
    and esophageal cancer, 875
    and gastric cancer, 888–889, 891
    and idiopathic thrombocytopenic purpura, 489
    and MALT lymphoma, 637, 638, 639–640
Helixor, 1213t
HELLP syndrome, 494
Helmet cells, 275
Hemangioma(s)
    in Kassabach-Merritt syndrome, 295–296, 296f
    liver, 123, 124f
    vs. melanoma, 308t
Hemarthrosis, 265, 266b
    in hemophilia A, 498, 499, 499f
Hematemesis, 106b, 144
Hematocrit
    decreased. See Anemia.
    in erythrocytosis, 256
Hematologic disorders, myelodysplasia after, 568
Hematologic manifestation(s), of cancer, 1166–1172, 1167b
    anemia as, 1166–1168, 1167f, 1168f
    cold agglutinins and cryoglobulinemia as, 1170–1171, 1171f
    hypereosinophilic syndrome as, 1170
    monoclonal gammopathies as, 1171–1172, 1171f
    polycythemia as, 1168
    thrombocytosis and thrombocytopenia as, 1169–1170

Waldenström's macroglobulinemia as, 1172
    white blood cell abnormalities as, 1168, 1169t
Hematoma(s), 266b
    subungual, 308t, 309–310
Hematopoiesis, 566, 567f
    extramedullary, in idiopathic myelofibrosis, 707
Hematopoietic growth factors. See Growth factor(s).
Hematopoietic progenitor cell transfusions, 437–438, 438t
Hematopoietic stem cell(s), in myelodysplasia, 566–567
Hematopoietic stem cell toxins, myelodysplasia due to, 568–569, 569t
Hematopoietic stem cell transplantation (HSCT), 391–414. See also Bone marrow transplantation.
    allogeneic, 391, 392–397
        advantages and disadvantages of, 394, 398t
        autologous vs., 398t
        conditioning regimens for, 393, 394–396, 395t, 396t
        for Hodgkin's disease, 627
        for leukemia
            acute lymphoblastic, 559
            acute myeloid, 536, 537–539, 538t, 540t
            chronic lymphocytic, 696
            chronic myeloid, 683–684
        for multiple myeloma, 592
        for myelodysplastic syndrome, 575b, 578
        for non-Hodgkin's lymphoma, 643–644
        graft-versus-host disease due to, 391, 396–397
        graft-versus-tumor effect in, 394
        identification of donor for, 392–393
        nonmyeloablative, 394
        principles underlying, 393–394
        sources of cells for, 391–392, 392t
    autologous, 391, 397–398, 399t
        for Hodgkin's disease, 627
        for leukemia
            acute lymphoblastic, 559
            acute myeloid, 536, 539, 539t, 540t
            chronic myeloid, 684
        for multiple myeloma, 589b, 591–592
        for non-Hodgkin's lymphoma, 643, 652
    blood products with, 438t
    complications after, 403–405
    defined, 556t
    expected response to, 437
    fever of unknown origin due to, 11–13, 12b
    for aplastic anemia, 395, 395t, 413–414, 413t
    for breast cancer, 414
    for Hodgkin's disease, 399t, 410–411, 411f, 627–628
    for leukemia, 399t
        acute lymphoblastic, 408–409, 409f, 559
        acute myeloid, 405–408, 406f–407f, 536–540, 538t–540t
        chronic lymphocytic, 696
        chronic myeloid, 409–410, 683–684
    for multiple myeloma, 399t, 412–413, 413f, 589b, 591–592
    for myelodysplastic syndromes, 408, 575b, 578
    for non-Hodgkin's lymphoma, 399t, 411–412, 411f
        intermediate-grade, 652
        low-grade, 643–644
    immunologic considerations for, 437–438
    in children, 400
    indications for, 437
    infections after
        bacterial, 400
        fungal, 400–401
        Pneumocystis carinii, 403
        viral, 401–403
    myeloid growth factors for, 425–427, 426t, 427t
    patient evaluation for, 398–400
    psychosocial issues with, 399, 405
    second malignancies after, 404–405
    sources of cells for, 391–392, 392t
    syngeneic, 391, 392t
    types of, 391

Hematuria, 173–178
　asymptomatic microscopic, 174
　defined, 173
　differential diagnosis of, 173, 173b, 174t
　due to bladder cancer, 842
　evaluation of, 175–176, 175f, 176b, 177f
　flank pain with, 174–175
　general considerations for, 173
　gross, 175, 176–178, 176b
　history of, 174–175
　initial, 175
　management of, 176–178, 176b
　prevalence of, 173
　risk factors for significant urologic disease
　　with, 174, 174t
　runner's, 174
　terminal, 175
　total, 175
　urine dipstick testing for, 173–174
Hemianopsia, due to cranial neuropathy, 29t
Hemiparesis, postictal, 1064
Hemobilia, 146
Hemochromatosis, 210–211, 211b
Hemodialysis, for hyperkalemia, 1189
Hemoglobin
　decreased. See Anemia.
　in erythrocytosis, 256
　indices for, 234–235, 235t
　mean corpuscular, 234
　normal values for, 232
　structure and gene locus for, 458, 458f
Hemoglobin Bart's, 459
Hemoglobin C disease, 275f
Hemoglobin content, of reticulocytes, 207
Hemoglobin S (Hb S), 275, 275f, 462
Hemoglobinopathy(ies), 456t, 458–466, 458f. See
　　also Sickle-cell disease;
　　Thalassemia.
Hemoglobinuria, paroxysmal nocturnal,
　　448–450, 468–469
　diagnosis of, 240, 456t, 469
　pancytopenia due to, 254, 469
　pathogenesis of, 448–449
　pathophysiology of, 468–469
　treatment for, 449–450, 449f, 469
Hemolysis
　alloimmune, 470t
　drug-induced immune, 470t, 471, 472t
　hyperbilirubinemia due to, 197
Hemolytic anemia, 238–240, 239f, 240f
　autoimmune, 233t, 469–472
　　classification of, 469, 470t
　　cold, 470t, 471–472, 472f
　　diagnosis of, 238, 456t, 469–470, 471f
　　due to cancer, 1168, 1168f
　　in chronic lymphocytic leukemia, 689
　　red blood cell abnormalities in, 276, 276f,
　　　469, 470f
　　signs and symptoms of, 469
　　warm, 470–471, 470t, 472f, 473b
　due to cancer, 1167–1168, 1168f
　evaluation of, 240b
　in sickle-cell disease, 464t
　microangiopathic, 238–240, 492, 492f
　nonimmune-mediated, 238
　transfusion support of, 434b
　warm autoimmune, 470–471, 470t, 472f,
　　473b
Hemolytic transfusion reactions, 438–439
Hemolytic uremic syndrome (HUS), 239, 274
Hemoperitoneum, 146
Hemophagocytic syndrome, in peripheral T-cell
　　lymphoma, 667
Hemophilia A, 498–501
　classification of, 498
　clinical manifestations of, 498–499, 499f
　differential diagnosis of, 498–499
　joint disease in, 409, 499, 499f, 502b
　laboratory evaluation of, 499
　management of, 499–501, 500b, 501f, 502b
　pathogenesis of, 498
　presentation of, 266, 267, 269, 270
　prevalence of, 498
　subcutaneous hemorrhage in, 295f
　with factor VIII alloantibody inhibitors,
　　501–504, 503b, 503f
Hemophilia B, 266, 267, 268, 270, 504
Hemophilia C, 267, 270, 504–505, 505b

Hemoptysis, 106–108, 106b, 107t
　due to lung cancer, 961
　in dying patient, 1255–1256
HemoQuantReq test, 210
Hemorrhage(s)
　elevated platelet count after, 229
　epidural, 1080
　gastrointestinal. See Gastrointestinal (GI)
　　bleeding.
　in dying patient, 1255–1256
　in myelodysplasia, 575b
　in surgical patient, 510
　intramuscular, 499
　subarachnoid, 157–158, 159
　subcutaneous, 295, 295f
　vaginal. See Vaginal bleeding.
Hemorrhagic cystitis, 173, 176, 177
Hemorrhoids, and colorectal cancer, 926
Hemostasis, 498
Hemostatic disorders, vaginal bleeding due to,
　　184, 186b
Henoch-Schönlein purpura, 298
Heparin, for venous thromboembolism, 514–515,
　　515t
　in pregnancy, 516
　with cancer, 1182
　with central venous catheter, 1183
Heparin-induced osteoporosis, 518
Heparin-induced thrombocytopenia, 303,
　　487–488, 488t, 517–518
Hepatic. See also Liver.
Hepatic artery infusion (HAI), 369–370
　for hepatocellular carcinoma, 902–903
　for islet cell tumors, 918
Hepatic dysfunction, chemotherapy with, 356t
Hepatic hydrothorax, 87
Hepatic metastasis, 117–119, 118f–120f, 119t
　hepatic artery infusion for, 369–370
　of breast cancer, 751t
　of carcinoid tumors, 1137
　of colorectal cancer, 118f, 927
　of lung cancer
　　non–small cell, 962
　　small cell, 946, 952
　of melanoma, 1087, 1101f
　staging laparoscopy of, 365
Hepatic vein thrombosis, due to polycythemia
　　vera, 702
Hepatitis
　lymphadenopathy due to, 214
　pancytopenia due to, 253
Hepatitis B virus (HBV), and hepatocellular
　　carcinoma, 899, 903
Hepatitis C virus (HCV)
　and hepatocellular carcinoma, 899
　with hemophilia A, 500b
Hepatobiliary cancer(s), 899–906
　biliary, 903–905, 905b
　gallbladder, 905–906
　primary liver cancer as, 899–903, 901t
Hepatobiliary disease, obstructive, pruritus due
　　to, 14
Hepatocellular adenoma, 125–126, 125f
Hepatocellular carcinoma (HCC), 899–903, 901t
　clinical evaluation of, 900
　clinical presentation of, 899–900
　erythrocytosis due to, 260, 261f
　follow-up evaluation of, 903
　GI bleeding due to, 144–145, 146
　imaging of, 119–120, 120t, 121f, 900
　prevention of, 903
　risk factors for, 899
　staging, prognostic features, and outcomes
　　for, 900–902, 901t
　treatment for, 902–903
Hepatomegaly
　in idiopathic myelofibrosis, 706
　in polycythemia vera, 702–703
Hepatosplenic gamma/delta T-cell lymphoma,
　　668–669, 670
HER-2/neu, in breast cancer, 721–722, 722f,
　　724b
　locally invasive, 745
　prognosis with, 751
　trastuzumab and, 345, 378, 758
Herb, defined, 1211
Herbal medicine, 1211–1212, 1213–1215, 1213t,
　　1214t

Herceptin (trastuzumab), 331f, 342t, 345, 378
　for metastatic breast cancer, 756t, 757t, 758
Hereditary breast/ovarian cancer (HBOC), 1194,
　　1194t, 1195, 1197
Hereditary cancer, 1193–1207. See also Genetic
　　basis.
　key features of, 1193, 1194t
　mechanisms of, 1193–1207
　types of, 1193, 1194t
Hereditary cutaneous melanoma, 1201
Hereditary diffuse gastric cancer, 1194t,
　　1201–1202
Hereditary elliptocytosis, 468
Hereditary hemorrhagic telangiectasia, 295, 295f
Hereditary nonpolyposis colon cancer (HNPCC),
　　921–922, 1200–1201
　Amsterdam criteria for, 1200–1201
　and endometrial cancer, 783
　Bethesda guidelines for, 1201, 1201t
　clinical characteristics of, 1200
　epidemiology of, 921
　genetic basis for, 921, 1194, 1194t, 1200
　management of, 1201
　prognosis for, 921–922
　prophylactic surgery for, 371–372
　variants of, 1201
Hereditary papillary renal cancer, 1194t
Hereditary spherocytosis (HS), 456t, 468
Herniated disk, 160–161, 1080
Herpes simplex virus (HSV)
　febrile neutropenia due to, 1173, 1177b,
　　1178
　with hematopoietic stem cell transplantation,
　　401
Herpes simplex virus–thymidine kinase (HSV-
　　TK), in gene therapy, 383
Herpes zoster
　febrile neutropenia due to, 1173, 1177b,
　　1178
　spinal radiculopathy or myelopathy due to,
　　159t, 161, 162, 162t
　with hematopoietic stem cell transplantation,
　　402–403
Herpesvirus, and Kaposi's sarcoma, 1158–1159
HES. See Hypereosinophilic syndrome (HES).
Hexagonal phase phospholipid assay, 269
Hexamethylmelamine, 333t
Hexose-monophosphate shunt, 466, 466f
HFE gene, 211, 211b
Hiccups, 1252
High colonic therapy, 1221t
High-grade squamous intraepithelial lesion
　　(HSIL), 769
Highly active antiretroviral therapy (HAART),
　　1155
　and Kaposi's sarcoma, 1160
　and non-Hodgkin's lymphoma, 1155, 1156,
　　1157, 1158
Hilar adenopathy, 94–97, 95f, 96f, 97b, 217
Hispanic cancer patient, 1230–1231
Histiocytoma, malignant fibrous, 154, 1029t,
　　1032–1033, 1039t, 1040
Histology, for cancer of unknown origin, 314,
　　315t
Histoplasmosis
　of lung, 966
　superior vena cava syndrome due to, 100
HIV. See Human immunodeficiency virus (HIV).
HLA (human leukocyte antigen)–matched sibling
　　transplantation, for acute myeloid
　　leukemia, 537, 538t
HLA (human leukocyte antigen) typing, 392–393
hMLH1 gene, 1201
hMSH2 gene, 1201
HNPCC. See Hereditary nonpolyposis colon
　　cancer (HNPCC).
Hoarseness, 50–56
　ancillary testing for, 53–54
　defined, 50
　diagnosis of, 52t
　differential diagnosis of, 52t
　direct laryngoscopy for, 55, 56b
　due to lung cancer, 961
　　small cell, 945–946
　electromyography/electroglottography for,
　　54–55
　etiology of, 50–51, 51f, 51t–53t, 52f
　history of, 51–53

Hoarseness, (*Continued*)
    imaging for, 54
    management of, 55–56
    physical examination for, 53
    rigid endoscopy for, 55
    videostroboscopy for, 54
Hodgkin, Sir Thomas, 615
Hodgkin's cells, 608f, 609, 610
Hodgkin's disease (HD), 615–630
    classical, 610–611, 610t, 618, 618t
    classification of, 617–618, 618t
    clinical presentation of, 616–617, 616t
    diagnosis of, 609–611, 610t, 612, 617–619
    eosinophilia due to, 249
    epidemiology of, 615–616
    Epstein-Barr virus and, 616
    extranodal, 617
    follow-up evaluations for, 626–628
    hematopoietic stem cell transplantation for, 399t, 410–411, 411f
    historical background of, 615
    HIV-related, 628
    immunologic impairment in, 629
    in pregnancy, 628–629
    infradiaphragmatic, 628
    long-term complications in, 629–630
    lymphadenopathy due to, 214, 216
    lymphocyte depletion, 610–611, 618
    lymphocyte-rich, 618
    mixed cellularity, 610, 618
    nodular lymphocyte predominant, 610t, 611, 612
    nodular sclerosis, 610, 618t
    prognostic factors for, 620–621
    pruritus due to, 16, 17b
    relapse of, 627–628
    secondary malignancies in, 629
    staging of, 619–620, 619t
    superior vena cava syndrome in, 99
    treatment of, 621–626, 621b
        cardiovascular complications of, 629–630
        chemotherapy for, 621b, 622–625, 624t
        combined modality, 625–626
        hematopoietic stem cell transplantation for, 627–628
        pulmonary complications of, 630
        radiation therapy for, 622
        secondary non-Hodgkin's lymphoma after, 618–619, 629
        with large mediastinal mass, 626
    with large mediastinal mass, 626
Homeopathy, 1221t
Homocysteine, fasting plasma levels of, 289b
Homonymous hemianopsia, due to cranial neuropathy, 29t
Hormonal deficiencies, due to pituitary adenoma, 1140–1141, 1142t
Hormonal excesses, due to pituitary adenoma, 1141, 1142t
Hormonal therapy
    for breast cancer, 751–756, 753t, 754t, 755f
    for pancreatic cancer, 916–917
    for prostate cancer, 867, 869–871, 872
    for renal cell cancer, 834
Hormone receptor status, of breast cancer, 721, 723b
Hormone replacement therapy (HRT)
    after breast cancer, 765, 766b
    and endometrial cancer, 782, 789
Horner's syndrome, due to lung cancer, 961
Hospice, 1256–1259, 1257t
Hot flashes, after breast cancer, 765, 766b
Howell-Jolly bodies, 229, 230b, 243, 272b, 277, 277f
Hoxsey, 1214t
HPC1 gene, in prostate cancer, 1203
HPCX gene, in prostate cancer, 1203
HPV. *See* Human papillomavirus (HPV).
HRT (hormone replacement therapy)
    after breast cancer, 765, 766b
    and endometrial cancer, 782, 789
HS (hereditary spherocytosis), 456t, 468
HSCT. *See* Hematopoietic stem cell transplantation (HSCT).
HSIL (high-grade squamous intraepithelial lesion), 769
HSPs (heat shock proteins), in vaccine therapy, 381

HSV (herpes simplex virus)
    febrile neutropenia due to, 1173, 1177b, 1178
    with hematopoietic stem cell transplantation, 401
HSV-TK (herpes simplex virus–thymidine kinase), in gene therapy, 383
5-HT³ receptor antagonists, for nausea and vomiting, 1251
HTLV-1 (human T-cell lymphotropic virus 1), 550, 672–673
HTLV-1 (human T-cell lymphotropic virus 1)–associated myelopathy (HAM), 673
Hu antigen, in small cell lung cancer, 947–948
Human anti-mouse antibodies (HAMA), 379
β-human chorionic gonadotropin (β-hCG)
    in gestational trophoblastic tumors, 810, 811–812
    in molar pregnancy, 806
Human immunodeficiency virus (HIV)
    anal carcinoma with, 938
    hemophilia A with, 500b
    Hodgkin's disease with, 628
    idiopathic thrombocytopenic purpura with, 492
    Kaposi's sarcoma with, 1158–1161, 1159t
    lymphadenopathy due to, 214
    neutropenia due to, 245
    non-Hodgkin's lymphoma with, 650, 1155–1158
    pancytopenia due to, 252, 253
    posttransplant lymphoproliferative disease with, 1161–1164, 1162t, 1163b
Human leukocyte antigen (HLA)–matched sibling transplantation, for acute myeloid leukemia, 537, 538t
Human leukocyte antigen (HLA) typing, 392–393
Human papillomavirus (HPV)
    and anal carcinoma, 938
    and cervical cancer, 770
    and vaginal cancer, 779
    and vulvar cancer, 776b
Human T-cell lymphotropic virus 1 (HTLV-1), 550, 672–673
Human T-cell lymphotropic virus 1 (HTLV-1)–associated myelopathy (HAM), 673
Humate-P, for von Willebrand's disease, 506
Hurthle cell carcinoma, 1119, 1120–1121
HUS (hemolytic uremic syndrome), 239, 274
Hutchinson sign, pseudo-, 310f
Hycamtin. *See* Topotecan (Hycamtin).
Hycoscyamine (Levsin SL), for death rattle, 1254t, 1255
Hydatidiform moles, 804–806, 805t, 807, 807b
Hydration
    of dying patient, 1255
    with interferon-alpha therapy of melanoma, 1096b
Hydrazine sulfate, 1217t, 1218–1219
Hydrocephalus, headache due to, 20t, 21, 21t, 22t
Hydrocodone, for pain, 1245
Hydrocortisone
    for acute lymphoblastic leukemia, 560
    for Burkitt's leukemia/lymphoma, 562t
Hydromorphone (Dilaudid), for pain, 1245, 1246, 1246t, 1247b, 1247t, 1254t
Hydrops fetalis, 459, 459t
Hydrothorax, hepatic, 87
Hydroxyurea, 336t, 355t
    for chronic myeloid leukemia, 680
    for myelodysplasia, 576
    for sickle-cell crisis, 465–466
Hydroxyzine (Vistaril), 1227, 1227b
Hyoscyamine, for nausea and vomiting, 1252t
Hyperbilirubinemia, 196–199
    causes of, 196–197, 197f
    due to anemia, 232, 233t, 240b
    due to biliary cancer, 903
    due to biliary tract obstruction, 198
    due to cholestasis
        extrahepatic, 198–199
        intrahepatic, 199
    due to defective glucuronide conjugation, 198

    due to hemolysis, 197
    due to increased direct bilirubin, 198–199
    due to increased indirect bilirubin, 197–198
    due to ineffective erythropoiesis, 197–198
    low-grade, 198b
    neonatal, 198
    protracted, 197b
Hypercalcemia, 191–194
    differential diagnosis of, 191, 192t
    in adult T-cell leukemia/lymphoma, 674
    in breast cancer, 760–761
    in multiple myeloma, 582, 584
    in non–small cell lung cancer, 963
    in renal cell cancer, 828
    mechanisms of, 192
    of malignancy, 191, 192–193, 193t
    plasma calcium determinations for, 192
    prevalence of, 191
    signs and symptoms of, 193
    therapy for, 193–194, 194t
Hypereosinophilic syndrome (HES)
    due to cancer, 1170
    idiopathic, 249–250
    pruritus due to, 16
Hyperfibrinolysis, 271
    in liver disease, 508
Hyperfractionation, 323, 327
Hypergammaglobulinemic purpura, 299, 300f
Hypergastrinemia, with gastric carcinoids, 1133
Hyperimmunoglobulin E syndrome, 478
Hyperkalemia, due to tumor lysis syndrome, 1188–1189, 1189t
Hyperleukocytosis, in acute myeloid leukemia, 529, 532t
Hyperoxygenation therapy, 1221t
Hyperparathyroidism, hypercalcemia due to, 191
Hyperphosphatemia, due to tumor lysis syndrome, 1189, 1189t
Hyperprolactinemia, 1140
Hypersplenism, 137
    pancytopenia due to, 252t, 253
Hyperthyroidism, due to pituitary adenoma, 1142t
Hypertrophic pulmonary osteoarthropathy, in non–small cell lung cancer, 963
Hyperuricemia, due to tumor lysis syndrome, 1187–1188, 1189t
Hyperviscosity syndrome
    headache due to, 21t, 22, 22t
    in chronic myeloid leukemia, 677b
    in multiple myeloma, 582, 583, 584–585
    in Waldenström's macroglobulinemia, 597
Hypnosis, for pain management, 1244
Hypocalcemia, due to tumor lysis syndrome, 1189–1190, 1189t
Hypochromia, in myelodysplasia, 572t
Hypofibrinogenemia, in liver disease, 508
Hypogammaglobulinemia, 202–203, 202t
    due to thymoma, 984
    in chronic lymphocytic leukemia, 689
Hypoglossal nerve deficit, 30t
Hypogonadism, due to pituitary adenoma, 1139
Hypokalemia, in acute myeloid leukemia, 530
Hypopharyngeal cancer, 1004–1005
Hypophosphatemia, in acute myeloid leukemia, 530
Hypothyroidism, after hematopoietic stem cell transplantation, 404
Hypouricemia, in acute myeloid leukemia, 530
Hysterectomy
    for cervical cancer, 772, 773b, 774f
    for endometrial cancer, 786
    for gestational trophoblastic tumor, 810
    for molar pregnancy, 806

I

Ibritumomab tiuxetan (Zevalin), for non-Hodgkin's lymphoma, 653
Ibuprofen (Motrin)
    for cachexia, 8
    for pain, 1245t
    with interferon-alpha therapy of melanoma, 1096b
Idarubicin (4-demethoxy-daunorubicin), 337t, 350
    for acute myeloid leukemia, 533, 535t
Idiopathic hypereosinophilic syndrome, 249–250
Idiopathic thrombocytopenic purpura (ITP), 488–492, 490f
IFN. *See* Interferon(s) (IFN).

Ifosfamide, 333t, 355t
 for Burkitt's leukemia/lymphoma, 562t
 for cervical cancer, 775t
 for Ewing's sarcoma, 1034–1035
 for germ-cell tumors, 820, 821b
 for head and neck cancer, 1008t
 for soft tissue sarcoma, 1044
 for thymoma, 989t
Ig (immunoglobulin), 200, 377–378
 intravenous. *See* Intravenous
   immunoglobulins.
 normal range of, 201t
IGF (insulin-like growth factor)
 and prostate cancer, 860
 biologic therapy using, 376
IL. *See* Interleukin(s) (IL).
Ileal carcinoid, 1134f
Imaging studies
 for back pain, 158–159
 for bowel obstruction, 111, 111f
 for cancer of unknown primary, 1149
 for cranial neuropathy, 28
 for dyspnea, 77
 for encephalopathy, 34
 for headache, 20f, 21, 21b
 for hematuria, 175–176, 175f, 177f
 for hemoptysis, 107
 for hilar and mediastinal adenopathy, 94–95,
   95f, 96f
 for hoarseness, 54
 for pleural effusion, 88
 for seizures, 24–25, 24f
 for venous thromboembolic disease,
   287–289, 287f–289f, 1181, 1181f
 of adrenocortical masses, 170f, 1129–1130
 of brain metastases, 1065–1066, 1066f, 1067f
 of breast mass, 59–60, 61f, 62f, 65–66,
   67f–68f
 of epidural cancer, 1079–1081, 1079f, 1080f
 of mesothelioma, 991, 992f
 of multiple myeloma, 587–588, 588f
 of neck mass, 46–47
 of non–small cell lung cancer, 966
 of pancreatic cancer, 911–913
 of pathologic fractures, 152, 152f
 of pituitary adenoma, 1140, 1141f
 of salivary gland carcinoma, 1019f,
   1020–1021, 1020f
 of soft-tissue mass, 1041
 of solitary pulmonary nodule, 81, 83b
 of testicular mass, 180–182
 of thymoma, 985, 985f
 of thyroid carcinoma, 1124
 of thyroid nodule, 1117–1118, 1118f
Imatinib mesylate (STI-571, Gleevec), 356
 for chronic myeloid leukemia, 410, 685,
   685b
 for gastrointestinal stomal tumors,
   1044–1045
Imidazotetrazines, 332t
Imipramine (Tofranil), 1227b
 for neuropathic pain, 1249t
Immune hemolytic anemia, 233t
Immune-mediated diseases, lymphadenopathy
   due to, 214
Immuno-augmentative therapy, 1217t
Immunocompromised host, 1155–1164. *See also*
   Human immunodeficiency virus
   (HIV).
 Kaposi's sarcoma in, 1158–1161, 1159t
 non-Hodgkin's lymphomas in, 650,
   1155–1158
 posttransplant lymphoproliferative disease in,
   1161–1164, 1162t, 1163b
 suspicious brain lesion in, 1162b
Immunocytochemistry, for cancer of unknown
   origin, 314, 315t
Immunoglobulin(s) (Ig), 200, 377–378
 intravenous. *See* Intravenous
   immunoglobulins.
 normal range of, 201t
Immunoglobulin abnormalities, 200–205
 differential diagnosis of, 201–205, 202t
 due to amyloidosis, 205, 205b
 due to hypogammaglobulinemia, 202–203,
   202t
 due to monoclonal gammopathy, 200, 201f,
   202t, 203–205, 203b

due to multiple myeloma, 203, 204–205
due to plasmacytoma, 205
due to polyclonal gammopathy, 201–202,
   201f, 202t
due to Waldenström's macroglobulinemia,
   205
initial considerations in evaluation of, 200b
pathogenesis of, 200, 201f
Immunoglobulin deficiency, and gastric cancer,
   889
Immunologic impairment, in Hodgkin's disease,
   629
Immunomodulatory drugs, for multiple
   myeloma, 591
Immunophenotype
 defined, 556t
 of acute lymphoblastic leukemia, 552–553,
   553t
 of acute myeloid leukemia, 530
 of B-cell chronic lymphocytic leukemia/small
   lymphocytic lymphoma, 604,
   604t
 of Burkitt's lymphoma, 606–607
 of diffuse large B-cell lymphoma, 606
 of follicular lymphoma, 607, 608f
 of low-grade lymphomas, 636, 637t
 of lymphoma, 602
 of marginal zone lymphoma, 605–606
 of peripheral T-cell lymphoma, 608–609, 670
Immunosuppression
 and skin cancer, 1105
 for aplastic anemia
   acute severe, 444–446, 444t, 446f
   moderate, 446–447
 for hematopoietic stem cell transplantation
   allogeneic, 393, 394–396, 395f, 396f
   autologous, 397–399, 399t
Immunotherapy
 for non-Hodgkin's lymphoma, 642–643
 for renal cell cancer, 834–838, 835t, 836t,
   837f, 838f, 838t
 for superficial bladder cancer, 846, 847b
Immunothrombocytopenia purpura, 224f
Impedance plethysmography, for deep vein
   thrombosis, 287
Impotence
 after hematopoietic stem cell transplantation,
   404
 due to radical prostatectomy, 866
Inclusions, in anemia, 236t, 237f
Incontinence, due to radical prostatectomy, 866
Indian rhubarb root, 1215
Indirect antiglobulin test, 470, 471f
Indomethacin (Indocin)
 for pain, 1244, 1245t
 with interferon-alpha therapy of melanoma,
   1096f
Induction therapy
 defined, 556t
 for leukemia
   acute lymphoblastic, 556–558, 557t–559t
   acute myeloid, 531t, 533–534, 535t
   relapsed or refractory, 541–542, 541f,
     542t
   acute promyelocytic, 545b
 for myelodysplasia, 576–578
 for non–small cell lung cancer, 970f
Indwelling catheters, thromboembolic disease
   with, 1182–1184, 1183f
Infection(s)
 bacterial
   back pain due to, 158–159, 159t,
     161–162, 162t
   in multiple myeloma, 582, 584, 592
   with hematopoietic stem cell
     transplantation, 400
 elevated platelet count due to, 229
 fungal (mycotic)
   fever of unknown origin due to, 11
   with hematopoietic stem cell
     transplantation, 400–401
 granulocyte count and, 1173, 1174f
 in chronic lymphocytic leukemia, 689
 in multiple myeloma, 582, 584, 592
 in sickle-cell disease, 463–464, 464t
 lymphadenopathy due to, 214, 214t
 neutropenia due to, 244–245, 245t
 opportunistic, encephalopathy due to, 35

peripheral smear abnormalities due to, 281f,
   282
Pneumocystis carinii
 febrile neutropenia due to, 1174
 with hematopoietic stem cell
   transplantation, 403
 recurrent, 475, 476f
 vascular cutaneous manifestations of, 297,
   297f, 298f
 viral, with hematopoietic stem cell
   transplantation, 401–403
 with hematopoietic stem cell transplantation,
   400–403
 with thymoma, 984–985
Infectious mononucleosis
 atypical lymphocytes in, 279, 279f
 lymphocytosis due to, 247, 247f
InFeD (iron dextran), 456b
Inferior vena cava, interruption of, 1184–1185
Infertility, after hematopoietic stem cell
   transplantation, 404
Inflammation, elevated platelet count due to,
   229
Inflammatory bowel disease, and colorectal
   cancer, 922, 922f
Infraclavicular lymph nodes, breast cancer
   metastasis to, 718
Inguinal adenopathy, 215t, 217, 219
INR (International Normalized Ratio), for
   warfarin, 506, 507, 516–517
Insomnia, 1227b, 1253
Insulin, for hyperkalemia, 1189
Insulin-like growth factor (IGF), biologic therapy
   using, 376
Insulin-like growth factor 1 (IGF-1), and prostate
   cancer, 860
Insulinoma, 1134t, 1135, 1135t, 1136, 1136t
Intensification therapy. *See* Intensive
   consolidation chemotherapy.
Intensive consolidation chemotherapy
 defined, 556t
 for acute lymphoblastic leukemia, 557t,
   558
 for acute myeloid leukemia, 534–536, 536t,
   537f, 539–540, 540t
Interferon(s) (IFN)
 biologic therapy using, 376, 377t
 for chronic lymphocytic leukemia, 696
Interferon α (IFN-α, Intron A)
 biologic therapy using, 376, 377, 377t
 for adult T-cell leukemia/lymphoma, 674
 for carcinoid tumors, 1137
 for chronic myeloid leukemia, 681–682
 for Epstein-Barr virus, 1163
 for essential thrombocythemia, 712
 for hairy cell leukemia, 698
 for head and neck cancer, 1013–1014, 1013t,
   1015
 for low-grade non-Hodgkin's lymphoma,
   641–642
 for melanoma, 1094–1095, 1096b, 1097,
   1098
 for mesothelioma, 996, 996t, 997
 for renal cell cancer, 834–835, 835t
 for squamous cell carcinoma, 1112
 for superficial bladder cancer, 846
Interferon α2, for multiple myeloma, 590
Interferon α2b, for giant cell tumors of bone,
   1036
Interferon β (IFN-β)
 biologic therapy using, 376, 377t
 for mesothelioma, 996, 996t
Interferon õ (IFN-õ)
 biologic therapy using, 376, 377t
 for mesothelioma, 992, 996, 996t, 997
Interleukin(s) (IL), biologic therapy using, 376,
   377t
Interleukin-1 (IL-1), in cachexia, 5
Interleukin-2 (IL-2)
 biologic therapy using, 376, 377
 for adult T-cell leukemia/lymphoma, 675
 for melanoma, 1097, 1098–1100, 1098f
 for mesothelioma, 996, 996t
 for renal cell cancer, 835–838, 835t, 836t,
   837f, 838f, 838t, 839b
 key functions of, 377t
Interleukin-2 (IL-2) receptor, 346–347
Interleukin-4 (IL-4), key functions of, 377t

Interleukin-6 (IL-6)
in multiple myeloma, 582
key functions of, 377t
Interleukin-8 (IL-8), key functions of, 377t
Interleukin-11 (IL-11)
biologic therapy using, 376
for acute myeloid leukemia, 532
key functions of, 377t
therapeutic use of, 429
Interleukin-18 (IL-18), key functions of, 377t
Internal mammary lymph nodes, breast cancer
metastasis to, 718
International Normalized Ratio (INR), for
warfarin, 506, 507, 516–517
International Prognostic Scoring System (IPSS)
for lymphoma
intermediate-grade, 650–651, 651t
low-grade, 639
for myelodysplasia, 566, 573–575, 574f, 574t
Interstitial fibrosis, bleomycin-induced, 630
Interval cytoreduction, for ovarian cancer, 799
Interventional radiologic procedures, for liver
tumors, 116
Intervertebral disk herniation, 160–161, 1080
Intestinal obstruction. See Bowel obstruction.
Intestinal T-cell lymphoma, enteropathy-type,
669, 670
Intra-abdominal catastrophe, 146
Intra-alveolar spread, of non–small cell lung
cancer, 962
Intracaval filters, for venous thromboembolism,
519
Intracavitary therapy
for ascites, 132
for mesothelioma, 995–996
Intracellular receptors, 331
Intracranial bleeding, in hemophilia A, 498
Intracranial pressure, increased
due to brain metastases, 1069b
due to brain tumor, 1049–1050, 1050t
Intrahepatic cholangiocarcinoma, 120–122, 121f,
122f
Intralesional injection, for basal cell carcinoma,
1107
Intramuscular hemorrhages, in hemophilia A,
499
Intraoperative radiation therapy, 368
and peritoneal chemotherapy, 368–369
Intraperitoneal chemotherapy, 368–369
for ascites, 132
for gastric cancer, 897–898
for ovarian cancer, 796
Intrathoracic pressure, and headache, 21b
Intravenous immunoglobulins
for chronic lymphocytic leukemia, 689–690
for idiopathic thrombocytopenic purpura,
489, 490, 490f, 491
for multiple myeloma, 592
for posttransfusion purpura, 486b
Intravenous pyelogram (IVP), for hematuria, 175
Intravenous urography, for renal cell cancer, 829
Intravesical therapy, for superficial bladder
cancer, 844–846, 848b
Intron. See Interferon α (IFN-α, Intron A).
Invasion/metastasis inhibitors, 331f
Invasive mole, 807
Inverse planning, for radiation therapy, 326
Inverted-Y field, 622
Involved field, 622
Iodinated contrast agents, for liver imaging, 117
Iodine-131, for thyroid carcinoma, 1122–1123
Ionizing radiation
energy of, 321, 322f
external vs. internal, 321–322
interaction of cells with, 322–323
interaction of tissues and organs with, 323
leukemia due to
acute lymphoblastic, 550
acute myeloid, 523
measurement of, 321
myelodysplasia due to, 569, 569t
IPSS. See International Prognostic Scoring System
(IPSS).
Iressa, for colorectal cancer, 930
Irinotecan (Camptosar, CPT-11), 339t, 352
for cervical cancer, 775t
for colorectal cancer, 929–930
for esophageal cancer, 878, 878t

for gastric cancer, 895, 895t, 896t
for lung cancer
non–small cell, 971t
small cell, 951
Irish's node, in gastric cancer, 890
Iron chelation therapy
for myelodysplasia, 575b
for thalassemia, 460b, 462b
Iron content
serum, 208, 209t, 237
tissue, 210
Iron deficiency, 455, 456t
biochemical indicators of, 208–210
bone marrow aspirate and biopsy for, 234b
cutaneous changes in, 232, 233t
diagnosis of, 237–238, 455
due to blood loss, 210
due to cancer, 1166
due to colorectal cancer, 926, 926t
elevated platelet count due to, 229
pathogenesis of, 207, 455
prevalence of, 455
red blood cells in, 274, 276
symptoms of, 233t
therapy for, 455, 456b
Iron deficient erythropoiesis, 207–208
Iron dextran (InFeD), 456b
Iron overload
biochemical indicators of, 208–210
genetic testing for, 210–211, 211b
therapy of, 452
Iron polysaccharide (Niferex), 456b
Iron replacement therapy, 455, 456b
Iron studies, 208–210, 209b
Iron supplements, for paroxysmal nocturnal
hemoglobinuria, 449
Iron-binding capacity, 208
Iscador, 1213t
Islet cell tumors, 917–918
Isolated limb perfusion, for melanoma, 1095
Isorel, 1213t
ITP (idiopathic thrombocytopenic purpura),
488–492, 490f
IVP (intravenous pyelogram), for hematuria,
175

J
Jaundice. See Hyperbilirubinemia.
Job syndrome, 478
Jogger's nipple, 73
Joint disease, in hemophilia A, 409, 499, 499f,
502b

K
Kaposi's sarcoma, 1158–1161
clinical evaluation of, 1159
clinical presentation of, 301, 301f, 1159
epidemiology of, 1158
HAART and, 1155
pathology and pathogenesis of, 1158–1159
staging, prognostic features, and outcome of,
1159–1160, 1159t
treatment for, 1160–1161
Karnofsky performance status
in brain metastases, 1064
in non–small cell lung cancer, 965
Kassabach-Merritt syndrome, cutaneous
manifestations of, 295–296, 296f
Kayexalate (polystyrene sulfonate), for
hyperkalemia, 1189
Kelp, 1215
Keplinger, Klaus, 1214
Keppra (levotiracetam), for seizures, 25t
Keratoacanthoma, 1109, 1110f, 1111
Keratoconjunctivitis sicca, after hematopoietic
stem cell transplantation, 404
Keratosis
actinic, 1108, 1111
seborrheic, 308t, 310f
Ketoconazole
for adrenal cancer, 1131
for prostate cancer, 872
Ketoprofen, for pain, 1245t
Ketorolac tromethamine (Toradol), for pain,
1244, 1245t
Kidney(s). See also under Renal.
lymphoma of, 168
transitional cell cancer of, 830–831

Ki-1–positive lymphoma, 609
anaplastic, 655–656
Ki-67, in breast cancer, 722
Klatskin's tumor, 121, 904
Klebsiella pneumoniae, febrile neutropenia due to,
1173
Klonopin. See Clonazepam (Klonopin).
Krebs, Ernst
Jr., 1217t, 1219–1220
Sr., 1217t, 1219–1220
Krukenberg's tumor, in gastric cancer, 890
Kubler-Ross, Elisabeth, 1256
Kyphoplasty, for skeletal complications of
multiple myeloma, 593

L
L cells, 608f, 611
Laboratory testing
for anemia, 233–237, 235f, 235t, 236t,
237f
for brain metastases, 1066
for deep vein thrombosis, 285–287
for hilar and mediastinal adenopathy, 96
for hypercalcemia, 193
for iron deficiency and iron overload,
207–210, 209b
for neck mass, 47
for non–small cell lung cancer, 967
for pancreatic cancer, 911
for pancytopenia, 253–254, 254t, 255f
for pathologic fractures, 152
for pelvic mass, 189
for thymoma, 986
for venous thromboembolic disease,
285–287, 1181–1182
Lactate dehydrogenase (LDH), in small cell lung
cancer, 950
Lactation, breast masses during, 62–63
Lactic acidosis, in acute myeloid leukemia, 530
Lactotroph adenomas, 1140
Lacunar cells, 608f, 610
LAD-1 (leukocyte adhesion deficiency-1),
478–479
Laetrile, 1217t, 1219–1220
LAKs (lymphokine-activated killer cells)
for mesothelioma, 996t
for renal cell cancer, 835–836
Lambert-Eaton myasthenic syndrome, 37
in small cell lung cancer, 948
Laminaria digitata, 1215
Laminectomy, for epidural cancer, 1082
Lamotrigine (Lamictal), for seizures, 25t
Lane, William, 1217t, 1220
LAP (leukocyte alkaline phosphatase), in reactive
leukocytosis, 242, 243f
Lapacho, 1213t
Laparoscopic resection, 368
Laparoscopy
of esophageal cancer, 877
staging, 365–366
Laparotomy, for ovarian cancer, 793
Large bowel obstruction, 109–110, 110t,
111–113
Large-cell carcinoma, of lung, 969
Larrea divericata, 1213t
Laryngeal cancer, 1002–1004, 1003t
hoarseness due to, 50, 51, 51f, 55
Laryngeal nerve
left recurrent, in small cell lung cancer,
945–946
surgery-related injury to, 53t
Laryngeal papilloma, 51t
Laryngectomy, for laryngeal cancer, 1002–1003
Laryngitis
reflux, 51t
viral, 51t
Laryngoscopy, for hoarseness, 55, 56b
Lasix. See Furosemide (Lasix).
Latex agglutination test, for deep vein
thrombosis, 285
LCIS (lobular carcinoma in situ), 726, 733–735,
734f
LDH (lactate dehydrogenase), in small cell lung
cancer, 950
Lead poisoning, 277
Leg ulcers, in anemia, 233
Leiomyomata, pelvic masses due to, 188–189
Leiomyosarcoma, 789, 1039t, 1040

lenograstim. *See* Granulocyte colony-stimulating factor (G-CSF, lenograstim, Filgrastim).
Lentiginosis, benign penile or vulvar, 311
Lentigo, 308t
Lepirudin, for heparin-induced thrombocytopenia, 487–488, 488t
Leptomeningeal metastases
  encephalopathy due to, 34t, 35
  of small cell lung cancer, 946
Leser-Trelat sign
  in gastric cancer, 890
  in ovarian carcinoma, 792
Letrozole (Femara), 341t, 347
  for metastatic breast cancer, 753t, 754–755, 754t
Leucovorin
  for Burkitt's leukemia/lymphoma, 562t
  for cancer of unknown primary, 1151b, 1153b
  for colorectal cancer, 929
  for esophageal cancer, 878
  for gastric cancer, 896t, 897f
  for mesothelioma, 995t
Leukemia
  acute lymphoblastic. *See* Acute lymphoblastic leukemia (ALL).
  acute lymphocytic, 280, 281f
    febrile neutropenia in, 1174
    headache with, 21t
    myeloid growth factors for, 424–425, 425t
  acute myeloid/myelogenous. *See* Acute myeloid leukemia (AML).
  acute promyelocytic
    all-trans retinoic acid for, 344, 543, 544t, 545b
    arsenic trioxide for, 544–545, 545t
    hematopoietic stem cell transplantation for, 405–408, 406f–407f
    relapsed or refractory, 543–544
    treatment of, 543–545, 543t–545t, 545b
    unique biologic features of, 543, 543t
  B-cell
    chronic lymphocytic, 603–604, 604f, 604t
    precursor (acute) lymphoblastic, 601–603
    prolymphocytic, 696–697
  Burkitt's, 550, 552, 559t, 561, 562t
  chronic lymphocytic. *See* Chronic lymphocytic leukemia (CLL).
  chronic myeloid. *See* Chronic myeloid leukemia (CML).
  chronic myelomonocytic, 570, 572, 576
  chronic neutrophilic, 244
  core binding factor, 525, 528t
  cranial neuropathies due to, 28t
  due to multiple myeloma treatment, 585
  due to polycythemia vera, 705
  epidural, 1083
  hairy cell, 248, 248f, 253, 697–698, 698b
  headache with, 21t
  hematopoietic stem cell transplantation for, 399t
  mixed lineage, 526–527, 562–563
  peripheral blood smear in, 279–280, 279f–281f
  prolymphocytic, 248, 689, 696–697
  pruritus due to, 16
  T-cell
    adult, 248, 550, 672–675, 673t
    precursor (acute) lymphoblastic, 601–602
    prolymphocytic, 697
Leukemia cutis, in acute myeloid leukemia, 528–529
Leukemoid reactions, 242–243, 243f
Leukocyte abnormality(ies), 241–250
  eosinophilia as, 249–250
  lymphocytosis as, 246–249, 247f, 247t, 248f
  monocytosis and monocytopenia as, 249
  neutropenia as, 244–246, 245t, 246f
  neutrophilia as, 241–244, 241t, 242f–244f
Leukocyte adhesion deficiency-1 (LAD-1), 478–479
Leukocyte alkaline phosphatase (LAP), in reactive leukocytosis, 242, 243f
Leukocytoclastic vasculitis, 299f
Leukocytosis
  drug-related, 243
  in polycythemia vera, 705

reactive neutrophilic, 241–242, 242f, 242t, 243f
  smoking-related, 243
Leukoerythroblastic reaction, 242
Leukopenia, due to cancer, 1168
Leukostasis, in acute myeloid leukemia, 529
Leuprolide, 341t
  for prostate cancer, 870
Levamisole, for colorectal cancer, 930–931, 931f
LeVeen shunt, for ascites, 131, 133, 133t
Levorphanol, for pain, 1246t, 1247t
Levotiracetam (Keppra), for seizures, 25t
Levsin SL (hyoscyamine), for death rattle, 1254t, 1255
LFS. *See* Li-Fraumeni syndrome (LFS).
LH (luteinizing hormone) deficiency, due to pituitary adenoma, 1142
LHRH. *See* Luteinizing hormone–releasing hormone (LHRH).
Libido, altered, 1235, 1238–1239
Lichen aureus, 300, 301f
Lichen sclerosis et atrophicus, of vulva, 776b, 776f
Lidocaine, for dysuria, 1256
LIFE (light-induced fluorescence endoscopy) device, 967
Lifestyle changes, for breast cancer, 765–767
Li-Fraumeni syndrome (LFS)
  brain tumors in, 1049
  genetic basis for, 1194, 1194t, 1197
  leukemia in, 551
  soft tissue sarcoma in, 1040
Light-induced fluorescence endoscopy (LIFE) device, 967
Linear accelerator, for radiation therapy, 321–322, 322f
Linitis plastica, in gastric cancer, 888
Lip cancer, 1007
Lipid therapy, 1221t
Liposarcoma, 1039, 1039t, 1040
Liposomal doxorubicin (Doxil), 350
  for ovarian cancer, 802
Listeria infection, febrile neutropenia due to, 1174, 1175
Lithium carbonate, 1227b
  neutrophilia due to, 243
Live cell therapy, 1217t
Liver, 115–127, 116t. *See also under* Hepatic.
  benign cystic lesions of, 116t
  benign focal lesions of, 122–126
  benign solid lesions of, 116t
  biliary cystadenoma of, 123, 125f
  focal nodular hyperplasia of, 124–125, 125f
  hepatocellular adenoma of, 125–126, 125f
  hepatocellular carcinoma of, 119–120, 120t, 121f
  hypervascular tumors of, 117, 119t
  hypodense lesions of, 117, 119t
  imaging of
    contrast materials for, 115, 117
    guidelines for, 127b
    manifestations of lesions in, 116–117
    modalities for, 115–116
  intrahepatic cholangiocarcinoma of, 120–122, 121f, 122f
  malignant tumors of, 116t
  metastasis to. *See* Hepatic metastasis.
  segmental anatomy of, 126, 126f
  veno-occlusive disease of, 1180–1181
Liver cancer, 899–903, 901t. *See also* Hepatocellular carcinoma (HCC).
  clinical evaluation of, 900
  clinical presentation of, 899–900
  follow-up evaluation of, 903
  prevention of, 903
  risk factors for, 899
  staging, prognostic features, and outcomes for, 900–902, 901t
  treatment for, 902–903
Liver cysts, 122–123, 123f
Liver disease, coagulopathy of, 269, 507–508
Liver function tests, in erythrocytosis, 259
Liver hemangiomas, 123, 124f
Liver metastasis. *See* Hepatic metastasis.
Liver transplantation
  for hepatocellular carcinoma, 902
  for islet cell tumors, 918

Liver tumors, ascites due to, 131
Livingston, Virginia C., 1217t
Livingston-Wheeler regimen, 1217t
Lobectomy, for non–small cell lung cancer, 970, 974
Lobular carcinoma in situ (LCIS), 726, 733–735, 734f
Local excision, for anal carcinoma, 941
Löffler's syndrome, 249
Lomustine (CCNU), 334t
  for high-grade gliomas, 1053, 1054b
Loop diuretics
  for ascites, 131
  for hypercalcemia, 193, 194t
Lorazepam (Ativan)
  for agitation, 1255
  for anxiety, 1227, 1227b, 1254t
  for brain metastases, 1069b
  for delirium, 1248, 1248t
  for nausea and vomiting, 1251
  for refractory pain, 1256t
Low-grade squamous intraepithelial lesion (LSIL), 769
Low-molecular-weight heparin, for venous thromboembolism, 515, 515t
Lumbar puncture
  for encephalopathy, 34
  for peripheral neuropathy, 39t
Lumpectomy
  for ductal carcinoma in situ, 729–731, 730b, 731t, 732t
  for locally invasive breast cancer, 737
Lung cancer
  diagnosis of solitary pulmonary nodule as. *See* Solitary pulmonary nodule.
  hilar and mediastinal adenopathy in, 94, 95f, 96f
  non–small cell, 958–979
    asymptomatic, 960
    brain metastases of, 1073
    carcinogenesis of, 958–960
    clinical evaluation of, 965–968, 967b
    clinical presentation of, 960–963, 962t
    cranial neuropathies due to, 28t
    epidemiology of, 958, 959f, 959t
    extrathoracic metastasis of, 961–962, 975–976, 975t, 976b, 976f, 977f
    headache with, 21t
    oncologic emergencies due to, 963
    paraneoplastic syndromes in, 962–963, 962t
    pathology of, 968–969, 968t
    prevention of, 970f, 976–978, 977b
    prognostic factors for, 965, 969–970
    screening for, 978–979, 978t
    staging of, 963–965, 964f, 965f
    treatment of
      by disease stage, 973–976, 975t, 976b, 976f, 977f
      chemotherapy for, 970, 970f, 971–973, 971t, 975t, 974–976
      combined method therapy for, 972–973
      general principles for, 970, 970f
      photodynamic therapy for, 971
      radiation therapy for, 970, 970f, 971, 972–973
      surgery for, 970–971, 970f, 974
  pleural effusion due to, 87, 89–90
  small cell, 943–955
    brain metastases due to, 1073
    clinical evaluation of, 948–950, 949f
    clinical presentation of, 944–946, 945t, 946f
    cranial neuropathies due to, 28t
    epidemiology of, 943
    extensive-stage, 948–950, 949f, 950–952, 951b, 952f
    follow-up evaluation for, 955
    growth pattern of, 944, 945f
    headache with, 21t
    histologic classification of, 944, 944f
    limited-stage, 948–950, 949f, 952b, 953
    metastatic, 946, 950
    paraneoplastic syndromes with, 944, 946–948
    pathology of, 943–944, 945f
    prognosis for, 950

Lung cancer (*Continued*)
  small cell, (*Continued*)
    prophylactic cranial irradiation for, 953, 954–955
    relapsed and refractory, 953–954
    staging of, 948–950, 949f
    treatment of, 950–955
      chemotherapy for, 950–951, 951b, 952b, 952f, 953
      for extensive-stage disease, 950–952, 951b, 952f
      for limited-stage disease, 952b, 953
      for patients with poor performance status, 953
      for relapsed and refractory disease, 953–954
      palliative, 954
      radiation therapy for, 951b, 952, 952b, 953, 954
      surgical, 953
      toxicity of, 954–955
    superior vena cava syndrome in, 99
Lung metastases
  cranial neuropathies in, 27
  of breast cancer, 751t
  of melanoma, 1087
Lupus anticoagulant, 269, 289, 289b
Lupus erythematosus, systemic
  pancytopenia due to, 253
  vascular cutaneous manifestations of, 299
Luteinizing hormone (LH) deficiency, due to pituitary adenoma, 1142t
Luteinizing hormone–releasing hormone (LHRH), 332t
Luteinizing hormone–releasing hormone (LHRH) agonists, for prostate cancer, 869, 870, 872
Luteinizing hormone–releasing hormone (LHRH) analogs, for locally invasive breast cancer, 741–742
Lymph node(s)
  axillary, in breast cancer, 718, 719, 720t
  carcinoma metastatic to, 216
  drainage areas of specific, 215t
  infraclavicular, breast cancer metastasis to, 718
  internal mammary, breast cancer metastasis to, 718
  matting of, 216
  normal size of, 213
  regional
    in breast cancer staging, 716t, 717–719, 717t
    in melanoma, 1092–1093
  sentinel
    in breast cancer, 718
    in gastrointestinal cancer, 366
    in melanoma, 1093–1094, 1094f, 1095b
  supraclavicular, breast cancer metastasis to, 718–719
Lymph node biopsy
  for breast cancer, 718
    ductal carcinoma in situ, 730b
  for gastrointestinal cancer, 366
  for Hodgkin's disease, 617
  for melanoma, 1093–1094, 1094f, 1095b
  pitfalls of, 218–219, 219b
Lymph node metastases, 216
  neck mass due to, 44–45, 48f
  of melanoma, 1087f, 1090–1091, 1090t
Lymphadenectomy, for gastric cancer, 893–894
Lymphadenopathy, 213–219
  abdominal or retroperitoneal, 217
  axillary, 215t, 216, 217
  causes of, 214t
  cervical, 214–216, 215t
  defined, 213
  diagnostic algorithm for, 217, 218f
  epitrochlear, 215t
  generalized, 214, 217
  hilar and mediastinal, 94–97, 95f, 96f, 97b, 217
  history of, 214, 215t, 216t
  inguinal, 215t, 217, 218–219
  localized, 213–214
  nonspecific, 213
  physical examination for, 214–216

pitfalls in lymph node sampling for, 218–219, 219b
  preauricular, 215t
  submental, 215t
  suboccipital, 215t
  supraclavicular, 214–217, 215t
  symptoms of, 214
Lymphangitic spread, of non–small cell lung cancer, 962
Lymphatic mapping, in melanoma, 1092, 1092f
Lymphatic obstruction, pleural effusion due to, 76
Lymphedema, due to breast cancer treatment, 763
Lymphoblastic leukemia
  acute. *See* Acute lymphoblastic leukemia (ALL).
  precursor B-cell, 601–602
  precursor T-cell, 601–602
Lymphoblastic lymphoma, 656
  precursor B-cell, 601–602
  precursor T-cell, 601–602, 604f
  with diffuse pattern, 604f
Lymphocyte(s), granular, 246, 246f
Lymphocytic leukemia, chronic. *See* Chronic lymphocytic leukemia (CLL).
Lymphocytosis, 246–249
  absolute, 247, 247t
  atypical, 246–247, 247f
  causes of, 247, 247t
  due to clonal lymphocyte disorders, 247–248, 247t, 248f
  due to other clonal lymphoid disorders, 238f, 248
  relative, 246
Lymphoid antigen, 314
Lymphoid markers, aberrant expression of, in acute myeloid leukemia, 530
Lymphoid neoplasms, classification of, 601, 602t
Lymphoid precursor cells, neoplasms of, 601–609
Lymphokine-activated killer cells (LAKs)
  for mesothelioma, 996t
  for renal cell cancer, 835–836
Lymphoma
  anaplastic large-cell, 608f, 609, 612, 655–656, 668
  angiocentric, 669
  B-cell
    diffuse large, 604f, 606
    marginal zone, 604f, 605–606
    precursor lymphoblastic, 601–602
    rituximab for, 345–346
    small lymphocytic, 603–604, 604f, 604t, 612
    types of, 603
  biologic therapy for, 378
  bone marrow biopsy in, 255f
  breast, 663
  Burkitt's, 656–657
    diagnosis of, 552, 604f, 606–607, 612
    etiology of, 550
    treatment for, 562t
  Burkitt's-like, 656–657
  CD30-positive, 609
  central nervous system, 655, 662, 662b, 1053–1054, 1055f
  classification of, 601, 602t, 611–613
  composite, 618
  cranial neuropathies due to, 27, 27t
  diagnosis of, 601–609, 603b
  DNA analysis of, 603b
  eosinophilia due to, 249
  epidural, 1079f, 1083
  flow cytometry analysis of, 603b
  follicular, 248, 248f, 607, 608f
    low-grade, 636–637, 637t
  gastrointestinal, 654–655, 654t, 662
  headache with, 21t
  hematopoietic stem cell transplantation for, 399t, 411–412, 411f
  hilar and mediastinal adenopathy in, 94–95, 96f
  histopathology of, 603b
  immunophenotyping of, 602
  in elderly, 653
  in Waldeyer's ring, 638, 650
  Ki-1–positive, 609
  lymphadenopathy due to, 214, 216

lymphoblastic, 656
mantle cell, 248, 653–654
  diagnosis of, 604f, 605, 612
  hematopoietic stem cell transplantation for, 411
marginal zone
  diagnosis of, 604f, 605–606, 612
  extranodal, 604f, 637
  low-grade, 637–638, 637t
  nodal, 604f, 637–638
mucosal associated lymphoid tissue
  clinical evaluation of, 638
  defined, 637
  gastrointestinal, 637, 638, 639–640, 662
  treatment for, 639–640
NK/T-cell, extranodal, nasal type, 669, 670
non-Hodgkin's. *See* Non-Hodgkin's lymphoma (NHL).
of cervix, 771
of kidney, 168
orbital, 662–663
pancreatic, 918
pancytopenia due to, 253
pathologic fractures due to, 154
pruritus due to, 16, 17b
rituximab for, 346
sinus, 662
small lymphocytic, 636, 637t
splenomegaly in, 137b
superior vena cava syndrome in, 99
T-cell
  adult, 248, 672–675, 673t
  anaplastic large, 668
  angioimmunoblastic, 668, 670
  cutaneous, 664–667
    anaplastic, 668
    clinical presentation of, 665, 665f, 666f
    epidemiology of, 664
    pathophysiology of, 664–665
    staging and prognosis for, 665–666
    treatment for, 344–345, 347, 666–667
  enteropathy-type intestinal, 669, 670
  hepatosplenic gamma/delta, 668–669, 670
  peripheral, 664–671
    classification of, 664, 665t
    clinical evaluation of, 670
    clinical presentation of, 667–668, 667t, 668t
    defined, 664
    diagnosis of, 607–609, 608f, 612
    mycosis fungoides and Sèzary syndrome as, 664–667, 665f, 666f
    prognostic features and outcome for, 670
    treatment for, 670–671
    types of, 668–670
  unspecified, 607–609, 669
  precursor lymphoblastic, 601–602, 604f
  subcutaneous panniculitis-like, 669
  testicular, 662
  thyroid, 663, 1126–1127
  Waldeyer's ring, 638, 650, 662
Lymphoproliferative disease, posttransplant. *See* Posttransplant lymphoproliferative disease (PTLPD).
Lymphoproliferative disorders, clonal, 247–248, 247t, 248f
Lymphoscintigraphy, in melanoma, 1092, 1092f
Lynch syndrome. *See* Hereditary nonpolyposis colon cancer (HNPCC).

M

M (myeloma) proteins, 587
MACOP-B regimen, for non-Hodgkin's lymphoma, 651t, 652
Macroadenoma, pituitary, 1139–1140, 1141f
Macrobiotics, 1221t
Macrocytosis, 272b
  in myelodysplasia, 572t
  with pancytopenia, 253
Macroglobulinemia, 596–598, 596t
  monoclonal, 596, 596t
  Waldenström's, 248, 597–598
    due to cancer, 1172
    immunoglobulin abnormalities due to, 205

Macro-ovalocytes, 277, 277f
Magnetic resonance angiography (MRA)
  of brain tumor, 1050
  of neck mass, 46–47
Magnetic resonance imaging (MRI)
  for back pain, 158–159
  for cranial neuropathy, 28
  for encephalopathy, 34
  for seizures, 24–25, 24f
  of adrenocortical masses, 1129–1130
  of brain metastases, 1065–1066, 1066f
  of brain tumor, 1050
  of breast mass, 65–66, 69f
  of endometrial cancer, 784, 785f
  of epidural cancer, 1079–1080, 1079f, 1080f
  of glioblastoma, 1053f
  of head and neck cancer, 1000
  of liver, 115, 116–119, 120f, 127
  of mesothelioma, 991
  of multiple myeloma, 588
  of neck mass, 46–47
  of pancreatic cancer, 912
  of pituitary adenoma, 1140, 1141f
  of renal cell cancer, 830, 830f
  of salivary gland carcinoma, 1021, 1021f
  of soft-tissue mass, 1041
  of solid renal masses, 167f
Magnification views, of breast, 65
Maintenance therapy
  defined, 556t
  for acute lymphoblastic leukemia, 557t,
    558–559
Majocchi's pigmented purpuric eruption, 300,
    300f
Major depressive disorder, 1225
Malaria, pancytopenia due to, 252
Male anabolic hormones
  for aplastic anemia, 448
  for Fanconi's anemia, 450
Male sexual dysfunction, 1235–1239
  after hematopoietic stem cell transplantation,
    404
  classification of, 1235
  etiology of, 1235–1236, 1236t
  evaluation of, 1235–1237, 1237b
  history of, 1235–1236
  medications and, 1236
  physical examination for, 1236–1237
  treatment for, 1237–1239, 1238b, 1238f
Malignant fibrous histiocytoma, 154, 1029t,
    1032–1033, 1039t, 1040
Malignant lymphoma. See Lymphoma.
Malignant melanoma. See Melanoma.
Malpractice litigation, for breast cancer, 60b
MALT lymphoma. See Mucosal associated
    lymphoid tissue (MALT)
    lymphoma.
Mammary lymph nodes, internal, breast cancer
    metastasis to, 718
Mammography
  abnormal findings on, 65–70
    additional diagnostic imaging studies for,
      65–66, 68f, 69f
    biopsy for, 66–70
    classification of, 65, 66t
    examples of, 67f–68f
    short-interval follow-up for, 66
  compression views in, 65, 68f
  degree of suspicion on, 65, 66t
  during pregnancy, 59
  magnification view on, 65
  of breast carcinoma
    ductal in situ, 730b
    infiltrating ductal, 61, 62f, 67f, 68f
    inflammatory, 67f
    medullary, 67f
  of cyst, 60f, 69f
  of fibroadenoma, 61f, 67f
  screening, 65–70
  spot compression, 65, 68f
Mangofodipir trisodium, for liver imaging, 117
Mannitol
  for brain metastases, 1069b
  for epidural cancer, 1081
Mantle cell lymphoma, 248, 653–654
  diagnosis of, 604f, 605, 612
  hematopoietic stem cell transplantation for,
    412

Mantle field, 622
Mantle field radiation therapy, for Hodgkin's
    disease, 626
MAP (mitogen-activated protein) kinases, in cell
    signaling, 386
Marfan syndrome, cutaneous manifestations of,
    296
Marginal zone lymphoma
  diagnosis of, 604f, 605–606, 612
  extranodal, 604f, 637
  low-grade, 637–638, 637t
  nodal, 604f, 637–638
Marimastat, in antiangiogenic therapy, 385
Marrow fibrosis
  in idiopathic myelofibrosis, 707, 709
  in myeloproliferative disorders, 702b
Marrow karyotype studies, for erythrocytosis,
    261
Masoka Staging System, for thymoma, 986, 987t
Mastectomy
  for ductal carcinoma in situ, 729
  prophylactic, 1196–1197
  reconstructive surgery after, 763–764
Mastitis, periductal, 74
Matched unrelated donor (MUD)
    transplantation, for acute myeloid
    leukemia, 538
Matrix metalloproteinases (MMPs), in
    antiangiogenic therapy, 384, 385
Matting, of lymph nodes, 216
May-Hegglin anomaly, 270
m-BACOD regimen, for non-Hodgkin's
    lymphoma
  AIDS-related, 1157
  intermediate-grade, 651–652, 651t
MBV (mixed bacterial vaccines), 1217t
MDR (multidrug resistance), defined, 556t
MDR-1 (multidrug resistance) gene
  in acute myeloid leukemia, 528
  in gene therapy, 383
MDS (myelodysplastic syndrome). See
    Myelodysplasia.
Mean corpuscular hemoglobin, 234
Mean corpuscular hemoglobin concentration,
    234
Mean corpuscular volume (MCV), 234
  in anemia, 1166
  in pancytopenia, 253
Mechanical bowel preparation, 112
Mechlorethamine, 332t
Meclizine (Bonine, Antivert), for nausea and
    vomiting, 1252t
Mediastinal adenopathy, 94–97, 95f, 96f, 97b,
    217
Mediastinal fibrosis, superior vena cava
    syndrome due to, 100
Mediastinal germ-cell tumors, 822b
Mediastinal lymph nodes, in non–small cell lung
    cancer, 965f
Mediastinoscopy
  for esophageal cancer, 876
  for non–small cell lung cancer, 967
  for superior vena cava syndrome, 103
Medical decision making, 1232
Medicare Hospice Benefit, 1256, 1257
Medroxyprogesterone acetate (Depo-Provera),
    for cachexia, 6–7
Medulloblastoma, 1055
  with hereditary nonpolyposis colorectal
    cancer, 1201
Megakaryocytic abnormalities, in myelodysplasia,
    570t, 571f
Megaloblastic anemia
  hyperbilirubinemia due to, 197–198
  mean corpuscular volume in, 235
Megestrol acetate (Megace), 342t
  for breast cancer, 753t, 754t, 755
  for cachexia, 6–7, 7t
  for endometrial cancer, 788
  for pancreatic cancer, 917
  for prostate cancer, 872
  for renal cell cancer, 834
Melanoma, 1085–1100
  adjuvant therapy for, 1094–1095, 1096b
  amelanotic, 306
  biologic therapy for, 1094–1095, 1096b,
    1097–1100, 1098f, 1099f
  biopsy of, 311–312

chemotherapy for, 1097–1100, 1099b, 1099f
  classification of, 1088, 1088t, 1089t
  clinical evaluation of, 1088
  clinical presentation of, 305, 306f, 306t, 307f,
    1086–1088, 1086t
  conjunctival, 310–311
  cranial neuropathies due to, 28t
  cutaneous, 1086
  differential diagnosis of, 305–308, 307f, 308t,
    309f, 310f
  epidemiology of, 1085–1086
  familial, 1194t, 1202
  follow-up evaluation for, 1100, 1100t
  genetic basis for, 1086, 1194t, 1202
  in unusual locations, 308–311, 312b
  local recurrence of, 1094
  lymph node management in, 1091–1094,
    1092f, 1093b
  metastatic
    adrenal, 1088
    classification of, 1090
    clinical presentation of, 1086–1088,
      1087f
    common distant sites of, 1087–1088,
      1095t
    in-transit, 1086, 1090, 1094
    lymph node, 1087f, 1090–1091, 1090t
    renal, 1087f, 1088
    satellite, 1086
    surgery for, 1097b
    systemic therapy for, 1097–1100, 1098f,
      1099f
    to bone, 1087
    to brain, 1074–1075, 1087–1088, 1087f,
      1100b
    to gastrointestinal tract, 1087–1088,
      1087f
    to liver, 1087, 1099f
    to lung, 1087
  mucosal, 1086
  noncutaneous primary, 1086
  of cervix, 778
  of genitalia, 311
  of unknown origin, 314
  oral mucosal, 311
  radiation therapy for, 1095
  risk factors for, 305, 306t, 1085–1086
  screening for, 305, 307t
  sentinel node biopsy for, 1093b
  staging and prognosis for, 1088–1091,
    1088t–1090t
  subungual, 309, 310f, 312b
  surgical management of, 1091–1094, 1091t,
    1092f, 1097b
  temozolomide for, 348, 1100b
  ulceration of, 1090, 1090t
Melatonin, for cachexia, 8
Melena, 145
Meloxicam, for pain, 1244
Melphalan, 333t
  for multiple myeloma, 588, 589b
  in conditioning regimen for hematopoietic
    stem cell transplantation
    allogeneic, 395, 395f, 396f
    autologous, 399t
  toxicities of, 396f
Membrane receptors, 342t, 345–347
MEN. See Multiple endocrine neoplasia (MEN).
Mendelian risk, 1204
Menetrier's disease, and gastric cancer, 889
Meningiomas, 1055, 1057f
  seizures due to, 23, 25
Meningismus, 157, 159t, 161, 162t
Meningitis
  carcinomatous, due to metastatic breast
    cancer, 751t
  headache due to, 20t
  leukemic, in acute myeloid leukemia, 529
Meningococcemia, vascular cutaneous
    manifestations of, 297f
Menopause, with breast cancer, 765, 766b
Menses, heavy, 266b
Mental status changes, due to brain metastases,
    1062–1063, 1065, 1065t
Meperidine, for pain, 1246, 1247t
Mercaptopurine, 336t
  for acute lymphoblastic leukemia, 557t, 558t
  for acute promyelocytic leukemia, 545b

Merkel cell carcinoma, 1104, 1113–1114, 1113f
Mesenteric cysts, pelvic mass due to, 189t
Mesna, for Burkitt's leukemia/lymphoma, 562t
Mesothelioma, 991–997
    biologic and targeted therapies for, 996–997,
        996t
    chemotherapy for, 995, 995t
    clinical evaluation of, 991, 992f
    clinical presentation of, 991
    diagnosis and pathology of, 992, 993t
    early intervention for, 992
    epidemiology of, 991
    immunohistochemistry of, 992, 993t
    intracavitary therapies for, 995–996
    neoadjuvant therapies for, 997
    pleural effusion due to, 93
    postoperative therapies for, 997
    prognosis and staging for, 992, 993t, 994,
        995t
    radiotherapy for, 994–995
    surgical options for, 992–994, 994f, 995t
Metabolic abnormalities, in acute myeloid
        leukemia, 530, 532
Metabolic changes, in cachexia, 3–5, 4t
Metabolic encephalopathy, 32, 34t
Metastasis(es)
    adrenal
        of melanoma, 1088
        of non–small cell lung cancer, 961, 964
    bone (skeletal). See also Pathologic fractures.
        of breast cancer, 151f, 155f, 255f, 751t,
            760–761
        of melanoma, 1087
        of non–small cell lung cancer, 961, 966
        of small cell lung cancer, 946
        pancytopenia due to, 253
    brain. See Brain metastasis.
    calvarial, headache due to, 21, 21t, 22, 22t
    central nervous system, of non–small cell
            lung cancer, 961–962
    cranial neuropathies due to, 28, 28t
    epidural, pain due to, 1243
    hepatic, 117–119, 118f–120f, 119t
        hepatic artery infusion for, 368–369
        of breast cancer, 751t
        of carcinoid syndrome, 1137
        of colorectal cancer, 118f, 927
        of lung cancer
            non–small cell, 962
            small cell, 946
        of melanoma, 1087, 1099f
        staging laparoscopy of, 365
    hoarseness due to, 51
    leptomeningeal
        encephalopathy due to, 34t, 35
        of small cell lung cancer, 946
    lymph node, 216
        neck mass due to, 44–45, 48f
        of melanoma, 1087f, 1090–1091, 1090t
    pituitary gland, of small cell lung cancer, 946
    renal, 168, 830
        of melanoma, 1087f, 1088
    seizures due to, 23
Metastasis inhibitors, 331f
Metastatic anal carcinoma, 941
Metastatic basal cell carcinoma, 1106
Metastatic bladder cancer, 853, 855b
Metastatic breast cancer, 750–762
    approach to solitary sites of, 761b
    chemotherapy for, 756–760, 756t
        high-dose, 758
        in older women, 758
        suggested approach to, 759–760, 759f
        vs. hormonal therapy, 755
        with capecitabine, 756t, 758
        with doxorubicin and taxanes, 756–758,
            756t, 757t
        with trastuzumab, 756t, 758
    clinical trials for, 761–762
    factors in management of, 750, 751f
    future of treatment of, 762
    hormonal treatment of, 751–756, 753t, 754t,
        755f
    incidence of, 750
    micro-, 718
        in ductal carcinoma in situ, 726–727
    natural history of, 750
    of unknown origin, 316

    presentation of, 750, 751t
    prognostic and predictive factors in, 750–751,
        752t
    psychosocial aspects and symptom
            management for, 761
    pure estrogen antagonist for, 754
    spinal cord compression due to, 160f, 751t,
        760
    to axillary lymph nodes, 718, 719, 720t
    to bone, 151f, 154f, 255f, 751t, 760–761
    to brain, 751t, 1073–1074
    to nonaxillary lymph nodes, 718–719
Metastatic cancer of unknown primary, 313–316
    biological behavior of, 315
    clinical evaluation of, 313–314
    defined, 313
    pathology of, 314–315, 315t
    treatment for, 316, 316b
Metastatic carcinoid tumors, 1134, 1134f,
        1136–1137
Metastatic cervical cancer, 774–775, 775t
Metastatic colorectal cancer, 118f, 927, 929–930
Metastatic endometrial cancer, 786t
Metastatic Ewing's sarcoma, 1035, 1035f
Metastatic germ-cell tumors
    management of, 817–821, 819b, 819t,
        820b–822b
    pattern of nodal spread for, 814, 814f
Metastatic laryngeal cancer, 1004
Metastatic lung cancer
    non–small cell, 961–962, 975–976, 975t,
        976b, 976f, 977f
    small cell, 946, 950
    to brain, 1073
Metastatic melanoma
    adrenal, 1088
    classification of, 1090
    clinical presentation of, 1086–1088, 1087f
    common distant sites of, 1087–1088, 1095t
    in-transit, 1086, 1090, 1094
    lymph node, 1087f, 1090–1091, 1090t
    renal, 1087f, 1088
    satellite, 1086
    surgery for, 1097b
    systemic therapy for, 1097–1100, 1098f,
        1099f
    to bone, 1087
    to brain, 1074–1075, 1099b
    to gastrointestinal tract, 1087–1088, 1087f
    to liver, 1087, 1099f
    to lung, 1087
Metastatic nasopharyngeal cancer, 1010
Metastatic neuroendocrine tumors, 1136–1137
Metastatic oral cavity cancer, 1007–1008, 1008t
Metastatic osteosarcoma, 1030, 1031–1032
Metastatic ovarian cancer, 792, 792f, 793, 795
Metastatic pancreatic cancer, 916–917
Metastatic pancreatic endocrine tumors, 120f,
        1137
Metastatic persistent gestational trophoblastic
            tumor, 807–808, 808t, 810–811
Metastatic prostate cancer, 863–864, 873
Metastatic renal cell cancer
    chemotherapy/hormonal therapy for, 834,
        834t
    debulking nephrectomy for, 833, 833b
    immunotherapy for, 834–838, 835t, 836t,
        837f, 838t, 838f
    radiation therapy for, 838
    to bone, 150f, 151f
Metastatic salivary gland carcinoma, 1019, 1020,
        1023–1024, 1024f
Metastatic small cell lung cancer, 946
Metastatic soft tissue sarcoma, 1044–1045
Metastatic squamous cell carcinoma, 1111
Metastatic testicular cancer, 817–821, 819b, 819t,
        820b–822b
Metastatic vaginal cancer, 780
Methadone, for pain, 1246, 1246t
Methotrexate, 335t, 355t
    for acute lymphoblastic leukemia, 556, 557t,
        558t, 560, 561
    for acute promyelocytic leukemia, 545b
    for bladder cancer, 853, 854
    for Burkitt's leukemia/lymphoma, 562t
    for CNS lymphoma, 1054, 1056b
    for esophageal cancer, 878
    for gastric cancer, 895t, 896t

    for gestational trophoblastic tumor, 809–811,
        810t
    for graft-versus-host disease, 396
        prophylactic use of, 447
    for head and neck cancer, 1008t
    for locally invasive breast cancer, 742
    for mesothelioma, 995t, 996t, 997
    for osteosarcoma, 1030
    pulmonary toxicity due to, 78t
Methotrimeprazine
    for delirium, 1254t
    for nausea and vomiting, 1252t
Methyl-CCNU (semustine), 334t
Methylmelamines, 333t
Methylphenidate (Ritalin), 1227b
    for opioid-related sedation, 1248
Methylprednisolone
    for graft-versus-host disease, 396
    for idiopathic thrombocytopenic purpura,
        491
Metoclopramide, for nausea and vomiting,
        1252t
Metronomic therapy, 354
MF (mycosis fungoides), 664–667, 665f
    pruritus due to, 16
MGUS (monoclonal gammopathy of
            undetermined significance),
            203–204, 581, 586–587, 586t
Microadenoma, pituitary, 1139, 1140
Microangiopathic hemolytic anemia, 492, 492f
Microdochectomy, 72–73
Microsatellite instability, 1194, 1200
Microspherocytes, 240b, 275
Microtubules, 352
    drugs that stabilize, 340t, 352–353
Microvascular thrombosis, in essential
            thrombocythemia, 711, 712
Microvessel density, with cancer of unknown
            primary, 1148
Midazolam (Versed)
    for delirium, 1248f, 1254t, 1255
    for dyspnea, 1254t
    for myoclonus, 1256
    for refractory pain, 1256t
Migraine headache, 20t
Minimal residual disease (MRD), defined, 556t
Minimantle field, 622
Mini-mental state exam (MMSE), with brain
            metastases, 1065, 1065t
Mirtazapine, 1227, 1227b
Misoprostol, with NSAIDs, 1244
Mistletoe, 1213t
Mitogen-activated protein (MAP) kinases, in cell
            signaling, 386
Mitomycin, 334t
    for anal carcinoma, 949
    for breast cancer, 757t
    for cervical cancer, 775t
    for esophageal cancer, 878, 878t, 882, 883
    for gastric cancer, 895t, 896t
    for mesothelioma, 995t, 996, 996t, 997, 997t
    for superficial bladder cancer, 844
Mitotane, for adrenal cancer, 1130–1131, 1131b
Mitotic apparatus, drugs that affect, 332t, 352
Mitotic index, in breast cancer, 722
Mitoxantrone, 338t, 351
    for acute myeloid leukemia, 533, 535t
    for prostate cancer, 872, 873t
Mixed bacterial vaccines (MBV), 1217t
Mixed lineage leukemia (MLL), 526–528,
        562–563
MLC (multileaf collimator), for radiation therapy,
        322, 322f
MLH1 gene, 1200
MMPs (matrix metalloproteinases), in
            antiangiogenic therapy, 384, 385
MMSE (mini-mental state exam), with brain
            metastases, 1065, 1065t
Mohs surgery
    for basal cell carcinoma, 1107
    for Merkel cell carcinoma, 1114
    for squamous cell carcinoma, 1111
Molar pregnancy, 804–806, 805t, 807, 807b, 811
Molecular complete remission, defined, 556t
Molecular markers, for second primary cancers
            of head and neck, 1012–1013
Molecular studies, for cancer of unknown origin,
            314–315, 315t

molgramostim. *See* Granulocyte-macrophage colony-stimulating factor (GM-CSF, sargramostim, molgramostim).
Monoclonal antibodies, 342t, 345–347
  biologic therapy with, 377–379, 378t, 385, 387
  for chronic lymphocytic leukemia, 696
  for colorectal cancer, 930
  for non-Hodgkin's lymphoma
    intermediate-grade, 652–653
    low-grade, 642–643
Monoclonal gammopathy(ies), 581–598
  amyloidosis as, 205, 205b, 595–596
  defined, 581
  differential diagnosis of, 202t, 203–205, 203b, 586t
  due to cancer, 1171–1172, 1171f
  due to multiple myeloma, 203, 204–205
  due to plasmacytoma, 205
  due to Waldenström's macroglobulinemia, 205
  hypogammaglobulinemia due to, 203
  macroglobulinemia as, 596–598, 596t
  multiple myeloma as. *See* Multiple myeloma.
  peripheral neuropathy due to, 36, 40
  serum protein electrophoresis of, 200, 201f
Monoclonal gammopathy of undetermined significance (MGUS), 203–204, 581, 586–587, 586t
Monoclonal protein (M-protein), 201, 201f, 203–204
Monocytoid cells, 604f
Monocytopenia, 249
Monocytosis, 249
  due to cancer, 1168
Mononeuropathy multiplex, 37
Mononucleosis, infectious
  atypical lymphocytes in, 279, 279f
  lymphocytosis due to, 247, 247f
MOPP regimen, for Hodgkin's disease, 623, 624t, 625
MOPP/ABV hybrid regimen, for Hodgkin's disease, 623, 624t, 625
Morphine
  for dying patient, 1254–1255, 1254t
  for dyspnea, 79, 1254t
  for pain, 1245, 1246, 1246t, 1247b, 1247t
  pruritus due to, 15
Motrin. *See* Ibuprofen (Motrin).
Mouth cancer, 1006–1008, 1008t
M-protein (monoclonal protein), 201, 201f, 203–204
MRA (magnetic resonance angiography)
  of brain tumor, 1050
  of neck mass, 46–47
MRD (minimal residual disease), defined, 556t
MRI. *See* Magnetic resonance imaging (MRI).
MSH2 gene, 1200
MSH6 gene, 1200
M-spikes, due to cancer, 1171–1172, 1171f
MTS1 gene, in familial melanoma, 1201
Mucinous ovarian carcinoma, 795f, 796
Mucormycosis, febrile neutropenia due to, 1177b, 1177f
Mucosal associated lymphoid tissue (MALT) lymphoma
  clinical evaluation of, 638
  defined, 637
  gastrointestinal, 637, 638, 639–640, 662
  therapy for, 639–640
Mucositis, 1249–1250
MUD (matched unrelated donor) transplantation, for acute myeloid leukemia, 538
Muir-Torre syndrome, 1201
Multidrug resistance (MDR), defined, 556t
Multidrug resistance (MDR-1) gene
  in acute myeloid leukemia, 528
  in gene therapy, 383
Multileaf collimator (MLC), for radiation therapy, 322, 322f
Multiple endocrine neoplasia (MEN)
  genetic basis for, 1194t, 1198–1199
  pancreatic endocrine tumors with, 1135
  thyroid carcinoma with, 1125
Multiple hamartoma syndrome, 1194, 1194t, 1197–1198

Multiple myeloma, 581–595
  amyloidosis with, 582, 596
  asymptomatic, 204, 586, 586t
  clinical evaluation of, 585–586
  clinical presentation of, 582–583
  complications of, 583–585, 585t
    treatment of, 592–593
  defined, 581
  differential diagnosis of, 586–588, 586t, 587f, 588f
  epidemiology of, 581
  etiology of, 581
  febrile neutropenia in, 1174
  headache with, 21t
  hematopoietic stem cell transplantation for, 399t, 412–413, 413f
  immunoglobulin abnormalities due to, 204–205
  pathogenesis of, 581–582
  plasmacytomas and, 593–595
  POEMS syndrome in, 583, 593
  prognosis for, 583, 583t
  relapsed and refractory, 590
  smoldering, 204, 586, 586t
  spinal cord compression due to, 160f
  staging system for, 593, 593t
  therapy of, 588–592, 589b
Mumps orchitis, 182
Munchausen's by proxy, 506
Munchausen's syndrome, 506
Muscle tension dysphonia, 51t
Music therapy, for pain management, 1244
Mutations, 1193–1194
Myasthenia gravis, 37
  due to thymoma, 983–984
Mycosis fungoides (MF), 664–667, 665f
  pruritus due to, 16
Mycotic infections
  fever of unknown origin due to, 11
  with hematopoietic stem cell transplantation, 400–401
Myeloblasts, in acute myeloid leukemia, 530
Myelodysplasia, 566–578
  after hematopoietic stem cell transplantation, 405, 523, 523t
  anemia due to, 569, 569t, 575b
  bleeding due to, 575b
  classification of, 566, 572–573, 572t, 573t
  clinical evaluation of, 566, 570–572
  clinical presentation of, 569–570, 569t, 570t, 571f, 572t
  defined, 566
  due to multiple myeloma treatment, 585, 585t
  etiology of, 568–569, 568t, 569t
  follow-up evaluation for, 578
  hyperbilirubinemia due to, 197–198
  incidence of, 567, 568f
  mean corpuscular volume in, 235
  natural history of, 575
  overview of, 566
  pancytopenia due to, 253, 254, 255
  pathobiology of, 566–567, 567f
  prognostic scoring systems for, 573–575, 574f, 574t
  red blood cells in, 276
  risk factors for, 568–569, 568t
  secondary, 568–569, 569t
  therapy-related, 568–569, 569t
  thrombocythemia due to, 227–230, 229t, 230b
  thrombocytopenia due to, 569t, 571f, 575b
  treatment of, 575–578, 575b, 577f
    erythropoietin for, 421
    hematopoietic stem cell transplantation for, 407–408, 575b, 578
    intensive therapy in, 576–578
    low-intensity therapy in, 576, 577f
    myeloid growth factors for, 427–428, 428b
    supportive care in, 575b
Myelodysplastic syndrome (MDS). *See* Myelodysplasia.
Myelofibrosis, idiopathic (primary), 706–709
  clinical evaluation of, 706–707, 707f, 708t
  clinical presentation of, 244, 706
  epidemiology of, 706
  etiology of, 702b, 706, 706t

  follow-up evaluation for, 709
  staging, prognostic features, and outcomes for, 707–708, 708t
  treatment for, 708–709
Myelography
  for back pain, 159
  for epidural cancer, 1080
Myeloid growth factors, 421–428
  enhanced antimicrobial function with, 423–424, 424t
  for acute lymphocytic leukemia, 424–425, 425t
  for acute myeloid leukemia, 421–424, 421t–425t, 426b
  for chemotherapy-induced neutropenia, 428
  for myelodysplasia, 427–428, 428b
  recruitment of cells into S-phase of cell cycle with, 424, 425t
  reduced period of neutropenia with, 421–423, 422t, 423t, 425–426, 426t
  uses of, 421, 421t
  with stem cell transplantation, 425–427, 426t, 427t
Myeloid leukemia
  acute. *See* Acute myeloid leukemia (AML).
  chronic. *See* Chronic myeloid leukemia (CML).
Myeloid metaplasia
  agnogenic. *See* Myelofibrosis, idiopathic (primary).
  in myeloproliferative disorders, 702b
  in polycythemia vera, 705
  with myelofibrosis. *See* Myelofibrosis, idiopathic.
Myelolipoma, adrenal, 170, 170f
Myeloma
  extramedullary, 586t
  multiple. *See* Multiple myeloma.
Myeloma (M) proteins, 587
Myelomonocytic leukemia, chronic, 570, 572, 5756
Myelopathy, 158
  herpes zoster spinal, 159t, 161, 162, 162t
Myeloperoxidase, in acute myeloid leukemia, 530
Myelophthisis, 278
  pancytopenia due to, 252t
Myeloproliferative disorders
  clinical notes on, 702b
  defined, 676
  platelet abnormalities in, 280–282
  platelet count in, 227–230, 227b, 229t, 230b
Myelosuppression, due to therapy for small cell lung cancer, 954
Mylotarg (gemtuzumab ozogomicin), 342t, 346
  for acute myeloid leukemia, 346, 542
Myocardial involvement, in lung cancer, 961
Myoclonus, 1256
Myopathies, 37
Myxoma, atrial, fever due to, 9

N
N-acetyl-cysteine, for head and neck cancer, 1014, 1014t
Naessons, Gaston, 1217t
Nail changes, in anemia, 232–233
Nailbed lesions, 309, 310f, 312b
Naloxone (Narcan), 1248
Nandrolone decanoate
  for aplastic anemia, 448
  for Fanconi's anemia, 450
NAPDH oxidase, in chronic granulomatous disease, 480
α-Naphthyl butyrate esterase, in acute myeloid leukemia, 530
Naproxen (Naprosyn)
  for pain, 1245t
  with interferon-alpha therapy of melanoma, 1096b
Narcan (naloxone), 1248
Narcotics. *See* Opioid analgesics.
Nasal T/NK-cell lymphoma, 669, 670
Nasopharyngeal cancer, 1008–1010, 1009t
Nasturtium officinale, 1215
National Hospice Organization (NHO), 1256

Nausea
  anticipatory, 1250
  chemotherapy-induced, 1250–1251, 1251t,
      1252t
  due to opioids, 1248
  due to therapy for small cell lung cancer, 954
Navelbine. See Vinorelbine (Navelbine).
  for renal cell cancer, 834t
Neck cancer. See Head and neck cancer.
Neck dissection, for oropharyngeal cancer, 1006b
Neck mass(es), 43–48
  algorithm for evaluation of, 45f
  congenital, 43, 44t
  diagnostic tests for, 46–48, 48f
  differential diagnosis of, 43, 44t
  due to benign neoplasms, 43, 44t
  due to malignant neoplasms, 43, 44t
  due to metastatic lymph nodes, 44–45
  history of, 43–45
  inflammatory, 43, 44t
  physical examination of, 45–46, 46f
Nefazodone (Serzone), 1227, 1227b
Neisseria meningitides, febrile neutropenia due to,
      1175
Neoadjuvant therapy
  for bladder cancer, 854–855, 855b
  for esophageal cancer, 879–880, 881t
  for gastric cancer, 897
  for mesothelioma, 997
  for non–small cell lung cancer, 975
  for pancreatic cancer, 915
  for soft tissue sarcoma, 1045
Neonatal alloimmune thrombocytopenia, 494
Neonatal jaundice, 198
Nephrectomy, for renal cell cancer, 832–833,
      833b
Nerve biopsy, for peripheral neuropathy, 37, 39t
Nerve compression, due to lung cancer, 961
Nerve conduction studies, for peripheral
      neuropathy, 39t
Nerve sheath tumors, malignant, 1040
Neuritis, cervical, headache due to, 20t
Neuroblastoma, epidural, 1080f
Neuroendocrine carcinoma, of unknown origin,
      1152b
Neuroendocrine tumors, 1133–1137
  carcinoid, 1133–1135
      appendiceal, 1134t, 1135
      bronchial, 1133, 1134t
      clinical presentation of, 1134t
      gastric, 1133–1134, 1134t
      hormone levels in, 1135t
      metastatic, 1134, 1134f, 1137
      of small intestine, 1134–1135, 1134f,
          1134t
      rectal, 1134t, 1135
      treatment for, 1136–1137, 1136t
  cervical, 770–771
  metastatic, 1136–1137
  pancreatic, 917–918, 1135–1136
      clinical presentation of, 1134t,
          1135–1136
      epidemiology of, 1135
      hormone levels in, 1135t
      localization of, 1135, 1136
      metastatic, 120f, 1137
      pathology of, 909
      treatment for, 917–918, 1136, 1136t,
          1137
  pathophysiology of, 1133
Neuroepidermal tumors, 315
Neurofibromatosis, 1040, 1049, 1194t
Neurofibrosarcoma, 1039f
Neuroforaminal stenosis, 161
Neuroimaging
  for back pain, 158–159
  for encephalopathy, 34
  for headache, 20f, 21, 21b
  for seizures, 24–25, 24f
Neurokinin-1 receptor antagonists, for nausea
      and vomiting, 1251
Neurologic signs and symptoms
  headache with, 21b
  of lung cancer, 947–948
  of multiple myeloma, 585
  of Waldenström's macroglobulinemia,
      597–598
  with back pain, 157–158, 162–163

Neurolytic techniques, for pain, 1249
Neuromuscular junction disorders, 37
Neuronopathy, 37
Neurontin (gabapentin)
  for neuropathic pain, 1248, 1249t
  for seizures, 25t
Neuropathy(ies)
  autonomic, 37
  axonal, 36–37
  causes of, 36–37, 36t, 40
  clinical features of, 36, 36t
  compression, 40
  cranial. See Cranial neuropathy(ies).
  differential diagnosis of, 37
  evaluation of, 37, 38f, 39b, 39t
  idiopathic, 40
  management of, 40, 40b
  paraneoplastic vasculitic, 37
  peripheral, 36–40
  sensory, 37
Neuropsychological impairment, due to
      prophylactic cranial irradiation,
      954–955
Neutrons, in radiation therapy, 321
Neutropenia, 244–246, 245t, 246f
  acute, 245
  chemotherapy-induced, myeloid growth
      factors for, 428
  chronic, 246f
  cyclic, 477
  defined, 1174
  drug-induced, 245
      myeloid growth factors for, 428
  due to infection, 244–245, 245t
  due to myelodysplasia, 569, 569t
  due to therapy for small cell lung cancer, 954
  "ethnic," 246
  febrile. See Febrile neutropenia.
  in acute lymphoblastic leukemia, 551
  in acute myeloid leukemia, 532, 532t
      myeloid growth factors for, 421–423,
          422t, 423t
  in stem cell transplantation, myeloid growth
      factors for, 425–426, 426t
  mild, 246
  severe congenital, 475–477, 477f, 477t
Neutrophil(s)
  hypolobated, hypogranulated, in
      myelodysplasia, 571f, 572t
  toxic granulation of, 272b, 278, 278f
Neutrophil motility, disorders of, 477–478, 478t
Neutrophilia, 241–244, 241t, 242f–244f
  drug-related, 243
  due to cancer, 1168
  familial, 243
  postsplenectomy, 243
  with splenomegaly or peripheral blood
      myeloid immaturity, 243–244,
          243f, 244f
Neutrophilic leukocytosis, 241–242, 242f, 242t
Nevoid basal cell carcinoma syndrome, 1194t,
      1202–1203
Nevus(i)
  benign, 307f, 308t, 309f
  biopsy of, 308, 311–312
  blue, 308t
  compound
      benign, 307f, 308t
      dysplastic, 309f
  congenital, 309f
  halo, 309f
  junctional, 308t
NF-1 gene, 1040
NHL. See Non-Hodgkin's lymphoma (NHL).
NHO (National Hospice Organization), 1256
Niehans, Paul, 1217t
Niferex (iron polysaccharide), 456b
Nilutamide (Nilandron), 341t, 344
  for prostate cancer, 870
Nipple, jogger's, 73
Nipple discharge, 71–74
  benign, 71
  bloody, 71, 72
      in pregnancy, 73
  diagnostic evaluation of, 72
  ductography and cytology for, 72
  due to duct ectasia/periductal mastitis, 74
  due to galactorrhea, 71

  due to irritation, 73
  due to Paget's disease, 73–74
  due to papilloma, 73
  malignant, 71, 72–73
  pathologic, 72
  physical examination for, 72
  physiologic, 71
  surgical evaluation of, 72–73
  types of, 71
Nipple irritation, 73
Nitrates, and gastric cancer, 889
Nitrites, and gastric cancer, 889
Nitrogen mustard, 332t, 333t, 348
  for Hodgkin's disease, 623
  for mycosis fungoides and Sézary syndrome,
      666
Nitrosoureas, 332t, 333t–334t
NK/T-cell lymphoma, extranodal, nasal type,
      669, 670
Nocturnal headache, 21, 21b
Nodal marginal zone lymphoma, 604f
Nodule(s)
  solitary pulmonary, 81–86
      biopsy of, 85–86
      calcifications in, 81, 83b, 84, 84f
      cavitation of, 83
      chest radiography of, 81, 83b
      computed tomography of, 81–84, 83t, 84t
          enhanced, 84–85
      contours and margins of, 82–83, 83f
      defined, 81, 82f
      density of, 83–84, 84f
      differential diagnosis of, 81, 82t
      fat in, 84
      indeterminate, 81, 85b
      positron emission tomography imaging
          of, 85, 85f
      size of, 81, 82
      vascular and bronchial relationships of,
          83, 84f
      vs. mass, 81
  thyroid
      benign, 1118–1119
      clinical presentation of, 1117
      evaluation of, 1117–1118, 1118f
      risk factors for carcinoma with, 1117,
          1118t
  vocal, 51t
Nolvadex. See Tamoxifen (Nolvadex).
Non-Hodgkin's lymphoma (NHL). See also
      Lymphoma.
  biologic therapy for, 378
  cranial neuropathies due to, 27, 28t
  diagnosis of, 649
  eosinophilia due to, 249
  epidemiology of, 636, 648
  Epstein-Barr virus and, 648–649, 1155–1156
  extranodal, 660–663
      clinical evaluation of, 661
      clinical presentation of, 660
      defined, 660
      etiology of, 660
      follow-up evaluation for, 663
      sites of, 660, 661f
      staging and prognosis for, 661
      treatment for, 661–663, 662b
  follow-up evaluation of, 644
  gastrointestinal, 654–655, 654t
  headache with, 21t
  hematopoietic stem cell transplantation for,
      399t, 411–412, 411f, 643–644
  high-grade, 649, 656–657
  intermediate-grade, 649, 650–656
      clinical presentation and evaluation of,
          649
      follow-up evaluation for, 652
      gastrointestinal, 654–655, 654t
      in elderly, 653
      KI-1+ anaplastic, 655–656
      mantle cell, 653–654
      primary central nervous system, 655
      staging of, 650–651, 650t
      treatment for, 652–653
  low-grade, 636–645
      classification of, 636, 637t
      clinical evaluation of, 638
      clinical presentation of, 636–638
      follicular, 636–637, 637t

Non-Hodgkin's lymphoma (NHL). (Continued)
  low-grade, (Continued)
    marginal zone, 637–638, 637t
    pathology of, 636, 637t
    prognostic factors in, 638–639
    small lymphocytic, 636, 637t
    staging of, 638–639, 638t
    treatment of, 639–644
      chemotherapy in, 641, 642t, 643,
        643t
      choice of initial therapy for, 641–643,
        642t, 643t
      hematopoietic stem cell
        transplantation in, 643–644
      immunization therapy in, 642–643
      in advanced-stage disease, 640, 640f
      in early-stage disease, 639–640
      interferon-α in, 641–642
      late sequelae of, 645
      monoclonal antibodies in, 642
      observation without, 640–641
      radiation therapy in, 639
  lymphadenopathy due to, 214, 216
  pruritus due to, 16, 17b
  risk factors for, 636, 637t
  rituximab for, 346
  secondary, 618–619, 629
  splenomegaly in, 137b
  superior vena cava syndrome in, 99, 649
  with HIV infection, 650, 1155–1158
Nonmyeloablative hematopoietic stem cell
    transplantation, 394
  for acute myeloid leukemia, 537–538
Nonmyeloablative therapy, as conditioning
    regimen for hematopoietic stem
    cell transplantation, 395, 395t
Nonseminomatous germ-cell tumor (NSGCT),
    815–817, 817t, 819b, 820b
Non–small cell lung cancer. See Lung cancer,
    non–small cell.
Nonsteroidal anti-inflammatory drugs (NSAIDs)
  for pain, 1244–1245, 1245t
  for prevention of colorectal cancer, 924
  with interferon-alpha therapy of melanoma,
    1096b
Nonsteroidal inhibitors, 754
Nonverbal behavior, 1231
Nortriptyline, for neuropathic pain, 1249t
NSAIDs (nonsteroidal anti-inflammatory drugs)
  for pain, 1244–1245, 1245t
  for prevention of colorectal cancer, 924
  with interferon-alpha therapy of melanoma,
    1096b
NSGCT (nonseminomatous germ-cell tumor),
    815–817, 817t, 819b, 820b
Nuclear medicine studies
  of breast mass, 66
  of liver, 116
Nucleic acid synthesis inhibitors, 332t,
    335t–336t, 347–350
Nutrition. See also Diet.
  total parenteral, 6, 365
Nutritional assessment, for gastrointestinal
    oncologic surgery, 364–365, 364t
Nutritional deficiencies, and esophageal cancer,
    875–876
Nutritional management, of cachexia, 5–6
Nutritional metabolic therapy, 1221t

O

OAF (osteoclast activating factor), in multiple
    myeloma, 583
Obstructive hepatobiliary disease, pruritus due
    to, 14
Octreotide
  for carcinoid tumors, 1136–1137
  for islet cell tumors, 917–918
  for nausea and vomiting, 1252t, 1256
  for pancreatic endocrine tumors, 1136
Oculomotor nerve deficit, 29t
Ogilvie, William, 110
Ogilvie's syndrome, 110
Olanzapine (Zyprexa), 1227b
  for nausea and vomiting, 1252t
Older adults
  acute myeloid leukemia in
    prognosis for, 528
    treatment of, 540–541

advanced cervical cancer in, 774b
lymphoma in, 653
metastatic breast cancer in, 758
myelodysplasia in, 567, 568f
opioid analgesics in, 1246–1247
Olfactory nerve deficit, 29t
Oligoastrocytomas, 1051
  anaplastic, 1052
Oligodendrogliomas, 1051
  anaplastic, 1052
  seizures due to, 23
Oligonucleotides, reverse complementary
    ("antisense"), 383
Omega-3 fatty acids, for cachexia, 7
Omental "cake," due to ovarian carcinoma, 792,
    792f
Omeprazole, with NSAIDs, 1244
Oncocytoma, 167
  renal cell, 826, 826t, 831
Oncofetal proteins, 378
Oncogenes, 380
  with cancer of unknown primary, 1148
Ondansetron
  for cachexia, 8
  for nausea and vomiting, 954, 1251, 1252t
  with interferon-alpha therapy of melanoma,
    1096b
Ontak (denileukin diftitox), 342t, 346–347
Oophorectomy, for metastatic breast cancer, 753t
Open biopsy, of breast mass, 63–64, 70
Ophthalmologic problems, after hematopoietic
    stem cell transplantation, 404
Opioid addiction, 1246
Opioid analgesics
  for back pain, 162
  for dying patient, 1254–1255
  for pain, 1245–1248, 1246t–1248t, 1247b
  in elderly, 1246–1247
  pruritus due to, 15
  side effects of, 1247–1248, 1248t
Opioid conversions, 1247, 1247b
Opioid equianalgesic doses, 1247, 1247t
Opportunistic infections, encephalopathy due to,
    35
Optic nerve deficit, 29t
Oral cavity cancer, 1006–1008, 1008t
Oral contraceptives, and endometrial cancer, 783
Oral discomfort, 1249–1250
Oral hygiene, 1249
Orbital chloromas, in acute myeloid leukemia,
    529, 529f
Orbital lymphoma, 662–663
Orchiectomy, for prostate cancer, 869
Orchitis, mumps, 182
Organ preservation, and radiation therapy,
    327–328
Organotherapy, 1217t
Oropharyngeal cancer, 1005–1006, 1006b
Orthopedic problems, after hematopoietic stem
    cell transplantation, 404
Orthotopic liver transplantation, for
    hepatocellular carcinoma, 902
OSI-774, 387
Osler, Sir William, 703
Osteoarthropathy, hypertrophic pulmonary, in
    non–small cell lung cancer, 963
Osteoblastoma, 154
Osteoclast activating factor (OAF), in multiple
    myeloma, 583
Osteogenesis imperfecta, cutaneous
    manifestations of, 296
Osteomyelitis, vertebral, 161
Osteoporosis
  after hematopoietic stem cell transplantation,
    404
  and breast cancer, 767
  heparin-induced, 518
Osteoporotic vertebral compression fracture, 160,
    162f
Osteoprotegerin, for skeletal complications of
    multiple myeloma, 593
Osteosarcoma, 1028–1032
  classification of, 1029t
  clinical features of, 1028–1029, 1029f, 1029t
  epidemiology of, 1028
  etiology of, 1028
  follow-up for, 1032
  metastatic, 1030, 1031–1032

pathologic fractures due to, 152f, 154
prognostic factors for, 1029–1030
staging of, 1030
treatment of, 1030–1031, 1030f
Ovarian ablation
  for locally invasive breast cancer, 741–742
  for metastatic breast cancer, 753t
Ovarian cancer, 791–802
  ascites due to, 128, 129f, 132
  CA-125 in, 796, 799–801, 800b
  chemotherapy for, 796–799, 797b, 801–802
  clinical evaluation of, 793–794, 793f
  clinical presentation of, 792–793, 792f
  epidemiology of, 791
  familial, 791–792
  genetic testing for, 791–792
  hereditary breast cancer and, 1194, 1194t,
    1195, 1197
  histology of, 795–796, 795f, 795t
  metastases of unknown origin due to, 316
  metastatic, 792, 792f, 793, 795
  pelvic mass due to, 187–188, 188f
  postoperative treatment for, 796–799, 797b
  prognostic factors and outcome for, 796,
    796t
  relapse of, 799–802, 800b
  screening for, 1197
  staging of, 794–795, 794t
  vaginal bleeding due to, 187, 187f
Ovarian cyst, complex, 793, 793f
Oxaliplatin, 335t, 348
  for colorectal cancer, 930
  for esophageal cancer, 878
  as gastric cancer, 896t
Oxcarbazepine (Trileptal), for seizures, 25t, 26b
Oxidant stress, agent associated with, 467, 467t
Oxidative therapy, 1221t
Oxycodone
  for dying patient, 1254t
  for pain, 1245, 1246, 1246t, 1247t
  pruritus due to, 15
Oxydology, 1221t
Oxygen dissociation curve, in erythrocytosis,
    263
Oxygen saturation, in erythrocytosis, 258–259
Oxygen treatments, 1221t
Oxygenation, of tumor, 354
Oxymedicine, 1221t
Oxymetholone
  for aplastic anemia, 448
  for Fanconi's anemia, 450
Oxymorphone, for pain, 1246t

P
p16
  in antiangiogenic therapy, 385
  in familial melanoma, 1201
p21, 382
p53, 382
  in antiangiogenic therapy, 385
  in cancer of unknown primary, 1148
  in cell signaling, 386
  in cervical cancer, 770
  in head and neck cancer, 1008t
  in skin cancer, 1105
Packed red blood cell transfusions, 431–433,
    432f, 433f, 434b, 435f
Paclitaxel (Taxol), 340t, 352–353, 356t
  for bladder cancer, 853–854
  for breast cancer
    locally invasive, 739
    metastatic, 756t, 757, 757t
  for cancer of unknown primary, 1150t,
    1151b, 1153b
  for cervical cancer, 775t
  for esophageal cancer, 878, 878t
  for gastric cancer, 895t, 896t
  for germ-cell tumors, 820, 821b
  for head and neck cancer, 1008t
  for Kaposi's sarcoma, 1160
  for non–small cell lung cancer, 971t, 972,
    976b, 976f, 977f
  for oral cavity cancer, 1008
  for ovarian cancer, 796–799, 797b, 801–802
  for prostate cancer, 872, 873t
  for renal cell cancer, 834t
  side effects of, 798–799
"Pagetoid" cells, in lobular carcinoma in situ, 734

Paget's disease
    nipple discharge in, 73–74
    of vulva, 778
Pain
    assessment of, 1240–1243, 1241f, 1242t
    back. See Back pain.
    bone, due to pathologic fracture, 150
    breakthrough, 1241, 1254t
    cancer-related, 1243
    delirium and, 1242
    end-of-dose, 1241
    facial, due to cranial neuropathy, 29t
    in final days, 1254–1255, 1254t
    incident, 1241
    neuropathic, 1242t, 1243
        adjuvant agents for, 1248–1249, 1249t
    nociceptive, 1242t
    postmastectomy, 1242–1243
    postthoracotomy, 1243
    procedure-related, 1243
    quality of, 1241, 1242t
    somatic, 1242t
    spontaneous, 1241
    therapy-related, 1242–1243
    visceral, 1242t
Pain diaries, 1241
Pain intensity scale, 1241, 1241f
Pain management
    adjuvant agents for, 1248–1249, 1249t
    anesthetic/neurolytic techniques for, 1249
    bisphosphonates for, 1249
    cognitive-behavioral interventions for,
        1244
    in final days, 1254–1255, 1254t
    nonpharmacologic, 1243–1244
    NSAIDs for, 1244–1245, 1245t
    opioids for, 1245–1248, 1246t–1248t,
        1247b
    pharmacologic, 1244–1249
    radiation therapy for, 1249
    radiopharmaceuticals for, 1249
    sedation in, 1256, 1256t
    WHO analgesic ladder for, 1244–1246
Palliation
    for esophageal cancer, 879
    for gallbladder cancer, 906
    for gastric cancer, 894
    for lung cancer
        non–small cell, 970f, 971
        small cell, 954
Pamidronate (Aredia)
    for hypercalcemia, 194, 194t
        in metastatic breast cancer, 760
    for pain, 1249
    for skeletal complications of multiple
        myeloma, 592–593
    for thyroid carcinoma, 1123
Pancoast's syndrome, 961
Pancoast's tumors, 961
Pancreatectomy
    for gastric cancer, 894
    for pancreatic cancer, 915
Pancreatic cancer, 908–918
    adjuvant therapy for, 915
    biology of, 910, 910t
    biopsy of, 913
    chemotherapy for, 915, 916
    diagnostic evaluation of, 911–913, 912f, 913f
    ductal, 910–917
    endocrine, 909, 917–918
    epidemiology of, 908–909, 909t
    genetic factors in, 908–909, 910, 910t
    hormonal therapy for, 916–917
    imaging of, 911–913
    liver metastasis from, 118f
    localized but unresectable, 915–916
    lymphomas as, 918
    management of, 914–917
    metastatic, 916–917
    neoadjuvant therapy for, 915
    pathology of, 909–910, 909t
    presenting symptoms and signs of, 910–911,
        911t
    radiation therapy for, 915–916
    resectable, 914–915
    risk factors for, 908–909, 909t
    sarcomas as, 918
    staging of, 914, 914t

stenting of biliary duct for, 916
    supportive care and symptom management
        for, 917, 917t
Pancreatic cholera, 1135
Pancreatic endocrine tumors, 917–918,
        1135–1136
    classification of, 917
    clinical presentation of, 1134t, 1135–1136
    epidemiology of, 1135
    hormone levels in, 1135t
    localization of, 1136
    metastatic, 120f, 1137
        to liver, 120f
    pathology of, 909
    treatment for, 917–918, 1136, 1136t, 1137
Pancreatic enzymes, for pancreatic cancer, 917
Pancreatoblastomas, 910
Pancreaticoduodenectomy, for pancreatic cancer,
        914–915
Pancreatitis, and pancreatic cancer, 908
Pancytopenia, 251–255
    autoimmune, 253
    causes of, 252–254, 252t
    defined, 251, 251t
    emergency management of, 252b
    history and physical examination for,
        251–253
    laboratory testing for, 253–255, 254t, 255f
    pathogenesis of, 251
    symptoms of, 251
Panendoscopy, for neck mass, 47–48
Panic attacks, 1226, 1227b
Panic disorder, 1226
Panniculitis-like T-cell lymphoma, subcutaneous,
        669
Pap smear
    for vaginal bleeding, 185, 186
    of cervical cancer, 770
Papillary adenocarcinoma, of lung, 968
Papillary renal cell cancer, 825, 826–827, 826t,
        827f
Papillary serous carcinoma
    endometrial, 788, 788t
    of peritoneum, 1153b
Papillary serous cystadenocarcinoma, ovarian,
        795, 795f, 795t
Papilledema, due to cranial neuropathy, 29t
Papilloma
    laryngeal, 51t
    nipple discharge due to, 73
Papillomavirus. See Human papillomavirus
        (HPV).
Pappenheimer bodies, 277
Para-aortic field, 622
Paracentesis, for ascites, 129–131, 132, 133
Paralysis, vocal cord, 51, 51t, 52f, 52t, 54
    causes of, 51t, 52f, 52t
    defined, 51
    diagnosis of, 54
    management of, 56
Paraneoplastic limbic encephalitis, 34t, 35
Paraneoplastic syndromes
    due to thymoma, 983–984, 984f, 984t
    encephalopathy due to, 35
    in hepatocellular carcinoma, 900
    in lung cancer
        non–small cell, 962–963, 962t
        small cell, 944, 946–948
    in renal cell cancer, 828, 828t
    peripheral neuropathy due to, 40
Paraneoplastic vasculitic neuropathy, 37
Parapneumonic effusion, 87
Paraprotein, 201, 201f, 203–204
Parathormone, in calcium homeostasis, 192
Parathormone-related protein (PTHrP), in
        hypercalcemia of malignancy,
        192, 193t
Parenteral nutrition, for cachexia, 6
Parotid gland carcinoma, 46f, 1018–1019, 1020f,
        1021f
Parotidectomy, 1024
Paroxetine (Paxil)
    for depression, 1227, 1227b, 1228
    for hot flashes, 766b
Paroxysmal nocturnal hemoglobinuria (PNH),
        448–450, 468–469
    diagnosis of, 240, 456t, 469
    pancytopenia due to, 254

pathogenesis of, 448–449
    pathophysiology of, 468–469
    treatment for, 449–450, 449f, 469
Partial thromboplastin time (PTT), 268f
    prolongation of, 266–267, 267t
Parvovirus infection, bone marrow failure due
        to, 451
Pathologic fractures, 149–155
    causes of, 150–152, 151t
    clinical evaluation of, 149b, 152–153, 152b,
        152f
    definitive treatment of, 153–154, 154f, 155f
    issues to explore with, 149–150
    presenting features of, 150, 150f, 151f
    primary management of, 153
Patient education, 1232, 1258
Pau d'arco, 1213t
Pauling, Linus, 1216
Pautrier microabscesses, 664
Paxil (paroxetine)
    for depression, 1227, 1227b, 1228
    for hot flashes, 766b
PCACP gene, in prostate cancer, 1203
PCNSL (primary central nervous system
        lymphoma), 1053–1054, 1055f,
        1056b
PC-SPES, 1214t
    for prostate cancer, 872
PCV. See Polycythemia vera (PCV).
Pediatric patients. See Children.
Pegylated doxorubicin (Doxil), for multiple
        myeloma, 590
Pegylated recombinant human megakaryocytic
        growth and development factor
        (PEG-rHuMGDF), for acute
        myeloid leukemia, 533
Pelger-Huet cells, 230b, 238, 239f, 245, 270,
        278–279, 279f
Pelvic mass, 187–190
    differential diagnosis of, 187–189, 189t
    etiology of, 187, 188f
    evaluation of, 189, 190f
    management of, 190
    physiologic, 188
Pelvic ultrasound, for vaginal bleeding, 186
Pemberton's sign, 101
Pemetrexed, for mesothelioma, 995, 995t
Penile injections, 1238
Penile lentiginosis, 311
Penile prosthesis, 1238
Pentaerythritol tetranitrate (PTEN), 387
Pentobarbital
    for brain metastases, 1069b
    for refractory pain, 1256t
Pentostatin (2-deoxycoformycin), 336t, 355t
    for hairy cell leukemia, 698
Pentoxifylline, for cachexia, 8
PEP-CK (phosphoenol pyruvate carboxykinase),
        1219
Peptic ulcer disease
    GI bleeding due to, 144
    in polycythemia vera, 702
Percent saturation, 209t
Percutaneous endoscopic gastrostomy, for
        cachexia, 6
Percutaneous pericardiocentesis, 77, 79
Percutaneous stent, for superior vena cava
        syndrome, 103–104
Percutaneous transhepatic cholangiography
        (PTC), for biliary cancer, 903,
        905b
Performance status, in non–small cell lung
        cancer, 965
Pericardial effusion, dyspnea due to, 76
Pericardial involvement, in lung cancer, 961
Pericardiocentesis, percutaneous, 77, 79
Periductal mastitis, 74
Perifollicular purpura, 296, 297f
Perineum, as source of vaginal bleeding, 185t
Peripheral blood myeloid immaturity,
        neutrophilia with, 243–244, 243f,
        244f
Peripheral blood progenitor cells, mobilization of,
        myeloid growth factors for, 427,
        427t
Peripheral blood smear, 272–282
    for anemia, 235, 236t, 237f
    general approach to, 272–273, 272b, 273f

Peripheral blood smear, (Continued)
    in chronic lymphocytic leukemia, 690, 690f
    in myelodysplasia, 570, 570t, 571f, 572t
    infection as cause of abnormalities in, 282
    platelet abnormalities on, 280–282, 281f
    red cell abnormalities on, 273–277,
        274f–276f
        in anemias, 272b, 276–277, 277f
    red cell inclusions on, 277, 277f, 278f
    rouleaux formation on, 272, 273f
    white blood cell abnormalities on, 277–280,
        278f–281f
Peripheral neuropathy, 36–40
    causes of, 36–37, 36t, 40
    clinical features of, 36, 36t
    differential diagnosis of, 37
    due to paclitaxel and carboplatin, 798–799
    evaluation of, 37, 38f, 39b, 39t
    in multiple myeloma, 585
    management of, 40, 40b
Peripheral T-cell lymphoma, 664–671
    classification of, 664, 665t
    clinical evaluation of, 670
    clinical presentation of, 667–668, 667t, 668t
    defined, 664
    diagnosis of, 607–609, 608f, 612
    mycosis fungoides and Sézary syndrome as,
        664–667, 665f, 666f
    prognostic features and outcome for, 670
    treatment for, 670–671
    types of, 668–670
    unspecified, 607–609, 669
Peritoneal carcinomatosis, of unknown origin,
    1153b
Peritoneal chemotherapy, 368–369
Peritoneal lavage, 365–366
Peritoneal serous cancers, primary, 791
Peritoneovenous shunt, for ascites, 131, 133,
    133f
Peritonitis, infectious, ascites due to, 131
Pernicious anemia, 233t, 455–457
    and gastric cancer, 888
Persistent gestational trophoblastic tumors,
    807–811
    clinical presentation of, 807
    diagnosis and staging of, 807–809, 808t, 809t
    metastatic, 807–808, 808t, 810–811
    molar pregnancy and, 807, 807b
    nonmetastatic, 809–810, 809f, 810t
    treatment for, 809–811, 809f, 810t
Personalismo, 1230
PET. See Positron emission tomography (PET).
Petechiae, 294, 294f
Ph (Philadelphia chromosome), 243, 678–679,
    679f
Ph (Philadelphia chromosome)–positive acute
    lymphoblastic leukemia, 561–562
Phagocytosis, in chronic granulomatous disease,
    480
Phantom choriocarcinoma, 811–812
Phantom hCG syndrome, 811–812
Phenergan (promethazine), for nausea and
    vomiting, 1256
Phenobarbital
    for refractory pain, 1256t
    for seizures, 25t
Phenothiazines, for nausea and vomiting, 1251
Phenytoin
    for brain metastases, 1069, 1069b
    for neuropathic pain, 1248, 1249t
    for seizures, 25t, 26b
Pheochromocytoma, 169, 170–171
    and thyroid carcinoma, 1125
Philadelphia chromosome (Ph), 243, 678–679,
    679f
Philadelphia chromosome (Ph)–positive acute
    lymphoblastic leukemia, 561–562
Phlebitis, superficial, 283
Phlebotomy, for polycythemia vera, 702b,
    704–705
Phobias, 1226
PhosLo (calcium acetate), for
    hyperphosphatemia, 1189
Phosphatidylinositol glycan class A (PIG-A) gene,
    469
Phosphoenol pyruvate carboxykinase (PEP-CK),
    1219
Phospholipase C, in cell signaling, 386

Phosphorous, for hypercalcemia, 194
Photodynamic therapy, for non–small cell lung
    cancer, 971
Photoelectric effect, 321
Photons, in radiation therapy, 321
Phrenic nerve entrapment, due to lung cancer,
    961
Physical status, functional classification of, 363t
Physician-patient working relationship,
    1231–1233, 1232b
Physiologic jaundice, 198
PI3-kinase, 387
PIG-A (phosphatidylinositol glycan class A) gene,
    469
Pigmented basal cell carcinoma, 308t
Pigmented dermatofibroma, 308t
Pigmented skin lesions, 305–312
    algorithm for evaluation of, 307t
    biopsy of, 308, 311–312
    evaluation of, 305–308, 307f, 308t, 309f,
        310f
    in unusual locations, 308–311, 312b
    management of, 305, 307t
    risk factors for melanoma with, 305, 306b
    screening for, 305, 307t
    suspicious features of, 305, 306f, 306t,
        307f
Pigmented squamous cell carcinoma, 308t
Pilocytic astrocytomas, 1051
Pituitary adenoma, 1139–1142
    clinical evaluation of, 1140–1141, 1141f
    clinical presentation of, 1139–1140
    corticotroph, 1140, 1142t
    epidemiology of, 1139
    galactorrhea due to, 71
    gonadotroph, 1140, 1142t
    hormonal findings with, 1139, 1140–1141,
        1142t
    lactotroph, 1140, 1142t
    macro-, 1139–1140, 1141f, 1142t
    micro-, 1139, 1140, 1142t
    nonsecretory, 1139–1140, 1142t
    secretory, 1140
    somatotroph, 1140, 1142t
    thyrotroph, 1140, 1142t
    treatment of, 1141–1142, 1142t
    types and relative frequency of, 1139–1140,
        1140t
Pituitary apoplexy, 1140
Pituitary gland metastases, of small cell lung
    cancer, 946
Pituitary tumor, therapy considerations for,
    1143b
Placebo effect, with pruritus, 16
Placental site trophoblastic tumor (PSTT), 807,
    811
Planning target volume (PTV), 324
Plasma, immunology of, 437, 437t
Plasma exchange, for thrombotic
    thrombocytopenic purpura, 492,
    493
Plasma transfusions, 432t, 436–437, 437t
Plasmacytoma(s), 154
    and multiple myeloma, 586t, 593–595
    immunoglobulin abnormalities due to, 205
    soft-tissue, 154
    solitary, of bone, 586t, 593–595
Plasmapheresis
    for pure red cell aplasia, 450
    for warm antibody autoimmune hemolytic
        anemia, 473b
Plasminogen activators and inhibitors, in breast
    cancer, 723
Platelet(s)
    continuous infusions of, 436
    decreased production of, 225, 225t, 485–
        487
    defined, 485
    fresh, 436
    human leukocyte antigen–matched and
        cross-matched, 436, 452
    immunology of, 434–435
    in anemia, 236t
    increased destruction of, 225–226, 225t,
        487
    refractoriness of, 435–436
    single-donor, 436
    structure of, 485

Platelet abnormalities, 485–495. See also
        Thrombocytopenia.
    causes of, 485, 486b
    functional, 267, 270–271, 494–495
    morphologic, 253, 280–282, 281f
Platelet clumps, 281f, 282
Platelet counts
    fetal, 491–492
    high. See Thrombocythemia; Thrombocytosis.
    low. See Thrombocytopenia.
    normal, 221
Platelet factor 4, in antiangiogenic therapy, 385
Platelet satellitism, 281f, 282
Platelet thrombus formation, 485
Platelet transfusions, 432t, 434–436
    for acquired platelet function disorders, 495
    for acute myeloid leukemia, 533
    for bone marrow failure syndrome, 451–452
    for idiopathic thrombocytopenic purpura,
        491
    for myelodysplasia, 575b
    for thrombocytopenia, 486
Platinating agents (platinum analogues), 332t,
        335t, 348
Pleomorphic carcinoma, of lung, 968t, 969
Plethora, in erythrocytosis, 257, 258f
Plethysmography, impedance, for deep vein
        thrombosis, 287
Pleural biopsy, 77
Pleural catheter, chronic indwelling, 92–93, 92f
Pleural effusion(s), 87–93
    benign, 87, 88t, 89, 89t
    biopsy of, 89
    causes of, 87, 88t
    chest tube for, 90–91
    chronic indwelling pleural catheter for,
        92–93, 92f
    decortication and radical surgery for, 93
    differential diagnosis of, 87–89, 88t, 89t
    dyspnea due to, 75–76, 77, 79
    fluid analysis for, 89, 89t
    imaging studies of, 88
    in lung cancer, 960
        small cell, 954
    in superior vena cava syndrome, 101
    interventional procedures for, 88–89
    malignant, 87, 88t, 89–93, 89t, 91f, 92f, 975
    management of, 89–93, 90f–92f
    pathogenesis of, 87
    pleurodesis for, 91–92, 91f
    therapeutic thoracentesis for, 88–89, 91f
Pleural metastases, of breast cancer, 751t
Pleurectomy, for mesothelioma, 993–994
Pleurodesis, 79
    for mesothelioma, 992–993
    for pleural effusion, 91–92, 91f
Pleuroscopy, for mesothelioma, 992–993
Plexopathy, 37
Plicamycin, for hypercalcemia, 194, 194t
PLL (prolymphocytic leukemia), 248, 689,
        696–697
PMS1 gene, 1200
PMS2 gene, 1200
PNET (primitive neuroectodermal tumors),
        1029t, 1034, 1040, 1045
Pneumococcus infection, febrile neutropenia due
        to, 1174, 1175
Pneumocystis carinii
    febrile neutropenia due to, 1174
    with hematopoietic stem cell transplantation,
        403
Pneumonectomy
    extrapleural, for mesothelioma, 991f, 994,
        994f
    for non–small cell lung cancer, 970–971, 974
    radical pleural, for pleural effusion, 93
Pneumonitis
    due to treatment for Hodgkin's disease, 630
    radiation, in small cell lung cancer, 955
PNH. See Paroxysmal nocturnal hemoglobinuria
        (PNH).
POEMS syndrome, 583, 593, 594
Poikilocytosis, 274
Polychromatophilia, 237f, 275, 275f
Polyclonal gammopathy, 201–202, 201f, 202t
Polycythemia. See also Erythrocytosis.
    defined, 256
    due to cancer, 1168

Polycythemia vera (PCV), 701–706. *See also* Erythrocytosis.
  bone marrow aspiration and biopsy for, 261, 262f
  burst-forming unit erythroid assays for, 261–262
  clinical evaluation of, 259t, 702–704, 703t
  clinical presentation of, 701–702, 702b
  c-mpl in, 262
  complete blood count in, 258
  complications of, 704t
  epidemiology of, 701
  follow-up evaluation for, 706
  GI bleeding due to, 145
  in pregnancy, 704
  marrow karyotype studies for, 261
  neutrophilia due to, 244
  pruritus due to, 15, 17b
  PRV-1 expression in, 262–263
  serum erythropoietin in, 260
  signs and symptoms of, 257–258, 258f, 258t, 259f
  splenomegaly in, 258, 259f, 260, 261f
  staging, prognostic features, and outcome of, 704
  treatment of, 702b, 704–705, 704t
Polymerized microtubules, drugs that stabilize, 340t, 352–353
Polyneuropathy, in Waldenström's macroglobulinemia, 597–598
Polyp(s)
  adenomatous, and colorectal cancer, 923–924, 923f, 924f
  colonic, GI bleeding due to, 145
  gastric adenomatous, and gastric cancer, 889
  urethral, hematuria due to, 174t
Polyposis, familial adenomatous, 1199–1200
  and colorectal cancer, 921, 1199–1200
  genetic basis for, 1194t
  prophylactic surgery for, 371–372
Polyprenoic acid, for hepatocellular carcinoma, 903
Polystyrene sulfonate (Kayexalate), for hyperkalemia, 1189
Popcorn cells, 608f, 611
Positron emission tomography (PET)
  of cancer of unknown primary, 1149
  of esophageal cancer, 877, 883
  of gastric cancer, 891
  of germ-cell tumors, 814
  of mesothelioma, 991
  of non–small cell lung cancer, 966
  of pancreatic cancer, 913
Positron emission tomography–fluorodeoxyglucose (PET-FDG) imaging
  of liver, 116
  of solitary pulmonary nodule, 85, 85f
Postictal hemiparesis, 1064
Postmastectomy syndrome, 1242–1243
Postphlebitic syndrome, 289
Postremission therapy
  for acute lymphoblastic leukemia, 558
  for acute myeloid leukemia, 531t, 534–540
Postthoracotomy pain, 1243
Posttransfusion purpura, 486b
Posttransplant lymphoproliferative disease (PTLPD), 1161–1164, 1163b
  classification of, 1161, 1162t
  clinical evaluation of, 1162–1163
  clinical presentation of, 1161
  epidemiology of, 1161
  pathology of, 1161–1162
  prevention of, 1164
  risk factors for, 1161
  therapy for, 1163–1164, 1163b
Posttraumatic stress disorder (PTSD), 1226, 1227b
Potassium-sparing diuretics, for ascites, 131
PPoma, 1134t, 1136
PPSC (primary peritoneal serous cancers), 791
Preauricular adenopathy, 215t
Precursor B-cell lymphoblastic leukemia, 601–602
Precursor B-cell lymphoblastic lymphoma, 601–602
Precursor T-cell lymphoblastic leukemia, 601–602

Precursor T-cell lymphoblastic lymphoma, 601–602, 604f
Prednisone
  for acute lymphoblastic leukemia, 557t, 558t
  for aplastic anemia, acute severe, 445
  for Burkitt's leukemia/lymphoma, 562t
  for cachexia, 7
  for hypercalcemia, 194t
  for idiopathic thrombocytopenic purpura, 489, 490f, 491, 492
  for multiple myeloma, 588, 589b
  for neuropathic pain, 1249t
  for paroxysmal nocturnal hemoglobinuria, 449
  for prostate cancer, 872, 873t
  for pure red cell aplasia, 450
  for thymoma, 989t
  for warm antibody autoimmune hemolytic anemia, 473b
Pregnancy
  bloody nipple discharge in, 73
  breast masses in, 62–63
  Hodgkin's disease in, 628–629
  idiopathic thrombocytopenic purpura in, 491–492
  molar, 804–806, 805t, 807, 807b, 811
  pelvic mass in, 188
  polycythemia vera in, 704
  thrombocytopenia in, 493–494
  vaginal bleeding in, 184–185, 185f
  venous thromboembolism in, 516–517
Prematurity, anemia of, 420–421
Preoperative chemoradiotherapy, for esophageal cancer, 881–883
Preoperative chemotherapy
  for esophageal cancer, 879, 880–881, 881f, 881t
  for osteosarcoma, 1031
Pressure sores, 1252–1253
Prevention
  of colorectal cancer, 924, 924t
  of non–small cell lung cancer, 970f, 976–978, 977b
  of posttransplant lymphoproliferative disease, 1164
  of prostate cancer, 860–861
  of thromboembolic disease, 1183–1185
Primary central nervous system lymphoma (PCNSL), 1053–1054, 1055f, 1056b
Primary peritoneal serous cancers (PPSC), 791
Primary purpura fulminans, 301–302, 302f
Primary tumor, in breast cancer staging, 715–717, 716t
Priming therapy, with myeloid growth factors, 424, 425t
Primitive neuroectodermal tumors (PNET), 1029t, 1034, 1040, 1045
Procarbazine, for high-grade gliomas, 1053, 1054b
Prochlorperazine, with interferon-alpha therapy of melanoma, 1096b
Prochlorperazine (Compazine), for nausea and vomiting, 1251t, 1252t
Progesterone, for cachexia, 6–7
Progesterone receptors, in breast cancer, 721
Progestin(s), 342t
  for endometrial cancer, 786, 787–788
  for metastatic breast cancer, 753t, 755
Programmed cell death, in radiation therapy, 323
Projectile vomiting, headache with, 21b
Prolactin deficiency, due to pituitary adenoma, 1142t
Prolactin excess, due to pituitary adenoma, 1142t
Prolactin levels, in galactorrhea, 71
Prolactinomas, 1140
Proliferative indices, for breast cancer, 722–723
Prolymphocytic leukemia (PLL), 248, 689, 696–697
ProMACE-CytaBOM regimen, for non-Hodgkin's lymphoma, intermediate-grade, 651t, 652
Promethazine (Phenergan), for nausea and vomiting, 1256
Promyelocytic leukemia, acute. *See* Acute promyelocytic leukemia.

Prophylactic cranial irradiation, for small cell lung cancer, 953, 954–955
Prophylactic gastrointestinal cancer surgery, 371–372
Prophylactic mastectomy, 1196–1197
Prophylactic salpingo-oophorectomy, 1197
Prophylaxis
  antiemetic, 1250, 1251t
  for febrile neutropenia, 1178
  for hyperuricemia, 1187
  for seizures, 25
Propionic acids, for pain, 1245t
Propofol, for brain metastases, 1069b
Prostate acid phosphatase. *See* Prostate-specific antigen (PSA).
Prostate cancer, 859–873
  androgen-independent, 871–873, 873t
  antiandrogens for, 344
  brachytherapy for, 868
  chemotherapy for, 872–873, 873t
  clinical presentations of, 862–863
  cranial neuropathies in, 27, 28t
  epidemiology of, 859–860
  genetics of, 860, 1202
  headache with, 21t
  hormonal therapy for, 867, 869–871, 872
  metastatic, 863–864, 873
  newly diagnosed
    clinical evaluation of, 863–864, 863b
    primary therapy for, 865–869
  prevention of, 860–861
  radiation therapy for, 867–868, 867t, 873
  radical prostatectomy for, 866–867, 866t
  risk factors for, 860
  screening for, 864–865, 865t
  staging of, 861–862, 861t, 862t
  watchful waiting for, 863b, 868–869
Prostatectomy, for prostate cancer, 866–867, 866t
Prostate-specific antigen (PSA), 290, 861, 862t, 864
Protamine sulfate, for heparin-induced bleeding, 517
Protein C assay, 289, 289b
Protein C resistance, activated, 289b
Protein S assay, 289b
Protein spike, 201, 201f, 203–204
Proteolysis-inducing factor, in cachexia, 4–5
Prothrombic risk factors, with idiopathic deep vein thrombosis, 289–290, 290t
Prothrombin G20210A mutation, 289b
Prothrombin time, 268f
  prolongation of, 266–267, 267t
Proto-oncogenes, 382
Protoporphyrin levels, 210
Prozac (fluoxetine), 1227, 1227b
  for hot flashes, 766b
Prudden, John F., 1217t, 1220–1221
Pruritus
  aquagenic, 15
    in polycythemia vera, 705
  changes in skin due to scratching from, 16, 17f
  diagnostic considerations in, 17b
  due to allergic drug reactions, 15
  due to cancer, 16, 17b
  due to central nervous system effects, 15
  due to chronic renal disease, 14–15
  due to hypereosinophilic syndromes, 16
  due to leukemia, 16
  due to lymphomas, 16, 17b
  due to mycosis fungoides, 16
  due to myeloproliferative disorders, 702b
  due to obstructive hepatobiliary disease, 14
  due to opioids, 15
  due to polycythemia vera, 15, 17b, 705
  general therapeutic considerations for, 16–17
  systemic causes of, 14–17, 15t
PRV-1 expression, in erythrocytosis, 262–263
PS-341, for multiple myeloma, 591
PSA (prostate-specific antigen), 290, 861, 862t, 864
Psammoma bodies
  in lung cancer, 968
  in ovarian cancer, 795, 795f
Psammoma calcifications, 728
Pseudallescheria boydii, febrile neutropenia due to, 1177b

Pseudo-Gaucher cells, in chronic myeloid leukemia, 677
Pseudo-Hutchinson sign, 310f
Pseudomonas aeruginosa, febrile neutropenia due to, 1173, 1174, 1174f
"Pseudopods," 305
Pseudoxanthoma elasticum, cutaneous manifestations of, 296
Psoralen-activated ultraviolet light irradiation (PUVA)
    for graft-*versus*-host disease, 397
    for mycosis fungoides and Sézary syndrome, 666
PSTT (placental site trophoblastic tumor), 807, 811
Psychiatric disorders, 1224–1226, 1226b
    medication options for, 1227–1228, 1227b
Psychogenic purpura, 300, 300f
Psychological assessment, for pain, 1241–1242
Psychological counseling, for pain management, 1244
Psychological disorders, 1224–1226, 1226b
    medication options for, 1227–1228, 1227b
Psychological distress, 1224–1231
Psychomotor seizures, 23
Psychosocial issue(s), 1224–1233
    adjustment to cancer diagnosis as, 1224, 1225b
    depressive and anxiety disorders as, 1224–1226, 1226b, 1233b
    ethnic and cultural issues as, 1230–1231
    for caregiver, 1228–1229
    for children, 1229–1230, 1230b, 1233
    for family, 1228–1230, 1228b
    medication options for, 1227–1228, 1227b
    physician-patient working relationship as, 1231–1233, 1232b
    psychological distress as, 1224–1231
    with brain tumors, 1058
    with breast cancer, 761, 767, 767t
    with hematopoietic stem cell transplantation, 399, 405
Psychotic symptoms, 1227b
PTC (percutaneous transhepatic cholangiography), for biliary cancer, 903, 905b
PTC gene, in nevoid basal cell carcinoma, 1201
PTCH gene, in skin cancer, 1105
PTEN (pentaerythritol tetranitrate), 387
PTEN gene, 1194, 1198
PTHrP (parathormone-related protein), in hypercalcemia of malignancy, 192, 193t
PTLPD. *See* Posttransplant lymphoproliferative disease (PTLPD).
PTSD (posttraumatic stress disorder), 1226, 1227b
PTT (partial thromboplastin time), 268f
    prolongation of, 266–267, 267t
PTV (planning target volume), 324
Pulmonary complications, of Hodgkin's disease, 630
Pulmonary contrast angiography, 287
Pulmonary embolectomy, 514t, 519
Pulmonary embolism
    clinical features predicting probability of, 284–285, 285t
    diagnosis of
        algorithm for, 286f, 513f
        clinical assessment for, 284–285
        laboratory testing for, 285–287
        objective tests for, 287–289, 288f, 289f, 512–513, 513f
    risk factors for, 289–290, 289b
    thrombolytic therapy for, 514t, 518–519
Pulmonary endarterectomy, 514t, 519
Pulmonary infection, due to lung cancer, 961
Pulmonary nodule, solitary, 81–86
    biopsy of, 85–86
    calcifications in, 81, 83b, 84, 84f
    cavitation of, 83
    chest radiography of, 81, 83b
    computed tomography of, 81–84, 83t, 84t
        enhanced, 84–85
    contours and margins of, 82–83, 83f
    defined, 81, 82f
    density of, 83–84, 84f
    differential diagnosis of, 81, 82t
    fat in, 84
    indeterminate, 85b

positron emission tomography imaging of, 85, 85f
    size of, 81, 82
    vascular and bronchial relationships of, 83, 84f
    vs. mass, 81
Pulmonary toxicity, drug-induced, dyspnea due to, 76–77, 78t
Punch biopsy
    for peripheral neuropathy, 39t
    of vulva, 776b, 776f, 777f
Pure estrogen antagonists, for metastatic breast cancer, 754
Pure red cell aplasia, 450–451
    due to cancer, 1167
    due to chronic lymphocytic leukemia, 690
    due to thymoma, 984
Pure white cell aplasia, 451
Purine analogues, 332t, 336t
    for hairy cell leukemia, 698
Purpura, 294, 294f
    autoimmune (idiopathic) thrombocytopenic, 488–492, 490f
    factitious, 268
    fulminans, 301–302, 302f
    Gaugerot-Blum, 300
    "glove and socks" papular, 300
    Henoch-Schönlein, 298
    hypergammaglobulinemic, 299, 300f
    perifollicular, 296, 297f
    posttransfusion, 486b
    psychogenic, 300, 300f
    senile, 296–297, 297f, 298f
    stasis, 301, 301f
    thrombotic thrombocytopenic
        clinical presentation of, 239, 269, 492
        diagnosis of, 492
        etiology of, 492
        red blood cell abnormalities in, 274–275, 492f
        relapsing, 269b
        therapy for, 492–493
    "wet" *vs.* "dry," 222
PUVA (psoralen-activated ultraviolet light irradiation)
    for graft-*versus*-host disease, 397
    for mycosis fungoides and Sézary syndrome, 666
Pyelogram
    intravenous, for hematuria, 175
    retrograde, for hematuria, 177f
Pyrimidine analogues, 332t, 335t

Q
Quetiapine (Seroquel), 1227b

R
RA (refractory anemia), 572, 573
Rad, 321
"Radial streaming," 305
Radiation
    energy of, 321, 322f
    external *vs.* internal, 321–322
    for meningiomas, 1055
    interaction of cells with, 322–323
    interaction of tissues and organs with, 323
    measurement of, 321
Radiation cystitis, 173, 176, 177
Radiation exposure
    acute lymphoblastic leukemia due to, 550
    acute myeloid leukemia due to, 523
    myelodysplasia due to, 569, 569t
    thyroid carcinoma due to, 1120
Radiation oncology, 321
Radiation pneumonitis, in small cell lung cancer, 955
"Radiation recall," with anthracyclines, 350
Radiation therapy, 321–329
    and organ preservation, 327–328
    and pancreatic cancer, 908
    as adjuvant therapy, 327–328, 328t
    as conditioning regimen for hematopoietic stem cell transplantation
        allogeneic, 395, 395t, 396t
        autologous, 399
    automated dose optimization (inverse planning) for, 326
    beam arrangement for, 325–326, 325f, 326f
    cellular effect of, 322–323

clinical applications of, 326–328, 328t
    dose distribution for, 325–326, 326f
    dose volume histograms for, 326, 326f
    for adrenal cancer, 1130
    for anal carcinoma, 939–941
    for basal cell carcinoma, 1107
    for biliary cancer, 904–905
    for bladder cancer, 846
    for brain metastases, 1069, 1070–1072, 1071t, 1072t
    for brain tumors, 1051
    for breast cancer
        ductal carcinoma in situ, 730b, 731–732, 731f, 732t
        locally invasive, 737–738, 743t
    for cervical cancer, 772, 773b, 773t
    for CNS lymphoma, 1054, 1056b
    for colorectal cancer, 932–933
    for endometrial cancer, 787
    for epidural cancer, 1081–1082, 1083
    for esophageal cancer, 877–878
        locally advanced, 884b
        neoadjuvant, 879–880, 881t
        palliative, 879
        preoperative, 881–883
        vs. surgery, 884
        with chemotherapy, 881–883, 883f, 884
    for Ewing's sarcoma, 1035
    for gastric cancer, 894–895, 896–897, 897f, 897t
    for germ-cell tumor, 823
    for gestational trophoblastic tumor, 811
    for gliomas
        high-grade, 1053, 1054b
        low-grade, 1051, 1052b
    for hemoptysis, 108
    for Hodgkin's disease, 622, 625–626
    for laryngeal cancer, 1002, 1003, 1003t
    for lung cancer
        non–small cell, 970, 970f, 971, 972–973, 974
        small cell, 951b, 952, 952b, 953, 954
    for lymphoma
        intermediate-grade, 651
        low-grade, 639
    for melanoma, 1095
    for Merkel cell carcinoma, 1114
    for mesothelioma, 994–995
    for mycosis fungoides, 666
    for nasopharyngeal cancer, 1009
    for oral cavity cancer, 1007
    for oropharyngeal cancer, 1006, 1006b
    for pain, 1249
    for palliation of symptoms, 328
    for pancreatic cancer, 915–916
    for pituitary adenoma, 1141–1142
    for prostate cancer, 867–868, 867t, 873
    for renal cell cancer, 838
    for salivary gland carcinoma, 1022, 1023
    for seminoma, 815, 817t
    for soft tissue sarcoma, 1044, 1045
    for squamous cell carcinoma, 1111–1112
    for superior vena cava syndrome, 103
    for thymoma, 987–988
    for thyroid carcinoma
        differentiated, 1123
        medullary, 1126
    for vaginal cancer, 779
    fractionation for, 323, 326, 327
    future of, 328–329
    in oncologic emergencies, 328
    intraoperative, 368
        and peritoneal chemotherapy, 368–369
    methods of administration of, 321–322, 322f
    neutropenia due to, 245
    pancytopenia due to, 253
    peripheral neuropathy due to, 40
    photons and electrons in, 321
    preoperative *vs.* postoperative, 328, 328t
    pulmonary toxicity due to, 76–77, 78t
    reason for efficacy of, 323
    second malignancies in, 322
    side effects of, 323
    surgical management of complications of, 371
    tissue and organ effects of, 323
    treatment planning for, 323–326, 324f–326f
    treatment simulator for, 324, 324f
    treatment strategies for, 327–328, 328t
    with curative intent, 327

Radiation Therapy Oncology Group (RTOG)
    Recursive Partitioning Tree, 1067, 1067f
Radiculopathy
    herpes zoster spinal, 159t, 161, 162, 162t
    in multiple myeloma, 585
Radiofrequency hyperthermia, for hepatocellular carcinoma, 902
Radiographic assessment. See Imaging studies.
Radioimmune-guided surgery, 366–367
Radioiodine therapy, for thyroid carcinoma, 1122–1123
Radionuclide imaging
    for epidural cancer, 1080–1081
    for thyroid nodule, 1117
Radiopharmaceuticals, for pain, 1249
RAEB (refractory anemia with excess blasts), 572
RAEB-T (refractory anemia with excess blasts in transformation), 523, 572
Rai system, for chronic lymphocytic leukemia, 691–692, 692t
Raloxifene (Evista), 341t, 344
Ranitidine, with interferon-alpha therapy of melanoma, 1096b
RANK ligand, in multiple myeloma, 583–584
Rapamycin, 387
RARα (retinoic acid receptor α) gene, in acute myeloid leukemia, 525
RARS (refractory anemia with ring sideroblasts), 572, 573
ras oncogene, 386–387
    in cancer of unknown primary, 1148
    in head and neck cancer, 1008t
RB (retinoblastoma) gene, in cervical cancer, 770
Rb protein, 382, 386
Rb1 gene, 1040, 1193, 1203
RBCs. See Red blood cell(s) (RBCs).
RDW (red cell distribution width), 235, 272b
Reactive neutrophilic leukocytosis, 241–242, 242f, 242t
REAL (Revised European-American Lymphoma) classification, 601, 611, 636, 664
    for peripheral T-cell lymphoma, 664
Recombinant vaccines, 381
Reconstructive surgery, after mastectomy, 763–764
Rectal bleeding, 145–146
    due to colorectal cancer, 926, 926t
Rectal cancer, 931–932. See also Colorectal cancer.
Rectal carcinoid tumors, 1134t, 1135
Rectum, obstruction of, 110t
Red blood cell(s) (RBCs)
    agglutination of, 272, 273f
    hypochromic, 273, 274f
    immunology of, 432–433
    in anemia, 236t, 237f
    in iron deficient erythropoiesis, 207
    in pancytopenia, 253
    normal, 273, 273f
    normochromic, 273
    nucleated, 253, 275, 277
Red blood cell (RBC) aplasia, 240, 240b
    pure, 450–451
        due to cancer, 1167
        due to thymoma, 984
        in chronic lymphocytic leukemia, 690
Red blood cell (RBC) disorder(s), 455–473, 456t
    anemia of chronic disease as, 456t, 457–458
    autoimmune hemolytic anemias as, 456t, 469–472, 470f, 470t
        cold, 470t, 471–472, 472f
        warm, 470–471, 470t, 472f, 473b
    due to cancer, 1166–1168, 1167f, 1168f, 1169t
    due to vitamin B12 deficiency, 455–457, 456t
    folate deficiency as, 455–457, 456t
    glucose-6-phosphate dehydrogenase deficiency as, 456t, 466–468, 466f, 467f, 467t
    hemoglobinopathies as, 456t, 458–466, 458f
    hereditary elliptocytosis as, 468
    hereditary spherocytosis as, 456t, 468
    in myelodysplasia, 570t
    iron deficiency anemia as, 455, 456b, 456t
    membrane abnormalities as, 456t, 468–469
    on peripheral smear, 273–277, 274f–276f

paroxysmal nocturnal hemoglobinuria as, 456t, 468–469
    sickle-cell disease as, 456t, 462–466, 462f, 463f, 463t, 464b, 464t, 465b
    α-thalassemia as, 456t, 458–459, 459t
    β-thalassemia as, 456t, 459–462, 460b, 461f, 461t, 462b
Red blood cell (RBC) inclusions, on peripheral smear, 277, 277f, 278f
Red blood cell (RBC) indices, 273
    for anemia, 234–235, 235f, 235t
Red blood cell (RBC) transfusions, 431–433, 432t, 433f, 434b, 435f
    for bone marrow failure syndrome, 451
    for myelodysplasia, 575b
Red cell distribution width (RDW), 235, 272b
Red cell mass
    in erythrocytosis, 256
    in polycythemia vera, 703
Red clover, 1215
Reed, Dorothy, 629
Reed-Sternberg (R-S) cells, 608f, 609, 610, 611
Reflux laryngitis, 51t
Refractory anemia (RA), 572, 573
Refractory anemia with excess blasts (RAEB), 572
Refractory anemia with excess blasts in transformation (RAEB-T), 523, 572
Refractory anemia with ring sideroblasts (RARS), 572, 573
Refractory disease, defined, 556t
Regional lymph nodes
    in breast cancer staging, 716t, 717–719, 717t
    in melanoma, 1092–1093
Reinduction therapy, for acute myeloid leukemia, 541–542, 541f, 542t
Reinke's edema, 51t
Relapsed disease, defined, 556t
Relaxation, for pain management, 1244
Release disease, 270
rem (roentgen equivalent in man), 321
Remission, cytogenetic or molecular complete, defined, 556t
Remission consolidation therapy. See Intensive consolidation chemotherapy.
Remission induction therapy. See Induction therapy.
Remnant ablation, for thyroid carcinoma, 1122
Renal angiomyolipoma, 167, 168f
Renal cell cancer, 825–839
    chromophobe, 825–826, 826t, 827f, 831
    clear-cell, 825, 826, 826t, 827f
    clinical evaluation of, 828–831, 829f, 830f
    clinical presentation of, 828, 828t
    collecting duct, 826, 826t, 827–828, 827f
    cranial neuropathies due to, 28t
    diagnosis of, 167, 167f
    epidemiology of, 825
    erythrocytosis due to, 259–260, 260f
    follow-up evaluation of, 838–839, 839b
    genetics of, 826–828
    headache with, 21t
    hematuria due to, 173, 173b
    hereditary papillary, 1194t
    histologic subtypes of, 825–826, 826t, 827f
    metastatic
        chemotherapy/hormonal therapy for, 834, 834t
        debulking nephrectomy for, 833, 833b
        immunotherapy for, 834–838, 835t, 836t, 837f, 838f, 838t
        radiation therapy for, 838
        to bone, 150f, 151f
    oncocytoma form of, 826, 826t, 831
    papillary, 825, 826–827, 826t, 827f
    paraneoplastic syndromes with, 828, 828t
    risk factors for, 825
    sarcomatoid, 827f
    staging, prognostic features, and outcome of, 831–832, 831t, 832t
    treatment of, 832–838
        chemotherapy/hormonal therapy for, 834, 834t
        immunotherapy for, 834–838, 835t, 836t, 837f, 838f, 838t
        radiation therapy for, 838
        surgery for, 832–833, 833b
Renal cysts, 165–166, 166f, 166t

Renal disease
    chemotherapy with, 355t
    chronic, pruritus due to, 14–15
    hemostatic abnormalities of, 508, 509b
Renal failure
    erythropoietin for, 419–420
    in multiple myeloma, 584
Renal function tests, in erythrocytosis, 259
Renal masses
    cystic, 165–166, 166f, 166t
    diagnosis of, 165–168
    incidence of, 165
    signs and symptoms of, 165
    solid, 166–168, 167f, 168f
Renal metastases, 168, 830
    of melanoma, 1087f, 1088
Renal pelvis, primary neoplasms of, 168
Renal trauma, hematuria due to, 174t
Renal vascular disease, hematuria due to, 174t
Rendu-Osler-Weber syndrome, 295, 295f
Rescue therapy, in acute lymphoblastic leukemia, 563–564
Resection
    extent of, 367
    laparoscopic, 368
Respeto, 1230
Respiratory complications, of hematopoietic stem cell transplantation, 403
Respiratory obstruction, in superior vena cava syndrome, 101
Respiratory symptoms, 1251–1252
Restless leg syndrome, 1253
Restlessness, in final days, 1255
Restoril (temazepam), 1227b
    for insomnia, 1253
RET mutation, 1199
Reticulin fibrosis, in idiopathic myelofibrosis, 707
Reticulocyte(s), 275, 275f
    hemoglobin content of, 207
    in anemia, 235, 237f, 238f
    in iron deficient erythropoiesis, 207
    residual RNA in, 277, 278f
Reticulocyte count
    in anemia, 235
        increased, 238–240, 239f, 240f
        reduced, 240
    in pancytopenia, 253
Reticulocyte response, in myelodysplasia, 572t
Retinal changes, in polycythemia vera, 258f
Retinoblastoma, 1040
    genetic basis for, 1193, 1194t, 1203
Retinoblastoma (RB) gene, in cervical cancer, 770
Retinoic acid receptor α (RARα) gene, in acute myeloid leukemia, 525
Retinoic acid receptor modulators, 332t, 344–345
Retinoic acid syndrome, 543, 544t
Retinoids
    for head and neck cancer, 1013–1015, 1013t, 1014f
    for lung cancer, 977–978
    for squamous cell carcinoma, 1112
Retinyl palmitate, for head and neck cancer, 1014, 1014t
Retrograde ejaculation, 1239
Retrograde pyelogram, for hematuria, 177f
Retroperitoneal adenopathy, 217
Retroperitoneal germ-cell tumors, 822b
Retroperitoneal lymph node dissection (RPLND), for nonseminoma, 815–817, 818, 822
Retroviral vectors, for gene therapy, 383, 383t
Reverse complementary oligonucleotides, 383
Revici therapy, 1221t
Revised European-American Lymphoma (REAL) classification, 601, 611, 636, 664
    for peripheral T-cell lymphoma, 664
Rh system, 432–433, 435f
Rhabdomyosarcoma, 1039, 1039t, 1040
    of unknown origin, 314
Rheum officinale, 1215
Rheumatoid vasculitis, 299, 299f
Richter's syndrome, 689
Ring sideroblasts, 276
    in myelodysplasia, 571f, 572
    refractory anemia with, 572, 573
Risk assessment
    for gastrointestinal oncologic surgery, 362–364, 363t, 364t
    models for, 1204–1205

Risk factors
  for acute myeloid leukemia, 522–523, 522f, 523f
  for bladder cancer, 850
  for brain tumors, 1049
  for breast cancer, 59
    ductal carcinoma in situ, 727
  for endometrial cancer, 782–783
  for febrile neutropenia, 1174–1175
  for gastric cancer, 888–890, 888t
  for melanoma, 305, 306t
  for myelodysplasia, 568–569, 568t
  for non-Hodgkin's lymphoma, 636, 637t
  for pancreatic cancer, 908–909, 909t
  for posttransplant lymphoproliferative disease, 1161
  for prostate cancer, 860
  for renal cell cancer, 825
  for salivary gland carcinoma, 1018
  for significant urologic disease with hematuria, 174, 174t
  for thromboembolic disease, 1179
  for thrombosis with thrombocythemia, 227
  for thyroid carcinoma, 1117, 1118t
    papillary, 1120
  for tumor lysis syndrome, 1187, 1188t
  for vaginal cancer, 779
  for vulvar cancer, 775
  prothrombic, 289–290, 289b
Risperidone (Risperdal), 1227b
Ristocetin cofactor assay, 267, 269
Ritalin (methylphenidate), 1227b
  for opioid-related sedation, 1248
Rituximab (Rituxan), 378
  for B-cell lymphoma, 345–346
  for chronic lymphocytic leukemia, 345–346, 690, 696
  for Hodgkin's disease, 627–628
  for non-Hodgkin's lymphoma, 346
    intermediate-grade, 652
    low-grade, 642, 642t
  for posttransplant lymphoproliferative disease, 1164
Rocky Mountain spotted fever, vascular cutaneous manifestations of, 298f
Roentgen equivalent in man (rem), 321
Rofecoxib (Vioxx), for pain, 1244
Rouleaux formation, 272, 273f
Round cell neoplasms, 1038–1039
RPLND (retroperitoneal lymph node dissection), for nonseminoma, 815–817, 818, 822
R-S (Reed-Sternberg) cells, 608f, 609, 610, 611
RTOG (Radiation Therapy Oncology Group) Recursive Partitioning Tree, 1067, 1067f
Rumex acetosella, 1214
Runner's hematuria, 174

S
Salicylates, for pain, 1244, 1245t
Saline, for hypercalcemia, 193, 194t
Salivary gland carcinoma, 1017–1025
  clinical evaluation of, 1019–1021, 1020f, 1021f
  clinical presentation of, 1018–1019, 1018t, 1019f
  epidemiology of, 1017–1018
  follow-up evaluation for, 1025
  histologic variants of, 1017, 1018t
  metastatic, 1019, 1020, 1023–1024, 1024f
  of major *vs.* minor glands, 1018–1019, 1018t, 1019f
  risk factors for, 1018
  staging, prognostic features, and outcomes of, 1021–1022, 1022t
  treatment of, 1022–1025, 1023f, 1024f
Salmonella infection, febrile neutropenia due to, 1174
Salpingo-oophorectomy, prophylactic, 1197
Salsalate, for pain, 1245t
Salt restriction, for ascites, 131
Salvage therapy
  for ductal carcinoma in situ, 732, 732f
  for esophageal cancer, 884b
  for germ-cell tumors, 820
  for testicular cancer, 820

Sarcoidosis, hilar and mediastinal adenopathy in, 94, 95f
Sarcoma(s)
  angio-, 1039t, 1041
  bone, 1027–1036
    classification of, 1027, 1028t
    diagnosis of, 1027
    incidence of, 1027
    malignant fibrous histiocytoma as, 1029t, 1032–1033
    small-cell, 1035
    staging of, 1027, 1028t
  chondro-, 1029t, 1033–1034, 1033f, 1033t
  Ewing's, 154, 315, 1029t, 1034–1035, 1034f, 1035f
  fibro-, 1039t, 1040
  granulocytic, in acute myeloid leukemia, 529, 529f
  Kaposi's, 1158–1161
    clinical evaluation of, 1159
    clinical presentation of, 301, 301f, 1159
    epidemiology of, 1158
    HAART and, 1155
    pathology and pathogenesis of, 1158–1159
    staging, prognostic features, and outcome of, 1159–1160, 1159t
    treatment for, 1160–1161
  leiomyo-, 1039t, 1040
  lipo-, 1039, 1039t, 1040
  neurofibro-, 1039t
  of unknown origin, 314, 315
  osteo-, 1028–1032, 1029f, 1029t, 1030f
  pancreatic, 918
  rhabdo-, 1039, 1039t, 1040
  soft tissue, 1038–1045
    biopsy of, 1041
    childhood, 1038, 1039, 1040, 1041, 1042, 1043
    clinical presentation of, 1040–1041
    epidemiology of, 1040
    etiology of, 1040
    histologic grading of, 1039–1040
    imaging of, 1041
    pathology of, 1038–1040, 1039t
    round cell, 1038–1039
    spindle cell, 1039
    staging and prognosis for, 1041–1043, 1042t
    therapy for, 1043–1045
  synovio-, 1039t
  uterine, 789, 789t
Sarcomatoid carcinoma, of head and neck, 1000
Sarcomatoid renal cell cancer, 827f
Sargramostim. *See* Granulocyte-macrophage colony-stimulating factor (GM-CSF, sargramostim, molgramostim).
Scedosporium prolificans, febrile neutropenia due to, 1177b
Schaumberg's progressive pigmentary dermatosis, 300, 300f
Schistocytes, 238–239, 240b, 274, 274f
Schwannoma, 1039t
SCLC (small cell lung cancer). *See* Lung cancer, small cell.
Scleroderma, vascular cutaneous manifestations of, 299
Scopolamine
  for death rattle, 1254t, 1255
  for nausea and vomiting, 1252t
Scott syndrome, 270
Screening
  for breast cancer, 62f, 65, 67f–69f, 1196t
  for colorectal cancer, 924–926, 925t
  for endometrial cancer, 784
  for familial melanoma, 1201
  for gastric cancer, 891–892
  for genetic cancer predisposition, 1206–1207, 1206b, 1206t
  for hematuria, 173–174
  for hereditary nonpolyposis colorectal cancer, 1201
  for lung cancer, 978–979, 978t
  for melanoma, 305, 307t
  for ovarian cancer, 1197
  for prostate cancer, 864–865, 865t
Screening mammography, 65–70

Scrotal swelling. *See* Testicular mass.
SCT (stem cell transplantation). *See* Hematopoietic stem cell transplantation (HSCT).
Scurvy, vascular cutaneous manifestations of, 296, 297f
Seborrheic keratosis, 308t, 310f
Second malignancy(ies)
  acute myeloid leukemia as, 522–523, 522f, 523f, 528
  after breast cancer, 764–765
  after hematopoietic stem cell transplantation, 405
  in chronic lymphocytic leukemia, 690
  in Hodgkin's disease, 618–619, 629
  of head and neck, 1012–1015, 1013t, 1014t
  with thymoma, 984, 989
Sedation
  of dying patient, 1256, 1256t
  opioid-related, 1248
Segmental resection, for non–small cell lung cancer, 971, 974
Seizures, 23–26
  due to brain metastases, 1064, 1069b
  due to brain tumor, 23, 24–25, 24f, 1057–1058
  grand mal, 23
  headache after, 23, 24f
  history of, 23–24, 24f
  neurologic examination and diagnostic studies for, 24–25, 24f
  partial, 23
    complex, 23, 1064
    simple, 23, 1064
  prevalence of, 23
  prophylaxis for, 25
  psychomotor, 23
  psychosocial issues with, 25–26
  tonic-clonic, 23
  treatment for, 25–26, 25t, 26b
Selective estrogen receptor modulators (SERMs), 340t–341t, 343–344
  for breast cancer, 740
  for hot flashes, 766b
Selective tyrosine kinase inhibitors, 331f
Selenium, 1216t
  and esophageal cancer, 875–876
  and lung cancer, 978
  and prostate cancer, 861
Seminal emission, failure of, 1239
Seminoma, 815, 817t, 819b, 820b
  cranial neuropathies due to, 28t
Semustine (methyl-CCNU), 334t
Senile purpura, 296–297, 297f, 298f
Sensory neuropathy, 37
Sentinel lymph node biopsy
  for breast cancer, 718
  for gastrointestinal cancer, 366
  for melanoma, 1092–1094, 1092f, 1093b
SERMs (selective estrogen receptor modulators), 340t–341t, 343–344
  for breast cancer, 740
  for hot flashes, 766b
Seroquel (quetiapine), 1227b
Serous cystadenocarcinoma, ovarian papillary, 795, 795f, 795t
Serous cystadenoma, ovarian, 793, 793f
Sertraline (Zoloft), 1227, 1227b, 1228
Serum ferritin, 208–210, 209t, 211b
Serum protein electrophoresis, for immunoglobulin abnormalities, 205, 206f
Serum transferrin receptor, 209–210
Serzone (nefazodone), 1227, 1227b
714-X, 1217t
Sexual dysfunction
  after hematopoietic stem cell transplantation, 404
  male. *See* Male sexual dysfunction.
Sézary cells, 665, 666f
Sézary syndrome (SS), 664–667, 666f
Shared antigens, in vaccine therapy, 381
Shark cartilage, 1217t, 1220–1221
Sheep sorrel, 1214
Sheridan, James V., 1217t
Shilling's test, 457
Shoulder weakness, due to cranial neuropathy, 30t, 31

SIADH (syndrome of inappropriate antidiuretic
        hormone secretion), in lung
        cancer
    non–small cell, 963
    small cell, 947
Sibling donor, 392t
Sibling transplantation, human leukocyte
        antigen–matched, for acute
        myeloid leukemia, 537, 538t
Sickle cell(s), 275, 275f
Sickle-cell disease, 462–466, 464t
    anemia in, 240
    categories of, 462, 463t
    complications of, 462–465, 464t
    laboratory findings in, 456t
    painful crises in, 465–466, 465b
    pathophysiology of, 462–463, 463f
    red cell abnormalities in, 274, 275f, 462,
        462f
    symptoms of, 233t
    transfusion in, 464b
Sickle-cell trait, 463t
Sideroblast(s), ring, 276
    in myelodysplasia, 571f, 572
    refractory anemia with, 572, 573
Sideroblastic anemias, 276
Siderocytes, 277
Sigmoidoscopy, flexible, for colorectal cancer,
        925
Signal transduction modulators, 340t–342t
Sildenafil, 1237–1238, 1238f
Silver nitrate, for hematuria, 177–178
Simpatia, 1230
Sinonasal carcinoma, 1018, 1019
Sinus lymphoma, 662
Sister Mary Joseph node, in gastric cancer,
        890
Skeletal metastases
    of breast cancer, 151f, 154f, 255f, 751t,
        760–761
    of lung cancer
        non–small cell, 961, 966
        small cell, 946
    of melanoma, 1087
    of multiple myeloma, 582, 585, 592–593
    pancytopenia due to, 253
    pathologic fractures due to. See Pathologic
        fractures.
Skin cancer, 1104–1114
    basal cell carcinoma as, 1105–1108
        clinical evaluation of, 1106, 1106f
        clinical presentation of, 1105–1106
        follow-up evaluation of, 1107–1108
        low-risk vs. high-risk, 1106, 1108t
        metastatic, 1106
        nodular, 1105–1106
        of vulva, 778
        pathogenesis of, 1104–1105
        pigmented, 308t, 1106
        recurrence of, 1107–1108, 1108t
        risk factors for recurrence of, 1106,
            1108t
        sclerosing, 1106
        staging of, 1106, 1107t
        superficial, 1106
        treatment for, 1106–1107, 1109f
        ulcerated, 1106f
    epidemiology of, 1104
    melanoma as. See Melanoma.
    Merkel cell carcinoma as, 1104, 1105,
        1113–1114, 1113f
    pathogenesis of, 1104–1105
    squamous cell carcinoma as, 1108–1113
        adenoid (acantholytic), 1111
        adenosquamous (mucin-producing),
            1111
        clear-cell, 1111
        clinical evaluation of, 1110
        clinical presentation of, 1108–1109,
            1109f, 1110f
        desmoplastic, 1111
        follow-up evaluation for, 1113
        high-risk, 1111–1112
        low-risk, 1111
        metastatic, 1111
        pathogenesis of, 1104–1105
        recurrence of, 1110
        spindle-cell, 1111

staging, prognostic features, and
        outcomes of, 1107t, 1110–1111
    treatment of, 1111–1113, 1112f
    variants of, 1108–1109, 1111
    types of, 1104, 1105t
Skin lesions, pigmented. See Pigmented skin
        lesions.
Skin manifestations, of bleeding and
        thromboembolic disorders. See
        Cutaneous manifestations, of
        bleeding and thromboembolic
        disorders.
Skin sparing, 321, 322f
Skull radiographs, in multiple myeloma, 588,
        588f
SLE (systemic lupus erythematosus)
    pancytopenia due to, 253
    vascular cutaneous manifestations of, 299
Sleep apnea syndrome, erythrocytosis due to,
        259
Slippery elm, 1215
Small bowel obstruction, 109, 110t, 111, 112
Small cell carcinoma, of esophagus, 885
Small cell fragments, 275
Small cell lung cancer (SCLC). See Lung cancer,
        small cell.
Small cell sarcomas, 1034, 1038–1039
Small intestine, carcinoid tumors of, 1134–1135,
        1134f, 1134t
Small lymphocytic lymphoma, B-cell, 603–604,
        604f, 604t
Smoking. See Cigarette smoking.
Smoldering multiple myeloma (SMM), 204, 586,
        586t
SMS (superior mediastinal syndrome), 100
Smudge cells, 279
Social assessment, for pain, 1241–1242
Social workers, 1258
Soft palate tumors, 1005
Soft tissue sarcoma, 1038–1045
    biopsy of, 1041
    childhood, 1038, 1039, 1040, 1041, 1042,
        1043
    clinical presentation of, 1040–1041
    epidemiology of, 1040
    etiology of, 1040
    histologic grading of, 1039–1040
    imaging of, 1041
    pathology of, 1038–1040, 1039t
    round cell, 1034, 1038–1039
    spindle cell, 1039
    staging and prognosis for, 1041–1043, 1042t
    therapy for, 1043–1045
Soft-tissue plasmacytoma (STP), 595
Solitary pulmonary nodule, 81–86
    biopsy of, 85–86, 967b
    calcifications in, 81, 83b, 84, 84f
    cavitation of, 83
    chest radiography of, 81, 83b
    computed tomography of, 81–84, 83t, 84t
        enhanced, 84–85
    contours and margins of, 82–83, 83f
    defined, 81, 82f
    density of, 83–84, 84f
    differential diagnosis of, 81, 82t
    due to metastatic breast cancer, 761b
    fat in, 84
    indeterminate, 85b
    positron emission tomography imaging of,
        85, 85f
    size of, 81, 82
    surgical resection of, 967b
    vascular and bronchial relationships of, 83,
        84f
    vs. mass, 81
Somatic mutations, 1193–1194
Somatostatin analogs
    for carcinoid tumors, 1136–1137
    for islet cell tumors, 917–918
    for pancreatic endocrine tumors, 1136
Somatostatinoma, 1134t, 1136
Sonography. See Ultrasonography.
Sopcak, Edward, 1217t
Spasmodic dysphonia, 51t
Sperm banking, for Hodgkin's disease, 622–623
S-phase, recruitment of cells into, with myeloid
        growth factors, 424, 425t
S-phase fraction, in breast cancer, 722

Spherocytes, 276, 276f
    in chronic lymphocytic leukemia, 279–280
    in immune-mediated hemolytic anemia,
        1168, 1168f
Spherocytosis, hereditary, 456t, 468
Spider angiomata, 297
Spinal cord compression
    by metastatic tumor, 159–160, 159t, 160f,
        162t
        of breast cancer, 160f, 751t, 760
        of lung cancer, 946
    clinical manifestations of, 1078–1079
    due to epidural tumor. See Epidural tumors.
    due to germ-cell tumor, 822b
    radiation therapy for, 328
Spinal cord damage, 1080
Spinal myelopathy, herpes zoster, 159t, 161, 162,
        162t
Spinal radiculopathy, herpes zoster, 159t, 161,
        162, 162t
Spinal stability, 1077, 1078f
Spinal stenosis, 161
Spindle cell tumors, 1039
Spine
    degenerative disease of, 159t, 160–161, 162t
    pathologic fractures of, 150, 151f
    spondylosis of, 161
Spiral computed tomography, 288–289, 289f
    of liver, 115
Spiritual assessment, for pain, 1242
Spiritual counseling, for pain management, 1244
Spironolactone, for ascites, 131
Splenectomy
    elevated platelet count after, 229
    febrile neutropenia after, 1175
    fever of unknown origin after, 10, 10b
    for chronic lymphocytic leukemia, 690, 696
    for gastric cancer, 894
    for hairy cell leukemia, 698
    for idiopathic thrombocytopenic purpura,
        490, 490f, 491, 492
    for pancreatic cancer, 915
    for polycythemia vera, 702
    for splenomegaly, 138
    for warm antibody autoimmune hemolytic
        anemia, 473b
    neutrophilia after, 243
Splenic aspiration and biopsy, for splenomegaly,
        138
Splenomegaly, 135–138
    and hypersplenism, 137
    bone marrow aspiration and biopsy for,
        137–138
    clinical evaluation of, 135, 136f, 137b
    clinical presentation of, 135
    differential diagnosis of, 135–136, 136t
    due to anemia, 232, 233t
    in essential thrombocythemia, 710
    in idiopathic myelofibrosis, 706, 708–709
    in polycythemia vera, 258, 259f, 260, 261f,
        702, 705
    neutropenia due to, 246
    neutrophilia with, 243–244, 243f, 244f
    pancytopenia due to, 252–253
    splenic aspiration and biopsy for, 138
    thrombocytopenia due to, 225
    with filling defects, 135, 136f
Spondylosis, of spine, 161
Spot compression, of breast, 65, 68f
Spur cells, 276, 277f
Squamous cell carcinoma, 1108–1113
    adenoid (acantholytic), 1111
    adenosquamous (mucin-producing), 1111
    clear-cell, 1111
    clinical evaluation of, 1110
    clinical presentation of, 1108–1109, 1109f,
        1110f
    desmoplastic, 1111
    follow-up evaluation for, 1113
    high-risk, 1111–1112
    low-risk, 1111
    metastatic, 1111
        to lymph node in neck, 48f
    of bladder, 850
    of cervix, 770, 770f, 774–775
    of head and neck, 999–1010
    of lung, 968, 968t
    of unknown origin, 1151b

Squamous cell carcinoma, (Continued)
  of vagina, 779
  pathogenesis of, 1104–1105
  pigmented, 308t
  recurrence of, 1110
  spindle-cell, 1111
  staging, prognostic features, and outcomes
      of, 1107t, 1110–1111
  superior vena cava syndrome due to, 100f
  treatment of, 1111–1113, 1112f
  variants of, 1108–1109, 1111
Squamous intraepithelial lesions, low-grade and
    high-grade, 769
SS (Sézary syndrome), 664–667, 666f
Staging
  of adrenal carcinoma, 1130
  of AIDS-related lymphoma, 1156
  of anal carcinoma, 939, 940t
  of basal cell carcinoma, 1106, 1107t
  of biliary cancer, 904
  of bladder cancer
    muscle-invasive, 851, 852t
    superficial, 843–844, 843f, 844t
  of bone sarcomas, 1027, 1028t
  of brain metastases, 1066–1068
  of brain tumor, 1051, 1051t
  of breast cancer, 715–719, 716t, 717t
    primary tumor in, 715–717, 716t
    regional lymph nodes in, 716t, 717–719,
        717t
  of cervical cancer, 771–772, 771t
  of chondrosarcoma, 1033
  of colorectal cancer, 927, 927f, 928t
  of endometrial cancer, 784–786, 785t–787t
  of esophageal cancer, 876–877, 876f, 877f,
      884b
  of Ewing's sarcoma, 1034
  of gallbladder cancer, 906
  of gastric cancer, 892–893, 892t, 893t
  of gastrointestinal cancer, 365–366
  of germ-cell tumors, 815, 816t
  of head and neck cancer, 1001–1002, 1001t
  of hepatocellular carcinoma, 900–902, 901t
  of idiopathic myelofibrosis, 707–708, 708t
  of Kaposi's sarcoma, 1159–1160, 1159t
  of lung cancer
    non–small cell, 963–965, 964f, 965f
    small cell, 948–949, 949f
  of malignant fibrous histiocytoma, 1032
  of melanoma, 1088–1091, 1088t–1090t
  of Merkel cell carcinoma, 1107t, 1113–1114
  of mesothelioma, 992, 993t, 994, 995t
  of osteosarcoma, 1030
  of ovarian cancer, 794–795, 794t
  of pancreatic cancer, 914, 914t
  of persistent gestational trophoblastic tumors,
      807–809, 808t, 809t
  of prostate cancer, 861–862, 861t, 862t
  of renal cell cancer, 831–832, 831t
  of salivary gland carcinoma, 1021–1022, 1022t
  of soft tissue sarcoma, 1041–1043, 1042t
  of squamous cell carcinoma, 1107t,
      1110–1111
  of thymoma, 986–987, 986t, 987t
  of thyroid carcinoma, 1119, 1119t
    differentiated, 1121
    medullary, 1125–1126
  of vaginal cancer, 779, 780f, 780t
  of vulvar cancer, 777–778, 777t
Staging laparoscopy, 365–366
Stanford V regimen, for Hodgkin's disease,
    623–625, 624t
Staphylococcus aureus, febrile neutropenia due to,
    1173, 1174
Staphylococcus epidermidis, febrile neutropenia due
    to, 1173
Starvation, vs. cachexia, 3–4, 4t
Stasis purpura, 301, 301f
Stauffer's syndrome, in renal cell cancer, 828
Steiner, Rudolph, 1213t
Stem cell(s), in gene therapy, 384
Stem cell transplantation (SCT). See
    Hematopoietic stem cell
    transplantation (HSCT).
Stenting
  biliary duct
    for biliary cancer, 905b
    for pancreatic cancer, 916

esophageal, 142–143
  percutaneous, for superior vena cava
      syndrome, 103–104
Stereotactic surgery, for pituitary adenoma, 1142
Sterility, after hematopoietic stem cell
      transplantation, 404
Steroid(s). See Corticosteroid(s).
Steroidal inactivators, 754
STI-571 (imatinib mesylate), 356
  for chronic myeloid leukemia, 410, 685,
      685b
  for gastrointestinal stomal tumors,
      1044–1045
Stomach cancer. See Gastric cancer.
Stomatocytes, 275
Storage pool disease, 270
STP (soft-tissue plasmacytoma), 595
Streptococcus bovis
  febrile neutropenia due to, 1174
  septicemia due to, and colorectal cancer, 923
Streptozocin, 334t, 355t
  for neuroendocrine tumors, 1137
Stroke, in sickle-cell disease, 464–465
Stromal sarcomas, uterine, 789
Subarachnoid bleeding, 157–158, 159
Subclavian vein thrombosis, catheter-associated,
      1184
Subcutaneous hemorrhage, 295, 295f
Subcutaneous panniculitis-like T-cell lymphoma,
      669
Sublethal damage repair, 323
Sublingual gland carcinoma, 1018, 1019
Submandibular gland carcinoma, 1018, 1019
Submental adenopathy, 215t
Suboccipital adenopathy, 215t
Subungual hematoma, 308t, 309–310
Subungual lesions, 309, 310f, 312b
Sucrose hemolysis test, 469
Suicidal thoughts, 1225
"Suicide genes," 382, 383
Suicide inhibitors, 754
Sulindac, for pain, 1245t
Superficial thrombophlebitis, 283, 1184
Superior mediastinal syndrome (SMS), 100
Superior vena cava (SVC), anatomy of, 98, 99f
Superior vena cava (SVC) syndrome, 98–105
  anticoagulation for, 104
  as oncologic emergency, 98, 101
  causes of, 99–100, 99t
  clinical presentation of, 100–101, 100f
  defined, 98
  diagnostic evaluation of, 101, 101f, 102f
  due to hilar and mediastinal adenopathy, 95,
      96f
  due to lung cancer
    non–small cell, 961
    small cell, 945, 946f, 952
  due to non-Hodgkin's lymphoma, 99, 649
  evaluation of, 103
  prognosis for, 104
  radiation therapy for, 328
  supportive care for, 104
  treatment for, 103–104
  venous thromboembolic disease with, 1182
  with previously known malignancy, 102
Superparamagnetic iron oxide particles, for liver
      imaging, 117
Superwarfarins, coagulation disorders due to,
      265, 268, 507, 507f, 508b
Supportive care
  for acute myeloid leukemia, 531–533, 532t
  for adrenal cancer, 1131
  for gastric cancer, 895–896, 896t
  for myelodysplasia, 575b
  for pancreatic cancer, 917, 917t
  for superior vena cava syndrome, 104
Supraclavicular adenopathy, 214–217, 215t
Supraclavicular lymph nodes, breast cancer
      metastasis to, 718–719
Surgery
  excessive bleeding after, 265, 266b
  for adrenal cancer, 1130
  for anal carcinoma, 939, 941–942
  for basal cell carcinoma, 1106–1107
  for biliary tract cancers, 904
  for bladder cancer
    muscle-invasive, 851
    superficial, 844

for brain metastases, 1071–1073, 1072t
  for breast cancer
    ductal carcinoma in situ, 729–732, 730b,
        731t, 732f
    locally invasive, 737–738
    metastatic, 761b
  for cervical cancer, 771, 772, 773b, 776f
  for chondrosarcoma, 1033–1034
  for colorectal cancer, 928–929, 932
  for endometrial cancer, 784–787
  for epidural cancer, 1082
  for esophageal cancer, 877–878
  for gastric cancer, 893–894, 894t
  for hypopharyngeal cancer, 1003
  for laryngeal cancer, 1002–1003
  for liver cancer, 902
  for lung cancer
    non–small cell, 970–971, 970f, 974
    small cell, 953
  for melanoma, 1091–1094, 1091t, 1092f,
      1097b
  for Merkel cell carcinoma, 1114
  for mesothelioma, 992–994, 994f, 995t
  for molar pregnancy, 806
  for oral cavity cancer, 1007
  for oropharyngeal cancer, 1005–1006
  for ovarian cancer, 797b
  for pancreatic cancer, 914–915
  for pituitary adenoma, 1141
  for prostate cancer, 865–867, 866t
  for renal cell cancer, 832–833, 833b
  for salivary gland carcinoma, 1022–1023,
      1024–1025
  for soft tissue sarcomas, 1043–1044
  for squamous cell carcinoma, 1111–1112
  for testicular cancer, 815, 818–820, 821
  for thymoma, 987
  for thyroid carcinoma
    differentiated, 1121–1122
    medullary, 1126
  for vaginal cancer, 779
  for vulvar cancer, 777–778
  gastrointestinal oncologic. See Gastrointestinal
      (GI) oncologic surgery.
Surgical margins
  for basal cell carcinoma, 1107
  for melanoma, 1091, 1091t
Surgical patient, bleeding in, 510
SVC. See Superior vena cava (SVC).
Swallowing difficulty, due to cranial neuropathy,
      30t, 31
Sweating, gustatory, 1024
Syndrome of ectopic corticotropin secretion, in
      small cell lung cancer, 948
Syndrome of inappropriate antidiuretic hormone
      secretion (SIADH), in lung cancer
    non–small cell, 963
    small cell, 947
Syngeneic hematopoietic stem cell
      transplantation, 391, 392t
Synovectomy, for joint disease in hemophilia A,
      502b
Synoviosarcoma, 1039t
Systemic lupus erythematosus (SLE)
  pancytopenia due to, 253
  vascular cutaneous manifestations of, 299

T
T cell depletion, for graft-versus-host disease, 396
Tabebuia impetiginosa, 1213t
Tachycardia, due to pulmonary embolism,
      284–285
Tachypnea, due to pulmonary embolism,
      284–285
Tacrolimus, for graft-versus-host disease, 396,
      397
Taheebo, 1213t
Talc pleurodesis, for pleural effusion, 91f, 92
Tamoxifen (Nolvadex), 331–343, 340t
  and endometrial cancer, 782–783
  for breast cancer
    ductal carcinoma in situ, 733, 733f
    lobular carcinoma in situ, 735
    locally invasive, 739, 740–742, 743t
    metastatic, 752–754, 753t, 754t
    with GnRH agonist, 755
  for hepatocellular carcinoma, 902
  for melanoma, 1097–1098

TAR (thrombocytopenia with absent radius) syndrome, 222
Tarceva, for colorectal cancer, 930
Target cells, 274f, 275, 275f
Targeted therapies, 387, 394–395
Targretin (bexarotene), 344–345
Tattoo, 308t
Taxanes, 332t, 340t, 352–353
    for breast cancer
        locally invasive, 739
        metastatic, 756–758, 756t, 757t
    for gastric cancer, 895, 895t
Taxol. See Paclitaxel (Taxol).
Taxotere. See Docetaxel (Taxotere).
TBI. See Total body irradiation (TBI).
TCC (transitional cell carcinoma)
    of bladder, 842, 850, 855b
    of kidneys, 830–831
T-cell leukemia
    adult, 248, 550, 672–675, 673t
    precursor (acute) lymphoblastic, 601–602
    prolymphocytic, 697
T-cell lymphoma
    adult, 248
    anaplastic large, 668
    angioimmunoblastic, 668, 670
    cutaneous, 664–667
        anaplastic, 668
        clinical presentation of, 665, 665f, 666f
        epidemiology of, 664
        pathophysiology of, 664–665
        staging and prognosis for, 665–666
        treatment for, 666–667
            bexarotene in, 344–345
            denileukin in, 347
    enteropathy-type intestinal, 669, 670
    hepatosplenic gamma/delta, 668–669, 670
    peripheral, 664–671
        classification of, 664, 665t
        clinical evaluation of, 670
        clinical presentation of, 667–668, 667t, 668t
        defined, 664
        diagnosis of, 607–609, 608f, 612
        mycosis fungoides and Sézary syndrome as, 664–667, 665f, 666f
        prognostic features and outcome for, 670
        treatment for, 670–671
        types of, 668–670
        unspecified, 607–609, 669
    precursor lymphoblastic, 601–602, 604f
    subcutaneous panniculitis-like, 669
Teardrop cells, 274, 274f, 707f, 1167, 1167f
Tegretol. See Carbamazepine (Tegretol, Carbatrol).
Telangiectasia
    ataxia, 296
    hereditary hemorrhagic, 295, 295f
    in CREST syndrome, 297, 298f
Teletherapy, 321
Temazepam (Restoril), 1227b
    for insomnia, 1253
Temozolomide, 334t, 348
    for high-grade gliomas, 1053
    for melanoma, 348, 1099b
Temporal arteritis, headache due to, 20t
Teniposide, 338t, 350
    for brain metastases, 1073
TENS (transcutaneous electrical nerve stimulation), for pain management, 1244
Terazocin, for urinary retention, 1247
Testicular biopsy, 182
Testicular cancer, 813–823
    clinical evaluation of, 180, 813–814, 814f
    clinical presentation of, 813
    cryptorchidism and, 179–180
    imaging of, 814
    management of, 815–821
        for advanced metastatic disease, 817–821, 819b, 819t, 820b–822b
        for low-stage germ-cell tumors, 815–817, 817t, 818b
        for nonseminoma, 815–817, 817t, 818b
        for relapse, 821b
        for seminoma, 815, 817t
        initial, 814b
        postchemotherapy surgery in, 818–819

salvage chemotherapy in, 820
sequelae of, 821–823
surgery in salvage setting for, 820–821
with good-risk disease, 818, 819b
with intermediate- and poor-risk disease, 818, 820b
    metastatic
        management
            of, 817–821, 819b, 819t, 820b–822b
            pattern of nodal spread for, 814, 814f
            to brain, 1075
        pathology of, 814–815, 815t
        staging of, 815, 816t
Testicular lymphoma, 662
Testicular mass, 179–183
    approach to patient with, 182–183
    causes of, 179
    extra-, 179, 180b, 183
    general considerations with, 179, 180b
    history of, 179–180
    imaging of, 180–182
    intra-, 179, 180b, 182
    laboratory evaluation for, 180
    pain with, 182–183
    physical examination for, 180, 181f
Testicular torsion, 180, 182
Testosterone, and prostate cancer, 860
Testosterone supplementation, 1238–1239
Tetracycline, for pleural effusion, 92
Thalassemia(s), 233t, 237, 278, 458–462
α-Thalassemia, 456t, 458–459, 459t
β-Thalassemia, 459–462
    classification of, 460, 461t
    epidemiology of, 459
    intermedia, 275f, 460, 461f, 461t
    laboratory findings in, 456t
    major, 460, 461t
    pathogenesis of, 459–460
    pathophysiology of, 460, 461f
    treatment for, 460b, 461–462, 462b
β-Thalassemia trait, 460b, 461t
Thalidomide
    for cachexia, 7
    for multiple myeloma, 589b, 590
    in antiangiogenic therapy, 385
Thioguanine, 336t
    for acute lymphoblastic leukemia, 557t
    for acute myeloid leukemia, 535t
Thiopental, for refractory pain, 1256t
Thiotepa, 333t, 356t
    for superficial bladder cancer, 844
Thoracentesis
    diagnostic, 77
    therapeutic, for pleural effusion, 88–89, 91t
Thoracoscopy
    for non–small cell lung cancer, 967–968
    for solitary pulmonary nodule, 86
Thoracotomy, for solitary pulmonary nodule, 86
Thorazine (chlorpromazine)
    for delirium, 1248, 1248t, 1254t, 1255
    for dyspnea, 1254t
Thrombasthenia, Glanzmann's, 270, 494
Thrombectomy, 514t, 519
Thrombocythemia, 226–230
    and thrombosis risk, 227
    criteria for evaluation of, 227b
    defined, 227
    essential, 709–712
        chromosomal abnormalities in, 709–710
        clinical evaluation of, 710–711
        clinical presentation of, 710
        diagnostic criteria for, 710t
        differential diagnosis of, 709, 709t
        epidemiology of, 709
        follow-up evaluation for, 712
        in pregnancy, 712
        platelet count in, 227, 229, 281f
        staging, prognostic features, and outcomes for, 711
        treatment for, 711–712
    etiology of, 229–230, 229t
    history of, 227–228, 230b
    in hospitalized medical/surgical patients, 228
    in outpatients, 228–229
    physical examination for, 228, 230b
    symptoms of, 227
Thrombocytopathies, 267, 270–271
Thrombocytopenia, 221–226, 485–494

antiplatelet antibody testing for, 224
bleeding risk of, 221
bone marrow analysis for, 224, 224f, 226b
cause of, 224–226, 225t
complete evaluation of, 226b
criteria for evaluation of, 222–224, 223b
dilutional, 224–225
drug-induced, 222, 487–488, 488t
due to artifactual or cell counter abnormalities, 224, 226f
due to cancer, 1169–1170
due to decreased platelet production, 225, 225t, 485–487
due to increased platelet destruction, 225–226, 225t, 487
due to myelodysplasia, 569t, 571f, 575b
due to posttransfusion purpura, 486b
due to splenomegaly, 225
emergency evaluation of, 223
heparin-induced, 303, 487–488, 488t, 517–518
history of, 222, 226b
in leukemia
    acute lymphoblastic, 551
    acute myeloid, 532t, 533
    chronic lymphocytic, 689
in pregnancy, 493–494
neonatal alloimmune, 494
pathogenesis of, 224–226, 225t, 226f, 485
petechiae in, 294f
physical examination for, 222, 226b
splenomegaly with, 137b
symptoms of, 221–222
vaginal bleeding due to, 186b
Thrombocytopenia with absent radius (TAR) syndrome, 222
Thrombocytopenic purpura
    autoimmune (idiopathic), 488–492, 490f
    thrombotic
        clinical presentation of, 239, 269, 492
        diagnosis of, 492
        etiology of, 492
        red blood cell abnormalities in, 274–275, 492f
        relapsing, 269b
        therapy for, 492–493
Thrombocytosis, 226–230, 485
    and thrombosis risk, 227
    criteria for evaluation of, 227b
    defined, 226
    due to cancer, 1169–1170
    etiology of, 229–230, 229t, 709t
    familial, 230
    history of, 227–228, 230b
    in hospitalized medical/surgical patients, 228
    in outpatients, 228–229
    in polycythemia vera, 705
    physical examination for, 228, 230b
    reactive, 228, 229–230, 229t, 230b
    rebound, 229–230
    symptoms of, 227
Thromboembolic disease
    cutaneous manifestations of. See Cutaneous manifestations, of bleeding and thromboembolic disorders.
    due to cancer, 1179–1185
        clinical presentation and diagnosis of, 1181–1182, 1181f
        etiology and natural history of, 1179–1181
        prevention of, 1183–1185
        recurrent, 1182
        risk factors for, 1179
        treatment of, 1182
    venous. See Venous thromboembolic disease.
    with brain tumors, 1058
    with central venous catheters, 1182–1184, 1183f
    with high-dose chemotherapy, 1180–1181
    with indwelling catheters, 1182–1184, 1183f
    with superior vena cava syndrome, 1182
Thrombolytic therapy, for pulmonary embolism, 514t, 518–519
Thrombophilia, screening for, 289–290, 289b
Thrombophlebitis, superficial, 283, 1184
Thromboplastin time, partial, 268f
    prolongation of, 266–267, 267t
Thrombopoiesis, ineffective, 225

Thrombopoietic growth factor, 429
Thrombopoietin (TPO), 429
Thrombosis
    elevated platelet count and risk of, 227
    recurrent, 289
Thrombospondin-1 (TSP-1), in antiangiogenic
        therapy, 385
Thrombotic events, in paroxysmal nocturnal
        hemoglobinuria, 450
Thrombotic thrombocytopenic purpura (TTP)
    clinical presentation of, 239, 269, 492
    diagnosis of, 492
    etiology of, 492
    red blood cell abnormalities in, 274–275,
        492f
    relapsing, 269b
    therapy for, 492–493
Thymic carcinoma, 983, 986, 986t, 987, 987t
Thymidine-labeling index (TLI), in breast cancer,
        723
Thymidylate synthase, 367
Thymoma, 983–990
    clinical evaluation of, 985–986, 985f
    clinical presentation of, 983
    epidemiology of, 983
    follow-up care for, 989
    histology of, 986, 986t
    infections with, 984–985
    late sequelae of, 989–990
    locally invasive, 987–988
    noninvasive, 987
    paraneoplastic syndromes due to, 983–984,
        984f, 984t
    recurrent advanced, 989
    second malignancies with, 984, 989
    staging of, 986–987, 986t, 987t
    superior vena cava syndrome due to, 99
    treatment for, 987–989, 988f, 989t
    unresectable/locally advanced, 988–989
Thyroglobulin, with thyroid carcinoma,
        1123–1124
Thyroid adenoma, 1117, 1121
Thyroid biopsy, 1118
Thyroid carcinoma, 1117–1126
    anaplastic, 1118t, 1124–1125
    clinical presentation of, 1117, 1118t
    differential diagnosis of, 1118–1119
    differentiated
        characteristics of, 1119–1121, 1119t, 1120f
        epidemiology of, 1117, 1118t, 1119, 1120
        follow-up for, 1123–1124
        recurrence of, 1121
        staging and prognosis for, 1121
        treatment of, 1121–1124, 1122b
    epidemiology of, 1117, 1118t
    evaluation of, 1117–1118, 1118f
    follicular
        biopsy of, 1118
        characteristics of, 1119–1121, 1119t
        epidemiology of, 1118t, 1119
        follow-up for, 1123–1124
        staging and prognosis for, 1121
        treatment of, 1121–1124
    Hürthle cell, 1119, 1120–1121
    medullary, 1118t, 1125–1126
        familial, 1125, 1198–1199, 1198t
        sporadic, 1125
    papillary
        biopsy of, 1118
        characteristics of, 1119–1120, 1119t,
            1120f
        epidemiology of, 1117, 1118t, 1120
        follow-up for, 1123–1124
        risk factors for, 1120
        staging and prognosis for, 1121
        treatment of, 1121–1124, 1122b
    recurrent, 1121, 1124, 1126
    risk factors for, 1117, 1118t
    staging of, 1119, 1119t, 1121, 1125–1126
    types of, 1117, 1118t
    undifferentiated, 1118t, 1124–1125
Thyroid cysts, 1119
Thyroid function abnormalities, after
        hematopoietic stem cell
        transplantation, 404
Thyroid hormone therapy, for thyroid
        carcinoma, 1123
Thyroid lobectomy, 1121
Thyroid lymphoma, 663, 1126–1127

Thyroid nodule
    benign, 1118–1119
    clinical presentation of, 1117
    evaluation of, 1117–1118, 1118f
    risk factors for carcinoma with, 1117, 1118t
Thyroidectomy, 1121–1122, 1126
Thyrotropin (TSH), serum, 1117
Thyrotropin (TSH) deficiency, due to pituitary
        adenoma, 1142t
Thyroxine, for thyroid carcinoma, 1123
Tiagabine (Gabitril), for seizures, 25t
TIBC (total iron-binding capacity), 208, 209t
Tibia
    adamantinoma of, 154f
    giant cell tumor of tibia, 153f
Tinzaparin, for venous thromboembolism, 515t
Tissue factor, and thromboembolic disease, 1179
Tissue-specific proteins, in vaccine therapy, 380
TLI (thymidine-labeling index), in breast cancer,
        723
TNF. See Tumor necrosis factor (TNF).
T/NK-cell lymphoma, extranodal, nasal type,
        669, 670
TNM staging. See Staging.
TNP-470, in antiangiogenic therapy, 385
Tobacco. See Cigarette smoking.
Todd's paralysis, 1064
Tofranil (imipramine), 1227b
    for neuropathic pain, 1249t
Tolmetin, for pain, 1245t
Tongue tumors, 1005, 1007
Tongue weakness, due to cranial neuropathy,
        30t, 31
Tonic-clonic seizures, 23
Tonsillar fossa tumors, 1005
Tooth extraction, bleeding after, 265, 266b
Topiramate (Topamax), for seizures, 25t
Topoisomerase inhibitors, 332t, 337t–339t,
        349–352, 349f, 351f
    myelodysplasia due to, 569, 569t
Topotecan (Hycamtin), 339t, 351–352, 355t
    for head and neck cancer, 1008t
    for non–small cell lung cancer, 971t, 972
    for ovarian cancer, 802
    for soft tissue sarcoma, 1044
Toradol (ketorolac tromethamine), for pain,
        1244, 1245t
Toremifene (Fareston), 340t, 343–344
Tositumomab (Bexxar), for non-Hodgkin's
        lymphoma, intermediate-grade,
        653
Total body irradiation (TBI)
    as conditioning regimen for hematopoietic
        stem cell transplantation
        allogeneic, 395, 395t, 396t
        autologous, 399t
    toxicities of, 396t
Total iron-binding capacity (TIBC), 208, 209t
Total lymphoid irradiation, for Hodgkin's disease,
        622
Total nodal irradiation, for Hodgkin's disease, 622
Total parenteral nutrition (TPN), 6, 365
Toxic granulation
    in neutrophilic leukocytosis, 241–242, 242f
    of neutrophils, 272b, 278, 278f
Toxic-metabolic encephalopathy, due to brain
        metastases, 1063
Toxins, pancytopenia due to, 252
TP53 gene, 1194
TPN (total parenteral nutrition), 6, 365
TPO (thrombopoietin), 429
Trachea, adenoid cystic carcinoma of, 969
Tramadol, for pain, 1245
Transcutaneous electrical nerve stimulation (TENS),
        for pain management, 1244
Transdermal fentanyl, for pain, 1245–1246,
        1246t, 1254t
Transferrin, serum receptor for, 209–210
Transferrin saturation, 208
Transfusion medicine. See Blood transfusions.
Transfusion reactions, 438–439
Transitional cell carcinoma (TCC)
    of bladder, 842, 850, 855b
    of kidneys, 830–831
Transplantation
    hematopoietic stem cell. See Hematopoietic
        stem cell transplantation (HSCT).
    lymphoproliferative disease after, 1161–1164,
        1162t, 1163b

Transrectal ultrasound (TRUS), for prostate
        cancer, 864
Transsphenoidal resection, of pituitary adenoma,
        1141
Transthoracic needle biopsy, of solitary
        pulmonary nodule, 86
Trans-urethral resection of bladder tumor
        (TURB), 844
Transvaginal sonography
    of endometrial cancer, 784
    of ovarian cancer, 793, 793f
Tranxene (clorazepate), for seizures, 25t
Trastuzumab (Herceptin), 331f, 342t, 345, 378
    for metastatic breast cancer, 756t, 757t,
        758
Trazodone (Desyrel), 1227b
Treatment simulator, in radiation therapy, 324,
        324f
Tretinoin (all-trans retinoic acid), 344
    for acute promyelocytic leukemia, 543, 544t,
        545b
Triazenes, 332t, 334t
Triazinate, for gastric cancer, 895t
Triazolam (Halcion), 1227b
    for insomnia, 1253
Tricyclic antidepressants, for neuropathic pain,
        1248, 1249t
Trifolium pratense, 1215
Trigeminal nerve deficit, 29t
Trileptal (oxcarbazepine), for seizures, 25t, 26b
Trilisate, for pain, 1244
Trimethoprim/sulfamethoxazole, with multiple
        myeloma, 592
Trimetrexate, for mesothelioma, 995t
Trochlear nerve deficit, 29t
Trophoblastic embolization, 806
Trophoblastic tumors, 804–812
    epidemiology of, 804
    long-term follow-up after, 811
    molar pregnancy (hydatidiform moles) as,
        804–806, 805t, 807, 807b, 811
    persistent gestational, 807–811
        clinical presentation of, 807
        diagnosis and staging of, 807–809, 808t,
            809t
        metastatic, 807–808, 808t, 810–811
        molar pregnancy and, 807b
        nonmetastatic, 809–810, 809f, 810t
        treatment for, 809–811, 809f, 810t
    placental site, 811
    subsequent pregnancy experience after,
        811
    surveillance following chemotherapy for,
        811
    terminology for, 804
    vaginal bleeding due to, 184–185, 185f
    vs. phantom hCG syndrome, 811–812
Tropical spastic paresis (TSP), 673
Tropisetron, for nausea and vomiting, 1251,
        1252t
Trousseau's syndrome, 287
    in gastric cancer, 890
    in ovarian carcinoma, 792
    in renal cell cancer, 828
Trumpet bush, 1213t
TRUS (transrectal ultrasound), for prostate
        cancer, 864
TSH (thyrotropin), serum, 1117
TSH (thyrotropin) deficiency, due to pituitary
        adenoma, 1142t
TSP (tropical spastic paresis), 673
TSP-1 (thrombospondin-1), in antiangiogenic
        therapy, 385
TTP. See Thrombotic thrombocytopenic purpura
        (TTP).
Tuberculosis
    febrile neutropenia due to, 1174
    pancytopenia due to, 253
Tuberous sclerosis, 1040, 1049
Tumor lysis syndrome, 1187–1190, 1188t
    corticosteroid-induced, 218–219
    hyperkalemia due to, 1188–1189, 1189t
    hyperphosphatemia due to, 1189, 1189t
    hyperuricemia due to, 1187–1188, 1189t
    hypocalcemia due to, 1189–1190, 1189t
    in acute myeloid leukemia, 530, 532, 532t
    pathogenesis of, 1187
    risk factors for, 1187, 1188t
    signs and symptoms of, 1187–1190, 1189t

Tumor markers, 367, 367t
Tumor necrosis factor (TNF)
  biologic therapy using, 376, 377, 377t
  for mesothelioma, 996t
  in cachexia, 4
Tumor suppressor genes, 382
  in cancer of unknown primary, 1148
  in skin cancer, 1105
Tumor vaccines, 331f, 379–382, 380t
Tumor-associated antigens, 380–382, 380f
TURB (trans-urethral resection of bladder
    tumor), 844
Turcot's syndrome, 921, 1049
Turmoil, 1224, 1225b
Twin, identical, as stem cell donor, 392t
Tyrosine kinase inhibitors, 387
  selective, 331f
Tyrosine kinase receptors, 386

U
Ubiquinone, 1216t
UFT (uracil-tegafur), for gastric cancer, 895t
Ulcer(s)
  leg, in anemia, 233
  peptic, GI bleeding due to, 144
Ulceration
  of basal cell carcinoma, 1106f
  of melanoma, 1090, 1090t
Ulcerative colitis
  and colorectal cancer, 922, 922f
  prophylactic surgery for, 372
Ulmus fulva, 1215
Ultrasonography
  endoscopic
    of esophageal cancer, 876, 877f
    of pancreatic cancer, 913
  for erythrocytosis, 259–260, 260f, 261f
  for vaginal bleeding, 186
  of breast mass, 65, 69f
    due to cyst, 69f
    due to ductal carcinoma, 62f
    due to fibroadenoma, 61f
  of deep vein thrombosis, 287, 287f, 288, 511
  of endometrial cancer, 784
  of liver, 115–116, 118f, 119
  of ovarian cancer, 793, 793f
  of pelvic mass, 189
  of prostate cancer, 864
  of renal cell cancer, 829–830
  of testicular mass, 180–182
  of thyroid nodule, 1117–1118, 1118f
Ultraviolet light, and skin cancer, 1104
Umbilical cord transplantation, 392t, 393
  for acute myeloid leukemia, 539
Una de gato, 1213–1214, 1213t
Uncaria tomentosa, 1213–1214, 1213t
Uncoupling proteins, in cachexia, 4
Unique antigens, in vaccine therapy, 381
Unorthodox treatment(s), 1209–1223
  aloe as, 1213t
  antineoplastons as, 1217–1218, 1217t
  cancell as, 1217t
  cat's claw as, 1213–1214, 1213t
  cellular, 1217t
  chaparral as, 1213t
  chelation therapy as, 1221t
  classification of, 1213, 1213t
  coenzyme Q-10 as, 1216t
  Coley toxins as, 1217t
  defined, 1209
  detoxification enemas as, 1221t
  detoxification-fasting as, 1221t
  dietary supplements as, 1212, 1213–1217,
      1213t, 1214t, 1216t
  dimethyl sulfoxide as, 1217t
  discussion of, 1221–1223
  essiac as, 1214–1215, 1214t
  garlic as, 1213t
  Gerson therapy as, 1221t
  green tea as, 1213t
  herbal, 1211–1212, 1213–1215, 1213t, 1214t
  homeopathy as, 1221t
  how to approach patients interested in, 1211
  hoxsey as, 1213t
  hydrazine sulfate as, 1217t, 1218–1219
  immuno-augmentative therapy as, 1217t
  laetrile as, 1217t, 1219–1220
  Livingston-Wheeler regimen as, 1217t
  macrobiotics as, 1221t

  mistletoe as, 1213t
  nutritional metabolic therapy as, 1221t
  oxygen therapy as, 1221t
  pau d'arco as, 1213t
  PC-SPES as, 1214t
  pharmacologic and biologic, 1217–1221,
      1217t
  reasons that patients seek, 1210
  Revici therapy as, 1221t
  risks of, 1210–1211
  selenium as, 1216t
  714-X as, 1217t
  shark cartilage as, 1217t, 1220–1221
  vitamin A as, 1216t
  vitamin C as, 1215–1217, 1216t
  vitamin E as, 1216t
Uracil-tegafur (UFT), for gastric cancer, 895t
Ureterosigmoidoscopy, and colorectal cancer,
    922–923
Urethral polyps, hematuria due to, 174t
Urethritis, hematuria due to, 174t
Urinary incontinence, due to radical
    prostatectomy, 866
Urinary protein analysis, for multiple myeloma,
    587
Urinary retention, due to opioids, 1247
Urine cytology, for hematuria, 175, 176b
Urine dipstick testing, for hematuria, 173–174
Urine tests, for peripheral neuropathy, 39t
Urography, intravenous, of renal cell cancer, 829
Urokinase, for clot formation in central venous
    catheter, 1184
Urokinase-type plasminogen activator, in breast
    cancer, 723
Uterine leiomyomata, pelvic masses due to,
    188–189
Uterine sarcomas, 789, 789t
Uterus, as source of vaginal bleeding, 185t, 186

V
Vaccine therapy, 331f, 379–382, 380t
Vacuum erection devices, 1238
VAD. See Dexamethasone.
Vagina, as source of vaginal bleeding, 185
Vaginal bleeding, 184–187
  differential diagnosis of, 184–185, 185f, 185t
  due to endometrial cancer, 186, 783
  etiology of, 184
  evaluation of, 185–187
  in children, 186–187
  management of, 187, 187f
  postmenopausal, 186
  premenopausal, 186
Vaginal cancer, 778–780
  clear-cell, 779
  clinical presentation and staging of, 779,
      780f, 780t
  epidemiology of, 778–779
  metastatic, 780
  risk factors for, 779
  squamous cell, 779
  treatment for, 779–780
Vagus nerve, surgery-related injury to, 53t
Vagus nerve deficit, 30t
Valproate (Depakote, Depakene), 1227b
  for seizures, 25t, 26b
Valrubicin, for superficial bladder cancer, 844
Varicella-zoster infection, with hematopoietic
    stem cell transplantation,
    402–403
Varices, GI bleeding due to, 144
Varicoceles, 180
Vascular access, in acute myeloid leukemia, 532t
Vascular disorders, cutaneous manifestations of,
    295–299, 295f–300f
Vascular endothelial growth factor (VEGF), 354
  in multiple myeloma, 582
Vasculitis(itides), cutaneous manifestations of,
    298–299, 298f–300f
Vasoactive intestinal peptide (VIP)oma, 1134t,
    1135, 1136t
Vaso-occlusion, in sickle-cell disease, 463, 464t,
    465–466, 465b
Vasopressin deficiency, due to pituitary adenoma,
    1142t
Vector delivery systems, for gene therapy,
    382–383, 383t
VEGF (vascular endothelial growth factor), 354
  in multiple myeloma, 582

Vena cava. See Inferior vena cava; Superior vena
    cava (SVC).
Vena caval interruption devices, 1184–1185
Venlafaxine, for hot flashes, 766b
Venography, contrast, for deep vein thrombosis,
    287, 511–512
Veno-occlusive disease (VOD)
  due to cytotoxic agents, 395–396, 1180–1181
  hepatic, 1180–1181
Venous limb gangrene, 302–303
Venous thrombectomy, 514t, 519
Venous thromboembolic disease, 511–519
  clinical manifestations of, 283–290, 1181
  diagnosis of
    approach to, 512t, 513t
    clinical assessment for, 283–285, 284f,
        284t, 285t, 286f
    laboratory tests for, 285–287, 1181–1182
    objective tests for, 287–289, 287f–289f,
        511–513, 1181, 1181f
  due to cancer, 1179–1185
    clinical presentation and diagnosis of,
        1181–1182, 1181f
    etiology and natural history of,
        1179–1181
    prevention of, 1185
    recurrent, 1182
    risk factors for, 1179
    treatment of, 1182
  due to essential thrombocythemia, 711
  due to polycythemia vera, 702
  elevated platelet count and risk of, 227
  in thrombophilic patient, 289b
  recurrent, 512
  risk factors for, 289–290, 290t
  treatment of, 514–519
    acute pulmonary embolectomy for, 514t,
        519
    anticoagulant therapy for, 514–518, 514t,
        515t, 516f, 518f
    in pregnancy, 516–517
    intracaval filters for, 519
    pulmonary endarterectomy for, 514t
    thrombolytic therapy for, 514t, 518–519
    venous thrombectomy for, 514t, 519
  with central venous catheters, 1182–1184,
      1183f
  with high-dose chemotherapy, 1180–1181
  with indwelling catheters, 1182–1184, 1183f
  with superior vena cava syndrome, 1182
Ventilation-perfusion lung scans, 287–288, 288f
Verrucous carcinoma
  of cervix, 770
  of head and neck, 1000
Versed. See Midazolam (Versed).
Vertebral compression fractures, 160, 162t
  in multiple myeloma, 582, 585, 592–593
Vertebral osteomyelitis, 161
Vertigo, 1252t
  due to cranial neuropathy, 30t, 31
Vesanoid (all-trans retinoic acid), 344
  for acute promyelocytic leukemia, 543, 544t,
      545b
Vestibular nerve deficit, 30t
VHL (von Hippel-Lindau) disease, 826, 832,
    1194t, 1203
Videostroboscopy, for hoarseness, 54
Vinblastine, 340t, 353, 356t
  for bladder cancer, 853, 854
  for breast cancer, 757t
  for esophageal cancer, 878t, 881t
  for germ-cell tumors, 821b, 822
  for non–small cell lung cancer, 973
  for prostate cancer, 873t
  for renal cell cancer, 834, 834t, 837
Vinca alkaloids, 332t, 340t, 353, 356t
  for idiopathic thrombocytopenic purpura,
      490
Vincristine, 340t, 353, 356t
  for acute lymphoblastic leukemia, 557t, 558t
  for Burkitt's leukemia/lymphoma, 562t
  for cervical cancer, 775t
  for Ewing's sarcoma, 1035
  for high-grade gliomas, 1053, 1054b
  for Kaposi's sarcoma, 1160
  for multiple myeloma, 588–589, 589b
  for osteosarcoma, 1030
  for small cell lung cancer, 951
  for thymoma, 989t

Vindesine, for esophageal cancer, 878t
Vindoline, 353
Vinorelbine (Navelbine), 340t, 353, 356t
    for esophageal cancer, 878t
    for head and neck cancer, 1008t
    for mesothelioma, 995t
    for metastatic breast cancer, 756t
    for non–small cell lung cancer, 971t, 972
Vioxx (rofecoxib), for pain, 1244
VIPoma, 1134t, 1135, 1136t
Viral infections, with hematopoietic stem cell
        transplantation, 401–403
Viral proteins, in vaccine therapy, 380
Viral vectors, for gene therapy, 383, 383t
Virchow's node, in gastric cancer, 890
Virchow's triad, in renal cell cancer, 828
Viruses
    acute lymphoblastic leukemia due to,
            550–551
    acute myeloid leukemia due to, 523
Viscum album, 1213t
Vision, double, due to cranial neuropathy, 29t,
        31
Vistaril (hydroxyzine), 1227, 1227b
Visual analog scale, 1241, 1241f
Vitamin A, 1216t
    for head and neck cancer, 1013t
Vitamin B$_{12}$, in erythrocytosis, 259
Vitamin B$_{12}$ deficiency, 233t, 238, 277, 455–457,
        456t
Vitamin B17, 1217t, 1219–1220
Vitamin C, 1215–1217, 1216t
    for Chédiak-Higashi syndrome, 479
Vitamin E, 1216t
    and prostate cancer, 861
    for hot flashes, 766b
    for lung cancer, 978
Vitamin K, for warfarin-induced bleeding, 517
Vitamin K antagonists, coagulation disorders due
        to, 506–507, 507f, 508b
Vitamin K deficiency, 265, 267–268
Vitiligo, due to interleukin-2 for melanoma,
        1098f
Vocal abuse, 50, 52
Vocal fold paralysis
    causes of, 51, 52f, 52t
    defined, 51
    diagnosis of, 54
    management of, 56
Vocal hygiene, 55
Vocal nodules, 51t
VOD (veno-occlusive disease)
    due to cytotoxic agents, 395–396, 1180–1181
    hepatic, 1180–1181
Voice quality, 50, 52t
Voice therapy, 55–56
Vomiting
    anticipatory, 1250
    chemotherapy-induced, 1250–1251, 1251t,
            1252t
    due to opioids, 1248
    due to therapy for small cell lung cancer, 954
    projectile, headache with, 21b
Von Hippel-Lindau (VHL) disease, 826, 832,
        1194t, 1203
von Willebrand disease, 267, 269, 270, 505–
        506
    vaginal bleeding due to, 184, 186b
von Willebrand factor receptor, 485
    defects in, 494

von Willebrand variant type 2 Normandy (2N),
        499, 505
VP-16. *See* Etoposide (VP-16).
Vulva
    as source of vaginal bleeding, 185, 185t
    lichen sclerosis et atrophicus of, 776b, 776f
    Paget's disease of, 778
Vulvar cancer, 775–778
    clinical presentation of, 776
    diagnostic evaluation of, 776–777, 776b,
            776f, 777f
    epidemiology of, 775
    follow-up evaluation for, 778
    recurrent, 778
    risk factors for, 775–776
    staging and prognosis for, 777–778, 777t
    treatment for, 778
Vulvar intraepithelial neoplasia, 778
Vulvar lentiginosis, 311

W

WAIHA (warm autoimmune hemolytic anemia),
        470–471, 470t, 472f, 473b
    transfusion support of, 434b
Waldenström's macroglobulinemia, 248, 597–598
    due to cancer, 1172
    immunoglobulin abnormalities due to, 205
Waldeyer's ring lymphoma, 638, 650, 662
Warburg, Otto, 1218
Warburg phenomenon, 966
Warfarin
    coagulation disorders due to, 265, 268,
            506–507, 507f, 508b, 517
    for heparin-induced thrombocytopenia, 488
    for venous thromboembolism, 515–516
        with cancer, 1182
    International Normalized Ratio (INR) for,
            506, 507, 515–516
    skin necrosis due to, 302, 302f, 518, 518f
Warm autoimmune hemolytic anemia (WAIHA),
        470–471, 470t, 472f, 473b
    transfusion support of, 434b
Watchful waiting, for prostate cancer, 863b,
        868–869
Watercress, 1215
WBC(s). *See* White blood cell(s) (WBCs).
WBRT (whole-brain radiation therapy), 1069,
        1070–1072, 1071t, 1072t
WBXRT, for melanoma, 1099b
WDHA syndrome, 1135
Weakness
    due to brain metastases, 1063
    due to epidural tumor, 1078
    management of, 1253–1254
Wegener's granulomatosis, 299f
Weight loss, 3–8
    differential diagnosis of, 4b
    for breast cancer, 767
    pathogenesis of, 3–5, 4b, 4t
    therapy for, 5–8, 5t, 7t
Wellbutrin-SR (bupropion), 1227b
Well's syndrome, 249
Wernicke's encephalopathy, 35b
Whipple procedure, 904
Whipple's triad, in insulinoma, 1135
White blood cell(s) (WBCs), in anemia, 236t
White blood cell (WBC) aplasia, pure, 451
White blood cell (WBC) count, 278
    in chronic myeloid leukemia, 676–677,
            677b

White blood cell (WBC) differential count, 253,
        278
White blood cell (WBC) disorders
    due to cancer and cancer treatment, 1168,
            1169t
    hereditary, 475–483, 476f
        Chédiak-Higashi syndrome as, 479–480,
                480f
        chronic granulomatous disease as,
                480–483, 482t, 483t
        cyclic neutropenia as, 477
        hyperimmunoglobulin E syndrome as,
                478
        leukocyte adhesion deficiency as,
                478–479
        of neutrophil motility, 477–478, 478t
        severe congenital neutropenia as,
                475–477, 477f, 477t
    in myelodysplasia, 570t
    on peripheral smear, 277–280, 278f–281f
WHO. *See* World Health Organization (WHO).
Whole-brain radiation therapy (WBRT), 1069,
        1070–1072, 1071t, 1072t
Wide local excision
    for melanoma, 1091, 1091t
    for Merkel cell carcinoma, 1114
Wilms' tumor gene, 1194t
    in acute myeloid leukemia, 528
World Health Organization (WHO) analgesic
        ladder, 1244–1246
World Health Organization (WHO)
        classification
    of acute lymphoblastic leukemia, 552
    of acute myeloid leukemia, 523, 525t
    of Hodgkin's disease, 617–618, 618t
    of lymphoid neoplasms, 601, 602t, 611
    of myelodysplasia, 573
    of non-Hodgkin's lymphoma, 636
    of peripheral T-cell lymphoma, 664, 665t

X

Xanax. *See* Alprazolam (Xanax).
Xeloda (capecitabine), 335t, 348–349
    for metastatic breast cancer, 756t, 757t, 758
Xerostomia, 1250
X-ray simulator, in radiation therapy, 324, 324f

Z

Zarontin (ethosuximide), for seizures, 25t
ZD1839, 387
Zenker's diverticulum, 140
Zevalin (ibritumomab tiuxetan), for non-
        Hodgkin's lymphoma, 653
Zidovudine, for adult T-cell leukemia/lymphoma,
        674
Zoladex. *See* Goserelin acetate (Zoladex).
Zoledronic acid (Zometa)
    for hypercalcemia, 194, 194t
        in metastatic breast cancer, 760–761
    for skeletal complications of multiple
            myeloma, 593
Zollinger-Ellison syndrome, gastric carcinoids in,
        1133
Zoloft (sertraline), 1227, 1227b, 1228
Zolpidem (Ambien), 1227b
Zone electrophoresis, for immunoglobulin
        abnormalities, 205, 206f
Zonisamide (Zonegran), for seizures, 25t
Zyprexa (olanzapine), 1227b
    for nausea and vomiting, 1252t